Textbook of Palliative Medicine

Textbook of Palliative Medicine

Edited by

Eduardo Bruera MD
Professor and Chair, Department of Palliative Care and
Rehabilitation Medicine, U.T. MD Anderson Cancer Center,
Houston, Texas, USA

Irene J Higginson BMed Sci BMBS FFPHM PhD FRCP
Professor and Head of Department, Department of
Palliative Care, Policy and Rehabilitation, King's College
London, UK; Scientific Director, The Cicely Saunders
Foundation, UK

Carla Ripamonti MD
Head, Day-Hospital and Outpatient Clinic of Pain Therapy
and Palliative Care, Rehabilitation and Palliative Care
Operative Unit, National Cancer Institute, Milan, Italy

Charles F von Gunten MD PhD
Director, Center for Palliative Studies, San Diego Hospice
and Palliative Care, San Diego, California, USA

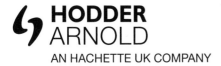

**HODDER
ARNOLD**
AN HACHETTE UK COMPANY

First published in Great Britain in 2006.
This paperback edition first published in 2009 by
Hodder Arnold, an imprint of Hodder Education, an Hachette UK company
338 Euston Road, London NW1 3BH

http://www.hoddereducation.com

Hachette Livre UK's policy is to use papers that are natural, renewable and recyclable products and made from wood grown in sustainable forests. The logging and manufacturing processes are expected to conform to the environmental regulations of the country of origin.

Whilst the advice and information in this book are believed to be true and accurate at the date of going to press, neither the author[s] nor the publisher can accept any legal responsibility or liability for any errors or omissions that may be made. In particular, (but without limiting the generality of the preceding disclaimer) every effort has been made to check drug dosages; however it is still possible that errors have been missed. Furthermore, dosage schedules are constantly being revised and new side-effects recognized. For these reasons the reader is strongly urged to consult the drug companies' printed instructions before administering any of the drugs recommended in this book.

British Library Cataloguing in Publication Data
A catalogue record for this book is available from the British Library

Library of Congress Cataloging-in-Publication Data
A catalog record for this book is available from the Library of Congress

ISBN: 978 0 340 966 242

1 2 3 4 5 6 7 8 9 10

Commissioning Editor: Sarah Burrows
Project Editor: Naomi Wilkinson
Production Controller: Joanna Walker
Cover Design: Georgina Hewitt

Typeset in 10/12 pts Minion by Charon Tec Ltd (A Macmillan Company), Chennai, India
www.charontec.com
Printed and bound in the UK by MPG Books, Bodwin, Cornwall.
Text printed on FSC accredited material

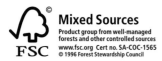

Mixed Sources
Product group from well-managed forests and other controlled sources
www.fsc.org Cert no. SA-COC-1565
© 1996 Forest Stewardship Council
FSC

What do you think about this book? Or any other Hodder Arnold title?
Please send your comments to www.hoddereducation.com

To Ed, Sofia and Sebastian

EB

To Kathleen and Leslie Higginson

IH

To Andrea, Francesca, Maria, Felice, Dario, Maddalena, and Fausto Ripamonti

CR

Dedicated to the staff and benefactors of San Diego Hospice and Palliative Care for
pursuing the mission of the academic hospice

CVG

Contents

Review drugs + receptors

Contributors

Jennifer Abbey MA
Pre-Doctoral Research Fellow
Department of Psychiatry and Behavioral Sciences
Memorial Sloan–Kettering Department of Psychiatry
and Cancer Center
New York
USA

Madhuri Are MD
Assistant Professor
and
Director of Pain Fellowship
Department of Anesthesiology and Pain Medicine
The University of Texas MD Anderson Cancer Center
Houston, Texas
USA

Elizabeth A Barnes MD, FRCPC, ABHPM
Toronto Sunnybrook Regional Cancer Centre
and
Assistant Professor
Department of Radiation Oncology
University of Toronto
Toronto
Canada

Sharon Baxter MSW
Executive Director
Canadian Hospice Palliative Care Association
Saint-Vincent Hospital
Ottawa, Ontario
Canada

Estela Beale MD
Associate Professor, Pediatrics – Patient Care
The University of Texas MD Anderson Cancer Center
Houston, Texas
USA

Marilu P Berry PhD
Licensed Psychologist
Houston, Texas
USA

Mauro Bianchi MD
Department of Pharmacology
School of Medicine
University of Milan
Milan
Italy

Heidi Blumhuber MBA
Executive Officer EAPC
National Cancer Institute of Milan
Milan
Italy

Cathryn Bogan MB
Specialist Registrar in Palliative Medicine
Marymount Hospice
St Patrick's Hospital
Cork, Ireland

Cara Bondly MD
Fellow
Department of Oncology
Mayo Clinic College of Medicine
Rochester, Minnesota
USA

Jeanette A Boohene MD
Fellow in Palliative Care
The University of Texas MD Anderson Cancer Center
Houston, Texas
USA

Sara Booth FRCP, FFARCSI
Macmillan Consultant in Palliative Medicine
Lead Clinician for Palliative Medicine
Cambridge Universities Foundation Trust
Cambridge
UK

Roni Borenstein BS
Research Associate
Department of Psychiatry and Behavioral Sciences
Memorial Sloan–Kettering Cancer Center
New York
USA

William Breitbart MD
Professor of Psychiatry
Weill Medical College of Cornell University
and
Chief
Psychiatry Service, Department of Psychiatry and
Behavioral Sciences
and
Attending Psychiatrist
Pain and Palliative Care Service
Department of Neurology
Memorial Sloan–Kettering Cancer Center
New York
USA

Eduardo Bruera MD
Professor and Chair
Department of Palliative Care and Rehabilitation Medicine
The University of Texas MD Anderson Cancer Center
Houston, Texas
USA

Rachel Burman MA, FRCP
Consultant and Honorary Senior Lecturer in Palliative Care
King's College Hospital NHS Trust
Department of Palliative Care and Policy
King's College London
Weston Education Centre
London
UK

Allen W Burton MD
Associate Professor
Section Chief of Cancer Pain Management
The University of Texas MD Anderson Cancer Center
Department of Anesthesiology
Houston, Texas
USA

Shirley H Bush MBBS, DCH, MRCGP, Dip Pall Med, FAChPM
Staff Specialist in Palliative Care
McCulloch House, Palliative Care Unit
Monash Medical Centre
and
Honorary Lecturer
Faculty of Medicine, Nursing and Health Sciences
Monash University
Clayton, Victoria
Australia

Augusto T Caraceni MD
Medical Director Hospice 'Virgilio Floriani'
Rehabilitation and Palliative Care Unit
National Cancer Institute of Milan
Milan
Italy

David Casarett MD, MA
Center for Health Equity Research and Promotion at the
Philadelphia VAMC
Assistant Professor, Division of Geriatrics University of
Pennsylvania
Philadelphia, Pennsylvania
USA

J Brian Cassel PhD
Senior Analyst
VCU Massey Cancer Center
Richmond, Virginia
USA

Carlos Centeno MD, PhD
Equipo de Medicina Paliativa
Clínica Universitaria
Universidad de Navarra
Pamplona
Spain

Eric L Chang MD
Associate Professor
The University of Texas MD Anderson Cancer Center
Houston, Texas
USA

Victor T Chang MD
Associate Professor of Medicine
UMDNJ
Section Hematology/Oncology (III)
VA New Jersey Health Care System
East Orange, New Jersey
USA

Nathan I Cherny MBBS, FRACP
Director Cancer Pain and Palliative Medicine
Department of Medical Oncology
Shaare Zedek Medical Center
Jerusalem
Israel

Harvey Max Chochinov OM, MD, PhD, FRCPC
Professor and Canada Research Chair in Palliative Care
Director, Manitoba Palliative Care Research Unit
Cancer Care
Winnipeg, Manitoba
Canada

Edward Chow MBBS, MSc, FRCPC
Associate Professor
Department of Radiation Oncology
Toronto Sunnybrook Regional Cancer Centre
University of Toronto
Toronto, Ontario
Canada

Alexie Cintron MD, MPH
Instructor
Brookdale Department of Geriatrics and Adult Development
Mount Sinai School of Medicine
New York
USA

David Clark PhD
International Observatory on End of Life Care
Institute for Health Research
Alexandra Square
Lancaster University
Lancaster
UK

Josephine M Clayton MB BS, FRACP, FAChPM, PhD
Clinical Lecturer
Central Clinical School (Medicine)
University of Sydney
and
Staff Specialist in Palliative Medicine
Sacred Heart Palliative Care Service
St Vincent's Hospital
Sydney
Australia

S Robin Cohen BSc, MSc, PhD
Research Director and Assistant Professor
Division of Palliative Care
Departments of Oncology and Medicine
McGill University
Jewish General Hospital
Centre for Patient Care and Family Support
Montreal
Canada

Lorenzo Cohen MD
Associate Professor
Integrative Medicine Program
Departments of Behavioral Science and Palliative Care
The University of Texas MD Anderson Cancer Center
Houston, Texas
USA

Massimo Costantini MD
Unit of Clinical Epidemiology
National Cancer Institute
Genova
Italy

Kerry S Courneya PhD
Professor and Canada Research Chair in
Physical Activity and Cancer
Faculty of Physical Education
University of Alberta
Edmonton, Alberta
Canada

Finella Craig MBBS, BSc, MRCP
Consultant in Paediatric Palliative Care
Great Ormond Street Hospital
London
UK

J Randall Curtis MD, MPH
Professor of Medicine
Division of Pulmonary and Critical Care
University of Washington
Harborview Medical Center
Seattle, Washington
USA

Shalini Dalal MD
Assistant Professor
Department of Palliative Care and Rehabilitation Medicine
The University of Texas MD Anderson Cancer Center
Houston, Texas
USA

Mellar P Davis MD, FCCP
Director of Research
The Harry R Horvitz Center for Palliative Medicine
Cleveland Clinic Foundation
Cleveland, Ohio
USA

Franco de Conno MD, FRCP
Director
Division Rehabilitation and Palliative Care
National Cancer Institute of Milan
Milan
Italy

Liliana De Lima MHA
Executive Director
International Association for Hospice and Palliative Care
Houston, Texas
USA

Egidio Del Fabbro MD
Assistant Professor
Department of Palliative Care and Rehabilitation Medicine
The University of Texas MD Anderson Cancer Center
Houston, Texas
USA

María Luisa del Valle MD, PhD
Servicio de Oncología
Hospital Universitario de Valladolid
Valladolid
Spain

Mary Devins MB BCh, BAO, DCH, MRCPI(Paeds), Dip Pall Med
Specialist Registrar in Paediatrics
Children's University Hospital
Dublin
Republic of Ireland

Eileen S Donovan PT, MEd
Rehabilitation Staff Educator
The University of Texas MD Anderson Cancer Center
Houston, Texas
USA

Edward R Duncan BA, MRCP
Cardiovascular Division
School of Medicine
King's College London
London
UK

Solvig Ekblad PhD
Associate Professor
IPM
Karolinska Institutet
Stockholm
Sweden

Badi El Osta MD
Fellow in Palliative Care and Rehabilitation Medicine
Department of Palliative Care and Rehabilitation Medicine
The University of Texas MD Anderson Cancer Center
Houston, Texas
USA

Linda Emanuel MD, PhD
Professor of Medicine
and
Principal
The EPEC Project
and
Director
The Buehler Center on Aging
Northwestern University Medicine School
Chicago, Illinois
USA

Bette Emery BSW, RSW
Tertiary Palliative Care Unit
Grey Nuns Community Hospital
Edmonton Alberta
Canada

Jørgen Eriksen MD
H:S Multidisciplinary Pain Centre
Rigshospitalet
Copenhagen
Denmark

D Scott Ernst MD, FRPCC
Associate Professor of Clinical Medicine
Division of Hematology/Oncology
Miller School of Medicine
University of Miami
Miami, Florida
USA

Nada Fadul MD
The University of Texas MD Anderson Cancer Center
Houston, Texas
USA

Robin L Fainsinger MD
Professor
Division of Palliative Care Medicine,
Department of Oncology, University of Alberta
Edmonton, Alberta
Canada

Frank D Ferris MD
Clinical Professor
Department of Family and Preventative Medicine and
Department of Medicine
University of California, San Diego School of Medicine
San Diego CA
and
Medical Director
Palliative Care Standards/Outcome Measures
San Diego Hospice & Palliative Care
San Diego CA
USA
and
Assistant Professor, Adjunct
Department of Family and Community Medicine
and
Member
Joint Center for Bioethics
University of Toronto
Toronto, Ontario
Canada

Ilora G Finlay
Professor of Palliative Medicine
Cardiff University
and
Consultant in Palliative Medicine
Velindre Hospital
Cardiff
UK

Michael J Fisch MD, MPH
Associate Professor
Section of General Oncology
Division of Cancer Medicine
The University of Texas MD Anderson Cancer Center
Houston, Texas
USA

Fabio Formaglio MD
Neurologist and Pain Specialist
Senior Staff Pain Medicine Center
Scientific Institute and Hospital San Raffaele
Milan
Italy

Miriam Friedlander MD
Instructor
Psychiatry Service
Department of Psychiatry and Behavioral Sciences
Memorial Sloan–Kettering Cancer Center
New York
USA

Kathryn G Froiland MSN, RN, CNS, AOCN, CWOCN
Oncology Clinical Educator
Glaxo Smith Kline Inc.
Houston, Texas
USA

Fabio Fulfaro MD
Operative Unit of Medical Oncology
University of Palermo
Italy

Carl Johan Fürst MD, PhD
Associate Professor
Stockholms Sjukhem Foundation
Stockholm
Sweden

Flavio Fusco MD
Palliative Care Unit
Department of Geriatric Care
Genoa
Italy

Bruno Gagnon MD, MSc
Palliative Care Medicine, Department of Oncology
McGill University and Division of Clinical Epidemiology
Royal Victoria Hospital,
Montreal, Quebec
Canada

Romayne Gallagher MD, CCFP
Clinical Professor
Division of Palliative Care
University of British Columbia
Vancouver, British Columbia
Canada

Claudia Gamondi MD
Department of Palliative Care
IOSI Oncology Institute of Southern Switzerland
Palliative Care Service
Lugano-Viganello
Switzerland

Christopher Gibson PhD
Research Coordinator
Psychiatry Service
Department of Psychiatry and Behavioral Sciences
Memorial Sloan–Kettering Cancer Center
New York
USA

Ann Goldman MBBS, FRCP, FRCPCH
Consultant in Palliative Care
Great Ormond Street Hospital
London
UK

Ying Guo MD
Assistant Professor
Department of Palliative Care and Rehabilitation Medicine
The University of Texas MD Anderson Cancer Center
Houston, Texas
USA

Richard D W Hain MBBS, MSC, MD, MRCP, FRCPCH
Senior Lecturer in Paediatric Palliative Medicine
and
Honorary Consultant Paediatric Oncologist
Department of Child Health
Cardiff School of Medicine
University Hospital of Wales
Cardiff
UK

Samuel J Hassenbusch III MD, PhD
Professor
Department of Neurosurgery
The University of Texas MD Anderson Cancer Center
Houston, Texas
USA

Irene J Higginson BMed Sci, BMBS, FFPHM, PhD FRCP
Professor of Palliative Care and Policy
King's College London
and
Scientific Director
The Cicely Saunders Foundation
Weston Education Centre
London
UK

Robert E Hirschtick MD
Assistant Professor of Medicine
Department of Medicine
Division of General Internal Medicine
Feinberg School of Medicine
Northwestern University
Chicago, Illinois
USA

Winford E Holland PhD
Houston, Texas
USA

Nicole Iannarone BA
Research Associate
Department of Psychiatry and Behavioral Sciences
Memorial Sloan-Kettering Cancer Center
New York
USA

Nora A Janjan MD, FACP, FACR
Professor of Radiation Oncology
The University of Texas MD Anderson Cancer Center
Houston, Texas
USA

Aminah Jatoi MD
Associate Professor of Oncology
Mayo Clinic College of Medicine
Rochester, Minnesota
USA

Anthony F Jerant MD
Associate Professor
Department of Family and Community Medicine
University of California Davis School of Medicine
Sacramento, CA
USA

Jennifer Kapo MD
Assistant Professor of Clinical Medicine
Division of Geriatric Medicine
Department of Medicine
University of Pennsylvania
and
Attending Physician
Palliative Care Service
Philadelphia Veteran's Administration
Philadelphia, Pennsylvania
USA

Louise Kashuba RN, BSCN
Tertiary Palliative Care Unit
Grey Nuns Community Hospital
Edmonton Alberta
Canada

John J Kavanagh MD
Department of Gynecologic Medical Oncology
The University of Texas MD Anderson Cancer Center
Houston, Texas
USA

Mark T Kearney MD, MRCP
Department of Cardiology
School of Medicine
King's College London
London
UK

Jeremy Keen MD, FRCPE
Consultant Physician in Palliative Care
Highland Hospice
Ness House
Inverness
UK

Kenneth L Kirsh PhD
Assistant Professor
Pharmacy Practice and Science
University of Kentucky
Lexington, Kentucky
USA

David W Kissane MD, MPM, FRANZCP, FAChPM
Alfred P. Sloan Chair
Attending Psychiatrist, and Chairman
Department of Psychiatry and Behavioral Sciences
and
Professor of Psychiatry
Weill Medical College of Cornell University
New York
USA

Jonathan Koffman BA (Hons), MSc
Lecturer in Palliative Care
Department of Palliative Care, Policy and Rehabilitation
King's College London
Weston Education Centre
London
UK

Benedict Konzen MD
Assistant Professor
Department of Palliative Care and Rehabilitation Medicine
The University of Texas MD Anderson Cancer Center
Houston, Texas
USA

Andreas Kopf MD
Director
Pain Unit, Department of Anaesthesiology and Intensive Care
Charité
Freie Universitaet Berlin
Berlin
Germany

Linda J Kristjanson RN, BN, MN, PhD
The Cancer Council Western Australia Chair of Palliative Care
School of Nursing, Midwifery and Postgraduate Medicine
Edith Cowan University
Joondalup, Western Australia
Australia

Marco Lacerenza MD
Neurologist and Pain Specialist
Senior Staff Pain Medicine Center
Scientific Institute and Hospital San Raffaele
Milan
Italy

J Norelle Lickiss AO, MD, FRCP(Edin), FRACP, FAChPM
Clinical Professor (Medicine)
University of Sydney
Sydney Institute of Palliative Medicine
Royal Prince Alfred Hospital, Camperdown
and

Consultant in Palliative Medicine
Royal Hospital for Women
Randwick
New South Wales
Australia

Victoria Lidstone
Specialist Registrar
South Wales
UK

Jon H Loge MD
Associate Professor at the Unit for Applied Clinical Research
The Norwegian University for Science and Technology
Trondheim
and
Consultant at the Centre for Palliative Medicine
Department of Oncology
Ulleval University Hospital
Oslo
Norway

David Lussier MD, FRCPC
Division of Geriatric Medicine
McGill University Health Center
Assistant Professor of Medicine
McGill University
Montreal
Canada

Joanne Lynn MD, MA, MS
Director
The Palliative Care Policy Center RAND
Arlington, Virginia
USA

Neil MacDonald CM, MD, FRCPC, FRCP(Edin)
Director
Cancer Nutrition-Rehabilitation Programme
McGill University Department of Oncology
Montreal, Québec
Canada

Karen Macmillan RN, BScN
Tertiary Palliative Care Unit
Grey Nuns Community Hospital
Edmonton, Alberta
Canada

Marco Maltoni MD
Palliative Care Unit
Oncology Department
Morgagni-Pierantoni Hospital
Forlì
Italy

Anita Mahajan MD
Assistant Professor
Radiation Oncology

The University of Texas MD Anderson Cancer Center
Houston, Texas
USA

Paolo Marchettini MD
Neurologist and Orthopaedic Surgeon Specialist
Director Pain Medicine Center
Scientific Institute and Hospital San Raffaele
Milan
Italy

Sue Marsden MBBS, FRANZCR, FAChPM
Senior Staff Specialist Palliative Medicine
Palliative Care Services
Illawarra Area Health
New South Wales
Australia

Pamela R Massey PT, MS
Director
Rehabilitation Services
The University of Texas MD Anderson Cancer Center
Houston, Texas
USA

Susan McClement RN, PhD
Assistant Professor
Faculty of Nursing
University of Manitoba
and
Research Associate
Manitoba Palliative Care Research Unit, Cancer Care
Manitoba
Canada

Margaret L McNeely MSc
Faculty of Physical Education
University of Alberta
Edmonton, Alberta
Canada

Diane E Meier MD
Director
The Lilian and Benjamin Hertzberg Palliative
Care Institute
and
Professor
Brookdale Department of Geriatrics and
Adult Development
and
Catherine Gaisman Professor of Medical Ethics
and
Director
Center to Advance Palliative Care
Mount Sinai School of Medicine
New York
USA

Sebastiano Mercadante MD
Chairman
Anesthesia and Intensive Care Unit and Pain Relief and
Palliative Care Unit
La Maddalena Cancer Center
and
Palliative Medicine
University of Palermo
Palermo
Italy

Anne Merriman MBE, FRCP
Director of Policy and International Programmes
Hospice Africa
Kampala
Uganda

Frederick J Meyers MD
Department of Internal Medicine
and Medical Director
Hospice and Home Health
University of California, Davis
Sacramento, California
USA

Kimberley Miller MD, FRCP(C)
Clinical Fellow
Department of Psychiatry and Behavioral Sciences,
Memorial Sloan–Kettering Cancer Center
New York
USA

Angela Miser
Associate Specialist in Paediatric Oncology
Children's Hospital of Wales
Cardiff
UK

Caterina Modonesi MD
Palliative Care Unit
Oncology Department
Morgagni-Pierantoni Hospital
Forlì
Italy

Fliss Murtagh MBBS, MRCGP, MSc
Research Training Fellow
Department of Palliative Care, Policy and Rehabilitation
King's College London
Weston Education Centre
London
UK

Sarah Myers MPH
Quality Improvement Consultant
Cincinnati Children's Hospital Medical Center
Cincinnati, Ohio
USA

Rudolph M Navari MD
Associate Dean
College of Science
and
Director
Walther Cancer Research Center
University of Notre Dame
Notre Dame, Indiana
USA

Cheryl L Nekolaichuk PhD
Assistant Professor
Division of Palliative Care Medicine
Department of Oncology
University of Alberta
Edmonton, Alberta
Canada

Hans Neuenschwander MD
Chief
Department of Palliative Care
IOSI Oncology Institute of Southern Switzerland
Palliative Care Service
Lugano-Viganello
Switzerland

Simon I R Noble
Senior Lecturer in Palliative Medicine
Cardiff University
and
Consultant in Palliative Medicine
Royal Gwent Hospital
Newport
UK

Diane M Novy PhD
Professor
Department of Anesthesiology
The University of Texas MD Anderson Cancer Center
Houston, Texas
USA

Joseph F O'Neill MD, MS, MPH
President and Chief Executive Officer
The Immune Response Corporation
Carlsbad, California
USA

Doreen Oneschuk MD
Associate Professor
Division of Palliative Medicine
Department of Oncology
University of Alberta
Edmonton, Alberta
Canada

Ellen A Pace RN, MSN
Palliative Care and Rehabilitation Medicine
The University of Texas MD Anderson Cancer Center
Houston, Texas
USA

Steven D Passik PhD
Associate Attending Psychologist
Memorial Sloan-Kettering Cancer Center
and
Associate Professor of Psychiatry
Cornell University College of Medicine
New York
USA

Carolyn J Peddle BSc
Faculty of Physical Education
University of Alberta
Edmonton, Alberta
Canada

Phillip C Phan MD
Assistant Professor
Director of Interventional Pain Management
Department of Anesthesiology and Pain Medicine
The University of Texas MD Anderson Cancer Center
Houston, Texas
USA

Russell K Portenoy MD
Chairman
Department of Pain Medicine and Palliative Care
Beth Israel Medical Center
and
Professor of Neurology
Albert Einstein College of Medicine
Bronx, New York
USA

Paula S Province BS
Visiting Scholar
Walther Cancer Research Center
University of Notre Dame
Notre Dame, Indiana
USA

Victoria H Raveis PhD
Associate Professor
Clinical Sociomedical Sciences
and
Co-Director
Center for the Psychosocial Study of Health and Illness
Columbia University
Mailman School of Public Health
New York
USA

Suresh K Reddy MD, FFARCS
Director of Fellowship Program
Department of Palliative Care and Rehabilitation Medicine
The University of Texas MD Anderson Cancer Center
Houston, Texas
USA

Carla Ripamonti MD
Medical Director
Day-Hospital and Outpatient Clinic of Pain Therapy and
Palliative Care
Rehabilitation and Palliative Care Operative Unit
National Cancer Institute
Milan
Italy

Graeme Rocker MHSc, DM
Professor of Medicine
Dalhousie University
Halifax, Nova Scotia
Canada

Javier Rocafort
Coordinator of the Regional Palliative Care Program of
Extremadura
Spain

Nancy C Russell MPH
Assistant Epidemiologist II
Integrative Medicine Program, Department of Palliative Care
The University of Texas MD Anderson Cancer Center
Houston, Texas
USA

True Ryndes ANP, MPH
President and CEO
National Hospice Work Group
Vice-President for Public Policy and Advocacy
San Diego Hospice and Palliative Care
San Diego, California
USA

Steffen Schmidt MD
Department of Anaesthesiology and Intensive Care
Charité
Freie Universitaet Berlin
Berlin
Germany

Hsien-Yeang Seow BS
Quality Improvement Coordinator
The Palliative Care Policy Center
RAND
Arlington, Virginia
USA

Ajay M Shah MD, FRCP
BHF Chair of Cardiology
and
Head of Cardiovascular Division
School of Medicine
King's College London
London
UK

Rosalie Shaw BA, BEd, MBBS, FRACMA, FAChPM
Department of Palliative Medicine
National Cancer Centre
Singapore
Republic of Singapore

Ki Shin MD
Assistant Professor
Department of Palliative Care and Rehabilitation Medicine
The University of Texas MD Anderson Cancer Center
Houston, Texas
USA

Fabio Simonetti
Neurology Unit
Rehabilitation and Palliative Care Unit
National Cancer Institute of Milan
Milan
Italy

Per Sjøgren MD
Multidisciplinary Pain Centre
Rigshospitalet
Copenhagen
Denmark

Thomas J Smith MD, FACP
Chair
Hematology-Oncology and Palliative Care
VCU Massey Cancer Center
Richmond, Virginia
USA

Pasquale Spinelli
National Cancer Institute of Milan
Milan
Italy

Daniele Stagno MD
Service de Psychiatrie de Liaison
C H U V
Lausanne
Switzerland

Christoph Stein MD
Professor and Chair
Department of Anesthesiology

Freie Universitaet Berlin
Berlin
Germany

Wendy M Stein MD
Associate Professor of Medicine/Geriatrics
University of California, San Diego
USA

Fritz Stiefel MD
Médcin Chef
CHUV Service de Psychiatrie de Liaison
Lausanne
Switzerland

Peter Strang MD, PhD
Professor in Palliative Medicine
Department of Oncology and Pathology
Karolinska Institute
Stockholm
Sweden

Susan Strang SRN, PhD, Minister
Department of Clinical Neuroscience and Rehabilitation
The Sahlgrenska Academy
Göteborg University
Sweden

Catherine Sweeney MB
Research Officer/Medical Tutor
Marymount Hospice
St Patrick's Hospital
Cork
Ireland

Paulina Taboada MD, PhD
Executive Director
Center for Bioethics
Pontificia Catholic University of Chile
Santiago
Chile

Yoko Tarumi MD
Assistant Professor
Division of Palliative Care Medicine
Department of Oncology
University of Alberta
Edmonton, Alberta
Canada

Martin H N Tattersall MB, BChir, MSc, FRCP, FRACP, MD
Professor of Cancer Medicine
University of Sydney
and
Director
Medical Psychology Research Unit

University of Sydney
Sydney
Australia

Lia Teloni MD
Rehabilitation Medicine Specialist
Junior Staff Pain Medicine Center
Scientific Institute and Hospital San Raffaele
Milan
Italy

Joan M Teno MD, MS
Professor
Community Health and Medicine
Center for Gerontology and Health Care Research
Brown University
Providence, RI
USA

Jay R Thomas MD, PhD
Associate Clinical Professor of Medicine
Center for Palliative Studies
San Diego Hospice & Palliative Care
Affiliate of University of California, San Diego
School of Medicine
San Diego, California
USA

Tabitha Thomas MRCP
Specialist Registrar in Palliative Medicine
Addenbrookes Hospital
Cambridge
UK

Andrew Thorns MA, FRCP
Consultant in Palliative Medicine
Pilgrims Hospices and the University of Kent
Margate
UK

James A Tulsky MD
Director
Center for Palliative Care
and
Professor of Medicine
Duke University
Durham VA Medical Center
Durham, North Carolina
USA

Mary L S Vachon RN, PhD
Psychotherapist and Consultant in Private Practice
and
Professor
Departments of Psychiatry and Public Health Science
University of Toronto
and

Clinical Consultant
Wellspring
Toronto, Ontario
Canada

Jeffrey K H Vallance MA
Faculty of Physical Education
University of Alberta
Edmonton, Alberta
Canada

Ernesto Vignaroli MD
Department of Palliative Care and Rehabilitation Medicine
The University of Texas MD Anderson Cancer Center
Houston, Texas
USA

Charles F von Gunten MD, PhD
Director
Center for Palliative Studies
San Diego Hospice & Palliative Care
and
Associate Clinical Professor of Medicine
University of California, San Diego
School of Medicine
San Diego, California
USA

Jamie H Von Roenn MD
Professor of Medicine
Department of Medicine
Division of Hematology/Oncology
Feinberg School of Medicine and Robert H Lurie Comprehensive Cancer Center of Northwestern University
and
Medical Director
Palliative Care and Home Hospice Program
Northwestern Memorial Hospital
Chicago, Illinois
USA

Rosemary Wade MBBS, MRCGP
Consultant in Palliative Medicine
West Suffolk Hospital
Bury St Edmunds
UK

Xipeng Wang MD
Department of Gynecologic Medical Oncology
The University of Texas MD Anderson Cancer Center
Houston, Texas
USA

Sharon Watanabe MD, FRCPC
Associate Professor
Division of Palliative Care Medicine
Department of Oncology
University of Alberta
Edmonton, Alberta
Canada

Roberto Wenk MD
Director
Argentinean Palliative Care Program – FEMEBA Foundation
Belgrano
San Nicolas
Argentina

Gary Wolch MD, CCFP
Clinical Adjunct Professor
University of Western Ontario
London, Ontario
Canada

R Cameron Wolf PhD, MSc
Senior Technical Advisor for Monitoring and Evaluation
US Agency for International Development
Office of HIV/AIDS
Global Health Bureau
Washington, DC
USA

Sriram Yennurajalingam MD
Assistant Professor
Department of Palliative Care and Rehabilitation Medicine
The University of Texas MD Anderson Cancer Center
Houston, Texas
USA

Donna S Zhukovsky MD, FACP
Associate Professor
Department of Palliative Care and Rehabilitation Medicine
The University of Texas MD Anderson Cancer Center
Houston, Texas
USA

Dedication to Dr Cicely Saunders
OM DBE FRCP FRCN FRCS

The purpose of this Textbook of Palliative Medicine is to disseminate the specialist knowledge of palliative medicine to all who wish to learn about it. Yet, to be a competent practitioner, knowledge is not enough. The ability to apply palliative medicine knowledge at a specialist level requires two things: a role model and precepted practice. For thousands of years, physicians have learned in an apprenticeship fashion under the tutelage of wise role models.

A singular individual who was a role model to thousands and a pioneer in palliative medicine was Dr Cicely Saunders. Born June 22, 1918, she first encountered the unmet needs of patients with far advanced cancer while working as a social worker in a busy surgical ward. Initially trained as a nurse, she had moved on to social work because of a bad back. Her encounter with real patients, with real needs for symptom control and psychological, social and spritual support led her to train as a physician in order to further pursue the work. With unmatched zeal and professional focus, she pioneered the interdisciplinary team-based approach we now know as palliative care. Some have observed that, with training in nursing, social work and medicine, and with an evangelical Christian background, Dr Saunders was in herself the first interdisciplinary palliative care team.

In pursuing interdisciplinary patient care, education and research into the needs of dying patients, Dr Saunders founded the modern hospice movement. As part of that movement, she founded St Christopher's Hospice in south suburban London, UK to be an academic hospice. The care provided, the physicians and other health professionals trained, and the research conducted there has changed health care around the world. She died July 14, 2005 knowing that she had left a legacy of a changed way of caring for both the living and the dying.

We dedicate this textbook to Dr Saunders in the year after her death in hope that it will play an important role in disseminating this knowledge to yet more generations of people around the world who want to understand the principles and practice of palliative medicine.

EB
IH
CR
CvG

Preface

Palliative medicine emerged in the United Kingdom during the 1960s as a response to the unmet needs of terminally ill patients and their families. This initially British initiative became progressively a global movement. The original community-based services were followed by programs of increasing complexity in secondary and tertiary hospitals and comprehensive cancer centers. Educational initiatives became progressively more sophisticated, ultimately resulting in palliative medicine becoming a full medical specialty. Research in many of the complex problems faced by patients and families has provided a growing body of knowledge on how to conduct our clinical care, education, organization and governance.

Our book has attempted to reflect the growth of our area of knowledge from a global perspective. Internationally recognized leaders have been asked to apply their first-hand knowledge in summarizing the principal issues in our discipline.

Palliative medicine covers a wide variety of subjects ranging from pharmacological interventions to historical, bioethical, and spiritual issues. This state of the art book cohesively addresses the full range of disciplines regularly involved in palliative medicine. We have attempted to produce a scholarly but accessible text following a user friendly format while respecting the needs of specific authors to deviate from the more traditional biomedical format when their area of content required them to do so.

We believe that this book will become a very useful resource for physicians, nurses, and other health care professionals involved in the clinical, academic, and administrative aspects of palliative care delivery worldwide.

EB
IH
CR
CvG

List of abbreviations

5-HT	5-hydroxytryptamine
6MWT	6-minute walk test (also 12MWT, 2 MWT)
ACE	angiotensin-converting enzyme
ACTH	adrenocorticotropic hormone
ADH	antidiuretic hormone
ADL	activities of daily living
AECOPD	acute exacerbations of chronic obstructive pulmonary disease
AgRP	Agouti-related peptide
AGS	American Geriatrics Society
AHA	American Heart Association
AIDS	acquired immune deficiency syndrome
ALCP	Latin American Association for Palliative Care (*Asociación Latinoamericana de Cuidados Paliativos*)
ALF	assisted living facility
ALS	amyotrophic lateral sclerosis
AMDA	American Medical Directors' Association
ANP	advanced nurse practitioner
APCA	African Palliative Care Association
APHN	Asia Pacific Hospice Palliative Care Network
APM	Association of Palliative Medicine
AP–PC line	anterior commissure–posterior commissure line
AS	actual survival
ASCO	American Society of Clinical Oncology
AUC	area under the curve
ARV	antiretroviral (drug)
BDI	Beck Depression Inventory
BMI	body mass index
BODE	body mass index, the degree of airflow obstruction, dyspnea scores, and exercise capacity
BPI	Brief Pain Inventory
BSI	bone scan index
BTS	British Thoracic Society
CACS	cancer anorexia-cachexia syndrome
CAM	Confusion Assessment Method
CAM	complementary and alternative medicine
CAPC	Center to Advance Palliative Care
CAPD	chronic ambulatory peritoneal dialysis
CB	cannabinoid (receptor)
CBT	cognitive–behavioral therapy
CCOG	Cancer Care Ontario Guidelines
CDP	complex decongestive physiotherapy
CES-D	Center for Epidemiologic Studies on Depression (scale)
CFS	chronic fatigue syndrome
CGRP	calcitonin gene-related peptide
CHF	congestive heart failure
CHPCA	Canadian Hospice Palliative Care Association
CIHR	Canadian Institutes of Health Research
CIVI	continuous intravenous infusion
CNS	central nervous system
COPD	chronic obstructive pulmonary disease
COREC	Central Office of Research Ethics Committees
COX-2	cyclooxygenase 2
CPAC	Center to Advance Palliative Care
CPR	cardiopulmonary resuscitation
CPS	Clinical Prediction of Survival
CRF	cancer-related fatigue
CRF	corticotrophin releasing factor
CRH	corticotrophin-releasing hormone
CRPS	complex regional pain syndrome
CSF	cerebrospinal fluid
CSI	continuous subcutaneous infusion
CT	computed tomography
CTZ	chemoreceptor trigger zone
DIC	disseminated intravascular coagulation
DLT	decongestive lymphatic therapy
DNR	do not resuscitate
DRG	diagnosis-related group
DSM	Diagnostic and Statistic Manual of Mental Disorders
DSM-IV	Diagnostic and Statistical Manual 4th edition
DVT	deep vein thrombosis
EACA	ε-aminocaproic acid
EAPC	European Association for Palliative Care
ECOG	Eastern Cooperative Oncology Group
EEG	electroencephalogram
EFAT	Edmonton Functional Assessment Tool
EFPPEC	Educating Future Physicians in Palliative and End-of-Life Care Project
EORTC	European Organization for Research and Treatment of Cancer
EPA	eicosapentaenoic acid
EPEC	Education in Palliative and End-of-life Care
ERCP	endoscopic retrograde cholangiopancreatography
ERPCP	Edmonton Regional Palliative Care Program
ESAS	Edmonton Symptom Assessment Scale
ESRD	end-stage renal disease
ESS	Edmonton Staging Score

EUS	endoscopic ultrasonography	MC-R	melanocortin receptor
FACIT-F	Functional Assessment for Chronic Illness Therapy – Fatigue	MD clinic	multidisciplinary symptom control and palliative care clinic
FAST	Functional Assessment Staging	MDAS	Memorial Delirium Assessment Scale
FEV$_1$	forced expiratory volume in 1 second	MDS	minimum data set
FFGT	Family Focused Grief Therapy	MFI-20	Multidimensional Fatigue Inventory
FHSSA	Foundation for Hospices in Sub-Saharan Africa	MLD	manual lymph drainage
(F)NHTR	(febrile) nonhemolytic transfusion reaction	MMSE	Mini-Mental State Examination
FQ	Fatigue Questionnaire	MMSQ	Mini-Mental State Questionnaire
FVC	forced vital capacity	MQOL	McGill Quality of Life Questionnaire
GABA	γ-aminobutyric acid	MRCP	magnetic resonance cholangiopancreatography
GDS	Geriatric Depression Scale	MRI	magnetic resonance imaging
GHQ	General Health Questionnaire	MSAS	Memorial Symptom Assessment Scale
GMP	good manufacturing practice	MSH	melanocyte-stimulating hormone
HAART	highly active antiretroviral therapy	MSKCC	Memorial Sloan–Kettering Cancer Center
HADS	Hospital Anxiety Depression Scale	NCCAM	National Center for Complementary and Alternative Medicine
HASA	Hospice Association of South Africa	NCCN	National Comprehensive Cancer Network
HBI	half-body irradiation	NCI	National Cancer Institute
hCG	human chorionic gonadotropin	NCSE	nonconvulsive status epilepticus
HCM	hypercalcemia of malignancy	NF-κB	nuclear factor kappa B
HDAT	Home Death Assessment Tool	NHO	National Hospice Organization
HIV	human immunodeficiency virus	NHPCO	National Hospice and Palliative Care Organization
HPCA	Hospice Palliative Care Association of South Africa	NHS	National Health Service
HRQOL	health-related quality of life	NIPPV	noninvasive positive pressure ventilation
HRT	hormone replacement therapy	NIV	noninvasive mechanical ventilation
HU	Hounsfield Units	NMDA	N-methyl-D-aspartate
IADL	instrumental activities of daily living	NMS	neuroleptic malignant syndrome
IAHPC	International Association for Hospice and Palliative Care	NNRTI	non-nucleoside reverse transcriptase inhibitors
IARC	International Agency for Research on Cancer	NNT	number need to treat
ICC	item-characteristic curve	NSCLC	nonsmall cell lung cancer
ICR	Institute of Cancer Research	NVR	nausea, vomiting, and retching
ICU	intensive care unit	NYHA	New York Heart Association
ICV	intracerebroventricular	OCCAM	Office of Cancer Complementary and Alternative Medicine
IL	interleukin		
IM	intramuscular	OIN	opioid-induced neurotoxicity
IMRT	intensity modulated radiation therapy	OPG	osteoprotegerin
INCB	International Narcotics Control Board	OSI	Open Society Institute
IOELC	International Observatory in End of Life Care	OTFC	oral transmucosal fentanyl citrate
IPT	interpersonal psychotherapy	PAC	project advisory committee
IRB	institutional review board	PAINAD	Pain Assessment in Advanced Dementia
IRT	item response theory	PAMPFF	Programa Argentino de Medicina Paliativa – Fundacion FEMEBA
IT	information technology		
IV	intravenous	PaP	Palliative Prognostic (Score)
JCAHO	Joint Commission of the Accreditation of Healthcare Organizations	PCA	patient-controlled analgesia
		PCCT	palliative care consultation team
JCMHT	Joint Committee on Higher Medical Training	PCDH	palliative care day hospitals
KPS	Karnofsky Performance Scale	PCIN	patient-controlled intranasal
LAS	lymphangioscintigraphy	PCU	palliative care unit
LMF	lipid-mobilizing factor	PDCH	palliative care day hospital
LOS	length of stay	PDIA	Project on Death in America
LSP	lumbosacral plexopathy	PEAT	Palliative Education Assessment Tool for Medical Education
M3G	morphine-3-glucuronide		
M6G	morphine-6-glucuronide	PEP	preexposure prophylaxis
MAR	medication administration record	PHC	palliative home care
MBO	malignant bowel obstruction	PHN	postherpetic neuralgia

PHPTH	primary hyperparathyroidism	SE	status epilepticus
PI	protease inhibitor	SF-36	Medical Outcome Survey Short Form 36
PIF	proteolysis-inducing factor	SLFC	sublingual fentanyl citrate
POLST	Physician Orders for Life-Sustaining Treatment	SMWT	self-paced minute walk test
PPI	Palliative Prognostic Index	SRE	skeletal-related events
PPS	Palliative Performance Score	SRT	spinoreticular tract
PS	performance status	SSRI	selective serotonin reuptake inhibitor
PSQI	Pittsburgh Sleep Quality Index	STT	spinothalamic tract
PTC	percutaneous transhepatic cholangiography	SUPPORT	Study to Understand Prognosis and Preferences for Outcomes and Treatments
PTH	parathyroid hormone		
PTHrP	parathyroid hormone-related protein	SVCS	superior vena cava syndrome
PVG/PAG	periventricular gray/periaqueductal gray	TCA	tricyclic antidepressant
QALY	quality-adjusted life year	THC	tetrahydrocannabinol
QELCC	Quality End-of-Life Care Coalition	TNF	tumor necrosis factor
QI	quality improvement	TPCU	tertiary palliative care unit
QOL	quality of life	TTS	transdermal therapeutic system
QTc	rate-corrected QT	VAS	visual analog scale
RANKL	receptor activator of nuclear factor κB-ligand	VEGF	vascular endothelial growth factor
REC	research ethics committee	VNRS	visual numerical rating scale
RSC	Research Steering Committee	VRS	verbal rating scale
RSCL	Rotterdam Symptom Checklist	vs.	versus
RTOG	Radiation Therapy Oncology Group	WBRT	whole-brain radiotherapy
SCEI	Simultaneous Care Educational Intervention	WHO	World Health Organization
SCLC	small cell lung cancer	ZAG	Zn-α_2-glycoprotein
SDS	Symptom Distress Scale		

Reference annotation and evidence scores

REFERENCE ANNOTATION

The reference lists are annotated, where appropriate, to guide readers to primary articles, key review papers, and management guidelines, as follows:

- ● Seminal primary article
- ◆ Key review paper
- ✳ First formal publication of a management guideline

We hope that this feature will render extensive lists of references more useful to the reader and will help to encourage self-directed learning among both trainees and practicing physicians.

EVIDENCE SCORES

Supporting evidence has been graded in the main body of the text for each clinical intervention as follows:

- ✳✳✳   Systematic review or meta-analysis
- ✳✳   One or more well-designed randomized controlled trials
- ✳   Nonrandomized controlled trials, cohort study, etc.

PART 1

The development of palliative medicine

The development of palliative medicine in the UK and Ireland

DAVID CLARK

INTRODUCTION

This chapter offers a brief history of palliative medicine in two of the countries where it gained rapid strides in the course of the later years of the twentieth century. It begins, however, by recognizing the nineteenth century legacy which was inherited by those later pioneers of the modern field who first carved out an area of sustained medical interest in the care of the dying. The chapter goes on to show how in the UK and Ireland, palliative medicine grew out of the activities of the voluntary hospice movement, how it built on the work of a small number of activists who had to struggle against indifference if not hostility and how, relatively quickly, it gained recognition from the medical establishment as a legitimate field of specialization. Of course, such developments have not been without their tensions, and the chapter concludes with some discussion of the argument surrounding the medicalization of death, the role of palliative medicine within it, and also the likely future of a specialty that makes its main focus the management of complex symptoms at the end of life.

NINETEENTH CENTURY BEGINNINGS

As the nineteenth century advanced, many industrialized countries saw the beginnings of an epidemiological transition wherein a shift took place in the dominant causes of death: from fatal infectious diseases of rapid progression, to chronic and life-threatening diseases of longer duration. As this transition became more marked, the departure from life for many people became an extended and sometimes uneven process. Consequently, people called 'the dying' began to emerge more clearly as a social category; and over time, the most common place to end one's life began to shift from the domestic home to some form of institution. For the first time in history special institutions were formed, often the work of religious orders or religiously motivated philanthropists, that were uniquely concerned with the care of dying people. Several of these were established in Cork, London, and Dublin in the closing decades of the nineteenth century and the beginning of the twentieth century.[1,2]

Another important antecedent to modern palliative medicine in the UK and Ireland at this time can be seen in the writings of key physicians and nurses who began to draw attention to the needs of dying patients. Outstanding among these in the UK context was the English physician, William Munk,[3] who has been described by one historian of the period as 'the most influential Victorian writer on the care of the dying'.[4] In 1887, exactly 100 years before palliative medicine was recognized as a specialty in the UK, Munk published a detailed treatise, 105 pages in length, on the care of the dying.[5] It was entitled *Euthanasia: or, Medical Treatment in Aid of an Easy Death*. In this work Munk uses the word 'euthanasia' in its classic sense to describe the goal of the physician in helping the sufferer to a more comfortable death. His work can be viewed as a precursor to the modern medical textbooks on the care of the dying that came to proliferate over a 100 years later.

In general Munk's book was favorably reviewed in a range of medical journals at the time (see for example, *British Medical Journal* 1861; **ii**: 231–2; *British Medical Journal* 1884; **i**: 1155–7; *Dublin Journal of Medical Science* 1884; **78**: 38–9). *The Lancet* printed a glowing account of *Euthanasia* calling it a 'treatise by a thoughtful and experienced physician' and supporting fully both Munk's aim in bringing the subject to the notice of the medical profession and his execution of important instruction in the medical management of the dying.[6] In 1888 it was also reviewed favorably by the famous Canadian physician William Osler, who praised its many valuable suggestions to practitioners and sound advice as to the medical management of the dying.[7] Indeed it has been argued that *Euthanasia* remained the authoritative text on medical care of the dying for the next 30 years,[4] but its influence was at best patchy and did not last beyond Munk's own generation. By 1926 the American physician Arthur Macdonald was still calling for a scientific study of death which would enhance the sum of knowledge and enable 'a general picture of the dying time, based upon a sufficient number of observations and with instruments of precision where possible' so that fear of death would be diminished and pain eliminated.[8] And as late as 1935 his fellow countryman, Alfred Worcester was arguing that the previous half-century had seen a deterioration in related medical practice, rather than progress, in the art of caring for the dying.[9]

Unfortunately this trickle of medical writings on the care of the dying found little interest in UK and Ireland in the decades following their publication and there is no evidence that they had an influence in the institutional homes for terminal care which were being created in the same period. If they did, it was insufficient to set in train any broader movement of reform; for the time being these writers and the founders of the homes remained isolated from one another and there was an absence of the kind of synergy which could lead to more widespread change.

A TWENTIETH CENTURY SEA CHANGE

In fact, it was not until the 1950s that some broader concerns about improving care at the end of life did begin to surface in the UK. This began when attention focused in a sustained way on the medical 'neglect' of the dying. Four particular innovations can be identified.[10] First, a shift took place within the professional literature of care of the dying, from idiosyncratic anecdote to systematic observation. New studies, by doctors, social workers, and social scientists provided evidence about the social and clinical aspects of dying in contemporary society. By the early 1960s leading articles in *The Lancet* and *British Medical Journal* were drawing on the evidence of research to suggest ways in which terminal care could be promoted and arguments for euthanasia (as medicalized killing) might be countered. Second, a new view of dying began to emerge which sought to foster concepts of personal dignity, autonomy, and meaning at the end of life. Enormous scope was opened up here for refining ideas about the dying process and exploring the extent to which patients should and did know about their terminal condition. Third, an active rather than a passive approach to the

care of the dying was promoted with increasing vigor. Within this, the fatalistic resignation of the doctor ('There is nothing more we can do') was supplanted by a determination to find new and imaginative ways to continue caring up to the end of life, and indeed beyond it, in the care of the bereaved. Fourth, a growing recognition of the interdependency of mental and physical distress created the potential for a more embodied notion of suffering, thus constituting a profound challenge to the body–mind dualism upon which so much medical practice of the period was predicated.

One particularly important development was a national survey carried out by a joint committee of the Marie Curie Memorial and the Queen's Institute of District Nursing, and chaired by the surgeon Ronald Raven.[11] The Marie Curie Memorial had been established in 1948 and held among its objects the promotion of the welfare and relief of patients with cancer. The joint committee first met in 1950 with the purpose of investigating the needs of domiciliary cancer sufferers and its report was published 2 years later. District nurses in 179 out of the 193 local authorities collected data on 7050 people living at home with cancer. They considered that 2195 were enduring a severe degree of suffering at the time they were visited. The report concluded with a series of recommendations, including the need for more residential and convalescent homes; the importance of better information for cancer sufferers; and greater provision of night nursing, home helps, and equipment. Within a year of the report's publication, the Marie Curie Memorial itself had begun opening homes for terminally ill cancer patients. In 1958 this was further extended by the provision of a night nursing service; and by the early 1960s 24 authorities in the provinces and 15 London district nursing areas were being served by over 200 Marie Curie nurses.[12] There is no evidence, however, of any systematic response to the report from elsewhere within the health and welfare system.

A second report, prepared by Dr H L Glyn Hughes at the request of the Calouste Gulbenkian Foundation was based on inquiries carried out between November 1957 and December 1958, and was published in 1960.[13] It contained a description of current provision for the care of the dying, together with recommendations for development. Like the joint committee, Glyn Hughes, himself a former army doctor, gave considerable attention to the social conditions of the terminally ill, but his report was more wide ranging in character and gave greater prominence to matters of policy and service organization. The report showed that two-fifths of all deaths in 1956 occurred in National Health Service (NHS) hospitals, with under a half of all deaths taking place in the home. Almost 46 000 cancer deaths (approximately a third of the total) took place at home and it was considered that many of these should have required continuous medical and nursing care. Similar needs were thought to be in evidence among some of the 121 000 who died at home from diseases of the circulatory system.

Overall Glyn Hughes estimated that some 270 000 people in need of 'skilled terminal care' died each year outside NHS hospitals. While dying at home was seen as the preferred alternative for most patients, Glyn Hughes stressed the importance of calculating the total number of inpatient beds which would be needed for terminal care. He was eager to stress the value of special terminal care beds within the curtilage of acute hospitals. At the same time the independent homes for the dying which did exist should develop closer links with hospital services to reduce their isolation.

Like bookends at the start and finish of the decade the reports of the joint committee and of Glyn Hughes had highlighted the deficiencies of terminal care in the welfare state of the 1950s. The joint national cancer survey committee had drawn attention to the abject social and economic conditions of many older people suffering with advanced cancer. Glyn Hughes had revealed the absence of a serious policy commitment to terminal care provision; indeed his recommendations highlighted the need for voluntary and for-profit organizations to work in conjunction with the NHS to achieve the necessary results.

During the same period and into the early 1960s a number of studies appeared that threw further light on the problems of terminally ill people in the UK. These included Margaret Bailey's survey of patients with incurable lung cancer conducted at the Brompton and Royal Marsden hospitals[14] as well as a study of delayed help seeking among patients with cancer, which noted that: 'The fact of palliative treatment is not understood, and hospitals appear to be trying to cure all their patients and failing in a high proportion of cases'.[15] Notable also was the early psychiatric work of Colin Murray Parkes on bereavement and mental illness.[16] By the mid-1960s research papers by Eric Wilkes, the Derbyshire general practitioner who later founded St Luke's Hospice in Sheffield, were appearing on terminal cancer at home[17,18] and in the second of these it was observed: 'There seems to be no valid reason why hospital provision for terminal care is so inadequate, or for the National Health Service to lean so heavily on the few Curie Foundation Homes and the devoted but over-worked religious institutions specialising in this work'. Closely associated with these research endeavors was Dr John Hinton, who had qualified in psychiatry from London's Maudsley Hospital in 1958. As a trainee doctor he had developed an interest in the psychiatric problems of terminally ill patients. His paper on the physical and mental distress of the dying was written in 1962 and published the following year, based on research conducted at a teaching hospital in 1959–61.[19] Hinton pointed out the need for more carefully designed research studies relating to terminal care and the need to get beyond anecdotal commentary. He noted in a 1964 editorial in the *Journal of Chronic Diseases* that: 'The large number of articles in which remembered experience is distilled into advice on the management of dying awesomely overshadows the few papers attempting to measure the degree of success or failure of treatment'.[20]

Hinton was inclined to a conversational approach to data collection and his 1963 research paper is based on interviews with 102 patients thought unlikely to live for more than 6 months, with controls. The dying group were more commonly depressed and anxious and half were aware that their illness might be fatal. Physical distress was more prevalent in those with heart or renal failure (57 percent) than those with malignancies (37 percent) and was in general more severe and unrelieved for longer within the dying group. The work was praised in an editorial in the *British Medical Journal*.[21]

In particular, however, it was the growing activities of Cicely Saunders, first developed in St Joseph's Hospice in Hackney, East London, that were to prove most consequential, for it was she who began to forge a peculiarly modern philosophy of terminal care combining a powerful religious and moral conviction alongside a rigorous approach to observation, research and clinical innovation. Through systematic attention to patient narratives and by listening carefully to stories of illness, disease and suffering, she evolved the concept of 'total pain'.[22] This view of pain moved beyond the physical to encompass the social, emotional, even spiritual aspects of suffering – captured so comprehensively by the patient who told her: 'All of me is wrong'.[23] But this was also linked to a hard-headed approach to pain management. Her message was simple: 'constant pain needs constant control'.[24] In a ground-breaking series of papers published in the late 1950s and early 1960s,[25] Cicely Saunders demonstrated that powerful analgesics could be used safely and with confidence. Despite considerable medical skepticism at the time,[26] she argued that if a method of regular giving of analgesia was employed, then pain could be prevented in advance, rather than alleviated once it had become established and the appropriate drug regimen was to work progressively, from mild, to moderate to strong.

When Cicely Saunders founded St Christopher's Hospice, in South London, in 1967, it quickly became a source of inspiration to others. As the first 'modern' hospice, it was at the time unique in combining three key principles: excellent clinical care, education, and research. It therefore differed significantly from the rather more modest goals of the other homes for the dying which had preceded it and sought to establish itself as no less than a center of excellence in a new field of care.

In particular, St Christopher's was associated with some major clinical and organizational studies that did a great deal to advance the field. Much of the former focused on the science of pain control and the underlying pharmacokinetic mechanisms at work in the administration of strong opioids. It began with close scrutiny of some of the methods of pain relief favored within the early hospices and terminal care homes, in particular the use of the so-called 'Brompton Cocktail',[27] which had been gaining popularity throughout the twentieth century and had appeared in print for the first time in the 1950s – a mixture of morphine hydrochloride, cocaine hydrochloride, alcohol, syrup, and chloroform water but with many local variants and names. Cicely Saunders, in her early writings, was eager to promote this rather exotic mixture but it was the St Christopher's research fellow Robert Twycross who set out to scrutinize it in detail, in what became a series of classical studies, among the first of their kind to be undertaken in the hospice setting. He concluded that the Brompton Cocktail was no more than a traditional British way of administering oral morphine to cancer patients in pain and urged that its use should be quietly abandoned in favor of simpler approaches.[28] But the actions of morphine, the development of new approaches to its administration and the teaching of healthcare professionals about its appropriate use alongside other analgesics and adjuvant drugs – all of these became a rich territory of both research and teaching in the modern hospice and palliative care context. Of particular importance was the work that compared the actions of morphine and diamorphine. Here Twycross reported a controlled crossover trial between the two drugs and showed that given regularly at individually optimized doses in an elixir with cocaine and a phenothiazine there was no clinically observable difference between the drugs.[29] As diamorphine was at that time (and remains) unlicensed for medical purposes in most countries, this was an important finding. Following these results, in 1977, St Christopher's changed its practice and morphine was prescribed for all oral narcotic medication, amounting to some two-thirds of doses given.[30]

Evaluation research at St Christopher's began before the first patient was admitted. The psychiatrist Dr Colin Murray Parkes embarked upon his detailed study of the memories of the carers of dying patients in the locality as the hospice opened and over time built up a cohort of cases. This consisted of 276 married patients under the age of 65 years who died of cancer in two London boroughs, 49 of whom were still under active treatment at the time of death; although the length of time after the end of such treatment varied greatly, the median length of stay for terminal care was 9 weeks. Parkes divided these patients into 'home based', including in this group all who died within a week of a final hospital admission, 'hospital based', and 'St Christopher's based'. He found much unrelieved pain, whether the patient died in a hospital or at home. As patients came into the study he was able to show that people with serious pain problems were referred from the start to the hospice and were largely relieved.[31] The study was repeated 10 years later as part of the ongoing evaluation of the work of the hospice. Although pain and symptom control improved in the hospital setting over time, psychosocial needs and continuity of care continued to be better approached in the hospice.[32]

The success of St Christopher's was phenomenal and it soon became the stimulus for an expansive phase of hospice development. In the UK there was a golden period of hospice expansion which peaked in the 1980s, when about 10 new hospices came into existence each year. But the ideals and practices developed in the hospices were also being disseminated into other settings, so that by the mid-1990s there were over 1000 specialist Macmillan nurses working in palliative care in the UK, approximately 400 home care teams, and over 200 day care and 200 hospital-based services as well as some 5000 Marie Curie nurses providing care in the home. From the outset, ideas developed at St Christopher's were applied differently in other places. Within a few decades therefore it had been accepted that the principles of hospice care could be practiced in many settings: in specialist inpatient units, but also in home care and day care services. Indeed hospital units and support teams were established that brought the new thinking about the care of the dying and those with advanced disease into the very heartlands of acute medicine. In 2004 there were 196 inpatient units in the UK, comprising 2730 beds, albeit just 19 percent of which were within the NHS with the remainder under the governance of independent hospices. There was also a large array of other services: home care (n = 341); day care (n = 237); hospital-based (n = 324); hospice at home (n = 97).[33] The UK has a population of 60 441 457 (July 2005 estimate). Its age structure is as follows: 0–14 years, 17.7 percent; 15–64 years, 66.5 percent; 65 years and over, 15.8 percent (male 4 063 357/female 5 472 683). The rate of death is 10.18 deaths/1000 population. Life expectancy at birth is 75.94 years (males) and 80.96 years (females). The principal ethnic groups, as derived from the 2001 census, are: white (English 83.6 percent, Scottish 8.6 percent, Welsh 4.9 percent, Northern Irish 2.9 percent) 92.1 percent; black 2 percent, Indian 1.8 percent, Pakistani 1.3 percent, mixed 1.2 percent, other 1.6 percent.

The expansion of hospice and palliative care quite quickly led to important considerations of workforce training and development. Even by the 1980s a growing cadre of doctors was developing an interest in the care of terminally ill patients and their families. While many had transferred into this work in mid or even late career, others were interested in dedicating an entire professional life to it. But without more formal recognition, the pathways into and routes through a training program for specialized work in the care of the dying, remained unclear.

SPECIALIZATION

In the context of this expansive period of hospice development in the 1980s, three factors conjoined to build a platform for the broad consolidation of the new field of activity: a medical association was formed to support its practitioners; a scientific journal was established; and recognition was given to palliative medicine as an area of specialization. (The following section draws on oral history interviews conducted by the author with Dr Gillian Ford [June 6, 1996] and Dr Derek Doyle [December 28, 1995 and February 13, 1996], as part of the hospice history program of the

International Observatory on End of Life Care, Lancaster University.)

By 1985, plans were being developed in the UK for the creation of an association to represent the interests of physicians working in palliative care. Cicely Saunders wrote enthusiastically about it to Edinburgh doctor and independent hospice pioneer Derek Doyle[34] who together with Robert Twycross and Richard Hillier (both of whom had developed hospice services within the context of the NHS) made up a key group of early protagonists. Following some early discussion about whether the term 'hospice' should appear in the name, the group soon came to be known as the Association for Palliative Medicine for Great Britain and Ireland. The executive committee of the new association quickly became aware of a paper written by the then Deputy Chief Medical Officer for England, Gillian Ford, in which she outlined the potential for this new field of medicine to gain recognition as a specialty in its own right. Discussions got underway with a number of key committees within the Royal Colleges, including the Intercollegiate Committee on Oncology and ideas were developed about how a training program for the field could be put together. It proved that the most influential group in this regard was the Joint Committee on Higher Medical Training (JCHMT). At the time, a growing number of universities and medical schools were calling on those working in hospices to teach students about pain control and about communications issues, although at that stage no formal curriculum on palliative medicine existed. Gillian Ford, a long-time friend of Cicely Saunders and close associate of St Christopher's, prepared a paper for the JCHMT and at the same time encouraged the chairman of the Specialty Advisory Committee in General Medicine and other senior medical colleagues to visit St Christopher's for an appreciation of the work being done there. These senior medical colleagues found themselves impressed by the research of Robert Twycross on the actions of morphine and diamorphine[29] and by Colin Murray Parkes' evaluations of the impact of hospice care.[35] There was also considerable interest in the multidisciplinary approach that was being adopted at the hospice and the way in which the efforts of the team were focused on the 'total pain' of the patient, seen in a multifactorial light. Yet there was still a sense up to the late 1970s and early 1980s that the constituent elements of what came to be called specialist palliative care, had not yet been teased out. This made for difficulties in devising a training program for what at that time were known as the senior registrar years within medical training. It was also necessary to determine the specific background experience that would be necessary for entry into the new field.

The outcome of these deliberations was enormously important for the history of palliative care in the UK and Ireland, and arguably much further afield too. In 1987 palliative medicine was established as a subspecialty of general medicine, initially on a 7-year 'novitiate', which once successfully concluded, led to the creation of a specialty in its

own right. Indeed the specialty broke new ground in accepting as an appropriate qualification for entry, membership of the Royal Colleges of Physicians, Radiology, and Anaesthetics; initially membership of the Royal College of General Practitioners was not a recognized mode of entry, though considerable protest and further campaigning led to its recognition within a few years.

At the same time as these wider developments were taking place, discussions were also underway about the creation of a journal to publish research, reviews, and debate relating to the work of the new field. Following some discussion about its name (again revolving around whether the word 'hospice' should be included) and orientation, the first issue was published in 1987. It bore the title *Palliative Medicine*, under which a 'strap line' appeared on the cover stating: *a multi-professional journal*. The wording was crucial and did a fair amount to antagonize colleagues in other professions, but the message was clear: medical practitioners had seized hold of the new field of caring for those with advanced disease at the end of life and over time, the medical model would exert a growing influence on thinking and practice.

Developments in Ireland took a similar path when in 1989 the first post of consultant physician in palliative medicine was created in the form of a joint appointment between Our Lady's Hospice and St Vincent's University Hospital, Dublin. Then in the mid-1990s, the Irish Medical Council considered the inclusion of palliative medicine in its list of recognized specialties. Such recognition required evidence of a significant corpus of knowledge specific to palliative medicine, over and above that which would be within the competence of any registered medical practitioner, as well as the existence of a recognized body to oversee developments in the new specialty, including training and education. The Minister for Health and Children approved the inclusion of palliative medicine among the list of recognized Irish medical specialties in June 1995.[36]

Within an intensive period of activity lasting just a few years, both the UK and Ireland had succeeded in establishing palliative care as a medical specialty, with a training program leading to consultant status. Arrangements for representing the interests of the field were now in place and an appropriate scientific journal had been established. Subsequently there was considerable expansion in the palliative medicine workforce.

A survey of the membership of the Association of Palliative Medicine (APM) in 2004[37] revealed that 58.1 percent were in full-time appointments in palliative medicine and 70.4 percent of the workforce was female. There were 325 consultants, 49 associate specialists, and 78 staff grade postholders as well as 160 specialist registrars, of which 83 percent were women. Some 60 consultants held honorary NHS contracts, but despite an APM recommendation, there were few NHS consultants holding honorary contracts with hospices. In Ireland specifically there were in 2005 seven consultant physicians in palliative medicine, with seven further consultant posts in the process of being filled.[38]

Trainees in palliative medicine undertake a 4-year program of professional development, which involves periods of 'rotation' through a variety of care settings – hospital based and community services, as well as hospices and departments of oncology. Most take advantage of a period for research, sometimes linked to academic departments, though numbers undertaking research degrees for MD and PhD appear to remain rather low.

Such expansion in the infrastructure of palliative medicine has been made possible by wider service developments and policy changes. During the 1970s and 1980s, as we have seen, a major program of hospice expansion had taken place in the UK, gaining wide geographical coverage. The expansion in charitable hospices was also reflected in a growing number of NHS inpatient units, although the ratio between the two has remained fairly constant at roughly 3:1. Indeed it is the 'mixed economy' of care between the nongovernment and government sectors that is such a distinct hallmark of the development of palliative care in the UK and Ireland. From the later 1980s onwards, hospice and palliative care services in the UK also benefited from special government funding streams, enabling the consolidation and expansion of provision and providing ring-fenced monies initially for independent hospices and then for palliative care more generally.[39] There were some other specific policy innovations at this time. In 1992 an expert group of physicians and nurses reported to the UK Minister of Health and was instrumental in making a case for palliative care to be provided on the basis of need, rather than diagnosis; the report called for wider education in palliative care for all health professionals and greater emphasis on matching services to needs identified at the population level.[40] Three years later the Expert Advisory Group on Cancer produced what came to be know as the 'Calman Hine Report' on the commissioning of cancer services in England and Wales.[41] It was crucial in giving a prominent place to palliative care within the different tiers of cancer care provision and in giving guidance on the staffing levels required in relation to a population of specific size. The report was seized upon by the palliative medicine community as an opportunity for development.

In the early 1990s the UK also saw the creation of the first university chair in the palliative care field. A professor in palliative medicine was appointed to it and this set the tone for subsequent academic developments, which tended to focus on the clinical disciplines. By 2005 there were in the UK some nine chairs in medicine and nursing relating to palliative care as well as three chairs occupied by social scientists with a major interest in the field. The academic departments of palliative medicine have developed varied cultures and strands of interest. In some cases the emphasis has been predominantly on clinical studies focused on pain and symptom management. In others there has been a leaning towards matters of policy, service organization, and evaluation. Social science perspectives have had considerable prominence in some departments, focusing around wider questions of social inequality, cultural values, ethnicity, spirituality, and the psychosocial dimensions of palliative care. The perspectives of the medical humanities have also been visible. A major boost to development came in 2005 with the creation of two major research collaboratives in supportive and palliative care supported by a consortium of funders coordinated through the National Cancer Research Institute. These will combine the efforts of multiple academic groups, along with a variety of other partners to advance the field and build the future infrastructure for research.

Other developments have also taken place in the education of healthcare professionals in matters relating to palliative care. During the 1980s and 1990s the curricula of medical and nursing schools as well as courses for occupational therapists and physiotherapists, social workers, and others began to include elements on the principles and practices of palliative care. A comparative survey to determine the presence of end-of-life issues in the undergraduate medical school curricula of the UK and USA found almost universal coverage of dying, death, and bereavement, and most addressed the topic of palliative care. Hospice involvement was found in 96 percent of UK medical schools.[42] Similarly, a survey of senior tutors coordinating entry level degree and diploma nursing courses showed that diploma students received a mean of 7.8 hours and degree students 12.2 hours of teaching in palliative care, compared with the mean of 20 hours of teaching offered to undergraduate medical students in the UK.[43] A 2002 study sought to examine changes in formal teaching about death, dying, and bereavement in undergraduate medical education in UK medical schools and was based on earlier surveys conducted in 1983 and 1994. It found that the amount of such teaching varied widely and appeared in the curriculum in a variety of aspects, times, and places. Specialists in palliative medicine, general practitioners, and nurse specialists were most frequently involved in teaching, with decreased involvement of nonpractitioners since 1983. Most schools covered a wide range of topics, with all addressing attitudes towards death and dying and symptom relief in advanced terminal illness. Some schools used terminally ill patients directly in their teaching and most included hospice participation. Changes in undergraduate medical education, especially in terms of more integrated curricula, mean that for many schools, palliative care teaching is integrated into learning in other areas. This should help students apply their palliative care learning to other contexts. The increase in teaching about the management of physical symptoms that had occurred since the previous surveys seemed to reflect the establishment of palliative medicine as a specialty and the current emphasis within palliative care practice in the UK.[44]

Such achievements have often been looked upon with admiration by others elsewhere, but palliative care in the UK and Ireland continues to face many challenges. In the British context, a health committee of the House of Commons reporting in 2004 took a critical view of palliative care provision. Its 30 key points included concerns about the lack of early referral to palliative care, the limited potential for those wishing to die at home to be enabled to do so, the continuing problem of matching provision to need, the concern that acceptance of the current diversity of provision could also entail tolerance of continued inequity – particularly in relation to age, ethnicity, and complex needs, and the lack of access to palliative care on the part of patients with diseases other than cancer. It also urged the Royal Colleges to ensure that training in palliative care becomes part of continuing professional development, and to consider making such modules a mandatory requirement for revalidation. Notably, the committee applauded the Government's ambition to double the number of palliative care consultants by 2015 based on the figures for 2002 – a point seen as particularly important in relation to the growing needs for palliative care resulting from population aging and a rising incidence of chronic disease and comorbidities. The findings of the committee provide an important agenda for UK palliative care development in the first decade of the twenty first century.

SPECIALIZATION AND ITS DISCONTENTS

In the early years modern hospice and palliative care in the UK and Ireland had many of the qualities of a social movement supported by wider forces. This movement may well have contributed to a new openness about death and bereavement which was in evidence in the late twentieth century. The first person ever to be seen dying on television in the UK, for example, was a patient in the care of an Irish hospice.[45] The hospice movement condemned the neglect of the dying in society and called for high quality pain and symptom management for all who needed it. At the same time it sought to reconstruct death as a natural phenomenon, rather than a clinical failure and marshaled practical and moral argument to oppose those in favor of euthanasia.

At the same time specialty recognition can be seen as a turning point in hospice and palliative care history.[46] For some, specialization is seen as the key to integration of palliative care into the mainstream health system and a major platform from which to develop an 'evidence-based' model of practice and organization that is crucial to long-term viability. Others mourn the loss of the early ideals of the hospice movement and condemn the emphasis upon physical symptoms at the expense of psychosocial and spiritual concerns. In short, there have been claims that forces of medicalization and routinization[47] are at work or even that the putative 'holism' of palliative care philosophy masks a new, more subtle form of surveillance of the dying and bereaved in modern society.[22] Even by the early 1990s, one Irish palliative medicine physician could raise concerns about palliative medicine developing into a specialty narrowly bounded by the practice of 'symptomatology' and thereby failing to create the conditions for deeper, personal 'healing'.[48]

In a later work he went on to emphasize the need for palliative medicine to draw upon Greek traditions associated with Asklepian healing and for these to be integrated with the modern science of symptom control.[49] As the specialty develops, its medical attention tends to focus on pain and symptom management as a bounded set of problems within the relief of suffering – giving weight to the charge of creeping medicalization. At the same time it is precisely in this biomedical area of palliative care that measurable and striking successes are to be found in the use of pain relieving and symptom controlling technologies, some of which seem not yet to have percolated into the wider healthcare system.

By the end of the twentieth century a growing commitment to the evidence base was emerging in palliative medicine, although several reviewers found this still a rather fragile enterprise and made claims for the particular problems faced by palliative care in assessing its practice by such means.[50,51] Two forces for expansion were, however, clearly visible. First was the impetus to move palliative care further upstream in the disease progression, thereby seeking integration with curative and rehabilitation therapies and shifting the focus beyond terminal care and the final stages of life. Second there was a growing interest in extending the benefits of palliative care to those with diseases other than cancer, to make 'palliative care for all' a reality. The new specialty was therefore delicately poised. For some, such integration with the wider system was a *sine qua non* for success; for others it marked the entry into a risky phase of new development in which early ideals might be compromised.

In the UK and Ireland hospice care and palliative care have a shared and brief history. The evolution of one into the other marks far more than a simple change of nomenclature. It signifies a transition which, if successful, could ensure that the benefits of a model of care previously available to just a few people at the end of life will in time be extended to all who need it, regardless of diagnosis, stage of disease, social situation, or means. Much remains to be done, however, if that goal is to be achieved.

Key learning points

- Some evidence of interest in the care of the dying began to develop in the late nineteenth century, but its influence was limited in extent.

- By the mid-twentieth century attention was beginning to focus on the social denial of death and medical neglect of the dying.

- As the new field of hospice care emerged a multidisciplinary approach to pain and symptom management was promoted.

- Attention was also given to the wider definition of suffering: physical, psychological, social, spiritual.

- A tripartite model of hospice care emerged: clinical care, education, and research.
- Modes of care delivery began to diversify.
- Specialty recognition was achieved for palliative medicine and the workforce grew accordingly.
- Palliative medicine sought to extend care to earlier stages of the disease progression and to nonmalignant disease.
- Attention focused on the establishment of an evidence base.
- While the development of the specialty of palliative medicine has been widely welcomed, there are some concerns about the medicalization of care at the end of life and the role of palliative medicine within the process.

REFERENCES

1   Humphreys C. 'Waiting for the last summons': the establishment of the first hospices in England 1878–1914. *Mortality* 2001; **6**: 146–66.

◆ 2   Clark D. History, gender and culture in the rise of palliative care. In: Payne S, Seymour J, Ingleton C, eds. *Palliative Care Nursing: Principles and Evidence For Practice.* Buckingham: Open University Press, 2004: 39–54.

3   Hughes N, Clark D. 'A thoughtful and experienced physician': William Munk and the care of the dying in late Victorian England. *J Palliat Med* 2004; **7**: 703–10.

4   Jalland P. *Death in the Victorian Family.* Oxford: Oxford University Press, 1996.

● 5   Munk W. *Euthanasia: or, Medical Treatment in Aid of an Easy Death.* London: Longmans, Green and Co, 1887.

6   Reviews and Notices of books. *Lancet* 1888; January 7: 21–2.

7   Cushing H. *The Life of Sir William Osler.* Oxford: Oxford University Press, 1940.

8   Macdonald A. The study of death in man [letter]. *Lancet* 1926; September 18: 624.

● 9   Worcester A. *The Care of the Aged, the Dying and the Dead.* Springfield, Illinois: Charles C Thomas, 1935.

10   Clark D. Cradled to the grave? Pre-conditions for the hospice movement in the UK, 1948–67. *Mortality* 1999; **4**: 225–47.

11   Joint National Cancer Survey Committee of the Marie Curie Memorial and the Queen's Institute of District Nursing. *Report on a National Survey Concerning Patients with Cancer Nursed at Home.* Chairman, Ronald Raven. London, 1952.

12   Gough-Thomas J. Day and night nursing for cancer patients. *District Nurs* 1962; November: 174–5.

13   Glyn Hughes HL. *Peace at the Last. A Survey of Terminal Care in the United Kingdom.* London: The Calouste Gulbenkian Foundation, 1960.

14   Bailey M. A survey of the social needs of patients with incurable lung cancer. *Almoner* 1959; **11**: 379–7.

15   Aitken-Swan J, Paterson R. The cancer patient: delay in help seeking. *Br Med J* 1955; **i**: 623–31.

16   Parkes CM. Recent bereavement as a cause of mental illness. *Br J Psychiatry* 1964; **110**: 198–204.

17   Wilkes E. Cancer outside hospital. *Lancet* 1964; June 20: 1379–81.

18   Wilkes E. Terminal cancer at home. *Lancet* 1965; **i**: 799–801.

19   Hinton J. The physical and mental distress of the dying. *Q J Med* 1963; **125**: 1–20.

20   Hinton J. Problems in the care of the dying. *J Chronic Dis* 1964; **17**: 201–5.

21   Distress in dying [leading article]. *Br Med J* 1963; August **17**: 400–1.

◆ 22   Clark D. 'Total pain', disciplinary power and the body in the work of Cicely Saunders 1958–67. *Soc Sci Med* 1999; **49**: 727–36.

23   Saunders C. Care of patients suffering from terminal illness at St Joseph's Hospice, Hackney, London. *Nurs Mirror* 1964; February 14: vii–x.

24   Saunders C. Drug treatment in the terminal stages of cancer. *Curr Med Drugs* 1960; July 1: 16–28.

◆ 25   Clark D. An annotated bibliography of the publications of Cicely Saunders – 1. 1958–67. *Palliat Med* 1998; **12**: 181–93.

26   Faull C, Nicholson A. Taking the myths out of the magic: establishing the use of opioids in the management of cancer pain. In: Meldrum ML, ed. *Opioids and Pain Relief: A Historical Perspective.* Seattle: IASP Press, 2003: 111–30.

27   Clark D. The rise and demise of the 'Brompton Cocktail'. In: Meldrum ML, ed. *Opioids and Pain Relief: A Historical Perspective.* Seattle: IASP Press, 2003: 85–98.

28   Twycross R. The Brompton Cocktail. In: Bonica JJ, Ventafridda V, eds. *Advances in Pain Research and Therapy, Vol 2.* New York: Raven Press, 1979.

● 29   Twycross RG. Choice of strong analgesic in terminal cancer: diamorphine or morphine? *J Int Assoc Stud Pain* 1977; **3**: 93–104.

30   Saunders C. Current views on pain relief and terminal care. In: Swerdlow M, ed. *The Therapy of Pain.* Lancaster: MTP Press, 1981: 251–41.

31   Murray Parkes CM. Home or hospital? Terminal care as seen by surviving spouses. *J R Coll Gen Pract* 1978; **28**: 29–30.

32   Murray Parkes CM, Parkes J. 'Hospice' versus 'hospital' care–re-evaluation after 10 years as seen by surviving spouses. *Postgrad Med J* 1984; **60**: 38–42.

33   National Council for Palliative Care. *Minimum Data Sets Project Update.* London: National Council for Palliative Care, February 2005.

34   Cicely Saunders to Derek Doyle, October 15, 1985. In: Clark D, ed. *Cicely Saunders. Founder of the Hospice Movement. Selected Letters 1959–1999.* Oxford: Oxford University Press, 2002: 262.

● 35   Murray Parkes C, Parkes J. Hospice versus hospital care – re-evaluation after ten years as seen by surviving spouses. *Postgrad Med J* 1979; **60**: 120–4.

36   O'Brien T, Clark D. A national plan for palliative care – the Irish experience. In: Ling J, O'Siorain L, eds. *Palliative Care in Ireland.* Maidenhead: Open University Press, 2005: 3–18.

37   Association for Palliative Medicine of Great Britain and Ireland *Reports from Medical Workforce Database 2004.* Southampton: APM, 2004.

38   Department of Health and Children. Palliative care in Ireland. Available at: www.dohc.ie/public/information/cancer_services/palliative_care.html (accessed August 17, 2005).

◆ 39   Clark D. Seymour J. *Reflections on Palliative Care. Sociological and Policy Perspectives.* Buckingham: Open University Press, 1999.

40 Standing Medical Advisory Committee/Standing Nursing and Midwifery Advisory Committee. *The Principles and Provision of Palliative Care.* London: HMSO, 1992.

41 Expert Advisory Group on Cancer. *A Policy Framework for the Commissioning of Cancer Services.* London: Department of Health and Welsh Office, 1995.

42 Dickinson GE, Field D. Teaching end-of-life issues: current status in United Kingdom and United States medical schools. *Am J Hosp Palliat Care* 2002; **19**:181–6.

43 Lloyd-Williams M, Field D. Are undergraduate nurses taught palliative care during their training? *Nurse Educ Today* 2002; **22**: 589–92.

44 Field D, Wee B. Preparation for palliative care: teaching about death, dying and bereavement in UK medical schools 2000–2001. *Med Educ* 2002; **36**: 561–7.

45 Neuberger J. Death on camera. *BMJ* 1998; **316**: 1100.

46 Fordham S, Dowrick C, May C. Palliative medicine: is it really specialist territory? *J R Soc Med* 1998; **91**: 568–72.

47 Hoy A. Routinisation and medicalisation. *Eur J Palliat Care* 1999; **6**: 178.

● 48 Kearney M. Palliative medicine – just another specialty? *Palliat Med* 1992; **6**: 39–46.

49 Kearney M. *A Place of Healing. Working with Suffering in Living and Dying.* Oxford: Oxford University Press, 2000.

50 Higginson I. Evidence based palliative care. *BMJ* 1999; **319**: 462–3.

51 Keeley D. Rigorous assessment of palliative care revisited. Wisdom and compassion are needed when evidence is lacking. *BMJ* 1999; **319**: 1447–8.

The development of palliative medicine in Europe

FRANCO DE CONNO, HEIDI BLUMHUBER, JAVIER ROCAFORT

INTRODUCTION

First of all it is important to consider what exactly constitutes 'Europe'. The World Health Organization (WHO) describes Europe as representing 52 different countries.[1] The Council of Europe, the oldest political European organization, has 46 member states.[2] The European Union linked 15 independent nations until 2004, when this number increased to 25.[3] These three different definitions of Europe clearly illustrate the diversity of 'Europe': countries with different languages, history, cultures, economies, and education and healthcare systems.

This variety is also reflected in the organization and development of palliative care in Europe. It is still impossible to talk about common development in Europe, but it is possible to present some snapshots and details that give an idea about palliative care in Europe. Of the 53 countries listed in Table 2.1, 34 countries[4] can be identified as having at least one palliative care association at the national level. Yet among these 34 countries there are distinct differences. The UK has six different palliative care associations (four for professionals, one common research society, and one umbrella organization). France and Italy have one multiprofessional association each (Société Française d'Accompagnement et de soins Palliatifs [SFAP] and Società Italiana di Cure Palliative [SICP], respectively) that collaborates closely with a federation of the supporting volunteer associations (Jusqu'à la mort accompagner la vie [JALMALV] and Federazione Cure Palliative Onlus [FCP]). In Germany there is the German Palliative Care Society, mainly formed of physicians, and a hospice association. In the Netherlands, the national association the called the 'Network of Palliative Care Services'. Belgium has different palliative care associations catering for the different languages spoken in the country, whereas in Switzerland there is one multiprofessional national association for professionals speaking any of the three languages of the country.

HISTORY

The development of modern palliative care started in the 1960s with the hospice movement in the UK, offering continuous care for incurable patients. Dame Cicely Saunders introduced this change with her vision of holistic medicine, combining a humanistic and sensitive approach to continuing care with the use of recent knowledge and advanced techniques in symptom control. For some years palliative care remained the 'exclusive property' of the UK.

In the rest of Europe two events were significant for development of palliative care. The first was the dissemination of WHO's *Cancer Pain Relief* in 1986.[5] This booklet, and its validation study, induced a change in the interest paid to the problem of cancer pain and heralded an increase in the consumption of opioids. Through attention to pain, an awareness of the multifaceted problems and needs of the patients with advanced disease crept into the daily practice of many healthcare professionals. Another significant event was the first international congress organized in Milan, Italy, thanks to the initiative of Professor Vittorio Ventafridda and the Floriani Foundation. As a consequence, the European Association for Palliative Care (EAPC) was created in December 1988, with the aim to increase awareness and promote the development and dissemination of palliative

Table 2.1 *Countries in Europe with national palliative care associations (NPCAs)*

Group	No.	Country	NPCA	Entry in Council of Europe	WHO
European Union until 2004	1	Austria	Yes	April 16, 1956	WHO
	2	Belgium	Yes	May 05, 1949	WHO
	3	Denmark	Yes	May 05, 1949	WHO
	4	Finland	Yes	May 05, 1989	WHO
	5	France	Yes	May 05, 1949	WHO
	6	Germany	Yes	July 13, 1950	WHO
	7	Greece	Yes	August 09, 1949	WHO
	8	Ireland	Yes	May 05, 1949	WHO
	9	Italy	Yes	May 05, 1949	WHO
	10	Luxembourg	Yes	May 05, 1949	WHO
	11	Netherlands	Yes	May 05, 1949	WHO
	12	Portugal	Yes	September 22, 1976	WHO
	13	Spain	Yes	November 24, 1977	WHO
	14	Sweden	Yes	May 05, 1949	WHO
	15	United Kingdom	Yes	May 05, 1949	WHO
European Union from 2004	16	Cyprus	Yes	May 24, 1961	WHO
	17	Czech Republic		June 30, 1993	WHO
	18	Estonia		May 14, 1993	WHO
	19	Hungary	Yes	November 06, 1990	WHO
	20	Latvia		February 10, 1995	WHO
	21	Lithuania	Yes	May 14, 1993	WHO
	22	Malta		April 29, 1965	WHO
	23	Poland	Yes	November 26, 1991	WHO
	24	Slovakia	Yes	June 30, 1993	WHO
	25	Slovenia	Yes	May 14, 1993	WHO
Application to join European Union	26	Bulgaria	Yes	May 07, 1992	WHO
	27	Croatia	Yes	November 06, 1996	WHO
	28	Romania	Yes	October 07, 1993	WHO
	29	Turkey		August 09, 1949	WHO
NOT European Union but part of Council of Europe	30	Albania	Yes	July 13, 1995	WHO
	31	Andorra		November 10, 1994	WHO
	32	Armenia		January 25, 2001	WHO
	33	Azerbaijan		January 25, 2001	WHO
	34	Bosnia and Herzegovina	Yes	April 24, 2002	WHO
	35	Georgia		April 27, 1999	WHO
	36	Iceland	Yes	March 07, 1950	WHO
	37	Liechtenstein		November 23, 1978	
	38	Moldova	Yes	July 13, 1995	WHO
	39	Norway	Yes	May 05, 1949	WHO
	40	Russian Federation	Yes	February 28, 1996	WHO
	41	San Marino		November 16, 1988	WHO
	42	Serbia and Montenegro		April 03, 2003	WHO
	43	Switzerland	Yes	May 06, 1963	WHO
	44	The former Yugoslav Republic of Macedonia	Yes	November, 09 1995	WHO
	45	Ukraine	Yes	November 09, 1995	WHO

(Continued)

Table 2.1   *(Continued)*

Group	No.	Country	NPCA	Entry in Council of Europe	WHO
NOT Council of	46	Belarus			WHO
Europe but listed as	47	Israel	Yes		WHO
European Region by	48	Kazakhstan			WHO
the WHO	49	Kyrgyzstan			WHO
	50	Monaco			WHO
	51	Tajikistan			WHO
	52	Turkmenistan			WHO
	53	Uzbekistan			WHO

WHO, World Health Organization.

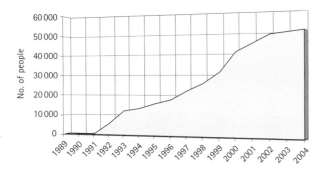

Figure 2.1   *European Association for Palliative Care: people represented 1989–2004. Reproduced with permission from the EAPC.*

care at scientific, clinical, and social levels. This could be best achieved through the implementation of existing knowledge, training of those who, at any level, are involved with the care of patients with incurable and advanced disease, and promotion of study and research (offering patronage to scientific and educational events promoting the dissemination and development of palliative care). In addition, the promotion and sponsorship of publications or periodicals concerning palliative care was endorsed, bringing together those who study and practice the disciplines involved in the care of patients with advanced disease (doctors, nurses, social workers, psychologists and volunteers). Finally, it was hoped that the EAPC would unify the national palliative care organizations and establish an international network for the exchange of expertise and addressing the ethical problems associated with the care of terminally ill patients.

In 1992 the first national palliative care associations joined the EAPC collectively and in 2004, the association became a federation with 31 associations from 22 countries representing a movement of about 50 000 persons (Figs 2.1 and 2.2).

THE EAPC DEFINITION OF PALLIATIVE CARE

In 1998, on the occasion of the revision of the bylaws to ratify its status as a 'nonprofit' organization (EAPC Onlus),

the EAPC also revised its definition of palliative care, first set out in Spring 1989 and published in the EAPC newsletter of that year:[6]

> 3. Palliative care is the active, total care of the patients whose disease is not responsive to curative treatment. Control of pain, of other symptoms, and of social, psychological and spiritual problems is paramount.

> 4. Palliative care is interdisciplinary in its approach and encompasses the patient, the family and the community in its scope. In a sense, palliative care is to offer the most basic concept of care – that of providing for the needs of the patient wherever he or she is cared for, either at home or in the hospital.

> 5. Palliative care affirms life and regards dying as a normal process; it neither hastens nor postpones death. It sets out to preserve the best possible quality of life until death.

RECOGNITION OF PALLIATIVE MEDICINE/ CARE BY GOVERNMENTAL BODIES

In 1998 the EAPC was awarded the status of nongovernmental organization (NGO) of the Council of Europe. In June 1999 the Parliamentary Assembly of the Council of Europe adopted a document on the: 'Protection of the human rights and dignity of the terminally ill and the dying'.[7] This document mentions and underlines the need for palliative care. Toward the end of 2003, the Council of Europe released a second document entitled 'Recommendation REC 24 (2003) of the Committee of Ministers to member states on the organisation of palliative care',[8] which was approved and adopted on by all ministers of health. In 2004, the EAPC promoted a project for the translation and dissemination of those recommendations in many different languages.

Delivery of palliative care

In view of the strategic developments taking place in the healthcare systems in Europe, we consider it timely to cite the

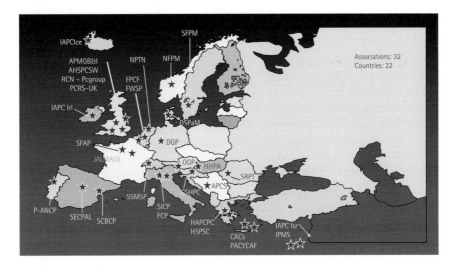

AHSPCSW	Association of Hospice and Specialist Palliative Care Social Workers	JALMALV	Fédération JALMALV
APMGB	Association for Palliative Medicine of Great Britain and Ireland	NFPM	Norwegian Association for Palliative Medicine
CACS	Cyprus Anti-Cancer Society	NPTN	Netherlands Palliative Care Network for Terminally Ill Patients
CSHPC	Croatian Society for Hospice and Palliative Care	OPG	Österreichische Palliativgesellschaft (Austrian Society for Palliative Care)
DGP	Deutsche Gesellschaft für Palliativmedizin		
DSPaM	Danish Society of Palliative Medicine	PACYCAF	Cyprus Association of Cancer Patients and Friends
FBSP	Fédération Bruxelloise Pluraliste de Soins Pallliatifs et Continus	P-ANCP	Associação Nacional de Cuid. Paliativos
		PCRS-UK	Palliative Care Research Society UK
FCP	Federazione Cure Palliative	RCN – Pcgroup	Royal College of Nursing – Palliative Nursing Group
FPCF	Federation Palliative Care Flanders	SAPC	Sarajevo Association of Palliative Care
FWSP	Fédération Wallonne des Soins Palliatifs	SCBCP	Soc. Catalano-Balear de Cures Palliatves
HAPCPC	Hellenic Association for Pain Control and Palliative Care	SECPAL	Soc. Española de Cuidados Paliativos
		SFAP	Société Française d'Accompagnement et de Soins Palliatifs
HHPA	Hungarian Hospice Association		
HSPSC	Hellenic Society of Palliative-Symptomatic Care	SFPM	Swedish Association for Palliative Care
IAPC Ice	Icelandic Association for Palliative Care	SICP	Società Italiana di Cure Palliative
IAPC Irl	Irish Association for Palliative Care	SRPT	The Romanian Society of Palliatology & Thanatology
IPAC Isr	Israel Association of Palliative Care	SSMSP	Société Suisse de Médecine et de Soins Palliatifs

Figure 2.2   *National associations – collective members of the European Association for Palliative Care, 2004. Reproduced with permission from the EAPC.*

following items from the above mentioned document (repro-duced from CM(2003)130 Addendum[9] with permission).

Settings

67. Palliative care takes place in the following settings:
  – home
  – nursing home
  – home for the elderly
  – hospital
  – hospice

Services

71. A distinction is useful between non-specialist and special-ist palliative care services. Non-specialist or conventional services provide palliative care without making this into their core business. They include: district nursing services, general practitioners, home care teams, general internal medicine wards, and nursing homes.

72. The large majority of palliative care is, and will probably always be, provided by non-specialist services. In many cases, non-specialised professionals provide the care without the intervention of specialists; in many other cases, specialised intervention may be needed in the context of non-specialist care, while in a small proportion of the cases, specialists will need to take over the care entirely.

73. Non-specialised services also include services that are involved only incidentally, such as radiology and radiotherapy departments, surgery. Such services sometimes have waiting lists that may be especially detrimental to palliative care patients because of their short remaining life span in which they could benefit from the treatment. Therefore, the con-cept of a 'palliative bus lane', involving preferential access for palliative patients, has been proposed.

74. A specific area where the concept of palliative care has received increased attention over the last years, is the intensive care unit.

75. Non-specialists may build up sufficient experience in rel-atively uncomplicated palliative care but, due to the limited number of palliative patients they see (in the Netherlands, for example, general practitioners on average see between 2–6 [*sic*] palliative care patients per year), the experience with complex palliative care cannot be acquired. Experiments with easily accessible consultation services show good possibilities

of support for non-specialised professionals while the patient can remain within their care.

76. Specialised services denote services fully devoted to palliative care, whose teams are specially trained in this area of care. Such services do not take the place of the care provided by front-line professionals (home care, hospital or rehabilitation facilities), but support and complement such care according to the needs identified and the complexity of the situation. Wherever they are, patients must be able, if necessary, to access such services at all times and without delay.

77. The most common services are specialist in-patient units, hospital palliative care teams, home care teams, day care facilities, hospitalisation at the home, and out patient clinics.

78. There is very little good evidence as to what type of palliative care services are preferred by patients. In a review, Wilkinson *et al.* noticed a trend toward greater satisfaction with specialised services, both in hospitals and in the community, as compared to general hospitals. (Wilkinson *et al.* 1999). Again, these results should be interpreted with caution.

79. Non-specialist services include the following:
   - informal caregivers
   - volunteers (?)
   - district nurses
   - general practitioners
   - non-palliative care specialists.

80. Specialist palliative care services are those services with palliative care as there [*sic*] core activity. They will require a higher level of professional skills from trained staff and a high staff/patient ratio. Such services should be available in all care settings and should be able to support a patient wherever the patient may be: at home, in hospital, in residential care, in nursing home, in day centres, in out-patients or in a specialist palliative care unit. Specialised palliative care services also have an important role in supporting other health care professionals in the delivery of palliative care services at hospital and community level. All health care professionals should be able to access, advise [*sic*] and support from specialised palliative care providers when required.

81. The key characteristics of a specialist palliative care services have been described by the National Council for Hospice and Specialist Palliative Care Services in the United Kingdom and are endorsed by the National Advisory Committee on Palliative Care (Ireland). These are summarised as follows:

   - the provision of physical, psychological, social and spiritual support, with a mix of skills delivered through a multi-professional, collaborative team approach;
   - at least the lead person in each professional group within the multi-professional team should be a trained and acknowledged specialist in palliative care;
   - patients and families are supported and involved in management plans;
   - patients are encouraged to express their preference about where they wish to be cared for and where they wish to die;

   - carers and families are supported through the illness into bereavement, and the needs of the bereaved are recognised and addressed;
   - there is cooperation and collaboration with primary health care professionals, hospital and home care services to support patients wherever they might be;
   - the contribution of volunteers is recognised and valued;
   - the service has either indirectly or directly a recognised academic external educational role and in-service education provision;
   - standards are set for the education and training provided;
   - quality assurance programmes are in place and are constantly used to review practice;
   - clinical audit and research programmes exist to evaluate treatment and outcome;
   - staff support arrangements exist which are appropriate to meet the needs of those working in specialist palliative care, whether fulltime or part-time.

We can summarize the characteristics described in the above citation as follows:

- A hospital-based palliative unit (specialist) can be composed of:
   – Ambulatory service (outpatients)
   – Day hospital (day care)
   – Beds (inpatients)
   – Intra-hospital consultation team
   – Home care team or home care support teams
- Hospices (free-standing) can be composed of:
   – Day hospital (day care)
   – Beds (inpatients)
- Home care can be delivered by:
   – Specialized teams
   – Support teams
   – General practitioners
- Nursing homes
- Homes for elderly people (long-term inpatients)

NATIONAL LEGISLATIONS

With the exception of the two documents of the Council of Europe, there is no unified European policy for the implementation of palliative care. In 2003, the EAPC decided to organize a survey on the situation of palliative care in each European country, with the aim to collect reliable information on the delivery of and to explain the current organization of hospice and palliative care in Europe, taking into account political, social, healthcare policy and related factors. This project will be carried out in form of a task force chaired by the Spanish EAPC Board Member Carlos Centeno Cortes, in collaboration with other institutions. From the literature review, the first step of the work of this task carried out by Javier Rocafort, we present an example of the data (see Appendix 2.1 for data sources) collected about the legislation of five different countries (Boxes 2.1–2.5).

Box 2.1 Palliative care in Belgium

Political system: Constitutional monarchy
Capital city: Brussels
Total area: 30 158 km^2
Population: 10.2 million
Currency: Euro
Laws:

- July 15, 1994: Law on the organization of palliative care units in hospitals, with the scope of symptom control, and psychological and bereavement support

- July 21, 1994: Law stating that employees can request unpaid leave of 2 years to care for a family member with an incurable (terminal) disease and receive economical support from the state

- October 30, 1996: Law defining need of 10 palliative care beds per 10 000 inhabitants

- June 15, 1997: Law defining that all geriatric nursing homes with more than 60 beds must have a palliative care unit

- July 15, 1997: Law about implementation of hospital consultation teams with the scope to develop attitudes and disseminate knowledge about palliative care in all hospital caregivers

- July 15, 1997: Law for the creation of regional bodies to coordinate delivery of palliative care. One body for an area of between 300 000 and 1 000 000 inhabitants

- October 13, 1998: Law defining need of one home care team with two nurses and one doctor for 100 patients (per 300 000 inhabitants)

Box 2.2 Palliative care in France

Political system: Republic
Capital city: Paris
Total area: 550 000 km^2
Population: 60.4 million
Currency: Euro
Laws:

- 1986: Law on the creation of at least one palliative care unit in each 'department' (French province)

- November 1994: A high-ranked commissioner of the health ministry identified pain as one of the most important problems in France. Law obliges the health institutions to organize better for the control of pain of their patients

- September 1995: Ethical code includes an item about the relief of suffering

- 1999: Establishment of a 3-year national program for the implementation of palliative care in the healthcare system with a financial budget of €58 million. This program also included that employees can request unpaid leave of 3 months to care for a family member with an incurable (terminal) disease and officially recognized the role of volunteers in palliative care

- 2002: Establishment of a second 3-year national program with the following aims: establishment of home care, guaranteeing a palliative care unit of 10 beds in at least one university hospital in each French region, and organization of a campaign to raise the awareness of the population

---

EDUCATION

In an editorial in *Palliative Medicine*[10] and the *European Journal of Palliative Care*[11] Phil Larkin (Chair of the Nursing Education taskforce of the EAPC) reported:

> One of the most difficult dilemmas for the palliative care educator is to achieve some kind of standardisation across programmes. In Ireland, for example, the proliferation of hospice centres providing essentially the same course led to some agreements about what should take place, why, when and where. In a small country like the Republic of Ireland, such national initiatives are possible. Compare the example of Switzerland with three official languages and the need for simultaneous translation in triplicate. The education recommendations of the Swiss National Palliative Care Society (SSMSP) are a credit to the ability to transcend linguistic challenges. Yet, the need for some form of guideline to set a common ground for educational preparation is now necessary for all disciplines involved in the delivery of high-quality palliative care.

In 1997, the EAPC proposed that the collective member associations in each country should create a national education network, which would link with the EAPC education network. The proposal from the EAPC Board of Directors was to establish minimal recommendations for training in palliative care for both nurses and doctors, and also to identify those training skills most appropriate for palliative care educators. The EAPC has, over the last two years, tried to unify the European voice of palliative care through its initiative 'one voice, one vision'. The creation of task force initiatives to address some of the key issues which pertain to this watchword included the project described here – a proposal to offer some kind of guidelines for the future development of palliative nurse education. This report entitled 'A Guide for the Development of Palliative Nurse Education in Europe' is the culmination of a three-year collaborative project, finally agreed in November 2003.

Box 2.3 Palliative care in Hungary

Political system: Republic
Capital city: Budapest
Total area: 93 000 km^2
Population: 10.2 million
Currency: Forint
Laws:

- 1997: New healthcare legislation includes the concept of palliative care and informed consent

Box 2.4 Palliative care in Italy

Political system: Republic
Capital city: Rome
Total area: 301 263 km^2
Population: 57.6 million
Currency: Euro
Laws:

- 1996: Creation of the Ministerial Commission for the definition of palliative care and its development in Italy

- 1998: Health Ministry recognizes an official palliative care curriculum and the need for at least one hospice per region

- February 1999: Ministerial decree that allocates governmental funding of €200 million for the opening of 200 palliative care units

Box 2.5 Palliative care in Spain

Political system: Constitutional monarchy
Capital city: Madrid
Total area: 504 782 km^2
Population: 39.4 million
Currency: Euro
Laws:

- 1990: The government of the region of Catalonia passes law on healthcare that includes palliative care
- 1991: Second law of Catalonia including palliative care
- 1994: Spanish healthcare system recognizes the existence of government-funded palliative care units, private palliative care units, and a combination of both

The comments and the full recommendations are published on the EAPC website (www.eapcnet.org/; click on EAPC Publications, and then on Education).

The EAPC considers education of palliative medicine at university of utmost importance for the future of palliative care. During 2003, Marilène Filbet (EAPC Vice President 2003–05 and President from 2005) carried out a survey on the state of education for physicians in Europe. A questionnaire was distributed. Among the questions asked, the following two were deemed the most important:

- Do you have a national program for training in palliative care for medical students in your country or state?
- Do you have a specialty in palliative care?

See Table 2.2 for the replies from 12 countries.

Following the survey the EAPC decided to create a taskforce on medical education of physicians to elaborate the European recommendations for the palliative care curricula for physicians for the three levels:

- A (undergraduate)
- B (post graduate, e.g., masters or special courses)
- C (specialist training)

The group chaired by Dr Marilène Filbet represents a broad spectrum of medical practitioners involved in the preparation and delivery of medical education throughout Europe. The curricula recommendations will be published on the EAPC website (section education in 2006).

Table 2.2 *Palliative care training for physicians: EAPC Questionnaire result*

	National program	Specialty
Belgium	No	No
Cyprus	No	No
Finland	Yes	No
France	Yes (100 hours)	Not yet, but many diplomas
Germany	Yes	Yes
Hungary	Yes (24 hours)	No
Ireland	No	No (national document)
Italy	Yes	No
Norway	No	Yes
Spain	Yes	Yes
Switzerland	No	Yes
UK	No	Yes

EAPC, European Association for Palliative Care.

CHALLENGES FOR PALLIATIVE CARE IN EUROPE

We envisage three major challenges for Europe.

Palliative care delivery

Europe is facing an important demographic change. The United Nations forecast for European countries for 2020 is that 26–32 percent of the population will be over the age of 60 years.[12] This situation implies a range of difficulties for the near future: changing epidemiology of disease, increasing age of caregivers, financial implications for healthcare systems, and the range of settings for care. The Recommendation REC 24 (2003)[8] of the Committee of Ministers of the Council of Europe has not given any particular attention to this. To highlight this problem the WHO has published two booklets (*Better Palliative Care for Older People*[13] and *The Solid Facts*[14]) which were the result of an expert meeting organized by the Floriani Foundation, Milano, and coordinated by Irene Higginson.

Education

Palliative care needs to become a specialty in as many European countries as possible. It was as early as 1988 when Calman[14] wrote that 'A well defined discipline:

- has a clearly defined body of knowledge
- has full-time specialists
- has sufficient patients who require the services of an expert in the area
- has technical procedures which can only be carried out by specialists
- has clear training programmes (plus special qualifications in the subject)
- is seen to have value by patients, the public, and other professionals.'

Palliative care fulfils all these requirements but still is a specialty only in the UK and Ireland. Higher professional training in the UK requires 4 years at senior registrar level:

- Obligatory: 2 years full time in a specialist unit which has a full range of services (inpatient beds, outpatient clinics, home care, bereavement)
- Recommended: an elective period of research or special experience in some aspect of palliative medicine.

Research

Research in palliative care is a complex and controversial subject and is not easy to realize. Physicians and nurses do not want to involve patients in trials, as they believe that the burden placed on the patient will be too high. But in modern medicine a new specialty will develop only if it is supported by scientific evidence to justify its aims and means. Clinical trials enable us to evaluate new treatment options. Obviously research in palliative care is not limited to clinical trials. We also need to enhance research, social assistance, psychiatry, psychology, the approach toward death, bereavement and grief, and healthcare policy and organization. The Board of Directors of the EAPC consider research a key issue for the future of palliative care and therefore decided in 1996 to put together a steering group with the aim of establishing a research network. When the Research Steering Committee (RSC) was first established, it felt it was premature to establish a network with the aim of carrying out multicenter and multinational studies. The committee decided to make use of the considerable information and knowledge that already existed among palliative care experts. Since its creation the group has organized 12 expert working groups on a variety of topics for which a common European position or recommendations are needed. For these, experts were invited from various fields in addition to members of the RSC. The results of the work of eight groups have been published, one of them in six languages, and have been made available to the EAPC members. These are listed below.

Klepstad P, Kaasa S, Cherny N, *et al.*; Research Steering Committee of the EAPC. Pain and pain treatments in European palliative care units. A cross-sectional survey from the European Association for Palliative Care Research Network. *Palliat Med* 2005; **19**: 477–84.

Caraceni A, Cherny N, Fainsinger R, *et al.* Pain measurement tools and methods in clinic research in palliative care: recommendations of an Expert Working Group of the EAPC. *J Pain Symptom Manage* 2002; **23**: 239–55.

Mercadante S, Radbruch L, Caraceni A, *et al.*; Steering Committee of the European Association for Palliative Care (EAPC) Research Network. Episodic (breakthrough) pain: consensus conference of an expert working group of the European Association for Palliative Care. *Cancer* 2002; **94**: 832–9.

Stiefel F, Die Trill M, Berney A *et al.* Depression in palliative care: a pragmatic report of an expert working group of the European Association for Palliative Care. *Support Care Cancer* 2001; **9**: 477–88.

Cherny N, Ripamonti C, Pereira J, *et al.*; Expert Working Group of the European Association of Palliative Care Network. Strategies to manage the adverse effects of oral morphine. An evidence-based report. *J Clin Oncol* 2001; **19**: 2542–54.

Ripamonti C, Twycross R, Baines M, *et al.* Clinical practice recommendations for the management of bowel obstruction in patients with end-stage cancer. *Support Care Cancer* 2001; **9**: 223–33.

Hanks GW, Conno F, Cherny N, Expert Working Group of the Research Network of the European Association for Palliative

Care. Morphine and alternative opioids in cancer pain: the EAPC recommendations. *Br J Cancer* 2001; 84: 587–93.

2001 WHO guidelines on cancer pain management: report on international application and current appraisal (in collaboration with Excerpta Medica), 5th Congress of the EAPC, 13 September 1997, London.

The RSC has obtained the right to upload five of the papers in PDF format to be available from our website (www. eapcnet.org/researchNetwork/resnetpublications.asp). (Access to this webpage requires registration with the EAPC.) One paper is ready for publication and another is in preparation.

The RSC has also organized panels and seminars for the fifth, sixth, seventh, and eighth congresses of the EAPC and other conferences.

FORUMS ON RESEARCH IN PALLIATIVE CARE

The RSC held its first forum on research and development for selected groups of carers interested in research in Berlin on December 7–10, 2000 (report available at: www.eapcnet.org/congresses/berlin2000.html). The second forum was held in Lyon, France, on May 23–25, 2002 (report available at: www.eapcnet.org/congresses/lyon2002.html) and the third at Stresa, Lago Maggiore, Italy, on June 4–6, 2004 (report available at: www.eapcnet.org/congresses/research2004.html). The fourth forum was held in Venice, Italy, on May 25–28, 2006.

OTHER RSC ACTIVITIES

The RSC has participated in two Expressions of Interest to the European Community (see www.eapcnet.org/researchNetwork/researchprojects.asp) and has submitted an application for funding to the European Community, which was accepted but with conditions that could not be realized. It organized a cross-sectional survey with two main aims: to create a network of European palliative care centers and services to introduce them to collaborative research and to obtain descriptive data of the practice of palliative care across Europe. At the conclusion of this survey, the Research Network intends to undertake multicenter research. The preliminary results of the survey were presented during the first Research and Development Conference in Berlin. Further results were presented in the session about the activities of the Research Network in Palermo on April 2, 2001. One paper has been published and is available in PDF format from the EAPC website. Others are ready for publication and we are in the process of analyzing the datasets for further papers.

The RSC is in the process of organizing its first European multicenter study: European Pharmacogenetic Opioid Study, which will generate data on clinical characteristics and measures, and serum concentrations of opioids, and collect biological material for pharmacogenetic analysis in an attempt to answer several research questions.

The establishment of a bio-bank for genetic studies has given the study group unique possibilities to explore hypotheses generated by genetic findings related to the pharmacogenetics of analgesics and the genetics of pain.

Key learning points

- The countries making up the continent of Europe have diverse cultures and languages, history, economies, and education and healthcare systems. There is also great diversity of legislation in the different countries.
- The development of modern palliative care started in the 1960s with the hospice movement in the UK by Dame Cicely Saunders but for several years this was limited to the UK.
- In the past 15 years, there has been rapid development of the movement of palliative care in Europe and the EAPC was created in December 1988 and is now a federation of nonprofit organizations. Recently, the EAPC revised its definition of palliative care to include total care of the terminally ill patients to preserve the best possible quality of life until death.
- Palliative care associations in European countries are different in the different countries.
- In 2003 the Council of Europe released recommendations of the delivery of palliative care in Europe. These are available on the Council's website and encompass hospital-based palliative care, hospices, home care, nursing homes and homes for elderly people.
- Several European countries have passed legislation in relation to palliative care.
- Europe faces challenges not only in the appropriate delivery of palliative care but also education of professionals delivering the care and research.
- The RSC has made huge efforts to improve and enhance research in palliative care. Several papers have been published and many projects currently are underway.

REFERENCES

1   World Health Organization Regional Office for Europe website, 2005 (see www.euro.who.int/countryinformation).
2   Council of Europe. About the Council of Europe, 2005. Available at: www.coe.int/T/E/Com/About_COE/ (accessed December 2005).
3   Europa website. The EU at a glance. Available at: europa.eu.int/abc/index_en.htm# (accessed December 2005).
4   European Association of Palliative Care. www.eapcnet.org
5   World Health Organization. *Cancer Pain Relief.* Geneva: WHO, 1986.
6   European Association of Palliative Care. EAPC By-laws (English). Available at www.eapcnet.org/about/bylaws.html (accessed December 20, 2005).

7　Parliamentary Assembly, Council of Europe. Protection of the human rights and dignity of the terminally ill and the dying. Document No. 1418. Available at: http://assembly.coe.int/Documents/AdoptedText/ta99/EREC1418.htm (accessed December 20, 2005).

8　Council of Europe. Social cohesion and quality of life. Recommendation REC 24 (2003) of the Committee of Ministers to member states on the organisation of palliative care and explanatory memorandum. Available at: www.coe.int/T/E/Social_Cohesion/Health/Recommendations/Rec(2003)24.asp (accessed December 20, 2005).

9　Council of Europe. Social cohesion and quality of life. Ministers' Deputies CM Documents, CM(2003)130 Addendum (restricted) 15 October 2003. Available at: www.coe.int/T/E/Social_Cohesion/Health/Recommendations/Rec%282003%2924%20Expl.%20Mem..asp#TopOfPage (accessed December 20, 2005).

10　de Vlieger M, Gorchs N, Larkin PJ, Porchet F. Palliative nurse education: towards a common language. *Palliat Med* 2004; **18**: 401–3.

11　de Vlieger M, Gorchs N, Larkin PJ, Porchet F. Palliative nurse education: towards a common language. *Eur J Palliat Care* 2004; **11**: 135–8.

12　United Nations Population Division. *World Population Prospects Population Database*. New York: United Nations Population Division 2002. Available at: http://esa.un.org/unpp/index.asp (accessed December 2005).

13　WHO Europe (Davies E, Higginson I, eds). *Better Palliative Care for Older People*. Geneva: WHO, 2004; supported by the Floriani Foundation.

14　WHO Europe (Davies E, Higginson I, eds). *The Solid Facts. Palliative Care*. Geneva: WHO, 2004; supported by the Floriani Foundation.

15　Calman KC. Palliative medicine: on the way to becoming a recognized discipline. *J Palliat Care* 1988; **4**: 12–14.

APPENDIX 2.1

Data sources: special laws, inquiries, papers

Recommendation REC 24 (2003) of the Committee of Ministers to member states on the organisation of palliative care. (Adopted by the Committee of Ministers on November 12, 2003 at the 860th meeting of the Ministers' deputies; see reference 8.)

Arrêté royal du 21 julliet 1994 fixant les critères d'application de la pause carrière pour soins palliatifs.

Arrêté royal du 15 julliet modifiant l'arrêté royal du 23 octobre 1964 portant fixation des norms auzquelles les hÙpitaux et leurs services doivent répondre.

Arrêté royal du 30 octobre 1996 modifiant l'arrêté royal du 21 décembre 1977 fixant les critères d'application pour la programmation des différents types de services hospitaliers.

Arrêté royal du 13 octobre 1998 déterminant les critères minimums auxquels doivent répondre les conventions entre les équipes d'accompagnement multidisciplinaires de soins palliatifs et le Comité de Assurance institute auprès du Service de soins de santé de'Institut National d'Assurance Maladie Invalidité.

Arrêté royal du 15 juillet 1997 fixant les norms auxquelles une function hospitalière de soins palliatifs doit répondre pour être agrees et Arrêté royal du 15 julliet 1997 rendant certaines disposition de la loi sur les hôpitaux coordonée le 7 ao°t 1987 applicables û la function de soins palliatifs.

Arrêté royal de 15 juillet 1997 modifiant l'arrêté royal du 2 décembre 1982 fixant les norms pur l'agrégation des maisons de repos et de soins.

Arrêté royal du 19 juin 1997 fixant les subsides allouées au associations en matière de soins palliatifs.

Arrêté royal du 16 décembre 1997 modifiant l'Arrêté royal du 19 juin 1997 fixant les norms auxquelles une association en matière de soins palliatifs doi répondre pour être agree.

Arrêté royal du 19 juin 1997 fixant les norms auxquelles une association en matière de soins palliatifs doit répondre pour être agree.

Vainio A. Treatment of terminal cancer pain in France: a questionnaire study. *Pain* 1995; **62**: 155–62.

Larue F, Fontaine A, Brasseur L, Neuwirth L. France: Status of cancer pain and palliative care. *J Pain Symptom Manage* 1996; **12**: 106–8.

Filbet M. Putting the plans for French palliative care into action. *Eur J Palliat Care* 2003; **10**: 24–5.

Muszbek K, Toldy-Schedel E. Hungary: palliative care – a new challenge. *J Pain Symptom Manage* 2002; **24**: 188–90.

Wright M, Clark D. The development of terminal care in Budapest, Hungary. *Eur J Palliat Care* 2003; **9**: 247–50.

Gazzetta ufficiale della Repubblica Italiana. Decreto-legge 28 dicembre 1998–450.

Gazzetta ufficiale della Repubblica Italiana. Legge 26 febbraio 1999–39.

Ventafridda V. Italy: status of cancer pain and palliative care. *J Pain Symptom Manage* 2002; **24**: 194–6.

Legge no. 39 of 26 february 1999: Disposizioni per assicurare interventi urgenti di attuazione del Piano Sanitario Nazionale 1998–2000. Gazzetta Ufficiale (Ser gen) no. 48 (February 27, 1999).

Gazzetta ufficiale della Repubblica Italiana. Decreto del Presidente del Consiglio dei Ministri 20 gennaio 2000.

Gazzetta ufficiale della Repubblica Italiana. Legge 8 gennaio 2001–12.

de Vlieger M, Gorchs N, Larkin PJ, Porchet F. Palliative nurse education: towards a common language. *Palliat Med* 2004; **18**: 401–3.

de Vlieger M, Gorchs N, Larkin PJ, Porchet F. Palliative nurse education: towards a common language. *Eur J Palliat Care* 2004; **11**: 135–8.

The development of palliative care in Canada

NEIL MACDONALD

INTRODUCTION

Relating an account of Canadian palliative care is risky, particularly when the historian has been involved in some of these activities, thus magnifying the possibility of bias. One may be fairly criticized for the failure to account adequately for the fine work of colleagues and groups not mentioned in the history, perhaps only because of the author's lack of familiarity with their work, or because of the lack of a readily available written record.

THE TWIN PARENTS

It is easy to trace the roots of Canadian palliative care; they clearly are evident in the seminal activities of Dr Balfour Mount and Dr David Skelton in the mid 1970s. The first Canadian programs were started within a month of each other in 1974. Dr Skelton opened a 'terminal care unit' at St Boniface Hospital in Winnipeg. Shortly thereafter the 'palliative care unit' at the Royal Victoria Hospital in Montreal was launched; from the start it encompassed an inpatient ward, a consult service, a coordinated home care program, and a bereavement service.

St Boniface, a teaching hospital of the University of Manitoba, is a part of the Grey Nuns Hospital network. The Grey Nuns is a religious order which has a long tradition of pioneering hospital and healthcare in Canada. Originally centered in Montreal, the sisters moved in concert with the original settlers of the Canadian West, starting hospitals which were often the only sources of healthcare in the developing towns and regions of the then Canadian frontier. Because of their long history of compassionate care, twinned with a record for innovation, they naturally became leaders in the palliative care field. Following upon their Winnipeg enterprise, the Grey Nuns organized the first inpatient palliative care unit in Edmonton in 1982, again led by Dr Skelton who had moved to the University of Alberta to head a new academic geriatric center.

At St Boniface Dr Skelton was joined by Dr Paul Henteleff in 1975, who took on the directorship of the terminal care unit. St Boniface continues to be an exemplary model of community palliative care linked with a first rate teaching hospital inpatient unit. One notices a strong continuum of leadership, Dr Henteleff served for 17 years, followed by Dr Deborah Dudgeon (now the director of the program at Queens' University in Kingston), and currently Dr Mike Harlos.

The Royal Victoria Hospital is a secular institution, its origin stemming from the support and drive of the men who built the Canadian Pacific Railway, which was the first railroad to traverse Canadian land, thus opening the west and securing the northern Pacific coast as a part of Canada. Reflecting the strong Scottish presence in Montreal and Canada as a whole – if the Scots did not 'invent the modern world'[1] they certainly influenced much of the nonfrancophone culture of Canada – the 'Vic' was modeled on the Edinburgh Royal Infirmary, and became one of the principal adult teaching hospitals of McGill University.

Herein lies an important point which strongly influenced Canadian palliative care – both of the founding hospitals were academic institutions. Elsewhere in the world palliative care usually started outside of the milieu of academic medicine, and only now is achieving presence and credibility within medical schools. Canada had a 'leg up' in these endeavors because of early acceptance of palliative care by academic colleagues in leadership positions. For example, at the Royal Victoria Hospital, the chairs of surgery and urology and the Director of Nursing sponsored a participant observation on the care of dying patients, a study which in part involved the experiences of a cadaverous appearing, albeit healthy, anthropologist passing as a patient with a cancer of the pancreas.[2] This participant observational study compared patient contacts occurring in the Royal Victoria Hospital Palliative Care Unit and a surgical ward. On the Unit both patient-to-staff and patient-to-patient contacts were considerably higher:[3] this study provided convincing evidence of the effects of palliative care. Based on this 'patient's' hospital encounters, coupled with other relevant studies, Dr Mount made a powerful case for his visionary palliative care program.

At that time Dr Mount was a happily and fully engaged urological oncologist with recent personal experience (a germ cell tumor of the testicle) which no doubt concentrated his thinking on the transience of life and the needs of people during their final passage. In the course of carrying out his initial work, Dr Mount encountered the studies of Elizabeth Kübler-Ross and through her writing learned of the work of Dame Cicely Saunders in London, England. Dr Mount contacted Dame Cicely, and arranged to work with her; a lifetime friendship was soon established. On his return to Montreal, Dr Mount set out to incorporate the principles espoused by Dame Cicely and her colleagues in a hospital-based program with consequent major impact on the life and culture of one of the world's premier teaching hospitals.

Dr Mount soon recognized that he needed a team to meet the expectations which he had established. In 1974 Dr Ina Cummings Ajemian, a highly regarded family physician in the community served as first clinical director. Soon thereafter (1975), another gifted family physician, Dr John Scott, joined the team. Dr Ajemian and Dr Scott in subsequent years held leadership positions in other parts of Canada; Dr Ajemian as Head of the Dalhousie Palliative Care Program, and Dr Scott as Director of the Elizabeth Bruyère Program in Ottawa.

PALLIATIVE CARE: THE ORIGIN OF THIS TERM FOR HOSPICE CARE

Initially a 'hospice program' was planned for the Royal Victoria Hospital. Francophone friends reminded Dr Mount the word 'hospice' had a pejorative connotation in French, conveying a feeling of disengagement from life and termination of hope. Shaving, for some of us a daily ritual, has some merits – while engaged in this onerous task one morning, Dr Mount reflected on the advice he had received

and thought of alternative titles. The phrase 'palliative care' jumped into his mind. Soon at the Royal Victoria Hospital one spoke of the 'Royal Victoria Hospital palliative care program'. Although initially Dr Mount encountered resistance from his respected British mentors, the phrase, conveying a sense of continuing improvement of the quality of existence, came into general global acceptance.

CANADIAN PALLIATIVE CARE SERVICES

Certain features of the Canadian programs are worthy of attention for their potential worldwide influence. Among these one may include team development and the comprehensive home care concept.

Team development

At McGill, Dr Ajemian proved highly adept at putting into practice the team concept initially conceived by Dr Mount. A nonhierarchical team was created, including nurses, psychologists, psychiatrists, music therapists, social workers, physical and occupational therapists, pastoral care workers, pet therapists, grief counselors, and an exceptional team of volunteers. From a distance I was particularly impressed with the Royal Victoria Hospital volunteer program, which placed highly trained volunteers in positions of direct meaningful patient contact, and provided a place at the team table for them. Over time the wisdom of this move became manifest, as it was clear that many patients and families could identify and communicate more openly, in some instances, with the volunteers, while the richness of the volunteer experience enabled the Royal Victoria Hospital to attract a particularly diverse and talented volunteer cadre.

Comprehensive home care

Canada enjoys a healthcare system with full public support for hospital and physician services, and partial support (varying from province to province) for home care, other professional services, and outpatient pharmaceuticals. Home care services are regionalized within large urban/rural districts. This system sets the table for innovative whole population palliative home care programs. A number of Canadian cities now have whole population home care coverage; I will mention two specific programs whose experience and guidance have had major influence throughout Canada.

THE VICTORIA HOSPICE

The influential Victoria Hospice program operates in a small Canadian city without a medical school. It has enjoyed strong leadership throughout the full course of its history (Dr Michael Downing was the first director, and continues in that role), and it has pioneered a number of community palliative care initiatives which are now widely represented in Canada, in some good part thanks to Victoria. These include:

- Establishment of home services and an inpatient palliative care unit within one organization from the onset of the program in September 1980.
- Development of a unique traveling home chart, facilitating interaction with local physicians.
- In 1989 Victoria pioneered the use of a 'palliative response team' created to provide 24-hour acute care service facilitated by the use of an in-home palliative care drug kit.
- The rate of home death for patients served by the Victoria program continues in the 40–50 percent range.
- The Victoria Hospice approach has had a substantive effect on hospice and palliative care development in British Columbia, a province with over 100 programs today. Aside from personal example and skillful program review which has demonstrated the benefits inherent in their approach, the Victoria program is renowned for its publication of excellent educational guides for both professionals and patients which are widely used and copied throughout Canada.

THE EDMONTON PROGRAM

With a population of 900 000, Edmonton is one of the largest cities in the world with a city-wide coordinated palliative care program. A city-wide home care program was in place in the late 1980s, but there were gaps in the links between institutional activities and the home care system. In 1994, Dr Eduardo Bruera put together an imaginative proposal for a coordinated home care program. On introduction, the program was able to demonstrate a comprehensive approach to the care of palliative care patients at no increased cost to the public purse. This initiative illustrates the benefits of marrying palliative care research and service.[4] The widespread community use of subcutaneous techniques for drug administration, assessment of patient needs, and innovative therapies pioneered by Edmonton colleagues enabled them to predict with confidence that they could successfully link the home and institution in a cost-effective program.[5]

LA MAISON MICHEL-SARRAZIN

La Maison Michel-Sarrazin, a 15-bed inpatient facility in Quebec City, occupies a unique niche in Canadian palliative care. The Quebec City area is almost completely francophone. Maison Michel-Sarrazin has had a major influence on the development of palliative care in the province of Quebec where the population is primarily French speaking. In keeping with its mandate over the years, it has developed written principles which have been published and widely disseminated in Quebec. It is a teaching institution of l'Université de Laval. The founding director, Dr Louis Dionne was an influential surgeon in that faculty, and well respected throughout Canada. Among other areas of interest, colleagues at la Maison Michel-Sarrazin are spearheading Canadian research in changes in cognitive function associated with illnesses related to advanced cancer.

WHY NO PALLIATIVE CARE SPECIALTY?

Canada stands unique as a home for sophisticated palliative care which has failed to develop a formal specialty in the field. The Royal College of Physicians and Surgeons (Canada) controls specialty development and educational practice. It decided to not act upon a plan presented to the College in 1995 by a representative group of Canadian academic palliative care physicians, which it did acknowledge to be one of the strongest submissions in many years. As a participant in discussions on the proposal, I recall spirited debate with representatives of the sister college, the Canadian College of Family Physicians, which controls family practice educational policy. Anything for peace in the house, or so seemed the perplexing decision of the Royal College. It backed away from support for a fully articulated specialty, and acquiesced to the family practice proposal for a 1-year training program which offers successful candidates a certificate but no true specialty status.

In my view, the decision of the Royal College has grievously hurt Canadian palliative care. Our burgeoning role within medical schools was set back, our ability to sit as equals at the table with academic peers was hampered, our profile as specialists with defined skills and responsibilities was diminished and the creation of well-defined palliative care posts has been limited. To their credit, certain centers with strong leadership and sympathetic deans and hospital administrators have overcome these handicaps.

PALLIATIVE CARE RESEARCH

Canada has a rich pedigree of palliative care research. Except for a few national trials sponsored by the Clinical Trials Unit of the National Cancer Institute this work was primarily localized to a few centers. The major granting agencies showed little initiative in sponsoring palliative care research, and tended to follow, year after year, traditional funding approaches. The story changed dramatically with the inauguration of a major research agency funded by the federal government, the Canadian Institutes of Health Research (CIHR) in June 2000. The CIHR has a mandate to 'foster research relating to the four pillars of health research': basic, clinical, health services and policy, and the health of populations. It was established as a federation of distinct institutes, one of which is the Institute of Cancer Research (ICR).

The scientific director of the ICR is a prominent biochemist (Dr Phil Branton) who has the ability to embrace promising lines of research, traditional and otherwise. With his guidance, the ICR set out to address the task of identifying cancer research priorities in Canada, particularly those which are currently underfunded. Following the completion of a comprehensive national advisory process, the ICR winnowed the list of priority areas to six, and to the surprise of many, palliative and end-of-life care emerged as the top priority area selected for special CIHR funding.

One may conjecture on how this came about, but two themes are clearly apparent:

1 The CIHR–ICR adapted the World Health Organization definition of palliative care which emphasized the importance of prevention (a concept readily understood by cancer researchers) and, most importantly, included the consideration of human suffering. 'Suffering' is a highly evocative word; regardless of whether one's interest lies, with the genome or at the bedside, all can understand that in life's short passage control of suffering is of great import.
2 The CIHR stresses the importance of cross-disciplinary research, and although traditionally associated with cancer care, palliative care clearly is relevant across the broad field of geriatrics and chronic diseases.

The CIHR inaugurated a dedicated pilot research program; it also provided support for a network of training programs in palliative care research. The largest initiative, entitled 'Palliative Care – New Emerging Teams' was established to create a series of palliative care research networks across the country. Ten networks have been awarded grants totaling Can$1 500 000 each over 5 years. The nature of these teams, which include colleagues from virtually every Canadian university, vary from those concerned with physical symptoms (a pain consortium and a group interested in anorexia-cachexia are funded) to many dealing with delivery of palliative care services and whole patient care issues.

Palliative care colleagues in all countries have often complained that their research work has been stifled by cynical, uninformed reviewers sitting on grants panels whose interests lay elsewhere. The CIHR addressed this concern through the establishment of dedicated palliative care review panels including colleagues from other countries to avoid conflict of interest.

Quality of life research

The McGill research program is perhaps best known for innovative quality of life studies. The work of Mount, Cohen, and their associates has clearly demonstrated that there is much more to quality of life at the end of life than simple physical wellbeing. Dr Mount frequently quotes, with conviction, his contact with patients who, with severe limitations, have stated that the last period of their life was also 'the best year of my life'. Drs Mount and Cohen called our attention to the importance of the spiritual/existential domain and the related importance of developing a sense of meaning as one encounters their final illness, a gift that can be enhanced if professional colleagues recognize and sustain patient–family spiritual interests.

The fruits of their research include the McGill Quality of Life Instrument[6,7] which stresses the importance of an existential/spiritual domain, and in 1999 the inauguration of the McGill Programs in Integrated Whole Person Care. This program has the objective to examine the effect of the inner life on healthcare outcomes.

Dr Mount, who once again faced his own mortality following a successfully treated experience with squamous cell carcinoma of the esophagus, recently penned a thoughtful 'personal narrative' called 'The existential moment'.[8] In it he states 'In accompanying those who are dying over the past quarter century I have come to view life as a spiritual experience, that is to say, a search for meaning purpose and personal connection, to something greater and more enduring than the self'. This view has imbued the Royal Victoria Hospital program throughout its existence, and has had a major impact on global palliative care.

Symptom control research

Amongst Canadian centers, Edmonton has been a leader in this field. Dr Helen Hayes, an Edmonton family physician, pioneered early research on hypodermoclysis, a useful technique for delivering both parenteral drugs and fluids in a cost-effective fashion. The Cross Cancer Institute – University of Alberta university hospital palliative care research program flowered with the recruitment of Dr Eduardo Bruera in 1984. Originally joining the program as a Fellow, within a few months he was clearly taking the lead in the development of palliative care research in Edmonton. Areas of particular interest included opioid studies, drug delivery, hydration, dyspnea, appetite, gastric emptying, and delirium. The Edmonton team was among the first to identify aberrations in autonomic function as a contributor to many common symptoms.

Dr Bruera created one of the more creative international research groups, including colleagues from a number of Central and South American countries.

Psychosocial research

For some years, an influential nursing research program at the University of Manitoba studied the palliative care needs of patients and families; work which has stimulated similar research in other centers. Dr Leslie Degner and her collaborator, Dr Linda Kristjanson, have served as mentors for many nurse researchers in addition to their seminal contributions to the palliative care/family care literature.

Dr Harvey Chochinov, a disciple of Dr Jimmie Holland (Memorial Sloan-Kettering Cancer Center), returned to

Winnipeg as a Soros/Open Society Fellow and launched a series of studies in the 1990s that have increased our understanding of the unique features of depression at the end of life. His work has both improved our management of depression and informed the continuing discussion on euthanasia and physician-assisted suicide. More recently Dr Chochinov has published insightful work on 'Dignity,'[9] what it means and how it may be maintained (see also Chapter 13).

PALLIATIVE CARE EDUCATION

The Royal Victoria Hospital program from its inception has been a nidus for education, both locally and at a distance. The 1980 Royal Victoria Hospital manual on palliative hospice care was an early influential guide for programs developing in various parts of the world. Perhaps reflecting a personal cultural interest, Dr Mount has always stressed the use of film in teaching. A series of excellent productions, of which *The Last Days of Living* and *On the Edge of Being* are best known, have been widely used around the world.

Arguably the largest international palliative care gathering has been sponsored by the McGill Program since 1976. The biennial International Congress on the Care of the Terminally Ill enjoyed its fifteenth session in the fall of 2004, a meeting which was attended over 5 days by in excess of 1300 registrants from 35 countries of the world. In both of the Canadian founding languages, the congresses successfully integrated sessions on psychosocial issues with those on basic and clinical research, clinical care and teaching, together with team development.

The Canadian curriculum

In 1990, representatives from all 16 Canadian medical schools together developed a palliative care curriculum, in the hope that this cooperative effort would strengthen the respective efforts in their schools to advance palliative medicine education. The product of their work, the Canadian Palliative Care Curriculum, first published in 1991, is one of the first global curricula in our field. The group who developed this curriculum found other initiatives on which it wished to work together, and formally incorporated itself as a National Educational Committee, which continues to exist under the aegis of the Canadian Society of Palliative Care Physicians. In 1997 the committee updated the Canadian Palliative Care Curriculum and published it with an illustrative *Case-Based Manual*.[10] Each case is designed to illustrate the various curricular points. Arrangements were made for a class in each of the Canadian medical schools to be provided with a copy of the manual, a project which continued for a number of years, and, one hopes, with federal government support, will continue. The committee has completed regular surveys on the status of palliative care education in each of the Canadian medical schools. One

hopes that these published reports have helped the deans and curriculum committees to note discrepancies which exist between schools and to take positive action.[11,12]

Currently a major national initiative entitled 'Educating Future Physicians in Palliative and End-of-Life Care' (EFPPEC) is going forward. Its overarching goal is to ensure that by the year 2008 all undergraduate medical students in clinical postgraduate training in Canada's (now 17) schools will be competent relative to their level of training at the completion of that training. Success is probable, as the project enjoys the strong support of the Association of the Faculties of Medicine of Canada.

The first palliative care fellowships came into being in the 1980s in Edmonton and Ottawa. The former has personal meaning for me as it was funded by Mr Overton, a man of modest means who owned a small confectionery in North Calgary, which as a child I frequented, though not always to the owner's delight. Mr Overton did not have a family, but obviously invested well. In his will I was named as the major beneficiary on the understanding that the funds would be used to support palliative care. With private support, other centers added fellowships in subsequent years. With the approval of the College of Family Practice and the Royal College, formal, publicly supported fellowship programs were established in the late 1990s. By the end of the 2005 academic year 68 trainees had completed these fellowships, and there are currently only 16 people in 12 programs across the country. A gap clearly exists between the numbers of trainees, the availability of positions, remuneration for positions, and the needs of the people.

PALLIATIVE CARE – A UNIVERSITY DISCIPLINE

In 1987, with support from the Alberta Cancer Board, the University of Alberta established the first Canadian chair in palliative medicine. Chairs have subsequently been established at three other Canadian schools (McGill, Ottawa, and Toronto). University divisions of palliative medicine are present, by name or in practice, in every Canadian faculty of medicine. The siting of these divisions within university departments seems to relate to the disciplines that offered early support. Many are in departments of either oncology or family medicine. Surprisingly, with only a few exceptions, departments of internal medicine have not been leaders in welcoming and cherishing palliative medicine.

GOVERNMENT INITIATIVES IN PALLIATIVE CARE

The Canadian Senate, an appointed body, formed a committee which framed a report on euthanasia and physician-assisted suicide,[13] *Of Life and Death*, in 1995. This report did not endorse euthanasia, rather it made recommendations for action to improve palliative care services in

Canada. Five years later another Senate committee tabled a follow-up report *Quality End-of-Life Care: the Right of Every Canadian* which added new recommendations related to support for family caregivers, access to home care, pharmacare, and suggestions for greater emphasis on education and research. In what must be a unique decision, shortly after the above report was tabled, the Prime Minister of Canada appointed a Senator, Sharon Carstairs, to be a cabinet minister with special responsibility for palliative care. Under her aegis, a secretariat on palliative and end-of-life care was established which formed a series of national working groups to advise the federal government on palliative care issues. A number of tangible results are already apparent from this federal initiative, including:

- a decision by the Canadian government to establish a formal policy streamlining disability support application for dying patients
- an online directory of Canadian hospice and palliative care services
- a government decision to ensure that 'Canadians can provide compassionate care to a gravely ill or dying child, spouse or parent without putting at risk their income or job'. Workers can now take a temporary absence from work to provide support. The compassionate care benefit is a reality, but is not uniformly applied in each province because of required changes in provincial legislation
- the establishment of a Canada research chair for palliative care (awarded to Dr Harvey Chochinov) and support for one of Dr Chochinov's initiatives, the Canadian Virtual Hospice.

In concert with the Canadian Council on Health Services Accreditation, an agreement was reached on standards for palliative and end-of-life care that encompass all healthcare facilities as well as volunteer organizations to provide this care. At the provincial level, various provinces have taken the lead in specific support of research and physician education. In some cases there is provincial funding dedicated to palliative care. Victoria demonstrates a support mix which is not uncommon across the country – it receives 65 percent of its budget through the Provincial Health Plan, and is expected to find 35 percent from private donations.

Commonly, the care facilities – physician and nursing services – receive public support, but to a variable extent private monies are required for other team members, and for research and education.

SELECT CANADIAN COOPERATIVE PALLIATIVE CARE INITIATIVES

Canada, the second largest land mass in the world with a population spread across four and a half time zones, may not naturally lend itself to national cooperative activities.

Notwithstanding geography, highly successful national organizations (notably the Canadian Hospice and Palliative Care Association and the Canadian Society of Palliative Care Physicians) now exist. Three national projects with international connotations include:

- The *Journal of Palliative Care*. This is our 'made in Canada' international journal. Under the consistent guidance of a single editorial team (Dr David Roy, Electa Baril, and Suzanne St Amour) since its first issue in 1985, the *Journal* has presented the best of Canadian palliative care work, accompanied by many articles from international authors. Although we now have many palliative care publications in the international community, the *Journal of Palliative Care*, one of the first, remains one of the best.
- The Pallium Project. The federal government has provided funding for the 'Pallium Project', aimed at improving the care of patients with advanced illness in rural and remote Canadian communities. This project, cosponsored by the Alberta Cancer Board, and under the direction of Dr José Pereira of the University of Calgary, will coordinate activities and provide a central resource for training people in distant areas of Canada with particular emphasis on health professionals in the Prairie Provinces and the vast northern lands.
- The Canadian Virtual Hospice. Launched in 2004, the Canadian Virtual Hospice is an interactive network designed to promote information, exchange communication, and mutual support among patients, friends and family, health providers, researchers, and palliative care volunteers. It consists of four websites directed toward patients, family, and friends, healthcare providers, and volunteers. One may use a website for specific information or as a two-way resource to share thoughts, ask questions, and learn from the experience of others.[14] This project, directed by Dr Harvey Chochinov, was initially supported by the federal Secretariat on end-of-life care. Other partners include Cancer Care Manitoba and a number of other provincial and city of Winnipeg agencies.

CONCLUSION

The history of Canadian palliative care resembles not a smooth flowing, gradually expanding stream; rather it is more like the rapidly flowing, occasionally turbulent, ever progressing rivers characteristic of the Canadian landscape. Canadian palliative care contributions are, in this parochial Canadian's view, disproportionately large in relation to its modest population. A history is a tale of events and the people who moved these events. Some extraordinary women and men have painted Canada's, all things considered, intricate but bright and positive landscape. One hopes that the examples cited in this review of Canada's palliative care life suitably honor the thousands of Canadians, only a few of whom are named, who have selflessly built and advanced this field.

Key learning points

- The appellation 'palliative care' was coined in Canada by Dr Balfour Mount.

- Palliative care started in academic institutions, thus enabling research and education initiatives at an earlier time than otherwise would have been possible.

- Canadian colleges of family medicine and specialty associations decided not to support palliative care as a specialty, opting for shorter training periods providing physicians with hospital/university certificates.

- In 1991, Canadians wrote one of the first national palliative care curricula, subsequently updated twice in association with a case-based textbook (*Palliative Medicine – A Case-Based Manual*) which illustrates the curriculum guidelines.

- The Institute of Cancer Research of the major Canadian research agency (CIHR) endorsed palliative care as the top priority for dedicated research funds in 2003, following up with an investment of more than Can$15 000 000, and the introduction of specific palliative care review panels.

- Led by examples in Edmonton and Victoria, several large urban areas in Canada have comprehensive palliative care programs linking home and hospitals.

- The national government of Canada has a dedicated palliative care initiative, as do many of the provincial health agencies.

REFERENCES

1 Herman A. *How the Scots Invented the Modern World: the True Story of how Western Europe's poorest Nation Created Our World and Everything in It*. New York: Crown Publishers, 2001.

2 Buckingham RW III, Lack SA, Mount BM, *et al*. Living with the dying: use of the technique of participant observation. *Can Med Assoc J* 1976; **115**: 1211–15.

3 Murray WB, Buckingham RW III. Implications of participant observation in medical studies. *Can Med Assoc J* 1976; **115**: 1187–90.

4 *Regional Palliative Care Program Annual Report April 1, 2000 – March 31, 2002*. Alberta: Capital Health Alberta, 2003.

5 Brenneis C, Bruera E. Models for the delivery of palliative care: the Canadian model. In: Bruera E, Portenoy RK, eds. *Topics in Palliative Care, Volume 5*. New York: Oxford University Press, 2001.

6 Cohen SR, Mount BM, Strobel MG, Bui F. The McGill Quality of Life Questionnaire: a measure of quality of life appropriate for people with advanced disease. a preliminary study of validity and acceptablity. *Palliat Med* 1995; **9**: 207–19.

7 Cohen SR, Mount BM, Tomas J, Mount L. Existential well-being is an important determinant of quality of life: evidence from the McGill Quality of Life Questionnaire. *Cancer* 1996; **77**: 576–86.

8 Mount BM. A personal narrative: the existential moment. *Palliat Support Care* 2003; **1**: 1–4.

9 Chochinov HM, Hack T, Hassard T, *et al*. Dignity and psychotherapeutic considerations in end-of-life care. *J Palliat Care* 2004; **20**: 134–42.

10 MacDonald N, ed. *Palliative Medicine – A Case-Based Manual*. Oxford: Oxford University Press, 1998.

11 MacDonald N, Boisvert M, Dudgeon D, Hagen N. The Canadian Palliative Care Education Group. *J Palliat Care* 2000; **16**: 13–15.

12 Oneschuk D, MacDonald N, Jung H. A pilot survey of medical students' perspectives on their educational exposure to palliative care in two Canadian cities. *Palliat Med* 2002; **5**: 353–61.

13 *Of Life and Death – Final Report 1995*. The Special Committee on Euthanasia and Assisted Suicide. Ottawa: Government of Canada Publications, 1995.

14 Chochinov HM, Stern A. The Canadian Virtual Hospice www.virtualhospice.ca. *J Palliat Care* 2004; **20**: 5–6.

The development of palliative medicine in the USA

TRUE RYNDES, CHARLES F VON GUNTEN

INTRODUCTION

The development of palliative medicine, the physician discipline working as part of the larger interdisciplinary field of palliative care, can be viewed in three distinct phases in the USA. The first phase lasted until the work of Dr Kübler-Ross and Dr Cicely Saunders became known. The second phase saw the development of hospice programs across the country. The third phase, in which we now find ourselves, is characterized by the development of a distinct and officially recognized subspecialty of medicine. This chapter will discuss each of these phases to the extent that their history is known either in the published literature or in the memories of those who experienced them. We will mainly focus on the physician component of this history which is the remit of this chapter. While we highlight seminal events in the development of hospice and palliative care in the USA, we purposely do not fully describe the larger history and vast army of contemporary pioneers due to space constraints.

EARLY HISTORY

In the USA as elsewhere in the Western world, dying was a routine part of life until the mid-twentieth century when it became medicalized.[1] Dr William Osler reported on the first large series of dying patients during his time at the hospital he helped to found at Johns Hopkins Medical School in Baltimore, Maryland.[2] Interestingly, he found that the majority of deaths he observed were not painful. Osler is also reported to have said that morphine was 'God's own medicine'. In his famous textbook *Principles and Practice of Medicine*, there is no specific mention of the care of the

dying, though Cushing reports an anecdote involving Sir William's exceptionally sensitive care of a dying child.[3]

Osler, who firmly based his practice in study of the history of medicine, was presumably referring to what little was written. A British monograph from 1701 refers to the curative and palliative uses of opium as a 'noble panacea'.[4] In 1890 Dr Herbert Snow published a text on the palliative treatment of terminal cancer, with an appendix on the use of the opium pipe.[5] Yet, while the term 'palliate' appears in the title of a medical paper as early as 1802 in England,[6] there was relatively little in the textbooks of medicine, or in formal medical training, to guide physicians in addressing the array of symptoms and issues associated with the care of the dying patient.

In 1935, Harvard physician Alfred Worcester published three lectures on 'The Care of the Aged, the Dying and the Dead,' intending them to serve as outlines of what medical students should be taught because of the 'unpardonable' shifting of care for the dying to nurses and sorrowing relatives.[7] (pp. 342–3) The text was circulated during the early days of the hospice movement in the USA, in part because of its thorough clinical observations and procedural recommendations (referencing Sir Henry Halford, Sir William Temple, the Soeurs Augustines, and Florence Nightingale) and in part because of its specific injunctions that younger physicians not allow science to distract them from the art of medical practice and the

> indispensable qualifications of the physician: tact and courtesy . . . sympathy and devotion . . . [for] in the practice of our art it often matters little what medicine is given, but matters much that we give ourselves with our pills.

The care of the dying as a special or particular focus of activity was carried out in a small number of homes beginning in the nineteenth century, much like has been described in France, Ireland, Scotland, and England.[8] All of them had Christian roots. They were founded and run by religious orders devoted to the sick dying as a demonstration of their faith. No particular physician component was identified. Rather, they appear to have been founded from a nursing perspective.

One early example in the USA is the Dominican Sisters of Hawthorne.[9] Rose Hawthorne, the daughter of the American novelist Nathaniel Hawthorne, took a 3-month nursing course at New York's Cancer Hospital, then moved into a three-room cold-water flat on New York City's Lower East Side and began to nurse the poor with incurable cancer. She took the religious name of Sister Alphonsa and founded a Roman Catholic order called the Dominican Congregation of St Rose of Lima, later called the Servants of Relief for Incurable Cancer. In imitation of St Rose of Lima, the order 'strives to give their lives to prayer and compassionate service to Jesus, who comes to them in every patient'. In 1901 Sister Alphonsa opened Rosary Hill Home in Hawthorne, New York (now the mother home of the order) as an inpatient facility to care for the dying.[10] The order is now called the Dominican Sisters of Hawthorne and operates six homes in five states.[10] One of the authors worked in their house in Fall River, Massachusetts from 1971 to 1975.

Another example is Calvary Hospital in New York City. In 1899, a small group of widows began caring for destitute women with terminal diseases. They were inspired by the work of Madame Jeanne Garnier in Lyons, France, who founded several homes for the dying poor she called hospices or *Calvaires*, beginning in 1842.[11] These widows first worked out of their own homes, then in two townhouses in Greenwich Village before moving to the Bronx in 1915. The House of Calvary was renamed Calvary Hospital in 1969. Several Roman Catholic religious orders have served Calvary Hospital over the years, but the organization was never owned or run by a specific religious order.[12]

This is not to say that physicians were unaware of the issues facing the dying during this period. However, in the USA, as elsewhere in Europe, the scientific method was introduced in the late nineteenth century as a way out of the fog of anecdote and quackery that passed for contemporary healthcare. Dr William Osler, writing in the late nineteenth century said 90 percent of the pharmacopeia could be thrown out and the worse it would be for the fish. The new idea was that human suffering stemmed from disease. If one could but understand the disease, the suffering would be stopped.

The second world war marked the beginning of the US federal government's unprecedented financial commitment to the expansion of medicine, medical research, and mental health services as well as to the construction and development of hospitals as the primary site of healthcare. In 1945 the research budget for the National Institute for Health was US$180 000. In 1948 the National Institute for Health, advocating a categorical approach to research and treatment of disease, became the National Institutes for Health, with the creation of the National Heart Institute. Two years later the budget had grown to US$46.3 million.[7] (pp. 358–9) The percentage of doctors describing themselves as full time specialists grew from 24 percent in 1940 to 69 percent in 1966.[13 (p. 6)] As advances in medical science were made, the dispassionate, scientific, mechanistic approach to patient problems ironically fostered the unintended consequence where the patient was treated as a disassembled bystander bearing the disease. Patients who complied submissively with 'the system' were deemed 'good' patients and those who sought a high degree of interactivity with their care providers, and challenged routines were often dubbed 'problem patients', deviant and uncooperative.[14] Furthermore, medicine adopted a near sacred duty to combat all the known causes of death.[15]

Organizational theorist William Starbuck has noted that organizations and their environments perform in a fashion described by scientists as 'co-evolution', that is, 'evolving simultaneously toward better fit for each other'.[16] Thus, it could be said that as the practice of medicine in the USA more greatly valued determinism and prediction in the post-war period, the environment changed, causing a need for compensatory medical care embodied in the palliative competencies of hospice care. Some long time observers of this process have referred to this shift as 'a return to good medicine',[17] a medicine that embraces the medical arts, along with appropriate and tailored use of therapeutics, as expressed in the twentieth century by physicians Alfred Worcester, Charles Aring, Eric Cassell, and Ira Byock.[17–19] Although 'good medicine' may sound trite, this evolutionary step heralds a shift in the meaning of the term 'palliate'. Where palliative treatments were formerly advocated to 'cloak' or 'hide' symptoms, newer palliative approaches actually address the etiology of the symptoms and/or modify the disease, not promising cure but the prospect of reduced symptom burden or longer life expectancy.

AFTER 1970

The success of the growing investment in medical research in the first half of the twentieth century produced unprecedented scientific discoveries and a change in the pattern of illness in the second. In the beginning of the twentieth century, Americans usually died of infectious diseases or trauma. This may explain why there was so little attention to it by physicians – it happened quickly. By the second half of the century, Americans were living longer and dying primarily of atherosclerotic diseases (myocardial infarctions, stroke, congestive heart failure) and cancer. Instead of death occurring quickly (in days) there was a new period of 'dying' that occurred over weeks to years. The paradigm of the scientific method was developed to counter the causes of death of the early part of the century, such as pneumococcal pneumonia. From this point of view, the change in patterns of death without a change in the scientific method leads directly to the physician to perceive death as a medical failure. Suffering, with its physical, psychologic, social, and spiritual components, was the result of the failure of the scientific method. Like most jests, the following statement, appearing in 1975, reflected an uncomfortable element of truth:[20]

> If only patients could leave their damaged physical vessels at the hospital for repair, while taking their social and emotional selves home.

By the end of the 1960s, a lively discussion about American attitudes and practices related to death can be discerned.[13 (p. 6)] For example, empirical research had demonstrated that patients with terminal illness did want to talk about death when they were given the opportunity to do so.[21] The publication of *On Death and Dying* by Dr Elizabeth Kübler-Ross in 1969 capped this period with a fortuitous combination of media exposure and timely substance.[22] A remarkable feature of her work was that she interviewed real patients facing death in teaching sessions with other students in a manner similar to that used in teaching other medical subjects. More important, probably, was that Dr Kübler-Ross was a highly effective speaker and was soon making personal appearances throughout the USA.

Another charismatic physician speaker in the USA at this period was Dr Cicely Saunders. She founded St Christopher's Hospice in a southern suburb of London, England, in 1967 as the culmination of nearly 20 years of direct observation of the care of terminally ill people. She had been publishing and speaking about her ideas about modern hospice care since the late 1950s. The work of Dr Cicely Saunders and her colleagues at St Christopher's Hospice in London reached the ears of many Americans like so many seeds on fertile ground – ground that was in part prepared by Dr Kübler-Ross. A particularly significant aspect of Kübler-Ross's presentations was the response of nurses,[13 (p. 7)] whom many credit, along with social workers and occasional lay persons, as the true force behind the modern hospice movement in the USA. The dialog opened by Kübler-Ross helped to give recognition to what they had experienced, and helped coalesce some of the anger they felt at how 'modern' health care approached the care of the dying.

For a short but eventful period of time, death became the media's darling. This exaggerated attention was manifest in newspapers, magazines, television, and public presentations. Two early programs were established during this time. In 1974, Florence Wald, then Dean of the School of Nursing at Yale University in New Haven, Connecticut, led the founding of the Connecticut Hospice with advice from Dr Saunders[23] and two others. Dr William Lamers, a psychiatrist who pioneered much of the early interactions between hospices and medical schools as medical director of one of the country's first hospice programs, Hospice of Marin, wrote, 'When we gathered in New Haven to talk about hospice care, Dr Bal Mount of Montreal and I were the only two doctors there,' crediting Dr Mount, a urologic surgeon from the Royal Victoria Hospital in Montreal, as 'the true hospice pioneer on this continent' (T Ryndes, personal communication, 2004). Dr Sylvia Lack, a young physician who had just completed training in hospice medicine at St Christopher's was soon recruited to be the medical professional. Connecticut Hospice played a seminal role in the development of hospice care in the USA. In contrast, in New York City, a consulting team began working throughout St Luke's Hospital in 1974, the same year that Connecticut Hospice was founded. In contrast with Connecticut Hospice, this nurse-led team provided support only in the hospital for dying patients in a scattered-bed model.[24]

A grass-roots 'hospice movement' started in the USA at this time, resulting in the founding of a large number of hospice programs. In contrast with the 'flagship' program in New Haven, local circumstances varied greatly. Hospice advocates had to develop positive collaborations as 'outsiders' to the established healthcare system rather than as a part of the system itself. Advocates were united by a vision of care that was defined by a departure from the types of situation that had been increasingly criticized – the patient either subjected to invasive but useless medical care or virtually abandoned. Physicians who played notable local and national activist roles included Tom Licht (Wisconsin), Dan Hadlock (Florida), Bob Brown (Minnesota), and pediatric hematologist/oncologist Doris Howell (Philadelphia and San Diego). Despite the roles that some physicians played, the hospice movement was perceived by the dominant medical system as anti-medical, and countercultural. Those working in hospices at the time do not disown these perspectives, but remember it as a time that was more anti-pain and anti-suffering than anti-medical.

In response to the enthusiasm but lack of consensus on common principles for hospice care in the USA, the Connecticut Hospice in New Haven sponsored a meeting for American and Canadian hospice advocates. From this meeting eventually emerged the National Hospice Organization (NHO). They developed a set of proposed standards and criteria which have been revised at least four times and expanded considerably since they were first developed.[25]

THE NATIONAL HOSPICE STUDY

The National Hospice Demonstration Project was a research study funded by the US federal government to study hospice care in the USA.[13 (p. 6)] The study aimed to select hospices from each of three models that had emerged in the USA:

- Hospital hospice programs. The majority only had a dedicated inpatient unit without a significant home care component

- Home health agency hospice programs without a dedicated hospice inpatient unit
- Independent hospice programs exclusively serving terminally ill patients, with or without a special inpatient unit, staffed primarily by volunteers (professional and lay).

The Health Care Financing Administration chose 26 existing hospice programs as demonstration projects out of 233 applicants in late 1979 and provided them with funding for their work. The chosen hospice programs were located in 16 states. A comparison sample of 14 hospice programs were chosen from among the three types as controls who did not receive federal demonstration project funding. The chosen hospices were not randomly selected. During the course of the National Hospice Study, 13 374 patients were admitted to participating demonstration and nondemonstration hospice programs between 1980 and 1982. Broadly, the study showed that patients who chose hospice care did not suffer any deprivation of care, often (although not always) required a lower level of expenditure, and had usually been able to spend more time at home.

THE MEDICARE HOSPICE BENEFIT

Interestingly, the US Congress enacted legislation in 1982 authorizing a hospice care benefit to all beneficiaries of the federal healthcare plan designed to cover the hospital needs of people over the age of 65 and those with disabilities. They did this while the National Hospice Study was still in progress. However, the findings were consulted in the subsequent development of the regulations that implemented the congressional action.

The standards and criteria that had been developed by the National Hospice Organization received enough dissemination and favorable reaction in the US Congress that they became part of the Medicare Hospice Benefit. This broad benefit led to rapid growth of hospice care in the USA. This federal funding led to the establishment of a hospice industry in the USA – a group of organizations that receive 80 percent of their funding under the terms of this federal legislation.

Briefly, in order for hospice care to be covered under the Medicare Hospice Benefit, two broad criteria must be met. First, the patient must have a prognosis of less than 6 months (later changed to less than 6 months if the disease follows its usual course) as determined by two physicians. Second, the care of the terminal illness must be palliative. Once a patient is eligible and elects hospice care, the hospice agency receives a fixed amount of money per patient per day for care. In the USA, this was the first federal example of a managed care plan where the hospice agency carried the 'risk' for caring for the population of patients rather than being reimbursed on a cost basis as was the standard for Medicare coverage.

Hospice programs had to have a medical director, but, under Medicare guidelines, the role explicitly did not include direct patient care. The model was that the patient's primary care physician would continue to serve as the patient's physician with the support of the hospice team.

THE PATH TO A SUBSPECIALTY IN PALLIATIVE MEDICINE

As in other areas of medicine, formal recognition by organized medicine enhances professionalism by creating practice standards and well-defined competencies within a specified domain of knowledge and/or practice. In palliative medicine, these competencies center on relief of suffering, promotion of quality of life for patients and families in the context of life-threatening illness, and promotion of the development and growth possible at the end of life. Subspecialists are needed to provide advanced care for patients and families whose needs exceed the capabilities of generalist or other specialist physicians. Subspecialists also have larger responsibilities to the field. They provide training and education, spearhead quality improvement initiatives and undertake the research that will ultimately yield the evidence on which general medical practice should be based. Formal recognition of the unique competencies of physicians practicing palliative medicine by the larger 'house' of medicine lays the foundation for sustained, long-term excellence by establishing credibility and facilitating the recruitment of the 'best and brightest' into the field. The path to formal recognition of the physician component of palliative care began to develop after hospice care grew rapidly with US federal funding.

Dr Kathleen Foley was an early pioneer.[26] A neurologist at Memorial Sloan-Kettering Cancer Hospital in New York, she both researched and advocated for better pain management as part of cancer care. Many of the physicians who trained with her as fellows in pain management have gone on to leadership roles in palliative medicine. For example, in 1987, Dr T Declan Walsh was recruited to the Cleveland Clinic to establish a palliative medicine program as part of the oncology division at the clinic. His program was unique in the USA in that it was a physician-led program that was hospital and healthcare system based.[27] Dr Walsh had received his training at St Christopher's Hospice in London as well as Memorial-Sloan Kettering in New York City. The program initially provided hospital consultation and an outpatient clinic.

Dr Josefina Magno, founder and medical director of Hospice of Southeast Michigan, formed the International Hospice Institute in 1978 as a forum for education and dissemination of research findings.[28] It was also to be a forum for mutual support. In 1988, she instituted the Academy of Hospice Physicians comprising 125 physicians who gathered in Estes Park Colorado at one of the meetings. The group subsequently became independent and changed its name to the American Academy of Hospice and Palliative Medicine. It has become the professional association for physicians practicing palliative medicine in the USA.

In 1993, Dr David Weissman established a consultation service at the Medical College of Wisconsin in Milwaukee.[29] He subsequently described the elements of palliative medicine consultation.[30] That same year, Dr Charles von Gunten established a consultation service at Northwestern Memorial Hospital in Chicago that was organizationally linked with a 10-bed acute palliative care unit and a hospice program. Their models led to rapid dissemination to other hospitals in the USA.[31]

Progress toward a recognized specialty took an important step forward in 1997 when the Institute of Medicine (IOM), an independent and influential body that advises the US Congress, highlighted deficiencies in the healthcare system's approach to end-of-life care and called for the development of professional expertise in palliative medicine in the USA to make this knowledge widely available in US healthcare.[32] The IOM report recognized the benefits formal recognition of palliative medicine would confer, stating that a formal specialty would:

- 'focus attention more powerfully on an existing knowledge base that is both insufficiently understood and inadequately applied and that is in need of further growth
- recognize more explicitly and publicly that palliative care is an appropriate goal of medicine
- conform to the value and recognition structure of medical professionals – providing credibility with peers (and perhaps patients and others) as a source of knowledge, guidance, and referral
- attract leaders to the field, and
- nurture the development of the field and its knowledge base.'

Palliative medicine needs to be integrated throughout the care system.[33] Primary palliative medicine is the responsibility of all physicians. This includes basic approaches to the relief of suffering and improving quality of life for the whole person and his or her family. Secondary palliative medicine is the responsibility of specialists and hospital or community based palliative care or hospice programs. The role of the secondary specialist or program is to provide consultation and assist the managing service. Tertiary palliative medicine is the province of academic centers where new knowledge is created through research, and new knowledge is disseminated through education. In addition, tertiary palliative medicine centers are likely to care for the most challenging cases.

The need for palliative care at the end of life has been reinforced in concurring opinions from the US Supreme Court that refused to recognize a constitutional right to assisted suicide.[34] The American College of Physicians and the American Board of Internal Medicine have both called for general physician competency in the care of persons with terminal illness.[35,36] Efforts are also underway to improve the skills of practitioners and to introduce palliative medicine training into physician education.[37–41]

Significant philanthropic funding spurred the development of palliative medicine. The Robert Wood Johnson Foundation, under the project direction of Rosemary Gibson and Victoria Weisfeld, invested US$95 million between 1997 and 2004 in projects aimed at improving end-of-life care. The project that most influenced the physician component was the Education for Physicians on End-of-life Care (EPEC) Project led by Drs Linda Emanuel, Frank D Ferris, and Charles F von Gunten. Initially developed in conjunction with the American Medical Association (AMA), the project convened leaders in the field to assemble a core curriculum in palliative medicine and disseminate it through a train-the-trainer dissemination model. The project was successful in reaching its educational targets,[42] but there were several unanticipated effects of the project. First, the AMA's imprimatur lent legitimacy to a cadre of EPEC trainers who felt encouraged to volunteer to teach the material at educational programs in their home institutions and advocate for curriculum change in their medical schools and residency programs. Second, in a survey of palliative medicine physicians, the majority said that the EPEC Project was their entry into the field.[43]

The Robert Wood Johnson Foundation also sponsored the Center to Advance Palliative Care (CAPC), initially led by Drs Christine Cassel and Diane Meier. The focus of this national center was to advance palliative care in hospitals and health systems. Dr Cassel had played an instrumental role in the recognition of geriatrics as a subspecialty 20 years earlier and held leadership positions in organized medicine in the USA.

Another major philanthropic spur was the Project on Death in America (PDIA). The Open Society Institute (funded by George Soros) invested US$45 million between 1994 and 2003 in a variety of projects to 'change the culture of dying' in the USA. One of those projects, the PDIA Faculty Scholars Program led by Dr Susan D Block, aimed to develop academic leaders in palliative medicine in the nation's medical schools. By the conclusion of the US$15 million project, the 89 PDIA faculty scholars had in turn been successful in attracting US$115 million in grants and awards from federal and other finding sources. Many PDIA scholars are now in leadership positions in the nation's medical schools, residency programs, and the committees that are shaping the specialty.

The combination of EPEC (a program of physician education), CAPC (a program to advance the practice of palliative medicine in hospitals and health systems), and the PDIA scholars (a program to develop academic physician leaders) can be viewed as a strategy to stimulate an evolution in American healthcare more rapidly than it would otherwise take. The strategy appears to be working. In 2004, the American Board of Internal Medicine convened a summit of all member boards of the American Board of Medical Specialties to consider an application to formally recognize palliative medicine. Formal recognition is seen as likely.

This strategy has not occurred without strain. The development of palliative medicine could be seen as a bid for physician domination of a field that values interdisciplinary team care using a bio-psycho-socio-spiritual model. Some also worry that widespread dissemination of palliative medicine throughout the healthcare system will lead to a dilution or co-option of some essential essence of good palliative care. For instance, skeptics fear that hospital-based palliative care services will be less likely to help patients return to their own homes and will be more likely to overuse diagnostic tests and procedures. In addition, palliative care as part of the US$200 billion dollar healthcare industry might swamp the US$9 billion hospice industry in terms of power and influence. Finally, some predict that the emergence of a cadre of academic palliative medicine specialists will engender a town–gown rift between community-based clinicians (primarily hospice medical directors – often part time and often volunteer or virtually volunteer) and fellowship-trained specialists practicing within the academic medical center.

These concerns are neither unique to palliative medicine nor inevitable. Subspecialization *per se* neither increases nor decreases the likelihood of these outcomes occurring. The root causes for these potential problems must be sought and prevented or redressed. They do not mitigate the driving rationale for professionalization of a field of new knowledge and practice of importance to the health of the public. In addition, the formal recognition of palliative medicine may lead to a broader change within the culture of medicine where 'whole person care' and the relief of suffering are combined with efforts to cure disease.

Key learning points

- In the USA, the history of palliative care prior to the 1970s mirrors that of England with a few homes for the dying operated from religious commitment.

- Dr Elizabeth Kübler-Ross, a psychiatrist, popularized the experience of dying patients through public appearances describing the results of her communication research beginning in the late 1960s.

- Dr Cicely Saunders, founder of St Christopher's Hospice in London, England, was a charismatic speaker and sparked interest among healthcare professionals in the early 1970s in the USA.

- A large number of hospice programs were formed in the second half of the 1970s in the USA, both hospital and community based.

- The US government funded a hospice demonstration project from 1980 to 1982.

- The US government instituted a funding benefit for Medicare patients (mostly over age 65) with terminal illnesses who were cared for mostly at home by family in 1982. This funding stream led to a large increase in the number of hospice programs, particularly community based.

- The path to a recognized physician specialty began in the late 1970s with the formation of a specialty association of hospice physicians.

REFERENCES

1   Aries P. *Western Attitudes Toward Death From the Middle Ages to the Present.* Baltimore: Johns Hopkins University Press, 1974: 76.

2   Hinohara S. Sir William Osler's philosophy on death. *Ann Intern Med* 1993; **118**: 638–42.

3   Cushing H. *The Life of Sir William Osler.* London: Oxford University Press, 1940.

4   Jones J. *The mysteries of opium revealed. I. Gives an account of the name, make, choice, effects, etc., of opium. II. Proves all former opinions of its operations to be meer chimera's. III. Demonstrates what its true cause is; by which he easily and mechanically explains all (even its most mysterious) effects. IV. Shews its noxious principle, and how to separate it; there by rendering it a safe, and noble panacea; whereof, V. He shews the palliative and curative use* [monograph]. London, 1701.

5   Snow HL. *The Palliative Treatment of Incurable Cancer; With an Appendix on the Use of the Opium-pipe.* London: Churchill, 1890.

6   Reece R. *The medical guide, for the use of the clergy, heads of families, and seminaries, and junior practitioners in medicine; comprising a complete modern dispensatory, and a practical treatise on the distinguishing symptoms, causes, prevention, cure, and palliation.* London, 1802.

7   Starr P. *The Social Transformation of American Medicine.* New York: Basic Books, 1982.

8   Saunders C. History of Hospice Care. In: Doyle D, Hanks G, MacDonald N, eds. *Oxford Textbook of Palliative Medicine*, 2nd ed. Oxford: Oxford University Press, 1998.

9   Eldritch Press. Nathaniel Hawthorne, 1804–1864. www.eldritchpress.org/nh/rose.html (accessed October 4, 2004).

10   The Dominic Sisters of Hawthorne. www.hawthorne-dominicans.org (accessed October 4, 2004).

11   Saunders C. Foreword. In: Doyle D, Hanks G, MacDonald N, eds. *Oxford Textbook of Palliative Medicine*, 2nd ed. Oxford: Oxford University Press, 1998: vi.

12   Calvary Hospital. www.calvaryhospital.org (accessed October 4, 2004).

13   Mor V, Greer DS, Kastenbaum R. The hospice experiment: an alternative in terminal care. In: Mor V, Greer DS, Kastenbaum R, eds. *The Hospice Experiment.* Baltimore: Johns Hopkins University Press, 1988.

14   Raps CS, Peterson C, Jonas M. Patient behavior in hospitals: helplessness, reactance or both? *J Pers Soc Pyschol* 1982; **42**: 1036–41.

15   Callahan D. Death and the research imperative. *N Engl J Med* 2000; **342**: 654–6.

16   Starbuck WH. Organizations and their environments. In: Dunnette MD, ed. *Handbook of Industrial and Organizational Psychology.* New York: Rand, 1976: 1069–123.

17   Aring CD. *The Understanding Physician*. Detroit, MI: Wayne State University Press, 1971.

18   Cassell, EJ. *The Nature of Suffering and the Goals of Medicine*. New York: Oxford University Press, 1991.

19   Byock I, Caplan A, Snyder L. Beyond Symptom Management – Physician Roles and Responsibility in Palliative Care; for the American College of Physicians – American Society of Internal Medicine, End-of-Life Care Consensus Panel, 2001.

20   Lorber J. Good patients and problem patients: conformity and deviance in a general hospital. *J Health Soc Behav* 1975; **16**: 213–25.

21   Ptacek JT, Eberhardt TL. Breaking bad news. A review of the literature. *JAMA* 1996; **14**: 496–502.

22   Kübler-Ross E. *On Death and Dying: What the Dying Have to Teach Doctors, Nurses, Clergy and Their Own Families*. New York: Macmillan Publishing, 1969.

23   Wald FS, Foster Z, Wald JH. The hospice movement as a health care reform. *Nurs Outlook* 1980; **28**: 173–8.

24   O'Neill WM, O'Connor P, Latimer EJ. Hospital palliative care services: three models in three countries. *J Pain Symptom Manage* 1992; **7**: 406–13.

25   *Hospice Standards*. Arlington, VA: National Hospice Organization, 1979.

26   Foley K. Advancing palliative care in the United States. *Palliat Med* 2003; **17**: 89–91.

27   Walsh TD. Continuing care in a medical center: the Cleveland Clinic Foundation palliative care service. *J Pain Symptom Manage* 1990; **5**: 273–8.

28   Holman GH, Forman WB. On the 10th anniversary of the organization of the American Academy of Hospice and Palliative Medicine (AAHPM): the first 10 years. *Am J Hosp Palliat Care*. 2001; **18**: 275–8.

29   Weissman DE, Griffie J. Weissman Integration of palliative medicine at the Medical College of Wisconsin 1990–1996. *J Pain Symptom Manage* 1998; **15**: 195–207.

30   Weissman DE. Consultation in palliative medicine. *Arch Intern Med* 1997; **157**: 733–7.

31   von Gunten CF, Martinez J. A program of hospice and palliative care in a private, non-profit US teaching hospital. *J Palliat Med* 1998; **1**: 265–75.

32   Field MJ, Cassel CK, eds. *Approaching Death: Improving Care at the End of Life*. Washington, DC: National Academy Press, 1997.

33   von Gunten CF. Secondary and tertiary palliative care in US hospitals. *JAMA* 2002; **287**: 875–81.

34   US Supreme Court. No 95–1858, 96–110. Justice O'Connor, Justice Stevens concurring opinions

35   Caring for the Dying: Identification and Promotion of Physician Competency-Educational Resource Document. Philadelphia: American Board of Internal Medicine, 1996.

36   Program Requirement for Residency Education in Internal Medicine. Philadelphia: American Board of Internal Medicine, 1998.

37   Billings JA, Block S. Palliative care in undergraduate medical education. *JAMA* 1997; **278**: 733–43.

38   Block, SD, Bernier, GM, Crawley LM, *et al.* Incorporating palliative care into primary care education. *J Gen Intern Med* 1998; **13**: 768–73.

39   Barnard D, Quill T, Hafferty F, *et al.* Preparing the ground: contributions of the pre-clinical years to medical education for care near the end-of-life. *Acad Med* 1999; **74**: 499–505.

40   Meier DE, Morrison RS, Cassel CK. Improving palliative care. *Ann Intern Med* 1997; **127**: 225–30.

41   Arnold R. The challenges of integrating palliative care into postgraduate training. *J Palliat Med* 2003; **5**: 801–7.

42   Robinson K, Sutton S, von Gunten CF, *et al.* Assessment of The Education for Physicians on End-of-life Care (EPEC) Project. *J Palliat Med* 2004; **7**: 637–45.

43   Cohen B, Salsberg, E. The supply, demand and use of palliative care physicians in the United States. A report prepared for the Bureau of HIV/AIDS, Health Resources and Services Administration. Center for Health Workforce Studies, School of Public Health, University at Albany, September 2002. http://chws.albany.edu (accessed December 2002).

4

The development of palliative medicine in Latin America

ROBERTO WENK

INTRODUCTION

The purpose of this chapter is to describe the development of palliative care in Latin America, accepting that the information could be incomplete because there are scarce updated regional data. The issues in Latin America that will be described here may be similar to those present in other developing countries.

THE REGION

The Latin American region has a total population of 510 million and is made up of 35 countries. Although the region is challenged by common economic, political, and cultural factors, there are differences between the countries and states or cities of the same country: size, natural resources, per capita income, resources allocated to health, development, technical expertise, how the people live, health system, stage of epidemiological transition, etc.[1,2]

The challenging difficulties that are common to all the countries despite the above mentioned heterogeneity underpin the serious deficiencies in the way that most of the health systems care for dying people. Many Latin American patients with advanced incurable diseases suffer in the final stages of their lives and die badly.[3,4]

HISTORICAL OVERVIEW

During 1981–85 several physicians in various Latin American countries started treating pain and other symptoms in patients with advanced cancer. Most of them were anesthesiologists concerned about how to improve the care of these patients. This interest generated a bidirectional flow of professionals – from Latin America to Canada, Italy, UK, and USA to find appropriate models of care, and from other countries to Latin America to teach the World Health Organization (WHO) model for pain and symptom control.[5,6] From different WHO collaborative centers, E Bruera, M Baynes, C Cleeland, K Foley, N Koyle, J Stjernsward, R Twycross, and V Ventafridda came to Latin America to teach.

A new perspective about the care of patients with advanced cancer began to grow in the region. As a result of this activity different professionals started to provide palliative care in different countries while promoting and teaching its concepts. They were from different disciplines, mostly volunteers, working at first independently and alone but then in teams based in their community or in their own hospitals. Their successes were the result of personal motivation and the time and resources dedicated to the development of assistance programs adapted to the needs and limitations of each country. They had different resources and opportunities, they varied in their capabilities to care for the dying patients and their families, and their funds came from multiple sources: charity, grants, research protocols, teaching, international subsidies, etc.[7,8]

This development 'on the ground' generated focal activity and initially operated at the level of motivated healthcare professionals who directly provided patient care. It was a time and energy consuming model, but an effective one. The impact of these individual initiatives stimulated action by the health authorities and generated growing interest in the community and among health personnel, which in turn resulted in the expansion of palliative care to programs of greater complexity.[9]

The programs and their activities highlighted two issues: the need for a practical and effective way to improve the quality of care at the end of life, and the deficiencies in the assistance provided to dying patients and their families. They demonstrated inadequacies in practice and identified different barriers to palliative care.

The key to success for these changes lay with the program leaders: their efforts, which were followed shortly by other people, had two primary goals:

- to recruit individuals from the community to work in palliative care with limited resources
- to recruit individuals from diverse organizations (governmental, professional, academic, etc.) to build partnerships with diverse resources and skills.

Their efforts had a profoundly positive impact: while seeding palliative care teams, they let the public learn about the benefit of adequate end-of-life care and provided health authorities with information about needs and possible interventions. In some cases the ongoing persuasive recruiting activity resulted in the development of national or regional palliative care associations, and in other cases it resulted in national official palliative care programs.

CURRENT STATUS

Despite the progress made in the past 20 years, there is evidence that in general the quality of life during the dying process is poor, with fragmented assistance resulting in uncontrolled suffering, poor communication between professionals, patients and families, and a great burden on family caregivers.[7] Most of the regional health systems fail to provide appropriate care for dying patients; the failures are clinical, educational, organizational, and ethical.

As a rule, adequate care of the dying is determined by the characteristics and interrelations of the health system, the health professionals and the patient–family unit. Each of them has unique characteristics that, after superimposing and/or mixing, define the guidelines for care.[10] To evaluate the current status of palliative care and the factors that modulate its development in Latin America, it is necessary to describe the different interrelated issues that affect the need and the delivery of palliative care.

Health systems

In spite of the experiences of regional programs with demonstrable positive results, and the availability of international guidelines, with the exception of a few countries care of the dying is not a public health priority and given low importance compared with preventive and curative services.[11]

Many Latin American countries offer some kind of palliative care services, but they are often minimal and access to these is limited. Fragmentation is the key characteristic of the available care: different disciplines interact in a non-organized way, sometimes cooperating but sometimes competing. The three structural factors discussed below can help us to understand the situation.

INSUFFICIENT SUPPORT OF THE HEALTH AUTHORITIES

There are reported national programs in only Chile, Colombia, Costa Rica, Cuba, the Dominican Republic, and Mexico (Latin America is made up of 35 countries).[12] Only three of these (Chile, Costa Rica, and Cuba) provide palliative care throughout the country; in the others the effective activity has not yet started. The difference between active and inactive programs may be that in the former the programs derive from official 'top down'[13] well-established plans based on assessments of the needs with a commitment to make changes. In Chile's program it is known how many teams, what kinds of professional, and how much medication, etc. are needed to have an integrated net of services for caring for patients in different settings across the country.[14] In the rest of the countries the programs are developing as described in the historical overview above.

Data from a survey of 566 professionals from Argentina, Brazil, Cuba, Mexico, and Peru[12] indicated that 70 percent of them considered that palliative care is not a priority in the health policies of their country. Data provided by 17 palliative care leaders of different Latin America countries (Ongoing surveys, personal communication, 2004) indicates that in 80 percent of the countries palliative care is not yet recognized as a discipline, and it is not included by mandate in either the free public health system or the private health system.

FINANCIAL CHALLENGES

Governments fail to allocate resources where they would be most beneficial. They are struggling with underfunding to solve different problems like lack of infrastructure and assistance centers, control of infectious diseases, prenatal assistance, undernourishment, etc. Yet their payment mechanisms reward life-prolonging interventions, even when futile.[15] The health systems have not yet matched and aligned financial incentives with better standards of care, namely palliative care. This situation is reinforced by the lack of capability to quantify the costs of palliative care, so that these costs cannot be compared with other health costs and potential cost savings cannot be documented.

BARRIERS TO OPIOID AVAILABILITY AND ACCESSIBILITY

Some countries have changed their policies with increase in the use of opioids, but in most countries this is below the global mean of 6.5 mg per capita.[16] Reasons for the well-documented underutilization are: the high cost of opioids and restrictive regulations for their use. There is good availability of different opioids, but the high price of most of them compared with the mean monthly income in the region acts as a barrier to their access and utilization.[17,18] In addition, there are outdated and nonscientific prescribing regulations that restrict the use of potent analgesics: 50 percent of the 566 professionals surveyed[12] (see above) considered them as barriers to utilization, and the Pan American Health Organization (PAHO) has identified definite barriers to opioid use in Colombia, Peru, Mexico, Argentina, and Costa Rica.[19,20]

The Latin America health authorities must intervene to make palliative care accessible to everyone through plans with a three-pronged approach:

- improving the economic, organizational, legal, and clinical environment
- educating professionals in end-of-life care
- educating the people about their right to demand high-quality assistance at the end of the life.

Willingness to modify policies can be perceived in some countries, but making the necessary changes is a slow process due to the inertial resistance in the systems and a lack of interest in individuals at different decision making levels.[9] Although these factors may be found throughout the world, their negative impact is greater in Latin America due to the poor socioeconomic health of the region.

Health professionals

Health professionals are focusing on the idea of a good death and are slowly becoming interested in the care of people at the end of life. This new perception of the dying process has not changed the situation in the region as yet: although there is limited information on the proportion of patients who receive palliative care, it can be estimated to be lower than 5 percent. The different factors discussed below can help us to understand the regional situation.

PROGRAMS AND TEAMS

In most Latin American countries the health authorities have not yet adopted palliative care with standards of assistance, and programs vary between cities and among themselves. The programs are more or less well developed with operational differences related to their degree of development; they are based either in the community or in hospitals, some involve one or more institutions within the same community and a few extend to the whole state. They operate in different settings and each program has unique experiences with regard to its creativity, persistence, and adaptability to changes in its environment. These programs provide treatment to the majority of cancer patients.

In general most palliative care programs provide partial care:[21] teams consisting of one or two disciplines with part-time commitment, with mixed or exclusive home or outpatient care, distance care[22] and institutional activity, but no specific facilities (mobile advisory teams without own beds). Full palliative care programs with dedicated inter-disciplinary teams providing 24 × 7 care in the consulting room, at home, and in day care, and hospitalization (with own beds) is not the rule.

In large cities, where 97 percent of the palliative care is primarily available,[12] a few health systems provide complete palliative care. In small cities and rural areas, where only 3 percent of the palliative care is available, all patients receive partial palliative care.

MODELS OF CARE

The traditional medical model is prevalent in the region: for many of the dying, quality of life is secondary to excessive medical interventions that too often are futile and sometimes expensive. The patients suffer needlessly both from errors of omission (they do not receive palliative care) and from errors of commission (they receive futile treatments); it is common to see 'curative' treatments being administered that are not beneficial for the patients, nor always in accordance with their wishes. There are multiple reasons for this situation:

- Most of the decisions about offering and providing treatments are not based on cost–benefit ratio and do not consider the patient's quality of life.
- Physicians favor the principle of beneficence rather than the principle of autonomy and adopt a paternalistic behavior with little regard to patient's preferences.
- There is poor communication between physicians and patients and their families that in some cases blocks the disclosure of diagnostic and prognostic information: physicians and/or families are likely to believe that the bad news should be withheld from patients and thus impede their ability to be decision makers in their own care. In other cases, in the absence of complete information about treatment options patients or their families demand useless or counterproductive treatments or cannot refuse what they see to be futile and/or painful treatments.
- Lack of education and awareness of ethical issues and the fragmentation of care complicate the necessary coordination and continuity of care needed to make ethical clinical decisions toward care that is adapted to the individual patient's and his or her family's needs and wishes.

EDUCATION

Undergraduate and graduate education does not adequately prepare health professionals to recognize the final stages of illnesses or to provide effective interventions. Their education and training fail to provide them with the attitudes, knowledge, and skills required to provide good care for the dying patient. Teaching for graduate health professionals is different, sometimes inadequate. Instruction with specifically structured content and curricula with clinical practice are limited; learning from tutors along with structured assessments is undervalued. As palliative care is still not recognized as a specialty, there are no residency requirements and licensure examinations.

Of the 566 professionals surveyed (see above) 70 percent considered that palliative care is not a priority in health education and that professionals do not have enough knowledge about symptom evaluation and control;[12] 90 percent of the 17 surveyed practitioners indicated that palliative care is not included in undergraduate education and only 15 percent knew about the possibility of graduate clinical training under tutor guidance; they also reported that possibilities for training are, in decreasing order: courses with lectures, self-capacitating and distance learning (Ongoing surveys, personal communication, 2004).

Many of the deficiencies in the practice of palliative care are based in these failures in education:

- professionals without adequate training provide inadequate services
- different professionals with different training performing the same task (i.e. nurse auxiliaries vs. professional nurses; psychologists vs. counselors) without a uniform standard of care
- inadequate communication skills (making it difficult to discuss end-of-life issues)
- training not including experience in interactive multiprofessional work (making teamworking difficult).

This situation is worsened by the lack of standards in each discipline for self-evaluating the quality of the work and by the difficulty in acknowledging the incapabilities.

The healthcare community is slowly accepting the responsibility for educating itself about end-of-life care issues. Some programs offer teaching opportunities with definite objectives and methods that target practice, improved teamwork, and problem solving, i.e. courses with a significant content of clinical practice and fellowships in clinical units to use and reinforce teamwork and reasoning skills.

LACK OF REWARDS AND INCENTIVES

In many countries palliative care is still not recognized as a medical discipline and palliative care teams and programs are difficult to finance because most of the health systems do not pay, or underpay, for their services. This makes sustainability an issue that has been solved (in most countries) with different approaches: resources from charity, working for free on a volunteer basis, and care paid by the patient (when

it is possible) or by the health coverage (some accept palliative care and pay for it). Most teams, if not all, can deliver assistance because of their high volunteer/paid personnel ratio. This situation can be longstanding and stable with regard to team interventions delivered by nonprofessional volunteers, but the professional volunteer's services are time limited. Professional volunteers usually join a palliative care team because they are both interested in this new discipline and wish to learn its practice. During the time of volunteer work their earnings come from their disciplines, but after some years most of them wish to shift to palliative care as their main discipline. If the team cannot pay for their work, as it usually happens, they withdraw from the team activity. The result is teams with cyclic staffing and effectiveness and trained professionals who do not have adequate job opportunities in this underrecognized and unpaid discipline.

Payment mechanisms for the care of dying patients impede the efficient and effective use of the limited health resources to improve quality of life. The pattern and quality of care is negatively influenced by the unbalanced reimbursement and provider time ratio: financing mechanisms encourage the overuse of procedural services and the underprovision of time consuming services such as palliative care. It is easier and more profitable for a physician to hospitalize a patient or start an aggressive and often ineffectual treatment that may prolong dying process, than to invest time creating consensus about therapeutic alternatives or discussing the dying process.

Health authorities must revise financing and payment mechanisms to encourage good end-of-life care and stop undertreatment or overtreatment of those approaching death.

Patients and families

The care of patients with advanced cancer and their families also depends on both where they live and their resources (effective health coverage and/or money). There are only three Latin American countries (Chile, Cuba, and Costa Rica) with palliative care programs that have reported provision of effective care throughout the country to most of the population (e.g. Chile reports that there are 41 palliative care teams in the whole of the country).[23] What is happening in most of the other countries? There are four different scenarios:

1 *Patients living in a large city with resources.* These patients have the possibility of accessing top interdisciplinary healthcare adapted to the individual patient's needs: at the office, at home, or during stay in hospital. (Resources and living in a large city do not guarantee effective palliative care.)
2 *Patients living in a large city without resources.* These patients have the limited possibility of receiving care in public hospitals. (Not all hospitals have palliative care

teams nor can all the teams provide all the treatment options.)

3 *Patients living in a small city or in a rural area with resources.* If moving to a large city these patients have the same possibilities as the patients in scenario 1.

4 *Patients living in a small city or in a rural area without resources.* These patients have the possibility of receiving some kind of care, characterized by poor control of symptoms.

The difficult, negative health situation of scenarios 2 and 4 is due to and amplified by poverty generated by Latin America's socioeconomic crisis: 200 million people (36 percent) live below the poverty level.[1] Medical, nursing, and social services are not available to them. Assistance and palliative care are often inaccessible and unaffordable, resulting in considerable suffering due to both lack of basic essentials for care and access to symptom control medication. Many people live in absolute poverty with unmet physical needs: without suitable food, drinking water, electricity, indoor toilets, etc., and for some needs are better met in hospital than at home. They spend their last days (sometimes weeks and months) in healthcare institutions under the care of professionals without instruction in palliative care.

Some of the deficiencies in the healthcare systems are solved by the informal care systems that play a central role for many if not most patients and families. Extended families (people with a legal, social, or biological relationship with the patient) collaborate in the care of the patient at home but they become burdened by the difficulty of caring, their lack of knowledge, the lack of drugs in the home, and their fear of not knowing what to do when the patient deteriorates.[24] In the community, voluntary groups and religious communities develop networks to help in the care of patients at home or in hospital by visiting regularly and providing food, medicines, or money. As in other developing regions of the world finding the money for outpatient consultations, medicines, transportation, and paying the funeral is a top ranked task.[25,26]

Notwithstanding even the huge efforts of different groups and institutions, the health situation of patients and families at the end of life is poor. They must be able to expect and receive efficient and skillful care. Educating them about palliative care, a shared responsibility of health professionals and the media, will encourage them to report suffering and to demand palliative care. Increased consumer demand is a powerful factor with the potential for reducing barriers through 'sensitizing' health providers and policy makers.[27]

LOOKING FORWARD

In Latin America, palliative care is impossible to stop because there is growing evidence that it is useful. Every year, in every country, many palliative care teams are formed.

Palliative care health professionals now acknowledge the two basic needs: adequate regional palliative care and changes in the systems of care and individual actions. The new perception of the poor health situation of the dying facilitated the consensus and the urgency to act to satisfy their needs: professionals from different countries funded the Latin American Palliative Care Association (Asociación Latino Americana de Cuidado Paliativo, ALCP) on April 23, 2001, in Buenos Aires, Argentina. The mission of this not-for-profit organization is

> to promote the development of palliative care in Latin America and the Caribbean by communication and integration of all those interested in helping improve the quality of life of patients with incurable progressive diseases as well as their families.

The ALCP has not yet found the way to obtain enough funds to be completely functional, but it has managed to launch three different tools:

- *Latin American congresses.* There is a demonstrable positive tendency to share experiences and results of assistance in regional meetings. The first congress in San Nicolas, Argentina, in 1990, brought together 35 people from seven countries. The last congress, held in Montevideo, Uruguay, in 2004, was attended by 284 people from diverse disciplines and 18 countries.
- *Circular of the ALCP (newsletter).* This is a free electronic monthly or bimonthly publication in Spanish and Portuguese. At present there are 1450 subscribers in 14 countries.
- *Website* (www.cuidadospaliativos.org). This is intended to disseminate information and collaborate in the development of support networks.

One of roles of the ALCP is to help in the identification of real or potential barriers to palliative care in the region and in individual countries. Some of them have been identified and others are suspected; after they are documented and understood different actions can be taken to reduce their impact. There is a need for information to aid in understanding the different professional, organizational, and cultural issues involved to guide the development of palliative care. The ALCP is the tool that will allow palliative care to develop in accordance with regional needs.

Key learning points

- Countries in the Latin American region face several common challenges that underpin the serious deficiencies in the way that most of the health systems care for dying people.

- In the 1980s a growing awareness of the need for treating pain and other symptoms in patients with advanced cancer resulted in visits from several international leaders in the field to Latin America to teach the WHO model for pain and symptom control.

- The first practitioners of palliative care in Latin America were from different disciplines, mostly volunteers, working at first independently and alone but then in teams based in their community or in their own hospitals.

- Despite the progress made in the past 20 years, there is evidence that in general the quality of life during the dying process is poor, with fragmented assistance resulting in uncontrolled suffering, poor communication between professionals, patients and families, and a great burden on family caregivers.

- Many Latin American countries offer some kind of palliative care services, but they are often minimal and access is limited. Only three (Chile, Costa Rica, and Cuba) provide palliative care throughout the country.

- Health systems face insufficient support of the health authorities, financial challenges, and barriers to opioid availability and accessibility.

- Health professionals and patients and their families face the challenges of lack of education, awareness, robust models of care, and standard programs, and payment mechanisms that impede the delivery of efficient and effective care.

- Despite the challenges palliative care continues to grow in Latin America and the ALCP will play a significant role in its future development.

REFERENCES

◆ 1   United Nations Development Programme. *Human Development Report, 2003.* New York: Oxford University Press, 2003. Website: http://www.undp.org/

◆ 2   Luna F, Van Delden JJM. Is physician-assisted death only for developing countries? Latin America as a case study. *J Palliat Care* 2004; **20**: 155–62.

◆ 3   Wenk R, Bertolino M. Argentina: Palliative care status 2002. *J Pain Symptom Manage* 2002; **24**: 166–9.

◆ 4   Wenk R, Ochoa J. Argentina: status of cancer pain and palliative care. *J Pain Symptom Manage* 1996; **12**: 97–8.

✱ 5   World Health Organization. *Cancer Pain Relief.* Geneva: WHO, 1986.

✱ 6   World Health Organization Expert Committee. *Cancer Pain Relief and Palliative Care.* Geneva: WHO, 1990.

◆ 7   Bruera E. Palliative care in Latin America. *J Pain Symptom Manage* 1993; **8**: 365–8.

◆ 8   Bruera E, Sweeney C. Palliative care models: International perspectives. *J Palliat Med* 2002; **5**: 319–27.

◆ 9   Wenk R, Bertolino M. Models of delivery of palliative care in developing countries: the Argentine model. In: Bruera E, Portenoy R, eds. *Cultural Issues in Palliative Care, Topics in Palliative Care.* New York: Oxford University Press 2001: 39–51.

✱ 10 Committee on Care at the End of Life, Division of Health Care Services, Institute of Medicine. Field MJ, Cassel CK, eds. *Approaching Death: Improving Care at the End of Life.* Washington, DC: National Academy Press, 1997.

◆ 11 DeLima L. Cuidados paliativos en países en desarrollo: retos y recursos. II Congreso de la Asociación Latinoamericana de Cuidados Paliativos, VIII Curso Latinoamericano de Medicina y Cuidados Paliativos, Montevideo, Uruguay, 2004.

● 12 Torres I. *Determinants of Quality of Advanced Cancer Care in Latin America – A Look at Five Countries: Argentina, Brazil, Cuba, Mexico and Peru.* Texas: University of Texas, School of Public Health, 2004. Doctoral dissertation.

◆ 13 Bruera E. Practical tips for health care professionals planning to teach in the developing world. In: Bruera E, DeLima L, Wenk R, Farr W, eds. *Palliative Care in the Developing World: Principles and Practice.* Houston, TX: IAHPC Press, 2004.

◆ 14 Derio L, Delgado C, Fuentes P, *et al.* Perfil de las mujeres con cancer de mama avanzado cervicouterino y de mama. 1999–2002, Chile. II Congreso de la Asociación Latinoamericana de Cuidados Paliativos, VIII Curso Latinoamericano de Medicina y Cuidados Paliativos, Montevideo, Uruguay, 2004.

◆ 15 Wenk R, Marti G. Palliative care in Argentina: deep changes are necessary for its effective implementation. *Palliat Med* 1996; **10**: 263–4.

◆ 16 Joranson DE. Improving availability of opioid pain medications: Testing the principle of balance in Latin America. *Innovations in End-of-Life Care* 2003; **5**(1). Available at: www.edc.org/ lastacts (accessed December 10, 2005).

◆ 17 De Lima L, Sweeney C, Palmer L, Bruera E. Potent analgesics are more expensive for patients in developing countries: a comparative study. Poster presentation at the International Association for the Study of Pain (IASP) 10th World Congress on Pain, San Diego, August 2002.

● 18 Wenk R, Bertolino M, DeLima L. Analgésicos opioides en Latinoamérica: la barrera de accesibilidad supera la de disponibilidad. *Medicina Paliativa* 2004; **11**: 148–51.

◆ 19 De Lima L, Bruera E, Joranson DE, *et al.* Opioid availability in Latin America: The Santo Domingo Report, progress since the Declaration of Florianapolis. *J Pain Symptom Manage* 1997; **13**: 213–19.

◆ 20 Stjernswärd J, Bruera E, Joranson DE, *et al.* Opioid availability in Latin America: The declaration of Florianopolis. *J Pain Symptom Manage* 1995; **10**: 233–6.

◆ 21 Latimer, EJ. The ethics of partial palliative care. *J Palliat Care* 1994; **10**: 107–10.

● 22 Wenk R, Monti C, Bertolino M. Asistencia a distancia: mejor o peor que nada? *Medicina Paliativa* 2003; **10**: 136–41.

◆ 23 Gobierno de Chile, Ministerio de Salud. Available at: www.minsal.cl/ (accessed December 10, 2005).

◆ 24 Bruera E, DeLima L, Wenk R, Farr W, eds. *Palliative Care in the Developing World: Principles and Practice.* Houston, TX: IAHPC Press, 2004.

◆ 25 Olweny C. Ethics of palliative care medicine: palliative care for the rich nations only! *J Palliat Care* 1994; **10**: 17–22.

◆ 26 Haines A, Heath I, Smith R. Joining together to combat poverty. *BMJ* 2000; **320**: 1–2.

◆ 27 Smith R. A good death. An important aim for health services and for us all. *BMJ* 2000; **320**: 129–30.

5

The development of palliative medicine in Africa

ANNE MERRIMAN

INTRODUCTION

In June 2004, the African Palliative Care Association (APCA) was launched officially in Arusha, Tanzania, during its first annual general meeting and conference.[1] Twenty-two African countries attended. This was amazing progress since 1994, when only four countries (Zimbabwe, South Africa, Kenya, and Uganda) had established palliative care in sub-Saharan Africa. Also in 2004, Zimbabwe celebrated 25 years of palliative care. It was the first country in Africa to commence palliative care in the 1970s, according to the concepts developed through the modern hospice movement (Table 5.1).

This chapter explores the slow start, and then the mushrooming of interest over 10 years in palliative care. Its findings must be seen in conjunction with the economic and social history of the African countries during this time. Of the 46 countries in Africa, by 2005, 26 have shown interest in palliative care including those with established care (five

Table 5.1 *Development of palliative care in Africa*

Year	Palliative care commenced
1979	Zimbabwe
1982	South Africa
1989	Kenya
1993	Uganda
1994–99	Zambia, Botswana, Swaziland, Nigeria
2000–04	Tanzania, Malawi, Ghana, Sierra Leone, Lesotho

countries) and those with early initiations without morphine and essential drugs or training in place (10 countries).

The importance of an accurate definition of palliative care in the African context

The African definition of palliative care, as in other contexts, is:

- The active total care of patients whose disease is not responsive to curative treatment.
- Control of pain and of other symptoms and of psychologic, social and spiritual problems is paramount.
- The goal is achievement of the best possible quality of life for patients and their families.

Palliative care combines supportive care (present in support home care teams before the advent of palliative care) and pain and symptom control using the methods researched since 1967. But the following are *not* palliative care:

- Supportive care *without* pain and symptom control using the researched methods. This is only **support care**.
- Pain and symptom control without supportive and holistic care: this is anesthesiology.

These distinctions are important in Africa today. With donors now funding palliative care, many organizations with supportive care or home care are claiming they offer palliative care. However, they do not have trained health professionals or the affordable medications that have made pain and symptom control possible at affordable prices. This approach is lowering standards. Donors and service providers as well as governments need to be aware of this problem.

Pain and symptom control are now being grafted onto supportive care programs in Africa. Supportive care has always been there in Africa, similar to the support Dame Cicely (Fig. 5.1) found in the UK while deciding to research pain and symptom control before St Christopher's was established (Dame Cicely Saunders, personal communication, June 2003). But in Africa pain control was absent. This is only possible when the knowledge of palliative methods of pain control are taught and practiced. Morphine, the main drug recommended by the World Health Organization (WHO) for severe pain control has not been available (or affordable) in a form that could be used in the home.

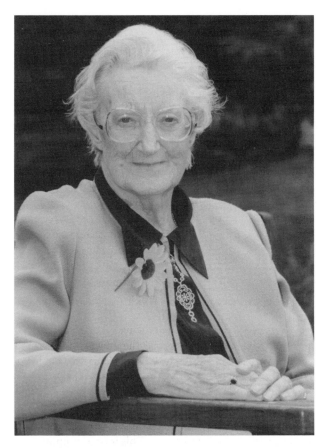

Figure 5.1 *Dame Cicely Saunders, founder of the modern hospice movement which introduced researched pain and symptom control as a basis for peace at the end of life.*

THE FIRST HOSPICES IN AFRICA: ESTABLISHED WITH THE NEEDS OF THE WHITE POPULATIONS IN MIND

Zimbabwe (Zimbabwe, Country Report, p 10, Eunice Garanganga, personal communication, September 2004)

In 1977, a young white girl, Frances, died in Zimbabwe, in severe pain from cancer. Her mother, Maureen Butterfield, hearing about St Christopher's Hospice in London, went there to see if she could prevent this suffering from continuing in Zimbabwe. This first move toward palliative care in Africa resulted in the opening of Island Hospice in Harare in 1979. Island Hospice was dedicated to home care and did not have an inpatient facility.

Initially created with the intention of meeting the needs of all Zimbabweans, it was mostly accepted and used by the white community with a large bereavement service and mainly older patients. The Island Hospice model gradually became more acceptable to the African community. In 1986 they took their first acquired immune deficiency syndrome (AIDS) patients in the program and have continued to do this. Island Hospice was modeled very much along the lines of the British hospice model but adapted to the needs of a mixed community. For example, in 1993, we found that Island Hospice had 9 nurses, 9 social workers, 9 cars, and no doctor for the home care service. About 75 percent of the patients were from the indigenous communities. The bereavement service had grown significantly, primarily due to traumatic deaths, and formed the major part of the social workers' work. Many staff at that time were white Zimbabweans. The attached doctor was advisory and attended case conferences only, seldom visiting a patient. The nurses were prescribing morphine with the support of their doctor (J Hunt, personal communication, September 2004). They were doing wonderful work, and had access to oral morphine allowing them to keep their patients comfortable. Training was in place. The hospice had expanded to other branches throughout Zimbabwe and was already networking with support teams to bring in palliative care.

Sadly, since the recent decline in the economy of Zimbabwe, the hospice is floundering for want of materials, which it cannot afford because of the decline in the value of the Zimbabwean dollar. Morphine is often not available. However those trained in palliative care are continuing to do all they can for their patients, are actively taking part in training both within Zimbabwe and other African countries and are active members of the APCA.

Most staff are now indigenous Zimbabweans, although filling and maintaining positions is becoming increasingly difficult. Many health professionals are lured away to organizations and other countries offering much better conditions than this hospice can afford. This is an example of how economic and political circumstances in a country can affect a humanitarian service.

South Africa[2]

South Africa was the second country in Africa to introduce palliative care. South Africa was brought into the fold of sub-Saharan Africa only since the cessation of apartheid in 1995. However, apartheid has left its mark on the South Africa of today. There is still a wide divide between the Caucasian races and others, although this divide is narrowing. The holistic approach to palliative care in South Africa reveals some terrible problems related to poverty, poor housing, drug and alcohol abuse and sexual promiscuity. More recently, an escalating human immunodeficiency virus (HIV) epidemic has added to the woes. Many of the problems in South Africa are comparable to the problems found in the poorer areas of the developed world and their origins can be found in the social development of the country.

The inspiration for founding hospice and palliative care in South Africa came from Chris Dare (Brief history of the Hospice Palliative Care Association of South Africa, Kath Defillippi, personal communication, 2004), who was in the same choir as Dame Cicely Saunders in London (Dr Mary Baines, personal communication, 2005). She was greatly inspired by the work of Cicely Saunders and how it had changed the face of suffering among patients in London. A physiotherapist, she decided to follow Cicely Saunders' example and become a doctor with the aim of commencing palliative care in South Africa. In 1979, while still a medical student at University of Cape Town, she persuaded Professor J P van Niekerk, Dean of Studies at the University, to invite Dame Cicely to Capetown to speak about her work. This eventually led to the opening of the first inpatient hospice in South Africa, St Luke's Hospice, Capetown, on February 1, 1983. This extended to a community service in 1992, and the service has grown rapidly to meet the needs of the HIV/AIDS epidemic.

Meanwhile, the example of St Luke's was taken up in many areas of South Africa. By the year 2000 there were 40 hospices established, 5 regional hospice associations and a national association (Hospice Association of South Africa [HASA]) was commenced in 1987. This national organization has set up standards, advocacy, and education and has been a resource both within and beyond South Africa.

HOSPICES SET UP WITH THE INDIGENOUS AFRICAN POPULATION IN MIND

Sociocultural aspects of sub-Saharan Africa

Sub-Saharan Africa above South Africa, has, on the whole, kept a stronger African heritage. Cultural beliefs come into play when approaching death, which are often a mix of African religious beliefs and the beliefs of religions (Christianity and Muslim mainly) new to the African scene (by 'new' meaning 100 years). This has meant that palliative care needs to be adjusted to each country and to the belief systems and felt needs of patients and families.

Nairobi Hospice

In 1988, the wife of a BBC correspondent, Ruth Wooldridge, watched helplessly as a Kenyan teacher returned home from hospital with a diagnosis of terminal cancer and proceeded to die with the family trying to care for her while she suffered terrible pain and symptoms without assistance. Ruth was a nurse and although not trained in palliative care, she knew that there was an answer to this problem; indeed she had witnessed hospice care in South Africa while with her husband in a previous posting.

Ruth started to find supporters for a foundation called Nairobi Hospice Charitable Trust (NHCT). In 1989, they had employed a senior nurse, Brigid Sirengo, who was working with Jane Moore, a volunteer nurse from UK. They were then working by candlelight in a small hut, while a pre-fabricated building was being set up adjacent to and on land belonging to Kenyatta Hospital (the government teaching hospital). They were already running a small service and had a Board in place, but did not have access to oral morphine. First through contacts overseas and later through the negotiations and advocacy to the Ministry of Health by Professor E Kasili, oncologist and Chairman of the Board of Nairobi Hospice, with the Ministry of Health, oral morphine was obtained, and I took up post as their first medical director in 1990. A training program was also established.[3] At Nairobi Hospice I was overwhelmed with the severe suffering we were seeing among patients dying in the community, with or without previous hospital consultation. Indeed the suffering of the African, with scant curable treatment, is the worst in the world both for cancer and for AIDS.

Nairobi Hospice has continued to carry out pioneer work in service and in training throughout Kenya. It provides patients with cancer a home care service and consultation in Kenyatta Hospital and other hospitals. In the last 2 years they have expanded their care to HIV/AIDS patients. New hospices came up slowly, with the first a branch of Nairobi Hospice commencing in 1993 (Nyeri Hospice). Most of the new services have started due to individual efforts. Today, there are small services in different parts of the country, some as part of an outreach program from hospitals and others as home care programs.

Hospice Africa Uganda

Uganda was the fourth country in Africa to embrace palliative care. There was a felt need for an African hospice that would have the hospice spirit of hospitality without bureaucracy and that would combine culturally acceptable practices and act as a model for other and poorer African countries.[4] After a feasibility study in three of the seven countries requesting hospice care, Uganda was chosen because of its track record of integrity in handling aid, the severity of the AIDS epidemic, and the willingness of the Ministry of Health to import morphine powder and support the service.

Fazal Mbaraka and I were the initial pioneers of this work. Fazal, a Kenyan of Pakistani origin was a nurse trained in palliative care at Nairobi Hospice. Sadly during the pioneer period, Fazal's father was murdered in Eldoret, Kenya. This resulted in Fazal having to return to Kenya in early 1994 to support her family. By that time we already had a training program in Makerere University medical school and had identified our first Ugandan pioneer nurse, Rose Kiwanuka. Hospice Africa Uganda commenced with three objectives:

1 To provide a palliative care service to patients and families, within a 20 km radius of the hospice and to promote this care throughout Uganda.
2 To provide education programs in palliative medicine, for health professionals at undergraduate and postgraduate levels throughout Uganda so that this form of care can be available to all in need.
3 To encourage the initiation/consolidation of palliative care in other African countries, by providing a facility at Hospice Uganda for training, and experience of palliative care working in the African context.

For the first 5 years, the priority was to simultaneously set up the service and the teaching. Teaching in the medical schools in Makerere University and later Mbarara University, was gradually producing doctors and nurses who understood the concepts of palliative care and could teach others. However, support from the Ministry of Health (MoH) was often difficult to maintain. Some senior physicians, due to earlier teaching, were unaware of the modern research on pain and symptom control and the recognition of palliative medicine as a specialty by the Royal College of Physicians (UK) in 1987.

In 1998, following a conference for senior MoH officials and those managing cancer and AIDS, initiated by the Hospice, the MoH agreed to form a committee to review the role of palliative care for Uganda. As a result of this, in 2000, Uganda became the first country in Africa to include palliative care as an essential service for all in Uganda as part of the 5-year Strategic Health Plan. This essential service came under AIDS, not cancer. Cancer in this country, where life expectancy was only 39 years, (now increased to 45), was not one of the top 10 causes of death; HIV/AIDS was the cause behind most deaths.

By 2000 the three priorities for a palliative care service in an African country were present in Uganda: drug availability, education and government support (Fig. 5.2).[5–8]

Generating government support to other African countries: 2000–2004

In 2000, the first funding was made available to support our third objective (see above). The training and support

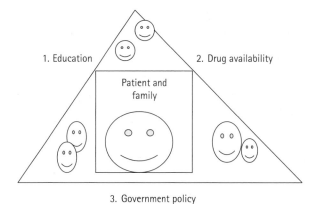

Figure 5.2 *The World Health Organization (WHO) three priorities for a new service in palliative care. Note that the patient and family are at the center of care. Adapted (to include the patient and family as the centre of care) from WHO.*[9]

was offered to teams in Tanzania, through ORCI (Ocean Road Cancer Institute) and PASADA (a comprehensive HIV/AIDS support organization under the Catholic Archdiocese) in Dar es Salaam. Through this experience we developed a three-pronged plan for assisting countries in Africa.

1 Assessment of need, guided by those on the ground requesting assistance.
2 Advocacy with our team and initiators of palliative care in the country to the MoH regarding the importation of powdered morphine for affordable pain relief.
3 Introduction of palliative care training for those who would prescribe medications using the WHO guidelines. We could not envisage the introduction of morphine without this special training being in place. If palliative care is wrongly used, it can cause more pain and discourage health workers in its use as an effective means of care. The introduction of standards is therefore essential from the start.

The advocacy to the governments was successful in Tanzania and Malawi. Powdered and affordable oral morphine was imported for the first time.

Role of the WHO: the public health approach

In 2001, the WHO[10,11] commenced its initiative to assist five African countries. The organization commenced a work which brought experience in Africa to four further countries by introducing country palliative care teams, research in situation analysis and needs of patients and carers in the community with a view to persuading governments to support palliative care and to legalize procurement of essential drugs including morphine.

In the following years this approach was brought from Hospice Africa Uganda in partnership with Diana, Princess of Wales Memorial Fund, to Malawi, Zambia, Ethiopia, and Ghana. Further requests are coming from all over Africa, and have increased since the first conference and annual general meeting of the APCA in June 2004 in Arusha, Tanzania.

PALLIATIVE CARE IN AFRICA AND DRUG AVAILABILITY

In line with most other developing countries, African countries had gradually decreased their requests for class A drugs, particularly morphine, because they were afraid of a back lash from drug trafficking laws (David Joranson at the WHO Collaborating Centre in Wisconsin, USA, personal communication over many years). In 2000, the WHO[12] pointed out the need for balance in narcotic control laws, so that patients would not be denied pain relief due to archaic laws. At Hospice Africa Uganda, more than 7000 patients have received pain control using morphine, without diversion or abuse of drugs.[13] This has been confirmed in other developing countries.[14]

At present, morphine solution reconstituted in a pharmacy, costs less than half a loaf of bread for the average patient to be free of pain for 10 days. The other medications (22 on our essential drug list) are affordable and usually available in any African country. This is a forceful advocacy statement for governments in fear of economic implications of palliative care.

However, there is a further problem in countries with few doctors. Doctors are still the only prescribers for class A drugs, such as morphine. Uganda recognized this problem and in 2004 changed the law so that nurses and clinical officers, who have undergone a 9-month training program in Clinical Palliative Care and are registered with the MoH, can prescribe morphine. It is hoped that this first will be taken up in other African countries.

Nigeria

Nigeria was visited in 1993 by the initiators of Hospice Africa, Mbaraka Fazal, and the author. Nigeria was among several countries that had requested that the model hospice might be in their country. In Lagos that year, a pioneer group was headed by Mrs Fatumnbi and Professor Duncan, a retired radiotherapist. Mrs Fatumnbi had been inspired by her visit to St Christopher's Hospice in London the previous year, and her meeting with Dame Cicely. They were very keen that Nigeria would be the country where we would commence and as we visited the MoH and other teaching centers in Lagos, Ibadan we realized that the problem of corruption was so bad that donors were reluctant to

support nongovernmental organizations, especially new ventures. The MoH promised to bring in powdered morphine, but this was not followed through after we left the country, much to the disappointment of the pioneers.

Today, this same group has registered Hospice Nigeria in Lagos, there is a teaching section in the undergraduate curriculum in University College Hospital (UCH), Ibadan, but it still has no affordable and available oral morphine for control of pain. The government is yet to take on this need. Nigeria is a huge country. I am aware of one or more small groups trying to commence palliative care, but it takes full time commitment by someone with fire in the belly (often due to a personal experience of the need having been fulfilled).

An Advocacy APCA visit to Nigeria in January 2005 brought great interest from many highly positioned medical and nursing leaders in the UCH Ibadan and beyond. Advocacy is now again being brought to the present government and teaching with a community home-based care service is planned for later this year in Ibadan itself.

Note added in proof: Nigeria and Cameroon now have morphine available for use in palliative care since February 2006.

PROBLEMS EXPERIENCED IN INTRODUCING PALLIATIVE CARE

The many problems that have yet to be addressed in the different African countries are as follows:

- How do you bring medications to a patient in pain when they do not have enough to eat? This happens in many countries with extremes of poverty, such as Ethiopia and Malawi.
- How do you ask nurses who come into work hungry in the mornings to bring food to their patients without assisting them and their own families?
- The majority of African patients want to die in their own homes.[15] However some of the laws in African countries were designed by and for sophisticated Western colonialists who occupied the African countries, and have not changed since independence. For example, in Zambia, the law says that if a patient dies in the home the body has to be carried to a doctor (usually in the nearest hospital) to be certified dead. This brings a huge cost to the family in the transport of a dead body. There is also a shortage of doctors in Zambia, as in many poorer African countries, due to a 'brain drain'. Thus families prefer patients to die in a hospital or institution where there is a doctor available.

No doubt as we continue this form of assistance, other hindrances will be discovered and of course this emphasizes the fact that palliative care services must be adapted to the cultural, social, and economic needs of each country.

ROLE OF PALLIATIVE CARE ASSOCIATIONS IN AFRICA

With the registration and recognition of the APCA in June 2004, the role of palliative care associations throughout Africa is highlighted. The APCA aims to:[16]

- promote standards for the quality provision of hospice and palliative care services for adults and children
- be an advocate to Governments for affordable and appropriate palliative care to be incorporated into the whole spectrum of healthcare services
- promote the availability of palliative care drugs for all in need
- encourage the establishment of national palliative care associations in all African countries
- encourage sharing among such associations
- promote training programs suitable to African countries
- make standard guidelines for training at different levels.

This brings tremendous hope to bring together all the expertise now available within Africa. The national palliative care associations have led the way, particularly in South Africa (Hospice and Palliative Care Association of South Africa, [HPCASA]) and Uganda (Palliative Care Association of Uganda [PCAU]), by providing forums for continuing medical education and sharing among palliative care teams and isolated trained personnel. They now have a continental parent organization to support them.

SUPRA-SAHARAN AFRICA

In countries north of the Sahara, development has been mainly associated with the Islamic religion and governments affiliated to this religion. Although these countries have been oil rich for many years and oncology is far advanced, there has been little development in palliative care. We cannot find any palliative care models in these countries although there is a great interest there at present.

WHERE ARE WE TODAY AND WHERE DO WE GO FROM HERE?

We need to maintain up-to-date information on all African countries, e.g. the stage of development of palliative care in each country:

- Country with no palliative care
- Country with some but not all three priorities in place
- All three priorities in place adapted to the needs in your own country

As we move palliative care into the Francophone and Portuguese speaking countries, we need training materials in these languages as well as books for carers in the vernacular languages. How can we scale up to have the best care for our patients and families the centre of our philosophy? Every step to bring comfort and peace at the end of life in the African situation is appreciated.

This is our challenge in Africa over the next 20 years. The way forward is hopeful but it will take a lot of dedication and attention to detail to reach even the poorest with modern palliative care.

ROLE OF MONITORING AND EVALUATION[17]

With palliative care having been provided for up to 25 years now in Africa there are rich resources being recorded. Every service now needs to measure outputs and needs in their own setting. Monitoring and evaluation is now part of all aspects of palliative care. Not only are papers becoming more frequent, tapping on the experiences to date, but also audit with computerized data has come to Uganda and other countries, which many can learn from. The African culture is much better at handling grief and bereavement than most of the developed world. There are many reasons for this but there are lessons to be learnt. There are also differences in metabolic handling of medications and tolerance to pain that need further research as well and research into the best and most economically acceptable ways to deliver quality palliative care. Africa is still trailing behind some countries in evaluation. However, effective auditing has begun and will continue …

Key learning points

- An accurate definition of palliative care is essential to maintain standards throughout Africa.

- Suffering from cancer, AIDS and other noncurable diseases is greater in Africa than anywhere in the world because of lack of resources.

- Palliative care using the researched methods of Dame Cicely Saunders, in Africa, is now affordable to the poorest with introduction of training, drug availability and government will.

- Africa has the greatest need of palliative care because of the HIV/AIDS epidemic and is meeting the challenge on the back of the epidemic.

- There has been rapid growth of palliative care in Africa since 1990. Monitoring and evaluation of this work to date can bring a wealth of experience to those just starting.

- Each country needs its own form of palliative care because of cultural, economic, and social needs which must be met at the end of life.

- Palliative care associations in Africa have a large part to play in setting standards, training, and advocacy.

- African governments need to ensure availability of affordable oral morphine and other medications to bring humanitarian relief in line with the human right of freedom from pain.

REFERENCES

1 Defilippi K, Downing J, Merriman A, Clark D. A palliative care association for the whole of Africa. *Palliat Med* 2004; **18**: 583–4.

2 van Nierkerk JP. Recollections in *The Hospice Movement in South Africa, a Brief History*. South Africa: Hospice Association of South Africa, December 2000: 1.

3 Merriman A. *Handbook of International Geriatric Medicine*. Singapore: PG Publishing, 1989: 182.

4 Merriman A. Living while dying. *Contact* October 1991: no 122, Christian Medical Commission, Geneva.

5 Stjernsward J. Uganda: initiating a government public health approach to pain relief and palliative care. *J Pain Symptom Manage* 2002; **24**: 257–64.

6 Livingstone H. Pain relief in the developing world: the experience of hospice Africa-Uganda. *J Pain Palliat Care Pharmacother* 2003; **17**: 107–18.

7 Ramsay S. Leading the way in African home-based palliative care. Free oral morphine has allowed expansion of model home-based palliative care in Uganda. *Lancet* 2003; **362**: 1812–13.

8 Jagwe JG, Barnard D. The introduction of palliative care in Uganda. *J Palliat Med* 2002; **5**: 160–3.

9 World Health Organization. *National Cancer Control Programmes: Policies and Managerial Guidelines*. Geneva: WHO, 1995.

10 Sepulveda C, Habiyambere V, Amandua J, *et al*. Quality care at the end of life in Africa. *BMJ* 2003; **327**: 209–13.

11 Olweny C, Sepulveda C, Merriman A, *et al*. Desirable services and guidelines for the treatment and palliative care of HIV disease patients with cancer in Africa: a World Health Organization consultation. *J Palliat Care* 2003; **19**: 198–205.

12 World Health Organization. *Achieving Balance in Narcotic Control*. Geneva: WHO, 2001. Ref. WHO/EDM/QSM/2000.4.

13 Logie DE, Harding R. An evaluation of a morphine public health programme for cancer and AIDS pain relief in Sub-Saharan Africa. *BMC Public Health* 2005; **5**: 82.

14 Rajagopal MR, Joranson D. A follow-up of 1723 patients treatment with oral morphine on outpatient home care basis for two years showed no incidence of misuse or diversion. *Lancet* 2001; **358**: 2001.

15 Kikule Ekiria. A good death in Uganda: survey of needs for palliative care for terminally ill people in urban areas. *BMJ* 2003; **327**: 192–4.

16 African Palliative Care Association. Constitution as at June 2004.

17 Harding R, Higginson IJ. Palliative care in sub-Saharan Africa. *Lancet* 2005; **365**: 1971–7.

6

The development of palliative medicine in Australia/New Zealand

J NORELLE LICKISS

INTRODUCTION

Australia is the outcome of an ongoing human conversation[1] which began over 60 000 years ago, incorporated Anglo-Saxon and Celtic elements from 1788 onwards, Chinese from mid-nineteenth century (the 'gold rush') and subsequently, especially from the mid-twentieth century onward, contributions from almost every part of the earth. Australians are all immigrants,[2] for even the first indigenous peoples came by boat from across the sea: some came willingly, others were forced to come (as convicts) – until the mid-nineteenth century, and, especially since the second world war, some came as refugees. So, people in Australia have been approaching death and caring for each other for over 60 000 years, in diverse ways. There has been sparse documentation of these matters, though a constant presence of death, if not dying, in Australian art and literature,[3] but there is increasing professional interest (Pollard B. Dr Fred Gunz and the First Five Years of the Palliative Care Association of New South Wales, unpublished manuscript).[4,5] Developments in palliative medicine and of palliative care in Australia in the last 30 years may be the fruits of disquiet, a little reminiscent of patterns articulated by Kuhn,[6] associated with paradigm shifts.

The care and concern for dying persons in the early years of British settlement in Sydney from 1788 onward was quite appalling: grave illness and deaths of convicts at sea during the long voyage from England, and soon after arrival, at what is now Sydney harbor, appeared to have been met with barbarity by today's standards.[7] Serious discrimination was manifest with respect to marginalized, indigent, and dying persons late in the nineteenth century,[8] yet subsequent medical history indicates a continual pattern involving concerned doctors of integrity and other humanitarians seeking to improve the health and welfare of the people.

The early Australian colonies were set up at a time of rapid secularization in Britain, and Kellehear records that during the first 100 years of European settlement Australians began to see their death as a failure of health and not a natural or divine outcome of life. Little is documented, however, about details of the care of the dying. Institutions for the care of the dying, and especially the dying poor, were established in the nineteenth century and early or mid-twentieth century by Christian organizations: Sacred Heart Hospice, Homes of Peace, and later Calvary Hospital in Sydney, Bethlehem Hospice in Victoria, and Mt Olivet Hospital in Brisbane, Queensland. These explicitly religious initiatives were complemented by the medical schools and teaching hospitals established in the mid-nineteenth century in Sydney and Melbourne: there is explicit mention of the concern for the poor in hospital documents.

John Rickard, writing at the time of the commemoration of 200 years of European settlement, wrote tellingly that[9]

a culture should be identified not so much by any sense of shared values, which may be artificially induced, as by the means it develops to reconcile or at least to accommodate the dissonant forces within it.

The multicultural conversation of Australia embodies not only ethnic diversity but many other forms of cultural difference, with patterns of emphasis in the conversation varying enormously across diverse places: metropolitan (inner, outer) regional, rural, desert ... and across the socio-economic spectrum. Cultural differences – and tensions – go far beyond customs surrounding death. Other matters need to be considered and respected; for example, patterns of interpersonal responsibility, modes of decision making and communication, caring styles, responses to loss/grieving, and bereavement customs. ... All but the indigenous people in Australia are in a sense 'displaced', with complex cultural roots and current cultural affiliations. English, although widely understood, is the second language (and not usually spoken at home) by over a third of population of major cities like Sydney.

Care of the other involves (at some period of life) most people past childhood (and even children in some circumstances): being human involves sociality, interpersonal bonds, social responsibilities. The philosophical basis of the duty of care is not law, or contract, but the call of the other.[10] People caring for each other (well or poorly) is, everywhere in Australia as elsewhere, the fundamental stratum of what has come to be known as palliative care. People with family or neighborhood bonds for one reason or another need assistance from others including, when available, health professionals. What has changed over the last 30 years in Australia is the nature, competence, and organization of the professional help available to support the family or neighborhood carers. Professional assistance with respect to palliative care in Australia is carried out by clinical staff within the whole healthcare system. The quality of such care depends enormously upon attitude, competence, and efficiency of staff involved as well as organizational factors. But there is no doubt that the burden (and privilege) of palliative care in Australia is dispersed very widely, and the whole population is increasingly in focus.[11]

The recently increased attention to improving care for those with progressive disease and approaching death, so apparent in the UK from the mid-twentieth century[12] and in the USA more recently[13] dates from the early 1970s in Australia. Several brief accounts exist of some aspects of the development of palliative care in Australia[14–16] with further major works in progress. But it is necessary to emphasize that many of the elements within the umbrella term 'palliative care' developed and remain principally outside specialist palliative care services (for example, oncology services, pain services/centers, bereavement services, palliative care within intensive care services, psychooncology, and so on): this trend is obvious in the two largest cities (Sydney and Melbourne) but is perceptible elsewhere. The history of the recent development of palliative care in Australia is truly the history of improvements within the whole health care system ... and the stirrings were obvious in the early 1970s, in widely separated parts of Australia, even though the term 'palliative care' was rarely used. The first national multidisciplinary palliative care meeting was held in Canberra in 1989, organized on behalf of the Medical Oncology Group of Australia (MOGA) by Dr Roger Woodruff of Melbourne. The 1-day meeting for the first time brought together doctors, nurses and allied health professionals to discuss the range of issues facing the emerging specialty of palliative care.[17]

Specialist palliative care services are now available in some form in most areas of Australia to assist, when requested, other clinical staff in various aspects of care.[18] The national (Commonwealth) government is explicitly involved, with inclusion of palliative care matters in policy and planning documents, and financial allocations, with devolution of responsibilities to the states for administration.[19] Palliative Care Australia, representing the palliative care associations (multidisciplinary) of each state, is in dialog with the national government on these matters, and has commissioned several valuable projects, including for example, a national census of palliative care services in 1998.[20] The National Health and Medical Research Council is investing targeted funds in both palliative care research and capacity building in palliative care nationally. This includes project grants for research, bursaries for postgraduate research studies and workshops on research. The national government has also produced a handbook on palliative care and the ethics of research. There has been a concerted effort to collect and make available all the completed but unpublished research and scoping that has been done in Australia since 1980 (www.caresearch.com.au). The Chapter of Palliative Medicine (within the Royal Australasian College of Physicians) has now over 200 Fellows (mostly Foundation Fellows) and around 15 supervised trainees. There has been explicit interest in provision of palliative care for children (especially in New South Wales [NSW]), and a recent major document[21] is part of a national strategy to improve all aspects of nursing home care.

Palliative medicine is part of the curriculum for medical schools throughout Australia although patterns of education vary and documentation is scanty. Postgraduate education in palliative medicine, and clinical training for skills enhancement or for progression to specialist status are now available in most states, again, with varying patterns of training and emphases, reflecting local factors. A national curriculum for palliative care in all health sciences is under consideration.

There are major differences between the states with respect to many indices – from ethnicity, to economic status, and to prevailing ethos. Much is related to geographical factors and population levels, but historical factors still have much influence.

NEW SOUTH WALES

In the early 1970s in NSW and Tasmania (historically closely related to Sydney), two academic hematologists, Fred Gunz in Sydney, then Director of the Kanamatsu Research Institute Sydney Hospital, and Albert Baikie,

Foundation Professor of Medicine, University of Tasmania 1967–75, previously in University of Melbourne and originally from Glasgow, co-authors of a major text on leukemia, urged that improvement needed to occur in the care of patients with progressive disease approaching death. These two eminent men were influential as well as innovative: Gunz laid the groundwork for palliative care service development in NSW (Pollard B. Dr Fred Gunz and the First Five Years of the Palliative Care Association of New South Wales, unpublished manuscript).[22] Anesthetists in Sydney – Dwyer (St Vincent's Hospital), Pollard (Concord Repatriation General Hospital), and Laird, internist (Royal Prince Alfred Hospital) – were instrumental in setting up palliative care services in the three teaching hospitals in Sydney by 1982 (around the time of an influential visit by Balfour Mount of Canada). In the mid-1980s decisions were made under the guidance of senior clinicians to restructure the service at Royal Prince Alfred Hospital: a steady evolution of the palliative care service was facilitated.[23]

From the late 1980s there was a focus in Sydney on clinical training for doctors especially through the Sydney Institute of Palliative Medicine (SIPM), based in Royal Prince Alfred Hospital (University of Sydney) and Prince of Wales Hospital (University of New South Wales), with their associated community services and inpatient units. Three domains of clinical experience were available for trainee posts: community, inpatient beds, and hospital consultancies.[24] The concept of these elements under one administration was adopted as the service model for NSW Area-based Palliative Care Services. The NSW Palliative Care Association, NSW Society of Palliative Medicine and the Sydney Institute of Palliative Medicine have continued to be active in education, planning and support for specialist palliative care services, and increasingly in cognate research involving major public funding.

Collaborative research (some with international links) is in progress in areas such as prognosis, care of patients with cardiac failure and communication, in addition to more traditional areas of inquiry. Postgraduates training in internal medicine (Royal Australian College of Physicians [RACP]) commonly undertake 3–6-month terms in clinical palliative medicine as part of their preparation for the RACP examination preceding various strands of advanced training: over 200 registrars (including British registrars) have occupied SIPM posts, either for skills enhancement or for specialist training. Many of the latter were examined by Geoffrey Hanks (UK), who served as external examiner to SIPM for nearly two decades. Particular emphasis in Sydney has been given to the need for recognition of the need for improvements in palliative care in acute hospitals.[25] The recent emergence of doctorate candidates marks a new phase in the development of academic palliative medicine in NSW.

Over the past 15 years in NSW, the University of Sydney and University of NSW fostered the development of medicine not by establishing university-funded chairs, but by conferring professorial status on senior clinicians. The University of Newcastle established a Chair in the 1980s and this has been crucial in the development of a cohesive palliative care service in the Hunter River region of NSW. Undergraduate medical education in palliative medicine within University of Sydney, University of NSW, and University of Newcastle has been undertaken for over a decade, with increasing formalization over time.

The situation in NSW continues to be challenging not only in the complex cities such as Sydney but also in the sparsely populated rural areas: staff (especially nurses) capable of adapting ideas and practices to the local situations are the sturdy backbone of palliative care in such circumstances, but inequities of resource levels in NSW and adequate provision for professional education and training need urgent attention.

VICTORIA

In Victoria several recent landmark events and strands of activity are noteworthy, building on the efforts of the period prior to 1970. Details of the impressive development of specialist palliative care services in Victoria, which have been largely community based, have been detailed by Redpath, one of the key figures in the whole process.[16] It is noteworthy that an inquiry into issues related to dying with dignity, held in Victoria in 1987[26] gave added impetus to coordinated improvements in palliative care, and led to law which enshrined the right to refuse treatment.

In the late 1970s the first community-based palliative care service, delivering specialist palliative care in patients' own homes was set up by City Mission. A nurse-led palliative care service was established at the Repatriation Hospital in 1988, closely followed in 1989 by the first multidisciplinary hospital-based palliative care service, established at the Austin Hospital.[27]

The University of Melbourne introduced a postgraduate diploma in 1996 and established a chair in palliative medicine. Elsewhere in Melbourne in the 1990s, chairs were also established in Monash and Latrobe University. Melbourne-based academic nurses have also been active in research regarding palliative care – with chairs established relevant to palliative care. Medical education with respect to palliative medicine and palliative care has been well documented by Melbourne-based clinicians.[28]

Palliative care services are well established in the Melbourne teaching hospitals, including the largest cancer center. Melbourne has centralized radiotherapy services in the Peter MacCallum Hospital, and therefore also a tendency to centralization of other aspects of oncology. The first steps were taken in 1980 by Dr Walter Moon who set up a pain clinic for inpatients and outpatients at the Peter MacCallum Hospital, reflecting again the growing concern in Australia during the period 1975–80, to improve seriously neglected dimensions of care. A senior radiotherapist, Dr Ruth Redpath, undertook extensive community consultations, and encouraged the development of community palliative care in Melbourne and elsewhere in Victoria. Peter MacCallum Cancer Centre (as it is now known), a teaching hospital of the University of Melbourne, has currently a significant multidisciplinary palliative care department with consultative responsibilities within the hospital as well as educational activities (undergraduates, including a 1 week full time attachment, and post graduates), with a special interest in psychooncology, and research programs (including PhD programs) in association with the University of Melbourne.

QUEENSLAND

Queensland is a state with one major city, Brisbane (the capital) several smaller cities, and a large hinterland. Administration is largely concentrated in Brisbane. Mt Olivet, Brisbane, a Catholic institution administered by the Sisters of Charity (like St Vincent's Sydney and St Vincent's Melbourne), was established in the mid-twentieth century (1957), but planned for the preceding 20 years. It was the result of a collaboration of two surgeons, a benefactor, the government and the vision of the Sisters of Charity. It was for many years the only recognized provider of palliative care services in Queensland, and a major contributor to the introduction of contemporary ideas of palliative care into the Queensland scene. Throughout the period of rapid development of palliative care services in several parts of Queensland in 1990s, Mt Olivet has remained a major provider of specialist services, with a 28-bed inpatient unit and formal home care service, and an active focus for education of doctors, especially general practitioners.

In 1992 the Queensland Cancer Fund, a charity, funded the establishment of a palliative care service in Mater Hospital, a teaching hospital of the University of Queensland, and also a service in Townsville, a northern Queensland city. The Queensland Health Department soon followed this initiative, establishing many other services in the south east of Queensland. Another teaching hospital in Brisbane (Prince Charles Hospital) was the site for a 16-bed unit, and provision was made for several other hospital-based inpatient palliative care units. In the city of Ipswich, not far from Brisbane, half of the cost of the establishment of the local hospice is funded by the local meat works – an unusual pattern of collaboration in any area of healthcare in Australia. Palliative care throughout the areas of Queensland distant from major centers continues to be the responsibility of the mainstream health services, assisted where feasible, by the small number of personnel within specialist services.

In Australia, the major teaching hospitals are public (government funded), but private hospitals play an important role in the care of patients with private insurance. In Queensland (as in several other states) the private sector has also established palliative care consultancies at several hospitals. This trend may be expected to strengthen in Australia in the next decade, especially if the concept of mixed management or parallel care becomes more widespread.

Multidisciplinary research in Queensland related to palliative care has been impressive over the last decade reflecting a wide range of interests, including ethical, social and spiritual matters. The University of Queensland has recently (2003) appointed a Professor of Palliative Care based in the Mater Hospital Brisbane, an encouragement to the Brisbane-based Centre for Palliative Care Research and Education.

SOUTH AUSTRALIA

South Australia, especially through the work and encouragement of Ian Maddocks, and more recently his successor, David Currow, has contributed significantly to the development of specialist palliative care services in Australia. Urban Adelaide lends itself to a logical and orderly development of hospital and associated community services (guided by wise leaders), and undergraduate medical education was given due emphasis. Distance learning, organized as a masters program, based in the International Institute of Hospice Studies, has assisted many professionals in Australia and elsewhere to enhance their skills and move into the practice of palliative care. Useful population-based studies, as well as institution-based studies have broadened the focus of studies of palliative care needs. It is noteworthy also that in South Australia, as in other Australian states, leading oncologists contribute significantly to support and investigation of issues relevant to palliative care. There was early recognition of the needs of patients with conditions other than cancer, notably cardiac and neurological conditions.

South Australia contributed significantly to developments in the legal situation. In South Australia, 'Do Not Resuscitate' orders are usually not written, rather, documentation for 'Good Palliative Care' is the norm in appropriate circumstances and the practice is currently under review.

WESTERN AUSTRALIA

In Western Australia, a state with the population much concentrated in the capital Perth, nurses played a crucial role in the development of specialist palliative care services. In the late 1970s oncology nurses at the Royal Perth Hospital were instrumental in arranging for Dame Cicely Saunders to give a lecture in Perth, and this proved a catalyst. Joy Brand, a nurse in an academic position, Rosalie Shaw (a medical graduate who had also been a nurse) and Douglas Macadam (the first medical director of the community-based Silver Chain Nursing service) were highly significant in those crucial years around 1980. The Cancer Council of Western Australia supported the community-based developments. Other influential doctors and nurses were supportive, and the specialist palliative care services in Perth developed in an orderly and comprehensive manner, with later involvement of the major acute hospitals. In the 1980s, Hollywood, a Veterans hospital, developed under the direction of Rosalie Shaw, an inpatient palliative care unit with significant influence on undergraduate medical education. Dr Shaw subsequently was invited to Singapore to assist in the development of palliative care services in that city and subsequently became Executive Director of the Asian Pacific Hospice and Palliative Care Network.

In the 1990s, the appointment of a nurse researcher Linda Kristjanson as Professor of Palliative Care at Edith Cowan University, led to Perth becoming a significant Australian focus for research activities and for leading impressive projects for improving practice (for example, the recently launched guidelines for palliative care for older people in residential care).[21]

TASMANIA

Tasmania, the smallest state, has a history intimately connected with Sydney. Hobart, the capital, prides itself on having a branch of the Royal Society (the first outside London). A medical school was planned for Hobart in 1854, to be of 3 years' duration with lectures in anatomy, chemistry, and the natural sciences as well as Latin and French, English, and History. There had already been apprentices trained by surgeons in Hobart since 1826. The plan for a medical school was abandoned (because the UK Royal Colleges insisted on 100, instead of the readily available 30, inpatients to be available for teaching). Palliative medicine had no place in training then, despite the prevailing high mortality in the Australian colonies. But in 1974 the University of Tasmania, under the guidance of Professor Albert Baikie, was the first Australian medical school to introduce teaching in clinical palliative medicine (called then 'clinical aspects of the care of the dying') as part of clinical studies (with relevant examination questions), with some joint teaching of medical and nursing students. The teaching of clinical ethics in the University of Tasmania undergraduate curriculum in the 1970s frequently included matter (in case-based format) directly related to palliative care.

The cancer services of Tasmania, developed under the guidance of Baikie, from 1967 until his untimely death in 1975, were, from the beginning, comprehensive, patient-centered, and explicitly multidisciplinary. Although the word 'palliative care' was not used, the elements of palliative care were embedded in the mainstream cancer services. Other clinical services were also deliberately comprehensive, encouraged by and supported by the conjunction of academic clinical staff with private specialists and general practitioners, as well as health administrators.

Collaboration between clinicians, government and the community has been significant in the further development of specialist palliative care services in Tasmania. As in

Queensland, a benefactor was also helpful, but consistent community interest reflects the value system of the island state. Service reviews by independent persons have served to guide the services toward sustainability as well as quality. Gradually, a well-resourced statewide specialist palliative care service evolved, with excellent facilities, multidisciplinary service provision in all areas – city and rural areas – with presence in all hospitals, excellent inpatient units, and availability of consultants to nursing homes, as well as organized home care service provision.

AUSTRALIAN CAPITAL TERRITORY AND NORTHERN TERRITORY

The territories of Australia – the Australian Capital Territory (Canberra) and the Northern Territory – have diverse histories with respect to the evolution of palliative care service. Nurses have for many years been crucial in caring for patients at home in both regions. Palliative medicine provision (in the form of palliative medicine specialists) commenced in Canberra in the early 1990s and more recently in Darwin/Northern Territory.

In Canberra, the palliative care service is well developed with a comprehensive community service and a purpose-built hospice. The oncology departments of the Canberra Hospital have strongly supported action and research regarding the care of patients with advanced disease.

The heated debate in the mid-1990s and short-lived legislation permitting euthanasia in the Northern Territory accelerated the development of specialist services in that territory. Darwin, the only city in the Northern Territory (total population 200 000), became a world center of interest in 1995 with the passage of the first legislation in the world to permit euthanasia. The Rights of the Terminally Ill Act (ROTI) was passed into law in late 1995 and was accompanied by a Bill to increase palliative care funding in the Northern Territory from about Aus\$100 000 to close to 1 million dollars per annum. The ROTI Bill was revoked by the Federal Parliament in 1997 amid much controversy over the intrusion of the Australian Government into Territory affairs: the status of the area as a Territory (not a state) had legal implications. There were seven euthanasia deaths recorded in the time the law was in place[29] and there were also clinical problems associated with the Act.[30]

A specialist palliative care program was commenced in 1989 with the appointment of two palliative care nurses working within the community nursing network. A voluntary board of interested stakeholders was established and continued to function with oversight of the program. Two palliative care teams were established in the Northern Territory, one in Darwin covering the 'top end' (population about 150 000) and one in Alice Springs (population about 50 000) but recruitment of doctors with expertise in palliative medicine proved difficult. An inpatient unit (hospice) was opened in 2005.

The rural and remote area of the Northern Territory encompasses some 200 aboriginal communities, many of which had their own language. The aboriginal communities account for between 25 percent and 30 percent of the total Northern Territory population, with the acute hospital population being up to 65 percent aboriginal. An aboriginal health worker position was created in 1998 (the first in palliative care in Australia), which enhanced the effectiveness of palliative care in the rural and remote aboriginal communities and eventually led to the development of an 'indigenous palliative care model' based on research funded by the National Health and Medical Research Council.

Documentation (even complete) of landmark events is not history. The history of the development of palliative medicine (to be a little more focused) in Australia is above all a history of ideas, and of their expression in diverse contexts. We know something of the values, dreams, courage, and tenacity of the colonial doctors who upheld (on the whole) the best traditions of Western medicine and contributed richly to the transformation of fairly chaotic colonies into modern communities – they had their counterparts elsewhere. We know little of the intellectual constructs, the ideas, the views of the indigenous people prior to European settlement, but we have a rich legacy of art, dance, bush craft, and stories. Proust, in his remarkable compendium of some of the material relating to the history of medicine in Australia,[31] documents some of what is known about aboriginal traditional medicine – ideas about causation of serious disease, the role of traditional healers (combining role of priest and physician). Blackwell[32] recounts that there is little aboriginal literature concerning death and dying, reflecting the importance and secrecy attached to death and dying, but papers by experienced palliative medicine practitioners are appearing.[33,34] Indigenous doctors, now numerous in Australia, with a professorial appointment in University of Melbourne, may assist in articulating and clarifying some of the rich ideas about dying – as well as living – which have flourished in indigenous communities – despite (or possibly because of) their profound experience of loss and grief over the last two centuries and continuing high mortality in some sectors of indigenous life in Australia.

For the rest, Manning Clark, historian, author of a six-volume history of Australia, considered that there were 'three different visions of God and man which Australians bought to the conversation which is Australia: Catholic Christendom, Protestant Christianity and the Enlightenment'.[35] A quarter of a century later he would have to make explicit mention of Buddhism (the fastest growing religion in Australia), and the many other ethnic and spiritual traditions long present in persons and institutions such as Judaism, Bahai, Islam, and the increasing strength of secular expressions of values (and of spiritual matters). Philosophical trends in Australia are not only heirs (or traces) of the Enlightenment: the conversation is very complex, the interplay of ideas vigorous, and both the shape and the content of the discussion vary markedly across the continent, and

within regions. Grand narratives from traditional cultures, and from communities from which Australians come, do not always appear to hold. Ideas are welcomed but tested and accepted or rejected or modified, on the whole courteously, but without grace or favor with respect to their origin.

WHAT DOES THIS MEAN FOR PALLIATIVE CARE?

The British hospice movement, especially embodied in Dame Cicely Saunders, has had profound influence in many parts of the world – and Australia is no exception. Several of the individuals who were influential during the 1970s and 1980s in raising the profile of the care of patients with incurable and especially progressive disease, and particularly when approaching death, had some personal contact with St Christopher's Hospice, London, and often with Dame Cicely in person. Ideas of St Christopher's found fertile soil in which to flourish, soil prepared by men such as Gunz and Baikie, influenced by other strands of thought and experience. Further, the way ideas took root in Australia was influenced subsequently by persons appointed to responsible positions – by their personality, background, medical discipline, resource levels and the environment in which they encountered their patients. Community care patterns are obviously closely influenced by local circumstances, but even the shape of clinical practice in hospitals differs from hospital to hospital, even within one state, as trainees in palliative medicine testify. Diversity in thought and practice is a hallmark of Australian life and the medical environment.

Some of the ideas held to be central by the UK hospice movement have been modified in some parts of Australia: for example, conditions from which patients suffer (with acquired immune deficiency syndrome [AIDS] patients readily seen in consultations and admitted if necessary to palliative care units), the contexts in which patients are seen, the acceptance of episodic involvement and of parallel care, the acceptance of mainstreaming of palliative care, the pattern of funding (government not charity), the concept of team (with specialists in palliative care being members of several teams), the secular basis of service (rather than religious), even the apparently compromising concept of a 'good enough death'.[36]

Documentation is available concerning the processes involved in specialist palliative medicine consultancy and palliative care services in several contexts – community, inpatient units, hospitals. However, outcome evaluation is not extensive – and will become less so in the future as (requested) input of specialist palliative care personnel (singly or as a team) becomes simply part of the common mainstream healthcare effort. The quality of palliative care as a whole may be measurable (best by its recipients), rather than the input of distinct services such as oncology services, specialist palliative care services, bereavement services, pain services, psychooncology services, etc. The whole is more important than any part.

Have the original ideas of the British hospice movement been betrayed? Or are we seeing the fruits Dame Cecily dreamed of – the incorporation of the core (not peripheral) ideas of palliative care into mainstream, public funded healthcare? These core (not peripheral) ideas are surely:

- Respect for the individuality and the uniqueness of each person.
- Recognition of the significance of the last phase of life – and the value of an individual usually knowing of his or her existential situation.
- The acceptance of the value of the weak in society – and the recognition that a society can be judged by its care of the most vulnerable.
- The understanding of the contribution of essential persons of different professional backgrounds, as well as family, friends, (all only as needed) in improving the quality of life of very ill persons – but with respect for the privacy of individuals and their places of care or residence.

Many in Australia, including this author, would not agree that palliative care should be considered as a social movement[37] but these core ideas are not contested.

WHAT OF THE FUTURE?

The problems of the present are, mainly, those of mismatch, the failure of resources to match inevitably increasing, legitimate needs as the population ages (with rising cancer rates, and multiple morbidity becoming more common), and as anti-disease therapies which control disease (but do not cure) may prolong the time span of serious illness, and morbidity. Increasing competence in palliative care of professionals outside specialist palliative care services may reduce the pressure on the latter by 'heightening the bar', raising the threshold at which personnel from a specialist palliative care service are needed. It is true, however, that the more professionals learn about palliative care, the more they become aware of needs of patients and families previously not noted or given little attention, and the possibilities for improvements in care. If this is true, there may be increased call for specialists in aspects of palliative care – medicine, nursing, or social work to assist with specific matters – and a high level of competence would be expected. Or will specialist palliative care services in Australia become unnecessary if skills enhancement of all other clinicians proceed? Probably not: rather, strengthening and expansion is planned and government support appears firm.

Will specialist palliative medicine survive in its present form in Australia? This is more worthy of discussion. The ratio of palliative medicine specialists to oncologists in Australia is less than 20 percent and a similar ratio applies to

trainees following the program of the RACP Chapter of Palliative Medicine. Many oncologists, without specific training in palliative medicine but with increasing expertise, do explicitly undertake palliative care for hospitalized and ambulant patients as part of their responsibilities. In view of the large numbers of oncologists in Australia, this trend may increase with respect to patients with cancer. Or it may be that consultant physicians (internists) wishing to practice palliative medicine especially in hospitals will undertake training in oncology and include a significant period in palliative medicine as the optional (elective) section of advanced training. Or palliative medicine consultants (and even palliative care services) may focus more in the problems of patients with diseases other than cancer, leaving palliative care with respect to patients with cancer more and more in the hands of oncologists. This would, however, also require structural and administrative changes with respect to some aspects of care (notably with respect to community services), and to training programs (in oncology as well as palliative medicine).

Resource allocation will be a critical factor. The current clinical caseload of most palliative medicine consultants and specialists mitigates against a flourishing academic activity of appropriate physicians, although several are courageously undertaking significant research. Financial incentives for research in palliative care related matters are plentiful now, but personnel to grasp the opportunities are relatively few. Experienced formally trained palliative medicine consultants or specialists with academic ability, are to be seen to be moving into fields removed somewhat from the clinical scene of one-to-one medicine for a large part of their time. But palliative medicine is primarily a highly personalized, indeed intersubjective activity. The tendency to objectification of the patients, and the blurring of individual differences even for research or planning purposes, needs careful scrutiny… or there may be a new wave of protest (as well as sadness).

Ethical issues (hopefully not medicolegal issues) will always be part of the stuff of palliative care; and there is a case for more rigor in training in clinical ethics. Palliative medicine specialists are, in general, aware of manifold ethical dimensions of everyday practice and seek to exercise clinical wisdom. End-of-life care is, everywhere, ethically complex – for the folding up of life is as complex as the living of it.

Public debate concerning euthanasia (at its height in the mid-1990s) is not a major feature of the Australian conversation in the early twenty-first century. However, disquiet concerning the quality of care, especially the elderly and about decisions made concerning end-of-life care, do surface from time to time in the media, and much more frequently in private conversations. There is well-based fear not of euthanasia but of life being prolonged (especially in hospitals) beyond the patient's wishes, and advance directives, though promoted now in primary care and by some geriatricians, are not in common use in hospital practice. It appears that despite excellent Australian writing on this theme[38] a balance has not yet been struck at least in some large metropolitan hospitals between a passion to affirm life – 'save' life where possible by all means possible – and a commitment not to obstruct death, but rather to care competently and comfort the patient and significant others as the end of life draws near. There is much to learn and to do, especially in hospitals, and hopefully palliative care services will have a role as agents of change.

NEW ZEALAND

New Zealand is a cohesive nation (population 3.8 million) with a longstanding interest in medical issues of community significance. The steps leading to the present situation are outlined by MacLeod.[39]

The first (inpatient) hospice in New Zealand, Mary Potter Hospice in Wellington, was opened in 1979, closely followed by Te Omanga Hospice and St Joseph's Mercy Hospice in Auckland. Little has been published concerning the climate of ideas and debate which preceded and undoubtedly prompted the foundation of these institutions, mainly Christian in inspiration. New Zealand has two major ethnic configurations: the indigenous Maori population and Anglo/Saxon/Celtic New Zealanders. The marked ethnic diversity of Australia (especially its large cities) is far less obvious in New Zealand.

Palliative medicine teaching has been limited in medical schools in New Zealand, but there is a well established liaison between the Mary Potter Hospice and the University. A Chair in Palliative Care was established at the Dunedin School of Medicine within the University of Otago in 2003. A national strategy for New Zealand is now in place, with now 37 hospice and around 40 palliative care services set up throughout the country.

The Australia and New Zealand Society for Palliative Medicine has been supportive of the development of palliative medicine in New Zealand. There is support for specialist palliative care from the community and from government, but it is clear that leadership given by a small group of influential clinicians, has – as in Australia – been crucial. There are 25 fellows of the Chapter of Palliative Medicine within the Royal Australasian College of Physicians. These influential senior clinicians in New Zealand have given particular attention to several matters relevant to specialist palliative care: for example, palliative care of patients with neurological disease and the psychiatric dimensions of palliative care.

The differences between Australia and New Zealand are predictable once the vast differences in size, distances between population centers, and patterns of migration and resultant cultural mix as well as political nuances are kept in mind. There has been excellent cooperation between the two countries to ensure that different emphases, attitudes, problems, and possibilities are articulated and understood, with the contribution of each contributing to the improved care of the people … the endpoint surely of all common endeavor.

CONCLUSION

Palliative medicine, as a component of palliative care, is a privilege, sometimes burdensome, sometimes painful, but a privilege nevertheless. If a society can be judged by its care of the weak – and palliative medicine attends to humankind in weakness – palliative medicine, far from being marginal, may be at the heart of the discipline and practice of medicine. There is much to be improved in the care of the dying 'down under'[40] and the whole community everywhere must be involved … but this task may make or remake Australia as it struggles for its soul.

Key learning points

- Australia is an ancient land, with humans caring for each other for over 60 000 years, but with dramatic changes in modes of life and death since the British settlement in the 1790s, and with increasing ethnic and cultural diversity.

- Recent developments in palliative care in Australia reflected Christian influences in the late nineteenth century and early twentieth century (first hospices), supplemented in the late twentieth century (from the 1970s) by broad humanitarian leadership given by leading academics and clinicians.

- It is accepted that palliative care is not a charity-funded optional extra, but part of mainstream care. Governments, national and state, have since the late 1980s given firm support concerning the need for specialist palliative care services and/or professionals to be available to improve palliative care given through the healthcare system, but deficiencies remain, despite extensive efforts. Palliative Care Australia monitors and coordinates many programs and projects.

- New Zealand is a more cohesive nation, with less cultural diversity than Australia, and progress has been steady.

- Outcome measures with regard to the quality of care as a whole remain inadequate, and despite current initiatives the care of institutionalized older people in the last phase of life needs much improvement.

- Research in various aspects of palliative care is being fostered by government.

ACKNOWLEDGMENTS

The assistance of colleagues in various parts of Australia is gratefully acknowledged, notably, David Currow (South Australia), Paul Dunne (Tasmania), Judi Greaves (Western Australia), Rod Macleod (New Zealand), Brian Pollard

(New South Wales), Robert Raynor (Northern Territory), Odette Spruyt and Roger Woodruff (Victoria), Bruce Stafford and Patricia Treston (Queensland).

REFERENCES

1 Thornhill J. *Making Australia. Exploring our National Conversation.* Newtown: Millennium Books, 1992.

2 Jupp J, ed. *The Australian People*, 2nd ed. Cambridge: Cambridge University Press, 2001.

3 Kellehear A. The changing face of dying in Australia. *Med J Aust* 2001; **175**: 508–10.

4 Kellehear A, ed. *Death and Dying in Australia.* Oxford: Oxford University Press, 2000.

5 Lewis MJ. *Medicine and the Care of the Dying: A Modern History.* New York: Oxford University Press, 2006.

6 Kuhn T. *The Structure of Scientific Revolutions.* Chicago: University of Chicago Press, 1962.

7 Flannery T. *The Birth of Sydney.* Melbourne: Text Publishing, 1999: 100.

8 Evans R. The hidden colonists: deviance and social control in colonial Queensland. In: Roe J, ed. *Social Policy in Australia, Some Perspectives 1901–1975.* Australia: Cassel, 1976: 74–100.

9 Rickard J. Quoted in Thornhill J. *Making Australia: Exploring Our National Conversation.* Newtown: Millennium Books, 1992: 8.

10 Manderson D. Unpublished lecture. Tenth Annual Symposium, Sydney Institute of Palliative Medicine, Sydney, March 2001.

11 Currow DC, Abernethy AP, Fazekas BS. Specialist palliative care needs of whole populations: a feasibility study using a novel approach. *Palliat Med* 2004; **18**: 239–47.

12 Clark D. Cradled to the grave? Terminal care in the United Kingdom, 1948–67. *Mortality* 1999; **4**: 225–47.

13 Field MJ, Cassel CK, eds. *Approaching Death: Improving Care at the End of Life.* Washington DC: National Academy Press, 1997.

14 Lickiss JN. Australia: status of cancer pain and palliative care. *J Pain Symptom Manage* 1993; **8**: 388–94.

15 Currow D. Australia: state of palliative service provision 2002. *J Pain Symptom Manage* 2002; **24**: 170–2.

16 Redpath R. Palliative care in Australia. In: Ramadge J, Aranda S, eds. *Australian Nursing Practice and Palliative Care: Its Origins, Evolution and Future.* Deakin: Royal College of Nursing Australia. Professional Development Series No. 9. 1–16.

17 Woodruff RK, ed. Palliative care for the 1990s. Proceedings of a multidisciplinary meeting conducted by the Medical Oncology Group of Australia, April 1989, Asperula, Melbourne, 1989.

18 Currow DC, Nightingale EM. 'A planning guide': developing a consensus document for palliative care service provision. *Med J Aust* 2003; **179**: S23–S25.

19 The National Palliative Care Program. www.palliativecare.gov.au (accessed October 6, 2005).

20 Palliative Care Australia. *Reporting a National Census of Palliative Care Service, 1998.* Canberra: Palliative Care Australia, 1999.

21 Australian Government Department of Health and Ageing. *Guidelines for a Palliative Approach in Residential Aged Care.* Canberra: Rural Health and Palliative Care Branch, Australian Government Department of Health and Ageing, 2004.

22 Gunz FW. What next in the care of the dying patient with cancer? *Med J Aust* 1987; **147**: 2–3.

23 Lickiss JN, Glare PA, Turner K, *et al.* Palliative care in Central Sydney: The Royal Prince Alfred Hospital as catalyst and integrator. *J Palliat Care* 1993; **9**: 33–42.

24 Turner K, Lickiss JN. Postgraduate training in palliative medicine: the experience of the Sydney Institute of Palliative Medicine. *Palliat Med* 1997; **11**: 389–94.

25 Glare P, Auret KA, Aggarwal G, *et al.* The interface between palliative medicine and specialists in acute-care hospitals: boundaries, bridges and challenges. *Med J Aust* 2003; **179**: S29–S31.

26 Parliament of Victoria. Social Development Committee 1987. Inquiry into options for dying with dignity report, second and final report. Melbourne: Parliament of Victoria.

27 Chan A, Woodruff RK. Palliative care in a general teaching hospital. 1 Assessment of Needs. *Med J Aust* 1991; **155**: 597–9.

28 Buchanan J, Millership R, Zalcberg J, *et al.* Medical education in palliative care. *Med J Aust* 1990; **152**: 27–9.

29 Kissane DW, Street A, Nitschke P. Seven deaths in Darwin: case studies under the Rights of the Terminally Ill Act, Northern Territory, Australia. *Lancet* 1998; **352**: 1097–102.

30 Street A, Kissane DW. Dispensing death, desiring death: an exploration of medical roles and patient motivation during the period of legalized euthanasia in Australia. *J Death Dying* 1999–2000; **40**: 231–48.

31 Proust AJ. A companion of the history of medicine in Australia 1788–1939. Canberra: A J Proust, 2003.

32 Blackwell N. Cultural issues in indigenous Australian peoples. In: Doyle D, Hanks GW, MacDonald N, eds. *Oxford Textbook of Palliative Medicine*, 2nd ed. Oxford: Oxford University Press, 1998: 799–801.

33 Fried O. Providing palliative care for Aboriginal patients. *Aust Fam Physician* 2000; **29**: 1035–8.

34 Maddocks I, Raynor RG. Issues in palliative care for indigenous communities. *Med J Aust* 2003; **179**: S17–S19.

35 Clark M. Quoted in Thornhill J. *Making Australia: Exploring Our National Conversation.* Newtown: Millennium Books, 1992: 9.

36 McNamara B. Good enough death: autonomy and choice in Australian palliative care. *Soc Sci Med* 2004; **58**: 929–38.

37 Elsey B. Hospice and palliative care a new social movement: a case illustration from South Australia. *J Palliat Care* 1998; **14**: 38–46.

38 Fisher MM, Raper RF. Withdrawing and withholding treatment in intensive care. Part 1. Social and ethical dimensions. *Med J Aust* 1990; **153**: 217–20.

39 MacLeod R. A national strategy for palliative care in New Zealand. *J Palliat Med* 2001; **4**: 70–4.

40 Hardy JR, Vora R. A good death down under. *Intern Med J* 2004; **34**: 450.

7

The development of palliative medicine in Asia

ROSALIE SHAW

INTRODUCTION

The development of palliative care in Asia has been hampered by poverty, lack of resources, the need to address more urgent healthcare needs, issues relating to the availability of opioids, and the unwillingness in many cultures to discuss issues surrounding death and dying. Asia covers about a third of the world's land mass and three-fifths of the world population. The eastern and southern part of this vast continent and the islands to the east of its coastal boundaries can be subdivided into three regions:

- East Asia – China, including Hong Kong, Taiwan, Mongolia, Korea, and Japan
- Southeast Asia – Myanmar, Thailand, Cambodia, Laos, Vietnam, Malaysia, Brunei, Singapore, Indonesia, and the Philippines
- South Asia – India, Pakistan, Bangladesh, Sri Lanka, Nepal, and Bhutan.

Within this region there is great diversity of race, language, religion, and culture as well as economic and political systems. Many countries are grappling with ways to provide basic healthcare in rapidly expanding and congested cities, as well as in isolated rural areas where infant and maternal death rates are high. Infectious disease is still a major cause of illness, and the incidence of cancer is rising. Healthcare staff, especially nurses, often have relatively poor status and very poor remuneration.[1] In most countries, traditional medicines are widely used, either instead of or concurrently with Western medicine.

There is wide variation in the level of development of palliative care services. In some countries (Japan, Taiwan, Hong Kong, and Singapore) services are relatively well developed with trained professional staff and with part or full government funding. However, in many countries, dedicated and committed individuals are struggling to establish credibility and to find resources for hospital-based and home care programs. The following sections review the development in different parts of Asia.

EAST ASIA

Korea

In East Asia the concept of hospice was introduced as early as 1965 when an order of Catholic nuns opened a clinic in Seoul in South Korea.[2] However, following 1982 when hospice services were started by Dr Kyung-Shik Lee at Kangnam St Mary's Hospital, expansion was gradual until a World Health Organization Collaborating Centre for Hospice Palliative Care was established in 1995 at the Catholic University of Korea, College of Nursing. This center has had an important role in the training of professional hospice nurses. By 1996, 90 percent of nursing colleges were teaching hospice palliative care.[3]

There are now more than 100 hospice programs in South Korea. Of these about 37 percent are nongovernmental organizations and 31 percent are in university hospitals. However, few doctors wish to train in the area of palliative medicine, which is not yet recognized as a medical specialty. Although slow-release preparations of morphine are available at government hospitals, there are still no oral immediate-release preparations of morphine available for titration or for the management of breakthrough pain.

Three umbrella hospice organizations have been important in raising public and professional awareness: the Korean Hospice Association (established in 1991), the Korean

Catholic Hospice Association (1992) and the Korean Society for Hospice and Palliative Care (1998). The sixth Asia Pacific Hospice Conference in March 2005 hosted by the Korean Society for Hospice and Palliative Care with 1200 local and international participants gave an impetus to the development of palliative medicine and will further advocacy for palliative care to be eligible for National Health Insurance funding in Korea. A 2-year pilot project was initiated by the government in 2003 to decide on a model of palliative care suitable for Korea so that national policies can be formulated.

Japan

Palliative care was brought to Japan in 1973 when Dr Tetsuo Kashiwagi returned from psychiatry training in the USA and set up an Organized Care of the Dying Patient (OCDP) team at the Yodogawa Christian Hospital, Osaka. Eleven years later a 23-bed inpatient hospice ward was opened at that hospital. By then the first inpatient hospice had been set up 3 years earlier at Serai Mikatabara General Hospital in Hamamatsu, in Shizuoka Prefecture. The first independent freestanding hospice, the Peace House Hospice, was opened in 1993 in Kanagawa Prefecture.

A landmark in the development of hospices in Japan was the publication in 1989 of a report on care of the dying patient by the Ministry of Health. This report resulted in National Health Insurance funding for accredited palliative care units from 1990. At that time there were only three hospices and one palliative care center in Japan. By the end of 2004 there were 131 government-approved hospice and palliative care units with 2449 beds. However, despite this rapid development, it is estimated that only 4.4 percent of cancer deaths occur in palliative care settings (inpatient or at home). In 2000 only 2.3 percent of patients being cared for by palliative care services died at home.[4] Patients are often not told the diagnosis or prognosis, hospice home care services are not well developed, and reimbursement for medical expenses is less for care at home than for care in a hospital.

Several organizations support hospice programs in Japan. The Japanese Association of Hospice and Palliative Care Units (now Hospice Palliative Care Japan) was registered in 1991, the Japan Society for Palliative Medicine in 1996, and more recently the Japan Hospice Palliative Care Foundation was established in 2001. The Japan Society for Palliative Medicine now has over 1200 members. However, palliative medicine is not yet recognized as a specialized area of medicine. The Japanese Association for Clinical Research on Death and Dying has also played a key role in the spread of the hospice movement in Japan since 1977.

People's Republic of China

In the People's Republic of China there had been interest in hospices since 1987 when two nurses from Tianjin Cancer Institute and Hospital (TCIH) went to the Royal Marsden Hospital in London for training in oncology. On their return in 1989 a five-bed palliative care unit was opened at the TCIH. A National Hospice Society was formed in Tianjin in 1992.[5] In the same year the Ministry of Health proposed a program to improve cancer pain relief in China. This included changes in policy to increase analgesic availability and training for healthcare professionals.[6] This was followed by many training programs and seminars at local and national levels and hundreds of hospice and palliative care units were started in hospitals or by licensed private companies.[7]

In 2000 a national network of hospice home care programs was set up by the Li Ka Shing Foundation, which is based in Hong Kong. Following the success of a pilot project in Shantou in Guangdong, the Foundation has been providing funding for hospice home care programs in 20 major hospitals in 16 provinces throughout China.

Hong Kong

In Hong Kong the first palliative care team was formed in 1982 in Our Lady of Maryknoll Hospital. Subsequently, in response to the perceived need for better care for terminally ill patients, the Society for the Promotion of Hospice Care was established in 1986. Six years later the Society secured funding to open Bradbury Hospice, a 26-bed independent inpatient hospice in Shatin. The Hospital Authority of Hong Kong took over management of five hospice units in 1991, established six more in the next 3 years and took over Bradbury Hospice in 1995. This recognition of the role of the hospice in healthcare was a key milestone in the development of hospices in Hong Kong.

There are now 11 palliative care services in Hong Kong under the Hospital Authority. All except Bradbury Hospice are located in hospitals. In 2003 restructuring of healthcare services into clusters resulted in the closure of Nam Long Hospital, a 200-bed inpatient unit. Palliative care services from Nam Long Hospital were then transferred to Grantham Hospital. Efforts are now being made to form consultative teams in general hospitals, to enhance liaison with nursing homes, and to encourage home care services.[8]

The Society for the Promotion of Hospice Care continues to play a major role in promoting public education and providing specialized professional training. The Jessie and Thomas Tam Centre, opened by the Society in 1997 as a bereavement counseling, and education and resource center, has been one of the major projects of the Society.

Professional organizations have been important in the development of palliative medicine in Hong Kong. Palliative medicine achieved specialty status under the Hong Kong College of Physicians in 1998. This was largely due to the efforts of the Hong Kong Society of Palliative Medicine, now the academic body of palliative medicine specialists. Since 1997 the Hong Kong Hospice Nurses' Association has also been active in training and research.

Taiwan

The concept of palliative care first began to attract interest in Taiwan in 1983 when Chantal Co-Shi Chao returned from a nurse PhD program in USA and organized a volunteer hospice home care program in Taipei. However, it was not until 1990 that the first inpatient hospice ward was opened by Dr David Chang and Dr Enoch Lai in Mackay Memorial Hospital. By 2000 this had evolved into a custom-built palliative care center with 63 beds, administrative offices, education facilities, and accommodation for students and faculty.

The Taiwan government became involved in palliative care in 1995 and this led to the setting of standards for inpatient and home care, and the development of guidelines for pain control. National Health Insurance reimbursement was introduced in 2000 for services accredited by the Taiwan Academy of Hospice Palliative Medicine and the Department of Health. This had been preceded earlier that year by the passage of legislation 'The Hospice Palliative Medical Act' which established the patient's right to sign a 'do not resuscitate' order, to choose palliative care, and to designate power of attorney for healthcare. The Act was amended in 2002 to allow for the withdrawal of life-sustaining devices for terminally ill patients.

Three foundations with religious affiliation have been important for the development of palliative care in Taiwan: the Hospice Foundation of Taiwan (established in 1990), the Catholic Sanapax Medical-Social Service Foundation (1993), and the Buddhist Lotus Hospice Care Foundation (1994). The Taiwan Hospice Organization has also been a unifying body for hospice volunteers and profession staff since 1995.

From 1990 the Hospice Foundation of Taiwan has been providing education and training. A multidisciplinary program was started in 1993 and revised in 1999. By 2003 a total of 1767 healthcare professionals had registered for the three-level program. The Taiwan Academy of Hospice Palliative Medicine was established in 1999 and in 2001 palliative medicine was accepted as a medical sub-specialty. By 2003, 172 physicians had been certified as palliative medicine specialists and 14 palliative care units had qualified as teaching units for the residency program. The majority of palliative care physicians have prior certification in family medicine.

By 2004 there were 29 hospice inpatient units with a total of 448 beds. However, it is estimated that less than 20 percent of cancer deaths receive palliative care. The National Cancer Control Program launched in 2003 has included the expansion of palliative care in its 5-year plan. The goal is to increase the coverage of terminally ill cancer patients to 50 percent and to improve the care of patients in nonhospice wards by introducing the concept of shared care.

Mongolia

Development in Mongolia has been more recent. A 10-bed palliative care unit was opened in the National Cancer Centre in 2000 with support from the Soros Foundation. In 2002 the Palliative Care Association of Mongolia was formed with 16 members. By 2005 there were two inpatient units with a total of 20 beds and two home care programs in Ulaan Bataar, all medical schools had teaching in palliative care and palliative medicine had been accepted as a medical specialty.[9]

SOUTHEAST ASIA

Singapore

Singapore has the most comprehensive palliative care services in Southeast Asia. However, early development was hampered by fears that hospices would be death houses like those that – until the 1980s – had sheltered the destitute dying in the back streets of Chinatown. The first 16 hospice beds were set aside in 1985 by the Canossian Sisters at St Joseph's Home. Subsequently, a volunteer hospice group under the Singapore Cancer Centre began providing home care in 1987.[10] In 1988 the Franciscan Missionaries of the Divine Motherhood at Assisi Home allocated 12 beds for hospice care and 4 years later the convent was remodeled to provide 35 beds.

In 1989 the first International Asia Pacific Hospice Conference with 250 participants from 10 countries was a major impetus for hospice development in Singapore and the region. This was followed later that year by the registration of the Hospice Care Association as an independent charity. This organization became the major provider of hospice home care in Singapore. An independent 40-bed inpatient hospice, Dover Park Hospice, was opened in 1995 in a custom-built facility shared with the Hospice Care Association.

When the Singapore Hospice Council was registered in 1995 as the umbrella body for hospice charities it took over public and professional education as well as advocacy with government. It also organized the second International Asia Pacific Hospice Conference in 1996 with Dame Cicely Saunders as keynote speaker and 550 participants from 22 countries.

Partial government funding was provided for hospice inpatient care from 1994 and for home care from 1996. In 2002 the policy was revised and funding is now provided only after means testing of the patient and family. In 2004 community hospice service providers received 2802 new referrals. This represents 74.9 percent of cancer deaths and 19.4 percent of total deaths.[11]

The establishment of a department of palliative medicine at the new National Cancer Centre in 1999 marked another milestone in hospice development in Singapore. This department provides consultancy and outpatient clinics for Singapore General Hospital and Kandang Kerbau Women's and Children's Hospital, as well as the National

Cancer Centre. Since 2002 all medical students from the National University of Singapore have had a 1-day palliative care posting. The Nanyang Polytechnic took the first students for the 1-year Advanced Diploma of Health Sciences (Palliative Care) in 2004.

There are now four inpatient hospices with 125 beds, five home care services, two hospice day care centers and four major hospitals with consultative teams. However, despite the success of the programs it is difficult to recruit medical staff. Efforts are being made to have palliative medicine recognized as a specialty so that there is an accredited training pathway for physicians who are interested in palliative care.

Malaysia

In Malaysia palliative care has developed along two streams: hospice home care provided by non-profit charity organizations and hospital-based palliative care units. In late 1991 home care programs were started by Hospis Malaysia in Kuala Lumpur and by Dato' John Cardosa and Dato' Dr T Devaraj of the National Cancer Society of Malaysia, Penang Branch, the organization that hosted the first hospice conference in Penang in 1993.[12]

The establishment of the palliative care unit at Queen Elizabeth II Hospital in Kota Kinabalu, Sabah, in 1995 was a landmark for hospice development in Malaysia. This unit, set up by Dr Ranjit Mathew Oommen, a surgeon at that hospital, initially had four beds but later expanded to 10 beds. A volunteer group (the Palliative Care Association of Kota Kinabalu) was formed to support patients who were discharged from the unit. This close association between the government hospital and the nongovernment organization providing home care in the community was seen by the Malaysian government as a suitable model for palliative care in Malaysia, and in 1997 the Department of Health announced that by 2000 all government hospitals were to have either a palliative care unit of at least six beds or a palliative care team.

By 2001 there were 11 palliative care units and 49 palliative care teams in government hospitals. In 2004, 20 organizations were providing hospice home care and there were two independent inpatient hospices that had opened in Penang in 2001, each with eight beds. However, despite this development, it is estimated that there is only about 20 percent coverage of cancer deaths and few patients with non-cancer diagnoses are referred for palliative care. In many hospitals the medical care in palliative care units is assigned to junior staff who have no formal training in palliative care and little interest in this area of medicine. Most palliative care services are in urban areas and, although attempts are being made to introduce the principles of palliative care to rural health workers, there is still an unmet need in rural areas.

The Malaysian Hospice Council was set up as the coordinating body for hospice nongovernment organizations in 1998. An annual congress hosted by a different state each year has provided a forum for education and networking. Although some physicians have undertaken distance-learning diploma courses from universities in Australia and UK, these are not recognized by the Medical Board as a specialist qualification. However, in February 2005, the Ministry of Health announced that an accredited training program for palliative medicine would be established.

The Philippines, Indonesia, Thailand, Vietnam, and Myanmar

In other countries in Southeast Asia development has been more sporadic. In the Philippines palliative care was integrated into the Family Health Care Program at Philippine General Hospital in 1989, and in 1991 the Philippine Cancer Society began a hospice home care program. The first National Convention on Hospice Palliative Care was held in Manila in 1995 with Dr Josephina Magno as guest speaker.

There are currently 16 organizations providing palliative care, mainly in or near Manila. These are mostly volunteer-run programs funded by charity. Apart from the Fellowship program at the Philippine General Hospital there are few training programs and palliative medicine is not recognized as a medical specialty. The formation of the National Hospice Palliative Care Council of the Philippines in 2004 is seen as an important step toward better coordination of services and advocacy of palliative care in the Philippines.

In Indonesia palliative care services have been established in Surabaya and in Jakarta since 1992. There are currently six centers providing palliative care: two in Jakarta, one in Surabaya, one in Denpasar, Bali, one in Yogyakarta and one in Makassar, South Sulawesi. These are hospital-based consultancy services with outpatient clinics and home care outreach. However, coverage is poor and accessibility to opioids outside the hospitals continues to be a problem. The Indonesian Palliative Society established in 2000 continues to hold a yearly meeting.

In Thailand, in 1996, a home care program was set up as a demonstration model in the National Cancer Institute in Bangkok, and in 1998 a 16-bed hospice was opened at the Mahavajiralongkorn Cancer Centre in Thanyaburi under the direction of Dr Tanadej Sinthusake. The first palliative care conference was held in 2004 in Hatyai where a consultative team had been operating in the Songklanagarind Hospital from 1999 and where palliative medicine was introduced into the undergraduate curriculum at the Prince of Songkla University Medical Faculty in 2001. A national professional hospice organization was formed in early 2005.

In Vietnam, since 1996 funding has been provided by Ms Elaine Magruder from Volunteers International, an American-based organization, for professional education in Ho Chi Minh City, Hanoi, and Hue, and for doctors and nurses to visit palliative care programs in Australia and USA. Other courses have been provided by experts from Australia, USA, and Singapore. At present there are three palliative care units in Vietnam: one in Cho Ray Hospital in Ho Chi Minh City (25 beds established in 2003), one in the Hue General Hospital in Central Vietnam (10 beds established in 2001), and one in the National Cancer Institute in Hanoi (40 beds established in 2000). Since 2005, a 3-year Train-the-Trainers project for doctors and nurses in Ho Chi Minh City, Hue, and Hanoi is being funded by the Singapore International Foundation.

In Myanmar two 40-bed independent inpatient hospices have been established by a private charity, the U Hla Tun Hospice (Cancer) Foundation, one in Yangon and one in Mandalay. Another is to be built in Taunggyi. However, there has been no further development of home care or hospital consultancy. Oral morphine is not available in Myanmar.

SOUTH ASIA

The first Indian hospice, Shanti Avadna, opened in Mumbai in 1986. Subsequently, other independent hospices were built and some hospitals established pain clinics and home care services. However, the development in South Asia has been largely centered in the southern Indian state of Kerala where 64 of the known 87 palliative care services in India are to be found.[13]

Dr M R Rajapopal, Dr Suresh Kumar, and others have attempted to develop a model of care adapted to the Indian situation where most patients are in late stage of disease when diagnosed, where there is shortage of resources, and where patients prefer to be cared for at home. In 1986 a pain and palliative care clinic was started in the Regional Cancer Centre in Trivandrum, Kerala. This was followed in 1993 by the registration of a nongovernment organization, the Pain and Palliative Care Society and the opening of a Pain and Palliative Care Clinic at the Calicut Medical College. The focus was on outpatient management of pain using trained volunteers for nursing and administrative duties, empowering families to provide care at home, and development of a network of clinics funded by the local community.[14]

The Pain and Palliative Care Clinic was declared a World Health Organization demonstration project in 1996 and became a major teaching resource for physicians in India and nearby countries including Nepal. In 2003 this function was taken over by the Institute of Palliative Medicine opened in Calicut (now Kozhikode) with accommodation for students and faculty as well as an inpatient facility with 40 beds. A 6-week intensive Basic Certificate Course in Palliative Medicine is recognized by the Edith Cowan University in Australia and students who compete the certificate course are eligible for three of the six study units of the postgraduate diploma offered by the University. In 2004 the Institute of Palliative Medicine launched a 1-year post-graduate fellowship program in palliative medicine. The AIIMS Hospital in Cochin now offers a 2-year diploma in pain and palliative medicine as well as a 6-week certificate course. The Indian

Association of Palliative Care, established in 1994, holds a conference in a different state each year.

FUTURE ISSUES

In Asia two issues continue to cause concern: the resistance to the use of opioids for symptom management and the reluctance to disclose diagnosis and prognosis to the patient. Only in Hong Kong, Taiwan, Japan, Singapore, the Philippines, Malaysia and in some states of India is oral morphine readily available for pain management. Barriers at every level limit access to cheap oral opioids and, even when available, doctors are disinclined to prescribe and families are reluctant to take the medication because of fear of addiction or toxic side effects.[15] Much public and professional education is needed before better pain management can be achieved.

In many countries in East and Southeast Asia, families are often unwilling to inform patients of a cancer diagnosis or of a poor prognosis. Doctors follow the wishes of the family even when the patient is asking for more information.[16,17] Reasons given are that the patient will not understand the information or will become depressed after disclosure.[18] This issue of truth telling creates conflict for professional caregivers, especially when there is need to obtain informed consent for investigative or treatment interventions.

The Asia Pacific Hospice Palliative Care Network (APHN) was established in 2001 to promote networking among those involved in palliative care in the region. By the fifth annual general meeting in 2005 the APHN had recruited 831 members from 26 countries (697 individual members and 134 organizational members). A visiting faculty scheme encourages experts from more developed countries to visit countries where services are being established and a directory of palliative care organizations in the region is published every 2 years with an updated copy on the APHN website (www.aphn.org).[19] The concept of APHN as a regional organization grew out of discussions during the first Asia Pacific Hospice Conference in Singapore in 1989 and the APHN is now having an increasing role in the conferences that are held biennially. The seventh conference will be held in Manila in 2007.

Even though the need for palliative care is becoming more widely accepted both by the public and healthcare professionals, there is still great variation in the quality of services and the coverage of patients in need. The lack of manpower and funding continues to limit the scope of services in many countries. Only in Hong Kong, Taiwan, Mongolia, and Malaysia has palliative medicine been accepted as a medical specialty. Underlying the struggle to have palliative medicine acknowledged as an accredited specialist field is the recognition that only when there is a trained workforce and a clear career path will it be possible to provide services for the growing numbers of patients with end-stage disease.

Professional education in palliative care is still sporadic and relies heavily on overseas faculty and distance-learning courses from UK and Australia. Little research has been published in English language journals apart from the work of Cecilia Lai-Wan Chan and her colleagues at the Hong Kong University. The extent of relevant research in non-English speaking countries such as Japan, Taiwan, and Korea is not known.

Key learning points

- The hospice concept was first introduced into Korea in 1965 and into Japan in 1973.

- National hospice and palliative care organizations have played an important role in the development of palliative care in Asia.

- Continuing resistance by patients, families and healthcare professionals to the use of opioids for symptom management contributes to the nonavailability of oral morphine in many countries.

- Reluctance by families to disclose diagnosis and prognosis to patients creates conflict for professional caregivers.

- Recruitment of medical staff is hindered by the lack of a clear career path with specialist accreditation.

REFERENCES

1 Maddocks I. Teaching palliative care in east Asia. *Palliat Med* 2000; **14**: 535–7.
2 Chung Y. Progress in palliative care in Korea: a nurse viewpoint. *Prog Palliat Care* 2000; **8**: 12–16.
3 Choi ES, Ro YS, Han SS, *et al.* A study on the curriculum development for the professional hospice nurse. *Korean J Acad Nur* 1998; **28**: 1027–35.
4 Ida E, Miyachi M, Uemura M, *et al.* Current status of hospice cancer deaths both in-patient and at home (1995–2000), and prospects of home care services in Japan. *Palliat Med* 2002; **16**: 179–84.
5 Ying W, Paice JA. People's Republic of China. In: Ferrell BR and Coyle N, eds. *Textbook of Palliative Nursing*. Oxford: Oxford University Press, 2001; 727–30.
6 Hong Z, Gu WP, Joranson DE, Cleeland C. People's Republic of China: status of cancer pain and palliative care. *J Pain Symptom Manage* 1996; **12**: 124–6.
7 Wang XS, Li TD, Yu SY, *et al.* China: status of pain and palliative care. *J Pain Symptom Manage* 2002; **24**: 177–9.
8 Sham MKM. Pain relief and palliative care in Hong Kong. *J Pain Palliat Care Pharmacother* 2003; **17**: 65–73.
9 Davaasuren O. Mongolia: the present situation and future of palliative care. *J Pain Symptom Manage* 2002; **24**: 208–10.
10 Goh CR, Shaw RJ. Evolution of hospice home care service in Singapore. *Ann Acad Med Singapore* 1994; **23**: 275–81.
11 Goh CR. Care of the dying – whose job is it anyway? *Singapore Med J* 2005; **6**: 205.
12 Lim RBL. Palliative care in Malaysia: a decade of progress and going strong. *J Pain Palliat Care Pharmacother* 2003; **17**: 77–85.
13 *Directory 2005*. Asia Pacific Hospice Palliative Care Network. Singapore, 2005; 16–26.
14 Rajagopal MR, Palat G. Kerala, India: status of cancer pain relief and palliative care. *J Pain Symptom Manage* 2002; **24**: 191–3.
15 Joranson D, Rajagopal MR, Gilson AM. Improving access to opioid analgesics for palliative care in India. *J Pain Symptom Manage* 2002; **24**: 152–9.
16 Mizuno M, Onishi C, Ouishi F. Truth disclosure of cancer diagnoses and its influence on bereaved Japanese families. *Cancer Nurs* 2002; **25**: 396–403.
17 Wang XS. End-of-life care in urban areas of China: a survey of 60 oncology clinicians. *J Pain Symptom Manage* 2004; **27**: 125–32.
18 Kawakami S, Arai G, Ueda K, *et al.* Physician's attitudes towards disclosure of cancer diagnosis to elderly patients: a report from Tokyo, Japan. *Arch Gerontol Geriatr* 2001; **33**: 29–36.
19 Goh CR. The Asia Pacific Hospice Palliative Care Network: a network of individuals and organisations. *J Pain Symptom Manage* 2002; **24**: 128–33.

8

Palliative care versus palliative medicine

EDUARDO BRUERA, ELLEN A PACE

INTRODUCTION

The development of palliative medicine in different regions of the world has been discussed in Chapters 1–7 of this book. In Chapter 1 David Clark discusses the origins of the modern hospice movement in the UK, and the other chapters discuss the progressive integration of these principles to other areas of the world.

Palliative care programs have three distinct characteristics:

- *Multidimensional assessment and management.* This includes the assessment and management of a large number of physical symptoms, psychosocial distress, and functional, spiritual, financial, and family concerns.
- *Interdisciplinary care.* This includes the pivotal role of a team including physicians, nurses, social workers, pastoral care, occupational therapy and physiotherapy, pharmacists, counselors, dieticians, and volunteers who work together in an integrated fashion for the delivery of care.
- *Emphasis on caring for patients and their families.* In the first palliative care programs it was realized that the majority of physical and emotional care near the end of life is provided by the patient's family. Thus programs were developed that aimed to support those families with counseling, education, respite, and bereavement care.

Physicians have had a major role in the development of palliative care programs in the UK and other areas of the world. They came from multiple specialties including family medicine, oncology, pain medicine, surgery, neurology, psychiatry, and geriatrics. These physicians integrated with the other medical disciplines to establish palliative care teams in programs that were mostly based in the community.

During the first two decades of the development of palliative care there was an impressive and global expansion of clinical programs. It soon became clear that some of the most seriously ill patients died in acute care hospitals and cancer centers, and palliative care programs progressively expanded from the periphery into major academic centers. The body of knowledge of palliative care started to progressively develop and the need for research became apparent. The growth in clinical programs, the variety of settings where palliative care was delivered, and the expanding body of knowledge and need for research led a number of physicians in the UK, Australia, and Canada to advocate for the development of the specialty of palliative medicine.

THE EMERGING MEDICAL SPECIALTY

During the late 1980s and early 1990s there was a strong debate regarding the potential advantages and disadvantages of palliative medicine as a specialty. In many countries around the world this debate continues. Box 8.1 summarizes some of the arguments for and against the development of

---

Box 8.1 Perceived advantages and disadvantages of palliative medicine specialists

Perceived advantages

- Access to specialist training
- Development of a career path
- Protected time for academic orientation
- Increased credibility among other medical professionals
- Access to acute care hospitals, cancer centers, and universities

a palliative medicine specialty.[1–3] At the present time palliative medicine has achieved specialty or subspecialty status in the UK, Canada, and Australia. In addition, there are active efforts to establish palliative medicine as a subspecialty in the USA, many European countries, and a number of countries in Latin America and Asia.

The original heated debate that accompanied the establishment of palliative medicine as a specialty in the UK in 1987 has continued in all other countries where the effort has been made to develop this specialty. Most of the debate has been centered around how to maintain the three main principles of palliative care delivery and how to avoid excessive medicalization of palliative care, but at the same time being able to make a major contribution to the body of knowledge by appropriate research and contributing to the education of future generations of physicians and other healthcare professionals.

The only nation where the specialty of palliative medicine has existed long enough to allow for some evaluation of its impact is the UK. David Clark, in Chapter 1, eloquently summarizes the current debate and also the major growth in the medical components of palliative care including education and research, which have resulted from the emergence of palliative medicine in the UK. The consensus among physician groups in most of the world is that the development of the specialty of palliative medicine is of great importance for the further development of the field, particularly in acute care institutions and universities.

THE ROLE OF PALLIATIVE MEDICINE

Figure 8.1 illustrates the main disciplines involved in the palliative circle of care. Each of these disciplines is responsible for developing its own body of knowledge and for contributing to the integration of this body of knowledge with that of the other disciplines within the circle. The effective growth of each of these disciplines and the successful interaction results in the collective body of knowledge of palliative care being increased, that is then provided to patients and families. In this theoretical model palliative medicine is the medical component of the multidimensional and interdisciplinary domain known as palliative care.

Figure 8.2 summarizes some of the most important contributors to the body of knowledge of palliative medicine. These contributors have not only included subspecialties of medicine but a large contribution to the palliative medicine knowledge has also been made by disciplines such as nursing, rehabilitation, psychology, social work, pastoral care, and nutrition. It is desirable to have representatives of these disciplines as part of the research and education in palliative

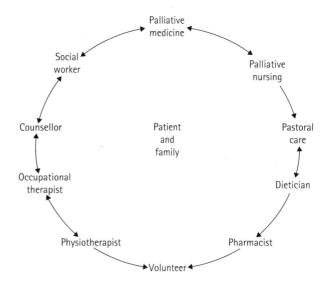

Figure 8.1 *The palliative circle of care.*

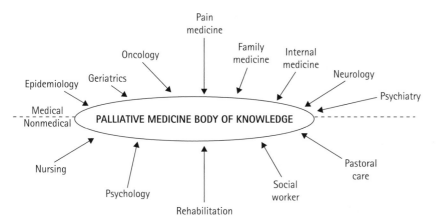

Figure 8.2 *The main medical and nonmedical disciplines that have influenced the body of knowledge in palliative medicine.*

care. It is likely that with the regular interaction as part of the palliative care circle these disciplines will continue to influence the growth of palliative medicine in the future.

Box 8.2 summarizes the role of palliative medicine specialists in the areas of clinical, educational, and research palliative care delivery. Palliative medicine specialists are not necessarily expected to see all patients with progressive, incurable diseases or their families. In most cases the physician in charge of the primary care of the patient, either their family physician (such as in Canada, the UK, Australia[4]) or their primary specialist (such as in USA,[5,6] most of continental Europe, and the developing world[7,8]) can deliver the principles of palliative care assessment and management. These primary care physicians can access a number of other palliative care disciplines for the patient including nursing, social work, pastoral care, counseling, rehabilitation, or volunteer services.

When patients present with physical or psychosocial distress that can not be appropriately controlled by their primary care physician, the palliative medicine specialist can be involved in secondary care. They can provide episodic care, such as consultations or collaborative care by following up with the patient in an integrated manner with the primary physician.[9,10] The palliative medicine specialist will then be able to access all other members of the palliative care team as required.

Box 8.2 The roles of the palliative medicine specialist (PMS)

Clinical

- Primary palliative care: by family physicians and primary specialists
- Secondary palliative care: PMS – episodic care (consultation)
- Collaborative care (joint follow-up)
- Tertiary palliative care: PMS – primary care (palliative care unit)

Education

- Undergraduate and postgraduate training of other physicians
- Palliative medicine specialty training
- Continuing medical education

Research

- Development of new assessment and management interventions
- Audit
- Epidemiological research
- Translational research

A small percentage of patients are severely distressed, and this requires that the palliative medicine specialist becomes the primary care physician. This will take place both in the ambulatory care setting and particularly in palliative care units.[11–13] In many cases the most important contribution of the palliative medicine specialist is to provide the sophisticated assessment and correct management plan that will help the team develop the most effective interventions.

These different levels of delivery of palliative care by palliative medicine specialists are not different from the role of other medical specialists in the management of different diseases. For example, it would not be reasonable to expect that cardiologists should be in charge of delivering primary care of all patients with arterial hypertension or that endocrinologists should be in charge of the primary care of all patients with type 2 diabetes. In most countries in the world their own primary care physician provides the majority of care for these patients. However, the specialist is available for consultation for a major proportion of these patients and for primary delivery of care in the most refractory situations.

The degree of use of the palliative medicine specialist as a consultant will be linked to the level of expertise of the primary physician. Some primary physicians will have acquired enough education and experience in palliative care to be able to resolve a large proportion of clinical problems whereas others will have a much lower threshold for consultation. The best monitoring for the appropriate utilization of palliative medicine specialty services will be the level of physical and psychosocial distress in patients and families in each institution and/or region.

Palliative medicine specialists are extremely important for undergraduate and postgraduate education.[14–17] They are also responsible for the continuing medical education of those primary care physicians already working in the community. The adoption of new assessments, pharmacological and nonpharmacological interventions by primary care physicians will heavily depend on the clinical and educational leadership of palliative medicine specialists in every community. Physicians adopt new diagnostic tests, medications, and procedures mostly as a result of the clinical leadership and education of those who have specialized in these specific areas of knowledge.[18]

Finally, palliative medicine specialists are responsible for the development of the body of knowledge that will result in changes in the assessment and treatment of patients and families. Although most physicians will use analgesics, antiemetics, and drugs for the management of delirium on a regular basis, there is a huge need for a small number of specialists with great dedication to the discovery of new assessments and treatments for pain, emesis, and delirium in palliative care. Individuals who are fully focused on palliative care research will ensure that there is progress in this field.

In summary, palliative medicine specialists are able to deliver clinical care to those patients and families with the most difficult problems, to educate colleagues about the appropriate delivery of palliative care, and to actively conduct research on new developments in assessment and management of clinical problems. Ideally, a significant proportion of palliative medicine specialists should operate within academically organized departments in medical schools. Such departments already exist in a number of universities in the UK, North America, and Europe. The university affiliation will allow palliative medicine specialists to have the necessary protected time for conducting academic activities, the possibility to influence the development of undergraduate and postgraduate curriculum, and the possibility to establish research teams by interacting with experts in methodology, content, and biostatistics affiliated with different universities.

CONCLUSIONS

Since the establishment of the specialty of palliative medicine in the UK in 1987 similar efforts have been made in a number of countries. Palliative medicine specialists have been instrumental in the development of scientific organizations and meetings, peer-reviewed journals, textbooks, and in the development of a curriculum for the undergraduate and postgraduate teaching of palliative medicine for physicians. These specialists have also linked with other healthcare professionals and volunteers to maintain the multidimensional and interdisciplinary nature of palliative care.

The nature and content of the teaching curriculum, the financial viability of the different palliative specialist positions in different countries, and the overall body of knowledge are not completely defined for this young medical specialty. As palliative medicine is progressively adopted by acute care facilities and academic institutions the need for palliative medicine specialist is likely to grow exponentially during the next decade in most of the world.

Key learning points

- Palliative care programs have three main characteristics: multidimensional assessment and management, interdisciplinary care, and emphasis on the patient and their families.

- Palliative medicine was initially established as a specialty in the UK in 1987.

- Palliative medicine specialists integrate with multiple other disciplines in the delivery of palliative care.

- Palliative medicine specialists provide clinical care in the most complex situations, graduate and postgraduate education, and research.

REFERENCES

1 Fordham S, Dowrick C, May C. Palliative medicine: Is it really specialist territory? *J R Soc Med* 1998; **91**: 568–72.

2 Hoy A. Routinisation and medicalisation. *Eur J Palliat Care* 1998; **6**: 178.

● 3 Kearney M. Palliative medicine – just another specialty? *Palliat Med* 1992; **6**: 39–46.

● 4 Brenneis C, Bruera E. Models for the delivery of palliative care: The Canadian Model. In: Bruera E, Portenoy RK, eds. *Topics in Palliative Care* Vol 5. Oxford: Oxford University Press, 2001: 3–23.

5 Morrison RS, Meier DE. Clinical practice. Palliative care. *N Engl J Med* 2004; **350**: 2582–90.

6 White KR, Cochran CE, Patel UB. Hospital provision of end-of-life services: who, what, and where? *Med Care* 2002; **40**: 17–25.

7 Centeno C, Gomez-Sancho M. Models for the delivery of palliative care: The Spanish Model. In: Bruera E, Portenoy RK, eds. *Topics in Palliative Care* Vol 5. Oxford: Oxford University Press, 2001: 25–38.

8 Wenk R, Bertolino M. Models for the delivery of palliative care in developing countries: The Argentine Model. In: Bruera E, Portenoy RK, eds. *Topics in Palliative Care* Vol 5. Oxford: Oxford University Press, 2001: 39–54.

9 Jenkins CA, Scarfe A, Bruera E. Integration of palliative care with alternative medicine in patients who have refused curative therapy: a report of two cases. *J Palliat Care* 1998; **14**: 55–9.

10 Kutner JS, Metcalfe T, Vu KO, et al. Implementation of an ad hoc hospital-based palliative care consult service. *J Pain Symptom Manage* 2004; **28**: 526–8.

● 11 Elsayem A, Swint K, Fisch MJ, et al. Palliative care inpatient service in a comprehensive cancer center: clinical and financial outcomes. *J Clin Oncol* 2004; **22**: 2008–14.

● 12 Strasser F, Sweeney C, Willey J, et al. Impact of a half-day multidisciplinary symptom control and palliative care outpatient clinic in a comprehensive cancer center on recommendations, symptom intensity, and patient satisfaction: a retrospective descriptive study. *J Pain Symptom Manage* 2004; **28**: 481–91.

● 13 Bruera E, Neumann C, Brenneis C, Quan H. Frequency of symptom distress and poor prognostic indicators in palliative cancer patients admitted to a tertiary palliative care unit, hospices, and acute care hospitals. *J Palliat Care* 2002; **16**: 16–21.

14 Legrand SB, Walsh D, Nelson KA, Davis MP. A syllabus for fellowship education in palliative medicine. *Am J Hosp Palliat Care* 2003; **20**: 279–89.

15 Oneschuk D. Undergraduate medical palliative care education: a new Canadian perspective. *J Palliat Med* 2002; **5**: 43–7.

16 Oneschuk D, Fainsinger R, Hanson J, Bruera E. Assessment and knowledge in palliative care in second year family medicine residents. *J Pain Symptom Manage* 1997; **14**: 265–73.

17 Oneschuk D, Hanson J, Bruera E. An international study of undergraduate medical education in palliative medicine. *J Pain Symptom Manage* 2000; **20**: 174–9.

18 Rodgers EM. *Adoption of Innovation Theory: Diffusion of Innovation*, 4th ed. New York: Free Press, 1995.

WEB RESOURCES

Edmonton Regional Palliative Care Program: www.palliative.org
International Association of Hospice Care: www.hospicecare.com

9

Palliative care as a public health issue

JOSEPH F O'NEILL, R CAMERON WOLF

INTRODUCTION

Palliative care is an important public health issue that has been markedly shaped over the past 20 years by the changes in society, especially the acquired immune deficiency syndrome (AIDS) pandemic and aging in many countries. With the emergence of human immunodeficiency virus (HIV)/AIDS, and the ever-increasing need to mobilize communities, adopt prevention measures, and increase access to services, an integrated public health model that spans the continuum of the illness and addresses not only clinical, but also material, psychosocial, and spiritual needs of the patient is needed. The discipline of palliative care offers, in addition to addressing pain and suffering and improving quality of life, an important means of meeting this need.

WHAT IS A PUBLIC HEALTH ISSUE?

The European Observatory on Health Systems and Policies defines public health as 'the science and art of promoting health, prevention disease, and prolonging life through organized efforts of society'.[1] The US Institute of Medicine further defines the role of public health as:[2]

what we as a society do collectively to assure the conditions in which people can be healthy. This requires that continuing and emerging threats to the health of the public be successfully countered. These threats include immediate crises, such as the AIDS epidemic, enduring problems, such as

injuries and chronic illness, and growing challenges, such as the aging of our population. . . . These and many other problems raise in common the need to protect the nation's health through effective, organized, and sustained efforts led by the public sector.

In a broader vein, the Public Health in the Americas Initiative, sponsored by the World Health Organization (WHO), the Pan American Health Organization, and others defines public health as:[3a]

a collective action of State and Civil Society to protect and improve the health of individuals. It is a notion that goes beyond population or community-based interventions and includes the responsibility of ensuring access by citizens to quality health care. It does not approach public health as an academic discipline but rather as an interdisciplinary social practice.

These and other definitions recognize that public health is targeted at communities and accomplished through social and political action, which distinguishes the field from, for example, clinical care where the target of activity is the individual patient or family. Public health actions have included the establishment of municipal health authorities, sanitation departments, new healthcare practices, community and professional education, research, reform of public laws impacting on health, and many other societal interventions.

The definition of what constitutes a public health issue has evolved with time. In its earliest Western incarnation after John Snow closed the famous London water pump and ended a cholera outbreak, public health's purview did not extend much beyond what is now considered basic infectious disease epidemiology. As, however, understanding of the determinants of health have become more sophisticated so has the perspective of public health practice. Disciplines of sociology, economics, psychology, nutrition, anthropology, and others are now considered by many to be important in understanding the health of individuals and, hence, populations and societies. The Acheson report commissioned by the UK Minister of Public Health to review and summarize health inequalities and to recommend priority areas for policy development and interventions to reduce them, noted that their work was based on a 'socioeconomic model of health' that recognized that the main determinants of health could be described as layers of environmental and social influence over the fixed individual constitutional factors.[3b] Similarly, the US Institute of Medicine in its seminal report on the future of public health defined health as a 'public good' because 'many aspects of human potential such as employment, social relationships, and political participation are contingent upon it.'[4] One area of action identified by this report was to adopt a population health approach that considers multiple determinants of health.

PALLIATIVE CARE AS A PUBLIC HEALTH ISSUE

As a health issue that significantly impacts a large number of people, that is amenable to population-based and public sector interventions, and that has the potential to reduce suffering on a massive scale, end-of-life care is an important public health issue. The discipline of palliative care, with its understanding of the interrelationships between physical, spiritual, emotional, and practical domains of human existence and suffering, fits quite comfortably into an approach to population health that recognizes multiple determinants of health and enduring health problems. It has made this philosophy the cornerstone of clinical practice for decades.

Palliative care encompasses, but extends far beyond, end-of-life care. The WHO has defined palliative care as:[5]

> an approach which improves quality of life of patients and their families facing life-threatening illness through the prevention and relief of suffering by means of early identification and impeccable assessment and treatment of pain and other problems, physical, psychological and spiritual.

A palliative approach then should be applied along all stages of serious illness regardless of the immediacy of death. To do otherwise can rightly be considered a failure to provide quality care. In this light, the public health mandate of palliative care becomes even larger and more complex: The target for palliative interventions is not just the result of a calculation based on incidence of death but, rather, on prevalence of life-threatening and serious disease in a defined population or geographical area.

PALLIATIVE CARE IN THE DEVELOPED VERSUS THE DEVELOPING REGIONS OF THE WORLD

Global trends

Between 2002 and 2050 the world's population is expected to grow from 6.4 billion to 8.9 billion and the 50 poorest countries will triple in size.[6] By 2050, however, the population of the developed world will have been in decline for 20 years.[7] Therefore, all of the world population increase will be in the developing world. The WHO estimates that there were 57 million deaths in 2002,[8] 85 percent of which occurred in the developing world. Assuming that each death affects five other people, end-of-life issues are estimated to affect about 5 percent of the world's population each year.[9]

The world's aging population brings palliative care to the forefront in disease management. Today, the world's population of those who are 60 years and above is 600 million, and by 2050 this number will reach 2 billion. Eighty percent of these people will be living in the developing world.[10] Aging is associated with increased incidence of chronic noncommunicable diseases including cancer, cardiovascular disease, and other conditions.[11] As recent guidance from the WHO demonstrates,[11,12] increased longevity in many countries brings with it an increase in chronic diseases as a cause of death and older people who can have complex, multiple conditions. It can be difficult to diagnose with certainty any one disease as the main cause of death, as many older people have several conditions together that might all contribute to death and to symptoms. Indeed, it is estimated that 22.4 million people are living with cancer today and that 12.6 percent of all deaths are caused by cancer.[13] There is evidence in some countries that access to palliative and hospice care is less among older people than their younger counterparts.[11] This is another example of where palliative care is a public health issue, which is concerned with ensuring access to care according to need.

An important global trend that has affected the need for palliative care is the HIV/AIDS pandemic. Some 38 million are people now living with HIV/AIDS, 2.1 million of whom are children under the age of 15 years. In 2003 there were 4.8 million new infections and 2.9 million AIDS deaths, of which 490 000 were of children. In total, the epidemic has claimed 23 million lives and is expected to take an additional 22 million by the end of the first decade of the twenty-first century.[14]

Global inequities

The burden of illness requiring palliative care is disproportionately borne by the developing world – regions least able to mount an effective response. Only 1.6 million of the 38 million estimated to be living with HIV today live in high-income countries. Approximately 10 percent of the world's population lives in sub-Saharan Africa, a region that is home to nearly two-thirds of all persons living with HIV. Explosive trends in HIV prevalence are expected in China, India, and Russia.[15] The US National Intelligence Council has projected that China will have 10–15 million cases of AIDS and India 20–25 million cases by 2010.[16]

Similarly, more than half the world's cancer burden (numbers of cases and deaths) is now borne by the developing world.[17] The 2003 World Cancer Report[13] further documents that:

- In wealthy countries, approximately 50 percent of patients with diagnosed cancer die compared with 80 percent of patients in the developing world.
- More than 80 percent of deaths from cervical cancer occur in developing countries.
- The occurrence of breast cancer in developed countries is >300/100 000 population per year compared to <1500/100 000 in developing countries.
- In wealthy countries chronic infections (such as hepatitis B and C, human papilloma virus, and *Helicobacter pylori* infections) are implicated in 8 percent of all malignancies compared with 23 percent in the developing world.
- Tobacco use remains a global concern and if current rates of use persist will cause 10 million deaths a year by 2005.[18] Moreover, in both developing and developed countries it is the poorest people who tend to smoke the most, and who bear most of the disease burden.[19]

Countries that shoulder the bulk of the world's disease burden and that have the greatest need for palliative care services are fiscally the least well equipped to act to provide it. The World Bank estimates that in 2001, 1.1 billion people consumed less than US$1 per day and 2.7 billion people less than US$2 per day.[20] Variation in spending on health between the developed and developing regions of the world is dramatic: an analysis of 1998 expenditures showed that Africa spent an estimated US$82 per capita per year on health (5.1 percent gross domestic product [GDP]); South Asia spent US$92 per capita per year (4.4 percent GDP) and the Organization for Economic Co-operation

and Development (OECD) countries expended US$2078 per capita per year (9.7 percent GDP).[16]

Only 58 percent of sub-Saharan Africans have access to clean water and 42 percent of the world's population do not have their basic sanitation needs met.[21] Hunger and malnutrition remain the number one risk to global health.[22] It is estimated that there are 800 million undernourished people in the world, that one out of four children are underweight and that, in 2002, 6 million children died from nutritional deficiencies.[19]

The implications of these global inequities are profound. Poverty correlates with disease and disease causes poverty – a vicious cycle resulting in higher and higher levels of suffering and morbidity. Projections of the economic costs of infectious diseases in Africa, for example, have held that for some countries economic growth could be reduced by as much as 25 percent in 20 years.[23] At a time when more health resources are needed than ever before, economies stand in danger of contracting as a result of the deterioration of their population's health and hence will become even less able to respond.

Social and cultural trends

Under the best and most stable of circumstances provision of palliative care requires a wide range of human and fiscal resources. Trained medical professionals are necessary – so are informal caregivers, spiritual healers, families, good nutrition, clean environments, good communication systems, access to medications, transportation, shelter, and, perhaps most important of all, peaceful societies.

In the developed world where populations are aging and rates of fertility have decreased, the availability of caregivers and people who pay for care (generally through taxes or private insurance pools) will decrease relative to the numbers who need care (see Fig. 9.1).[11] In the USA, between August 1999 and September 2000, more than 54 million people – 27 percent of the adult population – served as informal caregivers for people with chronic illnesses or disabilities.[24] A study of the economics of informal caregiving in the USA in 1997 valued it at US$196 billion, an amount equivalent to

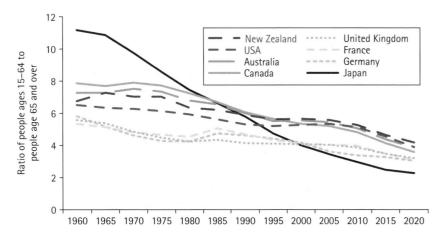

Figure 9.1 *The number of working-age people for every elderly person 1960–2020. Source: Better Palliative Care for Older People.[11] Redrawn with the permission of the editors. Original data from Anderson GF, Hussey PS. Health and Population Aging: A Multinational Comparison. New York: Commonwealth Fund, 1999.*

18 percent of total healthcare spending.[25] This relative level of support cannot be relied on to continue in the face of demographic shifts. The cost to society of supplanting these services will add to the already escalating demands on health resources.

In the developing regions of the world a variety of trends can be expected to impact on the ability to deliver palliative care. The impact of the HIV/AIDS epidemic on family, and hence social stability, is significant. Since 2000, 3.8 million African children have lost one or both parents to the epidemic and by 2010 sub-Saharan Africa will be home to an estimated 50 million such orphans. In 11 African countries, one in seven children are orphans. UNICEF estimates that there are 87.6 million orphans (from all causes) in Asia and 12.4 million in Latin America and the Caribbean.[26]

Social instability is exacerbated by trends in urbanization. Nearly 180 000 people are added to the world's cities each day and it is expected that 60 percent of the world's population will live in urban areas by 2030.[27] In addition, political instability and war in and of themselves cause suffering and hamper the ability of society to mobilize around human service needs such as palliative and end-of-life care. Largely as a result of war and instability there are now some 20.8 million refugees, asylum seekers, internally displaced persons and others of concern.[28] These populations are at high risk for disease, malnutrition, and death.

PALLIATIVE CARE AND THE AIDS EXPERIENCE

The concept of palliative care grew out of pain relief and comfort measures for cancer patients, wherein the traditional trajectory of illness was through a linear projection of diagnosis, growing severity of illness, and death. However, the AIDS epidemic has challenged traditional ideas of end-of-life care, as the trajectory of living and dying in this population has become highly variable and unpredictable. The introduction of antiretroviral drugs (ARVs) to combat HIV has resulted in a wide range of disease progressions, potential complications, and ultimately, survival. An individual's health may improve, then worsen, and then improve again before a terminal state of disease is reached. Some individuals may not respond to ARVs, others may be diagnosed late in the disease, and yet others may never have received treatment, especially those in resource-poor international settings. Therefore, the traditional trajectory of illness through a linear projection is not always an appropriate model for people with AIDS. Moreover, patients using ARVs may experience many other symptoms, including unpleasant side effects of treatment or opportunistic infections. As a result of the variable course of AIDS and its associated symptoms, palliative care in these patients becomes a balance between acute treatment and chronic symptoms and conditions.[29] For many, AIDS more closely resembles a chronic disease than a terminal illness.

Palliative care has been defined as:[30]

patient- and family-centered care, which optimizes quality of life by active anticipation, prevention, and treatment of suffering. Respectful and trusting relationships are the foundation used by the interdisciplinary team throughout the continuum of illness to address physical, intellectual, emotional, social and spiritual needs and facilitate patient autonomy, access to information, and choice.

The term 'continuum of illness' is a critical part of this definition, and implores public health models to integrate palliative care into the continuum of prevention, diagnosis, and treatment of a disease. Providing palliative care within the continuum of illness has many implications, especially in resource-poor settings. Pain control and symptom management may be given along with curative therapy or when curative therapy is absent. Traditional medicines and spirituality can be, and often are, an important component of a palliative approach.

The burden of grief is compounded among people living with AIDS, families and communities that have experienced losses of many loved ones and, at times, stigma and discrimination from their neighbors.[31,32] This has led to community mobilization of support and advocacy groups. Critical to the definition of palliative care is the inclusion of addressing psychosocial needs in this population. Several factors are important in optimizing clinical outcomes in patients with AIDS. These factors include a wide range of hard-to-control socioeconomic as well as personal characteristics: an understanding of the disease process; empowerment in relation to personal health; a safe place to live; freedom from pain and distressing symptoms; adequate nutrition; treatment for substance abuse, depression, and other mental illness; hope; adequate help of friends, family, and other caregivers, especially when functional status is diminished and disease progression is ongoing. These challenges can be met successfully by using a palliative care framework to approach the patient, providers, caregivers, family, loved ones, and the healthcare system. Conversely, the benefits of community mobilization around palliative care can enhance public health by increasing access to health education, prevention, and care services.

A PUBLIC HEALTH APPROACH TO SUSTAINING PALLIATIVE CARE

In practical terms, a public health approach to making it possible for everyone who needs quality palliative care to receive it must involve a range of activities. The WHO has identified three elements as necessary to further sustainable palliative care:[33,34]

● governmental policy – establishing national policies, making sure that palliative care is harmonized with national health and social service agendas

- education – of health professionals, the public, and media, policy makers, and others
- ensuring access to pain medications.

A public health approach would additionally emphasize the important role of research, and development of a strong evidence base from which to build programs and policies. The responsibility for these activities will vary from society to society, but each in its own way is necessary. Political commitment is a prerequisite for effective action. This, in turn, depends upon community awareness and mobilization. In all cases sensitivity to various cultural perspectives and norms is essential.

Governmental policies: national strategies for palliative care

Government policies can obstruct, permit, or promote an environment that enables palliative care to flourish. Examples can be found of each approach. Relatively few governments have established national strategies promoting palliative care. An outstanding example of forward leaning policy can be found in Uganda. In its Health Sector Strategic Plan 2000/02–2004/05 the Ministry of Health has classified palliative care as 'essential'[35] and has identified indicators, verification measures, and operational activities needed to achieve the goal of increased access to palliative care. The government of Canada has moved in a similar direction by establishing a Secretariat on Palliative and End of Life Care. This group was established by the Canadian government as 'a first step toward creating a Canadian strategy for end-of-life care, including palliative care.'[36]

Strategies like those adopted by Uganda and envisioned by Canada are invaluable in that they provide national leadership, provide a focus for the various activities that comprise a public health response, and set goals and outcome measures for palliative care. Even in the absence of a formal national strategy, however, there is much that the public sector can accomplish. Although the US Public Health Service has not developed a domestic strategy for palliative care, for example, it has promulgated guidelines for pain management,[37] and has made palliative care a key element of its global HIV/AIDS strategy.[38]

A national palliative care strategy must be harmonized with other national health approaches. This is particularly important in relation to national AIDS and cancer programs and with initiatives supporting home- and community-based care. The Canadian Palliative Care Association has developed guidelines for developing palliative care standards[39] that can serve as guidance for the process of strategy development.

FINANCING AND REIMBURSEMENT

Adequate reimbursement for palliative care services is essential if access is to grow. Resources available for healthcare are limited even in the wealthiest societies – finding the appropriate mix of curative and palliative investments is an ongoing challenge for public health policy makers. There is a range of approaches to public financing of palliative care services. In the UK, for example, palliative care, including hospice care, is funded as part of the mix of health services supported by the National Health Service. In contrast, in the USA, public resources do not generally support palliative care apart from the Medicare Hospice Benefit – a mechanism that focuses on care for those who have been determined to have less than 6 months to live. This has had the effect of making integration of palliative care across earlier stages of illness difficult. In many parts of the world, palliative care is only made available through private charitable organizations or international donors.[40]

Although public support through strategic planning, financing, consumer protection, and quality assurance is critical to the expansion of quality palliative care, it is essential that government policies create an environment that allows private sector creativity, participation, and leadership in health policy and program development. Most advances in palliative care and the hospice movement, in the developed and developing world, have begun in nongovernmental organizations and the private sector. Important examples can be found at every point along the way from Dame Saunders' seminal work at St Christopher's Hospice in London in 1967 to the formation of the African Palliative Care Association in 2004.[41]

CONSUMER PROTECTION AND QUALITY ASSURANCE

Development of standards of care and exercise of oversight to ensure that they are met and applied equitably and consistently are important public health responsibilities. In some cases such oversight is conducted through governmental associations. For example, in the USA, the Medicare Hospice Benefit also requires hospices to conduct comprehensive assessments of the quality of care provided.[42] In Uganda, the Ministry of Health has established detailed specifications for implementing palliative care in the healthcare system.[43] Oversight is also conducted through private voluntary associations. For example, in the USA the National Hospice and Palliative Care Organization has developed standards of care for hospice programs that have been widely promulgated.[44] Similarly, the Canadian Hospice and Palliative Care Association developed standards of practice for hospice and palliative care to guide the development of national standards of care.[45] Accreditation programs exist in many countries and typically operate nationally. In the USA, these programs include the Joint Commission on Accreditation of Healthcare Organizations,[46,47] the Community Healthcare Accreditation Program,[48] and the Accreditation Commission for Health Care.[49]

Education

Educational efforts must be directed to the general public, media, policy makers, business leaders, and community leaders as well as to health professionals and others who come into contact with the sick. Public education is necessary to mobilize communities, prompt advocacy, offer hope, and make people aware that there are better ways to approach illness and death than is generally expected. In the USA an initiative supported by the Robert Woods Johnson Foundation, called 'Last Acts', has used various forms of media and outreach to focus on 'educating the lay public, informing medical and health care professionals and promoting social change and policy reform as a means for developing quality care for people nearing the end of life'.[50]

Although education has been a primary focus of the palliative care movement, there is much room for improvement. The need for palliative care education was probably most clearly demonstrated in a 1995 US study that found that over a 5-year period about half of 9105 terminally ill patients being cared for in teaching hospitals spent their dying days in moderate or severe pain.[51] Several studies since then have also documented the poor state of palliative care both in regard to inadequate management of pain or other symptoms[52,53] and in regard to inadequate palliative care education.[54–60] Fortunately, training in palliative care has been identified as a priority over the past decade, and there have been significant increases in the time devoted to palliative care in the basic training of doctors and nurses.[61,62]

Important professional training initiatives are underway in many parts of the world. These range from the creation of academic departments and funded faculty positions in palliative care through distance-based learning programs to practical hands-on training in clinical settings. There will always be a need for specialized palliative care training, but it is important that palliative care education becomes part of the fundamental educational package offered to aspiring health professionals as palliative care is a complementary, not an alternative, therapy. To this end, in 2000 the Liaison Committee on Medical Education, the accrediting board for medical schools in the USA, mandated that every school's curriculum was to include end-of-life care.[63] In an effort to increase the availability of palliative care to all patients with limited prognosis, an International Working Group convened by the European School of Oncology has promulgated the use of both specialized palliative care provided by trained palliative specialists and basic palliative care provided by all healthcare professionals.[64]

The WHO's 1990 report, *Cancer Pain Relief and Palliative Care*,[65] identified several areas that professional education should include: training on attitudes, beliefs and values conducive to a palliative care approach (including ethics, multidisciplinary approaches, personal attitudes toward death and illness, and multidimensional aspects of illness); knowledge base (communication skills, pathophysiology of common symptoms, assessment and management of pain and symptoms, psychological and spiritual needs and their treatment, family and caregiver issues, community resources, and bereavement); and skills (goal setting, care plan development, and monitoring of management).

Ensuring access to medications

Crucial to the successful implementation of an effective palliative care program is a national policy to ensure that drugs are available to care for patients requiring palliative care, especially those used for pain management. The WHO has developed a method of relieving cancer pain that is effective in about 90 percent of these patients.[60] The WHO also recommends this method for people with AIDS because no distinction is made between patients with cancer and patients with AIDS. The WHO guidelines incorporate a stepwise approach whereby the clinician is advised to match a patient's reported pain intensity with the potency of the analgesic to be prescribed (see Chapter 48). As pain increases from mild to moderate or severe, so the medication suggested increases from nonopioids with or with-out an adjuvant medication to opioids or stronger opioids, possibly with this adjuvant medication. Morphine is generally regarded as the gold standard analgesic to control pain that is greater than mild severity, but its availability is sometimes restricted, especially in developing parts of the world (see, for example, Chapters 4, 5 and 7).

The primary obstacles to the availability of these drugs are regulatory and policy obstacles and lack of infrastructure necessary to ensure that these drugs are not misused or diverted. Moreover, in many parts of the world, only doctors can prescribe these drugs. In areas where there are few doctors, access to pain medications becomes especially problematic. Therefore, in these areas, it is imperative that nurses and general practitioners be properly trained and enabled to prescribe opioids. Uganda provides a commendable example of a country that has overcome the obstacle of morphine prescribing only by physicians. Based on a law that allowed midwives to prescribe pethidine (meperidine) for labor, a statute was altered that allowed nurses who are qualified in palliative care to administer morphine. At least one palliative care nurse specialist, who has been trained for 9 months by Hospice Uganda, is planned to be available to prescribe morphine in each district and each district referral hospital.[66] The issue of diversion of these medications to the black market and their subsequent misuse must be taken seriously. Mechanisms to monitor these medications through enhanced drug logistics and supply systems is a critical public health function. Again, we have a synergistic effect of enhanced public health benefiting improved palliative care.

Research

Clearly, tracking the scope of pain and suffering should be a vital concern that benefits public health and the public good. There is a clear need to develop an evidence base for policy and programs. Documentation of chronic illness, pain and symptoms and their management through epidemiological and demographic and health surveys should be integral in both developed and developing countries. Research is needed to identify salient characteristics of successful palliative care programs. Studies must be performed that describe and analyze practice, policy, and advocacy to inform future developments and research for building programs that achieve the varied goals of palliative care, that is, achieving the best quality of life for patients and their families.

To minimize risk of failure, it is important that new or expanding palliative care projects in developing countries understand both the successes and failures of existing programs.[67] Several key issues have recently been identified as research topics for investigation, including: availability of pain relieving drugs, pain and symptom control, access to services, education and training, identification of relevant needs and determination of outcomes for care at the community level, and evaluation of the impact of education of policy makers and program directors about palliative care.[68] Given the magnitude of palliative care required by people living in developing regions of the world, programs must also consider coverage and not simply strive to provide high-quality care to a few patients.

ADDRESSING PALLIATIVE CARE THROUGH AN EXPANDING PUBLIC HEALTH PARADIGM

Public health focuses on health promotion and prevention of disease and has often seen pain and suffering as removed from the public health paradigm, to be addressed by tertiary care in a biomedical/clinical model. Although the WHO[69] and various scholars[70] have long argued a broadening of the concept of health to include how well people are able to perform their daily tasks, only recently has daily functioning begun to be included routinely in the assessment of people's health status through measures of health-related quality of life. Simple measures have been tested and adapted for use in resource-poor settings.[71–73] Investigators are going beyond the traditional paradigm that views health only in terms of adherence to or deviation from physical or biochemical markers. Instead, they are including in their assessment of health, people's own reports of their sense of wellbeing and their ability to perform valued social roles.[74,75] Therefore, pain and suffering should be measured through epidemiological and social science methods, as a critical health condition that should be tracked just as we track infectious diseases. By expanding the public health paradigm to include and promote palliative care, we further the goals of

public health – prevention of disease and prolonging life in society. A redefined model of palliative care is not only applicable to the AIDS epidemic. As life expectancy increases and medical advances are being made, people are living longer with chronic diseases. Therefore, an integrated model of palliative care has practical and pragmatic implications for public health universally. Marginalizing those in need of palliative care services to clinical specialists or ignoring them entirely creates a society in dire need of public health action and intervention.

Key learning points

- Palliative care is an important public health issue that has been markedly shaped over the past 20 years by the AIDS pandemic.

- With the emergence of HIV/AIDS, and the ever-increasing need to mobilize communities, adopt prevention measures, and increase access to services, an integrated public health model that spans the continuum of the illness and addresses not only clinical, but also material, psychosocial and spiritual needs of the patient is needed.

- The WHO has identified three elements as necessary to further sustainable palliative care:[35,36] governmental policy (establishing national policies, making sure that palliative care is harmonized with national health and social service agendas); education (of health professionals, the public, and media, policy makers, and others); and ensuring access to pain medications. A public health approach would additionally emphasize the important role of research, and development of a strong evidence base from which to build programs and policies.

- Pain and suffering should be measured through epidemiological and social science methods, as a critical health condition that should be tracked just as we track infectious diseases.

- By expanding the public health paradigm to include and promote palliative care, we further the goals of public health – prevention of disease and prolonging life in society.

- Therefore, an integrated model of palliative care has practical and pragmatic implications for public health universally.

- Marginalizing those in need of palliative care services to clinical specialists or ignoring them entirely creates a society in dire need of public health action and intervention.

REFERENCES

1   European Observatory on Health Systems and Policies. www. euro.who.int/observatory/glossary/toppage?phrase=public+ health (accessed 10 June 2006).

2 National Academy of Sciences. *The Future of Public Health*. Washington, DC: National Academies Press, 2004. Available at: www.nap.edu (accessed 10 June 2006).

3a Pan American Health Organization/World Health Organization, Centers for Disease Control and Prevention, Centro Latino Americano de Investigación en Sistemas de Salud. Public Health in the Americas. Instrument for Performance Measurement of Essential Public Health Functions. www.phppo.cdc.gov/dphsdr/whoccphp/documents/Instrument.doc (accessed 10 June 2006).

3b Acheson Report: www.archive.official-documents.co.uk/document/doh/ih/synopsis.htm (accessed 11 June 2006).

4 National Academy of Sciences. *The Future of Public Health in the 21st Century*. National Academies Press, 2003. Accessed online at www.nap.edu (accessed 10 June 2006).

5 Sepulvada C, Marlin A, Yoshida T, Ullrich A. The World Health Organization's global perspective. *J Pain Symptom Manage* 2002; **24**: 91–6.

6 UNFPA. State of the world population 2004: journalists' press kit. Available at: www.unfpa.org/swp/2004/presskit/summary.htm (accessed 10 June 2006).

7 United Nations Population Division. *World Population Prospects. The 2002 Revision Highlights*. United Nations, 2003. Available at: www.un.org/esa/population/publications/wpp2002/WPP2002-HIGHLIGHTSrev1.PDF (accessed 10 June 2006).

8 United Nations Population Division. *World Population Prospects. The 2004 Revision Population Database*. United Nations, 2005. Available at: http://esa.un.org/unpp/index.asp?panel=2 (accessed 10 June 2006).

9 Singer PA, Bowman KW. Quality end-of-life care: a global perspective. *BMC Palliat Care* 2002; **1**: 4.

10 World Health Organization. World Health Organization launches new initiative to address the health needs of a rapidly ageing population, 2004. Available at: www.who.int/mediacentre/news/releases/2004/pr60/en/ (accessed 10 June 2006).

11 Davies E, Higginson IJ. *Better Palliative Care for Older People*. Denmark: World Health Organization, 2004.

12 Davies E, Higginson IJ. *Palliative Care: The Solid Facts*. Denmark: World Health Organization, 2004.

13 World Health Organization, International Union Against Cancer. *Global Action Against Cancer*. Geneva: WHO and IUCC. Available at: www.who.int/cancer/media/en/788.pdf (accessed 10 June 2006).

14 Joint United Nations Programme on AIDS. *Executive Summary. 2004 Report on the Global Epidemic AIDS*. Available at: www.unaids.org/bangkok2004/GAR2004_html/ExecSummary_en/Execsumm_en.pdf (accessed 10 June 2006).

15 National Intelligence Council. The Next Wave of HIV/AIDS: Nigeria, Ethiopia, Russia, India, and China, 2002. Available at: www.aegis.org/news/usis/2004/us040209.html (accessed 11 June 2006).

16 Poullier J-P, Hernandez P, Kawabata K, Savedoff WD. Patterns of Global Health Expenditures: Results for 191 Countries. Geneva: WHO, 2002, EIP/HFS/FAR Discussion Paper No. 51. Available at: www3.who.int/whosis/discussion_papers/pdf/paper51.pdf (accessed 11 June 2006).

17 World Health Organization. Global cancer rates could increase by 50% to 15 million by 2020. Available at: www.who.int/mediacentre/news/releases/2003/pr27/en/print.html (accessed 11 June 2006).

18 World Health Organization. Tobacco Free Initiative. Available at: www.who.int/tobacco/about/en (accessed 11 June 2006).

19 World Health Organization. The World Health Organization says that tobacco is bad economics all around, 2004. Available at: www.who.int/mediacentre/news/releases/2004/pr36/en/ (accessed 11 June 2006).

20 http://web.worldbank.org/WBSITE/EXTERNAL/TOPICS/EXTPOVERTY/EXTPA/0,contentMDK:20153855~menuPK:435040~pagePK:148956~piPK:216618~theSitePK:430367,00.html (accessed 11 June 2006).

21 *Sydney Morning Herald*. Clean water – simply astounding, 2004. Available at: www.smh.com.au/articles/2004/08/27/1093518095772.html?from=storyrhs&oneclick=true (accessed 11 June 2006).

22 World Food Programme. Available at: www.wfp.org/aboutwfp/facts/hunger_facts.asp (accessed 11 June 2006).

23 www.iaen.org/impact/stovboll.pdf (accessed 11 June 2006).

24 National Family Caregivers Association. *54 million Americans involved in family caregiving last year – double the previously reported figure*, 2000. Available at: www.thefamilycaregiver.org/who/stats.cmf#1 (accessed 11 June 2006).

25 Arno PS, Levine C, Memmott MM. The economic value of informal caregiving. *Health Aff* 1999; **18**: 182–8.

26 UNICEF. Available at: www.unicef.org/publications/cob_layout6-013.pdf

27 World Bank Group. Urbanization & Cities: Facts & Figures, 2001. Available at: www.worldbank.org/urban/facts.html (accessed 11 June 2006).

28 Available at: www.unhcr.org/cgi-bin/texis/vtx/basics (accessed 12 July 2006).

29 UNAIDS. AIDS: palliative care: UNAIDS technical update. Available at: www.unaids.org (accessed November 8, 2004).

30 O'Neill JF, Selwyn PA, Schietinger H, eds. *A Clinical Guide to Supportive and Palliative Care for HIV/AIDS*. Rockville, MD: US Department of Health and Human Services, 2003.

31 Williams A, Tumwekwase G. Multiple impacts of the HIV/AIDS epidemic on the aged in rural Uganda. *J Cross Cult Gerontol* 2001; **16**: 221–36.

32 Sikkema KJ, Kalichman SC, Hoffmann R, *et al.* Coping strategies and emotional wellbeing among HIV-infected men and women experiencing AIDS-related bereavement. *AIDS Care* 2000; **12**: 613–24.

33 Bigelow G, Hollinger J. Grief and AIDS: surviving catastrophic multiple loss. *Hosp J* 1996; **11**: 83–96.

34 Stjernsward J, Clark D. Palliative medicine – a global perspective. In: Doyle D, Hanks G, Cherny N, Calman K, eds. *Oxford Textbook of Palliative Medicine*, 3rd ed. Oxford: Oxford University Press, 2004.

35 Jagwe JG, Barnard D. The introduction of palliative care in Uganda. *J Palliat Med* 2002; **5**: 160–3.

36 www.hc-sc.gc.ca/hcs-sss/alt_formats/hpb-dgps/pdf/pubs/2005-strateg-palliat/2005-strateg-palliat_e.pdf (accessed 11 June 2006).

37 Agency for Health Care Policy and Research. *Management of Cancer Pain: Clinical Practice Guideline No. 9*. Rockville, MD: US Department of Health and Human Services, 1994. Available at: www.painresearch.utah.edu/cancerpain/guidelineF.html (accessed 13 July 2006).

38 Office of the United States Global AIDS Coordinator in collaboration with the United States Departments of State (including the United States Agency for International Development), Defense, Commerce, Labor, Health and Human

Services (including the Centers for Disease Control and Prevention, the Food and Drug Administration, the Health Resources and Services Administration, the National Institutes of Health, and the Office of Global Health Affairs); and the Peace Corps. *The President's Emergency Plan for AIDS Relief. US Five-Year Global HIV/AIDS Strategy.* Washington, DC: Office of the United States Global AIDS Coordinator, 2004. Available at: www.state.gov/documents/organization/29831.pdf (accessed 11 June 2006).

39 Ferris FD, Cummings I, eds. *Palliative Care: Towards Standardized Principles of Practice.* Ottawa, Ontario: Canadian Palliative Care Association, 1995.

40 O'Neill J, Higginson IJ. HIV/AIDS in the age of palliative care. Foreword. *J R Soc Med* 2001; **94**: 429.

41 African Palliative Care Association. The inaugural conference of the African Palliative Care Association (APCA). Overview – They came in their numbers!! Available at: www.soros.org/initiatives/pdia/articles_publications/publications/inaugural_20040806/apca.pdf (accessed 11 June 2006).

42 Health Care Financing Administration. *Code of Federal Regulations, Part 418 – Hospice Care. (Revised 10/1/97).* Washington, DC: US Government Printing Office, 1997.

43 Ministry of Health, Republic of Uganda. *National Sector Strategic Plan 2000/02–2004/05.* Kampala: Ministry of Health, 2000.

44 National Hospice and Palliative Care Organization. *Standards of Practice for Hospice Programs.* Alexandria, VA: National Hospice and Palliative Care Organization, 2000.

45 Ferris FD, Balfour HM, Bowen K, *et al.* A model to guide patient and family care: based on nationally accepted principles and norms of practice. *J Pain Symptom Manage* 2002: **24**: 106–23.

46 Joint Commission on Accreditation of Healthcare Organizations. *Framework for Improving Performance.* Oakbrook Terrace, IL: JCAHO, 1994.

47 Joint Commission on Accreditation of Healthcare Organizations. *2001–2002 Comprehensive Accreditation Manual for Home Care.* Oakbrook Terrace, Il: JCAHO, 2001.

48 Community Health Accreditation Program, Inc. *Standards of Excellence.* New York: Community Health Accreditation Program, 1997.

49 Accreditation Commission for Health Care. *Hospice Standards,* 2nd ed. Raleigh, NC: Accreditation Commission for Health Care, 2003.

50 Last Acts Partnership. Available at: www.lastactspartnership.org (accessed 11 June 2006).

51 The SUPPORT Principal Investigators. A controlled trial to improve care for seriously ill hospitalized patients. The study to understand prognoses and preferences for outcomes and risks of treatments (SUPPORT). *JAMA* 1995; **274**: 1591–8.

52 Cascinu S, Giordani P, Agostinelli R, *et al.* Pain and its treatment in hospitalized patients with metastatic cancer. *Support Care Cancer* 2003; **11**: 587–92.

53 Norval DA. Symptoms and sites of pain experienced by AIDS patients. *S Afr Med J* 2004; **94**: 450–4.

54 McMillan SC, Tittle M, Hagan S, *et al.* Knowledge and attitudes of nurses in veterans hospitals about pain management in patients with cancer. *Oncol Nurs Forum* 2000; **27**: 1415–23.

55 White KR, Coyne PJ, Patel UB. Are nurses adequately prepared for end-of-life care? *J Nurs Scholarsh* 2001; **33**: 147–51.

56 Van Niekerk LM, Martin F. Tasmanian nurses' knowledge of pain management. *Int J Nurs Stud* 2001; **38**: 141–52.

57 Lai YH, Chen ML, Tsai LY, *et al.* Are nurses prepared to manage cancer pain? A national survey of nurses' knowledge about pain control in Taiwan. *J Pain Symptom Manage* 2003; **26**: 1016–25.

58 Tse MM, Chan BS. Knowledge and attitudes in pain management: Hong Kong nurses' perspective. *J Pain Palliat Care Pharmacother* 2004; **18**: 47–58.

59 Heath DL. Nurses' knowledge and attitudes concerning pain management in an Australian hospital. *Aust J Adv Nurs* 1998; **16**: 15–8.

60 Farber NJ, Urban SY, Collier VU, *et al.* Frequency and perceived competence in providing palliative care to terminally ill patients: a survey of primary care physicians. *J Pain Symptom Manage* 2004; **28**: 364–72.

61 Hillier R, Wee B. From cradle to grave: palliative medicine education in the UK. *J R Soc Med* 2001; **94**: 468–71.

62 Field MJ, Cassel CK, eds. *Approaching Death: Improved Care at the End of Life. Report from the Institute of Medicine Committee on Care at the End of Life.* Washington DC: National Academy Press, 1997.

63 LCME Accreditation Standards. Liaison Committee on Medical Education accreditation standards, 2001. Available at: www.lcme.org/standard.htm (accessed November 8, 2004).

64 Ahmedzai SH, Costa A, Blengini C, *et al.* A new international framework for palliative care. *Eur J Cancer* 2004; **40**: 2192–200.

65 World Health Organization. *Cancer Pain Relief and Palliative Care.* Geneva: World Health Organization, 1990.

66 Merriman A. Uganda: current status of palliative care. *J Pain Symptom Manage* 2002; **24**: 252–6.

67 Higginson IJ, Bruera E. Do we need palliative care audit in developing countries? *Palliat Med* 2002; **16**: 546–7.

68 Harding R, Stewart K, Marconi K, *et al.* Current HIV/AIDS end-of-life care in sub-Saharan Africa: a survey of models, services, challenges and priorities. *BMC Public Health* 2003; **3**: 33–8.

69 World Health Organization. *The Constitution of the World Health Organization.* Geneva: World Health Organization, 1948.

70 DuBos R. *Man Adapting.* New Haven: Yale University Press, 1959.

71 Mast TC, Kigozi G, Wabwire-Mangen F, *et al.* Cultural adaptation, reliability, validity and feasibility of the MOS-HIV Health Survey to measure quality of life in rural Uganda. *Program and Abstracts of the 13th International AIDS Conference, July 9–14, 2000.* Durban, South Africa.

72 Kemerer V, Malitz F, Wolf RC, *et al.* A toolkit of patient-reported outcomes to evaluate care for people with HIV/AIDS in resource constrained settings. *Proceedings of the XV International AIDS Conference, July 11–16, 2004.* Bangkok, Thailand. Abstract 11200.

73 Wolf RC, Butler de Lister M, Weise G, *et al.* Piloting palliative care assessment methods in the Dominican Republic. *Proceedings of the XV International AIDS Conference, July 11–16, 2004.* Bangkok, Thailand. Abstract ThPeE8002.

74 Levine S. The changing terrains in medical sociology: Emergency concern with quality of life. *J Health Soc Behav* 1987; **28**: 1–6.

75 Ware J. *SF-36 Health Survey Manual and Interpretation Guide.* Boston: Nimrod Press, 1993.

10

The future of palliative medicine

CHARLES F VON GUNTEN, IRENE J HIGGINSON

INTRODUCTION

A reliable forecast for the future requires a hard look at the present. Therefore, we have structured this chapter in three parts. First, we broadly summarize the current state of palliative medicine in the world. Details of the development of palliative medicine in various parts of the world have been described in other chapters in this textbook. Second, we summarize the case for a future that rests on a response to three features: the needs of patients and families, demographic changes, and the physician's role in palliative medicine as a distinct subspecialty. Last, we describe the challenges that palliative medicine must face in the future if it is to prosper.

PALLIATIVE MEDICINE NOW

The current state of the field of palliative medicine can be summarized as highly variable. In some countries, such as Australia, Canada, Ireland, New Zealand and the UK, the field is a recognized specialty with organized programs for clinical care, education, and research. In the rest of the industrialized world, including the USA, a broad program of clinical care has emerged without the official recognition that grounds the discipline in the academic foundation of healthcare. In the poorest nations, the name is unknown and the most basic tools for the relief of suffering are unavailable.

One way to look at this is from an institutional change model. In such a model, an innovation (such as palliative medicine) is developed in one location (such as England) and then gradually spreads to other institutions as its merits become known. There is good evidence for this. Hospice Information reports that from a handful of hospices worldwide in the 1970s and 1980s the number of hospices and palliative care programs have grown to involve every continent of the world in around 100 countries. The total number of hospice or palliative care initiatives is in excess of 8000 and include hospice inpatient units, hospital-based palliative care services, community-based teams and day care centers. Unfortunately, change has been slow. In England 96 000 new patients were cared for by palliative home care teams in 2003–04, and 27 000 died in an in-patient hospice or palliative care unit: 95 percent of these patients had cancer. In the same year the number of cancer deaths in England was around 140 000, suggesting that around 65 percent of patients with cancer receive care from a palliative care/hospice home care team, and 18 percent die in a hospice. Over 100 000 new patients are seen by hospital palliative care teams each year, some of these go on to receive home care and/or hospice care. Hospital palliative care teams see more patients with noncancer conditions – on average around 11 percent of patients, but this ranges from 0 percent to almost 40 percent.[1] In the USA, nearly 25 percent of those who die receive hospice care, mostly in their homes.

Another way to look at the current state of affairs is from an economic point of view. Those countries that have most developed palliative care are comparatively wealthy countries where palliative care is paid for after other services are covered. In contrast, in poorer countries where it hasn't yet developed, healthcare funds are spent in other ways. In this world view, any money spent on palliative care in developing countries can be construed as a failure to provide the standard healthcare available in other countries. In other words, patients who can't get standard healthcare are given morphine in order to ease their otherwise preventable death.

Finally, the development of palliative medicine can be viewed from a public health point of view. An argument can be made that the most significant healthcare developments of the past century relate to health promotion (e.g. nutrition), prevention (e.g. sanitation, smoking cessation), and palliation (e.g. pain relief). In this model, palliative medicine is a basic approach to healthcare that even the poorest countries can assure their citizens.

THE FUTURE OF PALLIATIVE MEDICINE

The future of palliative medicine rests on the responses to three features.

Meeting patient and family needs

People with serious chronic illness, and their families, experience a remarkably similar set of needs that are relatively independent of the specific disease or diseases from which they suffer. These can be categorized in the physical, psychological (emotional), social (practical), and spiritual (existential) domains. The prevalence of symptoms such as pain, breathlessness, and fatigue ranges from 50 percent to 80 percent.[2] Psychological conditions such as depression and anxiety affect both patient and family. The social domain includes family and community relationships and support and the need for services be provided. This includes the patient's and family's need for information and training. Finally, the spiritual or existential domain involves the search for meaning and is often affected by serious illness.

Fortunately, there is growing evidence that palliative care is an effective response to these needs. When pain and symptoms are controlled, information is shared, family and caregivers are supported, and services are coordinated, healthcare outcomes are improved at reasonable cost.

Responding to demographic changes

People in both the developed and developing world are aging and live longer. The proportion of those living more than 65 years into very old age is also increasing rapidly. The pattern of disease from which these people die is now characterized by chronic progressive illnesses, including the frailty syndrome of advanced age. This means there will be more people needing healthcare toward the end of life.

At the same time as there is growth in the numbers of people who need care, there is a decrease in the number of both formal and informal caregivers. Innovative ways of providing care are needed. One component of that plan is palliative care.

Developing a unique physician role

The development of the palliative medicine role within the multiprofessional teams who deliver palliative care within hospitals, inpatient units, nursing facilities, or patient's homes is a significant development of the past 50 years. The future of palliative medicine rests on the strength of the case for the field as a distinct specialty. The specialty of palliative medicine has moved from an emerging discipline to a recognized area of expertise in part of the world. It is formally recognized as a distinct specialty in Great Britain, Ireland, Australia, and Canada (see Chapter 8). Its formal recognition is under active review in the USA.[3,4] We can expect similar recognition in other countries for the following reasons.

A DISTINCT BODY OF KNOWLEDGE

A distinct body of scientific knowledge in palliative medicine has accumulated over the past 40 years. The emergence of specialized journals, well-regarded textbooks, and formal curricula are all indicators. This textbook is but one repository. That knowledge is expressed in a variety of scientific and academic endeavors. For instance, the Cochrane Collaborative has a pain, palliative care and supportive care review group which has produced over 50 reviews and over 40 protocols.[5–10] In 2004, the UK government published guidance from the National Institute for Clinical Excellence on supportive and palliative care in cancer.[11] The guidance had reviewed the evidence for the effectiveness in 13 areas of supportive and palliative care, including communication, information, psychological support, specialist palliative care, end-of-life, care and rehabilitation.[12] Also in 2004, the National Consensus Project for Quality Palliative Care published clinical practice guidelines for quality palliative care based on an extensive evidence review and consensus process with the major US palliative care organizations.[13] Addressing the needs of policy makers, the World Health Organization (WHO) European Office produced evidence-based guidance on palliative care in two complementary booklets: *Palliative Care: The Solid Facts*[14] dealt with general palliative care issues, future needs, and evidence, and *Better Palliative Care for Older People*[15] dealt with the need to address the demographic changes in society and take a public health approach to palliative care. Most recently, the US National Institutes of Health conducted a state-of-the-science conference in December 2004. The literature review for the conference covered over 16 000 references,[16] and built on previous references.

The major skills central to palliative medicine are the assessment and management of physical, psychological, and spiritual suffering faced by patients with life-limiting illnesses and their families. Communication and teamwork are also critical skills in palliative medicine.

PUBLICATION OF SCHOLARLY RESEARCH

New knowledge is being discovered at an expanding rate. Research in the area of palliative medicine appears in at least nine international specialized peer-reviewed journals: *Journal of Palliative Care* (Canada), *Journal of Pain and Symptom Management* (including supportive and palliative care,

USA), *Journal of Palliative Medicine* (USA), *American Journal of Hospice and Palliative Care* (USA), *Palliative Medicine* (UK), *Palliative and Supportive Care* (USA), *Progress in Palliative Care* (Australia), *BMC Palliative Care* (a new web-based rapid publication from biomedcentral. com, an international group), *Supportive Care in Cancer* (Switzerland), and the *European Journal of Palliative Care* (UK). More than one curriculum for palliative medicine has been published.[17–20] Models to guide clinical palliative care have been disseminated[21] and a number of well-regarded textbooks are now available,[22–24] of which the *Oxford Textbook of Palliative Care* is now in its third edition. In fact, Oxford University Press now has a specific division for palliative care, with 96 current offerings (www.oup.com/us/catalog/general/subject/Medicine/PalliativeMedicine/?view =usa; accessed October 27, 2004).

GRADUATE MEDICAL EDUCATION

New specialties are characterized by defined training programs that prepare the holder of an undergraduate medical degree for independent practice. In the UK, individuals begin the 4-year training program in palliative medicine once they have completed their medical degree and around 3 years in general medical posts, including hospital medicine. The Association for Palliative Medicine of Great Britain and Ireland has over 800 members and there are 177 qualified doctors training in the 4-year program to become specialists in palliative medicine (personal communication, S Richards, Association for Palliative Medicine, November 2005). In the USA, there are 47 fellowship programs in operation with a total of 97 physicians in training[25,26] (www.AAHPM.org/fellowship/directory.html; accessed August 21, 2003).

PROFESSIONAL ASSOCIATIONS

New specialties are also characterized by professional associations. The American Academy of Hospice and Palliative Medicine (AAHPM) is the professional association for physicians in palliative medicine in the US. The AAHPM currently has 1900 physician members (AAHPM, personal communication, October 22, 2004). The Association for Palliative Medicine of Great Britain and Ireland has over 800 members. The European Association for Palliative Care is a membership organization composed, in part, by members of the national associations of countries throughout western and central Europe. Similar associations have formed in southeast Asia.

PRACTICE PATTERNS AND PROFESSIONAL ROLE

The 1997 Institute of Medicine report, *Approaching Death: Improving Care at the End of Life*, delineated a three-tiered structure for professional competence:[18]

1 A basic level of competence in the care of the dying patient for all practitioners.

2 An expected level of palliative and humanistic skills considerably beyond this basic level.
3 A cadre of superlative professionals to develop and provide exemplary care for those approaching death, to guide others in the delivery of such care, and to generate new knowledge to improve care of the dying.

These three levels correspond to the primary, secondary, and tertiary levels around which medical care is commonly organized. Primary palliative care (a term used mainly in the USA; in the UK and Europe the term used is 'the palliative care approach') is the responsibility of all physicians. This includes basic approaches to the relief of suffering and improving quality of life for the whole person and his or her family. Secondary palliative care is the responsibility of specialists and hospital or community based palliative care or hospice programs. The role of the secondary specialist or program is to provide consultation and assist the managing service. Tertiary palliative care is the province of academic centers where new knowledge is created through research, and new knowledge is disseminated through education, as well as providing a clinical service. The major competencies of the specialist level palliative medicine practitioner can be summarized under the broad patient-centered goals of:

- relief of symptoms and suffering
- promotion of quality of life for patients and families in the context of life-threatening illness
- promotion of the development and growth possible at the end of life.

While the knowledge domains and skills of palliative medicine overlap to some extent with the knowledge, attitudes, and skills that characterize other disciplines that care for patients with advanced illnesses, the specialty practice of palliative medicine is distinguished from other disciplines by its focus on the common features and symptoms associated with life-limiting disease. Palliative medicine reaches across many disease categories and organ systems to concentrate on relieving the burden of illness.

The palliative medicine specialist acquires and applies:

- a higher level of clinical expertise in addressing the multidimensional needs of patients with life-threatening illnesses, including a practical skill set in symptom control interventions
- a high level of expertise in both clinical and nonclinical issues related to death and dying
- a commitment to an interdisciplinary team approach
- the strong focus on the patient and family as the unit of care.

The specialist level competency required of practitioners in palliative medicine complements the core competency that should be maintained by other disciplines.

The majority of palliative medicine physicians practice as hospice medical directors and/or as hospital-based consultants. There are now more than 3200 hospice programs in the USA (www.nhpco.org/files/public/Facts_Figures_Jan_03.pdf; accessed August 21, 2003). Medicare-certified hospices are required to have a paid or volunteer staff medical director. The National and Hospice Palliative Care Organization (NHPCO) recently began an initiative to encourage member hospices to strengthen the role and competency of hospice medical directors.[27] Interest in hospital-based palliative care programs is also growing. The Center to Advance Palliative Care states that 800 hospitals now offer palliative care services and the number appears to be increasing by about 20 percent annually.[28] The Center for Workforce Studies at the State University of New York documented that physicians currently working within palliative medicine support formal recognition of the field.[29]

CHALLENGES FOR THE FUTURE

There are a number of challenges that confront the future of the field. These include the response of healthcare policy makers, the definition of the boundaries of the specialty, and the training of the new physicians who are needed.

Healthcare policy

The future of palliative medicine requires a social and political impetus that is beyond the scope of medicine and firmly in the sphere of government. For palliative medicine to prosper, healthcare policy must place much greater emphasis on the care of people of all ages who are living with and dying from a range of serious chronic diseases. The structure of health care *as if* these prevalent illnesses are acute and curable must be changed. Therefore, publicly funded palliative care services as a core part of health care is needed; it cannot be an 'add-on extra'. Those services must meet the needs in the rural and urban community dwelling public as well as in nursing homes and hospitals, including intensive care. Those services must be based on need rather than on specific diseases or prognosis. Finally, healthcare policy must provide for the development of new knowledge through research. Despite the prevalence of palliative care need, national research budgets are paltry. Surely we don't want to be using the same tools in 50 years that we have now.

Professional boundaries

A significant issue that confronts the future of the field is whether it focuses on a condition (the dying patient) or relates to a broader set of competencies that can be integrated across the spectrum of serious and chronic illness. The roots of palliative medicine in hospice care for the dying would lend itself to the former. The experience of hospital-based and outpatient office based palliative medicine physicians suggests that the skills are more broadly applicable than just for the dying.

Palliative medicine is practiced within the context of a team. Some would say it cannot be practiced without a team. Yet, the broad interdisciplinary nature of palliative medicine makes it more challenging to define the boundaries of the specialty than for those with a disease focus (such as oncology), an organ focus (such as cardiology) or a technical skill (such as surgery). As with other fields, there are areas of overlap with other specialties and subspecialties. Delineating and negotiating those boundaries is an important aspect of the maturation of the discipline. There is little argument that palliative medicine is primarily a consulting specialty to the other primary disciplines. There is no agenda, expressed or implied, that all suffering and dying patients be cared for by physicians board certified in palliative medicine.

Developing new and appropriate models of care in response to the different trajectories of illness and diseases

Although the symptom and problem profiles of patients with different chronic progressive conditions are similar, the trajectory of diseases is likely to vary. In addition, caring for older people, an increasing part of the palliative care population, has specific challenges – notably iatrogenic disease, multiple pathologies, and difficulties in prognostication. The early models of palliative care may have to evolve to care for these patients. In particular the model of consultation and palliative care offered for periods throughout the illness, rather than at a particular prognostic point, may have to develop. It will be a challenge for palliative medicine to develop and test such models of care, while maintaining existing services.

Fundraising and/or remaining part of statutory funded care

Currently much of palliative care is provided within the voluntary sector and not for profit organizations. These have a continued battle to raise funds to stand still – and provide a continued service to the community. The charitable sector is set to become more competitive in years to come and is subject to fluctuations in response to economic changes. Becoming part of the statutory sector or receiving increased statutory funds removes some of the freedom of previously voluntary units, although it provides more security. Achieving the right balance here can be a challenge, especially as national charity organizations in some countries (e.g. the charity commission in the UK) provide guidance that charities should not undertake tasks which should be provided by statutory services. Perhaps more and more the role of charitable organizations will be to innovate and discover better treatments and ways to care, while they advocate for the statutory sector to pick up the funding of the services they have proved, through good research, is effective and cost-effective.

Training

Another challenge to the field is to build enough capacity within training programs to train the next generation of specialists. The current interest in developing training programs is heartening, but financial resources are scarce and competition for them is strong. In England, palliative care posts go unfilled for want of trained specialists. In the USA, where the field is only emerging, a similar shortage is emerging. There is no reason to think this won't be the case in other countries unless the field is recognized and sufficient capacity built into the nation's programs for training medical professionals. There is an inherent challenge here, because the field needs the best dedicated and bright clinicians, who have undergone sufficient training. Therefore, a balance needs to be struck between filling posts and filling them with sufficiently experienced and qualified individuals who have the ability to deliver the services and development needed.

Palliative medicine clinicians often find themselves in leadership roles and so have to not only provide clinical care, but also be versed in managing and motivating staff, strategically developing their services and often negotiating contracts and teaching other doctors. Burnout is likely to be a problem in palliative care, especially if clinicians are isolated and asked to cover services 24 hours, without backup or peer support, as well as to deal with issues of staff management and service development. Equally, problems can arise in academic posts, where filling posts with individuals without sufficiently robust track records or from fields outside of palliative medicine, can lead to loss of respect for the field or a distraction of effort away from palliative medicine patients.

Research

A major challenge for the future of palliative medicine is to become a strong specialty for the future. Knowledge has to be a central key to this. If the specialty is to make a real contribution to the future care of patients and families then the evidence base for the treatment of many symptoms and problems needs to be improved. Unfortunately research has been relatively neglected in the past. There has been inadequate funding in all countries, a hesitancy on the part of some ethics committees and institutional review boards to fully support research, and a reluctance of some staff, who entered the specialty because they felt it did not involve research. There are problems too because of the nature of research in palliative care, which is often difficult because of ethical concerns, the intangible nature of many aspects to be measured (e.g. fatigue, quality of life, quality of death) and the fact that patients are ill and difficult to interview. They may live for unpredictable times. Weighed against this we should recognize that there have been enormous achievements in research in palliative medicine in the past decades, despite these problems and the lack of resources. This is a tribute to the few centers and individuals who are researching the field. In the future, an improved training in appraising and participating in research is needed for doctors and nurses entering the field. It is not expected that everyone will conduct research, but all will need to appraise it, and may increasingly be part of large studies organized in tertiary centers.

SUMMARY

In summary, there can be a bright future for palliative medicine. There is widespread need within society and this is set to increase in the future. There is now a body of good quality evidence showing that palliative medicine within palliative care programs can meet the need. The challenge is clear. The field needs to grow to sufficient size to be a sustainable response. It also needs to develop mechanisms to meet the challenge of the changing population, and in particular the increase in the older population and changed trajectory of illness, it needs to continually improve the caliber and skills of those in the field, through training, and to invest substantially in discovering and testing better methods of care and treatment.

Key learning points

- Palliative medicine is highly variable in the world.

- The evidence base supports the effectiveness of palliative care.

- The demographic changes in the world's populations (living longer with more chronic ultimately fatal disease) require expanded palliative care services.

- The development of a unique palliative medicine role for the physician within multiprofessional teams is a phenomenon likely to develop in most countries.

- Expanding clinical services to meet the needs of patients and families will require both modifications in patterns of care as well as expansion of the numbers of trained physicians and other professionals needed to provide palliative care.

REFERENCES

- 1 National Council for Palliative Care. *National Survey of Patient Activity Data for Specialist Palliative Care Services.* London: National Council for Palliative Care, 2005.
- 2 Solano JP, Gomes B, Higginson IJ. A comparison of symptom prevalence in far advanced cancer, AIDS, heart disease, chronic obstructive pulmonary disease (COPD) and renal disease. *J Pain Symptom Manage* 2006; **31**: 58–69.

3   von Gunten CF, Lupu D. Development of a medical subspecialty in palliative medicine: progress report. *J Palliat Med* 2004; **7**: 209–19.

4   Foley K. Advancing palliative care in the United States. *Palliat Med* 2003; **17**: 89–91.

◆ 5   http://www.consensus.nih.gov/2004/2004EndofLifeCare. 505024html.htm (accessed May 11, 2006).

◆ 6   The Cochrane Pain, Palliative Care and Supportive Care Group (PaPaS) website. http://www.jr2.ox.ac.uk/cochrane/ (accessed October 26, 2004).

7   JAMA patient page. Decisions about end-of-life care. *JAMA* 2000; **284**: 2550.

8   JAMA & Archives. End-of-life Care/ Palliative Medicine. http://jama.ama-assn.org/cgi/collection/endoflife_care_ palliative_medicine (accessed October 27, 2004).

◆ 9   Morrison RS, Meier DE. Clinical practice. Palliative care. *N Engl J Med* 2004; **350**: 2582–90.

10   Cochrane Pain, Palliative Care And Supportive Care Group. Abstracts of Cochrane Reviews. *Cochrane Library* Issue 2, 2005. http://www.cochrane.org/cochrane/revabstr/ SYMPTAbstractIndex.htm (accessed October 27, 2004).

✱ 11   National Institute of Clinical Excellence (NICE). *Improving Supportive and Palliative Care for Adults With Cancer – The Manual.* London: NICE, 2004.

◆ 12   Gysels M, Higginson IJ. I*mproving Supportive and Palliative Care for adults With Cancer: Research Evidence.* London: NICE, 2004. Available at: www.nice.org.uk/pdf/ csgsresearchevidence.pdf (accessed October 26, 2004).

✱ 13   National Consensus Project for Quality Palliative Care. *Clinical Practice Guidelines for Quality Palliative Care.* 2004.

14   Davies E, Higginson IJ. *Palliative Care: The Solid Facts.* Denmark: World Health Organization, 2004.

15   Davies E, Higginson IJ. *Better Palliative Care for Older People.* Denmark: World Health Organization, 2004.

16   State of the Science. *J Palliat Med* 2005; 9(Suppl 1).

17   Billings JA, Block SD, Finn JW, *et al.* Initial voluntary program standards for fellowship training in palliative medicine. *J Palliat Med* 2002; **5**: 23–33.

◆ 18   Field MJ, Cassel CK, eds. *Approaching Death: Improving Care at the End of Life.* Washington, DC: National Academy Press, 1997: 208.

◆ 19   Emanuel LL, von Gunten CF, Ferris FD, eds. The Education for Physicians on End-of-life Care (EPEC) Curriculum, 1999. Available at: www.epec.net (accessed October 26, 2004).

20   Schonwetter RS, Hawke W, Knight CF, eds. *Hospice and Palliative Medicine Core Curriculum and Review Syllabus.* American Academy of Hospice and Palliative Medicine. Dubuque IO: Kendall/Hunt Publishing Company, 1999.

21   Ferris F, Balfour H, Bowen K, *et al.* A model to guide patient and family care. Based on nationally accepted principles and norms of practice. *J Pain Symptom Manage* 2002; **24**: 106–23.

22   Berger AM, Portenoy RK, Weissman DE. *Principles and Practice of Palliative Care and Supportive Oncology.* Philadelphia: Lippincott-Raven, 2002.

23   Doyle D, Hanks GW, MacDonald N, eds. *Oxford Textbook of Palliative Medicine,* 3rd ed. Oxford: Oxford University Press, 2003.

24   Portenoy RK, Bruera EB, eds. *Topics in Palliative Care,* Vol 5. New York: Oxford University Press, 2001.

25   Billings JA. Palliative medicine fellowship programs in the United States: Year 2000 survey. *J Palliat Med* 2000; **3**: 391–6.

26   von Gunten CF, Sloan P, Portenoy R, Schonwetter R. Physician board certification in hospice and palliative medicine. *J Palliat Med* 2000; **3**:441–7.

27   National and Hospice Palliative Care Organization. Providing direct billable physician services to hospice patients: An opportunity to upgrade the medical component of hospice care. Alexandria, VA: NHPCO, 2003.

28   Pan CS, Morrison RS, Meier DE, *et al.* How prevalent are hospital-based palliative care programs? Status report and future directions. *J Palliat Med* 2001; **4**: 315–24.

29   Cohen B, Salsberg E. The supply, demand and use of palliative care physicians in the United States. A report prepared for the Bureau of HIV/AIDS, Health Resources and Services Administration. Albany, NY: Center for Health Workforce Studies, School of Public Health, University at Albany, September 2002 (http://chws.albany.edu).

PART 2

Bioethics

11

Principles of bioethics in palliative care

PAULINA TABOADA

INTRODUCTION

Ethical challenges in palliative medicine do not substantially differ from those encountered in other areas of medicine.[1,2] Nevertheless, the recognition of the needs of patients at the end of life demands some moral attitudes, skills, and knowledge that enable adequate decision making in relation to the unique sources of suffering encountered in the dying and their relatives.[3]

> Simply stated, ethical issues in palliative care center around decisions which will enable us to satisfy the criteria for a peaceful death, dignified and assisted by a helpful society.
> Roy and MacDonald, p. 97[3]

Hence, two basic moral attitudes belong to the very essence of palliative medicine:

1 An unconditional respect for human life and dignity even in situations of extreme weakness.
2 The acceptance of human finitude and death.[4]

In this context, other moral attitudes also acquire a special relevance, such as the virtues of truthfulness, prudence, and compassion.[5]

When dealing with concrete moral challenges in the care for terminally ill patients, the application of adequate methods for the systematization of ethical problems (Box 11.1) as well as basic knowledge of some ethical principles may help healthcare professionals.[5–11] In this chapter I shall briefly unfold the basic content of some of the ethical principles that are specially relevant in palliative care (Box 11.2). However, I will emphasize that the fundamental moral attitudes and virtues orienting healthcare professionals when caring for the dying are actually more important than the mere application of ethical principles to particular situations.[4,5,12]

Box 11.1 Systematization of the ethical analysis of clinical cases

1 Define the specific ethical dilemma/s
2 Refer to the ethical principles involved
3 Collect and analyze the 'ethically relevant' clinical information
4 Review alternative courses of action
5 Formulate an ethical solution
6 Consider the best way of implementing the solution

Box 11.2 Ethical principles specially relevant in palliative care

The four basic principles of contemporary bioethics:

- Nonmaleficence
- Beneficence
- Autonomy
- Justice

Other traditional principles generally acknowledged in medical ethics:

- Respect for human life and death
- Therapeutic proportionality
- Double effect
- Truthfulness in communication
- Prevention
- Nonabandonment

ETHICAL PRINCIPLES RELEVANT IN PALLIATIVE CARE

The four basic principles of contemporary bioethics

Beneficence and nonmaleficence have traditionally been the leading principles of medical ethics.[13] They correspond to the first and most general ethical intuition: do the good and avoid the bad (*bonum est faciendum, malum vitandi*). Hence Hippocrates thought that the first medical duty is to benefit or at least 'not to harm' (*primum non nocere*). Moreover, he deduced from this general duty a number of concrete consequences reflected in the Hippocratic Oath. For many centuries the Hippocratic tradition was taken for granted by the medical profession. Ethical principles and values contained in the Hippocratic Oath were applied to solve ethical dilemmas in medical practice without any further questioning of their origin or validity.

With the influence of positivism, this way of doing medical ethics was questioned and regarded as 'naive'. Ross' establishment of *prima facie* duties and its incorporation to ethical analysis was considered as a more 'scientific' approach to ethics, at least in the Anglo-Saxon world.[14] As a result of the application of this approach to medical ethics a trend arose known as *principlism*. This approach claims the existence of four self-evident ethical principles that serve to represent and codify the main values underlying medical ethics: nonmaleficence, beneficence, autonomy, and justice:[15]

- Nonmaleficence – do not harm (minimize the harm).
- Beneficence – do good (always act in the patient's best interest).
- Autonomy – acknowledge the patient's rights to self-determination.
- Justice – allocate healthcare resources equitably, according to need.

It is interesting to note that the principle of autonomy – not contained in the Hippocratic tradition – entered medical ethics much later as part of this system of *prima facie* principles devised to deal with moral pluralism.

Although to some extent useful, the principlist approach to solving moral dilemmas in medical praxis has not been exempt from contradictions and criticisms.[16–18] For instance, the concrete content of the so-called 'four basic principles of bioethics' is neither clearly specified nor secured, since the principlist approach does not provide an anthropological foundation for them. Moreover, in this system each principle is given equal weight. Thus, if two or more of the four basic principles conflict with each other this approach does not provide a clear-cut answer as to which of them should be given priority. In the Anglo-Saxon world, the general tendency is to grant moral hegemony to the principle of autonomy. According to this approach, the priority among principles can be definitively established only when the detailed circumstances of the particular situation are known. It therefore entails the risks of situation ethics.

To solve these difficulties, Gracia proposed that the four principles of bioethics should be placed on two levels, based on the distinction between *perfect* and *imperfect* moral duties.[19–22] This approach is known as *specified principlism*. Perfect duties are moral minimums or negative prescriptions, which ought to be respected always, regardless of the circumstances. According to Gracia nonmaleficence and justice belong to this category. Imperfect duties are ethical maximums or positive prescriptions that allow different degrees of fulfillment and Gracia lists beneficence and autonomy among the latter.

A number of other authors have also criticized principlism. Indeed Pellegrino, for instance, states that current bioethics is undergoing an 'anti-principlist' crisis.[13] Faced with this sort of 'crisis' of contemporary bioethics and looking toward the future, Pellegrino proposed virtue ethics.[23,24] Virtue theory as applied to medicine emphasizes that physicians should acquire good traits of character more than just learning about moral theories and principles.[25] Thus ethical inquiry in particular issues asks about the way in which a good person – a good physician in our case – would act if he or she were confronted with a similar situation.

Presently, a trend is opening in ethics toward a renewed discovery of the value of the person (*personalism*).[26–30] According to this approach, it is not duty as duty, or law as law, or principles as principles, or utility as utility, etc. that defines the content of moral obligations – as has been suggested by other major ethical trends. Personalism proposes that it is rather the dignity and the ontological structure of the person that defines the content of our moral duties.[26] The core of moral reasoning is derived here from the statement that the proper addressee for a moral subject is a concrete person. Hence, the most basic norm of morality is: *Persona est affirmanda propter seipsam et propter dignitatem suam* (the person shall be affirmed because of herself and because of her dignity).[26,28] In other words, the clue for the resolution of ethical dilemmas in medicine is the respect due to each individual person as person, which presupposes a proper understanding of the 'ontological structure' of the person.[26]

Summing up the above discussion, nowadays, besides principlism there are several other major approaches to medical ethics.[31–33] As some healthcare professionals are not familiar with either their essential content or with their potential contributions to clinical decision making, the interested reader is referred to summaries of the main trends in contemporary bioethics (Box 11.3) published elsewhere.[5,13,31]

Other traditional ethical principles especially relevant in palliative care

Besides the abovementioned four basic principles of bioethics, a number of other traditional ethical principles can be applied to solve ethical challenges in the care for the

Box 11.3 Main trends in contemporary bioethics

- Hippocratic tradition
- Principlism
- Utilitarianism
- Kantian ethics
- Casuistry
- Relational and feminist ethics
- Virtue ethics
- Personalism

dying.[4] I shall refer here mainly to the principles of respect for human life and death, therapeutic proportionality, double effect, and truthfulness in communication.

RESPECT FOR HUMAN LIFE AND DEATH

The duty to respect and promote human life and health is a basic ethical imperative in relation to the self and to others. In palliative care the ethical question arising is: How can this basic ethical principle be applied in the context of dying persons? In defining the specific goals of palliative care, the World Health Organization states that palliative care affirms life and regards dying as a normal process, neither hastening nor postponing death.[34] This definition corresponds to a conception of the so-called 'right to die with dignity' not simply as a right to die, but rather as a right to live one's life to the end. In other words, it refers to the right to be assisted by others in the dying process.[35] Hence, the main idea is that the human process of dying poses certain ethical demands for medical professionals as well as for society as such. Palliative care is conceived as a concrete and active answer to these ethical demands.[36]

To answer the question about what constitutes an appropriate use of medical resources in the care of a dying person presupposes adopting a moral attitude toward imminent death and an understanding of the meaning of the so-called 'good death'.[37,38] There seems to be general agreement about the fact that an artificially prolonged agony is contrary to the dignity of the dying person. The Judeo-Christian tradition, for instance, affirms the existence of a *moral duty to accept death* and regards the so-called 'medicalization of death' as an ethically wrong medical praxis.[39,40] But it is also well known that – in contradistinction to the way in which most proponents of euthanasia and medically assisted suicide understand the expression 'right to die with dignity' nowadays[41–44] – the Judeo-Christian tradition absolutely excludes the possibility of intentionally taking one's own life and/or helping others to do so. According to this tradition, the *right to die with dignity* is considered as a constitutive part of the *right to live*.[39,40]

To speak about a *good* or a *bad* death presupposes an understanding of the human act of dying as an act in which human freedom can be exercised, at least to a certain extent.[29,38,45] Nevertheless, it seems quite evident that dying is not something we can decide about. (The classical moral distinction between physical and moral acts expresses that the mere physical realization of an act (*actus homini*) does not necessarily coincide with the realization of a moral act. Only an action in which human freedom is exercised (*actus humanus*) can be morally qualified.[29,45]) We are not able to choose whether we want to die. But in spite of the inevitability of death proper to the human condition, we are actually free to choose an attitude of acceptance or rebellion in the face of imminent death. Elizabeth Kübler-Ross, for instance, describes five kinds of emotional reactions observed in patients facing death: anger, denial and isolation, pact or negotiation, depression, and acceptance.[46] The existence of various types of attitude toward inevitable death suggests the possibility of exercising personal freedom, at least to a certain extent. Indeed, we are free to adopt an attitude of acceptance or of rebellion in the face of unavoidable death. And it is precisely this inner attitude toward imminent death that becomes ethically relevant for a conception of a 'good' and a 'bad' death.[37,38]

Death certainly has deep cultural, moral, and religious meanings (reference 37 and Dekkers W. Images of death and dying. Unpublished manuscript). Hence, cultural, moral, and religious views of death shape what is considered to be an appropriate behavior toward both the dying person and his or her family. The orientation toward cure that characterizes contemporary medicine may encourage aggressive treatment – even if not clinically appropriate and/or contrary to the patient's wishes – to avoid any perception of under-treatment.[47] To be involved in such a cultural trend, as well as its opposite, i.e. the growing acceptance of the practice of euthanasia and physician-assisted suicide, may impose grave moral dilemmas on dying persons, not allowing them to die in the way they consider to be the right one.[48] Indeed, clinical surveys have shown that healthcare workers too often fall into the temptation of using all available technology to avoid imminent death.[47] They seem to have special difficulties in accepting human finitude and death.

PRINCIPLE OF THERAPEUTIC PROPORTIONALITY

No one is obliged to use all available medical interventions, rather only those offering a reasonable benefit/risk ratio. A more difficult question is whether one can refuse medical interventions in spite of their potential benefits or accept treatments for which the risks are still high or not yet well known. In these situations we are confronted with the question about the limits of our moral obligation to pursue healthcare. In an attempt to distinguish morally obligatory from nonobligatory medical interventions, a conceptual distinction between 'ordinary' and 'extraordinary' means has been proposed.[40,49]

The content of this traditional moral teaching is presently better known as the principle of therapeutic proportionality.[40] This principle states the moral obligation to provide a patient those treatments that fulfill a relation of due proportion between the means to be employed and the expected results. Medical interventions in situations in which this relation does not hold are considered 'disproportionate' (previously referred to as 'extraordinary') and regarded as morally nonobligatory. Hence, to verify whether a given medical intervention is morally mandatory one has to carefully judge the utility of this intervention in the context of the patient's concrete circumstances. It is important to note that the utility/futility has to be referred to the patient's overall clinical evolution and not merely to some isolated physiological effects. Also the risks and 'burdens' associated with the intervention should be carefully taken into account, understanding the notion of 'burden' in its widest sense, that is, including physical, psychologic, spiritual, humane, familial, social, financial, etc. distress.[49]

Judgments about therapeutic proportionality are relative to an individual's unique situation. Nevertheless, this does not mean that they are merely subjective. In fact, to be legitimate, proportionality judgments need to be grounded in an objective state of affairs regarding the clinical condition and the present state of medical art. From a medical point of view, some of the elements that always need to be taken into account to judge the proportionality of a given intervention are the certainty of the clinical diagnosis, the utility/futility of the intervention, the risks and side effects of the different therapeutic alternatives, and the accuracy of the prognosis. Evidence-based data become relevant, even though it is evident that a moral obligation cannot be sufficiently grounded in statistical probabilities.[50,51]

Moreover, judgments about therapeutic proportionality cannot be considered as the result of a mere cost/benefit equation. The way in which the different elements involved in therapeutic proportionality have to be weighted needs to be guided by the virtue of prudence. I am using the word 'prudence' here in its traditional philosophical understanding, that is, the ability to be practically wise or to exercise the right choice in a particular case in the light of moral universal knowledge. In other words, I am not referring to the contemporary understanding of 'prudence' as 'rational self-interest', but rather to the classic moral virtue of knowing what should be done and avoided in concrete situations.[48,49] And the moral relevance of proportionality judgments guided by the virtue of prudence is that the implementation of interventions judged as 'proportionate' is morally obligatory. This means that to omit them would represent an act of euthanasia by omission (sometimes referred to as 'passive euthanasia').

PRINCIPLE OF DOUBLE EFFECT IN PAIN MANAGEMENT AND SEDATION

There are various situations in normal daily life in which one cannot do the good without also causing undesired bad side effects. The traditional ethical principle of double effect sets the ethical criteria for the legitimacy of actions that have well-known, unavoidable, bad side effects.[26,40,52] This principle also sheds light on various ethical dilemmas in palliative care, for instance, when using opioids or sedatives in terminally ill patients, knowing that they *may* negatively affect the patient's state of awareness, blood pressure and respiration. Sometimes, the fear that the occurrence of these adverse effects may hasten the patient's death poses ethical dilemmas to the patient, relatives and even to healthcare professionals, who doubt whether this might represent a form of euthanasia (referred to as 'indirect euthanasia'). In this context, it is important to remember that adequate use of opioids is not necessarily associated with the occurrence of such feared side effects. But even if the undesired effects do occur, the principle of double effect helps to recognize the patients in whom the use of these drugs may be morally legitimate in spite of the risks. Provided that other pain killers have been tried and shown as inefficient in the control of pain, and if opioids are used in the right way and dose, then the use of opioids would represent the only possible way of benefiting the patient and their use is therefore morally justified. Indeed, the principle of double effect states that actions with both good and bad effects are ethically legitimate only if certain conditions are simultaneously fulfilled:[26,40,52]

- The action performed is not itself morally evil.
- The good effect is not caused by the evil effect.
- Only the good effects are directly intended; the bad effects are not intended but only tolerated (as unavoidable).
- There is a due proportion between the good and bad effects.

Thus, the double effect doctrine forbids the achievement of good ends by wrong means. It forbids doctors to relieve the distress of dying patients by killing them, but permits the use of drugs which relieve the distress of the dying, even when they may incidentally hasten an imminent death.

This principle similarly applies to the sedation of terminally ill patients.[53–56] If we consider the actual exercise of mental faculties to be objectively good for the person, then it would be morally wrong to deprive someone of the use of these faculties without a sufficient reason. Hence for sedation to be morally legitimate, the four conditions of the principle of double effect must be fulfilled. It would be morally wrong to sedate a person if there is not a good reason for it. Unfortunately, healthcare professionals are not always completely aware of the seriousness of this issue. Sometimes the scarcity of medical personnel and other related circumstances become the reason for sedating patients. This is a morally intolerable situation.

TRUTHFULNESS IN COMMUNICATION

Perhaps one of the most frequent ethical challenges in palliative care is the question of truthfulness with terminally ill patients.[57,58] Reluctance to share the truth about diagnosis and/or prognosis with the patient is frequently associated with family pressures related to cultural backgrounds. While medical professionals usually consider truth disclosure to be part of their duty of beneficence and respect for autonomy, relatives sometimes regard truth disclosure as being harmful for the patient. Seemingly, what is beneficent for some appears to be maleficent for others. This contrast in moral perspectives underlies some ethical dilemmas in palliative care.

Usually, a family's request not to disclose the truth to the patient is based on the assumption that truth disclosure will induce serious anxiety and depression, causing real harm to the patient.[59] Indeed, detailed disclosure has been shown to increase anxiety in the short term.[60] Nevertheless, follow-up surveys reveal that the excess anxiety dissipates within a few weeks, whereas the effects of limited information on psychological adjustment may persist.[61] Evasion and lying isolate patients behind either a wall of words or a wall of silence that prevents a therapeutic sharing of their fears, anxieties, and other concerns.

If a physician believes that it is not possible to offer good care without prior commitment to openness and honesty and goes on communicating the clinical information to the patient against the family's desire, he or she may be accused of an 'assault of truth', i.e. of imposing the truth on a patient.[62] The risk thereby is to interfere with the patient's coping mechanisms, as determined by his/her personality or cultural background. In fact, we know that within some ethnic groups the delegation of authority with regard to medical decision making is culturally implicit.[63] Under these circumstances, disclosure of a serious diagnosis to a patient by the physician can be regarded as a socially unacceptable behavior and an untactful act, because the family is considered to have the right to be informed first. In this cultural context an 'assault of truth' may cause irreversible damage to the physician–patient relationship as well as to the physician–family relationship. In such situations, the physician may perceive an apparent dichotomy between holding to the principle of autonomy and respecting the pluralism of different cultures. Nevertheless, a deeper understanding of the meaning of autonomy may help solve the apparent moral dilemma.

As Pellegrino states, the principle of autonomy is grounded in respect for the person and the acknowledgment that as rational beings we have the unique capability to make reasoned choices.[64] Through these choices we plan and live lives for which we are morally accountable. Inhibiting an individual's capability to make these choices is a violation of his or her integrity as a person and thus a maleficent act. Autonomy, therefore, is not in fundamental opposition to beneficence as is too often supposed, but in congruence with it.

Moreover, truth-telling goes far beyond providing mere information.[65] Truth is not just the opposite of lies, not just the sum of correct statements, but a reciprocal state in the patient–physician relationship. Deception appears to be harmful, because it may destroy the foundations of the interpersonal relationship that allows a doctor to 'do good' (beneficence). Thus respect for both autonomy and truth-telling can be regarded as intrinsic beneficent medical acts.

Competent human beings, however, also can freely choose the communication and decision making style they prefer. There are indeed different styles of decision making that can be – in principle – equally respectful for patient's autonomy. One may be called a 'patient-based model' and the other a 'family-based style'. If patients express the desire for personal involvement in the decision making process, they have the right to be informed in spite of the explicit requests of their relatives, who in such a case would in fact be violating the patient's right to autonomy. To respect the patient's autonomous choice it is mandatory to explore carefully his or her preferences with regard to communication and decision making style.

Hence in spite of cultural and ethnic diversities, respect for autonomy can still be said to be valid and universal principle in relation to truth disclosure because it is based on what it is to be a person and in the respect due to each person as a person ('personalist principle').[28] What actually varies among different ethnic groups and cultures is the way in which the respect for a person's freedom is best exercised with regard to communication and decision making styles. The uniformity of a family-based decision-making style within a given culture may suggest that delegation of decision making to family members is an expectation of the sick person that does not need to be made explicit in individual cases. This assumption cannot be taken for granted. The present trend toward globalization may result in a patient's appropriation of values different from the ones that are considered typical for his or her cultural background. One cannot assume that a given patient will prefer one style to the other just because he or she belongs to a given culture or ethnic group. Thus, the physician should tactfully explore the preferences of the individual patient with regard to communication and decision making styles.

FINAL REFLECTIONS

The peculiar needs and features of patients at the end of life demand from healthcare workers – even more explicitly than in other areas of medicine – some fundamental moral attitudes and virtues. These attitudes are an unconditional respect for human life and dignity as well as the acceptance of human finitude. To discover what appropriate palliative care is, a physician shall be dedicated to providing competent medical services with compassion and respect for human dignity.[66] This statement summarizes three central virtues in the praxis of palliative care: medical expertise, compassion, and respect for the dignity of the person – even in situations of extreme debility and suffering. Indeed, these virtues are tightly interconnected. A genuinely compassionate attitude allows healthcare professionals to identify the concrete way in which medical expertise has to be applied to truly respect the dignity of each person, especially in situations of extreme weakness and unavoidable death.

The term 'compassion' is commonly understood as synonymous of pity. Nevertheless, it can be better defined as 'the virtue by which we have a sympathetic consciousness of sharing the distress and suffering of another person and on that basis are inclined to offer assistance in alleviating and/or living through that suffering. Hence, there are two key elements in defining compassion: (1) an ability and willingness to enter into another's situation deeply enough to gain knowledge of the person's experience of suffering; and (2) a virtue characterized by the desire to alleviate the person's suffering or, if that is not possible, to be supportive by living through it vicariously.[67] Compassion – understood as a moral virtue – entails the willingness to effectively alleviate a person's sufferings. Hence, it demands unfolding the corresponding expertise or 'know-how'.

Human suffering at the end of life has different causes. Thus medical interventions aimed at alleviating suffering in terminally ill patients cannot be narrowly understood as just those having the potential to produce certain physiological effects on the person's body. This is doubtless an important goal of end-of-life care, but the medical commitment toward a dying person goes far further than the body. Indeed, a peculiar cause of human suffering at the end of life is the person's natural fear of imminent death, and healthcare workers should develop a special sensitivity toward this aspect, permitting their patients to reflect on their moral duty to accept death and to receive the necessary psychological and spiritual assistance, if they want. This will require – among other things – to preserve the patient's state of consciousness, as long as the clinical condition and the therapeutic goals allow it.

If compassion is primarily directed to the person in virtue of his or her sufferings and only secondarily to the sufferings, then we can draw another practical conclusion. In situations of extreme and prolonged suffering a truly compassionate attitude will prevent a healthcare provider from the temptation of accelerating death to alleviate their patient's sufferings. To end the life of a person cannot be an act of true compassion, because such an act would eliminate the very object of compassion: the person. On the contrary, a compassionate attitude allows healthcare providers to recognize the way in which their competent medical knowledge can be best used to palliate the person's sufferings in a way that truly respects each person's life and dignity, even in the events surrounding an unavoidable death.

Key learning points

Some ethical principles are especially relevant in palliative care (see Box 11.2). Besides the so-called four basic principles of bioethics (nonmaleficence, beneficence, autonomy, and justice), a number of other traditional ethical principles can be applied to solve ethical challenges in the care for the dying. These include the principles of respect for human life and death, therapeutic proportionality, double effect, and truthfulness in communication. Fundamental moral attitudes and virtues that help orientate healthcare professionals when caring for the dying are far more important than the mere application of ethical principles.

REFERENCES

◆ 1 Twycross R. Palliative care. In: Brokow D, Lehman J, eds. *Encyclopedia of Applied Ethics*, Vol. 3. New York: Academic Press, 1998: 419–33.

● 2 Kuuppelomäki M, Lauri S. Ethical dilemmas in the care of patients with incurable cancer. *Nurs Ethics* 1998; **5**: 283–93.

◆ 3 Roy D, MacDonald N. Ethical issues in palliative care. In: Doyle D, Hanks GW, MacDonald N, eds. *Oxford Textbook of Palliative Care*, 2nd ed. Oxford: Oxford University Press, 1998: 97–138.

● 4 Taboada P. Ethical issues in palliative care. In: Bruera E, De Lima L, Wenk R, Farr W, eds. *Palliative Care in the Developing World. Principles and Practice*. Houston: IAHPC Press, 2004: 39–51.

● 5 Taboada P, Bruera E. Ethical decision-making on communication in palliative cancer care: a personalist approach. *Support Cancer Care* 2001; **9**: 335–43.

● 6 Taboada P. Ética Clínica: Principios básicos y modelo de análisis. *Boletín Escuela de Medicina PUC* 1998; **27**: 7–13.

◆ 7 Lavados M, Serani A. *Etica Clínica. Fundamentos y aplicaciones*. Santiago: Ediciones Universidad Católica, 1993.

● 8 Pellegrino ED, Hart RJ, Henderson SR, *et al.* Relevance and utility of courses in medical ethics. A survey of physician's perceptions. *JAMA* 1985; **253**: 49–53.

● 9 McClung JA, Kamer RS, DeLuca M, Barber HJ. Evaluation of a medical ethics consultation service: opinions of patients and health care providers. *Am J Med* 1996; **100**: 456–60.

◆ 10 Pence GE. *Classical Cases in Medical Ethics: Accounts of the Cases that Have Shaped Medical Ethics*, 2nd ed. Boston: McGraw Hill, 1995.

● 11 Lo B, Schroeder S. Frequency of ethical dilemmas in a medical inpatient service. *Arch Intern Med* 1981; **141**: 1062–4.

◆ 12 Taboada P. What is appropriate intensive care? In: Cherry M, Engelhardt HT, eds. *Allocating Scarce Medical Resources. Roman Catholic Perspectives*. Washington DC: Georgetown University Press, 2002.

◆ 13 Pellegrino ED. The metamorphosis of medical ethics. A 30-year retrospective. *JAMA* 1993; **269**: 1158–62.

◆ 14 Ross WD. *The Right and the Good*. Indianapolis: Hackett Publishing Company, 1988.

◆ 15 Beauchamp T, Childress J. *Principles of Biomedical Ethics*, 5th ed. Oxford: Oxford University Press, 2001.

● 16 Clouser KD, Gert B. A critique of principlism. *J Med Philos* 1990; **15**: 219–36.

● 17 Brody B. Philosophical critique of bioethics. *J Med Philos* 1990; **15**: 161–78.

● 18 DeGrazia D. Moving forward in bioethical theory: theories, cases, and specified principlism. *J Med Philos* 1992; **17**: 511–39.

◆ 19 Gracia D. *Fundamentos de Bioética*. Madrid: Eudema, 1989.

◆ 20 Gracia D. *Fundamentación y Enseñanza de la Bioética.* Estudios de Bioética 1. Santa Fe de Bogotá: El Buho, 1998.

◆ 21 Gracia D. *Bioética Clínica.* Estudios de Bioética 2. Santa Fe de Bogotá: El Buho, 1998.

◆ 22 Gracia, D. *Ética en los confines de la vida.* Estudios de Bioética 3. Santa Fe de Bogotá: El Buho, 1998.

◆ 23 Pellegrino ED. Toward a virtue-based normative ethics for the health care professions. *Kennedy Inst Ethics J* 1995; **5**: 253–77.

◆ 24 Pellegrino ED. Virtue-based ethics: natural and theological. In: Pellegrino ED, Thomasma D. *The Christian Virtues in Medical Practice.* Washington, DC: Georgetown University Press, 1996: 6–28.

◆ 25 MacIntyre A. *After Virtue: A Study in Moral Theory.* Notre Dame, IN: University of Notre Dame Press, 1984.

◆ 26 Sgreccia E. *Manual de Bioética.* México DF: Diana, 1996.

◆ 27 Spaemann R. *Personen. Der Unterschied zwischen Jemand und Etwas.* Stuttgart: Klett-Cotta, 1996.

◆ 28 Wojtyla K, Szostek A, Styczen T. *Der Streit um den Menschen. Personaler Anspruch des Sittlichen.* Kevelaer: Butzon & Bercker, 1979.

◆ 29 Wojtyla K. *The Acting Person.* Dordrecht: Reidel, 1980.

◆ 30 Wojtyla K. *Person and Community. Selected Essays.* [Transl. by Th. Sandok.] New York: Peter Lang, 1993.

◆ 31 Levi BH. Four approaches to doing ethics. *J Med Philos* 1996; **21**: 7–39.

● 32 Sherwin S. Feminist and medical ethics: two different approaches to contextual ethics. *Hypatia* 1989; **4**: 52–72.

● 33 Waren V. Feminist directions in medical ethics. *Hypatia* 1989; **4**: 73–87.

◆ 34 World Health Organization. *Cancer Pain Relief and Palliative Care. Report of a WHO Expert Committee.* WHO Technical Report Series, No 804. Geneva: WHO, 1990.

◆ 35 Blanco LG. *Muerte digna. Consideraciones bioético-jurídicas.* Buenos Aires: Editorial Ad Hoc, 1997.

◆ 36 Saunders C. Foreword. In: Doyle D, Hanks GWC, MacDonald N, eds. *Oxford Textbook of Palliative Medicine.* Oxford: Oxford University Press, 1998: v–ix.

◆ 37 Laín Entralgo P. *Antropología Médica.* Barcelona: Salvat, 1958.

◆ 38 Pieper J. Tod und Unsterblichkeit. In: Pieper J. *Schriften zur philosophischen Anthropologie und Ethik: Grundstrukturen menschlicher Existenz.* Hamburg: Meiner Verlag, 1997: 280–397.

◆ 39 Juan Pablo II. Encíclica Evangelium Vitae. In: *El don de la vida. Textos del Magisterio de la Iglesia sobre Bioética.* Madrid: BAC, 1996: 619–779.

◆ 40 Pontifical Council for Pastoral Assistance to Health Care Workers. *Charter for Health Care Workers.* Vatican City: Vatican Press, 1995.

● 41 Materstvedt LJ, Kaasa S. Euthanasia and physician-assisted suicide in Scandinavia – via a conceptual suggestion regarding international research in relation to the phenomena. *Palliat Mede* 2002; **16**: 17–32.

● 42 Jochemsen H, Keown J. Voluntary euthanasia under control? further empirical evidence from the Netherlands. *J Med Ethics* 1999; **25**: 16–21.

● 43 Onwuteaka-Philipsen B, Van der Heide A, Koper D, *et al.* Euthanasia and other end-of-life decisions in the Netherlands in 1990, 1995, and 2001. *Lancet* 2003; **362**: 395–9.

● 44 Brock DW. Forgoing food and water: is it killing? In: Lynn J, ed. *By No Extraordinary Means: The Choice to Forgo Life-Sustaining Food and Water.* Bloomington: Indiana University Press, 1989: 25–39.

◆ 45 Santo Tomás de Aquino. *Suma de Teología* (I-II, q. 6–21). Madrid: BAC, 2001.

◆ 46 Kübler-Ross E. *Sobre la muerte y los moribundos.* Barcelona: Grijalbo, 1969.

● 47 Study to Understand Prognosis and Preferences of Outcomes and Risks of Treatments (SUPPORT), 1995.

◆ 48 Cherry M, Engelhardt HT. *Allocating Scarce Medical Resources. Roman Catholic Perspectives.* Washington DC: Georgetown University Press, 2002.

◆ 49 Wildes K. Conserving life and conserving means: lead us not into temptation. *Philos Med* 1995: 51

● 50 Evidence-Based Medicine Working Group. Evidence-based medicine. a new approach to teaching the practice of medicine. *JAMA* 1992; **268**: 2420–5.

● 51 Petersen S. Time for evidence based medical education. *BMJ* 1999; **318**: 1223–4.

● 52 Boyle J. Double-effect and a certain type of embryotomy. *Irish Theol Q* 1977; **4**: 3003–318.

● 53 Sykes N, Thorns A. The use of opioids and sedatives at the end of life. *Lancet Oncol* 2003; **4**: 312–18.

● 54 Morita T, Tsuneto S, Shima Y. Definition of sedation for symptom relief: a systematic literature review and proposal of operational criteria. *J Pain Symptom Manage* 2002; **24**: 447–53.

● 55 Muller-Busch C, Andres I, Jehser T. Sedation in palliative care – a critical analysis of 7 years experience. *BMC Palliative Care* 2003; **2**: 1–9.

● 56 Morita T, Hirai K, Akechi T. Similarity and difference among standard medical care, palliative sedation therapy and euthanasia: a multidimensional scaling analysis on physicians' and general population's opinions. *J Pain Symptom Manage* 2003; **25**: 357–62.

● 57 Surbone A. Truth telling to the patient. *JAMA* 1992; **268**: 1661–2.

● 58 Simes RJ, Tattersal MHN, Coates AS, *et al.* Randomized comparison of procedures for obtaining informed consent in clinical trials of treatment for cancer. *BMJ* 1986; **293**: 1065–8.

● 59 Levine C, Zuckermann C. The trouble with families: toward an ethic of accommodation. *Ann Intern Med* 1999; **130**: 148–52.

● 60 Fallowfield LJ, Baum M, Maguire GP. Addressing the psychological needs of the conservatively treated cancer patient: discussion paper. *J R Soc Med* 1987; **80**: 995–7.

● 61 Devlen J, Maguire P, Phillips P, Crowther D. Psychological problems associated with diagnosis and treatment of lymphomas. II. Prospective Study. *BMJ* 1987; **295**: 955–7.

● 62 Buttow N, Dunn S, Tattersall HN. Denial, misinformation, and the 'assault of truth'. In: Portenoy RK, Bruera E, eds. *Topics in Palliative Care*, Vol. 1. New York: Oxford University Press, 1997: 263–78.

● 63 Ali NS, Khalil HZ, Yousef W. A comparison of American and Egyptian cancer patients' attitudes and unmet needs. *Cancer Nurs* 1993; **16**: 193–203.

● 64 Pellegrino ED. Is truth telling to the patient a cultural artifact? *JAMA* 1992; **268**: 1734–5.

● 65 Freedman B. Offering truth. One ethical approach to the uninformed cancer patient. *Arch Intern Med* 1993; **153**: 572–6.

◆ 66 American Medical Association. *Principles of Medical Ethics.* Chicago, IL: AMA, 1981.

◆ 67 Dougherty Ch, Purtilo R. Physicians' duty of compassion. *Camb Q Healthc Ethics* 1995; **4**: 426–33.

12

Ethics in the practice of palliative care

JAMES A TULSKY

INTRODUCTION

Excellent palliative care demands careful attention to diagnostic, prognostic, and therapeutic challenges. The palliative care clinician must demonstrate sensitivity to psychosocial and spiritual concerns, and thoughtful, empathic communication with patients and families. Yet, even when these are done with superb skill, patients and providers will still find that the pathway of life-limiting illness presents ethical dilemmas. Some are subtle and, perhaps, not recognized. Other dilemmas are easily apparent. This chapter discusses several of the more common and vexing ethical issues that arise in care of patients at the end of life. These include truth-telling, when and how to engage in advance care planning, requests for ineffective/unproved treatment and limitation of potentially beneficial treatments, and, finally, consideration of aggressive measures for treating terminal pain and suffering.

The following case raises each of these dilemmas. The case is not unusual and the problems are not profound. However, the problems are common and reflect thorny issues that arise in the real daily practice of palliative care.

SK was a 68-year-old, retired, Korean born university professor who was admitted to the hospital with pneumonia and chest pain. A chest computed tomography (CT) scan revealed a 4 cm lesion obstructing the right upper bronchus and several rib lesions suspicious for malignancy. As the physician approached the patient's hospital room he was pulled aside by Mr K's son and daughter who wished to know the result of the CT scan. They request that the doctor not share the results with their father if it means he may have cancer.

DISCLOSURE AND TRUTH-TELLING

Truth-telling is fundamental to respectful patient care and a necessary component of informed consent. By fully including patients in all decision making, healthcare providers honor patient autonomy. Truth-telling also engenders trust in physicians and the profession and is desired by most patients. Surveys consistently show that most patients wish to receive as much information as possible,[1,2] perhaps as a way to cope with uncertainty.[3,4] In one typical survey of 2850 British patients, over 1000 of them receiving palliative care, nearly 90 percent, stated they would like to be told most or all information about their illness.[5] Yet, patients also wish to have an individualized approach to receiving bad news and discussing prognosis that does not necessarily share all of the information at one time or in the same way.[6] In most Western societies, it is common practice to answer patients' questions honestly and to share relevant information about their medical condition, prognosis, and therapeutic options. However, significant variation exists worldwide.[7,8]

The above work suggests that most patients prefer to participate in decision making but to receive a physician's advice regarding recommended options. Physicians must find the balance between conveying the ambiguity that clouds medical practice and helping patients find the best options for them. There are many good arguments for giving full information to patients.[5] Information allows patients to plan their futures and to make decisions. Lack of information may heighten their fear and anxiety, as the truth is often not as bad as what might be imagined, and they may lose the opportunity to achieve important goals prior to death. In addition, the secrecy and collusion necessary to withhold information may present a significant challenge to providers and families.

Nevertheless, even the most forthright physicians raise questions about the limits of disclosure. When patients don't ask, how much should healthcare providers tell? For example, when starting a new medication doctors rarely describe all of the possible side effects. They judge that this would not be helpful and, instead, mention only the most common, most serious, or most relevant side effects. Disclosure of serious diagnoses and their repercussions appears to be handled similarly. Physicians do not always share prognosis, and when they do, they tend to bias optimistically.[9]

Although withholding information or providing an overly optimistic assessment of illness may be deceptive, legitimate reasons for the practice also exist. Patients may find it too difficult to hear bad news, or may consciously defer all decision making to their families. Although such perspectives may challenge notions of patient autonomy, in fact autonomy dictates that patients also have the right to not hear or to defer responsibility to others.

Cultural issues also play a role. In many societies decision making is localized in the family and individual autonomy is not recognized. Blackhall *et al.* surveyed members of four distinct ethnic groups in the USA and found widely disparate perspectives on whether a patient should be told about a diagnosis of metastatic cancer. Only 47 percent of first generation Korean Americans and 65 percent of first generation Mexican Americans believed that patients should be told, whereas European Americans (87 percent) and African Americans (88 percent) were more likely to want to hear this news directly themselves.[10] In some cultures the delivery of bad news may determine how patients confront illness and being told the wrong information can cause harm. For example, in Navajo society, the concept of 'hozho', or living in beauty, may be violated by statements that are viewed as negative.[11] Such observations imply that, in different cultures, personal autonomy carries different levels of importance. That said, patients' preferences are not simply a reflection of their ethnic background. In Mr K's case, we might expect that Mr K has an approximately 50 percent likelihood of wanting the physician to honor his family's request and to tell the news only to them. However, there exists an equal likelihood that he would want to be told the news himself, and there are no identifiable predictors of such preferences.

In this context, some have argued for 'necessary collusion', or the need to delay disclosure of some specific prognostic information from patients to help maintain their hope.[12] This perspective does not advocate withholding information that is requested, but rather allowing the information to unfold only as requested or needed by the patient in a 'measured series of forecasts'. This perspective appears to strike a common ground that protects those patients who do not want too much information. However, it also risks withholding information from those who would want it, and makes assumptions about patients' needs or preferences that cannot be ascertained simply.

Therefore, a better resolution may be for the clinician to ask patients directly, 'How much information are you interested in hearing about your illness? Patients can declare clearly what they wish to hear and patients will receive only the amount of information they desire. Rather than waiting until the moment that more bad news presents itself, this question is well worth asking early in the care of any patient with serious illness, and certainly at the time of conducting diagnostic and prognostic tests.

ADVANCE CARE PLANNING

> Mr K was treated for his pneumonia and a biopsy revealed nonsmall cell lung cancer, metastatic to rib. He received radiation to his lung and ribs and felt much better. He was seen 6 weeks later in his doctor's office, and the physician wondered whether this was a good opportunity to begin advance care planning.

Advance care planning is the process by which patients, together with their families and healthcare providers, consider their values and goals, and articulate preferences for future care.[13] Written advance directives formalize these preferences and include living wills or other statements of patients' preferences, as well as durable powers of attorney for healthcare, which name healthcare proxies. Do not resuscitate (DNR) orders are written by physicians to operationalize one specific set of preferences articulated by patients and their proxies. In recent years, advance care planning has been promoted widely in the USA and other countries, particularly in response to high-profile cases in which patients in vegetative state have been kept alive despite a presumption that such treatment violated their preferences.[14]

Although it could refer simply to signing a form in a lawyer's or doctor's office, ideally advance care planning creates an opportunity for patients to explore their own values, beliefs, and attitudes regarding quality of life and medical interventions, particularly as they think about the end of their life. Patients may speak with loved ones, physicians, spiritual advisers, and others during the process. This reflective work can help patients make important decisions about issues that may come up even when they still have the capacity to make decisions. When a patient loses decision-making capacity, physicians and loved ones who have been involved in the advance care planning process may feel that they know the patient's goals and values better. This allows them to make medical decisions that are likely to be consistent with the patient's values and preferences.

Advance care planning accomplishes a variety of goals for patients and families.[15] First, patients may use the process to clarify their own values and to consider how these affect their feelings about care at the end of life. Second, patients can learn more about what they can expect as they face the end of life and about various options for life-sustaining treatment and palliative care. Third, they can gain a sense of control over their medical care and their future, obtaining reassurance that they will die in a manner that is consistent with their preferences. Finally, patients may increase the probability that loved ones and healthcare providers will make decisions in accordance with their values and goals.

Advance care planning may serve other goals, not directly related to medical treatments.[15] Patients may wish to relieve loved ones of the burden of decision making and to protect loved ones from having to watch a drawn-out dying process. Patients also may use the process to prepare themselves for death. Advance care planning may help one reflect more deeply about one's life, its meaning and its goals. Patients may reflect on relationships with loved ones, 'unfinished business', and fears about future disability and loss of independence. In this way, advance care planning may improve patients' feelings of life completion and satisfaction with their treatment in their final days. Advance care planning appears to increase patient satisfaction and, possibly, the quality of death and dying.[16,17]

When a patient's illness has progressed to its final stages, healthcare providers can use the groundwork from these earlier discussions to make specific plans about what is to be done when the inevitable worsening occurs. Among other things, the patient and the healthcare providers can decide the following: Should an ambulance be called? Should the patient come to the hospital? Which life-prolonging treatments should be employed and which should be forgone? Are there particular treatments aimed at symptomatic relief that should be employed?

Healthcare providers have their own reasons for wanting to engage their patients in advance care planning.[15] First, providers may use these discussions to reassure patients that their wishes will be respected. This can enhance a sense of trust. Second, providers may hope that advance directives will help to decrease conflict among family members and between family members and the healthcare team when the patient is seriously ill. Finally, they may hope that advance directives will assist them in making difficult decisions when the patient has lost decision-making capacity.

Physicians are often reluctant to raise the subject with their patients, and often do so later than patients may desire.[18] They may be under overwhelming time constraints. They may have never been trained to discuss this issue and are not sure how to introduce the topic. They may be worried that they will give patients the impression that they are 'giving up' on them or that they think they will die soon. If they have focused in past discussions on interventions rather than patient values and goals, they may have found these discussions frustrating and unhelpful.

Time constraints are difficult to overcome. Physicians could dedicate visits to discussing advance directives; but insurance companies may not pay for such a visit, and many patients may not wish to make a separate trip to the doctor for this purpose. The use of booklets and other tools to introduce the concepts involved in advance care planning may help physicians efficiently use their time to answer specific questions patients may have and to guide patients through the process. Enlisting nurses and social workers to help patients with the advance care planning process may also help.

Although physicians are often worried that patients will be put off by a discussion about advance care plans, surveys show that most patients want to discuss these issues early in the course of their disease, and that they think that the doctor should bring up the topic. Nevertheless, there will be some patients who are not ready to discuss advance directives. Healthcare providers must be sensitive to these patients. Advance care planning is a process that should be offered to patients, not forced upon them. The root cause of much of a physician's reluctance stems from lack of training in how to have these discussions. With training, physicians can feel more comfortable having these discussions, can learn how to deal with a patient's emotional responses, and can have effective discussions that the physician will find truly helpful in caring for patients.

Unfortunately, with few exceptions, the introduction of advance directives has had little demonstrated impact on actual resuscitation events.[19–26] This may be because of several reasons. Discussions often do not occur or are not recorded in ways that may have a lasting effect.[27] Some of the barriers to successful implementation have been procedural when, for example, documents are not available when needed. More importantly, problems arise with deciding in advance about specific interventions,[28] the adequacy of communication,[29] the willingness of healthcare providers to follow patients' preferences,[24,27] and patient and family misunderstandings about the process. Despite these limitations, written advance directives are useful when there is disagreement within a family, conflict between the family and healthcare team, or when the patient assigns a nontraditional family member (for example, a friend or same-sex partner) as the surrogate. In the USA, if the patient's preferences are known and understood by the family and team through an oral advance directive, in most states the written document is superfluous.

Entering these conversations may feel awkward, but if they are viewed as conversations about hopes, fears, and goals rather than decisions for specific preferences, they may be easier to engage. For example, Mr K could be asked how he has been doing since his hospitalization. What was it like to learn of his diagnosis, and how does this make him feel about the future? The clinician can empathize with his emotions and ask about specific concerns he has looking forward. By careful exploration of patients' values, healthcare providers can help patients discover their preferences. This expanded view of advance care planning allows people to think about their mortality and legacy. From such discussions, healthcare providers can help patients consider specifically whether there are certain treatments that they might wish to forgo, and to think about the circumstances under which they might forgo them.

REQUESTS FOR UNPROVEN OR INEFFECTIVE TREATMENTS

Mr K chose to undergo chemotherapy and received carboplatin and gemcitabine. However, he experienced a significant decline in his renal function and his tumor progressed. He then tried pemetrexed but was hospitalized with neutropenia and fever. Again he had no response and wished to try something else. He was given erlotinib, but he could not tolerate the diarrhea. At this point his oncologist told him that there were no more proven treatments left and that she would not suggest more treatment, given his age and poor responses to previous agents. Mr K asked, 'Isn't there any more chemotherapy? What about an experimental drug or laetrile?'

Desperate patients seek desperate measures. Mr K has exhausted the proved treatments for his cancer and, even though he has experienced significant side effects from his treatment, he does not want to die and is willing to consider other options. Such options generally fall into two categories, clinical trials of promising, but unproven therapies and alternative treatments generally considered ineffective by the mainstream medical community.

Phase I clinical trials are conducted to ascertain the safety of experimental therapies prior to testing for efficacy. Such studies are not meant to be therapeutic and, historically, approximately 5 percent of patients enrolled in such trials of cancer agents achieve a response.[30,31] Nevertheless, most patients enroll with the intent of achieving therapeutic benefit.[32,33] Some have questioned whether this represents a failure of informed consent. Increasingly it is recognized that patients choosing to enroll in phase I trials may have different values from those who do not enroll. Although they understand the prognostic data presented to them, they maintain a more optimistic perspective and believe that they will be the ones to gain benefit.[34,35] In fact, many now argue that hospice care and phase I trials should coexist simultaneously.[36,37] In contrast, requests for alternative, ineffective treatments are viewed differently. Some of these treatments may fall into a category similar to agents used in established clinical trials, but the majority are far less accepted and sometimes considered quackery. Although belief systems vary among patients and clinicians, the primary issue here is one of informed consent and trying to be sure that patients do not encounter more harm than good in reaching out to such treatments.

When receiving requests for unproven or ineffective therapy, physicians should counsel patients openly and not hesitate to give an opinion based upon their knowledge of the intervention and the patient's values. It is important to acknowledge the patient's affect and recognize that requests for unproven or ineffective treatments are frequent proxies for patient distress and difficulty coping with impending death. A common pitfall is responding to such distress by offering more therapy rather than engaging the patient's emotional state. Similarly, others may tell patients that 'We'll wait until you're stronger and can take the chemo then', knowing fully well that the patient will never meet such a goal. A more productive technique to use in this situation is the 'wish' statement.[38] By letting patients know that 'I wish I had more effective treatment to offer you', clinicians can both align themselves with patients, while implicitly acknowledging that this goal cannot be met.

In these settings, clinicians struggle to promote hope in the patient with advanced disease and to support a positive outlook.[1] Incorrectly, they fear that discussing death may distress patients.[9,39–42] As a result doctors frequently convey overly optimistic prognoses or do not give this information at all.[43] Fearing the loss of hope, patients frequently cope by expressing denial, and may be unwilling to hear what is said.[44] Not unexpectedly, patients with more optimistic assessments of their own prognosis are more likely to choose aggressive therapies at the end of life.[45,46]

Physicians should recognize that it is not their job to 'correct' the patient's hope for an unrealistic outcome.[47] Hope is the framework within which patients construct their future.[48] It may be a desire for a particular outcome, or it may be, more broadly, trust or reliance. The key question is whether the patient's construction of hope is interfering with appropriate planning and behavior. Clinicians, at their best, can provide an empathic, reflective presence that will help patients to marshal and draw strength from their existing resources. Together, the physician and the patient can 'hope for the best but prepare for the worst'.[49] Helping the patient and family manage their hope and their resources in a realistic way may leave the family in the best possible shape after their loss.

LIMITATION OF TREATMENT

Mr K became progressively more debilitated. He decided not to pursue unproven therapies and accepted a palliative approach to care, including a DNR order. He was spending an increasing amount of his time in bed and developed a fever and cough. He stopped eating and drinking. His family wondered whether he had pneumonia again and asked if he could receive antibiotics. In addition, they questioned whether a feeding tube should be placed or if an intravenous drip would be helpful.

Even when patients have elected to pursue a palliative approach to care, they and their care providers may struggle over the exact limitations of treatment. They may wonder whether treatments such as feeding tubes and intravenous fluids provide comfort, and if their trade-off in treatment burden is worthwhile. Antibiotics are particularly interesting because they tend to be among the least refused of medical interventions.[50,51] Their use is high even in palliative care units, where they are administered to as many as 30–40 percent of patients with comfort care plans.[52–54] The literature suggests that antibiotics can play a role in symptom relief, yet must be balanced against the burdens of needles, side effects, and cost.[52,53] In the case of Mr K, pneumonia may be his terminal event, with or without the use of antibiotics. He and his family will need to decide whether intravenous antibiotics are worth a trip to the hospital, or even whether it is worth trying to administer them at home intramuscularly or orally. His symptoms of cough and fever can be managed with antitussives and antipyretics – it is not clear if adding another few days or weeks to his life will meet his goals at this point. Such decisions become highly individualized with no correct answers.

Tube feeding has not shown a significant benefit for most patients with terminal illness.[55,56] Therefore, there is less controversy on medical grounds. In contrast, considerable debate exists about the benefits of artificial hydration. Recent evidence suggests that subcutaneous hydration can alleviate common symptoms of terminal illness with minimal burden.[57] Guidelines established by the European Association for Palliative Care recommend a three-step approach:[58]

- Step I – includes assessment of a variety of clinical factors.
- Step II – involves an assessment of pros and cons to establish a well-defined goal of therapy and endpoint.
- Step III – requires periodic reevaluation of the decision.

OPTIONS OF LAST RESORT

Mr K's illness progressed and he was bed-bound with fluctuating consciousness. His required large quantities of opioids for pain and dyspnea. His daughter was concerned that the medication might hasten his death, and was resisting the hospice nurse's suggestion to increase the dose further. But his son felt that Mr K had completed all he needed to do and was just lingering uncomfortably. He wanted to know how much longer he would continue to live and if there was anything that could be done to stop the waiting.

One of the major barriers to aggressive symptom management at the end of life is the fear of hastening death. Many clinicians and families are unsure where pain control stops and euthanasia begins. Moral clarity on these issues is critically important to ensure that no inappropriate boundaries are overridden and to give reassurance to ethical providers who are working hard to take the best care of patients.[59]

In situations such as Mr K's, clinicians generally rely on the principle of double-effect to justify their actions. This centuries-old ethical framework allows one to perform beneficial actions with potentially harmful consequences as long as four requirements are met:[60]

- The act itself must not be immoral.
- The act must be undertaken only with the intention of achieving the possible good effect, without intending the possible bad effect even though it may be foreseen.
- The act does not bring about the possible good effect by means of the possible bad effect.
- The act is undertaken for a proportionately grave reason. (Or, stated otherwise, the good effect must outweigh the bad effect.)

The principle of double-effect has been useful in medical practice generally and palliative care in particular. This is because it helps many physicians overcome barriers to prescribing adequate pain relief, and it provides a legal defense for opioid prescriptions at the end of life.[61] At the same time, the principle also allows the community to continue to reinforce prohibitions against directly and intentionally causing death.

Several problems exist with double-effect.[62] It can be difficult to distinguish between intended and foreseen consequences, particularly regarding death at the end of life. Conscientious clinicians not sure of their actions may be tormented by the outcome. Furthermore, the principle of double-effect prioritizes the absolute prohibition against patient death over patient autonomy. Advocates applaud the principle for exactly this reason. Yet those who wish to allow greater flexibility for ending patient suffering at the end of life find double-effect to be constraining.

One practice, termed terminal or palliative sedation, links two acceptable acts in a controversial way. Patients are deeply sedated (double-effect), yet receive no hydration or nutrition (withdrawal of life-sustaining therapy). This intervention is intended for dying patients who have unbearable symptoms unresponsive to other therapies.[63] In the Netherlands, and perhaps elsewhere, the practice precedes a substantial number of deaths.[64] In the USA and most other countries it still remains rare. Because death is certain if sedation is not withdrawn, some people view this as a form of euthanasia, particularly those who believe in an absolute prohibition of hastening death.[65] Yet there is a growing consensus in favor of the practice under appropriate circumstances, and it is legal in the USA and many other countries. Concerns remain about potential abuses,[66] yet the necessity of a team provides some safeguards.

With regard to hastening death, other practices exist, and a detailed discussion of their history, merits, and risks is beyond the scope of this chapter. Briefly, these would include voluntary stopping of eating and drinking, assisted suicide, and euthanasia. Any competent patient who is approaching the end of life and confronting overwhelming suffering may choose to voluntarily stop eating and drinking.[59] This difficult and potentially unpleasant option takes tremendous conviction.[67] Nevertheless, some take advantage of this because it is legal in most jurisdictions and there is a growing ethical consensus in support of the practice. Furthermore, it does not require physician involvement, which removes a significant barrier.

In contrast with voluntarily stopping eating and drinking, which has received relatively little attention, physician-assisted suicide has been at the center of considerable controversy, including decisions by the US Supreme Court. In the USA and many European nations there is a majority public support for this practice,[68–70] yet considerable controversy exists over its appropriateness.[71,72] Currently, the practice is legal in only one state in the USA, and in one European nation, although it is tacitly approved in others. The practice requires a competent patient – perceived as a safeguard to abuse and somewhat distancing the agency of physicians, which many prefer.

Euthanasia is the practice whereby someone other than the patient, usually a physician, administers a lethal agent to directly hasten a death. This practice is perceived differently in different countries.[73] In the USA, euthanasia is distinguished from physician-assisted suicide and no ethical consensus exists.[68] It is illegal everywhere and likely to be prosecuted. In the Netherlands, Belgium, and some other countries, the public response to the two practices is fairly similar and more accepting. From a practical perspective, euthanasia does not require a competent patient, which has raised concerns about safeguards to abuses of vulnerable patients.[74]

The debate about assisted dying has played out in the press, courts and legislatures. Yet, in the end, individual patients, families and healthcare providers confront real-life situations that must be resolved within the constraints of individual moral values and the law. As Mr K lay dying, his daughter might have been reassured by being told that the aggressive use of opioids is entirely within the accepted standard of care, as the intent is focused on controlling the patient's pain and other symptoms. The son's position is also understandable. It is difficult to sit at such a vigil and wait for a patient to die. In most settings, directly hastening a patient's death will not be an option. Nevertheless, nothing more needed to be done to extend Mr K life, such as giving nutrition, hydration, or antibiotics. All efforts should be focused on the patient's comfort, and helping the family find meaning during the last moments.

CONCLUSION

Ethical challenges lie in the paths of all patients, families, and healthcare providers dealing with a life-limiting illness. At different points in an illness, these may range from truth telling to requests for assisted dying. Healthcare providers must enter into such issues without assumptions about patient preferences and with an open mind to learn the underlying issues. Careful listening, clear thinking about the ethical issues at stake and empathic communication will help resolve most such dilemmas.

Key learning points

- Truth telling engenders trust and is a central aspect of good palliative care, yet patients very considerably in their preferences for information.

- Patients should be asked how much information they wish to receive early in the course of an illness so that their preferences can be known and honored.

- Advance care planning serves multiple goals for patients, families, and healthcare providers in addition to communicating preferences for future treatment.

- Patients value discussions of advance care planning, but clinicians must initiate them.

- Clinicians should recognize that requests for unproven or ineffective therapies may reflect patient distress and respond accordingly to their emotional state, not just the underlying question.

- When considering limiting therapies such as antibiotics and artificial nutrition or hydration, patients, families, and providers should assess clinical factors, the pros and cons of therapy, and make a plan with well-defined endpoints.

- The principle of double-effect justifies most aggressive therapies for symptom control at the end of life.

- More aggressive options such as terminal sedation and assisted dying must be considered in light of patient values and the local laws.

REFERENCES

1 Butow PN, Dowsett S, Hagerty R, Tattersall MH. Communicating prognosis to patients with metastatic disease: what do they really want to know? *Support Care Cancer* 2002; **10**: 161–8.

2 Ende J, Kazis L, Ash A, Moskowitz MA. Measuring patients' desire for autonomy: decision making and information-seeking preferences among medical patients. *J Gen Intern Med* 1989; **4**: 23–30.

3 Bruera E, Sweeney C, Calder K, *et al.* Patient preferences versus physician perceptions of treatment decisions in cancer care. *J Clin Oncol* 2001; **19**: 2883–5.

● 4 Heyland DK, Tranmer J, O'Callaghan CJ, Gafni A. The seriously ill hospitalized patient: preferred role in end-of-life decision making? *J Crit Care* 2003; **18**: 3–10.

5   Fallowfield LJ, Jenkins VA, Beveridge HA. Truth may hurt but deceit hurts more: communication in palliative care. *Palliat Med* 2002; **16**: 297–303.

6   Hagerty RG, Butow PN, Ellis PM, *et al.* Communicating with realism and hope: incurable cancer patients' views on the disclosure of prognosis. *J Clin Oncol* 2005; **23**: 1278–88.

7   Bruera E, Neumann CM, Mazzocato C, *et al.* Attitudes and beliefs of palliative care physicians regarding communication with terminally ill cancer patients. *Palliat Med* 2000; **14**: 287–98.

8   Peretti-Watel P, Bendiane MK, Obadia Y, *et al.* Disclosure of prognosis to terminally ill patients: attitudes and practices among French physicians. *J Palliat Med* 2005; **8**: 280–90.

◆   9   Christakis NA. *Death Foretold: Prophecy and Prognosis in Medical Care.* Chicago: University of Chicago Press, 2000.

● 10   Blackhall LJ, Murphy ST, Frank G, *et al.* Ethnicity and attitudes toward patient autonomy. *JAMA* 1995; **274**: 820–5.

● 11   Carrese JA, Rhodes LA. Western bioethics on the Navajo reservation. Benefit or harm? *JAMA* 1995; **274**: 826–9.

12   Helft PR. Necessary collusion: prognostic communication with advanced cancer patients. *J Clin Oncol* 2005; **23**: 3146–50.

13   Fischer GS, Tulsky JA, Arnold RM. Advance directives. In: Post SG, ed. *Encyclopedia of Bioethics*, 3rd ed. New York: Macmillan Reference USA, 2004.

14   Lo B, Steinbrook R. Beyond the Cruzan case: the U.S. Supreme Court and medical practice. *Ann Intern Med* 1991; **114**: 895–901.

15   Singer PA, Martin DK, Lavery JV, *et al.* Reconceptualizing advance care planning from the patient's perspective. *Arch Intern Med* 1998; **158**: 879–84.

16   Curtis JR, Patrick DL, Engelberg RA, *et al.* A measure of the quality of dying and death. Initial validation using after-death interviews with family members. *J Pain Symptom Manage* 2002; **24**: 17–31.

17   Tierney WM, Dexter PR, Gramelspacher GP, *et al.* The effect of discussions about advance directives on patients' satisfaction with primary care. *J Gen Intern Med* 2001; **16**: 32–40.

18   Johnston SC, Pfeifer MP, McNutt R. The discussion about advance directives. Patient and physician opinions regarding when and how it should be conducted. End of Life Study Group. *Arch Intern Med* 1995; **155**: 1025–30.

19   Baker DW, Einstadter D, Husak S, Cebul RD. Changes in the use of do-not-resuscitate orders after implementation of the Patient Self-Determination Act. *J Gen Intern Med* 2003; **18**: 343–9.

20   Yates JL, Glick HR. The failed Patient Self-Determination Act and policy alternatives for the right to die. *J Aging Soc Policy* 1997; **9**: 29–50.

● 21   Danis M, Southerland LI, Garrett JM, *et al.* A prospective study of advance directives for life-sustaining care. *N Engl J Med* 1991; **324**: 882–8.

22   Ditto PH, Danks JH, Smucker WD, *et al.* Advance directives as acts of communication: a randomized controlled trial. *Arch Intern Med* 2001; **161**: 421–30.

◆ 23   Hanson L, Tulsky J, Danis M. Can clinical interventions change care at the end of life? *Ann Intern Med* 1997; **126**: 381–8.

● 24   SUPPORT Principal Investigators. A controlled trial to improve care for seriously ill hospitalized patients. The study to understand prognoses and preferences for outcomes and risks of treatments (SUPPORT). *JAMA* 1995; **274**: 1591–8.

25   Teno J, Lynn J, Wenger N, *et al.* Advance directives for seriously ill hospitalized patients: effectiveness with the patient self-determination act and the SUPPORT intervention. SUPPORT Investigators. Study to Understand Prognoses and Preferences for Outcomes and Risks of Treatment. *J Am Geriatr Soc* 1997; **45**: 500–7.

26   Molloy DW, Guyatt GH, Russo R, *et al.* Systematic implementation of an advance directive program in nursing homes: a randomized controlled trial. *JAMA* 2000; **283**: 1437–44.

27   Hofmann JC, Wenger NS, Davis RB, *et al.* Patient preferences for communication with physicians about end-of-life decisions. SUPPORT Investigators. Study to Understand Prognoses and Preference for Outcomes and Risks of Treatment. *Ann Intern Med* 1997; **127**: 1–12.

28   Brett AS. Limitations of listing specific medical interventions in advance directives. *JAMA* 1991; **266**: 825–8.

● 29   Tulsky JA, Fischer GS, Rose MR, Arnold RM. Opening the black box: how do physicians communicate about advance directives? *Ann Intern Med* 1998; **129**: 441–9.

30   Smith TL, Lee JJ, Kantarjian HM, *et al.* Design and results of phase I cancer clinical trials: three-year experience at M.D. Anderson Cancer Center. *J Clin Oncol* 1996; **14**: 287–95.

31   Von Hoff DD, Turner J. Response rates, duration of response, and dose response effects in phase I studies of antineoplastics. *Invest New Drugs* 1991; **9**: 115–22.

32   Daugherty C, Ratain MJ, Grochowski E, *et al.* Perceptions of cancer patients and their physicians involved in phase I trials. *J Clin Oncol* 1995; **13**: 1062–72.

33   Meropol NJ, Weinfurt KP, Burnett CB, *et al.* Perceptions of patients and physicians regarding phase I cancer clinical trials: implications for physician-patient communication. *J Clin Oncol* 2003; **21**: 2589–96.

34   Weinfurt KP, Sulmasy DP, Schulman KA, Meropol NJ. Patient expectations of benefit from phase I clinical trials: linguistic considerations in diagnosing a therapeutic misconception. *Theor Med Bioeth* 2003; **24**: 329–44.

◆ 35   Agrawal M, Emanuel EJ. Ethics of phase 1 oncology studies: reexamining the arguments and data. *JAMA* 2003; **290**: 1075–82.

36   Byock I, Miles SH. Hospice benefits and phase I cancer trials. *Ann Intern Med* 2003; **138**: 335–7.

37   Casarett DJ, Karlawish JH, Henry MI, Hirschman KB. Must patients with advanced cancer choose between a Phase I trial and hospice? *Cancer* 2002; **95**: 1601–4.

38   Quill TE, Arnold RM, Platt F. 'I wish things were different': expressing wishes in response to loss, futility, and unrealistic hopes. *Ann Intern Med* 2001; **135**: 551–5.

39   Delvecchio MJ, Good BJ, Schaffer C, Lind SE. American oncology and the discourse on hope. *Cult Med Psychiatry* 1990; **14**: 59–79.

40   Herth K. Fostering hope in terminally-ill people. *J Adv Nurs* 1990; **15**: 1250–9.

41   Koopmeiners L, Post-White J, Gutknecht S, *et al.* How healthcare professionals contribute to hope in patients with cancer. *Oncol Nurs Forum* 1997; **24**: 1507–13.

42   Wenrich MD, Curtis JR, Shannon SE, *et al.* Communicating with dying patients within the spectrum of medical care from terminal diagnosis to death. *Arch Intern Med* 2001; **161**: 868–74.

● 43 Lamont EB, Christakis NA. Prognostic disclosure to patients with cancer near the end of life. *Ann Intern Med* 2001; **134**: 1096–105.

44 Kreitler S. Denial in cancer patients. *Cancer Invest* 1999; **17**: 514–34.

45 Murphy DJ, Burrows D, Santilli S, *et al.* The influence of the probability of survival on patients' preferences regarding cardiopulmonary resuscitation. *N Engl J Med* 1994; **330**: 545–9.

46 Weeks JC, Cook EF, O'Day SJ, *et al.* Relationship between cancer patients' predictions of prognosis and their treatment preferences. *JAMA* 1998; **279**: 1709–14.

47 Tulsky JA. Hope and hubris. *J Palliat Med* 2002; **5**: 339–41.

48 Tulsky JA. Beyond advance directives: importance of communication skills at the end of life. *JAMA* 2005; **294**: 359–65.

49 Back AL, Arnold RM, Quill TE. Hope for the best, and prepare for the worst. *Ann Intern Med* 2003; **138**: 439–43.

50 Ahronheim JC, Morrison RS, Baskin SA, *et al.* Treatment of the dying in the acute care hospital. Advanced dementia and metastatic cancer. *Arch Intern Med* 1996; **156**: 2094–100.

51 Ghusn HF, Teasdale TA, Skelly JR. Limiting treatment in nursing homes: knowledge and attitudes of nursing home medical directors. *J Am Geriatr Soc* 1995; **43**: 1131–4.

52 Chen LK, Chou YC, Hsu PS, *et al.* Antibiotic prescription for fever episodes in hospice patients. *Support Care Cancer* 2002; **10**: 538–41.

53 Clayton J, Fardell B, Hutton-Potts J, *et al.* Parenteral antibiotics in a palliative care unit: prospective analysis of current practice. *Palliat Med* 2003; **17**: 44–8.

54 Pereira J, Watanabe S, Wolch G. A retrospective review of the frequency of infections and patterns of antibiotic utilization on a palliative care unit. *J Pain Symptom Manage* 1998; **16**: 374–81.

55 Finucane TE, Christmas C, Travis K. Tube feeding in patients with advanced dementia: a review of the evidence. *JAMA* 1999; **282**: 1365–70.

56 Rabeneck L, Wray NP, Petersen NJ. Long-term outcomes of patients receiving percutaneous endoscopic gastrostomy tubes. *J Gen Intern Med* 1996; **11**: 287–93.

57 Bruera E, Sala R, Rico MA, *et al.* Effects of parenteral hydration in terminally ill cancer patients: a preliminary study. *J Clin Oncol* 2005; **23**: 2366–71.

✱ 58 Bozzetti F, Amadori D, Bruera E, *et al.* Guidelines on artificial nutrition versus hydration in terminal cancer patients. European Association for Palliative Care. *Nutrition* 1996; **12**: 163–7.

◆ 59 Quill TE, Lo B, Brock DW. Palliative options of last resort: a comparison of voluntarily stopping eating and drinking, terminal sedation, physician-assisted suicide, and voluntary active euthanasia. *JAMA* 1997; **278**: 2099–104.

60 Sulmasy DP, Pellegrino ED. The rule of double effect: clearing up the double talk. *Arch Intern Med* 1999; **159**: 545–50.

61 Meisel A, Snyder L, Quill T, American College of Physicians – American Society of Internal Medicine End-of-Life Care Consensus P. Seven legal barriers to end-of-life care: myths, realities, and grains of truth. *JAMA* 2000; **284**: 2495–501.

62 Quill TE, Dresser R, Brock DW. The rule of double effect – a critique of its role in end-of-life decision making. *N Engl J Med* 1997; **337**: 1768–71.

63 Lo B, Rubenfeld G. Palliative sedation in dying patients: 'we turn to it when everything else hasn't worked'. *JAMA* 2005; **294**: 1810–16.

64 Rietjens JA, van der Heide A, Vrakking AM, *et al.* Physician reports of terminal sedation without hydration or nutrition for patients nearing death in the Netherlands. *Ann Intern Med* 2004; **141**: 178–85.

65 Jansen LA, Sulmasy DP. Sedation, alimentation, hydration, and equivocation: careful conversation about care at the end of life. *Ann Intern Med* 2002; **136**: 845–9.

66 Gillick MR. Terminal sedation: an acceptable exit strategy? *Ann Intern Med* 2004; **141**: 236–7.

67 Eddy DM. A piece of my mind. A conversation with my mother. *JAMA* 1994; **272**: 179–81.

68 Blendon RJ, Szalay US, Knox RA. Should physicians aid their patients in dying? The public perspective. *JAMA* 1992; **267**: 2658–62.

69 Emanuel EJ, Fairclough DL, Emanuel LL. Attitudes and desires related to euthanasia and physician-assisted suicide among terminally ill patients and their caregivers. *JAMA* 2000; **284**: 2460–8.

● 70 van der Heide A, Deliens L, Faisst K, *et al.* End-of-life decision-making in six European countries: descriptive study. *Lancet* 2003; **362**: 345–50.

71 Foley KM. Competent care for the dying instead of physician-assisted suicide. *N Engl J Med* 1997; **336**: 54–8.

72 Quill TE, Lee BC, Nunn S. Palliative treatments of last resort: choosing the least harmful alternative. University of Pennsylvania Center for Bioethics Assisted Suicide Consensus Panel. *Ann Intern Med* 2000; **132**: 488–93.

73 Willems DL, Daniels ER, van der Wal G, *et al.* Attitudes and practices concerning the end of life: a comparison between physicians from the United States and from the Netherlands. *Arch Intern Med* 2000; **160**: 63–8.

74 Hendin H, Rutenfrans C, Zylicz Z. Physician-assisted suicide and euthanasia in the Netherlands. Lessons from the Dutch. *JAMA* 1997; **277**: 1720–2.

13

Dignity in palliative care

SUSAN E McCLEMENT, HARVEY M CHOCHINOV

INTRODUCTION

Scholars from various disciplines are directing increased attention toward understanding the concept of dignity, and its specific application to end-of-life care. Such understanding is neither readily nor easily achieved, so long as conceptual clarity of the term dignity remains elusive. Tension exists in trying to provide care that honors both individual patient conceptions of dignity, and societal constraints on choices concerning a dignified life and death.[1,2] No doubt, ongoing debate and dialog among academics, researchers, and practitioners will enrich our future understanding regarding the issue of dignity in end-of-life care. However, it is within the present morass of complexity and ambiguity characterizing dignity that those providing end-of-life care to the terminally ill must practice their craft.

The work presented here does not purport to be an exhaustive treatise on dignity. Rather, the purpose of this chapter is to examine some of the salient issues healthcare providers must grapple with when notions of dignity in the provision of end-of-life care are invoked. First, conceptual challenges identified in the literature related to the term dignity will be presented. Next, the salience of dignity in discussions regarding end-of-life care will be examined. Finally, empirical work examining the issue of dignity in end-of-life care will be presented, along with suggestions for future dignity-related research.

CONCEPTUAL CHALLENGES: DEFINING DIGNITY

The concept of dignity is ubiquitous, figuring prominently in discussions of bioethics, human rights documents, codes of research involving human subjects, patients' bill of rights, and decision making in end-of-life care.[3–8] Despite its widespread use, however, the concept of dignity is poorly understood, and consensus regarding both its meaning and utility in end-of-life discussions has yet to be realized.[9–12] The importance of conducting research into the construct of dignity was highlighted in the final report of a Special Committee of the Senate of Canada, mandated to explore the social, ethical, and legal aspects of euthanasia and assisted suicide.[13] That committee concluded health professionals cannot fully understand requests for assisted death and fears about loss of dignity if the construct remains vaguely defined. Far more than an academic exercise, clarification of the concept of dignity is important because our understanding of it appears to guide both healthcare providers and the public about the way they attend to the dying.

Dictionary definitions provide a starting point from which to begin to understand what dignity means. The word dignity is derived from the Latin *dignus* meaning 'worthy'.[14] Webster's *Dictionary* defines dignity as: 'worth or excellence; nobility of manner; quality of commanding esteem, high office, or rank'.[15] Defined in this way, dignity evokes notions of worth, honor, and esteem.[16] It is not clear from these definitions what one is worthy of. There is a tacit suggestion that evaluations of dignity involve a comparative process, however, specification regarding who confers evaluations or judgments of being worthy or esteemed is not clear.[12,17]

Synonyms for dignity include words like self-respect, self-esteem, poise, and pride,[18] suggesting that the concept is a broad one encompassing several meanings. Such 'umbrella' terms are typically difficult to define and operationalize.[19] Because the concept of dignity is not readily amenable to precise theoretical or operational definition, replacing it in favor of other concepts that appear to have greater definitional precision is tempting.[20] However, alternative concepts such as 'autonomy' are imbued with ambiguity as well.[7] Mere word substitutions, then, will not produce the sought after clarity.

One approach used to clarify the meaning of words is the process of concept analysis; a formal linguistic strategy that facilitates examination of the defining attributes or characteristics of a concept.[19] It is a process used to determine similarities and differences between concepts, and create tentative theoretical and operational definitions.[21] Concept analyses of the term dignity can be found in the literature. Mairis[22] examined dictionary and thesaurus definitions of dignity as well as personal definitions of dignity offered by nursing students and healthcare professionals. Critical attributes of dignity emerging from her work included notions of maintenance of self-respect, self-esteem, and appreciation of what dignity means to the individual. The theoretical definition arising from this concept analysis suggests that dignity exists when individuals are able to exert control over their behavior, surroundings, and the way they are treated by others. Central to this definition is the capability of the person to be able to understand information and make decisions.

Haddock's[17] concept analysis defines dignity as 'an individual's ability to feel important and valuable in relation to others, communicate this to others, and be treated as such by others in contexts which are perceived as threatening' (p. 930). This theoretical definition speaks to the dynamic subjective nature of dignity, the processes involved in maintaining self-regard amid threatening situations or circumstances, and the interpersonal nature of dignity.

Dignity, as defined by Justice Iacobucci of the Supreme Court of Canada speaks to the self-respect and self-worth that individuals or groups feel. This definition is concerned with physical and psychological integrity and empowerment.[23] It not only injects the notion of capacity for self-determination into the concept of dignity, but also evokes what would appear to be critical attributes of dignity, such as autonomy, privacy, reputation, self-image, and intrinsic worth.[22,23] Such a broad range of alternative notions subsumed within this characterization of dignity, while capturing the complexity of the concept, makes definitional precision problematic. And like the theoretical definitions arising from the process of concept analyses of dignity, this characterization, while heuristic, lacks an empirical foundation.

What contributes to the ambiguity surrounding the term dignity? First, dignity seems to be closely intertwined with our ideas about autonomy, with both terms often referred to 'in the same breath'.[24] The equating of human dignity with autonomy is not new and can be traced to the writings of eighteenth century philosopher Immanuel Kant. Kant argued that human beings have an intrinsic worth – that is dignity – because they are rational agents capable of setting their own goals and making their own decisions. Following Kant's reasoning, the basic moral worth of every human being resides in the human capacity for rational choice.[25,26]

The pervasive tendency to equate dignity with autonomy is troublesome, for it assumes that individuals lacking the capacity for autonomous thought also lack human dignity.[27]

Some authors have attempted to effect the distinction between autonomy and dignity by examining the ways in which dignity is used in ordinary discourse. Pullman[7] asserts that the language of dignity embraces two distinct conceptualizations of the word. Basic dignity is the fundamental moral notion that speaks to the intrinsic worth of all human beings. In contrast, personal dignity refers to norms of dignity of the individual or subgroup of individuals.[7] Personal dignity is constructed through complex processes of social interaction and evaluation, and is socially and individually referenced.[7,12] Moreover, given that considerations of what counts as dignified treatment or behavior is variable between individuals and across groups over time, personal dignity should be viewed as a transient rather than an ascribed notion.[7]

Proulx and Jacelon's[28] contention that the concept of dignity rests in a dichotomy, consisting of both internal and external components, echoes Pullman's[7] assertion. Internal aspects of dignity speak to the inherent worth ascribed to all human beings, which is uniquely expressed in their life stories.[28–30] External aspects of dignity are connected to and vary with what matters to the individual person and includes such factors as physical comfort, autonomy, meaningfulness, spirituality, and interpersonal connectedness. This later conceptualization speaks to the subjective way in which individuals discern what is dignified for themselves and for others, and the ways in which dignity is socially constructed.[9]

There is consensus in the literature that dignity is a complex and multifaceted concept. However, the data sources informing definitions of dignity in the context of end-of-life care have largely failed to include an emic, or insider's perspective. Consequently, our understanding of dignity towards the end of life has been largely devoid of the voices of those best qualified to speak about it – terminally ill patients themselves. A patient-centered approach to understanding dignity provides guidance to those caring for the dying regarding what constitutes dignity enhancing or dignity eroding actions.[31] Examining dignity in end-of-life care from this perspective, and making what is tacit more explicit, should reveal dimensions of dignity that are not captured in the existing literature.

THE IMPORTANCE OF THE NOTION OF DIGNITY

Confusion in the literature related to definitions of the term 'dignity', have resulted in some authors characterizing the concept as 'ambiguous', 'euphemistic', 'subterfuge-creating', 'useless', and 'cliché'.[8,12,20,32] While the concept of dignity currently enjoys neither definitional specificity nor consensual meaning,[9,10] there does appear to be agreement that dignity is foundational to the provision of quality end-of-life care.[33] Indeed, the link between providing palliative care and enabling patients to maintain their dignity is a perspective that Macklin[12] (p. 214) suggests proponents of palliative care are 'wont to emphasize'.

The importance of palliative care being philosophically rooted in an acknowledgment of the inherent dignity of the individuals has been expressed in the literature,[34] and dignity has been identified as one of the five basic requirements that must be satisfied in caring for dying patients.[35] The basic tenets of palliative care, including symptom management, spiritual and psychological wellbeing, and care of the family unit may all be summarized under the goal of helping patients die with dignity.[36–38] When the preservation of dignity becomes the clear goal of palliation, care options expand well beyond the symptom management paradigm and encompass the physical, psychologic, social, spiritual and existential aspects of the patient's terminal experience.[36] Dignity is thus a relevant concept in discussions regarding care of the terminally ill, in that it provides an overarching framework that may guide the physician, patient, and family in discussing and defining the objectives of care at the end of life.[39]

Considerations of helping patients to die with dignity is not, however, the sole purview of advocates of palliative care. Appeals to dignity are frequently invoked as the ultimate justification for euthanasia and assisted suicide – approaches to care of the dying diametrically opposed to the principles and practices of palliative care. For example, both the hospice movement and the Hemlock Society invoke the ideal of dying with dignity in defense of their opposing perspectives.[7,31,40,41] That dignity is used to defend and justify diametrically opposed actions and practices, seems to be predicated on the notion that for some, assisted death is consonant with, and the epitome of, respect for autonomy. This explains why in some circles, the term 'death with dignity' has become synonymous with the right to assisted suicide and euthanasia.[42] For others, however, such actions constitute the ultimate indignity.[43]

That 'loss of dignity' was the most common response of physicians when asked why their patients' had selected euthanasia or some form of self-assisted suicide clearly underscores the importance of better understanding the concept of dignity in end-of-life care.[44] In a Dutch nationwide study on euthanasia and other medical decisions concerning the end of life, loss of dignity was cited by physicians in 57 percent of cases, followed by pain (46 percent), unworthy dying (46 percent), social dependency (33 percent), and tiredness of life (23 percent). Research conducted by Back and colleagues[45] examining physician-assisted suicide and euthanasia in Washington State found that physicians of 207 patients who expressed a preference for hastened death reported that a loss of dignity was a concern for 72 percent of these patients.

A study conducted by Seale and Addington-Hall[46] explored differences in preferences for hastened death between cancer patients and patients with cardiac disease, stroke, and respiratory disease. Approximately 25 percent of the 'significant others' indicated that they would have preferred that the patient die sooner in his or her illness trajectory. Twenty-five percent of respondents also said that the patients themselves had expressed a desire for hastened death. Although these studies provide important insights into healthcare provider and family member perspectives, they did not solicit input from patients directly concerning this issue. Therefore, our understanding regarding patient experiences is incomplete.

Research has been conducted examining the types of physical and psychological concerns that may prompt terminally ill individuals to desire a hastened death. There is some suggestion in the literature that severe pain can result in a heightened desire for death. In their study of terminally ill cancer patients, Chochinov and colleagues[47] found that 75 percent of patients who had a significant desire for hastened death experienced moderate to severe pain, compared with 46 percent of patients with mild or no pain. Similarly, Rosenfeld and associates'[48] research examining interest in physician-assisted suicide among terminally ill patients with acquired immune deficiency syndrome (AIDS) found that pain intensity contributed significantly to the prediction of desire for death in those patients with pain.

Evidence also exists that depression contributes significantly to a desire for death among terminally ill patients. In a review of literature pertaining to physical and psychological distress associate with a desire for early death, Chochinov and Wilson[49] concluded that clinical depression, poor pain control, and low social support are significantly related to desires for hastened death, and that the degree of distress in these individuals is frequently very high. In an examination of desire for death in terminally ill patients, it was found that 8.5 percent of patients reported at least a moderate desire for death that was consistent over time. Slightly more than half of the patients (55 percent) reported no desire for early death and 36 percent of patients reported intermittent desire for early death. Follow-up interviews 2 weeks later indicated that four out of six of the original 17 patients with at least a moderate desire for death had changed their minds. This finding demonstrates that even strong desires for early death can change over a relatively short period of time. Given that requests for euthanasia in the Netherlands are usually satisfied within 2 weeks of the patient's request, efforts to explicate the factors that contribute to a desire for early death must be a continued foci of research.

In their review of terminally ill patients' requests for hastened death, Block and Billings[50] emphasized the importance of detailing the clinical determinants and the meaning of the request for early death, so that the therapeutic options offered by care providers may be broadened. Variables considered important in shaping patients' decisions to hasten death include symptom control, social support, psychological distress, and the meaning of life and suffering. Clearly, the psychological context within which a fear of lost dignity is fostered needs to be understood empirically. Systematic examination and description of those factors identified by the patient as prompting requests for hastened death provide a solid foundation from which caregivers might implement dignity preserving or bolstering interventions.

Central to the arguments for and against death hastening measures are notions of what constitutes a 'good death' – an experience within which notions of dignity appear to be embedded.[51] Emanuel and Emanuel[52] have examined the construct of a 'good death', describing a detailed framework for this event. Though not empirically validated, these researchers synthesized the dying experience as a process with four critical components including fixed patient characteristics, mutable elements of the patient's experiences, interventions that are available, and overall outcome.

Steinhauser and colleagues[53] used a cross-section stratified random national survey to collect information from patients, families, and healthcare practitioners, with an aim to identifying factors that were most important to them at the end of life. Factors identified by participants include pain and symptom management, preparation for death, decisions about treatment preferences, and being treated in a holistic fashion. Relevant strategies for addressing these factors were not identified in the study.

Turner and colleagues[54] sought to measure dignity in 50 terminally ill patients being cared for in an integrated palliative care service during the final 72 hours of life by focusing on symptom control, level of functioning, and negative events and situations that might compromise dignity. The limitations of this work include inconsistency and confusion regarding the ways in which these criteria were measured, and sole reliance on healthcare provider perspectives in assessing dignity.

EMPIRICAL WORK

Empirical literature examining the concept of dignity in end-of-life care, although limited, is instructive. Street and Kissane's[9*] discourse analysis of palliative patient and family case studies provides insights about how dying people feel about their bodies and the care they receive at the end of life. Results from their work help to further dimensionalize our understanding of dignity as it relates to the embodied experience of dying, and the ways in which abjection of the body might serve as a source of shame and disgust for the terminally ill. Their findings regarding the reciprocal, relational nature of dignity serve as a poignant reminder that patient's perceptions of worth are greatly influenced by the ways in which care providers communicate with and care for them.

Enes[20*] conducted a phenomenological study examining the meaning of dignity from the perspectives of patients, relatives, and healthcare providers in a hospice inpatient unit in England. Thematic analysis arising from this work suggests that dignity concerns issues of relationship and belonging; having control; being human in terms of having

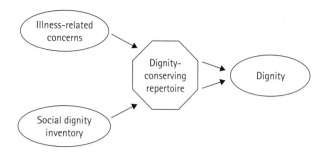

Figure 13.1 *The dignity-conserving model of care.*

rights and being worthy of respect; and maintaining the individual self. Patients, families and healthcare providers, while in agreement regarding the various facets of dignity, placed their emphases differently. For example, whereas healthcare providers emphasized issues of control and privacy, relatives emphasized issues of relationship and humanity. These findings speak to the need for, and challenges inherent in, trying to balance the multiple needs of care recipients and providers.

Chochinov and colleagues have been engaged in a program of research using a combination of qualitative and quantitative research methods to arrive at an understanding of the concept of dignity from the perspective of the terminally ill patient, and to identify various factors that support or erode a patient's sense of dignity.[55*] Inductive analysis of qualitative interviews conducted with 50 palliative cancer patients resulted in the generation of an empirically derived model of dignity in the terminally ill, and direction regarding dignity-conserving care[56*] (Fig. 13.1).

The model suggests that patient perceptions of dignity are related to and influenced by three major thematic areas:

- Illness-related concerns, i.e. those issues deriving from the illness that relate to one's level of independence and symptom experiences
- The patient's dignity-conserving repertoire, i.e. the personal approaches that individuals use to maintain their sense of dignity, and the internally held views or perspectives of their inherent qualities
- Social dignity inventory, i.e. factors external to the patient that influence the quality of his or her interactions with others that may bolster or undermine the person's sense of dignity (Table 13.1).

Quantitative data were collected in conjunction with the qualitative work to examine how various demographic and disease-specific variables were related to the issue of dignity in the terminally ill. A cohort of just over 200 terminally ill cancer patients were asked to rate their sense of dignity and complete measures of psychological wellbeing. Nearly half of the patients in the sample indicated they experienced some, or occasional, dignity-related concerns. Compared with those patients whose dignity was intact, patients with significant dignity-related concerns reported that they had increased pain, decreased quality of life, difficulty with bowel

Table 13.1   *Summary of major categories, themes, and subthemes arising from qualitative work examining the construct of dignity from the perspective of the terminally ill*

Illness–related concerns	Dignity-conserving repertoire	Social dignity inventory
Symptom distress	Dignity-conserving perspectives	Social issues/relationship dynamics affecting dignity
Physical distress	Continuity of self	Privacy boundaries
Psychological distress	Role preservation	Social support
medical uncertainty	Generativity/legacy	Burden to others
death anxiety	Maintenance of pride	Aftermath concerns
	Hopefulness	
	Autonomy/control	
	Acceptance	
	Resilience/fighting spirit	
Level of independence	Dignity-conserving practices	
Cognitive acuity	Living in the moment	
Functional capacity	Maintaining normalcy	
	Seeking spiritual comfort	

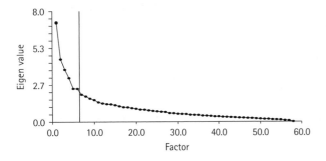

Figure 13.2   *Scree plot (see text for details).*

functioning, and were dependent on others [for bathing, dressing and incontinence issues]. These patients also reported a loss of will to live, increased desire for death, depression, hopelessness, and anxiety.[36*] The association between appearance (or the perception of how patients believe themselves to be seen or appreciated by others) and dignity, leads to the assertion that 'the reflection patients see of themselves in the eye of the beholder [care provider] needs to be one that is affirming of their sense of dignity'.[57]

Factor analysis of these data revealed six primary factors with Eigen values ranging from 7.19 to 2.39 (Fig. 13.2). This six factor solution accounted for 40.5 percent of the variance and included distinct aspects of the dying patient's experience: pain, intimate dependence, hopelessness/depression, informal support network, formal support network, and quality of life.[58*] This factor structure supports the model that arose from the qualitative work. Logistic regression analysis retaining those factors identified as being most malleable to palliative care intervention resulted in a highly significant two factor model that included hopelessness/depression and intimate dependency needs.[58*]

Some may argue that the model fails to resolve or dispel confusion around dignity's lack of definitional specificity. What every facet of the model has in common, however, is that each of the domains of concern identified within it

have been raised by terminally ill individuals as having a bearing on their sense of dignity.[33] As such, the dignity model provides an empirically derived theoretical framework which aids our understanding of the notion of dignity in those nearing death. We believe that the model of dignity-conserving care described here represents a new model of end-of-life care that may lead to enhanced palliation and new possibilities in care of the dying. Practical clinical considerations as to how healthcare providers might begin to apply dignity-conserving care approaches in practice are outlined in Table 13.2.

In addition to enhancing our understanding of dignity in those approaching death and providing a foundation upon which to both understand how a dying patient may experience a waning of their dignity, the dignity model also provides direction for how to construct dignity enhancing interventions for patients nearing death.[55] One such intervention is a brief psychotherapeutic intervention called dignity therapy that Chochinov and colleagues have developed and piloted tested. This approach comprises tape-recorded sessions, which give terminally ill patients the opportunity to speak to aspects of life they feel proudest of, things they feel are, or were most meaningful, the personal history they would most want remembered, or words they might provide in the service of helping to look after their soon to be bereft loved ones. These sessions are transcribed, edited, and returned to the patient, thereby bolstering patients' sense of purpose, meaning, and worth. Engagement in this empathic, therapeutic process provides patients tangible evidence that their thoughts and words have continued value. The creation of a 'generativity document' offers comfort in knowing that something of their personhood will transcend beyond the time of death. Preliminary findings suggesting this to be a viable way to address suffering and distress at the end of life has provided the basis for a National Institutes of Health funded international control trial of this novel end-of-life intervention.

Table 13.2 *Application of the dignity model to practice*

Illness–related concerns	Directions for practice
Symptom distress	
Physical distress	Baseline and ongoing assessment of physical and psychological symptoms
Psychological distress	
medical uncertainty	Provision of timely relevant information about the illness and plan of care
death anxiety	Exploration of concerns associated with illness progression
Level of independence	
Cognitive acuity	Baseline and ongoing assessment of cognitive functioning
	Vigilance in detection and treatment of delirium
Functional capacity	Baseline and ongoing assessment of ability to carry out activities of daily living
	Referrals to occupational and physiotherapy as appropriate
	Provision of supports needed to maintain independence (e.g. walker, raised toilet seat)
	Involvement in decision making regarding plan of care, as desired by patient

Dignity-conserving repertoire	Directions for practice
Continuity of self	Communication with patient about those facets of life not affected by their disease
	Learn about the patient's biography, attending to those aspect of life that he or she values most
Role preservation	Exploration of roles important to the patient
	Facilitation of role enactment within limitations of patient's illness
Maintenance of pride	Discussion with patient about those aspects of their life that they are most proud of
	Professional demeanor in provision of care
Hopefulness	Talk with the patient about what is still possible, despite illness limitations
	Encourage redefining of goals and expectations
Autonomy/control	Assess patient's perceived level of control, and explore preference regarding level of involvement in care decisions and planning
	Where possible, provide choices
Generativity/legacy	Facilitate life review, or other activities that foster the sharing of memories that are meaningful to patient
Acceptance	Explore the impact of the illness for the patient
	Appreciate the dynamism of the process of responding to a life-threatening illness
	Support patient in his or her outlook
Resilience/fighting spirit	Identify and promote patient participation in those interactions/activities that are most meaningful, given limited life expectancy

FUTURE DIRECTIONS

The empirical work conducted to date examining the concept of dignity in end-of-life care is still in its early stages. What is clear, however, is that the conceptual challenges related to defining dignity are not easily solved. The multifaceted, dynamic, and subjective nature of the concept seem to preclude exploration of the dignity experience using narrow definitions.[20] This suggests the need for researchers to understand and apply dignity in specific contexts in which it can be 'unpacked'.[31]

There is increasing appreciation for the need of palliative care that is both culturally sensitive and addresses the needs of individuals living with life-limiting illnesses apart from cancer.[59,60] As regards dignity research, future work could include exploration of the concept of dignity from the perspective of diverse cultural groups, various specific vulnerable populations, and those with nonmalignant conditions. Empirical work in these areas would inform us about the currency and relevance of the term dignity in other cultures, and help explicate nuances of dignity and dignity-conserving care that may be disease or group specific.

Little is known regarding the impact of terminal illness on perceptions and experience of dignity from the perspective of family members of the terminally ill. Research documents family members who perceive deficits in their terminally ill relative's care, experience changes in their own physical health and family functioning.[61] Therefore, the provision of care appraised by family as dignity eroding may impact on significant family outcomes. Accessing the perspectives of family members regarding the nature of dignified care of the dying is thus an important first step in meeting their care satisfaction needs.

Research has identified that the attributes of dignity may be emphasized or de-emphasized depending on the needs of the individual.[20] This finding speaks to the dynamic nature of dignity and suggests that longitudinal work indexing patient experiences of dignity across the illness trajectory is warranted. Such longitudinal work may reveal differences in threats to dignity experienced in early versus advanced stages of disease, and help explicate a range of dignity-enhancing strategies that patients use over time.

CONCLUSION

Becker[62] asserts that a significant psychological factor affecting terminally ill people is the compromising of their perceived personal dignity. Palliative care has been characterized as care that 'honors and protects those who are dying, and conveys by word and action that dignity resides in people'.[63] (p. 1) Palliative care practitioners thus ought to be concerned with the issue of patient dignity and to best support it in the delivery of end-of-life care. In particular, those involved in care of the dying need to understand what dignity means to the recipients of care, bearing in mind the various issues subsumed within dignity related concerns. Such understanding will arm healthcare providers with a range of patient-centered approaches and interventions, aimed at achieving humane care for individuals approaching the end of life.

Key learning points

- Dignity is a complex and multifaceted concept making it difficult to define and operationalize.

- Dignity is foundational to the provision of quality end-of-life care.

- Until recently, an understanding of dignity in end of life has largely been devoid of the voices of terminally ill patients.

- When the preservation of dignity becomes the clear goal of palliation, care options expand well beyond the symptom management paradigm and encompass the physical, psychologic, social, spiritual, and existential aspects of the patient's terminal experience.

- A patient-centered approach to understanding dignity provides guidance to those caring for the dying regarding what constitutes dignity-enhancing or dignity-eroding actions.

REFERENCES

1 Sampio L. To die with dignity. *Soc Sci Med* 1992; **35**: 433–41.
2 Badcott D. The basis and relevance of emotional dignity. *Med Health Care Philos* 2003; **6**: 123–31.
3 Macklin R. Yet another guideline? The UNESCO draft. *Developing World Bioeth* 2005; **5**: 244–50.
4 Sullivan AD, Hedberg K, Fleming DW. Legalized physician-assisted suicide in Oregon: the second year. *N Engl J Med* 2000; **342**: 598–604.
5 Leichtentritt RD, Rettig KD. Values underlying end-of-life decisions: a qualitative approach. *Health Soc Work* 2001; **26**: 150–9.
6 Stolberg SD. Human dignity and disease, disability, suffering: a philosophical contribution to the euthanasia and assisted suicide debate. *Humane Med* 1995; **11**: 144–7.
7 Pullman D. Death, dignity, and moral nonsense. *J Palliat Care* 2004; **20**: 171–8.
8 Lynch A. Death without dignity. *Ann R Coll Phys Surg Can* 1982; **15**: 117–22.
9 Street AF, Kissane DW. Constructions of dignity in end-of-life care. *J Palliat Care* 2001; **17**: 93–101.
10 deRave, L. Dignity and integrity at the end of life. *Int J Palliat Nurs* 1996; **2**: 71–6.
11 Coope CM. Death with dignity. *Hasting Cent Rep* 1997; **27**: 37–8.
12 Macklin R. Reflections on the Human Dignity Symposium: Is dignity a useless concept? *J Palliat Care* 2004; **20**: 212–16.
13 Senate of Canada. *On Life and Death. A Report of the Special Senate Committee on Euthanasia and Assisted Suicide*. Ottawa, ON: Minister of Supply and Services Canada, June 1995.
14 Sykes JB (ed.) *The Concise Oxford Dictionary of Current English*. Oxford: Clarendon Press, 1988.
15 *Merriam-Webster Dictionary*. Merriam-Webster OnLine. www.m-w.com/ (accessed September 2005).
16 Chochinov HM. Dignity-conserving care: A new model for palliative care. *JAMA* 2002; **287**: 2253–60.
17 Haddock J. Toward further clarification of the concept 'dignity'. *J Adv Nurs* 1996; **24**: 924–31.
18 Chapman RL. *Roget's International Thesaurus*, 4th ed. Toronto: Fitzhenry & Whiteside, 1977.
19 Walker LO, Avant KC. *Strategies for Theory Construction in Nursing*. Norwalk, CT: Appleton & Lange, 1988.
20 Enes SP. An exploration of dignity in palliative care. *Palliat Med* 2003; **17**: 263–9.
21 McCormack B. Intuition: concept analysis and application to curriculum development. 1. Concept analysis. *J Clin Nurs* 1992; **1**: 339–44.
22 Mairis ED. Concept clarification in professional practice – dignity. *J Adv Nurs* 1994; **19**: 947–53.
23 Downie J. Unilateral withholding and withdrawal of potentially life-sustaining treatment: a violation of dignity under the law. *J Palliat Care* 2004; **20**: 143–9.
24 Pullman D. The ethics of autonomy and dignity in long term care. *Can J Aging* 1999; **18**: 26–46.
25 Rachels J. *The Elements of Moral Philosophy*, 2nd ed. New York: McGraw-Hill, 1993: 127–38.
26 Grassian V. *Moral Reasoning: Ethical Theory and Some Contemporary Moral Problems*, 2nd ed. Englewood Cliffs, NJ: Prentice Hall, 1992: 83–98.
27 Meyer MJ. Dignity, death and modern virtue. *Am Philos Q* **32**: 45–55.
28 Proulx K, Jacelon C. Dying with dignity: The good patient versus the good death. *Am J Hospice Palliat Med* 2004; **21**; 116–20.
29 Holstein M. Reflections on death and dying. *Acad Med* 1997; **27**: 848–55.

30 Moody H. Why dignity in old age matters. *J Gerontol Soc Work* 1998; **29**: 13–38.

31 McDonald, M. Dignity at the end of our days: Personal, familial, and cultural location. *J Palliat Care* 2004; **20**: 163–70.

32 Caulfield T. Human cloning laws, human dignity and the poverty of the policy making dialogue. *BMC Med Ethics* 2003; **4**: E3.

33 Chochinov HM. Defending dignity. *Palliat Support Care* 2003; **1**: 307–8.

34 Latimer E. Caring for seriously ill and dying patients: the philosophy and ethics. *Can Med Assoc J* 1991; **144**: 859.

35 Geyman JP. Dying and death of a family member. *J Fam Pract* 1983; **17**: 125–34.

● 36 Chochinov HM, Hack T, Hassard T, *et al.* Dignity in the terminally ill: a cross-sectional, cohort study. *Lancet* 2002; **360**: 2026–30.

37 Ambiven M. Dying with dignity. *World Health Forum* 1991; **12**: 375–81.

38 Madan TN. Dying with dignity. *Soc Sci Med* 1992; **35**: 425–32.

39 Quill TE. Perspectives on care at the close of life: initiating end-of-life discussions with seriously ill patients: addressing the 'elephant in the room'. *JAMA* 2000; **284**: 2502–7.

40 Wanzer SH, Federman DD, Adelstein SJ, *et al.* The physician's responsibility toward hopelessly ill patients. A second look. *N Engl J Med* 1989; **320**: 844–9.

41 Wilson JK, Fox E, Kamakahi JJ. Who is fighting for the right to die? Older women's participation in the Hemlock Society. *Health Care Women Int* 1998; **19**: 365–80.

42 Ganzini L, Nelson HD, Lee MA, *et al.* Oregon physicians' attitudes about and experiences with end-of-life care since the passage of the Oregon Death with Dignity Act. *JAMA* 2001; **285**: 2363–9.

43 Simpson E. Harms to dignity, bioethics, and the scope of biolaw. *J Palliat Care* 2004; **20**: 185–93.

● 44 Van der Mass PJ, van Delden JJM, Pijnenborg L, Looman CWN. Euthanasia and other medical decisions concerning the end of life. *Lancet* 1991; **338**: 669–74.

45 Back AL, Wallace JI, Starks HE, *et al.* Physician-assisted suicide and euthanasia in Washington state: Patient requests and physician responses. *JAMA* 1996; **275**:919–925.

46 Seale C, Addington-Hall J. Euthanasia: Why people want to die earlier. *Soc Sci Med* 1994; **39**: 647–54.

● 47 Chochinov HM, Wilson KG, Enns M, *et al.* Desire for death in the terminally ill. *Am J Psychiatry* 1995; **152**: 185–91.

48 Rosenfeld B, Krivo S, Breitbart W, Chochinov HM. Suicide, assisted suicide, an euthanasia in the terminally ill.

In: Chochinov HM, Brietbart W, eds. *Handbook of Psychiatry in Palliative Medicine*. Oxford: Oxford University Press, 2000: 51–62.

49 Chochinov HM, Wilson KG. The euthanasia debate: attitudes, practices and psychiatric considerations. *Can J Psychiatry* 1995; **40**: 593–602.

50 Block SD, Billings JA. Patient requests to hasten death: evaluation and management in terminal care. *Arch Intern Med* 1994; **154**: 2039–47.

51 Payne SA, Langley-Evans A, Hillier R. Perceptions of a 'good' death: a comparative study of the views of hospice staff and patients. *Palliat Med* 1996; **10**: 307–12.

52 Emanuel EJ, Emanuel LL. The promise of a good death. *Lancet* 1998; **351**: Suppl 2:SII21–SII29.

53 Steinhauser KE, Christakis NA, Clipp EC, *et al.* Factors considered important at the end of life by patients, family, physicians, and other care providers. *JAMA* 2000; **284**: 2476–82.

54 Turner K, Chye R, Aggarwal G, *et al.* Dignity in Dying: a preliminary study of patients in the last three days of life. *J Palliat Care* 1996; **12**: 7–13.

● 55 McClement SE, Chochinov HM, Hack TF, *et al.* Dignity-conserving care: application of research findings to practice. *Int J Palliat Nurs* 2004; **10**: 173–9.

● 56 Chochinov HM, Hack T, McClement S, *et al.* Dignity in the terminally ill: a developing empirical model. *Soc Sci Med* 2002; **54**: 433–43.

57 Chochinov HM. Dignity and the eye of the beholder. *J Clin Oncol* 2004; **22**: 1336–40.

● 58 Hack TF, Chochinov HM, Hasaard T, *et al.* Defining dignity in terminally ill cancer patients: a factor-analytic approach. *Psychooncology* 2004; **13**:700–8.

59 Addington-Hall JM, Higginson I. *Palliative Care for Non-cancer Patients*. Oxford: Oxford University Press, 2001.

60 Pickett M. Cultural awareness of in the context of terminal illness. *Cancer Nurs* 1993; **16**: 102–6.

61 Kristjanson LJ, Solan JA, Dudgeon D, Adaskin E. Family members' perceptions of palliative cancer care: predictors of family functioning and family members' health. *J Palliat Care* 1996; **12**: 10–20.

62 Becker R. How will I cope?: Psychological aspects of advanced illness. In: Kinghorn S, Gamlin R, eds. *Palliative Nursing: Bringing Comfort and Hope*. Edinburgh: Bailliere Tindall, 2001.

63 Field MJ, Cassel CK, eds. *Approaching Death: Improving Care at the End of Life/Committee on Care at the End of Life*. Washington: National Academy Press, 1997.

PART 3

The problems and challenges of global reach

14

Transcultural palliative care

CARL JOHAN FÜRST, SOLVIG EKBLAD

TRANSCULTURAL PERSPECTIVES ON DEVELOPMENT OF PALLIATIVE CARE

> Challenging assumptions based on one's own culture is essential to the development of knowledge and insight into others.[1]

There has been rapid development in palliative care in many countries during the past decades, as witnessed in clinical practice, organization, education, and research. This development has been diverse, depending on the local culture and traditions and the context of the care being delivered.[2–4] The many organizational models for end-of-life care around the world and the meaning of and terminology used in different countries mirror some of these variations.[5,6] The World Health Organization (WHO) 2002 definitions reflect a broadening concept of palliative care as compared with the previous WHO definition of 1990 but still do not specifically address cultural issues.[7–9]

Transcultural palliative care deals with the understanding and evaluation of cultural factors in advanced disease and end-of-life care. It takes into account the different cultural, religious, ethnic, and ethical value systems, and it bridges the gap between different cultural contexts by a more fulfilling communication between the care providers and patients and their families. For patients from immigrant populations, transcultural palliative care takes a dual perspective of the norms of the prevailing culture and of the minority group to which the patient belongs. This is relevant in palliative care services in all parts of the world.

Models of palliative care which have been developed in wealthier societies are not easily transferred to societies where there is poverty, extended family structure, and insufficient health infrastructure. There is a need to adjust to local social and culture contexts.[10] At the same time, spiritual care, which plays an essential part in relief of suffering and pain, is just as important in developing countries where comfort and medical resources are limited.[11] In addition, it should be borne in mind that the basic needs and wishes of patients from ethnic minorities in palliative care are common to all human beings and independent of cultural background.[3] Patients from ethnic minorities try to fit in with the dominant culture, which provides another argument against stereotypical cultural care not being appropriate.[12]

Thus, on the whole, transcultural palliative care includes knowledge of the practices and rites of different religions and cultures and is sensitive to the specific needs of minority groups. The term is used synonymously with intercultural and multicultural care.[13] A cultural perspective may also mean that palliative care can pass on its values to institutions, organizations, or education programs. One of the main findings from reflections from focus groups' interviews with hospice staff regarding cultural challenges in end-of-life care was that 'to better understand other cultures it is important to raise awareness about the staff's own culture and to pay attention to culture especially in the context of the individual'.[14]

In parallel with the development of palliative care the world has experienced unrivaled advancements in medical technology and pharmacology, giving rise not only to hope for new possibilities but also to unrealistic expectations of cure and survival. Another factor that has influenced the development of palliative care has been the needs of patients with nonmalignant diseases.[9] Generally, the prevalence of chronic and life-threatening illnesses has increased due to the aging of populations in many developed countries.[9,15]

We are witnessing a change in social structures, toward smaller numbers of informal caregivers. Families look different, are becoming smaller, and are often dispersed. The pressures of a demanding society often influence the family structure and divorce rates are increasing in many countries. At the same time societies and families have lost many of the rites and rituals that were often based on religion or historical traditions. In the past these served as a support during life events such as dying and bereavement.

The acquired immune deficiency syndrome (AIDS) epidemic, in particular in the developing countries, especially has left large groups of children with little adult support and at risk for disease and early death. At the same time, Western countries have witnessed increasing numbers of immigrants from developing countries, war-ravaged regions, and totalitarian regimes, putting new ethical demands on good quality care at the end of life.

CULTURAL COMPETENCE AND EFFECTIVE COMMUNICATION SKILLS

Culture is a process by which activities acquire moral and emotional meaning for individuals.[16] In the twenty-first century, human beings are interconnected globally in the virtual and physical worlds. From this it follows that traditional definitions of culture are now challenged by globalization, which has led to differences within a cultural setting that may equal or exceed the dissimilarities between cultures.[17]

Cultural competence refers to a clinician's knowledge of various cultures and their ability to apply this knowledge to patient care.[18,19] This competence demands a dual stance: first the clinician's own perspective and then the perspective of the patient and family members. The issues that need to be dealt with by all palliative care clinicians irrespective of their background professions is illustrated by the example case in Box 14.1 and in the proposed assessment model (Box 14.2). The ability to communicate effectively gives the clinician an insight of the ethnic minority patient's immediate medical and psychosocial needs.

Box 14.1 A transcultural assessment

Sophia is 43 years old and mother of three children between the ages of 12 and 19 years. She left Iraq with her husband and children 10 years ago. Sophia was diagnosed as having acute leukemia 2 years ago and has been through several chemotherapy regimens including a bone marrow transplant. She is newly admitted to your hospice from the hematology department. Her blood values and general weakness prevent further chemotherapy. She knows only a few words in your language. Her husband and his brother speak your language to some extent and try to act as

interpreters. Mostly they talk and answer on behalf of Sophia. Sophia is prescribed intravenous nutrition, blood platelets when required, and erythropoietin, and is on intravenous antibiotics because of recent septicemia. Your impression is that Sophia is nearing death and is experiencing severe anxiety. The relatives are expecting a brief stay at the hospice before a new course of chemotherapy.

Questions

- How would you handle the situation?

- What more information do you need?

- Are there differences between the perspectives of the different professionals in the caring team?

Box 14.2 A transcultural assessment model: attitudes, skills, and knowledge of transcultural palliative care

Attitudes – issues to reflect upon:

- Assumptions based on one's own culture and possible prejudices

- Your general standpoints on nutrition and fluids, personal care, drugs including smoking and alcohol, alternative treatments such as traditional medicine, anticancer treatment in end-of-life care

- Beliefs, attitudes and values regarding: diseases and prognosis, death customs and bereavement; patient-centered or authority-centered care; expectations of care by patient, family and staff

Skills – issues to be dealt with:

- Social hierarchical structure, family patterns

- Identify adaptations already made by the patient

- Modification of emphasis in teaching, e.g. targeting one of the parents or an elder family member to obtain accurate information and deliver education such as in home care

- Being supportive toward **religious beliefs** as well as toward profane attitudes

- Appropriately adapt communication and behavior according to family structures, communication patterns, and styles, based on cultural influences

Knowledge – issues you need to know about:

- Beliefs and practices related to illness and health, basic habits around dying, death and bereavement in relation to the major religions

- Where to find 'up-to-date information' on religious and cultural habits

- Biological variations, e.g. genetic variation in susceptibility to disease

- Impact of earlier, untreated, traumatic life events during the terminal stage of life

Organizational issues:

- Space, e.g. for patients and relatives to visit and pray if they wish

- Environmental factors, e.g. food, presence of religious artefacts

- Contacts with religious representatives

Barriers to cultural competence can be in relation to the care providers and to health systems.[18,19] The former barriers arise when individual providers lack knowledge of their patients' cultural practices and beliefs or when providers' beliefs differ from those of their patients. Those who expect their patients to respond as they themselves would to issues such as medical decision making, artificial nutrition and hydration, and death and mourning, will be unprepared when patients respond differently. System-related barriers exist because most facilities have not been designed for cultural diversity, favoring instead a 'one-size-fits-all' approach to care. For example: Can a Buddhist family stay long enough with the dead body of a relative to allow for the spirit to leave by the open window?

Thus, culturally tailored care is an important quality factor,[20] but stereotypical cultural care may be inappropriate, since micro-cultural differences and individual diversifications within cultures are common. When needs are not obvious it is necessary to specifically explore the cultural aspects of care.

THE INDIVIDUAL AND THE FAMILY

The focus for palliative care should be centered on the needs of the unique person and patient whose autonomy and values the staff seeks to respect. At the end of life, everyone should be treated with the same respect, independent of religious, cultural, language, and ethnic background. The fundamental ethical principle is the patient's right to die in the way he or she wants to, regardless of his or her condition, lifestyle, culture, beliefs, and educational background. A culturally competent and ethical decision-making model is based on human rights and the use of ethical principles that include values and assumptions of the patients.

Patient autonomy is a key issue in the interface between the patient-centered care that is common in many Western societies and the cultures where the family and community have a more important role and function as advocates for the patient. In some cultures, the welfare of the community takes precedence over individual life, e.g. Korean Americans and Mexican Americans have been shown to be more in favor of the family making decisions on end-of-life issues than African Americans and European Americans.[21] In reality, decisions are often made by consensus.[22]

It is common to use an empirical ethical analysis that is based on patient autonomy. Other common and relevant ethical principles of Western cultures include the concepts of nonmaleficence, beneficence, and justice. In European philosophy there is sometimes a belief in absolute ethical principles that are the basis of morals. The two moral principles of nonmaleficence and justice are often seen as absolute.[2] Two other important principles are 'sanctity of life' and 'absence of suffering'.

BREAKING BAD NEWS

I will always prefer not to know, or to know as little as possible. No human being knows when he is going to arrive in this world, therefore I believe that his natural state is also not to know when he will depart.[2]

The ethical dilemma of giving diagnostic information or requesting informed consent for a medical procedure from a patient wishing to remain ignorant challenges the physician to balance respect for the patient's attitude with information which could be beneficial. Truth telling or breaking bad news, as well as communication about impending death, has to be seen in this context .[23–25] The nature and the amount of information given to patients with cancer is still approached differently, depending on the country and culture.[26–31] An important ethical question from a transcultural perspective is: What ethical justification can support the withholding of information or the giving of information to patients about their terminal illness? Culturally competent communication about death and dying is increasingly important once biomedical intervention is shown to fail to cure.

In many cultures, families of the patients still generally prefer to receive the information first. They can then filter the information to the patient. Their often-cited reasons for this include fear that the truth will cause the patient to lose hope, they need to protect the patient from bad news, and a strong religious belief.[32] However, effective communication about terminal prognosis allows patients and families to have realistic hope.[33] An example is the expression of parents' self-assumed duty to protect their child from knowing about a terminal prognosis. To carry out this family obligation, relatives should create a caring environment in which the patient does not have any unnecessary psychological burdens. Conflict occurs when the beliefs and wishes of family members differ from those of the patient, the team members, or both. If the patient desires and is capable of understanding full disclosure, the ethical challenge for the physician is whether to respect the patient's wishes or to follow the cultural views of the family members which may be different. The focus needs to be the quality of life of the patient,[34] and among the team's responsibilities is helping the family to understand the patient's need for information and teaching them that hope can prevail when life comes to an end.[18,35,36]

DIFFERENCES IN VIEWS WITHIN THE PROFESSIONAL CARING TEAM AND BETWEEN THE TEAM AND THE PATIENT AND FAMILY

Patients' needs may be expressed by themselves, by a family member or by a member of staff. These medical and psychosocial needs must be recognized by the team and be thoroughly discussed. Frustration may occur in the team when views of the patient, family and team differ with regard to acceptance of treatment, for example, of pain and other symptoms. Perceptions of the ethical challenges involved may differ and there may be difficulty in communication about the problems. The challenge is understanding each other's perceptions of the problem. If successful collaboration based on shared trust is to be achieved, which will include the participation and empowerment of patients and their families in decision making, the caring team needs to be sensitive to the unique values of each patient, be empathetic, and have the ability to communicate.

Patients and families may be used to a hierarchical healthcare system and may therefore have difficulties dealing with the democratic values of the palliative care team approach. Some male patients may get a feeling of degradation if seen by a female doctor and vice versa, e.g. a female patient being seen by a male gynecologist.[37] Another issue can be the age of the doctor. Older patients may be critical of younger doctors and the doctors may have to demonstrate the required knowledge in order to be trusted.

Access to a professional interpreter is an important right of patients. There may be some resistance on the part of the family members, who prefer to do the translation themselves. A professional interpreter can draw attention to unexpressed signals that may give important information to the staff, for example: Does the patient understand the questions? How does the patient formulate the answers? Are the answers direct? However, patients may be unwilling to talk about delicate matters through a professional interpreter, even when the interpreter is from the same country, region or ethnic group as the patient. In spite of the fact that the interpreter will give assurance about professional secrecy, the patient or the family may not be fully trustful. The personal attitude and professionalism of the interpreter have a large influence on their ability to communicate and facilitate the meeting.[38,39]

Communication problems, hierarchical processes, uncertainty, scarce resources and competing values are the usual causes for moral dilemmas in healthcare. Physicians and nurses responsible for making medical decisions in end-of-life care can experience moral distress. Every team will have different needs and difficulties when encountering suffering and trying to make the best possible decisions and handling the situation.[40] Some of these dilemmas are listed in Box 14.3.

Box 14.3 Issues causing moral distress in transcultural palliative care

- Communication: breaking bad news; role of interpreter; patient/family; role of different team members

- Uncertainty: role of doctor, role of medical treatment, 'false' hope

- Scarce resources: setting priorities for staff, medicine, hospice/hospital beds

- Competing values and hierarchical processes: Whose values and beliefs are the focus?

RELIGION

The religious map in many countries has changed during the last 20 years. There is a profane wind in several modern (including Western) countries and religious rites and traditions are getting less important. Another large change is the growing number of Muslims, making Islam an important religion in several Western countries. Likewise, due to refugee immigration many Catholics and orthodox Christians have gone to the Lutheran countries of northern Europe.

How a patient identifies him or herself in terms of religious belief usually affects their perceptions of health and healthcare up to the end of their lives. Grief is influenced by the cultural meaning that every culture lends to death and loss.[20] The many different death rituals sometimes have a gender implication. For example it is the Muslim norm that members of the same gender wash the diseased body.[41] A common spiritual belief in some religions is that the body must be as intact and unblemished as possible to facilitate the spirit's course through subsequent incarnations or rest. Box 14.4 gives a checklist of important culturally or religiously dependent practices and rituals. The purpose of this chapter is not to give detailed information about different religions, but to emphasize that it is the responsibility of the team to assess the individual preferences of the patient and their family.

With regard to the immediate handling of the body after death, health professionals need to respect the wishes and, if possible beforehand, gather information from relatives and a religious representative concerning restrictions on who (i.e. gender) will close the eyes and mouth of the deceased adult patient, straighten the legs, and for example, for a Muslim patient, put the face and feet in a specific direction, taking into consideration the location of Mecca.[42]

Box 14.4 Checklist of questions concerning cultural and religious practices and rituals. Individual preferences and concerns should always be considered

- *Fasting*: Christmas, before Easter, Ramadan, before funeral, fluids only

- *Dietary practices*: Vegetarian, flesh, meat, shellfish, no fermented, alcohol, kosher

- *Treatment*: Patient versus family, staff of same sex, no handshake, alternative treatment or approach, traditional medicine, shamanism

- *Professional interpreter*: same sex, same religion, local dialect, trust

- *Autopsy*: different levels of restriction, no organs taken

- *The dead body*: rituals, washing, dressing, same sex, cremation, burial, time constraints, bury in home country or host country

In addition, washing and shrouding procedures may also be related to religion and customs regarding death. If the patient had no relatives, usually the religious community will arrange the prescribed rituals if desired.

Organ transplantation, although uncommon in palliative oncology care situations, is another issue which may not be allowed due to religious beliefs and therefore it is always of importance that the family of the deceased patient is given the information in a sensitive manner and accurately with due respect, i.e. the family has a choice. In several religions there is a custom to bury the deceased as soon as possible and cremation is usually avoided, for example in Judaism and Islam.[41,43] This may become a problem if death occurs during a holiday in a foreign country, giving rise to anxiety among the relatives. Under such circumstances, a rapid release of the dead body prevents unnecessary and prolonged distress to the bereaved family and friends.[42] In Islam, as a sign of respect for the deceased, the grieving relatives will not eat until the funeral. In Islam, the woman's role is to mourn and the husband's duty is to protect his wife.

Bereavement is the objective state of having lost an important, significant person. Grief, on the other hand, is the emotional reaction following a bereavement. Mourning is the behavioral reaction, reflections that a society expects will follow a bereavement. Family members may have more or less appropriate networks for support and sharing during the care and mourning process. An example of a supportive network is the Jewish practice of 'shiva'. The bereaved family stays at home for some days after the death. Family and friends bring food and help with the necessities of life. Such support may enhance the healing process for the family members.

VULNERABLE INDIVIDUALS

Asylum seekers and refugees with a past history of trauma are displaced from their homelands to new environments. It is hard to die as a stranger in a strange land. These patients have often lost their past and old ways of life, their friends and their own people. So much is destroyed by war and, with the onset of palliative care, much of this will never be regained. To settle in the new host country, refugees need to make many changes, and old ways are not always helpful in the event of advanced disease. A life-threatening disease is likely to bring back suppressed memories of atrocities and of other terrible events. Unresolved traumatic life events may evolve into reactions of a psychiatric nature, such as psychoses, which need to be distinguished from development of actual psychiatric disease and from expected reactions to trauma and crisis. Survivors of the holocaust or concentration camps from the second world war may have severe difficulties in coping at the end of life and may even develop psychotic symptoms. Also, dying prisoners who are confined or are illegal immigrants or who are not permitted to spend their last days in a hospice outside the prison need special attention. It is a challenge to bring competent palliative care to dying prisoners.[44]

It is a challenge in communication having to tell a pregnant mother from an ethnic minority, who is infected with HIV/AIDS that she is at great risk of delivering a baby with life-limiting illness. With regard to the loss of a child, mourning is again related to culture and religious customs. Empowerment of parents including spiritual support, which is often neglected but is of importance to prevent unnecessary suffering.[45] For example, an Islamic family may be reminded that children are innocent and pure and as such assured paradise.[46]

Key learning points

- Transcultural aspects need to be included in palliative care.
- Cultural awareness, self-knowledge, and cultural competence are necessary tools for the palliative care team.
- Opposing ethical values and cultural norms may give rise to moral distress.
- Communication difficulties between staff, patient and family or within the professional caring team need to be resolved.
- Transcultural assessment should be made following a proposed structural model.
- Transcultural aspects of palliative care should be included in education and training.

REFERENCES

1 Jensen R. Cross-cultural perspectives in palliative care. *J Pain Palliat Care Pharmacother* 2003; **17**: 223–9.

2 Núnez Olarte JM, Guillén DG. Cultural issues and ethical dilemmas in palliative and end-of-life care in Spain. *Cancer Control* 2001; **8**: 46–54.

3 Voltz R, Akabayashi A, Reese C, *et al.* Organization and patients' perception of palliative care: a crosscultural comparison. *Palliat Med* 1997; **11**: 351–7.

4 Clark D. The International Observatory on End of Life Care: a new initiative to support palliative care development around the world. *J Pain Palliat Care Pharmacother* 2003; **17**: 231–8.

5 Rajagopal MR, Venkateswaran C. Palliative care in India: successes and limitations. *J Pain Palliat Care Pharmacother* 2003; **17**: 121–8.

6 Kikule E. A good death in Uganda: survey of needs for palliative care for terminally ill people in urban areas. *BMJ* 2003; **327**: 192–4.

7 World Health Organization. *Cancer, Pain Relief and Palliative Care. Report of a WHO Expert Committee*. Geneva: World Health Organization, 1990.

8 World Health Organization. *National Cancer Control Programmes: Policies and Managerial Guidelines*, 2nd ed. Geneva: World Helath Organization, 2002.

9 Davis E, Higginson IJ, eds. *The Solid Facts. Palliative Care*. Copenhagen: World Health Organization, Europe Region, 2004.

10 Pampallona S, Bollini P. Palliative care in developing countries: why research is needed. *J Pain Palliat Care Pharmacother* 2003; **17**: 171–82.

11 Lunn JS. Spiritual care in a multi-religious context. *J Pain Palliat Care Pharmacother* 2003; **17**: 153–66.

12 Diver F, Molassiotis A, Weeks L. The palliative care needs of ethnic minority patients attending day-care centre: a qualitative study. *Int J Palliat Nurs* 2003; **9**: 389–96.

13 Ekstrand L. Multicultural education. In: Husén T, Postlethwaite T, eds. *The International Encyclopedia of Education*. Oxford: Pergamon Press, 1994: 3960–70.

14 Abdullah SN. Towards an individualized client's care: implication for education. The transcultural approach. *J Adv Nurs* 1995; **22**: 715–20.

15 Davis E, Higginson IJ, eds. *Better Palliative Care for Older People*. Copenhagen: World Health Organization, Europe Region, 2004.

16 Kleinman A. Culture and depression. *N Engl J Med* 2004; **351**: 951–3.

17 Duffy ME. A critique of cultural education in nursing. *J Adv Nurs* 2001; **36**: 487–95.

18 Mazanec P, Tyler M. How ethnicity, age, and spirituality affect decisions when death is imminent. *Home Healthcare Nurse* 2004; **22**: 317–26.

19 McNeil C. Culture: the impact on health care. *J Cancer Educ* 1990; **5**: 13–16.

20 Mystakidou K, Tsilika E, Parpa E, *et al.* A Greek perspective on concepts of death and expression of grief, with implications for practice. *Int J Palliat Nurs* 2003; **9**: 534–7.

21 Blackhall LJ, Murphy ST, Frank G, *et al.* Ethnicity and attitudes toward patient autonomy. *JAMA* 1995; **274**: 820–5.

22 Kagawa-Singer M. The cultural context of death rituals and mourning practices. *Oncol Nurs Forum* 1998; **25**: 1752–6.

23 Surbone A. Information, truth and communication. For an interpretation of truth telling practices throughout the world. *Ann N Y Acad Sci* 1997; **809**: 7–16.

24 Butow PN, Tattershall MH, Goldstein D. Communication with cancer patients in culturally diverse societies. *Ann N Y Acad Sci* 1997; **809**: 317–29.

25 Surbone A. Persisting differences in truth telling throughout the world. *Support Care Cancer* 2004; **12**: 143–6.

26 Levy LM. Communication with the cancer patient in Zimbabwe. *Ann N Y Acad Sci* 1997; **809**: 133–41.

27 Faria SL, Souhami F, Souhami L. Communication with the cancer patient: information and truth in Brazil. *Ann N Y Acad Sci* 1997; **809**: 163–71.

28 Ghavamzadeh A, Bahar B. Communication with the cancer patient in Iran. *Ann N Y Acad Sci* 1997; **809**: 261–5.

29 Younge D, Moreau P, Ezzat A, Gray A. Communication with cancer patients in Saudi Arabia. *Ann N Y Acad Sci* 1997; **809**: 309–16.

30 Annunziata MA. Ethics of relationships: from communication to conversation. *Ann N Y Acad Sci* 1997; **809**: 400–10.

31 Mystakidou K, Parpa E, Tsilika E, *et al.* Cancer information disclosure in different cultural contexts. *Support Care Cancer* 2004; **12**: 147–54.

32 Ozdogan M, Samur M, Sat Bozcuk H, *et al.* 'Do not tell': what factors affect relatives' attitudes to honest disclosure of diagnoses to cancer patients? *Support Care Cancer* 2004; **12**: 497–502.

33 Hu W, Chiu T, Chuang R, Chen C. Solving family-related barriers to truthfulness in cases of terminal cancer in Taiwan. *Cancer Nurs* 2002; **25**: 486–92.

34 Bozuk H, Erdogan V, Eken C, *et al.* Does awareness of diagnosis make any difference to quality of life? *Support Care Cancer* 2002; **10**: 51–7.

35 Sabbioni MEE. Informing cancer patients: whose truth matters? *Ann N Y Acad Sci* 1997; **809**: 508–13.

36 Fallowfield L. Truth sometimes hurts but deceit hurts more. *Ann N Y Acad Sci* 1997; **809**: 525–36.

37 Rizk DE, El-Zubeir MA, Al-Dhaheri AM, *et al.* Determinants of women's choice of their obstetrician and gynecologist provider in the UAE. *Acta Obstet Gynecol Scand* 2005; **84**: 48–53.

38 Phelan M, Parkman S. How to do it: work with an interpreter. *BMJ* 1995; **311**: 555–7.

39 Kaufert JM, Putsch RW, Lavallee M. Experience of aboriginal health interpreters in mediation of conflicting values in end-of-life decision making. *Int J Circumpolar Health* 1998; **57**(Suppl 1): 43–8.

40 Oberle K, Hughes D. Doctors' and nurses' perceptions of ethical problems in end-of-life decisions. *J Adv Nurs* 2001; **33**: 707–15.

41 Lawrence P, Rozmus C. Culturally sensitive care of the Muslim patient. *J Transcult Nurs* 2001; **12**: 228–33.

42 Gatrad R, Sheikh A. Palliative care for Muslims and issues after death. *Int J Palliat Nurs* 2002; **8**: 594–7.

43 Bonura D, Fender M, Roesler M, Pacquiao D. Culturally congruent end-of-life care for Jewish patients and their families. *J Transcult Nurs* 2001; **12**: 211–20.

44 Lum K. Palliative care behind bars: the New Zealand prison hospice experience. *J Pain Palliat Care Pharmacother* 2003; **17**: 131–8.

45 Davies B, Brenner P, Orloff S, *et al.* Addressing spirituality in pediatric hospice and palliative care. *J Palliat Care* 2002; **18**: 59–67.

46 Tarazi N. *The Child in Islam*. Indiana: ATP, 1995: 84–7.

15

Palliative care: global situation and initiatives

LILIANA DE LIMA

GLOBAL SITUATION

The World Health Organization (WHO) estimates that 56.5 million deaths occurred worldwide in 2001. Approximately 76 percent of these deaths occurred in developing countries, where over three-fourths of the people in the world live. According to the data, the main causes of the total mortality for that year were the following:[1***]

- Noncommunicable conditions, including cancers and cardiovascular diseases – 58.5 percent
- Communicable diseases, including acquired immune deficiency syndrome (AIDS), maternal and perinatal conditions and nutritional deficiencies – 32.5 percent
- Intentional and unintentional injuries – 9 percent

In the past decade, infectious diseases such as malaria, dengue, tuberculosis, and cholera have caused over a fourth of the cumulative deaths in developing nations. In addition, approximately 8 percent of the adult population is infected with the human immunodeficiency virus (HIV) virus in sub-Saharan Africa, and global AIDS deaths totaled 3.1 million during 2003.[2***] Cancer is among the major noncommunicable causes of death worldwide and accounted for 12.6 percent of the total deaths in 2001.[1***] The International Agency for Research on Cancer (IARC) projects that global cancer rates will increase by 50 percent from 10 million new cases worldwide in 2000 to 15 million new cases in 2020, primarily due to the aging of population and increases in smoking. Fifty percent of the world's new cancer cases and deaths occur in developing nations and approximately 80 percent of these cancer patients are already incurable at the time of diagnosis.

Access to palliative care

Palliative care includes the management of symptoms and provision of spiritual and psychosocial support to patients and their families from the moment of diagnosis, throughout the course of the disease. Palliative care can be provided simply and inexpensively in tertiary care facilities, community health centers, and at home. However, access to pain relief and palliative care services is often limited, even in developed countries due to a lack of political will, insufficient information and education, and excessive regulation of opioids.

A recent study on advanced cancer care in Latin America of 667 physicians demonstrated that most of the care given to persons with advanced cancer is in hospitals as compared with other facilities or at home, whereas the majority of cancer deaths take place at home. The study also identified the following top barriers to cancer pain management as reported by the respondents: (i) inadequate staff knowledge of pain management; (ii) patients' inability to pay for services or analgesics; (iii) inadequate pain assessment; and (iv) excessive state/legal regulations of prescribing opioids.[3**]

Morphine as an indicator of access to palliative care

For several years, morphine consumption has been used as an indicator of adequate access to pain relief, one of the cornerstones of palliative care. In 1986, the WHO and its Expert Committee on Cancer Pain Relief and Active Supportive Care developed the *WHO Analgesic Ladder*[4**] for the relief of cancer pain. The method relies on the permanent availability of opioid analgesics, including morphine, codeine, and others. The *WHO Ladder* has been widely disseminated throughout the world. Still, opioid analgesics are insufficiently available, especially in developing countries, and prescription of morphine is limited to a small percentage of physicians and is unavailable in many countries of the world.

The International Narcotics Control Board (INCB) collects the consumption data yearly from government reports.[5] While supply of narcotic drugs for medical purposes remains inadequate, the consumption trends recorded by INCB indicate improvement. The global consumption of morphine has been doubling every 5 years since 1984. In 2002 global consumption amounted for 27.3 tons.[6] The trend is, however, mainly due to increasing consumption in a few countries. For 2002, 82 percent of the total global consumption of morphine occurred in six countries: USA, France, Canada, Germany, United Kingdom, and Australia; the remaining 18 percent was consumed in the other 133 countries for which data are available. There are 51 developing countries for which there is no registered morphine consumption at all.[5]

In the study of advanced cancer care in Latin America mentioned in the section above, over 80 percent of the respondents reported either good or excellent availability of the main nonopioid analgesics and adjuvants in their practice settings. In contrast, the availability of both short- and long-acting opioid analgesics varied greatly across by nations, practice settings, and by specific medication.[7]** The great majority of the countries reported difficulties in access and excessively strict regulations on the use of controlled substances. Other studies have confirmed similar results in the availability and accessibility to potent analgesics and limitations to palliative care in different regions of the world.[8–11]

Socioeconomic and cultural aspects

The developing world varies greatly from country to country and region to region. There are a limited number of excellent facilities in developing countries with the latest technology and medications capable of delivering care similar to that of the developed countries, but the majority of the population does not have access to these institutions, and are cared for in facilities with limited resources. Patients in extremely resource-poor settings pose different challenges which need to be taken into account when developing palliative care programs and strategies.

Palliative care is often perceived as part of the Christian movement. However, there are many palliative care programs and hospices in Islamic, Hindu, Jewish, and Buddhist regions of the world. The main concepts of palliative care – respect for the individual, compassionate care, holistic approach, and the incorporation of the relatives and family members as part of the care team – can be applied to all religions and faiths.

Cultural aspects play a significant role in the provision of care. Research has shown there are major differences in attitudes and beliefs regarding issues such as communication, the role of patients and families in the decision making process, amount of information disclosed in the diagnosis and prognosis, spiritual aspects, discussion of end-of-life issues and other related topics.[12,13] Professionals need to be aware that there is a need for recognition of these differences, especially in multicultural environments, or when traveling abroad to teach or work in another country.

Palliative care for patients in the developing world

The modern palliative care movement originated during the 1960s in the UK as a response to the unmet need of patients with terminal conditions and their families. This movement soon became global and there are now hospices and palliative care units in many countries around the world.

A large body of knowledge has emerged on the assessment and management of the physical and psychosocial problems that occur in patients who develop cancer and other progressive incurable illnesses. The overwhelming majority of the available written material refers to the delivery of palliative care for diseases that occur mostly in the developed world and using resources mostly available in developed countries. But patients in developing countries die younger and of conditions different to those in the developed world. In addition, there are socioeconomic and cultural issues that pose particular challenges for the healthcare team. Communication, disclosure of the diagnosis, active participation in the decision making and treatment, discussion of end-of-life issues and other matters are all influenced by the context in which these occur. Recent publications address these issues and highlight the importance of a global approach sensitive to the different conditions, cultures, and settings. Some of these include *Palliative Care in the Developing World: Principles and Practice*[14] and *Pain and Palliative Care in the Developing World and Marginalized Populations: A Global Challenge*.[15] These publications not only cover treatment of diseases common in developing countries, but also cultural and ethical principles affecting care of patients with varied religious beliefs, ethnical groups, and backgrounds.

GLOBAL INITIATIVES

The World Health Organization

The WHO World Cancer Report calls on all countries to establish comprehensive national cancer control programs aimed at reducing the incidence of cancer through primary prevention; providing earlier diagnosis and curative treatments; and improving the quality of life for patients with cancer and their families through the delivery of adequate palliative care and pain relief.[16]

AFRICA PROJECT ON PALLIATIVE CARE

Palliative care is one of the three main priorities of the WHO Program on Cancer Control (PCC) and is included in the agenda of several other WHO programs.[17] The WHO Program on Cancer Control in collaboration with the WHO Departments of Care for HIV-AIDS, governmental and intergovernmental agencies, nongovernmental organizations and the WHO Regional Office for Africa (AFRO) developed an initiative to strengthen palliative care in southern African countries. The project, called 'A Community Health Approach to Palliative Care for HIV and Cancer Patients in Africa' is being implemented in five countries – Botswana, Ethiopia, Tanzania, Uganda, and Zimbabwe.[18]

The main goal of this project is to contribute to the improvement of the quality of life for cancer and HIV/AIDS patients in southern African countries by facilitating and strengthening the initiation and development of palliative care programs with a public health approach. These programs provide pain relief and holistic care to an increasing proportion of patients with advanced HIV/AIDS.

The specific objectives are:

- To develop/reinforce palliative care programs with a public health approach in response to the needs and gaps identified, considering:
  - a holistic approach to palliative care, giving special emphasis to pain relief
  - a systemic approach to program implementation which considers policy development, provision of care, drug availability, training, and education in the context of HIV/AIDS and cancer health problems
  - integration with the existing health system, involving all levels of care with special emphasis on home-based care
  - a team approach at the organizational and care levels
  - the elements for good quality performance: improving access, acceptability, efficiency, effectiveness, etc.
- To advocate for drug availability and policy development among the governments of the participating countries
- To develop a network among the participating countries that will:
  - promote exchange of information and collaboration
  - advocate for the integration of such programs into national strategic plans for health and social services.

The first part of this project has been completed and WHO is seeking funds to continue with the second phase. Additional information about this project can be found in the Palliative Care Page on the WHO website (www.who.int/cancer/palliative/africanproject/en/).

WHO COLLABORATING CENTERS IN PAIN RELIEF AND PALLIATIVE CARE

The WHO collaborating center forms part of an inter-institutional collaborative network set up by WHO in support of its program at the country, inter-country, regional, interregional, and global levels. The Collaborating Centers in Pain Relief and Palliative Care are a resource for the Organization, professionals, policy makers, and the public in current and relevant issues in the field.[19] One particular collaborating center which has been very active in the field of opioid availability and policy is the WHO Collaborating Center for Policy and Communications in Cancer Care. The center specializes in the assessment of barriers in national approaches to opioid analgesic regulations, seeks to make opioids available for medical and scientific use, maintains a global communication network for the WHO Cancer Pain Relief and Palliative Care Program, and provides assistance to initiatives or country projects regarding palliative care, especially those concerning advocacy for drug availability and policy development. The center is located at the Pain and Policy Studies Group, University of Wisconsin Medical School, Comprehensive Cancer Center at Madison, WI, USA. The center has a website (www.medsch.wisc.edu/painpolicy) which lists several reports on opioid use, policies, and documents which are very useful to palliative care workers, legislators and government representatives from around the world.

The International Association for Hospice and Palliative Care (IAHPC)

The IAHPC is a not-for-profit membership-based organization dedicated to the development and the improvement of palliative care worldwide. The organization works with associations, agencies, and individuals, to improve communications and access to resources, as well as to foster opportunities in education and training. The IAHPC's Board of Directors is composed of recognized leaders in palliative care from 16 different countries.

PROGRAMS

In the last 4 years the IAHPC has become an organization recognized by its leadership and ability to improve the delivery of palliative and hospice care through its teaching and support programs.[20] These include:

- Traveling Fellowship Program: This program covers the cost of travel of an individual who has been invited to teach in a developing country for at least 2 weeks. From 1999 to date, 35 individuals have traveled to programs in 25 different countries.
- Traveling Scholarship Program: The Traveling Scholarship Program provides financial support to individuals from developing countries to cover the cost of travel to an international meeting or congress. They are selected for their outstanding leadership capabilities and past accomplishments in palliative and hospice care.
- Annual Recognition Awards Program: The Annual Awards are given in three categories – individual,

institutional, and university – as recognition to outstanding effort and work in the development, promotion and dissemination of palliative care practices and knowledge.

- Faculty Development Program: The main objective of this program is to promote formal education in healthcare institutions by funding faculty palliative care positions for nurses or physicians in developing countries.
- Clearing House Program: IAHPC has sent more than 4000 kg of donated journals and books to individuals, hospices, institutions, and libraries in developing countries.

The IAHPC website at www.hospicecare.com has more than 2500 pages of information with free universal access to all readers from around the world. IAHPC continues to work and support individuals, agencies, institutions and schools interested in the promotion and dissemination of palliative care.

The International Observatory in End-of-Life Care (IOELC)

The IOELC is located at Lancaster University, UK, within the Institute for Health Research.[21] The IOELC works with a team of researchers and in partnership with colleagues and organizations in many parts of the world. The Observatory concentrates on two streams of activity: global analysis of palliative care development; and historical, sociological and ethical studies of hospice and palliative care in specific contexts.

In addition to the Observatory's project-based research and development program it also houses the digital and paper archives of its Hospice History Program and contains an extensive collection of current reference materials.

The IOELC has done a major review of hospice and palliative care in eastern Europe, Central Asia and western Europe, including current initiatives and history of its development. A review of Africa and Latin America is under way.

OBJECTIVES

- To provide clear and accessible research-based information on hospice and palliative care provision in the international context, incorporating public health, demographic, epidemiologic and healthcare systems analysis as well as ethnographic, historical, and ethical perspectives.
- To disseminate this information through the Observatory website and through published articles, monographs, reports, CDs and other media, in ways that facilitate cross-national comparative analysis and stimulate practical development.
- To undertake primary research studies and reviews to generate such information.

- To develop a small grants program to support academic work relating to the aims of the Observatory in resource-poor regions.
- To work in partnership with key organizations and individuals, nationally and internationally, in order to foster a sense of inclusion and participation in the work of the Observatory.

The IOELC has a growing network of collaborators across several countries and continents and already has key links in India and South America, as well as eastern Europe, Central Asia and Africa. Additional information about the Observatory can be found on its website (www.eolc-observatory.net/).

World Hospice and Palliative Care Day

World Hospice and Palliative Care Day is a new unified day of action to celebrate and support hospice and palliative care around the world. It has been developed in association with Voices for Hospices and hospice and palliative care associations worldwide.[22] The initial date to celebrate the World Hospice and Palliative Care Day is set for 8 October 2005, and will hopefully become an annual global event. Activities will take place worldwide and a collective global voice comprising individuals and associations will raise awareness and understanding of the need and importance of hospice and palliative care.

REGIONAL INITIATIVES

European Association for Palliative Care (EAPC)

The EAPC was established on December 1988, with 42 founding members after an important initiative by Professor Vittorio Ventafridda and the Floriani Foundation. The aim of the EAPC is to promote palliative care in Europe and to act as a focus for all of those who work, or have an interest, in the field of palliative care at the scientific, clinical, and social levels.[23] Since 1990, the Head Office of EAPC has been based at the Division of Rehabilitation and Palliative Care in the National Cancer Institute in Milan, Italy. By 2004, EAPC counted individual members in 40 countries, with collective members from 30 national associations in 20 European countries, representing a movement of some 5000 healthcare workers and volunteers working or interested in palliative care.

AIMS OF EAPC

- Promote the implementation of existing knowledge; train those who at any level are involved with the care of patients and families affected by incurable and advanced disease; and promote study and research.

- Bring together those who study and practice the disciplines involved in the care of patients and families affected by advanced disease (doctors, nurses, social workers, psychologists and volunteers).
- Promote and sponsor publications or periodicals concerning palliative care.
- Unify national palliative care organizations and establish an international network for the exchange of information and expertise.
- Address the ethical problems associated with the care of terminally ill patients

INITIATIVES OF THE EAPC

The EAPC website (www.eapcnet.org) has become a crucial communication tool to update on the latest developments and report in detail on the activities of EAPC.

The *European Journal of Palliative Care* is the journal of the EAPC. It is a multidisciplinary journal, published six times a year in both English and French. The journal concentrates on reviews and current awareness of palliative care on the European scene. *Palliative Medicine* is the leading peer-reviewed research journal of palliative care in Europe. It is published eight times a year and the printed version, with online access to the back issues of the last 5 years, is available by subscription.

The 'Research Network' has organized 11 expert working groups on a variety of topics for which a common European position or recommendations are needed. By the end of 2003, the results of the work of seven groups had been published, one of them in six languages. One of the priorities of the EAPC for the future is the support of development of palliative care in eastern Europe.[24] In 2001 the EAPC coordination center was established at Stockholm's Sjukhem Foundation in Sweden, which hosts and supports the center locally.

EAPC TASKFORCES (PROJECTS)

- The EAPC Ethics Task Force on Palliative Care and Euthanasia: The paper is available on the Web (www.eapcnet.org/projects/ethics.asp) in English, French, Italian, and Hungarian.
- EAPC Taskforce on Palliative Care Standards: A goal of this taskforce is to identify the needs for a European standard and create a checklist that anyone can follow.
- EAPC Taskforce on Palliative Care Development in Europe: This taskforce is in collaboration with EAPC Onlus; the IOELC; Help the Hospices and IAHPC, with the aim to achieve an overall vision of the care activity and development of palliative care teams in Europe.
- Taskforce on Palliative Care for Children: The goal of this taskforce is to enhance the opportunities for knowledge exchange between adult and pediatric palliative care physicians.
- Taskforce on Nursing Education: This taskforce was convened to develop recommendations for palliative

nurse education in Europe. Recommendations will be published on the EAPC Website.
- Survey on Medical Education: This taskforce was convened to carry out a survey on the state of the art of education for physicians in Europe.
- Taskforce on Medical Education: This taskforce was convened to create recommendations for curricula for medical education.

EAPC CONGRESSES AND FORUMS

Since 1990 the EAPC has organized nine European congresses and three research forums with the participation of individuals from countries of Europe and other regions of the world. The tenth congress of EAPC is scheduled for June 2007 in Budapest, Hungary. The fourth research forum of the EAPC is scheduled for May 2006 in Venice, Italy.

African Palliative Care Association (APCA)

The APCA was founded in 2003 to help support and promote the development of palliative care and palliative care professionals throughout Africa. Members include professionals, individuals with a special interest in the promotion of palliative care, and national and local palliative care associations/programs. APCA recently held its inaugural conference in Arusha, Tanzania, and a new journal was created.[25] Additional information about this meeting and the association can be found on the internet (www.hospicecare.com/newsletter2004/aug04/regional-africa.htm).

OBJECTIVES

- To promote the availability of palliative care for all in need.
- To encourage governments in sub-Saharan Africa to support affordable and appropriate palliative care which is incorporated into the whole spectrum of healthcare services.
- To promote the availability of palliative care drugs for all in need.
- To encourage the establishment of national palliative care associations in all African countries.
- To promote palliative care training programs suitable for sub-Saharan African countries.
- To develop standard guidelines for training and care at different levels of health professional and care providers.

Hospice Palliative Care Association of South Africa (HPCA)

The HPCA was established in South Africa in 1988. Its mission is to provide a holistic and individually tailored palliative care service to all who require such a service, irrespective of the ability to pay.[26]

The Hospice Association of South Africa (now the HPCA) has been providing palliative care through an ever-developing network of hospices throughout South Africa, Botswana, Swaziland, and Zimbabwe, since 1989. The Hospice Association of South Africa developed the Short Course in Palliative Nursing for Professional Nurses in 1994, which is accredited by the South African Nursing Council. Member hospices provided palliative care for 2900 patients in 2002–03, supported their families into the bereavement period, and provided training for 3000 professional and lay people in various aspects of palliative care. Six thousand AIDS orphans were supported in the bereavement programs. With the increasing number of children infected and affected by HIV/AIDS, the need for pediatric palliative care has been highlighted. A national survey revealed a lack of training curricula in this discipline for members of the multidisciplinary team. The HPCA received a grant from the Diana, Princess of Wales Memorial Fund to develop a curriculum for training doctors, nurses, social workers, and other members of the multidisciplinary team, in accordance with the National Qualifications Framework. This is in the process of development with input from role players from around South Africa. Additional information can be found in the website (www.hospicepalliativecaresa.co.za/index.htm).

Foundation for Hospices in Sub-Saharan Africa (FHSSA)

The FHSSA mission is to support organizations in their provision of hospice and palliative care in sub-Saharan Africa.[27] The foundation is partnered with the National Hospice and Palliative Care Organization (NHPCO) in USA.[28] The FHSSA was incorporated in November 1999 and the 21-member Board of Directors included individuals representing a variety of hospice, AIDS service, and medical disciplines from the USA.

An international consultation, which involved both Africans and Americans, was held in 2000 to map out a strategic plan for the FHSSA's efforts. The consultation produced a strategy paper for hospice and palliative care development in the sub-Saharan region. Action recommendations for funding were approved and supported by standards for African programs seeking assistance. These program standards were modified from those adopted by the Hospice Association of South Africa for its members.

In addition, the FHSSA's International Advisory Council is a multinational body whose members help advise the FHSSA on international efforts to raise awareness of the African hospice movement. The FHSSA has a website (http://fhssa.org/).

Asia Pacific Hospice Palliative Care Network (APHN)

The APHN has been established to link all those who are interested in developing hospice and palliative programs in Asia and the Pacific. There are now more than 700 members. Sixteen percent of these are organizations that have joined as organizational members; the rest are individuals who are working with some of the 500 hospices and palliative care services in the Asia Pacific region.[29] The APHN evolved over a series of meetings between March 1995 and March 2001 when the organization was registered in Singapore. Although the Secretariat has been established in Singapore, the APHN is a regional organization with 14 founding sectors.

OBJECTIVES[30]

- To facilitate the development of hospice and palliative care programs.
- To promote professional and public education in palliative care.
- To enhance communication and dissemination of information among members.
- To foster research and collaborative activities.
- To encourage cooperation with other relevant professional and public organizations.

Additional information about the organization and its activities is available on the internet (www.aphn.org/).

Latin American Association for Palliative Care (*Asociación Latinoamericana de Cuidados Paliativos*; ALCP)

The ALCP was recently incorporated as a legal entity, but for more than 14 years, several Latin American palliative care workers have been meeting every 2 years to discuss problems, review recent developments and establish networks of support. For some years, the participants voiced their interest in establishing a formal organization to represent the needs and goals of the region.

The mission of the ALCP is to promote the development of palliative care in Latin America and the Caribbean by integrating of all those interested in helping improve the quality of life of patients with incurable progressive diseases as well as their families.[31] The Association recognizes palliative care as 'the active total care of patients and their families by a multi-professional team when the patients' disease is no longer responsive to the curative treatment'. Control of pain, of other symptoms, and of psychologic, social and spiritual problems is paramount.

OBJECTIVES

- To associate all those who are interested in caring for patients with incurable diseases and their families.
- To promote regional information exchange of experiences to strengthen the existing programs and help in the development of new programs.
- To promote the implementation of existing available knowledge, study and research.

- To develop a basic system to be adapted and applied in every country for the accreditation of institutions and the certification of health personnel of different disciplines.
- To collaborate with its members in:
  - their relationships with the community and the sanitary authorities
  - the identification and planning of the best healthcare model for their country or region
  - the development of systems of economic retribution applicable to their country
  - the development of norms of quality applicable to their country
  - the procurement of resources
  - training of healthcare personnel
  - obtaining regional information to identify needs and collaborate in the design of strategic plans based on this information
  - publishing guidelines and papers in Spanish and Portuguese
  - providing information on educational activities for healthcare professionals, patients, legislators, and the general public
  - supporting initiatives for changes in public health policies which seek to endorse and ensure adequate palliative care
  - promoting the necessary changes in policies and regulations to ensure that the necessary drugs for pain relief and other symptoms are available in all countries, in rural and urban regions.

THE LATIN-AMERICAN CONGRESSES

The Regional meetings serve as a venue where participants share experiences, disseminate new information, and establish a network of colleagues around the world. The meetings started in 1998 and have been going on every 2 years. The next congress will take place in 2006 in Venezuela.

CIRCULAR OF THE ALCP (NEWSLETTER)

The circular is a free electronic monthly or bi-monthly publication in Spanish and Portuguese. It is sent via e-mail to more than 2000 readers in the region. The publication is available on the internet (www.cuidadospaliativos.org/circular/index.html).

WEBSITE

The ALCP website (www.cuidadospaliativos.org) provides the regional colleagues a tool for the dissemination of information and for the development of support networks.

Open Society Institute (OSI)

The Open Society Institute (OSI) is a private operating and grant making foundation based in New York City that serves as the hub of the Soros Foundations Network, a group of autonomous foundations and organizations in more than 50 countries.[32] OSI and the network implement a range of initiatives that aim to promote open societies by shaping government policy and supporting education, media, public health, and human and women's rights, as well as social, legal, and economic reform. In the last years OSI has played a crucial role in providing support and funding to palliative care initiatives and hospices mainly in eastern Europe and Africa.

NATIONAL ASSOCIATIONS WITH INTERNATIONAL PROGRAMS AND INITIATIVES

National Hospice and Palliative Care Organization (NHPCO)

The NHPCO is the largest nonprofit membership organization representing hospice and palliative care programs and professionals in the United States.[33] The organization is committed to improving end-of-life care and expanding access to hospice care with the goal of profoundly enhancing quality of life for people dying in America and their loved ones.

The NHPCO, founded in 1978 as the National Hospice Organization, changed its name in February 2000. With headquarters in Alexandria, VA, USA, the organization advocates for the terminally ill and their families. It also develops public and professional educational programs and materials to enhance understanding and availability of hospice and palliative care; convenes frequent meetings and symposia on emerging issues; provides technical informational resources to its membership; conducts research; monitors Congressional and regulatory activities; and works closely with other organizations that share an interest in end-of-life care.

The NHPCO works collaboratively with existing organizations and individuals who are advancing hospice and palliative care in several regions of the world. It has recently joined forces with the FHSSA to support the development of hospice care in Africa. The *Journal of Pain and Symptom Management* has recently been named as the official journal of NHPCO.[34]

UK Forum for Hospice and Palliative Care Worldwide

The UK Forum for Hospice and Palliative Care Worldwide is the national umbrella and representative body for organizations and individuals working in the UK to support hospice and palliative care services overseas. The Forum is established within Help the Hospices with the goal of promoting a national, strategic, and collective response in the UK to hospice and palliative care services overseas.[35]

ACTIVITIES OF THE FORUM

- Development of a UK network of people and organizations interested in working in hospice and palliative care overseas.
- Creating a funding structure to support hospices overseas.
- Facilitating twinning arrangements among hospices in the UK and abroad.
- Providing support for training and education for individuals in developing countries.
- Promoting advocacy and dissemination of information.

Worldwide Palliative Care News

The aim of this service is to provide information and sign-posting of information sources to international palliative care workers and to their counterparts based in the UK. The service is managed by Hospice Information Service and the UK Forum for Hospice and Palliative Care Worldwide which aims to keep people involved in international projects informed about funding opportunities, twinning, publications, disease information, policy, and practice.

LESSONS LEARNED FROM THE GLOBAL SITUATION

Thanks to the advancements in technology, the palliative care community around the world is now able to establish and maintain communication on a global scale. Many initiatives were isolated in their efforts, and knowledge of developments in other countries was scarce and limited. E-mail and the internet have had a huge impact in our ability to stay connected and disseminate information. Some of the most important lessons learned from the global situation are:

- Currently many resources, funding organizations, and professional associations are reaching out to individuals and programs around the world. In this process, it is necessary to keep our focus and avoid duplication of efforts. Each one of the organizations and initiatives described in this chapter has a clear mandate. Our ability to maintain this will keep us from using resources in doing what others may have better experience about and knowledge. This may have a devastating effect and can become quite confusing to individuals and local governments. Ideally, efforts should be coordinated among agencies to ensure maximal effect and better use of resources.

- The best global strategy is by cooperation rather than competition. With the advent of technology and the ability to communicate rapidly, the exchange of ideas and mutual collaboration among agencies and programs is the key to success. Having a unified front of specialized organizations collaborating in achieving the goal of improving access to hospice and palliative care is important as a strategy. Advocacy campaigns, calls for policy changes, integration of palliative care in the mainstream of care have a greater chance of being heard if it comes in a single, loud voice. Several examples of success of mutual collaboration among programs, organizations and individuals include the Declaration of Florianopolis,[36] the Santo Domingo Progress Report,[37] and the recent Korea Declaration.[38]

- At the country level, it is important to support multiple local initiatives as a strategy to develop palliative care worldwide. The provision of training, support, information, and funding to various programs maximizes the chances of success and minimizes risks.

- It is crucial to settle realistic goals for each program or initiative. The goals that may be applicable in Latin American countries can not be applied to Middle Eastern, Eastern European or North American countries. When establishing objectives for a program, taking into account its cultural and ethnical values is critical for an effective use of resources.

- Cultural differences and beliefs need to be remembered when establishing strategies for countries. Issues such as communication, decision making, spiritual beliefs and many others vary greatly from group to group. The communication bridge must be established in order to be able to establish effective programs.

CONCLUSION

Development of palliative care in the world has been an increasing trend in the past few decades. This has been largely the result of the commitment of extraordinary individuals and the financial support provided by generous donors and organizations. Many patients are now benefiting from hospice and palliative care services in developed countries, but services in developing countries are scarce and fragile and more is needed to guarantee their permanence and survival.

Education needs to be incorporated in the undergraduate medical and nursing curricula to guarantee the provision of services by a large body of healthcare providers, especially in developing countries. Services and medications need to be subsidized for those who are unable to pay and should be incorporated in the public healthcare systems and reimbursement plans for providers.

More studies are needed on the status of palliative and hospice care services in the world and should be the focus of future research projects. Many organizations such as the ones described in this chapter have made an enormous effort and have had a large impact in the development of palliative care globally.

Key learning points

- There were about 57 million deaths in 2001, of which almost 80 percent occurred in the developing world. A large number of patients around the globe can benefit from palliative care.

- Palliative care includes the management of symptoms and provision of spiritual and psychosocial support to patients and their families from the moment of diagnosis, throughout the course of the disease.

- Palliative care can be provided simply and inexpensively in tertiary care facilities, community health centers, and at home. However, access to pain relief and palliative care services is often limited, even in developed countries, due to a lack of political will, insufficient information and education, and excessive regulation of opioids.

- The WHO World Cancer Report calls on all countries to establish comprehensive national cancer control programs aimed at reducing the incidence of cancer through primary prevention; providing earlier diagnosis and curative treatments; and improving the quality of life for cancer patients and their families through the delivery of adequate palliative care and pain relief.

Global initiatives

- 'A Community Health Approach to Palliative Care for HIV and Cancer Patients in Africa' from the WHO Program on Cancer Control in collaboration with the WHO Departments of Care for HIV-AIDS.

- International Association for Hospice and Palliative Care programs to support efforts mainly in developing countries and to increase knowledge and awareness of the needs of patients and healthcare providers.

- International Observatory in End of Life Care: The Observatory concentrates on global analysis of palliative care development – historical, sociological, and ethical studies of hospice and palliative care in specific contexts.

- World Hospice and Palliative Care Day: Day of action to increase awareness and celebrate and support hospice and palliative care around the world. Developed in association with Voices for Hospices and hospice and palliative care associations worldwide. Initial day set for 8 October 2005.

Regional initiatives:

- The European Association for Palliative Care (EAPC)
- African Palliative Care Association (APCA)
- Hospice Palliative Care Association of South Africa (HPCA)
- Foundation for Hospices in Sub-Saharan Africa (FHSSA)
- Asia Pacific Hospice Network (APHN)
- Latin American Association for Palliative Care (ALCP)
- Open Society Institute (OSI)

National Associations with international programs and initiatives:

- National Hospice and Palliative Care Organization (NHPCO)
- UK Forum for Hospice and Palliative Care Worldwide

A global palliative care initiative needs to be developed through the collaboration of the organizations, individuals, and programs which have the expertise and knowledge needed for success. This strategy avoids duplication of efforts and maximizes chances of success. Global strategies need to take in consideration the cultural and social differences among patient populations and ethnic groups. Communication issues, disclosure of information and treatment practices need to be tailored to the needs and resources of each country.

REFERENCES

● 1   World Health Organization. *The World Health Report 2002: Reducing Risks, Promoting Healthy Life.* Geneva: WHO, 2002.
● 2   UNAIDS/WHO. *AIDS Epidemic Update, December 2004.* Geneva: UNAIDS/WHO, 2004.
● 3   Torres I, Wang XS, Palos G, Gning I, *et al.* Advanced cancer care in Latin America and the Caribbean: A survey of healthcare professionals. Presented at the American Public Health Association Conference, Atlanta, GA, USA, 22 October 2002.
✱ 4   *World Health Organization Cancer Pain Relief and Palliative Care: Report of a WHO Expert Committee.* (Technical Report Series No. 804), Geneva: WHO, 1990.
   5   International Narcotics Control Board. *Availability of Opiates for Medical Needs.* Special Report prepared pursuant to Economic and Social Council Resolutions 1990/31 and 1991/43. Vienna: INCB, 1996.
   6   International Narcotics Control Board. Consumption of the Principal Narcotic Drugs. In: *Narcotic Drugs. Estimated World Requirements for 2004 and Statistics for 2002.* Vienna: INCB, 2004.
● 7   Torres I, Wang, XS, Palos G, Jones P, *et al.* Physicians' perceptions of barriers to optimal cancer pain management: preliminary findings of a survey on advanced cancer care in Latin America and the Caribbean. Presented at the 21st Annual Scientific Meeting of the American Pain Society, Baltimore, MD. March 15–16, 2002.

● 8   Livingstone H. Pain relief in the developing world: the experience of hospice Africa-Uganda. *J Pain Palliat Care Pharmacother* 2003; **17**: 107–18.

● 9   Rajagopal MR. The challenges of palliative care in India. *Natl Med J India* 2001; **14**: 65–7.

● 10   Mosoiu D. Romania: cancer pain and palliative care. *J Pain Symptom Manage* 2002; **24**: 225–7.

● 11   Harding R, Stewart K, Marconi K, O'Neill JF, *et al.* Current HIV/AIDS end-of-life care in sub-Saharan Africa: a survey of models, services, challenges and priorities. *BMC Public Health* 2003; **3**: 33

12   Levorato A, Stiefel F, Mazzocato C, Bruera E. Communications with terminal cancer patients in palliative care: are there differences between nurses and physicians? *Support Care Cancer* 2003; **9**: 420–7.

13   Bruera E, Neumann CM, Mazzocato C, Steifel F, Sala R. Attitudes and beliefs of palliative care physicians regarding communication with terminally ill cancer patients. *Palliat Med* 2000; **14**: 287–98.

14   Bruera E, De Lima L, Wenk R, Farr W, eds. *Palliative Care in the Developing World: Principles and Practice.* Houston: IAHPC Press, 2004.

15   Rajagopal MR, Mazza D, Lipman AG, eds. *Pain and Palliative Care in the Developing World and Marginalized Populations: A Global Challenge.* Binghamtom, USA: Haworth Press, 2003.

✱ 16   World Health Organization. *Cancer Control Program: Policies and Managerial Guidelines.* Geneva: WHO 2002.

● 17   Sepulveda C, Marlin A, Yoshida T, Ullrich A. Palliative care: the World Health Organization's global perspective. *J Pain Symptom Manage* 2002; **24**: 91–6.

18   World Health Organization. A Community Health Approach to Palliative Care for HIV and Cancer Patients in Africa. Retrieved from: www.who.int/cancer/palliative/africanproject/en/ (1 December 2004).

19   World Health Organization. World Health Organization Collaborating Centers in Palliative Care. Retrieved from: http://whocc.who.int/result_index.asp?s_search_string=.~CE%60^cancer/^/%60/~&tsl_pagesize= 10000&tsl_presentation_style=2&tsl_report_sort=1 (30 April 2005).

● 20   De Lima L, Bruera E, Woodruff R. The International Association for Hospice and Palliative Care: international activities and future initiatives. *J Pain Palliat Care Pharmacother* 2003; **17**: 31–7.

● 21   Clark D. The International Observatory on End of Life Care: a new initiative to support palliative care development around the world. *J Pain Palliat Care Pharmacother* 2003; **17**: 231–8.

22   World Hospice and Palliative Care Day. Retrieved from: www.worldday.org/index.asp (30 April 2005).

● 23   Blumhuber H, Kaasa S, De Conno F. The European Association for Palliative Care. *J Pain Symptom Manage* 2002; **24**: 124–7.

● 24   Fürst CJ. The European Association for Palliative Care Initiative in Eastern Europe. *J Pain Symptom Manage* 2002; **24**: 134–5.

25   Regional News: African Palliative Care Association (APCA): Inaugural Conference in Arusha, Tanzania. *IAHPC Newsletter,* August, 2004. Available at: www.hospicecare.com/newsletter2004/aug04/regional-africa.htm

● 26   Gwyther E. South Africa: the status of palliative care. *J Pain Symptom Manage* 2002; **24**: 236–8.

27   Foundation for Hospices in Sub-Saharan Africa (FHSSA). Retrieved from: www.fhssa.org/i4a/pages/index.cfm?pageid=1 (12 November 2004).

28   NHPCO Partners with Foundation for Hospices in Sub-Saharan Africa, Inc. (Press Release). Retrieved from: www.nhpco.org/i4a/pages/index.cfm?pageid=3845&openpage = 3845 (2 December 2004).

● 29   Goh CR. The Asia Pacific Hospice Palliative Care Network: a network for individuals and organizations. *J Pain Symptom Manage* 2002; **24**: 128–33.

30   APHN. Information retrieved from: www.aphn.org/ (23 September 2004)

31   Colleau S. Creation of the Latin American Association for Palliative Care. *Cancer Pain Release* 2002; **15**: 3.

32   Open Society Institute. Information retrieved from: www.soros.org/about (22 September 2004).

33   National Hospice and Palliative Care Organization. Information retrieved from: www.nhpco.org (15 November 2004).

34   Schumacher JD, Portenoy R, Connor SR, Joranson DE. Editorial. *J Pain Symptom Manage* 2004; **28**: 193.

35   UK Forum for Hospice and Palliative Care Worldwide. Retrieved from: www.helpthehospices.org.uk/international/index.asp?submenu=1 (30 April 2005).

36   Stjernsward J, Bruera E, Joranson D, Allende S, *et al.* Opioid Availability in Latin America: The Declaration of Florianopolis. *J Pain Symptom Manage* 1995; **10**: 3, 233–7.

37   De Lima L, Bruera E, Joranson D, *et al.* Opioid availability in Latin America: the Santo Domingo Report. Progress since the Declaration of Florianopolis. *J Pain Symptom Manage* 1997; **13**: 4.

38   Korea Declaration. Retrieved from: www.hpc-associations.net (30 April 2005).

PART 4

Education

16

Undergraduate education

DOREEN ONESCHUK

INTRODUCTION

An aim of undergraduate education in palliative medicine is to cultivate competencies in the care of patients with advanced diseases. Encouragingly, medical student surveys reveal that competencies in the areas of attitude, skills, and knowledge can be acquired and fostered by well-developed undergraduate palliative medicine programs with students requesting increased instruction in palliative and end-of-life care. Less positive is the knowledge that students display deficiencies in competency at the time of completing their undergraduate education.[1-10]

This chapter reviews the status of undergraduate palliative medicine education in multiple countries, identified barriers and deficiencies in palliative medicine education, recommended changes, how to develop and implement these changes, and national strategies in progress in palliative medicine education.

WHERE ARE WE NOW

To understand better where changes need to be made and how to implement these changes, we need to know where we are now. Many countries have conducted surveys updating the status of palliative medicine in their country and universities.

Canada

A 2001–02 Canadian survey of the 16 medical schools identified that compared with a similar but less comprehensive international survey completed in 1997, only minor changes have occurred in undergraduate palliative medicine education in Canada. The majority of palliative medicine teaching occurs in the preclinical years of medical school, with supervised patient encounters occurring primarily during electives. The median number of instructional hours increased from 6 to 10 hours. Three-quarters of the schools indicated that learning objectives are identified, although the coverage of palliative medicine topics is inconsistent across curricula. The majority of schools use a combination of lectures and small group/problem-based learning. More than half the schools have an academic division or department of palliative medicine, although faculty with protected time are few in number. Student evaluation methods also vary, with only one school using simulated patients.[11,12]

USA

Between 1975 and 2000, palliative medicine education in the USA had increased slightly. In a 2000 survey, palliative care was directly addressed in 87 percent of medical schools responding and the majority of students were exposed to a hospice patient. The number of schools 'not formally offering anything on dying and death' went down from 13 percent in 1975 to 0 percent in 2000. The average number of teaching hours was about 14 hours. Of 19 end-of-life curricular topics listed, eight topics were identified as being taught by at least 80 of the 112 medical schools. Several of the schools noted that they introduce students to terminally ill patients and their families in rotating clerkships, whereas others indicated that the topic is integrated throughout their curriculum. The majority of schools used seminar/small group discussions and lecture mode of presentation. A multidisciplinary team approach increasingly is the mode of presenting the material in the curriculum.[13]

UK and western Europe

In a 2000–01 UK survey, changes since 1994 involved an increase in the use of role play and a decrease in the use of simulated patients in favor of using dying patients. The mean number of taught hours was 20 compared with overall means of 6 hours in 1983 and 13 hours in 1994. The greatest change since the 1994 survey involved the increased use of nurse specialists in palliative medicine. Assessment and evaluation of palliative medicine learning was still not commonplace. A number of schools were planning on increasing their teaching hours.[14] A 2001 survey of palliative medicine teaching in Irish medical schools identified that in no school is teaching centrally coordinated. All five medical schools in Ireland provide formal teaching in palliative medicine and the majority of topics in the suggested curriculum are being taught. A wide range of departments provide teaching. Most teaching occurs in the clinical years and by didactic lecture. Some teaching occurs in the hospice setting. An extremely low percentage of students participate in elective rotations and assessments are not required in order to advance.[15] In a review of undergraduate medical education in palliative medicine in Ireland, the UK, and Europe from 2002, European undergraduate education in palliative medicine was noted to be underdeveloped.[16] Results of a survey of physicians from Germany, Austria, Switzerland, Great Britain, Denmark and France, revealed that less than 50 percent of the European students receive education in palliative medicine. Whereas 51 percent of the physicians in Great Britain felt sufficiently prepared for the task of caring for the dying, less than 25 percent in all other countries felt the same.[17]

Australia

In most Australian medical schools, concepts of palliative medicine are taught but instruction in this area is still limited, with emphasis on the pathophysiology of disease and its treatment. Medical students are not systematically prepared to assess the clinical and psychological factors. There is a lack of attention to skills in communication, shared decision making, and self-reflection, and minimal interdisciplinary education.[18,19]

AREAS OF DEFICIENCIES, BARRIERS, AND RECOMMENDATIONS

The following are identified deficiencies and barriers in undergraduate palliative medicine education with accompanying recommendations for educational development.[11,20–23]

- Training is largely preclinical and elective.
  Recommendation: Care at the end of life should be taught as a core professional task throughout the continuum of medical education. Training should occur in the clinical years since this is where key attitudes and life long practice patterns are learned.
- Education focuses primarily on knowledge rather than on attitudes or skills.
  Recommendation: Key content areas should be addressed with emphasis on humanistic attitudes and communication skills.
- Limited opportunity for or promotion of self-reflection.
  Recommendation: Students should be encouraged to reflect on personal attitudes about their work.
- Limited involvement and emphasis on an interdisciplinary model of care.
  Recommendation: In all phases of training, students should be exposed to dying patients and interdisciplinary teams of clinicians and other healthcare professionals who are skilled in palliative medicine and can model humanistic functions of medicine.
- Underutilization of hospice settings and home care as teaching venues and aids.
  Recommendation: The best learning grows out of direct experiences with patients and families, particularly when students have an opportunity to follow patients longitudinally.
- Lower profile of palliative medicine compared with other specialties and negative informal teaching. In the 'hidden curriculum'[24,25] death is perceived as representing a medical failure, dying patients are not seen as good 'teaching cases', and students and residents receive little emotional support in dealing with their often disturbing encounters.
  Recommendation: Students should be encouraged to develop positive feelings about dying patients and their families and the role of the physician in terminal care.
- Lack of student assessment and evaluation.
  Recommendation: Student competence in managing prototypical clinical settings related to death should be evaluated using state of the art methods.
- Limited faculty time and lack of faculty role models who often have limited training in palliative medicine.
  Recommendation: Hire and train more educators to provide and demonstrate state of the art palliative care. These educators are needed to serve as role models and teachers. Students need to see physicians offering excellent medical care to dying people and their families, finding meaning in their work, and modeling ideal behaviors and skills.
- Limited financial support from the universities.
  Recommendation: Resources need to be available to implement changes.

DEVELOPING A CURRICULUM

Strategic planning at a national and local level is often required to successfully create and implement curricular reform. Defining an outline or using recommended steps can aid this process, bearing in mind the uniqueness of each school and the need to individually adapt the process to each school.

To begin, a local champion or faculty committee leader should be identified in each school who would assemble an interdisciplinary committee that would be involved in curricular development. Members of the group could include individual course directors and instructors, undergraduate curriculum committee members, and medical students. Students can be very persuasive in eliciting faculty support for curricular change; their feedback and enthusiasm can help sustain the momentum of change.[26]

Needs assessment

One of the first tasks of the group would be to review the curriculum to identify what is being taught well and how to fill in the significant gaps. This can be achieved by conducting a needs assessment.[27] This is considered fundamental to change the process and the most important step in promoting change. A needs assessment evaluates the educational need for a curriculum, possible content, and instructional strategies. It also provides information so that appropriate and realistic implementation and evaluation plans can be developed based on the needs and resources of a particular institution.[28] It lays the foundation for curriculum design, implementation, and evaluation by answering questions about the clinical and educational needs of patients, families, and learners, available and needed resources, and potential political and logistical problems. Information can be gathered and organized into three categories:[29]

1 what is lacking
2 what is available
3 what would be needed to improve the clinical services or educational climate.

Methods of identifying course content include the Delphi technique, nominal group analysis, and single expert opinions.[30] The Palliative Education Assessment Tool for Medical Education (PEAT) is a flexible self-assessment tool that can be used to examine all required courses in the entire curriculum to uncover those areas where specific aspects of palliative care are taught, including those that are often considered 'hidden'.[31,32]

From the outset, it is beneficial to garner support from administrative staff such as deans and associate deans, pivotal committees that govern medical school content, and affiliated accrediting bodies. Carefully prepared, concise presentations to these individuals related to the need for education and/or awareness of national recommendations for curricular reform can be beneficial.[31,33]

Objectives and goals

Probably the most important determinant of the success or failure of a new curriculum is whether the objectives are clearly spelled out and are realistic. The objectives form the basis upon which the evaluation is designed and provide a clear message of accountability for the teachers, learners, and administrators who will review the curriculum's effectiveness.[29]

A key to writing useful educational objectives is to make them specific and measurable.[34] Objectives should contain five basic elements – *Who* will do *how* much *how* well of *what* by *when*? (Box 16.1).

Box 16.1 Types of objective[27]

- Learners' objectives – include objectives that relate to learning in the cognitive, affective, and psychomotor domains

- Process objectives – relate to the implementation of the curriculum. They may indicate the degree of participation that is expected from the learners and indicate the expected response of learners or faculty to a curriculum

- Outcome objectives – relate to potential outcomes, or effects of a curriculum beyond those delineated in the learners' and process objectives

---

Goals provide desired overall direction for a curriculum. An important and difficult task in curriculum development is to develop a manageable number of specific measurable objectives that do the following: interpret the goals; focus and prioritize curricular components that are critical to the realization of the goals and encourage creativity and flexibility; and nonspecified learning relevant to the curriculum's goals.[27]

Many countries and programs have existing palliative care curricula that include established objectives and goals. These could be used as a resource by newly developing programs. They include the core curriculum from the Association for Palliative Medicine for Great Britain and Ireland (1993),[5,35] the Canadian Palliative Care Undergraduate Curriculum (1991) that is presently being revised,[36] the Australian Multidisciplinary Undergraduate Palliative Care Curriculum Project,[19,37] and the American Board of Internal Medicine.[38]

Educational strategies

It is helpful to keep the following general principles in mind when considering educational methods for the curriculum:[27,39]

- maintain congruence between objectives and methods
- use multiple educational materials and instructional methods and

- choose educational methods that are feasible in terms of resources.

Adult learning principles espouse that adults learn effectively by being actively involved in a problem oriented approach because it promotes intrinsic interest and fosters the activation and elaboration of prior knowledge.[40] Attention to prior experience and to individualized approaches can enhance the learner's participation and understanding.[41]

Methods used to achieve knowledge objectives include lectures, assigned reading, small group discussions, programmed learning or problem solving exercises. When it works well, discussion can allow students to negotiate meanings, express themselves in the language of the subject, and establish closer contact with academic staff than more formal methods permit. Discussion can also develop the more instrumental skills of listening, presenting ideas, persuading, and working as part of a team. Discussion in small groups can or should give students the chance to monitor their own learning and thus gain a degree of self-direction and independence in their studies.[42] In problem-based learning, students use 'triggers' from the problem case or scenario to define their own learning objectives. They do independent, self-directed study before returning to the group to discuss and refine their acquired knowledge. Problem-based learning can be thought of as a small group teaching method that combines the acquisition of knowledge with the development of generic skills and attitudes.[43] Information technology now allows development of interactive exercises and distance learning.[39] Web-based conferencing tools hold promise for educators because of their flexibility and accessibility; not only do they have the potential to enhance discussion already taking place in the classroom and facilitate interactions among students and instructors in a course, but they also provide a platform for distributed learning. In other words, learners are able to learn during times and at venues that are convenient to them.[44] Methods for achieving affective objectives include exposure to readings, discussions, and experiences or views of others; facilitation of openness, introspection, and reflection; and role models.[27]

The current psychological concept 'attitude' has been defined as 'a learned predisposition to respond in a consistently favorable or unfavorable manner with respect to a given object'.[45] Attitudes can be difficult to measure, let alone change. Some undesirable attitudes are based in insufficient knowledge and will change as knowledge is expanded in a particular area. Other attitudes may be based in insufficient skill or lack of confidence. Attitudinal change requires exposure to knowledge, experiences, or the views of respected others that contradict undesired and confirm desired attitudes. Probably more than any other learning objective, attitudinal change is helped by the use of facilitation techniques with individuals and with groups that promote openness, introspection, and reflection. Properly facilitated small group discussions can also promote changes in attitudes by bringing into awareness the interests, attitudes, values, and feelings of learners and by making them available for discussion.[27]

Behavior objectives can be achieved by removal of performance barriers, provision of resources that facilitate performance, and behavioral reinforcements.[39] Instructional strategies for skills objectives include supervised clinical experiences, simulations (artificial models, role plays, standardized patients) and reviews of videotaped clinical encounters.[39] The learning of skills can be facilitated when:[27]

- learners receive an introduction to the skills by didactic presentations, demonstration, and discussion
- have the opportunity to practice the skills
- have the opportunity to reflect upon their performance
- receive feedback on their performance
- repeat the cycle of discussion, practice, reflection, and feedback until mastery is achieved.

Research has shown that students acquire skills best when they are taught in an experiential format and that using case histories and speaking to patients and relatives are all powerful learning tools.[46] Students have commented that the pedagogic technique of 'participant observation' has the effect of removing a defensive stance to the treatment of individual patients, allowing students to be more honest in their assessment of the efficacy of the palliative measures patients actually receive.[47–49] A comprehensive understanding and approach to death, dying, and bereavement is enhanced when students are exposed to the perspectives of multiple disciplines working together.[50] Students should participate in collaborative, longitudinal hospice and nursing home experiences, including interdisciplinary team meetings, patient home visits, telephone contact with patients and families and hospice nurses.[51] With the Structured Clinical Instruction Module (SCIM), an instructional tool, students rotate though a group of stations learning about different aspects of one major topic such as cancer pain; this learning technique involves the use of simulated and actual cancer patients.[52]

Implementation

The following is a checklist for implementation of a curriculum: identify resources, obtain support, develop an administrative mechanism to support the curriculum, anticipate and address barriers, and plan to introduce the curriculum.[27] Most educators would favor palliative medicine integration into the preexisting curricula in both the preclinical and clinical years,[25] the thinking being that there is considerable competition for curriculum time and an additional isolated curriculum in palliative medicine is probably unrealistic.[53] However, others favor stand alone blocks or courses taught by palliative medicine physicians and others who regularly work with dying patients.[54]

Faculty recruitment and training is essential to ensure quality of training and institutionalization of the educational program.[33] Supervising physicians often have no training in caring for a dying patient and are generally unaware of what they do not know about good end-of-life care.[20] Providing faculty with clear course and teaching outlines ensures uniformity of content delivered specific to objectives of the course.[33] Faculty will often require new teaching skills and knowledge to successfully implement new instructional approaches. Many faculty are limited in their experience in curricular change and an educational consultant may be of benefit.[29] However, if expert consultants are employed, that must be utilized judiciously; staff must not become overly reliant on outside consultants.[26]

The importance of securing funding and support for dedicated time and resources as early as possible in the development cannot be emphasized enough.[29] Internal support may be found among the faculty administration or students and external power alliances may be forged with other medical schools, foundations, unions, professional associations, or community, state or federal governing bodies. Developing the training programs and providing the faculty with release time to acquire new competencies requires support from school leadership at all levels – from dean to department head to faculty leaders.[26] The curriculum committee should be kept informed of trends in state of the art practices in end-of-life education and suggest ways to adapt these practices to local conditions.[55,56]

Evaluation and feedback

Without adequate evaluation, educators will be uncertain whether they have attained the stated goals and objectives.[25,27] The purpose of evaluation is to:

- ensure teaching is meeting students' learning needs
- identify areas where teaching can be improved
- inform the allocation of faculty resources
- provide feedback and encouragement for teachers
- support applications for promotion by teachers
- identify and articulate what is valued by medical schools
- facilitate development of the curriculum.

Similar to curriculum design and implementation, faculty coordinating teaching should consider having colleagues with expertise in evaluation methodology help in this effort from the outset.[25] Planners should demonstrate that different examiners (interrater reliability) or the same examiners over time (intrarater reliability) consistently classify each outcome.[39] The Cancer Pain Objective Structured Clinical Examination is an example of a performance-based tool designed to test individual skills in the essential components of cancer pain assessment and management.[57,58] Finally, the curriculum will need to be disseminated and will require ongoing maintenance and enhancement over the years.[27]

NATIONAL STRATEGIES IN PROGRESS

The Liaison Committee for Medical Education (LCME) which accredits Canadian and US medical schools recognized the importance of physician competence in end-of-life care with a requirement that all accredited US and Canadian medical schools include end-of-life care in their curricula.[59] However, like most such requirements, the LCME does not tell the schools the way they should meet the requirement. Fortunately, a number of efforts are underway, although the best way to accomplish this goal remains to be established.

A Canadian national strategy is titled 'Educating Future Physicians in Palliative and End-of-Life Care' (EFPPEC). This multi-tiered project (www.efppec.ca) will strive to bring palliative medicine education to undergraduate medical students and clinical postgraduate trainees in all Canadian medical schools so that they will graduate with competencies in these areas. There will be emphasis on interdisciplinary education and the development and implementation of core competencies.

In the US, there is no national policy that governs the curricula in the 125 medical schools in the country beyond the requirement for accreditation by the LCME. However, a curriculum called the 'Education for Physicians in End-of-life Care' (EPEC) project was developed in conjunction with the American Medical Association to target practicing physicians and has had a broad reach in medical education.[60] It provided the impetus for a national approach to the subject. The curriculum has been used and adapted by many medical schools in their attempts to meet the LCME requirements.[61]

The Australian Department of Health and Ageing was recently awarded a tender to undertake the National Multidisciplinary Undergraduate Palliative Care Curriculum Project (see www.anzspm.org.au) to promote inclusion of palliative care and its principles and practice into all healthcare training. It will develop a set of educational resources for undergraduate courses and identify strategies to encourage the uptake of palliative care principles and associated resources within tertiary education.

Key learning points

- Undergraduate palliative medicine education remains underdeveloped in many countries.

- Areas of deficiencies and barriers for undergraduate palliative medicine education have been identified with recommendations for change.

- Curricular development is best implemented using a step-wise structured approach.

- This step-wise approach should include needs assessment, development of objectives and goals, educational strategies, implementation, dissemination, and evaluation.

- Numerous countries are in the process of developing national strategies to improve and foster undergraduate palliative medicine education.

REFERENCES

1 Weissman DE, Dahl JL. Attitudes about cancer pain: a survey of Wisconsin's first-year medical students. *J Pain Symptom Manage* 1990; **5**: 345–9.

2 Fraser HC, Kutner JS, Pfeifer MP. Senior medical students' perceptions of the adequacy of education on end-of-life issues. *J Palliat Med* 2001; **4**: 337–43.

3 Ogle KS, Mavis B, Rohrer J. Graduating medical students' competencies and educational experiences in palliative care. *J Pain Symptom Manage* 1997; **14**: 280–5.

4 Weissman DE, Ambuel B, Norton AJ, *et al.* A survey of competencies and concerns in end-of-life care for physician trainees. *J Pain Symptom Manage* 1998; **15**: 82–90.

5 Charlton R, Smith G. Perceived skills in palliative medicine of newly qualified doctors in the UK. *J Palliat Care* 2000; **16**: 27–32.

6 Ury WA, Berkman CS, Weber CM, *et al.* Assessing medical students' training in end-of-life communication: a survey of interns at one urban teaching hospital. *Acad Med* 2003; **78**: 530–7.

7 Oneschuk D, MacDonald N, Bagshaw S, *et al.* A pilot survey of medical students' perspectives on their educational exposure to palliative care in two Canadian universities. *J Palliat Med* 2002; **5**: 353–8.

8 Weinstein SM, Laux LF, Thornby JI, *et al.* Medical students' attitudes toward pain and the use of opioid analgesics: implications for changing medical school curriculum. *South Med J* 2000; **93**: 472–8.

9 Ferrini R, Klein JL. The effect of community hospice rotation on self-reported knowledge, attitudes and skills of third-year medical students. Medical Education Online. www.meded-online.org/res00011.htm (accessed June 2004).

10 Lloyd-Williams M, Dogra N. Caring for dying patients-what are the attitudes of medical students. *Support Care Cancer* 2003; **11**: 696–9.

11 Oneschuk D, Moloughney B, Jones-McLean E, Challis A. The status of undergraduate palliative medicine education in Canada: A 2001 Survey. *J Palliat Care* 2004; **20**: 32–7.

● 12 Oneschuk D, Hanson J, Bruera E. An international survey of undergraduate medical education in palliative medicine. *J Pain Symptom Manage* 2000; **20**: 174–9.

13 Dickinson GE. A quarter century of end-of-life issues in U.S. medical schools. *Death Studies* 2002; **26**: 635–46.

14 Field D, Wee B. Preparation for palliative care: teaching about death, dying and bereavement in UK medical schools 2000–2001. *Med Educ* 2002; **36**: 561–7.

15 Dowling S, Broomfield D. Undergraduate teaching in palliative care in Irish medical schools: a questionnaire survey. *Med Educ* 2003; **37**: 455–7.

16 Dowling S, Broomfield D. Ireland, the UK and Europe: a review of undergraduate medical education in palliative care. *Irish Med J* 2002; **95**: 215–16.

17 Herzler M, Franze T, Dietze F, Asadullah K. Dealing with the issue 'caring of the dying' in medical education – results of a survey of 592 European physicians. *Med Educ* 2000; **34**: 146–7.

18 Barton MB, Simons RG. A survey of cancer curricula in Australian and New Zealand medical schools in 1997. *Med J Aust* 1999; **170**: 225–7.

19 Glare PA, Virik K. Can we do better in end-of-life care? The mixed management model and palliative Care. *Med J Aust* 2001; **175**: 530–3.

● 20 Weissman DE. Cancer pain as a model for the training of physicians in palliative Care. In: Portenoy RK, Bruera E, eds. *Topics in Palliative Care* Vol 4. Oxford: Oxford University Press, 2000: 119–29.

● 21 Simpson DE. National Consensus Conference on Medical Education for Care Near the End of Life: Executive Summary. *J Palliat Med* 2000; **3**: 87–91.

22 Block SD. Medical education in end-of-life care: the status of reform. *J Palliat Med* 2002; **5**: 243–8.

● 23 Billings JA, Block S. Palliative care in undergraduate medical education. status report and future directions 1997; **278**: 733–8.

24 Hafferty FW. Beyond curriculum reform: confronting medicine's hidden curriculum. *Acad Med* 1998; **73**: 403–7.

● 25 Nelson W, Angoff J, Binder E, *et al.* Goals and strategies for teaching death and dying in medical schools. *J Palliat Med* 2000; **3**: 7–16.

● 26 Bland CJ, Starnaman S, Wersal L, *et al.* Curricular change in medical schools: how to succeed. *Acad Med* 2000; **75**: 575–94.

● 27 Kern DE, Thomas PA, Howard DM, Bass EB. *Curriculum Development for Medical Education.* Baltimore: Johns Hopkins University Press, 1998.

28 Ury WA, Reznich CB, Weber CM. A needs assessment for a palliative care curriculum. *J Pain Symptom Manage* 2000; **20**: 408–16.

29 Ury WA, Arnold RM, Tulsky JA. Palliative care curriculum development: a model for a content and process-based approach. *J Palliat Med* 2002; **5**: 539–48.

30 Lloyd-Jones G, Ellershaw J, Wilkinsons S, Bligh JG. The use of multidisciplinary consensus groups in the planning phase of an integrated problem-based curriculum. *Med Educ* 1998; **32**: 278–82.

31 Meekin SA, Klein JE, Fleischman AR, Fins JJ. Development of a palliative education assessment tool for medical student education. *Acad Med* 2000; **75**: 986–92.

32 Wood EB, Meekin SA, Fins JJ, Fleischman AR. Enhancing palliative care education in medical schools curricula: implementation of the Palliative Education Assessment Tool. *Acad Med* 2002; **77**: 285–91.

33 Ross DD, Fraser HC, Kutner JS. Institutionalization of a palliative and end-of-life care educational program in a medical school curriculum. *J Palliat Med* 2001; **4**: 512–18.

34 Prideaux D. ABC of learning and teaching in medicine. Curriculum design. *BMJ* 2003; **326**: 268–70.

35 Field D. Education for palliative care: formal education about death, dying and bereavement in UK medical schools in 1983 and 1994. *Med Educ* 1995; **29**: 414–19.

36 MacDonald N, Mount B, Boston W, Scott JF. The Canadian Palliative Care Undergraduate Curriculum. *J Cancer Educ* 1993; **8**: 197–201.

37 Australia and New Zealand Society of Palliative Medicine. Undergraduate curriculum. Available at: www.anzspm.org.au/education/ugc (accessed June 2004).

38 American Board of Internal Medicine. *End-of-Life Patient Care Project: Caring for the dying: Identification and Promotion of Physician Competency.* Philadelphia: ABIM, 1996.

● 39 Green ML. Identifying, appraising, and implementing medical education curricula: a guide for medical educators. *Ann Intern Med* 2001; **135**: 889–96.

40 Maughan TS, Finlay IG, Webster DJ. Portfolio learning with cancer patients: an integrated module in undergraduate medical education. *Clin Oncol* 2001; **13**: 44–9.

41 Mularski RA, Bascom P, Osborne ML. Educational agendas for interdisciplinary end-of-life curricula. *Crit Care Med* 2001; **29**(Suppl): N16–N23.

42 Jaques D. ABC of learning and teaching in medicine. Teaching small groups. *BMJ* 2003; **326**: 492–4.

43 Wood DF. ABC of learning and teaching in medicine. Problem based learning. *BMJ* 2003; **326**: 328–30.

44 Pereira J, Murzyn T. Integrating the 'new' with the 'traditional': an innovative education model. *J Palliat Med* 2001; **4**: 31–7.

45 Olthuis G, Dekkers W. Medical education, palliative care and moral attitude: some objectives and future perspectives. *Med Educ* 2003; **37**: 928–3.

46 Lloyd-Williams M, Carter YH. Can medical education extend palliative care? *Palliat Med* 2003; **17**: 640–2.

47 Fins JJ, Gentilesco BJ, Carver A, *et al.* Reflective practice and palliative care education: a clerkship responds to the informal and hidden curricula. *Acad Med* 2003; **78**: 307–12.

48 Wear D. 'Face-to-face with It': Medical students' narratives about their end-of-life education. *Acad Med* 2002; **77**: 271–7.

49 Klein S. The effects of the participation of patients with cancer in teaching communication skills to medical undergraduates: a randomised study with follow-up after 2 years. *Eur J Cancer* 1999; **35**: 1448–56.

50 Billings JA, Ferris FD, MacDonald N, *et al.* The role of palliative care in the home in medical education: report from a national consensus conference. *J Palliat Med* 2001; **4**: 361–71.

51 Block SD, Bernier GM, Crawley LM, *et al.* Incorporating palliative care into primary care education. *J Gen Intern Med* 1998; **13**: 768–73.

52 Plymale MA, Sloan PA, Johnson M. Cancer pain education: the use of a structured clinical instruction module to enhance learning among medical students. *J Pain Symptom Manage* 2000; **20**: 4–11.

53 Charlton RC, Smith GD. Undergraduate palliative medicine education detailed in university prospectuses and websites. *Aust Fam Physician* 2001; **30**: 528.

54 Schulman-Green D. How do physicians learn to provide palliative care? *J Palliat Care* 2003; **19**: 246–52.

55 Barnard D, Quill R, Hafferty FW, *et al.* Preparing the ground: contributions of the preclinical years to medical education for care near the end of life. *Acad Med* 1999; **74**: 499–505.

56 Quill TE, Dannefer E, Markakis K, *et al.* An integrated biopsychosocial approach to palliative care training for medical students. *J Palliat Med* 2003; **6**: 365–80.

57 Sloan PA, Plymale MA, Johnson M, *et al.* Cancer pain management skills among medical students: the development of a Cancer Pain Objective Structured Clinical Examination. *J Pain Symptom Manage* 2001; **21**: 298–306.

58 Sloan PA, Plymale M, LaFountain P, *et al.* Equipping medical students to manage cancer pain: A comparison of three educational methods. *J Pain Symptom Manage* 2004; **27**: 333–42.

59 Liaison Committee on Medical Education. Functions and structure of a medical school. Standards for accreditation of medical education programs leading to the M.D. degree. Available at: www.lcme.org/functions2003march.pdf, p. 8 (accessed May 16, 2003).

60 Robinson K, Sutton S, von Gunten CF, *et al.* Assessment of the Education for Physicians on End-of-life Care (EPEC) Project. *J Palliat Med* 2004; **7**: 637–45.

61 Porter-Williamson K, von Gunten CF, Garman K, *et al.* Improving knowledge in palliative medicine with a required hospice rotation for third-year medical students. *Acad Med* 2004; **79**: 777–82.

17

Graduate education

ILORA G FINLAY, SIMON I R NOBLE

INTRODUCTION

Healthcare professionals are likely to be involved soon after graduation in the care of patients with life-threatening illness and facing death. An awareness of the problems of these patients, highlighted by the media focus on hospice and palliative care, has created awareness of educational needs for all healthcare professionals. After graduation, in many parts of the world, such education will be building on an undergraduate foundation. Even today, many graduating professionals have an inappropriate fear of prescribing opioids, and are unaware of some of the core methods of symptom control and of ways of encouraging patients to communicate. In postgraduate learning the focus switches from the need to pass examinations to the need to provide competent care for an individual patient. This drive to education from the need to learn is the most important feature of postgraduate education. Although terminology differs around the world, medical learning shares commonalities with respect to stages of training. After a period of school-based learning follows a period of apprenticeship. For those embarking on specialist training, this apprenticeship may continue for longer until a level of competency is achieved, enabling the individual to practice unsupervised. For the purposes of this chapter, the term 'graduate education' refers to training that occurs following the initial apprenticeship, at the point of embarking on a specialist career in palliative medicine. In countries where fully qualified general or family practitioners have an interest in palliative medicine, the term 'graduate education' would appropriately describe their ongoing learning.

DOMAINS OF LEARNING

A graduate program needs to focus around the four key domains in learning:[1]

- Knowledge and understanding
- Skills and competencies
- Attitudes and professional behavior
- Personal and professional development.

Objective assessment of these competencies is easier in the first two domains (knowledge and understanding, and skills and competencies) than the others, although the importance of attitude and professional behavior should be an underpinning ethos in any graduate program. Different teaching methods cover different domains, so a mixture of methods is required. A didactic lecture may impart facts and increase 'knowledge' but understanding does not develop until the application and facts to the clinical scenario is explored and understood. Without understanding, cold 'facts' may be applied inappropriately or even dangerously to a clinical situation. Similarly, communication skills training will not correct a poor underlying attitude to clinical practice; attitude difficulties may emerge during teaching sessions and must be separately addressed. Before a change can occur, learners need to have insight into why their attitudes appear appropriate, understand the fundamental reasons within themselves behind their behavior and also inherently wish to change. Much work has been done on the way that people change behaviors.[2] Those who feel there is nothing wrong with their attitude or approach may have not even begun to contemplate the need to change. It is only by moving from this precontemplation stage toward contemplating that their attitude may be a barrier to effective practice that they can begin to address areas where change in behavior or in their lifestyle could improve their effectiveness. Many problems of teamworking are linked to attitudinal difficulties; the course tutorials and small group work often reveal such difficulties. However it may be the course administrative and secretarial staffs who are aware first of a student's aggressive or awkward approach.

Learning outcomes on a graduate program are driven by the core competencies that have to be attained, and therefore assessed, by the end of the program. However, as graduate learning is usually driven by a powerful 'need to learn' it is useful to allow the graduates to set their own learning needs and outcomes that they can specify as they go through a program and reflect on what they are learning.[3] Such learning outcomes, particularly when defined by the graduate, may not be easily assessed within the context of the graduate course itself. This will apply particularly to practical skills, such as draining a pleural effusion, although an imaginative curriculum will allow such assessment from the student's work place to be fed into the overall assessment on the program. In addition, the learning needs may be determined by current knowledge and skills as compared to required competencies as applied to the learner's clinical practice. Palliative care graduate programs have been shown to improve knowledge and skills in fellows training in hematooncology,[4*] geriatrics,[5*] and critical care[6*] although their core level of knowledge prior to training varied. In addition small studies have demonstrated the benefits of palliative care education in internal medicine house staff and trainees.[7*,8*,9*,10*] However, there is little evidence that these improved skills are sustained or that reported changes in attitude are applied in the clinical setting.

ADULT LEARNING

Adult learning styles will determine how different graduates learn on a course.[11] Adults are more likely to learn if they wish to learn. Learning must be purposeful, voluntary and the course must provide clear goals and objectives. Adults learn much better when actively participating in learning rather than as passive listeners to a series of didactic lectures. Feedback on any work undertaken is essential and adult learners should be encouraged at all times to be reflective in the way that they approach a topic. Clear goals of learning or learning outcomes should state explicitly the skills and competencies that the learner is expected to be able to demonstrate.

REFLECTIVE PRACTICE

Reflective practice was described in the early 1930s, but the most celebrated description by Donald Schön has only become integrated into course design during the last two decades.[12] Reflection involves thinking about what we are doing, developing insight into our own approaches to a problem, analyzing the way that we tackle the problem and looking critically at the outcome. It then involves reflecting on that process, paying particular attention to what will be learnt at the end of it. Questions that the learner might ask include:

- What features do I notice when I recognize this situation?
- What are the criteria by which I make this judgment?
- What procedures am I enacting when I perform this skill?
- How am I framing the problem that I am trying to solve?

The learner also needs to think about and draw on related knowledge and experiences to be able to criticize, restructure and apply these principles for further learning. Schön calls this type of thinking 'Reflection on action'. This review of past experiences leads to a critical analysis of what led us to change our way of practice; sometimes reflection during the course of a process (reflection in action) involves modifications while dealing with a problem. It is very important that reflection is encouraged in a nonthreatening way so the learner does not become demoralized. Although mistakes or unsatisfactory outcomes often provide the best stimuli for learning, such events need to be handled sensitively and appropriately. Much learning can be effectively undertaken by reflecting on ordinary situations as they arise, thereby building on good practice. This can be particularly important for the learner who lacks confidence. When mistakes have occurred the learner should be encouraged to reflect on what they would do differently next time, rather than on what they did wrong.

In palliative care, the clinical situation is often extremely complex and many different ways of approaching the problem can have effective, or ineffective, outcomes. Emotionally charged situations can leave the palliative care learner feeling inadequate, upset and sometimes with unrealistic expectations of him or herself as a practitioner. Greenwood has been particularly critical of Schön's module because it failed to recognize the importance of reflection *before* action.[13] In palliative care such a reflective approach before acting integrates all previous experiences, with acquired knowledge and understanding, to empower the practitioner to behave differently to previously.

Boud defines reflection as 'an important human activity in which people recapture their experience, think about it, mull it over and evaluate it'.[14] Here, the reflection focuses on the individual's experience, involving both cognition and feelings as the two are closely interrelated and interact. Feelings, which may be 'positive' or 'negative', will prompt an individual to behave differently at the initial stage of reflecting, so Boud postulates that the individual encounters an experience, responds and at the same time starts to reflect. By returning later to recall what has happened, replaying the experience and reevaluating, additional processes occur:

1 Association – where new experiences relate to existing knowledge and understanding.
2 Integration – where the learner seeks relationship between the new information and what is already known.
3 Validation – where the learner determines validity of his/her feelings in response and the ideas that have resulted from it.
4 Appropriation – where the learner takes ownership of this knowledge and integrates it into long-term learning, to be used in future clinical practice.

These reflective processes underpin changes in behavior. They can be very powerful and underpin many of the teaching methods used for teaching graduates; these will be dealt with later in the chapter.

THE ROLE OF A TUTOR IN A GRADUATE PROGRAM

For the purposes of this chapter, a 'tutor' is defined as a person who facilitates the learning process. This term can be considered synonymous with mentor, teacher, or facilitator. All tutors need clear guidance about what is expected of them, and the time frame in which they are expected to be tutoring. They also need to be clear about the styles of tutoring that will encourage learners and styles that should be avoided as they lead to demoralization. Tutors need to be clear that they should operate within bounds of confidentiality, and explicitly explain to a student issues that would be shared with the course organizers/course directors. Where students are being tutored in groups, confidentiality of the group discussions becomes important and each member of the group must be treated with respect. Each member should have time to participate and care should be taken that no one member of the group dominates. The most effective teaching occurs in a safe environment where the individual feels supported and good practice is reinforced. However, sometimes, where individuals lack insight, the tutor may have to speak one to one with the student to help that student identify particular problems, which they are having. Such difficult conversations should be held outside the group setting.

Pendleton's method (Box 17.1) of feedback provides a useful set of rules by which feedback should be given.[15] It is a particularly useful method of feedback in a small group setting but can be adapted for one-to-one feedback by replacing feedback from other learners with comments from the tutor themselves.

Box 17.1 Pendleton's method of feedback

- Asking the learner what they felt they did well or were particularly happy with

- Learner/tutor feedback – what they feel went well

- Asking the learner what they felt could be improved

- Learner/tutor feedback – what they feel could be improved

THE INDIVIDUAL STUDENT'S SITUATION

In selecting graduates for a training program, it is important to know what has motivated the student to come forward and wish to learn. Some may have been told in their appraisal that they must go on a course to improve, while others may be motivated through their own, often bad, experience within their own friends or family, or a professional situation where they felt that their practice was substandard. Students also come from a wide range of clinical situations. Whereas in western Europe and the USA, libraries, journals and internet abound, in many third world and developing countries there are no journals in libraries and the internet is unreliable or nonexistent.

It is also important to know about the practice conditions of learners. Although it can be useful for learners to be exposed to a wide range of ways of practicing, including some high-tech interventions, for those practicing in much more primitive conditions most of their meaningful understanding and competency development will occur in relation to techniques and actions that they can instigate in their own work environment. This is consistent with the principle of justice,[16] which requires that each patient have the best treatment within the resources available, but also the professional is responsible for the just allocation of resources (equity).

REFLECTIVE CASE STUDY (PORTFOLIO LEARNING)

Reflective learning on an individual case can be a powerful teaching tool. The learner's everyday practice offers many stimuli for reflection as they go about their daily work, noting interesting or challenging situations as they occur. Many palliative care teams now use protected time for reflective practice in small groups. This can be successful within uniprofessional and interprofessional groups, providing it is conducted in a safe, nonthreatening environment, paying particular attention to confidentiality within the group. It can also be a powerful tool within the realms of team support and clinical supervision.

One of the most useful tools to capture and record reflection and personal development is portfolio learning. Portfolio learning is designed to provide a chronological record of the learning process of the student. The learning process is self-directed; the learner chooses the areas within a subject of particular interest. In the context of graduate education, this enables each learner to meet their own individual learning objectives. For example, a student who identifies a need to develop skills in the management of neuropathic pain can focus on this topic, while another colleague may concentrate on mouth care.

This style of learning varies greatly from the technical rational style encountered at most undergraduate schools. Those unaccustomed to this learning style will require gentle support and supervision. As reflective practice and portfolio and problem-based learning become more widespread within undergraduate curricula, graduates will become comfortable with this style of professional development. The beauty and simplicity of a reflective portfolio, which allows the learner to determine format, learning objectives, and emphasis to the learner may be seen by some as too unstructured and challenging. Most physicians are new to the relative lack of prescribed formal structure in the portfolio. Depending upon the experience of the educational supervisor, even the method of presenting the portfolio can be relaxed if the reasons are clear. The learner should be encouraged to develop the portfolio (Box 17.2) in a way similar to an artist's portfolio, reflecting their freedom of creativity in presentation.

Box 17.2 Most successful portfolios consist of the following elements, which are interrelated and cross-referenced[17]

- Factual case histories around which the learning usually occurs

- References to diverse sources, e.g. textbook reading, literature search, lay press, conversations with colleagues

- A record of the clinician's own decision-making processes including details of decisions made and how the learner came to them

- Documentation as to how the learner felt at the time, sources of stress or doubts are as useful as the outcome since the personal feelings of the learner will influence how they were able to approach a problem

---

- Ethical considerations

- Illustrative items such as photographs, drawings, quotations, poetry, etc., may clarify points being made. Care must be taken over anonymization and permission from the patient for such items to be used

- Some form of indexing is important, so the learner and supervisor can follow the learning process and refer to specific items at a later date

---

The self-directed learning portfolio acts as a tool for learning and as evidence to the supervisor that learning has taken place. The format of the portfolio can vary widely, allowing creative expression by the learner. Formative assessment between the supervisor and student in an informal setting is essential for learners to have feedback on their progress. It enables the supervisor to give constructive feedback to the student and provide support, especially to those new to the concept of portfolio learning. Summative assessment can help the student identify areas for future learning. Examples of marking schedules are given in Tables 17.1 and 17.2; these are for guidance only as the learning process needs to be as flexible and adaptable as possible.

The supervisor will be aware that some factual clinical details of the portfolio cannot be verified or crosschecked, as the reader will not know patients or episodes described. However, it is better to base a leaning portfolio around real cases and events rather than a fabricated scenario, since the learner will gain more from reflection on action with which they have first hand experience. The suggested marking schedules attribute only a small proportion of marks to the description of the case, awarding the majority of marks to evidence that learning has occurred. Social and personal issues in the case history balance the biological evolution of the disease process. The marking scheme reflects the importance placed upon teamworking within palliative care and the supervisor should actively encourage an appreciation of this if it is felt to be lacking in the portfolio.

For the graduate learner, a portfolio gives an excellent opportunity to focus experience. It can act as documentation

Table 17.1 *Summative portfolio mark schedule*

Contextual description of case	5%
Biologic issues of the case	5%
Individual issues of the case	5%
Teamworking	10%
Clarity of presentation	10%
Decision-making logic	20%
Attribution of evidence	20%
Critical analysis	15%
Index and discretionary marks	10%
Total	**100%**

Table 17.2 *Learners' guidance*

Academic background	15%
Display appropriate use of academic literature/ research, other influences in learning	
Coverage of topic (total 40%)	
Biology of the disease	10%
The natural history of the disease	
Screening and diagnosis	
Staging and disease progression	
Impact of cancer	10%
Psychological response to disease and the importance of honest communication	
Social impact of disease on patients and their families/carers	
Spiritual response to the diagnosis	
Clinical management	10%
Treatment options and how decisions are made	
Symptom control	
Coordinated care	10%
Multidisciplinary teamworking	
Response to loss and bereavement	
Approach to patient and problems	10%
Warmth	
Caring	
Empathy	
Respect	
Humanity	
Holistic assessment and management	25%
Communication and personal insight	10%
Physical, psychological, social, and spiritual assessment	
Ability to engage and talk to patients and their carers about their experience and develop a relationship with them	
Display insight into their own emotional reactions to difficult and sad situations	
Patient responses	5%
Identification of the patients problems, hopes, and fears	
Critical analysis of care	10%
Process of evaluating the efficacy of care from both the medical and patient perspective	
Display evidence of clear critical analysis and synthesis of issues	
Commitment	10%
Throughout the course, the student should have displayed commitment to learning in tutorials and in self-directed learning time	

of learning objectives, recording clinical situations commonly faced and areas of difficulty. For the supervisor it helps identify any topics requiring further experience or teaching. Often small group tutorials can be organized around subjects identified by several learners, all in a position to contribute in this environment with experiences to reflect upon and share.

Portfolio learning should be viewed as a dynamic, fluid learning process, which should ideally continue as long as the individual keeps learning. As all medical professionals become more accountable and are required to give evidence of continuing learning, the portfolio may become a more prominent educational tool within the whole of medicine, not just palliative care. The portfolio provides a unique opportunity for learning to occur in the wider context of the humanities. Relevant facets are incorporated and cross-referenced, giving validity to the learned experience described by others through art or literature.

COMMUNICATION SKILLS

The importance of communication skills is widely recognized in palliative care. Communication problems faced by graduates working in cancer medicine are not resolved by time and clinical experience,[18**] and there is strong evidence that training courses significantly improve key communication skills.[19***] It seems insidious to allow any professional to graduate from a course in palliative care without having ascertained that they have developed the appropriate communication skills to deal with the complex difficulties that will be encountered in clinical practice.[20]

Palliative care consultations are often the most challenging, since they may involve breaking bad news and talking about dying and loss.[21] Intrusive observation of such sensitive consultations, with recording devices or the presence of additional observers, may disrupt the flow of the consultation and hinder the patient's openness within discussions. Since the palliative care consultation is potentially difficult and may have wide ramifications if badly handled, the trainer must create a safe learning environment where the trainee can feel comfortable making mistakes without repercussions and protect potentially vulnerable patients. It necessarily follows that the use of real patients is not always appropriate.

Role play

Role play, using either actors or colleagues as patients, has long been established as a useful tool for developing communication skills.[22] It is best done as a small group of learners with one or more trained facilitators. It is important to keep the groups small enough to ensure that everyone has the opportunity to role play in the time allocated. People are initially wary of role play since, for many, it is unlike any other training they may have encountered. Maintaining a small group will help them feel more comfortable in the process.

Role play allows people to train for situations they rarely encounter but need to be ready for. The skills for breaking bad news or dealing with anger are best learned prior to encounter in practice. In the real world, one will not get a second opportunity to tackle a difficult consultation from scratch over and over again. Role play affords the learner this luxury.

There are several basic principles that should underpin any such learning session:

- Clearly established rules of role play
- Strict adherence to confidentiality
- Safe environment
- Avoidance of role playing situations that are potentially distressing for learners
- Option to call 'time-out' at any point
- Opportunity for all learners to participate
- Nonconfrontational feedback
- Time for those involved to 'come out of role' after a session
- Review of learning points and de-brief at end of each session.

Feedback can be given in several different ways. Pendleton's method[15] is one of the safest ways to give feedback singly or involving other participants and has been discussed earlier in the chapter (see Box 17.1). This approach to feedback has the merit of first highlighting what was done well, thereby reinforcing good practice and offering positive suggestions for improvement. Those members of the group who are not role playing should take an active part in the appraisal system, to observe and learn from peers. More recently the Calgary–Cambridge approach to communication skills teaching has been developed as a facilitation tool.[22] It encourages a far more agenda-led approach to communication skills, encouraging learners to focus those specific areas of the consultation they otherwise avoid through lack of confidence.

The skills to facilitate such sessions are sophisticated, so training is strongly recommended before embarking on this teaching style. Most learning of value will occur from the role play itself and the feedback session, but summative assessment can highlight particular areas of weakness. Selected videotaped consultations can complement role play. Box 17.3 illustrates a suggested marking scheme for the palliative care consultation. Marks are given in each section out of 10, 5 being the pass mark.

Box 17.3 Summative marking schedule for palliative care consultation

- Puts patient at ease
- Establishes problems sufficiently to erect hypothesis
- Prioritizes problems/hypothesis
- Checks back on problem list agreement
- Elicits fears/concerns
- Elicits beliefs/concepts/attitudes
- Establishes physical/psychosocial relationship of complaints
- Explores physical issues appropriately
- Evolves plan acceptable to patient
- Checks back that plan is understood/agreed
- Overall – nonverbals facilitate
- Overall – verbals appropriate
- Overall – patient appears comfortable/safe
- Overall – respects patient's pace
- Overall – closes interview well

TEACHING ETHICS

Ethical dilemmas abound in care of patients at the end of life. Ethical decision making is never straightforward, so mastering reflection will help the learner function better within zones of indeterminate practice or as Schön[12] describes it as 'the swamp'. Ethical decision making needs a sound understanding of the principles of autonomy, beneficence, nonmaleficence, and justice within the patient's clinical context.[16] Gillon has also highlighted the wide issues around each decision, which require the clinician to reflect on the 'scope' of application of the decision-making process and its outcomes.[23] Although a formal lecture may appear useful to inform, the complex decision making around each case requires ongoing reflection in action by both tutor and learner.

THE HUMANITIES AS AN EDUCATIONAL TOOL

Graduate training in palliative medicine should address not only the clinical and psychosocial needs of the patients and relatives but also those of the professional. A purely biomedical education cannot equip someone in their early twenties to understand the reactions of a bereaved person, the behavior of someone receiving bad news, or the devastation of a long-term disability.[24] The past decade has seen an increasing role for the arts and humanities in education although there is no consensus about which disciplines constitute the field of medical humanities. While the humanities have clear established roles in patient care and an emerging place in undergraduate education, graduate training remains an area of particular challenge. Art and poetry therapy are widely used to enable patients contemplate their own response to illness. A number of medical schools encourage the use of humanities such as art and literature within undergraduate special study modules.[25] However, variable access to expert support in what some will find an unfamiliar area of learning is likely to be a problem in graduate education for the foreseeable future. Like all areas of education, clear learning objectives need to be identified and appropriate assessment of learners and evaluation of facilitators undertaken.

There are three main areas of graduate education in palliative medicine that medical humanities can best address – namely reflection, connection, and support. Reflection enables learners to review their own feelings, practice, and experience, allowing insight into the strengths and weaknesses of their own practice. The response of physicians to a dying patient is more than just a scientific answer to a biomedical question. Recognition of one's own needs and values is essential if physicians are to move beyond their own concerns and place those of the patient at the forefront of their endeavors. Reflection on films, literature, art, and poetry may afford physicians an insight into the doctor–patient relationship not given in the biomedical approach to learning. Most graduate learners in their twenties have little personal experience of suffering and bereavement. An ability to connect with patients and their relatives will be essential in the delivery of patient-centered holistic care. Observing how doctors are portrayed in popular culture gives valuable insights into the expectations and fears that patients have of doctors, and doctors have of themselves.[26] Finally, graduate learners may draw on the medical humanities for their own personal development and support. Stress-related illness of professionals in this area of medicine is well documented and the use of the humanities addresses an ongoing need.

INFORMATION TECHNOLOGY AND INTERNET LEARNING

Progress within information technology (IT) has made a huge impact on the provision of healthcare across the world. The use of e-mail correspondence, computerized patient notes, and digital storage of radiology and patient information initiatives are likely to be ubiquitous applications of IT development within the next few years.

Distance learning postgraduate courses have traditionally been organized as a correspondence course, with course packs delivered regularly and completed assignments duly returned. Some of these courses have now adapted toward web-based learning, where learners are able to, course packs online, with links to relevant articles. E-mail allows students direct access to tutors for guidance and submission of assignments. Web-based chat rooms for students encourage informal sharing of ideas, avoiding the distance learner studying in isolation. The benefits of web-based learning are clear, with reduction in stationary costs, administration time, and

removal of the delay of postage, which for many distance learners can be considerable. More importantly it allows professionals from diverse localities and cultures to learn alongside each other, sharing ideas and experiences under the supervision of a suitably qualified facilitator. There appears to be an expanding role for videoconferencing in palliative care education.[27*,28*] Still in its infancy, learners tend to prefer face-to-face teaching to videoconferencing especially for learning about sensitive subjects. However, research suggests that learning outcomes are similar for both modalities.[29*]

An increasing number of journals are now available online although many require a subscription. In addition to accessing online journals, the ubiquitous personal computer has accommodated the publication of major textbooks on CD-ROM.

Although there are clear opportunities for learning by the internet and IT, it is important that these are focused appropriately and not instigated for the sake of progress. Videoconferencing may link learners across the globe but should never be considered as a complete alternative to traditional conferences, since opportunities to learn informally, develop new ideas, and network will be lost.

DETERMINING THE MARKET

Budget programs can provide learning at different levels. There are some core competencies in care that cut across all professional groups and can be taught in an interdisciplinary setting. Others are discipline specific and some relate to specialized or specialist level practice, so although core level learners should be aware of these, they do not need to have an indepth understanding of higher specialist levels of learning.

Interprofessional learning does not occur by simply putting people in the same room together. It becomes important that individuals can define their own common core skills and responsibilities and recognize the competencies that exist in others. Topics such as bereavement will be seen to be core to all those working in palliative care and is best dealt with in an interprofessional learning environment. However some aspects such as the management of spinal cord compression will vary from professional to professional. The physiotherapist or nurse may be the professional to recognize imminent spinal cord compression, the oncologist will instigate the investigation and indepth management, whereas the nursing aspects and rehabilitation aspects will revert to those initially involved in recognizing the problem, with the additional occupational therapy input.

ORGANIZING A GRADUATE PROGRAM

Whenever a graduate program is organized, there are three distinct phases that need to be addressed: needs assessment and precourse planning, course delivery, and finally assessment after the course to allow modification and confirm that the course met its own aims and objectives.

Careful precourse planning is essential; fundamental decisions about the course must be made: in particular the curriculum and format of the course. Planning should not be done by one individual in isolation, but rather with the involvement of a committee of potential course tutors/ facilitators. Once the course has been established, the committee should invite student representatives to contribute.

The curriculum, specific expected learning outcomes, and course delivery should take account of the needs of the learners and the resources available to meet them.[30*] Graduates have different levels of knowledge and experience of palliative medicine. Some may be general practitioners or specialists wishing to expand their palliative medicine skills whereas others may be following a specialist career in palliative medicine. The number of learners intended on the course and their geographical location will have significant impact on resources and course delivery. Distance learning and Web-based courses are more practical for a cohort of learners from a wide geographical distribution but this will have resource implications.

Many countries have a core curriculum of learning needs and descriptors of competencies that need to be achieved during the course.[31–35] Several courses based upon these competencies have run successfully within the UK, with the Cardiff course training over 900 postgraduates to diploma level within 15 years of activity. Although curricula that have been developed by national organizations can serve as 'guideposts' they may not address the specific needs and culture of an individual.[36*] Nevertheless, a survey of 263 clinicians from a wide variety of clinical, geographic, and cultural backgrounds suggests that the elements of such core curricula are of high relevance to their clinical practice.[37*] Learners considered areas of particular importance to include communication skills, multiprofessional teamworking and psychological aspects of care, subjects that lend themselves best to reflective practice and role play.

Resource allocation and availability will affect the course format. Distance learning courses require dedicated administrative staff and a cohort of course tutors. Some core competencies cannot be facilitated or assessed by distance learning and require face-to-face tutorials. Many distance-learning courses include residential weekends to address communication skills and allow group discussion on challenging topics; administrative staff salaries, teaching honoraria and venue costs all need to be considered.

Delivering a course that encompasses a multiprofessional holistic patient-focused approach to care holds many challenges, especially since some of the core competencies and methods of assessment do not lend themselves well to the didactic exam-focused way many doctors are used to learning by. It is likely that most will be new to reflective practice, portfolio learning, and using the humanities as a learning tool. Role play in communication skills training is often met with trepidation, usually manifest as resistance. The role of experienced, skilled facilitators/tutors cannot

be underemphasized to provide the support and input inevitably required, particularly at the beginning of the course.

Any teaching program needs regular evaluation to ensure it is educationally effective. The course must respond to the changing and individual needs of participants, provide competent teaching in theory and practice, and enable students to make a difference in their clinical practice.[38*] Structured feedback should be incorporated throughout the course, giving opportunities for learners and tutors alike to contribute to the continuing development of the venture. Feedback should be collated annually and reviewed by the planning committee, allowing time to act on areas in need of change. Student representatives should be encouraged to participate in this process and liaise directly with fellow learners.

POSTGRADUATE RESEARCH TRAINING

Some graduates may wish to pursue higher research degree training. There are various forms of research degree available, including masters in science (MSc), the Commonwealth doctor of medicine (MD), and doctor of philosophy (PhD). A research degree involves the presentation of a thesis on a research topic in a field of interest appropriate to an individual's training needs. Apart from a wish to improve research skills, a higher research degree is considered in other specialties to be associated with better job prospects. Within palliative care, higher research degrees serve four functions:[39]

- extending personal scholarship
- generating knowledge
- training for the individual
- contributing to the growth of the specialty.

Individuals with higher degrees are likely to be involved in research in the future[40*,41*] and to obtain research funding.[42*] To commence on such a training program, the candidate needs to demonstrate a sound knowledge base in palliative care and proficiency in research methodology. To demonstrate these, prospective candidates will need evidence of basic training within the specialty and involvement in related research. Several masters courses will only enroll candidates once they have achieved qualification to diploma level or will encompass training to diploma standard within the first year of enrollment. It usual for such teaching programs to train the candidate in research methodology at the initial stages of the course.

The likelihood of candidates obtaining a higher research degree does not lie solely upon their own attributes and commitment to the project. There are other essential requirements beyond their immediate control that must be fulfilled to obtain satisfactory completion:

- supervision
- environment conducive to undertaking research
- dedicated research time
- funding.

One of the major barriers to undertaking research in palliative care has been difficulties in obtaining appropriate supervision from senior colleagues.[43*] As a relatively young specialty, palliative care has fewer academic departments and hence available supervisors than other long-established specialties. Successful completion of higher research degrees is more likely to occur if the candidate has dedicated research time in a department with an ongoing research facility and some will need to access other specialties, e.g. oncology, to achieve this.[44] Since completion of a higher research degree is more likely with those in full-time research than part time, funding may be required to cover the trainee's salary as well as the running of the research project. Few charities within palliative care offer substantive grants to cover such costs and drug company research grants are lower than allocations for comparable ventures in other specialties. Consequently the majority of higher research degrees within palliative care are completed by part-time study.

CONCLUSION

As the specialty of palliative care expands so will the need to increase the education opportunities available to graduate healthcare professionals. The special nature of palliative medicine with holistic, multiprofessional patient-centered care necessitates what some will find new learning techniques, alien to the didactic method of training they are accustomed to. Communication skills, bereavement care, ethical decision making, and spiritual care may be better learned by role play and reflective practice. Distance-learning courses will facilitate the growing need for a geographically diverse group of professionals to learn together, particularly when facilitated by residential weekends and online. As well as gaining existing knowledge, it is important to encourage further the knowledge base of the specialty through research. Appropriately supervised and funded higher research training will advance knowledge and improve patient care through the twenty-first century.

Key learning points

- Postgraduate learning in palliative care offers challenges unique to medical specialties.

- Holistic multiprofessional learning may be unfamiliar to previous didactic learning experiences.

- Reflective practice and portfolio learning are excellent methods of adult learning.

- The internet, IT, and the humanities lend themselves well to palliative care learning.

- Communication skills training courses improve key communication skills.

- Completion of higher research degrees will improve the research base of palliative care in the future.

REFERENCES

● 1   Beard RM, Hartley J. *Teaching and Learning in Higher Education*. London: Paul Chapman, 1984.

◆ 2   Prochaska JO, Velicer WF. The transtheoretical model of health behavior change *Am J Health Promot* 1997; **12**: 38–48.

◆ 3   Grant J. Learning needs assessment. assessing the need. *BMJ* 2002; **324**: 156–9.

4   Gunten CF, Von Roenn JH, Gradishar W, Weitzman S. A hospice/palliative medicine rotation for fellows training in hematology-oncology. *J Cancer Educ* 1995; **10**: 200–2.

5   Montagnini M, Varkey B, DuthieE Jr. Palliative care education integrated into a geriatrics rotation for resident physicians. *J Palliat Med* 2004; **7**: 652–9.

6   DeVita MA, Arnold RM, Barnard D. Teaching palliative care to critical care medicine trainees. *Crit Care Med* 2003; **31**: 1257–62.

7   Hallenbeck JL, Bergen MR. A medical resident inpatient hospice rotation: experiences with dying and subsequent changes in attitudes and knowledge. *J Palliat Med* 1999; **2**: 197–208.

8   von Gunten CF, Mullan PB, Harrity S *et al*. Faculty, Center for Palliative Study. Residents from five training programs report improvements in knowledge, attitudes and skills after a rotation with a hospice program. *J Cancer Educ* 2003; **18**: 68–72.

9   von Gunten CF, Twaddle M, Preodor M, *et al*. Evidence of improved knowledge and skills after an elective rotation in a hospice and palliative care program for internal medicine residents. *Am J Hosp Palliat Care* 2005; **22**: 195–203.

10   von Roenn JH, Neely KJ, Curry RH, Weitzman SA. A curriculum in palliative care for internal medicine housestaff: a pilot project. *J Cancer Educ* 1988; **3**: 259–63.

● 11   Knowles M. *Self Directed Learning*. New York: Association Press, 1988.

● 12   Schön D. *Educating the Reflective Practitioner: Towards a New Design for Teaching and Learning in the Professions*. San Francisco: Jossey-Bass, 1987.

◆ 13   Greenwood J. The role of reflection in single and double loop learning. *J Adv Learning* 1998; **27**: 1048–53.

● 14   Boud D, Keogh R, Walker D. *Reflection: Turning Experience into Learning*. London: Kogan Page, 1985.

● 15   Pendleton D, Schofield T, Tate P, Havelock P. *The Consultation: An Approach to Learning and Teaching*. Oxford: Oxford University Press, 1984.

● 16   Beauchamp TL, Childress JF. *Principles of Biomedical Ethics*, 3rd ed. New York: Oxford University Press, 1989.

● 17   Finlay IG, Stott NCH, Marsh HM. Portfolio learning in palliative medicine. *Eur J Cancer Care* 1993; **2**: 41–3.

18   Fallowfield L, Jenkins V, Farewell V, *et al*. Efficacy of a cancer research UK communication skills training model for oncologists: a randomized controlled trial. *Lancet* 2002; **359**: 650–6.

19   Fellowes D, Wilkinson S, Moore P. Communication skills training for health care professionals working with cancer patients, their families and/or carers. *Cochrane Database Syst Rev* 2004:CD003751.

20   Finlay IG, Sarangi S. Oral medical discourse, communication skills and terminally ill patients. In: Brown K, ed. *Encyclopaedia of Language and Linguistics*, 2nd ed. Oxford: Elsevier, 2005.

● 21   Mansfield F. Supervised role-play in the teaching of the process of consultation. *Med Educ* 1991; **25**: 485–90.

● 22   Kurtz S, Silverman J, Draper J. *Teaching and Learning Communication Skills in Medicine*. Oxford: Radcliffe Medical Press, 1988.

● 23   Gillon R. Medical ethics: four principles plus attention to scope. *BMJ* 1994; **309**: 184–8.

24   Evans M, Finlay I, eds. *Medical Humanities*. London: BMJ Publishing Group, 2001.

25   Calman K. Literature in the education of the doctor. *Lancet* 1999; **29**: 1622–5.

26   Glasser B. From Kafka to casualty doctors and medicine in popular culture and the arts – a special studies module. *J Med Ethics: Med Humanities* 2001; **27**: 99–101.

27   Regnard C. Using videoconferencing in palliative care. *Palliat Med* 2000; **14**: 519–28.

28   Lynch J, Weaver L, Hall P, *et al.* Using telehealth technology to support CME in end-of-life care for community physicians in Ontario. *Telemed J E Health* 2004; **10**: 103–7.

29   van Boxell P, Anderson K, Regnard C. The effectiveness of palliative care education delivered by videoconferencing compared with face-to-face delivery. *Palliat Med* 2003; **17**: 344–58.

30   Ury WA, Arnold RM, Tulsky JA. Palliative care curriculum development: a model for a content and process-based approach. *J Palliat Med* 2002; **5**: 539–48.

31   Association for Palliative Medicine. *Palliative Medicine Curriculum*. Southampton: APM, 2002.

32   Irish Committee on Higher Medical Training. Curriculum for Higher Specialist Training in Palliative Medicine. Dublin: Royal College of Physicians of Ireland, 1997.

33   Royal Australasian College of Physicians. *Requirements for Physician Training (Mango Book). Vocational Training in Palliative Medicine for 2003*. Sydney: RACP, 2002.

34   Hong Kong College of Physicians. *Guidelines for Higher Physician Training*. Hong Kong: HKCP, 2002.

35   LeGrand SB, Walsh D, Nelson KA, Davis MP. A syllabus for fellowship education in palliative medicine. *Am J Hosp Palliat Care* 2003; **20**: 279–89.

36   Ury WA, Reznich CB, Weber CM. A needs assessment for a palliative care curriculum. *J Pain Symptom Manage* 2000; **20**: 408–16.

37   Rawlinson F, Finlay I. Assessing education in palliative medicine: development of a tool based on the Association for Palliative Medicine core curriculum. *Palliat Med* 2002; **16**: 51–5.

38   Kenny LJ. An evaluation-based model for palliative care education: making a difference to practice. *Int J Palliat Nurs* 2003; **9**: 189–94.

39   Higginson I, Corner J. Postgraduate research training: the PhD and MD thesis. *Palliat Med* 1996; **10**: 113–18.

40   Williams WO. A survey of doctorates by thesis among general practitioners in the British Isles from 1973 to 1988. *Br J Gen Pract* 1990; **40**: 491–4.

41   Pincus HA, Haviland MG, Dial TH, Hendryx MS. The relationship of postdoctoral research training to current research activities of faculty in academic departments of psychiatry. *Am J Psychiatry* 1995; **152**: 596–601.

42   Lee TH, Ognibene FP, Schwartz JS. Correlates of external research support among respondents to the 1990 American Federation for Clinical Research survey. *Clin Res* 1991; **39**: 135–44.

43   Stirling LC, Pegrum H, George R. A survey of education and research facilities for palliative medicine trainees in the United Kingdom. *Palliat Med* 2000; **14**: 37–52.

44   Quigley C. Postgraduate research training. *Palliat Med* 1996; **10**: 346.

18

Changing the norms of palliative care practice by changing the norms of education

LINDA EMANUEL

INTRODUCTION

Medical professionalism requires earnest adherence to optimal practices for patient care. Because of the potency of the medical armamentarium, the obligation to restrict medical practices to those that optimize patient care is a solemn duty.[1] Career-long learning and modification of practices in the light of new knowledge or new challenges are a necessary part of that duty.

In the past decades, medicine has generated hitherto unsurpassed capacities in symptom management, as is evident for instance from the chapters in this textbook. Medicine has, however, also struggled with a lost balance between the aim to cure and the need to ameliorate suffering. This imbalance occurred during the culture of scientific enthusiasm that had lost too much of the appropriate emphasis on whole-person context of illness-related suffering in favor of organ and molecular-based attention to diseases. It had overlooked quality-of-life issues and suitable care for those with chronic and serious or incurable illness and those engaged with the processes of inevitable death.[2]

It has therefore been a challenge to the profession to put in place sufficiently effective palliative care education that the balance of curative approaches with symptom management and a culture of care could be returned. The challenge was taken on at a time when the norms of medical education were entrenched in dry didactic methods even though research had demonstrated their minimal impact on practices. This chapter traces the efforts of one project in particular, as it coordinated its activities with that of

other projects, to do its part among other key programs in confronting this challenge.

ASSESSING THE CHALLENGE, SELECTING THE STRATEGY

The case-study project used here for illustrative purposes is the Education in Palliative and End-of-life Care (EPEC) Project. How did this project assess its circumstances as it designed its strategy?

Many studies have documented minimal impact on practices of carefully designed and implemented medical educational interventions.[3] More effective programs use multiple education methods and multiple interventions such as clinical reminders simultaneously.[4] Nonetheless, impact remains modest at best. Part of the problem is likely attributable to the fact that continuing medical education had become a ritualized process of information presentation. These forms of information delivery are not designed according to principles of adult education theory and are not much influenced by social science understandings of what can drive changes in social expectations and behavioral norms. A related, practical part of the problem was that it was not accepted in mainstream practices, so that multi-method approaches such as clinical reminders would realistically only be implemented *after* the field had gained acceptance. Given the enormity of the challenge that palliative care needed to rise to and the inadequacy of education as a vehicle for an immediate change, the field faced the stark choice between becoming highly creative or plodding forward with too little and too late. Choosing the former, palliative care has managed to bring about significant changes in a relatively short time, to the point that it has provided something of a model for other fields seeking to bring about changes in norms of practice.

Starting out in the mid 1990s, the EPEC Project took stock of what it could do best as one among other programs. It was situated, when it began, within a national physicians' organization serving all specialties that also had an international presence. So it chose as its mission to improve the skills of physicians from any discipline; and it aimed for a national and international scope. Aware that the focus on physicians might seem counter-cultural to the hospice and palliative care movement that emphasized the essential role of the interdisciplinary team, it nonetheless wanted to capitalize on its unique ability to reach physicians. It settled on a train-the-trainer approach that would allow physician trainers to reach not only other physicians but nonphysician clinicians.

Other features informing the strategy of the EPEC Project included the following. It would have to address the need to address norms among practicing clinicians, since it would take too long to wait for the gradual infiltration of change by incoming newly trained clinicians. Further, the existing practice norms that did not support palliative care would rapidly eliminate any learning among medical students if the norms were left unchanged. A strategy was needed to address the need for changed practice norms, especially since much of the knowledge that should have driven change was not new; that is, the knowledge was mostly available but not applied in practice. Another problem was presented by the perception that palliative care was nonreimbursable; this appeared to be impeding administrative support for palliative care services in mainstream medical practices. The question of which physicians to target came up early since there was a pressing need for palliative care in virtually all the existing specialties in medicine, whether surgery, cardiology, oncology, or general internal medicine. So the strategy for the project would have to allow for 'uptake' within the cultures of these diverse specialties. Regarding geographical location, palliative care was needed for great swatches of territory on the globe, especially where the human immunodeficiency virus (HIV)/ acquired immune deficiency syndrome (AIDS) epidemic had taken root. Finally, the strategy would have to fit with the national nature of the organization from which the program was being launched, and with the reality that one program could not cover the global needs in palliative care.

SITUATING A PROGRAM WITHIN A BROADER STRATEGY, RELIANT ON SOCIAL CHANGE THEORY

What successes the EPEC Project enjoyed were in great part made possible by the existence of a well-crafted and funded, national strategy created by the staff and board of the Robert Wood Johnson Foundation. Their approach was driven by the awareness that even a well-designed program, if it is in a hostile larger social context, will be hard pressed to succeed and even harder pressed to sustain its impact after funding is over.

The Robert Wood Johnson Foundation invited a proposal to create what became the EPEC Project as part of an overall, evolving strategy that included projects in nursing education (ELNEC), in training for physicians-in-residence (EPERC), in faculty development (provided by Harvard's Center for Palliative Care), to promote institutional palliative care programs (CAPC), to reach specific communities, for instance, the African–American community (APPEAL) and numerous projects for public education. Later on, when the time was right, support was also provided to the American Academy of Hospice and Palliative Medicine (AAHPM) to get it to a point where it could sustain specialty educational offerings. Reconstructed in retrospect, the strategy can be mapped approximately as in Figure 18.1.

Central to this strategy was a social marketing perspective for each major project that identified how to go about changing the social assumptions in the relevant sectors of

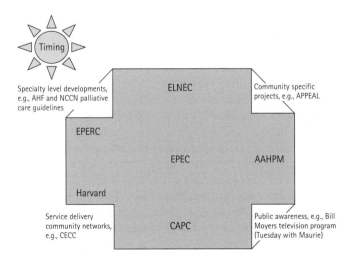

Figure 18.1 *Robert Wood Johnson Foundation strategic programming. AAHPM, American Academy of Hospice and Palliative Medicine; AHF, American Hospice Foundation; APPEAL, A Progressive Palliative Education Curriculum for Health Care for African-Americans at Life's End; CAPC, Center to Advance Palliative Care; CECC, Chicago End-of-Life Care Coalition; ELNEC, End-of-Life Nursing Education Consortium; EPEC, End-of-Life Care; EPERC, End of Life Physician Education Resource Center; NCCN, National Comprehensive Cancer Network.*

society about end-of-life care. Significant involvement of consultative opinion from a social marketing group contributed importantly to the design of several of the major projects. In this fashion, the social taboos and other behaviors of denial that surrounded dying in America at the time, were to be addressed and reversed to the point that a social movement could begin. The programs were also strongly encouraged to achieve programmatic self-sufficiency during their last stages of funding, so that their impact would be sustained after the end of grant funding.

This combination of Robert Wood Johnson Foundation strategies was coordinated with those of the few other funding agencies that were supportive of palliative and end-of-life care. Through meetings of the Grantmakers in End of Life Care and in other settings, the granting agencies were able to coordinate their efforts. All were assisted by the publication of the Institute of Medicine report that called for panoramic improvements in care near the end of life.[2] For instance, the Soros Foundation funded the Project on Death in America, which fostered the career development of young careerists with leadership potential by providing grants and a supportive setting for research and clinical projects in palliative care. Toward the end of the Robert Wood Johnson Foundation's major efforts in end-of-life care, other agencies such as the American Cancer Society, and agencies at the National Institutes of Health such as the National Cancer Institute, were being encouraged to take on funding of what had become successful projects that were nevertheless still being only cautiously accepted in the mainstream of medicine. Leaders had been successfully fostered and a Board of Hospice and Palliative Medicine had been established in association with the AAHPM, leading eventually to the recognition in 2005 of palliative care by the American Board of Medical Specialties as a discipline warranting its own Certificate of Additional Qualification.

Looking back on the decade between 1995 and 2005, the Robert Wood Johnson Foundation can fairly say that the culture of society transformed from one in which death was denied, the dying were shunned, and those who cared for the dying were given minimal support in the practice of medicine. It transformed to become a society in which palliative care has become almost fashionable; it is widely accepted that dying is a matter for open discussion in society and palliative care is a type of service that patients and families demand. Medical institutions throughout the USA are setting up and developing palliative care services, having accepted that every major multispecialty medical institution needs one.

MAXIMIZING DISSEMINATION

Train-the-trainer strategy

The choice of a national and potentially international scope for this project necessitated a highly effective dissemination strategy, especially given the expectation of modest funding. A dissemination format that had enjoyed success in nonmedical settings was the train-the-trainer approach. Effectiveness in bringing about broad social change through the impact of one thought leader through a few opinion leaders to a large number of people who then institutionalize the new norms is a model that has been effective since biblical times and before. It is also well suited to the medical culture, in that there is a strong cultural commitment to the 'see one, do one, teach one' approach in which skills are passed from one colleague to another.

At the same time, this approach was not a common one in medicine at the time that the EPEC Project began. It was an approach more often associated with low-skilled, nontechnical matters. After the initial risk of introducing an unfamiliar format associated if anything with low prestige, the advantage of novelty took over, and this approach seems to have enjoyed enough success that a 'tipping point' was reached so that many train-the-trainer programs in other areas are now also being implemented. It soon became desirable within the medical culture to be a certified EPEC Trainer. Although some other train-the-trainer programs have also enjoyed success, others have not. It may be that the train-the-trainer format just one feature in effective dissemination.

Leadership and professional grassroots buy-in

Attention to the social context and what would drive relatively rapid and sustainable social change was necessary. The platform from which the project was launched was, importantly, the most powerful national medical association, the American Medical Association. It was launched with buy-in and input from leaders in the political and clinical spheres of medicine.

The project chose to simultaneously involve clinicians at the grassroots level. An important mechanism for achieving buy-in at all of these diverse levels was to invite input into the project itself. The curriculum was drafted by a wide range of experts, and suggestions made by participants were taken very seriously in the production of the first edition of the curriculum. Suggestions are still taken at every conference and considered in every new edition of the curriculum.

The commitment of the hospice and palliative care fields to the interdisciplinary team drove a strong focus on how to be maximally inclusive without losing momentum. The difficult choice was made, as noted above, to target the project to physician education; one rationale was that nonphysicians would come to physician education programs but not the reverse. This approach acknowledged and even leveraged a social hierarchy within medicine that many members of the interdisciplinary team did not like. The thought was that it was already enough of a challenge to bring about a new popularity for palliative care without taking on additional challenges to social norms in medicine. As the implementation of the project was tracked, it emerged that most EPEC trainers did indeed teach a full range of clinicians, so the targeting strategy seemed to have been effective.[5]

Individual buy-in

Additional features of the social and cultural context of individual motivation were also considered so that physicians' identification with the program could be achieved. Curricular materials were made to be visually and technologically appealing; that is, the look-and-feel was designed to be meaningful and attractive, and the slides and trigger tapes state of the art. Both conferences and materials were initially provided for free as part of an outreach strategy, with a gradual progression to a cost-recovery nonprofit status kicking in only later. Perhaps most important in this regard, permission was given to the EPEC Trainer to modify the materials to suit his or her teaching style and his or her audience's needs. This allowed individual investment in and career advancement through this curriculum. Every Trainer was able to look and be polished and effective in their presentations when these materials were being used.

Widely applicable curriculum

In order to allow use of the curriculum by Trainers in a wide range of different settings, the curriculum was designed in a modular format. Thus, a 16-module curriculum could be presented in full at a several day conference, over a longer time in periodic presentations or in part at individual seminars or presentations. It was also designed to cover core material that all practitioners need command of. Perhaps also because it was effectively a national core curriculum, EPEC became a de facto normative standard for practice in palliative care.

Venues of discourse

Ultimately, the institutionalization process that moved the EPEC Project from a one-time grant-funded project to a kind of institution was inspired by and molded by its participants. Initially, feedback made clear that the project was satisfying an appetite for collegial connection; so requests for list servs and continuing advice as Trainers conducted their own teaching were readily granted. Soon, Trainers began to want to become members of the smaller group of Master Facilitators who were teaching the Trainers. To allow for that, we instituted a Professional Development Workshop in which principles of education were transmitted and participants learned and practiced teaching skills using the most effective teaching methods known to education that were also suitable for the medical context.

Virtual college

The result of these developments was a transition to something much more than a train-the-trainer program. The project became virtually a college, complete with layers of training opportunities, certification, ways to advance up through the layers, educational materials, and venues for participant socialization.

Tracking dissemination

The dissemination of EPEC teaching was estimated by an external group for a 1-year period between 1999 and 2000. They found that the *EPEC Curriculum* was well regarded and was perceived by most trainers to have provided great improvement in their knowledge and ability to teach end-of-life care. More than 90 percent of trainers were actively using the *Curriculum* to teach; the 184 trainers in the study were estimated to have taught ~ 120 000 professionals.[5] By extrapolation, it appears that by 2006 the EPEC Project has probably reached about 1 million professionals.

The partnership phase

The next step in the transition had partly to do with dissemination; it was necessary to move beyond the population of clinicians who were well disposed to the idea of palliative care into the population that was skeptical. It also had partly to do with the motivation to help move palliative care 'upstream' from the end of life to include the entire spectrum of illness, bringing the goal of optimizing quality of life to all patients. Both goals were addressed by the transition of the EPEC Project into a partnership phase. By collaborating with specialty societies and institutions, the project has become well positioned to make curricular adaptations with buy-in from the relevant group in medicine. Adaptations for specific communities, such as Roman Catholics or the African American communities, and for specialties such as oncology and emergency medicine are examples that already exist.[6] Dissemination in collaboration with the appropriate community is then possible. The same model has been used for adaptations of EPEC in other countries.

A sustainable, professional institution

To maintain programmatic integrity and reliable standards in the education associated with the project, the EPEC Project retains the exclusive prerogative of creating EPEC Trainers and owns the intellectual property on its materials. To continue the dissemination and accommodate adaptation to suit diverse audiences, automatic permission is granted to adapt the materials for educational, noncommercial purposes and a standard acknowledgment statement that users can apply to adapted material is provided. To allow for some cost recovery, teaching services are provided for a standard registration fee; costs for adaptation to new programs are covered by grants. The program is maintained within an academic medical institution on the same not-for-profit basis as other academic projects.

MAXIMIZING IMPACT

Change through education

Education theorists, lead by Davis, Dixon, and others, describe different layers of learning resulting in changes to norms of practice. First, attitudes are essential if suitable attention is to be given to the subject matter. Second, knowledge must be acquired. Third, skills that use the knowledge must be acquired. Fourth, behaviors that use the skills must be engaged. Fifth, the behaviors must have the intended outcome. Finally, changes must be brought about in society as a whole so that adjusted norms integrate and sustain the new behaviors and outcomes.[7]

Attitudes and knowledge change

To maximize the change in attitudes and knowledge, EPEC Trainers must use the most effective educational methods and materials possible. Experts in adult education and physician education in particular emphasize the need for several features. Adult education theory notes that the human mind can only take in a modest number of facts at a time if the facts are to be retained and used. After a period of about 45 minutes, the human mind needs to take a break. Visual aids are most effective if the information presented is simple and to the point, with minimal distracting material. At the same time, if the information can be presented through multiple channels – say visual and auditory – that is helpful. For clinicians time is precious so learning must make good use of their time. Like other adult learners clinicians are motivated to learn if they perceive a need. The use of data that identify need and the use of cases that illustrate a recognizable situation with human meaning in which clinical knowledge is needed can be very effective in generating the empathic feeling that in turn provides a teachable moment into which the curriculum can place its 'just-in-time' learning. These and other points guided the design of the curricular materials for EPEC. The resulting materials used accessible language, presented information in simple units, and used slides with clear points using a minimum of words. The modules were all accompanied by a trigger tape describing a case or something similar that would provide the human meaning and recognizable, emotionally and intellectually engaging context for learning.

To provide for the layers of teaching and learning roles in the train-the-trainer approach, materials were provided in the form of a participant's manual and a trainer's guide.

As the curricular content grew, portions were designated as core or optional. For specialty societies where the cultural norm was for more complex information, that was provided and information was identified by its level of evidence.[8]

Behaviors, skills, and practice norms

Among the effective teaching methods, one used above others in the EPEC Project was small-group role-play. The reason for this is that attitude and knowledge gains do not 'stick' without the experience of their implementation.

However, to cross the knowledge–practice chasm will take more than wide dissemination of well integrated attitude change, absorbed knowledge and preliminarily practiced new skills. Davis has recently illustrated again in a commentary on a particularly successful, integrated program of education and practice change, how complex it is to translate knowledge into practice.[9] Knowledge does not translate into practice change without suitable context and motivation. The next adaptations and editions of the EPEC curriculum are being designed so that learning objectives in each module are linked to identified clinical practices, and these clinical practices are in turn linked to measurable outcomes whenever possible. In this fashion, the new curricular materials will be positioned for implementation in systems that can promote and assess the translation of new knowledge into practice improvement. We anticipate that by linking learning to behavioral accountability in this fashion it may finally be possible to cross the boundaries between education and practice change.

MAXIMIZING EFFICIENCY

Long-term, sustainable change requires programs that are not only effective but also efficient and sustainable.

Investing in change agents and opinion leaders

One approach of the EPEC Project, along with that of others such as the Ian Anderson Project in Canada,[10] has been to first use small-group learning for those who will become change agents or opinion leaders.

In the case of the EPEC Project, immersion teaching to create trainers makes use of groups that are optimally sized at about 16 participants and are capped at 25. Although the cost of these immersion courses is large on a per-participant basis, when the Trainers have reached their end-users the cost can be calculated in terms of per-end-user, and the unit cost drops dramatically to about $10 per end-user, depending on the age of the program and other factors. Similarly, the 'capital outlay' involved in producing a curriculum that is of high enough quality that it will have enduring impact and wide appeal across disciplines and other social groupings is initially high. But the more the curriculum is used the more the per-user unit cost drops.

Distance learning

Another approach to maximizing efficiency in education is to allow for learning from a distance. Among the first palliative care education programs to be offered at a distance was one pioneered by Hospice Africa Uganda.[11] By combining in-person, immersion training with follow-up course work by mail (and later, when it became available, electronic communication), the educational center of Hospice Africa Uganda in Kampala was able to train palliative care leaders from many different African countries. The Pallium Project makes use of a similar paradigm, bringing educational opportunities to widely dispersed locations in Canada.[12]

The effectiveness of distance learning is not well studied. The EPEC Project will be comparing different modalities of distance learning in order to ascertain which types of program are most effective and which are most efficient for different settings. Highly sophisticated versions of learning will also soon be available. Simulations of clinical images are already in use for surgical and other types of education. Additional developments are anticipated.

CONCLUSION

Medicine had become a victim of its own success by the time the hospice and palliative care movement decided to construct a different road to care in which comfort and quality of existence are emphasized. The challenges to the educational arm of this movement were many and the power of traditional medical education was not sufficient for the task. By borrowing heavily from social change theory and adhering closely to proven but little used adult education practices, and by working as one among multiple coordinated projects, the EPEC Project was able to contribute its part to graduate medical education, until eventually the integration of palliative care practices into medical norms was happening throughout medicine. Key features of its design included its train-the-trainer structure with investment of intense education in a relatively small group of trainers; its modular, adaptable curriculum and emphasis on role play as a teaching method; and its establishment of a self-perpetuating college like structure. However, the most important determinant of what impact it has had is probably the synthesis of many effective approaches and collaborations, all occurring in the setting of collaborative projects that could reset the cultural expectations of medicine and society at large.

Key learning points

- Didactic information transfer is a small component of education that, on its own, effects minimal practice change.

- The attitudinal and social context are strong determinants of practice, and educational interventions should include efforts to adjust both to the educational goals.

- Empathic consideration of the relevant situations stimulates attitudinal change and information intake. Use of trigger tapes can facilitate suitable emotional involvement.

- Dissemination programs are most effective if they invest heavily in small groups of opinion leaders and change agents.

- Education programs that seek enduring changes in practice norms must be sustained for many years.

ACKNOWLEDGMENTS

The learning that contributed to the educational and social change approaches identified in this chapter came from many people. Major contributors to the overall perspective include, but are not limited to the following. Charles von Gunten, Frank Ferris, Jeanne Martinez, Joyce Newman, Yvonne Steinert, Sharyn Sutton, Joshua Hauser, Michael Preodor, and Larry Librach all contributed in major ways to the core EPEC Project. Miles Sheehan, Richard Payne, Jamie von Roenn, Tammie Quest, Joan Teno, and David Casarett all helped to pioneer adaptations of EPEC to specific groups in society or specialty groups in medicine. Kathryn Meshenberg brought management skills and essential patient perspective and Mike Meshenberg contributed the caregiver perspectives. Arthur Derse contributed legal expertise and experience in distance learning. RM Rajagopal, Vivek Khemka, Anne Merriman, Lydia Mpanga, and Ekie Kikule all helped to pioneer palliative care collaborative or EPEC-adapted education in India, Africa or both, building on excellent existing programs. David Weissman, Diane Meier, Betty Ferrel, and others contributed to the coordinated approach of the sibling programs that were funded by the Robert Wood Johnson Foundation. Rosemary Gibson and Vicky Weisfeld masterminded much of the coordinated approach at the Robert Wood Johnson Foundation. Kathy Foley, with the help of Mary Callaway, ran the Project on Death in America. All the master facilitators, many trainers and many end-users of the EPEC Project also contributed their suggestions. Michelle Grana, Elisa Roman, Emily Hagenmaier, Kami Chin, Sean Buchanon, and Mark Yoon currently keep the program in excellent shape. Daniel Duffy appreciated the need for palliative care to be recognized by the ABMS and help it to achieve specialty status. Not one single successful outcome of the effort to change the norms of education in palliative care could have been achieved without the extraordinary, collaborative approach of these and many other equally fine people.

REFERENCES

● 1 Wynia M, Latham S, Kao A, *et al.* Physician professionalism in society. *N Engl J Med* 1999; **341**: 1612–15.

● 2 Field MJ, Cassel CK, eds. *Approaching Death: Improving Care at the End of Life.* Washington, DC: Institute of Medicine, National Academy Press, 1997.

◆ 3 Davis DA, Thomson MA, Oxman AD, Haynes RB. Evidence for the effectiveness of CME. A review of 50 randomized controlled trials. *JAMA* 1992; **268**: 1111–17.

● 4 Tu K, Davis D. Can we alter physician behavior by educational methods? Lessons learned from studies of the management and follow-up of hypertension. *J Contin Educ Health Prof* 2002; **22**: 11–22.

● 5 Robinson K, Sutton S, von Gunten CF, *et al.* Assessment of the education for physicians on end-of-life Care (EPEC) curriculum. *J Palliat Med* 2004; **7**: 637–45.

✱ 6 The EPEC Project. www.epec.net (accessed June 23, 2006).

◆ 7 Davis D, Taylor-Vaisey AL. Two decades of Dixon: The question(s) of evaluating continuing education for the health professions. *J Contin Educ Health Prof* 1997; **17**: 207–13.

8 EPEC-O can be found at www.epec.net (accessed June 23, 2006).

● 9 Davis D. Clinical practice guidelines and the translation of knowledge: the science of continuing medical education. *Can Med Assoc J* 2000; **163**: 1278–9.

✱ 10 Ian Anderson Continuing Education Program in End-of Life Care, University of Toronto. www.cme.utoronto.ca/endoflife/.

11 Hospice Africa – Uganda. www.hospiceafrica.or.ug/(accessed June 23, 2006).

12 Kent H. Palliative Care: project to improve end-of-life support in Western Canada. *Can Med Assoc J* 2004; **170**: 1086.

19

Public education

SHARON BAXTER, ROMAYNE GALLAGHER

INTRODUCTION

Public education regarding hospice palliative care or end-of-life care has been growing steadily since the movement began 40 years ago. However, there is limited research on the process and outcomes of hospice palliative care education compared with other areas of health education and health promotion. The authors will refer to their experience in Canada as there is little published in this field of palliative medicine.

In Canada, the movement has developed under two names – hospice and palliative care. In a national consensus-building initiative it was decided to adopt the name 'hospice palliative care' to demonstrate that the principles were the same and to reduce confusion among the public and healthcare providers outside the movement.

There are several reasons to pursue public education regarding hospice palliative care:

- Advocacy
- Education of decision makers
- Awareness of hospice palliative care in the general population
- Education of patients and informal caregivers.

The hospice palliative care movement developed over time both within the healthcare system and at the community level, arising from the perceived 'medicalization' of dying. While the community as a whole has embraced the philosophy and practice of hospice palliative care, the healthcare system has not yet fully recognized hospice palliative care as an integral part of the care, including care delivered at the end of life. In addition, knowledge and skills development related to end-of-life care is ongoing in Canada and only recently has palliative medicine become a certified specialty. In 2002 Canada became the first nation to establish standards or norms of practice for hospice palliative care.[1] Advocates have continued to raise public awareness of hospice palliative care services, prompting healthcare systems and providers to educate themselves and effect change in the provision of these services. Ongoing advocacy and the education of decision makers have been essential in the movement of some provincial governments toward legislating hospice palliative care as a core healthcare service within their province.

Increased awareness of hospice palliative care within the general population has several benefits including assisting with advocacy strategies and encouraging preparation for future needs. It is fair to say that there is a public perception that dying is a painful and feared process and therefore little is expected of the healthcare system or providers when someone dies. This is demonstrated when examining pain management where research has shown that most people are satisfied with their pain management despite significantly unrelieved pain.[2] However, it is hoped that having an educated public will enable patients and caregivers to be effective advocates for themselves or their loved ones that they are caring for.

With healthcare systems becoming increasingly complex and having multiple options for care, there is a need for patients to be aware of how to access care and how to navigate the healthcare system. Options for care also entail knowing the rights of patients and families, especially concerning issues of refusal and withdrawal of therapy. Many patients already in the system are not aware of their options or rights as shown by a study of 728 outpatients in an Oregon internal medicine clinic.[3] Only 69 percent were aware of their right to refuse treatment and only 46 percent were aware of their right to the withdrawal of treatment. Interestingly, having an advanced directive in place did not predict for greater knowledge about rights with regard to treatment. A report on the informational needs of

Canadian caregivers[4] cited a number of learning and coping styles of patients and families as necessitating information being provided by oral communication supplemented by a variety of written or electronic media. Similar findings were discovered in a study of primary caregivers of Greek patients with cancer,[5] with those exhibiting high information needs being positively associated with a preference for cancer-specific printed material and negatively associated with satisfaction with the doctor's communication of information and affective behavior.

Lastly, there is a need to educate patients and caregivers who are in the midst of coping with a life-threatening illness. With the rise of chronic illness as a major cause of death, the role of the patient in their illness has dramatically changed. Since chronic diseases are ongoing, it is the patient who must undertake much of the therapy, make behavior changes and learn to cope with the changes that the illness brings. In addition, they must communicate with the healthcare providers and know how and when to access the system for treatment. In the latter stages of illness, informal caregivers take over much of this role. Much of the care in the last year of life occurs at home, according to research from the UK,[6] putting most of the responsibility on the patient and their caregivers. Thus there is a much greater need for education about signs and symptoms, symptom management, coping with illness, and acquiring help when it is needed.

Studies of caregivers have repeatedly noted unmet informational needs.[7] Most of the need for information is related to symptom management, how to care for someone who is dying, and what to expect in the dying process. The best people to provide this information are the healthcare providers which implies that the role of healthcare providers needs to change from that of a 'provider' to the additional roles of educator and collaborator.[8]

Theories of health behavior change

Mainstream health education has evolved dramatically over the last century. There has been a marked decline in infectious diseases in industrialized countries over the last 100 years. While medical knowledge and therapies have advanced tremendously, it is clear from population studies that the declines began before medical interventions such as antibiotics and vaccines were available.[9] It was the improvement in living conditions such as the wide availability of clean water, uncontaminated food, and separation of sewage in these nations that began the reduction in mortality. Heart disease became the major killer of people in these nations and remains so to this day. However, health educators began to see that much of the mortality and morbidity of heart disease and cancer was due to lifestyle factors such as smoking, sedentary lifestyle, and poor diet. Public health evolved into health promotion which combines education with political, regulatory, and system changes that act together to bring about a change in health behavior and disease.

At first glance it may seem a paradox that health promotion should apply to hospice palliative care, but the World Health Organization (WHO) in its Ottawa charter of 1986[10] defined health promotion as 'the process of enabling people to increase control over, and improve their health'. The same document goes on to speak of health in these terms:

> To reach a state of complete physical, mental and social well-being, an individual or group must be able to identify and to realize aspirations, to satisfy needs, and to change or cope with the environment. Health is, therefore, seen as a resource for everyday life, not the objective of living. Health is a positive concept emphasizing social and personal resources, as well as physical capacities. Therefore, health promotion is not just the responsibility of the health sector, but goes beyond healthy life-styles to well-being.

The charter saw three main prerequisites for health promotion: advocacy, enabling equity, and coordinated action between the health sector, government, voluntary sector, industry, and the media. These elements are all essential for equitable access to quality end-of-life care and thus the principles of health promotion are applicable to hospice palliative care.

Health promotion, as well as changing policy and services, also seeks to change individual attitudes and behaviors. Several models of psychological behavior have been developed to explain how behavior can be changed in an individual and a population. The theory of planned behavior was developed by Ajzen and has applied quite well to a number of behaviors in the field. The theory notes that there are three major influences on a person's intention to change their behavior: attitude toward the specific action, subjective norms of behavior around the issue, and perceived behavioral control. For example, applying the model to quitting smoking a person may develop an attitude that it is worthwhile to quit smoking as they will be healthier, fitter, and lower their chance of dying from a smoking-related illness. The subjective norms of behavior around smoking vary with culture and location and have changed dramatically over the past 50 years, becoming unacceptable in some countries and more acceptable in others. As an example of perceived control, a person may feel that they cannot control this behavior as they have too much stress or too much going on at work to quit smoking at this time. These factors act together to influence intention to change behavior and therefore on the behavior itself.

Adapting this model to hospice palliative care education makes it evident where the major challenges and opportunities are in health education regarding hospice palliative care.

Attitude toward specific behavior

An attitude toward a specific behavior depends upon the information given to the public. The individual weighs their vulnerability to the issue as well as the severity of its effect upon them in developing an attitude toward the issue. Most people perceive serious illness and/or dying as a painful and fearful process. Providing information to counteract this feeling based on what hospice palliative care can do for symptom relief and improving quality of life would be an effective way to present the case for people knowing about hospice palliative care. However, a person's vulnerability to this information likely depends upon their health status. If they have a chronic illness or are caring for someone who does, they are likely to feel quite vulnerable to the fear of a painful death and welcome information on ways in which they can prevent this.

Unfortunately, it cannot be assumed that all healthcare providers and health systems will automatically provide quality end-of-life care for the patient. Therefore, informing the public of what can be done using hospice palliative care services will result in improved overall care once those services are accessed.

Information needs to be provided in a way that the individual receiving it feels that it applies to him or her. However, giving people information that only generates fear (e.g. a painful death) does not change behavior unless the individual has a perception that they can do something about the issue.[11] A meta-analysis of fear appeals[12] indicates that fear appeals motivate positive behavioral change but also maladaptive fear control actions such as defensive avoidance or reactance. It appears that fear appeals must be accompanied by successful intervention messages. Therefore any information about unrelieved pain or symptoms must be accompanied by information about how to access hospice palliative care.

Subjective norms about the behavior

The norms regarding the open discussion of behaviors are dependent on culture. During the sixteenth and seventeenth centuries in Europe it was not uncommon to speak of death and dying openly, in fact there were prescribed practices for dying – the *artes moriendii*.[13] At the end of the nineteenth century, the customs of death changed with the rise of science and the decline of religion. Death became a hidden part of life and thus less acceptable to talk about. Even with the rise of the hospice palliative care movement and the pioneering work of Elisabeth Kübler-Ross in the 1970s there is still a societal reluctance to mention the words dying or death.

However, even in cultures where speaking openly of death or dying may be seen as disrespectful, there are times when speaking of death may be appropriate. For example, a local information fair about hospice palliative care presented in Chinatown in Vancouver, BC is well attended because there is attention to cultural details. The forum is held in the season of Ching Ming, when celebrating and remembering ancestors is commonly done. As well, the forum does not use the word 'death' or 'dying' in its title as this would not be considered appropriate.

Some cultures specifically celebrate death, as Mexico's Dia de los Muertos.[14] It is a festival held on 1/2 November and is a cultural blend of an Aztec festival dedicated to the dead with the Christian tradition of All Saints and All Souls days. During the festival the dead are welcomed back to the family home and commemorated. The festival is a social, festive occasion that is an important way of acknowledging the cycle of life and death as a natural part of human existence.

Perceived behavioral control

It makes intuitive sense that perceiving a capability to change behavior is extremely important in effecting an actual change in health-related behavior. Factors that influence this can be external to the person – factors they have no control over – or internal factors such as self-efficacy or belief in ability to control their circumstances. Factors such as lower education, depression, stress, and personal and situational factors can adversely influence an individual's perceived control.[15]

Death anxiety – the fear of the dying process or being dead – has been studied in a number of groups of people. Interestingly, death anxiety is not a function of illness alone, as older patients have less death anxiety and terminally ill patients' death anxiety varies according to interpersonal factors such as social support and personal resources such as coping styles and spiritual beliefs.[16] As well, higher death anxiety among physicians has been associated with more negative attitudes regarding dying patients.[17]

Public education regarding death and dying needs to be mindful of death anxiety. One way to avoid increasing death anxiety is to raise awareness of the ability of hospice palliative care to help meet the psychosocial and spiritual needs of the individual and their family. As well, highlighting the ability of people to transcend suffering – called 'post-traumatic growth' by researchers[18] – helps to reduce death anxiety and improve quality of life.

ISSUES CONCERNING PUBLIC EDUCATION

Canada is a country of 32 million people with approximately 235 000 deaths per year. In 2000 the Senate of Canada released a report that indicated that an estimated 5 percent of dying Canadians received hospice palliative care.[19] In 2004 it is estimated that this number has grown to less than 15 percent. A number of factors affect the slow growth of access to these services. Currently, Canada has less than 200 practicing palliative care physician specialists out of a total of almost 60 000 physicians. In Canada's 17 medical schools palliative care training is variable, ranging from a mandatory clinical rotation to classroom hours with elective rotations. As well, none of the 91 schools of nursing include hospice palliative care as a core curriculum component. It is apparent that Canada is not training enough hospice palliative care professionals to provide for an increase in programs and services.

This creates a dilemma concerning issues related to public education regarding hospice palliative care. Should the public be empowered to demand hospice palliative care programs and services that the healthcare system is not capable of providing in the near future? In Canada, the hospice palliative care community continues to advocate for increased programs and services at the same time as working with partner organizations to develop the necessary research and education that will be required in the future. Two examples of this include the recent designation of hospice palliative care nursing as a specialty within the Canadian Nurses Association (CNA) and the Educating Future Physicians in Palliative and End-of-Life Care Project (EFPPEC).

Under the leadership of the CNA standards and core competencies for nurses working in hospice palliative care were developed and the first set of certification exams were held in the spring of 2004. The EFPPEC Project is a 4-year project that began in February 2004. To date all 17 medical schools in Canada have agreed to participate in the project to create interdisciplinary hospice palliative care education curriculum over the next 4 years. This project is working to increase the skill level of graduating physicians in end-of-life care through the use of core competencies. Its goal is to have substantially more family physicians graduating with skills in hospice palliative care.

Making the case for public education

There is a strong case for the need for public education regarding programs and services available at the end of life. Canadians responded positively to the Commission on the Future of Health Care in Canada, indicating that the healthcare system's ability to provide good quality of life at the end of life is a priority.[20] Canadians in favor of hospice palliative care have also overwhelmingly reported (91 percent) that they feel it is important for patients in their last days to be comfortable and in familiar surroundings.[21]

In a 2004 Ipsos-Reid Survey[22] Canadians polled were asked to identify where hospice palliative care services were provided. Not surprisingly 80 percent identified long-term care facilities and/or nursing homes and 76 percent identified hospitals. However, 74 percent of respondents identified the patient's home as a setting of care. If three-quarters of Canadians think that end-of-life care is provided in the home then what is the healthcare system's requirement to address this?

The lack of sufficient research regarding hospice palliative care programs and services and related issues needs to be addressed if education of the public is to be effective. Three key issues which need to be addressed include:

- What does the current healthcare system currently provide with regard to end-of-life care?

- What programs and services does the general public want for themselves and their loved ones at the end of life?
- The economics of hospice palliative care services, i.e. are available hospice palliative care services less expensive than utilizing the current acute care system?

Educating decision makers

Governments are complex organizations where influencing decision making is often challenging. Governments are composed of both political and bureaucratic structures which both have a role in the policy development process. Often new programs and services are created by elected officials due to political pressures, however bureaucrats need to be involved in the development of these programs and services as they are critical to their successful implementation. A strong relationship with both levels of government is critically important.

How healthcare systems are funded varies from country to country. In Canada most of the funds required to pay for the Canadian healthcare system are provided by the federal government with the implementation and ongoing monitoring of health programs being overseen by the provincial or territorial governments. This relationship is complex and at times has been confrontational; however, in order to effect sustainable change an understanding of each player's strengths and weaknesses is necessary. A successful public education plan is based on finding the 'win-win' situation between the various levels of government including the community.

The first step in educating the decision makers is to have the appropriate research and data available; to have an understanding of the healthcare system; and to know what the public expects from the healthcare system. A draft plan outlining the services and programs that need to be developed or augmented is also helpful. Presentations regarding new programs or services can only be presented a limited number of times – it is imperative that organizations are prepared for their presentations by presenting well-thought-out options. Many times, it is the personal experiences of the decision makers that can also drive policy change, so personal experience coupled with an offering of workable options can be very successful in achieving change.

A well-planned multipronged approach is necessary to achieve change in service provision. Support from grassroots stakeholders is imperative because if stakeholders do not support the plan, it will not be supported. As an example, the HIV/AIDS movement in Canada has used the grassroots approach to community development and mobilization extremely well. The voice of People Living with HIV and AIDS has been front and center in all their public education responses.

In Canada, governments are recognized as wanting to act in the best interests of their citizens however they are not always sure what the best interest are. All levels of government depend on advice and input from experts to inform them of the issues and provide possible solutions.

Increasing public awareness of hospice palliative care

Increasing awareness of hospice palliative care services and programs to the general public is imperative. Canadian residents need to know that hospice palliative care is a group of services provided by an interdisciplinary team in a variety of settings (acute care hospital, long-term care facility, hospice or home) that provides care for persons approaching death so that the burdens of suffering, loneliness and grief are lessened. Reaching the public will be discussed under the Process section.

Educating patients and informal caregivers

As mentioned previously in this chapter there is much to be gained by providing education and information to both patients and informal caregivers.

THE PROCESS OF PUBLIC EDUCATION

Building momentum for hospice palliative care

With an aging population it has become apparent that there needs to be an increase in programming in end-of-life care. Data from a recent Statistics Canada report indicate that that the estimated number of deaths in Canada will increase by 40 percent by the year 2020.[23]

Leadership is imperative for sustainable gains. It is also critical that the group or groups leading this plan have the support of stakeholder groups. Division within the hospice palliative care community can undermine any possible gains so it is important to spend time building the partnerships and relationships within the community. It is also critical to have agreement on the key messages being used. A communication strategy needs to be developed for public education no matter which constituents are targeted. Tactics regarding how a communication strategy is implemented will vary depending on the target audience. Public education campaigns targeting the general public may include the following tactics:

- Public awareness campaigns
- Media – placement of personal stories and opinion and editorial articles
- Targeted brochures and pamphlets
- Internet and a campaign to encourage visits to pertinent web sites.

Public education campaigns targeting decision makers may include:

- Briefs and reports
- Presentations to government committees

- Meetings with key decision makers
- Letter writing campaigns
- Petitions.

Models of excellence

There are models of excellence outside the hospice palliative field that should be reviewed when developing a public education campaign. A particularly successful public education campaign in Canada was the *ParticipACTION* campaign. *ParticipACTION* was a campaign aimed at increasing the physical activity levels of school children and young adults. There were many lessons learned from campaigns such as this including the need to keep the campaign fresh, renewed, and sustained. It is also important to look at hospice palliative care campaigns taking place in other countries.

Networks and coalitions have proved useful in Canada, communicating messages to both the general public and to government. The Quality End-of-Life Care Coalition of Canada (QELCCC) established in December 2000 currently has 31 member organizations. QELCCC members represent national health professional organizations, disease-specific organizations, disability awareness organizations, seniors' organizations, and home care organizations and foundations. The QELCCC's main goal is to promote increased access to end-of-life care services for all Canadians. In September 2004 the Coalition published *Dying for Care*,[24] a status report on the state of end-of-life care in Canada that outlines areas of improvement. The Coalition believes it is the right of every Canadian to die with dignity, free of pain, surrounded by loved ones, in a setting of their choice.

The hospice palliative care community has much to learn from the human immunodeficiency virus (HIV)/acquired immune deficiency syndrome (AIDS) community. The HIV/AIDS community has over the last 20 years taken an unpopular health issue and has forced the public and government to act. It can be argued that funding levels for domestic HIV/ AIDS programs continues to be underresourced but on balance they have managed to raise the profile of the disease. Public education regarding hospice palliative care must keep in mind that today's society is death denying and therefore discussions regarding end-of-life issues are often suppressed.

In British Columbia a unique forum has been developed entitled: 'Making Death a Part of Life: a public forum on death and dying'.[25] This forum uses the trade show format with presentations and exhibitor booths featuring local hospice palliative care organizations and related businesses. Presentations deal with practical issues regarding caregiving, pain management, the biological processes of dying, and spiritual issues. The forum is held in a central venue and promoted through local media, hospice palliative care organizations and word of mouth. Funding for the event is generated from sponsorships with government, health authorities, and businesses. This format has been repeated in other areas of Canada (Winnipeg) as well as the USA and Germany.

OUTCOMES

Outcomes in public education are notoriously hard to measure. One reason for this is that outcomes must be focused on behavioral change evaluated in well-designed randomized controlled trials with standardized outcomes designed for use in the population being studied. So the diligence and experience required to achieve accurate measurement with outcomes that will be sensitive or specific enough to detect a difference is considerable. For example, a Cochrane review of self-management education for chronic obstructive pulmonary disease[26] showed inconclusive results with respect to health-related quality of life, but if a disease-specific instrument was used a better quality of life was seen in the intervention group. The follow-up must be sufficiently long for useful conclusions to be drawn from the studies.

Another major handicap to hospice palliative care outcomes research is that many patients will be too ill to complete questionnaires that are used to self-report. This suggests that those who are experiencing the most problems may be too ill to be included in data collection.[27] Proxy completion is known to have pitfalls as well.

However, there are some outcome studies that can serve as examples in the general healthcare field. Self-management is a common theme in the arthritis diseases. A Cochrane review of patient education interventions on health status in rheumatoid arthritis[28] showed that public education had short-term effects on disability, joint counts, patient global assessment, psychological status, and depression, but these faded after the first follow-up visit and no significant effects of patient education were found by the final visits.

Education interventions on the general population that only has a risk for a disease pose further challenges. A Cochrane review of counseling or education to modify risk factors for cardiovascular disease[29] showed no effect on the mortality rate of the disease. However, among high-risk patients such as those with hypertension, mortality did reduce with medication, counseling, and education. This seems to support the theory that the population must believe they are at serious risk to modify their behavior.

A search of the literature for studies on hospice palliative and end-of-life public education interventions revealed two studies on public attitudes on hospice palliative care and death and dying,[30,31] but educational outcomes seemed to be studied only on healthcare providers. This is likely due to the lack of attempts to undertake a public education intervention to promote thinking and planning for care at the end of life.

There is evidence that public attitudes to death and dying are changing in some countries. A campaign called *Living Lessons*[32] was initiated by a commercial industry foundation – The GlaxoSmithKline Foundation in Canada – in partnership with the Canadian Hospice Palliative Care Association. The campaign included a professionally conducted telephone survey of Canadians' awareness of hos-pice palliative care and what hospice palliative care entails. Additionally, the campaign developed resources to educate policy makers, healthcare providers, volunteers, and caregivers about hospice palliative care and the difference it can make in the living and dying process. This was done through various print media, press kits, and a website (www.living-lessons.org).

In 1997, in the first poll regarding the attitude of Canadians toward hospice palliative care, only 30 percent of Canadians had heard of palliative care.[21] The 2004 survey repeated similar questions and when asked, 60 percent of Canadians had heard of the term palliative care.[22] Fifty-one percent of those people who had heard of it were able to mention what the key attributes of hospice palliative care are.[22] These results indicate a dramatic change in awareness of hospice palliative care. There are numerous reasons that could be postulated for this, including the *Living Lessons* campaign, reports on end-of-life care by the Senate of Canada, as well as high profile legal cases that featured patients requesting the right to physician-assisted suicide. Twenty-five percent of Canadians in the 2004 survey reported that they or someone in their family had used hospice palliative care services.[22]

Canadians were also asked to identify services that they associated with hospice palliative care and the most common services were pain management and psychological support such as dealing with depression and anxiety. Sixty-four percent of Canadians identified hospice palliative care as being available to all people who are dying irrespective of illness.[22] The challenge for healthcare educators was that 90 percent of Canadians would go to their family physician for access to hospice palliative care information.[22] The startling piece of information was that whereas 83 percent felt it was important to discuss end-of-life care with their family, only 49 percent felt it was important to discuss it with their doctor and only 9 percent had actually done that.[22]

Although greater awareness is an excellent start in public education, ultimately the goal is to have increased awareness result in increased access, provision, and quality of end-of-life care. One way to ensure improved provision of care is to link hospice palliative care standards to healthcare facility accreditation. This process has begun in Canada with the Canadian Hospice Palliative Care Association (CHPCA) model[1] being used as a template for healthcare facility accreditation. Accreditation in Canada is a voluntary undertaking but it is customary for every healthcare facility to undergo accreditation approximately every 3–5 years. As well as establishing standards for healthcare facilities such as acute care facilities and residential facilities, standards are being developed which will apply to free-standing hospice facilities and it is expected that these facilities will begin the accreditation process in the next 3–5 years.

The ultimate measurement tool to determine if patients were receiving the care that they expect would be to use a hospice palliative outcome scale of which several have been developed and validated.[33-35] While these scales are subject to biases such as seen in people's satisfaction with pain management although there is still significant pain, they are likely the best indicators available at this time. It would be important to apply these scales to dying patients both in and out of hospice palliative care facilities in order to determine if all patients were receiving the symptom control and psycho-spiritual support they needed through consultative services. Other important outcomes would involve system capacity to handle all the people requiring and requesting hospice palliative care.

The hospice palliative care movement has much to learn from other public awareness and policy-changing campaigns that have pioneered policy change. The need for hospice palliative care must be treated as a public health issue where the public, patients, caregivers and decision-makers are educated about suffering at the end of life and how effective quality hospice palliative care can be in relieving suffering and enhancing the quality of life for the last stages of life. Strategic public education can be a very effective force to move the public, healthcare providers, and policy makers into providing quality care at the end of life.

Key learning points

- Public education is important in hospice palliative care around advocacy, education of decision makers, awareness of hospice palliative care in the general population, and education of patients and informal caregivers.

- As healthcare systems become more complex with multiple options for care there is a need for patients to be aware of how to access care and how to navigate the healthcare system.

- The WHO's Ottawa charter of 1986 defined health promotion as 'the process of enabling people to increase control over, and improve their health'.

- Educating healthcare decision makers is essential and is achieved by understanding the healthcare system and knowing what the public expects from the healthcare system and backing that up with appropriate research and data.

- Public education campaigns targeting the public may contain public awareness messages, media engagement, and targeted brochures and pamphlets and other materials.

- Models of excellence (HIV/AIDS movement) should be considered in creating public education campaigns.

- Outcomes in public education are hard to measure as considerable diligence and experience is required to achieve accurate measurement with outcomes that will be sensitive or specific enough to detect a difference.

REFERENCES

● 1 Ferris FD, Balfour HM, Bowen K, et al. A Model to Guide Hospice Palliative Care: Based on National Principles and Norms of Practice. Ottawa, ON: Canadian Hospice Palliative Care Association, 2002. Available at: www.chpca.net/publications_and_resources.htm (accessed Spetember 6, 2005).

2 Zhukovsky DS, Gorowski E, Hausdorff J, et al. Unmet analgesic needs in cancer patients. J Pain Symptom Manage 1995; 10: 113–19.

3 Silveira MJ, DiPiero A, Gerrity MS, Feudtner C. Patients' knowledge of options at the end of life: ignorance in the face of death. JAMA 2000; 284: 2483–8.

4 Secretariat on Palliative & End-of-Life Care, Health Canada. The Informational Needs of Informal Caregivers – From the Informal Caregiver's Perspective. Health Canada, Ottawa, Canada, 2004.

5 Iconomou G, Vagenakis AG, Kalofonos HP. The informational needs, satisfaction with communication, and psychological status of primary caregivers of cancer patients receiving chemotherapy. Support Care Cancer 2001; 9: 591–6.

6 Robbins M. Evaluating Palliative Care: Establishing the Evidence Base. Oxford: Oxford University Press, 1998.

7 Kristjanson L. The family as a unit of treatment. In: Portenoy R, Bruera E, eds. Topics in Palliative Care, Vol. 1. New York: Oxford University Press, 1997.

8 Holman H. Chronic disease – the need for a new clinical education. JAMA 2004; 292: 1057–9.

9 McKinlay JB, McKinlay SM. Medical measures and the decline of mortality. In: Conrad P, Kern R, eds. The Sociology of Health and Illness. New York: St Martins, 1981.

● 10 Ottawa Charter for Health Promotion. World Health Organization, 1986. www.who.int/hpr/NPH/docs/ottawa_charter_hp.pdf (accessed September 6, 2005).

11 Shani E, Ayalon A, Hammad IA, Sikron F. What picture is worth a thousand words? A comparative evaluation of a burn prevention programme by type of medium in Israel. Health Promot Int 2003; 18: 361–71.

12 Witte K, Allen M. A meta-analysis of fear appeals: implications for effective public health campaigns. Health Educ Behav 2000; 27: 591–615.

13 Aries P. The Hour of Our Death. New York: Alfred A Knopf, 1981.

14 Salvador RJ. What do Mexicans celebrate on the day of the dead? In: Morgan JD, Laungani P, eds. Death And Bereavement In The Americas. Death, Value And Meaning Series, Vol. II. Amityville NY: Baywood Publishing Co., 2003.

15 Reynolds N, Testa M, Marc L, et al. Factors influencing medication adherence beliefs and self-efficacy in persons naive to antiretroviral therapy: a multicenter, cross-sectional study. AIDS Behav 2004; 8: 141–50.

16 Neimeyer R, Wittkowski J, Moser R. Psychological research on death attitudes: an overview and evaluation. Death Studies 2004; 28: 309–40.

17 Kvale J, Berg L, Groff J, Lange G. Factors associated with residents' attitudes towards dying patients. Fam Med 1999; 31: 691–6.

18 Tedeschi R, Park C, Calhoun L, eds. Posttraumatic Growth: Positive Changes in the Aftermath of Crisis. Mahwah, NJ: Lawrence Erlbaum Assoc., 1998.

● 19   Carstairs S, Beaudoin G. *Quality End-of-Life Care: The Right of Every Canadian*. The Senate of Canada, 2000.

20   Romanow RJ (Commissioner) *Building on Values: The Future of Health Care in Canada*. Commission on the Future of Health Care in Canada, 2003.

21   Angus Reid Group. *Canadians' Perceptions of Hospice Care: Key Findings*. Submitted to GlaxoWellcome, 1997.

22   Ipsos-Reid. *Hospice Palliative Care Study: Final Report*. The GlaxoSmithKline Foundation and the Canadian Hospice Palliative Care Association, 2004.

23   George MV, Loh S, Verma RBP, Shin YE. *Population Projections for Canada, Provinces and Territories: 2000–2026 Statistics Canada*. Publication catalog no. 91-520-XIB, 2001: 124.

24   Quality End-of-Life Care Coalition. *Dying for Care: Status Report*. June, 2004.

25   Gallagher R. Using a trade show format to educate the public about death and survey public knowledge and needs about issues surrounding death and dying. *J Pain Symptom Manage* 2001; **21**: 52–8.

26   Monninkhof E, van der Valk P, van der Palen J, *et al.* Self-management education for chronic obstructive pulmonary disease (Cochrane Review). In: *Cochrane Library*, Issue 3, 2004.

◆ 27   Hearn J, Higginson I. Outcome measures in palliative care for advanced cancer patients: a review. In: Field D, Clark D, Corner J, Davis C, eds. *Researching Palliative Care*. Philadelphia: Open University Press, 2001.

28   Riemsma RP, Kirwan JR, Taal E, Rasker JJ. Patient education for adults with rheumatoid arthritis (Cochrane Review). In: *Cochrane Library*, Issue 3, 2004.

29   Ebrahim S, Davey Smith G. Multiple risk factor interventions for primary prevention of coronary heart disease. (Cochrane Review). In: *Cochrane Library*, Issue 3, 2004.

30   Di Mola G, Crisci M. Attitudes towards death and dying in a representative sample of the Italian population. *Palliat Med* 2001; **15**: 372–8.

31   Beuzart P, Ricci L, Ritzenhaler M, *et al.* An overview on palliative care and the end of life. Results of a survey conducted in a sample of the French population [article in French]. *Presse Med* 2003; **32**: 152–7.

32   The GlaxoSmithKline Foundation and the Canadian Hospice Palliative Care Association. *A Guide for Caregivers*, 2002.

33   Sulmasy D, McIlvane J. Patients' ratings of quality and satisfaction with care at the end of life. *Arch Intern Med* 2002; **162**: 2098–104.

● 34   Hearn J, Higginson I. Development and validation of a core outcome measure for palliative care: the palliative care outcome scale. Palliative Care Core Audit Project Advisory Group. *Qual Health Care* 1999; **8**: 219–27.

35   Morita T, Chihara S, Kashiwaga T. Quality Audit Committee of the Japanese Association of Hospice and Palliative Care Units. A scale to measure satisfaction of bereaved family receiving inpatient palliative care. *Palliat Med* 2002; **16**: 141–50.

PART 5

Research and audit

20

Challenges of research in palliative medicine

IRENE J HIGGINSON

INTRODUCTION

All research, whatever the field, faces scientific, practical, and ethical challenges. Palliative medicine is no exception.[1,2] Indeed the challenges in palliative medicine are often greater than those experienced in other fields of medical research because of the nature and complexity of the problems faced by patients and their families, the services they receive, the settings of care and way that patients' conditions can change dramatically in a short period of time. There is often a web of challenges that the investigator has to face. As much as possible, problems should be anticipated and prepared for in advance to minimize their effects. But this is not always possible, and sometimes problems must be dealt with as they arise. Often it requires great courage, skill and hard work to manage obstacles that can occur during the course of a study and to minimize the effect these have on the quality of the findings. Many of the challenges described here apply equally to clinical audits, quality assurance, and total quality management projects.[3] An audit where the design is not appropriate, or a quality assurance review that collects information from a biased sample of people, suffers from the same weaknesses and limitations as a research study with these problems.[4] The wealth of studies already conducted in palliative care and the evidence base to date demonstrate that successful research and audit are possible.[5,6]

SCIENTIFIC CHALLENGES

Scientific challenges are the most predictable difficulties to be faced in any study and should be planned for in advance. Careful piloting of the methods can test possible solutions,

and this may uncover further challenges that need to be planned for. A pilot will often consist of a small investigation, or series of investigations, to test specific components of study design and analysis. This may include, for example, testing the methods of recruitment to see how many patients can be recruited, testing the questionnaires to see how long they take and which are acceptable for patients, or the range of scores to calculate sample size.

Setting the aims and objectives and/or hypothesis or research question

All research is driven by a question or idea that the investigator wants to answer or better understand. Focusing one's ideas on what is to be explored, and what can be investigated in a study is an important step, requiring knowledge of clinical concerns, literature review (see Chapter 25), and self-discipline. It is better to decide to answer a question or explore an issue that can be achieved realistically within the resources and timescale available than to attempt to answer a whole multitude of questions that are very broad and cannot be covered within the scope of the study. Time spent refining the aims and objectives and then considering if these can be answered by the right study design is a fundamental step in any study (see also Chapter 22). In a study following a grounded theory method (in qualitative research) the process varies from that above, but guidance is available.[7]

Study design

Choosing the most appropriate design for a study's aims and objectives is then one of the most important decisions that any researcher can make.[8] Always the aims and research questions should lead the design. For example, there is no point attempting to test the efficacy of a new drug treatment by conducting a survey of patients' views of the drug. Such a survey may give interesting information about acceptability, side effects, actual use, and patient views, but it will not give information about efficacy (i.e. if the drug works better than the current best practice in controlled conditions). Chapter 22 outlines the different research designs and options for the researcher.

Certain study designs are problematic in palliative care, and perhaps the most often discussed is the randomized controlled trial (RCT). Some RCTs have experienced such severe problems that the trial failed to produce any results.[9] Nowadays RCTS, especially crossover trials for drug treatments in palliative care, are more often used,[10,11] although there can be difficulties with recruitment, attrition, and measurement (see below). However, trials of nondrug interventions often face additional difficulties in maintaining a difference between intervention and control, and because they are difficult to blind can have problems of contamination and disappointment (if patients feel they are not receiving a service they wish to receive).[12–14] There is a growing body of literature showing that, although the RCT is often regarded as the gold standard method in evaluative research, alternative quasi-experimental and observational methods can yield just as much, and sometimes more, useful results.[8,15,16] Some successful RCTs have been conducted, for example of communication skills training,[17] a nurse clinic for breathlessness,[18] community palliative care teams,[19,20] and a broader range of trial methods have been developed including cluster randomized trials,[21,22] wait list control groups (only possible among patients with longer life expectancy) and N of 1 trials.[23] Studying the designs of others, including those researching outside palliative care, and their successes and failings, can often provide useful guides.[24]

Increasingly mixed method study designs (combining quantitative and qualitative methods) are being used in health services and clinical research. These methods have much to offer to palliative care. The quantitative approaches can count numbers affected and provide external validity, whereas the qualitative methods can help to understand the more intangible aspects of symptoms, feelings, or treatment effects, and provide internal validity.[25–31]

Selection and recruitment

Many studies in palliative care, whatever the design, can have problems with patient selection and recruitment. Selection (or sampling) bias occurs when the group of patients selected for or included in the study is different from the total population of interest. For example, one may wish to study the management of pain in patients toward the end of life, but the way that one is able to recruit patients means that patients in the last week of life are excluded – because they could not participate in interviews, or for some other reason. There are many reasons why selection or sampling bias may occur, some of the common types and their effects are shown in Table 20.1. Chapter 21 considers the patient population in greater depth and the issues and problems of recruitment, including among disadvantaged groups.

Further, recruiting patients who are often quite ill, or carers who are distressed and/or bereaved can be difficult.[32] Many research studies assessing the efficacy of drug treatments have automatically excluded older people (even those over 65 years), and those with multiple pathologies, because of the difficulties of recruiting individuals who are ill. In palliative care, excluding people in these categories would remove almost the entire sample, leading to terrible selection bias (see Table 20.1). However, recruiting ill or frail people into research studies requires skill, time, and energy. It involves winning the hearts of professionals who may refer patients to the study, and interviewing patients and families in a way that makes them feel prepared to take part and continue to be involved. Jordhøy et al. and others have written useful guidance on methods of improving recruitment,[1,33] including ensuring staff awareness, and ensuring regular updates and feedback (see Chapter 25 for useful tips, and Chapter 21 for more information on selecting the patient population). In palliative care interviewers must be sensitive and flexible when attempting to recruit patients. There may need to be three or four visits to patients to secure one interview (because patients are ill, factors change, and patients may prefer the interviewer to come back at different time). In one recent study we conduced at King's College London among patients with advanced cancer, in one instance more than 10 contacts were required to secure a complete interview, despite the patient wishing to be involved in the study. That said, many patients in palliative care do wish to be involved in research, and to tell their story, particularly if they feel it may help others in their situation in the future.

A common challenge in palliative care is establishing suitable criteria for recruitment to the study. If prognosis is used, then past experience suggests that patients may be referred too late for the study. In one instance, when patients with a prognosis of less than 1 year were to be referred for the study, 1 in 4 patients had died before the interviewer could recruit them.[12] Teno has suggested the criteria of 'not being surprised if the patient had died within one year', which is likely to be more successful, but may not work in some cultures (J Teno, personal communication, 2004). Prognostication is difficult but a range of estimated survival is more likely to be correct than any absolute assessment.[34] Further work is improving our prognostic assessments by providing information on other relevant factors.[35] Other recruitment criteria, such as the nature of problems or functional assessment, or a combination of these, may also be needed[1,36] (see Chapters 21 and 25). Careful piloting may shed light on the most effective strategies and methods for recruiting research subjects, and the information and updates needed for staff and subjects.

Table 20.1   *Common biases (i.e. systematic rather than random errors) that can be encountered in palliative care research*[a]

Type of bias	Definition
Sampling bias	The inclusion of subjects that distorts the nature of those who would have been chosen by chance
Selection bias	The selection of subjects that distorts the nature of those who would have been chosen by chance, for example selection by nurses or doctors or patients suitable for interview. This can occur in many ways, but selection of any sample is likely to result in sample bias, especially in palliative care where patients may become too ill to contact, or may not be in contact with particular services from which patients are selected (e.g. clinic, hospital, primary care doctor), or may be excluded because staff feel they are too ill for interview
Nonresponse bias	The biasing of the sample due to the nature of those who do not respond being different from that of those who do respond, For example, relatives who are most distressed may (or may not) respond to a questionnaire
Attrition/dropout bias	The biasing of the sample due to subjects being lost to follow-up because they choose not to be involved in the study, or become too ill for interview, move away, or die. Some attrition bias is inevitable in palliative care
Missing data bias	The biasing of the responses due to some subjects not responding to some questions. For example, if the most distressed patients do not answer questions about depression. There is in effect a nonresponse by some of the sample to some of the questions
Measurement bias	The collection of data or measurements that distorts the nature of the data collected from its true state
Recall bias	The biasing of data collected because of inaccurate or varied recall, perhaps for some events more than others, or because of varied time (e.g. 1 year vs. 6 weeks) or events
Poor measurement tools, validity/ reliability	The use of measurement tools that introduce bias because they are not valid or reliable in certain situations, or among certain cultures
Digit preference bias	The use of measurement tools that introduce bias because respondents choose particular digits in their answers. For example, on a scale of 1–100 most people tend to use numbers that end in 0 (10, 20, etc)
Observer/ researcher's bias	The systematic error introduced by an expectation or belief on the part of the observer or researcher (this can be quite unconscious and is most common when researchers are not blinded to situations, although it can occur even then)
Subject bias	The systematic error introduced by an expectation or belief on the part of the research subject (this can be quite unconscious, and is most common when subjects are not blinded to situations, although it can occur even then)
Hawthorne effect	The change in behavior made by people (e.g. staff or patients) when they know they are being studied. The effect was first noticed in the Hawthorne plant of Western Electric. Production increased not as a consequence of actual changes in working conditions introduced by the plant's management but because management demonstrated interest in such improvements
Reporting bias	The reporting and publication of research findings in a way which distorts the dissemination of findings toward more positive or negative findings
Publication bias	The publication or nonpublication of research findings, depending on the nature and direction of the results. In general positive studies are more often published than negative ones
Language bias	The publication of research findings in a particular language, depending on the nature and direction of the results. Research findings in some languages, particularly English, are more accessible
Funding bias	The reporting of research findings, depending on how the results accord with the aspirations of the funding body. Further there may be considerable hidden bias in the nature of research supported, whereby certain investigations are not funded
Selective outcome reporting bias	The selective reporting of some outcomes but not others, depending on the nature and direction of the research findings. For example, positive findings are reported but a lot of negatives ones are not
Time lag reporting bias	The delayed (or rapid) publication of research findings, depending on the nature and direction of the results
Developed country bias	The publication of findings, depending on whether the authors were based in developed or in developing countries

[a]Main categories of bias are shown in italics, subcategories/causes of each type of bias are shown above. Note that over 100 different types of biases are known, but three main categories – sampling, measurement, and reporting – include most types.

Measurement, interviews, and data collection

The insurmountable challenge in palliative care research is to find measures that detect relevant changes and yet are suitable for very ill populations. This creates tension between attempting to capture detail by using long-standardized measures or conducting qualitative interviews and having short interviews with short measures and/or short qualitative interviews. In the end the researcher must balance the amount of information that can realistically, reliably, and validly be collected with the ideal needed. Often the plan of analysis is helpful here, as well as referring back to the aim, objectives, and/or hypothesis of the research. The analysis plan helps to clarify how the data will be used, and this in turn clarifies what needs to be collected.

There are now many hundreds of quality-of-life instruments and a range of palliative outcome scales that have been developed or validated specifically for palliative care. Chapter 23 provides more details of individual scales and outcome measurement. In addition, there are several books on quality-of-life assessment and reviews of the measures.[37-43] Therefore, there is every opportunity for the researcher and clinician to use validated and tested scales. Only if a thorough systematic review reveals that no suitable (or partially) suitable scale is available, should the researcher embark on developing a new scale.

Less frequently qualitative researchers publish their topic guides, which are generally developed for specific lines of inquiry. However such publication is useful, for conducting open qualitative interviews is a highly skilled activity. Listening to the tapes of, or reading or typing the transcripts of highly skilled qualitative interviews is very instructive.

In general interviews should be kept as short as possible, and in some instances the researcher should order the questions or scales so as to collect the more important information first. Missing data for some questions among some patients will be inevitable, and researchers should minimize this for the primary outcomes of their study. When patients become tired or do not wish to continue interview, the data collection should be terminated because collection will become unreliable if patients cannot concentrate. It may be necessary to complete the interview at a later date if the person is willing.

Missing data and attrition

Missing data in palliative care studies are inevitable. Data may be missing for individual questions (for example if the patient did not wish to answer a question or scale) or for individual subjects (for example in a longitudinal study, a patient may miss a follow-up interview because they are away or because of illness, or they may be lost to follow-up because they become too ill to participate in the study, or they die). The most important thing is to understand the reason for the missing data and in which subjects this

occurs. Any missing data may bias the results (see Table 20.1). Therefore missing data should never be ignored. In general missing data should be classified and explored in three categories:

- *Data missing completely at random.* There is no discernable pattern to the missing data with any variable in the data set.
- *Data missing at random,* There is no relation between the missingness of data with the outcome variables of interest, but there is a relation with one of the other variables which does not appear to be related to the exposure or outcome variable. For example in an evaluation of palliative day care, we found missingness was associated with whether patients had smoked or not, although there was no relation with pain, symptoms, quality of life, hope, diagnosis, or any clinical variable.
- *Data missing not at random.* The missingness of the data is associated with an important variable in the study, e.g. diagnosis, or importantly, with one of the outcome variables, e.g. quality of life.

The field of research into missing data and its effects is growing rapidly. New techniques are being developed (e.g. imputation and modeling) to handle missing data.[1,44,45] The old notion of just ignoring missing data is now rarely acceptable, unless there are minimal missing data. Any analysis conducted with missing data excluded from the analysis is in effect assuming that those subjects with missing data will give the same results as those with complete data. Thus there is an implicit imputation, even if the researcher has not formally carried this out. And even if it is missing completely at random, missing data will reduce the sample size, and may mean that the study becomes underpowered. Missing data should always be reported and understood. In palliative care the pattern of missing information can often say much about the sample and the subjects. If modeling or imputations are undertaken, then often several imputations are advisable, followed by a sensitivity analysis, to determine the effects of different approaches.

CLINICAL, ORGANIZATIONAL, AND PRACTICAL CHALLENGES

Challenges in this area can occur in all forms. There may be concerns among colleagues or reluctance to refer patients for studies in palliative care on the part of both specialists outside palliative care and those in the field. This may be because of concerns about the nature of the questions or a belief that palliative care equates with end-of-life care, and so patients should only be included in studies when they are very close to death. Interviews may have to be organized around clinical treatments. Patients may not clearly distinguish between new services or interventions and the research interview if both are introduced at the same time. The Hawthorne effect (see Table 20.1) is likely for a wide range of reasons.

In addition, there are many practical challenges to consider in a palliative care research project. One may need to travel to patients' homes to conduct interviews, and the nature of a home may make it difficult to ensure that patients and carers can be interviewed separately. Sometimes the only way to achieve separate patient and carer interviews is to have two interviewers, and even in some homes this is not possible. Travel time and costs must be accounted for.

During the course of any study things will change. New treatments or services may be introduced which may require a change in the recruitment or inclusion criteria. Staff in the clinical service will change, which may mean there is a need to educate the new staff. Even researchers on a study may leave because of being offered a post elsewhere, finding the work not as interesting as they thought, or they may fall ill. A common problem in palliative care research is if the researcher suffers a bereavement in the family and so begins to find interviewing difficult (see below). Senior investigators and research teams are often crucial here; they have seen this problem before and there may be several individuals who can help out with the study or who can at least speak with the funding body and others to let them know what is happening.

The potential effects of interviews on those conducting them should also be considered in terms of safely and emotional effects. When interviewing patients in the community the safety of interviews, especially in more deprived and dangerous areas, should be considered. Community clinical services may provide useful information. Using mobile phones, keeping lists of places/people to be visited, agreeing associates who will check whereabouts, and in difficult circumstances joint interviewing can be helpful. Conducting interviews, transcribing and even analyzing data (including collected by post) can also be potentially distressing for researchers, particularly those who do not have clinical experience to make them aware of services that might be available for others. Often a system of support – even if mutual within a department – is helpful. At times of particular stress, e.g. following a bereavement, for clinical staff it may be appropriate that the person should not conduct the interviews.

A project advisory committee (PAC) can also be helpful. The PAC usually comprises relevant clinical investigators, and depending on the scale of the project it may be small (two or three individuals) or for complex projects it may be large (involving several centers, representatives of the funding body, external experts, and users/patients). The PAC may be established by the funding body or by the investigators. It meets regularly and oversees the progress of the project, and provides a forum to discuss challenges as they arise, monitor research ethics, governance, and progress, and considers the relevance of findings to patients, policy, and practice.

A final practical challenge is obtaining funding for the study. Many funding bodies do not see palliative care as a priority, and many scientific assessors on grant awarding bodies are not aware of the specific outcome measures and methods needed. In Canada a specific palliative care program has been established within the national research boards and has international expert assessors. This is a good model for other countries, as only with specific programs dedicated to a field can the best studies be supported.

ANIMAL MODELS: ISSUES IN TRANSLATING FINDINGS TO PEOPLE

Often work with animal models involves the artificial inducement of the problem under study in the animals (e.g. the cancer is induced in the animal). Then the researchers measure parameters that they believe are sufficiently close to or reflect those of interest in humans. The animals are killed at a point when they are thought to be suffering. There are many challenges in animal model studies. Specific guidance exists in many countries regarding the welfare of animals, but it is beyond the scope of this chapter. Research using animal models requires a model sufficiently close to the situation experienced in humans to be developed in the animals. For example, to study hypertension, types of rat that develop high blood pressure have been bred. To study problems in cancer, the cancer is often artificially induced. One of the apparent problems is being able, in animals, to induce problems sufficiently similar to those faced by humans and to find ways to measure them. Caution is therefore needed when extrapolating from animal studies to human beings.

ETHICAL ISSUES AND DEALING WITH INSTITUTIONAL REVIEW BOARDS

The ethical challenges in palliative care research are wide ranging, and for this reason Chapter 24 deals with this subject in detail. Common ethical issues that can arise occur at the point of consent (ensuring that full information is given, and the time taken for consent in the interview), during the interview, when researchers may uncover problems that they feel they need to act on, and dealing with distressed individuals. Nevertheless, it is arguably unethical to make decisions for patients about whether or not they should be given the option of being involved in research if they wish. Institutional review boards (IRBs) or ethics committees will need to approve the research (and in many instances the audit) to be undertaken, and will required detailed project information. They will cover not only research among patients but also staff surveys and any action that is not part of routine good clinical practice. Allowing sufficient time during a study for the review is essential. Ethical committees and IRBs vary in their approach and are often not familiar with palliative care and survey research, and so may initially be reluctant to pass a study. Often considerable persistence and explanation is needed, although often their suggestions and advice improve the study. If in doubt about whether the study requires IRB approval it is sensible to take advice from the chair of the committee. Chapter 24 provides further guidance.

INVOLVING USERS IN RESEARCH

There is a growing view, on the part of many patients, families, caregivers, and research investigators that the involvement of patients and families/relevant others in research is helpful and good practice. Some charities that support research have user forums that help to decide on research priorities, questions, and the review of potential grants. For example, at King's College London, a study we have been conducting, funded by the Multiple Sclerosis Society (UK), was reviewed by users as well as scientific experts and is being monitored by a PAC involving users, scientific experts, and clinicians. A user chairs our PAC.

However, there can be particular challenges in involving users in palliative care research and audit – patients are often quite ill, may need special facilities, and cannot be recruited in all circumstances. Increasingly it is recognized that users involved in appraising research need some development or training, so that they can understand some of the concepts involved. This, and the course of a research study over 1–3 years, takes time. But it is completely unrealistic to expect palliative care patients to be involved for this period of time. Involving users who are not palliative care patients, for example involving cured cancer patients, can be problematic, because these users – although very familiar with some of the problems in care – have not experienced the specific issues faced by palliative care patients. Other proxies, such as bereaved relatives, or representatives from relevant patient bodies and in some instances relevant clinicians, may overcome this to some extent, but bring other challenges. However, the ways to involve users in palliative care needs more development and testing. Small and Rhodes' guide provides a good introduction.[46]

REPORTING THE RESULTS

Many challenges can arise in the final stage in a research project – reporting the results (see Table 20.1 and Chapter 25). It can be difficult to write-up the paper fully within the word limit required by many journals, and there is often a time lag between completing the study, analyzing the data and finally getting the paper out. However, dissemination is an important part of all research, different audiences should be considered, and a dissemination strategy should be developed in the original protocol.

CONCLUSION

There are many challenges in conducting research in palliative care, which mean that research in palliative care needs skills, training, effort, and links to those with expertise in dealing with such issues. Some of the challenges are similar to those in other fields (especially for example psychiatry and health services research), whereas other challenges are unique (for example the problem of attrition, issues of involving users). A growing number of units are becoming skilled and experienced in conducting research in palliative care, and have sufficient expertise and infrastructure to begin supporting others in their research training. In the future, bringing researchers, clinicians and users together – through collaboratives, rotations,[47] and ideally institutes devoted to palliative care – will help improve the infrastructure for researchers, especially new investigators. Successfully completed studies are rewarding for investigators and more importantly for patients and families. Research can begin to discover better and more effective, efficient, and humane ways of providing care and treatments to benefit patients and families.[48–50] But failed studies are demotivating for investigators and take valuable time away from patients, families, and clinical staff.[51,52] Good research in palliative care can overcome many of the challenges, although there is a need to find better ways to deal with some of the problems of recruitment, attrition, outcome measurement, and missing data.

Key learning points

- Research in palliative care faces a complex web of scientific, practical, organizational and clinical challenges.

- Many of these challenges are common to those faced in other fields, but some (e.g. attrition and missing data) are especially likely in palliative care.

- Scientific challenges include setting aims and objectives, study design, outcome measures, recruitment, follow-up, attrition, and dealing with missing data.

- Practical and other challenges include selling the project to others, interviewing patients in various settings and different contexts, managing changes in treatments and/or services and/or staff, ethical issues, and involving users.

- Many challenges can be avoided or their effects minimized by careful planning and piloting, developing a PAG and working in or with units that possess relevant palliative care research expertise and skills.

- Research is important to palliative care, to develop the knowledge and discover improved treatments and care.

REFERENCES

1 Jordhøy MS, Kaasa S, Fayers P, et al. Challenges in palliative care research; recruitment, attrition and compliance: experience from a randomized controlled trial. *Palliat Med* 1999; **13**: 299–310.

2 Penrod JD, Morrison RS. Challenges for palliative care research. *J Palliat Med* 2004; **7**: 398–402.

3 Higginson I. *Clinical Audit in Palliative Care*. Oxford: Radcliffe Medical Press, 1993.

4 Higginson I, McCarthy M. Evaluation of palliative care: steps to quality assurance? *Palliat Med* 1989; **3**: 267–74.

5 Gysels M, Higginson IJ. *Improving Supportive and Palliative Care for Adults with Cancer: Research Evidence*. London: National Institute of Clinical Excellence, 2004.

6 Harding R, Higginson IJ. What is the best way to help caregivers in cancer and palliative care? A systematic literature review of interventions and their effectiveness. *Palliat Med* 2002; **17**: 63–71.

7 Seale C. Classics revisited. Awareness of method: re-reading Glaser and Strauss. *Mortality* 1999; **4**: 195–202.

8 Bausewein C, Higginson IJ. Appropriate methods to assess the effectiveness and efficacy of treatments or interventions to control cancer pain. *J Palliat Med* 2004; **7**: 423–30.

9 McWhinney IR, Bass MJ, Donner A. Evaluation of a palliative care service: problems and pitfalls. *BMJ* 1994; **309**: 1340–2.

10 Bruera E, de Stoutz N, Velasco Leiva A, et al. Effects of oxygen on dyspnoea in hypoxaemic terminal-cancer patients. *Lancet* 1993; **342**: 13–14.

11 Sykes AJ, Kiltie AE, Stewart AL. Ondansetron versus a chlorpromazine and dexamethasone combination for the prevention of nausea and vomiting: a prospective, randomised study to assess efficacy, cost effectiveness and quality of life following single-fraction radiotherapy. *Support Care Cancer* 1997; **5**: 500–3.

12 Addington-Hall JM, MacDonald LD, Anderson HR, et al. Randomised controlled trial of effects of co-ordinating care for terminally ill cancer patients. *BMJ* 1992; **305**: 1317–22.

13 Grande GE, Todd CJ, Barclay SIG, Farquhar MC. A randomised controlled trial of a hospital at home service for the terminally ill. *Palliat Med* 2000; **14**: 375–85.

14 Hanks GW, Robbins M, Sharp D, et al. The imPaCT study: a randomised controlled trial to evaluate a hospital palliative care team. *Br J Cancer* 2002; **87**: 733–9.

15 Khaw K-T, Day N, Bingham S, Wareham N. Observational versus randomised trial evidence. *Lancet* 2004; **364**: 753–4.

16 McKee M, Britton A, Black N, McPherson K, et al. Interpreting the evidence: choosing between randomised and non-randomised studies. *BMJ* 1999; **319**: 312–15.

17 Fallowfield L, Jenkins V, Farewell V, et al. Efficacy of a cancer research UK communication skills training model for oncologists: a randomised controlled trial. *Lancet* 2002; **359**: 650–6.

18 Bredin M, Corner J, Krishnasamy M, et al. Multicentre randomised controlled trial of nursing intervention for breathlessness in patients with lung cancer. *BMJ* 1999; **318**: 901–4.

19 Zimmer JG, Groth Juncker A, McCusker J. Effects of a physician-led home care team on terminal care. *J Am Geriatr Soc* 1984; **32**: 288–92.

20 Zimmer JG, Groth Juncker A, McCusker J. A randomized controlled study of a home health care team. *Am J Public Health* 1985; **75**: 134–41.

21 Fowell A, Russell I, Johnstone R, et al. Cluster randomisation or randomised consent as an appropriate methodology for trials in palliative care: a feasibility study. *BMC Palliative Care* 2004; **3**: 1.

22 Torgerson DJ. Contamination in trials: is cluster randomisation the answer? *BMJ* 2001; **322**: 355–7.

23 Bruera E, Schoeller T, MacEachern T. Symptomatic benefit of supplemental oxygen in hypoxemic patients with terminal cancer: the use of the N of 1 randomized controlled trial. *J Pain Symptom Manage* 1992; **7**: 365–8.

24 Kapo J, Casarett D. Working to improve palliative care trials. *J Palliat Med* 2004; **7**: 395–7.

25 Corner J. In search of more complete answers to research questions: quantitative versus qualitative research methods: is there a way foward? *J Adv Nurs* 1991; **16**: 718–27.

26 Dale J, Shipman C, Lacock L, Davies M. Creating a shared vision of out of hours care: using rapid appraisal methods to create an interagency, community oriented, approach to service development. *BMJ* 1996; **312**: 1206–10.

27 Grande GE, Todd CJ, Barclay SI. Support needs in the last year of life: patient and carer dilemmas. *Palliat Med* 1997; **11**: 202–8.

28 Kristjanson LJ, Atwood J, Degner LF. Validity and reliability of the family inventory of needs (FIN): measuring the care needs of families of advanced cancer patients. *J Nurs Meas* 1995; **3**: 109–26.

29 Richardson A, Wilson Barnett J. *A Review of Nursing Research in Cancer and Palliative Care*. London: King's College London, School of Nursing 1997: 1–23.

30 Teno JM, Stevens M, Spernak S, Lynn J. Role of written advance directives in decision making: insights from qualitative and quantitative data. *J Gen Intern Med* 1998; **13**: 439–46.

31 Wallen GR, Berger A. Mixed methods: in search of truth in palliative care medicine. *J Palliat Med* 2004; **7**: 403–4.

32 Phipps E, Harris D, Braitman LE, Tester W, et al. Who enrolls in observational end of life research? Report from the cultural variations in approaches to end of life study. *J Palliat Med* 2005; **8**: 115–20.

33 Casarett D, Kassner CT, Kutner JS. Recruiting for research in hospice: feasibility of a research screening protocol. *J Palliat Med* 2004; **7**: 854–60.

34 Higginson IJ, Costantini M. Accuracy of prognosis estimates by four palliative care teams: a prospective cohort study. *BMC Palliative Care* 2002;**1**.

35 Vigano A, Donaldson N, Higginson IJ, et al. Quality of life and survival prediction in terminal cancer patients. A multicenter study. *Cancer* 2004; **101**: 1090–8.

36 Ling J, Hardy J, Penn K, Davis C. Evaluation of palliative care. Recruitment figures may be low. *BMJ* 1995; **310**: 125.

37 Bowling A. Choice of health indicator – the problem of measuring outcome. *Complement Medi Res* 1988; **2**: 43–63.

38 Bowling A. *Measuring Disease*. Milton Keynes: Open University Press, 1995.

39 Wilkin D, Hallam L, Doggett M. *Measures of Need and Outcome for Primary Health Care*. Oxford: Oxford University Press, 1992.

◆ 40 Carr AJ, Higginson IJ, Robinson PG. *Quality of Life*. London: BMJ Books, 2003.

41 Higginson IJ, Carr AJ. Measuring quality of life: Using quality of life measures in the clinical setting. *BMJ* 2001; **322**: 1297–300.

42 Paci E, Miccinesi G, Toscani F, *et al*. Quality of life assessment and outcome of palliative care. *J Pain Symptom Manage* 2001; **21**: 179–88.

43 Robinson PG, Carr AJ, Higginson IJ. How to choose a quality of life measure. In: Carr AJ, Higginson IJ, Robinson PG, eds. *Quality of Life*. London: BMJ Books, 2003: 88–100.

44 Neymark N, Kiebert W, Torfs K, *et al*. Methodological and statistical issues of quality of life (QoL) and economic evaluation in cancer clinical trials: report of a workshop. *Eur J Cancer* 1998; **34**: 1317–33.

45 Robinson PG, Donaldson N. Longitudinal analysis of quality of life data. In: Carr AJ, Robinson PG, Higginson IJ, eds. *Quality of Life*. London: BMJ Books, 2003: 101–12.

46 Small N, Rhodes P. *Too Ill To Talk? User Involvement and Palliative Care*. London: Routledge, 2000.

47 von Gunten CF, Von Roenn JH, Gradishar W, Weitzman S. A hospice/palliative medicine rotation for fellows training in hematology-oncology. *J Cancer Educ* 1995; **10**: 200–2.

48 Breitbart W, Bruera E, Chochinov H, Lynch M. Neuropsychiatric syndromes and psychological symptoms in patients with advanced cancer. *J Pain Symptom Manage* 1995; **10**: 131–41.

49 Corner J. Is there a research paradigm for palliative care? *Palliat Med* 1996; **10**: 201–8.

50 Ripamonti C. Management of dyspnea in advanced cancer patients [see comments]. *Support Care Cancer* 1999; **7**: 233–43.

51 Higginson I. Research degree supervision: lottery or lifebelt. *Critical Public Health* 1990; 42–7.

52 Higginson I, Corner J. Postgraduate research training: the PhD and MD thesis. *Palliat Med* 1996; **10**: 113–18.

21

The patient population: who are the subjects in palliative medicine research?

JENNIFER KAPO, DAVID CASARETT

INTRODUCTION

Although the volume of published research in palliative medicine has increased substantially in the past 20 years, there is still a need for high-quality, randomized trials to provide evidence for many palliative care interventions.[1–5] However, researchers face many barriers including the difficulty of defining precise outcomes, and the ethical issues that pertain to studying dying patients with the resultant scrutiny by institutional review boards.[6] These other challenges will be discussed in depth in Chapters 24 and 25. This chapter focuses on the additional challenge of defining the population to be studied, and will consider three key questions related to the palliative care population in research:

- Which patients should be included in palliative medicine research?
- What are the challenges of recruitment and retention of subjects in this population?
- What groups are currently underrepresented in palliative research, and how can these disparities be overcome?

WHICH PATIENTS SHOULD BE INCLUDED IN PALLIATIVE RESEARCH?

Researchers and clinicians appear to be in the process of redefining what characterizes a 'palliative care patient'. In the early stages of the field's development, attention was focused

primarily on patients near the end of life and their families. More recently, however, there has been a shift in the definition of palliative medicine from care only for the imminently dying to a larger population. Typically, palliative care now encompasses the care of persons who have chronic medical illnesses with physical, spiritual, and psychological symptoms in need of palliation, but who are not necessarily terminally ill.[7] Indeed, the most recent World Health Organization definition emphasizes palliative care's focus on improving quality of life rather than its focus on a particular patient population.

Therefore, there is reason to avoid definitions of the palliative care research population that are prognosis based. For instance, recruitment strategies that rely on prognostic inclusion criteria may exclude a group of healthier patients whose inclusion would have improved the generalizability of the study's results. In addition, investigators who use prognosis to define study eligibility must overcome substantial inaccuracies in the predictions even using the best available models as tools.[8*,9*] Finally, physicians are not only reluctant to make prognostic estimates, but also tend to overestimate life expectancy.[10*,11*] They may therefore be hesitant to refer their patients to palliative studies with a prognostic inclusion criterion.[12]

Instead, investigators might rely on a symptom or cluster of symptoms to identify the study population. This approach is particularly appropriate for randomized, controlled trials that aim to demonstrate the efficacy of an intervention. However, depending on the prevalence of the symptom, accrual may be very slow.[3,13,14*] Finally, a population defined in these terms may be heterogeneous, particularly if the symptom is commonly found in different disease states. For example, pain is associated with diverse conditions including cancer, osteoarthritis, and end-stage renal disease. Although one might logically include several of these conditions in a single study, the resulting heterogeneity may make analysis difficult.

Investigators may also define the study population using a single diagnosis. Although this may the best approach for studying many outcomes such as dyspnea related specifically to chronic obstructive pulmonary disease (COPD), focusing on one disease state may lead to limiting information applicable to other disease states. For example, although only a minority of all deaths in the USA are due to cancer, the majority of the existing palliative medicine research focuses on the care of patients with cancer. Cancer tends to follow an illness trajectory that is often more predictable than that of other diagnoses,[15*] and a substantial symptom burden is common at the end of life.[16–19] Although in some cases the results of studies that focus on one condition may be applicable to other conditions, this need not be the case. For instance, although the phenomenological experience of dyspnea may be similar for patients with cancer and patients with COPD, the mechanisms that produce dyspnea in these populations may be very different.

Another strategy for defining the palliative care population for research might rely on functional status. This approach is worth considering, first, because it is known that functional impairment may be closely linked to other symptoms such as fatigue, pain, and depression.[18,20–22] Therefore, investigators who rely on functional impairment as an inclusion criterion are likely to identify patients with a high prevalence of palliative care needs. Although this is a heterogeneous population, as a group they may have substantial disability and may benefit considerably from palliative interventions. Second, functional status can be assessed readily and with minimal clinical data. Thus eligibility criteria that are based on functional status offer a relatively straightforward way to identify potential study participants. However, not all patients at the end of life have functional impairment and frailty. In fact, many patients retain high levels of function until the last days of life.[15*] Therefore, focusing on functional status alone will both include patients with a good prognosis and will also exclude a significant number of patients who are near the end of life.

As detailed above, there are disadvantages and advantages to all of the strategies described. Different approaches have particular value when evaluating specific questions. For example randomized controlled trials generally require highly specific inclusion criteria such as symptom severity, functional status, and prognosis. However, a study designed to assess home care needs could use a more broad set of inclusion criteria, perhaps based on functional needs. Studies that use qualitative methods, for which precisely defined sample characteristics may not be essential, can often sample a broader and more heterogeneous population using more general inclusion criteria.

OTHER PALLIATIVE CARE POPULATIONS: FORMAL AND INFORMAL CAREGIVERS

Although the focus of palliative care research is typically on the patient, patients are surrounded by others who play a substantial role in their care. Therefore, it is also reasonable to consider these caregivers as potential subjects of palliative care research. For instance, a growing body of evidence points to the unique and significant stresses with associated morbidity that can be associated with caring for a loved one at the end of life.[23–29*] While the effects of caregiving are clear, their scope and reach are not, and it may be difficult to determine how to define a 'caregiver' for eligibility purposes (see Chapter 108). Similarly, the formal caregivers who comprise the interdisciplinary team (physicians, nurses, social workers, aids, chaplains, etc.) also need to be included as a part of the population to be studied. The team's decisions and actions are paramount to the delivery of quality palliative care. In addition, a wealth of information may be gained by studying the attitudes, beliefs, and practices of the providers who provide 'up-stream' care and eventually refer their patients for palliative care, or who wish to provide this care themselves.

Finally, both formal and informal caregivers experience grief and loss after a patient's death. These responses have been studied both for formal and informal caregivers, and it is clear that the effects of a patient's death can be both multifaceted and longlasting. Therefore, in defining the population that is relevant to palliative care research, both formal and informal caregivers should continue to be the focus of research even after the patient's death.[30–32]

CHALLENGES OF RECRUITMENT AND RETENTION

Recruitment for palliative care research may be limited both by patient and physician-specific barriers.[33] For instance, numerous patient characteristics impede research recruitment, including poor performance status, intense emotional strain, and uncontrolled symptoms. Together, these factors limit patients' ability to answer questions and to undergo repeated tests or examinations that are often required in research participation.[2,14] Patients may also have cognitive impairment that makes it difficult to communicate, which may impair their ability to provide adequate informed consent, to contribute valid and reliable self-reports, or both.

In addition, even among those patients who are eligible and approached to participate, a substantial proportion may decline to enroll for personal ('Not the right time', 'I need more time to think about it') and family-related reasons. In several studies this rate is reported to exceed 50 percent.[3*,34*] Finally, once patients are enrolled, dropout rates due to deteriorating health status, noncompliance with the treatment regimen, and death are high.[14,34] It is not uncommon for less than half of those enrolled to finish a trial.[7,8*,14]

Accrual to studies may also be delayed if healthcare providers are hesitant to refer their patients. Several researchers have documented their experiences and the challenges they face with recruiting patients.[3,33,35,36] Physicians may have trouble identifying patients who have poor prognosis,[10*] and they may be reluctant to express the possibility of a poor prognosis with a patient and/or their family for fear of causing psychological distress and harm.[11*,34] Physicians may be uncomfortable with the proposed research agenda, and fail to see the benefits of the study. For instance, some providers, such as home hospice clinicians, may have very strong preferences about valuable research and important research questions.[37*] An investigator whose research does not fit with these priorities faces additional challenges of recruitment. In addition, many providers have concerns that a patient referred to a palliative care study may not receive the highest quality care available. Patients and their families may be reluctant to enroll for similar reasons.[34*] Finally, providers may be concerned that asking their patients to participate in palliative medicine research is intrusive, particularly when patients are experiencing physical or emotional distress, or are near the end of life.[31,32]

IMPROVING RECRUITMENT AND RETENTION

Despite these perceived harms of enrolling in palliative medicine research, there is evidence to suggest that patients recognize several advantages of enrolling in trials, and that they may in fact derive benefit from research involvement, even at the end of life.[13,38–41*] For instance, patients may wish to enroll in research studies to benefit from close monitoring and attention provided by the research team. Others may hope for clinical benefit, even if none is expected. Patients also report humanistic benefits such as wanting to help others and wishing to 'give something back' to society, and to leave a legacy. Others report enrolling in trials as an expression of gratitude for the staff that provided care to them throughout the illness course.[34,39]

In order to improve enrollment and retention of subjects, several strategies have been proposed. One method is to capitalize on the potential benefits of study enrollment alluded to above. However, there is the possibility of creating an undue inducement to enroll if the patient feels that they need to enroll in a study to gain a treatment or evaluation to which they would not otherwise have access. Strategies to improve enrollment in trials have been the subject of several reviews and empirical studies.[33*,34,42,43*]

To improve recruitment, relationships must be forged with the referring doctors to build trust and enthusiasm for the study. One researcher suggests writing personal letters to care providers to engage them in the study and ask them to be a part of an advisory committee for the project.[42] Given the daunting challenges of recruitment, some trials may require specialized training of a person or persons who

are responsible for the recruitment process and are therefore committed to the success of the project. The numbers of patients enrolled can be increased by the efforts of a dedicated recruiter who is stationed in primary care providers' offices, and by advertising with flyers and public service announcements.[44] In addition, more specific recruitment interventions for subgroups of patients may be useful as well and are described below.

Preventing dropout and loss to follow-up is often more difficult in this population. However, three broad recommendations show promise. First, clinic visits for data collection should be limited in number and duration. Techniques of remote data collection are promising and, if widely adopted, have the potential to dramatically decrease the burdens associated with palliative research participation. Second, assessments and instruments used should be minimally burdensome and invasive. Last, if there is a high attrition rate during data collection the patients' and caregivers' opinions regarding the study should be elicited to determine if minor changes to the study protocol will keep patients from withdrawing from the study.

UNDERREPRESENTED POPULATIONS IN PALLIATIVE MEDICINE RESEARCH

As discussed in the preceding section, there are considerable challenges to the recruitment and retention of palliative care research subjects. Although this is true of the population taken as a whole, it is important to consider groups of patients who may be underrepresented in palliative medicine research. For example, there is a growing body of evidence that suggests that ethic minorities, in particular African Americans, as well as older patients have been underrepresented in research studies.[45–51] As a consequence, data from many clinical trials are extrapolated, often inappropriately, for application to older adults and those from ethnic minorities.[12,52–54]

Individuals from different countries and ethnic backgrounds have different preferences and needs for end-of-life care. Focusing only on Western, predominantly white patients will result in research conclusions which lack generalizability to all populations. Currently, there is a small, but growing body of research that is examining cultural differences in regards to attitudes, preferences, and care needs of those from different cultures at the end of life. However, there is an enormous need for further work in this area. For example, there is extensive evidence that African American patients are less willing to forgo life-sustaining treatment compared with white patients.[35,55–60*] Researchers from the UK have studied the differences in end-of-life preferences between native born white and black Caribbean patients. These studies suggest significant differences in the characteristics of informal caregivers, preferred location of death, acceptance of euthanasia, and reported symptom related distress; however, the authors conclude that there is a need for larger studies to fully describe these differences.[61-63] Hawaiian researchers have studied cancer evaluation and treatment strategies preferred by Native Hawaiians compared to Japanese, Filipino, Chinese, and white patients.[64-66] Failing to enroll patients from different ethnic and cultural groups will result in invalid conclusions in studies that have similar outcomes.

Research programs can improve the enrollment and retention of ethnic minority patients in studies if the researchers are aware of the knowledge gained from previous work that examines end-of-life care preferences of those from different ethic groups. For example, one researcher advocates that it might be best to address mistrust at the time of enrollment and/or follow-up by asking the patient directly, 'Is it difficult to trust a physician who is not (of the same background as you)'.[67] Another strategy includes stating explicitly that the team will work together with the patient and family to accomplish common goals.[68] In order to communicate effectively during recruitment and data collection, it may be particularly helpful to hire ethnically and culturally diverse research staff.[67]

CASE STUDY: EXAMPLE OF RECRUITING OLDER ADULTS IN PALLIATIVE CARE RESEARCH

Older adults are one important population that has traditionally been underrepresented in clinical research, including palliative care research. The most significant evidence of underrepresentation comes from oncology trials, which often exclude older adults despite the fact that most people with advanced cancer are elderly.[12,48*,49,53] As a result, clinicians who make treatment decisions need to rely on data that are extrapolated from studies of younger patients who may have better biological and physiological function, less comorbid diseases, and less polypharmacy.[52,54,69] Palliative care research, and particularly palliative care research that focuses on patients with cancer, may be following the same pattern, making this population a useful case study in the challenges of recruitment and potential solutions.

Perhaps the most significant barriers to including older adults in palliative care research are eligibility criteria that exclude patients with comorbid conditions. More generally, studies may exclude patients with hearing impairment, cognitive impairment, or those with functional impairment. As all of these are more common in older adults, these criteria create a *de facto* exclusion of this group.

Barriers to recruiting and retaining older adults in palliative care research may also come from providers. For instance, referring physicians may refuse to enroll older patients because they may perceive them to be too sick to participate, have too many comorbidities, or likely to benefit more from conventional therapies. They may also feel that the enrollment process is too time consuming, both for the patient and for themselves.[18*,50*] In fact, these sorts of barriers are not unique to recruitment of older patients, and are a magnified version of providers' reluctance to recruit patients who are near the end of life and perceived to be vulnerable.

Finally, patients and families may also be reluctant to enroll in research.[18,49-51,70] Common reasons not to enroll include: underlying comorbidities, concerns for potential toxicities, lack of social support, and excessive time for enrollment.[51] Several researchers note that older persons are particularly concerned with the added costs of treatment related to research protocols, including the treatment of adverse effects and the cost of travel to the evaluation appointments.[18,51] In addition, patients fear that the research will be inconvenient and take excessive time away from family and friends.[49] Again, these barriers are not unique to the recruitment of older adults. Concerns about risks and toxicity are common, and may be magnified in populations that harbor mistrust of the medical establishment.

Given these potential challenges to enrollment, several practical strategies have been proposed to improve enrollment of older adults. These strategies are a useful case study both because the challenges are not unique and because they require solutions that are multidimensional. Broadly, efforts to enhance recruitment of older adults, and indeed all underrepresented patient populations, can be grouped in three main categories: study-specific issues; provider-specific issues; and patient and family-specific issues. Each of these is discussed briefly below.

First, study-specific barriers to enrollment should be addressed in the earliest phases of a study's design. Inclusion criteria that are as broad as possible are ideal, and efforts should be undertaken to avoid study design features that may constitute a particularly significant barrier for some groups. Of course, broad inclusion criteria create other design challenges. For instance, by including older, more frail subjects, a prospective study may need to anticipate higher dropout rates. In addition, a study sample that is more heterogeneous may make it more difficult to detect main effects in an interventional trial. However, these and other difficulties should not by themselves prevent investigators from including a diverse patient population, but instead require careful attention and trade-offs in the early phases of study design.

Second, in order to address physician concerns regarding patients' comorbidities, researchers might design protocols that specifically target underrepresented populations (e.g. older adults, ethnic minorities, rural populations). Researchers need to find meaningful ways to communicate the importance of studying this group with the referring care providers. Involving the referring physicians as consultants during the design of the study may result in modifications of the protocol that will increase its appeal to the collaborators. In addition, training an efficient research recruiter with expertise in communication with older adults will limit burdens on the referring physician's time and efforts, and therefore increase their willingness to refer patients for enrollment in studies.[49]

Third, in order to address patient and family-specific barriers to study recruitment and enrollment, several overlapping strategies may be useful. For instance, one approach is to use an interdisciplinary research team including nurses, physicians, social workers, pharmacists and chaplains who can evaluate and care for the needs of study participants. This approach has been used successfully to increase recruitment and retention of older adults in clinical research[49,70] and offers promise for other underrepresented populations as well.

Others suggest designating a portion of the study budget to provide transportation to and from the study site, or providing interventions within the older person's home.[18] A portion of the budget should also be available to use to purchase the supplies needed to treat adverse effects that are the result of a study intervention. Given the importance that the family and caregivers frequently have in the care of older patients, the research staff may benefit from involving them in the study process. Finally, the time spent completing the study intervention should be kept to the minimum needed to be complete.[50]

CONCLUSION

Researchers are faced with many challenges in the identification, recruitment, enrollment, and retention of the population to be included in palliative medicine research. However, there is a growing body of evidence elucidating these challenges and defining targets for intervention to improve the quality of research and ultimately the care we provide to vulnerable and potentially under-served patients at the end of life. Further research is needed to determine the best interventions to improve the quality of recruitment and retention of patients, particularly those from different cultural and ethnic groups and older patients.

Key learning points

- Different approaches may have particular value when evaluating specific questions.
- Recruitment and retention of palliative care research subjects is subject to both patient and physician-specific barriers.
- Despite the challenges, there are several well-written guidelines to guide researchers.
- Ethnic minorities have traditionally been underrepresented in palliative care research.

- An understanding of the cultural differences in regards to the attitudes, preferences, and care needs of patients may help researchers design appropriate trials.
- Older persons are also underrepresented in palliative care research.
- Older persons may be excluded from enrollment due to medical comorbidities, concerns for toxicity, and declining functional status.
- Strategies that include education for the referring clinicians and the participation of a trained research coordinator with expertise in palliative medicine may increase the number of older patients enrolled in palliative medicine trials.

REFERENCES

◆ 1 Casarett DJ, Knebel A, Helmers K. Ethical challenges of palliative research. *J Pain Symptom Manage* 2003; **25**: S3–S5.

2 Grande GE, Todd CJ. Why are trials in palliative care so difficult? *Palliat Med* 2000; **14**: 69–74.

◆ 3 Rinck GC, van den Bos GA, Kleijnen J, *et al*. Methodologic issues in effectiveness research on palliative cancer care: a systematic review. *J Clin Oncol* 1697; **15**: 1697–707.

4 Corner J. A new forum for research, debate, and advice. *Palliat Med* 1996; **3**: 201–8.

◆ 5 Twycross RG. Research and palliative care: the pursuit of reliable knowledge. *Palliat Med* 1993; **7**: 175–7.

◆ 6 Krouse RS, Rosenfeld K, Grant M, *et al*. Palliative care research: issues and opportunities. *Cancer Epidemiol Biomarkers Prev* 2004; **13**: 337–9.

7 Meier DE. Variability in end of life care. *BMJ* 2004; **328**: 15.

● 8 Fox E, Landrum-McNiff K, Zhong Z, *et al*. Evaluation of prognostic criteria for determining hospice eligibility in patients with advanced lung, heart, or liver disease. SUPPORT Investigators. Study to Understand Prognoses and Preferences for Outcomes and Risks of Treatments. *JAMA* 1999; **282**: 1638–45.

● 9 Teno JM, Harrell FE Jr, Knaus W, *et al*. Prediction of survival for older hospitalized patients: the HELP survival model. Hospitalized Elderly Longitudinal Project. *J Am Geriatr Soc* 2000; **48**(5 Suppl).

● 10 Christakis NA, Lamont EB. Extent and determinants of error in doctors' prognoses in terminally ill patients: prospective cohort study. *BMJ* 2000; **320**: 469–72.

● 11 Lamont EB, Christakis NA. Prognostic disclosure to patients with cancer near the end of life. *Ann Intern Med* 2001; **134**: 1096–105.

12 van Agthoven M, *et al*. A review of recruitment criteria, patient characteristics and results of CHOP chemotherapy in prospective randomized phase III clinical trials for aggressive non-Hodgkin's lymphoma. *Hematol J* 2003; **4**: 399–409.

◆ 13 Mazzocato C, Sweeney C, Bruera E. Clinical research in palliative care: patient populations, symptoms, interventions and endpoints. *Palliat Med* 2001; **15**: 163–8.

◆ 14   Jordhoy MS, Kaasa S, Fayers P, et al. Challenges in palliative care research; recruitment, attrition and compliance: experience from a randomized controlled trial. Palliat Med 1999; 13: 299–310.

15   Lunney JR, Lynn J, Foley DJ, et al. Patterns of functional decline at the end of life. JAMA, 2003; 289: 2387–2392.

16   Lobchuk MM, Kristjanson L, Degner L, et al. Perceptions of symptom distress in lung cancer patients: Congruence between patients and primary family caregivers. J Pain Symptom Manage 1997; 14: 136–46.

17   Ventafridda V, Ripamonti C, DeConno F. Symptom prevalence and control during cancer patients' last days of life. J Palliat Care 1990; 6: 7–11.

18   Chang BH, Hendricks AM, Slawsky MT, Locastro JS. Patient recruitment to a randomized clinical trial of behavioral therapy for chronic heart failure. BMC Med Res Methodol 2004; 4: 17.

● 19   Lutz S, Norrell R, Bertucio C, et al. Symptom frequency and severity in patients with metastatic or locally recurrent lung cancer: a prospective study using the Lung Cancer Symptom Scale in a community hospital. J Palliat Med 2001; 4: 157–61.

20   Hallan S, Asberg A, Indredavik B, Wideroe TE. Quality of life after cerebrovascular stroke: a systematic study of patients' preferences for different functional outcomes. J Intern Med 1999; 246:309–16.

21   List M, Mumby P, Haraf D, et al. Performance and quality of life outcome in patients completing concomitant chemoradiotherapy protocols for head and neck cancer. Qual Life Res 1997; 6: 274–84.

● 22   Mor V. Cancer patients' quality of life over the disease course: lessons from the real world. J Chronic Dis 1987; 40: 535–44.

23   Vachon ML, Kristjanson L, Higginson I. Psychosocial issues in palliative care: the patient, the family, and the process and outcome of care. J Pain Symptom Manage 1995; 10: 142.

● 24   Lynn J, Teno JM, Phillips RS, et al. Perception by family members of the dying experience of older and seriously ill patients. SUPPORT Investigators. Study to Understand Prognoses and Preferences for Outcomes and Risks of Treatments. Ann Intern Med 1997; 126: 97–106.

25   Kristianson LJ, Sloan JA, Dudgeon D, Adaskin E. Family members' perceptions of palliative cancer care: predictors of family functioning and family members' health. J Palliat Care 1996; 12: 10–20.

26   Emanuel EJ, Fairclough DL, Slutsman J, et al. Assistance from family members, friends, paid care givers, and volunteers in the care of terminally ill patients. N Engl J Med 1999; 341: 956–63.

27   Steele RG. Needs of family caregivers of patients receiving home hospice care for cancer. Oncol Nurs Forum 1996: 823–8.

28   Chen ML. The generalizability of Caregiver Strain Index in family caregivers of cancer patients. Int J Nurs Stud 2002; 39: 823–9.

29   Haley WE, LaMonde LA, Han B, et al. Family caregiving in hospice: effects on psychological and health functioning among spousal caregivers of hospice patients with lung cancer or dementia. Hosp J 2001; 15: 1–18.

30   Rando T. Treatment of Complicated Mourning. Champaign, IL: Research Press, 1993.

◆ 31   Casarett D, Kutner JS, Abrahm J. Life after death: A practical approach to grief and bereavement. American College of

Physicians Consensus Paper. Ann Intern Med 2001; 128: 208–15.

32   Lenart SB, Bauer CG, Brighton DD, et al. Grief support for nursing staff in the ICU. J Nurs Staff Dev 1998; 14: 293–6.

◆ 33   Ewing G, Rogers M, Barclay S, et al. Recruiting patients into a primary care based study of palliative care: why is it so difficult? Palliat Med 2004; 18: 452–9.

34   Ross C, Cornbleet M. Attitudes of patients and staff to research in a palliative care specialist unit. Palliat Med 2003; 17: 491–7.

35   Blackhall LJ, Frank G, et al. Ethnicity and attitudes towards life sustaining technology. Soc Sci Med 1999; 48: 1779–89.

36   Crowley R, Casarett D. Patients' willingness to participate in symptom-related and disease-modifying research: results of a screening initiative in a palliative care clinic. Cancer 2003; 97: 2327–3.

● 37   Casarett D, Karlawish J, Hirschman K. Are hospices ready to participate in palliative care research? Results of a nationwide survey. J Palliat Med 2001; 5: 397–406.

◆ 38   Fine PG. Maximizing benefits and minimizing risks in palliative care research that involves patients near the end of life. J Pain Symptom Manage 2003; 25: S53–S62.

39   Penson RT, Joel SP, Roberts M, et al. The bioavailability and pharmacokinetics of subcutaneous, nebulized and oral morphine-6-glucuronide. Br J Clin Pharmacol 2002; 53: 347–54.

40   Hudson P. The experience of research participation for family caregivers of palliative care cancer patients. Int J Palliat Care Nurs 2003; (March): 120–3.

41   Casarett DJ, Sankar P, Karlawish J, et al. Obtaining informed consent for cancer pain research: do patients with advanced cancer and patients with chronic pain have different concern? J Pain Symptom Manage 2002; 24: 506–16.

42   Mazzocato C, Sweeney C, Bruera E. Clinical research in palliative care: choice of trial design. Palliat Med 2001; 15: 261–4.

◆ 43   Ling J, Rees E. What influences participation in clinical trials in palliative care in a cancer centre? Eur J Cancer 2000; 36: 621–6.

◆ 44   Karim K. Conducting research involving palliative medicine patients. Nurs Standard 2000; 15: 34–6.

◆ 45   Earl CE, Penney PJ. The significance of trust in the research consent process with African Americans. West J Nursing Res 2001; 23: 753–62.

46   Green BL, Partridge EE, Fouad MN, et al. African-American attitudes regarding cancer clinical trials and research studies: results from focus group methodology. Ethn Dis 2000; 10: 76–86.

47   Giuliano AR, Mokuau N, Hughes C, et al. Participation of minorities in cancer research: the influence of structural, cultural, and linguistic factors. Ann Clin Epidemiol, 2000; 10 (8 Suppl): S22–S34.

● 48   Hutchins LF, Unger JM, Crowley JJ, et al. Underrepresentation of patients 65 years of age or older in cancer-treatment trials. N Engl J Med 1999; 341: 2061–7.

◆ 49   Cassidy EL, Baird E, Sheikh JI. Recruitment and retention of elderly patients in clinical trials: issues and strategies. Am J Geriatr Psychiatry 2001; 9: 136–40.

50   Kornblith AB, Kemeny M, Peterson BL, et al. Cancer and Leukemia Group B. Survey of oncologists' perceptions of barriers to accrual of older patients with breast carcinoma to clinical trials. Cancer 2002; 95: 989–96.

51 Trimble E. Barriers to recruitment of older patients into breast cancer trials. *Cancer* 1994; **74**: 2208–14.

52 Britton A, McKee M, Black N, *et al.* Threats to applicability of randomised trials: exclusions and selective participation. *J Health Serv Res Policy* 1999; **4**: 112–21.

53 Cameron HJ, Williams BO. Clinical trials in the elderly. Should we do more? *Drugs Aging* 1996; **9**: 307–10.

54 John V, Mashru S, Lichtman S. Pharmacological factors influencing anticancer drug selection in the elderly. *Drugs Aging* 2003; **20**: 737–59.

55 Diringer M, Edwards DF, Aiyagari V, Hollingsworth H. Factor associated with withdrawal of mechanical ventilation in a neurology/neurosurgery intensive care unit. *Crit Care Med* 2001; **29**: 1792–7.

56 Eleazer G, Hornung CA, Egbert JR, *et al.* The relationship between ethnicity and advance directives in a frail, older population. *J Am Geriatr Soc* 1996; **44**: 938–43.

◆ 57 Phipps E, True G, Harris D, *et al.* Approaching the end of life: attitudes, preferences, and behaviors of African Americans and white patients and their family caregivers. *J Clin Oncol* 2003; **21**: 549–54.

58 McKinley ED, Garrett JM, Evans AT, Danis M. Differences in end-of-life decision making among black and white ambulatory cancer patients. *J Gen Intern Med* 1996; **11**: 651–6.

59 Caralis PV, Davis B, Wright K, Marcial E. The influence of ethnicity and race toward advance directives, life-prolonging treatments, and euthanasia. *J Clin Ethics* 1993; **4**: 155–65.

60 Murphy ST, Palmer JM, Azen S, *et al.* Ethnicity and advance care directives. *J Med Ethics* 1996: 108–17.

61 Koffman J, Higginson IJ. Dying to be home? Preferred location of death of first-generation black Caribbean and native-born white patients in the United Kingdom. *J Palliat Med* 2004; **7**: 628–36.

62 Koffman JS, Higginson IJ. Fit to care? A comparison of informal caregivers of first-generation Black Caribbeans and White dependants with advanced progressive disease in the UK. *Health Soc Care Comm* 2003; **11**: 528–36.

63 Higginson IJ, Koffman J. Attitudes to timeliness of death and euthanasia among first generation black Caribbean and white patients and their families living in the United Kingdom. *J Palliat Med* 2003; **6**: 245–9.

64 Braun KL. Do Hawaii residents support physician-assisted death? A comparison of five ethnic groups. *Hawaii Med J* 1998; **57**: 529–34.

65 Braun KL, Fong M, Gotay C, *et al.* Ethnicity and breast cancer in Hawaii: increased survival but continued disparity. *Ethn Dis* 2005; **15**: 453–60.

66 Braun KL, Fong M, Kaanoi ME, *et al.* Testing a culturally appropriate, theory-based intervention to improve colorectal cancer screening among Native Hawaiians. *Prev Med* 2005; **40**: 619–27.

67 Kagawa-Singer M, Blackhall LJ. Negotiating cross-cultural issues at the end of life: 'You got to go where he lives'. *JAMA* 2001; **286**: 2993–3001.

◆ 68 Crawley L, Payne R, Bolden J, *et al.*; Initiative to Improve Palliative and End-of-Life Care in the African American Community. Palliative and end-of-life care in the African American community. *JAMA* 2000; **284**: 2518–21.

◆ 69 Swift CG. The clinical pharmacology of ageing. *Br J Clin Pharmacol* 2003; **56**: 249–53.

70 Brown ML. Cancer patient care in clinical trials sponsored by the National Cancer Institute: what does it cost? *J Natl Cancer Inst* 1999; **91**: 818–19.

22

Study designs in palliative medicine

MASSIMO COSTANTINI

The question being asked determines the appropriate research architecture, strategy, and tactics to be used – not tradition, authority, experts, paradigms, or schools of thought.

Sackett and Wennberg (1997)[1]

INTRODUCTION

The objectives of this chapter are to define, discuss, and compare study designs commonly used for quantitative research in palliative care. Quantitative research uses the epidemiological approach to define and shape all the aspects of a study, including its design.

Epidemiology is the study of disease and health in human populations.[2] In palliative medicine we focus on at least two populations of interest: people at the end of their lives and their families. For both populations, 'the disease' is a multidimensional problem involving suffering, dignity, care needs, and quality of life.[3] Within these specific areas of interest, the general aims of epidemiological research in palliative medicine are:

- *to describe* needs and problems of people at the end of their lives and their families in terms of frequency, risk factors (frequency within groups), and trends
- *to explain* the causal relationships between the developing of a particular outcome and the presence of a study factor or exposure. The outcome in palliative medicine is one or more components of the multidimensional concept of quality of life, or other issues that, directly or indirectly, can help to better know and improve the quality of care. The study factors

(the exposure) are the potential determinants of the outcome. These include characteristics of the subject, of the disease, or of the environment

- *to assess the effectiveness of interventions* aimed at modifying the distribution of the problems in the population of interest by prevention of new occurrences, effective treatment of existing cases, or, in general terms, by improving quality of life of affected persons.

High-quality research is required to achieve these aims because of the unique challenges posed by studies focused on terminally ill patients. The choice of appropriate study design is probably the most important factor for the quality of a study. A study design can be defined as the strategy adopted to describe a problem (in descriptive designs), or to test hypotheses and evaluate strengths of associations (in analytical and experimental designs). Each study design has a particular methodology and can investigate particular aims (Table 22.1).

Epidemiological research makes use of observational, quasi-experimental and experimental studies. In observational studies there is no artificial manipulation of the study factors, and events and associations are described and analyzed as they naturally occur. Whenever there is an artificial manipulation of the study factor, the study is (i) experimental if the study factor is randomly allocated to study subjects, and (ii) quasi-experimental if the study factor is allocated without randomization.[2]

Any attempt to rank study designs according to their inherent value makes little sense, since it is the main objective that defines the most appropriate design for a specific study (see Table 22.1).[1] This chapter seeks to help the researcher to identify the most appropriate study design for answering a specific question.

Table 22.1   *Types and general aims of the principal study designs*

Study design	Method used	General aim
Cross-sectional	Observational	Descriptive – analytic
Retrospective cohort study	Observational	Analytic – descriptive
Prospective cohort study	Observational	Analytic – descriptive
Case–control	Observational	Analytic
Quasi-experimental	Experimental without randomization	Analytic
Experimental	Experimental with randomization	Analytic

STUDY DESIGNS

In all study designs, the investigator must be concerned with avoiding any effect or inference that tends to produce results which depart systematically from true values. In other words, the researcher should avoid any kind of bias at any stage of the study, from study design to publication of the results. More than 100 biases have been described.[4] A conceptually appealing classification identifies two general classes of systematic error. The first, selection bias, includes any error that arises in the process of identifying the study population. The second, information bias, refers to any error in the measurement of information on exposure or outcome.

Observational studies

There are three basic designs for observational studies: cross-sectional, case–control and cohort studies. The differences between them are related to the sampling frame and the time frame.

In a **cross-sectional study** subjects are selected from the target population at a particular point in time, regardless of their exposure and disease, and the associations among variables are evaluated.[2] This type of study can be conducted at a specific point in time (e.g. of pain at a specific date), at a fixed point during the course of events (e.g. of pain at hospice admission), or in a specific time window (e.g. of pain during the last month of life).

In a **case–control study** samples of subjects with (cases) and without (controls) a condition are identified, and the groups compared with respect to prior exposure to one or more study factors.[2] The validity of this design depends on the ability to draw valid samples of cases and controls from the target population. In palliative care, it is difficult to identify the whole population of palliative patients, and to appropriately sample cases and controls (for example, patients with and without a symptom). As a consequence, this design, seldom used in palliative care research, will not be discussed in this chapter.

In a **cohort study** (also called longitudinal study) samples of subjects with and without specific characteristics of exposure are followed forward in time from exposure to outcome, and the outcome in persons exposed to the study factor (exposed) is compared with the outcome in persons not exposed to the study factor (unexposed).[2] A cohort study can be done 'prospectively', where the study population is identified at the time the study starts, and then followed over a certain period to assess the outcome; or 'retrospectively', where the study population of exposed and unexposed is identified in the past and the occurrence of the outcome is evaluated in the period elapsed from the time when exposure was assessed to the present.

The choice of a retrospective or prospective design is based essentially on logistic and scientific considerations. Retrospective studies require much less time and resources, because all events have already occurred when the study is initiated. In palliative care, retrospective cohort studies are difficult to perform because information on exposure or outcomes is usually not available retrospectively. In at least two situations this design is possible and potentially useful. The first one refers to palliative care services that routinely assess quality of life using validated tools such the Palliative Outcome Scale as part of quality management programs.[5] In these cases, the 'historical database' of the service can be used to implement retrospective cohort studies. The second situation is for studies assessing 'hard outcomes', such as place of death, easy retrievable for all patients, also retrospectively. At least two limitations should be taken into account. First, data were collected for purposes other than research and their quality can be variable and is sometimes poor.[6] Second, as all information on potential confounders is not routinely collected, the results of the study need to be interpreted cautiously.

Experimental and quasi-experimental designs

In experimental and quasi-experimental designs an intervention is deliberately introduced to observe its effects (the artificial manipulation of the study factor). The general aim of these designs is to study the efficacy (or the effectiveness) of the intervention. Random allocation of the intervention between groups of patients discriminates experimental (with randomization) from quasi-experimental (without randomization) studies.[2] All quasi-experimental and experimental studies are, by definition, prospective.

QUASI-EXPERIMENTAL DESIGNS

A variety of quasi-experimental designs have been proposed: some are not very reliable, others, more sophisticated, allow in some situation a strong causal inference.[7] The validity of the study design depends on the degree of control that the researcher has over several elements of the study design such as the assignment of the patients to different treatments, the measurement of the outcomes, the choice of comparison groups, or the application and the scheduling of the treatment.[7]

In the classic non-equivalent groups design, the two (or more) groups are identified from convenience (patients of different services, hospitals, health districts) or according to their voluntary behavior. The researcher can also compare the subjects of the experimental group with subjects who received a different intervention for the same condition at a different time, generally an earlier period (so called historical controls). In these studies, the control group is selected to be as similar as possible to the intervention groups for all characteristics but the intervention. Matching or stratifying for relevant characteristics, or adjusting for baseline values of the outcomes can increase the comparability between groups.

These designs can prove severely biased when the subjects themselves determine the intervention they receive. People who choose a new therapy or to be followed by an experimental service are likely to be different for many characteristics related to the outcome of interest. Designs less amenable to selection bias are those in which the two groups are selected for factors not related to their preference for the intervention.

EXPERIMENTAL DESIGNS

In experimental studies the population of units selected for the study is split into two (or more) groups using randomization. This procedure ensures that chance alone determines the groups to which each unit is assigned. Each group is assigned to a different intervention, and outcomes in the groups are compared to infer the relative effects of the intervention(s).

Randomization implies that the probability of receiving each of the possible interventions under study is the same for each unit being entered into the study. Notably, this probability does not need to be the same for all interventions being compared. For instance, the researcher may decide to randomly assign 25 percent of the patients to the experimental intervention and 75 percent of the patient to the control (usually the standard intervention), for various reasons (convenience, costs, organizational problems, etc.). This approach is correct as long as these probabilities are the same for all subjects being entered into the study. Randomization is a powerful tool that, if appropriately used, protects the study by the risk of selection bias. Note that randomization does not guarantee that the two groups are identical, even in large samples. However, it does guarantee that the distribution of known and unknown characteristics in the two groups is determined by chance alone.

At least three experimental designs are used in palliative care research: the parallel group design, the crossover design, and the cluster randomization design. In the **parallel design** patients are randomly allocated to receive the intervention(s) of interest (the experimental group) and the best available treatment (the control group). Only if no effective treatment for the condition under study is available, the control group should receive either a placebo or no treatment.[8] In the **crossover trial** patients are given various treatments in sequence, with the aim of studying differences between these treatments.[9] In a randomized crossover trial patients are randomly allocated to different sequences of treatments. In the simplest design (AB/BA design), half of the patients are randomly allocated to receive treatment A followed by B, and half to receive the treatment B followed by A. In **cluster randomization**, the randomization unit is represented by groups of individuals (for instance, all patients of a given health district).[10] This means that all the individuals belonging to that group will receive the same treatment, and that different groups, at random, will receive different treatments.

STUDY AIMS

Descriptive studies

Descriptive studies describe 'patterns of problems occurrence' in relation to variables such as person, place, and time. In palliative care they have been used to describe needs and problems encountered by patients and their families during the advanced and terminal phase of disease.[11]

Two basic designs are used: **cross-sectional** and **longitudinal** studies. The first design, regarded as primarily descriptive, provides a snapshot of the health experience of a population at a given time. The simplest design is relatively inexpensive and quick as compared to longitudinal studies. If well designed, the results from the study sample can be generalized to the population of interest. Moreover, it provides estimates of the prevalence of all factors measured. Studies describing the proportion of patients with severe pain among hospitalized patients,[12] or the prevalence of severe communication problems among patients followed by palliative care services,[13] are classic descriptive studies. The cross-sectional design is not well suited to study rare problems. It has an inherent bias (usually referred to as length biased sampling), since it overrepresents subjects who have the problem for a long duration of time.

Longitudinal studies represent the best way to describe the natural history of a disease in terms of outcomes relevant to palliative care. The main advantage of a longitudinal design is that the individual development of the outcomes of interest over time can be studied. This approach is easy when the outcome variable is an irreversible endpoint. In palliative care most outcomes should be measured in the same individual on different occasions, and viewed in a dynamic prospective over time. To this purpose, a longitudinal design is the best choice, although statistical analysis of its results can be complex.[14]

Apart from the statistical problems, in longitudinal studies researchers deal with a number of methodological issues related to the validity of the results of their descriptive study. A descriptive study is valid in as much as it is able to describe what it intends to in the population from which the sample is drawn. Selection and information bias can compromise the ability of a study to provide information generalizable to the population of interest.[2]

Information bias is a particularly sensitive issue in palliative care, as it is difficult to measure without distortion the 'subjective point of view' of patients experiencing progressive functional and cognitive decline. As far as selection bias is concerned, there is a theoretical and practical difficulty in identifying the population of terminally ill patients in a specific geographical area. At least theoretically, patients with cancer can be identified when they enter the terminal phase of disease and assessed when they are still alive. For most patients dying from noncancer diseases, there is uncertainty about the course of disease, and even theoretically, it is impossible to avoid any selection bias. Also for patients with cancer, it is difficult to plan an unbiased population-based study (either cross-sectional or longitudinal) as these patients are followed by a number of health agencies in all possible different settings of care.

Retrospective studies have tried to overcome these problems using the 'after death' approach, where information is collected after the death of the patient from the non-professional person who attended the patient during the last period of life. This cross-sectional design (but similar in some characteristics to a retrospective cohort design) has been used in a number of influential studies[15–18] to estimate the multidimensional problems experienced by patients during their last period of life. The strength of this design lies in the possibility to evaluate a representative sample of patients with advanced and terminal disease, as the sample is built after deaths have occurred. So far, the most reliable estimates of patients needs during their last year of life derive from the 'after death surveys' conducted in UK between 1969 and 1995.[11] For example, according to these studies, it is possible to estimate that 84 percent of patients with cancer in the last year of life experience pain that requires treatment.[11]

This approach overcomes many of the problems of the studies performed directly on the patients, as it has been possible to generalize the results to the whole population of terminally ill patients. This approach has at least two weaknesses. First, in death certificates, the cause is often unreliable, especially for older patients, or incomplete, especially for noncancer deaths.[19] Second, the assessment of the outcomes from bereaved carers, usually several months after a patient's death, may result in a large distortion of the results.[20]

Analytical observational studies

Analytical studies are epidemiological investigations in which the association between a dependent variable (the outcome of interest) and one or more independent variables is evaluated, and possible cause–effect relations are assessed. Although some implicit or explicit type of comparison exists in all study designs, analytical studies are primarily planned for determining if the frequency of an outcome is different for people exposed to a study factor (exposed) from the frequency of the outcome in those not exposed to the factor (unexposed).

The presence of an association does not imply that the relation between variables is one of cause and effect. We can speak of causal association only when an induced change in the quantity of the study factor results in a corresponding change in the quantity of the outcome. In theory, causality can be definitely demonstrated only through appropriately designed experiments. As a consequence, in observational studies, assessing whether the observed association (or the lack of one) represents a cause–effect relation, is a matter of determining the likelihood that alternative explanations could account for the observed results. In this process, at least three explanations should be considered:

- the observed association could be due to the play of chance
- the association could be the result of a systematic error in the selection of the study subjects (selection bias) or in the assessment of exposure and/or the outcome (information bias)
- the association could be due to the effect of an extraneous factor associated with the study factor that independently affects the risk of outcome (confounding).

It is not possible to summarize in this chapter the long and often sophisticated discussions on the nature of causation and on the methods for identifying causal effects. On this topic, the Bradford–Hill criteria are very popular, and seem to provide a road map through a complicated territory[21,22] (Table 22.2). Although erroneously referred to as 'causal criteria', they simply offer a systematic approach, neither necessary nor sufficient, to infer causation from a statistical association observed in epidemiological data.

The same designs used for a descriptive purpose (cross-sectional and longitudinal) can be used to analyze associations between outcome(s) and possible causative factors. Since in cross-sectional studies, problems and their determinants are collected simultaneously, it is possible to assess a number of associations among them. Using such a design with an analytical intent is often at risk of bias because it is difficult to determine the temporal sequence of the association (if the determinant preceded or resulted from the problem). Cross-sectional designs can be considered for testing hypotheses of association when the determinants are fixed, such as gender, or unalterable over time, or to

Table 22.2   *Bradford–Hill criteria*

Strength	Strong association
Consistency	Repeated observations in different populations under different circumstances
Specificity	The cause leads to a single effect
Temporality	The cause precedes the effect in time
Biologic gradient	Monotonic (unidirectional) dose–response curve
Plausibility	Biological plausibility of the hypothesis
Coherence	The association does not conflict with what is known of the disease
Experimental evidence	Evidence from laboratory experiments on animals or from humans experiments
Analogy	Analogy with similar situations

Table 22.3   *Strengths and weaknesses of cohort (longitudinal) studies*

Strengths	Weaknesses
The best way to study the natural history of a disease and its determinants	Expensive and time consuming
Clear temporal sequence of exposure and outcome	Inefficient for rare outcomes
Possible to evaluate multiple outcomes arising from a single exposure	Selection bias is unavoidable
Efficient for studying rare exposures	
It is possible to estimate incidence and to calculate relative risk	

generate hypotheses of association that will be tested with longitudinal designs.

A well-designed and well-conducted longitudinal study allows a valid inference about risk factors influencing the outcome(s) of interest. A number of variants of the basic design can be used, sometimes difficult to design and analyze.[2] The most important weakness remains the unavoidable presence of a systematic distortion in the estimate of effect resulting from the manner in which subjects are selected for the study population (selection bias) (Table 22.3).

Studies to assess the effectiveness of an intervention

A fundamental objective of epidemiology in the area of palliative medicine is to produce knowledge that might be or is useful to prevent and control a patient's and family's problems during the terminal phase of disease.

Although the randomized clinical trial represents the gold standard for the assessment of the effectiveness of an intervention, observational and quasi-experimental designs can provide, with different degrees of feasibility, validity, and generalizability, useful information for establishing if (and to what extent) an intervention is effective both in clinical and in health services research. The feasibility of a trial depends on its acceptance by all the subjects involved into the research. Clinical staff may be not persuaded about the utility of subjecting very sick and dependent patients to any more experimentation. Patients are not interested in experiments, and randomization is often seen with suspect.[23] As a consequence, the trial could not be accepted, or recruitment could be too slow.

Two criteria are used to assess the quality of a trial: internal and external validity. The internal validity implies an accurate measurement of the effect apart from random errors, but all studies, including randomized ones, are subject to some type of bias. The procedure used to allocate subjects to the different treatments is the major source of bias. In all nonrandomized studies some selection bias is unavoidable, but in observational studies, and in poorly designed quasi-experimental studies where little or no control is possible on allocation procedures, the risk of selection bias is high. For example, in a retrospective study designed to determine whether a palliative home care team modified hospital utilization of patients with cancer in the last 6 months before death, the difference between the two groups (followed and not followed by the service) were significantly different, and the results suggested that the provision of home care reduced days in hospital.[24] Although the two groups were similar for most characteristics of the patients, we must consider that a selection bias could have affected the validity of the results. More specifically, there may have been differences between the groups, for example in the preference for place of care, which would independently affect hospitalization.

Another major source of bias in palliative care studies derives from the patients effectively analyzed for the outcome. In randomized clinical trials the principle of 'intention to treat' is recommended to preserve the internal validity. This approach should be extended, whenever possible, to all effectiveness studies. According to the 'intention to treat' principle, all randomized (or registered) patients should be included in the analyses of results, independent of their effective eligibility, of the received treatment, of the adherence and compliance to the treatments, and of the compliance to the assessments procedures. In palliative care research the attrition rate is usually high and the contamination by exposure (especially in health services research) frequent. Although the problem is common to all study designs, in

Table 22.4 *Differences between explanatory and pragmatic trials*

Explanatory design (the aim is efficacy)	Pragmatic design (the aim is effectiveness)
Selected patients	Patients as similar as possible to the common clinical practice
Sophisticated study protocol	Very simple study protocol
Intensive follow-up	Follow-up as in clinical practice
Multiple and complex endpoints	Simple endpoint (reflecting the benefit to the patient)
High-quality centers	Generic centers
Minimal sample size	Large sample size

nonrandomized studies it is often, mistakenly, considered less important.

External validity refers to the generalizability and applicability of study results. In this regard, an important distinction is that between the efficacy and the effectiveness of an intervention, because it defines the general aim of the study.[25] Efficacy is the extent to which a specific intervention produces a beneficial result under ideal conditions. Effectiveness assesses the same beneficial effect in the field, estimating if it does what it is intended to do for a defined population. The studies require different study designs: explanatory for assessing the efficacy, and pragmatic to assess the effectiveness of an intervention (Table 22.4).

Explanatory studies are aimed at providing the proof of principle that the intervention works (or does not work) under the most favorable conditions. As a consequence the study design is focused on detecting the maximum potential benefit (only trained and skilled centers, highly selected patients, intensive assessment of the outcomes). In these studies the internal validity must be carefully preserved. On the other hand, pragmatic studies are interested at assessing the effectiveness of the intervention in a scenario as similar as possible to everyday practice. As a consequence, patients and centers are not selected, the intervention and follow-up procedures not well codified, but the study reflects the common mistakes typical of every medical practice. In this perspective, the intention to treat approach in the analysis of the results of a study is crucial also to evaluate the true effectiveness of the intervention under study.

In clinical research, explanatory randomized studies (both the crossover and the classic parallel design) on selected patients should be considered as the first option to assess the efficacy of a new intervention. Problems in recruitment could be overcome by implementing collaborative networks of high-quality palliative care units. For these studies the internal validity is crucial, and, also if the planned sample size is not attained, they can be combined with other studies in a systematic review.

When the clinical question becomes more pragmatic, and refers to the ability of the intervention to work in clinical everyday practice, the best design is often a quasi-experimental or an observational study. Note that negative results from a pragmatic trial in the absence of evidence from explicative trials, may lead to the false conclusion that the treatment is not effective at all, and, as a consequence, to discard potentially useful practices.

For health services research the problem is more complicated. Most of the questions are intrinsically pragmatic, and pure randomized explanatory trials are very difficult to conceive. It is difficult to randomize selected series of patients, avoiding any contamination between the groups. To assess the effect of a service, a number of outcomes with their valid, reliable and sensitive tools should be available, and the best timing of the assessments clearly defined. Moreover, new activities are difficult to standardize, so that it is often difficult to be certain that the effect (or the lack of effect) is not due to the intrinsic quality of that specific team.

As a consequence, in the assessment of new services, one might consider the use of a cluster-randomized design, which recent studies report favorably as an alternative method for establishing evidence of effectiveness.[26] A second option is to consider a well-designed quasi-experimental trial, in which the researcher maintains the highest possible control over the elements of the study design, including, of course, the allocation of the subjects to different interventions.

CONCLUSIONS AND FUTURE PRIORITIES

In this chapter, the various study designs commonly used in palliative care research were reviewed and discussed in terms of feasibility, validity, and potential biases. Further methodological research is much needed in palliative care research and particularly in three critical areas:

- the validity of the 'after death' designs and their ability to produce an accurate portrait of the care provided to dying patients, recently questioned in a paper[27]
- advantages and disadvantages of quasi-experimental designs in palliative care research to assess the effectiveness of an intervention, and the identification of the study designs that can provide a high level of internal validity
- the differences between explanatory and pragmatic trials, and their relative role in palliative care research.

Key learning points

- As the design of a study is the strategy of answering a clinical or epidemiological question, it is the question that determines the appropriate study design.

- In studies regarded as primarily descriptive, selection and information bias (in different degrees according to the study design) can compromise the ability of the study to provide information generalizable to the population of interest.

- In analytical observational studies, the architecture of the study design should allow the researcher to assess if the observed associations represent a cause–effect relation, or if alternative explanations could account for the observed results (chance, bias, and confounding).

- Studies aimed at assessing the efficacy or the effectiveness of an intervention require different study designs: explanatory for assessing the efficacy, and pragmatic to assess the effectiveness.

- In clinical research, explanatory randomized studies should be the first option to assess the efficacy of a new intervention, followed by more pragmatic quasi-experimental or observational designs aimed at assessing the beneficial effect on the field.

- For health service research, the questions are intrinsically pragmatic, and pure explanatory trials difficult to conceive. Cluster randomized trials or quasi-experimental designs (with a high control over the elements of the study design) should be considered as the first option for the assessment of a new service.

- The perfect study design for answering a specific question is not always feasible, and often the choice will be based on a compromise between feasibility, validity, and generalizability.

REFERENCES

● 1   Sackett DL, Wennberg JE. Choosing the best research design for each question. *BMJ* 1997; **315**: 1636.

2   Kleinbaum DG, Kupper LL, Morgenstern H, eds. *Epidemiologic Research*. New York: Van Nostrand Reinhold, 1982.

3   Davies E, Higginson IJ, eds. *Palliative Care. The Solid Facts*. Geneva: World Health Organization, 2004.

◆ 4   Sackett DL. Bias in analytic research. *J Chronic Dis* 1979; **32**: 51–63.

5   Hearn J, Higginson HJ. Development and validation of the core outcome measure for palliative care: the palliative care outcome scale. *Qual Health Care* 1999; **8**: 219–27.

6   Johnson JC, Kerse NM, Gottlieb G, *et al.* Prospective versus retrospective methods of identifying patients with delirium. *J Am Geriatr Soc* 1992; **40**: 316–19.

◆ 7   Shadish WR, Cook TD, Campbell DT, eds. *Experimental and Quasi-experimental Designs*. Boston: Houghton Mifflin Company, 2002.

8   Meinert CL, Tonascia S, eds. *Clinical Trials: Design, Conduct, and Analysis*. New York: Oxford University Press, 1986.

◆ 9   Senn S, ed. *Cross-over Trials in Clinical Research*. London: John Wiley, 2002.

10   Campbell MJ, Donner A, Elbourne D. Design and analysis of cluster randomized trials. *Stat Med* 2001; **20**: 329–496.

◆ 11   Higginson IJ. Palliative and terminal care. In: Stevens A, Raftery J, eds. *Health Care Needs Assessment*. Oxford: Radcliff Medical Press, 1997.

12   Costantini M, Viterbori P, Flego G. Prevalence of pain in Italian hospitals: results of a regional cross-sectional survey. *J Pain Symptom Manage* 2002; **23**: 221–3.

13   Higginson IJ, Costantini M. Communication in End-of-Life Cancer care: a comparison of Team Assessment in three European countries. *J Clin Oncol* 2002; **20**: 3674–82.

14   Twisk JWR, eds. *Applied Longitudinal Data Analysis for Epidemiology*. Cambridge: Cambridge University Press, 2003.

● 15   Cartwright A, Hockley L, Anderson JL, eds. *Life Before Death*. London: Routledge and Kegan Paul, 1973.

16   Addington-Hall JM, McCarthy M. The Regional Study of Care for the Dying: methods and sample characteristics. *Palliat Med* 1995; **9**: 27–35.

17   Teno JM, Clarridge BR, Casey V, *et al.* Family perspectives on end-of-life care at the last place of care. *JAMA* 2004; **291**: 88–93.

18   Costantini M, Beccaro M, Merlo F. The last 3 months of life of Italian cancer patients. Methods, sample characteristics and response rate of the Italian Survey of the Dying of Cancer (ISDOC). *Palliat Med* 2005; **19**: 628–38.

19   Gau DW, Diehl AK. Disagreement among general practitioners regarding cause of death. *Br Med J (Clin Res Ed)* 1982; **284**: 239–41.

◆ 20   McPherson CJ, Addington-Hall JM. Judging the quality of care at the end of life: can proxies provide reliable information? *Soc Sci Med* 2003; **56**: 95–109.

21   Phillips CV, Goodman KJ. The missed lessons of Sir Austin Bradford Hill. *Epidemiol Perspect Innov* 2004; **1**: 3.

● 22   Hill AB. The environment and disease: association or causation? *Proc R Soc Med* 1965; **58**: 295–300.

23   Cook AM, Finlay IG, Butler-Keating RJ. Recruiting into palliative care trials: lessons learnt from a feasibility study. *Palliat Med* 2002; **16**: 163–5.

24   Costantini M, Higginson IJ, Boni L, *et al.* Effect of a palliative home care team on hospital admissions among patients with advanced cancer. *Palliat Med* 2003; **17**: 315–21.

● 25   Schwartz D, Lellouch J. Explanatory and pragmatic attitudes in therapeutical trials. *J Chronic Dis* 1967; **20**: 637–48.

26   Fowell A, Russell I, Johnstone R, *et al.* Cluster randomization or randomized consent as an appropriate methodology for trials in palliative care: a feasibility study. *BMC Palliat Care* 2004; **3**: 1.

27   Bach PB, Schrag D, Begg CB. Resurrecting treatment histories of dead patients. *JAMA* 2004; **292**: 2765–70.

23

Outcomes measurement in palliative care research

JOAN M TENO

WHY MEASURE OUTCOMES?

Key to achieving excellence in palliative medicine is a process of self-reflection that measures the end results of care. To not know the outcomes of care is simply not an acceptable medical practice. Without knowledge of the outcomes of care, the quality of care will not be improved. Excellent quality of care is only achieved through a process of ongoing research that examines the outcomes of palliative care programs and medical treatments, audits that help to shape quality improvement efforts to change medical practice, and publicly reported quality indicators. Auditing the quality of care is not just applicable to industrial nations. Rather, program evaluation is important in developing nations with limited resources.[1] While outcomes measures that examine new medications or other treatments are essential for the development of the evidence base of palliative medicine, the focus on this chapter will be on the use of measurement in health services research, quality improvement, and publicly reported quality indicators.

An outcome measure examines the 'end results' of care. The 'end results' are the impact of medical care on the dying person and/or family. For the seriously ill and aged, it is important for the measurement of the outcomes of care to acknowledge the important role of informal caregivers, usually close family members, and that medical care must attend to both the needs of seriously ill persons and those of their family. This view is ratified in the World Health Organization[2] definition of palliative medicine as achieving the best possible quality of life for dying patients *and* their families. Outcomes measures are the ultimate judge of the quality of care. Achieving those outcomes is based on ensuring that processes of care are in place to achieve the desired outcomes. A process measure examines what health providers 'do' for dying persons and their family. Often, process measures can be proxy for outcome measures that can only be examined years later (e.g. the treatment of hypertension and prevention of strokes). Ultimately, the quality of care is based on the outcomes of care. However, a focus on achieving quality of care is to ensure that correct processes of care are undertaken for the right patient.

The natural reaction of staff to outcome measurement is fear that the results will be misinterpreted that they are providing inadequate care. Often, that is hardly the case. Outcome measurement should not be used to 'punish' staff. The vast majority of people come to work every day to do the best possible job within the constraints of current healthcare systems. It is important that the use of outcome measurement is not used to blame staff. Rather, outcomes are the result of complex interactions. It is important that the people assessing the quality of care approach the examinations of outcomes from this perspective. For example, a local hospice found that 80 percent of decedents were dying in the hospital as opposed to at home. One interpretation of these results is the staff are not doing their job in providing adequate supportive care that allows a person to die at home. In this particular example, a further exploration of semi-structured interviews with the staff about the barriers to people dying at home revealed that all home deaths were being treated by the local authorities as potential homicide. Families had learned to avoid the embarrassment of having their loved ones' death be treated as a homicide investigation by insisting that the dying person was transferred to an acute care hospital. The solution is not blaming the staff but making changes to the system of care (e.g. developing an inpatient hospice unit, working with the police to change how expected home deaths are treated, etc.) to ensure that dying persons and their family are receiving medical care consistent with their needs and expectation. This is an important lesson. Achieving excellence in end-of-life care requires a critical examination of the systems and processes of care alongside the outcomes.

WHAT IS QUALITY OF CARE FOR SERIOUSLY ILL AND DYING PERSONS?

Having a serious illness that raises the possibility of mortality is unique and sentinels time of life, unlike any other time period. Consider the following two clinical cases and the implications for measuring the quality of care:

- A 45-year-old man presents with acute anterior wall myocardial infarction. One proposed measure of quality of care by the Center for Medicaid and Medicare Services, the branch of the US government that oversees healthcare services, is whether he is discharged with an aspirin.[3]
- For a person of the same age and gender with stage IV lung cancer, the development of quality indicators that examine both the outcomes and process of care is much more difficult. Not all persons will want active treatment. The vast majority of 45 year olds without a contraindication to aspirin would want to take it given the evidence of its efficacy. Seriously ill persons with lung cancer are faced with important trade-offs where their preferences are important for measuring the outcomes of care.[4]

The importance of patient preferences is reflected in the Institute of Medicine's proposed definition of quality of care as 'the degree in which health services for individuals and populations increase the likelihood of the *desired* health outcome and are consistent with current professional knowledge'[5]. Over the past century, the majority of deaths have been from chronic, progressive illnesses, often involving a decision that weighs the quality versus quantity of life. Despite the early stage of development of quality of measure, there is an evolving consensus regarding what are the key domains to examine the quality of care for seriously ill and/or dying persons (Table 23.1).

To date, various sources of evidence have been used to formulate definitions of quality of medical care for the seriously ill and dying. Professional bodies that rely on expert opinion, such as the National Hospice and Palliative Care Organization[8] or the Canadian Palliative Care Organization have proposed key domains and processes of care that define quality of palliative and/or hospice care. Newer proposed definitions of the quality of care have involved the input of consumers.[10,11] While there is agreement on many key domains, dying persons and their families provide a unique perspective that should be accounted for in definitions of quality of care. Based on experts and focus groups with dying persons and family members, Teno and colleagues have developed a model of quality medical care entitled patient-focused, family centered medical care (see Table 23.1).[10] Under this model, high-quality medical care is achieved when healthcare providers:

- provide the desired physical comfort and emotional support
- promote shared decision making, including advance care planning for future period of impaired decision-making capacity
- treat the dying person with dignity and respect
- attend to the needs of the family for information and skills in providing care for the dying person and support the family at a time prior to and after the patient's death
- coordinate care across settings of healthcare given the increasing fragmentation of the healthcare of the dying.

Over the past decade, a consensus has been emerging regarding what are the key domains to examine both the processes and outcomes of care. In the future, a linking of outcome and process measures to authoritative professional standards, such as the National Consensus Project in the USA,[12] will be critical to the evolution of measurement of quality of care for the seriously ill and dying.

WHAT ARE THE SOURCES OF INFORMATION TO JUDGE THE OUTCOMES OF CARE?

A key step in measuring the outcomes of care is the decision on what is the source of information to judge the outcomes of care. Each source has both advantages and limitations. Often, an audit will need to draw from multiple sources of information to provide a more comprehensive view of care of the seriously ill and dying. Among the available sources of information on the outcomes of the quality of care are:

- the medical record, e.g. one could examine whether patients in pain receive medications for pain
- administrative data, e.g. site of death based on death certificate data
- staff reports of the outcomes of care, e.g. pain noted on the minimum data set (MDS)
- interviews with dying persons and/or their families conducted prior to and after the patient's death
- independent assessment of the quality of care performed by experts.

Each involved trade-offs of strengths, limitations, and financial costs.

The medical record is a legal record that reflects healthcare providers' documentation of the patient's condition

Table 23.1 *Comparison of domains of experts, patients, family members, healthcare providers, and the combined model*

Expert opinion			Consumer opinion			Combined model
Emanuel and Emanuel[6]	IOM[7]	NHO Pathway[8]	Patients with HIV, renal failure on dialysis, and nursing home residents[9]	Patients, families, and healthcare providers	Bereaved family members[10]	New proposed conceptual model of patient-focused, family-centered medical care[10]
Physical symptoms	Overall quality of life	Safe and comfortable dying	Receiving adequate pain and symptom management	Pain and symptom management	Providing desired physical comfort	Provide desired level of physical comfort and emotional support
Psychological and cognitive symptoms	Physical wellbeing and functioning	Self-determined life closure	Avoiding inappropriate prolongation of the dying	Clear decision making	Achieving control over healthcare decisions and everyday decisions	Promote shared decision making
Social relationships and support	Psychosocial wellbeing and functioning	Effective grieving	Achieving sense of control	Preparation for death		Focus on the individual. This includes closure, respect, and patient dignity
Economic demands and care giving demands	Family wellbeing and perceptions		Relieving burdens	Completion	Burden of advocating for quality medical care	Attend to the needs of the family for information, increasing their confidence in helping with patient care and providing emotional support prior to and after the patient's death
Hopes and expectations			Strengthening relationships	Contributing to others	Educating on what to expect, and increasing confidence in providing care	Coordination and continuity of care
Spiritual and existential beliefs				Affirmation of the whole person	Emotional support prior to and after the patient's death	Informing and educating

IOM, Institute of Medicine; NHO, National Hospice Organization; HIV, human immunedeficiency virus.
Based on Teno *et al.*[10]

and treatment decisions. The absence of documentation of a process of care in a chart audit of medical record does provide valuable information, given the legal standard that if it is not documented, it was not done. However, the medical record does reflect that bias of a healthcare provider. For example, the documentation that discharged medications were reviewed with the patient and family may not indicate that the patient and family understood how properly to take the medications after discharge from the hospital.

Administrative data can range from information used for the purpose of billing to death certificate data. Similarly, these data sources reflect the perspective of the healthcare providers. However, these data are often available at minimal costs and can provide important overall descriptive information for program planning. For example, aggregate death certificate data can provide important information on the site of death that can allow for examining changes in

the location of death with time as well as differences among subpopulations such as leading cause of death, age groups, or ethnicity. This information, however, does not provide definitive information on the quality of care. It is important for tracking changes, and information on site of death can provide both hospice and palliative care programs with important information to strategize on where to provide services. For example, the state of Rhode Island, USA, went from twenty-fifth to second in the nation for nursing homes as the site of death.[13] This in itself may not indicate poor quality of care, but provides important information for healthcare providers regarding the importance of developing programs in nursing homes on care of the dying.

In the USA, all nursing homes are required to complete the Resident Assessment Instrument for every nursing home resident on admission, quarterly, and with significant changes in health status. Although the intent of this assessment is care planning, it represents an important source of information to examine some of the key domains. However, the important limitation similar to the other sources of data is ascertainment bias (e.g. pain is underreported when compared to an expert assessor of pain). Given the important role of patient preferences, surveys of dying persons and/or family provide an important source of information about the quality of care. There are important limitations of the typical satisfaction survey item that asks the respondent to rank a particular aspect of care on a scale from 'excellent' to 'poor'. The distribution is often skewed given the reluctance of respondents to use 'fair' or 'poor'. In addition, research has found that a respondent will rate that care is excellent despite reporting severe pain, reflecting the lowered expectations that the respondents have for the level of pain control that can be achieved among the dying. A third limitation is that the typical rating question does not provide information to guide improvement. Knowing that 85 percent of bereaved families rated an aspect of care as 'very good' does not provide information that allows the healthcare provider to improve. However, knowing that one in four people did not understand how to take their pain medications provides a target for improvement that has face validity. Such information can provide information that raises awareness of the opportunity to improve.

WHAT TOOL SHOULD BE USED?

Key to selecting a measurement tool is to first clearly state the goals of measurement. Table 23.2 notes that the audience, focus of measurement, evidence base to justify the use of the measure, and psychometric properties vary based on the intended use of an outcome measure. A measure as part

of an audit for a quality improvement intended audience is the teamworking on improving the quality of care, and the focus of measurement is to provide information that will help select the target for improvement, raise awareness of the opportunity to improve, and monitor whether the quality improvement effort is achieving its stated goals. A measure for public reporting (or accountability) is held to higher standards given the focus is to provide consumers and payers with information to select healthcare providers.[15] It is important that the chosen measure is under the control of that healthcare institution and the psychometric properties have been validated across multiple settings of care.

The selection or development of the measurement tool should receive careful consideration. Too often, researchers and persons conducting an audit ignore the critical steps of ensuring the reliability and validity of the chosen or developed measures. Reliability examines the reproducibility of the measure. Two different nurses using the same chart abstraction tool getting different results would indicate a concern with the reliability of the tool. Achieving reliability is a key step, but not sufficient evidence of the validity of a measurement tool. A measurement tool is valid if there is evidence that it measures the constructs that it purports to measure. Essentially, you are asking 'Is the tool measuring the "truth"?'. Often, there is not a 'gold standard' to judge the validity of the measurement tool. In that situation, the measurement tool should present evidence of the content or face validity, construct, and potentially criterion validity if a 'gold standard' exists.

The content validity essentially asks whether the measurement tool is examining the right constructs. To meet the goal of content validity there should be evidence that the development of the measurement tool was based on a systematic review of the literature, involved experts in the field, and that theoretical model informed the selection of items

Table 23.2 *Purpose of outcome measurements*

	Purpose of measure		
	---	---	---
	Research	Improvement	Accountability
Main audience	Science community	Quality improvement team and clinical staff	Payers; public
Focus of measurement	Knowledge	Understand care process	Comparison
Confidentiality	Very high	Very high	Purpose is to compare groups
Evidence base to justify use of the measure	Builds off existing evidence to generate new knowledge	Important	Extremely important in that proposed domain ought to be under control of that institution
Importance of psychometric properties	Extremely important to that research effort	Important within that setting	Valid and responsive across multiple settings

This table was adapted from Solberg *et al.*[15] and modified from *Journal of Pain and Symptom Management*, **17**, Teno JM, Byock I, Field MJ. Research agenda for developing measures to examine quality of care and quality of life of patients diagnosed with life-limiting illness. White paper from the Conference on Excellent Care at the End of Life through fast-tracking Audit, Standards, and Teamwork (EXCELFAST), September 28–30, 1997. 75–82, Copyright (1999) with permission from The US Cancer Pain Relief Committee.

to include in the outcome measure. Construct validity tests whether known relationships hold with the measurement tool. For example, a survey that examines patient perceptions of the process of care regarding pain management should have at least a moderate correlation with the respondents' overall satisfaction with pain management. Criterion validity examines whether the measure is associated with an accepted 'gold standard' or predicts future outcomes.

Over the past decade, there have been increasing numbers of measures to examine key outcome measures for the seriously ill or dying. Previously, a structured literature review was conducted by the staff at the Center to Improve Care of the Dying and Center for Gerontology and Health Care Research (see www.chcr.brown.edu/pcoc/toolkit.htm[16]) and updated by Lorenz and colleagues[17] for the National Institutes of Health conference on the State of the Science of End of Life Care in December 2004. Each key domain has several potential outcome measures with the majority of measures having psychometric properties reported. However, there are still two important areas for research. First, the responsiveness of measures is often not documented. Responsiveness examines the degree to which an intervention or historical event results in change in the outcome measure. For example, a change in policy regulation that limits access to opioids would be expected to result in different reports of bereaved family members regarding unmet needs for pain medications. Second, many of the instruments have been developed and validated in a population of English-speaking people only. Future research needs to examine whether the same constructs hold in different cultures and, when appropriate, have the instrument translated into other languages.

A common mistake in measurement is the attempt to examine every possible outcome. Rigorous data collection on a small number of items is far superior to any effort that collects a lot of items in a manner where there are concerns about the accuracy of the data collection. This can result in time consuming data collection and raises important concerns in terms of respondent burden, especially when one is interviewing seriously ill or dying persons. Parsimony is important. Winnowing should be based on the goals of measurement and the realization that examining multiple outcomes raises the possibility that one outcome will statistically significantly be based on chance alone. While time is one aspect of individual respondent burden, a second concern is the number of subjects on which data collection occurs. For the purpose of a quality improvement effort, a small number of cases collected from a random sample can provide enough data to guide efforts to select targets for and monitor the rate of improvement. The sample size for research or accountability should be based on the effect size that is required to be able to measure the level of statistical significance, and the probability that you want to be able to find that difference. Statistical software packages such nQuery Advisor 4.0 (Statistical Solutions, USA) allow for estimation of the sample size with these three parameters.

WHOSE OUTCOMES ARE MEASURED?

A key specification of any proposed outcome measure is choosing a numerator (e.g. the number of people with a moderate or excruciating level of pain) and denominator (e.g. all people who are not comatose). At face value, this can seem quite simplistic. However, the difficulty is determining who should be counted among the 'dying' or the denominator. This decision has important implications. Numerous studies have reported the limitation of physicians in prognostication[18] and that prognostic guidelines can be overly specific, but not sensitive.[19] Thus, careful consideration must be given to the specification of the sample. For the dying person, the last month of life often involves transitions in care and flare of symptoms such as pain, dyspnea, etc. Often, a dying person is not able to give interviews during the last month of life. One solution is the mortality follow-back survey that uses death certificates to determine the denominator and contact the next-of-kin. This represents an efficient data collection strategy with important, acknowledged limitations.[20] With this strategy, the denominator is clearly defined. However, family members more accurately report on factual information and their interactions with healthcare providers. Those observations are valuable. Families are less accurate in reports of symptoms and other subjective patient outcomes.[21] This limitation needs to be acknowledged, but one should not ignore the perceptions of bereaved family members. Dame Cicely Saunders, the founder of the modern hospice movement, eloquently stated, 'How people die remains in the memories of those who live on.'[22]

WHAT TO DO WITH CONFLICTING OUTCOME MEASURES?

Often a research effort involves examining multiple sources of data to evaluate an intervention, such as the palliative care team or to conduct an audit of the quality of care that a hospice delivers. Sometimes the results are in conflict. In my experience, this is more likely in an audit or quality improvement effort. For example, an audit of nursing home pain management may use the MDS (i.e. an assessment form completed by nursing home staff), chart review (e.g. whether a complete pain assessment was done on admission to the nursing home), and interviews with cognitively intact nursing home residents regarding their observations of staff efforts in their pain management. Often, these results are in apparent conflict. For example, a nursing home could have a 10 percent prevalence of moderate pain, with the chart review indicating that only 30 percent of residents had a complete pain assessment done on admission and 45 percent of the nursing home residents reporting that they had to wait too long for pain medications. The low prevalence of moderate pain seems in conflict with the other two results. However, this discrepancy is most likely explained by ascertainment bias, in that staff of the nursing home complete the MDS pain items and often, they under-report the pain. The other two indicators provide tangible opportunities for improvement. The goal should be that 100 percent of the people should have a complete pain assessment on admission with as low as possible number of nursing home residents reporting they have to wait too long for pain medication.

CONCLUSION

Knowledge and use of outcome measure is an important tool for healthcare providers with an interest in palliative and hospice medicine. Both process and outcome measures can provide important information to guide efforts to improve quality of care. Outcome measures are key to generating new scientific knowledge of the efficacy of medical treatments and interventions. Key steps to selection of a measure tool is to be clear on the goals of measures including the proposed definition of the quality of care, the proposed source of data, and consideration of the bias and perspective of the source of data. The choice of measurement tools should be based on knowledge of the reliability and validity of the measure. The mistake of collecting information about every possible outcome should be avoided. Rather, a focused data collection effort on a small number of subjects can provide valuable information for quality improvement efforts.

Key learning points

- Assessment of processes and outcomes is an important and essential part of examining the quality of palliative care in all settings.

- Consumer preferences are an important aspect of examining the quality of end-of-life care.

- Valid and reliable measures are needed whatever the purpose.

- Strengths and limitations of various sources of information need to be considered in the selection of measures and interpretation of results.

- Different purposes of measurement mean that different measures may need to be used.

- It is unwise and usually impractical to try to measure everything. Rather, a small amount of information collected on a random sample of subjects can guide quality improvement efforts.

REFERENCES

1 Higginson IJ, Bruera E. Do we need palliative care audit in developing countries? *Palliat Med* 2002; **16**: 546–7.

2 World Health Organization. *Cancer Pain Relief and Palliative Care: Report of a WHO Expert Committee*. Geneva: World Health Organization, 1990. Technical Report Series No. 804.

3 Jencks SF, Cuerdon T, Burwen DR, *et al*. Quality of medical care delivered to Medicare beneficiaries: A profile at state and national levels. *JAMA* 2000; **284**: 1670–6.

4 Teno JM. Putting the patient and family voice back into measuring the quality of care for the dying. *Hosp J* 1999; **14**: 167–76.

5 Institute of Medicine, Lohr KN, ed. *Medicare: A Strategy for Quality Assurance*. Washington, DC: National Academy Press, 1990.

6 Emanuel EJ, Emanuel LL. The promise of a good death. *Lancet* 1998; **351**(Suppl 2): SII21–SII29.

7 Institute Of Medicine. Committee on Care at the End of Life, Field MJ, Cassel CK, eds. *Approaching Death: Improving Care at the End of Life*. Washington, DC: National Academy Press, 1997.

8 National Hospice Organization. *A Pathway for Patients and Families Facing Terminal Illness: Self-Determined Life Closure, Safe Comfortable Dying and Effective Grieving*. Alexandria, VA: National Hospice Organization, 1997.

9 Singer PA, Martin DK, Kelner M. Quality end-of-life care: patients' perspectives. *JAMA* 1999; **281**: 163–8.

10 Teno JM, Casey VA, Welch L, Edgman-Levitan S. Patient-focused, family-centered end-of-life medical care: views of the guidelines and bereaved family members. *J Pain Symptom Manage Special Section on Measuring Quality of Care at Life's End II*. 2001; **22**: 738–51.

11 Steinhauser KE, Clipp EC, McNeilly M, *et al*. In search of a good death: observations of patients, families, and providers. *Ann Intern Med* 2000; **132**: 825–32.

12 National Consensus Steering Committee. Clinical Practice Guidelines for Quality Palliative Care. May, 2004. Available at: www.nationalconsensusproject.org/ (accessed October 12, 2005).

13 Teno JM. Facts on Dying: Brown Atlas Site of Death 1989–1997. Available at: www.chcr.brown.edu/dying/factsondying.htm (accessed February 26, 2004).

14 Teno JM, Byock I, Field MJ. Research agenda for developing measures to examine quality of care and quality of life of patients diagnosed with life-limiting illness. White paper from the Conference on Excellent Care at the End of Life through Fast-Tracking Audit, Standards, and Teamwork (EXCELFAST), September 28–30, 1997. *J Pain Symptom Manage* 1999; **17**: 75–82.

15 Solberg LI, Mosser G, McDonald S. The three faces of performance measurement: improvement, accountability, and research. *Jt Comm J Qual Improv* 1997; **23**: 135–47.

16 TIME: Toolkit of Instruments to Measure End-of-life care. www.chcr.brown.edu/pcoc/toolkit.htm (accessed October 6, 2005).

17 Lorenz K, Lynn J, Morton SC, *et al*. *End-of-Life Care and Outcomes. Summary, Evidence Report/Technology Assessment: Number 110. AHRQ Publication Number 05-E004-1, December 2004*. Rockville, MD: Agency for Healthcare Research and Quality, 2004. Available at www.ahrq.gov/clinic/epcsums/eolsum.htm (accessed October 13, 2005).

18 Teno JM, Coppola KM. For every numerator, you need a
    denominator: a simple statement but key to measuring the
    quality of care of the 'dying'. *J Pain Symptom Manage* 1999;
    17: 109–13.

19 Fox E, Landrum McNiff K, *et al.* Evaluation of prognostic
    criteria for determining hospice eligibility in patients with
    advanced lung, heart, or liver disease. SUPPORT Investigators.
    Study to Understand Prognoses and Preferences for Outcomes
    and Risks of Treatments. *JAMA* 1999; **282**: 1638–45.

20 Addington-Hall J, McPherson C. After-death interviews with
    surrogates/bereaved family members. some issues of validity.
    J Pain Symptom Manage 2001; **22**: 784–90.

21 McPherson C, Addington-Hall J. Judging the quality of care at
    the end of life: can proxies provide reliable information. *Soc Sci
    Med* 2003; **56**: 95–109.

22 Saunders C. Pain and impending death. In: Wall PD, Melzack R,
    eds. *Textbook of Pain*. Edinburgh: Churchill Livingstone, 1989:
    624–31.

24

Ethics in palliative care research

JONATHAN KOFFMAN, FLISS MURTAGH

INTRODUCTION

Palliative care has at its core not only the discipline of rigorous symptom control but also the need for patient-centered communication, holistic care of the patients and their families, the consideration of advance directives including patient preferences for place of care and death, and respect for spiritual and religious beliefs of patients and families.[1] Palliative care as a specialty remains unique in its contribution to patient and family care, but the fundamental ethical principles underpinning the conduct of medical research are identical to those in primary, secondary, and tertiary care. Where or how the research takes place should not affect the standards laid down in national and international guidelines such as the Declaration of Helsinki and the Belmont Report (as discussed later). However, the application of these guidelines, and their underlying principles, may have specific implications for particular types of research carried out in palliative care, and for the health and social care professionals involved. Given that palliative care is a relatively new specialty, the volume of research conducted is increasing. This includes exploration of disease groups and symptoms associated with advanced disease that are potentially amenable to palliative care intervention,[2–5] the context in which care is provided,[6–8] cost-effectiveness of service provision,[9] and provider effects, including how care is delivered and received by an increasingly diverse society.[10,11] The impact of the proliferation of 'evidence-based guidelines' for managing advanced disease is also an all-pervading concern.[12] These areas, among others, were the subject of a recent National Institutes of Health State-of-the-Science Conference in end-of-life care.[13]

One of the most useful issues raised by the State-of-the-Science Conference summary statement were the ethical concerns associated with palliative and end-of-life research.[13] Expansion of research in palliative care requires more than merely transposing traditional clinical trials, methods of health services research, or epidemiological methodologies into the specialty. New methods and research approaches need to be developed and refined to explore the complex clinical, psychosocial, and service and policy-related situations seen in palliative care. There has been some discussion of the theoretical and practical problems of research in palliative care and approaches to developing high-quality rigorous research[14–16] but less discussion of the ethical

---

Box 24.1 Key terms

- *Research* is defined as any form of disciplined inquiry that aims to contribute to a body of knowledge or theory

- *Research ethics* refers to the moral principles guiding research, from its inception through to completion and publication of results and beyond

- *Human participants* (or subjects) are defined as including living human beings, human beings who have recently died (cadavers, human remains and body parts), embryos and fetuses, human tissue and body fluids, and human data and records (such as, but not restricted to medical, genetic, financial, personnel, criminal, or administrative records and test results including scholastic achievements)

issues raised. Research in palliative care may raise different ethical questions to other specialties, including the nature of the study design, issues of consent, the balance of benefits versus the risks of involvement in research, what is considered a potential harm, and the importance of confidentiality. In this chapter we apply the historical perspective of ethics in relation to medical research to palliative care, appraise international codes that guide ethical frameworks in research, describe a practical approach to research ethics, and discuss important ethical challenges when undertaking palliative care research. Box 24.1 defines some key terms.

A HISTORICAL PERSPECTIVE ON RESEARCH ETHICS

There are historical reasons why the regulation of clinical and health research involving patients differs from the regulation of normal clinical practice. The horrific medical experiments conducted by a number of doctors under the Nazi regime led to the first internationally agreed guidelines on research involving people, the Nuremberg Code of 1947.[17] This consisted of 10 principles that were finally incorporated into the Declaration of Helsinki produced by the World Medical Association in 1964, an international body set up soon after the Second World War to represent doctors, and funded by national medical associations. The Declaration has been revised no less than five times since 1964, the last being in 2000, and a further note of clarification was added in 2002[18] (see Box 24.2).

Box 24.2 Extracts from the Declaration of Helsinki (2002) with particular considerations in palliative research (our italics)

1 The World Medical Association has developed the Declaration of Helsinki as a statement of ethical principles to provide guidance to physicians and other participants in medical research involving human subjects. Medical research involving human subjects includes research on identifiable human material or identifiable data.

5 In medical research on human subjects, considerations related to the well-being of the human subject should take precedence over the interests of science and society.

7 In current medical practice and in medical research, most prophylactic, diagnostic and therapeutic procedures involve *risks and burdens*.

---

10 It is the duty of the physician in medical research to protect the life, health, privacy, and dignity of the human subject.

13 The design and performance of each experimental procedure involving human subjects should be clearly formulated in an experimental protocol. This protocol should be submitted for *consideration, comment, guidance*, and where appropriate, *approval to a specially appointed ethical review committee, which must be independent of the investigator, the sponsor, or any other kind of undue influence*.

15 Medical research involving human subjects should be conducted only by scientifically qualified persons and under the supervision of a clinically competent medical person. *The responsibility for the human subject must always rest with a medically qualified person and never rest on the subject of the research, even though the subject has given consent.*

20 The subjects must be *volunteers and informed participants* in the research project.

29 The *benefits, risks, burdens*, and *effectiveness* of a new method should be tested against those of the best current prophylactic, diagnostic, and therapeutic methods. This does not exclude the use of placebo, or no treatment, in studies where no proven prophylactic, diagnostic, or therapeutic method exists.

30 At the conclusion of the study, every patient entered into the study should be assured of access to the *best proven prophylactic, diagnostic, and therapeutic methods identified by the study*.

Source: World Medical Association[18]

The Declaration has been significant in its influence in setting ethical standards for medical and human research.[19] However the latest version has not been without its critics. In particular, disagreement has focused on clauses 29 and 30 (see Box 24.2) and concern has been voiced about the potential exploitation of research subjects in developing countries.[20] These clauses have also been criticized for being too crude and absolute, and that they may even be damaging to the very research subjects they are intended to protect by unintentionally limiting research in those countries.[21] This has serious implications for palliative care research, and particularly for research that takes place in developing countries. The reasons for this include increasing evidence that double standards are frequently adopted in the quality of clinical trials that could never pass ethical muster in the sponsoring country.[22]

The current version of the Declaration has also been criticized for its overly expansive remit. It now includes all forms of medical research.[23] It has, for example, changed its designation from 'recommendations for doctors', to that of 'ethical principles for everybody involved in research'. Medical research in general, and palliative care research in particular, are frequently an interdisciplinary exercise, and there are times when research is either inadequately conceptualized or not addressed at all in the Declaration of Helsinki. The focus of the Declaration was originally, and still is, the *conduct of human experiments*: the frequent use of the term 'experimentation' in the current version of the Declaration is just one manifestation of this. Doll states that the Declaration only really applies to 'research in which patients are required to take drugs or have invasive procedures' (a relatively small part of palliative research) but that 'even here, however, some of the principles show a lack of understanding of what their effects would be if rigidly applied'.[23]

RESEARCH ETHICS COMMITTEES

The Declaration of Helsinki stipulates that any research involving any human subjects should be reviewed by a properly constituted research ethics committee (REC) or institutional review board (IRB). As a result, many countries throughout the world now have strict regulations governing the formation and procedure of such bodies. The Netherlands, Belgium, and the USA have specific legislation in this area.[24–26] Until recently, the UK adhered to a regulatory system controlled by government, but not by legislation.[27] Following implementation of the EU Clinical Trials Directive in 2004, UK research ethics committees now have a basis in law. Their accountability is also clearly defined: they are answerable to strategic health authorities in England and to the Central Office of Research Ethics Committees (COREC).

Both RECs and IRBs are responsible for ensuring that they act independently within their institutions. They must be free from bias and undue influence from the institution in which they are located, from the researchers whose proposals they consider and from the personal or financial interests of their members.[28] This independence is founded on its membership, on strict rules regarding conflict of interests and on regular monitoring of and accountability for decisions made. The membership of an REC or IRB must ensure that it has the range of expertise and the breadth of experience necessary to provide competent and rigorous review of the research proposals submitted to it, and to do so from a position that is independent of both the researchers and the institution in which it is located. They should be multidisciplinary and consist of both men and women, as well as reflecting other aspects of diversity within society.[29] There must also be members who have broad experience of and expertise in the areas of research regularly reviewed and who have the confidence and esteem of the research community. This can be problematic with palliative care research given the limited number of ethics committee members who have experience of such research. End-of-life care is typically characterized by a focus on symptom control with minimum interference and intervention. Many RECs and IRBs are reluctant to approve studies in this group of patients. It has been suggested that this might be so because of misconception that research studies may detract from the ethos of care, that studies are unlikely to be supported by previous good research in the field, and because of the perceived vulnerability of research participants. In addition, even when studies are approved, extensive gate-keeping by health professionals may create future barriers to recruitment.[30]

For all their good, RECS and IRBs are not without their critics. It has been stated that they are risk averse,[31] and that they concentrate disproportionately on the information about a study that will be given to potential participants.[32] This includes the manner in which consent is recorded (the expectation is usually a signed consent form for each participant) and the justification and special procedures required for studies involving children, or mentally incompetent or otherwise vulnerable adults. However, given the emphasis on the production of information sheets for clinical trials or other research, there are still some participants who do not fully understand the information they have been given as part of the procedure to obtain consent for their participation.[33,34] As with research involving children or other vulnerable patients,[35,36] the closer scrutiny of research involving patients with advanced disease may necessitate that palliative care researchers need to invest more time, effort, and ingenuity in developing consent procedures to gain approval for their studies.[37] This may bring benefits in the protection of patients, and it may also result in fewer evaluated interventions and services for these groups.

A PRACTICAL APPROACH TO RESEARCH ETHICS

Three broad areas of ethical concern outlined by Foster[38] have been identified in relation to research:

- Duty of care to research participants
- Respect for the rights and autonomy of research participants
- The scientific validity of the research (without which no research can be ethically justified).

These areas approximate to different moral and philosophical traditions. Duty of care derives from duty-based deontological thinking, which acknowledges that there are rules of conduct which ought to be followed, not because of the ends that are likely to be achieved, but by the nature of those involved and their inherent responsibilities. Respect for rights derives from rights-based deontological traditions, which recognize the right of each person to self-determination and autonomy. Emphasis on the scientific validity of research

Table 24.1   *Ethical principles guiding medical research*

Ethical principles derived from Beauchamp and Childress[39] and Gillon[40]	Ethical principles derived from the Belmont Report[41]
Respect for autonomy: This implies self-rule, but is probably better described as deliberated self-rule, a special attribute of all moral agents. If we have autonomy we can make our own decisions on the basis of deliberation. In healthcare, respecting people's autonomy has many *prima facie* implications. It requires consulting people and obtaining their agreement before we do things to them	**Respect for persons:** Incorporates at least two ethical convictions: first, that individuals should be treated as autonomous agents, and second, that persons with diminished autonomy are entitled to protection
Beneficence: Whenever healthcare professionals try to help others they inevitably risk harming them. Those who are committed to helping others must therefore consider the principles of beneficence and aim at producing net benefit over harm	**Beneficence:** Persons are treated in an ethical manner not only by respecting their decisions and protecting them from harm, but also by making efforts to secure their wellbeing. Such treatment falls under the principle of beneficence
Nonmaleficence: An obligation not to inflict harm intentionally, that is distinct from that of beneficence – an obligation to help others. In codes of medical practice the principle of nonmaleficence (*primum non nocere*) has been a fundamental tenet	**Justice:** Who ought to receive the benefits of research and bear its burdens? This is a question of justice, in the sense of 'fairness in distribution' or 'what is deserved.' An injustice occurs when some benefit to which a person is entitled is denied without good reason or when some burden is imposed unduly. Another way of conceiving the principle of justice is that equals ought to be treated equally
Justice: This is often regarded as being synonymous with fairness and can be summarized as the moral obligation to act on the basis of fair adjudication between competing claims	
Scope: There may be agreement about substantive moral commitments and *prima facie* moral obligations of respect for autonomy, beneficence, nonmaleficence, and justice. Yet there still may be disagreement about their scope of application, that is, about to whom do we owe these moral obligations	

draws on goal-based moral theory (consequentialism) which judges the moral worth according to predicted or actual outcomes. These different but complementary philosophical approaches have been used by Claire Foster to derive a framework for the consideration of research ethics,[38] and this can be a useful way to review any specific research project. Dilemmas or tensions which arise usually occur because of conflict between these different moral approaches; in palliative research it is particularly important to recognize the reasons why conflict arises, the moral arguments in support of each approach, and then aim to achieve an acceptable balance between these different ethical demands.

These three broad areas of ethical concern can more simply be viewed as based on key ethical principles[39,40] and each principle should be applied in the context of any one research study (Table 24.1). But ethical considerations should be wider than just the single research study or group of studies. Allocation of research resources, cost-effectiveness (of both research and the interventions evaluated), population benefit (and harm), and overall public health must all be considered, and here the concepts of justice and equity become important. The experience of individual research participants and the conduct of the researchers themselves are also important considerations, which introduce concepts of fidelity, trust, and truthfulness.

THE SPECIFIC ETHICAL CHALLENGES IN PALLIATIVE CARE RESEARCH

There has been extensive debate about whether research in palliative care raises ethical challenges unique to the specialty.[30,42] Particular ethical challenges in palliative research include research-related distress and the perceived vulnerability of participants; research burden for ill patients; consent and capacity issues; ensuring confidentiality and anonymity; and the methodological challenge of producing high-quality research, including the contribution of the randomized controlled trial (RCT).

Research-related distress and vulnerability of research participants

In Foster's ethical framework,[38] it is duty of care which requires that distress and vulnerability are given careful ethical consideration. It is often perceived that interviews, surveys, or questionnaires about end-of-life care may be distressing to those interviewed, whether patients or their unpaid informal caregivers. Indeed, patients with advanced disease often experience many distressing symptoms and are frequently fatigued, frail, depressed, and heavily dependent on others.[43–46] Questions therefore need to be raised regarding whether it is ethical to engage these patients in research at a time when they may wish to make use of their remaining time with their family and friends. Given that many of these patients will not stand to benefit directly from the research they are involved in it could be argued that it is unreasonable and unethical for them to offer their remaining time,[47] as well as a host of concerns that research in palliative care should be wary of including those patients with disease who are particularly vulnerable as they represent a captive audience.[48] Some have even suggested that research involving dying patients is, because of this vulnerability, ethically unacceptable.[49] Few would currently accept that position, and a contrary argument, that it is unethical *not* to undertake palliative research because this diminishes the ability to provide patients with a high standard of evidence-based care, is much more widely accepted. There is no doubt, however, that it is sensible to pay additional attention to the rights of palliative patients who take part in research, and the ways in which those rights will be protected, in the same way that other vulnerable groups such as the elderly or cognitively impaired are considered. This approach has been adopted in a number of countries, with, for example, the Office of Human Research Protections in the USA classifying terminally ill patients as a 'special class' for research purposes.[50] Incorporating the 'user voice' is another way to endeavor to protect the rights of vulnerable research participants, and to ensure that the patient perspective influences research goals.[51]

It has also been suggested that those patients who are cared for within inpatient hospice settings may believe that refusing to participate in a study may result in their discharge. Some patients may be experiencing severe pain and rely on healthcare professionals to administer pain relief in addition to tending to intimate care needs. It has therefore been suggested that this entirely appropriate reliance on healthcare professionals means that it is unethical to ask patients to participate in research because they may well feel coerced into doing so, or may be unwilling to give an honest appraisal of the care they have received.[52] Other evidence does not support this; on the contrary many patients and their informal caregivers are very willing to participate in research.[53–55] The reasons that may account for this include altruism, defined as a desire to increase a third party's welfare.[56] Other important interrelated factors may involve gaining a sense of purpose from participation, and finding the overall experience of being involved in research cathartic and helpful.[55,57]

Although post-bereavement research has been shown to carry a small risk of distress, this has been shown to be much less than expected, and this distress was often outweighed by the benefits of open discussion.[58] Seamark *et al.* have also demonstrated low levels of distress in post-bereavement interviews.[59]

Research burden: balancing risk against benefit

The risks and benefits of research in palliative care are often hard to assess comprehensively because of the limited preexisting evidence. The frequent heterogeneity of study populations also makes weighing up risk and benefit difficult. In general, palliative research participants are likely to be at greater overall risk, because of their advanced disease and the nature of end-of-life care.

As previously mentioned, RECS and IRBs have tended to be reluctant to permit palliative patients to be burdened, and professionals may 'gate-keep' to protect patients from research because of perceptions about their frailty and distress,[54] which concur with the perception of this research group as vulnerable, as discussed above.

Consent and capacity

Informed consent and the patients' capacity to consent are prerequisites if any research in palliative care is going to be conducted. Until recently, however, there has been little consideration or practical advice for palliative care research regarding the methodological challenges of informed consent.[60] There are reasons why consent deserves additional consideration in palliative care research. Patients involved in these studies are drawn from a population with a high prevalence of characteristics that make informed consent challenging, with those who enroll in palliative care studies often being seriously ill. These issues are important given that research ethics committees scrutinize the consent process very closely, particularly when a study involves patients near the end of life.

In order for consent to be valid, it must be informed, voluntary, and given by a research participant with full decision-making capacity. Research consent procedures need to be planned carefully, with detailed consideration of the expected prevalence of impaired capacity, and how capacity should be assessed. An important question is how extensive and detailed assessment of decision-making capacity should be. This depends to a large extent on the level of impairment of capacity expected within a study population, whether participants with impaired capacity will be included in or excluded from the research, and the risks and benefits associated with the research – higher risk demanding correspondingly greater effort to protect the rights of participants.[60] Palliative care patients often have high levels of cognitive impairment and hence potentially impaired capacity,[61] so exclusion from research is self-defeating. If a formal assessment of capacity is required (only likely in those studies associated with greater risk), then a number of tools have been developed, or modified,[62] to guide the decision-making process about which patients may be eligible for inclusion in a study (see Box 24.3).

Box 24.3 The MacArthur Competency Assessment Tool modified for clinical research (MacCAT-CR)

The MacCAT-CR consists of a series of scripted interview questions, divided into four sections that relate to four domains of decision-making capacity. The MacCAT-CR is scored on a scale of 0–2. Incorrect and correct responses are scored as 0 and 2, respectively. Responses that are difficult to interpret are scored as 1.

Understanding (total possible score = 26)
The subject understands:

- the purpose of the study is to test the effectiveness of a case-management intervention (2)
- the study lasts 1 year (2)
- the study requires two additional procedures (two questions) (4)
- the effectiveness of the intervention is unknown (2)
- not all subjects will receive the intervention (2)
- subjects who do not receive the intervention must complete surveys and undergo health evaluations (2)
- the intervention will be assigned at random (2)
- how the study results will benefit future patients (2)
- how subjects in the study may benefit (2)
- the study imposes two additional burdens (two questions) (4)
- subjects can refuse to participate or can withdraw from the study without penalty (2)

Appreciation (total possible score = 6)
The subject appreciates that he or she:

- would not be asked to be in the study solely for his or her personal benefit (2)
- would not be assigned to receive the intervention or not based on his or her needs (2)
- can refuse to participate or can withdraw from the study without penalty (2)

Reasoning (total possible score = 8)
The subject is able to:

- describe two reasonable consequences of participating in the study (2)
- compare the merits of participating versus not participating (2)
- give two examples of the impact of participating on his or her everyday life (2)
- express a choice that is consistent with the consequences that he or she has described (2)

Choice (total possible score = 2)

- The subject is able to express a choice about whether or not to enroll (2)

Reproduced with permission from Grisso et al.[62]

When a research subject does not have capacity, as is common in the last days or weeks of life, then several considerations are important.[63] First, ethical consideration of the research risks and benefits must be reevaluated in the context of lack of capacity; how much risk is the individual participant exposed to by participating, and is the overall likely benefit of the research substantial? Second, the precise role of a proxy, such as a relative, in the consent process must be considered. Third, incapacity is variable and not always total: a participant may be able to give consent at some level, and it is important to include this within the consent process. Lastly, alternative consent procedures might be necessary, especially in the final days of life, such as the advanced consent suggested by Rees and Hardy.[37]

Confidentiality and anonymity

Most clinical or health research involves collecting patient data, which should always be kept confidential and anonymous. Palliative care research is no exception. A researcher could be found negligent if reasonable precautions were not taken to ensure that all the information gained during a study was not stored in a secure manner or if the identity of a research subject was compromised. Further, information resulting from a part of a study should not be shared with a third party unless there is explicit consent of the research subject. This requirement is underpinned by the ethical principle of autonomy. In quantitative studies these obligations are more straightforward, with the use of unique identifying codes in place of names. In qualitative research, however, the data collection process requires more prolonged face-to-face contact, and makes researcher–participant anonymity more challenging. Pseudonyms can be used in place of actual names in written reports and publications. Participant confidentiality can be further protected through the omission of identifying of key contextual details and circumstances. However, the reality of small sample sizes and the detailed descriptions which accompanies this information may be recognizable to some readers familiar with the setting.

Ethical challenges among disadvantaged patient or population groups

Ill health, chronic diseases, high levels of comorbidity, polypharmacy, cognitive impairment, and fatigue frequently challenge or prevent an individual's ability to consent and then participate in palliative care research. However, there are other patient and population-related factors that may operate in isolation or in combination to further complicate this situation. These include very old patients, those with learning disabilities, and those from black and minority ethnic communities, to name just a few. It has been suggested that because of these difficulties these groups may be excluded from research or may be particularly vulnerable.[64–68]

Older people represent a heterogeneous group where competency and capacity vary considerably. Indeed many will have no problems with consent and will be able to participate in research. At a purely practical level, however, others may be excluded as a result of their inability to consent due to poor vision or as a result of hearing problems.[69] The type of research older people are invited to engage with also needs to be considered. It has been suggested that frail older people, who would probably not be competent for inclusion in a pharmaceutical trial because they may have difficulties understanding the extent of their involvement and possible implications for their health, may, however, still be eligible to participate in research if it involved noninvasive, semi-structured interviews, to discuss their experiences of advanced disease or service use.[70]

In the past, individuals with learning disabilities were sometimes chosen as research participants precisely because they were less capable of understanding what was being done to them and were less likely to object.[71] There are many different kinds and degrees of learning disability, and many patients, depending on the extent of the disability, will be able to consent on their own behalf. Ensuring that the consent is indeed informed may be more difficult and require special skills in conveying the relevant information, but it should be attempted wherever at all possible. Even if patients can give consent, it is always advisable for it to be witnessed by a relative.

To date, there has been very little published research about engaging patients from black and minority ethnic communities and refugees in palliative care research.[66] Since these population groups have traditionally been socially excluded from mainstream health services research they have been referred to as 'invisible' or 'elusive' populations. Their notable absence and unheard voices in research therefore reflects their position on the periphery of society.[72] Where they are identified and recruited, research considerations include those described above. Heterogeneity will be evident and naturally many will be able to consent. Those persons who do not possess adequate language skills either may be excluded from the research or may have to rely upon family members or advocates to translate for them. Given the many sensitivities associated with palliative care researchers need to be aware that confidentiality may become compromised, or in order to prevent this, the respondent, the family member, or advocate, may distort realities to protect privacy.

Methodological challenges and the use of RCTs

The type of research methodology employed during palliative care research poses interesting ethical questions. While quantitative studies often place considerable time and energy demands on dying patients, participation in qualitative studies, which frequently explore issues in considerable detail, may create an emotional burden for patients and their families.[73] Qualitative interactions often become highly personal and interpersonal, and in that context, may be even more intrusive than with quantitative approaches.[74] The researcher comes to know the interviewees in a more intimate manner. Interviews that raise issues such as terminal illness, suffering, and loss may bring research participants' feelings to the fore, feelings that may have been previously largely suppressed. These undisclosed problems may then be exposed with serious consequences. Johnson and Plant[75] and others[57] have reported that, in their interviews with cancer patients, participants sometime reported they were emotionally troubled as a result of reminders of their diagnosis, experienced upset feelings in response to talking about their illness, and began to question if their condition might be more serious than they had assumed.

Randomized controlled trials raise particular issues in palliative research. Traditionally, the RCT has been viewed as the gold standard for conducting clinical research.[76] Proponents of RCTs argue that where there is uncertainty, randomization minimizes the risks of exposure to unevaluated hazards. Although in select situations RCTs have been successfully employed in palliative care research, for example examining the management of pain,[77] breathlessness,[78] and the enhancement of advanced directives,[79] they are not without their problems[15] or ethical challenges.[80] Randomization can partially involve relinquishing individualized care and for some patients, the forgoing of potential benefits to new treatment or care. McWhinney and colleagues endeavored to minimize the potential of the latter[81] during an evaluation of a palliative care home support team based in an inpatient unit. Patients in the study group received a service immediately, whereas those in the control group received the service a month later. The two groups were then compared after a period of one month using measurement of symptoms levels and patients' quality of life. The trial however failed. The reasons advanced for this included high rates of attrition due to death, and low compliance rates due to very sick and weak patients. Knowing this, health professionals too may have been reluctant to cooperate with the study, discouraging recruitment.

CONCLUSION

The ethical issues in palliative care research need to be understood in the context of the historical background of research ethics, and the national and international frameworks which already exist to inform ethical standards in research. Having said this, both impose some constraints on present day palliative research, having been developed primarily for research in different contexts. Imaginative and intelligent ways to refine existing research methodologies, develop new ones, and to work with the vulnerabilities of palliative research participants need to be found. There are ways to respect patient autonomy, minimize harm, and reduce research burden. But these are not always easy to find, nor encouraged within existing structures for ethical review.

Key learning points

- Historically, research among human subjects was not governed by guiding ethical principles. This had catastrophic consequences.

- International guidelines, notably the Declaration of Helsinki, relating to health research now advocate ethical review, and RECs and IRBs are an almost worldwide phenomena.

- In many countries, RECs and IRBs now have a basis in law, their accountability is clearly defined and their performance regularly audited.

- Ethical regulation of medical research on humans provides essential reassurance that the risk of harm has been minimized for all participants.

- Palliative care research raises unique methodological and therefore ethical challenges. These include research-related distress and the perceived vulnerability of participants; research burden for ill patients; consent and capacity issues; ensuring confidentiality and anonymity; and the methodological challenge of producing high-quality research, including the contribution of the RCT.

REFERENCES

1 World Health Organization. *National Cancer Control Programmes: Policies and Managerial Guidelines*, 2nd ed. Geneva: World Health Organization, 2002.

2 Oneschuk D, Bruera E. The potential dangers of complementary therapy use in a patient with cancer. *J Palliat Care* 1999; **15**: 49–52.

3 Lan LK, Chidgey J, Addington-Hall JM, Hotopf M. Depression in palliative care: a systematic review. Part 2 Treatment. *Palliat Med* 2002; **16**: 279–84.

4 Ross JR, Saunders Y, Edmonds PM, *et al.* Systematic review of the role of bisphosphonates in metastatic disease: skeletal morbidity. *BMJ* 2005; **327**: 469–72.

5 Jones B, Finlay I, Ray A, Simpson B. Is there still a role for open cordotomy in cancer pain management? *J Pain Symptom Manage* 2003; **25**: 179–84.

6 Higginson IJ. It would be NICE to have more evidence? *Palliat Med* 2004; **18**: 85–6.

7 Higginson IJ, Finlay IG, Goodwin DM, *et al.* Is there evidence that palliative care teams alter end-of-life experiences of patients and their caregivers? *J Pain Symptom Manage* 2003; **25**: 150–68.

8 Salisbury C, Bosanquet N, Wilkinson EK, *et al.* The impact of different models of specialist palliative care on patient's quality of life: a systematic literature review. *Palliat Med* 1999; **13**: 3–17.

9 Douglas HR, Normand CE, Higginson IJ, et al; Palliative Day Care Project Group. Palliative day care: what does it cost to run a centre and does attendance affect use of other services? *Palliat Med* 2003; **17**: 628–37.

10 Koffman J, Higginson IJ. Accounts of carers' satisfaction with health care at the end of life: a comparison of first generation black Caribbeans and white patients with advanced disease. *Palliat Med* 2001; **15**: 337–45.

11 Tennstedt SL. Commentary on research design in end-of-life research: state of science. *Gerontologist* 2002; **42**: 99–103.

12 Sackett DL, Rosenberg WM, Gray JA, *et al.* Evidence based medicine: what it is and what it isn't [editorial]. *BMJ* 1996; **312**: 71–2.

13 NIH Consensus Development Programme. National Institutes of Health State-of-the-Science conference on improving end-of-life care, Draft statement (Dec 6–8, 2004). Bethesda, MD: NIH Consensus Development Programme, 2005.

14 Kassa S, De Conno F. Palliative care research. *Eur J Cancer* 2001; **37**: S153–S159.

15 Penrod JD, Morrison RS. Challenges in palliative care research. *J Palliat Med* 2004; **7**: 398–402.

16 George LK. Research design in end-of-life research: state of science. *Gerontologist* 2002; **42**: 86–98.

17 Nuremberg doctors trial: the Nuremberg Code 1947. *BMJ* 1996; **313**: 1448.

18 World Medical Association. *World Medical Association Declaration of Helsinki: Ethical Principles for Medical Research involving Human Subjects*. Ferney-Voltaire: World Medical Association, 2002.

● 19 Human D, Fluss SS. *The World Medical Association's Declaration of Helsinki: Historical and Contemporary Perspectives*. Ferney-Voltaire: World Medical Association, 2001.

20 Guenter D, Esparza J, Macklin R. Ethical considerations in the internatir: HIV vaccine trials: summary of a consultative process conducted by the joint United National Programme of HIV/AIDS (UNAIDS). *J Med Ethics* 2000; **26**: 37–43.

21 Tollman SM. What are the effects of the fifth revision of the *Declaration of Helsinki*? Fair partnerships support ethical research. *BMJ* 2001; **323**: 1417–19.

22 Lurie P. Unethical trials of interventions to reduce perinatal transmission of the human immunodeficiency virus in developing countries. *N Engl J Med* 1997; **337**: 853–6.

23 Doll R. What are the effects of the fifth revision of the *Declaration of Helsinki*? Research will be impeded. *BMJ* 2001; **323**: 1421–2.

24 Central Committee on Research Involving Human Subjects. EU Clinical Trial Directive in the Netherlands. Central Committee on Research Involving Human Subjects, 2005.

25 Ministere de la Same Publique et de 1'Environment. Arrete royal du 12 aout 1994 modifant 1'Arret6 royal du 23 Octobre 1964, fixant les normes auxelles les hospitaux et leurs services doivent repondre., Moniteur belge, 27 Septembre 1994. Belgium: Ministere de la Same Publique et de 1'Environment, 1994.

26 United States Department of Human and Human Services. Code of Federal Regulations Part 46. Protection of Human Subjects. United States Department of Human and Human Services, 2005.

27 Department of Health. Research Governance Framework for Health and Social Care. London: Department of Health, 2005.

28 Economic and Social Research Council. *Research Ethics Framework*. London: Economic and Social Research Council, 2005.

29 Gbolade BA. The recruitment and retention of members of black and other ethnic minority groups to NHS research ethics committees in the United Kingdom. *Res Ethics Rev* 2005; **1**: 27–31.

30 Riley J, Ross JR. Research into care at the end of life. *Lancet* 2005; **365**: 735–7.

31 Minnis HJ. Ethics review in research: Ethics committees are risk averse. *BMJ* 2004; **328**: 710–11.

32 Boyce M. Observational study of 353 applications to London multicentre research ethics committee 1997–2000. *BMJ* 2002; **325**: 1081.

33 Brown RF, Butow PN, Butt DG, *et al.* Developing ethical strategies to assist oncologists in seeking informed consent to cancer clinical trials. *Soc Sci Med* 2004; **58**: 379–90.

34 Gammelgaard A, Rossel P, Mortensen OS. Patients' perceptions of informed consent in acute myocardial infarction research: a Danish study. *Soc Sci Med* 2005; **58**: 2313–24.

35 Osborn DPJ, Fulford KWM. Psychiatric research: what ethical concerns do LRECs encounter? A postal survey. *J Med Ethics* 2003; **29**: 55–6.

36 Glasziou P, Chalmers I. Ethics review roulette: what can we learn? *BMJ* 2004; **328**: 121–2.

37 Rees E, Hardy J. Novel consent process for research in dying patients unable to give consent. *BMJ* 2003; **327**: 198.

38 Foster C. *The Ethics of Medical Research on Humans*. Cambridge: Cambridge University Press, 2001.

39 Beauchamp TL, Childress JF. *Principles of Biomedical Ethics*. Oxford: Oxford University Press, 1989.

40 Gillon R. Medical ethics: four principles plus attention to scope. *BMJ* 1994; **309**: 184–8.

41 The National Commission for the Protection of Human Subjects of Biomedical and Behavioral Research. *Belmont Report: Ethical Principles and Guidelines for the Protection of Human Subjects of Biomedical and Behavioral Research*. Washington: The National Commission for the Protection of Human Subjects of Biomedical and Behavioral Research, 1979.

42 Casarett DJ, Knebel A, Helmers K. Ethical challenges of palliative care research. *J Pain Symptom Manage* 2003; **25**: S3–S5.

43 Addington-Hall J, McCarthy M. Dying of cancer: results of a national population-based investigation. *Palliat Med* 1995; **9**: 295–305.

44 Lynn J, Teno JM, Phillips RS, *et al.* Dying experience of older and seriously ill patients: findings from the SUPPORT and HELP projects. *Ann Intern Med* 1997; **126**: 97–106.

45 Koffman J, Higginson IJ, Donaldson N. Symptom severity in advanced cancer, assessed in two ethnic groups by interviews with bereaved family members and friends. *J R Soc Med* 2003; **96**: 10–16.

46 Butters E, Higginson I, George R, *et al.* Assessing the symptoms, anxiety and practical needs of HIV/AIDS patients receiving palliative care. *Qual Life Res* 1992; **1**: 47–51.

47 Janssens R, Gordijn B. Clinical trials in palliative care: an ethical evaluation. *Patient Educ Couns* 2000; **41**: 55–62.

48 Raudonis BM. Ethical considerations in qualitative research with hospice patients. *Qual Health Res* 1992; **2**: 238–49.

49 De Raeve L. Ethical issues in palliative care research. *Palliat Med* 1994; **8**: 298–305.

50 Penslar RL. *Protecting Human Research Subjects: Institutional Review Board Guidebook*. Produced by The Poynter Center for the Study of Ethics and American Institutions, Indiana University, IN, for the United States Department of Health and Human Services, 2005.

51 Seymour J, Skilbeck J. Ethical considerations in researching user views. *Eur J Cancer Care (Engl)* 2002; **11**: 215–19.

52 Addington-Hall J. Research sensitivities to palliative care patients. *Eur J Cancer Care* 2002; **11**: 220–4.

53 Henderson M, Addington-Hall JM, Hotopf M. The willingness of palliative care patients to participate in research. *J Pain Symptom Manage* 2005; **29**: 116–17.

54 Ross C, Cornbleet M. Attitudes of patients and staff to research in a specialist palliative care unit. *Palliat Med* 2003; **17**: 491–7.

55 Emanuel EJ, Fairclough DL, Wolfe P, Emanuel LL. Talking with terminally ill patients and their caregivers about death, dying, and bereavement: is it stressful? Is it helpful? *Arch Intern Med* 2004; **164**: 1999–2004.

56 Batson CD. *The Altruism Question: Toward a Social and Psychological Answer*. New Jersey: Lawrence Erlbaum Associates Inc., 1991.

57 Davies EA, Hall SM, Clarke CR, *et al.* Do research interviews cause distress or interfere in management? Experience from a study of cancer patients. *J R Coll Phys Lond* 1998; **32**: 406–11.

58 Takesaka J, Crowley R, Casarett D. What is the risk of distress in palliative care survey research? *J Pain Symptom Manage* 2004; **28**: 593–8.

59 Seamark DA, Gilbert J, Lawrence CJ, Williams S. Are postbereavement research interviews distressing to carers? Lessons learned from palliative care research. *Palliat Med* 2000; **14**: 55–6.

60 Casarett DJ. Assessing decision-making capacity in the setting of palliative care research. *J Pain Symptom Manage* 2003; **25**: S6–S13.

61 Pereira J, Hanson J, Bruera E. The frequency and clinical course of cognitive impairment in patients with terminal cancer. *Cancer* 1997; **79**: 835–42.

62 Grisso T, Appelbaum PS, Hill-Fotouhi C. The MacCAT-T: a clinical tool to assess patients' capacities to make decisions. *Psychiatr Serv* 1997; **48**: 1415–19.

63 Karlawish JHT. Conducting research that involves subjects at the end of life who are unable to give consent. *J Pain Symptom Manage* 2003; **25**: S14–S24.

64 Regnard C, Mathews D, Gibson L, Clarke C. Difficulties in identifying distress and its causes in people with severe communication problems. *Int J Palliat Nurs* 2003; **9**: 173–6.

65 Chouliara Z, Kearny N, Worth A, Stott D. Challenges in conducting research with hospitalized older people with

cancer: drawing from the experience of an ongoing interview-based project. *Eur J Cancer* 2004; **13**: 409–15.

66 Gunaratnam Y. *Researching 'Race' and 'Ethnicity'*. London: Sage, 2003.

67 Koffman J, Camps J. No way in: including the excluded at the end of life. In: Payne S, Seymour J, Skilbeck J, Ingelton C, eds. *Palliative Care Nursing: Principles and Evidence for Practice*. Maidenhead: Open University Press, 2004.

68 Tuffrey-Wijne I. The palliative care needs of people with intellectual disabilities: a literature review. *Palliat Med* 2003; **17**: 55–62.

69 Gregson BA, Smith M, Lecouturier N, *et al.* Issues of recruitment and maintaining high response rates in a longitudinal study of older hospital patients in England–pathways through care study. *J Epidemiol Comm Health* 1997; **51**: 541–8.

70 Dubler NN. Legal judgments and informed consent in geriatric research. *J Am Geriatr Soc* 1987; **35**: 545–9.

71 Smith T. *Ethics in Medical Research*. Cambridge: Cambridge University Press, 1999.

72 Koffman J, Higginson IJ. Rights, needs and social exclusion in palliative care. In: Faull C, Carter Y, Daniels L, eds. *Handbook of Palliative Care*. London: Blackwell, 2005: 43–60.

73 Dean RA, McClement SE. Palliative care research: methodological and ethical challenges. *Int J Palliat Nurs* 2002; **8**: 376–80.

74 Froggatt KA, Field D, Bailey C, Krishnasamy M. Qualitative research in palliative care 1990–1999: a descriptive review. *Int J Palliat Nurs* 2003; **9**: 98–104.

75 Johnson B, Plant H. Collecting data from people with cancer and their families: what are the implications? In: de Raeve L, ed. *Nursing Research: An Ethical and Legal Appraisal*. London: Bailliere Tindall, 1996: 85–100.

76 Alderson P, Green S, Higgins JPT. *Cochrane Reviewers' Handbook*. Chichester: John Wiley & Sons, 2004.

77 Rowbotham MC, Twilling L, Davies PS, *et al.* Oral opioid therapy for chronic peripheral and central neuropathic pain. *N Engl J Med* 2003; **348**: 1223–32.

78 Bruera E, MacEachern T, Ripamonti C, Hanson J. Subcutaneous morphine for dyspnea in cancer patients. *Ann Intern Med* 2003; **119**: 907.

79 Meier DE, Fuss BR, O'Rourke D, *et al.* Marked improvement in recognition and completion of health care proxies. A randomized controlled trial of counseling by hospital representatives. *Arch Intern Med* 1996; **156**: 1227–32.

◆ 80 Snowdon C, Garcia J, Elbourne D. Making sense of randomization; responses of parents of critically ill babies to random allocation of treatment in a clinical trial. *Soc Sci Med* 1997; **45**: 1337–55.

◆ 81 McWhinney IR, Bass MJ, Donner A. Evaluation of a palliative care service: problems and pitfalls. *BMJ* 1994; **309**: 1340–2.

25

Practical tips for successful research in palliative care

EDUARDO BRUERA, ELLEN A PACE

INTRODUCTION

Palliative medicine emerged in the UK during the 1960s as a response to the unmet needs of terminally ill patients and their families. The development of this movement in the UK has been addressed in Chapter 1, and Chapters 2–7 have addressed the successful development of palliative medicine as a global discipline.

In most regions of the world palliative care did not emerge as a result of mainstream academia, rather it emerged as a number of 'bottom up' approaches on the fringes of the existing healthcare movement. This relative isolation allowed palliative clinical programs to successfully interact with their communities and to develop the basic principles of the disciplines. However, this isolation also made it difficult for palliative medicine groups to interact with academic groups including methodologists, biostatisticians, clinical trialists, epidemiologists, and other groups that are readily available to other content areas of healthcare.

Palliative medicine programs have a strong clinical commitment and limited access to protected time for research and research training.[1–3] For this reason our book has committed a considerable amount of space to chapters on the specific challenges of research, the patient population, the different research designs, outcomes, ethics in research, and the process of audit and quality improvement.

The purpose of this chapter is to discuss some practical issues that are not always available in methodology textbooks, but that are crucial to the success of research projects in palliative care. Most of the tips included in this book are the result of difficulties encountered by our and other research teams in the process of establishing a research program.

THE SETTING FOR PALLIATIVE CARE RESEARCH

Choosing the appropriate setting is of great importance and one of the main reasons why research projects fail. Box 25.1 summarizes what is important about the setting where research will take place.

Box 25.1 Understanding the research setting

- Clinical characteristics of patients

- Socioeconomic characteristics of patients and families

- Type of care provided

- Staffing arrangements

- Length of stay and/or frequency of patient follow-up

Appropriate understanding of the patient population requires not only the basic diagnosis and demographics but also many practical issues such as the level of literacy. (Several studies in the developing world could not be performed because they required patients to complete questionnaires they were not able to read. See also Chapter 21.) The inclusion of minorities may be difficult in some areas of the USA unless Spanish versions of questionnaires are available. The average length of stay of patients in the specific setting or average number of patient visits to outpatient settings is an important consideration to ensure that the study can be completed in time. In the case of studies on patients and families it is important to know how many patients are accompanied by a relative and in how many cases the relative lives with the patient. The percentage of patients unable to attend a scheduled outpatient visit ranges from 20 percent to 50 percent in most outpatient care settings and thus can have major impact on missing data for clinical studies. The ability for patients to communicate on the telephone for follow-up may be useful in recovering some of this missing information. The availability of rooms where interviews can be conducted and discussing arrangements for the research team in the inpatient or outpatient areas needs to be appropriately planned prior to study initiation. Otherwise it may be impossible to keep a patient in an examining room for assessments or consent, and there may not be staff available for notification when a patient becomes eligible for a study.

The types of treatment are of great importance. In many clinical trials there are criteria for eligibility including certain treatments. Appropriate understanding of these criteria will assist in determining how feasible a certain study will be. For example, in two clinical trials in patients with dyspnea, patient accrual was extremely difficult because although dyspnea is a frequent symptom in palliative care settings, the clinical trials required patients to be able to complete self-assessment questionnaires with excellent cognitive status and comply with complex research designs.[4,5] As a consequence, a large number of patients were identified but only a small number were able to actually enter the clinical trials. A clinical trial comparing methadone versus morphine as first-line opioid for cancer pain required simple assessments by patients with a common pain problem. However, the main difficulty in admitting and maintaining patients on this study was the requirement for very frequent follow-up assessments during the first week of treatment. Many of the centers were not able to conduct frequent assessments in the patients' home or admit the patients for a 1-week period.[6]

The idea for a study on the use of methylphenidate 'as needed' for the management of cancer-related fatigue emerged from the comments of a colleague who had observed excellent response of patients to this modality of administration.[7] The idea for a clinical trial of donepezil on the management of sedation and fatigue emerged from a letter to the editor submitted by a clinician who had observed improvement among patients receiving opioids when treated with donepezil.[8,9] A randomized controlled trial comparing methylphenidate 'as needed' with placebo emerged from the result of the pilot study by the same group.[10] These three examples emphasize the importance of publishing letters to the editor, based on observations or pilot projects. This is one of the ways in which colleagues can pick up important ideas from findings and translate them into useful research projects.

The research idea

In palliative care research ideas may emerge from a clinical observation, comments by colleagues, papers published in different journals, or previous research conducted by a group. Clinical research is most successful when it is investigator driven because investigators who are highly committed to a certain domain will be much more motivated to spend a considerable amount of extra time in pursuing this research in addition to other clinical and educational responsibilities.

One of the most difficult processes is that of turning a research idea into a well formulated hypothesis. Being able to frame the general idea into a very specific question is extremely important because this will frame the whole methodology of the project. It is important for researchers to have a conversation with a mentor at an early stage in the development of this early hypothesis. This will help them to immediately identify how feasible the whole project may be.

LITERATURE SEARCH

It is very important to read good-quality material but it is not necessary to read all material on a given subject. The literature search should consist of a number of recent high-quality reviews of the area as well as a number of recent original papers on the subject under study. This quick review of the literature will rapidly demonstrate if the investigator's hypothesis has already been appropriately studied or if it would be justifiable to proceed with further research on the subject. If there have been only one or two brief reports or letters to the editor with a small number of cases, this suggests that there is probably strong justification for the study. If the investigator finds no reference at all it is important to consider whether they are researching the correct literature on this subject.

The literature search has three main purposes:

- to provide an indepth understanding of the content area in which the investigator is planning to conduct research
- to be able to understand the methodology employed by other researchers
- to understand the main outcomes studied by previous researchers.

As much as possible the investigators should attempt to take advantage of previous knowledge and methodologies. This will save a great amount of time and also will increase the likelihood of publication of their findings since they can provide literature support for having followed a certain methodology.

The literature search is not only useful for justifying the project and applying to a research committee and/or granting agency, but it can also *per se* become a major publication and be extremely helpful to other readers. For example, the literature search concerning survival estimation used for the design of a clinical trial was also very useful when published as a systematic review.[11,12]

DEFINING THE RIGHT OUTCOMES

In palliative care outcomes are mostly subjective (i.e. symptom intensity, satisfaction with communication by patients and/or families, perceptions of quality of communication, etc.; see Chapter 23 for a full assessment of measures). These outcomes are much more likely to be subject to bias and therefore the nature of these outcomes will have major impact on the methodology used by the investigator.

In the study of a specific problem such as cachexia there may be a combination of outcomes highly unlikely to be influenced by patient or investigator bias (such as body weight and other nutritional findings), other outcomes that may have an intermediate risk of bias (such as daily energy intake), and a third group of outcomes that is highly subject to bias (such as anorexia, fatigue, etc.). Similar statements could be made for other physical and psychosocial symptoms. The timing for modification of variables may also differ dramatically (for example anorexia or fatigue can be modified by an intervention in hours whereas body weight may require weeks).

It is important to use a methodological approach that will best address the most important question and to try to keep it very simple as the likelihood of the completion of the study will be directly linked with the simplicity of the design. One of the most common mistakes is to attempt to address too many outcomes or one main outcome that is beyond the reach of the research team. In the case of cancer cachexia a clinical trial of megestrol acetate showed significant improvement in body weight but was of limited clinical relevance as the main outcome was to successfully reverse cachexia.[13] On the other hand, when clinical trials were conducted using a very simple subjective outcome such as appetite the same drug was found to be effective.[14,15]

ORGANIZING THE TEAM

The principal investigator will need to put together a research team. Box 25.2 summarizes the main members of the research team. The methodology expert will need to be an individual who may or may not work in the palliative care area but who is highly experienced in the use of the methodology for this research project, for example an expert in surveys, clinical trials, qualitative studies, etc. This individual will have a major role in helping the team choose the different

tools, the overall design, and refining the outcomes the principal investigator is currently considering.

Box 25.2 The research team

- Principal investigator
- Content expert
- Methodology expert
- Biostatistician
- Clinical expert
- Administrative expert

The statistician should be approached early during the process of consideration of a study. Even if the outcomes are likely to be mostly descriptive the statistician may have a crucial role in assisting the team in the best use of the existing data. The role of the statistician will become more prominent as the study becomes more complex. One of the most important roles of the statistician is to assist the investigators in calculating the sample size required. It may become clear early in the study that the number of patients required is too large for the setting where the investigator is planning to conduct the research. This will require the investigator to find a number of additional sites where data collection can take place. It is very important that this process takes place early in the research project so that so the individuals responsible for the other sites can become part of the research team during the process of defining the study.

The principal investigator may certainly be a content expert. It is always useful to have at least one more additional expert in the content under study. These experts are usually also familiar with many methodological issues and they can make suggestions based on their personal experience and the connections they have with other content experts. For example, in a study on cachexia a content expert may be aware of research being conducted by a colleague somewhere else and may be helpful in directly contacting this investigator for specific information about the rationale for a certain study or outcome.

Clinician experts include nurses, pharmacists, and other clinical colleagues. These individuals are essential for the success of any clinical study including trials, surveys, or qualitative studies. These individuals will be able to address many practical issues that are crucial for the success of the study. Clinical trials may be more apt to fail if patients receiving placebo have to make multiple hospital visits; if patients are required to take an excessive number of tablets; if questionnaires are too long and difficult to explain; and if there are a number of practical aspects regarding the setting of care that the principal investigator and other experts did not completely understand.

It is important for the investigators to remember that the current access to global communication by low-cost telephones and internet allows teams to function quite well and in real time from multiple locations. It is important to understand if the local requirement of the institutional review board (IRB) puts some limitations on the participation by distance co-investigators. Two important items need to be discussed very early in the process of planning the research:

- *Authorship.* This expectations of the different team members regarding authorship is an important issue to discuss in an open and friendly way. It may be possible to designate expected first authors and senior authors for presentation, publication of the main paper, as well as other secondary publications that may result from the study. A frank discussion regarding the different roles of the investigators will help prevent misunderstandings and unnecessary stress on the participants. This is the responsibility of the principal investigator.
- *Financial issues.* It is important to be open about any resources that may be obtained for conducting the study and how this will be distributed among the different participants. If an application is being made to a research granting agency or an industry sponsor all details regarding the financial arrangements need to be disclosed before the application is submitted. This will maintain the friendly and open environment throughout the project and will ensure collaboration for future projects.

It is important for the principal investigator to put together a successful research team and to understand that it is his or her ultimate responsibility to write the proposal.

Palliative care is a content area and researchers working in this area will need to use a variety of methodologies to better understand their areas of work. It is impossible for an investigator to become an expert on the methodology and biostatistics of all the different approaches. However, it should be expected that the principal investigator would have a basic understanding of methodologies and biostatistics to be able to appropriately communicate with these experts and be a resource for all areas of content.

WRITING THE PROTOCOL

The protocol should be written down in all cases, including case series and retrospective reviews. The process of writing the protocol will help the research team clarify ideas, to make sure that all aspects of the process are well outlined, and will clearly show the team if they are attempting to address too many issues. In general it is much more effective to address one aspect well rather than many aspects with a lower level of evidence. By its nature palliative care research takes place with patients and families who are facing multiple problems and therefore the likelihood of our interventions may be at best only partially successful. Complex and lengthy studies have a high chance of failure.

ADMINISTRATION OF THE STUDY

One of the main challenges is to obtain appropriate approval by the IRB. This may require the research team to make several modifications in their design, questionnaires, and consent forms. Understanding how the IRB operates, their main areas of expertise, and the wording they prefer to see in the research protocols and consent forms can prevent many problems. It is important that at least one member of the research team is familiar with the operation of the IRB and is able to provide advice about the way the protocol and consent forms should be written. In case of doubt it can be helpful to consult the chair of the IRB about specific aspects of the study before a full submission.

Once the study has been approved the investigators should meet regularly to see if there are any problems with the actual conduct of the study. Some of the most common problems include lack of patient accrual related to some of the eligibility criteria, missing data because of an excessively ambitious assessment method, patients who are unable to stay on in the study because of clinical and social issues, or unexpected side effects or distress by patients and families in the case of discussion of questionnaires (see Chapter 20). It is important to make very early adjustments in the criteria for eligibility or methods since each adjustment needs to be submitted to the IRB for consideration and this will take a considerable amount of time (see Chapters 20 and 24). It is also important to accept when studies can just not be completed so they can be completely rewritten in a more appropriate way.

PREPARATION OF THE MANUSCRIPT

Although the input of the whole research team is vital at this stage, the principal investigator should write the initial draft of the manuscript. This will provide the necessary leadership for all the other experts to contribute. It is essential to write concise manuscripts summarizing the main aspects of the study. If there is other information it could be prepared as additional reports for presentation at scientific meetings or as additional publications.

During the past 10 years there has been a major improvement in the number of peer-reviewed palliative medicine journals and in the number of scientific meetings where palliative medicine research can be presented. It is important to submit for publication all studies whether the results were encouraging or disappointing since this information can be invaluable to other researchers who are planning to conduct similar research. One should be flexible while responding to the comments from the reviewers and take advantage of these reviews as a way of improving the manuscript even if the journal has decided to reject the manuscript. Consideration to the reviewer's comments will result in a better manuscript to be submitted to the next journal.

Young investigators frequently feel disheartened by devastating comments from reviewers. Journal editors should take appropriate steps to protect authors from vicious comments by reviewers protected by anonymity. Investigators should never decide to discard the manuscript without consulting with an experienced mentor who may help put some of the comments from the reviewer in perspective. It is important to remember that 100 percent of the manuscripts that are not resubmitted will not get published. Resubmission will result in a higher success rate for publication if the investigator adequately addresses the reviewer's comments in the resubmission letter to the journal.

APPLYING FOR FUNDING

In many cases the only way a research project can be conducted is after the research team applies for funding. This is time consuming and slow but unfortunately there is no other way to conduct successful research than establishing a research team and completing grant applications. The methodology expert, biostatistician, and content expert will usually have considerable experience in grant writing and will be able to advise the investigator along the way. Most of the time it is most useful for the investigator to hold individual meetings with each of the members of the team rather than lengthy meetings involving the whole team assembled together. It is important to understand that each of the experts has limited time and that the investigator should use this time in the way that is most conducive to writing a successful application.

In most cases having some pilot data (see Chapter 20 regarding the importance of conducting a pilot study) will be essential for writing a grant application. This short pilot study may need to be conducted with no access to funding. A number of organizations/universities provide bridge money for conducting brief pilot studies that will lead to major grant applications. These granting committees usually require simple design outlines. The investigator may obtain considerable information about availability of philanthropical or bridge funding from the local research office of their university. It is important to arrange for a formal visit and consultation with the research director.

CONCLUSIONS

Palliative medicine is a young specialty. A large number of aspects of this discipline are not well understood. Almost all clinicians are capable of making a meaningful contribution by publishing their observations, case series, retrospective studies, and other more sophisticated research designs.

Perhaps the most important tip for an investigator is to put together a research team that can collaborate in a friendly and effective manner. This will ensure that not only is the research project successful but that the whole experience is highly enjoyable for all members of the research team.

Key learning points

- Choosing the appropriate setting for palliative care research is of great importance and is one of the main reasons why research projects fail.

- Clinical research is most successful when it is investigator driven.

- A thorough literature search is essential to complete prior to starting a research project to take advantage of previous knowledge and methodologies.

- In palliative care research the outcomes are mostly subjective (i.e. symptom intensity, etc.), and thus it is essential for the investigator to use a methodological approach that will address the most important question and keep the design of the study simple.

- Authorship and financial issues should be discussed early in the process of planning the research project.

- The research team should be able to collaborate in a friendly and effective manner to ensure the success of the research project

REFERENCES

1 Brenneis C, Bruera E. Models for the delivery of palliative care: The Canadian Model. In: Bruera E, Portenoy RK, eds. *Topics in Palliative Care* Vol 5. Oxford: Oxford University Press, 2001: 3–23.

2 Clark D. The development of palliative care in the UK and Ireland. In: Bruera E, Higginson IJ, Ripamonti R, von Gunten C. *Textbook of Palliative Medicine.* London: Hodder Arnold, 2006.

3 Ryndes, T. The development of palliative medicine in the USA. In: Bruera E, Higginson IJ, Ripamonti R, von Gunten C. *Textbook of Palliative Medicine.* London: Hodder Arnold, 2006.

4 Bruera E, de Stoutz N, Velasco-Leiva A, *et al.* Effects of oxygen on dyspnea in hyopoxaemic terminal-cancer patients. *Lancet* 1993; **342**: 13–14.

5 Bruera E, MacEachern T, Ripamonti C, Hanson J. Subcutaneous Morphine for dyspnea in cancer patients. *Ann Intern Med* 1993; **119**: 906–7.

6 Bruera E, Palmer JL, Bosnjak S, *et al.* Methadone versus morphine as a first-line strong opioids for cancer pain: a randomized, double-blind study. *J Clin Oncol* 2004; **22**: 185–92.

7 Bruera E, Driver L, Barnes EA, *et al.* Patient-controlled methylphenidate for the management of fatigue in patients with

advanced cancer: a preliminary report. *J Clin Oncol* 2003; **21**: 4439–43.

8   Slatkin N, Rhiner M. Treatment of opioid-induced delirium with acetylcholinesterase inhibitors: a case report. *J Pain Symptom Manage* 2004; **27**: 268–73.

9   Bruera E, Strasser F, Shen L, *et al.* The effect of donepezil on sedation and other symptoms in patients receiving opioids for cancer pain: a pilot study. *J Pain Symptom Manage* 2003; **26**: 1049–54.

10   Bruera E, Valero V, Driver L, *et al.* Patient-controlled methylphenidate for cancer fatigue: a double blind, randomized, placebo-controlled trial. *J Clin Oncol* 2005; **23**(16 Suppl): 740s.

11   Vigano A, Donaldson N, Higginson IJ, Bruera E. Quality of life and survival prediction in terminal cancer patients: a multicenter study. *Cancer* 2004; **101**: 1090–8.

12   Vigano A, Dorgan M, Buckingham J *et al.* Survival prediction in terminal cancer patients: a systematic review of the medical literature. *Palliat Med* 2000; **14**: 363–74.

13   Maltoni M, Nanni O, Scarpi E, *et al.* High-dose progestins for the treatment of cancer anorexia-cachexia syndrome: a systematic review of randomized clinical trials. *Ann Oncol* 2001; **12**: 289–300.

14   Bruera E, Macmillan K, Kuehn N, *et al.* A controlled trial of megestrol acetate on appetite, caloric intake, nutritional status, and other symptoms in patients with advanced cancer. *Cancer* 1990; **66**: 1279–82.

15   Bruera E, Ernst S, Hagen N, *et al.* Effectiveness of megestrol acetate in patients with advanced cancer: a randomized, double-blind, crossover study. *Cancer Prev Control* 1998; **2**: 74–8.

26

Audit and quality improvement in palliative care research

HSIEN-YEANG SEOW, SARAH MYERS, JOANNE LYNN

INTRODUCTION

High-quality care can mean better outcomes,[1] enhanced efficiency and patient safety,[2,3] and reduced disparities.[4,5] Traditionally, methods to improve quality of care have used formal research to guide reform. Formal research is key to identifying more effective pharmaceuticals or procedures but less effective in rapidly changing clinical practice. In discerning how to deliver optimal care to a specific patient population without incurring unacceptable costs, quality improvement can be superior.

WHAT IS AUDIT AND QUALITY IMPROVEMENT?

Quality improvement (QI) is an empirical, goal-oriented method of improving the performance of a system.[6] Not a new concept by any means, QI as applied to healthcare dates back to the Crimean War in 1854, when Florence Nightingale began keeping statistical records to reform the hospital and sanitary administration within the British army.[7] In recent years, QI has become pervasive within the healthcare system. QI allows clinicians to assess whether they are doing the right thing, with the right patients, at the right time – and if not, to make needed changes quickly.[8] Quality improvement models provide clinical teams with a structure for identifying areas ripe for improvement, strategies for identifying process improvements to test on a small scale, and tools for measuring progress toward reaching established goals. Generally, QI requires stating an aim, measuring success, and testing possible improvements.

Effective QI is an ongoing cycle that encourages ongoing organizational learning.[8–13] Quality improvement teams ideally begin by addressing discrete, narrow problems, but then expand their efforts in size and scope, moving from time-limited, focused tests of change to broad implementation of changes that their own data have proved to be effective.

Audit – a term most often used in Britain – is 'a continuous process whereby healthcare professionals review patient care against agreed standards and make changes, where necessary, to meet those standards'.[14] In essence, audit is similar to QI. One key difference is that the process is formalized and centralized by a governmental body, the National Health Service, and thus is a core function of the healthcare system. In the USA, private healthcare organizations embark upon and carry out QI efforts on their own initiative for the most part, in response to consumer or professional demand, outside standards, or business considerations. In the past several years, however, more and more healthcare organizations have been required to participate in QI by payers or by their accrediting bodies. Audit and QI can apply to any size population from the quality of care for a few patients daily[15] (often called clinical QI or audit initiatives) to implementing guidelines across a nation.[16]

AUDIT AND QUALITY IMPROVEMENT IN PALLIATIVE CARE

Palliative care 'aims to relieve suffering and improve quality of life for patients with advanced illness, and their families.'[17] Only recently have some healthcare organizations begun to incorporate formal and informal palliative care programs and services. In many nations, distinct palliative care programs are relatively new in the healthcare system, with palliative care services having previously been part of primary care, geriatrics, and hospice. This nascent field – with a dearth of well-established standards and guidelines – presents tremendous opportunities for QI. The opportunities reach all aspects of palliative care, including advance care planning, symptom management, and continuity and coordination of care.

A case study using one QI model

The following case study describes a team's application of QI.

A hospital serves a substantial number of oncology patients through their clinical trials program. Although their remission rate is high, there are generally around 60 deaths per year in the hospital. Nurses are frustrated because so many of these patients' families say that they would have preferred to die at home. Seeing an opportunity for improvement, a few colleagues express an interest in improving this outcome. Together, they analyze the potential causes of unwanted inhospital deaths and determine that (1) no-one is sure that staff are soliciting information about patients' preferred site of death, and (2) staff are uncomfortable with discussing this with patients who are pursuing aggressive cancer treatment.

First, the team develops a measurable aim: 'Within two months, we will have documented site-of-death preference for 100 percent of acute leukemia patients within 24 hours of admission'. They start small by targeting only one segment of the oncology patient population. However, by setting an aim of 100 percent within 2 months, they alert their colleagues they want to change current clinical practice quickly. To achieve this, they test several different methods:

- including a question regarding preferred site of death on the admission form

- instituting a social worker visit within the first 24 hours of admission, during which site of death would be one topic of discussion

- providing pamphlets regarding advance care planning in all patient rooms.

To learn from their efforts, a nurse will review the chart of two patients in the target population each week to look for documentation of site of death preference, and the team will review the results. Over the next 2 months, the team test out their ideas with a small number of new patients. They quickly realize that the direct question asked on the admission

form is well received and leads to an increase of documented preferences in the medical record. They also learn that staff are still avoiding talks about preferred site of death. Based on these results, they continue the intervention, add role-playing about preferred site of death conversations for staff, and start expanding both to all new admissions. They also continue to review charts to track their effectiveness.

Within 2 months, 100 percent of acute leukemia patients have a site of death preference noted in their chart within 24 hours of admission. Having achieved this process-oriented aim, the team sets an aim related to the actual outcome – increasing the number of patients for whom death occurs at their preferred site. Over the next several months, they set about testing changes and learning from their results.

In summary, the team identified a problem, stated an aim, tested ways to achieve their aim, measured their progress, and learned from their trials to modify current hospital practice and expand their efforts.

EXAMPLES FROM AROUND THE GLOBE

Quality improvement is applied to palliative care on large scale (e.g. national guidelines and care standards)[18–21] and small scale (e.g. clinical QI and audit initiatives).[15,22] The former is generally the purview of regulatory and oversight bodies and healthcare payors, both private and public. The latter often arises at the organizational level. A review of the experience of several countries and regions seeking to improve palliative care reveals a range of approaches in each domain. Below we highlight some examples of such approaches from around the globe though we do not imply that these examples are superior to those not addressed here.

National guidelines and care standards

Many countries have begun using national guidelines and policies to improve palliative care, often in the form of accreditation. A global study for the World Health Organization (WHO) in 2000 identified 36 nationwide healthcare accreditation programs.[23] Starting with the Joint Commission of the Accreditation of Healthcare Organizations (JCAHO) in the USA in 1951, the number of programs around the world has doubled every 5 years since 1990.[24] JCAHO in the USA accredits healthcare organizations in compliance with their quality standards. In 2000 JCAHO added pain management standards that address assessment and management of pain, education around effective pain management to patients and families, and continuous organizational improvement.[25,26] In 2004 JCAHO explicitly made advanced directives (addressing the patient's wishes related to end-of-life decisions) a part of the patient rights standards that hospitals and other healthcare organizations must adhere to.[27] Presently, nearly 16 000 healthcare providers – from small, rural clinics to expansive, complex healthcare networks – use JCAHO standards to improve their quality performance and how they provide care.[28]

Large-scale QI efforts have also been implemented in developing countries. The WHO is working with five African countries to improve the quality of life for patients with cancer and human immunodeficiency virus (HIV)/acquired immune deficiency syndrome (AIDS) by developing palliative care programs with a community health approach.[29] Key to this collaboration program is its emphasis on developing palliative care services and standards and attempting to integrate them into existing health systems and national strategic plans for health and social services. For instance, the WHO has defined a minimum standard of care for HIV patients with cancer in Africa.[30] The initial phase of the project identified improved care for dying patients using palliative care as a national concern. Using data to guide reforms, the project collected information concerning target countries' health systems performance and also assessed needs and gaps in patient care.

The first phase of the project found that terminally ill patients in the target countries had these key needs: relief of pain, accessible and affordable drugs, and financial support.[31] Suggested strategies to address these needs include: incorporating drugs in palliative care packages, focusing on home-based palliative care, and establishing national policies to support availability of analgesics. The second phase of the project calls for a 'stepwise approach to fill in the gaps, so that existing resources/initiatives are optimized', and specific pilot projects that use a 'methodology of problem solving and team learning'.[29] A survey of end-of-life programs in Africa already shows some successes in palliative care program development.[32] Of the programs surveyed, 85 percent reported government endorsement of their program, 94 percent had written goals and objectives, 90 percent had measurement indicators, 79 percent had guidelines for good practice in place, and 86 percent reported monitoring critical elements such as patient care and outcomes, patient and carer need, or place of death preferences.

Canada also established national initiatives and policies focused on creating care standards to improve end-of-life and palliative care. In June 2000, a Canadian Senate subcommittee produced a national end-of-life strategy.[33] The subcommittee noted as integral to ensuring integration of quality end-of-life care within the healthcare system specialized training for end-of-life interdisciplinary teams, increased research, and ongoing development of guidelines. The subcommittee recommended that the federal government, in collaboration with the provinces, develop a national strategy for end-of-life care, implement it within 5 years, and prepare an annual progress report. Additionally, the Canadian Hospice Palliative Care Association addressed national care standards in hospice and palliative care in 2002,

when it published the results of a 10-year consensus-building process to develop a national model to guide hospice and palliative care across the country.[34]

Clinical QI and audit initiatives

In contrast with the national projects described above, many QI and audit initiatives have been implemented at the healthcare system and organization level. There are also many examples of individuals and grouped audit initiatives and it is impossible to review them all. A large variety of individual topic based audits have led to improvements in practice for the management of individual symptoms, discharge planning, coordination, and education.[35–42] There has been the incorporation of outcome measures into clinical practice[35,43–45] (see also Chapter 23) and the use of these measures, e.g. the Palliative Outcome Scale, to help to audit care.

In nonspecialist palliative care settings, Dr Keri Thomas and the Macmillan Cancer Trust have developed the 'gold standards framework', which is 'a practice-based system to improve the organization and quality of palliative care services for patients who are at home in their last year of life'.[46] This framework gives providers seven 'gold standards' for care of patients: communication, coordination, control of symptoms, continuity out-of-hours, continued learning, carer support, and care in the dying phase. A key goal was to improve generalist palliative care to better dovetail with specialist palliative care, thereby enhancing continuity and coordination. The framework was implemented using QI models, and began with 12 family doctor practices.[47] Unpublished results suggested that between December 2001 and August 2002, indicators related to coordination had improved and there was an increase in the number of deaths taking place in the place preferred by patients.[48,49] A more detailed evaluation is underway.

Another example of local collaborative QI efforts with a national impact comes from the USA, where the RAND Palliative Care Policy Center has partnered with over 200 healthcare provider organizations through QI collaboratives.[15,50] A collaborative consists of multiple healthcare organizations working together for up to 2 years to improve a specific clinical or operational area, under the guidance of a panel of national experts. Following the collaborative model, teams quickly learn from one another, promising ideas are easily disseminated among teams, and in turn these teams spread proved interventions within their respective organizations. Past collaboratives have made significant improvements in various palliative care areas such as pain, advanced care planning, and dyspnea around the country.

Other local QI efforts have led to wide dissemination of knowledge, tools, and resources. The Beth Israel Medical Center Division of Palliative Care and Pain Medicine in the USA developed a free online manual and toolkit based on its own QI learning.[51] The online manual includes tools such as an interdisciplinary plan of care and a documentation tool for daily assessments and interventions so that goals such as reducing unnecessary interventions and minimizing symptom distress can be achieved.

FUTURE OF QUALITY IMPROVEMENT

Despite documentation of some successes resulting from QI applied to palliative care, there is substantial room for continued improvement. Recent WHO Europe reports state that challenges in palliative care remain in integrating with health services; educating health professionals, policy makers and the public; implementing improvements; and prioritizing palliative care research.[52,53] Moreover, a qualitative study of palliative care in a developed (Scotland) and developing (Kenya) country demonstrate that dying patients in developing countries still lack access to analgesics, medical support, equipment and facilities, basic necessities, and relief from great physical suffering, whereas patients in developing countries on the whole do not.[54] The study also shows however, that despite the availability of resources in the UK, people still have major areas of unmet needs.

The inertia of accepting current practice is difficult to overcome, and there are still insufficient forces driving continuous improvement, and barriers that need to be overcome.[43–45] Outlined below is a vision of the future of QI, building the case for its use as a widely adopted – and indeed sometimes required – method for change.

Building obligation and opportunities

All of those involved in the healthcare system – from the policy maker to each clinician – needs to honor the obligation to provide the best quality of care. That obligation involves not accepting substandard care and making small improvements in everyday clinical practice based on evidence. Financial incentives, such as performance linked to payment or accreditation can help foster this obligation to improve quality of care.[55,56] Moreover, we need to better develop opportunities to utilize QI in everyday practice. For example, healthcare contracts should mandate audit and evaluation, a plan to implement research findings,[57–60] and forethought about the scalability, replicability, and spread of the intervention.[61] Quality improvement should be a part of the education of any healthcare provider.

Monitoring quality and responding

Quality must be continually monitored on a large scale, such as through tracking adherence to national quality standards. By doing so, the national standards generate a feedback loop for quickly assessing which ideas are successful, which ones are not, and which require a mid-course

correction.[19] Integrating technology into the monitoring process, so that the information is timely, meaningful and actionable will be important. Furthermore, quality standards will help countries learn from each other through international comparisons,[62] alleviate the variation that exists among settings and geography,[63] fill in the missing gaps in knowledge as to which interventions are most effective in which settings, and help highlight the various factors for success.[64,65]

Publicizing benchmarks and supporting QI efforts

We need not only monitor quality but also to publicize the results. Standards that are simple and transparent will help get the public involved as an important advocate for change. Recognizing the exceptional facilities and revoking accreditation for those that fail to meet standards could be key to validating the efforts. Lastly, we must provide support to QI through knowledge and finance, nurture struggling facilities, and commit to teaching the QI process, so that an environment exists that allows good ideas to succeed and spread.

Not long ago, discovering the latest drug or publishing the newest procedure in the professional literature was seen as sufficient to change clinical practice. No-one believes that now. Deliberate, planned improvement activities are proving effective at changing practice. In order to build a care system that we can rely on and will serve us well at the end of life, we need to quickly acquire the skills that will allow us to learn from our current clinical practices, to improve upon it, and to disseminate the information broadly. Audit and QI can help us achieve that.

Key learning points

- Traditional methods to improve quality of care use formal research to guide reform, however, these methods are less effective for introducing rapid change in clinical practice.

- Quality improvement allows clinicians to assess whether they are doing the right thing, with the right patients, at the right time – and if not, to make needed changes quickly. Effective QI is an ongoing cycle that encourages ongoing organizational learning.

- Audit is similar to QI, the key difference being that in audit the process is formalized and centralized by a governmental body.

- All aspects of palliative care, including advance care planning, symptom management, and continuity and coordination of care, present tremendous opportunities for QI.

- Many countries have begun using national guidelines and policies to improve palliative care, often in the form of accreditation, e.g. JCAHO in the USA and the WHO's QI program in Africa involving a community health approach.

- An example of QI at the local health system level is the 'gold standards framework' approach in the UK. The gold standards arose from general practitioner (family doctor) practices trying to improve care for those in the dying phase and has since spread to hundreds of practices.

- Quality improvement has a growing role in improving palliative care. The future effectiveness of QI depends on several factors including building obligation and opportunities for QI; monitoring quality and responding; and publicizing benchmarks and supporting QI efforts.

REFERENCES

1   Institute of Medicine. Crossing the Quality Chasm: A New Health System for the 21st Century. Washington DC: National Academies Press, 2001.

2   Kohn LT, Corrigan JM, Donaldson MS, eds. To Err is Human: Building a Safer Health System. Washington DC: National Academies Press, 2000.

◆ 3   Chassin MR, Galvin RW. The urgent need to improve health care quality: Institute of Medicine National Roundtable on Health Care Quality. JAMA 1998; 11: 1000–5.

4   Collins KS, Hughes DL, Doty MM, et al. Diverse Communities, Common Concerns: Addressing Health Care Quality for Minority Americans. New York: The Commonwealth Fund, 2002.

5   Wennberg JE, Cooper M, eds. The Dartmouth Atlas of Health Care in the United States. Chicago: American Hospital Publishing, 1998.

6   Nolan K, Nolan T. Learning from quality improvement in healthcare systems. In: Mitchell BM, Lynn J, eds. Symptom Research: Methods and Opportunities. [Online textbook] Washington DC: National Institutes of Health, 2003. Available at: http://symptomresearch.nih.gov (accessed August 2004).

7   Goldie SM. Florence Nightingale: Letters from the Crimea 1854–1856. Manchester UK: Mandolin, 1997.

8   Higginson I. Clinical and organizational audit in palliative care. In: Doyle D, Hanks GWC, MacDonald N, eds. Oxford Textbook of Palliative Medicine, 2nd ed. New York: Oxford University Press, 1998.

● 9   Lynn J, Nolan K, Kabcenell A, et al. Reforming care for persons near the end of life: The promise of quality improvement. Ann Intern Med 2002; 2:117–22.

10   Berwick DM. Developing and testing changes in delivery of care. Ann Intern Med 1998; 128: 651–6.

11   Langley G, Nolan K, Nolan T, et al. The Improvement Book. San Francisco: Jossey-Boss, 1996.

12   Shaw CD. Medical Audit: A Hospital Handbook. London: King's Fund Centre, 1989.

● 13   Institute for Healthcare Improvement. Improvement Methods: How to Improve. Available at: http://ihi.org/IHI/Topics/Improvement/ImprovementMethods/HowToImprove (accessed September 2004).

14   Commission for Health Improvement. What is Clinical Audit? Available at: www.chi.gov.uk/eng/audit/about.shtml#00 (accessed September 2004).

● 15   Lynn J, Schuster JL, Kabcenell A. Improving Care for the End of Life: A Sourcebook for Health Care Managers and Clinicians. New York: Oxford Press, 2000.

✳ 16   National Institute for Clinical Excellence. Improving Supportive and Palliative Care for Adults With Cancer: The Manual. London: National Institute for Clinical Excellence, 2004.

17   Center to Advance Palliative Care. The Case for Hospital-based Palliative Care. New York: Mt. Sinai School of Medicine, 2004.

18   United Kingdom Parliament. The NHS Plan: A Plan for Investment: A Plan for Reform. CM; 4818-I. London: The Stationery Office, 2000.

19   McGlynn EA, Cassel CK, Leatherman ST, et al. Establishing national goals for quality improvement. Med Care 2003; 41 (1 Suppl): I16–I29.

◆ 20   National Committee for Quality Assurance. The State of Health Care Quality 2003: Industry Trends and Analysis. Washington DC: NCQA Publications, 2003.

21   Department of Health. NHS Performance Ratings: Acute Trusts, Specialist Trusts, Ambulance Trusts, Mental Health Trusts 2001/02. 2002. Available at: www.performance.doh.gov.uk/performanceratings/2002/national.html (September 2004).

● 22   Bookbinder M, Romer AL. Raising the standard of care for imminently dying patients using quality improvement. J Palliat Med 2002; 5: 635–44.

23   International Society for Quality in Healthcare. Global Review of Initiatives to Improve Quality in Health Care. Geneva: World Health Organization, 2003.

24   Shaw CD. Evaluating accreditation. Int J Qual Health Care 2003; 15: 455–6.

✳ 25   Joint Commission on Accreditation of Healthcare Organizations. Comprehensive Accreditation Manual for Hospitals. Oakbrook Terrace, IL: Joint Commission on Accreditation of Healthcare Organizations, 2001.

✳ 26   Joint Commission of the Accreditation of Healthcare Organizations. Improving the Quality of Pain Management Through Measurement and Action [monograph]. Oakland Terrace, IL: Joint Commissions Resources Inc, 2003.

✳ 27   Joint Commission on Accreditation of Healthcare Organizations. Ethics, Rights, and Responsibilities Standards for Hospitals. Oakbrook Terrace, IL: Joint Commission on Accreditation of Healthcare Organizations, 2004.

28   Joint Commission on Accreditation of Healthcare Organizations. Setting the Standard: The Joint Commission and Health Care Safety and Quality [brochure]. Oakbrook Terrace, IL: Joint Commission on Accreditation of Healthcare Organizations, 2003.

29   World Health Organization. Africa Project on Palliative Care: Project Description. 2003. Available at: www.who.int/cancer/palliative/projectproposal/en/ (accessed September 2004).

30   Minimum standard of care defined for HIV patients with cancer. Bull World Health Organ 2002; 80: 176.

31   Sepulveda C, Habiyambere V, Amandua J, et al. Quality care at the end of life in Africa. BMJ 2003; 327: 209–13.

32   Harding R, Stewart K, Marconi K, et al. Current HIV/AIDS end-of-life care in sub-Saharan Africa: a survey of models, services, challenges and priorities. BMC Public Health 2003; 3: 33.

33 Standing Senate Committee on Social Affairs, Science and Technology. *Quality End of Life Care: The Right of Every Canadian* [Report]. Ottawa ON: Library of Parliament, 2000. Available at: www.parl.gc.ca/36/2/parlbus/commbus/senate/com-e/upda-e/rep-e/repfinjun00-e.htm (accessed September 2004).

✳ 34 Ferris FD, Balfour HM, Bowen K, *et al. A Model to Guide Hospice Palliative Care*. Ottawa ON: Canadian Hospice Palliative Care Association, 2002. Available at: www.chpca.net/publications/norms_of_practice.htm (accessed September 2004).

35 Stevens AM, Gwilliam B, A'hern R, *et al.* Experience in the use of the palliative care outcome scale. *Support Care Cancer* 2005; **13**: 1027–34.

36 Moore S, Sherwin A. Improving patient access to healthcare professionals: a prospective audit evaluating the role of e-mail communication for patients with lung cancer. *Eur J Oncol Nurs* 2004; **8**: 350–4.

37 Lloyd-Williams M, Payne S. Can multidisciplinary guidelines improve the palliation of symptoms in the terminal phase of dementia? *Int J Palliat Nurs* 2002; **8**: 370–5.

38 Galvin J. An audit of pressure ulcer incidence in a palliative care setting. *Int J Palliat Nurs* 2002; **8**: 214–21.

39 Rawlinson F, Finlay I. Assessing education in palliative medicine: development of a tool based on the Association for Palliative Medicine core curriculum. *Palliat Med* 2002; **16**: 51–5.

40 Lee L, White V, Ball J, *et al.* An audit of oral care practice and staff knowledge in hospital palliative care. *Int J Palliat Nurs* 2001; **7**: 395–400.

41 Neo SH, Loh EC, Koo WH. An audit of morphine prescribing in a hospice. *Singapore Med J* 2001; **42**: 417–19.

◆ 42 Hearn J, Higginson IJ. Outcome measures in palliative care for advanced cancer patients: a review. *J Public Health Med.* 1997; **19**: 193–9.

43 Higginson I. Clinical audit and organizational audit in palliative care. *Cancer Surv* 1994; **21**: 233–45.

44 Dunckley M, Aspinal F, Addington-Hall JM, *et al.* A research study to identify facilitators and barriers to outcome measure implementation. *Int J Palliat Nurs* 2005; **11**: 218–25.

45 Hughes RA, Sinha A, Aspinal F, *et al.* What is the potential for the use of clinical outcome measures to be computerised? Findings from a qualitative research study. *Int J Health Care Qual Assur Inc Leaders Health Serv* 2004; **17**: 47–52.

✳ 46 Macmillan Cancer Relief. Gold standards framework, 2004. Available at: www.macmillan.org.uk/healthprofessionals/disppage.asp?id=2062 (accessed September 2004).

47 Thomas K. *The Gold Standards Framework Flyer: A Programme for Community Palliative Care*. UK: Macmillan Cancer Relief, 2004.

48 Lynn J, Myers S, Olsson M, *et al.* Learning lab: End of life and palliative care. Presented to the Institute for Healthcare Improvement National Forum, Orlando, FL, December 8, 2002.

49 Macmillan cancer relief. Latest news, 2004. Available at: www.macmillan.org.uk/healthprofessionals/disppage.asp?id=6875 (accessed September 2004).

● 50 Lynn J, Schall M, Milne C, *et al.* Quality improvements in end of life care: Insights from two collaboratives. *Jt Comm J Qual Improv* 2000; **26**: 254–67.

◆ 51 Beth Israel Continuum Health Partners Inc. Palliative Care for Advanced Disease (PCAD) Pathway: Unit Reference Manual [online manual]. Available at: www.stoppain.org/services_staff/pcad1.html (accessed September 2004).

◆ 52 Davies E, Higginson IJ, eds. *The Solid Facts: Palliative Care*. Denmark: World Health Organization Europe, 2004.

◆ 53 Davies E, Higginson IJ, eds. *Better Palliative Care for Older People*. Denmark: World Health Organization Europe, 2004.

54 Murray SA, Grant E, Grant A, Kendall M. Dying from cancer in developed and developing countries: lessons from two qualitative interview studies of patients and their carers. *BMJ* 2003; **326**: 368.

55 The Leapfrog Group. Rewarding Results Publications. Available at: www.leapfroggroup.org/RewardingResults/pubs.htm (accessed September 2004).

56 Bailit health purchasing and Sixth man consulting. *The Growing Case for Using Physician Incentives to Improve Health Care Quality*. Washington DC: National Health Care Purchasing Institute, 2001.

57 Haines A, Jones R. Implementing findings of research. *BMJ* 1994; **308**: 1488–92.

58 Clancy C. Health services research: from galvanizing attention to creating action. *Health Serv Res* 2003; **38**: 777–81.

◆ 59 Ferlie EB, Shortell SM. Improving the quality of health care in the United Kingdom and the United States: a framework for change. *Milbank Q* 2001; **79**: 281–315.

60 Stryer D, Clancy C. Boosting performance measure for measure. *BMJ* 2003; **326**: 1278–9.

61 Berwick DM. Lessons from developing nations on improving health care. *BMJ* 2004; **328**: 1124–9.

62 Marshall MN, Shekelle PG, McGlynn EA, *et al.* Can health care quality indicators be transferred between countries? *Qual Saf Health Care* 2003; **12**: 8–12.

◆ 63 Schuster MA, McGlynn EA, Brook RH. How good is the quality of health care in the United States? *Milbank Q* 1998; **76**: 517–63.

◆ 64 Wilson T, Berwick DM, Cleary PD. What do collaborative improvement projects do? Experience from seven countries. *Jt Comm J Qual Saf* 2003; **29**: 85–93.

65 Bradley EH, Webster TR, Baker D, *et al. Translating Research into Practice: Speeding the Adoption of Innovative Health Care Programs* [issue brief]. New York: Commonwealth Fund, 2004.

PART 6

Organization and governance

27

Standards of care

FRANK D FERRIS

WHY STANDARDS OF CARE?

With the successful implementation of modern medicine and public health, patients and their families are living for much longer with one or more life-threatening illnesses and multiple issues that can cause them suffering and adversely impact the quality of their lives. Today more than ever before there is an urgent need for palliative care, including hospice care, around the world. This is particularly true when access to therapies to treat the disease process and/or resources are limited.

To this end, patients and families are hoping that palliative care will 'relieve their suffering and improve the quality of their lives whether they are living with an advanced life-threatening illness, or are bereaved'.[1,2] They are hoping for a consistent approach to palliative care wherever they receive their care so they can maintain their health and the activities that bring them meaning and value for as long as possible.[3] They want to choose from therapeutic options appropriate for their context and goals of care.[4] They want help to navigate the healthcare system. They do not want to have multiple repeat assessments, mixed messages or fragmented care from many different healthcare providers who do not function as a team.[5,6] This is particularly true for older people, who may not have the energy, stamina, or friends or family members available to help them.

At the same time, clinicians want to know how to provide palliative care in a way that will produce the best results for their patients and families without adverse events, and may even prolong their lives. Administrators, policy makers, regulators, and funders want to know how to best integrate palliative care into their existing healthcare system in a manner that is ethical, legal, fundable, and provides a consistent experience for patients, families, healthcare organizations and systems, and ultimately, for their society within the available resources. They also want to ensure that the correct medications and therapies are available when and where the patient needs them, and that they are delivered safely, with the least risk of adverse events.

Today, there is increasing interest and value to develop standards of care for palliative care that provide clear definition and elaboration of:

- the practice of palliative care (a model to guide patient and family care) and the organizational structures and functions needed to provide it (a model to guide organizational development)
- the activities that are part of the process of providing palliative care (preferred practice guidelines)
- the data and documentation that clinicians should routinely collect (outcome measures)
- what palliative care realistically hopes to achieve, i.e. its goals or targets (standards of practice)
- strategies to review these outcomes so that the patient's, family's and society's experience will improve over time (performance improvement).

If growth in the number of palliative care programs occurs rapidly without widely accepted standards of care, there is a risk that clinicians and organizations will start services that address only some of the issues that patients and families face. Clinical practice may vary considerably with little or no sense of the impact of the care provided. Healthcare funders and policy makers may develop limited funding and service delivery models and regulations, which are barriers to good palliative care delivery, e.g. limit access to opioids.

INDUSTRY ANALOGY

Industry has long known that standardized approaches to facilitate consistency in products and services are invaluable. When a company wants to make an automobile, there are fixed expectations on the part of a consumer for what a car will do. Once a design is established, it is easy to reproduce the product.

Industry has refined the process of mass-producing a high-quality product. The industry uses an interactive process that includes regularly updated:

- needs assessments to find out what the customer wants/needs (both opinion and data driven)
- definition of the organizational strategic and business plan
- definition of the principal activities and the products the company will produce (through consensus, refined based on evidence); the goal is a high-quality product that is overall consistent, yet customized to the individual hopes, expectations, and needs of each individual customer
- measurement of their outcomes of process and products (fruits of their labor), e.g. through statistics, changes, resources used, risks
- review of their outcomes to improve their products and the process to create them.

Comparison between industry and palliative care

The development of plans of care for individual patients and families follows a similar process. Clinicians first identify each patient's and family's issues, expectations and goals of care using standardized approaches to functional inquiry, communication, and decision-making. Once their treatment priorities have been clarified, the interdisciplinary team plans and delivers the agreed-to medications, therapies, and care in the manner that has the greatest potential for benefit, and the least risk of adverse events based on best practice and treatment guidelines. Each visit, the team reassesses the patient's and family's status, issues, expectations, goals, treatment priorities, understanding, and satisfaction with the plan and treatments and revises them whenever necessary.

The most significant difference between palliative care and a manufactured product occurs in the outcome – the patient/customer satisfaction. A manufactured product is just what it appears to be. The manufacturer and customer can both examine it and determine whether it is satisfactory or not. The quality is easily measured. In addition, manufacturers compete in markets where consumers have access to information and choices, and can compare price and value across companies. Customers make choices based on subjective and objective evaluation of the product. If they make a bad choice, they tell their friends, sell the product, and buy something different.

Care, on the other hand, can be defined in one way by the health professionals who deliver it, and assessed quite differently by the patient/family who receives it. It is the perception of what is received, and not the care plan or vision of the health professionals, which determines patient/family satisfaction. If the patient or family does not like the care they are receiving, they may be able to change providers, but it might not be easy.

Paradigm shift

We are all familiar with the process of deciding what is in the best interests of the patient/family, deciding on a plan of care, implementing it, and assessing how well we have followed through with our plan. However, to deliver care effectively and improve patient/family satisfaction requires a dramatic re-focusing of our understanding, *a paradigm shift*. We must move away from autonomously making decisions and evaluating the quality of service we deliver, to a position where it is the satisfaction of the patient/family with the outcomes of the care they receive that determines success or failure.[7]

TYPES OF STANDARDS

Clinicians, administrators of healthcare organizations, funders, policy makers, regulators, and accreditors are all interested to know how palliative care will be delivered. As a result of their different perspectives (see Fig. 27.1), many different types of standards have been developed relative to the practice of palliative care. Examples are listed in Appendix 27.1. A regularly updated listing is available online (http://standards.cpsonline.info).

Well developed **organizational standards of practice** are of greatest importance to guide a consistent patient/family experience. Each healthcare organization should be developing standards of practice specific to the culture, environment, funding, and service delivery models in

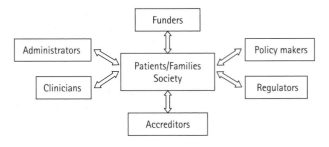

Figure 27.1 *Perspectives on palliative care practice. Redrawn with permission from Canadian Hospice Palliative Care Association, 2005.*

which it works. These standards describe the structure for their palliative care service(s), the issues they address, the process for providing care, the outcomes they measure, and their performance improvement strategies.

STANDARDS OF PROFESSIONAL CONDUCT

Individual disciplines on the interdisciplinary palliative care team may also develop standards of professional conduct that govern the professional behavior of their members. They often focus on maintaining the integrity of the profession. They address how a professional acts and define core competencies for the discipline.

MINIMUM STANDARDS

Policy makers and funders often define minimum standards that must be met before an organization can use the label 'palliative care service' and/or receive funding. As an example, the Medicare Hospice Conditions of Participation in the USA specify the minimum standards of practice for hospice organizations to be eligible to be reimbursed under the Medicare Hospice Benefit.[8]

LAWS

Policy makers and regulators may create laws to ensure that minimal standards of practice are enforceable, e.g. opioid control legislation specific to each country.

ACCREDITATION STANDARDS

Accreditation organizations focus on developing accreditation standards that can be used to examine and compare the activities and outcomes of many different healthcare organizations providing palliative care services. (As an example, the Canadian Council on Healthcare Services accreditation is currently developing modules to examine the delivery of palliative care services in acute and long-term care facilities, cancer clinics and home care programs across Canada.)

Central role of organizational standards of practice

Historically, most organizations that were part of the early grassroots hospice and palliative care movement were developed by people with passion and good will. There was minimal literature to guide consistent practice; each organization developed its own approaches to palliative care delivery; components of palliative care were frequently been left out, leaving gaps in the services available within a given geographical region; organizational standards of practice were frequently not been developed. As a result, patients and families experienced considerable variability in the services available to them, and the care they received.

Today, for there to be consistency in the palliative care experienced by patients and families, across an organization,

or across a geographical region, there needs to be a shared understanding by clinicians, administrators, and volunteers of the standards, preferred practice guidelines, data collection, and documentation strategies that the organization or the region has decided on. Ideally, each healthcare organization will develop its own standards of practice as it first evolves. Then, on a routine cyclic basis, it will review all of its standards to assess what is current and working well, and what is not working and needs modification, e.g. yearly.

If an organization's standards of practice are well known and understood by all staff, they will influence the language everyone uses, the values and principles guiding their activities, the issues they address, their approach to care planning and delivery, their management of resources, the data they collect, the documentation they keep, and the outcomes they achieve. Once the standards of practice have been subjected to review and updating, they will also stand up to external scrutiny when outsiders compare one organization with another, e.g. during accreditation.

DEVELOPING ORGANIZATIONAL STANDARDS OF PRACTICE

Whom to involve

Any process to improve the quality of palliative care being provided by an organization must engage everyone who will be involved in the process, i.e. clinicians, administrators, volunteers, and selected patients and families. When stakeholders are not involved in the development process, there may be little or no improvement in quality as people who don't know the content can't be expected to work with it. It is not advisable to delegate the process to a committee that then tells the rest of the organization how to improve their practice. Committee-based processes to develop standards of practice rarely change behaviors or patient/family experience as 'knowledge alone is insufficient for change'.[9]

Decision-making process

For there to be consistent high-quality palliative care, every individual in the organization will need to know, accept and agree to work with all elements of the final standards of practice that are pertinent to their day-to-day activities. Most people like to participate and have a say in developing any product. Ultimately, people who agree with a plan are much more likely to adhere to it, whereas people who don't agree with a plan, or don't have a chance to participate in building it, are much more likely to 'battle' the plan.

A carefully constructed consensus-based process based on a Delphi technique[10] is an ideal strategy to ensure that everyone has a working knowledge of the content and a chance to discuss and express their opinion about each issue. Groups need time to form, storm, and norm before they perform effectively.[11] A consensus-building process will encourage everyone to join at least one workgroup to work through the content. Ideally, the decision-making process will stimulate discussion among all stakeholders and increase their awareness of all aspects of palliative care practice and organizational development.

When constructing a consensus-building process, start by establishing (i) a quantitative and qualitative strategy to collect reviewers opinions of each of the major elements of the proposed model; (ii) the degree of agreement that will constitute consensus on numerical data (typically 70–80 percent); and (iii) the minimum number of contrary comments that will trigger modification of the content. Then, ensure that everyone who will participate agrees in advance to (i) share their opinions honestly and openly, (ii) listen to others, and (iii) work with the final product, even though they may not agree with all aspects of it. Also ensure that there is agreement on the values and principles guiding discussions and committee processes, e.g. honest, empathic, motived, professional, respectful, trustworthy.

To facilitate the process for each issue for which content is needed:

1 Constitute a small workgroup to draft content based on a review of the chosen model, e.g. the Canadian Hospice Palliative Care Association (CHPCA) model, existing literature, and committee opinion
2 Disseminate the draft to all organizational stakeholders and educate them about the content
3 Invite stakeholders to review and comment on the draft within a specified timeframe
4 Modify the draft based on the feedback
5 Ask stakeholders if they can agree to accept and work with the content; if not, make any necessary modifications and ask them again
6 Once consensus is reached, publish and disseminate the final content.

What approach

There are two possible approaches to developing organizational standards of practice:

- Develop independently: Each organization develops the process and content from scratch without using an existing model[1,2] to guide the process or provide content to review.
- Develop based on a model: Each organization uses a widely accepted model standard of care to (i) guide the process to develop its own standards of practice and (ii) provide content to review and adapt to the culture, environment, funding and service delivery models in which the organization works, rather than developing it from scratch.

The latter approach is faster and more efficient. If several organizations within a given geographical region base their process on the same model, there is much greater potential for consistency in practice and the experience for patients, families, organizations, and society across the region.

Based on what model

Already there are a number of widely accepted model standards of care that can be used by an organization to guide it through the process of developing standards of practice. The CHPCA's *Model to Guide Hospice Palliative Care: Based on National Principles and Norms of Practice* is one such widely accepted model.[1,2]

The CHPCA Model took 9 years to develop through three iterative consensus-building cycles based on a Delphi technique.[10] Hundreds of participants from across Canada representing thousands of stakeholders from their organizations reviewed the successive draft documents, participated in workshops, and provided their opinions. By 2001 there was >90 percent agreement on virtually all of more than 100 items (exceeding the goal of >75 percent agreement) and the model was published in both English and French in 2002. Already it has been endorsed by all 11 provincial hospice palliative care associations, the College of Family Physicians of Canada (http://www.cfpc.ca), the Royal College of Physicians and Surgeons of Canada (http://rcpsc.medical.org/), the Canadian Nurses Association (http://www.cna-nurses.ca/cna/), the Quality End-of-Life Care Coalition of Canada (http://www.chpca.net/quality_end-of-life_care_coalition_of_canada.htm), and the Canadian Strategy on Palliative and End of Life Care as the basis for a variety of national efforts in education, research, public awareness, and service delivery (see http://www.hc-sc.gc.ca/hcs-sss/pubs/caresoins/2005-strateg-palliat/index_e.html#4). The Canadian Medical Association (http://www.cma.ca) has supported it.

The model will be used in this chapter to illustrate the process, and its impact is detailed in Appendix 27.2. Other model standards of care are listed in Appendix 27.1. A regularly updated listing is available online (http://standards.cpsonline.info).

Clarify the framework

Once a model has been chosen, clarify the framework contained within the model so that all of the components are clear. Figure 27.2 presents the framework that is the basis for the CHPCA Model. It builds from the bottom up, and starts by specifying all of the components of standards of practice that are defined during the strategic planning process, including:

- the mission/vision of the organization
- definitions of the common language/terminology it uses
- values, foundational concepts and principles guiding its activities.

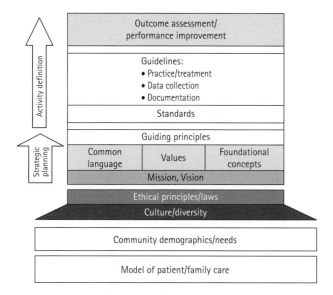

Figure 27.2 *Components of organizational standards of practice. Redrawn with permission from Canadian Hospice Palliative Care Association, 2002.*

It then specifies the components that are detailed for each principal activity and each issue the organization will address, including:

- standards that the organization is hoping to achieve
- practice and treatment guidelines
- data collection and documentation guidelines
- outcomes to measure
- performance improvement strategies.

Developmental steps

Once the participants have been selected, the process clarified, and a model to guide the process chosen, the following sequential steps are recommended as a strategy to build the standards of practice.

STEP 1: REVIEW THE ORGANIZATION'S STRATEGIC PLAN

Start by reviewing the organization's strategic plan.

Organizational focus

From the outset, remind all participants that the organization focuses on changing the experience of patients and families, not simply on providing care. To consider this perspective effectively, the CHPCA Model provides a model to guide patient and family care to help participants develop a shared understanding of the patient and family experience, the definition of palliative care, and the process for providing care to them.[1,2]

- Modern illness experience: Today, in the face of any illness process, most patients and families experience multiple issues that are the manifestations of the underlying disease process(es) or aging (e.g. symptoms, functional and psychosocial changes), and the predicaments of how to adjust and continue living life to the fullest given these new circumstances (see Fig. 27.3).[12–18] If not treated properly, many of these issues can cause considerable suffering, reduce the quality of their lives and have an adverse impact on their future.[19] Patients and families come to the healthcare system seeking help to address the issues that are bothering them.

- Definition of palliative care: To address these issues, the CHPCA Model states that 'palliative care aims to prevent and relieve suffering and promote quality of life'.[1,2] In 2002, the World Health Organization endorsed a more elaborate definition of palliative care:[20]

  Palliative care is an approach that improves the quality of life of patients and their families facing the problem associated with life-threatening illness, through the prevention and relief of suffering by means of early identification and impeccable assessment and treatment of pain and other problems, physical, psychosocial and spiritual.

- Process of providing palliative care: Over time, clinicians build a therapeutic relationship with patients and families through a series of sequential encounters (see Fig. 27.4). During each encounter, clinicians follow six essential steps to provide palliative care (see Fig. 27.5).

Environment in which the organization functions

For participants to consider all perspectives related to their organization, it will be important for them to understand the environment in which they provide care, including:

- the demographics of the population
- who the customers and stakeholders are
- what their unmet needs are
- the ethical principles that will be the foundation for their activities including autonomy, beneficence, nonmaleficence, justice, confidentiality, truth-telling and discrimination[21–24]
- the laws and regulations governing care in their jurisdiction.

Definition of the organization

After reviewing the strategic plan, participants should understand the organization's:

- Mission: A short statement of the organization's purpose, e.g. what it is, what it does, and in which geographical region. For example: 'The (named) program provides palliative care services and education to all patients and families within (named geographical region or health care district)'.

- Vision: A short statement of the organization's aspirations; what it hopes to become and achieve. For example: 'The (named) program will be the leading palliative care program providing clinical services to all

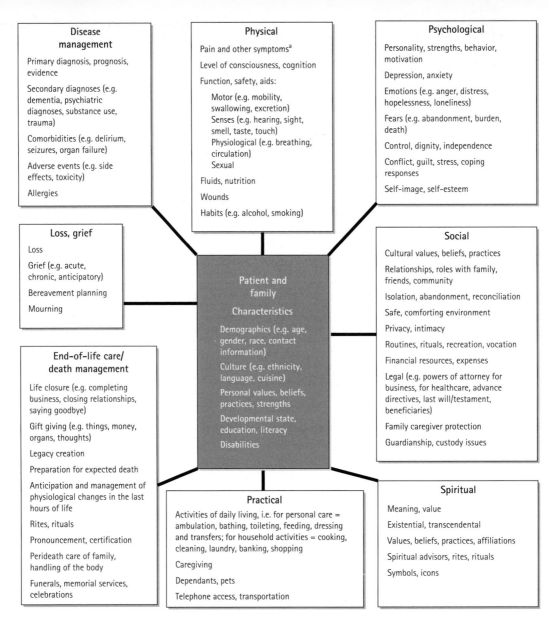

Disease management

Primary diagnosis, prognosis, evidence

Secondary diagnoses (e.g. dementia, psychiatric diagnoses, substance use, trauma)

Comorbidities (e.g. delirium, seizures, organ failure)

Adverse events (e.g. side effects, toxicity)

Allergies

Physical

Pain and other symptoms[a]

Level of consciousness, cognition

Function, safety, aids:

Motor (e.g. mobility, swallowing, excretion)
Senses (e.g. hearing, sight, smell, taste, touch)
Physiological (e.g. breathing, circulation)
Sexual

Fluids, nutrition

Wounds

Habits (e.g. alcohol, smoking)

Psychological

Personality, strengths, behavior, motivation

Depression, anxiety

Emotions (e.g. anger, distress, hopelessness, loneliness)

Fears (e.g. abandonment, burden, death)

Control, dignity, independence

Conflict, guilt, stress, coping responses

Self-image, self-esteem

Loss, grief

Loss

Grief (e.g. acute, chronic, anticipatory)

Bereavement planning

Mourning

Patient and family Characteristics

Demographics (e.g. age, gender, race, contact information)

Culture (e.g. ethnicity, language, cuisine)

Personal values, beliefs, practices, strengths

Developmental state, education, literacy

Disabilities

Social

Cultural values, beliefs, practices

Relationships, roles with family, friends, community

Isolation, abandonment, reconciliation

Safe, comforting environment

Privacy, intimacy

Routines, rituals, recreation, vocation

Financial resources, expenses

Legal (e.g. powers of attorney for business, for healthcare, advance directives, last will/testament, beneficiaries)

Family caregiver protection

Guardianship, custody issues

End-of-life care/ death management

Life closure (e.g. completing business, closing relationships, saying goodbye)

Gift giving (e.g. things, money, organs, thoughts)

Legacy creation

Preparation for expected death

Anticipation and management of physiological changes in the last hours of life

Rites, rituals

Pronouncement, certification

Perideath care of family, handling of the body

Funerals, memorial services, celebrations

Practical

Activities of daily living, i.e. for personal care = ambulation, bathing, toileting, feeding, dressing and transfers; for household activities = cooking, cleaning, laundry, banking, shopping

Caregiving

Dependants, pets

Telephone access, transportation

Spiritual

Meaning, value

Existential, transcendental

Values, beliefs, practices, affiliations

Spiritual advisors, rites, rituals

Symbols, icons

[a] Other common symptoms include, but are not limited to:
Cardio-respiratory – breathlessness, cough, edema, hiccups, apnea, agonal breathing patterns
Gastrointestinal – nausea, vomiting, constipation, obstipation, bowel obstruction, diarrhea, bloating, dysphagia, dyspepsia
Oral conditions – dry mouth, mucositis
Skin conditions – dry skin, nodules, pruritus, rashes
General – agitation, anorexia, cachexia, fatigue, weakness, bleeding, drowsiness, effusions (pleural, peritoneal), fever/chills, incontinence, insomnia, lymphedema, myoclonus, odor, prolapse, sweats, syncope, vertigo

Figure 27.3   *Multiple issues patients and families experience. Redrawn with permission from Canadian Hospice Palliative Care Association, 2002.*

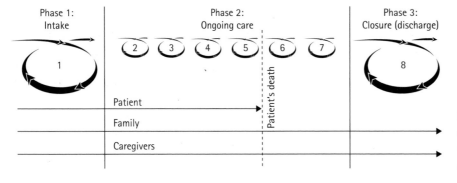

Figure 27.4   *Sequential encounters in a therapeutic relationship. Redrawn with permission from Canadian Hospice Palliative Care Association, 2002.*

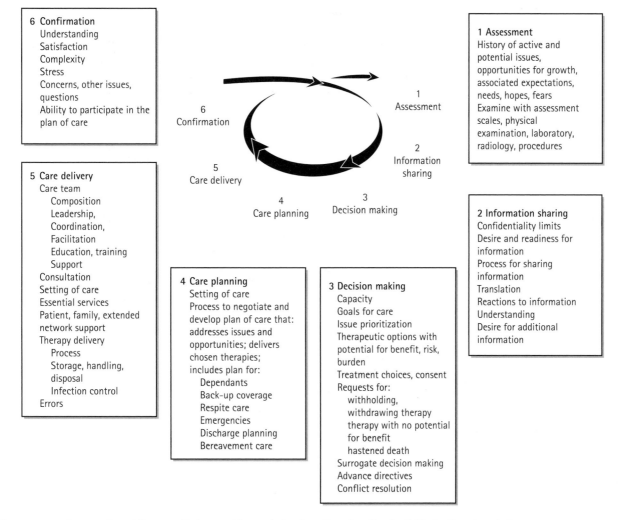

6 Confirmation
Understanding
Satisfaction
Complexity
Stress
Concerns, other issues,
questions
Ability to participate in the
plan of care

5 Care delivery
Care team
Composition
Leadership,
Coordination,
Facilitation
Education, training
Support
Consultation
Setting of care
Essential services
Patient, family, extended
network support
Therapy delivery
Process
Storage, handling,
disposal
Infection control
Errors

4 Care planning
Setting of care
Process to negotiate and
develop plan of care that:
addresses issues and
opportunities; delivers
chosen therapies;
includes plan for:
Dependants
Back-up coverage
Respite care
Emergencies
Discharge planning
Bereavement care

3 Decision making
Capacity
Goals for care
Issue prioritization
Therapeutic options with
potential for benefit, risk,
burden
Treatment choices, consent
Requests for:
withholding,
withdrawing therapy
therapy with no potential
for benefit
hastened death
Surrogate decision making
Advance directives
Conflict resolution

1 Assessment
History of active and
potential issues,
opportunities for growth,
associated expectations,
needs, hopes, fears
Examine with assessment
scales, physical
examination, laboratory,
radiology, procedures

2 Information sharing
Confidentiality limits
Desire and readiness for
information
Process for sharing
information
Translation
Reactions to information
Understanding
Desire for additional
information

6 Confirmation

1 Assessment

2 Information sharing

5 Care delivery

4 Care planning

3 Decision making

Figure 27.5   *Process of providing care. Redrawn with permission from Canadian Hospice Palliative Care Association, 2002.*

patients and families within (named geographical region or healthcare district) and a leader in palliative care education and research'.

- Common language: Definitions of the terminology commonly used by staff. A detailed lexicon is available in the CHPCA Model.
- Values: The fundamental beliefs on which organizational activities are based. Examples from the CHPCA Model include:[2 (p. 19)]
  - The intrinsic value of each person as an autonomous and unique individual.
  - Value of life, the natural process of death, and the fact that both provide opportunities for personal growth and self-actualization.
  - The need to address the suffering, expectations, needs, hopes and fears of patients and families.
  - Care is provided only when the patient and/or family are prepared to accept it.
  - Care is guided by quality of life as defined by the individual.
  - Caregivers enter into a therapeutic relationship with patients and families based on dignity and integrity.
  - A unified response to suffering strengthens communities.
- Foundational concepts: Concepts that underlie all activities. All healthcare organizations are built on: effective group dynamics/leadership; effective communication based on a common language; and effective strategies that aim to change the experience of patients, families, caregivers, and the communities in which they provide care.
- Guiding principles: The fundamental truths guiding all of the organization's activities. Principles frequently used by palliative care programs include patient/family focused, high quality, safe and effective, accessible, adequately resources, collaborative, knowledge based, advocacy based, research based, etc.
- Principal activities that the organization engages in: In addition to patient/family care, palliative care organizations often engage in education, research

and advocacy. They all need an administrative infrastructure to support their activities.

- Specific issues: Specific issues the organization addresses in each principal activity. For patient and family care this might include pain control, spiritual management, legacy creation, and the management of the symptoms during the last hours of life. For education, this might include orientation for staff, continuing education for community clinicians, volunteer training, and an introduction to palliative care for medical and nursing students.

STEP 2: DEVELOP CONTENT FOR THE STANDARDS OF PRACTICE

No organization will be able to develop all of the content for its standards of practice at one time. It will likely take months to years to develop all of the necessary standards, guidelines, and outcome measurement tools. Start by developing and prioritizing the list of issues that the organization will address in each area of activity. For the purposes of planning and developing standards of practice, the interrelationship of the therapeutic process with the issues faced by the patient can be illustrated as a simple table 'The Square of Care' (Fig. 27.6). As organizations implement their services, the table can be filled in to illustrate the specific issues for which standards, guidelines, and outcomes measurements have been developed. The gaps will indicate where work is still needed.

On the basis of preestablished priorities, workgroups can then develop standards, guidelines, and outcome measures for each issue the organization will address:

- Standards: These are criteria established for the measurement of quality, value, or extent.[25,26] They present the organization's process and outcome goals related to a particular issue. In a widely accepted model, e.g. the CHPCA Model, norms present the 'usual' or 'average' practice across many different organizations (see Fig. 27.7). They are less specific than the standards which each individual organization will

define based on their local environment, and funding and service delivery capabilities. Norms are also different from minimum or regulatory standards (which typically describe the 'floor' or minimum that is acceptable, e.g. the Medicare Hospice Benefit Conditions of Participation in the USA[27]). Many existing standards detail process. Only recently have there been attempts to look at outcome standards. An example of how standards can be developed from norms is presented in Appendix 27.3.

- Guidelines: These are systematically developed statements to assist decision making about appropriate strategies to manage specific circumstances.[25,28] Ideally, guidelines include details of the process to be followed, the data to be collected, and how to document the activity. Many organizations will want to develop two types of guideline: (i) practice guidelines that detail the essential steps to assess and manage a particular issues, e.g. pain; and (ii) treatment guidelines that detail the indications, steps for delivering a specific medication or therapy, e.g. morphine, and potential risks, e.g. drug interactions and adverse effects. Some organizations

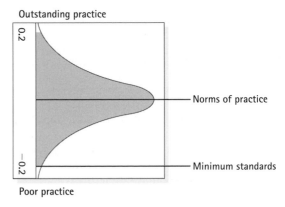

Figure 27.7 *Norms versus minimum standards. Redrawn with permission from Canadian Hospice Palliative Care Association, 2002.*

Domains of issues	Standards	Practice, data collection, documentation guidelines						Outcomes to measures	Performance improvement strategies
		1 Assess	2 Share information	3 Make decisions	4 Plan	5 Deliver	6 Confirm		
Disease management									
Physical									
Psychological									
Social									
Spiritual									
Practical									
End-of-life care/ death management									
Loss, grief									

Figure 27.6 *The square of care. Adapted from Canadian Hospice Palliative Care Association, 2002 with permission.*

will choose to develop specific disease management pathways, with or without standing orders. For sensitive issues, i.e. infection control, many organizations will develop very specific policies and procedures to guide care. For examples see Appendix 27.1.

- Outcome measures: These are the measurable end results or consequences of a specific action or essential step in a process, including effectiveness, resource utilization, risk, compliance and satisfaction. These can be simple measures to compare the change in a variable from day to day, e.g. the severity of a patient's pain today compared with yesterday. They can also be complex measures that capture overall performance of the organization related to a given issue, e.g. the percentage of patients with a pain severity score <5/10, 48 hours after admission to the program. For examples see Appendix 27.1.

STEP 3: IMPLEMENT THE STANDARDS OF PRACTICE

As each part of the model is developed and accepted by the staff, disseminate it throughout the organization. Modify staff orientation and continuing education activities to include the changes. Ask staff to practice to the new standards and guidelines, and measure their outcomes.

STEP 4: DEVELOP A PERFORMANCE IMPROVEMENT STRATEGY

Concurrently, every palliative care organization will want to choose specific outcomes to measure and review on a regular basis. Then, based on the results, specific strategies to improve staff's performance related to problematic activities can be implemented. The Plan-Do-Study-Act cycle is an excellent model to guide performance improvement strategies.[29,30] The document *Improving the Quality of Pain Management Through Measurement and Action* by the Joint Commission on the Accreditation of Healthcare Organizations is a wonderful example of a performance improvement strategy.[25]

SUMMARY

Standards of care are increasingly important for everyone involved in palliative care. By defining its principal activities, standards, practice and treatment guidelines and outcome measures, and developing a performance improvement strategy, a palliative care organization will set the stage to ensure that it changes the experience of patients and their families.

Although it is possible for individual organizations to define themselves independently, a regionally, nationally, or internationally accepted consensus-based 'model standard of care' can: expedite the process for all stakeholders; ensure

that the standards of care live from day to day; increase the possibility of consistency of the experience for patients and families regardless of the setting or the organization from which they receive care; and minimize risks of liability of adverse events. A number of models, standards and guidelines already exist to guide the development of sound approaches to the delivery of palliative care. At present, most are based on consensus opinion. With time, as the evidence supporting palliative care practice grows so will the strength of our service delivery models.

After all, isn't it true that: 'The standards of practice we create and the people we train will look after us when it's our turn to receive care. If it was your turn tomorrow, would you get the care you hoped for?'[31]

Key learning points

- There is a growing need for widely accepted standards of care to ensure that patients and families receive consistent, high-quality palliative care wherever they receive their care.

- It is the experience of the patient and family, and their satisfaction with the outcomes of the palliative care they received that matters, not how the care was delivered.

- There are many different types of standard, of which the most important is organizational standards of practice.

- Every organization needs to develop its own organizational standards of practice specific to the culture, environment, funding, and service delivery models in which it operates.

- When developing organizational standards of practice, involve everyone in the process who will participate directly or indirectly with providing care using an iterative consensus-building process

- Rather than building standards of practice from scratch, use a widely accepted model standard of care as a template to guide the process and provide content for participants to consider, e.g. the CHPCA *Model to Guide Hospice Palliative Care.*

- Start by reviewing the organization's strategic plan and the environment in which the organization operates.

- Once the principal functions and issues the organization addresses are clear, for each issue develop content sequentially, including process and outcome standards, practice and treatment guidelines, data collection and documentation guidelines, and outcomes to measure.

- As content becomes available for each issue, disseminate and implement it across the organization.

- Concurrently, review the measured outcome and develop a performance improvement strategy.

REFERENCES

● 1 Ferris F, Balfour H, Bowen K, *et al.* A model to guide patient and family care. Based on nationally accepted principles and norms of practice. *J Pain Symptom Manage* 2002; **24**: 106–23. Available at http://dx.doi.org/10.1016/S0885-3924(02)00468-2 (accessed December 15, 2005).

● 2 Ferris FD, Balfour HM, Bowen K, *et al. A Model to Guide Hospice Palliative Care.* Ottawa, ON: Canadian Hospice Palliative Care Association, March 2002. Available at www.chpca.net/publications/norms_of_practice.htm in English and www.acsp.net/publications_et_ressouces/normes.htm in French (accessed December 15, 2005).

3 Preamble to the Constitution of the World Health Organization as adopted by the International Health Conference, New York, 19–22 June, 1946; signed on 22 July 1946 by the representatives of 61 States (Official Records of the World Health Organization, no. 2, p. 100) and entered into force on 7 April 1948. See http://www.who.int/about/definition/en/ (accessed December 15, 2005).

4 Edgman-Levitan S, Cleary PD. What information do consumers want and need? *Health Affairs* 1996; **15**: 42–56.

5 Hall P, Weaver L. Interdisciplinary education and teamwork: a long and winding road. *Med Educ* 2001; **35**: 867–75.

6 Murray SA, Boyd K, Kendall M, *et al.* Dying of lung cancer or cardiac failure: prospective qualitative interview study of patients and careers in the community. *BMJ* 2002; **325**: 929.

7 Clemenhagen C. Patient satisfaction: the power of an untapped resource. *Can Med Assoc J* 1994; 150 : 1771–2.

8 Centers for Medicare & Medicaid Services. CMS Medicare Hospice Manual. Available at http://new.cms.hhs.gov/Manuals/PBM/itemdetail.asp?filterType=none&filterByDID=-99&sortByDID=1&sortOrder=ascending&itemID=CMS021912 (accessed December 15, 2005).

9 Ferris FD, von Gunten CF, Emanuel LL. Knowledge: insufficient for change. *J Palliat Med* 2001; **4**: 145–7. Available at http://dx.doi.org/10.1089/109662101750290164 (accessed December 15, 2005).

10 Polit DF, Hungler BP, eds. *Nursing Research.* Philadelphia: JB Lippincott, 1991: 356–7.

11 Tuckman B. Developmental sequence in small groups. *Psychol Bull* 1965; **63**: 384–99.

12 Emanuel LL, Alpert HR, Baldwin DC, Emanuel EJ. What terminally ill patients care about: toward a validated construct of patients' perspectives. *J Palliat Med* 2000; **3**: 419–31. Available at http://www.liebertonline.com/doi/abs/10.1089/jpm.2000.3.4.419 (accessed December 15, 2005).

13 Emanuel EJ, Emanuel LL. The promise of a good death. *Lancet* 1998; **351**: 21–9.

14 Gerteis M, Edgmam-Levitan S, Daley J, Delbanco TL, eds. *Through the Patient's Eyes: Understanding and Promoting Patient-Centered Care.* San Francisco: Jossy-Bass Publishers, 1993.

15 Singer PA, Martin DK, Kelner M. Quality end-of-life care: patients' perspectives. *JAMA* 1999; **281**: 163–8.

16 Steinhauser KE, Clipp EC, McNeilly M, *et al.* In search of a good death: observations of patients, families and providers. *Ann Intern Med* 2000; **132**: 825–32.

17 Steinhauser KE, Christakis NA, Clipp EC, *et al.* Factors considered important at the end of life by patients, family, physicians, and other care providers. *JAMA* 2000; **284**: 2476–82.

18 Steinhauser KE, Christakis NA, Clipp EC, *et al.* Preparing for the end of life: preferences of patients, families, physicians, and other care providers. *J Pain Symptom Manage* 2001; **22**: 727–37.

19 Covinsky KE, Goldman L, Cook EF, *et al.* The impact of serious illness on patients' families. SUPPORT Investigators. Study to Understand Prognoses and Preferences for Outcomes and Risks of Treatment. *JAMA* 1994; **272**: 1839–44.

20 WHO Definition of Palliative Care. Available at http://www.who.int/cancer/palliative/definition/en/ (accessed December 15, 2005).

21 Sepulveda C, Marlin A, Yoshida T, Ullrich A. Palliative Care: the World Health Organization's global perspective. *J Pain Symptom Manage* 2002; **24**: 91–6. Available at http://dx.doi.org/10.1016/ S0885-392400440-2 (accessed December 15, 2005).

22 *Canadian Medical Association Journal*, Bioethics for Clinicians Series. Available at http://www.cmaj.ca/cgi/collection/bioethics_for_clinicians_series (accessed December 15, 2005).

23 Baker RB, Caplan AL, Emanuel LL, Latham SR. *The American Medical Ethics Revolution.* Baltimore, MD: The Johns Hopkins University Press, 1999.

24 Beauchamp TL, Childress JF. *Principles of Medical Bioethics*, 5th ed. Oxford: Oxford University Press, 2001.

25 Joint Commission on the Accreditation of Healthcare Organizations. Improving the Quality of Pain Management Through Measurement and Action. Oakbrook Terrace, IL: Joint Commission on the Accreditation of Healthcare Organizations, 2003: 4. Available at http://www.jcaho.org/news±room/health±care±issues/pain_mono_jc.pdf.

26 Joint Commission on Accreditation of Healthcare Organizations. *Lexicon: A Dictionary of Health Care Terms, Organizations, and Acronyms*, 2nd ed. Oakbrook Terrace, IL: Joint Commission on the Accreditation of Healthcare Organizations, 1998.

27 Conditions of Participation, Hospice Care. Washington, DC: Health Care Financing Administration, US Department of Health and Human Services, Title 42, Chapter IV, Part 418. Viewable at: http://www.access.gpo.gov/nara/cfr/waisidx_00/42cfr418_00.html (accessed December 15, 2005).

28 Field MF, Lohr KN, eds, for the Committed to Advise the Public Health Service on Clinical Practice Guidelines, Institute of Medicine. *Clinical Practice Guidelines: Directions for a New Program.* Washington, DC: National Academy Press, 1990.

29 Langley GJ, Nolan KM, Nolan TW. The foundation of improvement. *Quality Progress* 1994:81–6.

◆ 30 Joint Commission on the Accreditation of Healthcare Organizations. Using performance improvement tools in health care settings: revised edition. Available at http://www.jcrinc.com/publications.asp?durki=753&site=4&return=78 (accessed December 15, 2005).

31 Ferris FD, in: Ferris FD, Balfour HM, Bowen K, *et al. A Model to Guide Hospice Palliative Care.* Ottawa, ON: Canadian Hospice Palliative Care Association, March 2002: Inside back cover. Available at www.chpca.net/publications/norms_of_practice.htm in English and www.acsp.net/publications_et_ressouces/ normes.htm in French (accessed December 15, 2005).

● 32 Hospice Palliative Care Nursing Standards of Practice. Ottawa, ON: Canadian Hospice Palliative Care Association,

2002. Available at http://www.chpca.net/interest_groups/ nurse.htm (accessed December 15, 2005).

33 Client Service Standards for the Volunteer Hospice Visiting Service. Toronto, ON: Hospice Association of Ontario. Available at http://www.hospice.on.ca/Publications/ publications.htm (accessed December 15, 2005).

34 2003 First Ministers' Accord on Health Care Renewal. Health Canada. Available at http://www.hc-sc.gc.ca/hcs-sss/delivery-prestation/fptcollab/2003accord/index_e.html (accessed December 15, 2005).

35 Ontario End-of-Life Care Strategy, October 2005. Available at http://ogov.newswire.ca/ontario/GPOE/2005/10/04/c7208. html?lmatch=&lang=_e.html (accessed December 15, 2005).

APPENDIX 27.1: SELECTED RESOURCES

Several regional and national organizations have already developed models, standards, and guidelines. These can be used to increase awareness of the importance of palliative care and guide the development of organizational standards of practice that guide palliative care practitioners and organizations. A regularly updated listing is available online (http://standards.cpsonline.info).

Models/norms/standards

AUSTRALIA

- Palliative Care Australia. *Standards for Providing Quality Palliative Care for all Australians.* Deacon West, ACT: Palliative Care Australia, 2005. Available at www.pallcare.org.au/Portals/9/docs/ Standards%20Palliative%20Care.pdf (accessed December 15, 2005).
- Quality Assurance Development Working Group 2. *Standards for Aged Care Facilities.* Ageing and Community Care Division, Department of Health and Aged Care, Commonwealth of Australia, 2000. Available at www.health.gov.au/acc/standard/facility/ sacfindx.htm (accessed December 15, 2005).

CANADA

- Ferris FD, Balfour HM, Bowen K, *et al.* A model to guide hospice palliative care. Ottawa, ON: Canadian Hospice Palliative Care Association, March 2002. Available at www.chpca.net/ publications/norms_of_practice.htm in English and www.acsp.net/ publications_et_ressouces/normes.htm in French (accessed December 15, 2005).
- The above is also available as: Ferris F, Balfour H, Bowen K, *et al.* A model to guide patient and family care. Based on nationally accepted principles and norms of practice. *J Pain Symptom Manage* 2002;24:106–23. Available at http://dx.doi.org/ 10.1016/S0885-3924(02)00468-2 (accessed December 15, 2005).
- CHPCA Nursing Standards Committee. *Hospice Palliative Care Nursing Standards of Practice.* Ottawa, ON: Canadian Hospice Palliative Care Association, 2002. Available at www.chpca.net/ interest_groups/nurse.htm (accessed December 15, 2005).

HUNGARY

Hungarian Hospice–Palliative Association. *Professional Guidelines. Palliative Care of Terminally Ill Cancer Patients,* 2nd ed. Budapest: Hungarian Hospice–Palliative Association, 2002. Available at www. hospice.hu/english/ hosp12_en.htm (accessed December 15, 2005).

ITALY

Recommendations and minimal prerequisites for palliative care in Italy (Societa italiana di Cure Palliative, Federazione Cure Palliative ONLUS). Available at www.fedcp.org/areanorma.asp? IDAreaNorma = 6 (accessed December 15, 2005).

NEW ZEALAND

The New Zealand Palliative Care Strategy. Wellington, NZ: Ministry of Health, 2001. See www.moh.govt.nz/moh. nsf/0/ b91ac89e05e74cb2cc256b6d0071b104?OpenDocument (accessed December 15, 2005).

SCOTLAND

Clinical Standards Board for Scotland and Scottish Partnership for Palliative Care. *Clinical Standards for Specialist Palliative Care,* 2002. Available at www.palliativecarescotland.org.uk/publications/ (accessed December 15, 2005).

Scottish Executive. *National Care Standards: Hospice Care,* 2002. Available at www.scotland.gov.uk/Resource/Doc/1095/0001719.pdf (accessed December 15, 2005).

SPAIN

Guide to Quality Criteria in Palliative Care. SECPAL Quality Group, 2002. Available from www.secpal.com/ (accessed December 15, 2005).

SWITZERLAND

Quality Standards, March 2001. Available in French, German and Italian from www.palliative.ch (accessed December 15, 2005).

UNITED KINGDOM

- NICE. *Improving Supportive and Palliative Care for Adults with Cancer.* London: NICE, 2004. Available at www.nice.org.uk/ Docref.asp?d = 110006 (accessed December 15, 2005).

UNITED STATES

- National Consensus Project for Quality Palliative Care. Clinical Practice Guidelines for Quality Palliative Care, 2004. Available at: www.nationalconsensusproject.org (accessed December 15, 2005).
- NASW. *Standards for Social Work Practice in Palliative and End-of-life Care.* Washington, DC: National Association of Social Workers, 2004. Available at www.socialworkers.org/practice/bereavement/ standards/default.asp (accessed December 15, 2005).
- Standards and Accreditation Committees. *Standards of Practice for Hospice Programs.* Alexandria, VA: National Hospice and Palliative Care Organization, 2000. Available at: http://eseries.nhpco.org/ eseries/source/Orders/index.cfm?task=3&CATEGORY=TECHMAT&

PRODUCT_TYPE=SALES&SKU=711077&DESCRIPTION=&FindSpec=standards&CFTOKEN=56192319&continue=1&SEARCH_TYPE=FIND (accessed December 15, 2005).

The Grace Project: End-of-life Care Standards of Practice in Correctional Settings. Alexandria, VA: Volunteers of America, 2001. Available at www2.edc.org/lastacts/archives/archivesMay00/standards.asp (accessed December 15, 2005).

Guidelines/tools

GENERAL

Fisher R, Ross MM, MacLean MJ. A Guide to End-of-Life Care for Seniors. See www.rgp.toronto.on.ca/iddg/eol.htm (accessed December 15, 2005).

National Comprehensive Cancer Network (NCCN) and the American Cancer Society. Advance Cancer and Palliative Care Treatment Guidelines for Patients – Version I, 2003. Available at www.nccn.org/patient_gls/_english/_palliative/index.htm (accessed December 15, 2005).

● Cochrane Pain, Palliative Care and Supportive Care Group (PaPaS). Abstracts of Cochrane Reviews. Available at: www.update-software.com/ abstracts/SYMPTAbstractIndex.htm (accessed December 15, 2005).

Hospice Organization and Palliative Experts (HOPE) of Wisconsin; Wisconsin Department of Health and Family Services (DHFS), Division of Supportive Living (DSL), Bureau of Quality Assurance (BQA); The Wisconsin Health Care Association; and The Wisconsin Association of Homes and Services for the Aging. *Guidelines for Care Coordination for Hospice Patients Who Reside in Nursing Homes.* Wisconsin Department of Health and Family Services, 2001. Available at http://dhfs.wisconsin.gov/rl_DSL/Publications/01042a.htm (accessed December 15, 2005).

● National Guideline Clearinghouse, Agency for Healthcare Research and Quality (US). See http://www.guideline.gov/ (accessed December 15, 2005).

Nixon M. Guidelines for medical care in long-term care facilities. *Can Fam Physician* 1994; 40: 1324–5.

CancerBACUP. UK Treatment Guidelines – Palliative Care. Available atwww.cancerbacup.org.uk/Healthprofessionals/Treatmentguidelines/Cancertreatments/Palliativecare (accessed December 15, 2005).

BEREAVEMENT

Palliative Care Australia. *Principles for the Provision of Bereavement Support.* Deacon West, ACT: Palliative Care Australia, 1998. Available at www.pallcare.org.au/Portals/9/docs/publications/bereavement.pdf (accessed December 15, 2005).

DEHYDRATION, FLUID MAINTENANCE

American Medical Directors Association. *Clinical Practice Guideline: Dehydration and Fluid Maintenance.* Columbia, MD: American Medical Directors Association, 2001. Available at www.amda.com/info/cpg/dehydration.htm (accessed December 15, 2005).

DEPRESSION

American Medical Directors Association. *Clinical Practice Guideline: Depression.* Columbia, MD: American Medical Directors

Association, 2003. Available at www.amda.com/info/cpg/depression.htm (accessed December 15, 2005).

DOCUMENTATION

Centers for Medicare & Medicaid Services. *Documentation Guidelines – Evaluation and Management Services.* Baltimore MD: Centers for Medicare & Medicaid Services 1997. Available at http://new.cms. hhs.gov/MedlearnProducts/downloads/Teaching-Physician-Brochure-9-29-04.pdf (accessed December 15, 2005).

HOME CARE

Houts PS, ed. *American College of Physicians Home Care Guide for Advanced Cancer.* American College of Physicians, 1997. Available at http://www.acponline.org/public/h_care/ (accessed December 15, 2005).

HOSPICE

Keay TJ, Schonwetter RS. Hospice care in the nursing home. *Am Fam Physician* 1998;57:491–4. Available at www.aafp.org/afp/980201ap/ keay.html (accessed December 15, 2005).

National Hospice and Palliative Care Organization. *Medical Guidelines For Determining Prognosis In Selected Non-Cancer Diseases – Second Edition.* Alexandria, VA: National Hospice and Palliative Care Organization, 1996. Available at http://eseries.nhpco.org/eseries/ source/Orders/index.cfm?task=3&CATEGORY=TECHMAT&PRODUCT_TYPE=SALES&SKU=713008&DESCRIPTION=&FindSpec=Medical%20Guidelines%20For%20Determining%20Prognosis%20&CFTOKEN=34453697&continue=1&SEARCH_TYPE=FIND (accessed December 15, 2005).

MEDICATIONS

Palliativedrugs.com. See http://www.palliativedrugs.com/ (accessed December 15, 2005).

MULTICULTURAL

Taylor A, Box M. Multicultural Palliative Care Guidelines. Palliative Care Council of South Australia, Inc., 1999. See www.pallcare.asn.au/mc/mccontents.html (accessed December 15, 2005).

PAIN

● AHCPR. *Clinical Practice Guideline: Management of Cancer Pain.* Bethesda, MD: US Department of Health and Human Services, Public Health Service, Agency for Health Care Policy and Research, 1994. Available at www.painresearch.utah.edu/cancerpain/guidelineF.html (accessed December 15, 2005).

American Medical Directors Association. *Clinical Practice Guideline: Pain Management in the Long Term Care Setting.* Columbia, MD: American Medical Directors Association, 2003. Available at (accessed December 15, 2005) www.amda.com/info/cpg/chronicpain.htm.

Hypermedia Assistant for Cancer Pain Management (HACPM, formerly Talaria). Available at http://www.painresearch.utah.edu/cancerpain/(accessed December 15, 2005).

◆ Joint Commission on the Accreditation of Healthcare Organizations. *Improving the Quality of Pain Management Through*

Measurement and Action. Oakbrook Terrace, IL: Joint Commission on the Accreditation of Healthcare Organizations, 2003. Available at www.jcaho.org/news±room/health±care±issues/pain_mono_jc.pdf (accessed December 15, 2005).

Pain and Policy Studies Group, University of Wisconsin Comprehensive Cancer Center. See www.medsch.wisc.edu/painpolicy/ index.htm (accessed December 15, 2005).

PRESSURE ULCERS

American Medical Directors Association. *Clinical Practice Guideline: Pressure Ulcers.* Columbia, MD: American Medical Directors Association, 1996. Available at www.amda.com/info/cpg/pressureulcer.htm (accessed December 15, 2005).

SOCIAL WORK

National Hospice and Palliative Care Organization. *Guidelines for Social Work in Hospice.* Alexandria, VA: National Hospice and Palliative Care Organization, 1994.

National Cancer Control Initiative. *Clinical Practice Guidelines for the Psychosocial Care of Adults with Cancer.* Carlton, Australia: National Cancer Control Initiative, 2003. Available at www.ncci.org.au/projects/psych/psychosocial_care.htm (accessed December 15, 2005).

URINARY INCONTINENCE

American Medical Directors Association. *Clinical Practice Guideline: Urinary Incontinence.* Columbia, MD: American Medical Directors Association, 1996. Available at www.amda.com/info/cpg/incontinence.htm (accessed December 15, 2005).

Curricula guiding practice

A Progressive Palliative Care Education Curriculum for the Care of African Americans at Life's End (APPEAL). New York, NY: Initiative to Improve Palliative Care for African Americans (IIPCA), 2003. Available at www.appealproject.org/ (accessed December 15, 2005).

Center to Advance Palliative Care. Educational strategies to increase the availability of quality palliative care services in hospitals and other health care settings for people with life-threatening illnesses, their families, and caregivers. Available at www.capc.org (accessed December 15, 2005).

Education on Palliative and End-of-life Care (EPEC) Project, 1999 and 2003.* Core competencies in palliative care for all healthcare practitioners is available at www.epec.net/ (accessed December 15, 2005). The EPEC Curriculum 1999 Participant's Handbook is available at http://www.epeconline.net/EPEC/Webpages/ph.cfm (accessed December 15, 2005).

EPEC-Oncology is available at http://www.epec.net (accessed December 15, 2005).

EPEC Roman Catholic is available at http://epeconline.net/EPEC/webpages/partnerrc.cfm (accessed December 15, 2005).

End of Life Nursing Education Consortium (ELNEC) Project. Core competencies in palliative care for nurses are available at www.aacn.nche.edu/elnec/ (accessed December 15, 2005).

Educating Future Physicians on Palliative/End of Life Care (EFPPEC). A project of the Association of Canadian Medical Colleges and the Canadian Hospice Palliative Care Association. Available at www.efppec.ca (accessed December 15, 2005).

End of Life/Palliative Education Resource Center (EPERC). An online community of educational scholars and resources to advance end-of-life/palliative care is available at www.eperc.mcw.edu/ (accessed December 15, 2005).

The Ian Anderson Continuing Education Program in End-of-Life Care. Core competencies in palliative care for all healthcare providers available at www.cme.utoronto.ca/endoflife/ (accessed December 15, 2005).

The Pallium Project. See http://www.pallium.ca/ (accessed December 15, 2005).

APPENDIX 27.2: IMPACT OF A WIDELY ACCEPTED MODEL

By providing 'one message, one voice', the CHPCA *Model to Guide Hospice Palliative Care* has already had significant impact since its publication in 2002, including:

- **Companion standards of care** have been developed by
  - Canadian Nurses Association to develop standards for nurses working in hospice palliative care and a process to certify them[32]
  - Hospice Association of Ontario to build standards for both volunteer hospice visiting services and community residential hospices,[33]
  - Canadian Network of Palliative Care for Children (CNPCC) to develop norms of practice for pediatric hospice palliative care (see http://cnpcc.ca/pages/documents.htm).
- **Patient/family care:** In 2003–04, the new Canada Health Accord included money to provide universal access to home-based care across Canada.[34] As part of this strategy, the Ontario Ministry of Health is increasing home-based palliative care across the province based on the CHPCA *Model*.[35] In 2005, Cancer Care Ontario made palliative care one of its four strategic thrusts. Implementation will be based on the CHPCA *Model*. Multiple palliative care programs and services are in the process of building their standards of practice based on the CHPCA *Model*.
- **Accreditation:** The Canadian Council on Health Services Accreditation is using it to develop accreditation standards for all healthcare agencies across the country, including acute and long-term care facilities, cancer clinics, homecare programs and hospice palliative care programs (see http://www.cchsa.ca).
- **Education:** The Educating Future Physicians in Palliative and End-of-Life Care Project is developing competencies for both undergraduate and graduate medical trainees (see http://www.efppec.ca). EPEC-O, the Education on Palliative and End-of-life Care for Oncology Project, is structured based on it (see http://www.epec.net).

● **Research:** The Canadian Institutes for Healthcare Research (CIHR) used it to guide palliative care research proposals (see http://www.cihr-irsc.gc.ca/e/22757.html).

APPENDIX 27.3: DEVELOPING STANDARDS FROM NORMS

Norms present the 'usual' or 'average' practice across many different organizations (see Fig. 27.7). They are less specific than the standards which each individual organization will define based on their local environment, and funding and service delivery capabilities. In the example in Table 27.1, norms for care delivery (on the left) become much specific standards for the delivery of pain management (on the right).

Table 27.1

Norm 5.13 from the CHPCA Model	Standards for pain delivery
All therapeutic interventions are delivered in a safe and timely manner that:	All pain management is delivered in a safe and timely manner:
is consistent with the organization's standards of practice and policies and procedures	90 percent of care plans follow the network's policies and procedures
optimizes their potential for benefit	The incidence of medication interactions and adverse events is <1 percent
minimizes the potential for medication interactions, adverse effects or burden	90 percent of patients and families express their acceptance of the therapies offered to manage their pain
is consistent with manufacturer's/supplier's instructions	50 percent of patients have pain <5/10 within 48 hours of admission
is acceptable to the patient and family	

28

The adoption of palliative care. The engineering of organizational change

WINFORD E HOLLAND

INTRODUCTION

Imagine that you have just been named to the faculty of a distinguished medical institution. Further imagine that you have been asked by the director of the institution to 'help us implement palliative care in our institution'. What would you do? How would you do it? With whom would you work? Whom might you avoid? What mis-steps would you want to avoid?

Hopefully many of the readers of this book will be asked exactly that question: 'Can you help us implement palliative care?' The goal of this chapter is to offer a framework for thinking about such an implementation as well as some practical tools that might be used to make such an implementation possible in a relatively short period of time.

ELEMENTS OF THE FRAMEWORK

Although most of us spend our time inside a large organization, we usually do not spend much time thinking about the organization. What is an organization? What is it made of? What do we mean when we talk about 'changing the organization'? When we say that we want to implement palliative care in an organization, what does that mean?

The following three subject areas can form a framework for envisioning and then changing an organization and how it operates:

1 *The organization as a mechanical system.* A large organization can be thought of as a mechanical system made up of concrete 'moving parts' – parts that can be altered to cause the organization to function in a different way, like delivering a new service such as palliative care to the institution's clients. As a metaphor, organizations can be thought of as 'theatre companies' performing in continuous 'plays'.

2 *The diffusion of innovation within a social organization.* Innovations – ideas that are new to an organization – diffuse through an institution in a patterned way over time, with some organization members far more inclined to adopt an innovation like palliative care than others.

3 *The role of leadership in creating change in an organization.* Leaders cause things to happen in an organization. Leaders take direct actions on the moving parts of an organization; they influence organization members to enable the organization to make changes like implementing palliative care on an institutional basis.

The following sections of this chapter will explore in more detail these three key framework ideas, providing both understanding as well as action steps that can be used to implement, or 'engineer', an innovation into an institution in an effective and efficient way. The last section of the chapter will 'pull it all together' to illustrate how the actions can be used for real-world implementation of palliative care.

THE ORGANIZATION AS MECHANICAL SYSTEM

Implementing a change ... like the introduction of palliative care ... requires us to know something about what an organization is from a structural or system point of view – the mechanics of organizations. In today's world of work, we must be able to do two things at the same time – to *use* the organization to get today's business done and *change* the organization so that we can be ready to do tomorrow's business.

Organizations as ongoing theatrical performances

We see an organization as an ongoing play, where organization members are cast and crew in a satisfying performance for clients/patients. Use of the scenario of changing plays from *Romeo and Juliet* to *My Fair Lady* as an example of what happens in organizational change is a helpful framework for managers and employees to easily grasp the changes involved in moving a theater company from one performance to another – from learning new scripts to changing costumes and sets, all the way to the full dress rehearsal before opening.

Once this theater metaphor is learned, our students of change management can use it to understand why many changes they have seen go awry! More importantly, it becomes easy to understand the *single most important concept* in organizational change – that organizations are structured, mechanical systems with concrete moving parts that must work and change together. Translating the theater metaphor to organizations, students can see the four primary structural elements:

- Vision – like the play's storyline and script
- Work processes – like the roles in the play
- Plant/equipment/tools – like costumes and sets
- Performance agreements – like contracts for actors

Although it is easy to comprehend the 'work process–role' and the 'plant/equipment/tools–props' connections, it does take some stretch to see that the 'agreements for performance', like actor contracts, are an attribute of the organization and not the 'employees–actors' themselves. In our experience, the most difficult part of organizational change for many companies is understanding that change is designed to alter the roles that people play in the organization, not to alter people themselves. Failure to grasp the idea that *change hinges on altering roles* and subsequent performance agreements that we make with employees is the most common downfall of organizational change.

For an organization to change, all four mechanical attributes of the organization (Fig. 28.1) must change – in concert – or there will be no change. Vision alteration, work process alterations, plant/equipment/tools alterations as well as performance agreement changes are all done in a social setting. All the alterations have to be done by people who are involved and committed to (i) making the alterations and (ii) working in the new organization after the alterations are made. Managing the people dynamics can

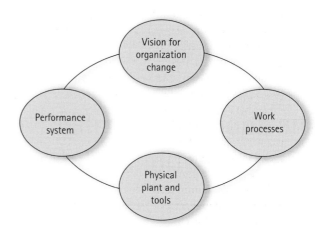

Figure 28.1   *Mechanical attributes of organizations.*

be challenging, but it is doable as long as leaders of the change understand the mechanical things that must be done to achieve organizational change.

The five requirements for engineering change

As discussed, the way any organization works at a given point in time is the direct and inescapable result of the configuration of the firm's Vision, work processes, physical plant, and performance system (agreements with employees and their competence to perform to those agreements). Just as in a mechanical system, the way the organization operates cannot change without a change in its key components.

Calling these needed alterations 'requirements' allows us to see change as a true engineering challenge. These four alterations, along with the development/communication of action plans, make up what we call the 'Five requirements for engineering change'. The critical part of organizational change is the unglamorous, detail-oriented, hard work of engineering.

REQUIREMENT 1: ENGINEERING AND COMMUNICATING THE CHANGE VISION

The first requirement of organizational change is to engineer a Vision of the organization's desired future that will be valid, complete, feasible, resourceable, and engaging. In this case, the detailed vision would include palliative care. Once detailed, the Vision should be tested with members of the organization to ensure that it is an understandable picture of the desired future. To ensure that the organization is positioned to really hear and digest the Vision, we construct a 'Case for Change' that describes in some detail the potential consequences of keeping the organization exactly the way it is now.

An institution bent on implementing palliative care would be able to describe a time in the near future when such care was an integral part of the organization's services, providing a real alternative to end-of-life care in an intensive-care facility. In addition, reasons for implementing palliative care, including benefits to patients, families, as well as institutional economics, should be clearly detailed.

Once the change Vision and the Case for palliative care are complete, the next step is to communicate with all organization members multiple times using multiple media. In today's world that means the institution's website as well as its internal communication programs. Palliative care brochures, signage, and even slogans, pins, and badges, could complement the face-to-face communication of the Vision.

Technically this communication requirement is not complete until all management levels have worked through the Vision and Case for Change and translated them into action terms for their level and function, as well as for their individual associates. The final step in this requirement is to test each employee's understanding of the translation of the palliative care Vision for his or her job. Without this test, leaders of the change can hardly know if they are ready to move on to the next requirements of altering the mechanical components of the organization.

Failure to translate the Vision and Case for Change would be like the director of a theater company who does not individualize the new play for each member of the cast and crew. Imagine trying to stage a new play without specific role assignments for each actor!

REQUIREMENTS 2–4: ENGINEERING THE ORGANIZATION'S MECHANICAL COMPONENTS

Requirements 2–4 call for the physical alteration of the institution's work processes, its physical plant/equipment/tools (PET), and the employee performance system. The first step in this alteration process is to inventory the organization's current components – work processes, PET, and performance agreements with employees – to identify those elements that will not be in sync with the palliative care Vision of the future organization. Once identified, each of the elements must be physically altered and tested. It is these alterations of the existing components, along with the addition of new work processes (e.g. billing procedures for palliative care), physical plant (e.g. dedicated palliative care beds), and performance agreements (e.g. job descriptions for personnel servicing palliative care beds) that will become the 'stuff' of the changed organization that will include palliative care.

Development and negotiation of new performance agreements for all affected managers and employees is critical at this point to ensure they are signed up for palliative care in the institution. Organizations and theater companies alike deal with the reality that some employees, or actors, will *not* elect to sign up for the change. Completing these alterations is akin to the work that must get done in the theater company to ensure that the new play is translated into individual roles and scripts for the newly assigned cast, that the new costumes and sets have been constructed, and that the actors have been put under formal contract and rehearsed for the new play.

The final step in each of these three requirements is to systematically dismantle or remove those elements that will not be a part of the new organization's structure. Old work processes, procedures, tools, and equipment will need to be removed from the workplace to ensure they will not be used again. This dismantling includes the often forgotten step of directly and formally cancelling any agreements with managers and employees for performance in the old organization. For example, we might want to verbally and in writing cancel the institutional procedure that assigns end-of-life patients to this intensive care unit or to that designated wing.

We want to cancel the agreements that our employee had for doing work the old way (without palliative care) now that they have already been signed up for doing work the new way (with palliative care as a mainstream service). This final dismantling is akin to the director removing all vestiges of the last play (old scripts, costumes, and props) to ensure that they will not be inadvertently used in the new production. Included in this dismantling step is the cancellation of any cast contracts that would have tied them to the old play.

REQUIREMENT 5: ENGINEERING ACTION PLANS FOR CHANGE WORK

Even though employees are clear on the Vision that is to be implemented, they need day-by-day or week-by-week action plans to guide them through the many steps of organizational change. Employees need an action plan that tells them 'What to do on Monday morning...' to go forward with the coordinated implementation of the new Vision.

These action plans must be a part of a critical path project management plan and master schedule that lays out all the engineering work to be done for the organizational change to embrace palliative care. Critical to the action planning requirement is the translation of action plans on a weekly or monthly basis for all involved managers and employees so that they are clear on their roles in (i) transitioning to the new organization and (ii) playing new or altered roles in that new organization. Failure to keep action plans updated and communicated would be like the director who does not lay out and communicate detailed plans and schedules for reading the new roles, signing contracts, fitting new costumes, or rigging new props.

The engineering challenge in this action planning requirement is to ensure that all of the required modifications to Vision, work processes, physical plant, and performance agreements have been done in a thorough, comprehensive manner. Although it may be a technical challenge to keep track of all of the needed alterations, particularly if the organization is large, it is technically not difficult to find out exactly where the organization is in organizational change.

Implementation planning is first and foremost a case of deciding exactly and precisely *what* alterations will be required in each of the components and then *how* the required alterations are to be made. The physical change piece is all about making the required alterations and ensuring that they were done … and done right.

Knowing where we are in engineering change to include palliative care is a matter of auditing the status of required alterations and dealing with the reality of what we find:

- Either work processes have been altered to include palliative care or they have not. New procedures that allow people to bill for palliative care have been written and distributed or they have not. The old processes and their supporting procedures have been dismantled/destroyed or they have not.
- Either new tools (beds devoted to palliative care) are assigned and working or they are not. Either the guidelines for operating the new palliative care suite have been written and distributed or they have not.
- And either the performance contract for each and every doctor, nurse, and administrator impacted by the introduction of palliative care has been altered and negotiated with them or it has not. Either each and every manager and employee has been trained on the new palliative care admission processes and new suite or they have not … and so on.

So ends this section of the framework that deals with the organization as a mechanical system, a system that can be literally engineered from one configuration to another. But organizations vary in their susceptibility to engineering, as explained in the next section.

THE DIFFUSION OF INNOVATION

The mechanical approach to leading an organization change like the introduction of palliative care is simple and straightforward to describe, but there are organizational situations in which it is an oversimplification. In professional organizations where there is a high degree of individual autonomy, another framework element has much to offer.

A major social study area for the past few decades has been the 'diffusion of innovation' – the way and rate something new to an individual or organization gets adopted by the members of the organization. The basic idea is that an innovation spreads rather slowly across a social system, like a healthcare institution, by traveling from member to member. Key elements of the diffusion theory include:

- *The innovation.* An idea or practice (like palliative care) that is perceived as new by individuals or the institution.
- *Communication channels.* The means by which messages about the innovation get from one individual to another (formal and informal communication

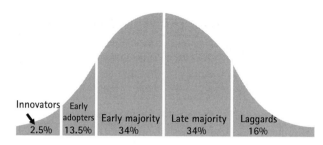

Figure 28.2 *Categories of adopters of innovations.*

between departments and members of the medical community).
- *Time.* The relative time an innovation takes to be adopted by an individual or group.
- *Social system.* A set of interrelated units (departments) that are engaged in accomplishing a common goal (providing healthcare to patients – the institutional goal).

In studying the diffusion process, researchers have been able to consistently identify individuals who have different rates of adoption. The by now classic categories of adopters are (Fig. 28.2):

- Innovators
- Early adopters
- Early majority
- Late majority
- Laggards

Several characteristics dominant in each category have been identified (Box 28.1).

Box 28.1 Characteristics of adopters by category

Innovators

- Venturesome; desire for the rash, the daring, and the risky

- Control of substantial financial resources to absorb possible loss from an unprofitable innovation

- Ability to understand and apply complex technical knowledge

- Ability to cope with a high degree of uncertainty about an innovation

Early adopters

- Integrated part of the local social system

- Greatest degree of opinion leadership in most systems

- Serve as role model for other members or society
- Respected by peers
- Successful

Early majority

- Interact frequently with peers
- Seldom hold positions of opinion leadership
- Deliberate before adopting a new idea
- Constitute a third of the members of a system

Late majority

- Pressure from peers
- Economic necessity
- Skeptical
- Cautious
- Constitute a third of the members of a system

Laggards

- Possess no opinion leadership
- Isolates
- Point of reference in the past
- Suspicious of innovations
- Innovation-decision process is lengthy
- Resources are limited

The practical significance of these categories has not been lost on the advertising and sales communities who routinely take advantage of innovator categories. Change leaders can also take advantage of the research by treating different populations within their institutions differently.

For example, when an innovation like palliative care is first introduced into a department or institution, healthcare professionals produce an 'adoption reaction'. Thinking simply, about a third of the community is likely to have an open, even positive reaction, while another third might have a very closed or even negative reaction. A middle third might be observable as those professionals who lean no way or the other, as if waiting for the next act. In fact, this middle third is likely to be doing just that … waiting to see how the introduction goes.

From the point of view of the change leader(s), working with the three communities takes very different levels of energy and produces varying degrees of results:

- First third (innovators and early adopters) – working with them is simple, straightforward, and positive.

Reasonable suggestions about palliative care and its adoption are heard, evaluated, and frequently acted on.
- Second third (majority adopters) – working with them is frequently frustrating since they are less into 'listening, trying, and evaluating ideas' than they are into 'watching the success' (or lack of success) of the first third.
- Third third (late majority and laggards) – working with this group is usually argumentative, frequently unfriendly, and sometimes downright nasty and unpleasant.

Change leaders assigned and/or committed to the implementation of palliative care have the choice of the populations they address. Diffusion of innovation research would suggest the tactic of working with the first third to gain as much implementation success as possible … and then allowing those in the first third do the job of influencing others through their own work and social channels.

LEADERSHIP IN ORGANIZATIONAL CHANGE

Organizational change does not happen without leadership … and lots of it! We have not seen success in change when the organization's leadership, at all levels, was unwilling to take responsibility for setting a direction or was lacking the courage and commitment needed to carry out that direction. Decisive leadership at the highest level of the organization is essential for successful change. The leader who is unable or unwilling to pick a new future for the organization, give that future some detail, and then steer toward that future is destined to keep the organization right where it is. The bottom line is simple: organizational change takes leadership … from both the boss and his or her collaborators (Fig. 28.3). The final word, however, is that the boss must be the one who brings the energy and excitement to organizational change along with the personal leadership to get his or her collaborators on board.

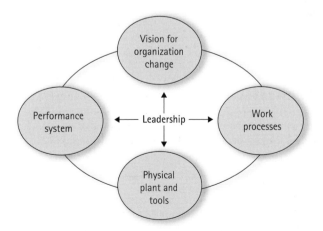

Figure 28.3 *Change leadership acts on the mechanical attributes of organizations.*

Three critical sources of leadership must be engaged for successful organizational change: the Chief Executive, key managers at the department level, and healthcare professionals. Each leadership source has a primary mission to accomplish in an organizational change to implement palliative care. The Chief Executive is the 'Chief Change Officer' for the organization. Period. No one else in the organization has the authority and stroke to make change happen. No one else has the legal responsibility for the enterprise. No one else can be held accountable for the performance of the organization before, during, and after organizational change. The primary Change Mission for the Chief Executive in organizational change is defining the future for the organization.

The Chief Executive's primary change mission is to develop (or select) the desired future for the organization and express it as the Vision that includes palliative care, just like the director's job is to select a script that will result in a successful play. In addition, the executive must resource with dollars and personal commitment the palliative care Vision as it is being implemented. The need to continuously resource the change initiative is because a change like the movement to palliative care is difficult, frustrating, and tiresome. It is critical for the Chief Executive to be personally visible and available while the organization is implementing the palliative care Vision.

The Chief Executive must also develop his/her own altered executive role as it will need to be played for palliative care to become a reality. Actions speak louder than words, but we are talking about something more than that. What the Chief Executive does on a day-to-day, week-to-week, and month-to-month basis must routinely include the Vision of palliative care if that Vision is to become a reality.

The Cadre of Management serves as the organization's source of energy and initiative for altering work processes, altering the physical plant, and altering the performance system to include palliative care. In this cadre will likely be the organization's departmental palliative care leader(s) who have taken on primary responsibility for day-to-day operations as well as guiding the implementation effort.

The organization's Cadre of managers is directly and personally responsible for completing the changes needed to get palliative care into operation. The Cadre's job is the 'Chief Change Communicator and Director' for their part of the institution. Their primary change mission is threefold:

- relentlessly communicate the palliative care Vision
- guide organizational healthcare professionals as they complete the organization's move to palliative including professional education and training
- develop their own altered management and professional roles as they will need to be played for palliative care to be a reality,

The healthcare professionals in the organization will do the majority of the Change Engineering needed to alter the organization's mechanical attributes. It is the workers who will physically do the detailed alternations needed in work processes and physical plant and develop the new organizational roles that enable palliative care. The primary change mission of the involved professionals must, however, be focused on the alteration and development of their own roles and skills needed for their success as a part of the palliative care Vision.

PULLING IT ALL TOGETHER ... A PALLIATIVE CARE SUCCESS STORY

Take for example, the introduction of palliative care at MD Anderson Cancer Center (MDACC) in Houston. The Chief Executive made the decision to move toward palliative care and hired a leading physician to come to Anderson and 'run the show'. Upon arrival, the newly appointed Palliative Care Department Head encountered stiff resistance and many logistical obstacles that were almost impossible to overcome. At the end of the first 18 months, progress in gaining acceptance of palliative care was very slow, and the third-third population of resisters had made themselves heard. The situation was uncomfortable enough for the Department Head to say 'that he felt like he had parachuted in behind enemy lines'.

In an effort to move the ball, MDACC retained the services of a change consultant to work directly with the Department Head and his palliative care team of department member physicians and administrators. The steps taken included the following:

- Instruction of and consultation with the palliative care team in the change concepts that are described in this paper. The Department Head stated that the consultations and training has 'opened a window into the world of organizations' that allowed to better see and understand the actions that he and his team needed to take.
- Decision of the palliative care team to 'ignore the third-third detractors' and to find and work with 'first-third' professionals only (i.e. working only with those who were relatively positive and eager to look at palliative care as a treatment alternative).
- Formation of a Palliative Care Steering Team made up of volunteer senior physicians/faculty members (all of whom were first-third).
- Arranging an early meeting/workshop of the Steering Committee to hear directly from the MDACC Chief Executive. The Chief Executive explained to the steering team his reason for moving the institution toward palliative, his reasons for selecting the Department Head and his vision of palliative care as a legitimate and important treatment modality for the institution.
- These key, friendly members helped establish a vision, mission, and strategic plan of action and not only provided extremely useful feedback but by the same process they were sold.

Table 28.1   *The Impact of Palliative Care Services on overall hospital mortality in a comprehensive cancer care center*

	1999	2000	2001	2002	2003	2004
Consultations prior to inpatient death Under services other than PCS	8	17	54	106	112	95
Inpatient death under primary care of the Palliative Care Service (PCS)	NA	NA	NA	54	123	169
Total number of patients accessing palliative care before death	8	17	54	160	235	264
Percent of patients accessing palliative care before death	1% (8/583)	3% (17/657)	8% (54/671)	24% (160/657)	35% (235/689)	35% (264/764)
Total number of palliative care inpatient visits (death and discharges)	800	1006	3396	5476	6489	6689

- This strategic plan was later moved upwards in the administration to convince senior management, and a process of continuous monitoring of the level of adoption of palliative care was established.
- The palliative care team and Steering Team worked directly with administrative officers of the institution to ensure that processes were in place to handle business and scheduling aspects of palliative care.
- With a palliative vision and strategic in place, the Department was able to launch communication and public relations programs, clinical education sessions, as well as consultations inside and outside MDACC. The focus on these programs initially focused on the first-third. As a result of positive acceptance by the first-third, members of the second-third began to sign up … and before long the first two-thirds were chiding members of the third-third as 'being behind the times'.
- The result of this was the large growth in referrals to the palliative care program that have succeeded in fully establishing it as a viable clinical and financial program. Note the rapid rate of palliative care consultations in Table 28.1.

The palliative care initiative has continued to increase in use and popularity with consultations continuing to increase and number and cost of deaths in internal care continue to decline. Blending the messages from the three framework elements is essential to effective change. The essential message of this chapter, therefore, is for leaders to:

- take strong, aggressive, visible action with/through the 'first-third' managers and professionals
- alter the mechanical attributes of the organization that will enact palliative care
- take leadership in healthcare organizations where individuals have high autonomy.

In summary, key to the success of the effective and efficient introduction of palliative care will be the continuing partnership between the committed chief executive and leaders in the management cadre. Dedicated action in the engineering framework described in this chapter … along with huge doses of 'blood, sweat, and tears'… should lead to another palliative care success story.

Key learning points

- The introduction of palliative care can be looked at as a mechanical problem that can be engineered … many moving parts must be identified and changed.
- Individuals have different rates of change acceptance … plan to work with the most eager supports of palliative care first.
- Changing an organization's way of operating requires aggressive, visible, hands-on leadership. The boss must want and support palliative care.
- Get the physical assets needed for palliative care in place early on so that the organization can see tangible organizational commitment.
- Involvement of professionals must be done at every step of the way. Involve them now to have them own palliative care later.

FURTHER READING

Davies S. *The Diffusion of Process Innovations.* Cambridge: Cambridge University Press, 1979.

Holland WE. *Change Is the Rule: Practical Actions for Change: On Target, On Time, and On Budget.* Chicago: Dearborn Trade Press, 2000.

Rogers EM. *Diffusion of Innovations.* New York: The Free Press, 1972.

Rogers EM. New product adoption and diffusion. *J Consumer Res* 1976: 290–301.

29

Cost avoidance and other financial outcomes for palliative care programs

J BRIAN CASSEL, THOMAS J SMITH

INTRODUCTION

Of all the imperatives and outcomes for palliative medicine and palliative care programs, one would hope that financial issues would rank as among the least important. Surely the other motivations for palliative care, and effects thereof – humanitarian, moral, ethical, clinical, to name a few – should be more important than costs and reimbursement. Be that as it may, financial questions are crucial for the success of palliative care, regardless of the country, system of healthcare, institutional values, and personal commitments of those involved.

Most physicians, nurses, and others who seek to begin or expand palliative care within a hospital or health system know that it will be necessary to make an accurate and compelling financial case for doing so. Clinical revenue is rarely sufficient to support the whole multidisciplinary team,[1] so palliative care teams have made their financial arguments around the notion of cost avoidance.

What do we know, given that the field is relatively new and rapidly growing? The literature to date provides two conflicting conclusions about the financial impact of palliative care. One is that palliative care has little or no impact on medical costs; 'palliative care appears to have roughly zero net effect on patient medical costs …' is how the outcome of a cost benefit analysis is described.[2] In contrast, we know from our own experience[3,4] and the success of other programs that palliative care programs are making a compelling financial case based on cost-avoidance, convincing their institutions to invest significant resources. For instance, based on their internal studies of pilot projects,[5] Kaiser

Permanente is now investing over US$2 million dollars to roll-out a home-based palliative care program for its entire southern California region (David Brumley, personal communication, 18 February 2005). Cost-avoidance data are integral to justify investments in hospital-based programs.[6]

The mixed conclusions result from different definitions of what is 'palliative care'. Boni-Saenz et al.[2] lump together hospice and palliative care, and their 'no savings' conclusion is based largely on the mixed evaluations of hospice costs in recent years, which now question the long-held assumption that hospice saves significant utilization and total costs. In contrast, our analyses of the financial impact of palliative care focus on an acute palliative care program that is not synonymous with hospice care.

Looking at how this hospice cost debate is playing out, one can surmise that the hospice movement in America today has become inexorably tied to the Medicare hospice benefit (and its inherent cost-avoidance foundation). Witness the cautionary statements issued by a hospice advocacy group, National Hospice and Palliative Care Organization (NHPCO), such as 'retrospective studies can be difficult to analyze and findings must be kept in perspective'[7] about a very strong study[8] which had indicated that hospice adds to healthcare costs for noncancer patients of all ages. NHPCO's own study[9] found no cost difference related to hospice enrollment for 12 out of 16 disease groups it studied ($P < 0.05$ with no correction for multiple tests). Of the four disease groups for which hospice use was related to cost differences, there was such a large increase in costs for stroke patients (US$12 331 per patient) that in equal numbers they would largely cancel out the savings found for the three disease groups that demonstrated cost savings: liver cancer, pancreatic cancer, and congestive heart failure (US$14 936 combined per patient).

Clearly, both studies call into question the assumption that the Medicare hospice benefit saves Medicare money in the long run. Like many observers we believe that the hospice movement in the USA has painted itself into a cost-avoidance corner. We would caution the field to avoid basing the rationale for palliative care solely on a cost-avoidance foundation. Rather, one should fully exploit existing data to understand when and how palliative care does avoid utilization and direct costs, and to honestly admit when it does not. After all, the main goal is better patient care, and cost-avoidance is just one means of convincing administrative leaders to invest resources toward that end.

UNDERSTANDING THE RELATION BETWEEN PALLIATIVE CARE PROCESSES AND FINANCIAL OUTCOMES

Palliative care rests on two philosophical foundations: (i) zero-tolerance of suffering, which provides the basis for its focus on symptom assessment and management; and

(ii) an acceptance of death and the dying process, which results in the comfort care alternative to relentless high-tech interventions aimed at extending life at any cost.

Thus palliative care programs show two *personae*: one that is concerned with preventing and ameliorating symptom distress for all patients at any point in their disease course; and another that is primarily focused on questioning, clarifying, and challenging the assumed life-extending goals of care at certain critical points in the disease process. A good multidisciplinary palliative care team will have expertise in both aspects and be recognized by other professionals throughout the institution for both strengths.

We contend that almost all cost savings will follow from the goal-setting aspect of palliative care, although better symptom management may prevent some emergency visits and inpatient admissions. See Table 29.1 for our summary of the relation between clinical and financial aspects of palliative care.

RELATIVE TO WHAT?

From a program evaluation perspective, the question of palliative care finances should be framed in terms of 'relative to what exists otherwise'. But dying patients and others

Table 29.1 *Palliative care program features that have possible financial outcomes*

Feature of palliative care program	Possible financial impact
Pain and symptom specialists alleviate and prevent suffering; best possible management of all symptoms	Within acute admission, small impact on individual length of stay and perhaps on likelihood of quick re-admission is possible. If achieved over longer period of time in home setting, may prevent emergency visits and inpatient admissions significantly
Team members clarify and possibly change goals of care when intensive care and procedures are not producing a marked improvement in patient disposition	If impact on goals of care is significant (e.g., moving patients from critical to acute care, or reducing orders for ancillary services such as diagnostics and drugs), then financial impact may be large. Financial impact will be negligible if the clinical impact is negligible
Presence of palliative care unit gives patient, families, and providers an attractive alternative kind of end-of-life care	May prevent escalation from acute to intensive care unit (ICU) level care. May encourage transfers from ICU to comfort care. If ICU beds are scarce, this may allow ICU beds to be used by other patients who are more likely to benefit from them – traumas, surgeries, etc.
Presence of, or quick access to, palliative care team in emergency department (ED); ED team may call palliative care for consult when patients present with late-stage disease for whom symptom management and comfort care is most appropriate	This prevents such patients from going to ICUs or other units and receiving procedures or testing from which they would probably not benefit. It is easier for palliative care to be included in goals of care at the time of admission, than for the palliative care team to facilitate a change of goals at some point during the admission
Multidisciplinary team that prevents and ameliorates physical, emotional, psychosocial, and spiritual distress	Patients and families who are highly satisfied with care are probably more likely to refer their friends, return when they themselves are sick, and perhaps donate money or volunteer their time
Palliative care team refers more patients, earlier, to hospice	May improve the length of stay in hospice, which may help hospice program to operate at higher margins. However, some evidence indicates that expanding use of hospice with some disease types may result in lower margins

who would benefit from palliative care may comprise 5 percent or less of most departments' admissions. With responsibility for them diffused across all providers, disciplines and cost centers, most hospital or health system administrators will have little understanding of the nature of their care and the costs and reimbursement thereof; the palliative-appropriate population is almost entirely 'under the radar' for administrative and clinical leaders in most institutions. One of the critical differences that palliative care programs make, clinically, is to halt that diffusion of responsibility, and to provide accountability for the nature and cost of the care of such patients. See Table 29.2 for a further analysis of the diffusion of responsibility, as well as the concept of diffusion of innovation. Both have implications for the financial aspects of palliative care.

One of the first steps, then, in planning for and evaluating palliative care programs is to assess the status quo before the team begins to change bedside practices, clinician education, and institutional culture. A series of leading questions are provided in Box 29.1 for such an assessment.

Delving into the baseline or status quo data on this issue is important not only for eventual program evaluation, but also for program development: it may help the nascent palliative care team better understand what they could change; and it may help administrators understand this unknown patient

---

Box 29.1 Ten questions to ask about patients dying in your institution before palliative care team begins

1   How many patients die in system each year?

2   What was their first location, department, admitting service, registration source?

3   What was their end location, department, discharging service, length of stay (LOS)?

4   What were all the locations and departments in between?

5   What were the diagnosis-related groups (DRGs), primary disease groups, and acuity?

6   What were the patients' demographics and history of utilization prior to last admission?

7   What was the quality of care?

8   If ICUs and intensive procedures were used, at what point during admission?

9   What were the costs of care – the total, pattern per day, kinds of cost drivers?

10 Were there any opportunities where a palliative care team could have made a difference?

Table 29.2 *Two 'Diffusions' relevant to palliative care and financial outcomes*

	Diffusion of responsibility	Diffusion of innovation
Source	Latane and Darley, 1968[10]	Rogers, 1995[11]
Concept	Knowing that others are available to take action reduces the likelihood that any given individual will take action. Problems remain unaddressed	Getting a good idea disseminated and adopted throughout a group is often harder than one thinks it should be. As the innovation is increasingly adopted, the baseline for evaluating impact moves and changes as well
Relevance	It is difficult to manage symptoms and clarify or change goals of care, and these tasks do not belong to any one specialty. Palliative care specialists may break the cycle of denial and inattention by taking responsibility, by refusing to pass the buck, by not assuming someone else will have the difficult conversations and tackle the intractable symptoms	One method of diffusing innovation is to get the new behavior adopted by opinion leaders such as chief residents. Palliative care teams have learned (sometimes the hard way) to ignore those physicians who would reject the innovations of palliative care, and to focus instead on those who are likely to be early adopters and who would also be persuasive change agents for their peers
Implications for financial aspects of program development and evaluation	Prior to the palliative care team's existence, no one in the institution has a good idea of the extent of suffering, futile intensive care, the cost of care for dying patients, etc. Thus palliative care teams must first generate the baseline data about the problem, both to garner support and to establish goals and benchmarks. Demonstrating the need for the program, and its effects, are equally important aspects of ongoing program development and evaluation	A goal of most palliative care teams is to educate other clinicians about symptom assessment and management, and goal clarification. Some take this one step further, and aim for institutional culture change. As these innovations become adopted and diffused throughout an organization, the baseline moves – the natural 'comparison groups' against whom we can measure the quality and cost of the palliative care patients are also improved. If the culture change is thorough and complete then it is difficult to say that patients treated by a palliative care team will look markedly different than those treated elsewhere. We can only hope.

population, and current costs. Conducting and sharing financial analyses on the target population – complex and dying patients (however defined in a given setting), may itself be an educational intervention for administrators and department chairs, whose attention may be drawn to that population for the very first time.

Before continuing with our examination of approaches to assessing palliative care, we should address the natural question: since palliative care is not concerned only with dying patients (and indeed some programs may studiously avoid focusing on death and dying), why focus so much analysis on patients who did die? Much palliative care research uses dying patients in analyses to provide an adequate comparison group, because they have the complexity of care (symptoms, psychosocial, family needs, goal clarification, etc.) that are typical of patients who would benefit from palliative care. And philosophically, if the palliative care team does not take responsibility for dying patients, who will? For these reasons, many studies of palliative care use patients who died as the population.

EVALUATING FINANCES OF PALLIATIVE CARE PROGRAMS

Informally, we would say that palliative care programs cannot be evaluated as 'silos' – evoking the image of a lone structure separate from others. Traditionally most business analyses in healthcare treat each department and program as a financial silo that must produce sufficient revenues to cover the costs of its treatments. In contrast, we contend that palliative care programs will have two populations of patients: those admitted directly to the palliative care units or services, and those transferred to palliative care from intensive upstream services such as neuroscience, oncology, and cardiology.

A 'silo' analysis is indeed appropriate for the former set of patients, at least as a start: care begins and ends under the control of the palliative care team, and all reimbursement for the case is attributable to the program itself. For patients transferred to palliative care at some point usually late in the admission, the question is, what cost differential does the palliative care program achieve for each day the patient is under its care, rather than standard care? What would have happened with those patients had the palliative program not existed? Because the goals and nature of the care on the palliative care unit (PCU) are dramatically different from those elsewhere in the hospital, the costs are generally much lower.

The lesson is deceptively simple. Palliative programs get at least half of their patients from upstream services, and have an institutional impact via cost avoidance rather than a local impact via revenue generation. At the heart of this issue is clarifying or changing goals of care so that patients who are not responding to curative or life-extending care (e.g. in intensive care units (ICUs)) are offered care that

focuses mostly or entirely on palliation, comfort and perhaps life closure.

INSIDE THE COST-AVOIDANCE CLAIMS OF PALLIATIVE CARE PROGRAMS

The most critical questions – and perhaps those least understood – about finances are those pertaining to cost avoidance, which is a result of comfort care goals, and that is what we will focus on in this section. We have organized this section by a series of questions.

1   Do palliative care interventions change the nature of the care provided, such that it is less intense, and therefore less costly?
    – Critical or intensive care is the site of a great deal of expensive, high-tech care for patients, some of whom do not benefit from this level of care. At the point when the care team and family recognize that comfort care would be more appropriate and beneficial for a given patient and family, the palliative care intervention can facilitate a profound change in the goals of care and thus the cost as well. In the inpatient setting, simply moving the patient from intensive to acute care can reduce the cost per day by hundreds of dollars. A typical pattern is shown in Figure 29.1, where we have disaggregated our patient population into those patients who were at high cost care, and compared them with patients whose care was already low cost.
    – However, one must not assume that just because a palliative care consult or other intervention has been done, that the care goals have been dramatically changed. As with any program evaluation, one must determine in each instance the nature, strength and penetration of the intervention (process evaluation), before assessing its impact (outcome evaluation).

2   What other financial implications are there for moving patients out of intensive care units, when they are no longer benefiting from that kind of care?
    – Most hospitals' bottlenecks occur in the ICU, and increased throughput at that critical juncture can allow for increased surgical admissions and fewer diversions. Surgeries are usually the most profitable treatment for hospitals to conduct, so anything that increases the hospital's ability to keep patients moving through its operating rooms is going to be beneficial to the bottom line. If a patient dies in the ICU after a 30-day stay, but the team knew on day 15 that the ICU was doing more harm than good for the patient and family from then on, how many other patients would have benefited from that ICU bed in the last 15 days? Does a Level 1 trauma center on diversion due to a full ICU serve its purpose, or might more patients benefit both from trauma care or transplantation of donated organs if there was no diversion?

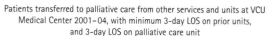

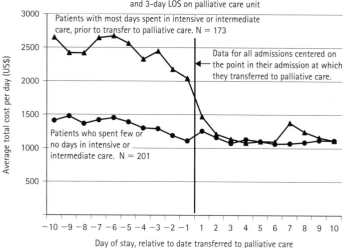

Figure 29.1 *Cost-avoidance analysis with patients transferred to palliative care. Total cost per day for patients transferred from the intensive care unit (ICU) or Intermediate (Step-Down) units to palliative care dedicated unit at Virginia Commonwealth University (VCU) Medical Center. Average daily cost data for 265 cases organized around common denominator of day of transfer to the palliative care unit (PCU). This is a within-patient analysis comparing costs before and after transfer to palliative care. LOS, length of stay.*

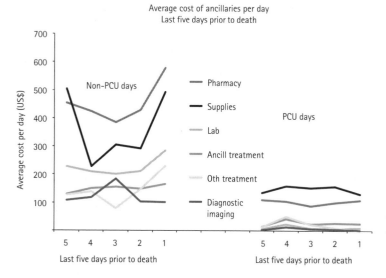

Figure 29.2 *Cost-avoidance analysis of days in palliative and nonpalliative settings. Cost per day, PCU versus acute medical-surgical cancer unit, last 5 days before death, at Virginia Commonwealth University (VCU) Medical Center. N = 133 patients, 65+ years old, cancer as primary diagnosis this admission, LOS at least 5 days, admission ended in death, in 2001–02. For the most part this is a between-groups analysis, although some patients (21 percent) transferred from non-PCU services to PCU during these last five days; the analysis is conducted at the 'day' level with each day coded as to location.*

3 What about patients who are already being treated in standard medical-surgical acute beds, and not in ICUs? Do palliative care programs still show an impact on ancillaries for such patients?

– This question was answered by the special study we did for the *Wall Street Journal*.[4] In that study we looked at the costs per day for patients who were 65+ years old, with a primary diagnosis of cancer, who died in the hospital, after an admission of at least 5 days. We used only the last 5 days prior to death so that it was the same time-frame for all patients. PCU patients' pharmacy costs were US$511 during those 5 days, compared with US$2267 for non-PCU patients; lab costs were US$56 versus US$1134; and radiology US$29 versus US$615. Supplies and other treatment costs showed similar differences. There was little difference in the room costs, as they were almost all in acute medical-surgical beds.

– Figure 29.2 shows the day-to-day pattern of costs for these ancillaries prior to death, not previously published. The costs spike for several categories on the last 2 days before death.

4 What about patients admitted directly into the PCU, rather than being transferred from another unit elsewhere in the hospital?

– Palliative care isn't just about changing an established goal of care, it is also about being in the right place to determine the course of care from the point of admission forward. Over the years, our palliative care program has established a closer and closer connection with the emergency department, where so many patients arrive for admission, and where the goals and level of care are determined on day 1. A palliative care consult can have a tremendous impact in that location by helping the emergency staff consider palliative care alternatives to intense, high-tech, life-extending or curative care. We believe that taking over control of care for appropriate patients right at the point of admission will be much easier for programs that have a dedicated unit, to which such patients can be sent, rather than a consult service only. At Virginia Commonwealth University (VCU), our direct admits to the PCU are profitable, as well as being at least one-half as costly per day as care in other units. These direct admissions have increased from just 32 cases in 2001 to 85 in 2004.

5 In typical hospitals, many patients who start to die are transferred from acute med-surg beds to ICUs, where the ensuing death takes place. Do hospitals with palliative care programs show less of that pattern?

– This would be a natural consequence, though not necessarily articulated as a goal, for mature palliative care programs, and is similar to the question of direct admissions at the point of the ED. As a palliative care team begins to have an impact on the culture of its institution, do clinicians begin to recognize *ahead of time* when using the ICU would be futile? Do they begin to accept that an ICU is not necessarily the place to achieve the best care, and a good death? We do not have data on clinicians' attitudes at VCU regarding this, but we do have data on 'escalation of acuity' that speak to this trend.

– In 2 years the number of adult cancer patients whose care trajectory went from acute to ICU, followed by death in the ICU, dropped from 27 to 12. Combined with fewer patients remaining in ICUs to die once they started there, our hospital has seen fewer such patients (adult cancer patients who die in the hospital) using the ICU at all during their final admission – from 40 percent in 1999 to 30 percent in 2003. There were no other interventions during this time that would explain this difference in care. This is the opposite of the trend toward higher intensity deaths in the USA documented by Barnato et al.[12]

6 Do home-based palliative care programs also show a reduced utilization and therefore cost?

– As mentioned in the introduction, the Tri-Central (California) Kaiser Permanente program has shown just that (for cancer and chronic obstructive pulmonary disease but not statistically significant for congestive heart failure).[5]

7 How are quality of care, the use of palliative care services, and cost of care all related?

– Few studies have been conducted to date that tie all of these pieces together. One intriguing study, however, was the benchmarking study conducted by the University Healthcare Consortium (UHC) using about 40 chart reviews each from 35 member institutions, for a total of 1596 cases. Most (90 percent) of these cases did not actually receive palliative care services but based on their selection criteria (certain DRGs, prior admissions, and LOS for target admission), were likely to be of the kind of complex, later-stage, typically high-symptom load patients for whom palliative care is thought to be most helpful. This study demonstrated three things: although care for most patients was sub-par, it was better for the 10 percent who received palliative care services; that the higher the quality, the lower the cost and LOS; and palliative care services were correlated with lower cost.[13] Thus, cost and quality are inversely correlated for all patients, and for those receiving palliative care, palliative care is correlated with higher quality and lower cost. About one-half of the difference in cost can be accounted for by the shorter LOS, while the remainder was due either to lower intensity or less use of ancillary services.

CONCLUSIONS AND FUTURE DIRECTIONS

Unlike biomedicine, health care finances are usually not measured in terms of confidence intervals and *P* values; business decisions are usually not made on the basis of experiments with patients randomly assigned to treatment conditions. Indeed, most internal assessments of program successes and failures are not documented and published. For these reasons, much of the data we have seen to date on palliative care financial outcomes, especially cost avoidance, range from anecdotal to correlational; most are based on nonscientifically designed data analyses.

The field would benefit from more research designs that assess inputs and outputs at a patient level or population level (rather than at an admission level) such as that employed by Brumley et al.[5] Also, we need prospective and longitudinal studies that can determine at which point for which patients palliative care is presented as an option and actually implemented. These kinds of research designs are especially important as the maturing movement of palliative care begins to address care from diagnosis forward, and not just a few hours or days before death.

We also look forward to multicenter studies that can assess whether consultative services have the same kind and degree of clinical and financial impact (or for the same kinds of patients) as dedicated units. Or, whether other aspects of program design are important, such as the degree of clinical control that the palliative care team has after their initial consultation. In such studies, we hope that the financial outcomes would be studied with as much rigor and interest as clinical effects.

Another research approach that will become more important in the next 5–10 years is whether incentives and disincentives provided by payors (e.g. extra payments for better symptom management) have an impact on the field of palliative care.

Key learning points

- The imperatives for palliative care include financial issues, but the main goal is better patient care.

- The evidence for cost avoidance in hospice is mixed.

- The evidence for cost avoidance in acute palliative care is sufficient for investment.

- The financial outcomes of palliative care programs are not limited to cost avoidance.

REFERENCES

◆ 1 von Gunten CF. Financing palliative care. *Clin Geriatr Med* 2004; **20**: 767–81.

● 2 Boni-Saenz AA, Dranove D, Emanuel LL, Lo Sasso AT. The price of palliative care: Toward a complete accounting of costs and benefits. *Clin Geriatr Med* 2005; **21**: 147–63.

● 3 Smith TJ, Coyne P, Cassel JB, *et al.* A high volume specialist palliative care unit and team may reduce in-hospital end of life care cost. *J Palliat Med* 2003; **6**: 699–705.

● 4 Naik G. Unlikely way to cut costs: Comfort the dying. *Wall Street J* 2004: A1.

● 5 Brumley RD, Enguidanos S, Cherin DA. Effectiveness of a home-based palliative care program for end-of-life. *J Palliat Med* 2003; **6**: 715–24.

6 Center to Advance Palliative Care. www.capc.org (accessed June 16, 2005).

7 NHPCO. Communications Memorandum Re: Article in *Annals of Internal Medicine*. Available at: www.nhpco.org/i4a/pages/Index.cfm?pageid=4214 (accessed June 16, 2005).

● 8 Campbell DE, Lynn J, Louis TA, Sugarman LR. Medicare program expenditures associated with hospice use. *Ann Intern Med* 2004; **140**: 269–77.

● 9 Pyenson B, Connor, S, Fitch K, Kinzbrunner B. Medicare cost in matched hospice and non-hospice cohorts. *J Pain Symptom Manage* 2004; **28**: 200–10.

10 Darley JM, Latane B. Bystander intervention in emergencies: Diffusion of responsibility. *J Pers Soc Psychol* 1968; **8**: 377–83.

11 Rogers EM. *Diffusion of Innovations*, 4th ed. New York: The Free Press, 1995.

● 12 Barnato AE, McClellan MB, Kagay CR, Garber AM. Trends in inpatient treatment intensity among Medicare beneficiaries at the end of life. *Health Serv Res* 2004; **39**: 363–75.

● 13 Maxwell T, Cuny J. The UHC palliative care benchmarking project. Annual Assembly of the American Academy of Hospice and Palliative Medicine, New Orleans, LA, 2005.

30

Organization and support of the interdisciplinary team

KAREN MACMILLAN, BETTE EMERY, LOUISE KASHUBA

INTRODUCTION

Palliative care encompasses the physical, psychosocial, and spiritual dimensions of the patient and family. The expertise of various healthcare professionals is necessary to manage their complex needs.[1–18] In this chapter the interdisciplinary team will be explored. Team composition, communication and collaboration strategies, and support and leadership for interdisciplinary teams will be outlined. Areas of required research will be identified. Interdisciplinary teams can provide care and support in all settings, however the focus will be on specialized palliative care units.

To discuss the organization and support requirements for professionals, terms need to be defined to foster a common understanding. Multiprofessional teams have existed since the early 1900s in the interests of achieving efficiency by reducing cost and minimizing interventions.[14] Multiprofessional teams are either multidisciplinary or interdisciplinary. There is a notable distinction between multidisciplinary and interdisciplinary teams.[4,14,17,19,20] Multidisciplinary teams consist of independent healthcare professionals who conduct independent assessments, planning, and provision of care with little communication or coordination with other team members. In a multidisciplinary team the physician traditionally prescribes the involvement of the other team members. Interdisciplinary teams, in contrast, function as collaborative units working together to establish common goals of care. Automatic referral is assumed for each team member; the professional, along with the rest of the interdisciplinary team, determines the focus of intervention. In order to provide care, the interdisciplinary team uses skills of communication, problem solving, and goal setting to enhance the collaborative nature of interaction between team members.

INTERDISCIPLINARY TEAM: COMPOSITION

There are many publications on the value of interdisciplinary teams in palliative care, however, there is a paucity of research to support this belief.[5,21–23] Although palliative patients and their families report satisfaction with the interdisciplinary approach,[24–28] there is an absence of substantive research to fully describe the benefits.[5,21–23,29] Systematic literature reviews, meta-analysis and meta-regression of published research on the effectiveness and impact of palliative care teams and models of care have been inconclusive.[5,21–23,30] Inherent problems with all of these studies exist because of the vulnerability of the terminally ill patients being studied and the lack of comprehensive outcome measures. Nevertheless, even with the poor quality of the studies, there is evidence that palliative care teams have a positive effect on patient symptoms, length of stay, patient/family satisfaction, and costs.[6,8,9,11,22,24–28,31–44,53]

Interdisciplinary teams can ensure comprehensive coordinated care. This requires time and financial resources in order to be successful.[14,45–48] Some question the costs associated with multiple disciplines and caution about the effectiveness and efficiency of too large a team.[48] Yet others have demonstrated that developments of comprehensive interdisciplinary palliative care programs/teams are cost effective in a variety of settings.[8,11,30,49] Again, there is limited research exploring team composition or team size based on patient caseloads.

Members of the interdisciplinary team may include:[3,6,8,12,16,17,50,53]

- Art therapists
- Dieticians
- Holistic health practitioners
- Music therapists
- Nurses
- Occupational therapists
- Pastoral/spiritual care
- Pharmacists
- Physicians
- Physiotherapists
- Psychiatrists
- Psychologists
- Recreation therapists
- Respiratory therapists
- Social workers
- Volunteers

Although all of these disciplines can add value to the patient and family experience, if resources are limited, choices must be made as to which disciplines will be part of the team. Many sources suggest a palliative care physician and a nurse as core members, with other team members added as determined by needs and resources.[9,31,38–40,51,52] The needs of the patient and family ultimately dictate which healthcare professionals are involved in their care. It is equally important that composition of the team reflects the needs of the patient group seen by the service. For example, a service that provides care for a large number of end-stage respiratory diseases might consider having a respiratory therapist as a permanent team member. Alternatively, if disciplines are not represented on the palliative care team, there needs to be a provision to consult them. Tracking the frequency of these referrals can support planning for team composition as programs expand and change.

INTERDISCIPLINARY COMMUNICATION AND COLLABORATION

Communication and collaboration are key aspects of any interdisciplinary team.[1,4,14,17,46,47,54] Each profession's education has unique vocabulary, similar problem solving strategies, and similar world views.[4] Members of each specialty and discipline have a theoretical basis through which they interpret and address issues that arise in their work.[4,55] Team members must excel at their competencies, be secure in their own disciplines, and be able to uphold their ideas.[20] Successful contributing members of an interdisciplinary team require skills beyond those typically acquired in their discipline-specific programs.

Roles within an interdisciplinary team are less well defined than traditional roles of healthcare workers in other settings. As roles often blur, it is important that team members feel secure, thus avoiding being undermined by these overlapping roles.[12] Role blurring can be problematic if it is not well understood and can lead to under or overutilization of team members. These situations can lead to resentment, burnout and team conflict. Poor communication is one of the major factors preventing effective interdisciplinary teamwork.[4] Exercises which clarify roles, professional competencies, perceptions, and expectations are valuable.[46]

Setting aside traditional roles is required to engage in creative dialog with each other. Each professional reviews the documentation completed by other team members, to clarify information, questions, and concerns prior to entering the patient's room. Patients should not have to repeatedly tell their stories if the team is effectively sharing information. This demonstrates courtesy and respect, as well as conserving the patient's energy. The use of discipline-specific language is discouraged, as plain language is important to enhance understanding and communication. It is recommended that all disciplines document in the same area of the health record. Documentation, including physician orders, must be supported by rationale to enhance understanding by all team members. Avoiding abbreviations enhances communications in documentation.

Team members need to respect, value, understand, and trust each other's contributions.[17,56,57] Effective conflict resolution will foster team growth and maturation. Methods to reach consensus, resolve conflict, and effectively communicate are essential. While allowing for individual differences, bridges are built by striving to understand others' perspectives and ways of doing things. Formal staff debriefing is helpful when case circumstances are particularly traumatic or there have been multiple deaths in a short period of time. If care did not go well, a clinical postmortem can identify ways to improve in the future.

Care planning is ongoing; formally with interdisciplinary team conferencing, and more informally between meetings as the need arises. Weekly team conferences enhance coordination of care with assessment, planning, and evaluation of patient care. This is an appropriate time for team members to identify individual responsibilities related to tasks and interventions.

Family conferences assist in directing care by updating medical information, formulating goals and planning discharge. Not all members of the interdisciplinary team participate in a family conference as having all of the professionals involved may overwhelm the patient and family. The goals of the family conference and the patient will dictate which team members attend. To ensure a comprehensive picture, it is helpful to elicit pertinent input about the patient's level of functioning from team members not attending the conference. When there is conflict a family conference may help to problem solve and/or support behavioral changes. Both team and family conferences may serve as a forum to exchange ideas, share information, set goals, develop care plans, and solve problems.

SUPPORT FOR THE INTERDISCIPLINARY TEAM

Individual team members and the interdisciplinary team require support to ensure the success of the team.[58] Team members must be clinically competent in their discipline and be committed to improving their practice through ongoing education. There needs to be recognition that each member will be at a different stage in his or her professional and personal development. Team members are encouraged to be involved in discipline-specific professional development activities such as participating in special interest groups, courses and reading professional journals.[54] Completing an oral presentation for educational rounds provides the team member a forum to present subjects relevant to their discipline and to other disciplines. These represent only a few of the many possibilities for professionals working in palliative care. The intense nature of work in palliative care, as with most high-demand specialty areas, requires diverse opportunities to reflect, grow, and find balance.[58] Support is necessary at the group level as well as at the individual level coming from within the group itself as well as from administration.

Support requirements of an interdisciplinary team are greater than a sum of the needs of the individuals. Within the work environment, the development of supportive, collaborative relationships is fundamental.[4,47,59] Factors for coping are planned orientation, ongoing education, administrative support, and an environment conducive to team building.[60]

Planning a comprehensive orientation for new staff extends beyond the organization's corporate orientation. The new team member must understand the roles of each discipline. When possible, a new team member overlaps with the team member they will replace. Time spent job shadowing prior to being independent allows scheduled time with a professional to answer questions and support the individual. Well-established teams can be daunting; therefore strategies to integrate a new team member need to be considered. Assigning a mentor may help. Those in remote areas need mentors to call for consultation and support. New programs should consider partnering with successful programs, as this can provide them with a wealth of knowledge and support.

Keeping abreast of developments in a cutting edge field can be challenging. A variety of palliative care texts, websites, professional peer-reviewed journals and subscriptions to listserves are available as resources for information for professionals. Journal clubs and weekly rounds are a structured means of advancing knowledge. By sharing an article or presentation the individual professional has the opportunity to discuss ideas with their colleagues to glean their perspective. Workshops and conferences are also educational but may be cost prohibitive. Distant learning or video conferencing may be more economical. Often availability of resources is not the problem; the limiting factor is time.

Commitment from administration for time and education opportunities as well as acknowledgment of interdisciplinary and individual projects contributes to the success of the team.[2,46,59,61] Adequate space for meetings and individual offices or workspaces in close proximity to one another can enhance teamwork and collaboration.[62] Space in offices that allow for counseling patients and their families may be required for team members such as the chaplain and social worker.

LEADING INTERDISCIPLINARY TEAMS

Program management is an ideal structure, given the unique composition and needs of the palliative care interdisciplinary team. This is a management structure in which groups of professionals with skills and expertise care for a specific population of patients. Co-leaders may be necessary for managing the team. It is common that the leaders are a nurse and physician; although any discipline with management expertise, education and skill could fill the nurse leader's role. The structure usually has physicians reporting to the physician leader and other disciplines reporting to the other co-leader (program manager).[63] The physician leader engages the palliative physicians to ensure their accountability and responsibility as team members. The program manager has the same responsibilities with all other disciplines. The program manager is also responsible for management activities such as budget, finance, hiring, operations, and administration of the program. The co-leaders provide vision and direction for future planning, as well as drive and support change. Since team members report to the program manager, there needs to be a mechanism for managing professional issues that is specific to each discipline.[63,64] Support and guidance may be necessary from a professional peer as well as the program manager.

Clearly defined and established mission, purpose, standards of care, values and goals to guide and support the interdisciplinary team are foundational concepts.[2,62,65] The involvement of team members in articulating these concepts is essential as this supports team development and future strategic planning. Strategic plans should be agreed upon by team members and revisited on a yearly basis. Consumer satisfaction surveys, outcome measurements and program evaluations may also shape the program's future directions.[34] Outcome measures chosen must reflect the goals of the program.

Commitment and ongoing support by senior administration is key to successful program management models of care delivery.[66] The leaders need to be clear on the direction of the program and be able to make decisions in order to achieve the team's agreed upon goals. The primary focus of the leaders is to serve the needs of the team, empower them in delivering care and advancing knowledge and skill in palliative care.[67,68]

One of the greatest barriers to an integrated team approach to end-of-life care is the structure of healthcare financing.[15] Physicians traditionally bill the healthcare system or the insurance company directly, whereas the program manager budgets for the other disciplines within the inter-disciplinary team.[15] System reimbursements for physicians ought to address the importance of spending adequate time with the patient and family, the need for family meet-ings and team meetings, as well as the appropriate utiliza-tion of costly interventions in terminal care. The cost of the palliative care interdisciplinary team must be justified to senior administration. A database to collect information that quantifies time and tasks performed by each discipline in providing care to patients assists this process. Team members must understand the significance of collecting and recording these data. This not only substantiates costs in the current program but also aids in projecting future resource requirements. Once the financial offsets are con-sidered, the interdisciplinary approach to palliative care is a cost effective program.[24,30,37,40,42] Leaders of palliative care interdisciplinary teams must be prepared to face the afore-mentioned administrative challenges by developing a strate-gic plan based on evidence and data analysis. Ensuring that the administrative needs of the program are addressed ulti-mately leads to a better functioning team that can more effectively provide care to the patient.

FUTURE DIRECTIONS IN RESEARCH

There are many unanswered questions related to interdisci-plinary teams in palliative care.[4,12,23,69] Examples of possi-ble research questions include:

- What outcomes need to be measured?
- Do interdisciplinary teams provide more holistic and effective care?
- How is palliative care best delivered?
- How are interdisciplinary teams best organized?
- Which disciplines are essential to a palliative care team?
- What size and composition of interdisciplinary teams are most cost effective?
- What environments and practice settings benefit from having an interdisciplinary team?
- Are members of interdisciplinary teams more satisfied with their work?

CONCLUSION

Successful teams value and support their members, have a commitment to improve communication, resolve disagree-ments, and provide services. Support for individuals within the team to pursue professional and personal growth is encouraged. A coordinated effort by administration and leadership is required to meet these needs. The key factors for the success of the palliative care interdisciplinary team are vision, leadership and coordinated delivery of care, respect-ful interactions, professional development, and competence.

Key learning points

- The composition of the interdisciplinary team in palliative care is determined by the unique needs of the patient population being served.

- Effective role blurring is essential for the coordinated delivery of care.

- Concentrated efforts to hone communication and collaboration skills are needed to facilitate team growth.

- Commitment at all levels of leadership is required for the interdisciplinary teams in palliative care to succeed.

REFERENCES

1   Lickiss JN, Turner KS, Pollock ML. The interdisciplinary team. In: Doyle D, Hanks G, Cherney M, Calman K, eds. *Oxford Textbook of Palliative Medicine*, 3rd ed. Oxford: Oxford University Press, 2003: 42–6.
2   McCallin A. Interdisciplinary team leadership: a revisionist approach for an old problem? *J Nurs Manage* 2003; **11**: 364–70.
3   Egan KA, Labyak MJ. Hospice care: a model for quality end-of-life care. In: Ferrell BR, Coyle N, eds. *Textbook of Palliative Nursing*. New York: Oxford University Press, 2001: 7–26.
● 4   Hall P, Weaver L. Interdisciplinary education and teamwork: a long and winding road. *Med Educ* 2001; **35**: 867–75.
5   Higginson IJ, Finlay IG, Goodwin DM, *et al.* Is there evidence that palliative care teams alter end-of-life experiences of patients and their caregivers? *J Pain Symptom Manage* 2003; **25**: 150–68.
6   Strasser F, Sweeney C, Willey J, *et al.* Impact of a half-day multidisciplinary symptom control and palliative care outpatient clinic in a comprehensive cancer center on recommendations, symptom intensity, and patient satisfaction: A retrospective descriptive study. *J Pain Symptom Manage* 2004; **27**: 481–91.
◆ 7   Hearn J, Higginson IJ. Do specialist palliative care teams improve outcomes for cancer patients? A systematic literature review. *Palliat Med* 1998; **12**: 317–32.
8   Bruera E, Michaud M, Vigano A. Multidisciplinary symptom control clinic in a cancer center: a retrospective study. *Support Care Cancer* 2001; **9**: 162–8.
9   Edmonds PM, Stuttaford JM, Penny J, *et al.* Do hospital palliative care teams improve symptom control? Use of a modified STAS as an evaluation tool. *Palliat Med* 1998; **12**: 345–52.
10   Hunt J, Keeley V, Cobb M, *et al.* A new quality assurance package for hospital palliative care teams: the Trent Hospice Audit Group model. *Br J Cancer* 2004; **91**: 248–53.
11   Bruera E, Sweeney C. The Development of palliative care at the University of Texas M.D. Anderson Cancer Center. *Support Care Cancer* 2001; **9**: 330–4.
12   Hockley J. Specialist palliative care within the acute hospital setting. *Acta Oncol* 1999; **38**: 491–4.
13   Sherman DW. End-of-life care: challenges and opportunities for health care professionals. *Hospice J* 1999; **14:** 109–21.

● 14 Fitzpatrick JJ. Building community: Developing skills for interprofessional health professions education and relationship-centered care. *J Nurse-Midwifery* 1998; **43**: 61–5.

15 Billings JA. Vicissitudes of the clinician-patient relationship in end-of-life care: recognizing the role for teams. *J Palliat Med* 2002; **5**: 295–300.

● 16 Ahmedzai SH, Costa A, Blengini C, *et al.* A new international framework for palliative care. *Eur J Cancer* 2004; **40**: 2192–200.

17 Crawford GB, Price SD. *Palliative care. Team working: palliative care as a model of interdisciplinary practice. Med J Aust* 2003; **179**(6 Suppl): S32–S34.

18 Kristjanson LJ, Toye C, Dawson S. New dimensions in palliative care: a palliative approach to neurodegenerative diseases and final illness in older people. *Med J Aust* 2003; **179**(6 Suppl): S41–S43.

19 Watson JM. President's message: from discipline specific to 'inter' to 'multi' to 'transdisciplinary' health care education and practice. *Nurs Health Care Perspect* 1996; **17**: 90–1.

20 Dyer JA. Multidisciplinary, interdisciplinary, and transdisciplinary educational models and nursing education. *Nurs Educ Perspect* 2003; **24**: 186–8.

21 Higginson IJ, Finlay I, Goodwin DM, *et al.* Do hospital-based palliative teams improve care for patients or families at the end of life? *J Pain Symptom Manage* 2002; **23**: 96–106.

◆ 22 Salisbury C, Bosanquet N, Wilkinson EK, *et al.* The impact of different models of specialist palliative care on patients' quality of life: a systematic literature review. *Palliat Med* 1999; **13**: 3–18.

23 Teno JM. Palliative care teams: self-reflection, past, present and future. *J Pain Symptom Manage* 2002; **23**: 94–5.

24 Hughes SL, Cummings J, Weaver F, *et al.* A randomized trial of the cost effectiveness of VA hospital-based home care for the terminally ill. *Health Serv Res* 1992; **26**: 801–17.

25 Viney LL, Walker BM, Robertson T, *et al.* Dying in palliative care units and in hospital: a comparison of the quality of life of terminal cancer patients. *J Consult Clin Psychol* 1994; **62**: 157–64.

26 Seale C, Kelly M. A comparison of hospice and hospital care for people who die: views of the surviving spouse. *Palliat Med* 1997; **11**: 93–100.

27 Higginson IJ, Wade AM, McCarthy M. Effectiveness of two palliative support teams. *J Public Health Med* 1992; **14**: 50–6.

28 Seale C. A comparison of hospice and conventional care. *Soc Sci Med* 1991; **32**: 147–52.

◆ 29 Wilkinson EK, Salisbury C, Bosanquet N, *et al.* Patient and carer preference for, and satisfaction with, specialist models of palliative care: a systematic literature review. *Palliat Med* 1999; **13**: 197–220.

30 Smith TJ, Coyne P, Cassel B, *et al.* A high-volume specialist palliative care unit and team may reduce in-hospital end-of-life care costs. *J Palliat Med* 2003; **6**: 699–705.

● 31 Addington-Hall JM, MacDonald LD, Anderson HR, *et al.* Randomised controlled trial of effects of coordinating care for terminally ill cancer patients. *BMJ* 1992; **305**: 1317–22.

32 Higginson I, Hearn J. A multicenter evaluation of cancer pain control by palliative care teams. *J Pain Symptom Manage* 1997; **14**: 29–35.

33 McQuillar R, Finlay I, Roberts D, *et al.* The provision of a palliative care service in a teaching hospital and subsequent evaluation of that service. *Palliat Med* 1996; **10**: 231–9.

34 Parkes CM, Parkes J. 'Hospice' versus 'hospital' care re-evaluation after 10 years as seen by surviving spouses. *Postgrad Med J* 1984; **60**: 120–4.

◆ 35 Hearn J, Higginson I. Outcome measures in palliative care for advanced cancer patients: a review. *J Public Health Med* 1997; **19**: 193–9.

36 McMillan SC, Mahon M. A study of quality of life of hospice patients on admission and at week 3. *Cancer Nurs* 1994; **17**: 52–60.

37 Tramarin A, Milocchi F, Tolley K. An economic evaluation of home-care assistance for AIDS patients: a pilot study in a town in northern Italy. *AIDS* 1992; **6**: 1377–83.

38 Ventafridda V, De Conno F, Ripamonti C. Quality-of-life assessment during a palliative care programme. *Ann Oncol* 1990; **1**: 415–20.

● 39 Ellershaw JE, Peat SJ, Boys LC. Assessing the effectiveness of a hospital palliative care team. *Palliat Med* 1995; **9**: 145–52.

● 40 Axelson B, Christensen SB. Evaluation of a hospital-based palliative care support service with particular regard to financial outcome measures. *Palliat Med* 1998; **12**: 41–9.

41 Higginson I, McCarthy M. Measuring terminal cancer: are pain and dyspnea controlled? *J R Soc Med* 1989; **82**: 264–7.

● 42 Raftery JP, Addington-Hall JM, MacDonald LD, *et al.* A randomized controlled trial of the cost-effectiveness of a district co-ordinating service for terminally ill cancer patients. *Palliat Med* 1996; **10**: 151–61.

● 43 Hockley J. Role of the hospital support team. *Br J Hosp Med* 1992; **48**: 250–3.

44 Hockley J. The development of a palliative care team at the Western General Hospital, Edinburgh. *Support Care Cancer* 1996; **4**: 77–81.

45 MacDonald N. Palliative care and primary care. *J Palliat Care* 2002; **23**: 58–9.

● 46 Mariano C. The case for interdisciplinary collaboration. *Nurs Outlook* 1989; **37**: 285–8.

47 Poulton BC, West MA. The determinants of effectiveness in primary health care teams. *J Interprofes Care* 1999; **13**: 7–18.

48 Wilson PR. Multidisciplinary … transdisciplinary … monodisciplinary … where are we going? *Clin J Pain* 1996; **12**: 253–4.

49 Bruera E, Neumann CM, Gagnon B, *et al.* Edmonton Regional Palliative Care Program impact on patterns of terminal cancer care. *Can Med Assoc J* 1999; **161**: 290–3.

50 Cummings I. The interdisciplinary team. In: Doyle D, Hanks G, MacDonald N, eds. *Oxford Textbook of Palliative Medicine.* Oxford: Oxford University Press, 1998.

● 51 Bruera E. Influence of the pain and symptom control team on the patterns of treatment of pain and other symptoms in a cancer center. *J Pain Symptom Manage* 1989; **4**: 112–16.

52 Stepans MB, Thompson CL, Buchanan ML. The role of the nurse on a transdisciplinary early intervention assessment team. *Public Health Nurs* 2002; **19**: 238–45.

53 Sommers LS, Marton KI, Barbaccia JC, Randolph J. Physician, nurse, and social work collaboration in primary care for chronically ill seniors. *Arch Intern Med* 2000; **160**: 1825–33.

54 Fountain MJ. Key roles and issues of the multidisciplinary team. *Semin Oncol Nurs* 1993; **9**: 25–31.

● 55 Clark PG. Values in health care professional socialization: implications for geriatric education in interdisciplinary teamwork. *Gerontologist* 1997; **37**: 441–51.

56   Hill A. Multiprofessional teamwork in hospital palliative care teams. *Int J Palliat Nurs* 1998; **4**: 214–21.

57   Antai-Otong D. Team building in a health care setting. *Am J Nurs* 1997; **97**: 48–51.

58   Maddix T, Pereira J. Reflecting on the work of palliative care. *J Palliat Med* 2001; **4**: 373–7.

59   Poulton BC, West MA. Effective multidisciplinary teamwork in primary health care. *J Adv Nurs* 1993; **18**: 918–26.

60   MacDonald N. Limits to multidisciplinary education. *J Palliat Care* 1996; **12**: 6.

61   Clark PG, Spence DL, Sheehan JL. A service/learning model for interdisciplinary teamwork in health and aging. *Gerontol Geriatr Educ* 1986; **6**: 3–16.

62   Robbins H, Finley M. Four myths about teams. In: *Why Teams Don't Work.* Available at: www.mfinley.com/articles/team-myths.htm (accessed September 8, 2005).

63   VanDeVelde-Coke S. Restructuring health agencies: from hierarchies to programs. In: Hibberd JM, Smith DL, eds.

Nursing Management in Canada. Toronto: WB Saunders Company, 1999: 135–55.

◆ 64   Tait A. Clinical governance in primary care: a literature review. *J Clin Nurs* 2004; **13**: 723–30.

65   Vachon M. Staff burnout: source, diagnosis, management and prevention. In: Bruera E, Portenoy R, eds. *Topics in Palliative Care.* New York: Oxford University Press, 1999: 247–93.

66   Peiro JM, Gonzalez-Roma V, Ramos J. The influence of work team climate on role, stress, tension, satisfaction and leadership perceptions. *Eur Rev Appl Psychol* 1992; **42**: 49–56.

67   Mendes IA, *et al.* The re-humanization of the executive nurse's job: a focus on the spiritual dimension. *Rev Latino-am Enfemangem* 2002; **10**: 401–7.

68   Howatson-Jones IL. The servant leader. *Nurs Manage* 2004; **11**: 20–5.

69   Higginson IJ, Finlay IG. Improving palliative care for cancer. *Lancet Oncol* 2003; **4**: 73–4.

31

Population-based needs assessment for patient and family care

IRENE J HIGGINSON, CHARLES F VON GUNTEN

INTRODUCTION

As palliative care services develop all across the globe, those planning and funding services for populations of people will seek to ensure that services are developed in a way to meet the needs of patients and families. This is a group of the population which is often least able to make their needs known – as Hinton said, 'the dissatisfied dead cannot noise abroad their concerns'. So it is often left to patient groups and professionals to advocate for them. Policy makers and planners responsible for the healthcare services to a population have to make decisions that involve a range of health services. One way to help to plan services is to undertake a population-based needs assessment. Thus, to negotiate with planning officers, governments and funders, and to develop services, those working in palliative medicine have to develop a good understanding of needs assessment.[1] This chapter explains the concepts of needs and shows various methods of needs assessment. It highlights some of the pitfalls and factors that should be considered in the different approaches. Needs assessment in this context takes as its starting point a community that requires palliative care, rather than individual patients. It is concerned with how many people need what types of service, and where and when. The assessment of an individual patient can occasionally be described as a needs assessment,[2] but this is a component of assessment for direct clinical care planning and is not considered here.

WHAT IS NEED?

Contributions to the definitions of need come from the fields of sociology, epidemiology, health economics, public health as well as from clinicians. Bradshaw outlined a 'taxonomy of social need'. This distinguished between:[3]

- felt need (what people want)
- expressed need (felt need turned into action)
- normative need (as defined by experts or professionals)
- comparative need (arising where similar populations receive different service levels).

Raised within these distinctions are the questions of:

- Who determines need (professional, politician, or public)?
- What are the influences of education and media in raising awareness about health problems?
- What are the cultural effects on need?

Social and cultural factors have an enormous impact on levels of morbidity and on health and the expression of health need.

CONCEPTS OF NEED, SUPPLY, AND DEMAND IN HEALTHCARE

The above definitions of need do not take account of whether there is an effective remedy or treatment (i.e. supply) that

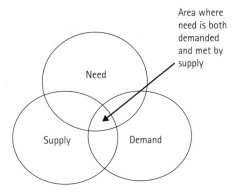

Figure 31.1   *Relationship between need, supply, and demand.*
Need = ability to benefit from healthcare.

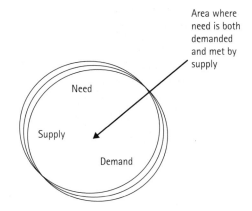

Figure 31.2   *Ideal relationship between need, supply, and demand.*

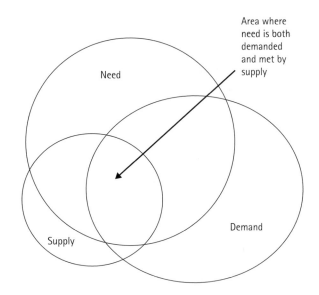

Figure 31.3   *Are the areas of need, supply, and demand of equal size? One hypothesis.*

can be provided for the problem experienced by the patient. Any assessment of the health needs of a community must take this into account. Thus needs assessment includes both the health problem (whether felt, expressed, normative, comparative, or a combination of these) and an effective humane and accessible remedy or treatment for this problem.[4] The remedy can include prevention, treatment, rehabilitation, and palliation. The modern epidemiological approaches to needs assessment take account of both health need and effective treatment.[5]

Demand in healthcare is a function of expressed need, although economists would define it as: 'What people would be willing to pay for in a market or might wish to use in a system of free health care'.[5] Demand, therefore, is influenced by the nature of information available to patients and to communities, the social and educational backgrounds, the media and the influence of doctors and nurses. Furthermore, for any patient or family, interpretation of information would be affected by the severity of his or her illness and his or her concern about that illness. The supply of health services has been influenced by historical patterns, political pressures, pressures from healthcare professionals, from the public, the media, and from patients.

Stevens and Raftery have argued that need for healthcare should be defined as: 'the population's ability to benefit from health care'.[5] They argue that need, supply and demand partly overlap but also differ. Figure 31.1 demonstrates the differences and overlap, and shows seven different potential situations.[5] In the central area, need is both demanded and supplied. However, there may be supply where there is no need, there may be care demanded but not needed, and there may be demand and supply without need. The aim of a needs assessment in this context is to bring the circles to overlap more closely (as in Fig. 31.2), so that need is demanded and supplied. However, this Stevens and Raftery hypothesis has one major flaw. It makes a rather simplistic assumption that need, demand, and supply are of equal size, and that reorganization of healthcare is a matter of lining up the need, demand, and supply. But in reality this is not likely to be the case. As part of the MSc in palliative care at King's College

London, students from different countries report how they feel need, demand, and supply are related and sized in their countries. Figure 31.3 shows one hypothesis, where supply is smaller than demand and need.

ALTERNATIVE APPROACHES TO NEEDS ASSESSMENT

Three main approaches to needs assessment have been developed. These can be used independently or in combination.

Comparative needs assessment

A comparative needs assessment contrasts the services received by a population in one area with those elsewhere. Thus if one area has, for example, 40 hospice beds per million population it might be seen as less well provided than an

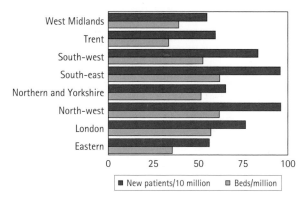

Figure 31.4   *An example of comparative needs assessment – comparing beds available. Beds per million population, new patients per 10 million population: health regions in England (2000). Redrawn with permission from Higginson,* Palliative Care for Londoners, *2001.[37]*

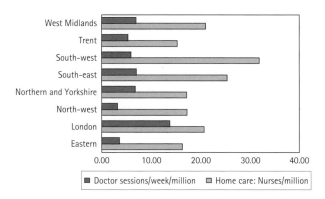

Figure 31.5   *An example of comparative needs assessment – comparing nurse and doctor sessions available. Home care nurses and doctor session per million population, England 2000. Redrawn with permission from Higginson,* Palliative Care for Londoners, *2001.[37]*

area with say 70 beds per million population. Figures 31.4 and 31.5 show examples of such a comparative assessment. However, such an assessment is clearly limited, as it does not take account of differences between the populations, nor of which model of care (more beds or more home nursing) is most effective for the population.

Corporate approach to needs assessment

The corporate approach to needs assessment is based on the demands, wishes, and alternative perspectives of interested parties including professionals, politicians, patients, and the public. A variety of interview schedules and tools in many areas of healthcare have been developed to aid this approach.[6] This approach commonly involves surveys of professionals,[7–9] and may also survey the public, patients,[10] or a combination of views (for example professionals and public).[11] Perhaps the most comprehensive instrument is that developed by Currow *et al.*, who surveyed 3027 randomly selected South Australians in 2000 on the need for,

uptake rate of, and satisfaction with specialist palliative care services. One in three people surveyed (n = 1069) indicated that someone 'close to them' had died of a terminal illness in the preceding 5 years. Of those who identified that a palliative service had not been used (38 percent, n = 403), reasons cited included family/friends provided the care (34 percent, n = 136) and the service was not wanted (21 percent, n = 86). Respondents with higher income and those with cancer were more likely to report that a specialist palliative care service had been used.[12] Currow *et al.*'s approach utilized the views of proxies, i.e. not directly the patients but bereaved carers or others. The corporate approach has the potential advantage of gauging the patient's (or their family's) perspectives and capturing expressed need. However, surveying only professionals captures only normative need. And there is the added problem that expressed need is determined by individual's understanding of services, which is dependent on the provision of information about palliative care. Such information can be highly varied both within and between countries, and should be considered when interpreting a corporate needs assessment.

Needs assessment reviews based on epidemiological data

The third approach to needs assessment is the epidemiologically based assessment. Epidemiological data have been applied in healthcare planning for many years.[4,13] Data on the incidence (the number of new cases arising in a given period) and prevalence (the total number of cases existing at one time) of diseases, and demographic information on population structure and likely changes, were used by healthcare planners to determine the extent and impact of health problems. Epidemiological studies are also concerned with the quality of measurements, including the validity and reliability of tests. Population comparisons are usually more clearly made using rates rather than crude numbers, often giving age- and sex-specific rates or standardized according to the national population.

The epidemiological approach to needs assessment[7] combines elements of epidemiology and health economics and is a triangulation of three components:

- incidence and/or prevalence
- health service effectiveness and cost-effectiveness
- information and views about existing services.
  Information allows funders and planners to determine the direction they wish to pursue in the future (see Fig. 31.6).

Because any needs assessment will usually make incremental rather than dramatic changes to existing services and because there is little information on effectiveness and prevalence, it is usually recommended that this approach is combined with the more simple comparative and corporate approaches described above. The main components of the epidemiologically based approach to needs assessment are shown in Table 31.1.

EPIDEMIOLOGICALLY BASED NEEDS ASSESSMENT FOR PALLIATIVE AND TERMINAL CARE

In an attempt to provide assistance for those planning and funding palliative care services, an epidemiologically based

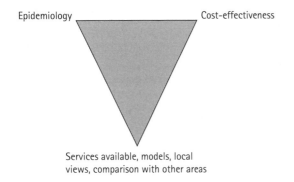

Epidemiology   Cost-effectiveness

Services available, models, local
views, comparison with other areas

Figure 31.6 *The three main components of the 'epidemiologically based' approach.*

needs assessment for palliative (and end of life) care was produced in the UK.[14] This provided standard definitions of palliative and end-of-life/terminal care and used national and local data on the incidence and prevalence of cancer, other diseases and likely symptoms to estimate the numbers of patients and families needing palliative care. The absolute numbers of patients dying from cancer and other diseases likely to have a palliative period are available from government statistical departments in many countries. Applying the prevalence of symptoms to this population gives estimates of the range of problems and the size of population needing care.

The protocol suggests that a standard population size is used, for example 1 million people. Within such a population, if the age and gender mix is similar to that of a developed country, there are approximately 2800 cancer deaths per year and 6900 other deaths, some of which may have a period of advancing progressive disease, when palliative care would be appropriate. Table 31.2 shows the number of deaths within a population during 1 year for the most common causes, and Tables 31.3 and 31.4 show the likely prevalence of problems for patients with cancer or patients with progressive nonmalignant diseases.

These prevalence data can then be contrasted with the numbers who are receiving different services in an area. For example, a needs assessment for the London region showed

Table 31.1 *Components of the epidemiological approach to needs assessment[5,14,37]*

Component	Description
Statement of the context of the problem	The problem in its context including labels attached to the disease or service, e.g. international classification of disease codes, healthcare resource groups. The context should relate the disease to the services it impinges upon
Subcategories	A division of the health problem into categories which are of value to purchasing, planning or providing healthcare. Often this is based on severity or type of problem presenting. Conventional, medical subcategories sometimes do not help
Prevalence and incidence	Prevalence and incidence data including that available for the subcategories described and/or need for treatment. It considers variations by age, sex, region, socioeconomic and ethnic status
Services available	Description of existing services defining the components, including the structures and processes as clearly as possible
Effectiveness and cost-effectiveness of services	The efficacy (benefits achieved under study – usually ideal conditions), effectiveness (the benefit achieved in the real world) and efficiency (output or outcome of healthcare per unit of money expended). Efficacy is considered first and the quality of the evidence is graded according to the strength of design of the studies. This is followed by a statement of the strength of recommendation to support or reject the use of the service or procedure based on the strength of the evidence
Models of care and local assessment	Alternative models of providing services to meet patients needs. For example, one model might be orientated towards prevention, one towards treatment and a third model towards education of existing staff. An appraisal of the models and their application in different social, geographical and healthcare settings is included Here local assessment of individual wishes or local data on the preferences/wishes of patients and families can be used. It may help to decide between the amounts of different models provided
Outcomes, targets, information and research	Outcome measures or targets which might prove useful in practice to monitor services plus other information and research needs

that in the over 7 million population there were 15 780 deaths from cancer each year, and of these it is estimated that 13 260 have pain; 12 200 patients received hospital support each year, and 11 700 home palliative care, suggesting that there may be reasonable but incomplete coverage (see Fig. 31.7). However, the proportion of noncancer patients with symptoms and who received services was much smaller (see Figs 31.7 and 31.8), suggesting a need to develop services for these groups of patients.

Current levels of use of specialist palliative care services can also be used to estimate need. However, this is really a comparative evaluation, and is really only as good as the

Table 31.2 *Number of deaths in the population during 1 year for the most common causes[14]*

Cause of death	Men	Women	Total
Neoplasms	1460	1340	2800
Circulatory system	2430	2620	5050
Respiratory system	600	630	1230
Chronic liver and cirrhosis	30	30	60
Nervous system and sense organs	90	90	180
Senile and presenile organic conditions	20	20	40
Endocrine, nutritional, metabolic, immunity	190	120	310
Total of these diseases	4820	4850	9670
Total deaths from all causes	5360	5640	11 000

Note: total population = 1 million, estimate for developed country.
Note: deaths in those aged under 28 days excluded.

Table 31.3 *Cancer patients: prevalence of problems (per 1 000 000 population, developed country context)[14]*

Symptom	% with symptom in last year of life[a]	Estimated number in each year
Pain	84	2357
Trouble with breathing	47	1318
Vomiting or feeling sick	51	1431
Sleeplessness	51	1431
Mental confusion	33	926
Depression	38	1065
Loss of appetite	71	1992
Constipation	47	1318
Bedsores	28	785
Loss of bladder control	37	1038
Loss of bowel control	25	701
Unpleasant smell	19	533
Severe family anxiety/worries	33	930
Severe patient anxiety/worries	25	700
Total deaths from cancer		2805

[a] Symptoms as per Cartwright[15] and Seale[16] studies, based on a random sample of deaths and using the reports of bereaved carers.
[b] Anxiety as per Field et al.,[17] Bennett and Corcoran,[18] Higginson et al.,[19] Addington Hall et al.[20]
Note: Patients usually have several symptoms.

Table 31.4 *Patients with progressive nonmalignant disease: prevalence of problems (per 1 000 000 population, developed country context)*

Symptom	% with symptom in last year of life[a]	Estimated number in each year
Pain	67	4599
Trouble with breathing	49	3363
Vomiting or feeling sick	27	1853
Sleeplessness	36	2471
Mental confusion	38	2608
Depression	36	2471
Loss of appetite	38	2608
Constipation	32	2196
Bedsores	14	961
Loss of bladder control	33	2265
Loss of bowel control	22	1510
Unpleasant smell	13	892
Severe family anxiety/worries[b]	33	2200
Severe patient anxiety/worries	25	1600
Total deaths from other causes, excluding accidents, injury, and suicide, and causes very unlikely to have a palliative period		6864

[a] As per Cartwright[15] and Seale[16] studies, based on a random sample of deaths and using the reports of bereaved carers.
[b] Anxiety as per Field et al.,[17] Bennett and Corcoran,[18] Higginson et al.,[19] Addington Hall et al.[20]
Note: Patients usually have several symptoms.

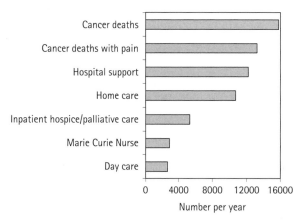

Figure 31.7 *Example 1 from* Palliative Care for Londoners, 2001. *Estimated yearly numbers of cancer deaths, cancer deaths with pain, and patients with cancer who receive different services in the London region. Redrawn with permission from Higginson,* Palliative Care for Londoners, 2001.[37]

estimated current levels of use. Such an approach maintains the status quo, although it may allow for comparison between areas. There are no really good estimates of 'correct' levels of use of palliative care. Estimates of the proportion of patients with cancer who need palliative care ranges from 15 percent to 80 percent, and are generally not based on good evidence. There are no comparative studies to show the effectiveness of provision at different levels, although there are good studies demonstrating the benefits of palliative care on symptom management and patient satisfaction, suggesting that most patients with cancer benefit.[21,22] The Australian survey discussed above suggested that less that 10 percent (86/1069) of people would not want palliative care services.[12]

INCORPORATING THE EVIDENCE BASE AND OTHER VIEWS

In addition to the data on prevalence of symptoms, an epidemiologically based needs assessment includes data on the effectiveness of different models of palliative care. Rather than attempt new systematic literature reviews, a variety of high quality systematic reviews and meta-analyses are available.[23–33] These show that specialist palliative care has

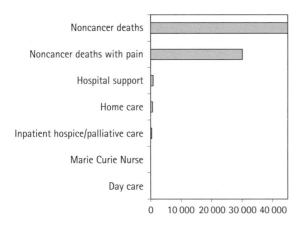

Figure 31.8 *Example 2 from* Palliative Care for Londoners, 2001. *Estimated yearly numbers of noncancer deaths, noncancer deaths with pain, and noncancer patients who receive different services in the London region. Redrawn with permission from Higginson, Palliative Care for Londoners, 2001.[37]*

benefits, particularly in terms of pain and symptom control and patient and carer satisfaction.[34,35] However, most evidence exists for specialist home care, and for inpatient palliative care, either with specialist beds in a freestanding unit or hospice, and/or advisory hospital teams, seeing patients on all wards (see Table 31.5).[23] Other components of palliative care, including day care, outpatient services and hospice at home have not yet been well evaluated. This evidence has now been used in several countries to plan for services and some evidence sources are available on the internet for free download for any groups wishing to use them.[23,32] However, much of the evidence is drawn from developing countries and the evidence base in African and developing countries is (for reasons clear in the chapters about those countries) not yet developed.[36]

Gaps identified between the epidemiological information on need and the services currently provided can then be appraised against the evidence and any comparative or corporate data. The gaps may also suggest lines of inquiry in a survey of patient, carer or professional views, e.g. would they prefer more home care, hospital support or inpatient care developed? This then suggests options for the future development of palliative care services.

LIMITATIONS OF NEEDS ASSESSMENT

Although the approach provides a useful model for examining health needs, it is based on assumptions that limit its conclusions:

- The overlapping circles of need, demand and supply shown in Fig 31.1 imply that if only need, demand, and supply can be lined up, then need and demand will be satisfied by supply. If demand and need are larger than supply, they cannot be met completely, even if improved alignment is of value. A needs assessment, where the supply of palliative care is limited, will lead to a demand for more resources, and health planners may not be prepared for this.
- The data available to undertake the needs assessment are often limited. Epidemiological studies have often been more concerned with the etiology of diseases than the scope for benefit or need for services. For this

Table 31.5 *Summary of evidence of the effectiveness of specialist palliative care services*[22,3,24,25,28,34]

Specialist palliative care service	Studies	Findings: compared with conventional care
Inpatient	1 RCT, >5 comparative, versus conventional care	Equal or improved symptoms, improved satisfaction
Multidisciplinary home care team	4 RCTs, >15 comparative, versus conventional care	Longer time at home, equal or improved symptoms, improved satisfaction
Multidisciplinary hospital team	1 RCT, >10 comparative observational studies	Symptoms and problems improve during care (as for home care and inpatient)

RCT, randomized controlled trial.

reason most of the epidemiological data are reliant on estimates from death registrations and estimates of the prevalence of symptoms in selected populations. Death registrations may not be available and can be inaccurate, especially among older people, where there may also be multiple causes of death. Such data do not take account of the trajectory of illness and the time period that services are needed for. Thus those undertaking the needs assessment must take these limitations into account when presenting the data.

- Effectiveness and cost-effectiveness studies may be carried out in communities different from that where the service is concerned. For example in palliative care, the well-designed randomized controlled trials were carried out in the USA and not the UK. Thus methods of needs assessment are needed for developing contexts, and require some further development.

- Effectiveness and cost-effectiveness are main components in an epidemiological approach. However, humanity, equity, acceptability, appropriateness, and accessibility are also essential in determining the quality of the service. However, it could be argued that without efficacy and effectiveness these are of no value (one would not want a humane service which had no effectiveness or was even harmful). Nevertheless, these are important components of care and, given that effectiveness data are often limited, excluding such components weakens the approach. A corporate assessment is often useful in exploring aspects of appropriateness, acceptability, and humanity, whereas a comparative assessment may throw light on accessibility. These approaches can be combined with the epidemiologically based needs assessment.

- The needs assessment approach was originally developed for disease-oriented single interventions, such as cataract surgery. Applying the model of needs assessment to care groups such as elderly people and, to some extent, to palliative care is more complex. There are multiple possible interventions and multiple possible needs within these populations. This limitation is evidenced by the aspects covered in the early needs assessments: diabetes mellitus, renal disease, coronary heart disease, cancer of the lung, colorectal cancer, hip replacement, hernia repair, prostatectomy, etc. More recently, however, needs assessments have addressed mental illness, dementia, learning difficulties, community child health services, and palliative care. However, the needs assessment in these contexts will tend to highlight a number of possible options, rather than, for example, the number of patients who require a particular operation.

CONCLUSIONS AND FUTURE ISSUES

The epidemiologically based needs assessment approach to planning palliative care services has emerged in the past decade. It has three main components: incidence and/or prevalence of a disease or condition; effectiveness and cost effectiveness of services; and review of existing services. It can be combined with corporate and comparative approaches to needs assessment. This information is combined and culminates in recommendations for particular procedures or interventions based on standard criteria for the quality of evidence and an appraisal of alternative models of care.

Because the approach is time-consuming and subject to limitations, some guidance is available, especially on the effectiveness of models of care and on incidence and prevalence guidance. However, there is a need to further develop approaches to needs assessment in developing countries and those where there is little palliative care. Ideally a template is needed, which can be applied to different settings. Presentation of the data to local groups (statutory and voluntary and at public meetings) can help to facilitate discussion about where services should develop in the future.

Key learning points

- There are four main elements of need: felt need, expressed need, normative need, and comparative need.

- Need, supply, and demand for services may not overlap.

- There are three common approaches to needs assessment, all of which have been used in palliative care.

- A comparative needs assessment determines need by a comparison of supply between areas.

- A corporate needs assessment determines needs by taking views from local stakeholders.

- Both of these approaches can tend to confirm the status quo, rather than identify groups who are missing out on care more fundamentally.

- An epidemiological approach to needs assessment examines the incidence and prevalence of problems, the effectiveness of services and the services available and views on these.

- The epidemiological approach can be combined with the comparative and corporate approaches.

REFERENCES

1   Clark D, Malson H, Small N, *et al.* Needs assessment and palliative care: the views of providers. *J Public Health Med* 1997; **19**: 437–42.
2   Osse BH, Vernooij MJ, Schade E, Grol RP. Towards a new clinical tool for needs assessment in the palliative care of cancer patients: the PNPC instrument. *J Pain Symptom Manage* 2004; **28**: 329–341.

● 3 Bradshaw JS. A taxonomy of social need. In: McLachlan G, ed. *Problems and Progress in Medical Care: Essays on Current Research.* Seventh series ed. Oxford: Oxford University Press, 1972.

4 McCarthy M. *Epidemiology and Policies for Health Planning.* London: King Edward's Hospital Fund for London, 1982.

● 5 Stevens A, Raftery J. Health care needs assessment. In: Stevens A, Raftery J, eds. *The Epidemiologically-Based Needs Assessment Reviews.* Oxford: Radcliffe Medical Press, 1994: 11–30.

6 Asadi-Lari M, Gray D. Health needs assessment tools: progress and potential. *Int J Technol Assess Health Care* 2005; **21**: 288–97.

7 Shipman C, Addington-Hall J, Richardson A, *et al.* Palliative care services in England: a survey of district nurses' views. *Br J Community Nurs* 2005; **10**: 381–6.

8 Shirai Y, Kawa M, Miyashita M, Kazuma K. Nurses' perception of adequacy of care for leukemia patients with distress during the incurable phase and related factors. *Leuk Res* 2005; **29**: 293–300.

9 Wotton K, Borbasi S, Redden M. When all else has failed: Nurses' perception of factors influencing palliative care for patients with end-stage heart failure. *J Cardiovasc Nurs* 2005; **20**: 18–25.

10 Skilbeck J, Mott L, Page H, *et al.* Palliative care in chronic obstructive airways disease: a needs assessment. *Palliat Med* 1998; **12**: 245–54.

11 Kwekkeboom K. A community needs assessment for palliative care services from a hospice organization. *J Palliat Med* 2005; **8**: 817–26.

● 12 Currow DC, Abernethy AP, Fazekas BS. Specialist palliative care needs of whole populations: a feasibility study using a novel approach. *Palliat Med* 2004; **18**: 239–47.

13 Knox D. *Epidemiology in Health Care Plannning.* Oxford: Oxford University Press, 1979.

✱ 14 Higginson I. *DHA Project: Research Programme. Epidemiologically-based Needs Assessment. Series 2: Palliative and Terminal Care.* London: NHS Executive, 1996.

● 15 Cartwright A. Changes in life and care in the year before death 1969–1987. *J Public Health Med* 1991; **13**: 81–7.

16 Seale C. A comparison of hospice and conventional care. *Soc Sci Med* 1991; **32**: 147–52.

17 Field D, Douglas C, Jagger C, Dand P. Terminal illness: views of patients and their lay carers. *Palliat Med* 1995; **9**: 45–54.

18 Bennett M, Corcoran G. The impact on community palliative care services of a hospital palliative care team. *Palliat Med* 1994; **8**: 237–44.

19 Higginson IJ, Wade AM, McCarthy M. Effectiveness of two palliative support teams. *J Public Health Med* 1992; **14**: 50–6.

20 Addington-Hall JM, MacDonald L, Anderson H, Freeling P. Dying from cancer: the views of bereaved family and the friends about the experiences of terminally ill patients. *Palliat Med* 1991; **5**: 207–14.

● 21 Higginson IJ, Hearn J. A multi-centre evaluation of cancer pain control by palliative care teams. *J Pain Symptom Manage* 1997; **14**: 29–35.

◆ 22 Higginson IJ, Finlay I, Goodwin DM, *et al.* Do hospital-based palliative teams improve care for patients or families at the end of life? *J Pain Symptom Manage* 2002; **23**: 96–106.

◆ 23 Gysels M, Higginson IJ. *Improving Supportive and Palliative Care for Adults with Cancer: Research Evidence.* London: National Institute of Clinical Excellence, 2004. Available at: www.nice.org.uk/page.aspx?0=11001 (accessed April 27, 2006).

24 Davies E, Higginson IJ. Communication, information and support for adults with malignant cerebral glioma: a systematic literature review. *Support Cancer Care* 2003; **11**: 21–9.

25 Harding R, Higginson IJ. What is the best way to help caregivers in cancer and palliative care? A systematic review of interventions and their effectiveness. *Palliat Med* 2003; **17**: 63–74.

26 Finlay IG, Higginson IJ, Goodwin DM, *et al.* Palliative care in hospital, hospice, at home: results from a systematic review. *Ann Oncol* 2002; **13**: 257–64.

27 Goodwin DM, Higginson IJ, Edwards AGK, *et al.* An evaluation of systematic reviews of palliative care services. *J Palliat Care* 2002; **18**: 77–83.

28 Davies E, Higginson IJ. Systematic review of specialist palliative day care for adults with cancer. *Support Cancer Care* 2005; **13**: 607–27.

29 Gruenewald DA, Higginson IJ, Vivat B, *et al.* Quality of life measures for the palliative care of people severely affected by multiple sclerosis: a systematic review. *Mult Scler* 2004; **10**: 690–704.

30 Gysels M, Richardson A, Higginson IJ. Communication training for health professionals who care for patients with cancer: a systematic review of effectiveness. *Support Care Cancer* 2004; **12**: 692–700.

31 Gysels M, Higginson IJ, Richardson A. Communication training for health professionals who care for patients with cancer: a systematic review of training methods. *Support Cancer Care* 2005; **13**: 356–66.

32 Lorenz KA, Asch SM, Yano EM, *et al.* Comparing strategies for United States veterans' mortality ascertainment. *Popul Health Metr* 2005; **3**: 2. Available at: www.pophealthmetrics.com/content/3/1/2 (accessed April 27, 2006).

33 Harding R, Easterbrook PE, Karus D, *et al.* Does palliative care improve outcomes for patients with HIV/AIDS? A systematic review of the evidence. *Sex Transm Infect* 2004; **81**: 14.

◆ 34 Higginson IJ, Finlay IG, Goodwin DM, *et al.* Is there evidence that palliative care teams alter end-of-life experiences of patients and their caregivers? *J Pain Symptom Manage* 2003; **25**: 150–68.

35 Hearn J, Feuer D, Higginson I, Sheldon T. Systematic reviews. *Palliat Med* 1999; **13**: 75–80.

● 36 Harding R, Higginson IJ. Palliative care in sub-Saharan Africa. *Lancet* 2005; **365**: 1971–8.

37 Higginson I. *Palliative Care for Londoners.* London: Department of Palliative Care and Policy, 2001.

32

The palliative care consult team

ALEXIE CINTRON, DIANE E MEIER

INTRODUCTION

Larger numbers of patients treated in hospitals are not imminently dying but are living with chronic and debilitating illnesses. In addition, virtually all persons with serious illness spend at least some time in a hospital, usually on multiple occasions, in the course of their disease or condition.[1] Unfortunately, hospital care of these patients is often characterized by untreated physical symptoms, poor communication between providers and patients, treatment decisions in conflict with prior stated preferences, treatments that may be more burdensome than beneficial, and poor care transition management. These patients need expert symptom management, communication and decision-making support, and care coordination. By addressing these needs, the palliative care consultation team (PCCT) aims to improve hospital care for patients living with serious illness.

In the USA, national initiatives have called for improved pain and symptom management and for psychologic, social, and spiritual support for patients and families living with serious illness.[2–10] Hospital-based palliative care programs of widely varying structures and composition have grown rapidly in number in recent years.[11–13] In a survey of 100 teaching hospitals in the USA published in 2001, researchers found that 26 percent of respondents had either a PCCT or a palliative care unit, and 7 percent had both.[12] Another survey of hospitals in the USA showed that 30 percent of respondents had a hospital-based palliative care service and another 20 percent had plans to establish one.[13] Although specialist-level palliative care is delivered through a range of clinical models, the predominant delivery model in the USA (outside of hospice) is the inpatient PCCT.[13,14] In this chapter, we describe the organization, operation, and outcomes assessment of the hospital-based PCCT. We also discuss the design and implementation of a successful hospital-based PCCT.

STRUCTURE OF THE PALLIATIVE CARE CONSULTATION TEAM

As described in the recently released National Consensus Project's *Clinical Practice Guidelines for Quality Palliative Care*,[4] palliative care is optimally delivered through an interdisciplinary team consisting of appropriately trained and credentialed physicians, nurses, and social workers with support and contributions from chaplains, rehabilitative experts, psychiatrists, and other professionals as indicated. However, individual institutions have adopted different models to provide palliative care in a manner that is feasible and sustainable according to the particular needs of these institutions. The PCCT is generally structured in one of two ways: the solo practitioner model or the full team model.

Solo practitioner model

In a solo practitioner model, the PCCT consists of a physician or advanced nurse practitioner (ANP) who provides an initial assessment of the patient's needs and communicates this assessment directly with the attending physician, the nursing staff, and the social work staff. The practitioner may or may not write patient orders. The physician or ANP then refers patients to needed services, discusses needs in conference, and communicates with clinicians. In addition, the practitioner assists patients and their families with clarification of goals of care, care plans, and advance directives. Finally, the palliative care physician or ANP develops protocols for patient care in conjunction with treatment teams and educates staff about palliative care and treatment protocols.

The solo palliative care practitioner must have access to and sufficient time allotted from social work, nursing, physical therapy, occupational therapy, and pharmacy to respond to referrals, all of which should be monitored for time requirements. The practitioner must spend time providing psychosocial support and symptom management to the patient, coordinating services, and teaching family and staff. The literature does not define the patient volume that the practitioner is able to handle, but reports from established programs suggest that a maximum comfortable caseload would consist of four new cases per day and an average daily census of 15 patients.

The advantages of the solo practitioner consultation model of palliative care are lower start-up costs and financial risk, opportunity to develop a program based on the existing patient population, lower threat to medical staff, and the ability to build on existing programs and services and use them whenever possible. The major disadvantage to this model is that the program and the care of highly complex cases rest on one discipline and one individual's shoulders. The patient volume can be quickly limited by workload.

Full team model

The full team model for the palliative care consultative service consists of a physician, an ANP or nurse, and a social worker. Everyone on the team is responsible for assessing and following patients referred by an attending physician. The team then provides advice to the primary physician based on the assessment and follow-up. Alternatively, the team may assume all or part of the care of the patient including writing patient orders. The team refers the patient to needed services, discharges the patient to appropriate settings, discusses needs in conference, and communicates with all care providers. For this model to be successful, the team must work in unison to coordinate the plan of care and to provide appropriate services.

As with the solo practitioner model, the team model should have access to and time allotted from social work, nursing, physical and occupational therapy, and pharmacy services. In contrast with the solo practitioner model, the patient volume threshold for the team model varies depending on whether patients are transferred to the team for complete management. Consequently, the team model may reach a larger number of patients compared to the solo practitioner model.

The team model has several advantages over the solo practitioner model. More providers on the team means more disciplines and more expertise are available to the patient and the hospital community and an ability to reach a large number of nurses and physicians through bedside and nursing station teaching and role modeling. The PCCT can also provide support and teaching to medical staff learning to implement new

skills and knowledge. The major disadvantage of the team approach to the PCCT is the added costs for a team with limited, or no, additional revenue beyond the physician's billing.

OPERATION OF THE PALLIATIVE CARE CONSULT SERVICE

The role of the PCCT is to assess the physical, psychologic, social, spiritual, and cultural needs of patients with advanced, life-threatening illness. The team then advises the consulting provider on how to address these needs. Why do primary providers request a palliative care consultation? What is the PCCT's approach?

Reasons for palliative care consultation

Studies characterizing the reasons for palliative care consults among different hospital settings have demonstrated that pain management and other symptom management were the predominant reasons for consultation, usually accounting for about 70–80 percent of palliative care consultations.[13,15–17] Other reasons for consultation included discharge planning,[13,15,17] organization of care,[16] establishing goals of care,[13] and end-of-life discussions.[15] The PCCT also provides psychosocial, spiritual, and bereavement support.[7,18–23] Finally, the PCCT provides help with care coordination and continuity.[18,24,25] While more than one reason for consultation was identified per patient in most consults,[15–17] after investigation, the number of problems subsequently identified by the PCCT tended to be higher than those initially reported by the primary care provider.[16]

The consultation process

Palliative care consults must be ordered by a physician, but nurses, or social workers may initiate a consult if approved by the attending physician.[26] The PCCT can also get involved in a case if the patient or the family request to be seen.[5] Once the consult has been ordered, the first task is to elicit the specific reasons for consultation from the primary care team.

The approach to the patient then begins with a comprehensive assessment of the patient and family including physical and psychological symptoms, as well as social, spiritual, and cultural aspects of care. Validated assessment instruments should be used whenever possible. The assessment is followed by the evaluation and management of symptoms.

Once the patient is comfortable, a discussion of realistic goals and overall goals of care can be held. The PCCT should elicit the patient's understanding of the disease and its treatment as well as the patient's opinion about what constitutes an acceptable quality of life. During this process, the PCCT can assist the primary care provider to communicate bad news and discuss the benefits and burdens of various treatments. Once goals of care are established, decision making regarding treatment options and advance directives can be pursued. At this time, the team should also encourage the patient to designate a healthcare proxy or durable power of attorney for healthcare to ensure continuity of decision making if and when the patient loses decisional capacity.

The team's approach to the family begins with identification of the patient's primary care giver and/or healthcare agent. With the patient's permission, the team can then elicit the family's understanding of the disease and its treatment and provide the primary caregiver and family with support and education about the patient's distress and symptom management, practical needs, and plans for the future. The PCCT typically coordinates a family meeting to discuss goals of care and further plans for care. An appropriate plan of care and discharge plan should take into account family support systems including their physical, emotional, and financial resources and should be consistent with the established goals of care.

Throughout this process, the PCCT maintains a close working relationship with the primary care team. This begins with good communication regarding the assessment and recommendations made, paying particular attention to the original reasons for the consultation. An attempt should be made to establish personal contact with the primary service rather than rely on communication by notes in the medical chart.[27] While the primary care service generally decides whether or not to implement the consult team's recommendations, the PCCT can seek to obtain permission from the primary service to implement certain interventions promptly to avoid unnecessary delay and suffering.[27] The consult team should encourage participation from the primary service at family meetings (especially important in teaching hospitals) and should educate staff regarding particular aspects of the patient's management and care plan.

Interaction with and engagement of nursing and support staff is key to the success of the palliative care consult. The consult team should, therefore, encourage participation from nursing and support staff in the formulation of the patient's care plan, educate the nursing and support staff about palliative care management issues specific to the patient, and provide the staff with bedside support regarding difficult patient situations and treatment decisions.

This consultation process is time consuming. One study reported that the median time spent in consultation was 60 minutes by the palliative care fellow and 30 minutes by the palliative care attending physician.[15] Another study reported that an initial consult of over 2 hours was common.[28] Moreover, the total time spent in consultation and follow-up – including review of the medical record, interviewing and examining the patient, meeting with the family and having discussions with the attending physician, nursing, social work, and other members of the primary care team – often exceeds 5 hours.[28] The process can therefore take several visits over several days. Most of the time spent during consultation is occupied by eliciting and giving information and providing counseling.[27,29]

IMPACT OF PALLIATIVE CARE CONSULT TEAMS

Few studies have specifically examined the impact of PCCTs on patient care. Among these studies, some have found that a PCCT makes an average of three to four recommendations per patient to consulting physicians.[17,27] Of these recommendations, over 90 percent are implemented.[27,28] This statistic is impressive in the light of the paucity of evidence demonstrating the impact of PCCT structures and processes on patient-related outcomes.

Various studies have shown that inpatient palliative care teams improve patient symptoms, particularly pain.[30*,31*] However, these studies have been small and observational. A pilot study conducted at Mount Sinai Medical Center in New York compared pain ratings for 463 cancer patients followed by the PCCT to 653 cancer patients not receiving palliative care. Palliative care patients were significantly more likely to be discharged from the hospital with no or mild pain (96 percent of patients) compared with cancer patients not receiving palliative care (84 percent of patients, $P < 0.001$). Similarly, compared with patients receiving palliative care, usual care patients were significantly more likely to be discharged from the hospital with moderate to severe nausea (14 vs. 2 percent, $P < 0.001$) and moderate to severe constipation (46 vs. 3 percent, $P < 0.001$) (R Sean Morrison, personal communication, June 12, 2004).

Other studies have examined the impact of PCCTs on establishment of goals of care. One such study demonstrated that goals of care were identified in about 85 percent of patients seen.[15] The most commonly cited goals of care were: improved symptom control, return home, receipt of hospice care, no further hospital admissions, and a comfortable death.[15] Another study showed that the PCCT conducted discussions with patients/families about prognosis and goals of care in about 94 percent of cases. After these discussions, there was a modification of the understanding of prognosis and goals of care in 87 percent of cases.[27*] PCCTs have also been effective in increasing discussion of advance directives, including discussion about a Do Not Resuscitate (DNR) order[15*,27*] and designation of a healthcare proxy.[27*] Some studies have associated palliative care consultation with reductions in resource utilization, hospital costs, and hospital and length of stay in the intensive care unit.[32*,33,34]

Regarding the impact of PCCTs on communication with patients and families about heir care, researchers at Mount Sinai Medical Center have surveyed relatives of patients who died in the hospital and received palliative care consultation (n = 14) or usual care (n = 13) (unpublished data, R Sean Morrison, personal communication (June 12, 2004). As compared with relatives of usual care patients, palliative care patients' relatives were more likely to report being informed about the patients' condition (64 vs. 46 percent), receiving the right amount of support (79 vs. 69 percent), and that a physician or nurse talked to them about how they might feel after their relative's death (91 vs. 62 percent). Another study showed that relatives of patients receiving palliative care consultation were more likely to report that doctors listened to them (100 vs. 86 percent), received the right amount of information regarding the patients' condition (100 vs. 85 percent), and were informed as to how the patients' pain would be managed (100 vs. 60 percent) compared with families of patients not receiving palliative care.[27*]

In summary, studies to date point to the benefits of palliative care services on patient care. Yet, while the number of hospital-based PCCTs have increased dramatically over the last two decades, most of what we know about the effectiveness of such programs comes from small studies of palliative care provided in individual hospital units, free-standing hospices, and at home. Most of these studies were observational and inadequately powered to detect clinically significant differences in outcomes such as the management of pain and other symptoms, analgesic prescribing, and service utilization. Systematic reviews[35–38***] have summarized these studies and suggest modest benefits for patients with life-limiting illness and their families from palliative care compared to usual medical care, but the effect of palliative care on family outcomes of satisfaction and anxiety was not significant.[35***] Clearly, further studies are necessary to demonstrate the clinical outcomes of palliative care programs and to delineate the key program structures and processes required to achieve them.

BARRIERS TO CONSULTATION AND UTILIZATION OF SERVICES

Perhaps the lack of empirical evidence supporting the use of PCCTs has led to their underutilization. Even when palliative care services are used, there is evidence that many referrals tend to occur late in the course of the patient's illness or hospital stay.[15] Another barrier to consultation in palliative care is the limited acceptance of the concept of palliative care consultation. This lack of acceptance has been attributed in part to cultural attitudes of inpatient hospitals, which focus on curative treatment and may view palliative care as tantamount to 'giving up' on this mission. This attitude is fueled in turn by confusion around the distinction between palliative care (medical care focused on relief of suffering offered simultaneously with all other appropriate therapies) and hospice care (care limited by statute to the terminally ill who are willing to give up life-prolonging treatments).[39] Even more compelling is the belief that requesting a palliative care consult signals a point in the course of the patient's illness when there is no more 'hope'. Primary physicians are therefore likely to request a consult only after the patient has

decided to forego further curative therapy rather than earlier in the course of serious, life-threatening illness when the patient could be experiencing significant symptom burden and social, psychologic, or spiritual distress.

Palliative care consultation has also been seen as threatening to some physicians who feel that many of the PCCT's recommendations overlap with care that, in theory, every physician should be able to provide for a patient.[26–28] Educating every physician in the basics of palliative medicine has been a goal of the Education on Palliative and End-of-life Care (EPEC) project, which has been sponsored by the American Medical Association and the Robert Wood Johnson Foundation.[6] However, at this time, physicians with special interest and training in palliative care possess attitudes, knowledge, and skills not yet shared by most physicians[26,27] and are equipped to handle the very time-consuming and complex interventions required by hospitalized patients with serious, life-threatening illness.[27,28] The reality is that the typical busy physician simply does not have time to devote the hours necessary in this high-intensity subset of their patients.

DESIGNING THE IDEAL PALLIATIVE CARE CONSULT SERVICE

The following segment provides some recommendations for structuring and running a PCCT. These recommendations are not meant to be exhaustive, but simply a starting point. The material for this section was obtained from the website (www.capc.org) for the Center to Advance Palliative Care (CAPC).[5] Further details on how to establish a successful, lasting, hospital-based palliative care program can be found in *A Guide to Building a Hospital-Based Palliative Care Program* published by CAPC.[40]

The design of a successful palliative care program tries to reflect the unique mission, needs, and constraints of the hospital it serves. The program design should address the type and volume of patients that will be served, how they will be referred, and the type of program and palliative care team that will care for them. The initial design may require modification once implementation begins, and it will likely require further adjustment as the program grows and evolves. A strong palliative care program adjusts to accommodate shifts in hospital priorities and patient needs. Such flexibility and responsiveness are required for programs to retain their base of support and to remain successful over time.

Administrative structure

The decision about how to administratively structure a program generally depends on how the program was initiated. For instance, if a clinical leader has spearheaded the palliative care initiative, the program usually is placed within the clinical specialty of that leader. There is no 'right' administrative home. Successful programs have been located in a range of settings including: oncology departments, geriatrics departments, intensive care units, scattered inpatient beds throughout a hospital, and in outpatient clinics. When deciding on the optimal administrative structure, the planning team should consider how best to support the program and respond to unintended consequences of the decision.

Program model

Just as there is no one solution as to the best program location, there is no single palliative care program model that works for all hospitals. Nevertheless, the program model must fit the needs and resources of the institution. Selecting the appropriate model may depend on hospital size, patient load, physician practice patterns and culture, bed availability, and other circumstances. For example, a physician-led team may work more effectively in a private practice or academic culture while a nurse-led team may be ideal in a more institutional or collaborative culture. The availability of trained palliative care staff often guides the choice between starting the program with a solo practitioner versus a full team. As more staff trained in palliative care become available and the demand for services from the PCCT increase in the institution, the program can transition from a solo practice to a full team model.

Referral and support sources

When designing a PCCT, planners should make a list of the best potential sources of referrals, clinician supporters, and targeted departments. To achieve this, the program should consider the following questions:

- What target populations does the program intend to serve?
- What clinical departments of the hospital have the greatest need for palliative care services?
- Where do most patients die within the hospital and service areas?
- Which departments of the hospital have palliative care supporters or clinicians who are likely to refer to a palliative care program?
- In what areas is palliative care strategically matched to departmental initiatives?

In addition, the program should consider creating a database of internal and external stakeholders such as managers, community health leaders, donors, and grateful families. These individuals should be updated on the progress of establishing a program, as they can be tapped for support and resources once the program is established.

Core clinical components and staffing requirements

Ideally, a PCCT should be an interdisciplinary team consisting of at least a physician, a nurse, and a social worker with appropriate training and education in palliative care. Other team members may include clergy, rehabilitation professionals, psychologists, and psychiatrists. The team should have skills and training in: complex medical evaluation, pain and symptom management, professional-to-patient communication, addressing difficult decisions about the goals of care, sophisticated discharge planning, and providing bereavement support. Due to fiscal constraints, this may be difficult to achieve. Therefore, many programs pursue a shared arrangement with the hospital's social work and pastoral care departments to provide the necessary services.

The team should provide a coordinated assessment and services adhering as closely as possible to accepted guidelines of care and/or accepted practice standards. In the USA, the National Consensus Project for Quality Palliative Care has identified eight domains as the framework for its clinical practice guidelines.[4] These domains include:

- Structure and processes of care
- Physical aspects of care
- Psychological and psychiatric aspects of care
- Social support
- Spiritual, religious, and existential aspects of care
- Cultural considerations
- Care of the imminently dying patient
- Ethics and the law

Proper adherence to these guidelines requires that members of the team have special training and/or work experience in palliative medicine, hospice, or nursing home settings, as well as familiarity with the demands and standards of the acute hospital culture.

Equally important is the team's ability to work well and communicate effectively with each other and with other healthcare professionals. Effective palliative care teams understand that the referring physician is their client. While their work directly benefits the patient, they understand that they must show a benefit to the clinicians treating that patient if they want to obtain future support and referrals. The PCCT supports and supplements other physicians' care of their most complex and seriously ill patients. Consultation educates clinicians about the benefits of palliative care, generates visibility and awareness of the program, and builds support for the services it provides.

Key learning points

- The role of the PCCT is to assess the physical, psychologic, social, spiritual, and cultural needs of patients with advanced illness. The team then advises the consulting provider on how best to address these needs, often operationalizing their recommendations upon the referring physician's request.

- The major reasons for palliative care consultation are to relieve pain and other symptoms, to establish communication about goals of care and provide support for complex decision making, to provide psychosocial, spiritual, and bereavement support, and to provide care coordination and continuity.

- A major barrier to palliative care consultation is the belief that recommendations made by the PCCT may overlap with care that every physician should be able to provide for a patient. However, at this time, physicians with special training in palliative care possess the time, attitudes, knowledge, and skills not yet shared by nor available to most physicians and are therefore better equipped to handle the very time-consuming and complex interventions required by hospitalized patients with advanced illness.

- Most of what we know about the effectiveness of palliative care programs comes from small, preliminary studies that suggest modest benefits of palliative care, particularly in alleviating pain and other symptoms. Further studies are necessary to demonstrate the clinical outcomes of palliative care consultation and to delineate the key program structures and processes required to achieve them.

- While the ideal PCCT should have an interdisciplinary team of physician, nurse, and social worker with appropriate training and education in palliative care, the design of a successful PCCT fully reflects the unique mission, needs, and constraints of the hospital it serves and adjusts to accommodate shifts in hospital priorities and patient needs.

REFERENCES

1 Dartmouth Atlas 2004. Available at: www.dartmouthatlas.net (accessed November 28, 2004).
2 American Academy of Hospice and Palliative Medicine. Mission Statement, Glenview, IL, 2001. Vol. 2001. Available at: www. aahpm.org (accessed November 28, 2004).
3 American Geriatrics Society. The care of dying patients: a position statement from the American Geriatrics Society. AGS Ethics Committee. *J Am Geriatr Soc* 1995; **43**: 577–8.
✱ 4 National Consensus Project for Quality Palliative Care. *Clinical Practice Guidelines for Quality Palliative Care.* Brooklyn, NY: National Consensus Project for Quality Palliative Care, 2004. Available at: www.nationalconsensusproject.org (accessed November 28, 2004).
5 Center to Advance Palliative Care. CAPC: The Center to Advance Palliative Care. Available at: www.capc.org (accessed October 19, 2004).
6 EPEC. The EPEC Project: Education on Palliative and End-of-life Care. Available at: http://www.epec.net (accessed October 19, 2004).
7 End of Life/Palliative Education Resource Center (EPERC). Milwaukee, WI, 2004. Available at: www.eperc.mcw.edu (accessed November 28, 2004).
✱ 8 American Pain Society Quality of Care Committee. Quality improvement guidelines for the treatment of acute pain and cancer pain. American Pain Society Quality of Care Committee. *JAMA* 1995; **274**: 1874–80.
9 American Board of Internal Medicine. *Caring for the Dying: Identification and Promotion of Physician Competency.* Educational Resource Document, 1996.
10 Joint Commission on Accreditation of Healthcare Organizations. *2002 Comprehensive Accreditation Manual for Hospitals: The Official Handbook (CAMH).* Oakbrook Terrace, IL: Joint Commission on Accreditation of Healthcare Organizations, 2002.
11 American Hospital Association. *AHA Hospital Statistics.* Chicago: American Hospital Association, 2004.
12 Billings J, Pantilat S. Survey of palliative care programs in United States teaching hospitals. *J Palliat Med* 2001; **4**: 309–14.
13 Pan CX, Morrison RS, Meier DE, *et al.* How prevalent are hospital-based palliative care programs? Status report and future directions. *J Palliat Med* 2001; **4**: 315–24.
14 von Gunten CF. Secondary and tertiary palliative care in US hospitals. *JAMA* 2002; **287**: 875–81.
15 Homsi J, Walsh D, Nelson KA, *et al.* The impact of a palliative medicine consultation service in medical oncology. *Support Care Cancer* 2002; **10**: 337–42.
16 Kuin A, Courtens AM, Deliens L, *et al.* Palliative care consultation in The Netherlands: a nationwide evaluation study. *J Pain Symptom Manage* 2004; **27**: 53–60.
17 Virik K, Glare P. Profile and evaluation of a palliative medicine consultation service within a tertiary teaching hospital in Sydney, Australia. *J Pain Symptom Manage* 2002; **23**: 17–25.
◆ 18 Morrison RS, Meier DE. Clinical practice. Palliative care. *N Engl J Med* 2004; **350**: 2582–90.
19 Block SD. Perspectives on care at the close of life. Psychological considerations, growth, and transcendence at the end of life: the art of the possible. *JAMA* 2001; **285**: 2898–905.
20 Bass D, Noelker L, Rechlin L. The moderating influence of service use on negative caregiving consequences. *J Gerontol B Psychol Sci Soc Sci* 1996; **51**: S121–31.
21 Levine C. The loneliness of the long-term care giver [see comments]. *N Engl J Med* 1999; **340**: 1587–90.
22 Billings J. What is palliative care? *J Palliat Med* 1998; **1**: 73–81.
23 Meier DE, Morrison RS, Cassel CK. Improving palliative care. *Ann Intern Med* 1997; **127**: 225–30.
24 Meier DE, Thar W, Jordon A, *et al.* Integrating case management and palliative care. *J Palliat Med* 2004; **7**: 121–36.
25 Bass D, Bowman K, Noelkes L. The influence of caregiving and bereavement support on adjusting to an older relative's death. *Gerontologist* 1991; **31**: 32–42.
26 Weissman D. Consultation in palliative medicine. *Arch Intern Med* 1997; **157**: 733–7.
27 Manfredi PL, Morrison RS, Morris J, *et al.* Palliative care consultations: how do they impact the care of hospitalized patients? *J Pain Symptom Manage* 2000; **20**: 166–73.
28 Warren SC, Emmett MK. Palliative care consultation in West Virginia. *W V Med J* 2002; **98**: 94–9.
29 von Gunten CF, Camden B, Neely KJ, *et al.* Prospective evaluation of referrals to a hospice/palliative medicine consultation service. *J Palliat Med* 1998; **1**: 45–53.
30 Edmonds PM, Stuttaford JM, Penny J, *et al.* Do hospital palliative care teams improve symptom control? Use of modified STAS as an evaluative tool. *Palliat Med* 1998; **12**: 345–51.
31 Ellershaw JE, Peat SJ, Boys LC. Assessing the effectiveness of a hospital palliative care team. *Palliat Med* 1995; **9**: 145–52.

32 Lilly CM, De Meo DL, Sonna LA, *et al.* An intensive communication intervention for the critically ill. *Am J Med* 2000; **109**: 469–75.

33 Campbell ML, Guzman JA. Impact of a proactive approach to improve end-of-life care in a medical ICU. *Chest* 2003; **123**: 266–71.

34 Bruera E, Neumann CM, Gagnon B, *et al.* The impact of a regional palliative care program on the cost of palliative care delivery. *J Palliat Med* 1999; **3**: 181–6.

◆ 35 Higginson IJ, Finlay IG, Goodwin DM, *et al.* Is there evidence that palliative care teams alter end-of-life experiences of patients and their caregivers? *J Pain Symptom Manage* 2003; **25**: 150–68.

36 Rinck GC, van den Bos GA, Kleijnen J, *et al.* Methodologic issues in effectiveness research on palliative cancer care: a systematic review. *J Clin Oncol* 1997; **15**: 1697–707.

37 Salisbury C, Bosanquet N, Wilkinson EK, *et al.* The impact of different models of specialist palliative care on patients' quality of life: a systematic literature review. *Palliat Med* 1999; **13**: 3–17.

◆ 38 Higginson IJ, Finlay I, Goodwin DM, *et al.* Do hospital-based palliative teams improve care for patients or families at the end of life? *J Pain Symptom Manage* 2002; **23**: 96–106.

39 Fischberg D, Meier DE. Palliative care in hospitals. *Clin Geriatr Med* 2004; **20**: 735–51.

40 Center to Advance Palliative Care. *A Guide to Building a Hospital-Based Palliative Care Program.* New York: CAPC, 2004. Available at www.capc.org (accessed November 28, 2004).

33

Models of palliative care delivery

BADI EL OSTA, EDUARDO BRUERA

INTRODUCTION

Palliative care delivery has changed considerably during the past 30 years. During the second half of the past century in North America, care of the terminally ill patients moved from the home, where most patients state that they would prefer to die,[1] to the hospital, where medical technology shifted the focus to prolonging life and avoiding death.

After a brief presentation of the different settings of palliative care delivery discussed elsewhere in this book, this chapter will attempt to provide an integrated vision for palliative care programs capable of delivering high rates of access and seamless care to patients in the palliative stage of their illness and to their families.

PATIENT AND FAMILY NEEDS

Palliative care is appropriate at every stage of the disease whether or not the patient is seeking curative treatment. By introducing palliative care earlier in the disease process, it becomes possible for healthcare professionals to detect subtle shifts that take place and help patients and their families to adapt to the disease progression, redefine goals of care, and reframe hope. Therefore, understanding patient and family needs and expectations is important for the patient's care. The lack of addressing their needs and expectations adequately leads to further distress and conflicts between patients, family members, and healthcare workers.[2]

Patients who are terminally ill may develop a number of devastating physical and psychological symptoms[3] that necessitate the need for access to a multidisciplinary palliative

Table 33.1 *Frequency of symptom distress and poor prognostic indicators in palliative care patients admitted to a TPCU, hospices, and acute care hospitals*

Symptom	TPCU	Acute care	Hospices
Pain (%)	75	48	57
Fatigue (%)	90	70	82
Nausea (%)	37	20	24
Depression (%)	59	43	45
Anxiety (%)	67	49	51
Drowsiness (%)	72	64	74
Appetite (%)	76	82	74
Wellbeing (%)	80	71	65
Shortness of breath (%)	50	32	38
Overall (%)	67	55	57

Reproduced from Bruera E, Neumann C, Brenneis C, Quan H. *J Pall Care* 2000; **16**(3): 16–21, with permission.

care service to achieve better symptom control, and psychosocial and spiritual support until death (Table 33.1). Patients need to have good symptom control for improved quality of life.[4] Among the symptoms at the end of life, fatigue has been reported to be the most common[3,4] and pain, depression, and anxiety to be the most distressing for patients with advanced cancer.[3]

Patients also expect to be treated with dignity and respect and not as a 'disease' and appreciate physicians who listen to them and allow them to express their personal concerns and feelings.[5] Most patients expect truth telling from their physician in an honest, timely, and sensitive manner as well as continuity of care and ability to participate in their plan of care, especially when more than one option is available.[3]

They need interdisciplinary help while coping with the physical, financial, psychosocial, and spiritual impact of their disease. Finally, most terminally ill patients prefer to live the remainder of their life as fully as possible, rather than marking time waiting to die.[5]

Helping families to meet their needs will also lead to an improvement in the patient's care. Informational needs have been identified as the most important among other needs.[6] Given et al.[7] identified three types of need for family members of a dying person: need for information regarding the disease; need for assistance with how to structure care activities; and continued guidance to alleviate stressors, burden, and associated depression. Families should be provided with clear information about physical care and comfort measures, what to expect and how to manage symptoms as the disease progresses, treatments and their side effects, patient's emotional response, and community resources. Families need assistance in monitoring and reporting symptoms, nutritional considerations, transportation, coordination of care, financial concerns, and in coping with escalation of care as the patient's disease status worsens, without forgetting their psychosocial needs as well as the respite care.

In conclusion, the interdisciplinary approach to patient and family needs leads to improvement in the patient's care and avoidance of a vicious circle of severe burnout and conflicts between the patient, the family, and the medical team. Effective communication secures the trusting partnership and help to ease their burden.[4]

INTERDISCIPLINARY CARE

Palliative care has been successful in borrowing ideas and techniques from other disciplines in healthcare, to meet the patients' and families' needs during the trajectory of their terminal illness. The timely referral to each discipline allows its members to carry out baseline assessment, monitor changes, and apply appropriate interventions that meet the physical, psychosocial, and spiritual needs of the patients and their families. The main disciplines involved in palliative care are: occupational therapy, physical therapy, music therapy, speech therapy, nutrition, pharmacy, clinical psychology (counseling), social work, and chaplaincy.[8]

In some settings (e.g. acute care hospitals), these disciplines are readily available. Therefore, outpatient facilities, inpatient hospices, acute palliative care units, and day hospitals should ideally be placed geographically within acute care facilities that already have these healthcare professionals available. If outpatient centers, inpatient hospices, and day hospitals operate elsewhere, it may be necessary to make the appropriate transportation arrangements to allow the different disciplines to see the patients in case these facilities don't have their own interdisciplinary team.

Interdisciplinary care may be difficult, if not impossible, to conduct at home or in a nursing home because of the cost of transportation of all the different disciplines to the patient's location. However, the possibility of video interactive techniques for the access to social worker, counselor, pastoral care, and other members of the interdisciplinary team may be a promising way to stay in touch with the patients and their families. These techniques have been used in psychiatry for various purposes.[9,10] Studies need to be done in palliative care telemedicine to assess cost effectiveness of these techniques as well as patients' and families' satisfaction. The best level of palliative care delivery consists of having multiple disciplines involved in each setting to provide care that meet the needs of patients and families. The subsequent sections of this chapter discuss the different settings of palliative care and their integration into a seamless network that every patient can access.

DIFFERENT SETTINGS FOR PALLIATIVE CARE DELIVERY

The home

Although most patients die in hospital or a nursing home, surveys indicate that more than 70 percent of people would prefer to die at home.[11] Despite the existence of different models internationally, palliative home care provides a patient the possibility of a quality of life and death at home, if that is the preferred place to spend his or her last days. This setting has its own advantages and limitations, and can be challenging as well as rewarding for the patient and the family. Wenk has discussed these issues in depth in Chapter 34.

At home, most patients have more autonomy, privacy, freedom, and feel safer than anywhere else.[12] The family can potentially anticipate the loss, have a better bereavement and familiarize with death by learning that death is a normal stage of life.[12] Care at home at the end of life can also reduce the cost of care: it prevents unnecessary admissions to acute hospital and skilled nursing facilities and avoids unnecessary use of the emergency department by having nurses (backed up by a palliative care specialist) on-call 24 hours per day, 7 days per week to provide a rapid response to changes in symptoms in the last days of life.[13] On the other hand, care at home may be difficult or impossible if the patient does not wish so; lives alone or far away; cannot afford the care expenses; needs higher skilled care; if the family is physically or emotionally tired, cannot deal with uncontrolled symptom or cannot provide the patient with 24-hour care; or if the home does not meet the minimal comfort needs.[14] When providing palliative home care, the team should be able to get early referrals, have access to an inpatient hospice unit for possible direct admission, provide medications and home equipment for the patient, be able to assess and control symptoms using universal tools, and document visits and phone calls on the patient's chart.

The responsible caregiver is the member of the family who is in better condition (health, relation, proximity and available time) to carry out and coordinate the care.[15] The education of the responsible caregiver must be done progressively, with simple verbal, written, audio- and/or video-taped instructions about how to administer medications, evaluate symptoms, diet, hydration, hygiene and evacuation, position and dressing changes, organize family tasks, and recognize death. To prevent frequent hospitalization, the responsible caregiver needs support with the guarantee of the best possible symptom control, the availability of the team, and access to easy admissions 24/7, establishing a caring plan and a schedule of activities, anticipating the changes that can occur in the patient's condition, and reducing doubts and uncertainty, and providing material resources.

Usually a month of care should include approximately two medical visits per week, two nursing visits per week, two psychology/counseling interviews for the patient and two for the family per month, and provision of oral and parenteral opioids analgesic. When the patient's condition is stable, medical and nursing visits can occur once weekly; in the terminal phase, one or more visits are needed per day. However, available services can vary dramatically in different areas of the world, particularly regarding access to medical care.

Volunteer collaboration increases both team activity and interaction with the community.[16] After their selection and training, volunteers can help in evaluating patients at home or on the phone, educate the responsible caregiver, offer practical support (housekeeping, transport, etc.), and be company for the patient and family.

The home hospice service enables patients to live at home in the last days of life. The demand for such services is expected to increase in the future because of the aging population.[17] This rapidly growing concept can be a source of ethical dilemmas.[18] It is very important to have a complete discussion with the patient and family regarding the choices and wishes of where to receive end-of-life care and get into an agreement within some principles with the possibility of changing choices at any time:[19] patients and families should be aware that palliative home care does not medicalize or technicalize the dying process, and it should not intrude on the privacy of their home or disturb the family life.[1]

Finally, it is unclear whether palliative home care produces savings by reduction of the expenses of both fragmented care and the use of high-tech interventions; however, in many cases the burden of cost shifts from the healthcare system to the caregiver.[12] Because nonprofessional caregiving is crucial to effective end-of-life care for patients who wish to die at home, early recognition of family distress, validation of their role, and effective communication by physicians may ease their burden and avoid physical illness, emotional distress, financial hardship, and early mortality in the caregivers.[20] If palliative home care is promoted and implemented, resources should be minimized for medications and maximized for responsible caregiver funding.

Palliative care outpatient centers

Patients with advanced cancer often develop devastating physical, psychosocial, and existential distress[21–25] associated with the disease or its treatment.[21,23,24] These symptoms cannot be controlled appropriately[22] in a standard setting based on a physician/nurse team with a waiting area and small private examining rooms, which do not allow interactions between different discipline members. Therefore, the multidisciplinary symptom control and palliative care (MD) clinics were developed to unify different disciplines in a team that combines their assessments and formulates a plan of care[21,22] that meet patients' and families' needs in the same visit and at the same place. The MD clinic helps patients and their families to avoid the distress generated by the visits of several offices located in different areas of a tertiary hospital, and by the waiting time before each appointment in order to receive a multidisciplinary assessment and management.

In their retrospective study, Strasser et al.[21] compared the assessment of 138 consecutive patients with advanced cancer referred to the MD clinic and 77 patients referred to a traditional pain and symptom management clinic. The two groups were similar in tumor type, demographics, and symptom burden. Patients of both clinics were evaluated using the same tools: Edmonton Symptom Assessment Scale[26] (ESAS), CAGE questionnaire,[27] and Mini-Mental State Questionnaire[28] (MMSQ). In addition to a physician and a nurse, the patient was assessed by a social worker, physical and occupational therapist, pharmacist, clinical nutritionist, pastoral care worker and a psychiatric nurse practitioner. The MD clinic has no waiting area and patients had their own private rooms with a full-sized bed and bathroom. After the patient's evaluation, the multidisciplinary team discussed the assessment, interventions, and recommendations in a team conference. The patient as well as his or her oncologist and primary care physician received a handwritten and audio-taped[29] form of the team conference. A follow-up visit was scheduled within 1–2 weeks after initial assessment[21] and monthly thereafter; otherwise, follow-ups were provided per patient or family needs at the MD clinic[21] or over the phone.[22] Patients from the MD clinic received a total of 1066 nonphysician recommendations (median 4 per patient, range 0–37) in a 5-hour assessment. Among 83 patients interviewed after the MD clinic visit, satisfaction was rated as excellent in the following areas: caring team members, adequate assessment, treatment plan, useful recommendations, and time spent. In contrast, the duration of the pain and symptom management clinic assessment, done only by a physician and a nurse, was 30–45 minutes. No nonphysician recommendations were given; instead, eight patients were referred to specialists in psychiatry, three to rehabilitation, and three to social work.[21]

In conclusion, the interventions of a interdisciplinary half-day symptom control and palliative care clinic can result in reduction of the physical and psychosocial distress of patients with advanced cancer,[21,22] large numbers of physician and nonphysician specific care recommendations,[21] and high levels of patient satisfaction.[21,22]

There are some specific characteristics of successful outpatient palliative care delivery:

- *'Just in time access'*. Patients need to access these consult programs without lengthy appointments or waiting times. It is important to encourage a 'drop-in' approach.
- *Physical facilities.* The rooms need to have enough space for a full-sized bed since palliative care patients are frequently severely symptomatic and cannot tolerate long period on examining tables. These rooms also need enough space for families to be able to sit comfortably with the patient. Privacy is important for the different discussions that take place.
- *Availability of team members.* A successful outpatient palliative care program requires rapid access to the different disciplines. Physicians and nurses are generally ineffective in identifying problems that require interdisciplinary interventions.[22] Therefore, palliative care patients and families should ideally be provided access to as many disciplines as possible during the course of an initial outpatient consultation. Further follow-up may not be required by all disciplines.

Day care hospitals

Day care hospitals were originally developed for the geriatric population[30] in response to a lack of continuity of care between acute hospitalization and long-term placement[31] and with a concept to lower the cost of care.[32–37] Later on, day hospitals extended to other specialties[38] including palliative care.

Day care hospitals vary in funding, facilities, and staff.[39] They are mainly funded by the private sector.[39–54] A third are attached to inpatient units, another third are attached to inpatient units with home care teams, and the last third are attached to a home care team alone or are freestanding.[39,46] Palliative care day hospitals (PCDH) are usually open 3–5 days a week and are mainly led and managed by nurses.[39,46,47] The day hospital staff is specialized in palliative care and includes physicians, bedside and clinical nurses, psychologists, social workers, physical and occupational therapists, chiropodists, dieticians, chaplains, managers, aromatherapists, hairdressers, and volunteers. A mixture of hospital bedrooms with private washrooms, clinic-type rooms, interview rooms, treatment rooms, and specific rooms with special research equipment is ideal. Sufficient space for patients and family members should be provided such as a waiting room, a kitchen, a private meeting room, etc. A unified, well-planned central working area for the staff increases efficiency of communication and should not replace separate offices to allow team members to perform their charting and telephone communications.

It is essential to plan a lounge area within the day hospital setting for the staff to rest while remaining accessible to patients and family needs during their resting time.

A PCDH provides palliative care assessment and management to patients with severe symptoms, existential distress, difficult family situation, regardless of their prognosis. It assumes a consult role for patients who are not in terminal phase of their illness, and a treating physician role with terminal patients with complex palliative care issues. It also provides family meetings, advanced care planning including clarification of code status, emergency consults within 48 hours, and specialized services to special populations (i.e. patients with lymphedema, wound care, methadone clinic, etc.). A PCDH coordinates referrals to other palliative care services and allows access to other disciplines available in a tertiary care hospital such as anesthesiologists, surgeons, oncologists, radiooncologists, skin care nurses, etc. PCDH should improve links between specialized services of the hospital, promote links with home care services and hospices through adequate referral, respond to home 'crisis' by giving support to home-based palliative care teams and by coordinating admissions to the day hospital or the inpatient unit to prevent terminally ill patients visits to the emergency room, provide phone consultations to physicians and nurses in the community regarding complex issues, and develop protocols of care with community services. The day hospital setting has been discussed in depth by Gagnon in Chapter 35.

Fifteen papers reported data from 12 observational studies of day care, 11 from the UK[41–54] and one from the USA,[40] and provided some information on the structure, process and outcomes of day care. Many qualitative studies found that most patients were highly satisfied and valued the social contact[41,44,48,50–53] and the opportunity to take part in activities that day care provided. Caregivers opinions was sought in one study:[53] the majority found care 'excellent' or 'good' and were 'greatly helped' by their day off. However, further studies are needed to provide conclusive evidence of improved symptom control, mainly pain,[41,43,44,53] and quality of life in PCDH as well evidence-based standards of care.[39]

The three settings discussed above, home care programs, outpatient centers, and day hospitals are part of the palliative care services available to patients who are still staying at home. In these settings, bus rounds[55,56] may be a useful mechanism for unifying criteria and sharing strategies for patient care as well as promoting continuing patient-based education in palliative care for physicians, nurses, and medical students in the community. They have been shown to be highly satisfactory from participants' perspective[56] with low overall cost.[55]

Consult teams in acute care facilities

Consult teams in acute care facilities act as a bridge between the 'palliative' and 'active' models[57,58] of care by providing access to palliative care services at a time when the patient is still receiving active treatment.

In a retrospective study, Jenkins et al.[57] reviewed the charts of 100 consecutive cancer patients who had been referred to a palliative care consult team within a tertiary acute care hospital during a 6-month period. The palliative care consult team consisted of a physician and a nurse trained in palliative care and available on a full-time basis. Demographic characteristics, including reason for admission and disease status upon admission, length of stay, length of time from consult to discharge, admission location, and code status on admission and discharge were recorded. Symptom acuity, cognitive status, and risk for substance abuse were evaluated respectively using the ESAS,[26] CAGE[27] questionnaire, and MMSQ.[28] Medications before and after the consult were compared to the recommended medications; compliance of the primary team with the consult team recommendations was assessed. Five patients were not palliative at the time of the consult. Only 46/95 (48 percent) were known to have untreatable cancer at the time of their admission. The CAGE questionnaire for alcoholism and the MMSQ were abnormal in 19/78 (24 percent) and 40/91 (44 percent), respectively. The most intense symptoms, as measured by the 100 mm scales of the ESAS were fatigue (72 ± 24), appetite (60 ± 32), and well-being (50 ± 29). Eighty-nine of the 95 patients were living at home prior to admission and 34/95 (36 percent) were able to return home. The median length of time between consultation and discharge was 6 days[57] (5 days in a recent study carried out by O'Mahony et al.[59]). Twenty patients died during hospitalization, 23 were transferred to a palliative care unit, and the remaining 18 were discharged to another hospital or long-term care facility. Two-thirds of the patients were on dimenhydrinate as anti-emetic by their primary team, 4 percent of the patients had neuroleptics ordered before the consult compared to 19 percent for whom neuroleptics were recommended, 22 percent of the patients were not prescribed opioids, and 54 percent were prescribed opioids on an as needed basis. The patient's physician complied with the palliative care consult team's recommendations in 122/137 cases (89 percent).

Hospitalization of terminally ill patients is a pivotal time in their disease course. In this study,[57] 52 percent learned that they were in the palliative phase during this hospitalization. The consult team was able to rapidly assess and treat patients, verify a terminal diagnosis and ensure that medical options have been exhausted. By providing alternative palliative care resources and placements options, the consult team helped in reducing the number of patients admitted to the hospital for social reasons,[57] hospital charges,[59] length of stay,[57,59] and inter-unit transfers.[59] Using the cited tools above,[26–28] the consult team was able to help the primary team in detecting missed delirium in about half of the patients, assessing and managing cancer pain as well opioid side effects, and other symptoms related to the cancer more effectively. The high rate of adherence to the consult team's recommendations[57,59] suggests that the primary team was able to incorporate palliative care approaches into the management of acute patients.

Higher adherence rate (>90 percent) was reported in a recent study carried out by O'Mahony et al. after evaluating data regarding 592 consecutive patients seen by their palliative care consult team during a 16-month period.[59]

Palliative care units

A tertiary palliative care unit (TPCU) is a distinct type of palliative care unit, designated for terminally ill patients who require intensive involvement of a specialist interdisciplinary team able to manage their complex problems. von Gunten defined it as an academic medical center where specialist knowledge for the most complex cases is practiced, researched and taught.[60]

Given the physical, psychosocial, and spiritual nature of the TPCU patient population complexity, the ideal location for such unit is in an acute care hospital that offers a full range of diagnostic and interventional procedures, support services, specialty and subspecialty consultation. The TPCU staffing includes palliative care specialists, nurse practitioners, registered nurses, research nurses, licensed practical nurses, nursing attendants, a chaplain, a social worker, a physical therapist, an occupational therapist, a pharmacist, a clinical dietician, a palliative care counselor, a clerk, and volunteers. The optimal unit size for staffing efficiency is 16–24 beds and the minimum size is 10–12 beds.[96] Watanabe and Macmillan have discussed in depth this setting in Chapter 37.

One example of TPCU is the Edmonton Regional Palliative Care Program (ERPCP) PCU in Canada.[62] The ERPCP is a publicly funded program that provides a comprehensive range of palliative care services, including home care and specialist consultation in the community, long-term care, hospices, ambulatory care and acute care settings. Its TPCU is located in an acute care teaching hospital and has 14 beds. Amenities include a patient smoking room, a family lounge, a kitchenette, a quiet room, and a conference room. Family members may stay overnight if they wish, and pets are allowed. Referrals are screened after direct patient's assessment by the palliative care consultants. Such patients are referred for acute symptom control, emotional and family distress, difficult discharge planning, and rehabilitation. As discussed in Chapter 37, the TPCU is intended to be a short-term place of care, until symptoms have stabilized sufficiently to allow discharge of the patient to another palliative care setting: the expected length of stay is less than 2 weeks. The goal of admission and its temporary nature should be discussed with the patients and their families. Most patients are asked to agree electively to a 'do-not-resuscitate' status prior to admission. Discussing 'do-not-resuscitate' status is a valuable opportunity to clarify the patient and family's understanding of the illness, prognosis, as well as goals of care.[63] The tools used daily for assessment are: ESAS,[26] CAGE questionnaire,[27] MMSQ,[28] Edmonton Staging System (ESS) for cancer pain,[64]

Edmonton Labeled Visual Information System[65] (ELVIS), Edmonton Functional Assessment Tool[66] (EFAT), Palliative Performance Score (PPS),[67] and constipation score.[68] A family conference coordinated by the social worker and attended by the team, the patient, family members, and friends whom the patient wishes to involve is often advisable to clarify goals and establish plans of care and further discharge to a more appropriate palliative care setting that will satisfy their needs. Patients have the option not to be present at the family conference.

For those patients who are discharged home, clear and timely communication with community healthcare providers (e.g. primary care physician, home care manager, pharmacist) is critical. Transfer to a hospice may pose a difficult transition for the patients and their families because of their need to adjust to a new environment and staff, and most importantly because they may view hospice as a lower level of care and feel a sense of abandonment.[69] These concerns may be alleviated by explaining to them that the fact that the patient does not require treatment in a TPCU is a positive outcome and that the option of coming back is possible if the symptoms exacerbate and the patient decides so.

The TPCU provides an excellent environment for research in which all the interdisciplinary team's medical members are expected to participate. Since patients are under direct care of the medical team, the process of screening and recruiting them for studies becomes easier. The TPCU of the Edmonton Regional Palliative Care Program receives undergraduate and postgraduate medical trainees from the University of Alberta on a regular basis. Clinical teaching is enhanced by journal club,[70] held three mornings a week, during which time relevant articles to palliative care are presented and discussed. Other educational activities include tests taken before and after the residents PCU rotation,[67] seminars, weekly grand rounds, and presentations from other specialists sharing their expertise as applied directly or indirectly to palliative care.

Inpatient hospices

Hospice is a model designed to provide care at the end of life. The goal of hospice is to palliate the suffering at the end of life by addressing the emotional, social, physical, and spiritual needs of patients and their families. The in-patient hospice care is the highest level of care within a hospice program. It is designated to control physical suffering and support family and patients when such care is not manageable at home. Described in depth by Keen in Chapter 36, the majority of inpatient hospices are staffed by at least one full-time physician trained in palliative medicine, nurses, physiotherapists, occupational therapists, social workers, chaplains, and offer bereavement support services. In addition to providing inpatient end-stage care, patients are admitted for symptom control, rehabilitation, and sometimes respite care.

Statistically, five independent factors were found to predict inpatient hospice care: pain in the last year of life, constipation, breast cancer, being under 85 year of age, and being dependent on others for help with activities of daily living for between 1 and 6 months before death.[71] Hinton demonstrated a higher rate of admission among patients receiving palliative home care over those who were living alone or with unfit relatives and those with breast cancer.[72] One study of data relating to cancer deaths showed that patients accessing palliative care services were significantly younger and had longer survival times from diagnosis.[73] An analysis of place of death of cancer patients demonstrated an increased likelihood of dying in a hospice if they lived close by.[74]

In the USA, cancer diagnosis accounted for 46 percent of hospice admissions during 2004 and noncancer diseases accounted for 64 percent: end-stage heart disease and dementia have been shown to be the two most common terminal illnesses.[75] Medicare, through Part A, limits in-patient hospice care reimbursement (US\$491.19/day in 2000).[76] The length of stay per hospice admission was 4–5 days and the median length of stay in 2004 was 22 days.[75] In the UK, the average length of stay in inpatient hospice was 13.5 days[77] compared to Canada where the average of stay was 44 days and the median length of stay was 22 days.[78] The principal problems triggering admission were mainly anorexia, weakness, and drowsiness.[3]

There is little good quality research measuring the contribution that inpatient hospice care makes to patient care. However, the studies at St Christopher's Hospice comparing hospice and hospital care from the viewpoint of the surviving spouse found a consistent impression of a better social and psychological environment within the hospice compared to the hospital.[79,80]

Consult teams in nursing homes

More than 25 percent of Americans die in a nursing home.[81] Considerable evidence indicates that nursing home residents do not receive optimal end-of-life care,[82,83] their pain is undertreated,[84] and they are often transferred to an acute care setting to receive aggressive rather than palliative treatment in the last weeks of life.[85,86] Therefore, families express dissatisfaction with the end-of-life care that their loved ones receive in nursing homes.[87] Hospice care may improve the quality of end-of-life care for nursing home residents, but it is underused by this population, in part because physicians are not aware of their patients' preferences.[82]

Casarett et al. carried out a randomized controlled trial of 205 nursing home residents and their surrogate decision makers in three US nursing homes to determine whether it is possible to increase hospice utilization and improve the quality of end-of-life care by identifying residents whose goals and preferences are consistent with hospice care.[82] A structured interview identified nursing home residents whose goals for care, treatment preferences, and palliative care needs made them appropriate for hospice care. Of the 205 residents, 107 were randomly assigned to receive the intervention, and 98 received usual care. Intervention residents were more likely than usual care residents to enroll in hospice within 30 days (21/107 [20 percent] vs. 1/98 [1 percent]; $P < 0.001$ [Fisher exact test]) and to enroll in hospice during the follow-up period (27/207 [25 percent] vs. 6/98 [6 percent]; $P < 0.001$). Intervention residents had fewer acute care admissions (mean: 0.28 vs. 0.49; $P = 0.04$ [Wilcoxon rank sum test]) and spent fewer days in an acute care setting (mean: 1.2 vs. 3.0; $P = 0.03$ [Wilcoxon rank sum test]). Families of intervention residents rated the resident's care more highly than did families of usual care residents (mean on a scale of 1–5: 4.1 vs. 2.5; $P = 0.04$ [Wilcoxon rank sum test]).

In conclusion, by increasing early access to hospice care in a nursing home setting by a simple and prompt communication intervention, pain will be better controlled, the use of inappropriate medications as well as physical restraints and acute hospital admissions will decrease, and family satisfaction with end-of-life care will increase.[82]

INTEGRATION OF CARE

Figure 33.1 summarizes the different components of palliative care delivery. The most important aspect of this model is the different arrows connecting the different settings of care. The flow of patients needs to be seamless and this is facilitated by using compatible assessment tools, similar treatment and counseling protocols, and frequent communication among the different teams, video-conferencing, regular teaching rounds, or bus rounds. However, the different settings do not need to have a unified ownership or administrative structure to be able to meet the goal of seamless patient and family care.

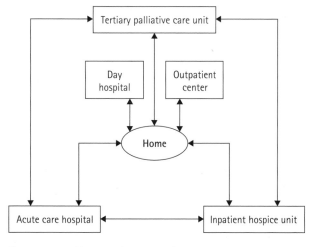

Figure 33.1 *Home as the center of palliative care delivery.*

During the past several decades, terminally ill patients were increasingly dying in acute care setting.[88–90] With the recent changes in healthcare, there is greater emphasis on providing care at home and supporting families to enable more home deaths.[90,91] Since home death may not be simple, practical or desirable in every family situation,[90–94] there is a need for an objective way to assess the viability of a home death in each family situation. Cantwell *et al.*[14] formulated a tool called the Home Death Assessment Tool (HDAT) as a result of a cohort study conducted to describe the relative role of predictors of home death in palliative care patients with advanced cancer. They created a simple questionnaire of five questions to assess the viability of a home death: patient and caregivers' desire for a home death, physician's support for a home death, presence of more than one caregiver, patient's environment, and sufficient financial resources. Ninety questionnaires were administered by home care coordinators and a follow-up questionnaire was administered to record the place of death. Of the 73 patients, 34 (47 percent) died at home and 39 (53 percent) died in a hospital or a hospice. Logistic regression identified a desire for home death by both the patient and the caregiver as the main predictive factor for a home death. The presence of more than one caregiver was also predictive of home death. The financial resources, in a private healthcare system, can determine also the feasibility of death at home. However, physician's support for a home death and patient's environment were not significant predictors of home death in Cantwell's study.

In that study, HDAT was highly specific in identifying patients who were not going to die at home but was not sensitive in identifying those who would die at home. It was used to guide the care coordinator in planning a home death and to increase the understanding among patient, family, and professional caregivers of what is required for a successful palliative care delivery at home.[14] If there are fewer than three positive answers, the home care coordinator should explore a different setting as a care plan.

Home death is not universal and has its limitations. Decreased support, symptom distress, and inability of the palliative home care and caregivers to meet the patients' needs make peaceful death at home impossible. Also, patients and caregivers can change their minds about their desire for a home death as their circumstances change.[16,94,95] In these cases, the patient has to be moved to a higher skilled setting. The role of day hospital team in this case is very important: it assures support for the palliative home care team and responds to home crisis within 48 hours, provides optimal care if possible, or helps coordinating a patient's disposition to the appropriate setting (specialized clinics, TPCUs, acute care hospitals, inpatient hospice units).

There are no systematic reviews of the effectiveness of palliative day care and no randomized controlled trials comparing this care with other settings.[39] There are no studies of referral into day care or the cost of this care.[39] Planned to provide a leadership role in promoting links between a tertiary care hospital and community services, the day care hospital should be for patients with terminal illness who are still receiving active treatment and for patients in their terminal phase who need rapid access to palliative care. Inpatient care can be delivered, in decreasing order of patient and family distress, at the TPCU, by consult teams in acute care hospitals, and in hospices. In a review of admission data for all patients discharged from the ERPCP from November 1, 1997 to October 31, 1998, patients with high symptom distress, positive screening for alcoholism, and poor prognostic indicators of cancer pain (ESS[64] > 0/5) were referred to TPCU, while those with lower level of distress, negative screening for alcoholism, and better prognostic indicators (ESS = 0) were treated in acute care hospitals, hospices, and the community.[3] The availability of a palliative care consult team allows patients access to palliative care at an early stage of their illness, when they are still receiving active treatment and when they are still candidates for cardiopulmonary resuscitation.[57] It has reduced significantly hospital charges[59] as well as length of stay,[57,59] inter-unit transfers,[59] and admissions for social reasons.[57]

In the USA, admissions to inpatient hospice are limited to a median of approximately 5 days. This length of stay is related to the need to deliver 80 percent of hospice care at home. Since the median length of inpatient hospice stay in the USA during 2004 was 22 days,[75] the median inpatient hospice stay per admission is approximately 5 days (20 percent of the yearly total stay). This duration is relatively shorter than in Canada or UK where its average is 44[78] and 13.5,[77] days respectively. Therefore admission to hospice in the USA may not be able to meet the patients' and families' needs, and referrals to higher skilled-setting would be the appropriate choice so patients can spend more time at home after discharge from a TPCU for example, and avoid recurrent admissions to inpatient hospice.

In the outpatient setting, the multidisciplinary symptom control and palliative care (MD) clinic allows a better integration of care between a cancer center and community-based physicians and nurses. It also allows patients access to multiple disciplines that are not available outside tertiary centers.[22] Home is considered the center of palliative care delivery since most patients and their families prefer to stay at home as long as possible,[1] and during all the early stages of the illness patients receive all their care while residing at home. From home, patient can be moved to an acute care hospital (e.g. patient develops hematemesis), admitted to a tertiary palliative care unit (e.g. control of severe symptoms or psychosocial distress), or even to an inpatient hospice unit in case the responsible caregiver becomes ill or needs a respite. Of note, patients can also be transferred from one setting to another within this model based on their needs as well as their family needs (e.g. after controlling an acute exacerbation of a right arm pain in a tertiary palliative care unit, a patient can be moved to an inpatient hospice unit while waiting for the caregiver to recover from a severe flu; the same or a different patient can be transferred from an inpatient hospice unit to an acute care hospital after a hip

fracture secondary to a fall from the bed; again, the same or a different patient can be transferred from a surgery floor to a tertiary palliative care unit if they develop a delirium that the surgeon cannot manage appropriately). In any of these settings, the discharge plan would be directed, if practical and desirable, toward returning the patient home to spend the last days surrounded by loved ones.

The two main issues in deciding the setting of care are the level of distress and available support. The patient's distress may be physical, psychosocial, or spiritual and can be measured with the ESAS, the MMSQ,[28] the McGill Quality of Life Questionnaire[96] (MQOL), the EFAT,[66] the PPS,[67] the constipation score,[68] and others. The level of support can be determined by the structure and function of the family, financial status, medical insurance, and overall physical condition of the home. If there's worsening of the physical and the psychosocial distress, the patient has to be transferred to an acute care hospital where he or she will have access to many disciplines (e.g. consult teams or tertiary palliative care unit). Once the distress is controlled, the patient can be moved to the community or home if he or she has good social and financial support. Otherwise, a transfer to an inpatient hospice unit would be more appropriate. If the distress could not be alleviated or the support could not be provided, the patient would not be able to return home and might die in an acute care hospital or in the inpatient hospice unit (Fig. 33.2).

In summary palliative care services should match the needs of patients and families. These services can be provided in an inpatient or outpatient setting. The inpatient care can be delivered in TPCUs, in acute care hospitals, and in the inpatient hospice units. The outpatient care can be delivered at home, in day hospitals, in nursing homes, or in MD clinics. No single palliative care program needs to have all these components. These settings can be owned by one institution or can have different owners to integrate palliative care delivery. Most importantly, every palliative care patient should be able to have access to any of these settings in a seamless way

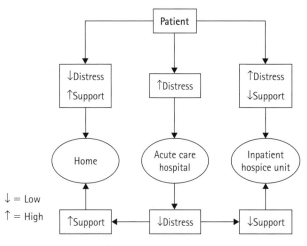

Figure 33.2 *Matching palliative care services to patient and family care needs.*

appropriate to their needs. To achieve a seamless network for delivery of care, palliative care programs should have the following resources: agreement between different settings, bus rounds, common assessment tools, common treatment guidelines, and regular communication (audio-visual: patient care and education).

CONCLUSION

In more than 30 years since the inception of the modern hospice movement, a number of clinical programs have emerged. These programs have demonstrated their value in a number of specific patient populations. One of the greater challenges has been to make it possible for patients in different regions of the world to access the system that is most appropriate to their needs (i.e. home care and day care hospitals versus inpatient hospices or inpatient acute care facilities). In addition, a setting that is appropriate for a patient at a particular time, i.e. the patient is comfortable at home with home care, may be inappropriate when there is complete family burnout or severe aggravation of symptoms distress.

One of the greatest challenges is to have a seamless care so that patients at any given time are able to receive palliative care in the setting that is most appropriate to their needs. There has been significant progress in recognizing that the different settings described in this chapter are complementary rather than competitive. There is still considerable need for research on the best way to integrate these different programs into a seamless network.

Key learning points

- Palliative care services should match the needs of patients and families.

- The interdisciplinary approach to patient and family needs leads to improvement in the patient's care and avoidance of a vicious circle of severe burnout and conflicts between the patient, the family, and the medical team.

- A multidisciplinary symptom control and palliative care clinic allows patients and their families to avoid the distress generated by the visits of several departments located in different areas of a tertiary hospital, and by the waiting time before each appointment to receive a multidisciplinary assessment and management.

- The inpatient care can be delivered in TPCUs, in acute care hospitals, and in the inpatient hospice units.

- The outpatient care can be delivered at home, in day hospitals, in nursing homes, or in MD clinics.

- Integration of the different settings into a seamless network is necessary for patients to be able to have access to any of these settings as appropriate for their needs.

REFERENCES

1 Lattimer EJ. Ethical decision-making in the care of the dying and its application to clinical practice. *J Pain Symptom Manage* 1991; **6**: 329–36.

2 Neuenschwander H, Bruera E, Cavalli F. Matching the clinical function and symptom status with the expectations of patients with advanced cancer, their families, and health care workers. *Support Care Cancer* 1997; **5**: 252–6.

◆ 3 Bruera E, Neumann C, Brenneis C, Quan H. Frequency of symptom distress and poor prognostic indicators in palliative cancer patients admitted to a tertiary palliative care unit, hospices, and acute care hospitals. *J Palliat Care* 2000; **16**: 16–21.

4 McMillan SC, Small BJ. Symptom distress and quality of life in patients with cancer newly admitted to hospice home care. *Oncol Nurs Forum* 2002; **29**: 1421–8.

5 Farber SJ, Egnew TR, Herman-Bertsch JL, *et al.* Issues in end-of-life care: patient, caregiver, and clinician perceptions. *J Palliat Med* 2003; **6**: 19–31.

6 Tringali CA. The needs of family members of cancer patients. *Oncol Nurs Forum* 1986; **13**: 65–70.

7 Given BA, Given CW, Kozachik S. Family support in advanced cancer. *Cancer J Clin* 2001; **51**: 213–31.

8 Doyle D, Hanks G, Cherny N, Calman K. *Oxford Textbook of Palliative Medicine*, 3rd ed. Oxford: Oxford University Press, 2004: 1033–84.

9 Pesamaa L, Ebeling H, Kuusimaki ML, *et al.* Videoconferencing in child and adolescent telepsychiatry: a systematic review of the literature. *J Telemed Telecare* 2004; **10**: 187–92.

◆ 10 Kuulasmaa A, Wahlberg KE, Kuusimaki ML. Videoconferencing in family therapy: a review. *J Telemed Telecare* 2004; **10**: 125–9.

11 Solloway M, LaFrance S, Bakitas M, Gerken M. A chart review of seven hundred eighty-two deaths in hospitals, nursing homes, and hospice/home care. *J Palliat Med* 2005; **8**: 789–96.

12 Wilkinson J. Ethical issues in palliative care. In: Doyle D, Hanks G, Cherny N, Calman K, eds. *Oxford Textbook of Palliative Medicine*. Oxford: Oxford University Press, 1993.

13 von Gunten CF, Martinez J. A program of hospice and palliative care in a private, nonprofit US Teaching Hospital. *J Palliat Med* 1998; **1**: 265–76.

◆ 14 Cantwell P, Turco S, Brenneis C, *et al.* Predictors of home death in palliative care cancer patients. *J Palliat Care* 2000; **16**: 23–8.

15 Neale B. Informal care and community care. In: Clark D, ed. *The Future for Palliative Care: Issues of Policy and Practice*. Buckingham: Open University Press, 1993: 52–67.

16 Claxton-Oldfield S, Jefferies J, Fawcet C, *et al.* Palliative care volunteers: why do they do it? *J Palliat Care* 2004; **20**: 78–84.

17 Tyrer F, Exley C. Receiving care at home at end of life: characteristics of patients receiving Hospice at Home care. *Fam Pract* 2005; **22**: 644–6.

18 Randall F, Downie RS. *Palliative Care Ethics, A Companion for All Specialties*. Oxford: Oxford Medical Publications, 1999.

19 Van Eys J. The ethics of palliative care. *J Palliat Care* 1991; **7**: 27–32.

20 Fleming DA. The burden of caregiving at the end-of-life. *Mo Med* 2003; **100**: 82–6.

◆ 21 Strasser F, Sweeney C, Willey J, *et al.* Impact of a half-day multidisciplinary symptom control and palliative care outpatient clinic in a comprehensive cancer center on recommendations, symptom intensity, and patient satisfaction: a retrospective descriptive study. *J Pain Symptom Manage* 2004; **27**: 481–91.

◆ 22 Bruera E, Michaud M, Vigano A, *et al.* Multidisciplinary symptom control clinic in a cancer center: a retrospective study. *Support Care Cancer* 2001; **9**: 162–8.

23 Walsh D, Donnelly S, Rybicki L. The symptoms of advanced cancer: relationship to age, gender, and performance status in 1,000 patients. *Support Care Cancer* 2000; **8**: 175–9.

24 Vainio A, Auvinen A. Prevalence of symptoms among patients with advanced cancer: an international collaborative study. Symptom Prevalence Group. *J Pain Symptom Manage* 1996; **12**: 3–10.

25 Bruera E. Symptom control in patients with cancer. *J Psychosoc Oncol* 1990; **8**: 47–73.

◆ 26 Bruera E, Kuehn N, Miller MJ, *et al.* The Edmonton Symptom Assessment System (ESAS): a simple method for the assessment of palliative care patients. *J Palliat Care* 1991; **7**: 6–9.

◆ 27 Ewing J. Detecting alcoholism: the CAGE Questionnaire. *JAMA* 1984; **252**: 1905–7.

◆ 28 Folstein MF, Folstein S, McHugh PR. 'Minimental state': a practical method for grading the cognitive state of patients for the clinician. *J Psychiatr Res* 1975; **12**: 189–98.

◆ 29 Bruera E, Pituskin E, Calder K, *et al.* The addition of an audiocassette recording of a consultation to written recommendations for patients with advanced cancer: A randomized, controlled trial. *Cancer* 1999; **86**: 2420–5.

30 Evans LK, Forciea MA, Yurkow J, Sochalski J. The geriatric day hospital. In: Katz PR, Kane RL, Mezey MD, eds. *Emerging Systems in Long-Term Care*. New York: Springer, 1999: 67–87.

31 Densen PM. Tracing the elderly through the health care system: An update. AHCPR 91–11 ed. Rockville, MD: Department of Health and Human Services, 1991.

32 Dekker R, Drost EA, Groothoff JW, *et al.* Effects of day-hospital rehabilitation in stroke patients: a review of randomized clinical trials. *Scand J Rehabil Med* 1998; **30**: 87–94.

33 Mor V, Stalker MZ, Gralla R, *et al.* Day hospital as an alternative to inpatient care for cancer patients: a random assignment trial. *J Clin Epidemiol* 1988; **41**: 771–85.

34 Rogge R. Diabetic day hospital in Wiesbaden: education and treatment under everyday conditions during job and leisure time. *Med Welt* 2000; **51**: 219–22.

35 Wisseler HM, Lautenschlager J, Leichner-Hennig R, Henrich H. Rheumatological day clinic in the Auerbach Clinic Dr. Vetter–Beginnings and initial experiences. *Aktuelle Rheumatol* 2003; **28**: 30–5.

36 Gill HS, Walter DB. The day hospital model of care for patients with medical and rehabilitative needs. *Hosp Technol Ser* 1996; **15**: 1–14.

37 Capomolla S, Febo O, Ceresa M, *et al.* Cost/utility ratio in chronic heart failure: comparison between heart failure management program delivered by day-hospital and usual care. *J Am Coll Cardiol* 2002; **40**: 1259–66.

38 Biem HJ, Cotton D, McNeil S, *et al.* Day medicine: an urgent internal medicine clinic and medical procedures suite. *Health Manage Forum* 2003; **16**: 17–23.

39 Davies E, Higginson IJ. Systematic review of specialist palliative day-care for adults with cancer. *Support Care Cancer* 2005; **13**: 607–27.

40 Thompson B. Hospice day care. *Am J Hosp Care* 1990; **7**: 28–30.

41 Wilkes E, Crowther AGO, Greaves CWKH. A different kind of day hospital – for patients with preterminal cancer and chronic disease. *BMJ* 1978; **2**: 1053–6.

42 Cockburn M, Twine J. A different kind of day unit. *Nurs Times* 1982; **78**: 1410–11.

43 Sharma K, Oliver D, Blatchford G, *et al.* Medical care in hospice day care. *J Palliat Care* 1993; **9**: 42–3.

44 Edwards A, Livingston H, Daley A. Does hospice day care need doctors? *Palliat Care Today* 1997; **6**: 36–7.

45 Kennett CE. Participation in a creative arts project can foster hope in hospice day care. *Palliat Med* 2000; **4**: 419–25.

46 Copp G, Richardson A, McDaid P, Marshall-Searson DA. A telephone survey of the provision of palliative day care services. *Palliat Med* 1998; **12**: 161–70.

47 Higginson IJ, Hearn J, Myers K, Naysmith A. Palliative day care: what do services do? *Palliat Med* 2000; **14**: 277–86.

48 Faulkner A, Higginson IJ, Heulwen E, *et al. Hospice Day Care: A Qualitative Study.* Sheffield: Help the Hospices and Trent Palliative Care, 1993.

49 Langley-Evans A, Payne S. Light-hearted death talk in a palliative day care context. *J Adv Nurs* 1987; **26**: 1091–7.

50 Douglas H-R, Higginson IJ, Myers K, Normand CE. Assessing structure, process and outcome in palliative day care: a pilot for a multi-centre trial. *Health Soc Care Community* 2000; **8**: 336–44.

51 Hopkinson JB, Hallet CE. Patients' perceptions of hospice day care: a phenomenological study. *Int J Nurs Stud* 2001; **38**: 117–25.

52 Lee L. Inter-professional working in hospice day care and the patients' experience of the service. *Int J Palliat Nurs* 2000; **8**: 389–400.

53 Goodwin DM, Higginson IJ, Myers K, *et al.* What is palliative day care? A patient perspective of five UK services. *Support Care Cancer* 2002; **10**: 556–62.

54 Goodwin DM, Higginson IJ, Myers K, *et al.* Effectiveness of palliative day care in improving pain, symptom control and quality of life. *J Pain Symptom Manage* 2003; **25**: 202–12.

◆ 55 Bruera E, Fornells H, Perez E, *et al.* Bus rounds for medical congresses on palliative care. *Support Care Cancer* 1998; **6**: 529–32.

◆ 56 Bruera E, Selmser P, Pereira J, Brenneis C. Bus rounds for palliative care education in the community. *CMAJ* 1997; **157**: 729–32.

57 Jenkins CA, Schulz M, Hanson J, Bruera E. Demographic, symptom, and medication profiles of cancer patients seen by a palliative care consult team in a tertiary referral hospital. *J Pain Symptom Manage* 2000; **19**: 174–84.

58 Fins JJ, Miller FG. A proposal to restructure hospital care for dying patients. *N Engl J Med* 1996; **334**: 1740–2.

◆ 59 O'Mahony S, Blank AE, Zallman L, Selwyn PA. The benefits of a hospital-based inpatient palliative care consultation service: preliminary outcome data. *J Palliat Med* 2005; **8**: 1033–9.

60 von Gunten CF. Secondary and tertiary palliative care in US hospitals. *JAMA* 2002; **287**: 875–81.

◆ 61 von Gunten CF, Ferris FD, Portenoy R, Glachen M, eds. *CAPC Manual: Everything You Wanted to Know About Developing a Palliative Care Program but Were Afraid to Ask*, 2001. Available at: www.capc.org/support-from-capc/capc_publications/ (accessed February 5, 2006).

62 Brenneis C, Bruera E. Models for the delivery of palliative care: the Canadian model. In: Bruera E, Portenoy RK, eds. *Topics in Palliative Care*, Vol 5. New York: Oxford University Press, 2001: 3–23.

63 von Gunten CF. Discussing do-not-resuscitate status. *J Clin Oncol* 2001; **19**: 1576–81.

64 Bruera E, Schoeller T, Wenk R, *et al.* A prospective multicenter assessment of the Edmonton Staging System for cancer pain. *J Pain Symptom Manage* 1995; **10**: 348–55.

♦ 65 Walker P, Nordell C, Neumann CM, Bruera E. Impact of the Edmonton Labeled Visual Information System on physician recall of metastatic cancer patient histories: a randomized controlled trial. *J Pain Symptom Manage* 2001; **21**: 4–11.

66 Kaasa T, Loomis J, Gillis K, *et al.* The Edmonton Functional Assessment Tool: preliminary development and evaluation for use in palliative care. *J Pain Symptom Manage* 1997; **13**: 10–19.

67 Oneschuk D, Fainsinger R, Hanson J, Bruera E. Assessment and knowledge in palliative care in second year family medicine residents. *J Pain Symptom Manage* 1998; **14**: 265–73.

♦ 68 Bruera E, Suarez-Almazor M, Velasco A, *et al.* The assessment of constipation in terminal cancer patients admitted to a palliative care unit: a retrospective review. *J Pain Symptom Manage* 1994; **9**: 515–19.

69 Maccabee J. The effect of transfer from a palliative care unit to nursing homes – are patients' and relatives' needs met? *Palliat Med* 1994; **8**: 211–14.

70 Mazuryk M, Daeninck P, Neumann CM, Bruera E. Daily journal club: an education tool in palliative care. *Palliat Med* 2002; **16**: 57–61.

71 Addington-Hall J, Altmann D, McCarthy M. Which terminally ill cancer patients receive hospice in-patient care? *Soc Sci Med* 1998; **46**: 1011–16.

72 Hinton J. Which patients with terminal cancer are admitted from home care? *Palliat Med* 1994; **8**: 197–210.

73 Gray JD, Forster DP. Factors associated with the utilization of specialist palliative care services: a population based study. *J Public Health Med* 1997; **19**: 464–9.

74 Gatrell AC, Harman J, Francis BJ, *et al.* Place of death: analysis of cancer deaths in part of North West England. *J Public Health Med* 2003; **25**: 53–8.

♦ 75 National Hospice and Palliative Care Organization. *Hospice Facts and Figures 2004.* www.nhpco.org (accessed November 19, 2005).

76 Elsayem A, Driver L, Bruera E. *Hospice Services. The MD Anderson Symptom Control and Palliative Care Handbook*, 2nd ed. 2003: 131–6.

77 Bradshaw PJ. Characteristics of clients referred to home, hospice and hospital palliative care services in Western Australia. *Palliat Med* 1993; **7**: 101–7.

78 Regional Palliative Care Program. *Annual Report April 1, 1996 to March 31, 1997.* Edmonton: Capital Health Authority, 1997.

79 Parkes CM, Parkes J. 'Hospice' versus 'hospital' care – re-evaluation after 10 years as seen by surviving spouses. *Postgrad Med J* 1984; **60**: 120–4.

80 Seale C, Kelly M. A comparison of hospice and hospital care for people who die: views of the surviving spouse. *Palliat Med* 1997; **11**: 93–100.

81 Teno J. *The Brown Atlas of Dying in the United States: 1989–2001.* Available at: www.chcr.brown.edu/dying/brownsodinfo.htm (accessed November 23, 2004).

82 Casarett D, Karlawish J, Morales K, *et al.* Improving the use of hospice services in nursing homes: a randomized controlled trial. *JAMA* 2005; **294**: 211–17.

83 Rice KN, Coleman EA, Fish R, *et al.* Factors influencing models of end-of-life care in nursing homes: results of a survey of nursing home administrators. *J Palliat Med* 2004; **7**: 668–75.

84 Bernabei R, Gambassi G, Lapane K, *et al.* Management of pain in elderly patients with cancer. *JAMA* 1998; **279**: 1877–82.

85 Levy CR, Fish R, Kramer AM. Site of death in the hospital versus nursing home of Medicare skilled nursing facility residents admitted under Medicare's Part A Benefit. *J Am Geriatr Soc* 2004; **52**: 1247–54.

86 Miller SC, Gozalo P, Mor V. Hospice enrollment and hospitalization of dying nursing home patients. *Am J Med* 2001; **111**: 38–44.

87 Teno J, Clarridge B, Casey V, *et al.* Family perspectives on end-of-life care at the last place of care. *JAMA* 2004; **291**: 88–93.

88 Thorpe G. Enabling more dying people to remain at home. *J Palliat Care* 2000; **16**: 23–8.

89 Mount BM, Ajemian I. The palliative care service integration in a general hospital. In: Ajemian I, Mount BM, eds. *The RVH Manual on Palliative/Hospice Care.* New York: Arno Press, 1980: 269–80.

90 Stajduhar KI, Davies B. Death at home: challenges for families and directions for the future. *J Palliat Care* 1998; **14**: 8–14.

91 McWhinney IR, Bass MJ, Orr V. Factors associated with location of death (home or hospital) of patients referred to a palliative care team. *CMAJ* 1995; **152**: 361–7.

92 Stephany TM. Place of death: home or hospital. *Home Health Nurse* 1992; **10**: 62.

93 Dudgeon DJ, Kristjanson L. Home versus hospital death: assessment of preferences and clinical challenges. *CMAJ* 1995; **152**: 337–40.

94 Doyle D. Domiciliary palliative care. In: Doyle D, Hanks G, MacDonald N, eds. *Oxford Textbook of Palliative Medicine.* New York: Oxford University Press, 1998: 957–63.

95 Hinton J. Can home care maintain an acceptable quality of life for patients with terminal cancer and their relatives? *Palliat Med* 1994; **8**: 183–96.

♦ 96 Cohen SR, Mount BM, Bruera E, *et al.* Validity of the McGill quality of life questionnaire in the palliative care setting: a multi-centre Canadian study demonstrating the importance of the existential domain. *Palliat Med* 1997; **11**: 3–23.

34

Palliative home care

ROBERTO WENK

INTRODUCTION

Most seriously sick patients prefer to stay at home during their final days; 50–80 percent elect to receive treatment and to die in their homes.[1] They prefer their homes to the unknown environment of a healthcare institution. However, there is a majority who die in the institution where they have been receiving care or treatment.[2]

Palliative care provides a way to change this situation. Its objective is to obtain the best possible quality of life for patients with incurable advanced illnesses, and for their families.[3] With palliative home care (PHC) all patients have the possibility to receive good quality care and die in their homes if that is the place where they would prefer to spend their last days. A growing number of patients are preferring PHC, and this is a great challenge because it is largely dependent upon the patients and their families, the health system, and the health professionals.[4]

This chapter analyzes different aspects of PHC based on the experience of the palliative care teams of the Pograma Argentino de Medicina Paliativa-Fundación FEMEBA (PAMP): CCP San Nicolas, UCP Sommer, and UCP Tornú. The methods described here may be similar to those present in other developing countries.

PALLIATIVE HOME CARE

Palliative home care is an option for patients who wish to be cared for at home and has three essential requirements: needs which can be met at home, a home where care can be provided, and a family to collaborate. Patients, families, professionals, and the public need to know about this option, its availability, and its limits; and they must also be aware that it can be challenging as well as rewarding for the patient and the family.

Advantages

The following factors regarding PHC are related to the fact that it enhances the patient's and family's independence and psychological wellbeing: the home is a place of familiarity and comfort without institutional regulations.[5]

- *Autonomy*. Patients stay with the family and plan their activity, rest, and diet. They can carry out some tasks at home and thus maintain their role.
- *Privacy*. Patients are not exposed to intrusive, at times unnecessary and not desired, medical activities. Nor are they exposed to the suffering of other patients.
- *Protection*. Patients are less exposed to therapeutic procedures, which are at times futile in incurable advanced diseases (intensive care, parenteral nutrition, etc.).
- *Better bereavement*. The family can anticipate the loss.
- *Less discomfort with death*. The death of a relative in the place where life was shared is a way to learn that death is a normal not unusual stage of life.

Saying that a patient spent the last days at home says little about the quality of life during that time. If PHC is efficient, symptom control is similar to that offered at an institution with palliative care; and better than that offered by an institution without palliative care.[6]

Disadvantages

With the patient at home there is only a partial return of the family equilibrium; finally the equilibrium is disturbed with the physical changes in the patient and the modifications of mood and behavior. The families facing the changes suffer, experience negative emotions (anxiety, fear, guilt, anger) and crisis and may develop psychological disorders.[7] There is considerable reduction of sleeping hours and activities, and families face economic hardships due to the increase in expenses (medication, healthcare personnel fees, etc.) and reduction of income (absence from or giving up work).[8]

The following patient and family factors make PHC difficult or not possible:

- Patient wishes to be hospitalized.
- Patient lives alone, with no family willing to provide care[†].
- Family members tired, no responsible adult, physically or emotionally weak, or dysfunctional.
- Home with unmet comfort needs (kitchen, running water, indoor toilets, electricity)[†].
- Situations that generate anxiety or family discomfort (convulsions, hemorrhages, smelly tumors, fecal incontinence).
- Frequent need of medical or nursing procedures.
- Hospital far away from patient's home.

BARRIERS TO DEVELOPMENT

The multiple barriers to the implementation of PHC are basically extensions of barriers to palliative care and can be discussed under the following headings according to the source of the barrier.

Health systems

Most public or private health systems include neither home care for chronic diseases nor palliative care.[9] With this background, plans to offer palliative care to different groups of patients are lacking with some exceptions and thus there are few PHC services available. The exceptions include a few health systems, mostly private and in small cities, that include PHC because the authorities became interested as a result of the positive results of local palliative care programs.

The lack of support from health authorities for PHC is the reason why most patients with incurable, advanced diseases spend their last days (sometimes weeks and months) in public or private institutions that guarantee available physicians, medication, technical resources, and some kind of symptom control; but these as a rule also provide medical interventions, which are often futile and expensive.[10]

[†] Main cause of long hospitalizations among the patients assisted by the UCP Sommer and UCP Tornú.

It is a contentious situation based on the failure to use resources efficiently and effectively: there is no budget assigned to PHC but admissions and aggressive treatments are encouraged. By supporting PHC the health system can offer an adequate solution to both the poor quality care of dying patients and the problem of maintaining full institutions with high assistance costs.

Professionals

There is no uniformity with regard to PHC: late referrals, treatment options not discussed with the patients and the families, poor symptom control, home visits without the necessary frequency, etc. characterize the care pattern. There is no difference among healthcare professionals from different disciplines in this respect – they have all neither learned about palliative care nor learned about the concepts of symptom control. They do not have experience in home care, and have difficulties in both team working and communicating with patients, families, and other team members.[11]

The reason for this situation is that palliative care is still not accepted as discipline, and as a consequence education and reimbursement for professionals are inconsistent. It is impossible to provide good home care with unpaid or underpaid professionals with incomplete training: it is more profitable and technically easier to hospitalize a patient.

Patients and families

Poverty challenges PCH. It cannot be effectively provided to patients who live in homes without kitchens, running water, indoor toilets, electricity, etc. It is also impossible if there is no public or charity support to pay for expenses related to care: medications, equipment, personal care items, transportation costs, and sometimes food.

The lack of public awareness about treatment options delays PHC: community education about the care they may expect can encourage patients to demand PHC, a possible powerful factor for its development.[12] There is a need to document these barriers to plan appropriate actions to reduce their impact and move community acceptance of the institutional care model to the background. Health systems require reforms to increase the availability and provision of PHC.

SPECIFIC ASPECTS OF PALLIATIVE HOME CARE

Models

For a better understanding of the different models of PHC the local development of palliative care is described in this section.

Ideal palliative care requires a complete team: (i) multiprofessional and interdisciplinary to treat the social, psychologic,

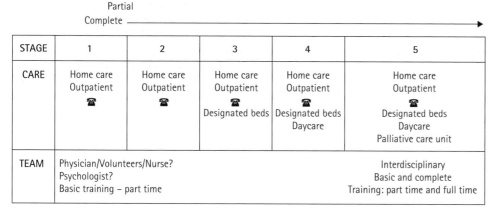

Figure 34.1 *Development stages of a palliative home care team.*

Few teams reach stage 5.

physical and existential problems according to the needs of the patients and their families, and (ii) activity adapted to the changing situations of the patient with 24 × 7 activity in the office, at home, and during day care or hospitalization. Universally, and especially in developing countries, comprehensive palliative care teams are not in majority; partial palliative care is the most common model of care in the final period.[13] In Argentina, almost all palliative care teams begin their activity in similar way: a group of volunteers (physicians, trained naïve personnel, nurse, psychologist) working in an institution or in the community, without specific planning, start the activity with outpatients. Then, with resources, they progress to develop a complete team. Figure 34.1 shows the development stages of a palliative care team in Argentina.

Each stage is a model providing palliative care based on the team's available resources; in all the stages there is home care, but of different complexity and effectiveness. In stage 1 home care is in the charge of the responsible caregiver (RC); the team works from the office and over the phone and does not come to the patient's home. In the other stages the care is still in charge of the RC, but home visits and care aid are added according to the team's capacity (personnel, time, transportation, etc.). The stages (and thus the models) are not static: activity is modified continuously with the development of the team and its changing characteristics. Different combinations of characteristics (Box 34.1) determine the complexity and the results of the PHC.

Examples

A team in stage 1 – community based with institutional support – offers care to outpatients. When patients cannot come (bad physical condition, long distances to travel, no transportation) 'distance' PHC is carried out: (i) the RC provides information about the condition of the patient, (ii) a presumptive diagnostic is made, (iii) the RC receives verbal and written instructions on specific techniques and takes care of the patient at home, (iv) when the patient gets worse he or she is hospitalized and cared for by other

---

Box 34.1 Characteristics of teams that influence palliative home care

- Institutional support (diagnostic and therapeutic resources)

- Availability of resources for home visits (vehicles/drivers)

- Number of disciplines

- Training

- Free care or paid care

- Dedication time/availability

---

professionals.[14] A team in stage 2 – community based with institutional support – offers care to outpatients and performs home visits. In out of office hours (nighttime, weekends) the institution's physicians collaborate in the care (they know the patient's clinical condition: the RC is provided with a summary of the clinical record, the medications in use and therapeutic suggestions in possible crisis).

- The UCP Sommer, in stage 5, in rural areas with resources for home visits: 60 percent of the patients die at home[‡].
- The UCP Tornú, in stage 5, in Buenos Aires city, without resources for home visits: 17 percent of the patients die at home[‡].
- The CCP San Nicolas offers paid palliative care to patients with health coverage. In this model, the team (2 physicians, 2 psychologists, and 2 nurses) are permanently available and assistance is completely delivered at home; 85 percent of the patients die at home[‡] cared for by the members of the team. Some members of the team (1 physician, 1 psychologist, and

3 trained persons; volunteer work) offer free palliative care to patients without resources one morning and one afternoon for a week at the office; when the patient deteriorates and cannot come to the office, he or she is hospitalized; 50 percent of the patients die in institution[‡], cared for by other professionals.

Team development can be optimized by:

- easier access to program by early referral
- availability of institutional beds for direct admissions
- medications from a specific *vademecum*
- equipment for comfort in the patient's home
- progressive development of:
  - care standards (symptom control, bereavement)
  - assessments tools
  - PHC chart
  - information systems
  - teaching protocols for team members
  - program audit.

THE RESPONSIBLE CAREGIVER

The availability of teams and resources do not guarantee the PHC. The family (persons with biologic, legal, or social relationship with the patient) plays a central role in all the treatments.[16] If these informal caregivers, who carry out a full time job without being paid, are integrated into the team, the majority of the patients can remain in their homes until death.

Steps in integrating the family

1 Evaluation of the family's capacity to care for the patient.
   - Do they wish to do it?
   - Can they understand and follow the indications for the treatment?
   - Will they be able to continue with their work?
   - Is the financial situation and the health coverage enough for the treatment expenses?
2 Identification of the RC.
   The RC is the member of the family who is in a better position (health, relation, proximity, and available time) to carry out and coordinate the care.[17] In one study[18¶] 81 percent of RCs were women, 54 percent were siblings, and 32 percent spouses or couples; the average age was 46 ± 15 years. In all the cases the RC was the same person throughout the treatment period.

3 Education of the RC.
   It must be done progressively, with simple verbal and written instructions about how to carry out home procedures. Key areas to cover are:
   - Administration of medications (i.e. following schedules, measuring syrups, placing suppositories, subcutaneous injections, etc.)
   - Symptom evaluation (vomiting, pain, dyspnea, cough, insomnia, constipation, and delirium) and recognition of their different aspects (Is it nausea or vomiting? How many times per day? For how long was the episode? Content?)
   - Diet and hydration
   - Control of evacuations
   - Hygiene (bath, oral cavity)
   - Changes of position, dressings
   - Organization of the family tasks
4 Recognition of the death.
   The RC has the information about the patient's physical condition and completes the necessary cycling of information for the care: he or she is the intermediary between the team and the family. In the study described above,[18] the RC reported little practical difficulty in carrying out the task (2.32 ± 3.5) and great satisfaction to have done it (8.9 ± 1.6) at the end of the treatment[¶].
5 Support for the RC.
   Lack of support is a frequent cause of patient hospitalization. The RC is supported by:
   - guaranteeing the maximum possible control of symptoms, the availability of the team and access to easy admission
   - establishing a caring plan and a schedule of activities
   - anticipating the changes that can occur in the patient's condition
   - reducing doubts and uncertainty about:
     - choice of the adequate therapeutic option
     - possibility of causing damage
     - medication (drugs and doses, when to increase the dose, fear of overdosing, undesirable effects)
     - meaning of new symptoms with negative impact (feeding difficulties, problems with breathing, pain, sleeping disorders, delirium, weakness, increase of dependence, mood changes) and how they will be corrected
     - operating dichotomies (personal needs versus those of the patient)
   - arranging measures to reduce the emotional load.
   The RC is part of the patient–family unit of treatment: they are clients with full-time tasks and responsibilities who need to be cared for.[19] In teams in stages 1 and 2 the RC is invited to psycho-educational meetings of 1–2 hours duration, every 2–4 weeks. In the meetings, coordinated by a psychologist, they can reflect upon issues, doubts are analyzed and resources are optimized.

[†]If admission is possible when the patient's symptoms are not controlled at home it can be assumed that the number and length of hospitalization are smaller, and the percentage of deaths in the institution is lesser when the PHC quality is greater; these data can be used as indirect indicators of the PHC efficacy.[15]

In more developed teams the RC is assisted during the visits to the office or during hospitalization. In the above mentioned study[18] the RC reported moderate emotional difficulty (5.7 ± 3.8) in carrying out the home care¶. They also reported a lot of suffering during the entire treatment, with no difference between the initial (7.5 ± 2.8) and final (8.4 ± 1.8) evaluations after a mean time of 39 ± 11 days. The causes of suffering were their own emotional situation, the emotional and physical condition of the patient, and the financial problems.

6 Providing material resources.

During PHC, resources must be provided; the public hospital and community are sources of medications, hospital beds, wheelchairs, urinals, commodes, walkers, etc. If possible, financial aid should also be offered to compensate for the increase of the family expenses and the reduction in income. In general the negative impact of the home care of a patient is underreported: in spite of the bad economic situation of the family, and of the limited aid that is given, no economic damages are reported. In the reported study[18] a mean 2.2 (±1.9) RCs reported sufficient family income during the treatment and 1.8 (±2.8) reported negative economic repercussions of the home care¶. Although a family's capacity for adaptation to adverse situations seems unlimited, it is a fact that the home care of a patient generates significant economic deterioration.

7 Symptom control.

Symptoms are controlled according to the criteria established by the World Health Organization (WHO).[3] The important issues are:

- *Medication.* In Argentina the high cost of commercial preparations of opioids is a barrier to adequate pain treatment.[20,21] The provision of opioids without charge or at low cost can be guaranteed with compound preparations (prepared by a pharmacist according to the national pharmacopeia in an individualized prescription) or generic preparations (products for which the patent has expired and thus can be manufactured and commercialized without restrictions of trademark) of aqueous solutions of morphine (6 g/mL), oxycodone (3 mg/mL) or methadone (1 mg/mL) for oral use, or aqueous solutions of morphine or oxycodone (10 mg/mL) for subcutaneous use. The same can be done to provide

dexamethasone, metoclopramide, hyoscine, bisacodyl, haloperidol, acetaminophen (paracetamol), etc.

- *Treatment monitoring.* The semi-structured evaluation of symptoms enables different team members (volunteer, nurse) to carry out uniform and regular monitoring of the treatment. This is especially important when patients remain for variable periods of time without medical evaluation (stages 1, 2, and 3). The information is obtained from:
  - the patient, on office or home visits. The PAMP uses a form to collect date and place of consultation, clinical disorders, symptoms (ESAS),[22] cognitive disorders, hydration, bowel movements, hospitalizations, route and doses of opioids, adjuvant drugs, diagnostic and therapeutic practices.
  - the RC, on an office visit or via telephone calls. The RC reports the patient's symptoms on a form that lists 22 symptoms; for 11 the options are yes/no and for 11 information on symptom intensity is recorded with a 4-point Likert scale.
- *Regulation of the interventions* that are prescribed and carried out to avoid 'hospitalization at home'. The following can be included:
  - administration of symptomatic medication
  - psychological interventions
  - lab tests
  - thoracic/peritoneal drainage, dressings, rectal maneuvers, physical therapy, electrocardiogram (EKG), chest/abdominal X-rays
  - subcutaneous administration of drugs
  - hypodermoclysis, blood transfusions, bladder catheterization, oxygen supplement, etc.

At the CCP San Nicolas the three most frequent therapeutic practices are subcutaneous infusion of drugs, enemas, and hypodermoclysis; the three most frequent diagnostic investigations are plain X-rays, echocardiography and EKG, and the six most frequent lab tests are complete blood count, creatinine, electrolytes, blood sugar, calcium and prothrombin time, and partial thromboplastin time.[23]

- *Psychological evaluation and assistance of the patient.* As this is not possible for all patients it is carried out:
  - when the patient comes to the office or during hospitalization
  - according to established criteria: the patient or a team member request it, risky situations, lack of adhesion to treatment, or anguish, sadness and insomnia with intensity over 6 in the 0–10 scale
  - with semistructured evaluation based on the Diagnostic and Statistical Manual (DSM)-IV axes system
  - With brief psychotherapeutic practices: analysis of problems, behavioral techniques, cognitive techniques, and relaxation techniques.

¶In the CCP San Nicolas the RCs of 50 consecutive patients were interviewed and aspects related to the caring task were evaluated: their suffering and their causes (Suffering Scale, MSKCC, NCI 1.0), the emotional and practical difficulties of the task (0–10 scale: 0 without difficulty, 10 maximum difficulty) and satisfaction with the caring task (0–10 scale: 0 dissatisfied; 10 maximum satisfaction), the sufficiency of family incomes during the home care (0–10 scale: 0 not enough for nothing, 10 permits savings), and the negative economic repercussions of the home care (0–10 scale: 0 none, 10 maximum).[19]

ECONOMIC ISSUES

It is unclear if palliative care produces savings by reduction of the expenses of both fragmented care and use of high-tech interventions; some studies do not show savings and others show up to 68 percent savings.[24] The direct cost of PHC is related to the intensity of the assistance, the number of professionals that intervene, and the use of therapeutic and diagnostic resources. PHC can produce savings by the reduction of the number and the length of the hospitalizations.[15]

The use of resources was registered in CCP San Nicolas (stage 2, exclusive home care) and UCP Tornú (during its stage 4, assistance only in office and hospitalization). Members of both teams have similar training and therapeutic approach; the patients have free access to the resources. When comparing the therapeutic and diagnostic resources used with cancer patients with similar initial clinical conditions the results showed that (i) there were no differences in the length of treatments, nor in the number of diagnostic investigations, therapeutic practices, lab tests and consultations with non-team healthcare professionals, and (ii) there were significant differences in hospitalization (proportion of patients and length of stay) and in the percentage of deaths at home (lower and higher, respectively, in CCP San Nicolas).

In our experience, PHC by a team that does not carry out diagnostic procedures or therapeutic measures without reasonable expectation of benefit and that incorporates a competent RC, requires resources similar to institutional care but can generate savings by reduction of the number and length of hospitalizations.

ASSISTANCE COSTS FOR A GIVEN TIME PERIOD

The items that generate the cost over a period of time are:

- Number of professional visits
- Diagnostic and therapeutic procedures
- Medication
- Medical supplies
- Medical equipment (i.e. wheelchairs, pneumatic mattresses, etc.)
- Operative expenses (i.e. vehicle, communication, distance to the home, secretary, office setup, etc.)

If each team member determines the utilization average of each item and knows the value of each one, it is simple to structure the assistance costs for a period of time.

The CCP San Nicolas charges the PHC by modules of assistance that have the same cost for all the patients. The items that are considered in the cost of 1 month's assistance are: 2 medical visits per week (a), 2 nursing visits per week (a), 4 psychology/counseling interviews per month (b) and provision of oral and parenteral opioids analgesic (c). The module includes regular and on-call medical and nurse home visits in a 20 km radius area, and excludes hospitalization, all the drugs except opioids analgesics, oxygen, life support measures, palliative radiotherapy and chemotherapy, diagnostic investigations, lab tests, and medical supplies and equipment.

(a) – one per week at the beginning, with patients in stable clinical condition and controlled symptoms; one or more per day in the final period; each visit in the covered area demands 2 hours in average.
(b) – two per month for the patient and two for the family.
(c) – average daily oral dose: methadone 30 mg and three morphine 30 mg rescue doses, or their equivalent parenteral doses.

THE VOLUNTEER'S ROLE

Volunteers from different professions and social groups play an essential role in palliative care: few teams could offer quality end-of-life care without their collaboration; they increase both team activity and interaction with the community.[25] After the volunteers are convened, interviewed, selected and specifically trained to work with patients and families, they can take on different tasks in all the development stages of palliative care, but with greater importance in stages 1 and 2. The tasks which have an impact on the PHC are:

- Semi-structured evaluation of the patient, at home and by phone
- RC education
- Massages, diet, hygiene
- Practical support (transfers, housekeeping activities, purchases)
- Recreation (company, walks)

ETHICAL ASPECTS

Palliative home care is a relatively new but rapidly growing concept that redefines care; thus it can be the source of ethical dilemmas.[26] To avoid them, when making decisions the wishes, beliefs and values of patients and families must be considered within the frame of some principles.

INFORMED CHOICES

The choice of where to receive assistance at the end of life is important and worrying for patients and families. The options should be evaluated with correct and complete information, and the patient, the family and the team should agree the choice. Two tips are: adequate choices are impossible with incomplete or biased information, and it must be possible to change the choice.[27]

BENEFITS/BURDENS RATIO

Palliative care is a medical discipline that uses all available diagnostic and therapeutic practices, including high technology. In order to justify an intervention, its expected benefits must outweigh its burdens: the selection of each intervention in each unique situation must be based on the benefit/burden analysis. Practices with bad benefit/burden ratios that do not respect the proportionality principle (i.e. mechanical ventilation, vital monitoring, dialysis, parenteral nutrition) should not be offered or included in PHC plans.[26] PHC is different from 'hospitalization at home': it must not medicalize or technologize the dying process.

PRIVACY

Palliative home care should not be an intrusion in the privacy of the home and nor should it disturb the family life; to avoid those inconveniences a balanced plan of activity should be prepared considering the needs and the operating/organizing capacity of the family.[28]

COSTS

The choice of the place of care should be made without the pressures of economic factors (the goal of the PHC is not to reduce costs but to improve the quality of life) and it is probable that there can be savings for the health system, but it should not be forgotten that it represents an economic burden for the family. If PHC is promoted and implemented resources must be provided: as a minimum to provide medication (i.e. opioids) and a maximum to assign funds to the RC; it is a fact that in most cases the burden of cost shifts from the healthcare system to the caregiver.[29]

Key learning points

- Teams must start and maintain for the longest possible time, with the best possible quality, the process of assistance at home. PHC is not a high-technology approach, but it is a sophisticated approach considering the number of factors that determine its outcomes and results. Both issues make it a challenge. But it is also a source of satisfaction: if good-quality PHC is achieved, the patient receives the best possible care.

- It is important to have a better understanding of the practice, strengths, and limitations of PHC to promote, with a strong base, this approach to care that contributes to patient and family wellbeing.

REFERENCES

◆ 1 Doyle D. The provision of palliative care. In: Doyle D, Hanks G, MacDonald N, eds. *Oxford Textbook of Palliative Medicine*, 2nd ed. Oxford: Oxford University Press, 1998.

◆ 2 Field D, James N. Where and how people die. In: Clark D, ed. *The Future for Palliative Care: Issues of Policy and Practice.* Buckingham: Open University Press, 1993: 6–18.

✳ 3 World Health Organization Expert Committee. *Cancer Pain Relief and Palliative Care.* Geneva: WHO, 1990.

✳ 4 Field MJ, Cassel CK, eds. *Approaching Death: Improving Care at the End of Life.* Washington DC: Committee on Care at the End of Life, Division of Health Care Services, Institute of Medicine; National Academy Press, 1997.

◆ 5 Stajduhar K, Davies B. Death at home: Challenges for families and directions for the future. *J Palliat Care* 1998; **14**: 8–14.

◆ 6 Singer PA, Bowman KW. Quality care at the end of life. *BMJ* 2002; **324**: 1291–2.

◆ 7 Vachon M. Psychosocial needs of patients and families. *J Palliat Care* 1998; **14**: 49–56, 208–12.

◆ 8 Kinsella G, Cooper B, Picton C, Murtagh D. A review of the measurement of caregiver and family burden in palliative care. *J Palliat Care* 1998; **14**: 37–45.

◆ 9 Wenk R, Marti G. Palliative Care in Argentina: deep changes are necessary for its effective implementation. *Palliat Med* 1996; **10**: 263–4.

◆ 10 American Academy of Hospice and Palliative Medicine. *Unipac One: the Hospice/palliative Medicine Approach to End-of-life Care.* Iowa: Kendall/Hunt Publishing Company, 1998.

◆ 11 Ferrell B. Integration of pain education in home care. *J Palliat Care* 1998; **14**: 62–8.

◆ 12 DeLima L. Cuidados paliativos en países en desarrollo: retos y recursos. II Congreso de la Asociación Latinoamericana de Cuidados Paliativos VII Curso Latinoamericano de Medicina y Cuidados Paliativos, Montevideo, Uruguay, 2004.

◆ 13 Latimer E. The ethics of partial palliative care. *J Palliat Care* 1994; **10**: 107–10.

◆ 14 Wenk R, Monti C, Bertolino M. Asistencia a distancia: mejor o peor que nada? *Medicina Paliativa* 2003; **10**: 136–41.

◆ 15 Whynes D. Costs of palliative care. In: Clark D, Hockey F, Ahmedzai S, eds. *Facing Death: New Themes in Palliative Care.* Philadelphia: Open University Press, 1997.

◆ 16 Glajchen M. Role of the family caregivers in cancer pain management. *J Pain Symptom Manage* 2003; **26**: 644–54.

◆ 17 Neale B. Informal care, community care. In: Clark D, ed. *The Future for Palliative Care: Issues of Policy and Practice.* Buckingham: Open University Press, 1993: 52–67.

● 18 Wenk R, Monti C. El sufrimiento de los cuidadores responsacles. *Medicina Paliativa* 2005 (in press).

◆ 19 Brown P, Davies B, Martens N. Families in supportive care: Part II: Palliative care at home: A viable care setting. *J Palliat Care* 1990; **6**: 21–7.

● 20 Wenk R, Bertolino M, DeLima L. Analgésicos opioides en Latinoamérica: la barrera de accesibilidad supera la de disponibilidad. *Medicina Paliativa* 2004; **11**: 148–51.

● 21 Wenk R, Bertolino M. High opioids costs in Argentina: an availability barrier that can be overcome. *J Pain Symptom Manage* 2000; **20**: 81–2.

◆ 22 Bruera E, MacDonald S. Audit methods: The Edmonton System Assessment Sytem. In: Higginson I, ed. *Clinical Audit in Palliative Care.* Oxford: Radcliffe Medical Press, 1993.

● 23 Wenk R, Bertolino M. Direct medical costs of an Argentinian domiciliary palliative care model. *J Pain Symptom Manage* 2000; **20**: 162–4.

◆ 24 Robbins M. The economics of palliative medicine. In: Doyle D, Hanks G, MacDonald N, eds. *Oxford Textbook of Palliative Medicine*, 2nd ed. Oxford: Oxford University Press, 1998.

◆ 25 Claxton-Oldfield S, Jefferies J, Fawcet C *et al.* Palliative care volunteers: why do they do it? *J Palliat Care* 2004; **20**: 78–84.

✱ 26 Randall F, Downiw RS. *Palliative Care Ethics, A Companion for All Specialties.* Oxford: Oxford Medical Publications, 1999.

◆ 27 Van Eys J. The ethics of palliative care. *J Palliat Care* 1991; **7**: 27–32.

◆ 28 Lattimer E. Ethical decision-making in the care of the dying and and its application to clinical practice. *J Pain Symptom Manage* 1991; **6**: 329–36.

◆ 29 Wilkinson J. Ethical issues in palliative care. In: Doyle D, Hanks G, MacDonald N, eds. *Oxford Textbook of Palliative Medicine.* Oxford: Oxford University Press, 1993.

Day hospitals

BRUNO GAGNON

SETTING THE STAGE

Provision of palliative care services has been in constant evolution since the initiation of the modern hospice movement in 1960. At first, emphasis was put on inpatient beds in hospices or in hospital settings. Rapidly, homecare services, often in association with hospice settings, were developed to take palliative care expertise into the home and to allow the terminally ill to remain at home until death if at all possible and if desirable. The first Palliative Care Day Care, inspired by the experience of day care services provided to older and psychiatric patients, opened in 1975 at St Luke's hospice in Sheffield, UK, to support patients with pre-terminal cancer and chronic disease.[1] This experience was reproduced extensively in the UK and elsewhere around the world in countries such as the USA, Australia, Japan, and several European countries.[2] Situated within communities, these day centers aim at providing a link between homecare services and inpatients units[3] with special emphasis on providing support through social interaction, psychological support, and respite for caregivers, as well as offering expertise in monitoring and symptom control.[4] The efficacy of this latter role of symptom management and improvement in quality of life provided by specialist palliative day care, referring to facilities offering medical and nursing assessment of all patients, was evaluated in the UK by comparing 120 consecutive patients referred to five specialized palliative care day centers to 53 patients receiving routine palliative care services who did not attend day care.[5*] All patients were prospectively assessed through three different interviews (at baseline, at 6–8 weeks and at 12–15 weeks) using the McGill Quality of Life Questionnaire (MQOL) and the Palliative Care Outcome Scale. At baseline, the two groups differed as the day center group had a

lower score in the support domain of the MQOL than the comparison group ($P = 0.065$) and this latter group had marginally more severe pain at baseline ($P = 0.053$) and more severe symptoms at the second assessment ($P = 0.025$). This study was not conclusive in demonstrating improvement of quality of life of patients attending these facilities due to some methodological issues, mainly the limitations of the quality-of-life measures in identifying the effects of palliative day care. Further studies are needed to evaluate their clinical relevance.

A survey of palliative day care centers[6*] documented that these facilities were mostly situated within the community and had criteria for admitting patients to their services. These criteria often included being terminally ill or having active and progressive disease above their need for palliative interventions. These realities may in fact limit the access to palliative care by patients in need of such care who may not be in the terminal phase of their illness and/or are still mainly cared for in the hospital setting. Palliative care should be accessible to all cancer patients[7] as there is growing evidence that proper symptom management and psychological and existential support can be contributory in cancer control.[8] An example of the benefits associated with an early palliative care approach is the recent development in the treatment of cancer-associated anorexia-cachexia syndrome as a necessary element of cancer care.[9]

The concept of the day hospital was originally developed for the geriatric population. In 1951, the first geriatric day hospital was opened at Oxford, England,[10] in response to a lack of continuum of care between acute hospitalization and long-term placement.[11] By 1995, more than 400 day hospitals were implemented in the United Kingdom.[12*] Hospital based, these facilities operate 5 days a week but most patients visit only two to three times a week and service duration is usually up to 12 weeks.[13] These services have been defined as 'an outpatient facility where frail older patients can receive subacute or acute medical, nursing, social and/or rehabilitative services over any portion of a full day, with return visits as necessary'.[14] A systemic review of 12 controlled trials comparing day hospital care for older people to comprehensive, domiciliary, or no comprehensive care concluded that hospital day care seems to be an effective service with trends toward reduction in hospital bed use and placement in institutional care, but methodological problems with these trials limit the evaluation of the services.[15***] A recent economic evaluation of a day hospital in Canada, based on the data of 151 subjects, found that for every dollar invested in the geriatric day hospital program, the benefit for the healthcare system was Can$2.14 (95 percent confidence interval (CI) Can$1.72–2.56).[16**] By definition, a day hospital should be hospital based, however in the USA, although standard day hospitals do exist,[17,18] the Collaborative Assessment and Rehabilitation for Elders Program established a community-based center offering similar services as in a day hospital.[19] This initiative challenges the definition of the day hospital based on its location as similar services could be provided in the community.

Furthermore, during the same period, the concept of day hospital has also been developed for patients with mental illnesses. Psychiatric day hospitals usually offer services and care on a daily basis but a recent survey of five European countries found no consistent profile of structure and procedural features.[20*] For the purpose of a systematic review of the effectiveness of day care for people with severe mental disorders, day hospitals were defined as multidisciplinary day care facilities offering comprehensive psychiatric care.[21***] In these reviews, they identified nine randomized controlled trials (1568 patients). Day hospital treatment was feasible for between 23.2 percent and 37.5 percent of those admitted to inpatient care. As expected, day hospital patients spent fewer days in inpatient care and more days in day hospital than the control group, showed significantly faster improvement in mental status ($P = 0.006$) and they did not differ in readmission rates. Day hospital care was reported to be cheaper than inpatient care.

The desire to manage patients within lower cost settings led to the extension of day hospitals to other medical illnesses such as orthopedic surgery, laparoscopic surgery, stroke[22***] cancer,[23*] diabetes mellitus,[24] rheumatological diseases,[25] chronic obstructive pulmonary disease,[26] congestive heart failure,[27] and other illnesses.[28] Cost effectiveness remains the major issue for the most day hospital initiatives. For example, in stroke recovery where multiple trials have been carried out, the lack of a standardized definition of the concept of day hospital rehabilitation made it impossible to fully demonstrate effectiveness in hastening functional recovery and reducing outpatients visits among older stroke patients without additional cost.[22***] A randomized

trial comparing the effectiveness of a day hospital program to usual care, in 234 patients with congestive heart failure, demonstrated reduction in morbidity and mortality with a cost/utility ratio for the integration of the day hospital management of US$19 462 (95 percent CI US$13 904 to $34 048).[27**] Interestingly, day hospitals have also been established for the management of pain crisis related to sickle cell anemia with successful pain management and possible reduction of hospital admissions.[29*,30*]

With the desire to offer palliative care services to patients with advanced cancer but who are still receiving active oncology treatments and/or may be candidates for complex palliative care interventions necessitating the hospital setting, a palliative care day hospital (PCDH) was opened in 1998 at the Montreal General Hospital in Montreal, Canada. After 6 years of operation, we reviewed our experience using a Delphi method. Twenty-one members of our team participated in the review process: eight physicians, five nurses, two clinical nurses, two administrators, one psychologist, one pastoral person, one patient assistant, and one clerk. This chapter presents the conclusions of this review process.

MANDATES AND ROLES OF THE PALLIATIVE CARE DAY HOSPITAL

From the beginning, the PCDH was planned to provide a leadership role in promoting links between a tertiary care hospital and community services. Box 35.1 enumerates the different mandates assumed by the PCDH. Special emphasis was made to be all inclusive for patients in need of palliative care interventions during the whole disease trajectory from diagnosis to the terminal phase of their illness. At the present time, patients with a cancer diagnosis are mainly, but not exclusively, referred to the PCDH, as part of an initiative promoted in close collaboration with the oncology services. The PCDH offers services to patients who could not access such comprehensive palliative care without hospitalization due to the complexity of their clinical situation and their limited physical tolerance, and to less sick patients with difficult pain or other symptoms who then can receive, in a relaxed setting, specialized palliative care not available in the community. The PCDH rapidly evolved as a communication center between community services and tertiary hospital services. Being situated in a university teaching facility, the PCDH contributes to the development of academic excellence in palliative care through teaching and research.

Box 35.2 describes in more detail the specific roles assumed by the PCDH. The team acts as consultant to primary physicians by providing optimal palliative care assessment and specialized interventions. However, the reality of limited resources in the community, especially of physicians making home visits[31*] and the complexity of the clinical presentation warrants that the team should assume a more

Box 35.1 Mandates of the Day Hospital

- The Day Hospital provides palliative care services to patients with life-threatening illnesses, primarily cancer; due to the complexity of their symptoms and/or their psychosocial context, these patients could not be appropriately cared for without being hospitalized. Patients may still be receiving palliative chemotherapy and can be candidates for complex medical/surgical interventions to improve quality of life

- The Day Hospital provides specialized palliative care that is not available in the community or in other institutions. The goal of the Day Hospital is to improve the quality of life of patients and to support their families while allowing them to remain at home as long as possible

- The Day Hospital works as a coordination center between hospital services, including inpatient palliative care services, and community-based services such as homecare services and hospices to improve continuity of care and access to appropriate services according to patients' specific needs

- The Day Hospital, as part of the McGill Palliative Care Division, promotes academic excellence by participating in teaching and research

Box 35.2 Roles of the Palliative Care Day Hospital

Patient care

- Should provide optimal palliative care to patients with: severe symptoms, existential distress, difficult family situation, regardless of their prognosis

- Should assume a consultation role for patients who are not in terminal phase of their illness

- Should assume treating physician role with terminally ill patients only in special situations: complexity of palliative care issues and to supplement lack of resources in the community

- Should coordinate referrals to other palliative care services: pastoral, psychology, etc.

- Should organize advance care planning including clarification of code status

- Should provide emergency consultations within 48 hours

- Should coordinate special investigation and interventions to patients in the terminal phase of their illness and, in coordination with other hospital outpatient services, to patients receiving active treatment

- Should provide specialized services to special populations, for example patients with lymphedema or severe anorexia-cachexia syndrome

Coordination of services

- Should improve links between specialized services of the hospital, especially oncology services and community resources

- Should promote links with homecare services and hospices through adequate referral

- Should respond to home 'crisis' by giving support to home-based palliative care teams and by coordinating admission to the day hospital or the inpatient unit so as to prevent, if at all possible, visits to the emergency room by terminally ill patients

- Should provide phone consultations to physicians and nurses in the community regarding complex issues

- Should develop protocols of care with community services

Education

- Should educate colleagues in other disciplines within the hospital about Day Hospital mandates, resources available in the community and the process to link patients and family with community resources

- Should promote palliative care through teaching within the institution, in the community and at national and international congresses

- Should offer training sessions to physicians, nurses, social workers, and other specialized caregivers

- Should participate in teaching medical students, residents, fellows, and students of other healthcare disciplines

Research

- Should provide equivalent care to all palliative care patients including those participating in research

- Should collect baseline clinical and socio-demographic data for research purposes

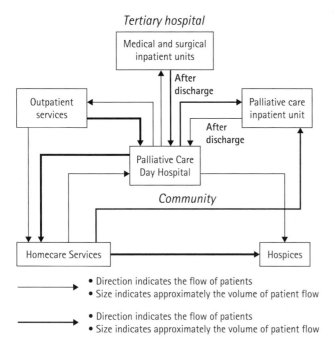

Tertiary hospital

Medical and surgical inpatient units

After discharge

Outpatient services

Palliative care inpatient unit

After discharge

Palliative Care Day Hospital

Community

Homecare Services

Hospices

- Direction indicates the flow of patients
- Size indicates approximately the volume of patient flow

- Direction indicates the flow of patients
- Size indicates approximately the volume of patient flow

Figure 35.1 *Links between the Palliative Care Day Hospital and other services.*

direct role in caring for this very sick population. The clinical condition of patients with advanced cancer can change drastically in a very short time and may mandate rapid interventions to adjust the plan of care. The PCDH can respond to such changes and provide support to the community by ensuring good coordination by communicating through phone calls with hospital and community services, by offering emergency visits to the day hospital and to other services within the hospital, and by coordinating admission to palliative care inpatient units. This coordination effort is an important component of the PCDH role and provides an important benefit to patients and caregivers.

Figure 35.1 illustrates the different links and the possible movement of patients between the places of care. While it was originally thought that most referrals to the PCDH would originate from community services for patients in need of specialized palliative care not available in the community, the experience demonstrated that most referrals came from other outpatient services within the hospital, such as oncology, radiooncology, and surgical clinics. Such a pattern of referrals is explained by the fact that cancer patients received care mainly through outpatient services of the hospital with minimal input from the community services until they reached the terminal phase of their illness.[31*] A possible explanation is that patients with cancer retain overall good physical function until late in the disease progression,[32,33*] and are therefore able to be cared for in outpatient clinics by cancer specialists. So, the PCDH evolved naturally into an evaluation, stabilization, and referring facility within the hospital for patients needing palliative care. Because they are located within the hospital, the PCDH team

members have access to the whole chart, previous investigations, and the technical support to rapidly assess and stabilize patients, and to provide community services with a complete palliative care evaluation and advanced care plan. However, the PCDH continues to provide valuable support to patients whose care has been assumed by community resources by providing ongoing reevaluations for complex situations and by offering specialized interventions.

The team members of the PCDH are all specialized in palliative care; they assume a leadership role in education and in research. Because the population of patients seen at the PCDH includes a spectrum of clinical conditions from early diagnosis to terminal phase of the illness within the same day, it is an ideal setting for teaching and research. Research with this population of patients is challenging due to the complexity and instability of their clinical situation. The PCDH provides a secure setting to patients with advanced disease, allowing them to contribute to the development of knowledge of palliative care by participating in research activities. Such participation offers to these patients, whose disease has often removed their social role, a sense that they are still contributing members of society.

PALLIATIVE CARE MULTIDISCIPLINARY TEAM

The basic team consists of physicians, bedside nurses, and a clinical nurse specialist in palliative care. Depending on the specific needs of individual patients, other members of the palliative care team such as the psychologist, social worker, physiotherapist, nutritionist, pharmacist, and pastoral care person will be involved in the care of the patient. Depending on the acuity of clinical situation and resources available in the community, a given patient may be evaluated the same day or at a later date by the members of the extended PCDH team or referred to services available in the community. Important elements of the team are also the unit clerk, patient attendee and the volunteers who provide an attentive ear and a helping hand during the stay of the patient in the unit. Creating an environment wherein patients can interact with staff and other patients is considered an important element of the therapeutic benefits of palliative care.[34*]

The PCDH makes it possible to access valuable highly specialized expertise available in a tertiary care hospital such as anesthesiologists, surgeons, oncologists, radiooncologists, psychiatrists, and other medical specialists, and also skincare nurses, stoma therapists, etc.

The day-to-day functioning of the Day Hospital

The daily functioning of the PCDH is based on a model of care delivered by a primary team composed of a bedside nurse and a physician. Box 35.3 presents their respective roles. As patients may be referred to the PCDH at any point

---

Box 35.3 Roles of the primary team members

Role of the Day Hospital physicians

- To take a complete history and physical including past history, cancer history, pain, and other important symptom issues

- To document diagnosis and prognosis

- To establish the priority of palliative care interventions: investigation, medication and therapeutic interventions, and referrals, in collaboration with the bedside nurse, to other team members

- To clarify the level of care and resuscitation status

- In collaboration with other team members, to establish advanced care planning: follow-up, admission, referral to hospice, etc.

- To call and to run family meetings

- To communicate information to treating physician

- To respond to phone consultations from the community related to medical issues

Role of bedside nurse

- Evaluation of the basic palliative care nursing including documentation of symptoms, performance status, cognitive testing, basic psychosocial assessment, drug profile and specific care issues such catheter, wounds, and stoma

- To establish a nursing care plan

- To teach patient and caregivers about proper use of medications, especially related to symptom management, and any other care issues

- To provide support to patients and families facing the palliative course of a disease

- To coordinate the involvement of the other team members from the PCDH or from the community

- To take an active role in the running of family meetings

- To organize and to coordinate care between the hospital and the community services to ensure continuum of care

- To assure support to community nurses

---

along their illness trajectory, the palliative care physician needs to clarify by communicating with the treating physician if necessary the exact diagnosis and prognosis to determine the level of involvement by the palliative care team and the need for follow-up. In some instances, palliative care interventions are limited in time until optimization of control of the symptoms before returning the patient to the treating physician. In most instances, the PCDH initiates care for patients receiving palliative oncology treatments and gradually assumes a growing role until assuming full care. This process involves a constant effort of communication to prevent confusion of roles and undue suffering to the patients and their caregivers. A challenging aspect of this process is the determination of level of care and resuscitation status. The treating physician has the primary responsibility in determining this important aspect of the care. In most situations, the PCDH team is called to help

patients and family to understand the meaning of a palliative care approach. By establishing a concrete advance care plan and by calling a family meeting, it is usually possible to have a smooth process that provides patients and caregivers with a sense of security and control over the situation. However, the PCDH team is at times confronted with distressed patients and family members who may not have fully understood the meaning of the information provided by the treating physicians. In these circumstances, it is useful to invite the treating physician to participate with the team in the family meeting. This approach has been extremely beneficial to this group of patients and has also revealed itself as a powerful tool to teach other specialists about the communication of bad news.

In view of better efficiency, the bedside nurse role is based on the concept of case management of the patient and family in relation with the environment. A thorough biologic, psychologic, social, and existential evaluation of the patient is carried out by the nurse. As most patients present with complex clinical situations, the use of specific tools like the Edmonton Symptom Assessment Scale[35] (ESAS) to document symptom profile; the palliative performance scale[36] to evaluate the physical performance status; Folstein's mini-mental questionnaire[37] to screen for cognitive failure; and a locally developed semi-structured nursing interview, assure completeness of the evaluation in a timely fashion. This basic evaluation is also a therapeutic intervention which allows patients and caregivers, often for the first time, the opportunity to freely express their needs and concerns and by this very process to develop a trustful relationship with the palliative care team. It is an invaluable part of the service offered by the PCDH.

After the initial assessment has been performed by the nurse and the physician, the clinical situation of the patient is discussed to establish the plan for the day regarding further investigations, therapeutic interventions and referrals to other team members. The stay in the PCDH offers a comfortable environment to patients and family and an opportunity for observation. As the day progresses, it is not rare that hidden issues are voiced by patients and family members as they develop trust in the team members. Usually, patients are in need first of symptom control before organization of the advanced care planning. The PCDH offers access to multiple services (see Box 35.4) that allow rapid management of distressing symptoms without the need for multiple visits. After the symptoms are managed optimally, usually accomplished within one to three visits to the PCDH, patients and family caregivers, and not rarely professional caregivers from the community, are called for a family meeting. This advanced care plan includes provision of homecare services, recommendations to follow in case of difficulties with symptom management or emergency situations, and steps to follow when death occurs. Of special mention, this plan includes, in case care could not be provided at home until death, a referral to one of the hospices or to the tertiary palliative care unit for patients with complex syndromes necessitating special expertise.

During this process or after patients have been referred to either the treating oncologist if still receiving active treatments, or to the community resources for terminal care, the PCDH remains a support resource through phone calls or emergency visits. In certain situations, especially with patients in severe pain or distressing situations, or when community resources are insufficient, the PCDH assures regular follow-up until death in collaboration with the community healthcare providers.

PHYSICAL SETTING

Because the PCDH serves patients with a wide range of clinical conditions from bed bound to fully ambulated,

---

Box 35.4 Services offered at the Day Hospital

Clinical services

1 Thorough palliative care assessment

2 Diagnostic tests including radiological imaging tests

3 Coordination and administration of treatments available in tertiary hospital:
   - Blood transfusions
   - Abdominal paracentesis, thoracocentesis, etc.
   - Anesthetic interventions
   - Radiotherapy for symptom control
   - Wound and stoma care

4 Teaching to patients and family caregivers:
   - Pain medication and other care issues
   - Community services available
   - Solutions to special distressing situations like major bleeding events[38]

5 Family meeting

6 Palliative care counseling services:
   - Psychologist
   - Pastoral care
   - Nutrition
   - Physiotherapy and ergotherapy

Specialized clinics

- Lymphedema clinic
- Cancer nutrition and rehabilitation clinic
- Cancer related cognitive failure clinic
- Neuropathic cancer pain/methadone clinic

---

from specific single issues such as weight loss or lymphedema, to multiple palliative care issues, the physical settings should be variable. Our experience shows that a mixture of hospital bedrooms with private washroom, clinic type rooms, interview rooms, treatment room, and specific rooms with special research equipment, is ideal. The exact number is determined by the volume of daily visits. Sufficient space for patients and family members to relax should be provided such as a waiting room, kitchen, etc. A specific meeting room for family meetings or private discussions is essential to keep privacy. A unified, but well thought out, well planned central working area for the staff increases efficiency of communication and should not replace separate offices to allow team members to perform their charting and telephone communication. Finally, it is essential to plan a lounge area within the day hospital setting for the staff to rest in while remaining accessible to respond to patients and family during their resting time.

INSTRUMENTAL IN ALLOWING PALLIATIVE CARE RESEARCH

The PCDH has become over the years an important setting to enable research with this fragile population. Thorough palliative care assessment and optimal symptom management assure that only patients with sufficient stable condition are offered the opportunity to participate in research protocols. Also, accessing patients and family members with palliative care needs earlier on during the illness trajectory has made it feasible to study ongoing changes in quality of life over a longer time-frame, as well as the occurrence of early cognitive failure, the value of nutritional and rehabilitation interventions when anorexia-cachexia is only beginning, new drugs for the treatment of cancer pain that require patients with longer survivals, etc. The PCDH physical setting and organization provide a supervised environment sometimes needed in specific research protocols. The establishment of specialized clinics (see Box 35.4) within the PCDH has allowed the development of expertise in specific fields of research.

THE PALLIATIVE CARE DAY HOSPITAL IN NUMBERS

In 1999, after 9 months of operation, we reviewed 154 new consecutive referrals to the PCDH over a period of 8 months.[39*] Table 35.1 gives the characteristics of the patients at the initial PCDH visit. The reduced representation of patients with breast cancer is explained by the limited number of women treated in our hospital. As expected, the majority of patients had advanced disease but we were agreeably surprised by the number of patients with regional disease in need of symptom control. While some patients were followed-up from the palliative care inpatient services, the great majority (77 percent) were new referrals to palliative care. The symptom profile as measured by the ESAS was characterized by fatigue, loss of appetite, and decreased wellbeing, for which 50 percent of patients scored their level of distress as moderate to severe (>40 on a visual analog scale from 0 mm = no symptom to 100 mm = worst symptom). Pain remained quite prevalent at 69 percent with 35 percent of these patients expressing moderate to severe pain. In fact most of these patients needed some opioid

Table 35.1 *Characteristics of patients at the initial day hospital visit (N = 154)*

		Percent
Age in years (mean ± SD)	65.6 ± 12	
Sex, M/F	93/61	60/40
Primary cancer diagnosis		
Lung	36	23
Genitourinary	45	29
Gastrointestinal	45	29
Breast	9	6
Others	19	12
Extent of cancer		
Metastatic	112	73
Locoregional	42	27
Referral source		
New consults to palliative care	118	77
Follow-up from palliative care inpatient consultation service	36	23
Symptom profile prevalence (out of 144 patients)		
Pain	99	69
Decreased level of activity	127	88
Nausea	51	35
Depressive mood	73	51
Anxiety	98	68
Drowsiness	86	60
Lost of appetite	117	81
Shortness of breath	74	51
Decrease in wellbeing	125	87
Type of pain medication		
None	25	16
Acetaminophen or non-steroidal anti-inflammatory drugs	21	14
Codeine ± acetaminophen	25	16
Oxycodone	4	3
Morphine	45	29
Hydromorphone	17	11
Fentanyl patch	11	7
Other	6	4
Morphine equivalent daily dose in mg (mean ± SD)	118 ± 80	

adjustments: initiation (15 percent), increase (20 percent) or switch to other opioids (12 percent). Table 35.2 provides a summary of the follow-up of these patients. These 154 patients were seen 469 times. For 12 percent of patients, a same-day admission to the palliative care inpatient unit was necessary at their first visit. For the majority of patients (74 percent), one to three visits were sufficient to optimize their comfort and to arrange community-based care. However, 26 percent of patients needed four or more visits to be cared for by the PCDH team. This group of patients is composed of patients with difficult symptoms or psychosocial issues, and of patients without access to a family physician in the

Table 35.2 *Characteristics of the follow-up of the day hospital patients*

	N	Percent
Total number of day hospital visits	469	100
Number of direct admissions to the palliative care inpatient service	58	12
Number of day hospital visits per patient		
1	54	35
2	39	25
3	21	14
4–7	24	16
8 or more	16	10
Patient follow-up at the end or the chart review		
Number of patients still alive	33	21
Lost to follow-up	25	16
Number of patients deceased	96	62
Place of death (96 deaths)		
Home	21	22
Acute palliative care unit	33	34
Hospice	20	21
Hospital beds	22	23
Length of follow-up for deceased patients median (10th and 90th percentiles)	54 (15, 125)	

community. During this period, the specialized clinics (see Box 35.4) were not yet organized. With these new specialized clinics, patients with more than three visits to the PCDH should represent a higher proportion of the PCDH workload. The majority of patients were seen 2–3 months before death.

The cost of the PCDH has not been fully evaluated. In Quebec, physicians working in such settings are paid a fixed salary. The nurses and other team members are paid out of the palliative care service total budget. Transportation from home to the PCDH hospital is usually covered by the patients or their family. For patients 65 years and older, ambulance transportation is usually paid by social programs. The return transportation from the PCDH to home by ambulance or adapted transportation, if necessary, is covered by the hospital.

Is the PCDH cost effective? This remains to be determined as it has not been decided which outcomes should be used. For example, even if the majority of patients are still referred late in their illness trajectory, what is the exact value of earlier symptom management, especially through our specialized clinics? From a pure health service research perspective, the benefit of enhanced communication between the cancer center and the community-based services would need to be evaluated; the value of rapid referral back to the specialized palliative care based at the PCDH could be difficult to quantify; the continuum of care from specialized oncology services and hospital-based palliative care to

homecare services would also need to be evaluated; the prevention of emergency room visits should be quantified; a reduction in the utilization of inpatient beds could lead to cost saving but should be supported by evidence of good quality of care at home, etc. Of note, the closest similar experience available has been the one of multidisciplinary symptom control clinics based at a cancer center. Two similar clinics, one in Canada and another in the USA, were partially evaluated and were found to be effective in improving symptom control and patient satisfaction.[40,41] However, cost-effectiveness was not evaluated.

CONCLUSION

Assuring access to optimal care to patients in need of palliative care remains a challenge. The creation of day hospitals within the tertiary hospitals or the cancer centers is a valuable option for patients with advanced cancer who are still receiving active care and for those in the terminal phase of their illness who need rapid access to palliative care due to their deteriorating medical condition. Such a model of care could easily be extended to other advanced, life-threatening illnesses such as chronic obstructive pulmonary disease, congestive heart failure, and neurologic degenerative diseases.

Key learning points

- Access to optimal palliative care remains limited to the very few.

- A PCDH can increase access to palliative care.

- The PCDH cares for patients earlier during their illness.

- The PCDH links the tertiary care center with the community resources.

- A basic medico-nursing team promotes efficiency and integration of care.

- The PCDH provides access to specialized palliative care techniques.

- The PCDH offers an ideal setting for end-of-life clinical research.

REFERENCES

- 1 Wilkes E, Crowther AG, Greaves CW. A different kind of day hospital – for patients with preterminal cancer and chronic disease. *BMJ* 1978; **2**: 1053–6.
- 2 Clark D, ten Have H, Janssens R. Common threads? Palliative care service developments in seven European countries. *Palliat Med* 2000; **14**: 479–90.
- 3 Fisher RA, McDais P. *Palliative Day Care.* London: Arnold, 1996.

◆ 4 Hearn J, Myers K. *Palliative Day Care in Practice*. Oxford: Oxford University Press, 2001.

● 5 Goodwin DM, Higginson IJ, Myers K, *et al*. Effectiveness of palliative day care in improving pain, symptom control, and quality of life. *J Pain Symptom Manage* 2003; **25**: 202–12.

● 6 Higginson IJ, Hearn J, Myers K, Naysmith A. Palliative day care: what do services do? Palliative Day Care Project Group. *Palliat Med* 2000; **14**: 277–86.

◆ 7 MacDonald N. Palliative care – an essential component of cancer control. *Can Med Assoc J* 1998; **158**: 1709–16.

◆ 8 MacDonald N. Palliative care – the fourth phase of cancer prevention. *Cancer Detect Prev* 1991; **15**: 253–5.

◆ 9 MacDonald N. Is there evidence for earlier intervention in cancer-associated weight loss? *J Support Oncol* 2003; **1**: 279–86.

10 Evans LK, Forciea MA, Yurkow J, Sochalski J. The geriatric day hospital. In: Katz PR, Kane RL, Mezey MD, eds. *Emerging Systems in Long-Term Care*. New York: Springer Publishing Company, Inc., 1999: 67–87.

11 Densen PM. *Tracing the Elderly Through the Health Care System: An Update*. AHCPR 911–1 ed. Rockville, MD: Department of Health and Human Services, 1991.

12 Brocklehurst J. Geriatric day hospitals. *Age Ageing* 1995; **24**: 89–90.

13 Brockelhurst JC. The development and present status of day hospitals. *Age Ageing* 1979; **8**(suppl): 76–9.

14 Siu AL, Morishita L, Blaustein J. Comprehensive geriatric assessment in a day hospital. *J Am Geriatr Soc* 1994; **42**: 1094–9.

15 Forster A, Young J, Langhorne P. Systematic review of day hospital care for elderly people. The Day Hospital Group. *BMJ* 1999; **318**: 837–41.

16 Tousignant M, Hebert R, Desrosiers J, Hollander MJ. Economic evaluation of a geriatric day hospital: cost-benefit analysis based on functional autonomy changes. *Age Ageing* 2003; **32**: 53–9.

17 Cummings V, Kerner JF, Arones S, Steinbock C. Day hospital service in rehabilitation medicine: an evaluation. *Arch Phys Med Rehabil* 1985; **66**: 86–91.

18 Lorenz EJ, Hamill CM, Oliver RC. The day hospital: An alternative to institutional care. *J Am Geriatr Soc* 1974; **22**: 316–20.

19 Eng C, Pedulla J, Eleazer GP, *et al*. Program of All-inclusive Care for the Elderly (PACE): an innovative model of integrated geriatric care and financing. *J Am Geriatr Soc* 1997; **45**: 223–32.

20 Kallert TW, Glockner M, Priebe S, *et al*. A comparison of psychiatric day hospitals in five European countries: implications of their diversity for day hospital research. *Soc Psychiatry Psychiatr Epidemiol* 2004; **39**: 777–88.

21 Marshall M, Crowther R, Almaraz-Serrano A, *et al*. Systematic reviews of the effectiveness of day care for people with severe mental disorders: acute day hospital versus admission; vocational rehabilitation; day hospital versus outpatient care. *Health Technol Assess* 2001; **5**: 1–75.

22 Dekker R, Drost EA, Groothoff JW, *et al*. Effects of day-hospital rehabilitation in stroke patients: a review of randomized clinical trials. *Scand J Rehabil Med* 1998; **30**: 87–94.

23 Mor V, Stalker MZ, Gralla R, *et al*. Day hospital as an alternative to inpatient care for cancer patients: a random assignment trial. *J Clin Epidemiol* 1988; **41**: 771–85.

24 Rogge R. Diabetic day hospital in Wiesbaden: education and treatment under everyday conditions during job and leisure time. *Medizinische Welt* 2000; **51**: 219–22.

25 Wisseler HM, Lautenschlager J, Leichner-Hennig R, Henrich H. Rheumatological day clinic in the Auerbach Clinic Dr. Vetter – Beginnings and initial experiences. *Aktuelle Rheumatol* 2003; **28**: 30–5.

26 Gill HS, Walter DB. The day hospital model of care for patients with medical and rehabilitative needs. *Hosp Technol Serv* 1996; **15**: 1–14.

27 Capomolla S, Febo O, Ceresa M, *et al*. Cost/utility ratio in chronic heart failure: comparison between heart failure management program delivered by day-hospital and usual care. *J Am Coll Cardiol* 2002; **40**: 1259–66.

28 Biem HJ, Cotton D, McNeil S, Boechler A, Gudmundson D. Day medicine: an urgent internal medicine clinic and medical procedures suite. *Healthcare Manage Forum* 2003; **16**: 17–23.

29 Benjamin LJ, Swinson GI, Nagel RL. Sickle cell anemia day hospital: an approach for the management of uncomplicated painful crises. *Blood* 2000; **95**: 1130–6.

30 Wright J, Bareford D, Wright C, *et al*. Day case management of sickle pain: 3 years experience in a UK sickle cell unit. *Br J Haematol* 2004; **126**: 878–80.

● 31 Gagnon B, Mayo NE, Hanley J, MacDonald N. Pattern of care at the end of life: does age make a difference in what happens to women with breast cancer? *J Clin Oncol* 2004; **22**: 3458–65.

● 32 Teno JM, Weitzen S, Fennell ML, Mor V. Dying trajectory in the last year of life: does cancer trajectory fit other diseases? *J Palliat Med* 2001; **4**: 457–64.

● 33 Lunney JR, Lynn J, Foley DJ, *et al*. Patterns of functional decline at the end of life. *JAMA* 2003; **289**: 2387–92.

● 34 Langley-Evans A, Payne S. Light-hearted death talk in a palliative day care context. *J Adv Nurs* 1997; **26**: 1091–7.

● 35 Bruera E, Kuehn N, Miller MJ, *et al*. The Edmonton Symptom Assessment System (ESAS): a simple method for the assessment of palliative care patients. *J Palliat Care* 1991; **7**: 6–9.

● 36 Anderson F, Downing GM, Hill J, *et al*. Palliative performance scale (PPS): a new tool. *J Palliat Care* 1996; **12**: 5–11.

● 37 Folstein MF, Folstein SE, Mchugh PR. Mini-Mental State – practical method for grading cognitive state of patients for clinician. *J Psychiatr Res* 1975; **12**: 189–98.

◆ 38 Gagnon B, Mancini I, Pereira J, Bruera E. Palliative management of bleeding events in advanced cancer patients. *J Palliat Care* 1998; **14**: 50–4.

39 Schreier G, Gagnon B, Lawlor K. The McGill University Health Center Palliative Care Day Hospital: A Unique Approach. Palliative Care Conference – Palliative Care in Different Cultures, Jerusalem, Israel, 19–23 March, 2000 [abstract].

40 Bruera E, Michaud M, Vigano A, *et al*. Multidisciplinary symptom control clinic in a cancer center: a retrospective study. *Support Care Cancer* 2001; **9**: 162–8.

41 Strasser F, Sweeney C, Willey J, *et al*. Impact of a half-day multidisciplinary symptom control and palliative care outpatient clinic in a comprehensive cancer center on recommendations, symptom intensity, and patient satisfaction: a retrospective descriptive study. *J Pain Symptom Manage* 2004; **27**: 481–91.

36

Inpatient hospices

JEREMY KEEN

EVOLUTION OF INPATIENT HOSPICES

The lineage of modern inpatient hospices is usually traced back to the medieval hospices that were initially 'guest-houses' (from the Latin, *hospitium*) run by religious orders for journeying pilgrims. These hospices inevitably became involved in the care of sick and dying travelers hoping for miraculous cures at the shrines to which they were heading. It is interesting to note that the words hospice, hospital, and hospitality are derived from the Latin, *hospes*, which has had different meanings as either 'guest/stranger' or 'host' at different times in history. This reflects the intimate relationship between carer and the 'cared-for' and was integral to the aspirations of the modern hospice movement.

The history of hospice evolution is punctuated by a series of remarkable individuals, mostly women, mostly with a religious conviction, who have sought to offer hospitality to the dying. Jeanne Garnier formed L'Association des Dames du Calvaire in Lyon in 1842, and opened a home for the dying the following year. The development of hospice and palliative care in Paris and New York can trace its lineage directly back to Jeanne Garnier and this first establishment in Lyon. As Superior of the Irish Sisters of Charity, Mary Aikenhead was instrumental in the opening of St Vincent's Hospital, Dublin, in 1834. Fulfilling her long-held ambition, the convent where she spent her final years became Our Lady's Hospice for the Dying in 1879. The Sisters of Charity opened St Joseph's Hospice in East London in 1905 and other hospices were to follow in Australia, Canada, and Scotland. During the period between 1879 and 1905 four other institutions opened in London specifically for the care of the 'dying poor' but did not call themselves hospices. St Luke's Home for the Dying Poor opened in 1893, was the only institution established by a doctor and its organization

of services and delivery of care was most closely linked to that developed in modern hospices. Although St Luke's employed lay nursing staff rather than those drawn from religious orders, as in the other establishments, the emphasis was still firmly on spiritual care. Dr Howard Barrett the founder of St Luke's wrote:

> It is much if we can render the last weeks and months less destitute of comfort, less tortured by pain. It is far more if through any instrumentality of ours some become humble followers of Christ.

Interested readers are directed to an excellent review of the development of hospices in the period 1878–1914.[1] The influence of St Luke's on the development of the 'modern hospice' is due in no small part to the time spent in St Luke's by Dame Cicely Saunders as a volunteer nurse. When planning St Christopher's Hospice, Dr Saunders stated:

> The name hospice, 'a resting place for travellers or pilgrims', was chosen because this will be something between a hospital and a home, with the skills of one and the hospitality, warmth, and the time of the other.

She sought to capture the hospitality of hospice but recognized that this was not enough on its own to ensure the optimal relief of suffering. Her vision for the model, upon which so many hospices in the UK and elsewhere are based, very much included aspirations toward research and the application of best evidence as an integral part of the provision of care.

After St Christopher's opened in 1967 there was a steady growth in the number of hospices opening in the UK and, internationally, a growth in the 'Hospice Movement' which has developed and adapted the philosophy of hospice care most often in a community setting rather than in institutions called 'hospices'. Hospice care in the USA is an obvious example of a community-based service with statistics for 2003 showing that only 3.4 percent of patient days in hospice care were spent as inpatients in a hospice and only 6.1 percent of deaths in hospice care occurred in an inpatient hospice unit.[2] The philosophy of hospice care was first formally introduced into the general hospital setting by Dr Balfour Mount, who, having spent time training at St Christopher's Hospice, established a 'Palliative Care' service in Montreal in 1975.

The rate at which new hospices (for adults) opened in the UK reached a peak during the late 1980s and early 1990s (Fig. 36.1) with the majority resulting from local community enthusiasm and support rather than NHS planning.[4] The overall numbers of hospices reached a plateau in the mid-1990s. The latest statistics (2005[5]) report 220 specialist palliative care units in the UK of which 64 are totally funded by the National Health Service (NHS), and are usually situated within acute hospitals, and the remainder are independent hospices. The NHS units tend to be smaller (mean of 10.4 beds compared with 16.0 beds in independent hospices) but have very similar levels of staffing, discharge rates, and lengths of stay. The population cared for within hospices also appears to have stabilized (Box 36.1) with little obvious change over many years with approximately 95 percent of patients having a diagnosis of cancer and 96 percent being of a white ethnic background. All independent hospices in the UK now tender their services to the NHS and in so doing receive contributions approximating to one-third of their total budget. The UK government is committed to increasing its contribution to care within the independent sector but with 'strings attached' to ensure equity of access regardless of, for example, diagnosis or ethnicity.[6] This is significant for although the majority of hospices have not excluded those with diagnoses other than cancer, they equally may not have actively advertised their services for this population.

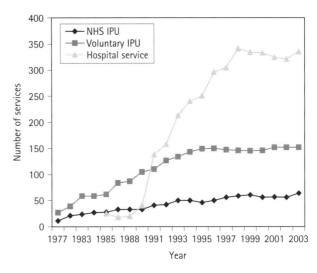

Figure 36.1   *The growth in numbers of inpatient hospices (IPUs) and hospital palliative care services in the UK (data taken from Hospice Information 2003[3]).*

Box 36.1   Inpatient hospices in the UK. Service provision 2003[3]

- Total number of adult hospices and palliative care units – 216

- Beds per million population (adults) – 51

- Beds per hospice (average)– 15

- Most common size – 10 beds

- Mean length of stay – 13.5 days

- Average discharge rate – 50 percent

In the UK the hospices have remained a focus of inpatient palliative care, research, and education. However, since the recognition of palliative medicine as a specialty by the Royal College of Physicians in 1987 and the proliferation of hospital-based services and academic departments of palliative medicine and care (see Fig. 36.1) the main focus, particularly in terms of research, has tended to shift toward the teaching hospital. This has increased awareness and acceptance of the specialty in mainstream medicine and nursing and eased the break from the perceived constraints of the hospices, by providing care for patients regardless of diagnosis and exploring 'supportive care' for patients at earlier stages of a disease process.[7,8]

Perhaps partly as a result of the recognition of palliative medicine as a specialty questions were raised as to the validity of hospices as separate institutions for the dying.[7] They were famously described as being 'too good to be true and too small to be useful'[9,10] and simply providing, to quote a general surgeon at a national meeting, 'designer deaths'. At the same time as voices outside the discipline were beginning to question hospice care, warnings were being issued from within the ranks.[11–13] Although the future of palliative and supportive care within mainstream hospital services seems to be assured, authors have continued to echo Professor David Clark's question: 'Whither the hospices?'.[14]

The development of hospices outwith the NHS, for the most part, facilitated the introduction and development of new models of care with an emphasis on an holistic approach dependent on true multidisciplinary teamworking. Features of these approaches, even the associated symbiotic 'niceness behavior' as recognized and defined by a recent study[15] are now found within mainstream medicine but, equally, increasing technology and issues of clinical governance have found their way back into the hospices. As the systems of care come closer together there is a danger that, for hospice care at least, the original concepts become lost in a drift toward medicalization and bureaucracy. However, the maintenance of independent institutions with little national governance or accountability brings with it the danger of inequitable delivery of services, little in the way of quality control and a lack of coordination in efforts to improve the delivery of care.[16,17]

As hospices struggle with their changing role in patient care, perhaps their origins will provide a key to their further evolution. The rate of development in knowledge of symptom control has not been matched by development (or rediscovery?) of spiritual care. Now perhaps, as at no other time in history, the spiritual needs of those suffering life-limiting illnesses, with little in the way of personal religious terms of reference or the distraction of overriding physical symptoms, are becoming obvious. To use the relative freedoms of independent institutions to maintain excellence in symptom control but also to address other aspects of suffering in a novel and creative fashion may be a way forward. This may begin to ease the tensions of some of those working in hospices who feel they have become part of 'just another specialty'.[13]

WHO IS ADMITTED TO A HOSPICE?

Figures for 2001–02 show that 41 000 people in the UK were admitted to a hospice for the first time.[3] Hospices had a total of 59 000 admissions with an estimated 29 000 people dying during their inpatient stay. In England and Wales 4.3 percent of all deaths occurred in 'freestanding' hospices[18] (the Office for National Statistics is unable to separate figures for Palliative Care Units within an acute NHS hospital). Of these deaths 96 percent were certified to be due to malignancy, which demonstrates no change in the population as defined by diagnosis over the 5 years from 1998 for which statistics were accessible. The age distribution of inpatients at time of death is portrayed in Figure 36.2. Data from England and Wales in 2002 demonstrate 15.7 percent of all cancer deaths occurring in freestanding hospices compared with 22.2 percent at home and 50 percent in NHS-run institutions (hospitals and some care homes) with the age distribution shown in Figure 36.3. If deaths in NHS-run palliative care units are accounted for then figures approximate to 19 percent of cancer deaths occurring in palliative care/hospice units.[3] This represents a continuation of a trend noted by Higginson in her analysis of English data between 1985 and 1994, toward an increase in deaths in hospice and overall decline in deaths at home.[19] She added in a subsequent study that the overall proportion of deaths at home hid variations dependent upon social and geographical parameters.[20*]

Douglas in his oft quoted 'Personal View' in the *BMJ* observed, among other accusations, that the independent hospice movement was inefficient in that it provided 'deluxe' care for a favored minority.[9] A review of data generated by the Regional Study of Care of the Dying sought to address the issue of which cancer patients, dying in 1990, received inpatient hospice care.[21*] Statistically, five factors were found to independently predict hospice inpatient care: having pain in the last year of life, having constipation, being dependent

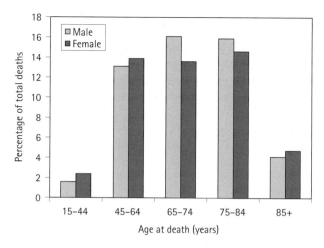

Figure 36.2 *Distribution of deaths in 2002 in independent hospices in the UK by age group. Data from Office for National Statistics.[18]*

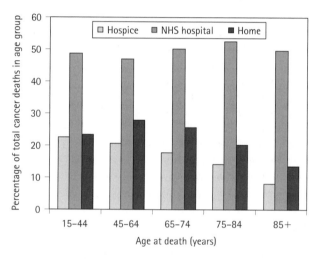

Figure 36.3 *Distribution of deaths from cancer in the UK in 2002 by place of death and age at time of death. Data from Office for National Statistics.[18]*

on others for help with activities of daily living for between 1 and 6 months before death, having breast cancer, and being under 85 years of age. Hinton demonstrated a higher rate of admission among patients receiving palliative home care in those who were living alone or with unfit relatives and those with breast cancer.[22] Patients and relatives felt that the principal problems triggering admission were most frequently, weakness, pain or depression, and anxiety. A further study of data relating to cancer deaths in 1991 compared those who had accessed any palliative care service, including home care, with those who had not.[23*] The group accessing palliative care services were significantly younger, had longer survival times from diagnosis and tended to have been referred from certain general practices. Although it may be that general practitioner referral patterns contribute to a recognized inequity of access to palliative care across the UK,[5,24*] geographical and historical factors are likely to be more important. An analysis of place of death of cancer patients in the North West of England demonstrated an increased likelihood of dying in a hospice if they lived close by.[25] Wood *et al.* have suggested a method of analyzing the provision of inpatient hospice care to a geographical region with particular reference to estimated level of demand, ease of accessibility in terms of 'drive-time', and levels of material deprivation.[26] In so doing the group was able to define an area within their region in which there was potential high demand, poor access, and high levels of deprivation, and which therefore merited a discussion of additional inpatient hospice provision.

A recent systematic review of access and referral to specialist palliative care found a lack of standardized criteria to guide referral.[27***] There are no national referral guidelines in the UK but most areas will have locally based guidance.[28]

The issue of the provision of hospice care for those with diagnoses other than cancer has been debated for several years now. Although many working within hospices would agree with the principle of broadening the diagnostic criteria for admission and are being encouraged to do so by the UK government there is little evidence that the hospice inpatient population is actually changing. This is likely to be a result of a perceived, and in some areas real, lack of skills and expertise among hospice staff in terms of assessing patients for admission and ongoing clinical management. There is, in addition, an ongoing perception that services will be overwhelmed by referrals. It is interesting to contrast the situation in the UK with the demographics of hospice care in the USA where only 49 percent of admissions carry a diagnosis of cancer. However, with Medicare funding only 20 days of hospice care the vast majority of patients referred are clearly in the final stages of their disease processes (35 per cent of patients die within 7 days of commencing hospice care).[2] The difficulty with prognosis in earlier stages of nonmalignant disorders has made hospices in the UK wary of potential long-term commitments and an ever-increasing rise in the number of patients 'on the books'. The introduction of NHS funding of care deemed 'palliative' in community-based care homes has focused awareness of the level of palliative care expertise that exists within these institutions. Educational initiatives are underway, some based in hospices, which not only afford support for the care homes but also allow a reverse flow of education back to the hospices in terms of the palliative care needs of the general population.[29]

WHAT DO HOSPICES PROVIDE?

The majority of hospices in the UK are staffed by at least one full time physician trained in palliative medicine, nurses, physiotherapists, occupational therapists, social workers and chaplains. Luxurious staffing levels in comparison to NHS hospitals ensure perhaps the most important aspect of care delivered to patients is the carer's time (1.88 trained nurses

per hospice bed is the national average). In addition to providing inpatient end-stage care, hospices accept admissions for symptom control, rehabilitation and often, but not always, respite care. Most inpatient hospices will also provide day care and run multidisciplinary outpatient services for general palliative care needs and increasingly symptom-specific clinics for the management of, for example, lymphedema and breathlessness. In the independent hospices particularly, both inpatients and day patients may be able to access complementary therapies and in some units art and music therapy. The majority of hospices offer bereavement support services. The hospice and its staff will also act as a resource for the community providing advice and education to health workers and carers, and practical support in terms of equipment loans.

ARE HOSPICES SUCCESSFUL?

Literature supporting the care afforded by hospices is sparse certainly in terms of strictly controlled studies of sound methodology. Despite this, however, the independent hospices, in which are to be found 68 percent of available hospice beds, continue to find funds from charitable giving and operate large armies of volunteers. A survey of 2000 members of the public drawn randomly from the population in the UK asked participants to rank 12 different areas of healthcare in order of priority.[30] Interestingly, 'special care and pain relief for people who are dying' was ranked second overall to 'treatments for children with life-threatening diseases', coming above such services as hip replacements, transplant surgery, community nursing and psychiatric services. The area of care ranked as the lowest priority was care for those over 75 years of age with acute life-threatening illness.

The measurement of influence upon an individual patient's experience of hospice care is both a personal (for the hospice worker) and institutional problem. Outcomes in palliative care have often been developed to justify the service and have examined parameters that are relatively easily measured, for example, time of response to a referral, waiting times for admission, and pain and symptom control assessments. The early studies by Parkes at St Christopher's Hospice were encouraging but the methodology of retrospective carer interviews has been questioned.[31,32] Nonetheless the carers of those in the hospice were much less anxious than those with relatives in hospital and, additionally, felt part of a 'family' in the hospice. It is of interest to note the implied improvement in hospital care noted in the 10-year period between the comparative studies and the resulting relatively minor perceived difference between hospital and hospice care. This finding, in terms of the surviving spouse's perception of physical symptom control, was confirmed in a later study.[33] This is somewhat discouraging of further attempts at evaluation for a service that remains in a continuing battle for financial support. The focus for hospices has shifted toward satisfying nationally approved standards of care that are for the most part derived from easily measurable components of service provision (e.g., QIS [NHS Quality Improvement Scotland] in Scotland). However, Needham and Newbury have recently attempted to give an evaluation of care, in an individual hospice, by assessing outcomes in terms of the achievement of individual goals set at the start of an admission by the patient, main carer, and hospice staff.[34*] Interestingly, the authors report a trend toward patients' and carers' goals of admission being more specific and functional compared with those of the staff that were more symptom or problem orientated. However, the large majority of goals evaluated from the three different perspectives were at least partially achieved in those patients discharged from hospice, with evaluations by carers and family of those dying proving difficult to obtain. More goals set by the staff were at least partially achieved than those goals set by patients or their main carers. This may reflect more realistic goal setting, optimistic assessments or possibly the relatively poor ability to identify patients' 'goals' demonstrated in an earlier study of hospice nurses.[35*] The words of Dame Cicely Saunders from over 20 years ago still need to be heeded:[36]

> No patient will thank you for much handholding or sympathetic counselling unless the things he or she perceives as the basics at that moment are attended to first.

The studies at St Christopher's Hospice comparing hospice and hospital care from the viewpoint of the surviving spouse found a consistent impression of a better social and psychological environment within the hospice compared to the hospital.[31,33*] A more recent study of patient and carer satisfaction suggested a greater influence on 'satisfaction with care' from perceived quality of life within hospice than from the presence of physical symptoms.[37*] This, as the authors observe, may reflect the general improvement over time in physical symptom control that is now occurring before admission to hospice.

If a person receiving palliative care is to be aided to 'live until he dies at his own maximum potential', again quoting Dame Cicely Saunders,[38] then this should be reflected in a wish within hospices to seek to maximize an individual's quality of life. A systematic review could find no evidence that inpatient hospices improved patient's quality of life[39***] but discussed the lack of good quality research and made suggestions of how outcomes may be assessed. However a more recent single study did suggest that quality of life improves after admission to a sample of palliative care units in Canada.[40*] However, the study quoted recognized its limitations with a mere 12 percent of admissions able to complete the study tool on admission, and only 8 percent a follow-up interview 1 week later. The study used the McGill Quality of Life Questionnaire (MQOL) and was able to show improvements in physical, psychological and existential domains. Earlier work by the same author demonstrated the importance of the 'meaningful existence' subscale of the MQOL in determining overall quality of life in palliative care.[41] The goal of improving quality of life particularly through addressing issues surrounding the preservation of a meaningful existence such as, for example the maintenance of dignity and personhood[42,43] may become an increasing focus of research and development in care in inpatient hospices in the future.

CONCLUSIONS

The modern hospice movement and the specialty of palliative care has revolutionized the approach to the care of those living and dying with incurable illness. Inpatient hospices modeled on St Christopher's Hospice are now to be found in all parts of the world, although it is hospice as a philosophy of care, in the community or hospital, that has been developed most widely.

Inpatient hospices have proved over the centuries to be institutions that have been visionary in terms of providing for gaps in the provision of care for others. The early medieval hospices spawned hospitals and later the modern hospices which very much maintained the central ethos of providing hospitality for the stranger with the spiritual dimension of care as critical to this process. The 'modern' hospice in the UK, with independence in terms of resources and management structure, enjoyed space for the development of true holistic care and the new specialty of palliative care. The control of physical symptoms in the first phase of modern hospice development proved to be of overriding importance, and necessarily so because, just as in the care of any individual patient, one cannot address psychospiritual issues to any depth in the setting of uncontrolled physical symptoms. However, with a slowing of the rate of new developments in physical symptom control, and with the aid of comprehensive education programs, often run by the hospices, clinicians other than specialists in palliative care are able to provide a very good level of symptom control. Often initially attracted into hospice work by these early major advancements in patient care, individual staff in the UK are now having to examine their role in patient care and are dealing with new stresses. This may be particularly pertinent for practitioners who are hospice based rather than hospital-based specialists in palliative care.

A recent observational study submitted for a PhD has noted that in a freestanding hospice patients were left alone for significant amounts of time and reminds us of the power of 'being with' as a fundamental of hospice care and hospitality (E Haraldsdottir, personal communication, 2004). So, it could be asked, has care in hospices become too medicalized so that the carer's time is consumed by too many medical interventions? Have hospices, by becoming specialist palliative care units, taken on too broad a spectrum of patients so that those who are dying and 'comfortable' are not afforded as much time as others? Do we feel helpless in the light of our patients' significant emotional and spiritual difficulties unmasked by good symptom control? In response to these sorts of questions there have been calls for 'hospice care' and 'palliative care' in the UK to proceed as distinct specialties,[44] in a somewhat similar fashion to the evolution of end-of-life care in North America.

The debate over the role and future of hospices has been ongoing since the early 1980s perhaps, in part, for reasons summed up eloquently by Torrens[45] as quoted by Small:[46]

> Early on it was clear who the villains and the heroes were, where the challenges lay, what were the pitfalls to be avoided. There was the good work and it was easy to devote one's life. . . . I think now we have passed that stage and ahead lie many diverse paths, many confusions of a subtler nature.

Now, nearly 25 years later, perhaps it is finally time for the hospices to admit their strengths and opportunities. The hospices do have the space, time and expertise to critically push forward psychological and particularly spiritual care. The acknowledgment of the existential dimension to suffering has always been fundamental to any definition of what hospices do and many authors have explored the approaches that can be taken within hospices and in palliative care. However, it is only now that, in general terms, patients have the relative freedom from physical symptoms and the hospices are perhaps mature enough to seriously explore these issues. If history is anything to go by this would only be good news for the hospitals and healthcare of tomorrow.

Key learning points

- Modern inpatient hospices evolved from institutions for the dying where spiritual care was paramount.

- There has been a phenomenal spread of the hospice movement and palliative care principally through the activity of early hospice practitioners.

- Significant developments in palliative and now supportive care are increasingly centered on the provision of care in mainstream hospitals.

- The value and role of inpatient hospice care has been questioned by the healthcare professions, but not by the lay public.

- There is little good quality research measuring the contribution inpatient hospice care makes to patient care.

- Recent research into the maintenance of personhood and dignity with an emphasis on the spiritual and psychological aspects of care may point the way to major areas of influence that inpatient hospices may have on palliative and general medical care in the future.

REFERENCES

◆ 1 Humphreys C. 'Waiting for the last summons': the establishment of the first hospices in England 1878–1914. *Mortality* 2001; **6**: 146–66.

2 National Hospice and Palliative Care Organization. Hospice facts and figures 2005. www.nhpco.org (accessed July 14, 2005).

3 Hospice Information. *Hospice and Palliative Care Facts and Figures 2003.* London: Hospice Information, 2003.

4 Clark D, Neale B, Heather P. Contracting for palliative care. *Soc Sci Med* 1995; **40**: 1193–202.

5 Hospice Information. *Hospice and Palliative Care Facts and Figures 2005.* London: Hospice Information, 2005.

6 HM Government UK. Government response to house of commons health committee report on palliative care. Fourth report of session 2003–4. London, HMSO, 2004.

7 National Institute for Clinical Excellence (NICE) *Improving Supportive and Palliative Care for Adults with Cancer (Cancer Service Guidance), 2004.* Published by National Institute for Clinical Excellence and King's College, London. Available at: www.nice.org.uk/page.aspx?o=110005 (accessed October 24, 2004).

8 Cherny NI, Catane R, Kosmodis P. ESMO takes a stand on supportive and palliative care. *Ann Oncol* 2003; **14**: 1335–7.

9 Douglas C. For all the saints. *BMJ* 1992; **304**: 479.

◆ 10 Seale CF. What happens in hospices: a review of research evidence. *Soc Sci Med* 1989; **28**: 551–9.

11 James N, Field D. The routinization of hospice: charisma and bureaucratization. *Soc Sci Med* 1992; **34**: 1363–75.

12 Scott JF. Palliative care 2000: what's stopping us? *J Palliat Care* 1992; **8**: 5–8.

● 13 Kearney M. Palliative medicine – just another specialty? *Palliat Med* 1992; **6**: 39–46.

14 Clark D. Whither the hospices? In Clark D, ed. *The Future for Palliative Care: Issues of Policy and Practice.* Open University Press, 1993:167–77.

● 15 Li S. 'Symbiotic niceness': constructing a therapeutic relationship in psychosocial palliative care. *Soc Sci Med* 2004; **58**: 2571–83.

16 Bradshaw PJ. Characteristics of clients referred to home, hospice and hospital palliative care services in Western Australia. *Palliat Med* 1993; **7**: 101–7.

◆ 17 Payne S. To supplant, supplement or support? Organisational issues for hospices. *Soc Sci Med* 1998; **46**: 1495–504.

18 Office for National Statistics. *Mortality Statistics 2002, Series DHT No. 29.* Office for National Statistics, London. Available at: www.statistics.gov.uk/downloads/theme_health/Dh2_29/DH2No29.pdf (accessed October 24, 2004).

◆ 19 Higginson IJ, Astin P, Dolan S. Where do cancer patients die? Ten-year trends in the place of death of cancer patients in England. *Palliat Med* 1998; **12**: 353–63.

20 Higginson IJ, Jarman B, Astin P, Dolan S. Do social factors affect where patients die: an analysis of 10 years of cancer deaths in England. *J Public Health Med* 1999; **21**: 22–8.

● 21 Addington-Hall J, Altmann D, McCarthy M. Which terminally ill cancer patients receive hospice in-patient care? *Soc Sci Med* 1998; **46**: 1011–16.

22 Hinton J. Which patients with terminal cancer are admitted from home care? *Palliat Med* 1994; **8**: 197–210.

23   Gray JD, Forster DP. Factors associated with the utilization of specialist palliative care services: a population based study. *J Public Health Med* 1997; **19**: 464–9.

24   Shipman C, Addington-Hall J, Barclay S, *et al.* How and why do GPs use specialist palliative care services? *Palliat Med* 2002; **16**: 241–6.

25   Gatrell AC, Harman J, Francis BJ, *et al.* Place of death: analysis of cancer deaths in part of North West England. *J Public Health Med* 2003; **25**: 53–8.

26   Wood DJ, Clark D, Gatrell AC. Equity of access to adult hospice inpatient care within north-west England. *Palliat Med* 2004; **18**: 543–9.

◆ 27   Ahmed N, Bestall JC, Ahmedzai SH, *et al.* Systematic review of the problems and issues of accessing specialist palliative care by patients, carers and health and social care professionals. *Palliat Med* 2004; **18**: 525–42.

28   Bennett M, Adam J, Alison D, *et al.* Leeds eligibility criteria for specialist palliative care services. *Palliat Med* 2000; **14**: 157–8.

29   Froggatt KA. Palliative care and nursing homes: where next? *Palliat Med* 2001; **15**: 42–8.

30   Bowling A. Health care rationing: the public's debate. *BMJ* 1996; **312**: 670–4.

● 31   Parkes CM, Parkes J. 'Hospice' versus 'hospital' care – re-evaluation after 10 years as seen by surviving spouses. *Postgrad Med J* 1984; **60**: 120–4.

32   Hinton J. How reliable are relatives' retrospective reports of terminal illness? Patients and relatives' accounts compared. *Soc Sci Med* 1996; **43**: 1229–36.

33   Seale C, Kelly M. A comparison of hospice and hospital care for people who die: views of the surviving spouse. *Palliat Med* 1997; **11**: 93–100.

● 34   Needham PR, Newbury J. Goal setting as a measure of outcome in palliative care. *Palliat Med* 2004; **18**: 444–51.

● 35   Heaven CM, Maguire P. Disclosure of concerns by hospice patients and their identification by nurses. *Palliat Med* 1997; **11**: 283–90.

36   Saunders C. The hospice: its meaning to patients and their physicians. *Hosp Prac (Off Ed)* 1981; **16**: 93–108.

37   Tierney RM, Horton SM, Hannan TJ, Tierney WM. Relationships between symptom relief, quality of life, and satisfaction with hospice care. *Palliat Med* 1998; **12**: 333–44.

38   Saunders C. Foreward. In Doyle D, Hanks G, MacDonald N, eds. *Oxford Textbook of Palliative Medicine*, 2nd ed. Oxford: Oxford University Press, 1998.

◆ 39   Salisbury C, Bosanquet N, Wilkinson EK, *et al.* The impact of different models of specialist palliative care on patients' quality of life: a systematic literature review. *Palliat Med* 1999; **13**: 3–17.

● 40   Cohen SR, Boston P, Mount BM, Porterfield P. Changes in quality of life following admission to palliative care units. *Palliat Med* 2001; **15**: 363–71.

41   Cohen SR, Mount BM, Strobel MG, Bui F. The McGill Quality of Life Questionnaire: a measure of quality of life appropriate for people with advanced disease. A preliminary study of validity and acceptability. *Palliat Med* 1995; **9**: 207–19.

● 42   Chochinov HM. Dignity-conserving care – a new model for palliative care: helping the patient feel valued. *JAMA* 2002; **287**: 2253–60.

43   Kabel A, Roberts D. Professionals' perceptions of maintaining personhood in hospice care. *Int J Palliat Nurs* 2003; **9**: 283–9.

44   Biswas B. The medicalization of dying: a nurse's view. In Clark D, ed. *The Future for Palliative Care: Issues of Policy and Practice.* Buckingham: Open University Press, 1993: 132–9.

45   Torrens P. Achievement, failure and the future: hospice analyzed. In Saunders C, Summers DH, Teller N, eds. *Hospice: The Living Idea.* London: Edward Arnold, 1981: 187–94.

46   Small N. HIV/AIDS: Lessons for policy and practice. In Clark D, ed. *The Future for Palliative Care: Issues of Policy and Practice.* Buckingham: Open University Press, 1993: 80–97.

37

The palliative care unit

SHARON WATANABE, KAREN MACMILLAN

INTRODUCTION

The term 'palliative care unit' usually applies to a group of beds designated for the care of patients with terminal illness, located in an acute care hospital. Various models of palliative care units are possible, depending on local needs, resources, system characteristics and philosophies of care. Potential options in the design of a palliative care unit are listed in Table 37.1, each of which presents advantages and disadvantages.[1] Reasons for admission to a palliative care unit may include symptom control, terminal care, respite care, special treatment and investigations, and rehabilitation.[2] However, the availability of diagnostics, procedures, support services and consultants in an acute care hospital makes palliative care units particularly suited to the care of patients with problems of a complex nature.

A tertiary palliative care unit is a distinct type of palliative care unit, defined as an 'academic medical (center) where specialist knowledge for the most complex cases is practiced, researched and taught'.[1] The purpose of this chapter is to describe and discuss the role, structure, and operation of a tertiary palliative care unit, using the authors' unit in Edmonton, Canada as an example.

CONTEXT

The Tertiary Palliative Care Unit (TPCU) in Edmonton is an integral component of the Capital Health Regional Palliative Care Program.[3] This publicly funded program provides a comprehensive range of palliative care services, including home care and specialist consultation in the community,

Table 37.1 *Options in the design of palliative care units*[1]

Design element	Options
Location	Inside/outside main hospital
Admission policy	Open (any physician)/closed (specialist only)
Visiting hours	Open/limited
Source of admissions	Direct from home/in-hospital transfer only
Range of procedures, tests, therapies	Unlimited/limited
Do-not-resuscitate status	Required/not required

long-term care, ambulatory care, and acute care settings. It also supports designated units in long-term care facilities (i.e. hospices) for patients who have a life expectancy of 2 months or less.

The TPCU is located in an acute care teaching hospital. It consists of 14 private rooms in a dedicated geographical area. Amenities include a patient smoking room, a family lounge, a kitchenette, a quiet room, and a conference room. Family members may stay overnight if they wish, and pets are allowed.

PATIENT SELECTION

Admission criteria for the TPCU are listed in Box 37.1. The role of the TPCU is to provide care for the subset of patients who have the most complex problems and who require the intensive involvement of a specialist interdisciplinary team. The problems may be in the physical, psychologic, social, or spiritual domains. Although no limitations are placed on diagnosis, the vast majority of patients have cancer as their primary illness. Unlike the hospice setting, life expectancy is not specified. However, the TPCU is intended as a temporary place of care, until symptoms have stabilized sufficiently to allow discharge to another setting. Patients are asked to agree to a 'do-not-resuscitate' status prior to admission; the pros and cons of this policy will be reviewed later in this chapter.

Box 37.1 Admission criteria for the Tertiary Palliative Care Unit, Edmonton, Canada

- Experiencing progressive disease where the focus of care is on comfort, not cure, and improving quality of life

- Requiring active care to alleviate distressing symptoms related to physical, psychosocial and spiritual needs

- Severe symptom problems for which management has not been successful in any of the other settings, and requiring intensive management

- Expected length of stay of approximately 2 weeks

- Over 18 years of age

- Accepting of do-not-resuscitate status

Referrals are screened by the palliative care consultants covering the various settings. The consultant determines, after direct assessment of the patient, whether or not a referral to the TPCU is indicated. The goals of admission to the TPCU and the temporary nature of the admission are discussed with the patient and family. The consultant is also responsible for confirming and documenting that the patient accepts a do-not-resuscitate status.

Once admission has been agreed upon, the patient's medical records are forwarded to the TPCU. The referrals are triaged to determine priority. Patients are usually scheduled for admission on weekday mornings. This allows sufficient time for a comprehensive assessment and discussion of the goals and plan of care with the patient and family. However, admissions for problems requiring urgent intervention can be accommodated 24 hours a day, 7 days a week.

STAFFING

Staffing of the TPCU is described in Table 37.2. The patients are admitted under the care of physicians who are specialists in palliative medicine, one of whom also assumes the medical

Table 37.2 *Staffing of the Tertiary Palliative Care Unit at Edmonton, Canada*

Type of staff	Full-time equivalent
Registered nurses	8.81 (2 per shift)
Licensed practical nurses	8.0 (2–4 per shift)
Nursing attendants	1.4 (1 per night shift)
Physicians	2.5
Chaplain	1.0
Social worker	1.0
Physical therapist	0.6
Occupational therapist	0.5
Dietician	0.2
Pharmacist	0.2
Clinical educator	1.0
Program manager	1.0
Unit clerks	1.7
Secretaries	1.6

administrative responsibilities. The nurses function in a team nursing model and work 8-hour shifts. The complexity of the patient population necessitates the inclusion of the chaplain, social worker, physical therapist, occupational therapist, pharmacist, and dietician as core members of the team. The program manager is charged with the organizational administrative responsibilities of the TPCU. The clinical educator arranges the admissions and supports the team's educational needs. The unit clerks, secretaries, and volunteers play an essential supporting role.

Other hospital support services, such as respiratory therapy, are frequently involved. The TPCU has a formal arrangement with an anesthesiology service at another acute care hospital for support for procedures such as spinal administration of analgesics. Patients are often referred to the regional cancer center for palliative oncological therapies. Other specialists may be accessed from within the hospital as needed.

ASSESSMENT

The tools routinely employed on the TPCU are listed in Table 37.3. Many were developed on the TPCU itself.[4-8] The tools have been adopted in all the settings of the Capital Health Regional Palliative Care Program.

The Edmonton Symptom Assessment System (ESAS) is a validated tool for measuring the intensity of common symptoms in palliative care patients.[4] Besides providing important clinical information on a daily basis, it has been successfully employed for audit purposes.[9] When patients are unable to complete the ESAS because of decreased level of consciousness, the families and nurses indicate their perceptions of patient comfort with the Edmonton Comfort Assessment Tool.[5] The Folstein Mini-Mental State Examination[10] is

Table 37.3 *Assessment tools used on the Tertiary Palliative Care Unit at Edmonton, Canada*

Tool	Domain measured	Team member responsible	Frequency
Edmonton Symptom Assessment System[5] (ESAS)	Intensity of common symptoms	Nurse	Daily
Edmonton Comfort Assessment Tool[6]	Overall patient comfort	Nurse	Daily (if patient unable to complete ESAS)
Folstein Mini-Mental State Examination[11]	Cognition	Physician	On admission and weekly
CAGE Questionnaire[13]	History of alcoholism	Physician	On admission
Edmonton Staging System for Cancer Pain[7]	Prognosis for achieving pain control	Physician	On admission
Edmonton Labeled Visual Information System[8]	Sites of disease	Physician	On admission
Edmonton Functional Assessment Tool[9]	Function	Occupational and physical therapist	On admission
Constipation score[15]	Quantity and location of retained stool	Physician	On admission and as needed
Morphine equivalent daily dose	Type, dose, and route of opioid	Physician	Daily
Palliative Performance Scale[17]	Performance status	Nurse	On admission

used because cognitive failure is an extremely common and potentially distressing complication in palliative care patients, but one that is easily missed without the use of a screening tool.[11] Identification of a history of alcoholism with an instrument such as the CAGE Questionnaire[12] is important because of this condition's underdiagnosis and association with poor pain outcomes.[13] The Edmonton Staging System for Cancer Pain is valuable for describing patient populations in terms of prognosis for achieving good pain control.[6] The Edmonton Labeled Visual Information System has been shown to improve physician recall of patient information.[7] The Edmonton Functional Assessment Tool measures 10 domains of function relevant to palliative patients.[8] As constipation is a frequent problem in this patient population, the constipation score is used to objectively quantify and locate stool, based on a plain abdominal radiograph.[14,15] The type, total dose, and route of opioid are recorded daily to track patient progress. The Palliative Performance Scale describes functional status and prognosis.[16]

WARD ROUTINE

At the beginning of the day, the nurses' observations of the patients during the preceding shifts are relayed to the medical team. The physicians then spend the morning assessing the patients and negotiating a plan of care for the day. Interaction with the team occurs on an ongoing basis. Once a week, a team conference is held, during which the admissions of the previous week are discussed in detail and a comprehensive management plan is formulated. The progress

of the other patients is also reviewed and plans adjusted accordingly.

While discussions with patients and families take place throughout the course of admission, a designated family conference is often advisable to clarify goals and establish plans of care. The conference is coordinated by the social worker and attended by the team, the patient, and all family members whom the patient wishes to involve.

DISCHARGE PLANNING

Approximately half of the patients admitted to the TPCU are eventually discharged to other settings. Some may be able to return home. Usually, a discharge home is preceded by a family conference that includes the homecare case manager. It is important that the patient and family understand who will be responsible for care once the discharge has taken place. The primary roles of the family physician and the homecare case manager are therefore emphasized. If the success of the discharge is in question, a trial discharge is recommended, whereby the patient's bed on the TPCU is retained for a few days in case the patient needs to return. Once the patient has been discharged, a medical summary is immediately sent to the family physician and to the homecare office. Patients whose symptoms have stabilized but who are unable to return home are usually transferred to a hospice.

Other patients remain on the TPCU until death. Some cannot be discharged because of progressive deterioration, whereas others have ongoing needs that cannot be met in any other setting. For example, hospices do not have the

Table 37.4   *Patient demographics in different palliative care settings*[22]

	TPCU	Acute care	Hospices	*P*-value
Number	164	674	516	NA
Mean age $\pm$ SD (years)	61 $\pm$ 14	68 $\pm$ 14	71 $\pm$ 13	<0.0001
Male (%)	79 (49)	313(47)	271 (53)	0.0713
Primary tumor (%)				
Gastrointestinal	35 (21)	208 (31)	102 (20)	<0.0001
Genitourinary	33 (20)	115 (17)	89 (17)	n.s.
Breast	19 (12)	34 (5)	40 (8)	0.0073
Lung	33 (20)	125 (19)	113 (22)	n.s.
Hematological	9 (5)	30 (4)	8 (2)	0.0082
Other cancer	4 (2)	50 (7)	110 (21)	<0.0001
Other diagnosis	21 (13)	59 (9)	33 (6)	0.0306
Unknown diagnosis	14 (9)	53 (7)	21 (4)	0.0166
CAGE $\geqslant$ 2 (%)	34/126 (27)	91/565 (16)	41/297 (14)	<0.0001
ESS** Stage 2 (%)	110/127 (87)	397/608 (65)	NA	<0.0001
Abnormal MMSQ* (%)	59/150 (39)	216/631 (34)	161/338 (48)	0.0002

*MMSQ, Mini-Mental State Questionnaire; ** ESS, Edmonton Staging System for Cancer Pain; n.s., not significant; TCPU, tertiary palliative care unit.
Modified from Bruera *et al.* Frequency of symptom distress and poor prognostic indicators in palliative cancer patients admitted to a tertiary palliative care unit, hospices, and acute care hospitals. *J Palliat Care* 2000 Autumn; **16**: 16–21,[22] with permission.

resources required to manage spinal analgesics, total parenteral nutrition, or respiratory care.

EDUCATION AND RESEARCH

All members of the team are expected to participate in education and research. Most of the physicians have appointments in the Division of Palliative Care Medicine of the Department of Oncology, University of Alberta.

The TPCU receives undergraduate and postgraduate medical trainees from the University of Alberta on a regular basis. A total of four residents and fellows may be accommodated at a given time. Family medicine residents undertake a mandatory 2-week palliative medicine rotation on the TPCU. An analysis of multiple choice question examinations given to family medicine residents at the beginning and the end of their palliative care rotations demonstrated a significant improvement in knowledge.[17] Oncology residents also spend part of their compulsory 4-week palliative medicine rotation on the TPCU. Residents in the 1-year palliative medicine program spend 6 months on the TPCU. Elective rotations are open to residents from other programs and to medical students. Learners from other disciplines such as nursing and social work are also welcome. The TPCU has a long history of training palliative care specialists from across Canada and around the world.

Clinical teaching is complemented by journal club, held three mornings per week, during which time articles with relevance to palliative care are presented and discussed. A survey revealed that a majority of trainees found this activity to be of value for education, clinical practice, and

development of critical appraisal skills.[18] Other educational activities include seminars and weekly program-wide rounds, which incorporate medical, interdisciplinary, and research topics. Presenters from other specialties are invited to share their expertise as applied directly or indirectly to palliative care, thus fostering the exchange of knowledge between different healthcare fields.

Funding for research on the TPCU is derived from a variety of sources. The priority given to this activity is reflected in the numerous examples of innovations in symptom assessment and treatment developed in this setting.[4–8,19–21]

OUTCOMES

Tables 37.4 and 37.5 compare the characteristics and symptoms of patients admitted to the TPCU, those assessed by the acute care consultation teams, and those admitted to the hospices.[22] Patients on the TPCU were significantly younger and had a significantly higher frequency of positive CAGE scores, poor prognosis for achieving good pain control, and severe symptoms. This suggests that patients were being appropriately selected for admission to this setting. An analysis of ESAS scores revealed an improvement in total symptom distress during the first 5 days of admission.[4]

In 2002, the total number of patients admitted to the TPCU represented 17 percent of all patients seen by the Capital Health Regional Palliative Care Program that year.[23] Median length of stay was 19 days and bed occupancy was 91 percent. Fifty-eight percent of patients died on the TPCU, while 24 percent and 13 percent were discharged to

Table 37.5 *Frequency of severe symptoms (ESAS ≥ 50/100) in different palliative care settings*

Symptom (%)	TPCU	Acute care	Hospices	P-value*
Pain	90/157 (57)	203/642 (32)	152/425 (36)	<0.0001
Activity	108/155 (70)	480/625 (77)	265/449 (59)	<0.0001
Nausea	38/153 (25)	65/638 (10)	56/382 (15)	<0.0001
Depression	65/149 (44)	155/568 (27)	115/408 (28)	0.0004
Anxiety	82/153 (54)	176/578 (30)	131/420 (31)	<0.0001
Drowsiness	82/155 (53)	281/623 (45)	217/434 (50)	0.1181
Appetite	102/153 (67)	428/617 (69)	265/444 (60)	0.0045
Wellbeing	90/148 (61)	266/536 (50)	192/422 (45)	0.0059
Shortness of breath	46/154 (30)	133/633 (21)	92/409 (22)	0.0621
Overall	703/1377 (51)	2187/5460 (40)	1485/3793 (39)	<0.0001

*P-values determined using chi-square test. Significance was accepted at the $P < 0.0055$ level to take into account the Bonferroni correction for multiple comparisons.
ESAS, Edmonton Symptom Assessment System; TCPU, tertiary palliative care unit.
Modified from Bruera *et al.* Frequency of symptom distress and poor prognostic indicators in palliative cancer patients admitted to a tertiary palliative care unit, hospices, and acute care hospitals. *J Palliat Care* 2000 Autumn; **16:** 16–21,[22] with permission.

the home and hospice settings, respectively. The annual budget for the TPCU is approximately Can$2 380 000, of which 88 percent is used to fund salaries (excluding physician salaries, which are paid from a separate source). Another 8 percent is directed toward drugs, while the remainder is allocated for supplies.

DISCUSSION

Tertiary palliative care units fulfill a unique clinical role in the continuum of care for patients with terminal illness. They are designed to care for patients with the most complex problems of a physical, psychologic, social, or spiritual nature. In a comprehensive, integrated palliative care program, approximately 15–20 percent of patients would be appropriate for admission to such a unit.

Given the complexity of the patient population, the ideal location for such a unit is in an acute care hospital that offers a full range of diagnostic and interventional procedures (e.g. magnetic resonance imaging (MRI), endoscopy), support services (e.g. respiratory therapy), and specialty and subspecialty consultation (e.g. anesthesiology, surgery, internal medicine, psychiatry). For units that admit cancer patients predominantly, access to oncological consultation and therapy is essential. Indeed, it is possible for such units to be situated in cancer centers, although access for patients with diagnoses other than cancer may be limited. In the opinion of some administrators, the optimal unit size for staffing efficiency is 16–24 beds and the minimum size is 10–12 beds.[24]

The issue of requiring a do-not-resuscitate status for admission to a palliative care unit is controversial. This policy is based on the finding that the chance of success of cardiopulmonary resuscitation, defined as survival to discharge from hospital, is nil in patients with metastatic cancer.[25] Agreement on this issue prior to admission lessens the chance of subsequent confusion about the overall goals of care. Furthermore, patients and families are spared the distress of experiencing or witnessing a resuscitation attempt. However, this policy may pose a barrier to care for those patients who could benefit from the unit's services but are not willing to accept a do-not-resuscitate status. Moreover, some palliative care specialists perceive that selected patients may be appropriate for resuscitation, depending on prognosis, quality of life, and the patient's wishes.[26] Whatever decision is made regarding policy, discussion of do-not-resuscitate status presents a valuable opportunity to clarify the patient's and family's understanding of the illness and prognosis, as well as goals of care.[27]

In order that the limited resources of the TPCU may be used for the appropriate patients, a process for screening referrals is required. Direct assessment of the patient by a palliative care consultant is preferred. Besides determining whether or not the patient's concerns warrant admission to this specialized setting, the consultant is able to prepare the patient and family for the type of care that will be provided on the unit. Meticulous communication between the referring and receiving teams is important for continuity of care and to minimize unnecessary duplication of assessments.

Given the complex nature of the patients' problems, a specialist interdisciplinary team is required. The team should comprise members who together can address the breadth of concerns of the patients and families referred to the TPCU. The Edmonton TPCU does not currently have a psychologist on the team, but one would be desirable. Consultants from other specialties also make a significant contribution to the care of patients on a TPCU.

A disciplined approach to assessment and documentation of patient and family concerns is essential for achieving the goals of admission. First, it is a fundamental step in identifying and characterizing the patient's issues. Second, it allows for tracking of the patient's course over time and outcomes of interventions. Third, it facilitates communication of the patient's situation to the various care providers involved. Finally, the data collected may be used for program management, quality assurance, and research. As much as possible, the tools should be validated, easy to understand, not burdensome to complete and clinically useful. Also, they should capture the multidimensional nature of patients' concerns. Ideally, the same tools should be used in all associated healthcare settings, as the use of a common language facilitates transfer of care between settings and allows for comparisons to be made among settings.[22,23] The acuity and complexity of the patients admitted to the TPCU necessitate frequent assessment, rapid adjustment of therapies, timely communication between team members, and careful coordination of efforts. The patient and family must be recognized as being central to the team.

In order that the TPCU beds remain readily accessible to patients requiring admission, an effective and proactive discharge planning process is required. Options for discharge depend on local resources. For those patients who are discharged home, clear and timely communication with community healthcare providers (e.g. primary care physician, homecare manager, pharmacist) is critical. Transfer to a hospice often poses a difficult transition for the patients and families, not only because of their need to adjust to a new environment and staff, but also because they may view hospice as a lower level of care and feel a sense of abandonment.[28] These concerns may be alleviated by noting that the fact that the patient no longer requires management on the TPCU is a positive outcome, providing reassurance that the patient's needs can be adequately met in hospice, and arranging for families to tour the hospice. Depending on the resources available outside the TPCU, there may also be patients who stay despite stable symptoms because their needs cannot be met in any other setting. Some of these patients may remain on the TPCU for a prolonged period of time.

As a setting for the management of the most complex cases, the TPCU has an inherent mandate to transfer its knowledge to others, as well as to advance the state of that knowledge. These roles are facilitated by locating the unit in a teaching hospital, and by appointing the staff to faculty positions in the university. The TPCU presents a number of advantages as a learning environment. It provides learners with the opportunity to be exposed to a broad range of problems in palliative care, to follow patients closely, to gain experience dealing with distressed families and to work with an interdisciplinary team, all under the direct supervision of experts in the field. The potential disadvantage is that the patients and problems encountered on the TPCU are highly selected and not necessarily representative of those encountered in other practice settings. Also, the interventions performed on the TPCU may not be transferable to other settings because of resource limitations. The TPCU

provides an environment that is well suited to the conduct of research. Since the patients are under the direct care of the team, the process of screening and recruiting for studies may be simpler. If the study involves medically complex interventions or monitoring, then this may be most readily achieved in an acute care setting such as the TPCU. Also, compared with patients admitted to hospices, patients on a TPCU are more likely to be cognitively intact.[23] On the other hand, patients on a TPCU have a greater degree of symptom distress and therefore may not be well enough to participate in studies. In addition, the results may not be generalizable to other palliative patient populations. Nonetheless, many patients admitted to palliative care units are willing to consider participation in clinical trials.[29]

A number of publications have reported variable symptom outcomes in patients admitted to individual palliative care units.[9,30–33] Generalizability of the data is uncertain, in part because the characteristics of these units are diverse or incompletely described. A prospective, multicenter study demonstrated that admission to palliative care units resulted in significant improvements in the physical, psychologic, and existential domains of quality of life.[34]

The economic impact of palliative care units has also been described. In a report from a 23-bed palliative care unit in a comprehensive cancer center, costs were shown to exceed revenues if length of stay was greater than 10 days. Also, cost was inversely proportional to patient census.[35] Analysis from a palliative care inpatient service in another comprehensive cancer center revealed that mean daily charges were 38 percent lower than in the rest of the hospital.[33] Both units are characterized by intensive interdisciplinary symptom management and discharge planning, high patient volumes, short lengths of stay and low mortality rates. Economic outcomes have been described for a different model of palliative care unit, located in an acute care facility but providing terminal care for patients with a variety of diagnoses. Charges and costs were 66 percent lower for days on the unit, compared with days in hospital prior to transfer to the unit, and almost 60 percent lower for patients who died on the unit versus matched controls who died elsewhere in the hospital.[36] Economic issues are of course influenced by the funding mechanisms particular to each healthcare system. For example, in the USA, the distinction between acute palliative care services and hospice services is essential for reimbursement purposes.[33]

CONCLUSION

By providing specialist interdisciplinary care for the most complex patients, tertiary palliative care units fulfill a unique and leading role in clinical care, education, and research within palliative care programs, healthcare systems and academic centers. Further study is needed to clarify the impact of such units on clinical, economic, and academic outcomes.

Key learning points

- Different models of palliative care units in acute care hospitals are possible.

- A TCPU admits patients with the most complex problems.

- The key roles of a TCPU are clinical care, education, and research.

- Effective use of a TCPU requires a process for selecting appropriate patients and for discharging them.

- Successful management of these patients requires a specialist interdisciplinary team and access to diagnostic and interventional procedures, support services and consultants.

- A disciplined approach to assessment and documentation is essential for achieving the goals of admission.

REFERENCES

◆ 1 von Gunten CF. Secondary and tertiary palliative care in US hospitals. *JAMA* 2002; **287**: 875–81.

2 Heedman P, Starkhammar H. Patterns of referral to a palliative care unit: an indicator of different attitudes toward the dying patient? *J Palliat Med* 2002; **5**: 101–6.

3 Brenneis C, Bruera E. Models for the delivery of palliative care: the Canadian model. In: Bruera E, Portenoy RK, eds. *Topics in Palliative Care*, Volume 5. New York: Oxford University Press, 2001: 3–23.

4 Bruera E, Kuehn N, Miller MJ, *et al.* The Edmonton Symptom Assessment System (ESAS): a simple method for the assessment of palliative care patients. *J Palliat Care* 1991; **7**: 6–9.

5 Bruera E, Sweeney C, Willey J, *et al.* Perception of discomfort by relatives and nurses in unresponsive terminally ill patients with cancer: a prospective study. *J Pain Symptom Manage* 2003; **26**: 818–26.

6 Bruera E, Schoeller T, Wenk R, *et al.* A prospective multicenter assessment of the Edmonton Staging System for cancer pain. *J Pain Symptom Manage* 1995; **10**: 348–55.

7 Walker P, Nordell C, Neumann CM, Bruera E. Impact of the Edmonton Labeled Visual Information System on physician recall of metastatic cancer patient histories: a randomized controlled trial. *J Pain Symptom Manage* 2001; **21**: 4–11.

8 Kaasa T, Loomis J, Gillis K, *et al.* The Edmonton Functional Assessment Tool: preliminary development and evaluation for use in palliative care. *J Pain Symptom Manage* 1997; **13**: 10–19.

9 Dudgeon DJ, Harlos M, Clinch JJ. The Edmonton Symptom Assessment Scale (ESAS) as an audit tool. *J Palliat Care* 1999; **15**: 14–19.

10 Folstein MF, Folstein S, McHugh PR. 'Mini-mental state': a practical method for grading the cognitive state of patients for the clinician. *J Psych Res* 1975; **12**: 189–98.

11 Bruera E, Miller L, McCallion J, *et al.* Cognitive failure in patients with terminal cancer: a prospective study. *J Pain Symptom Manage* 1992; **7**: 192–5.

12 Ewing J. Detecting alcoholism: the CAGE questionnaire. *JAMA* 1984; **252**: 1905–7.

13 Bruera E, Moyano J, Seifert L, *et al.* The frequency of alcoholism among patients with pain due to terminal cancer. *J Pain Symptom Manage* 1995; **10**: 599–603.

14 Starreveld JS, Pols MA, Van Wijk HJ, *et al.* The plain abdominal radiograph in the assessment of constipation. *Z Gastroenterol* 1990; **28**: 335–8.

15 Bruera E, Suarez-Almazor M, Velasco A, *et al.* The assessment of constipation in terminal cancer patients admitted to a palliative care unit: a retrospective review. *J Pain Symptom Manage* 1994; **9**: 515–19.

16 Anderson F, Downing GM, Hill J, *et al.* Palliative Performance Scale (PPS): a new tool. *J Palliat Care* 1996; **12**: 5–11.

17 Oneschuk D, Fainsinger R, Hanson J, Bruera E. Assessment and knowledge in palliative care in second year family medicine residents. *J Pain Symptom Manage* 1998; **14**: 265–73.

18 Mazuryk M, Daeninck P, Neumann CM, Bruera E. Daily journal club: an education tool in palliative care. *Palliat Med* 2002; **16**: 57–61.

19 Bruera E, Fainsinger R, MacEachern T, Hanson J. The use of methylphenidate in patients with incident cancer pain receiving regular opiates. A preliminary report. *Pain* 1992; **50**: 75–7.

20 Bruera E, de Stoutz N, Velasco-Leiva, *et al.* The effects of oxygen on the intensity of dyspnea in hypoxemic terminal cancer patients. *Lancet* 1993; **342**: 13–14.

21 de Stoutz ND, Bruera E, Suarez-Almazor M. Opioid rotation (OR) for toxicity reduction in terminal cancer patients. *J Pain Symptom Manage* 1995; **10**: 378–84.

● 22 Bruera E, Neumann C, Brenneis C, Quan H. Frequency of symptom distress and poor prognostic indicators in palliative cancer patients admitted to a tertiary palliative care unit, hospices, and acute care hospitals. *J Palliat Care* 2000; **16**: 16–21.

23 *Regional Palliative Care Program Annual Report April 1, 2002–March 31, 2003 and April 1, 2003–March 31, 2004.* 2005. Available at: www.palliative.org (accessed September 7, 2005).

24 von Gunten CF, Ferris FD, Portenoy R, Glachen M, eds. *CAPC Manual: Everything You Wanted to Know About Developing a Palliative Care Program but Were Afraid to Ask*, 2001. Available at: www.capcmssm.org (accessed September 7, 2005).

25 Faber-Langendoen K. Resuscitation of patients with metastatic cancer. Is transient benefit still futile? *Arch Intern Med* 1991; **151**: 235–9.

26 Thorns AR, Ellershaw JE. A survey of nursing and medical staff views on the use of cardiopulmonary resuscitation in the hospice. *Palliat Med* 1999; **13**: 225–32.

27 von Gunten CF. Discussing do-not-resuscitate status. *J Clin Oncol* 2001; **19**: 1576–81.

28 Maccabee J. The effect of transfer from a palliative care unit to nursing homes – are patients' and relatives' needs met? *Palliat Med* 1994; **8**: 211–14.

29 Ross C, Cornbleet M. Attitudes of patients and staff to research in a specialist palliative care unit. *Palliat Med* 2003; **17**: 491–7.

30 Rees E, Hardy J, Ling J, *et al.* The use of the Edmonton Symptom Assessment Scale (ESAS) within a palliative care unit in the UK. *Palliat Med* 1998; **12**: 75–82.

31   Lo RSK, Ding A, Chung TK, Woo J. Prospective study of symptom control in 133 cases of palliative care inpatients in Shatin Hospital. *Palliat Med* 1999; **13**: 335–40.

32   Mancini I, Lossignol D, Obiols M, *et al.* Supportive and palliative care: experience at the Institut Jules Bordet. *Support Care Cancer* 2002; **10**: 3–7.

33   Elsayem A, Swint K, Fisch M, *et al.* Palliative care inpatient service in a comprehensive cancer center: clinical and financial outcomes. *J Clin Oncol* 2004; **22**: 2008–14.

● 34   Cohen SR, Boston P, Mount BM, Porterfield P. Changes in quality of life following admission to palliative care units. *Palliat Med* 2001; **15**: 363–71.

35   Davis MP, Walsh D, Nelson KA, *et al.* The business of palliative medicine – Part 2: The economics of acute inpatient palliative medicine. *Am J Hospice Palliat Care* 2002; **19**: 89–95.

36   Smith TJ, Coyne P, Cassel B, *et al.* A high-volume specialist palliative care unit and team may reduce in-hospital end-of-life care costs. *J Palliat Med* 2003; **6**: 699–705.

38

Combined care models

FREDERICK J MEYERS, ANTHONY F JERANT

INTRODUCTION

Often considered synonymous with end-of-life care, palliative care is increasingly viewed as encompassing intensive supportive care throughout an illness. The World Health Organization (WHO) updated definition of palliative care includes relief of suffering throughout illness (not just at end of life) for adults and children.[1] The integration of intensive palliative care at transition points of illness – when psychosocial and family trauma is often greatest – has the potential to remedy glaring shortfalls in the quality of healthcare.[2] Conceptually, patients should not be asked to arbitrarily choose between disease directed and palliative care. Rather patients should be able to simultaneously receive both, when appropriate.

The physical discomfort often associated with illness or therapy combined with the emotional distress is the essence of suffering and of the rationale for palliative care throughout illness. Progressive palliative care responds to unique patient problems and progressively increases in intensity as illness progresses, often best addressed in-between illness exacerbations. In this chapter, we explore the concept of palliative care as a quintessential example of patient-centered care and discuss relevant skills for providing comprehensive, longitudinal palliative care. We also present promising process improvement models for integrating 'best practice' palliative care into daily primary care practice, cancer centers, and longitudinal care facilities.

PERSPECTIVE: CANCER

At the time of diagnosis, cancer generates a sense of vulnerability for virtually every patient, engendering fear, uncertainty, and significant new demands. In spite of this early trauma, the majority of adult patients with newly diagnosed cancer gradually adapt to the crisis of their diagnosis and related treatments.[3,4] The literature does not provide similar information for young adults[5*] nor for diverse populations, though psychosocial distress screening and problem-based data have demonstrated that patients of all ages have significant and clearly definable problems.[6***,7***] The study of the dynamic changes in the psychological response to cancer and appropriate interventions have expanded to include time points beyond the initial diagnosis.[8***] Survivorship begins on the day of diagnosis as cancer patients begin to redefine all aspects of their lives.

The effects of cancer reverberate throughout the family.[9,10] Families can exhibit significant variation in their ability to adapt and respond to the overall cancer experience. While a variation in family response exists, family members can experience increased anxiety and depression, disruptions in social roles, and diminished physical health with an escalation of somatic complaints.[11] Cancer generates demands that impose severe levels of stress that challenge even the most well-functioning family.[6,12] These struggles occur as families attempt to serve as the primary source of support for the patient, a buffer against stress, and a facilitator for effective decision making and problem solving.[13]

When family caregivers are incapacitated by their reactions to the cancer diagnosis and treatment, the healthcare team loses a significant resource in the overall care of the patient. Distress in the family undermines decision making and problem-solving skills.[14] Family members' capacity to be effective caregivers is related to family functioning along the dimensions of adaptability and cohesion. The level of family functioning may simply be inadequate to meet the caregiving expectations of the healthcare team. Nearly all families experience difficulties and problems if the role of caregiving is prolonged over time.[15*] Consequently, an imperative in cancer care has emerged to develop effective methods that enhance the problem-solving abilities of family caregivers to resolve difficulties related to the care of the patient outside the hospital during these critical transition points. The healthcare team is most challenged by patients and families who fail to adapt to the psychological and social problems of illness and living, often not manifest to the healthcare team until a crisis.

Quantitative or qualitative evidence of the benefit of the simultaneous provision of palliative care and disease-directed therapy has been difficult to demonstrate. Problems around patient selection, important and accurate measurements of quality of life and quality of care at baseline and after intervention, and an intervention that is consistent and reproducible may be the most important considerations. A simple efficacious example of a palliative care intervention that can be provided with disease directed therapy is the provision of an antidepressant medication.[16**] Two psychosocial or mental health interventions as models of beneficial supportive interventions have been reported.[17*,18]

Integration of palliative care into cancer centers: simultaneous care

Chemotherapy is commonly administered in the last 6 months of life and has had the dichotomous result of increasing hospice referral but reducing the duration of hospice services per family.[19] The use of cancer chemotherapy without curative intent is considered by some as a palliative intervention. Several randomized studies in prostate carcinoma have reported reduced pain in patients receiving chemotherapy compared with corticosteroids.[20] The quality-of-life metrics in one study were inclusive and may have shown overall benefit, though methodological problems with patient dropout prevent a definitive answer. In addition, follow-up was relatively brief with no sustained endpoints such as hospice referral and open to the criticism that the improved quality of life seen with chemotherapy without a real attempt to address suffering will disappear and show a final deterioration at end of life and lead to high risk grief.

Thus palliative chemotherapy is widespread but of unproved benefit compared with best supportive care and may degrade the reputation of the oncology community.[21] No one receives best supportive care because in oncology practice such care is usual care – a standard that is often deficient in pain relief and psychosocial support. Welcome calls to integrate comprehensive palliative care with disease directed therapy may set the stage for well-done studies that adhere to highest quality study design and outcome analysis.[22] Investigational cancer chemotherapy programs can serve as a model example for the integration of palliative care and disease directed therapy. Entry into investigational clinical trials, i.e. phase I and early phase II trials, should be an unmistakable sign that palliative care needs will be prominent. Cancer centers should be the epitome of palliative care provision, but most are not.

Concomitant with progressive disease, thousands of patients consult comprehensive cancer centers each year and receive technically outstanding, often protocol-governed care. The goals of these phase I and early phase II investigations are to define toxicity patterns, establish maximum tolerated dose, and if responses are seen, lead to advanced disease specific phase II and phase III trials. Any responses measured in phase I and early phase II trials rarely convert into prolonged survival for patients.

The clinical and ethical problem is well defined.[23,24] Cancer patients on investigational therapy are not treated with curative intent and need palliative care. The consequences of this cognitive dissonance between care planning and research had led to serious deficiencies in quality including late referral to hospice, unaddressed end-of-life issues, and patient family dissatisfaction including family caregiver stress and complicated bereavement issues. In addition, anecdotal evidence indicates that the clinical research mission is undermined as some patients forego participation in clinical trials because they perceive the loss of palliative options.

Why does this situation continue?

- The clinical research mission is central to oncology's efforts to reduce cancer mortality. However cancer centers and patients are unable to focus on both therapy and supportive care. The precepts of patient-centered care are obscured.
- The regulatory barrier in the USA that prevents simultaneous hospice care and disease therapy payments extends to the pre-hospice phase and separates the two care modalities, palliative care and disease-directed therapy. Interestingly, the criteria for hospice entry and investigational therapy entry are the same, advanced recurrent or refractory illness for which there is no proved therapy.
- Many advanced-stage cancer patients who make decisions to participate in cancer clinical trials are also characterized by a highly motivated personality. They feel that active treatment is best for them.[25] Other factors identified with enrollment may include altruism and the influence of the physician.[26] Patient expectations include a response to therapy despite consent forms that are explicit in stating otherwise,[27] a reduction in symptoms, and improved and increased communication with their physician.[28,29] Therapeutic efforts are often equated with superior quality of life and are measured against no other options. In contrast, patients and families believe palliative care is a passive choice, the equivalent of 'no care'.
- As a corollary, patients with advanced cancer overestimate their survival, making them more likely to choose 'life-extending' therapy over palliative care.[30] Patients and occasionally physicians have a distorted

view of intent and prognosis.[31] Studies of physician prognostication have documented that physicians were accurate in their estimate of survival yet were unable to effectively communicate the prognosis to patients. The bioethical implications of physicians' ability to foresee but not foretell has been explored.[32] The challenge, therefore, is not knowledge, but communication between patients, their families, and physicians.

- Healthcare providers lack training and role models in palliative care and systems do not support providers.
- Distress varies between patients and families and thus treatment strategies should vary.[33]
- Investigations are not done with clarity. An example of asking a clear question and developing a clear answer is the finding that consent forms for investigational therapy are not a barrier to effective palliative care.[27]

Despite these barriers, there are some recent developments suggesting progress in this area. For example, inpatient palliative care units deliver support to patients with life-threatening illness and advanced chronic diseases. Acceptance of the inpatient palliative care unit model has been enthusiastic and the model has also been associated with reduced hospitalization and post-hospitalization costs. Furthermore, the National Cancer Institute has also recently issued a call for research proposals in palliative care and has completed a consensus conference on improving end-of-life care.[34***]

In addition, the American Society of Clinical Oncology (ASCO) has developed several strategies to enhance the education of oncologists. For example, ASCO has issued a report that emphasized simultaneous caring of patients throughout illness.[35] ASCO has also modified the highly successful Education in Palliative and End-of-life Care (EPEC) program to an EPEC Oncology educational program. The organization also has included several sessions on palliative care at national meetings, and their publication *Journal of Clinical Oncology* has a section for original reports in supportive care

and a series 'The Tumor is not the Target' that features profound and comprehensive articles. The ASCO curriculum template includes the integration of palliative care in tumor types and a comprehensive list of topics such as supportive care, survivorship, psychosocial aspects, communication skills, and geriatric oncology.[36]

In addition to these clinical and educational developments, process improvement provides perhaps the most promising mechanism for improving end-of-life care, one that is advantageous for both patients and the institution. Process improvement involves a cyclic approach to improving clinical practice by assessing the problem, planning an approach, implementing the approach, and reassessing the problem with measurable endpoints.

We have designed a series of interventions in investigational therapy patients predicated on the process improvement approach. The goal was to evaluate the role of the simultaneous provision of palliative care, by an advanced practice home nurse and social worker, whereas the patients enrolled in the study also received disease-directed therapy (Fig. 38.1). Between 1998 and 2001 a homecare-based intervention was completed (Fig. 38.1a). In this nonrandomized study, no patient, family, or physician adverse events were observed and in fact the model was enthusiastically accepted.[37*] Quality-of-life endpoints were not improved but one quality-of-care endpoint, referral to hospice, was improved whereas another, number of cycles of chemotherapy was not changed.

These results were analyzed, psychometrics were enhanced, and the intervention was refined in an ongoing a multi-institutional randomized study (Fig. 38.1b). The Simultaneous Care Educational Intervention (SCEI) teaches patients and caregivers to work as an effective team to manage symptoms and distress by acquiring a set of problem-solving skills. The SCEI intervention is based on the substantial body of social problem solving research conducted primarily by D'Zurilla and Nezu.[38] Through their

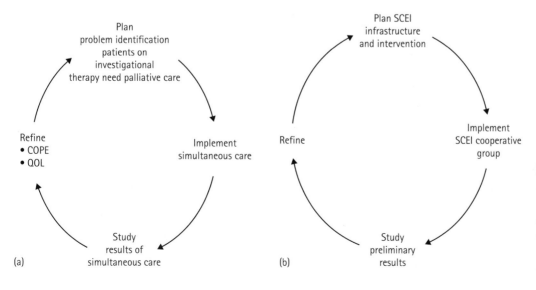

Figure 38.1
(a) Simultaneous care 1998–2001. (b) 2002 to present, QOL, quality of life; SCEI, Simultaneous Care Educational Intervention.

work, D'Zurilla and Nezu as well as others have developed conceptual frameworks for problem-solving therapy.[14,38] They have also conducted research that demonstrates that counseling caregivers who are under stress reduces their distress while increasing their problem-solving competence. This conceptual model has been applied successfully with a number of diverse health-related problems[39] including cancer.[3] Prior research has shown that problem-solving counseling of family caregivers has had beneficial effects, including lessened caregiver distress and reduced long-term depression in patients,[11] and is also highly appreciated by caregivers.[40]

Houts *et al.* have proposed a new conceptual model that adapts problem-solving counseling, and applies these principles in an educational format for family caregivers.[41] Houts' conceptual model has four components summarized by the acronym COPE for *Creativity, Optimism, Planning,* and *Expert* information. We employed the COPE operationalization of problem-solving education in our current study.

In summary, our study includes a simple and easily remembered framework for problem-solving counseling, a well defined patient population, robust psychometrics, and a randomized design powered for clinical significance. The intervention may be more ideal for patients at initial diagnosis and does not vary in intensity or type of intervention based upon baseline psychometric findings. The intervention is based on well established theory that translates to clinical research and, if successful, can readily be integrated into clinical practice.[42]

INTEGRATING PALLIATIVE CARE INTO 'MAINSTREAM' PRIMARY CARE PRACTICE

Does palliative care 'belong' in primary care practice? We and others[43,44] believe it does. The typical primary care physician only cares for 6–10 patients who die each year,[44] so if palliative care is conceptualized as a synonym for 'end-of-life care', then the role of the primary care provider in palliative care is indeed modest. However, when palliative care is viewed more broadly, to include early and ongoing communication regarding personal goals, effective discussions around the uncertainty of prognosis and outcome, and preferences for advanced directives, then the primary care provider is clearly integral to palliative care.[45]

Important barriers to greater integration of palliative care into primary care practice have been identified, including not only knowledge deficits but also attitudinal issues and practice structural barriers.[46] Most efforts to integrate palliative care into primary care practice have been focused exclusively on educating providers regarding technical topics (e.g. pain medication use). The underlying assumption is that primary care providers lack the clinical knowledge and skills to provide quality palliative care and that if these knowledge and skills deficits are corrected, palliative care will become an integral part of primary care practice.

While some research supports the idea that primary providers' palliative care knowledge base and skills may be suboptimal,[47] other research does not.[48] Furthermore, knowledge-oriented continuing medical education[49] and expert consultation[50*] interventions are generally ineffective in changing healthcare provider behaviors. Primary care provider communication behaviors and attitudes should be the primary targets linked to innovations in healthcare delivery processes and systems that facilitate delivery of palliative care.

Communication behavior changes: palliative care as patient–centered care

Primary providers are being encouraged to employ a patient-centered approach to healthcare. The patient-centered approach is generally preferred by patients compared to solely a disease-focused approach and may improve health outcomes.[51] Sociopolitical and ethical concerns[52] add to the considerable momentum for patient-centered care.[53] Mead and Bower recently outlined key components of a patient-centered approach to healthcare (Box 38.1).[54]

Box 38.1 Key facets of patient-centered care[54]

- A biopsychosocial perspective on medicine (e.g. exploring the illness experience as well as the disease)

- Understanding the patient as person

- Finding common ground regarding management of clinical concerns

- Enhancing the provider–patient relationship (fostering the therapeutic alliance)

- Understanding the provider as person

Exemplary palliative care can be considered as an example of ideal patient-centered care. For example, excellent communication is the *sine qua non* of effective palliative care.[55***] The manifestation of such communication is agreement on treatment and supportive care goals and on the evolution of those goals as disease progresses (finding common ground). The importance of recognizing transitions in illness and inpatients underscores the dynamic nature of palliative care, strengthening the provider–patient relationship over time. High patient family satisfaction with hospice programs may relate as much to coordination of care around patient and family concerns as symptom management.

The problem in the USA (as opposed to Canada, the UK, and some other countries) is that palliative care has traditionally been provided only by a small cadre of 'special' individuals and 'saved' for those actively dying, despite its potential for transforming the quality and process of care throughout the trajectory of illness. For example, in the USA, primary care providers do not generally have conversations with patients and families early in the illness trajectory regarding the prognosis and typical course of illness and the patient's goals for therapy and remaining life – in other words, 'patient-centered' communication. Such conversations enhance understanding of the patient as person, allow common ground to be reached for management, and foster the therapeutic alliance. Missed communication opportunities early in the illness trajectory – for example, at the point where a chronically ill elderly person first begins to suffer irreversible decline in basic and/or instrumental activities of daily living, a marker for limited life expectancy – contribute to quality-of-care shortfalls such as the high number of hospital intensive care unit deaths[56] and very late referrals to hospice.[57] Beginning these critical conversations from the outset of diagnosis or close to it could allow the level of dialog around palliative care to be at a much higher level and might reduce intensive care unit deaths and late hospice referrals.[58***]

Attitude changes: cultivating mindful practice

Cultivating mindful practice may be somewhat less familiar than the other patient-centered care concepts. 'Understanding the doctor as person' means consciously considering the influence of one's own personal qualities, values, experiences, and interaction style on the process and outcomes of care. In the patient-centered care model, provider and patient continually influence each other through their actions.[54] The provider's unconscious internal reactions and external responses to various patients and clinical problems may be clinically constructive (empathy) or counterproductive (patients who 'push buttons'). Counterproductive reactions and responses can only be modified, and constructive reactions therapeutically harnessed, when the physician becomes fully cognizant of them. Thus, in the patient-centered method, the provider must become conscious of cues to their emotional relationship with the patient as it unfolds, cultivating self-awareness during clinical encounters.[59]

Many hospice staff tend to welcome self-awareness, exploration and, contemplation of spiritual and existential issues. However, for some primary care providers, such issues are initially frightening, painful, and even 'draining'.[60] Powerful unprocessed provider emotional reactions and feelings such as incomplete grieving for a loved one, can lead to a lack of self-efficacy in situations that call for palliative care. Cultivation of a mindful approach to practice will be required for adept palliative care, preventing patient abandonment and increasing tolerance for the anxiety that can accompany care of the dying and their family. Practical

approaches to cultivating mindful practice include journaling and peer discussion groups.

Systems changes: supportive primary care processes

Another fundamental challenge to integrating palliative care into primary care is the problem of competing demands.[61] In one encounter primary care providers must prioritize acute and chronic illnesses, psychosocial issues, and preventive services. Even if primary providers feel a strong clinical imperative to address palliative care concerns in a longitudinal, proactive manner, they may find that retooling their practice habits is simply not feasible without structural changes in the health system.

One potential partial solution is to 'frame' the issue of palliative care in primary care within the context of the patient-centered care. The chronic care model, a systems redesign approach to the continuous quality improvement of chronic illness, is instructive.[62] Several key elements to the model include reorganization of healthcare, delivery system redesign, increased access to decision support and clinical information systems, an emphasis on patient self-management, and linking with community resources.

One specific approach that is more effective than usual care and might be emulated in 'mainstreaming' palliative care practices is the collaborative model of mental healthcare.[63**] Patients with various mental illnesses (including depression and panic disorder) are provided access to a care manager supervised by a psychiatrist and a primary care expert and offered education, care management, and support of the patient's primary care physician with antidepressant medication management. A brief psychotherapy for depression intervention is offered, Problem Solving Treatment in Primary Care.[64] Other key aspects of the model involves a stepped care approach, in which the intensity and type of therapy are targeted to need.[63**]

Considering the success of the collaborative depression care model alongside the generally disappointing results of a recent study attempting to incorporate expert palliative care team recommendations into primary care is instructive.[50] The investigators asserted that primary care providers had simply 'ignored' many of the team's well-informed and reasonable recommendations. In contrast, the collaborative care model provides a framework for overcoming attitudinal and systems-based barriers and offers a useful model for integrating palliative care into primary care.

INTEGRATING PALLIATIVE CARE INTO LONG-TERM CARE FACILITIES

Assisted living facilities (ALFs) are congregate elderly residential settings that provide or coordinate personal services, supervision, activities, and health-related services. There are about 1.5 million ALF beds in the USA, and demand is expected to grow as the population 'grays'. ALFs are an ideal setting in which to evaluate new models of palliative care. The elderly resident population is increasingly functionally impaired and frail. The 'typical' resident is an 80-year-old woman who needs assistance with two activities of daily living, and the estimated life-expectancy for people of this age and degree of frailty is less than 2 years.[65] Further, most residents suffer from multiple chronic illnesses for which accurate prognosis is difficult. The current approach of delaying palliative care until death is clearly imminent likely results in unnecessary, prolonged resident suffering.

We recently described a model – TLC – in ALFs that envisions palliative care as *Timely* and *Team*-oriented, *Longitudinal*, and *Collaborative* (including loved ones) and *Comprehensive*.[66] In a study evaluating palliative care improvement interventions grounded in the TLC model, no subjects were found to be eligible for hospice at baseline per National Hospice Organization criteria.[67*] Yet subjects' answers to two basic life values questions indicated a strong tendency to value maintaining the quality of remaining life over prolonging life at less than current quality. The TLC model has shown preliminary promise as a framework for improving palliative care in ALFs and might also be extended beyond the assisted living setting and applied to other populations of elderly patients, such as those in skilled nursing facilities and in the community.

Integrating palliative care into other settings

Failure to improve palliative care concomitant with intensive care because of late intervention is one of the lessons of the Study to Understand Prognoses and Preferences for Outcomes and Risks of Treatments (SUPPORT).[68**] Thoracic societies and palliative care experts have begun to campaign for improved palliative care within the ICU setting.[69,70] The emergence of a new intervention, inpatient palliative care consultation services, may overcome some of the barriers noted in the SUPPORT study and extend palliation earlier in patients with advanced chronic illness (www.capc.org). Position papers are available on the integration in many chronic illnesses including AIDS and neurodegenerative diseases (www.promotingexcellence.org).

Key learning points

Despite the variety among the palliative care innovations we have reviewed and the wide array of patient populations and clinical problems/conditions to which they have been applied, several common themes unify these 'best practice' approaches. They also serve as key learning points for those seeking to transform palliative care from a parallel system providing care to a small number of terminally ill patients by a handful of experts to an integral part of the longitudinal care delivered by all providers to each and every patient:

- a patient-centered philosophy, including a focus on tangible, measurable health outcomes that matter to patients and their families

- deployment across the trajectory of illness rather than solely when death is imminent

- a simultaneous care approach that recognizes that co-existence of palliative and disease-focused or curative measures ought to be the rule rather than the exception in the setting of chronic, slowly progressive illnesses with often unpredictable trajectories

- an emphasis on integration of palliative care into existing 'mainstream' clinical settings (e.g. primary care, cancer centers) using a systems-based, process improvement approach

- targeting care approaches to suit the needs of well-defined and relatively homogeneous patient subpopulations (e.g. assisted living residents)

- recognition of patients' family members as essential members the palliative care team

- incorporation of coaching and problem-solving training to improve patient self-care and family caregiver care self-efficacy and skills.

REFERENCES

◆ 1 Sepulveda C, Marlin A, Yoshida T, Ullrich A. Palliative Care: The World Health Organization's global perspective. *J Pain Symptom Manage* 2002; **24**: 91–6.

◆ 2 Committee on Quality Health Care in America. Institute of Medicine. *Crossing the Quality Chasm: A New Health System for the 21st Century.* Washington, DC: National Academy Press, 2001: 364.

3 Nezu AM, Nezu CM, Faddis S. *Helping Cancer Patients Cope: A Problem-solving Approach.* Washington, DC: American Psychological Association, 1998.

● 4 Weisman AD, Worden JW. The existential plight in cancer: significance of the first 100 days. *Int J Psychiatry Med* 1976; **7**: 1–15.

5 Zebrack BJ, Eshelman DA, Hudson MM, *et al.* Health care for childhood cancer survivors: insights and perspectives from a Delphi panel of young adult survivors of childhood cancer. *Cancer* 2004; **100**: 843–50.

6 Loscalzo MJ, Zabora JR. Care of the cancer patient: response of family and staff. In: Bruera E, Portenoy RK, eds. *Topics in Palliative Care.* New York: Oxford University Press, 1998.

◆ 7 Zabora JR, Loscalzo MJ. Psychosocial consequences of advanced disease. In: Portenoy RK, Weissman DE, Berger A, eds. *Principles and Practice of Supportive Oncology.* Philadelphia: Lippincott-Raven, 1998.

◆ 8 Holland JC. History of psycho-oncology: overcoming attitudinal and conceptual barriers. *Psychosomatic Med* 2002; **64**: 206–21.

9 Barakat LP, Kazak AE, Meadows AT, *et al.* Families surviving childhood cancer: a comparison of posttraumatic stress symptoms with families of healthy children. *J Pediatr Psychol* 1997; **22**: 843–59.

10 Toseland RW, Smith G, McCallion P. Supporting the 'family' in family caregiving. In: Smith G (ed.) *Enabling Aging Families: directions for practice and policy.* Newbury Park, CA: Sage Publications, 1995.

11 Toseland RW, Blanchard CG, McCallion P. A problem solving intervention for caregivers of cancer patients. *Soc Sci Med* 1995; **40**: 517–28.

12 Zabora JR, Smith ED. Family dysfunction and the cancer patient: early recognition and intervention. *Oncology (Huntingt)* 1991; **5**: 31–35; discussion 36, 38, 41.

13 Zabora JR, Smith ED, Baker F, *et al.* The family: the other side of bone marrow transplantation. *J Psychosoc Oncol* 1992; **10**: 35–46.

14 Nezu AM, Nezu CM, Houts PS, *et al.* Relevance of problem-solving therapy to psychosocial oncology. *J Psychosoc Oncol* 1999; **16**: 5–26.

15 Nezu AM. Efficacy of a problem-solving therapy approach for unipolar depression. *J Consult Clin Psychol* 1986; **54**: 196–202.

16 Fisch MJ, Loehrer PJ, Kristeller J, *et al.* Fluoxetine versus placebo in advanced cancer outpatients: a double-blinded trial of the Hoosier Oncology Group. *J Clin Oncol* 2003; **21**: 1937–43.

17 Watson M, Haviland JS, Greer S, *et al.* Influence of psychological response on survival in breast cancer: a population-based cohort study. *Lancet* 1999; **354**: 1331–6.

18 Spiegel D, Classen C, eds. *Group Therapy for Cancer Patients: a research based handbook of psychosocial care.* New York: Basic Books, 2000.

19 Emanuel EJ, Young-Xu Y, Levinsky NG, Gazelle G, Saynina O, Ash AS. Chemotherapy use among Medicare beneficiaries at the end of life. *Ann Intern Med* 2003; **138**: 639–43.

✱ 20 Canil CM, Tannock IF. Is there a role for chemotherapy in prostate cancer? *Br J Cancer* 2004; **27**: 1005–11.

21 Weissman DE, von Gunten CF. Oncology and hospice care community. *Oncology* 2004; **2**: 85–91.

22 Malin JL. Bridging the divide: integrating cancer-directed therapy and palliative care. *J Clin Oncol* 2004; **22**: 3438–40.

23 Agrawal M, Emanuel EJ. Ethics of phase 1 oncology studies: reexamining the arguments and data. *JAMA* 2003; **290**: 1075–82.

24 Agrawal M, Danis M. End-of-life care for terminally ill participants in clinical research. *J Palliat Med* 2002; **5**: 729–37.

25 Ferrell BR, Grant MM, Rhiner M, Padilla GV. Home care: maintaining quality of life for patient and family. *Oncology (Huntingt)* 1992; **6**: 136–40.

26 Daugherty C, Ratain MJ, Grochowski E, *et al.* Perceptions of cancer patients and their physicians involved in phase I trials. *J Clin Oncol* 1995; **13**: 1062–72.

27 Horng S, Emanuel EJ, Wilfond B, *et al.* Descriptions of benefits and risks in consent forms for phase 1 oncology trials. *N Engl J Med* 2002; **347**: 2134–40.

28 Jenkins V, Fallowfield L. Reasons for accepting or declining to participate in randomized clinical trials for cancer therapy. *Br J Cancer* 2000; **82**: 1783–8.

29 Yoder LH, O'Rourke TJ, Etnyre A, *et al.* Expectations and experiences of patients with cancer participating in phase I clinical trials. *Oncol Nurs Forum* 1997; **24**: 891–6.

30 Weeks JC, Cook EF, O'Day SJ, *et al.* Relationship between cancer patients' predictions of prognosis and their treatment preferences. *JAMA* 1998; **279**: 1709–14.

31 Joffe S, Cook EF, Cleary PD, *et al.* Quality of informed consent in cancer clinical trials: a cross-sectional survey. *Lancet* 2001; **358**: 1772–7.

32 Iwashyna TJ, Christakis NA. Physicians, patients, and prognosis. *West J Med* 2001; **174**: 253–4.

33 Clark MM, Bostwick JM, Rummans TA. Group and individual treatment strategies for distress in cancer patients. *Mayo Clin Proc* 2003; **78**: 1538–43.

◆ 34 Improving end-of-life care. National Institutes of Health State-of-the-Science Conference Statement, December 6–8, 2004. Available at: http://consensus.nih.gov/ta/024/ EoLfinal011805pdf.pdf (accessed April 2, 2005).

✱ 35 Cancer care during the last phase of life. ASCO Policy Statement, February 20, 1998. Available at: www.asco.org/ ac/1,1003,_12-002546,00.asp (accessed April 2, 2005).

36 Muss HB, Von Roenn J, Damon LE, *et al.* ACCO: ASCO Core Curriculum Outline. *J Clin Oncol* 2005; 23: 2049–77.

● 37 Meyers FJ, Linder J, Beckett L, *et al.* Simultaneous care: a model approach to the perceived conflict between investigational therapy and palliative care. *J Pain Symptom Manage* 2004; **28**: 548–56.

38 D'Zurilla TJ, Nezu AM. Social problem-solving in adults. In: Kendall P (ed.) *Cognitive Behavioral Research and Therapy.* New York: Academic Press, 1982.

39 Nezu AM, Nezu CM, Perri MG. *Problem-solving Therapy for Depression: Theory, Research, and Clinical Guidelines.* New York: Wiley, 1989.

40 Bucher JA, Loscalzo M, Zabora J, *et al.* Problem-solving cancer care education for patients and caregivers. *Cancer Pract* 2001; **9**: 66–70.

41 Houts PS, Nezu AM, Nezu CM, Bucher JA. The prepared family caregiver: a problem-solving approach to family caregiver education. *Patient Educ Couns* 1996; **27**: 63–73.

42 Sung NS, Crowley WF Jr, Genel M, *et al.* Central challenges facing the national clinical research enterprise. *JAMA* 2003; **289**: 1278–87.

43 Gwinn RB. Family physicians should be experts in palliative care. *Am Fam Physician* 2000; **61**: 636, 641–2.

◆ 44 Block SD, Bernier GM, Crawley LM, *et al.* Incorporating palliative care into primary care education. National Consensus Conference on Medical Education for Care Near the End of Life. *J Gen Intern Med* 1998; **13**: 768–73.

45 Back AL, Curtis JR. When does primary care turn into palliative care? *West J Med* 2001; **175**: 150–1.

46 Mitchell GK, Reymond EJ, McGrath BP. Palliative care: promoting general practice participation. *Med J Aust* 2004; **180**: 207–8.

47 Haines CS, Thomas Z. Assessing needs for palliative care education of primary care physicians: results of a mail survey. *J Palliat Care* 1993; **9**: 23–6.

48 Nowels D, Lee JT. Cancer pain management in home hospice settings: a comparison of primary care and oncologic physicians. *J Palliat Care* 1999; **15**: 5–9.

49 Davis DA, Thomson MA, Oxman AD, Haynes RB. Evidence for the effectiveness of CME. A review of 50 randomized controlled trials. *JAMA* 1992; **268**: 1111–17.

50 Rabow MW, Dibble SL, Pantilat SZ, McPhee SJ. The comprehensive care team: a controlled trial of outpatient palliative medicine consultation. *Arch Intern Med* 2004; **164**: 83–91.

51 Stewart M, Brown JB, Donner A, *et al*. The impact of patient-centered care on outcomes. *J Fam Pract* 2000; **49**: 796–804.

52 Sullivan M. The new subjective medicine: taking the patient's point of view on health care and health. *Soc Sci Med* 2003; **56**: 1595–604.

53 Continuing education. Bayer Institute for Health Care Communication. Available at: www.bayerinstitute.org/conted/index.htm (accessed December 3, 2003).

◆ 54 Mead N, Bower P. Patient-centredness: a conceptual framework and review of the empirical literature. *Soc Sci Med* 2000; **51**: 1087–110.

◆ 55 Morrison RS, Meier DE. Clinical practice. Palliative care. *N Engl J Med* 2004; **350**: 2582–90.

56 Angus DC, Barnato AE, Linde-Zwirble WT, *et al*. Use of intensive care at the end of life in the United States: an epidemiologic study. *Crit Care Med* 2004; **32**: 638–43.

● 57 Christakis NA, Escarce JJ. Survival of Medicare patients after enrollment in hospice programs. *N Engl J Med* 1996; **335**: 172–8.

58 Wennberg JE, Fisher ES, Stukel TA, *et al*. Use of hospitals, physician visits, and hospice care during last six months of life among cohorts loyal to highly respected hospitals in the United States. *BMJ* 2004; **328**: 607.

◆ 59 Epstein RM. Mindful practice. *JAMA* 1999; **282**: 833–9.

60 McWhinney IR, Stewart MA. Home care of dying patients. Family physicians' experience with a palliative care support team. *Can Fam Physician* 1994; **40**: 240–6.

● 61 Jaen CR, Stange KC, Nutting PA. Competing demands of primary care: a model for the delivery of clinical preventive services. *J Fam Pract* 1994; **38**: 166–71.

62 Robert Wood Johnson Foundation. Improving Chronic Illness Care. Available at: http://improvingchroniccare.org (accessed December 18, 2003).

✱ 63 Katon W, Von Korff M, Lin E, *et al*. Stepped collaborative care for primary care patients with persistent symptoms of depression: a randomized trial. *Arch Gen Psychiatry* 1999; **56**: 1109–15.

● 64 Unutzer J, Katon W, Callahan CM, *et al*. Collaborative care management of late-life depression in the primary care setting: a randomized controlled trial. *JAMA* 2002; **288**: 2836–45.

65 Walter LC, Covinsky KE. Cancer screening in elderly patients: a framework for individualized decision making. *JAMA* 2001; **285**: 2750–6.

66 Jerant AF, Azari RS, Nesbitt TS, Meyers FJ. The TLC model of palliative care in the elderly: preliminary application in the assisted living setting. *Am Fam Med* 2004; **2**: 54–60.

67 National Hospice Organization. *Medical Guidelines for Determining Prognosis in Selected Non-cancer Diseases*, 2nd ed. Arlington, Virginia: National Hospice Organization, 1996.

● 68 SUPPORT Investigators. A controlled trial to improve care for seriously ill hospitalized patients: the Study to Understand Prognoses and Preferences for Outcomes and Risks of Treatments (SUPPORT). *JAMA* 1995; **274**: 1591–8.

69 Carlet J, Thijs LG, Antonelli M, *et al*. Challenges in end-of-life care in the ICU. Statement of the 5th International Consensus Conference in Critical Care: Brussels, Belgium, April 2003. *Intensive Care Med* 2004; **30**: 770–84.

70 Danis M, Federman D, Fins JJ, *et al*. Incorporating palliative care into critical care education: principles, challenges, and opportunities. *Crit Care Med* 1999; **27**: 2005–13.

PART 7

Overview of assessment

39

Multidimensional assessment in palliative care

ERNESTO VIGNAROLI, EDUARDO BRUERA

INTRODUCTION

Palliative medicine aims to decrease symptom burden and alleviate psychosocial distress in patients and families. Suffering is a state of distress that occurs when the intactness or integrity of the person is threatened or disrupted. Much of this suffering is often left unaddressed when healthcare is focused on the *disease* rather than the *person* with the disease.[1]

A patient's experience of advanced illness is complex: from physical symptoms, to coping, financial concerns, caregiver burden, social and family changes, and spiritual concerns. These issues should be managed through an interdisciplinary approach, with the focus of care being the patient and the family rather than the disease. Physicians must work together with many other professionals, such as nurses, psychologists, chaplains, occupational therapists, physical therapists, nutritionists, social workers, pharmacists and volunteers, to provide care and support.[2] This enables a multidimensional evaluation that includes assessment of the patient's clinical and psychosocial characteristics, identification of specific prognostic factors related to symptoms, and the patient's self-reported symptom burden (Fig. 39.1).[3]

This chapter aims to bring together and summarize the different components of multidimensional bedside clinical assessment in palliative care and its importance for symptom control, quality of life, and decision making. The type of assessment tool and the intensity of assessment will vary according to the patient population (e.g. cancer patients, geriatric patients, etc.), the setting (palliative care unit, outpatients, home, etc.), and a variety of issues related to the

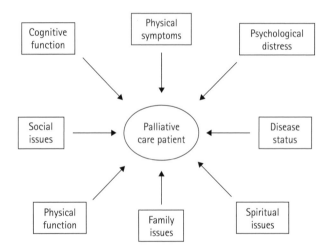

Figure 39.1 *Assessing the palliative care patient.*

team composition, culture, etc. The reader is referred to specific chapters in this book for a more comprehensive assessment and the use of specific tools for each particular symptom.

MULTIDIMENSIONAL ASSESSMENT

There are three steps in the experience of symptoms: production, perception, and expression. Production of a symptom is the process by which nociception occurs. In the case of cancer pain, for example, J receptor stimulation in the lung results in the production of dyspnea or the afferent stimulus from the gastrointestinal tract or central nervous system results in the production of nausea. Production can be significantly different in one individual to another and in different areas within the same individual (e.g. some patients have multiple bone metastases of which only one hurts). Perception is the process by which the symptom reaches the brain cortex. This can also differ significantly from one individual to another (in the case of pain, endorphins or descending inhibitory pathways can significantly confound the intensity of the pain perceived). Unfortunately, these two stages cannot be measured. Finally, the expression of the distress is the only measurable part of the experience and is a target of therapy. However, this stage can also vary from one individual to another due to beliefs about the symptom experience, intrapsychic factors such as depression or somatization, and even cultural factors.

In summary, although it is important to measure the intensity of a certain symptom such as pain, fatigue, or nausea, it is important to recognize that this intensity of expression does not have the same unidimensional value of, for example, blood glucose in of the control of diabetes, or blood pressure in the control of arterial hypertension. Interpreting the intensity of pain expression as being only the expression of nociception would deny that in addition to variability in nociception, there is a great variability in both perception and

expression. Rather, symptom expression should be interpreted as a multidimensional construct. In a given patient, a score of 8 out of 10 in pain intensity could be the result of nociception plus a certain level of somatization, coping chemically, and mild delirium. The multidimensional assessment should help in the recognition of the contribution of the different dimensions to the patient's symptom expression, and thereby assist in the planning of care. A purely unidimensional interpretation of intensity of pain would result in assuming that 100 percent success can be achieved with the simple use of higher and higher doses of analgesics. This simplistic approach could result in massive doses of opioids, opioid-related toxicity and excessive reliance on pharmacologic, as compared with nonpharmacologic, approaches to symptom control. A number of tools can be used to assess the contribution of different dimensions of the patient's symptom expression.[4–6] Figure 39.2 summarizes these steps with regard to the production of cancer pain. However, similar steps can be described for most other physical symptoms.

DISEASE STATUS

Patients are considered eligible for palliative care when they have a progressive life-threatening illness. It is therefore

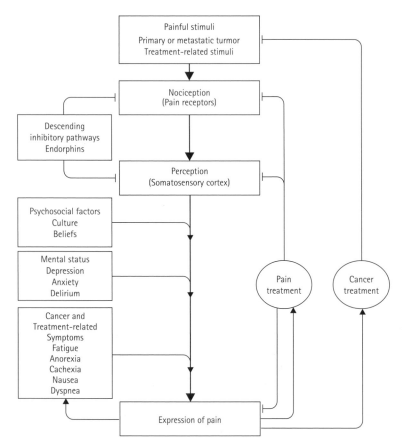

Figure 39.2 *Steps in the expression of cancer pain. Redrawn from Bruera and Kim. Cancer pain. JAMA 2003;**290**: 2476–9[6] with permission.*

important for the palliative care specialist to understand the stages of the underlying illness.

The initial step involves a complete medical history that reviews the disease diagnosis (cancer, acquired immune deficiency syndrome (AIDS), end-stage chronic obstructive pulmonary disease, congestive heart failure, or renal disease, etc.), the chronology of disease-related events, previous therapies, and all relevant medical, surgical, and psychiatric problems. A detailed history includes current and prior use of prescription and nonprescription drugs, 'alternative' medical therapies, drug allergies, and previous adverse reactions. The patient should be questioned about prior treatment modalities for each symptom and their perceived efficacy. Symptom assessment must include a thorough physical examination and review of the available laboratory and imaging data. Specific imaging, laboratory tests, or specialist referral may be appropriate to understand the pathophysiology of symptoms and their relationship to the disease.[7]

Walker *et al.*[8] developed and tested the Edmonton Labeled Visual Information System (ELVIS), a pictorial representation aimed at improving a physician's ability to comprehend and remember the basic details of the patient's disease status and prior treatments (Fig. 39.3). This instrument is a simple one-page line diagram that is used to graphically document the extent of disease in advanced cancer. It consists of two figures, of which one is used to document visceral and soft-tissue disease and the second, portraying the skeleton, is used to document bony disease. The diagrams are simple, and require the user to draw in, as necessary, sex-specific organs such as breasts, ovaries, the uterus, or testes, as well as other structures that have not been included. White space is provided to add labels to the visual representations and to document type and date of different treatments.

Palliative medicine specialists needs to be knowledgeable about the natural history and treatment of patients referred to their care. This allows for the appropriate recognition of

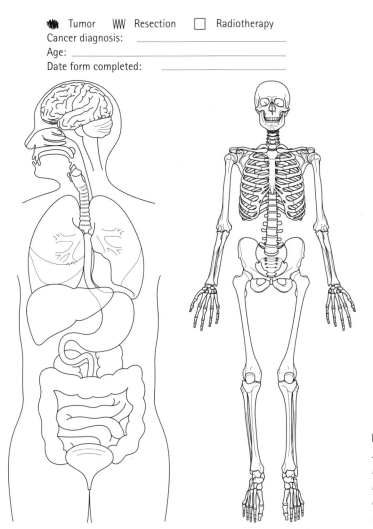

Figure 39.3 *The Edmonton Labeled Visual Information System (ELVIS). Redrawn from Walker et al. Impact of the Edmonton Labeled Visual Information System on physician recall of metastatic cancer patient histories. A randomized controlled trial.*[8] J Pain Symptom Manage *2001; 21: 4–11 with permission.*

patients referred to palliative care who might significantly benefit from life-prolonging, or occasionally even curative therapy. For example, a patient with advanced testicular cancer or Hodgkin disease may be severely symptomatic and appropriate for a palliative care referral. However, this patient should also immediately be referred to an oncologist because there is potentially curative therapy available. Similarly, a patient with opportunistic symptomatic infections related to AIDS with no history of previous triple antiviral therapy should be treated by the palliative care team in coordination with an AIDS specialist.

SYMPTOM ASSESSMENT

Symptoms are inherently subjective. They are perceptions, usually expressed by language.[9] Patient self-report is the primary source of information of symptom presence and severity. Communication is frequently difficult in terminally ill patients because of delirium or severe sedation due to drugs, metabolic abnormalities, infections, brain metastases, etc.[10] Proxies may be considered as an alternative or complementary source of information, especially during end-of-life care.[11] However, numerous studies have demonstrated that observer and patient assessments are not highly correlated, and that the accuracy of a clinician's assessment cannot be assumed.[12–14]

Healthcare providers often underestimate the severity of pain and other symptoms.[12,15] In studies of patients with terminal cancer assessed by healthcare workers as compared with the patients, agreement was higher for physical than psychological and cognitive symptoms, there was a greater agreement on absence rather than on the presence of a symptom,[10] and the variation in symptom scores was minimal when at least two individuals contributed in the assessment.[16]

Data about concordance of patient proxies' reports suggest that a patient's and their family members' reports of patient pain and performance status were highly correlated, although family members consistently reported more pain and disability.[13] Another study that assessed patients and their spouse caregivers suggests that caregivers agree with patients on objective measures with observable referents (e.g. ability to dress independently) but disagree with subjective aspects of patients' functioning (e.g. depression, fear of future, and confidence in treatment).[14]

Frequency of symptoms

Patients with advanced illnesses have an extraordinarily high frequency of physical and psychological complaints that impact on quality of life. Symptoms may vary with age, sex, primary tumor, and extent of disease.[17–21] In different studies[22–25] conducted in cancer patients referred to a palliative medicine program both as inpatients or outpatients the

median number of symptoms per patient was 11 (range 1–27). The 10 most prevalent symptoms were pain, lack of energy, dry mouth, dyspnea, feeling drowsy, anorexia, insomnia, feeling sad, constipation, and greater than 10 percent weight loss. The frequency of these 10 symptoms ranged from 50 percent to 84 percent. The most common symptoms were also the most severe. Gastrointestinal symptoms were also common in nongastrointestinal primary site cancers. Specific symptoms were influenced by age, sex, or performance status. For example, males had more dysphagia, hoarseness, >10 percent weight loss and sleep problems; females had more early satiety, nausea, vomiting, and anxiety. Vogl et al.[26] conducted a study in 504 AIDS outpatients and observed higher symptom distress and symptoms (mean number 16). The most prevalent symptoms were worrying, fatigue, sadness, and pain. Patients with intravenous drug use as an HIV transmission factor reported more symptoms and higher overall and physical symptom distress.

Assessment tools

In the process of instrument selection, the physician must carefully consider the goals of assessment and the practicality and acceptability of the assessment instrument by the terminally ill patient.[27] Simple assessment tools are the most appropriate for patients with advanced cancer. These patients may be weak and experiencing symptoms that make it difficult to complete a time-consuming and complex assessment tool.

Assessment tools are not only useful to diagnose and evaluate the intensity of the symptoms but also to monitor the effectiveness of therapy and to screen for side effects of medications. They play a role in the early identification of poor prognostic factors that can hamper the management of the symptoms of advanced cancer. Assessment tools should be used regularly, especially when patients experience new symptoms, an increase in the intensity of preexisting symptoms, or when therapy changes. The results should be documented in the patient's chart to ensure accuracy in the monitoring of the symptoms. The Memorial Symptom Assessment Scale[28] (MSAS), the Symptom Distress Scale[29] (SDS), the Rotterdam Symptom Checklist[30] (RSCL), and the Edmonton Symptom Assessment System[31] (ESAS) are examples of instruments that have been developed to monitor multiple symptoms in the setting of advanced cancer.

The ESAS is a concise, user-friendly, palliative care assessment tool that has been widely used in the clinical setting. It consists of a series of 10 visual analog scales that evaluate a mix of psychological and physical symptoms, in addition to a global sense of wellbeing[32] (Fig. 39.4). The visual analog scales are used by patients who are cognitively intact to rate symptoms from 0 to 10 and the resulting scores are then transferred to a graphical representation in the patient's chart. In patients with mild cognitive impairment, the ratings are

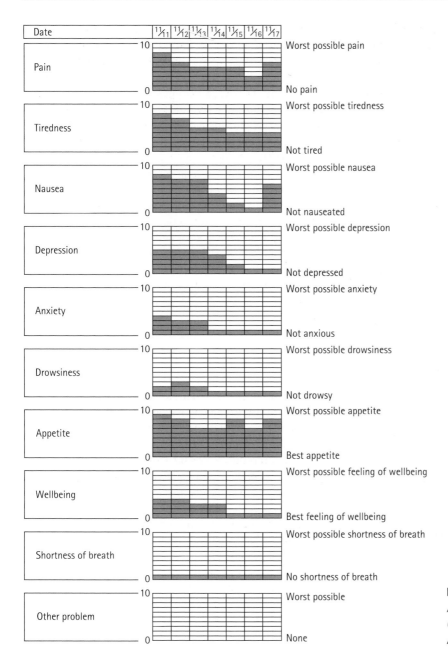

Figure 39.4 *The Edmonton Symptom Assessment System (ESAS). Adapted from Guidelines for using the Edmonton Symptom Assessment System (ESAS) with permission.[32]*

conducted in association with family or staff. For patients with moderate or severe cognitive impairment, especially during the last days of life, the family or staff provide the ratings.[33] Certain visual patterns which developed over time on the graphical display can alert the physician to the interdependence of the various symptoms and psychosocial influences. There appears to be a tendency for patients who experience psychosocial distress on a physical level consistently to rate many of their symptoms at a high level. Recognition of these patterns allows caregiving teams to be proactive and to focus on psychosocial influences as well as addressing the physical symptoms.

The validity and reliability of ESAS has recently been explored, and in advanced cancer it is apparent that it is a valid instrument.[34] The MSAS is a validated, patient-rated

instrument that assess the frequency, intensity, and distress level associated with 32 physical and psychological symptoms. It is mostly used in research settings[35,36] because it is lengthy and inconvenient to use on a regular basis. Recently, Chang *et al.* developed the Condensed Memorial Symptom Assessment Scale[37] (CMSAS), a 14-symptom instrument that contains both quality of life and survival information equivalent to the original 32 items. The symptoms identified by Chang *et al.* are also included in other widely used clinical symptom assessment instruments, such the ESAS, RSCL, and SDS. This report is also one of the first to demonstrate that scales from a shorter instrument can be predictive of survival, and that there is a core of symptoms that provide most of the information about health, quality of life and survival. The CMSAS needs to be further evaluated and validated and the optimal number of symptoms in this version are still under study.

ASSESSMENT OF DELIRIUM AND COGNITIVE IMPAIRMENT

The presence of cognitive impairment, whether as a result of delirium or dementia, presents a major impediment in the assessment of symptoms in patients with advanced disease.[38] Delirium is an important source of distress to patients, family members, and caregivers. Patient assessment becomes difficult, communication of patients with caregivers and family members is impaired, the patient's expression of their symptoms is usually increased, and they are usually unable to participate in their own care.[39] The frequency of delirium in patients with advanced cancer varies from 28 percent to 40 percent on admission.[40,41] Eventually, up to 83 percent of patients develop delirium in their final days, and 10–0 percent of them may require palliative terminal sedation.[42,43] In some studies delirium was not detected in 22–50 percent of the cases.[44]

The diagnosis of delirium is made on the basis of acute onset, fluctuation in course, reduced sensorium, attention deficit, and cognitive and perceptual disturbance, which occurs in the presence of an underlying organic derangement.[45] The Mini-Mental State Examination (MMSE)[46] is a widely used screening tool for cognitive impairment as a component of delirium. The cut-off points depend on formal education reached and age, and may vary for elderly people in different countries.[47,48] Other tools have been developed and validated for screening or monitoring the course of delirium, such as the Memorial Delirium Assessment Scale[49,50] (MDAS), the Delirium Rating Scale,[51,52] and the Confusion Assessment Method[53–55] (CAM). See Chapter 72 for the different uses of these assessment tools in delirium.

Based on the level of psychomotor activity, there are three subtypes of delirium: hyperactive, hypoactive, and mixed, which is the most frequent form of presentation.[56,57] Misdiagnoses of hypoactive delirium as depression or agitated delirium as anxiety disorder is not unusual. The emotional lability, disinhibition, and psychomotor agitation components of delirium are frequently interpreted as worsening pain by relatives, and sometimes by medical and nursing staff,[58] especially in the absence of any objective cognitive testing. Fainsinger et al.[59] described a 'destructive triangle' created as a result of the family's misinterpretation of the patient's delirium as pain, and their consequent desire for nursing and the physician's efforts to 'do something'. The doctor may be placed under pressure to relieve the patient and family's distress. This emotional overload may lead to an increase in the opioid dose and aggravate the agitation, in particular when the opioid is already implicated as a precipitant.[60] A multidimensional assessment in this setting will lead to cognitive testing and the recognition of delirium. This assessment may result in more appropriate interventions, such as opioid rotation or dose reduction, and prescription of a neuroleptic for the symptomatic treatment of delirium.[61]

Delirium can result in misinterpretation of symptoms and emotion expression, and conflict between the patient's family and healthcare professionals, or even among different healthcare professionals with regard to the patient's behavior. Once the diagnosis of delirium has been confirmed by a thorough medical assessment it is important to appropriately inform the different disciplines in the team about the presence of this syndrome because a number of pharmacologic, rehabilitation, and counseling interventions may be inappropriate in patients with severe cognitive failure or delirium. Education for the family will also be important to help them understand the inhibited expression of physical or emotional distress in a cognitively impaired or delirious patient.

ASSESSMENT OF PHYSICAL FUNCTION

The majority of patients with terminal illness have impaired ability to perform everyday functions during the various stages of the disease. Functional status is an independent predictor of survival.[62] It is also essential for planning the setting of care, which can be the home, hospice, or acute service.

The Karnofsky Performance Scale[63] (KPS) and the Eastern Cooperative Oncology Group[64] (ECOG) have been used widely in the assessment of physical function in cancer patients. The KPS is considered a 'gold standard' for assessment of functional status in cancer patients.[65,66] However, in patients with advanced cancer in palliative care setting assessments these instruments tend to generate clustering of scores at the extreme end of impairment. Consequently, newer instruments such as the Edmonton Functional Assessment Tool[67] (EFAT) and the Palliative Performance Scale[68] (PPS) have been developed. The EFAT includes domains such as pain, mental alertness, sensory function, communication, and respiratory function, in addition to domains that more directly reflect physical function, such as balance, mobility, wheelchair mobility, activity, activities of daily living, and dependence performance status. This information can give physicians prognostic information about the patient. For example, a bedridden patient with severe pain due to a pathological hip fracture has a much better potential for recovery than a patient bedridden due to cachexia and delirium. A revised version of the EFAT has recently been validated.[69] The PPS is essentially a modification of the KPS and assesses ambulation, activity, self-care, intake, and conscious level.[70]

An objective assessment of physical functioning constitutes part of the multidimensional symptom assessment in palliative care. Impairment in physical functioning and distressing physical symptoms such as pain have the potential to adversely affect psychosocial function.[71,72] Physical and occupational therapy assessments may reveal deficits and suggest interventions that can be essential to maintaining functional capacity, ensuring patient safety, conserving energy, and decreasing fatigue. A speech therapy assessment can provide valuable information regarding swallowing function, while a nutritional assessment by a dietician can aid in determining caloric intake.

The assessment of physical function in palliative medicine will allow for the identification of simple measures such as special wheelchairs, ramps if there are steps in the home, bathroom supplies, a trapeze for bed mobility, or the need for a formal rehabilitation approach. On the other hand, in some cases decreased function may be associated with conditions such as severe incidental pain, delirium, dyspnea with minimal efforts, or irreversible neurological damage and in these cases appropriate adaptation to the loss in function, and patient and family education will be the most appropriate course of action. Therefore, the assessment of physical function needs to be integrated with an understanding of the underlying disease status, symptom control, psychosocial distress, etc.

ASSESSMENT OF PSYCHOLOGICAL DISTRESS

The perception of different symptoms, such as pain or fatigue, may be accentuated by the emotional or psychological distress of the patient. Psychological distress impairs the patient's capacity for pleasure, meaning, and connection; erodes quality of life; amplifies pain and other symptoms;[73] reduces the patient's ability to do the emotional work of separating and saying good-bye; and causes anguish and worry among family members and friends. Finally, psychological distress, particularly depression, is a major risk for suicide and for requests to hasten death.[74] On the other hand, severe undertreated physical distress leads to severe psychological distress. Untreated or under-treated pain, nausea, dyspnea, or other uncomfortable physical symptoms can profoundly disturb mood, sleep, and make it impossible for patients to relate appropriately to their family and their healthcare professionals.

A psychological assessment should be done to evaluate mainly mood and coping. It is important for a team's members to become familiar with each of these areas, and to recognize when there are issues that need further assessment and/or intervention by another healthcare discipline.[2] Medical staff often fail to recognize and address psychological distress, and this impacts negatively on quality of life.[75]

Patients with terminal diseases have a variety of ways of coping with their diagnosis, including fear, anger, avoidance, denial, intellectualization, intense grieving, and existential questioning. The distinction is often difficult to make between the normal psychological burden that exists in relation to physical and psychological distress and certain aspects of psychopathology such as somatization, anxiety, adjustment

disorder, and depression.[58,76] In addition, physical symptoms of depression (such as fatigue, anorexia, sleep disturbance, etc.) may be attributable to the disease itself.

Numerous factors act as barriers to recognition and treatment of psychological symptoms. Both patients and clinicians believe that psychological distress is a normal feature of the dying process and fail to differentiate natural, existential distress from clinical depression. Physicians lack clinical knowledge and skills to identify depression, anxiety, and delirium, especially in terminally ill patients where the diagnostic clues are confounded by coexisting medical illness and appropriate sadness. Patients and clinicians often avoid exploration of psychological issues because of time constraints and concerns that such exploration will cause further distress. Physicians are reluctant to prescribe psychotropic agents, which can have additional adverse effects, and therefore may hesitate to diagnose a condition that they feel they cannot treat successfully. Finally, when caring for dying patients, physicians may feel a sense of hopelessness that can lead to therapeutic nihilism.[72,77]

Mood disorders

Studies conducted during the past decades have revealed that mood disorders are highly prevalent in oncology: figures ranged from 2 percent to 46 percent for anxiety, from 6 percent to 42 percent for depressive, and from 32 percent to 52 percent for adjustment disorders, depending on sample characteristics (e.g. stage of disease, outpatient or inpatient), mode of data collection (e.g. interviews vs. self-assessment) and diagnostic criteria (e.g. cut-off scores for determining pathological cases).[78–81]

The clinical interview is the gold standard for diagnosis of depression.[82,83] Chochinov et al.[84] found that the single question 'Are you depressed?' provides a sensitive and specific assessment of depression in terminally ill patients. Another useful question is: 'Have you often been bothered by having little interest or pleasure in doing things?' The first question targets mood, while the latter is an indicator of anhedonia.[85] A patient who responds affirmatively to any of these questions is likely to receive a diagnosis after a comprehensive interview.[86,87]

Patients who are at increased risk for developing psychiatric complications are those with low performance status, those receiving certain cancer treatments, and those with uncontrolled physical symptoms, functional limitations, lack of social support, and past history of psychiatric disorder, substance abuse, or family history of depression or suicide.[88,89]

Somatization

Somatization is broadly defined as the somatic manifestation of psychological distress. This should be distinguished from the 'somatization disorder' in the somatoform disorders section of Diagnostic and Statistical Manual (DSM)-IV.[90] Somatoform disorders are rare in cancer patients and have a restrictive set of criteria.[91,92] Somatization is closely related to depression, anxiety, personality disorders, and cognitive impairment.[93–95] Patients who somatize will have a tendency to express pain intensity as higher, will have poorly defined etiology after appropriate investigations, will describe pain 'all over the body', and derive little benefit (but often toxicity) from pharmacological treatment.[57,96] In addition to a history of affective disorder, a history of functional somatic syndromes[97] (e.g. chronic pelvic pain, irritable bowel syndrome, fibromyalgia, tension headache, chronic fatigue syndrome), and the simultaneous presence of multiple highly intense symptoms (high ESAS scores in multiple domains) are all signs suggestive of somatization. Because of the absence of a gold standard, the diagnosis of somatization is made based on a number of repeated observations, and after extensive discussion with the patient and family.[98]

Patients who somatize frequently express increased symptom intensity associated with stressors, and many patients are unaware of this coping mechanism. It is important to recognize that in most palliative care patients, somatization consists of the increased expression of a symptom for which there is a clear pathophysiological mechanism, rather than the expression of symptoms for which there is no demonstrable pathophysiology, as is the case for somatoform disorders.

Chemical coping

Patients who have a past or active history of substance abuse present a special problem for symptom management. Their history of abuse reflects maladaptive coping strategies, which frequently lead to excessive expression of symptomatology. In patients with pain, this is often misinterpreted as nociception and may lead to an escalation of opioids and opioid-induced neurotoxicity.[57] The frequency of addictive disorders in the USA ranges from 3 percent to 16 percent with the higher rates reflecting prevalence of alcoholism.[99,100] Our group[101] reported a positive CAGE (Cut down, Annoyed by criticism, experiencing Guilt, Eye-opener drink in the morning) score 2/4 or more in 27 percent of cancer patients who were admitted to a palliative care unit. The rates of alcoholism in cancer patients may also be higher, as alcohol use and abuse can play an etiological role in several types of malignant disease (e.g. head and neck or esophageal cancer). Opioid abuse and misuse are more likely to be seen in cancer patients with a history of drug or alcohol abuse.[102,103] The CAGE[104] alcohol questionnaire is frequently used as a brief screening tool for detection of alcohol abuse. A positive response to two of the four questions is indicative of alcohol dependence and may also indicate abuse of other substances.[97] The questions refer to lifetime experience and not to any specific or limited time-frames in the patient's history. To improve the validity of the CAGE results, the questionnaire should be completed as part of the initial assessment, in particular before asking the patients about amounts of alcohol or drugs ingested.[3,5]

In palliative care the importance of a diagnosis of chemical coping is not related to the consequences of using alcohol or drugs. It rather relates to the patient's coping strategies and the increased likelihood that patients may cope chemically using opioid analgesics prescribed for pain control, mostly due to sharing a similar 'reward brain pathway' with alcohol (endorphins play a role in both).[105,106] A number of studies have observed that a history of chemical coping is an independent poor prognostic factor for pain control using opioid analgesia.[107,108] Fainsinger et al. have recently confirmed in a study on 619 patients, the independent prognostic value of chemical coping as a predictor of poor analgesic response to opioids.[109]

FAMILY ASSESSMENT

Chronic illness from advanced disease impacts on all the family members. A patient's relationship with their world changes with the news that their lifespan has been defined, thus altering their family interactions. Although the family is traditionally defined by individuals of blood relationship, a broader definition of family is most appropriate, best defined as those individuals considered as family by the patient.[110,111]

The patient's role/s within the family, as a provider, a caregiver, a parent, a spouse, or a sexual partner, may be challenged. Therefore the particular issues and needs of family members, in addition to the patient, must also be assessed.[112] Furthermore, because care will be provided by family members in the home setting, the family should also be consulted and educated about the diagnosis, treatment options, the illness trajectory, symptom burden and treatment, and caregiving.[2,113]

A genogram or family tree facilitates the understanding of a particular family's structure and dynamics. It helps to identify the family structure in a clear and comprehensive way. It highlights relationships and strengths and weaknesses, and can often clarify some of the family norms around disease/illness and coping. Family communication patterns, roles, and coping methods are components of family functioning affected by the cancer. For example, family members frequently do not share their thoughts or concerns with one another in an effort to protect each other. These 'conspiracies of silence' may complicate coping, and they should be diagnosed and treated.[114]

Caring for a person with cancer is demanding and overwhelming and can be a stressful experience that may erode the physical and psychological health of the caregiver.[115] For example, caregivers who provide 24-hour day care often experience cumulative sleep disruption, and fatigue is common.[116]

Also, caregivers of patients with cancer-related pain report even higher levels of depression, tension, and mood disturbances than caregivers of pain-free patients.[117,118] Therefore, to address and manage these issues, these patients should be managed together with psychologists and social workers, and this is important to reduce the psychological distress of caregivers. The patient–family unit is expected to make decisions about treatment options, goals of care, advance directives, and finances. The importance of advance care planning for the patient and family is stressed and this is best addressed early in the course of illness and frequently reassessed. Early discussions regarding prognosis, likely course of the disease, events to anticipate, and clarifying advanced directives all can serve to mitigate subsequent dilemmas, and increase control and lessen angst.

The family assessment is particularly important for patients who will receive care at home. The willingness of the family to deliver care at home is the most important predictor of a home death.[119] Family members will be involved in all aspects of patient care at home including hygiene, repositioning, and administration of multiple medications. Knowledge of the family's structure and function will help physicians organize medications and other aspects of care. Ultimately, the level of family care available will be the main defining factor in discharging a patient back to the community or to an institution. Family meetings should be conducted in the majority of cases when a palliative care team discharges a patient home.

Involvement of family caregivers is essential for optimal treatment of cancer patients at the end of life, especially in ensuring treatment compliance, continuity of care, and social support.[120] For example, family members who fear drug addiction or respiratory depression may undermedicate a patient even though the patient is experiencing unrelieved pain.

SOCIAL ASSESSMENT

A number of socioeconomic factors have great influence on the expression of symptoms, psychosocial distress, family dynamics, and even overall access to healthcare professionals and medications. Socioeconomic status is one of the main predictors of home death,[121] and it is particularly important in countries where there is no universal access to healthcare such as the USA. However, socioeconomic status can also be an independent predictor of home death in other countries. The appropriate assessment of social and cultural needs will provide for better counseling, better planning of the site of care, enhanced communication, and even better adherence to pharmacological therapy. For example, patients with limited coverage for medications may not be able to afford some expensive opioid analgesics or antibiotics and it may be preferable to prescribe less expensive medications to ensure adherence to the treatment. Even

patients with adequate insurance incur substantial burdens related to uncovered services such as transportation or home care, lost salaries and work, household modifications, and alternative treatments.[122]

In some cases a simple social assessment will reveal that patients may benefit from a disabled parking sign, application for benefits, preparation of a will or funeral arrangements, or assistance with financial planning. These issues can greatly improve the quality of life for the patients and their communication with healthcare professionals and their family.

SPIRITUAL ASSESSMENT

Spiritual wellbeing is increasingly recognized as an important factor for patients with cancer and their caregivers. Spirituality can have a profound influence on the distress, ability to cope, and quality of life of seriously ill patients and their family caregivers. While religion is defined as a specific set of beliefs and practices associated with a recognized religious denomination, spirituality is a thought process or belief system that allows a person to experience a transcendent meaning in life, including the conviction that one is fulfilling a unique role and purpose in one's life.[123–125] Some studies have demonstrated the relationship between spiritual factors and lower levels of anxiety and distress, and between spirituality and experiencing a better quality of life.[126] Spiritual beliefs also may help patients and caregivers construct a meaningful framework for their illness and resultant suffering, and this may promote acceptance of the situation.[127]

Spiritual care can be provided not just by pastoral care workers. Most literature supports the idea that all individuals involved in palliative care, to the degree that they are willing and able to do so, be involved with the spiritual issues of their patients.[128] The most important way by which caregivers can promote good spiritual care of patients is listening. Taylor et al.[129] surveyed what patients with cancer and primary family caregivers expect from nurses with regard to having their spiritual needs addressed. Although some patients or caregivers do not want overt forms of spiritual care, many others are eager for them. Spiritual needs identified by participants in Taylor et al.'s study included kindness and respect, talking and listening, prayer, connecting with symmetry, authenticity, and physical presence; quality temporal nursing care; and mobilizing religious or spiritual resources.

Assessment of spirituality is important because on one hand those patients who use spirituality and/or religion as part of their coping skills can be encouraged to increase their use of these resources with the help of either supportive individuals within the palliative care team or their own community of faith. On the other hand, occasionally, a patient at the end of life may have a severe crisis from existential or spiritual distress resulting in severe psychological and/or physical symptom expression.[130] The identification of these issues may lead to appropriate spiritual support with improvement in symptom distress.

Clinical example

A 51-year-old man with nonsmall cell lung cancer, metastatic to lymph nodes and bone was referred to a palliative care service. He had been treated with cisplatinum and paclitaxel for three cycles with no response, and had received palliative radiation to the right hip, right lung, and associated mediastinum. Further disease progression was observed after second-line chemotherapy. He complained of increased chest wall pain for 2 weeks. The pain was sharp and stabbing, radiating from the anterior to the posterior chest wall on the right side. Intensity was 9/10. It was partially relieved with oxycodone ER 240 mg/day, hydro-morphone 48 mg/day, and oxycodone 40 mg as needed (approximately 160 mg/day). He also received temaze-pam 20 mg two tablets at bedtime, paroxetine 40 mg once daily, ondansetron 24 mg/day, and warfarin 1 mg daily. A unidimensional approach would have resulted in initially a large increase in the opioid dose followed by assessment in 3 days. In the multidimensional assessment high intensity levels of all symptoms were found in the ESAS (Fig. 39.5a). Other complaints included constipation (no bowel movement for last 3 days), sleep walking, confusion, myoclonus and hallucinations, and cough with white-to-clear colored sputum. The MMSE score was 23/30. The psychosocial history revealed that the patient was on disability benefits, and had a high school education. CAGE screening for alcoholism was 2/4. He was married for the second time and had a child from the previous marriage. His wife stated that she also had cancer. His daughter was supportive, but she had acquired immune deficiency syndrome (AIDS) and cervical cancer. Due to the symptoms and family issues, the patient was admitted to the palliative care unit. He underwent an opioid rotation to methadone because of the probable opioid-induced neurotoxicity (myoclonus, confusion, and hallucinations). Constipation was treated with senna and docusate. The dose of paroxetine was reduced and haloperidol was added for delirium. The patient and family were extensively counseled by the social worker, counselor, and pastoral care worker. After 3 days the patient showed significant symptom improvement (Fig. 39.5b). The oncologist commented that the patient was doing well, was maintaining an excellent performance status, and was interested in pursuing other treatment options.

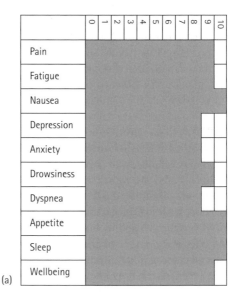

(a)

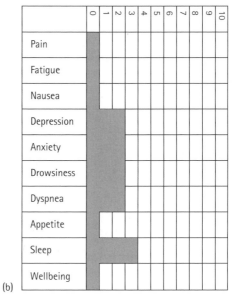

(b)

Figure 39.5 *Edmonton Symptom Assessment System (ESAS) for a 51-year old man with nonsmall cell lung cancer, showing (a) high scores for all symptoms and (b) significant improvement after 3 days of treatment.*

The clinical example above summarizes the importance of multidimensional assessment and the impact that this has on quality of life. This patient had symptoms of opioid-induce neurotoxicity and significant psychological distress, which exacerbated the expression of his symptoms, leading to increased opioid doses and aggravated confusion.

The assessment of the patient's severe pain and high opi-oid requirement within the context of all other symptoms and the family situation resulted in a dramatic change in the medical management. This rapid identification of multiple problems allowed for interdisciplinary management and rapid resolution of distress. It is important to practice disciplined multidimensional assessment of palliative care patients to be able to find unexpected abnormalities such as delirium, serious family difficulties, or multiple symptom distress. If the assessment only takes place in those cases in which problems are already suspected it is likely that a large number of patients with severe suffering will go undetected and untreated.

CONCLUSION

The traditional unidimensional model of assessment often equates symptom expression with symptom production. This approach has the potential for excessive reliance on pharmacological agents, with the likelihood of increases in toxicity, and under-utilization of nonpharmacological treatments. In turn, a multidimensional approach recognizes the interaction of many concurrent symptoms with one another and the influence of psychological distress, such as depression or somatization, and distress relating to financial, spiritual, and existential issues on symptom expression.

Recognition and relief of psychosocial and spiritual distress in terminally ill patients are among the fundamental principles of the multidisciplinary palliative care model, whose ultimate objective is the relief of symptoms and global patient distress, thereby helping to provide an optimal quality of life.

Key learning points

- Most palliative care patients suffer multiple physical and psychosocial symptoms.

- Symptom assessment needs to include the different dimensions that contribute to the production, perception, and expression of symptoms.

- Whenever possible, patients should be asked to score their symptoms.

- Mood disorders, somatization, and chemical coping have major influence on symptom expression.

- Social, spiritual, and family assessment is part of routine care in palliative medicine.

REFERENCES

1　Cassell EJ. Diagnosing suffering: a perspective. *Ann Intern Med* 1999; **131**: 31–4.

2　Muir JC, McDonagh A, Gooding N. Multidimensional patient assessment. In: Berger D, Portenoy RK, Weissman DE, eds. *Principles and Practice of Palliative Care and Supportive Oncology*, 2nd ed. Philadelphia, PA: Lippincott Williams & Wilkins, 2002: 653–60.

3　Elsayem A, Fish MJ. Assessment of pain and other symptoms. In: Elsayem A, Driver L, Bruera E, eds. *The MD Anderson Symptom Control and Palliative Care Handbook,* 2nd ed. The University of Texas-Houston Health Science Center, USA, 2002: 9–15.

4　Bruera E. Patient assessment in palliative cancer care. *Cancer Treat Rev* 1996; **22**(Suppl A): 3–12.

5　Kim HN, Bruera E, Jenkins R. Symptom control and palliative care. In: Cavalli F, Hansen HH, Kaye SB, eds. *Textbook of Medical Oncology*. Boca Raton, FL: Taylor & Francis, 2004: 353–70.

● 6　Bruera E, Kim HN. Cancer pain. *JAMA* 2003; **290**: 2476–9.

7　Ingham JM, Portenoy RK. Symptom assessment. In: Cherny NI, Foley KM, eds. *Hematology/Oncology Clinics of North America*. Philadelphia PA: WB Saunders, 1996; **10**: 21–40.

8　Walker P, Nordell C, Neumann CM, *et al.* Impact of the Edmonton Labeled Visual Information System on physician recall of metastatic cancer patient histories. A randomized controlled trial. *J Pain Symptom Manage* 2001; **21**: 4–11.

9　Ingham JM, Portenoy RK. The measurement of pain and other symptoms. In: Doyle D, Hanks G, Cherny N, Calman K, eds. *Oxford Textbook of Palliative Medicine*, 3th ed. Oxford: Oxford University Press, 2004: 167–84.

10　Zhukovsky DS, Abdullah O, Richardson M, *et al.* Clinical evaluation in advanced cancer. *Semin Oncol* 2000; **27**: 14–23.

11　Brunelli C, Constantini M, Di Guilio P, *et al.* Quality of life evaluation: when do terminal cancer patients and health care providers agree? *J Pain Symptom Manage* 1998; **15**: 149–50.

12　Grossman SA, Sheidler VR, Swedeen K, *et al.* Correlation of patient and caregiver ratings of cancer pain. *J Pain Symptom Manage* 1991; **6**: 53–7.

13　Elliott BA, Elliott TE, Murray DM, *et al.* Patients and family members: the role of knowledge and attitude in cancer pain. *J Pain Symptom Manage* 1996; **12**: 209–20.

14　Clipp EC, George LK. Patients with cancer and their spouse caregivers. Perceptions of illness experience. *Cancer* 1992; **69**: 1074–9.

● 15　Nekolaichuk CL, Bruera E, Spachynski K, *et al.* A comparison of patient and proxy symptom assessments in advanced cancer patients. *Palliat Med* 1999;13: 311–23.

● 16　Nekolaichuk CL, Maguire TO, Suarez-Almazor M, *et al.* Assessing the reliability of patient, nurse, and family caregiver symptom ratings in hospitalized advanced cancer patients. *J Clin Oncol* 1999; **17**: 3621–30.

17　Donnelly S, Walsh D. The symptoms of advanced cancer. *Semin Oncol* 1995; **22**(2 Suppl 3): 67–72.

18　Krech RL, Walsh D. Symptoms of pancreatic cancer. *J Pain Symptom Manage* 1991; **6**: 360–7.

19　Curtis EB, Krech R, Walsh TD. Common symptoms in patients with advanced cancer. *J Palliat Care* 1991; **7**: 25–9.

20　Komurcu S, Nelson KA, Walsh D, *et al.* Common symptoms in advanced cancer. *Semin Oncol* 2000; **27**: 24–33.

21　Reuben DB, Mor V, Hiris J. Clinical symptoms and length of survival in patients withterminal cancer. *Arch Intern Med* 1988; **148**: 1586–91.

22　Walsh D, Donnelly S, Rybicki L. The symptoms of advanced cancer: relationship to age, gender, and performance status in 1,000 patients. *Support Care Cancer* 2000; **8**: 175–9.

23　Portenoy RK, Thaler HT, Kornblith AB, *et al.* Symptom prevalence, characteristics and distress in a cancer population. *Qual Life Res* 1994; **3**: 183–9.

24　Chang VT, Hwang SS, Feuerman M, *et al.* Symptom and quality of life survey of medical oncology patients at a veterans affairs medical center: a role for symptom assessment. *Cancer* 2000; **88**: 1175–83.

25 Vainio A, Auvinen A. Prevalence of symptoms among patients with advanced cancer: an international collaborative study. Symptom Prevalence Group. *J Pain Symptom Manage* 1996; **12**: 3–10.

26 Vogl D, Rosenfeld B, Breitbart W, *et al.* Symptom prevalence, characteristics, and distress in AIDS outpatients. *J Pain Symptom Manage* 1999; **18**: 253–62.

◆ 27 Bruera E, Pereira J. Recent developments in palliative cancer care. *Acta Oncol* 1998; **37**: 749–57.

28 Portenoy RK, Thaler HT, Kornblith AB, *et al.* The Memorial Symptom Assessment Scale: an instrument for the evaluation of symptom prevalence, characteristics and distress. *Eur J Cancer* 1994; **30A**: 1326–36.

29 McCorkle R, Young K. Development of a symptom distress scale. *Cancer Nurs* 1978; **1**: 373–8.

30 de Haes JC, van Knippenberg FC, Neijt JP. Measuring psychological and physical distress in cancer patients: structure and application of the Rotterdam Symptom Checklist. *Br J Cancer* 1990; **62**: 1034–8.

31 Bruera E, Kuehn N, Miller MJ, *et al.* The Edmonton Symptom Assessment System (ESAS): a simple method for the assessment of palliative care patients. *J Palliat Care* 1991; **7**: 6–9.

32 Guidelines for using the Edmonton Symptom Assessment System (ESAS). Available at: www.palliative.org/PC/Assessment tools?easa.pdf (accessed on March 21, 2005).

33 Rees E, Hardy J, Ling J, *et al.* The use of the Edmonton Symptom Assessment Scale (ESAS) within a palliative care unit in the UK. *Palliat Med* 1998; **12**: 75–82.

● 34 Chang VT, Hwang SS, Feuerman M. Validation of the Edmonton Symptom Assessment Scale. *Cancer* 2000; **88**: 2164–71.

35 Chang VT, Hwang SS, Feuerman M, *et al.* The memorial symptom assessment scale short form (MSAS-SF). *Cancer* 2000; **89**: 1162–71.

36 Collins JJ, Devine TD, Dick GS, *et al.* The measurement of symptoms in young children with cancer: the validation of the Memorial Symptom Assessment Scale in children aged 7–12. *J Pain Symptom Manage* 2002; **23**: 10–16.

37 Chang VT, Hwang SS, Kasimis B, *et al.* Shorter symptom assessment instruments: the Condensed Memorial Symptom Assessment Scale (CMSAS). *Cancer Invest* 2004; **22**: 526–36.

◆ 38 Ingham J, Breitbart W. Epidemiology and clinical features of delirium. In: Portenoy RK, Bruera E, eds. *Topics in Palliative Care, Vol 1.* New York: Oxford University Press, 1997: 7–19.

◆ 39 Centeno C, Sanz A, Bruera E. Delirium in advanced cancer patients. *Palliat Med* 2004; **18**: 184–94.

● 40 Lawlor PG, Gagnon B, Mancini IL, *et al.* Occurrence, causes, and outcome of delirium in patients with advanced cancer: a prospective study. *Arch Intern Med* 2000; **160**: 786–94.

41 Minagawa H, Uchitomi Y, Yamawaki S, *et al.* Psychiatric morbidity in terminally ill cancer patients. A prospective study. *Cancer* 1996; **78**: 1131–7.

42 Bruera E, Miller L, McCallion J, *et al.* Cognitive failure in patients with terminal cancer: a prospective study. *J Pain Symptom Manage* 1992; **7**: 192–5.

43 Morita T, Tei Y, Tsunoda J, *et al.* Underlying pathologies and their associations with clinical features in terminal delirium of cancer patients. *J Pain Symptom Manage* 2001; **22**: 997–1006.

44 Inouye SK. The dilemma of delirium: clinical and research controversies regarding diagnosis and evaluation of delirium in hospitalized elderly medical patients. *Am J Med* 1994; **97**: 278–88.

45 American Psychiatric Association. Delirium, dementia and amnesic and other cognitive disorders. In: *Diagnostic and Statistical Manual of Mental Disorders*, 4th ed. Washington DC: American Psychiatric Association, 1994: 123–33.

46 Folstein MF, Folstein SE, McHugh PR. 'Mini-mental state'. A practical method for grading the cognitive state of patients for the clinician. *J Psychiatr Res* 1975; **12**: 189–98.

47 Lobo A, Saz P, Marcos G, *et al.* Revalidation and standardization of the cognition mini-exam (first Spanish version of the Mini-Mental Status Examination) in the general geriatric population. *Med Clin (Barc)* 1999; **112**: 767–74.

48 Hjermstad M, Loge JH, Kaasa S. Methods for assessment of cognitive failure and delirium in palliative care patients: implications for practice and research. *Palliat Med* 2004; **18**: 494–506.

49 Breitbart W, Rosenfeld B, Roth A, *et al.* The Memorial Delirium Assessment Scale. *J Pain Symptom Manage* 1997; **13**: 128–37.

● 50 Lawlor PG, Nekolaichuk C, Gagnon B, *et al.* Clinical utility, factor analysis, and further validation of the memorial delirium assessment scale in patients with advanced cancer: Assessing delirium in advanced cancer. *Cancer* 2000; **88**: 2859–67.

51 Trzepacz PT, Baker RW, Greenhouse J. A symptom rating scale for delirium. *Psychiatry Res* 1988; **23**: 89–97.

52 Gagnon P, Allard P, Masse B, *et al.* Delirium in terminal cancer: a prospective study using daily screening, early diagnosis, and continuous monitoring. *J Pain Symptom Manage* 2000; **19**: 412–26.

53 Inouye SK, van Dyck CH, Alessi CA, *et al.* Clarifying confusion: the confusion assessment method. A new method for detection of delirium. *Ann Intern Med* 1990; **113**: 941–8.

54 Fabbri RM, Moreira MA, Garrido R, *et al.* Validity and reliability of the Portuguese version of the Confusion Assessment Method (CAM) for the detection of delirium in the elderly. *Arq Neuropsiquiatr* 2001; **59**(2-A): 175–9.

55 Marcantonio ER, Flacker JM, Wright RJ, *et al.* Reducing delirium after hip fracture: a randomized trial. *J Am Geriatr Soc* 2001; **49**: 516–22.

56 Ross CA, Peyser CE, Shapiro I, *et al.* Delirium: phenomenologic and etiologic subtypes. *Int Psychogeriatr* 1991; **3**: 135–47.

57 Liptzin B, Levkoff SE. An empirical study of delirium subtypes. *Br J Psychiatry* 1992; **161**: 843–5.

58 Coyle N, Breitbart W, Weaver S, *et al.* Delirium as a contributing factor to 'crescendo' pain: three case reports. *J Pain Symptom Manage* 1994; **9**: 44–7.

59 Fainsinger RL, Tapper M, Bruera E. A perspective on the management of delirium in terminally ill patients on a palliative care unit. *J Palliat Care* 1993; **9**: 4–8.

60 Lawlor P, Walker P, Bruera E, *et al.* Severe opioid toxicity and somatization of psychosocial distress in a cancer patient with

a background of chemical dependence. *J Pain Symptom Manage* 1997; **13**: 356–61.

◆ 61 Lawlor PG. Multidimensional assessment: pain and palliative care. In: Bruera E, Portenoy RK, eds. *Cancer Pain.* New York: Cambridge University Press, 2003: 67–88.

● 62 Vigano A, Dorgan M, Buckingham J, *et al.* Survival prediction in terminal cancer patients: a systematic review of the medical literature. *Palliat Med* 2000; **14**: 363–74.

63 Yates JW, Chalmer B, McKegney FP. Evaluation of patients with advanced cancer using the Karnofsky performance status. *Cancer* 1980; **45**: 2220–4.

64 Osoba D, MacDonald N. Principles governing the use of cancer chemotherapy in palliative care. In: Doyle D, Hanks GWC, MacDonald N, eds. *Oxford Textbook of Palliative Medicine*, 2nd ed. Oxford: Oxford University Press, 1998:249–67.

65 Conill C, Verger E, Salamero M. Performance status assessment in cancer patients. *Cancer* 1990; **65**: 1864–6.

66 Mor V, Laliberte L, Morris JN, *et al.* The Karnofsky Performance Status Scale. An examination of its reliability and validity in a research setting. *Cancer* 1984; **53**: 2002–7.

67 Kaasa T, Loomis J, Gillis K, *et al.* The Edmonton Functional Assessment Tool: preliminary development and evaluation for use in palliative care. *J Pain Symptom Manage* 1997; **13**: 10–19.

68 Anderson F, Downing GM, Hill J, *et al.* Palliative performance scale (PPS): a new tool. *J Palliat Care* 1996; **12**: 5–11.

69 Kaasa T, Wessel J. The Edmonton Functional Assessment Tool: further development and validation for use in palliative care. *J Palliat Care* 2001; **17**: 5–11.

70 Virik K, Glare P. Validation of the palliative performance scale for inpatients admitted to a palliative care unit in Sydney, Australia**.** *J Pain Symptom Manage* 2002; **23**: 455–7.

71 Portenoy RK, Payne D, Jacobsen P. Breakthrough pain: characteristics and impact in patients with cancer pain. *Pain* 1999; **81**: 129–34.

72 Walsh D, Rybicki L, Nelson KA, *et al.* Symptoms and prognosis in advanced cancer. *Support Care Cancer* 2002; **10**: 385–8.

73 Breitbart W, Bruera E, Chochinov H, *et al.* Neuropsychiatric syndromes and psychological symptoms in patients with advanced cancer. *J Pain Symptom Manage* 1995; **10**: 131–41.

74 Chochinov HM, Wilson KG, Enns M, *et al.* Desire for death in the terminally ill. *Am J Psychiatry* 1995; **152**: 1185–91.

75 Breitbart W, Chochinov HM, Passik SD. In: Doyle D, Hanks G, Cherny N, Calman K, eds. *Oxford Textbook of Palliative Medicine*, 3th ed. Oxford: Oxford University Press, 2004: 746–71.

◆ 76 Block SD. Assessing and managing depression in the terminally ill patient. ACP-ASIM End-of-Life Care Consensus Panel. American College of Physicians – American Society of Internal Medicine. *Ann Intern Med* 2000; **132**: 209–18.

77 Block SD, Billings JA. Patient requests to hasten death. Evaluation and management in terminal care. *Arch Intern Med* 1994; **154**: 2039–47.

78 Bredart A, Didier F, Robertson C, *et al.* Psychological distress in cancer patients attending the European Institute of Oncology in Milan. *Oncology* 1999; **57**: 297–302.

79 Derogatis LR, Morrow GR, Fetting J, *et al.* The prevalence of psychiatric disorders among cancer patients. *JAMA* 1983; **249**: 751–7.

80 Razavi D, Delvaux N, Farvacques C, *et al.* Screening for adjustment disorders and major depressive disorders in cancer in-patients. *Br J Psychiatry* 1990; **156**: 79–83.

81 Ibbotson T, Maguire P, Selby P, *et al.* Screening for anxiety and depression in cancer patients: the effects of disease and treatment. *Eur J Cancer* 1994; **30A**: 37–40.

82 Koenig HG, Cohen HJ, Blazer DG, *et al.* A brief depression scale for use in the medically ill. *Int J Psychiatry Med* 1992; **22**: 183–95.

83 Gerety MB, Williams JW Jr, Mulrow CD, *et al.* Performance of case-finding tools for depression in the nursing home: influence of clinical and functional characteristics and selection of optimal threshold scores. *J Am Geriatr Soc* 1994; **42**: 1103–9.

● 84 Chochinov HM, Wilson KG, Enns M, *et al.* 'Are you depressed?' Screening for depression in the terminally ill. *Am J Psychiatry* 1997; **154**: 674–6.

85 Fisch MJ. Depression. In: Elsayem A, Driver L, Bruera E, eds. *The MD Anderson Symptom Control and Palliative Care Handbook,* 2nd ed. Houston: The University of Texas-Houston Health Science Center, 2002: 91–6.

86 Lloyd-Williams M, Spiller J, Ward J. Which depression screening tools should be used in palliative care? *Palliat Med* 2003; **17**: 40–3.

87 Whooley MA, Avins AL, Miranda J, *et al.* Case-finding instruments for depression. Two questions are as good as many. *J Gen Intern Med* 1997; **12**: 439–45.

88 Grassi L, Malacarne P, Maestri A, *et al.* Depression, psychosocial variables and occurrence of life events among patients with cancer. *J Affect Disord* 1997; **44**: 21–30.

89 Breitbart W. Identifying patients at risk for, and treatment of major psychiatric complications of cancer. *Support Care Cancer* 1995; **3**: 45–60.

90 American Psychiatric Association. Somatoform disorder. In: *Diagnostic and Statistical Manual of Mental Disorders*, 4th ed. Washington DC: American Psychiatric Association, 1994: 445–65.

91 Gureje O, Simon GE, Ustun TB, *et al.* Somatization in cross-cultural perspective: a World Health Organization study in primary care. *Am J Psychiatry* 1997; **154**: 989–95.

92 Lipowski ZJ. Somatization: the concept and its clinical application. *Am J Psychiatry* 1988; **145**: 1358–68.

93 Simon GE, VonKorff M, Piccinelli M, *et al.* An international study of the relation between somatic symptoms and depression. *N Engl J Med* 1999; **341**: 1329–35.

94 Chaturvedi SK, Maguire GP. Persistent somatization in cancer: a controlled follow-up study. *J Psychosom Res* 1998; **45**: 249–56.

95 Chaturvedi SK, Hopwood P, Maguire P. Non-organic somatic symptoms in cancer. *Eur J Cancer* 1993; **29A**: 1006–8.

96 Robinson K, Bruera E. The management of pain in patients with advanced cancer: the importance of multidimensional assessments. *J Palliat Care* 1995; **11**: 51–3.

97 Wessely S, White PD. There is only one functional somatic syndrome. *Br J Psychiatry* 2004; **185**: 95–6.

● 98 Daeninck PJ, Bruera E. Opioid use in cancer pain. Is a more liberal approach enhancing toxicity? *Acta Anaesthesiol Scand* 1999; **43**: 924–38.

99 O'Connor PG, Schottenfeld RS. Patients with alcohol problems. *N Engl J Med* 1998; **338**: 592–602.

100 Regier DA, Myers JK, Kramer M, *et al.* The NIMH Epidemiologic Catchment Area program. Historical context, major objectives, and study population characteristics. *Arch Gen Psychiatry* 1984; **41**: 934–41.

● 101 Bruera E, Moyano J, Seifert L, *et al.* The frequency of alcoholism among patients with pain due to terminal cancer. *J Pain Symptom Manage* 1995; **10**: 599–603.

102 Passik SD, Portenoy RK, Ricketts PL. Substance abuse issues in cancer patients. Part 1: Prevalence and diagnosis. *Oncology* 1998; **2**: 517–21.

103 McCorquodale S, De Faye B, Bruera E. Pain control in an alcoholic cancer patient. *J Pain Symptom Manage* 1993; **8**: 177–80.

104 Ewing JA. Detecting alcoholism. The CAGE questionnaire. *JAMA* 1984; **252**: 1905–7.

105 Oswald LM, Wand GS. Opioids and alcoholism. *Physiol Behav* 2004; **81**: 339–58.

106 Kiefer F, Wiedemann K. Neuroendocrine pathways of addictive behaviour. *Addict Biol* 2004; **9**: 205–12.

107 Bruera E, MacMillan K, Hanson J, *et al.* The Edmonton staging system for cancer pain: preliminary report. *Pain* 1989; **37**: 203–9.

108 Bruera E, Schoeller T, Wenk R, *et al.* A prospective multicenter assessment of the Edmonton staging system for cancer pain. *J Pain Symptom Manage* 1995; **10**: 348–55.

109 Faisinger RL, Nekolaichuk C, Lawlor P, *et al.* The revised Edmonton stating system for cancer pain. (Abstract #19) EAPC Abstracts. *Palliat Med* 2004; **18**: 307.

110 Ferrell BR, Ferrell BA, Rhiner M, *et al.* Family factors influencing cancer pain management. *Postgrad Med J* 1991; **67** (Suppl 2): S64–9.

111 Panke JT, Ferrell BR. Emotional problems in the family. In: Doyle D, Hanks G, Cherny N, Calman K, eds. *Oxford Textbook of Palliative Medicine*, 3rd ed. Oxford: Oxford University Press, 2004: 985–92.

112 Vachon ML. Psychosocial needs of patients and families. *J Palliat Care* 1998; **14**: 49–56.

113 Teno JM, Nelson HL, Lynn J. Advance care planning. Priorities for ethical and empirical research. *Hastings Cent Rep* 1994; **24**: S32–6.

114 Kristjanson LJ. The family as a unit of treatment. In Portenoy RK, Bruera E, eds. *Topics in Palliative Care.* Vol 1. Oxford: Oxford University Press, 1997: 245–62.

115 Glajchen M. The emerging role and needs of family caregivers in cancer care. *J Support Oncol* 2004; **2**: 145–55.

116 Schulz R, Beach SR. Caregiving as a risk factor for mortality: the Caregiver Health Effects Study. *JAMA* 1999; **282**: 2215–19.

117 Miaskowski C, Kragness L, Dibble S, *et al.* Differences in mood states, health status, and caregiver strain between family caregivers of oncology outpatients with and without cancer-related pain. *J Pain Symptom Manage* 1997; **13**: 138–47.

118 Haley WE, LaMonde LA, Han B, *et al.* Family caregiving in hospice: effects on psychological and health functioning among spousal caregivers of hospice patients with lung cancer or dementia. *Hosp J* 2001; **15**: 1–18.

● 119 Cantwell P, Turco S, Brenneis C, *et al.* Predictors of home death in palliative care cancer patients. *J Palliat Care* 2000; **16**: 23–8.

120 Warner JE. Involvement of families in pain control of terminally ill patients. *Hosp J* 1992; **8**: 155–70.

121 Higginson I, Webb D, Lessof L. Reducing hospital beds for patients with advanced cancer. *Lancet* 1994; **344**: 409.

122 Covinsky KE, Goldman L, Cook EF, *et al.* The impact of serious illness on patients' families. SUPPORT Investigators. Study to Understand Prognoses and Preferences for Outcomes and Risks of Treatment. *JAMA* 1994; **272**: 1839–44.

123 Karasu TB. Spiritual psychotherapy. *Am J Psychother* 1999; **53**: 143–62.

124 Kristeller JL, Zumbrun CS, Schilling RF. 'I would if I could': how oncologists and oncology nurses address spiritual distress in cancer patients. *Psychooncology* 1999; **8**: 451–8.

125 Puchalski CM. Spirituality and end-of-life care: a time for listening and caring. *J Palliat Med* 2002; **5**: 289–94.

126 Daaleman TP, VandeCreek L. Placing religion and spirituality in end-of-life care. *JAMA* 2000; **284**: 2514–17.

127 Koenig HG. Religious attitudes and practices of hospitalized medically ill older adults. *Int J Geriatr Psychiatry* 1998; **13**: 213–4.

128 International Work Group on Death, Dying, and Bereavement. A statement of assumptions and principles concerning education about death, dying, and bereavement. International Work Group on Death, Dying, and Bereavement. *Death Stud* 1992; **16**: 59–65.

129 Taylor EJ. Nurses caring for the spirit: patients with cancer and family caregiver expectations. *Oncol Nurs Forum* 2003; **30**: 585–90.

130 Macdonald SM, Sandmaier R, Fainsinger RL. Objective evaluation of spiritual care: a case report. *J Palliat Care* 1993; **9**: 47–9.

40

Tools for pain and symptom assessment in palliative care

VICTOR T CHANG

INTRODUCTION

The importance of symptoms was recognized by the convening of a National Institutes of Health (NIH) symposium to discuss the target symptoms of fatigue, pain, and depression.[1] All palliative care personnel assess and manage pain and symptoms.[2]

Why are tools needed? Advantages of the use of a tool are a certain regularity, and tabulation of their answers allows for data analysis and comparisons. Potential disadvantages of a tool are additional time and energy spent obtaining potentially irrelevant information, as well as resources required to store, track, and organize the data. The usefulness and interpretation of these tools in clinical practice is an area of ongoing research. While both symptom and quality-of-life tools emphasize patient-rated outcomes, symptom tools differ from quality-of-life instruments in emphasis on symptoms rather than general physical, social or emotional wellbeing.

FUNDAMENTALS OF SYMPTOM MEASUREMENT AND ASSESSMENT TOOLS

Biological underpinnings

Best understood for pain, the perceived intensity of a sensory stimulus is proportional to the rate of firing by sensory nerves, and the number of nerves which send impulses. Sensory impulses reach the cerebral cortex where they may be recognized, and trigger various responses such as evaluative (severity), affective (unpleasantness or distress), and behavioral (agitation).

Theoretical underpinnings of symptom instruments

CLINIMETRICS

Clinimetrics focuses on the quality of measurements in clinical medicine.[3] Descriptive statements (mensuration) are combined to express a numerical summary (quantification).[4] The descriptive statements are chosen on the basis of clinical relevance, usually by clinicians, and can be eclectic with a variety of symptoms, physical findings, and laboratory findings. An example is the Apgar score, where 5 items (heart rate, skin color, respiratory effort, muscle tone, reflex irritability) are combined to form a score to describe the condition of a newborn infant.[5]

PSYCHOMETRICS

The degree to which a respondent agrees with items (statements) allows an inference about whether the respondent has a particular, otherwise unmeasurable psychological state (latent trait), such as pain, anxiety or depression. Another analogy is the blind men describing an elephant. Each blind man is an item, and the latent trait is the elephant.

The extent of agreement between items is commonly determined with Likert scales, (e.g. not at all, a little bit, somewhat, quite a bit, very much). The intraclass correlation coefficient (Cronbach α) is a measure of self-consistency between the statements; α levels of 0.70 or greater are considered acceptable. Factor analyses and other statistical techniques are used to analyze the collection of statements to see whether they measure one factor, and are therefore unidimensional, or more than one factor. Longer instruments with more items are preferred to minimize variation, and maximize the Cronbach α.

ITEM RESPONSE THEORY (IRT)

In this very simplified explanation, IRT starts with the concept of item difficulty, the percentage of respondents who respond correctly to a test item. Similar to psychometrics, IRT tries to estimate a latent trait. The correspondence between the item difficulty and the latent trait is described by the item-characteristic curve (ICC), which is usually S shaped. Easier items are on the left of the trait scale, and more difficult items on the right. IRT models estimate the difficulty parameter for each item from questionnaire data, where the difficulty parameter is the trait level needed to answer the item correctly 50 percent of the time. The different kinds of IRT models differ in the numbers and types of parameter used to describe the ICC. The attractiveness of this approach lies in the potential improvements in symptom and other forms of assessment. These include shorter questionnaires, computerized adaptive testing, and comparisons of different instruments. Questionnaires will not be as dependent on variations in the population being tested. This is an area which should see much development in the future.[6]

Properties of symptom assessment instruments

VALIDITY, RELIABILITY

Validity means that the instrument measures what it claims to measure. Measures of validity include face validity (items are easy to understand), content validity, criterion validity, and construct validity. Content validity shows how the items in the instrument reflect what the instrument is trying to measure. For example, a pain instrument might include a rating of pain severity. Criterion validity is shown by correlation with other accepted measures of the symptom in question. Criterion validity can be demonstrated by expected agreement (convergent validity) or expected disagreement (divergent validity). Construct validity is an assessment of how well the instrument measures its goal.[7]

Reliability implies freedom from error, and is defined as the true variance divided by the true variance and variance from repeated administration of the instrument. Reliability can be measured by the degree of reproducibility (test–retest) and self-consistency (Cronbach α).[8]

RESPONSIVENESS

Responsiveness of the instrument to change has received increased attention recently, along with the notion of minimal clinically significant difference. Measures of clinically significant difference are important for sample size estimation in trials designed to improve symptom control or quality of life. They also illustrate the transformation of symptom instruments into outcome measures. Much of the work to date has been done with quality-of-life measures, where the minimal clinically important difference has been defined as 'the smallest difference in score in the domain of interest which patients perceive as beneficial and which would mandate, in the absence of troublesome side effects and excessive cost, a change in the patient's management'.[9]

Anchor-based and distribution-based methods have been used to define clinically important differences.[10] Anchor-based methods use established clinical criteria or patient ratings as ways to anchor interpretations of difference scores. An example is the Performance Status rating. Distribution-based methods rely upon the statistical aspects of the score distributions.[11] A half of the standard deviation may be a good approximation of the clinically significant difference.[12]

Instruments which are designed to evaluate the patient at a point in time may not be the optimal instruments for measuring changes.[13] An alternative approach has been the transition rating, a single item where the patient is asked to rate the change he or she perceives in the target measure. This can be expressed as a percentage, as a 7-point Likert scale ranging from very much worse to very much better, or on visual analog scales (VAS). Likert and VAS approaches were equivalent in one study.[14] While the ability of patients to remember their previous symptom status has been questioned, this approach is quick and sensitive, and corresponds to the usual clinical conversation between the patient and healthcare provider. The minimum difference has been estimated as 0.5 on a 7-point scale. The magnitude of the transition score is correlated with the pretreatment score.[15]

SCALES

Nominal scales have items that cannot be combined (e.g. list of pain descriptors). Ordinal scales have responses that can be ranked. Numerical scales ask the respondent to assign a number, and may be an interval scale or a ratio scale. In an interval scale, the difference between the scale values is a number, and linear transformations can be performed (e.g. conversion of temperature from Fahrenheit to Celsius). In a ratio scale, a zero point is present, and only multiplicative transformations can be performed (e.g. measures of length).[16]

DIMENSIONS

Symptoms have dimensions. A medical history will ask about the presence of a symptom, exacerbating and alleviating events, temporal variation, descriptors, and relief. A palliative symptom history can additionally include severity, frequency, duration, distress, effect on function, and associated meanings for the patient. Many of these terms are self-explanatory. It remains an open question as to how many dimensions are needed. Is one dimension enough? Severity tends to be the most dimension most commonly used, followed by distress. However, symptoms are not always categorized easily by one dimension. A patient who has breakthrough bone pain may have difficulty deciding whether the severity or frequency or both are important. This has led to interest in the use of multidimensional symptom instruments, such as the Memorial Symptom Assessment Scale.

To summarize, potentially important dimensions of a symptom include frequency, severity, distress, duration, and associated meanings.

TYPES OF RESPONSE CATEGORY

- Visual analog scales (VAS): The symptom of interest is represented by a straight line 10 cm long. Anchors are no symptom on one end, and worst on the other end. The patient marks off with a straight line the severity of the symptom. Horizontal and vertical VAS have been described. Visual analog scales are one of the oldest forms of symptom assessment approaches, and have the advantage of providing a continuous variable for subsequent analyses.[17] VAS have been used for many symptoms. Disadvantages include a tendency for the marks to bunch up in the middle, and physical problems with completing the form in patients with impaired eyesight and/or motor disability. Mechanical VAS have been described, where patients move a marker along the line.
- Numerical rating scale: Patients are asked to rate the symptom on a numerical scale, such as 0–5 or 0–10. However, not all patients are able to express themselves numerically. In one study, 10 percent of hospice patients were unable to use a numerical rating scale for pain.[18]
- Categorical rating scales: Patients are asked to categorize the symptom by severity or other attributes. These categories often are none, a little bit, somewhat, quite a bit, and very much in the Likert version. Other categories have also been described. This presents an alternative for patients who cannot give numerical values.
- Ranking: Patients are asked to rank symptoms in order of priority. This provides a different way of characterizing symptoms, and may help the interviewer set priorities for symptom control. Patients in palliative care may have many severe symptoms and may have difficulty ranking symptoms.
- Pictorial approaches: Best known examples include the FACES design for children,[19] and the use of symbols such as fire to characterize intensity. These approaches are appropriate in populations where the ability to read may be a barrier.
- Descriptors: Patients select from a list of adjectives to capture qualitative aspects of the symptoms.

SINGLE SYMPTOM VERSUS MULTISYMPTOM INSTRUMENTS

Many instruments are devoted to information about one symptom. Because palliative care patients may have multiple symptoms, instruments which assess multiple symptoms have been developed. A related question is how many symptoms should be routinely covered? By the time patients reach palliative care status, the stamina can last for 5–10 questions at most. Many symptoms – pain, tiredness, nausea, difficulty sleeping, drowsiness, dry mouth, shortness of breath, and sadness – are common to most of the multisymptom instruments.

MODE OF ADMINISTRATION

Tools can be administered by an interviewer or can be completed by the patient in a variety of ways (pen and paper, telephone, computer, internet, interactive voice response, perhaps text messaging in the future!).

SPECIFIC SYMPTOM INSTRUMENTS

A large number of instruments have been developed.

Appetite

- Visual analog scale: A 10 cm line, where the left represented no appetite and the right anchor is 100 percent appetite.[20]
- The Bristol-Meyers Cachexia Recovery Instrument (BACRI):[21] This is a 7-item VAS where patients rated their improvement in eating.
- The North Central Cancer Treatment Group Patient Questionnaire:[22] This has seven items and a VAS score for quality of life.
- The Functional Assessment of Appetite Cancer Therapy[23] Subscale has 12 items rated on a Likert score.

Constipation

The Constipation Assessment Scale is a validated 8-item scale for assessment of constipation in cancer patients.[24]

Delirium

- The Confusion Assessment Method (CAM)[25] is based upon Diagnostic and Statistical Manual (DSM)-III criteria and nonpsychiatrist clinicians can use an algorithm of four items – acute onset and fluctuating course, inattention, either altered level of consciousness or disorganized thinking. The CAM has been translated into Portuguese[26] and a version has been developed for patients in intensive care units (ICU).[27]

- The Delirium Rating Scale[28] is a 10-item instrument with clinician-rated symptoms. A revised longer 16-item version has been developed with improved sensitivity and specificity[29] The Delirium Rating Scale has been translated into Japanese[30] and validated for adolescents.[31]
- The Memorial Delirium Assessment Scale (MDAS)[32] is a 10-item tool which can be used for diagnosis, severity, and repeated assessments. A cut-off score of 13 is diagnostic, and a cut-off score of 7 has been proposed for advanced cancer patients in a palliative care setting.[33] The MDAS has been translated into Italian[34] and Japanese.[35]
- The Mini-Mental State Examination (MMSE)[36] was originally developed as a screening test for dementia, and has been used as a screen for other cognitive dysfunction. Norms should be adjusted for age and educational level.[37,38] The instrument has been translated into Chinese,[39] French,[40] Gujarati,[41] Hebrew,[42] Japanese,[43] Korean,[44] Sinhalese,[45] and Spanish.[46]

In a comparison of 12 different tools for delirium, the CAM was felt to be the best diagnostic tool and the Delirium Rating Scale best for screening symptom severity. The CAM-ICU was recommended for ICU patients and the MDAS for cancer patients.[47]

Depression

- Single-item VAS have correlated well with depression tools.[48]
- The Beck Depression Inventory[49] is a 21-item instrument where the patient rates the severity of attitudes and symptoms over a 1-week period. In 1996, the Beck Depression Inventory II was released to conform to the DSM-IV criteria. The Beck Depression Inventory has been translated into modern standard Arabic,[50] Chinese,[51] Japanese,[52] Russian,[53] and Spanish.[54]
- The Center for Epidemiologic Studies on Depression (CES-D)[55] is a validated instrument with 20 items and asks for patient-rated frequency and has been studied in cancer patients. The CES-D has been translated into Brazilian Portuguese,[56] Chinese,[57] Greek,[58] Japanese[59] Spanish,[60] and Turkish.[61] A 10-item version has been introduced.[62]
- The Geriatric Depression Scale (GDS)[63] is a 30-item instrument which can be administered by telephone[64] and has been translated into Chinese,[65] Hindi,[66]

Spanish,[67] and Swedish.[68] A GDS Short Form with 15 items has been validated[69] and translated into French,[70] Greek,[71] Korean,[72] and Spanish.[73] A shorter 5-item version has been reported[74] and translated into Chinese.[75] The GDS may not be valid in patients with moderate to severe dementia.

- The Hamilton Depression Rating Scale[76] is a 17-item severity rated scale and is widely used in trials of antidepressants. It has been translated into Chinese.[77] A 6-item version has been developed.[78]
- The Hospital Anxiety Depression Scale (HADS) is a validated instrument that has two subscales.[79,80] Patients rate frequency of symptoms for 14 items, seven related to anxiety and seven for depression. The HADS is widely used in Europe, and has been translated into Arabic,[81] Chinese,[82] French,[83] German,[84,85] Maltese,[86] Japanese,[86] and Spanish.[88]
- Screening questions: Single[89] and two question screens[90] have been validated.
- The Zung Self Rating Depression Scale is a 20-item instrument.[91] The Zung scale has been translated into Chinese,[92] Czech,[93] Dutch,[94] Finnish,[95] Greek,[96] studied in India,[97] and Spanish.[98] A shorter 12-item version has been translated into Dutch.[99] Both have been validated in ambulatory cancer patients.[100]

Common problems of these instruments are that as screening tools, the cut-off points have not been derived for palliative care patients, and that the patient's self-report may be influenced by stress and the desire to be socially acceptable.[101] In one literature review of depression screening tools for use in a palliative care population, the authors concluded that the single question 'Are you depressed' had the highest sensitivity and specificity, and identified cut-off values of 20 for the HADS, and 13 for the Edinburgh Postnatal Depression Scale.[102]

Dysphagia

Most studies have used an ordinal scale for measuring dysphagia in five categories: no symptoms, can take solids, can take soft food, can take liquids, cannot swallow at all. Many studies do not specify whether this is patient rated or observer rated.

Dyspnea

- The Borg scale measures symptoms with a vertical scale from 0 to 10 anchored by descriptive words, and requires an exertional test.[103]
- A VAS is a validated measure of dyspnea,[104] as is a numerical rating scale.[105]
- The Chronic Respiratory Questionnaire[106] and the St George's Respiratory Questionnaire[107] are quality-of-life instruments for patients with chronic obstructive

pulmonary disease (COPD), with an emphasis on dyspnea. The Chronic Respiratory Questionnaire has been translated into German,[108] Japanese,[109] and Spanish.[110] The St George's Respiratory Questionnaire has 50 items and has been translated into American English,[111] Chinese,[112] French,[113] Japanese, Polish,[114] Spanish,[115] and Swedish.[116] The minimal important difference for the St George's is estimated at 4 on a scale of 0–100.[117]

- The Baseline Dyspnea Index assesses functional impairment, magnitude of task, and magnitude of effort required to produce breathlessness and the Transition Dyspnea Index measures changes in these three components.[118] These instruments have been translated into German, Italian, Japanese, and Spanish.[119] A 1-point change in the Transition Dyspnea Index is clinically meaningful.[120]

Descriptions of many other instruments can be found in reviews (references 121–123).

Fatigue

- The Brief Fatigue Inventory assesses fatigue severity with a 0–10 numerical rating scales for worst and usual fatigue, and fatigue now, and has six interference items. It has been translated into Chinese,[124] German,[125] and Japanese.[126] In one study, worst fatigue ratings of 7–10 identified patients with severe fatigue.[127] In another study, a cut-off for worst fatigue of 3 or usual fatigue of 2 separated mild from moderate fatigue.[128]
- The Piper Revised Fatigue Scale[129] contains 22 items and four subscales: behavioral/severity, affective meaning, sensory and cognitive/mood. It has been translated into French[130] and Chinese.[131]
- The FACIT Fatigue module[132] is a 13-item subscale with Likert responses. An effect size for the FACT Fatigue subscale has been estimated to be between 0.51 and 0.89.[133]
- A single-item of distress from fatigue correlated well with responses to the Brief Fatigue Inventory and the FACIT Fatigue model.[134]
- The Schwartz Cancer Fatigue Scale is a 28-item instrument with four subscales: physical, emotional, cognitive, and temporal.[135] A minimal important clinical difference has been estimated to be 5, and per item 0.8.[136] A 6-item version with two subscales has also been developed.[137]

Nausea

The development of a solid accepted methodology for measuring chemotherapy-related nausea and vomiting, and response has helped advance the field of palliating–chemotherapy-related emesis. Nausea is measured with a VAS and vomiting is quantitated as the number of episodes in a 24-hour period.[138]

Pain

- VAS: A mark of more than 30 mm is more than mild pain.[139] A clinically significant change was estimated at 13 mm for patients with initial VAS scores of 34 mm, and 28 mm for patients with initial VAS scores greater than 67 mm.[140]
- Numerical rating scale of 0–10: Analysis of pain severity in a multinational sample suggests that 1–4 may be mild pain, 5–6 moderate pain, and 7–10 severe pain.[141] Changes in severity of 2 may correspond to a minimally clinically significant difference.[142,143]
- The Brief Pain Inventory (BPI)[144] and the BPI Short Form are widely used and validated pain instruments. The instrument contains a body diagram, numerical rating scale ratings of pain severity, relief, and interference with function. The BPI has been translated into Chinese,[145,146] German,[147] Greek,[148] Hindi,[149] Italian,[150] Japanese,[151] Norwegian,[152] Spanish,[153] and additional languages.[154]
- The McGill Pain Questionnaire[155] has a present pain intensity item, and 20 sets of descriptors to assess for sensory, affective, and evaluative components of pain. It has been translated into Amharic,[156] Arabic,[157] Chinese,[158] Danish[159,160] Dutch,[161] Finnish,[162] Flemish, French,[163] German[164,165] Greek,[166] Italian, Japanese,[167,168] Norwegian,[169] Polish, Slovak,[170] and Spanish.[171,172]
- The McGill Short Form has 17 items: present pain intensity, pain severity VAS, and ratings of 15 descriptors.[173] It has been translated into Czech,[174] Greek,[175] and Swedish.[176]
- The Memorial Pain Assessment Card[177] has one item for each of the dimensions of severity, mood, relief, and a set of descriptors.

Neuropathic pain scales have been developed where patients rate the presence and severity of pain descriptors. The purpose of these research scales has been to distinguish neuropathic from nociceptive pain: the Neuropathic Pain Scale,[178] the Leeds Assessment of Neuropathic Signs and Symptoms,[179] and the Neuropathic Pain Questionnaire.[180] The ongoing development of prognostic systems for staging pain, such as the Edmonton Staging System,[181,182] and the Cancer Pain Prognostic Scale,[183] provides a different kind of assessment. Readers interested in pain assessment may find references 184 and 185 helpful.

MULTIPLE SYMPTOM INSTRUMENTS

- The Symptom Distress Scale (SDS) introduced the concept of distress to symptom assessment.[186,187]

The SDS has 13 items, with 11 symptoms; pain and nausea are each assessed twice. Variations include the Adapted Symptom Distress Scale 2[188] and the Symptom Experience Scale.[189] The Adapted Symptom Distress Scale has 31 items for 14 symptoms, and includes symptom occurrence. The SDS has been translated into Chinese,[190] Dutch, Italian,[191] Korean,[192] Spanish, and Swedish.[193] It has been studied in patients receiving cancer chemotherapy, home care,[191] and a variety of other settings.

- The Edmonton Symptom Assessment Scale (ESAS)[194] is a validated 9-item VAS scale with eight symptoms and a wellbeing item;[195,196] a modification with a numerical rating scale has been introduced. A French[197] version has been developed. The ESAS has been studied in multiple settings, including hospice, palliative care consultation teams,[198] home care,[199] and the ICU.[200]

- The Lung Cancer Symptom Scale[201] has nine patient-rated items and five observer-rated items.

- The MD Anderson Symptom Inventory[202] was derived from hierarchical cluster analysis on patient responses. A core number of 14 items accounted for 64 percent of the variance in symptom distress. Patients are asked to rate the severity of 13 symptoms and six interference items with a numerical rating scale.

- The Memorial Symptom Assessment Scale (MSAS) is a validated patient-rated instrument in which patients rate symptom severity, distress, and frequency for 32 highly prevalent physical and psychological symptoms.[203,204] Each symptom is rated on a Likert scale and scored from 0 to 4 ranging from 'no symptom' to 'very much'. The MSAS subscales include: the Global Distress Index (GDI), the Physical Symptom distress (PHYS), the Psychological Symptom distress (PSYCH). In the MSAS Short Form, patients rate symptom distress for physical symptoms and symptom frequency for psychological symptoms.[205] In the condensed MSAS, the number of items has been reduced to 14.[206] The MSAS has been studied in cancer chemotherapy, hospital settings,[207] hospice,[208] ICU,[209] and longitudinal studies.[210] The minimal clinically significant difference has been estimated for the MSAS Short Form.[211] A children's version has been developed.[212]

- The Rotterdam Symptom Checklist[213] is a validated 34-item instrument where patients rate distress. A physical and a psychological symptom subscale are described. It has been translated into French[214] Italian,[215] Spanish,[216] and Turkish.[217] A modified version has been validated in an American population of cancer patients.[218] This instrument has been used extensively in European cancer chemotherapy trials and symptom intervention studies.

APPLICATIONS OF SYMPTOM INSTRUMENTS

- Audit: The review of processes of palliative care with the goal of improving quality is the goal of clinical and organizational audits. The process of symptom control, especially where effective treatments are available, such as pain, nausea, and depression, can be monitored with the use of symptom instruments.[219]

- Epidemiology and descriptive studies: Symptom surveys with the ESAS, MSAS, and other instruments have established that multiple symptoms are highly prevalent. Descriptive longitudinal studies with symptom instruments are now being reported.[220–222]

- Improvement of symptom recognition: In surveys of medical records, data concurrently gathered with the ESAS show that routine symptom assessment by doctors and nurses often misses data captured by the ESAS.[223,224] There is a growing consensus that the use of symptom instruments is feasible and contributes important information.

- Patient triage: The use of instruments to screen for symptoms, in particular depression, is an area of interest. A distress thermometer was successful in identifying patients with psychological distress.[225]

- Patient prioritization: One British study used data from a symptom checklist to suggest that patients with lung cancer or brain tumors should be high priority for specialist palliative care.[226] Another British study found differences in symptom patterns by service component of patients referred to a hospice inpatient service, a community team, a National Health Service (NHS) hospital support team, and an outpatient service, suggesting that different symptom management strategies may be needed for different patient groups.[227]

- Prognosis: Patient ratings of symptoms can add prognostic information. In studies of patients with cancer, individual symptoms as well as combinations of symptoms provide prognostic information in addition to that provided by the Karnofsky Performance Score.[228] Physical symptoms may carry more of the prognostic information.[229]

- Symptom clusters: Factor analyses with the MSAS, Rotterdam Symptom Check List, and the Canberra Symptom Scorecard[230] have shown two major groups of symptoms – physical and psychological symptoms. The use of multisymptom instruments is a logical step in establishing the presence of these clusters.[231]

- Quality control: Tools may also be important to the program as evidence for the quality of care given, where the act of symptom assessment is taken as the process. In this concept tools may be important as a way of evaluating the structure of the program.[232]

- Treatment outcome: Tools can serve by recording the outcomes of symptom management.

- Caregivers' and patients' ratings: Ideally, patients should be the source of information about symptoms, but become unable near the end of life. The role of caregivers or other proxies in symptom assessment has been an area of ongoing research and studied with symptom scales.[233,234]
- Relationship of symptoms to other aspects of palliative care, such as spirituality[235] and dignity.[236]

SPECIAL POPULATIONS

In patients who are unable to communicate, the ascertainment of symptoms becomes more difficult. This is especially true for the pediatric, geriatric and ICU populations. One approach for pain has been the development of behavioral measures of pain which can be recorded by observers. For children, behavioral scales include FLACC (*Face*, *Legs*, *Activity*, *Cry*, *Consolability*),[237] and for demented patients, the PainAD[238] and Pain Assessment for the Dementing Elderly.[239] This area has been recently reviewed.[239a] Pain behaviors have been described for ICU patients.[240]

PRACTICAL ISSUES

The selection of tools for pain and symptom assessment reflects a balance, as elsewhere, between what is possible and what is desirable. These considerations include the nature of the organization, and the uses to which the information from the tool will be put.

Research and practical tools

The difference between research and practical tools lies in their purpose and function (Table 40.1). Most instruments in use started out as research tools to better describe symptom(s). As such, these reflected concepts about the symptom, tended to be longer, studied healthier patients, were administered by research personnel. These studies have provided many insights into symptom epidemiology and their relationship to other aspects of patient experience, and demonstrated feasibility. In the clinical context, pragmatism is emphasized, and time and personnel are limited. As instruments are converted from research to clinical application, there is then an evolutionary pressure for the development of shorter and simpler instruments which can be rapidly administered and interpreted.

Patient stamina is decisive. Many terminally ill patients may be unable to answer more than a handful of questions. In one study of patients with terminal cancer at an American hospital, only half were able to complete one of the three instruments offered – the McGill Pain Questionnaire, the Memorial Pain Assessment Card, or the FACES Pain Rating Scale.[241] In a study of hospice inpatients, only 30 out of 71

Table 40.1 *Differences between research and practical tools*

Research	Practical
Comprehensive	Screening
Based upon specific theories	Empirical
Longer	Shorter
Wide choice of answers	Yes/No
Specific	Global
Multiple item	Single item
Patient rated	Observer rated

patients with pain were available to participate in a study where they were asked to answer a 6-item questionnaire about pain, with each item scaled from 0 to 10. The ratings were completed without difficulty and showed good reproducibility 1 hour later.[242]

Availability of instruments

In addition to the time-honored practice of contacting the developers of an instrument or finding the journal, many instruments may be viewed on websites. These include the American Thoracic Society website (www.atsqol.org), the Center to Advance Palliative Care (www.capc.org), the International Hospice Association (www.hospicecare.com), the MAPI Research Institute (www.mapi-research-inst.com, www.qolid.org), the Regional Palliative Care Program in Edmonton, Alberta (www.palliative.org), the Robert Wood Johnson Promoting Excellence in End of Life Care (www.promotingexcellence.org), and the toolkit of instruments to measure end-of-life care (www.chcr.brown.edu/pcoc/Physical.htm) Another source for symptom items can be quality-of-life instruments, such as the FACIT system,[243] the EORTC QLQ-C30,[244] or the RAI-PC.[245] The first two instruments have developed disease-related modules, have been translated into many languages, and contain symptom items.

Choosing an instrument

Criteria for an ideal pain instrument, as listed by Chapman and Syralja, apply to symptom instruments in general.[246] These criteria include:

- Minimal patient burden
- Understandable by patients
- Produce a wide range of scores
- Sensitive to interventions
- Demonstrate appropriate reliability and validity
- Availability of appropriate norms

Their principles of selection are equally applicable. These ultimately depend on the needs of the clinician and limitations of the patient population. The principles include:

- Define the goal of assessment (complexity of problem and information required).

- Decide which dimensions are appropriate for the problem at hand (severity, behavior, and function).
- Select subparts of instruments most suitable.
- Consider development of a clinical database – layout to be suitable for analyses.
- Consider automated data collection.
- Avoid too much data.
- Be sure the test instruments fit the patient population.
- Take care to collect responses to all items on the forms.[246]

Translation of instruments

Even within the same language, symptoms, and aspects of symptoms may be difficult to describe for the purposes of a symptom questionnaire (e.g. British vs. American English). These problems are magnified further when translations are attempted as different connotations may be associated with the symptom or the items in the second language. However, it may be easier to translate an instrument than to develop one. If the reader would like to translate an instrument, it is advisable to work with the group that developed the original instrument. The instrument is translated into the new language, then back translated into the original language by a second team, and then retranslated into the new language by a third team. After each translation, the instrument is reviewed again.[247]

Validation

In a new population, or with a new language, the tool should be validated. A representative sample of at least 40 patients should complete the tool, a reference tool known to be valid, and have their performance status and demographic data recorded. Practical aspects, such as ease of administration and comprehension should also be recorded. These data can then be analysed for validity.[248]

Implementation of tools

Principles of implementation by Higginson[249] are applicable to symptom tools. These include:

- Measures that form a part of treatment planning and evaluation are more likely to influence clinical decision making than monitoring alone.
- Are the symptoms relevant?
- How long does it take to complete
- Will it measure differences?
- Who will use the measures?
- Involve staff and patients.
- Plan and begin training in both the use of the measure and associated clinical skills.

I would add that a plan of action for symptom control should be in place or no improvements will result.

UNEXPLORED AREAS

Symptom monitoring

The combination of symptom tools and new computerized technology has led to the concept of symptom monitoring.[250] A symptom monitoring program could cover more areas of patient concern, aid in better understanding the relations between multiple symptoms, identify symptoms before they become severe, complement measures of tumor response, and assist in clinical decision making. Frequency of assessments is unknown. The role of caregiver-rated and healthcare–professional-rated symptoms for noncommunicative patients remains an area of investigation.

PROPOSE AN IDEAL TOOL PACKAGE WITH GOOD PSYCHOMETRIC PROPERTIES AND MINIMAL OVERLAP: HOW IS IT DONE AT CERTAIN CENTERS?

- MD Anderson Center, University of Texas, Houston, USA:[251] ESAS, MMSE, CAGE questionnaire,[252] Morphine Equivalent Daily Dose, Functional Impairment Measure[253]
- Institut Jules Bordet, Brussels, Belgium:[254] MMSE, MDAS, Edmonton Functional Assessment Tool,[255] ESAS
- University of Cologne, Germany:[256] MMSE, BPI, Medical Outcome Study Short Form-12[257]

How to select a tool

No instrument is perfect and the package depends upon the local needs of the patients (types of disease and prevalence of symptoms) and resources available to the staff (manpower, time) and purpose (research or practice or screening). Areas of practical interest at intake include the ability of the patient to make decisions, the presence of key symptoms, and a performance status rating. Additional instruments can be added depending upon the interest of the group. At follow-up, we need to screen for new symptoms, and determine if older symptoms have changed.

If the reader is planning to set up a palliative care program, it is better to select an available validated instrument (or module) and add items than to pick and choose items from different tools. The reader may wish to try out different tools on a few patients to see which one works best in terms of comprehension and ease of administration. Possible combinations are presented in Table 40.2.

Table 40.2   *Suggested use of the various assessment instruments*

	Better KPS Research	Worse KPS (KPS < 50 percent) Practice/Screening
Symptoms	RSCL, MSAS	ESAS, CMSAS, SDS
Pain	BPI, MPQ SF	Numeric rating scale
Depression	Depression instrument	Screening questions
Noncommunicative	PAINAD	PAINAD
Mental Status	CAM	CAM, MDAS

RSCL, Rotterdam Symptom Checklist; MSAS, Memorial Symptom Assessment Scale; BPI, Brief Pain Inventory; MPQ SF, McGill Pain Questionnaire Short Form; CAM, Confusion Assessment Method; ESAS, Edmonton Symptom Assessment Scale; CMSAS, Condensed MSAS; SDS, Symptom Distress Scale; MDAS, Memorial Delirium Assessment Scale; KPS, Karnofsky Performance Score.

Key learning points

- Many validated and reliable tools are available for many symptoms, as well as for multiple symptoms.

- Responsiveness is being established.

- The usefulness and validity of these tools in different populations requires further study.

- The items of the symptom instruments selected should be perceived as useful, easy to understand, easy to answer, and easy to interpret.

- Follow-up plans for symptom treatment should be developed.

- Symptom tools are versatile in their applications. The choice of symptom tools depends on the priorities set by the palliative care staff and the stamina of the patients.

- Application of these instruments to clinical care is the next challenge.

REFERENCES

◆ 1   Patrick DL, Ferketich SL, Frame PS, *et al.* National Institutes of Health State-of-the-Science Panel. National Institutes of Health State-of-the-Science Conference Statement: Symptom Management in Cancer: Pain, Depression, and Fatigue, July 15–7, 2002. *J Natl Cancer Inst* 2003; **95**: 1110–7.

✱ 2   National Consensus Project. *Clinical Practice Guidelines for Quality Palliative Care.* www.nationalconsensusproject.org (accessed September 7, 2005).

3   de Vet HCW, Terwee CB, Bouter LM. Current challenges in clinimetrics. *J Clin Epidemiol* 2003; **56**: 1137–41.

4   Feinstein AR. *Clinical epidemiology.* Philadelphia: WB Saunders Co, 1985.

5   Feinstein AR. Multi-item 'instruments' vs Virgina Apgar's principles of clinimetrics. *Arch Intern Med* 1999; **159**: 125–8.

6   Hays RD, Morales LS, Reise SP. Item response theory and health outcomes measurement in the 21st century. *Med Care* 2000; **38**(Suppl 2): 28–42.

7   Jensen MP. Questionnaire validation: a brief guide for readers of the research literature. *Clin J Pain* 2003; **19**: 345–52.

8   Pickering RM. Statistical aspects of measurement. *Palliative Med* 2002; **16**: 359–64.

9   Jaeschke R, Singer J, Guyatt GH. Measurement of health status: ascertaining the minimal clinically important difference. *Control Clin Trials* 1989; **10**: 407–15.

◆ 10   Guyatt GH, Osoba D, Wu AW, *et al.* Methods to explain the clinical significance of health status measures. *Mayo Clin Proc* 2002; **77**: 371–83.

◆ 11   Sprangers MA, Moinpour CM, Moynihan TJ, *et al.* Assessing meaningful change in quality of life over time: a users' guide for clinicians. *Mayo Clin Proc* 2002; **77**: 561–71.

12   Norman GR, Sloan JA, Wyrwich KW. Interpretation of changes in health-related quality of life: the remarkable universality of half a standard deviation. *Med Care* 2003; **41**: 582–92.

13   Kirshner B, Guyatt G. A methodological framework for assessing health indices. *J Chronic Dis* 1985; **38**: 27–36.

14   Guyatt GH, Townsend M, Berman LB, Keller JL. A comparison of Likert and visual analogue scales for measuring change in function. *J Chronic Dis* 1987; **40**: 1129–33.

15   Guyatt GH, Norman GR, Juniper EF, Griffith LE. A critical look at transition ratings. *J Clin Epidemiol* 2002; **55**: 900–8.

16   Killian KJ. The objective measurement of breathlessness. *Chest* 1985; **88** (suppl): 84S–90S.

17   McCormack HM, Horne DJ, Sheather S. Clinical applications of visual analogue scales. A critical review. *Psychol Med* 1988; **18**: 1007–19.

18   Sze FK, Chung TK, Wong E, *et al.* Pain in Chinese cancer patients under palliative care. *Palliative Med* 1998; **12**: 271–7.

19   Bieri D, Reeve RA, Champion GD, *et al.* The Faces Pain Scale for the self-assessment of the severity of pain experienced by children: development, initial validation, and preliminary investigation for ratio scale properties. *Pain* 1990; **41**: 139–50.

20   Coates A, Dillenbeck CF, McNeil DR *et al.* On the receiving end – II. Linear analogue self-assessment (LASA) in evaluation of aspects of the quality of life of cancer patients receiving therapy. *Eur J Cancer Clin Oncol* 1983; **19**: 1633–37.

21   Cella DF, von Roennn J, Lloyd S, Browder HP. The Bristol-Myers Anorexia/Cachexia Recovery Instrument (BACRI): a brief assessment of patients' subjective response to treatment for anorexia/cachexia. *Qual Life Res* 1995; **4**: 221–31.

22 Loprinzi CL, Sloan JA, Rowland KM, Jr. Methodologic issues regarding cancer anorexia/cachexia trials. In: Portenoy RK Bruera E, eds. *Research and Palliative Care: Methodologies and Outcomes.* New York: Oxford University Press, 2003: 25–40.

23 Ribaudo JM, Cella D, Hahn EA, *et al.* Re-validation and shortening of the Functional Assessment of Anorexia/ Cachexia Therapy (FAACT). *Qual Life Res* 2000; **9**: 1137–46.

24 McMillan SC, Williams FA. Validity and reliability of the Constipation Assessment Scale. *Cancer Nurs* 1989; **12**: 183–8.

● 25 Inouye SK, van Dyck CG, Alessi CA, *et al.* Clarifying confusion: the confusion assessment method. *Ann Intern Med* 1990; **113**: 941–8.

26 Fabbri RM, Moreira MA, Garrido R, Almeida OP. Validity and reliability of the Portuguese version of the Confusion Assessment Method (CAM) for the detection of delirium in the elderly. *Arq Neuropsiquiatr* 2001; **59**(2-A): 175–9.

27 Ely EW, Inouye SK, Bernard GR, *et al.* Delirium in mechanically ventilated patients: validity and reliability of the confusion assessment method for the intensive care unit (CAM-ICU). *JAMA* 2001; **286**: 2703–10.

28 Trzepacz PT, Baker RW, Greenhouse J. A symptom rating scale for delirium. *Psychiatric Res* 1988; **1**: 89–97.

29 Trzepacz PT, Mittal D, Torres R, *et al.* Validation of the Delirium Rating Scale-revised-98: comparison with the Delirium Rating Scale and the Cognitive Test for Delirium. *J Neuropsychiatry Clin Neurosci* 2001; **13**: 229–42.

30 Isse K, Uchiyama M, Tanaka K, *et al.* Delirium: clinical findings and its neuro-psychological etiology. *Rinsyo Seisin Yakuri* 1998; **1**: 1231–42.

31 Turkel SB. Braslow K, Tavare CH, Trzapacz PT. The delirium rating scale in children and adolescents. *Psychosomatics* 2003; **44**: 126–9.

● 32 Breitbart W, Rosenfeld B, Roth A, *et al.* The Memorial Delirium Assessment Scale. *J Pain Symptom Manage* 1997; **13**: 128–37.

33 Lawlor PG, Nekolaichuk C, Gagnon B, *et al.* Clinical utility, factor analysis, and further validation of the Memorial Delirium Assessment Scale in patients with advanced cancer: Assessing delirium in advanced cancer. *Cancer* 2000; **88**: 2859–67.

34 Grassi L, Caraceni A, Beltrami E, *et al.* Assessing delirium in cancer patients: the Italian versions of the Delirium Rating Scale and the Memorial Delirium Assessment Scale. *J Pain Symptom Manage* 2001; **21**: 59–68.

35 Matsuoka Y, Miyake Y, Arakaki H, *et al.* Clinical utility and validation of the Japanese version of the Memorial Delirium Assessment Scale in a psychogeriatric inpatient setting. *Gen Hosp Psychiatry* 2001; **23**: 36–40.

● 36 Folstein ME, Folstein SE, McHugh PR. Mini-Mental State. A practical method for grading the cognitive state of patients for the clinician. *J Psychiatr Res* 1975; **12**: 189–98.

37 Crum RM, Anthony JC, Bassett SS, Folstein MF. Population-based norms for the Mini-Mental State Examination by age and educational level. *JAMA* 1993; **269**: 2386–91.

38 Dufouil C, Clayton D, Brayne C, *et al.* Population norms for the MMSE in the very old: estimates based on longitudinal data. Mini-Mental State Examination. *Neurology* 2000; **55**: 1609–13.

39 Xu G, Meyer JS, Huang Y, *et al.* Adapting mini-mental status examination for dementia screening among illiterate or

minimally educated elderly Chinese. *Int J Geriatr Psychiatry* 2003; **18**: 609–16.

40 Derouesne C, Poitreneau J, Hugunot L, *et al.* Mini-Mental State Examination: a useful method for the evaluation of the cognitive status of patients by the clinician. Consensual French version. *Presse Med* 1999; **28**: 1141–8.

41 Lindesay J, Jagger C, Mlynkik-Szmid A, *et al.* The Mini-Mental State Examination (MMSE) in an elderly immigrant Gujarati population in the United Kingdom. *Int J Geriatr Psychiatry* 1997; **12**: 1155–67.

42 Werner P, Heinik J, Mendel A, *et al.* Examining the reliability and validity of the Hebrew version of the Mini Mental State Examination. *Aging (Milano)* 1999; **11**: 329–34.

43 Mori E, Mitani Y, Yamadori A. Usefulness of a Japanese version of the Mini-Mental State in neurological patients. *Shinkeishinrigaku* 1985; **1**: 82–90.

44 Jeong SK, Cho KH, Kim JM. The usefulness of the Korean version of modified Mini-Mental State Examination (MMSE) for dementia screening in community dwelling elderly people. *BMC Public Health* 2004; **4**: 31.

45 De Silva HA, Gunatilake SB. Mini Mental State Examination in Sinhalese: a sensitive test to screen for dementia in Sri Lanka. *Int J Geriatr Psychiatry* 2002; **17**: 134–9.

46 Lobo A, Saz P, Marcos G, Dia JL, *et al.* Revalidation and standardization of the cognition mini-exam (first Spanish version of the Mini-Mental Status Examination) in the general geriatric population. *Med Clin (Barc)* 1999; **112**: 767–74.

◆ 47 Schuurmans MJ, Deschamps PI, Markham SW, Shortridge-Baggett LM. The measurement of delirium: review of scales. *Res Theory Nursing Practice* 2003; **17**: 207–24.

48 Chochinov HM. Depression in the terminally ill: prevalence and measurement issues. In: Portenoy RK, Bruera E, eds. *Issues in Palliative Care Research.* New York: Oxford University Press, 2003; 189–202.

● 49 Beck AT. An inventory for measuring depression. *Arch Gen Psychiatry* 1961; **4**: 53–61.

50 Abdel-Khalek AM, Internal consistency of an Arabic adaptation of the Beck Depression Inventory in four Arab countries. *Psychol Rep* 1998; **82**: 264–6.

51 Zhang Y, Wei L, Gos L, *et al.* Applicability of the Chinese Beck Depression Inventory. *Compr Psychiatry* 1988; **29**: 484–9.

52 Kojima M, Furukawa TA, Takahashi H, *et al.* Cross-cultural validation of the Beck Depression Inventory-II in Japan. *Psychiatry Res* 2002; **110**: 291–9.

53 Andriushchenko AV, Drobizhev MIu, Dobrovol'skii AV. A comparative validation of the scale CES-D, BDI, and HADS(d) in diagnosis of depressive disorders in general practice. *Zh Nevrol Psikhiatr Im S S Korsakova* 2003; **103**: 11–8.

54 Penley JA, Wiebe JS, Nwosu A. Psychometric properties of the Spanish Beck Depression Inventory – II in a medical sample. *Psychol Assess* 2003; **15**: 569–77.

● 55 Radloff LS. The CES-D Scale: a self-report depression scale for research in the general population. *Appl Psychol Measurement* 1977; **1**: 385–401.

56 Da Silveria DX, Jorge MR. Reliability and factor structure of the Brazilian version of the Center for Epidemiologic Studies Depression. *Psychol Rep* 1998; **82**: 211–4.

57 Rankin SH, Galbraith ME, Johnson S. Reliability and validity data for a Chinese translation of the Center for Epidemiological Studies-Depression. *Psychol Rep* 1993; **73**(3 Pt 2): 1291–8.

58 Fountoulakis K, Iacovides A, Kleanthous S, *et al*. Reliability, validity and psychometric properties of the Greek translation of the Center for Epidemiological Studies-Depression (CES-D) scale. *BMC Psychiatry* 2001; **1**: 3 [Epub June 20, 2001].

59 Furukawa T, Hirai T, Kitamura T, Takahashi K. Application of the Center for Epidemiologic Studies Depression Scale among first-visit psychiatric patients: a new approach to improve its performance. *J Affective Disord* 1997; **46**: 1–13.

60 Soler J, Perez-Sola V, Puigdemont D, *et al*. Validation study of the Center for Epidemiological Studies-Depression of a Spanish population of patients with affective disorders. *Actas Luso Esp Neurol Psiquiatr Cienc Afines* 1997; **25**: 243–9.

61 Spijker J, van der Wurff FB, Poort EC, *et al*. Depression in first generation labour migrants in Western Europe: the utility of the Center for Epidemiologic Studies Depression Scale (CES-D). *Int J Geriatr Psychiatry* 2004; **19**: 538–44.

62 Irwin M, Artin KH, Oxman MN. Screening for depression in the older adult. Criterion validity of the 10-Item Center for Epidemiological Studies Depression Scale (CES-D). *Arch Intern Med* 1999; **159**: 1701–4.

● 63 Yesavage JA, Brink TL, Rose TL, *et al*. Development and validation of a geriatric depression screening scale: a preliminary report. *J Psychiatr Res* 1982–83; **17**: 37–49.

64 Burke WJ, Roccaforte WH, Wengel SP, *et al*. The reliability and validity of the Geriatric Depression Rating Scale administered by telephone. *J Am Geriatr Soc* 1995; **43**: 674–9.

65 Chan AC. Clinical validation of the Geriatric Depression Scale (GDS): Chinese version. *J Ageing Health* 1996; **8**: 238–53.

66 Ganguli M, Dube S, Johnston JM, *et al*. Depressive symptoms, cognitive impairment and functional impairment in a rural elderly population in India: a Hindi version of the geriatric depression scale (GDS-H). *Int J Geriatr Psychiatry* 1999; **14**: 807–20.

67 Fernandez-San Martin, Andrade C, Molina J, *et al*. Validation of the Spanish version of the geriatric depression scale (GDS) in primary care. *Int J Geriatr Psychiatry* 2002; **17**: 279–87.

68 Gottfries GG, Noltorp S, Norgaard N. Experience with a Swedish version of the Geriatric Depression Scale in primary care centres. *Int J Geriatr Psychiatry* 1997; **12**: 1029–34.

69 Lesher EL, Berryhill JS. Validation of the Geriatric Depression Scale Short Form among inpatients. *J Clin Psychol* 1994; **50**: 256–60.

70 Clement JP, Nassif RF, Leger JM, Marchan F. Development and contribution to the validation of a brief French version of the Yesavage Geriatric Depression Scale. *Encephale* 1997; **23**: 91–9.

71 Fountoulakis KN, Tsolaki M, Iacovides A, *et al*. The validation of the short form of the Geriatric Depression Scale (GDS) in Greece. *Aging* 1999; **11**: 367–72.

72 Jang Y, Small BJ, Haley WE. Cross-cultural comparability of the Geriatric Depression Scale: comparison between older Koreans and older Americans. *Aging Ment Health* 2001; **5**: 31–7.

73 Baker FM, Espino DV. A Spanish version of the geriatric depression scale in Mexican-American elders. *Int J Geriatr Psychiatry* 1997; **12**: 21–5.

74 Hoyl MT, Alessi CA, Harker JO, *et al*. Development and testing of a five-item version of the Geriatric Depression Scale. *J Am Geriatr Soc* 1999; **47**: 873–8.

75 Cheng ST, Chan AC. A brief version of the geriatric depression scale for the Chinese. *Psychol Assess* 2004; **16**: 182–6.

● 76 Hamilton M. Development of a rating scale for primary depressive illness. *Br J Soc Clin Psychol* 1967; **6**: 278–96.

77 Zheng YP, Zhao JP, Phillips M, *et al*. Validity and reliability of the Chinese Hamilton Depression Rating Scale. *Br J Psychiatry* 1988; **152**: 660–4.

78 O'Sullivan RL, Fava M, Agustin C, *et al*. Sensitivity of the six-item Hamilton Depression Rating Scale. *Acta Psychiatr Scand* 1997; **95**: 379–84.

● 79 Zigmond A, Snaith RP. The Hospital Anxiety Depression Scale. *Acta Psychiatric Scand* 1983; **67**: 367–70.

80 Johnston M, Pollard B, Hennessey P. Construct validation of the Hospital Anxiety and Depression Scale with clinical populations. *J Psychosom Res* 2000; **48**: 579–84.

81 El-Rufaie OE, Absood GH. Retesting the validity of the Arabic version of the Hospital Anxiety and Depression (HAD) scale in primary health care. *Soc Psychiatry Psychiatr Epidemiol* 1995; **30**: 26–31.

82 Leung CM, Wing YK, Kwong PK, *et al*. Validation of the Chinese-Cantonese version of the hospital anxiety and depression scale and comparison with the Hamilton Rating Scale of Depression. *Acta Psychiatr Scand* 1999; **100**: 456–61.

83 Lépine JP, Godchau M, Brun P, *et al*. Evaluation de l'anxiété et de la dépression chez des patients hospitalisés en médecine interne. *Ann Medico-Psychol* 1985; **143**: 175–89.

84 Herrmann C, Scholz KH, Kreuzer H. Psychologic screening of patients of a cardiologic acute care clinic with the German version of the Hospital Anxiety and Depression Scale. *Psychother Psychosom Med Psychol* 1991; **41**: 83–92.

85 Hinz A, Schwarz R. Anxiety and depression in the general population: normal values in the Hospital Anxiety and Depression Scale *Psychother Psychosom Med Psychol* 2001; **51**: 193–200.

86 Baldacchino DR, Bowman GS, Buhagiar A. Reliability testing of the hospital anxiety and depression (HAD) scale in the English, Maltese and back-translation versions. *Int J Nurs Stud* 2002; **39**: 207–14.

87 Higashi A, Yashiro H, Kiyota K, *et al*. Validation of the hospital anxiety and depression scale in a gastro-intestinal clinic. *Nippon Shokakibyo Gakkai Zasshi* 1996; **93**: 884–92.

88 Quintana JM, Padierna A, Esteban C, *et al*. Evaluation of the psychometric characteristics of the Spanish version of the Hospital Anxiety and Depression Scale. *Acta Psychiatr Scand* 2003; **107**: 216–21.

89 Chochinov HM, Wilson KG, Enns M, Lander S. 'Are you depressed?' Screening for depression in the terminally ill. *Am J Psychiatry* 1997; **154**: 674–6.

90 Whooley MA, Avins AL, Miranda J, Browner WS. Case-finding instruments for depression. Two questions are as good as many. *J Gen Intern Med* 1997; **12**: 439–45.

● 91 Zung WWK. A self-rating depression scale. *Arch Gen Psychiatry* 1965; **12**: 63–70.

92 Lee HC, Chiu HF, Wing YK, *et al*. The Zung Self-rating Depression Scale: screening for depression among the Hong Kong Chinese elderly. *J Geriatr Psychiatry Neurol* 1994; **7**: 216–20.

93 Kozeny J. Psychometric properties of the Zung Self-Rating Depression Scale. *Act Nerv Super (Praha)* 1987; **29**: 279–84.

94 Van Marwijk HW, van der Zwan AA, Mulder JD Jr. The family physician and depression in the elderly. A pilot study of prevalence of depressive symptoms and depression in the elderly in 2 family practices. *Tijdschr Gerontol Geriatr* 1991; **22**: 129–33.

95 Kivela SL, Pahkala K. Sex and age differences of factor pattern and reliability of the Zung Self-rating Depression Scale in a

Finnish elderly population. *Psychol Rep* 1986; **59**(2 Pt 1): 589–97.

96 Fountoulakis KN, Iacovides A, Samolis S, *et al.* Reliability, validity and psychometric properties of the Greek translation of the Zung Depression Rating Scale. *BMC Psychiatry* 2001; **1**: 6 [Epub October 20, 2001].

97 Master RS, Zung WW. Depressive symptoms in patients and normal subjects in India. *Arch Gen Psychiatry* 1977; **34**: 972–4.

98 Martinez KG, Guiot HM, Casas-Dolz I, *et al.* Applicability of the Zung Self-Rating Depression Scale in a general Puerto Rican population. *P R Health Sci J* 2003; **22**: 179–85.

99 Gosker CE, Berger H, Deelman BG. Depression in independently living elderly, a study with the Zung-12. *Tijdschr Gerontol Geriatr* 1994; **25**: 157–62.

100 Dugan W, McDonald MV, Passik SD *et al.* Use of the Zung Self Rating Depression Scale in cancer patients: feasibility as a screening tool. *Psychooncology* 1998; **7**: 483–93.

◆ 101 Stiefel F, Trill MD, Berney A, *et al.* Depression in palliative care: a pragmatic report from the Expert Working Group of the European Association for Palliative Care. *Support Care Cancer* 2001; **9**: 477–88.

102 Lloyd-Williams M, Spiller J, Ward J. Which depression screening tools should be used in palliative care? *Palliat Med* 2003; **17**: 40–3.

103 Borg G. *Borg's Perceived Exertion and Pain Scales.* Champaign: Human Kinetics, 1998.

104 Gift AG. Validation of a vertical visual analogue scale as a measure of clinical dyspnea. *Rehabil Nurs* 1989; **14**: 323–5.

105 Gift AG, Narsavage G. Validity of the numeric scale as a measure of dyspnea. *Am J Crit Care* 1998; **7**: 200–4.

106 Williams JE, Singh SJ, Sewell L, *et al.* Development of a self-reported Chronic Respiratory Questionnaire (CRQ-SR). *Thorax* 2001; **56**: 954–9.

107 Jones PW, Quirk FH, Baveystock CM, Littlejohns P. A self-complete measure of health status for chronic airflow limitation. The St.George's Respiratory Questionnaire. *Am Rev Respir Dis* 1992; **145**: 1321–7.

108 Puhan MA, Behnke M, Frey M, *et al.* Self-administration and interviewer-administration of the German Chronic Respiratory Questionnaire: instrument development and assessment of validity and reliability in two randomized studies. *Health Qual Life Outcomes* 2004; **2**: 1; www.hqlo.com/content/2/1/1.

109 Hajiro T, Nishimura K, Tsukino M, *et al.* Analysis of clinical methods used to evaluate dyspnea in patients with chronic obstructive pulmonary disease. *Am J Respir Crit Care Med* 1998; **158**: 1185–9.

110 Guell R, Casan P, Sangenis M, *et al.* Quality of life in patients with chronic respiratory disease: Spanish version of the Chronic Respiratory Questionnaire (CRQ). *Eur Respir J* 1998; **11**: 55–60.

111 Barr JT, Schumacher GE, Freeman S, *et al.* American translation, modification, and validation of the St. George's Respiratory Questionnaire. *Clin Ther* 2000; **22**: 1121–45.

112 Chan SL, Chan-Yeung MM, Ooi GC, *et al.* Validation of the Hong Kong Chinese version of the St. George Respiratory Questionnaire in patients with bronchiectasis. *Chest* 2002; **122**: 2030–7.

113 Bouchet C, Guillemin F, Hoang T, *et al* Validation of the St George's questionnaire for measuring the quality of life in patients with chronic obstructive pulmonary disease. *Rev Mal Respir* 1996; **13**: 43–6.

114 Kuzniar T, Patkowski J, Liebert J, *et al.* Validation of the Polish version of St George's respiratory questionnaire in patients with bronchial asthma. *Pneumonol Alergol Pol* 1999; **67**: 497–503.

115 Ferrer M, Alonso J, Prieto L, *et al.* Validity and reliability of the St George's Respiratory Questionnaire after adaptation to a different language and culture: the Spanish example. *Eur Respir J* 1996; **9**: 1160–6.

116 Engstrom CP, Persson LO, Larsson S, Sullivan M. Reliability and validity of a Swedish version of the St. George's Respiratory Questionnaire. *Eur Respir J* 1998; **11**: 61–6.

117 Schunemann HJ, Griffith L, Jaeschke R, *et al.* Evaluation of the minimal important difference for the feeling thermometer and the St. George's Respiratory Questionnaire in patients with chronic airflow obstruction. *J Clin Epidemiol* 2003; **56**: 1170–6.

118 Mahler DA, Weinberger DH, Wells CK, Feinstein AR. The measurement of dyspnea: contents, interobserver agreement, and physiologic correlates of two new clinical indexes. *Chest* 1984; **85**: 751–8.

119 Mahler DA, ed. *Dyspnea (Lung biology in health and disease).* New York: Marcel Dekker, 1998.

120 Witek TJ Jr, Mahler DA. Meaningful effect size and patterns of response of the transition dyspnea index. *J Clin Epidemiol* 2003; **56**: 248–55.

121 Van der Molen B. Dyspnoea: a study of measurement instruments for the assessment of dyspnea and their application for patients with advanced cancer. *J Adv Nurs* 1995; **22**: 948–56.

122 Mancini I, Body JJ. Assessment of dyspnea in advanced cancer patients. *Support Care Cancer* 1999; **7**: 229–32.

◆ 123 Meek PM, Lareau SC. Critical outcomes in pulmonary rehabilitation: Assessment and evaluation of dyspnea and fatigue. *J Rehabil Res Dev* 2003; **40** (Suppl 2): 13–24.

124 Wang XS, Hao XS, Wang Y, *et al.* Validation study of the Chinese version of the Brief Fatigue Inventory (BFI-C). *J Pain Symptom Manage* 2004; **27**: 322–32.

125 Radbruch L, Sabatowski R, Eisner F, *et al.* Validation of the German version of the Brief Fatigue Inventory. *J Pain Symptom Manage* 2003; **25**: 449–58.

126 Okuyama T, Wang XS, Akechi T, *et al.* Validation of the Japanese version of the Brief Fatigue Inventory. *J Pain Symptom Manage* 2003; **25**: 106–17.

127 Mendoza TR, Wang XS, Cleeland CS, *et al.* The rapid assessment of fatigue severity in cancer patients: use of the Brief Fatigue Inventory. *Cancer* 1999; **85**: 1186–96.

128 Hwang SS, Chang VT, Cogswell J, Kasimis BS. Clinical relevance of fatigue levels in cancer patients at a Veterans Administration Medical Center. *Cancer* 2002; **94**: 2481–9.

129 Piper BF, Dibble SL, Dodd MJ, *et al.* The revised Piper Fatigue Scale: psychometric evaluation in women with breast cancer. *Oncol Nurs Forum* 1998; **25**: 677–84.

130 Gledhill JA, Rodary C, Mahe C, Lizet C. French validation of the Piper Fatigue Scale. *Rech Soins Infirm* 2002; **68**: 50–65.

131 So WK, Dodgson J, Tai JW. Fatigue and quality of life among Chinese patients with hematologic malignancy after bone marrow transplantation. *Cancer Nurs* 2003; **26**: 211–19.

132 Yellen SB, Cella DF, Webster K, *et al.* Measuring fatigue and other anemia-related symptoms with the Functional Assessment of Cancer Therapy (FACT) measurement system. *J Pain Symptom Manage* 1997; **13**: 63–74.

133 Cella D, Zagari MJ, Vandoros C, *et al*. Epoeitin alfa treatment results in clinically significant improvements in quality of life in anemic cancer patients when referenced to the general population. *J Clin Oncol* 2003; **21**: 366–73.

134 Hwang SS, Chang VT, Kasimis BS. A comparison of three fatigue measures in veterans with cancer. *Cancer Investig* 2003; **21**: 363–73.

135 Schwartz AL. The Schwartz Cancer Fatigue Scale: testing reliability and validity. *Oncol Nurs Forum* 1998; **25**: 711–7.

136 Schwartz AL, Meek PM, Nail LM, *et al*. Measurement of fatigue determining minimally important differences. *J Clin Epidemiol* 2002; **55**: 239–44.

137 Schwartz A, Meek P. Additional construct validity of the Schwartz Cancer Fatigue Scale. *J Nurs Meas* 1999; **7**: 35–45.

◆ 138 Hesketh PJ, Gralla RJ, duBois A, *et al*. Methodology of antiemetic trials: response assessment, evaluation of new agents and definition of chemotherapy emetogenicity. *Support Care Cancer* 1998; **6**: 221–7.

139 Collins SL, Moore RA, McQuay HJ. The visual analogue pain intensity scale: what is moderate pain in millimeters? *Pain* 1997; **72**: 95–7.

140 Bird SB, Dickson EW. Clinically significant changes in pain along the visual analog scale. *Ann Emerg Med* 2001; **38**: 639–43.

141 Serlin RC, Mendoza TR, Nakamura Y, *et al*. When is cancer pain mild moderate or severe? Grading pain severity by its interference with function. *Pain* 1995; **61**: 277–84.

● 142 Farrar JT, Young JP Jr, LaMoreaux L, *et al*. Clinical importance of changes in chronic pain intensity measured on an 11-point numerical pain rating scale. *Pain* 2001; **94**: 149–58.

143 Farrar JT, Berlin JA, Strom BL. Clinically important changes in acute pain outcome measures: a validation study. *J Pain Symptom Manage* 2003; **25**: 406–11.

● 144 Daut RL, Cleeland CS, Flanery RC. Development of the Wisconsin Brief Pain Questionnaire to assess pain in cancer and other diseases. *Pain* 1983; **17**: 197–210.

145 Wang XS, Mendoza TR, Gao SZ, Cleeland CS. The Chinese version of the Brief Pain Inventory (BPI-C): its development and use in a study of cancer pain. *Pain* 1996; **67**: 407–16.

146 Ger LP, Ho ST, Sun WZ, *et al*. Validation of the Brief Pain Inventory in a Taiwanese population. *J Pain Symptom Manage* 1999; **18**: 316–22.

147 Radbruch L, Loick G, Kiencke P, *et al*. Validation of the German version of the Brief Pain Inventory. *J Pain Symptom Manage* 1999; **18**: 180–7.

148 Mystakidou K, Mendoza T, Tsilika E, *et al*. Greek Brief Pain Inventory: validation and utility in cancer pain. *Oncology* 2001; **60**: 35–42.

149 Saxena A, Mendoza T, Cleeland CS. The assessment of cancer pain in north India: the validation of the Hindi Brief Pain Inventory – BPI-H. *J Pain Symptom Manage* 1999; **17**: 27–41.

150 Caraceni A, Mendoza TR, Mencaglia E, *et al*. A validation study of an Italian version of the Brief Pain Inventory (Breve Questionario per la Valutazione del Dolore). *Pain* 1996; **65**: 87–92.

151 Uki J, Mendoza T, Cleeland C, Nakamura Y, Takeda F. A brief cancer pain assessment tool in Japanese: the utility of the Japanese Brief Pain Inventory BPI-J. *J Pain Symptom Manage* 1998; **16**: 364–73.

152 Klepstad P, Loge JH, Borchgrevink PC, *et al*. The Norwegian Brief Pain Inventory questionnaire: translation and validation in cancer pain patients. *J Pain Symptom Manage* 2002; **24**: 517–25.

153 Badia X, Muriel C, Gracia A, *et al*. Validation of the Spanish version of the Brief Pain Inventory in patients with oncological pain. *Med Clin (Barc)* 2003; **120**: 52–9.

154 MD Anderson Center. Symptom research. Available at: www.mdanderson.org/departments/PRG.

● 155 Melzack R. The McGill pain questionnaire.: Major properties and scoring methods. *Pain* 1975; **1**: 277–99.

156 Aboud FE, Hiwot MG, Arega A, *et al*. The McGill Pain Questionnaire in Amharic: Zwai Health Center patients' reports on the experience of pain. *Ethiop Med J* 2003; **41**: 45–61.

157 Harrison A. Arabic pain words. *Pain* 1988; **32**: 239–50.

158 Hui YL, Chen AC. Analysis of headache in a Chinese patient population. *Ma Zui Xue Za Zhi* 1989; **27**: 13–8.

159 Drewes AM, Helweg-Larsen S, Petersen P, *et al*. McGill Pain Questionnaire translated into Danish: experimental and clinical findings. *Clin J Pain* 1993; **9**: 80–7.

160 Perkins FM, Werner MU, Persson F, *et al*. Development and validation of a brief, descriptive Danish pain questionnaire (BDDPQ). *Acta Anesthesiol Scand* 2004; **48**: 486–90.

161 van der Kloot WA, Oostendorp RA, van der Meij J, van den Heuvel J. The Dutch version of the McGill pain questionnaire: a reliable pain questionnaire. *Ned Tijdschr Geneeskd* 1995; **139**: 669–73.

162 Ketovuori H, Pontinen PJ. A pain vocabulary in Finnish – The Finnish pain questionnaire *Pain* 1981; **11**: 247–53.

163 Boureau F, Luu M, Doubrere JF. Comparative study of the validity of four French McGill Pain Questionnaire (MPQ) versions. *Pain* 1992; **50**: 59–65.

164 Kiss I, Muller H, Able M. The McGill Pain Questionnaire – German version. A study on cancer pain. *Pain* 1987; **29**: 195–207.

165 Stein C, Mendl G. The German counterpart to McGill Pain Questionnaire. *Pain* 1988; **32**: 251–5.

166 Mystakidou K, Parpa E, Tsilika E, *et al*. Greek McGill Pain Questionnaire: validation and utility in cancer patients. *J Pain Symptom Manage* 2002; **24**: 379–87.

167 Hasegawa M, Hattori S, Mishima M, *et al*. The McGill Pain Questionnaire, Japanese version, reconsidered: confirming the theoretical structure. *Pain Res Manag* 2001; **6**: 173–80.

168 Satow A, Nakatani K, Taniguchi S. Japanese version of the MPQ and pentagon profile illustrated perceptual characteristics of pain. *Pain* 1989; **37**: 125–6.

169 Strand LI, Ljunggren AE. Different approximations of the McGill Pain Questionnaire in the Norwegian language: a discussion of content validity. *J Adv Nurs* 1997; **26**: 772–9.

170 Bartko D, Kondas M, Janco S. Quantification of pain in neurology. The Slovak version of the McGill-Melzack pain questionnaire. *Cesk Neurol Neurochir* 1984; **47**: 113–21.

171 Escalante A, Lichtenstein MJ, Rios N, Hazuda HP. Measuring chronic rheumatic pain in Mexican Americans: cross cultural adaptation of the McGill Pain Questionnaire. *J Clin Epidemiol* 1996; **49**: 1389–99.

172 Lazaro C, Caseras X, Whizar-Lugo VM, *et al*. Psychometric properties of a Spanish version of the McGill Pain Questionnaire in several Spanish-speaking countries. *Clin J Pain* 2001; **17**: 365–74.

173 Melzack R. The McGill Short Form Pain Questionnaire. *Pain* 1987; **30**: 191–7.

174 Solcova I, Jakoubek B, Sykora J, Hnik P. Characterization of vertebrogenic pain using the short form of the McGill Pain Questionnaire. *Cas Lek Cesk* 1990; **129**: 1611–14.

175 Georgoudis G, Oldham JA, Watson PJ. The development and validation of a Greek version of the short form McGill Pain Questionnaire. *Eur J Pain* 2000; **4**: 275–81.

176 Burckhardt CS, Bjelle A. A Swedish version of the short-form McGill Pain Questionnaire. *Scand J Rheumatol* 1994; **23**: 77–81.

● 177 Fishman B, Pasternak S, Wallenstein SL, *et al.* The Memorial Pain Assessment Card. A valid instrument for the evaluation of cancer pain. *Cancer* 1987; **60**: 1151–8.

178 Galer BS, Jensen MP. Development and preliminary validation of a pain measure specific to neuropathic pain: the Neuropathic Pain Scale. *Neurology* 1997; **48**: 332–6.

179 Bennett M. The LANSS pain scale: the Leeds assessment of neuropathic symptoms and signs. *Pain* 2001; **92**: 147–57.

180 Krause SJ, Backonja MM. Development of a Neuropathic Pain Questionnaire. *Clin J Pain* 2003; **19**: 306–14.

181 Bruera E, Macmillan K, Hanson J, *et al.* The Edmonton Staging System for cancer pain: preliminary report. *Pain* 1989; **37**: 203–9.

182 Bruera E, Schoeller T, Wenk R, *et al.* A prospective multicenter assessment of the Edmonton staging system for cancer pain. *J Pain Symptom Manage* 1995; **10**: 348–55.

183 Hwang SS, Chang VT, Fairclough DL, Kasimis BS. Development of a cancer pain prognostic scale. *J Pain Symptom Manage* 2002; **24**: 366–78.

◆ 184 Caraceni A, Cherny N, Fainsinger R, *et al.* Pain measurement tools and methods in clinical research in palliative care: recommendations of an Expert Working Group of the European Association of Palliative Care. *J Pain Symptom Manage* 2002; **23**: 239–55.

◆ 185 Turk DC, Melzack R. *Handbook of Pain Assessment*, 2nd ed. New York: The Guilford Press, 2001.

● 186 McCorkle R, Young K. Development of a symptom distress scale. *Cancer Nurs* 1978; **1**: 373–8.

187 McCorkle R, Cooley M, Shea JA. *A User's Manual for the Symptom Distress Scale*. Philadelphia: University of Pennsylvania, National Institute of Nursing Research, 1998.

188 Rhodes VA, McDanies RW, Homan SS, *et al.* An instrument to measure symptom experience. Symptom occurrence and symptom distress. *Cancer Nurs* 2000; **23**: 49–54.

189 Samarel N, Leddy SK, Greco K, *et al.* Development and testing of the Symptom experience scale. *J Pain Symptom Manage* 1996; **12**: 221–8.

190 Lai YH, Chang JT, Keefe FJ, *et al.* Symptom distress, catastrophic thinking, and hope in nasopharyngeal carcinoma patients. *Cancer Nurs* 2003; **26**: 485–93.

191 Persuelli C, Camporesi E, Colombo AM, Cucci M, Mazzoni G, Pac E. Quality-of-life assessment in a home care program for advanced cancer patients: a study using the Symptom Distress Scale. *J Pain Symptom Manage* 1993; **8**: 306–11.

192 Oh EG. Symptom experience in Korean adults with lung cancer. *J Pain Symptom Manage* 2004; **28**: 133–9. Tishelman C, Degner LF, Mueller B. Measuring symptom distress in patients with lung cancer. A pilot study of experienced intensity and importance of symptoms. *Cancer Nurs* 2000; **23**: 82–90.

193 Tishelman C, Degner LF, Mueller B. Measuring symptom distress in patients with lung cancer. A pilot study of experienced intensity and importance of symptoms. *Cancer Nurs* 2000; **23**: 82–90.

● 194 Bruera E, Kuehn N, Miller MJ, Selmser P, Macmillan K. The Edmonton Symptom Assessment System (ESAS): A simple method for the assessment of palliative care patients. *J Palliat Care* 1991; **7**: 6–9.

195 Philip J, Smith WB, Craft P, Lickiss N. Concurrent validity of the modified Edmonton Symptom Assessment System with the Rotterdam Symptom Checklist and the Brief Pain Inventory. *Support Care Cancer* 1998; **6**: 539–41.

196 Chang VT, Hwang SS, Feuerman M. Validation of the Edmonton Symptom Assessment Scale. *Cancer* 2000; **88**: 2164–71.

197 Pautex S, Berger A, Chatelain C, *et al.* Symptom assessment in elderly cancer patients receiving palliative care. *Crit Rev Oncol Hematol* 2002; **47**: 281–6.

198 Jenkins CA, Schulz M, Hanson J, Bruera E. Demographic, symptom, and medication profiles of cancer patients seen by a palliative care consult team in a tertiary referral hospital. *J Pain Symptom Manage* 2000; **19**: 174–84.

199 Heedman PA, Strang P. Pain and pain alleviation in hospital-based home care: demographic, biological and treatment factors. *Support Care Cancer* 2003; **11**: 35–40.

200 Nelson JE, Meier DE, Oei EJ, *et al.* Self-reported symptom experience of critically ill cancer patients receiving intensive care. *Crit Care Med* 2001; **29**: 277–82.

201 Hollen PJ, Gralla RJ, Kris MG, *et al.* Measurement of quality of life in patients with lung cancer in multicenter trials of new therapies. Psychometric assessment of the Lung Cancer Symptom Scale. *Cancer* 1994; **73**: 2087–98.

202 Cleeland CS, Mendoza TR, Wang XS, *et al.* Assessing symptom distress in cancer patients: the MD Anderson Symptom Inventory. *Cancer* 2000; **89**: 1634–46.

203 Portenoy RK, Thaler HT, Kornblith AB, *et al.* The Memorial Symptom Assessment Scale: an instrument for the evaluation of symptom prevalence, characteristics and distress. *Eur J Cancer* 1994; **30A**: 1326–36.

204 Chang VT, Hwang SS, Thaler HT, *et al.* The Memorial Symptom Assessment Scale. *Expert Rev Pharmacoeconomics Outcomes Res* 2004; **4**: 171–8.

205 Chang VT, Hwang SS, Feuerman M, *et al.* The memorial symptom assessment scale short form (MSAS-SF). *Cancer* 2000; **89**: 1162–71.

206 Chang VT, Hwang SS, Kasimis BS, Thaler HT. Shorter Symptom Assessment Instruments: The Condensed Memorial Symptom Assessment Scale (CMSAS). *Cancer Investig* 2004; **22**: 477–87.

207 Tranmer JE, Heyland D, Dudgeon D, *et al.* Measuring the symptom experience of seriously ill cancer and noncancer hospitalized patients near the end of life with the Memorial Symptom Assessment Scale. *J Pain Symptom Manage* 2003; **25**: 420–9.

208 McMillan SC, Small BJ. Symptom distress and quality of life in patients with cancer newly admitted to hospice care. *Oncol Nurs Forum* 2002; **29**: 1421–8.

209 Nelson JE, Meier DE, Litke A, *et al.* The symptom burden of chronic critical illness. *Crit Care Med* 2004; **32**: 1527–34.

210 Hwang SS, Chang VT, Fairclough DL, *et al.* Longitudinal quality of life in advanced cancer patients: pilot study results from a VA medical cancer center. *J Pain Symptom Manage* 2003; **25**: 225–35.

211 Chang VT, Hwang SS, Alejandro Y, *et al*. Clinically significant differences (CSD) in the Memorial Symptom Assessment Scale Short Form (MSAS-SF). *Proc ASCO* 2004; **23**: 792, [abstract 8269].

212 Collins JJ, Byrnes ME, Dunkel IJ, *et al*. The measurement of symptoms in children with cancer. *J Pain Symptom Manage* 2000; **19**: 363–77.

213 De Haes JCJM, van Knippenburg FCE, Nejit JP. Measuring psychological and physical distress in cancer patients: structure and application of the Rotterdam Symptom Checklist. *Br J Cancer* 1990; **62**: 1034–8.

214 Tchen N, Soubeyran P, Eghbali H, *et al*. Quality of life in patients with aggressive non-Hodgkin's lymphoma. Validation of the Medical Outcomes Study Short Form 20 and the Rotterdam Symptom Checklist in older patients. *Crit Rev Oncol Hematol* 2002; **43**: 219–26.

215 Paci E. Assessment of validity and clinical application of an Italian version of the Rotterdam Symptom Checklist. *Qual Life Res* 1992; **1**: 129–34.

216 Agra Y, Badia X. Evaluation of psychometric properties of the Spanish version of the Rotterdam Symptom Checklist to assess quality of life of cancer patients. *Rev Esp Salud Publica* 1999; **73**: 35–44.

217 Can G, Durna Z, Aydiner A. Assessment of fatigue in and care needs of Turkish women with breast cancer. *Cancer Nurs* 2004; **27**: 153–61.

218 Stein KD, Denniston M, Baker F, *et al*. Validation of a modified Rotterdam Symptom Checklist form with cancer patients in the United States. *J Pain Symptom Manage* 2003; **26**: 975–89.

219 Higginson IJ. Clinical and organizational audit in palliative medicine. In: Doyle D, Hanks G, Cherny NI, Calman K, eds. *Oxford Textbook of Palliative Medicine*, 3rd ed. Oxford: Oxford University Press, 2004: 184–96.

220 Hwang SS, Chang VT, Fairclough DL, *et al*. Longitudinal quality of life in advanced cancer patients: pilot study results from a VA medical cancer center. *J Pain Symptom Manage* 2003; **25**: 225–35.

221 Huang HY, Wilkie DJ, Chapman CR, Ting LL. Pain trajectory of Taiwanese with nasopharyngeal carcinoma over the course of radiation therapy. *J Pain Symptom Manage* 2003; **25**: 247–55.

222 Cella D, Pulliam J, Fuchs H, *et al*. Evaluation of pain associated with oral mucositis during the acute period after administration of high-dose chemotherapy. *Cancer* 2003; **98**: 406–12.

223 Stromgren AS, Groenvold M, Pedersen L, *et al*. Does the medical record cover the symptoms experienced by cancer patients in palliative care? A comparison of medical records against patient self rating. *J Pain Symptom Manage* 2001; **21**: 191–8.

224 Stromgren AS, Gorenvold M, Sorenson A, Andersen L. Symptom recognition in advanced cancer. A comparison of nursing records against patient self rating. *Acta Aneasthesiol Scand* 2001; **45**: 1080–5.

225 Roth AJ, Kornblith AB, Batel-Copel L, *et al*. Rapid screening for psychologic distress in men with prostate carcinoma: a pilot study. *Cancer* 1998; **82**: 1904–8.

226 Lidstone V, Butters E, Seed PT, *et al*. Symptoms and concerns amongst cancer outpatients: identifying the need for specialist palliative care. *Palliat Med* 2003; **17**: 588–95.

227 Potter J, Hami F, Bryan T, Quigley C. Symptoms in 400 patients referred to palliative care services: prevalence and patterns. *Palliat Med* 2003; **17**: 310–4.

228 Chang VT. The value of symptoms in prognosis of cancer patients. In: Bruera E, Portenoy RK, eds. *Topics in Palliative Care*, Vol. 4. New York: Oxford University Press, 2000: 23–54.

229 Vigano A, Donaldson N, Higginson IJ, *et al*. Quality of life and survival prediction in terminal cancer patients. *Cancer* 2004; **101**: 1090–8.

230 Barresi MJ, Shadbolt B, Byrne D, *et al*. The development of the Canberra symptom scorecard: a tool to monitor the physical symptoms of patients with advanced tumors. *BMC Cancer* 2003; **3**: 32.

231 Paice JA. Assessment of symptom clusters in patients with cancer. *J Natl Cancer Inst Monogr* 2004; **32**: 98–102.

232 Dudgeon DJ, Harlos M, Clinch JJ. The Edmonton Symptom Assessment Scale (ESAS) as an audit tool. *J Palliat Care* 1999; **15**: 14–9.

233 Lobchuk MM, Degner LF. Symptom experiences: perceptual accuracy between advanced-stage cancer patients and family caregivers in the home care setting. *J Clin Oncol* 2002; **20**: 3495–507.

234 Nekolaichuk CL, Maguire TO, Suarez-Almazor M, *et al*. Assessing the reliability of patient, nurse, and family caregiver symptom ratings in hospitalized advanced cancer patients. *J Clin Oncol* 1999; **17**: 3621–30.

235 Nelson CJ, Rosenfeld B, Brietbart W, Galietta M. Spirituality, religion and depression in the terminally ill. *Psychosomatics* 2002; **43**: 213–20.

236 Chochinov HM, Hack T, Hassard T, *et al*. Dignity in the terminally ill: a cross-sectional, cohort study. *Lancet* 2002; **360**: 2026–30.

237 Merkel SI, Voepel-Lewis T, Shayevitz JR, Malviya S. The FLACC: a behavioral scale for scoring postoperative pain in young children. *Pediatr Nurs* 1997; **23**: 293–7.

238 Warden V, Hurley AC, Volicer L. Development and psychometric validation of the Pain Assessment in Advanced Dementia (PAINAD) Scale. *J Am Dir Assoc* 2003; **4**: 9–15.

239 Villanueva MR, Smith TL, Erickson JS, *et al*. Pain Assessment for the Dementing Elderly (PADE): reliability and validity of a new measure. *J Am Med Dir Assoc* 2003; **4**: 1–8.

239a Herr K, Bjoro K, Decker S. Tools for assessment of pain in nonverbal older adults with dementia: a state-of-the-science review. *J Pain Symptom Manage* 2006; **31**: 170–92.

240 Puntillo KA, Morris AB, Thompson CL, *et al*. Pain behaviors observed during six common procedures: results from Thunder Project II. *Crit Care Med* 2004; **32**: 421–7.

241 Shannon MM, Ryan MA, D'Agostino N, Brescia FJ. Assessment of pain in advanced cancer patients. *J Pain Symptom Manage* 1995; **10**: 274–8.

242 Costello P, Wiseman J, Douglas I, *et al*. Assessing hospice inpatients with pain using numerical rating scales. *Palliative Med* 2001; **15**: 257–8.

◆ 243 Webster K, Cella D, Yost K. The Functional Assessment of Chronic Illness Therapy (FACIT) Measurement System: properties, applications, and interpretation. Review. *Health Qual Life Outcomes* 2003; **1**: 79. Available at: www.hqlo.com/content/1/1/79 (accessed).

● 244 Aaronson NK, Ahmedzai S, Bergman B, *et al*. The European Organization for Research and Treatment of Cancer QLQ-C30: a quality of life instrument for use in international clinical trials in oncology. *J Natl Cancer Inst* 1993; **85**: 365–76.

245   Steel K, Ljunggren G, Topinkova E, *et al.* The RAI-PC: an instrument for palliative care in all settings. *Am J Hosp Palliat Care* 2003; **20**: 211–9.

246   Chapman CR, Syralja. Measurement of pain, In: Loeser JD, ed. *Bonica's Management of Pain*, 3rd ed. New York: Lippincott, Williams and Wilkins, 2001: 310–28.

247   Guillemin F, Bombardier C, Beaton D. Cross-cultural adaptation of health-related quality of life measures: literature review and proposed guidelines. *J Clin Epidemiol* 1993; **46**: 1417–32.

248   Jensen MP. Questionnaire validation: a brief guide for readers of the research literature. *Clin J Pain* 2003; **19**: 345–52.

249   Higginson IJ, Carr AJ. Using quality of life measures in the clinical setting. *BMJ* 2001; **322**: 1297–300.

250   Soni M, Cella D, Masters G, *et al.* The validity and clinical utility of symptom monitoring in advanced lung cancer: a literature review. *Clinical Lung Cancer* 2002; **4**: 153–60.

251   Bruera E, Sweeney C. The development of palliative care at the University of Texas MD Anderson Cancer Center. *Support Care Cancer* 2001; **9**: 330–4.

252   Ewing JA. Detecting alcoholism: the CAGE questionnaire. *JAMA* 1984; **252**: 1905–7.

253   Keith RA, Granger CV, Hamilton BB, Sherman FS. The Functional Independence Measure; a new tool for rehabilitation. In: Eisenberg MG, Grzesiak RC, eds. *Advances in Clinical Rehabilitation.* New York: Springer, 1987: 18.

254   Mancini I, Lossignol D, Obiols M, *et al.* Supportive and palliative care: experience at the Institut Jules Bordet. *Support Care Cancer* 2001; **10**: 3–7.

255   Kaasa T, Loomis J, Gillis K, Bruera E, Hanson J. The Edmonton Functional Assessment Tool: preliminary development and evaluation for use in palliative care. *J Pain Symptom Manage* 1997; **13**: 10–19.

256   Radbruch L, Sabatowski R, Loick G, *et al.* Cognitive impairment and its influence on pain and symptom assessment in a palliative care unit: development of a Minimal Documentation System. *Palliat Med* 2000; **14**: 266–76.

257   Ware J Jr, Kosinski M, Keller SD. A 12-item Short Form Health Survey: construction of scales and preliminary tests of reliability and validity. *Med Care* 1996; **34**: 220–33.

41

Quality of life assessment in palliative care

S ROBIN COHEN

INTRODUCTION

The ultimate goal of palliative care is to optimize the quality of life (QOL) of people living with a life-threatening illness and that of their families. Assessment of QOL is therefore necessary if we are to provide the best care possible and ensure that we are eliminating unnecessary suffering. In this chapter I hope to clarify the concept of QOL at the end of life, and identify the questions that you must ask yourself before deciding how to best assess QOL in your particular situation.

WHAT IS QUALITY OF LIFE?

Quality of life remains an ill-defined concept, widely used but much argued about across and within disciplines.[1,2] Is QOL completely subjective, dependent only on a person's perception of their life situation, or does it also depend on the objective (directly observable) situation? Objective situations such as the availability of schools, or ability to safely walk the streets, are arguably important contributors to the QOL of the general population. However, I would argue that near the end of life, the world of the patient and even that of the family caregiver has shrunk, and the environmental setting that contributes to QOL is much more closely tied to the setting of care and healthcare system. Furthermore, I believe that the best definition of QOL for palliative care is *subjective well-being*, the key word being 'subjective'. How else can we explain that we may have two people in similar physical situations and close to death, but one judges their QOL to be good and cherishes each day,

while the other feels that life is not worth living? The psychological, sociological, and philosophical disciplines have debated the meaning of the term QOL for over half a century. Medicine, nursing, and allied health professions have adopted the term and considered QOL as an important outcome in many cases. However, in the healthcare setting, much less consideration has been given to the concept and it is often used without clarification.[1,3,4] Some published papers claiming to study QOL are in fact studying a single symptom such as pain or diarrhea, while others are truly trying to study subjective wellbeing. Health status is often mistakenly used as a surrogate term for QOL.

The term health-related QOL, which I and others consider a misnomer[1,5,6] was, depending on the point of view, developed to broaden the prevalent focus on physical health to also include physical and social functioning, as well as mental health, *or* to exclude from concern domains perceived as unrelated to healthcare, such as spirituality and life satisfaction. Whatever the reason for developing the concept of health-related QOL, it involves limiting the concept of QOL to certain aspects of the person whose QOL we want to assess. Whole person care is more than simply caring for all aspects of a person, it is also the recognition and understanding that all aspects of the person are interrelated, affecting one another. For this reason I believe that the concept of health-related QOL was created for the convenience of healthcare researchers with good intentions, but it is not a construct that has a match in reality. We cannot separate the physical, psychologic, and social aspects of the person from other essential parts, such as existential wellbeing or spirituality. Furthermore, good QOL is not simply the absence of problems, as it is often defined in health-related QOL measures. Quality of life is determined by the evaluation of both the positive and negative aspects of one's life, and the value or weight you put on each aspect.[6–14] A concrete example: if you are treating pain that originates in a trapped nerve, and the patient also happens to believe that pain is a test from God, if you do not address the person's belief regarding the pain being God's will, you are unlikely to get the pain under control using only medication unless you use a dose so large that the person has a very clouded sensorium.

If QOL results not only from external circumstances but from an interaction between those and the person whose QOL we are assessing, then there are many things that need to be taken into account. What follows is a partial list of what we should keep in mind when assessing QOL.

- *QOL is the discrepancy or gap between a person's expectations and their actual situation.*[15–17] This provides us with two means of improving QOL (or decreasing the gap): we can improve the actual situation (e.g. reduce pain) and we can decrease expectations where we cannot improve the actual situation (e.g. desire to retain full physical functional status).
- *Response shift or adaptation.* People have an amazing capacity to adapt to new and even difficult circumstances. This is a powerful way of coping with a difficult situation which is in large part out of your control. When evaluating their QOL, people may have (i) changed their internal standards (called recalibration), (ii) focused on areas in which they are doing better and de-emphasized the importance of areas in which they are not doing well (change in values); or (iii) changed what areas they call to mind when they answer 'How is your QOL?' (called reconceptualization).[14] The data from Kreitler et al.[18] are an excellent cross-sectional example of the power of adaptation. We are only beginning to learn how response shift may come about, and the situations in which it is most likely to occur. If we are truly interested in subjective wellbeing, and recognize QOL as a perception, then the fact that response shift or adaptation is affecting our assessment of QOL is not a problem. However, when we are determining the effect of a noncoping intervention on QOL, then if there is differential response shift in two groups we are comparing, it is often important to know how response shift or adaptation is affecting our assessment of QOL. If the group that received the intervention improves a lot and therefore does not make a response shift (there is no need to adapt, as the situation has improved), but the group that did not get the intervention had a large response shift over the month that the intervention was being given to the other group, and de-emphasized the importance of the area in which they were not doing well, the two groups may give similar assessments of their QOL. In the case of the intervention group, it will be because the situation has improved. In the case of the control group, it will be because they have changed their

expectations or evaluation of the situation. Both are coping well, but this will hide the effectiveness of the intervention. Within-subject crossover trials may also be greatly influenced by response shift, since the washout period does not 'wash out' any response shift.[19] We are still exploring how to measure response shift and take it into account when it is important to do so.[11,12,20,21] Note that response shift is not limited to QOL and is a factor in all self-report measures, such as for pain or fatigue. This must be taken into account when interpreting the results of most clinical trials. Some factors likely to influence the ability to adapt are listed below.

- Social comparison. The theory[22] is that a factor in how we judge our situation is how we compare ourselves to others (are we doing better or worse in comparison), and who we choose to compare ourselves to (people in the general population? People with the same disease who are doing better than we are? People with the same disease who are doing worse than we are?).[19,23,24]
- Personality characteristics such as optimism[19,25–27] and sense of self-efficacy.[28]
- Existential wellbeing. Being able to see yourself in this situation as still being a valuable part of something larger than yourself (e.g. the world; nature; God's plan) and finding meaning in life.[7,8,29]

REASONS FOR ASSESSING QUALITY OF LIFE

Be clear about your purpose in assessing QOL. It will help you decide how best to do it. Do you want to:

- distinguish between groups of people?
- determine changes in the QOL of a group of people over time?
- assess an individual's (patient, or family caregiver), or even family's QOL at a specific point in time?
- assess changes in an individual's QOL over time?

BASIC REQUIREMENTS FOR ASSESSING QUALITY OF LIFE

Content validity

Any assessment of QOL, whether for clinical purposes or research purposes, needs to have content validity: you need to be assessing QOL, and not some other construct (such as health status). There is not complete agreement in the literature as to which domains are important for the QOL of palliative care patients, but there is a general consensus that it includes at least the physical, psychologic, social/relationship, and existential/spiritual domains.[30] Interestingly, these are the same as those generated by children with cancer.[31] Other domains such as cognitive functioning,[8,32] environment,[8] and communication have been found to be important in some but not all studies.[8,30] When assessing QOL in different cultures, content validity needs to be assessed for each culture. It is not enough to know that the translation of the scale or interview is accurate and embraces the same concepts, it is necessary to be sure that the interview or questionnaire includes all the relevant content and only relevant content.

Acceptability/feasibility

Any assessment of QOL needs to be acceptable to the person whose QOL is being assessed. The questions must not be distressing. They may raise important feelings and even bring tears, but if these appear to be a welcome opening by the person to discuss important issues with the assessor, then I do not consider it distressing, provided they are given the opportunity to discuss these issues. I and others have informally noted that many palliative care patients find QOL assessments therapeutic. A formal study demonstrates this to be true for family caregivers as well.[33] The assessment must also be within the limits of the strength and other capabilities (e.g. reading) of the person whose QOL is being assessed.

Stability/test-retest reliability

When the person's or group's QOL is stable, the assessment should reflect that stability.

Responsiveness or sensitivity to change

When the person's or group's QOL changes, the assessment should reflect that change.

Interpretation of change

If QOL is being measured, so that a score is obtained, you need to know how to interpret a change in score. What amount of change in the scale is clinically meaningful to the patient? A statistically significant difference in scores between groups or over time is not necessarily an important one. Fortunately, recent work suggests that the minimal clinically important difference is similar across many QOL studies with different populations and represents about 0.2–0.5 standard deviations, or 5–10 percent of the scale range,[34] although it is always more reassuring if you have data available for the specific QOL instrument you are using. Can you put the change in scores into a clinically meaningful context (e.g. an improvement in score of 25 percent or 2 points on Psychological Subscale X corresponds to the difference between someone who is clinically depressed and someone who is not really enjoying every day but is not depressed)?

LEVEL AT WHICH TO ASSESS QUALITY OF LIFE

Quality of life can be assessed at different levels of detail.

1 Overall QOL.
2 Different areas or domains that contribute to QOL (e.g. physical; psychologic; social; existential).
3 Specific contributors to QOL (e.g. pain; anxiety about suffocating).

STANDARDIZED VERSUS INDIVIDUALIZED MEASURES

Standardized measures of QOL have fixed questions. Depending on the questionnaire, answers can be combined to obtain either a score for overall QOL, separate scores for different domains contributing to QOL, or both. In contrast, individualized QOL measures ask each person to name the areas of their life that are most important to their QOL, how satisfied they are in these areas, and the relative importance of each area named. Standardized measures can also include items asking people to rate the importance to them of various areas, but in practice these have been problematic.[35] Weighting the responses by the importance assigned to each area or question by each participant has not seemed to change the results when studying the QOL of groups of people, and it therefore is rarely used as it adds to participant burden.[36,37]

Because the specific contributors to QOL differ from person to person or for the same person over time, some argue it is not possible to measure QOL, or that if measurement is possible, it cannot be done using standardized measures.[38,39] I believe it depends on the purpose of QOL assessment. While the contributors to our QOL differ at the level of the specifics, at the level of domains, which can even be thought of as a deeper if less specific level, there is commonality among people and perhaps across cultures. For example, everyone wants to be physically comfortable, be neither depressed nor anxious, be comfortable with their place in the world, etc. This also remains to be tested. If this is the case, then standardized measures can be useful for measuring the QOL of groups, but may not be as useful as individualized measures for clinical care of individuals, where specific contributors to QOL may be of interest rather than wellbeing in domains. However, individualized measures have the drawback of not having everyone (or the same person over time) propose the same items as important to their QOL. Therefore, individualized measures provide a measure of overall QOL to compare across groups or for a group over time, but do not permit comparison of contributors to QOL at the level of domains, as not everyone will nominate the same domains. Since people may also change the weight assigned to different items in individualized questionnaires over time, interpretation of changes or differences in QOL scores on individualized measures is complex. If people are asked to nominate items at each assessment rather than using the ones they nominated at the first assessment, some sensitivity to change may be lost.[40] However, if forced to use the same items at both times, the individualization at the second time of measurement is somewhat adulterated. Furthermore, sometimes people do not propose a certain item as important to their QOL simply because they have forgotten to mention it.[41]

HOW DO YOU MEASURE QUALITY OF LIFE?

Here are some questions you must answer in order to decide how best to assess QOL for your purpose.

- *Am I interested in QOL or rather in a specific contributor to QOL?* If the latter (e.g. physical functioning), choose a measure of that contributor rather than of QOL (although if you also expect overall QOL to be affected, or QOL in several domains to be affected, you may decide to make these secondary measures).
- *What level of QOL information do I need?* You may only want an answer to the question: how is your QOL? However, for many purposes, more detailed information is required, and you will want to know in what domains the person is doing well, and in what domains they are doing poorly. This is especially important in palliative care, where there is an inevitable decline in some areas such as physical wellbeing, but there may be improvement in others such as relationships or existential wellbeing.[42–45] If you only measure overall QOL over time, it may remain steady despite large changes in different domains. In this case you would select either an instrument that has well-established subscales for different domains (standardized measure with psychometrically sound subscales) or one that allows the person to name the domains important to their QOL and rate their status in each one (individualized measure).
- *Am I interested in comparing groups of people?* If yes, do these people have the same disease or different diseases? If you are comparing groups of people with different diseases, do the contributors to QOL differ at the level at which you want to measure QOL? If not, you can use a standardized measure. If the contributors to QOL differ for the two groups at the level you are measuring, the content of a standardized measure will not be equally valid for both groups, and an individualized measure is required for validity. If the contributors to QOL are the same for both groups, do you need to compare at the level of domains (in which case you will need a standardized measure) or at the level of overall QOL (in which case you can choose either an individualized or standardized measure).

- *Do I need information regarding everyone in the group, or is it acceptable to have only information regarding people capable of completing a questionnaire?* If you are in the camp that agrees that QOL is subjective, then it is clear that the person whose QOL is being measured is the best person to rate their own QOL. However, the physical or cognitive status of many palliative care patients precludes them being able to participate in rating their QOL. In this case, proxy measures may be considered. Ideally, someone who knows the patient well will rate the patient's QOL on his or her behalf. This may be a member of the staff or the family. However, proxy measures are known to differ from the patient's own ratings, and the difference tends to be greatest for areas that are less concrete (such as existential wellbeing) and where the patient is doing poorly. Many studies have been conducted regarding proxy measures, and the results are not particularly consistent.[4,46–48] There is no perfect solution in palliative care. You will have to balance the limitations of using proxy measures against the limitation of assessing only those who are well enough to complete a questionnaire.
- *How do I interpret a change in scores?* Note that the clinical importance of a change in scores may not be represented by the same amount of change in the directions of improvement and deterioration. Sometimes relevant information is available for the instrument you are using, but at this time this information tends to be limited. For example, the difference in score between bad, average, and good days is known for the McGill Quality of Life Questionnaire.[29] However, if you expect a more subtle change due to your intervention of difference between groups, you may need to be creative and think of ways of asking the person completing the questionnaire to in some way directly rate the importance of the change or indicate what it means clinically (e.g. if measuring physical functioning, what can you do now that you could not do before?).[49–52] In addition, in some circumstances response shift must be taken into account.
- *Do I want to assess QOL to help a particular patient (or family caregiver)?* If so, do I just want an initial assessment, periodic assessments, or do I want to track change in QOL over time? Will the answers to a formal assessment be useful (e.g. the scores), or should I use the QOL instrument as a guide for what to ask, without focusing on the numbers generated? For clinical purposes, I do not think any measure can replace a *good* clinical interview, although this remains to be tested. However, QOL measures are helpful as an initial interview guide or to flag areas that need further attention.[53–56] If QOL measurement turns out to be clinically useful, much work needs to be done to address barriers to its use in this way.[57]
- *How much can I expect my participants to do?* Can they complete the questionnaires on their own – do they

have the strength, concentration, sight, and reading skills? Or do I need to plan for someone to help explain the process of completing the questionnaire and read the questions to them? If so, who should this person be? Is it better to be a research assistant not involved in the patient's care, or should it be a staff member? What bias does each choice introduce to the answer to my question? What is feasible?

- *Will response shift (adaptation) interfere with my interpretation of the answer, or is the extent to which it occurs irrelevant to my question?* If it is not relevant, it simply needs to be taken into account when interpreting your results. However, if a response shift may greatly influence your conclusions, ideally you would plan some way of measuring the degree of response shift to help you interpret your data.[11,12,20,21]

- *If assessing over time, how will I use the data from the different times of data collection? How will I handle the inevitable missing data?* There are many established ways of dealing with data missing completely at random. However, in palliative care most of our missing data is *not* missing at random (it is informatively censored): usually it is missing because the patient has become too ill to respond or has died, or the patient's deterioration means that the family caregiver no longer has time to complete the questionnaire. Some headway has been made recently in dealing with this situation,[58] and if conducting a study you should check the recent literature to see if new papers on the topic have been published as it is presently an active area of research.

- *What time-frame should the questions refer to?* It is important that your questions clearly indicate the time period that people are to consider when answering. QOL measures developed for the general population often refer to the past month, while those that are disease-specific often use a time-frame of the past week. I have used the time-frame of the past 2 days in the measures I have developed for palliative care[42–44,59,60] because I believe that QOL often changes so rapidly near the end of life that it is too difficult to determine QOL over a longer period of time. Even with a time-frame of 2 days, sometimes people are having to average over a very good day and a bad one. However, I feel that 2 days is a better time-frame than a shorter one, which would only give a brief snapshot, taking into consideration that our population is probably not up to answering more than one to three times a week.

WHERE TO FIND MORE SPECIFIC INFORMATION ABOUT QOL MEASUREMENT TOOLS

Several reviews of the QOL instruments in the palliative care setting have been published in the scientific literature.[59,61,62]

In addition, compendiums of QOL instruments can be purchased.[63,64] The McGill Quality of Life Questionnaire,[42–44] and Hospice Quality of Life Index[65] are examples of standardized QOL instruments used for palliative care patients. The Palliative Outcome Scale[66–67] and Memorial Symptom Assessment Scale[68] have extensive overlap with QOL measures and are well-developed. The more recent Quality of Life at the End of Life (QUAL-E) was in fact developed based on data regarding what is most important at the end of life and to the quality of dying (rather than QOL *per se*); but there is much overlap with the content of the QOL questionnaires developed for palliative care.[69,70] The Edmonton Symptom Assessment System is not a measure of QOL but is widely used in conjunction with QOL instruments when specific symptoms are also of interest.[71] The Schedule for Evaluation of Individualized Quality of Life – Direct Weighting[9] and Patient Generated Index[10] are examples of individualized QOL instruments that can be used for patients or family caregivers. The Caregiver Quality of Life-Cancer instrument,[72] Caregiver Quality of Life Index,[73] and Quality of Life in Life-Threatening illness-Caregiver Version[59,60] have been used to measure the QOL of family caregivers. A retrospective measure of the quality of death and dying is the Quality of Death and Dying Scale.[74]

THE FUTURE

I look forward to a future where patients and family caregivers will be described not only in terms of their disease and symptom status, but also in terms of their QOL. Only then can palliative care really be addressing whole person care.

Key learning points

- Improving QOL is the main goal of palliative care, therefore assessing it is critical if we want to understand the extent to which we are achieving our goals.

- QOL assessment provides an assessment of the whole person. QOL is a perception. It is not a specific set of external circumstances, but rather the interaction of the person with external and internal circumstances.

- QOL assessment involves assessing what enhances someone's QOL as well as what makes it worse.

- The 'best' way of assessing QOL will depend on your purpose in assessing it.

- There is no perfect way to assess QOL in palliative care. Choose the best way, or combination of ways, and be aware of its strengths and limitations.

REFERENCES

1   Gill TM, Feinstein AR. A critical appraisal of the quality of quality-of-life measurements. *JAMA* 1994; **172**: 619–31.

2   Gladis MM, Gosch EA, Dishuk NM, *et al.* Quality of life: Expanding the scope of clinical significance. *J Consult Clin Psychol* 1999; **67**: 320–31.

3   Hunt SM. The subjective health of older women: Measuring outcomes in relation to prevention. *Qual Life Res* 2000; **9**: 709–19.

◆ 4   George LK. Research design in end-of-life research: State of science. *Gerontologist* 2002; **Special Issue III**: 86–98.

● 5   Cohen SR, Mount BM. Quality of life in terminal illness: Defining and measuring subjective well-being in the dying. *J Palliat Care* 1992; **8**: 40–5.

● 6   Hunt SM. The problem of quality of life. *Qual Life Res* 1997; **6**: 205–12.

● 7   Folkman S. Positive psychological states and coping with severe stress. *Soc Sci Med* 1997; **45**: 1207–221.

8   Cohen SR, Leis A. What determines the quality of life of terminally ill cancer patients from their own perspective? *J Palliat Care* 2002; **18**: 48–58.

● 9   Waldron D, O'Boyle CA, Kearney M, *et al.* Quality of life measurement in advanced cancer: Assessing the individual. *J Clin Oncol* 1999; **17**: 3603–11.

10   Ruta DA, Garratt AM, Russell IT. Patient centred assessment of quality of life for patients with four common conditions. *Qual Health Care* 1999; **8**: 22–9.

11   Rapkin BD, Schwartz CE. Toward a theoretical model of quality of life appraisal: Implications of findings of studies of response shift. *Health Qual Life Outcomes* 2004; **2**: 14.

12   Schwartz CE, Rapkin BD. Reconsidering the psychometrics of quality of life assessment in light of response shift and appraisal. *Health Qual Life Outcomes* 2004; **2**: 16.

13   Ryff CD. Happiness is everything, or is it? Explorations on the meaning of psychological well-being. *J Personality Soc Psychol* 1989; **57**: 1069–81.

● 14   Sprangers MAG, Schwartz CE. Integrating response shift into health-related quality-of-life research. *Soc Sci Med* 1999; **48**: 1507–15.

● 15   Cantril H. *The Pattern of Human Concerns.* New Jersey: Rutgers University Press, 1965.

● 16   Campbell A, Converse PE, Rodgers WL. *The Quality of American Life.* New York: Russell Sage Foundation, 1976.

17   Calman KC. Quality of life in cancer patients: An hypothesis. *J Med Ethics* 1994; **10**: 124–7.

18   Kreitler S, Chaitchick S, Rapoport Y, *et al.* Life satisfaction and health in cancer patients, orthopedic patients and healthy individuals. *Soc Sci Med* 1993; **36**: 547–56.

19   Allison PJ, Locker D, Feine JS. Quality of Life: A dynamic construct. *Soc Sci Med* 1997; **45**: 221–30.

20   Lowy A, Bernhard J. Quantitive assessment of changes in patients' constructs of quality of life: An application of multilevel models. *Qual Life Res* 2004; **13**: 1177–85.

21   Bernhard J, Lowy A, Mathys N, Herrmann R, *et al.* Health related quality of life: A changing construct? *Qual Life Res* 2004; **13**: 1187–97.

● 22   Festinger L. A theory of social comparison processes. *Hum Relat* 1954; **7**: 117–40.

23   Wood JV. Theory and research concerning social comparison of personal attributes. *Psychol Bull* 1989; **106**: 231–48.

24   Gibbons F, McCoy SB. Self-esteem, similarity, and reaction to active versus passive downward comparison. *J Personality Soc Psychol* 1991; **60**: 414–24.

25   Wrosch C, Scheier MF. Personality and quality of life: The importance of optimism and goal adjustment. *Qual Life Res* 2003; **12**(Suppl. 1): 59–72.

26   Berterö C, Ek A-C. Quality of life of adults with acute leukaemia. *J Adv Nurs* 1993; **18**: 1346–53.

27   Yu CLM, Fielding R, Chan CLW. The mediating role of optimism on post-radiation quality of life in nasopharyngeal carcinoma. *Qual Life Res* 2003; **12**: 41–51.

28   Benight CC, Antoni MH, Kilbourn K, *et al.* Coping self-efficacy buffers psychological and physiological disturbances in HIV-infected men following a natural disaster. *Health Psychol* 1997; **16**: 248–55.

29   Cohen SR, Mount BM. Living with cancer: 'Good Days' and 'Bad Days' – What produces them? Can the McGill Quality of Life Questionnaire distinguish between them? *Cancer* 2000; **89**: 1854–65.

◆ 30   Cohen SR. Assessing quality of life in palliative care. In: Portenoy R, Bruera E, eds. *Issues in Palliative Care Research.* New York: Oxford University Press, 2003: 231–41.

31   Hinds PS, Gattuso JS, Fletcher A, *et al.* Quality of life as conveyed by pediatric patients with cancer. *Qual Life Res* 2004; **13**: 761–72.

32   Padilla GV, Ferrell B, Grant MM, Rhiner M. Defining the content domain of quality of life for cancer patients with pain. *Cancer Nurs* 1990; **13**: 108–15.

33   Hudson P. The experience of research participation for family caregivers of palliative care cancer patients. *Int J Palliat Nurs* 2003; **9**: 120–3.

● 34   Norman GR, Sloan JA, Wyrwich KW. Interpretation of changes in health related quality of life: The remarkable universality of half a standard deviation. *Med Care* 2003; **41**: 582–92.

35   Cella D. Manual of the Functional Assessment of Chronic Illness Therapy (FACIT) Measurement System. *FACIT Manual.* November 1997; Version 4.

36   Skevington SM, O'Connell KA, the WHOQOL Group. Can we identify the poorest quality of life? Assessing the importance of quality of life using the WHOQOL-100*. *Qual Life Res* 2004; **13**: 23–34.

37   Cella D. The Functional Assessment of Cancer Therapy-Anemia (FACT-An) Scale: A new tool for the assessment of outcomes in cancer anemia and fatigue. *Semin Hematol* 1997; **34**(Suppl 2): 13–19.

● 38   McGee HM, O'Boyle CA, Hickey A, *et al.* Assessing the quality of life of the individual: The SEIQoL with a healthy and gastroenterology unit population. *Psychol Med* 1991; **21**: 749–59.

39   Montazeri A, Gillis CR, McEwan J. Measuring quality of life in oncology: Is it worthwhile? *Eur J Cancer Care* 1996; **5**: 159–75.

40   Bayle B, Kemoun G, Migaud H, Thevenon A. Comparison of two modes of administration of a personalized quality of life scale in a longitudinal study of total hip arthroplasty. *Joint Bone Spine* 2000; **67**: 101–6.

41   Ahmed S, Mayo N, Corbière M, *et al.* Individualized health-related quality of life (HRQL) post-stroke: Revealing response shift. *Quality Life Res* 2003; **12**: 765.

42   Cohen SR, Mount BM, Tomas J, Mount L. Existential well-being is an important determinant of quality of life: Evidence

from the McGill Quality of Life Questionnaire. *Cancer* 1996; **77**: 576–86.

43 Cohen SR, Hassan SA, Lapointe BM, Mount BM. HIV Disease and AIDS: Increasing importance of the existential domain in determining quality of life as T4 cell counts decrease. *AIDS* 1996; **10**: 1421–7.

● 44 Cohen SR, Mount BM, Bruera E, Provost M, *et al.* Validity of the McGill Quality of Life Questionnaire in the palliative care setting. A multi-center Canadian study demonstrating the importance of the existential domain. *Palliat Med* 1997; **11**: 3–20.

45 Ringdal GI, Ringdal K, Kvinnsland S, Götestam KG. Quality of life of cancer patients with different prognoses. *Qual Life Res* 1994; **3**: 143–54.

◆ 46 Sneeuw KCA, Aaronson NK, Sprangers MAG, *et al.* Evaluating the quality of life of cancer patients: Assessments by patients, significant others, physicians and nurses. *Br J Cancer* 1999; **81**: 87–94

47 Horton R. Differences in assessment of symptoms and quality of life between patients with advanced cancer and their specialist palliative care nurses in a home care setting. *Palliat Med* 2002; **16**: 488–94.

◆ 48 McPherson CJ, Addington-Hall JM. Judging the quality of care at the end of life: Can proxies provide reliable information? *Soc Sci Med* 2002; **56**: 95–109.

49 Osoba D, Rodrigues G, Myles J, *et al.* Interpreting the significance of changes in health-related quality-of-life scores. *J Clin Oncol* 1998; **16**: 139–44.

50 Cella D, Hahn EA, Dineen K. Meaningful change in cancer-specific quality of life scores: Differences between improvement and worsening. *Qual Life Res* 2000; **11**: 207–21.

◆ 51 Cella D, Bullinger M, Scott C, *et al.* Group vs individual approaches to understanding the clinical significance of differences or changes in quality of life. *Mayo Clinic Proc* 2002; **77**: 384–92.

● 52 Guyatt GH, Osoba D, Wu AW, *et al.* Methods to explain the clinical significance of health status measures. *Mayo Clinic Proc* 2002; **77**: 371–83.

53 Finlay I, Pratheepawanit N, Salek S. Monitoring self-reported quality-of-life among patients attending a palliative medicine outpatient clinic. *Palliat Med* 2003; **17**: 83–4.

54 Higginson IJ, Carr AJ. Using quality of life measures in the clinical setting. *BMJ* 2001; **322**: 1297–300.

55 Eischens MJ, Elliot BA, Elliot TE. Two hospice quality of life surveys: A comparison. *Am J Hospice Palliative Care.* 1998; **15**: 143–8.

56 Hughes R, Aspinal F, Addington-Hall JM, *et al.* Professionals' views and experiences using outcome measures in palliative care. *Int J Palliat Nurs* 2003; **9**: 234–8.

57 Hughes R, Aspinal F, Addington-Hall JM, *et al.* It just didn't work: The realities of quality of life assessment in the English healthcare context. *Int J Nurs Stud* 2004; **41**: 705–12.

58 Fairclough DL. *Design and Analysis of Quality of Life Studies in Clinical Trials.* Boca Raton: Chapman & Hall, 2002.

59 Cohen SR. Defining and measuring quality of life in palliative care. In: Bruera E, Portenoy RK, eds. *Topics in Palliative Care.* New York: Oxford University Press, 2001; 137–56.

60 Cohen SR, Leis A, Porterfield P, *et al.* QOLLTI-F: A Measure of the QOL of Family Caregivers of Palliative Care Patients. Annual Meeting of the International Society for Quality of Life Research. Amsterdam, November 7–10, 2001. *Qual Life Res* 2001; **10**: 231.

61 Edwards B, Ung L. Quality of life instruments for caregivers of patients with cancer. *Cancer Nurs* 2002; **25**: 342–9.

62 Salek S, Pratheepawanit N, Finaly I, Luscombe D. The use of quality-of-life instruments in palliative care. *Eur J Palliat Care* 2002; **9**: 52–6.

63 Salek Sam. Compendium of Quality of Life Instruments 2004; **6** Euromed Communications Ltd.UK.,; e-mail: subs@ euromed.uk.com

64 MAPI Research Trust. www.mapi-research.fr ProQOLID. www.mapi-research.fr/t_03_serv_qoli.htm (accessed April 23, 2006).

● 65 McMillan SC, Mahon M. Measuring quality of life in hospice patients using a newly developed Hospice Quality of Life Index. *Qual Life Res* 1994; **3**: 437–47.

● 66 Hearn J, Higginson IJ. Development and validation of a core outcome measure for palliative care: The palliative care outcome scale. *Qual Health Care* 1999; **8**: 219–27.

67 Higginson I, Donaldson N. Relationship between three palliative care outcome scales. *Health Qual Life Outcomes* 2004; **2**: 68.

● 68 Portenoy RK, Thaler HT, Kornblith AB, *et al.* The Memorial Symptom Assessment Scale: An instrument for the evaluation of symptom prevalence, characteristics, and distress. *Eur J Cancer* 1994; **30A**: 1226–36.

69 Steinhauser KE, Clipp EC, Tulsky JA. Evolution in measuring the quality of dying. *J Palliat Med* 2002; **5**: 407–14.

● 70 Steinhauser KE, Bosworth HB, Clipp EC, *et al.* Initial assessment of a new instrument to measure quality of life at the end of life. *J Palliat Med* 2002; **6**: 829–41.

● 71 Bruera E, Kuehn N, Miller MJ, *et al.* The Edmonton Symptom Assessment System (ESAS): A simple method for the assessment of palliative care patients. *J. Palliat Care* 1991; **7**: 6–9.

● 72 Weitzner MA, Jacobsen PB, Wagner H Jr, *et al.* The Caregiver Quality of Life Index-Cancer (CQOLC) scale: Development and validation of an instrument to measure quality of life of the family caregiver of patients with cancer. *Qual Life Res* 1999; **8**: 55–63.

73 McMillan SC, Mahon M. The impact of hospice services on the quality of life primary caregivers. *Oncol Nurs Forum* 1994; **21**: 1189–95.

74 Randall CJ, Donald PL, Engelburg RA, *et al.* A measure of the quality of dying and death: Initial validation using after-death interviews with family members. *J Pain Symptom Manage* 2002; **24**: 17–31.

PART 8

Pain

42

Pathophysiology of chronic pain

SEBASTIANO MERCADANTE

INTRODUCTION

Pain is a normal consequence of tissue injury or of intense stimuli that produce tissue injury. Peripheral nerves transmit this information from the body tissues to the spinal cord, from where neurons relay the information to the brain and simultaneously trigger reflexes that withdraw the body part involved in the painful stimulus. The higher brain centers organize the appropriate behaviors that restore health by protecting and facilitating healing of the damaged body site. Pain tends to diminish as healing progresses. Thus in healthy individuals, pain serves highly adaptive, survival-oriented purposes. However, pain can occur as a consequence of dysfunction of the peripheral or central nervous system, or prolonged and intense stimuli from damaged tissues. The differences between acute and chronic pain include peripheral responses of the organism and central nervous system modifications induced by the chronic afferent volley of nociceptor activity.[1]

The clinical picture of cancer pain varies depending on the pathophysiological mechanism, which further depends on the characteristics and progression of disease, and the preferential sites of metastases. Traditionally, pain related to malignant disease has been classified as nociceptive-inflammatory (somatic and visceral) and neuropathic. Somatic and visceral pains involve direct activation of nociceptors, and these pains are often a complication of infiltration of tissue by tumor or tissue injury as a consequence of oncological treatments. Neuropathic pain may be a complication of injury to the peripheral or central nervous system. This type of pain is often poorly tolerated and difficult to control. In the chronic pain situation that occurs following injury, infection, or inflammation of peripheral nerves, sensory processing in the affected body region is grossly abnormal. Environmental stimuli that would normally not result in the sensation of pain now do so, and painful stimuli elicit exaggerated perceptions of pain. Finally, pain is frequently spontaneous, that is, no stimulus can be identified to account for the pain.

Although nociceptive and neuropathic pains depend on separate peripheral mechanisms, they are both significantly influenced by changes in central nervous system function. It is now clear that cancer pain is a more complex entity, particularly regarding the response to analgesics, where numerous factors play a role. However, it remains unclear whether cancer pain is a unique type of pain or merely a subtype of inflammatory or neuropathic pain, as in cancer pain models there are changes in transmitters commonly produced in either neuropathic or inflammatory pain states. In contrast with inflammatory and neuropathic animal models, in a model of cancer pain no detectable changes were found in substance P, calcitonin gene-related peptide, and other peptides in either primary afferent neurons or the spinal cord. The greatest change observed in the spinal cord in response to cancer pain was a massive astrogliosis without neuronal loss, an increase in the neuronal expression of c-*fos*, and an increase in the number of dynorphin-immunoreactive neurons in the spinal cord ipsilateral to the limb with cancer.[2] Thus, the classical distinction may be of value only from an educational point of view.

PHYSIOPATHOLOGY OF NOCICEPTIVE PAIN

No specific histological structure acts as a nociceptive receptor. Primary afferent sensory neurons are the gateway by which sensory information from peripheral tissues is transmitted. Aδ and C nociceptors have been clearly identified in fibers innervating somatic structures, but not in the viscera where the situation is even more complicated. In cutaneous tissue thermal, mechanical, and chemical stimuli that induce tissue damage activate unmyelinated polymodal transducers attached to Aδ and C fibers. Nearly all large-diameter myelinated A and B fibers normally conduct non-noxious stimuli. In contrast, most small-diameter sensory fibers (unmyelinated C fibers and finely myelinated Aδ fibers) are specialized sensory neurons, the main function of which is to detect and convert environmental stimuli, chemical or physical, into electrochemical signals that are transmitted to the central nervous system. As the intensity of the stimulus increases high-threshold receptors are involved. Various chemicals are released into damaged tissue cells. Sustained stimuli or damage to the nerve can alter the profile of several peptides such as substance P contained within primary afferents. Substance P is able to induce the production of nitric oxide, a vasodilator, and the degranulation of mast cells with further vasodilation and subsequent extravasation and release of bradykinin. Bradykinin is a powerful algogenic substance which also sensitizes nociceptors by means of prostaglandin E_2. Other factors, such as cytokines, are released after tissue damage under the influence of bradykinin. These substances have an important role in the inflammatory process. Although prostaglandins are weak algogens, they have a major role in the sensitization of nociceptors to other substances. The concerted effects of these mediators at the site of tissue damage underlie peripheral hyperalgesia, which accounts for much of the peripheral sensitization of nociceptors.[1]

Thus, a repeated and intense stimulus induces the release of several inflammatory mediators which reduce the threshold for activation, increase the response to a given stimulus, or induce the appearance of spontaneous activity. This sensitization of nociceptors is responsible for some features of hyperalgesia. Many inactive receptors may become excitable in conditions of inflammation and are recruited to amplify the stimuli in these circumstances. Sensory neurons may change their phenotype. Substance P, for example, binds and activates the neurokinin-1 receptor which is expressed by a subset of spinal cord neurons. Of interest, inflammation is able to unmask opioid receptors peripherally. Primary hyperalgesia involves increased sensitivity to noxious stimulation at the site of the injury and is mediated by peripheral mechanisms, whereas secondary hyperalgesia extends beyond the site of the injury and is related to central activity or sensitization. This latter is characterized by prolonged excitation of dorsal horn cells, resulting in an expansion of receptive fields of dorsal horn neurons. As a consequence of such sensitization the expression of c-*fos* in the superficial dorsal horn increases. Peripheral nerve injury leads to the abnormal expression of receptors and channels that may result in ectopic discharges from neurons.

After injury to somatic, visceral, and neural structures, there may be an alteration in the response of the autonomic nervous system, which may react by novel sprouting of sympathetic efferents and formation of rings around dorsal root ganglia. Central neural mechanisms are also involved, leading to a constellation of peripheral vasomotor and sudomotor changes.[3] Immune system cells, including macrophages, neutrophils, and T cells, either in the tumor mass or produced as a reaction, sensitize or directly excite primary afferent neurons. Local acidosis produced by cancer cells can activate or express further nociceptors. Moreover, tumor necrosis factors and inflammatory cells are able to express opioid receptors, which may influence the response to opioids due to initial sequestration first, and then by release of nitric oxide, known as hyperalgesic agent (see below).[4]

VISCERAL PAIN

The viscera have a complex peripheral nervous system, and different neurophysiological understandings of visceral pain have been reported. Unlike their cutaneous counterparts, visceral nociceptors do not appear to be a simple acute warning system. Many viscera are innervated by receptors that do not evoke conscious perception. Visceral nociceptors, however, have a wide range of responses, and may be activated in the presence of inflammation or tissue injury. Therefore, visceral afferents are considered polymodal, providing excitatory responses to different stimuli, including inflammation, stretching, and distension. Two distinct classes of nociceptive sensory receptors that innervate internal organs have been proposed:

- high-threshold receptors – mostly mechanical, activated by stimuli within the noxious range
- low-threshold receptors – activated in the range of stimulation intensity from innocuous to noxious.

According to this theory, high-threshold receptors contribute to the peripheral encoding of noxious events in the viscera. Other prolonged and intense stimuli, such as hypoxia or tissue inflammation, result in the sensitization of these receptors and bring into play previously silent receptors, normally unresponsive to innocuous stimuli. The activity of afferents and the excitability of dorsal horn neurons are increased with repeated or persistent stimuli due to a process of sensibilization of afferents, which occurs secondary to local release of chemical substances in damaged or ischemic tissues. A critical level of preceding activity in the afferents is required to induce facilitation of dorsal horn neuronal responses via central mechanisms.[5]

Neurons that transmit visceral sensory information to the spinal cord have cell bodies that reside in the dorsal root ganglia. These primary afferents travel through the paravertebral ganglia and the prevertebral ganglia and have sensory endings in the viscera themselves. These afferents occur in conjunction with motor fibers of parasympathetic and sympathetic nervous system. Most visceral afferents have relatively slow conduction velocities.

Visceral pain tends to be diffuse because of the absence of a separate visceral sensory pathway and a low proportion of visceral afferent nerve fibers compared with those of somatic origin. Thus, neurological mechanisms of visceral pain differ from those involved in somatic pain. The nature of referred pain is not clearly defined. Some spinal neurons are involved in the localization of pain and project to the brain, whereas another group of neurons has short ascending projections with collaterals into multiple spinal segments. The activation of visceral efferents should lead to changes in the excitability of multiple spinal units, including those responsible for somatic nociceptive sensory pathways, or direct activation of neurons receiving both visceral and somatic inputs. Alternatively, the brain may misinterpret activity in the viscerosomatic neurons. Convergent receptive fields are generally described as multidermatomal, centered in the dermatome corresponding to the spinal segment stimulated, and are significantly larger than the receptive fields of spinal neurons receiving only somatic input.[6,7] These observations explain why visceral pain is difficult to localize and is often referred to other areas of the body. Pain originating from any viscus cannot be easily differentiated from pain originating in another viscus, although some visceral pains are associated with specific etiologies, such as in the case of pancreatic pain or peptic ulcer pain.

Mechanic stimuli, such as torsion or traction of mesentery, distension of hollow organs, stretch of serosal and mucosal surfaces, and compression of some organs, produce pain in humans. These conditions are frequently observed in cancer patients with abdominal diseases and intraperitoneal masses. Human studies have revealed that pain is produced when the intraluminal pressure of hollow organs is maintained above certain pressure thresholds. Obstruction or inflammation within the biliary tract or pancreatic duct induces pain directly related to the increased intraluminal pressure with consequent inflammation, and release of pain-producing substances. Capsular stretch of liver due to cancer growth produces pain. Distension or traction on the gallbladder leads to deep epigastric pain, inspiratory distress, and vomiting. Spontaneous spasm of the sphincter of Oddi or that induced by morphine on the one hand leads to increases in pain sensation, resulting in a paradoxical opioid-induced pain. On the other hand, morphine and other opioids may counterbalance this effect, increasing the pressure threshold necessary to produce the sensation of pain due to distension of the biliary system.

Renal colic is usually secondary to ureteral obstruction and subsequent distension of the ureter and renal pelvis. This may be seen in circumstances in which an abdominal–pelvic mass compresses or invades the ureters, as often occurs in gynecological cancers. Reports of pain appear to be directly related to the compression of the urinary bladder. Bladder distension may also activate mechanisms related to the phenomenon of counter-irritation. Better localization of stimulus occurs when the disease extends to a somatically innervated structure such as the parietal peritoneum. Thus initially, visceral pain is poorly localized and dull because of the wide divergence of visceral afferents in the spinal cord. Poorly localized visceral pain becomes localized as visceral afferent input increases due to spinal facilitation or activation of visceral nociceptors. The greatest localization occurs when somatic structures such as the peritoneum become involved.

CHRONIC PAIN AND PLASTIC CHANGES OF THE CENTRAL NERVOUS SYSTEM

Chronic pain, regardless the initial etiology, produces important changes in the central nervous system. A prolonged stimulus from the periphery through either stimulation of nociceptors or ectopic firing after neural damage leads to repetitive activation of C fibers. This results in augmentation of activity in dorsal horn wide dynamic range neurons and a strong increase in the magnitude of the responses evoked by subsequent stimuli. Thus, increased input from injured neurons, ectopic nerve action potentials, and sensitization of nociceptors by the peripheral nerves produce tonic input to the spinal cord.

Central sensitization and a wind-up phenomenon at the spinal and supraspinal levels have been described to explain the pathophysiological background of chronic pain conditions due to persistent peripheral stimuli or nerve injury.[8] The existence of peripheral hyperalgesia has a bearing on the induction of central hypersensitivity in the spinal cord. The enhanced release of substance P and other neurokinins may provide the mechanisms by which the N-methyl-D-aspartate (NMDA) receptor for the excitatory amino acids becomes more easily activated. These transmitters cooperate to activate spinal cord neurons. The release of peptides such as substance P into the spinal cord on afferent stimulation removes the magnesium block of the channel of the NMDA receptor and thus allows glutamate to activate the NMDA receptor in the range of persistent pain states.[1] The ion channel for the NMDA receptor allows vast amounts of calcium to enter into the neurons, resulting in an amplification of the response underlying central hyperalgesia. The repetition of a constant intensity C fiber stimulus induces the phenomenon of wind-up, that is, the switch from a low level of pain-related activity to a high level without any change in the inputs arriving from the peripheral nerves. This results in prolongation and amplification of nociceptive activity even after the cessation of the peripheral input.

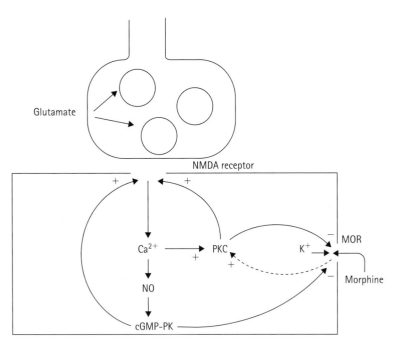

Figure 42.1 *Activation of N-methyl-D-aspartate (NMDA) receptors increases intracellular Ca²⁺ concentration and subsequent intracellular activation of protein kinase C (PKC) and nitric oxide (NO). Substrate phosphorylation by PKC or NO-mediated protein kinase may produce enhanced activity of glutamate receptor–Ca²⁺ complex, with development of hyperactive states. PKC and NO-mediated protein kinase actions may produce uncoupling of G-protein with mu opioid receptor (MOR), so reducing morphine anti-nociception.*

The activation of such receptors is involved in the development and maintenance of injury-induced central hyperactive states by initiating a variety of intracellular processes. These principally consist of an increase in intracellular calcium concentration, activation of protein kinase C (PKC) and the calcium–calmodulin-mediated production of nitric oxide, and, in a complex manner, lead to neuronal excitability. It has been suggested that feedback by nitric oxide increases the release of C fiber transmitters, further enhancing pain transmission. Protein kinase C translocation and nitric oxide production may enhance postsynaptic neuronal excitability, leading to the development of hyperactive states. Furthermore, PKC and nitric oxide may activate presynaptic NMDA receptors localized on primary afferent fibers by removing the magnesium blockade of the NMDA receptor. In so doing even small amounts of excitatory amino acid ligands may allow the opening of calcium channels, with further activation of a second pool of PKC (Fig. 42.1). Increases in intracellular calcium and activation of PKC also result in c-*fos* expression in postsynaptic dorsal horn neurons as well as in supraspinal areas. This is considered to be a third messenger, probably involved in encoding a variety of cellular responses that are responsible for the neural changes associated with hyperalgesia.[9] This has been demonstrated by similar time courses of c-*fos* expression and the development of hyperalgesia.[10] Whereas the entry of calcium can also activate phospholipases and lead to the spinal production of prostanoids, persistent activation of excitatory amino acid receptors within the spinal cord may contribute to central hyperexcitability. This is because irreversible morphological changes may occur with loss of function of spinal cord inhibitory interneurons. These excitotoxic processes may result in disinhibition phenomena, reinforcing the central hyperactivity state.[11]

Peripheral nerve injury also results in a number of dorsal horn effects, such as changes in the distribution and density of α-amino-3-hydroxy-5-methyl-4-isoxazole propionic acid receptors (better known as AMPA), releases of neurotrophins, sprouting of central terminals, and loss of inhibitory neurons containing γ-aminobutyric acid.[3] Mechanisms of normal synaptic transmission and intense and prolonged activation are shown in Figures 42.2 and 42.3. Similar mechanisms are presumably operating at the supraspinal level, although available data are less clear. Pain activates brain structures, such as the periaqueductal gray matter of the midbrain (which is involved in blood pressure regulation, respiration, vasomotor control and metabolic homeostasis) and the thalamus (which is a major relay in the transmission of nociceptive information). Prolonged activation of these structures can have a strong impact on psychological function, also inducing complex cognitive responses.

DESCENDING MODULATION OF NOCICEPTION

Brainstem descending pathways constitute a major mechanism for modulating nociceptive transmission at the spinal level. The rostral ventromedial medulla (RVM) includes the nucleus raphe magnus and adjacent lateral reticular formation. A biphasic descending modulation of nociception has been postulated, through the activation of facilitation and inhibition of nociceptive processes, consequent to activation of two types of cell group, 'on-cell' and 'off-cell', respectively. Descending pathways are activated by tissue injury to counteract the cascade of events that ultimately contribute to the development of inflammatory hyperalgesia. Opioidergic

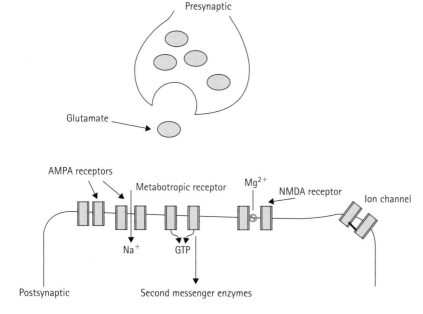

Figure 42.2 *Normal synaptic transmission: presynaptic activation produces exocytosis of glutamate, which binds to postsynaptic receptors: (i) AMPA receptors, leading to opening of Na^+ and K^+ channels, and resulting in depolarization; (ii) metabotropic receptors, causing the binding of GTP to G-proteins and activation of second messengers (protein kinase C, adenyl cyclase); and (iii) NMDA receptors, potentially opening ion channels. Mg^{2+} blocks the ion flux.*

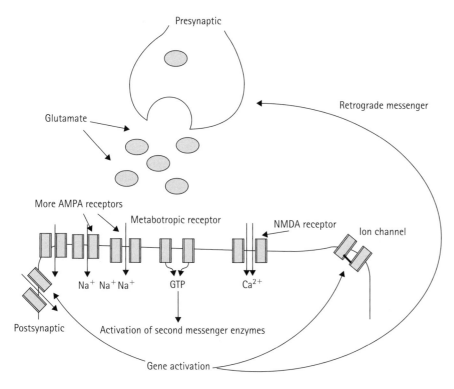

Figure 42.3 *Intense and prolonged activation causes abnormal release of glutamate. More AMPA receptors are activated, limiting the Mg^{2+} block on NMDA receptors. Ca^{2+} ions flow through these channels, interacting with the second messenger enzymes, resulting in more availability of AMPA receptors, as consequence of gene activation. Phosphorylation of ion channels makes the cell more excitable. Retrograde messengers also act on presynaptic nerve terminals causing the release of more glutamate.*

circuits are involved in descending inhibition of nociception, increasing the activity of the antinociception-inhibiting 'off-cells', and decreasing the activity of the nociceptive-facilitating 'on-cells' of the RVM. Studies suggest that descending serotonergic and noradrenergic pathways differently suppress the responses of spinal neurons.[12] The organization and functional significance of the facilitatory network is less known and is possibly involved in pro-nociceptive mechanisms. For example, prolonged administration of opioids induces neuroplastic changes resulting in enhanced ability of

cholecystokinin (CCK) to excite facilitatory pathways from the RVM, and/or upregulation of dynorphin levels, evoking release of excitatory transmitters from primary afferents (see below).[13] Ventrolateral periaqueductal gray matter could be one of the sites where the repeated administration of opioids induces opioid tolerance. There is evidence that endogenous or exogenous opioids lead to an enhancement of CCK activity, which in turn attenuates the antinociceptive effect of opioids and may be one of the mechanisms responsible for opioid tolerance.[14] The dynamic plasticity of descending pathways may render the system vulnerable and lead to pathological consequences.

CHRONIC PAIN STATES AND OPIOID ACTIVITY

Opioids inhibit or block excitation of dorsal horn cells by depressing firing through both presynaptic and postsynaptic inhibitory effects in the spinal cord.[15] The physiological targets of both exogenous and endogenous opioids are receptors coupled to G-proteins: μ, δ, and κ receptors. The acute effects of the opioids include inhibition of cAMP formation, activation of inward K^+ channels, and inhibition of voltage-gated Ca^{2+} channels. These lead to presynaptic hyperpolarization, inhibition of excitatory neurotransmitter release, and activation of descending antinociceptive pathways.[16] Opioid receptors undergo adaptations such as desensitization, downregulation, and internalization in response to agonist treatment. Molecular processes underlying desensitization are thought to include rapid uncoupling of the receptor from its G-protein by phosphorylation of the receptor or binding of accessory proteins, such as β-arrestin. Receptor internalization has been implicated in the process of dephosphorylation and the resensitization recycle of the receptor. After prolonged treatment loss of receptor protein, named downregulation, may occur, leading to increased degradation or decreased synthesis of the receptor. Opioids differ in their capability of inducing such molecular events.

Repeated administration of opioids produces a decrease in analgesia, an effect termed tolerance. In opioid tolerance, a functional decoupling of opioid receptors occurs by cellular mechanisms regulated by second messengers, in addition to downregulation of opioid receptors and adaptive behavioral changes.[17] Loss of opioid presynaptic receptors as a result of a peripheral nerve injury has been reported at the level of the dorsal horns. However clinically, the degree and the time course of tolerance are influenced by several factors, including drugs, dosing schedules, and routes of administration.[18]

Several factors common to neuropathic pain and tolerance have been found, although some central changes at spinal cord level typically present in neuropathic pain states are not found with chronic exposure to morphine. Activation of spinal cord NMDA receptors, PKC activation, and nitric oxide production are biochemical steps capable equally of leading to a state of hyperalgesia or the development of morphine tolerance.[10,15] Substrate phosphorylation by PKC and nitric oxide may result either in enduring enhancement of synaptic activity at spinal cord level[19] and decreasing the μ-receptor activity, uncoupling of G-protein with the μ receptor or facilitating its desensibilization.[17,20] Thus, the reduction of morphine analgesia induced by nerve injury may share a mechanism similar to that of morphine tolerance. Reduction of morphine antinociception occurs after hyperalgesia induced by nerve injury in the absence of daily exposure to morphine,[10] as nerve injury would produce a reduction of morphine nociception prior to exposure to morphine itself.

In other terms, it is possible that a sort of tolerance and/or hyperalgesia develops before exposure to morphine and a neuropathic pain state may be equivalent to that of the development of morphine tolerance or facilitating hyperalgesia with a consequent pro-nociceptive effect.[10,21] This is consistent with the clinical observation of increased opioid requirements in patients with neuropathic pain.[22,23] However, these neuroplastic changes may be distinct and divergent intracellular events may take place, as the expression of hyperalgesia is not necessarily associated with the expression of tolerance and vice versa. A single dose of MK-801, an inhibitor of NMDA receptors, has been shown to reduce hyperalgesia but not to enhance morphine antinociception.[10,17]

Prolonged opioid treatment not only results in a loss of opioid antinociceptive efficacy but also leads to activation of a pro-nociceptive system characterized by a reduction of nociceptive threshold.[24] It has been suggested that the concurrent expression of hyperalgesia during chronic opioid administration counteracts antinociception, producing an impression of tolerance due to compensatory neuronal hyperactivity. Descending facilitation at RVM level has been reported. This pro-nociceptive activity has been found to be associated with increases in expression of dynorphin in the spinal dorsal horn, which promotes the release of excitatory transmitters from primary afferent neurons.[25]

Other aspects of pain modulation have been reported. The reduction in receptor function is hypothesized to contribute to opioid tolerance. Opioid receptor are desensitized on the cell surface through a phosphorylation process. On the other hand, receptor internalization is now believed to contribute to resensitization through a dephosphorylation during endosomal stages.[26] An inverse relation between tolerance liability and μ-opioid receptor endocytosis has been shown. On the other hand the loss of response to opioid agonists upon long-term treatment seems to be the result of two partially overlapping processes: the gradual loss of inhibitory opioid signal transduction and an increase in excitatory signaling.[27] Chronic opioid agonist treatment simultaneously desensitizes the inhibitory effects of the opioids and augments the stimulatory signaling, possibly through a time-dependent alteration of the specificity of opioid–G-protein coupling. The supersensitivity of neurons to the excitatory effects of opioids seems to be to a GM1-ganglioside–mediated conversion of the opioid receptors from an inhibitory (Gi coupled) to an excitatory (Gs coupled) mode.[28] These changes cause a compensatory increase in cellular cAMP formation, due to an increased activity of PKC. This superactivation is manifested by an apparent desensitization of the inhibitory opioid signaling. Removal of the agonist unmasks an underlying sensitization of cAMP formation to stimulatory inputs. Clinically, this may occur in circumstances where, for different pharmacokinetic reasons, opioid concentrations significantly decrease at the receptor site, producing a sort of mini-withdrawal.

As it becomes clear that chronic pain, particularly cancer pain, is able to specifically modify the response of the central nervous system, recent data indicate a close relation between cancer disease and its metabolic and immunological consequences, and plastic changes of the central nervous system associated with the concomitant chronic administration of opioids, which require better knowledge of molecular events underlying such mechanisms. An integrated approach taking into account information from both experimental work and the bedside is advised.

Key learning points

- The clinical picture of cancer pain varies depending on the pathophysiological mechanism, which further depends on the characteristics and progression of disease, and the preferential sites of metastases. Although pain related to malignant disease can be classified as nociceptive-inflammatory and neuropathic, they are both significantly influenced by changes in central nervous system function.

- It is now clear that cancer pain is a more complex entity, particularly regarding the response to analgesics, where numerous factors play a role.

- Central sensitization and a wind-up phenomenon at the spinal and supraspinal level have been described to explain the pathophysiological background of chronic pain conditions.

- Brainstem descending pathways constitute a major mechanism for modulating nociceptive transmission at the spinal level. The dynamic plasticity of descending pathways may render the system vulnerable and lead to pathological consequences.

- Opioids produce inhibition or block excitation of dorsal horn cells within the spinal cord. Repeated administration of opioids produces a decrease in analgesia, an effect termed tolerance.

- There are several common factors in neuropathic pain and tolerance.

- Prolonged opioid treatment not only results in a loss of opioid antinociceptive efficacy, but also leads to activation of a pro-nociceptive system characterized by a reduction of nociceptive threshold.

REFERENCES

◆ 1 Besson JM. The neurobiology of pain. *Lancet* 1999; **353**: 1610–15.

● 2 Honorè P, Rogers SD, Schwei MJ, *et al.* Murine models of inflammatory, neuropathic and cancer pain each generates a unique set of neurochemical changes in the spinal cord and sensory neurons. *Neuroscience* 2000; **98**: 585–98.

◆ 3 Siddall PJ, Cousins MJ. Persistent pain as a disease entity: implications for clinical management. *Anesth Analg* 2004; **99**: 510–20.

◆ 4 Friedman R. Pain at the cellular level: the role of the cytokine tumor necrosis factor-a. *Reg Anesth Pain Med* 2000; **25**: 110–12.

◆ 5 Ness TJ, Gebhart GF. Visceral pain: a review of experimental studies. *Pain* 1990; **41**: 167–234.

◆ 6 Cervero F, Laird JMA. Visceral pain. *Lancet* 1999; **353**: 2145–8.

◆ 7 Giamberardino MA. Recent and forgotten aspects of visceral pain. *Eur J Pain* 1999; **3**: 77–92.

● 8 Woolf CJ, Thompson SW. The induction and maintenance of central sensitization is dependent on N-methyl-D-aspartic acid receptor activation: implications for the treatment of post-injury pain hypersensitivity states. *Pain* 1991; **44**: 293–9.

◆ 9 Coderre TJ, Katz J, Vaccarino AL, Melzack R. Contribution of central neuroplasticity to pathological pain: review of clinical and experimental evidence. *Pain* 1993; **52**: 259–85.

● 10 Mao J, Price D, Mayer DJ. Experimental mononeuropathy reduces the antinociceptive effects of morphine: implications for common intracellular mechanisms involved in morphine tolerance and neuropathic pain. *Pain* 1995; **61**: 353–64.

◆ 11 Dubner R. Neuronal plasticity and pain following peripheral tissue inflammation and nerve injury. In: Bond MR, Charlton JE, Woolf CJ, eds. *Pain Research and Clinical Management, Vol. 4, Proceedings of the VIth World Congress on Pain.* Amsterdam: Elsevier, 1991: 263–76.

◆ 12 Ren K, Zhuo M, Willis W. Multiplicity and plasticity of descending modulation of nociception: implications for persistent pain. In: Devor M, Rowbotham M, Wiesenfeld-Hallin Z, eds. *Proceedings of the 9th World Congress on Pain.* Seattle: IASP Press, 2000: 387–400.

◆ 13 Ossipov M, Lai J, Vanderah T, Porreca F. Induction of pain facilitation by sustained opioid exposure: relationship to opioid antinociceptive tolerance. *Life Sci* 2003; **73**: 783–800.

◆ 14 Tortorici V, Nogueira L, Salas R, Vanegas H. Involvement of local cholecystokinin in the tolerance induced by morphine microinjections into the periaqueductal gray of rats. *Pain* 2003; **102**: 9–16.

● 15 Mayer DJ, Mao J, Price DD. The development of morphine tolerance and dependence is associated with translocation of protein kinase C. *Pain* 1995; **61**: 365–74.

◆ 16 Varga EV, Yamamura Hi, Rubenzik, *et al.* Molecular mechanisms of excitatory signaling upon chronic opioid agonist treatment. *Life Sci* 2003; **74**: 299–311.

● 17 Trujillo KA, Akil H. Inhibition of morphine tolerance and dependence by the NMDA receptor antagonist MK-801. *Science* 1991; **251**: 85–7.

● 18 Mercadante S, Portenoy RK. Opioid poorly responsive cancer pain. Part 2. Basic mechanisms that could shift dose-response for analgesia. *J Pain Symptom Manage* 2001; **21**: 255–64.

● 19 Chen L, Huang LYM. Protein kinase C reduces Mg^{2+} block of NMDA-receptor channels as a mechanism of modulation. *Nature* 1992; **356**: 521–3.

◆ 20 Collin E, Cesselin F. Neurobiological mechanisms of opioid tolerance and dependence. *Clin Pharmacol* 1991; **14**: 465–88.

◆ 21 Basbaum AI. Insights into the development of opioid tolerance. *Pain* 1995; **61**: 349–52.

● 22 Portenoy RK, Foley KM, Inturrisi CE. The nature of opioid responsiveness and its implications for neuropathic pain: new

hypothesis derived from studies of opioid infusions. *Pain* 1990;
43: 273–86.

23 Mercadante S, Dardanoni G, Salvaggio L, *et al.* Monitoring of
opioid therapy in advanced cancer patients. *J Pain Symptom
Manage* 1997; **13**: 204–12.

◆ 24 Mao J. Opioid-induced abnormal pain sensitivity: implications
in clinical opioid therapy. *Pain* 2002; **100**: 213–17.

◆ 25 Vanderah TW, Ossipov MH, Lai J, *et al.* Mechanisms of opioid-
induced pain and antinociceptive tolerance: descending
facilitation and spinal dynorphin. *Pain* 2001; **92**: 5–9.

● 26 He L, Fong J, von Zastrow M, Whistler JL. Regulation of opioid
receptor trafficking and morphine tolerance by receptor
oligomerization. *Cell* 2002; **25**: 271–82.

◆ 27 Ueda H, Inoue M, Mizuno K. New approaches to study the
development of morphine tolerance and dependence. *Life Sci*
2003; **74**: 313–20.

● 28 Crain SM, Shen KF. Antagonists of excitatory opioid receptor
functions enhance morphine's analgesic potency and
attenuate opioid tolerance/dependence liability. *Pain* 2000;
84: 121–31.

43

Causes and mechanisms of pain in palliative care patients

SURESH K REDDY

INTRODUCTION

Pain due to cancer is one of the most common symptoms experienced by palliative care patients, as shown by many studies in this patient population.[1,2,3*] The consequences of undertreatment of pain are daunting, yet pain is underdiagnosed and undertreated for many reasons.[4*,5*] One of the main reasons for undertreatment of pain in patients with cancer continues to be a lack of appropriate pain assessment.[6*,7*] In cancer, pain is predominantly caused by the tumor and its consequences. Other reasons include treatment side effects and coexisting pain conditions[3,8] (Box 43.1). In noncancer situations pain may result from chronic degenerative disorders of the spine and joints:[9*10*,11*] central pain because of spinal cord injury, and neuropathic pain due to metabolic, infective and other causes[12,*13*,14*] (Box 43.2).

Box 43.1 Common clinical pain syndromes and their causes

Tumor pain

- Bone pain due to metastasis (somatic pain) from breast, prostate, and other cancers

- Plexopathy pain (neuropathic pain) due to Pancoast's tumor/pelvic tumor

- Abdominal pain (visceral pain) due to pancreatic cancer and liver metastasis

- Chest wall pain due to mesothelioma (somatic and neuropathic pain)

Cancer treatment pain

- Postchemotherapy pain syndromes

- Peripheral neuropathy due to cisplatin and paclitaxel

Post-irradiation pain syndromes

- Chronic throat pain due to radiation-induced mucositis

- Chronic abdominal pain due to radiation-induced enteritis in fistulas

- Radiation-induced plexopathy pain

Postsurgical pain syndromes

- Postmastectomy pain syndrome

- Postradical neck dissection pain syndrome

- Phantom limb pain syndrome

Noncancer pain

- Chronic low back pain due to degenerative process in the spine

- Pain secondary to osteoarthritis and rheumatoid arthritis

- Migraine headaches

Box 43.2 Noncancer pain syndromes

Headache

- Migraine
- Tension-type headache
- Cluster headache
- Miscellaneous

Facial pain

- Trigeminal neuralgia
- Temporomandibular joint pain
- Glossopharyngeal neuralgia
- Postherpetic neuralgia (PHN)
- Myofascial pain syndromes

Neck pain

- Diskogenic radicular pain
- Whiplash injury pain syndrome
- Cervicogenic pain
- Facet joint pain syndrome

Thoracic pain syndromes

- Costochondritis
- Intercostal neuralgia
- PHN
- Facet joint pain syndrome
- Chronic shoulder pain: frozen shoulder; rotator cuff tear

Abdominal pain

- Chronic pancreatitis
- Chronic peptic ulcer disease
- Postcholecystectomy syndrome
- Crohn disease
- Irritable bowel syndrome

Pelvic pain

- Chronic interstitial cystitis
- Chronic testicular pain
- Chronic prostatitis pain
- Chronic pelvic pain from inflammatory pelvic disease
- Endometriosis-related pain syndromes

Low back and lower extremity pain

- Central pain
- Lumbosacral spine disease: myofascial; diskogenic; osteoporotic; facet joint pain syndrome
- Peripheral vascular disease and ischemic pain syndrome
- Dorsal tunnel syndrome
- Complex regional pain syndrome
- Phantom limb pain

Medical diseases causing pain

- Chronic fatigue syndrome
- Sickle cell disease
- Peripheral neuropathy pain (e.g. diabetes)
- Rheumatoid arthritis, multiple sclerosis, osteoarthritis

HIV/AIDS pain syndromes

- Headache (e.g. cryptococcal meningitis)
- Oral cavity pain secondary to candidiasis, herpes simplex, or Kaposi sarcoma
- Chest pain secondary to candidal esophagitis
- Chronic abdominal pain from infections such as cryptosporidiosis, cytomegalovirus, cholecystitis, pancreatitis
- Pain syndromes related to Kaposi sarcoma
- Neuropathic pain syndromes (e.g. predominantly sensory neuropathy, myelopathy, radicular pain from Guillain–Barré syndrome)

Pain results from the activation of nociceptors by a variety of chemical mediators released from damaged cells. The mediators include potassium, serotonin, bradykinin, and histamine, and usually associated with the redness and swelling of inflammation. In addition, cells may be sensitized by other substances such prostaglandins, leukotrienes, and substance P. Sensitization can extend to areas away from the original damage, resulting in hypersensitivity of the area.

Cancer pain can occur after activation of peripheral nociceptors (somatic and visceral 'nociceptive' pain) or by direct injury to peripheral or central nervous structures (neuropathic or 'deafferentation' pain). In addition, both nociceptive and neuropathic pain may be modified by involvement of the sympathetic nervous system, resulting in sympathetically maintained pain (SMP) or complex regional pain syndrome type 1 (CRPS). Each of these painful states has somewhat unique clinical characteristics which may aid in its identification and directed treatment. A key step, therefore, in the evaluation of a cancer patient with pain, is to elicit a careful history of the quality, nature, and location of perceived pain, as the descriptors may provide valuable clues to the etiology of the complaint.

Somatic pain results from involvement of bone and muscle structures. Metastatic bone disease is the most common pain syndrome in patients with cancer. Myelinated and unmyelinated afferent fibers are present in bone, and their density is greatest in the periosteum. Prostaglandins play a multifactorial role in the etiology of bone pain. Prostaglandin concentrations are increased at sites of bone metastasis.[15*] In addition, prostaglandins are now known to mediate osteolytic and osteoclastic metastatic bone changes. Prostaglandin E_2 is known to sensitize nociceptors and produce hyperalgesia. These observations have resulted in steroidal and nonsteroidal anti-inflammatory drugs (NSAIDs) as important therapy for metastatic bone pain. Reports suggest that NSAIDs are uniquely effective.[16**]

Visceral pain is also common in patients with cancer, and presumably results from stretching or distending or from the production of an inflammatory response and the release of analgesic substances in the vicinity of nociceptors. Visceral pain is commonly referred to cutaneous sites, which can mislead the examiner, particularly since those cutaneous sites may be tender to palpation. This property likely results from convergence of visceral and somatic afferent information onto common neuronal pools in the dorsal horn of the spinal cord.[17*] Neuropathic pain from neural injury such as brachial plexus infiltration by tumor is often severe. The pain is described as paroxysms of burning or electric-shocklike sensations which may result, at least in part, from spontaneous discharges in the peripheral and central nervous systems.

Somatic, visceral, and deafferentation pain may be modified by the sympathetic nervous system. Sympathetically maintained pain is often suspected when pain is severe in intensity (even after relatively trivial tissue insults) and described as burning in quality, with associated features of allodynia, hyperpathia, brawny edema, and osteoporosis.[18*] Several mechanisms involving both peripheral and central nervous systems have been postulated to explain SMP. For example, one peripheral mechanism may be the development of ephaptic connections at sites of tissue injury such that efferent sympathetic impulses produce activation of afferent nociceptive pathways. Others have postulated that traumatic injury to peripheral tissues may produce sensitization of spinal cord nociceptive neurons, which may then be secondarily activated by efferent sympathetic activity.

It is common for patients with cancer to present with mixtures of the pain types described above. Furthermore, the pattern of pain intensity is often not constant, but rather includes episodes of pain exacerbations on a background of continuous pain, called 'breakthrough' pain (see Chapter 54).[19*]

SPECIFIC PAIN SYNDROMES IN PATIENTS WITH CANCER

There are several specific pain syndromes that may present difficult diagnostic and therapeutic problems, of which the palliative care specialist needs to be aware of during the evaluation of the cancer patient with pain.[20*] The characteristic clinical features of these syndromes are summarized in Box 43.3 and discussed below. Please note that notable but short-lived pain syndromes, such as mucositis, that complicate chemotherapy and radiation therapy, and the acute pain associated with diagnostic and therapeutic procedures, such as bone marrow aspiration are not included in Box 43.3.

Box 43.3 Clinical characteristics of intractable pain syndromes

- Tumor-related infiltration of bone – acute and chronic nociceptive pain

- Skull-base metastasis – severe head pain (usually referred to vertex or occiput) with associated cranial nerve deficits. Bone scan and plain films of the skull may show normal findings

- Vertebral metastasis – significant risk of associated spinal cord compression. Of patients with back pain and vertebral body metastasis, 30 percent will eventually develop epidural spinal cord compression, and pain alone may precede root or spinal cord signs by many months

- Pelvis and long bones – risk of pathological fracture with weight-bearing activities; orthopedic consultation helpful

- Tumor-related infiltration of nerve – acute and chronic neuropathic pain

- Brachial/lumbosacral plexopathy – may occur by contiguous spread of tumor or by hematogenous dissemination; radiographic studies helpful to distinguish from radiation-induced plexopathy

- Spinal cord compression – neurological emergency requiring prompt treatment with corticosteroids, radiation therapy, and/or surgery

- Meningeal carcinomatosis – headache and meningeal signs. Causes significant pain in about 15 percent of patients

- Visceral tumor infiltration – acute and chronic visceral pain that is poorly localized and widely referred. Common examples include pancreatic carcinoma, liver metastasis, pleural effusion

- Therapy-related post-surgical pain – chronic pain that persists well beyond healing of the incision and may or may not be associated with recurrent disease

- After thoracotomy – may be associated with recurrent tumor or may occur as a chronic intercostals neuralgia

- After mastectomy – occurs in 5 percent of women; more common in women undergoing modified radical procedure with axillary dissection; intercostal brachioradial neuralgia is one cause

- After radical neck surgery – mechanisms unclear; chronic infection may play a role

- After amputation – stump pain and phantom phenomena are common; role of preventive analgesic and anesthetic therapies are under investigation

TUMOR INFILTRATION OF BONE

Pain from invasion of bone by either primary or metastatic tumor is the most common cause of pain in patients with cancer. Several important pain syndromes are often misdiagnosed because physicians are unfamiliar with the characteristic signs and symptoms, and plain X-rays of the involved areas may show normal findings.

The pathophysiology of metastatic bone pain is poorly understood. Although most patients with bone metastasis report pain, a large proportion of patients with radiographic evidence of disease deny pain. This has been best studied in breast cancer,[21*] but is also true in prostate cancer. Tumor growth in bone may produce pain by several mechanisms:

- Relatively rapid growth causing expansion of the marrow space and increased interosseal pressure (beyond 50 mmHg). In theory, this may activate mechanoreceptive nociceptors in bone. In addition, elevation or invasion of the periosteum may also activate nociceptors that innervate this structure.
- Weakening of the bone leading to fractures.
- Edema and inflammation associated with tumor growth in bone may liberate chemical mediators that activate nociceptors.
- Recent data regarding mechanisms of bone destruction emphasize that osteoclasts may be stimulated by a

number of humoral factors associated with tumors. For example, carcinomas may secrete prostaglandins,[15*] which would have the dual role of activating osteoclasts and sensitizing nociceptors. These observations have provided a rationale for the use of corticosteroids and NSAIDs for the management of metastatic bone pain.[22**]

Metastatic bone pain is often associated with neurological dysfunction because of the close anatomical relations between the brain and cranial nerves and the skull vault, and the spinal cord and its roots and the vertebral column. Therefore, characteristic clinical syndromes may be identified by the site of bony involvement, the coexistence of mechanical instability secondary to fractures, and neurological dysfunction caused by tumor infiltration of contiguous neurological structures. Bone metastasis to the hip and pelvis often produces local pain that is exacerbated by movement, especially when weight bearing. In addition to palliative radiotherapy, this type of 'incident pain' may require specific orthopedic interventions.

Spread of cancer to the vertebral bodies and calvarium, especially the base of the skull, often produces distinctive neurological syndromes. These are important to recognize early because prompt initiation of antitumor treatments, especially radiation, may avoid neurological impairment. For example, local and radicular back or neck pain is the predominant symptom in epidural spinal cord compression complicating vertebral body metastasis in these locations. Pain may be the only symptom of impending spinal cord compression, and often precedes motor weakness and bowel or bladder incontinence by days or weeks. The spinal cord is compromised by growth of the tumor in an anterior direction from the vertebral body. Irreversible spinal cord injury may occur when the vascular supply is compromised as a result of severe compression. Thoracic spine vertebral body metastases often produce bilateral radicular pain and sensory symptoms (a 'bandlike' squeezing sensation across the upper abdomen or chest) because of the close proximity of the thoracic nerve roots to the vertebral body. On the other hand, metastases in the cervical or lumbar spine may produce unilateral pain and sensory loss as the vertebral bodies are wider in these areas and lateral extension of the tumor may compress only one root at the time.

Skull metastasis

Spread of tumor to the calvarium may produce neurological symptoms by two mechanisms. Metastases to the skull vault which grow to compress the sagittal sinus may produce a syndrome of severe headache with associated papilledema and seizures caused by elevation in the intracranial pressure. If untreated, focal neurological deficits may occur secondary to venous infarction of the brain. The cause of metastatic sagittal sinus occlusion is usually obvious, and is easily confirmed by magnetic resonance imaging (MRI) of the brain. The gadolinium-enhanced MRI will not only demonstrate the tumor metastasis, but will also demonstrate the blood clot in the sagittal sinus. It is noteworthy that nonmetastatic sagittal sinus occlusion may also occur in prostate cancer as a complication of a hypercoagulable state induced by diethylstibestrol treatment.

Tumor metastasis to the base of the skull may also produce distinct neurological syndromes.[23*] Bone metastasis to this portion of the skull often produces severe headache referred to the top of the head or the occiput. Also, single or multiple cranial nerve palsies usually accompany basal skull metastasis. For example, clival metastasis often compresses the hypoglossal nerve producing unilateral weakness of the tongue and deviation of the tongue to the side of the lesion when protruded from the mouth. Bone metastasis to the middle cranial fossa may compress and infiltrate the facial nerve, producing ipsilateral weakness of the upper and lower face. Tumor invasion of the jugular foramen will produce severe head pain with associated dysphagia, dysphonia and hoarseness caused by dysfunction of the glossopharyngeal and vagal nerves, which exit the skull base through this foramen. Involvement of foramen ovale may result in compression of trigeminal nerve leading to facial pain.

Small lesions at the skull base may not be visible on plain X-rays or bone scans. It is mandatory that computed tomography (CT) scans with bone windows and 5 mm sections are done to demonstrate the tumor. It is sometimes necessary to do MRI scans of the base of the skull when CT scans are negative.[20*] Radiation therapy directed to the base of the skull is the preferred treatment. Again, prompt recognition of these syndromes and aggressive treatment is indicated to prevent irreversible cranial nerve palsies that often produce devastating neurological impairments.

Cervical spine metastasis

Metastatic disease involving the odontoid process of the axis (first cervical vertebral body) results in a pathological fracture. Secondary subluxation occurs and results in spinal cord or brainstem compression. The symptoms are usually severe neck pain radiating to the posterior aspect of the skull to the vertex, exacerbated by movement. The diagnostic evaluation may require MRI, as plain X-rays and bone scans may not show the problem. Imaging procedures must be carried out carefully to ensure spinal stability.

Pain in C5–6 is characterized by a constant dull aching pain radiating bilaterally to both shoulders with tenderness to percussion over the spinous process. Radicular pain in a C7–8 distribution occurs most commonly unilaterally in the posterior arm, elbow, and ulnar aspect of the hand. Paresthesias and numbness in the fourth and fifth fingers, progressive hand and triceps weakness are the neurological signs. Horner syndrome suggests paraspinal involvement. The diagnostic evaluation must be done carefully. Plain X-rays are often negative since this area is visualized poorly

in these, and CT or preferably MRI scans are necessary to define metastatic disease.

Thoracic spine metastasis

The onset of back pain in association with bandlike tightening across the chest or upper abdominal or radicular arm or leg pain may be the first sign of impending spinal cord compression. Motor and sensory loss occurs later, and autonomic disturbances producing bladder and bowel incontinence occur later still. Thus the evaluation of the patient should begin at the onset of pain for the best chance to preserve motor and sphincteric function. This should include plain X-rays of the entire spine, focused on the symptomatic area, and an MRI. This is necessary because there is about a 15 percent incidence of another epidural lesion.[24*] Corticosteroid therapy should be started even before the radiological evaluation, since this may decrease pain and protect the spinal cord from further compression caused by edema from the tumor or radiotherapy. Even if metastatic disease is found on plain spine films, the MRI should be done to define the extent of tumor invasion in the epidural space because this will influence the size of the radiation therapy ports and will determine the dose and duration of corticosteroid therapy. If anterior vertebral body subluxation has occurred and there is bony compression of the spinal cord, surgical decompression is indicated should the patient's medical condition permit. This is usually followed by radiation therapy. Surgery is usually not attempted as a primary modality of treatment because the results of radiation therapy and corticosteroid treatment are usually equal to surgical decompression.[24*] This is especially true if a simple posterior decompressive laminectomy is done. However, if patients have recurrent spinal cord compression in a previously irradiated port, then an anterior spinal approach with removal of tumor from the vertebral body, decompression of tumor from the spinal canal, and restructuring of the vertebral body with methyl methacrylate should be considered.[25*]

Lumbar spine and sacral metastasis

Dull and aching mid-back pain exacerbated by lying or sitting and relieved by standing is the usual presenting complaint of L1 metastasis. Pain may be referred to the hip, both paraspinal lumbosacral areas and referred pain to the sacroiliac joint or superior iliac crest. Aching pain in the low back or coccygeal region exacerbated by lying or sitting, relieved by walking is the common complaint with sacral metastases. Associated symptoms include perianal sensory loss, bowel and bladder dysfunction, and impotence.

Local invasion of tumor from the pelvis into the sacrum may produce the syndrome of perineal pain, which is often difficult to manage. This syndrome is characterized by local pain in the buttocks and perirectal area, which is often accentuated by pressure on the perineal region such as that caused by sitting or lying prone. In its most extreme form, the patient cannot sit to eat meals or lie flat to sleep, and may spend much of their time standing. Because of the critical role of the parasympathetic sacral innervation to normal bladder and rectal sphincter function, continence is impaired early in the course of this syndrome, perhaps even before significant weakness can be discerned in the legs.

TUMOR INFILTRATION OR TRAUMA TO PERIPHERAL NERVE, PLEXUS, ROOT, AND SPINAL CORD

These syndromes present with radicular pain in the neck, chest, or trunk and the differential diagnosis includes tumor infiltration of the peripheral nerves, and surgical injury, partial, complete or secondary to direct surgical interruption or traction, and nerve compression secondary to musculoskeletal imbalance, diabetic peripheral neuropathy, acute herpes zoster and PHN.

Pain is characterized by constant burning pain with hypoesthesia and dysesthesia in an area of sensory loss. The most common causes are tumor compression in the paravertebral or retroperitoneal area or in association with metastatic tumor in rib causing intercostal nerve infiltration. Pain is usually the first sign of tumor infiltration of nerve and presents as either a local, radicular, or referred pain. Local and radicular pain is seen with tumor infiltration or compression of nerve peripheral to the paraspinal region, whereas referred pain with or without a radicular component is seen with tumor infiltration of the paraspinal region and more proximal areas. Associated autonomic dysfunction causing loss of sweating and loss of axonal flair response to pin scratch can help define the site of the nerve compression or infiltration. The pain is characterized initially by a dull, aching sensation with tenderness to percussion in the distribution of the nerve. Mild paresthesia or dysesthesia can occur as the next sensory symptom followed by the late appearance of motor symptoms and signs.

As tumor invades the perineurium or compresses nerve externally, the nature of the pain changes to a burning, dysesthetic sensation. A careful neurological examination followed by a CT scan to define the site of nerve compression is the diagnostic procedure of choice. Electromyography (EMG) can help to define the site of nerve involvement but it is not diagnostic. Rib erosion and retroperitoneal and paraspinal soft tissue masses are the most common associated findings. In patients with paraspinal tumor, MRI scanning is often necessary to exclude epidural extension. Antitumor therapy is the first-line therapy when possible, but interim pain management with analgesics is almost always necessary. Steroids may provide a useful diagnostic test, and provide both anti-inflammatory and antitumor effects, or may act to reduce local swelling, and secondarily to relieve pain.

Brachial plexopathy

Brachial plexopathy in patients with cancer may occur by metastatic spread of tumor to the plexus or radiation injury producing transient sensory and motor symptoms. More prolonged neurological dysfunction may result from previous radiation therapy to a port which has included the plexus, involvement of the plexus by radiation-induced tumor such as malignant schwannoma or fibrosarcoma, and trauma to the plexus during surgery and anesthesia.

Tumor infiltration and radiation injury are the most common causes.[26*] A review of 100 cases suggested that there are reliable clinical signs and symptoms to distinguish metastatic plexopathy from radiation injury. The characteristics of the pain are quite different and a useful distinguishing clinical sign.[26] Magnetic resonance imaging has been advocated as a better means to image the brachial plexus,[27*] and may be a useful means to diagnose metastatic brachial plexopathy. Rarely biopsy of the brachial plexus may be necessary to distinguish from radiation fibrosis versus a recurrent tumor or a new primary tumor.[28*] However, biopsy is not always definitive.

Metastases to the brachial plexus most commonly involves the lower cords of the brachial plexus, giving rise to neurological signs and symptoms in the distribution of the C8, T1 roots. In contrast, radiation plexopathy most commonly involves the upper cords of the plexus, predominantly in the distribution of the C5–C7 roots. Severe pain is most commonly associated with metastatic plexopathy, and Horner syndrome is more commonly associated with metastatic plexopathy than radiation plexopathy. A significant number of patients with metastatic plexopathy show epidural extension of disease. A primary tumor of the lung, the presence of Horner syndrome, or involvement of the whole plexus should alert the physician to the possibility of epidural extension and warrants immediate MRI. Neither a negative surgical biopsy nor observation for several years for other metastases rules out recurrence of tumor or a new primary tumor.[28*]

Brachial plexopathy in Pancoast tumors

Brachial plexopathy in Pancoast tumor, as described by Kanner et al.[29*] is an integral part of the disease. Pain in the distribution of C8–T1 is an early sign and is part of the clinical diagnosis of Pancoast syndrome. Pain is the most reliable sign to follow as it closely reflects progression of disease and may be the only sign of epidural cord compression. Plain X-rays and bone scans are not reliable diagnostic tests for this disorder and MRI yields the most important diagnostic information. As many as 50 percent of patients develop epidural cord compression, with pain being the earliest and most consistent clinical symptom. In patients who present with Pancoast syndrome and involvement of the brachial plexus, the initial diagnostic workup should include MRI to determine the extent of tumor infiltration. Initial antitumor surgery should be directed at radial removal of all the local tumor and secondary treatment with external radiation therapy and brachytherapy.[30*]

The Pancoast syndrome is commonly misdiagnosed and confused with cervical disk disease, which appears in less than 5 percent of patients in a C8–Tl distribution.

Lumbosacral plexopathy

Lumbosacral plexus tumor infiltration most commonly occurs in genitourinary, gynecological, and colonic cancers. Pain varies with the site of plexus involvement. Radicular pain occurs in L1–L3 distribution (i.e. anterior thigh and groin) or down the posterior aspect of the leg to the heel when in an L5–S1 distribution. In some instances, there is only referred pain without local pain over the plexus. Common referred points are the anterior thigh, knee, and lateral aspect of the calf. These areas are commonly painful but the origin of the pain is in the plexus. Pain is the earliest symptom, followed later by complaints of paresthesia, numbness, dysesthesia leading to motor and sensory loss.

Jaeckle et al.[31*] have described the clinical symptoms and natural history of this disorder in a review of 85 patients with lumbosacral plexopathy. In this study the pain was noted to be of three types: local in 72 of 85 patients, radicular in 72 of 85 patients, and referred in 37 of 85 patients. Local pain in the sacrum or sciatic notch occurred in 59 percent of patients followed by low back pain in 27 percent and pain in the groin or lower abdominal quadrant in 21 percent. Referred pain to the hip or flank occurred in patients with upper plexus lesions whereas pain in the ankle or the foot occurred in patients with a lower plexopathy. Typically the pain precedes objective sensory, motor, and autonomic signs for weeks to months, with a mean of 3 months. Also, initially the CT scan may be negative. Unilateral and bilateral plexopathy with significant motor weakness is commonly associated with epidural extension and both CT and MRI are necessary to define the extent of tumor infiltration and/or epidural compression. Plain X-rays are not often helpful because the lumbosacral plexus lies within the substance of the psoas muscle and is not radiodense.

Pain occurs in 40 percent of patients with leptomeningeal metastases[32*] and is of two types:

- headache with or without neck stiffness
- back pain localized to the low back and buttock regions.

There may be associated confusion, delirium, cranial nerve palsies, radiculopathy, and myelopathy. Diagnostic workup should include MRI, with contrast to determine enhancement in the basal subarachnoid cisterns and to rule out hydrocephalus; MRI to rule out bulk disease on nerve roots which might require focal radiation therapy; and a lumbar puncture to determine cerebrospinal fluid (CSF) glucose, protein, cell count, cytology, and biochemical markers.

PAIN SYNDROMES ASSOCIATED WITH CANCER THERAPY

This category includes those clinical pain syndromes that occur in the course of or subsequent to treatment of cancer patients with the common modalities of surgery, chemotherapy, or radiation therapy.

Post-surgical injury to peripheral nerves

Four distinct pain syndromes involving the peripheral nerves occur following surgery in patients with cancer.

POST-THORACOTOMY PAIN

This pain occurs in the distribution of an intercostal nerve following surgical interruption or injury. The intercostal neurovascular bundle courses along a groove in the inferior border of the rib. Traction on the ribs and rib resection are the common causes of nerve injury during a surgical procedure on the chest. Kanner et al.[29*] prospectively followed 126 consecutive patients undergoing thoracotomy and defined several groups of patients. In the majority (79 patients) immediate postoperative pain was reduced at approximately 2 months, but in 13 of the 79 patients recurrence of the pain occurred. Recurrence of tumor in the distribution of the intercostal nerves was the cause of recurrent pain. The immediate postoperative pain is characterized by an aching sensation in the distribution of the incision with sensory loss with or without autonomic changes. There is often exquisite point tenderness at the most medial and apical point of the scar with a specific trigger point. In another group (20 of the 126 patients) pain persisted following the thoracotomy and increased in intensity during the follow-up period. In this group of patients, local recurrence of disease and/or infection were the most common causes of increasing pain. In the third group, 18 of the 126 patients had stable or decreasing pain which resolved over time and did not represent a difficult management problem.

Thus persistent or recurrent pain in the distribution of the thoracotomy scar in patients with cancer is commonly associated with recurrent tumor. However, a small number of patients will have a traumatic neuroma at the site of their previous thoracotomy scar, but this should not be the initial consideration in evaluating such cancer patients.

POST-MASTECTOMY PAIN

Post-mastectomy pain occurs in the posterior arm, axilla, and anterior chest wall following any surgical procedure on the breast from lumpectomy to radical mastectomy.[33*] It may be more likely to occur from axillary dissection and lymph node dissection.[34*] There is marked anatomical variation in the size and distribution of the intercostal brachial nerve accounting for its variable appearance of this syndrome in patients undergoing mastectomy. The pain results from interruption of the intercostal brachial nerve, a cutaneous sensory branch of T1 – T2. The pain may occur immediately following the surgical procedure but as late as six months following surgery. It is characterized as a tight, constricting, burning pain in the posterior aspect of the arm and axilla radiating across the anterior chest wall. The pain is exacerbated by movement of the arm and relieved by immobilization of the arm. Patients often posture the arm in a flexed position close to the chest wall and are at risk to develop a frozen shoulder syndrome if adequate pain and post-surgical rehabilitation are not implemented early on.

Approximately 5 percent of women undergoing surgical procedures on the breast develop the syndrome. The nature of the pain and the clinical symptomatology should readily distinguish it from tumor infiltration of the brachial plexus. The syndrome appears to occur more commonly in patients with postoperative complications who are at risk for local fibrosis in and about the nerve following surgery, following wound infection or seroma. Typically a trigger point in the axilla or on the anterior chest wall may be found and this is usually the site of the traumatic neuroma. Breast reconstruction does not alter the tight, constricting sensation in the anterior chest wall that is associated with this syndrome.

AFTER RADICAL NECK SURGERY

Prospective studies of pain after radical neck dissection are lacking. In any patient in whom the pain occurs late, i.e. several months following the surgical procedure, and particularly any pain occurring several years following the surgical procedure, re-evaluation is necessary to exclude recurrence of tumor.

POST-AMPUTATION PAIN

Loss of a body part is often followed by psychological adjustment, which may include a grief reaction.[35*] The physiological phenomena of nonpainful and painful phantom sensations referred to the missing part, pain in the scar region after limb amputation, and involuntary motor activity also occur. Many patients note more sensations in the distal phantom limb or in the nipple of the phantom breast. A phantom visceral organ may be associated with functional sensations, e.g. the urge to urinate or defecate.

There are a few reports on the course of post-amputation pain in malignant disease. In a study of 17 patients with cancer who underwent forequarter amputation, none of the seven survivors had pain requiring the use of analgesics after an average of 69 months follow-up.[36*] Larger surveys of post-mastectomy patients reveal that at least 10 percent experience chronic phantom breast pain, more than is generally believed.[37*] Increasing pain in the cancer amputee may signify disease progression or recurrence.[38*,39*]

Chemotherapy-related pain syndromes

Painful dysesthesias follow treatment with several chemotherapeutic agents, in particular, the vinca alkaloid drugs such as vincristine and vinblastine. Cisplatin and taxol are also toxic to peripheral nerve.[40*,41*] These agents produce a symmetrical polyneuropathy as a result of a subacute with chronic axonopathy. Pain is usually localized to the hands and feet, and is characterized as burning pain exacerbated by superficial stimuli, which improves as the drug is withdrawn. Aseptic necrosis of the humeral and more commonly femoral head is a known complication of chronic steroid therapy.[42*] Pain in the shoulder and knee or leg is the common presenting complaint, with X-ray changes occurring several weeks to months after the onset of pain. The bone scan and MRI are the most useful diagnostic procedure.

Post-herpetic neuralgia[43*] can be thought of as a post-chemotherapy pain syndrome since immunocompromised patients are at risk for acute zoster infection or a recurrence of latent zoster. Persisting pain after healing of the cutaneous eruption of herpes zoster infection has generally three components:

- a continuous burning pain in the area of sensory loss
- painful dysesthesias
- intermittent shocklike pain.

Older patients are at greater risk of this complication.

Post-radiation therapy pain

These syndromes are becoming less common as the sophistication with which radiation therapy portals are planned decreases the likelihood of radiation overdose to tissues and spares surrounding normal tissues. Nonetheless, radiation fibrosis of peripheral neural structures such as the brachial and lumbar plexus still occurs, and radionecrosis of bone is occasionally seen.

Radiation fibrosis of the brachial plexus was discussed previously. Pain occurring in the leg from radiation fibrosis of the lumbar plexus is characterized by the late onset of pain in the course of progressive motor and sensory changes in the leg.[44*,45*] Lymphedema, a previous history of radiation therapy, myokymia on EMG, and X-ray changes demonstrating radiation necrosis of bone may help to establish this diagnosis.

Pain is an early symptom in 15 percent of patients with radiation myelopathy.[46*,47*] Some patients may have the Lhermitte sign, signifying transient demyelination in the posterior columns, which does not necessarily predict the development of myelopathy. Pain may be localized to the area of spinal cord damage or may be a referred pain with dysesthesias below the level of injury. The neurological symptoms and signs often start as Brown–Séquard syndrome, a lateral hemisection of the cord, such that pain and temperature sensation are lost contralateral to the side of weakness.

Position and vibration sensation are lost ipsilateral to the side of weakness. The incidence of myelopathy increases with increasing radiation exposure, and approaches 50 percent with 1500 ret exposure. The latency from completion of radiation to the onset of symptoms of myelopathy ranges from 5 to 30 months, with an average of 14 months in most series.

A painful enlarging mass in an area of previous irradiation suggests a radiation-induced peripheral nerve tumor.[48*],[49*],[50*],[51*] In one study, seven of nine patients who developed radiation-induced nerve tumors presented with pain and progressive neurological deficit with a palpable mass involving the brachial of lumbar plexus; these nine patients developed their tumors 4–20 years following radiation therapy. Neurofibromatosis is associated with an increased risk for the development of radiation-induced peripheral nerve tumors.[48*]

NONCANCER PAIN SYNDROMES AND MECHANISMS

Like cancer pain syndromes, noncancer pain syndromes may be nociceptive or neuropathic in nature. Internists and family physicians deal with common degenerative, musculoskeletal pain syndromes along with specialist assessment as indicated. Palliative care specialists are likely to encounter pain in patients with human immunodeficiency virus (HIV) infection/acquired immune deficiency syndrome (AIDS).

Human immunodeficiency virus and pain

Pain is a common symptom in HIV and AIDS patients. With the increasing burden of this disease in Africa and Asia, palliative care specialists are likely to encounter these pain syndromes. Pain syndromes encountered in HIV and AIDS are diverse in nature and etiology. The most common pain syndromes include painful sensory peripheral neuropathy, pain due to extensive Kaposi sarcoma, headache, oral and pharyngeal pain, abdominal pain, chest pain, arthralgias and myalgias, and painful dermatological conditions.[52*],[53*],[54*],[55*],[56*],[57] Hewitt and colleagues in 1997 demonstrated that although pains of a neuropathic nature (e.g. polyneuropathies, radiculopathies) certainly comprise a large proportion of pain syndromes encountered in AIDS patients, pains of a somatic and/or visceral nature are also common clinical problems.[56*] The etiology of pain syndromes seen in HIV disease can be categorized into three types:

- those directly related to HIV infection or consequences of immunosuppression
- those due to AIDS therapies
- those unrelated to AIDS or AIDS therapies.

In studies to date, approximately 45 percent of pain syndromes encountered are directly related to HIV infection or consequences of immunosuppression; 15–30 percent are due to therapies for HIV- or AIDS-related conditions and to diagnostic procedures; and the remaining 25–40 percent are unrelated to HIV or its therapies.[54*],[56*]

Oropharyngeal pain

Oral cavity and throat pain is common, accounting for approximately 20 percent of the pain syndromes encountered in one study.[58*] Common sources of oral cavity pain are candidiasis, necrotizing gingivitis, and dental abscesses and ulcerations caused by herpes simplex virus (HSV), cytomegalovirus (CMV), Epstein–Barr virus (EBV), atypical and typical mycobacterial infection, cryptococcal infection, or histoplasmosis. Frequently no infectious agent can be identified and painful recurrent aphthous ulcers (RAU) are encountered.[59*]

Esophageal pain

Many HIV/AIDS patients experience dysphagia or odynophagia, most commonly caused by esophageal candidiasis. Ulcerative esophagitis is usually a result of CMV infection but can be idiopathic. Infectious causes of esophagitis include HIV, papovavirus, HSV, EBV, *Mycobacterium*, *Cryptosporidium*, and *Pneumocystis carinii*. Kaposi sarcoma and lymphoma have both been reported to invade the esophagus, resulting in dysphagia, pain, and ulceration.[59*] Nonsteroidal medications as well as zidovudine and zalcitabine have been implicated in esophagitis.

Abdominal pain

The abdomen is the primary site of pain in 12–25 percent of patients with HIV disease.[60*] Infectious causes of abdominal pain predominate, and include: cryptosporidiosis, *Shigella*, *Salmonella*, and *Campylobacter enteritis*, CMV ileitis and mycobacterial infection (MAI). Perforation of the small and large intestine secondary to CMV infection has been described.[61*] Repeated intussusception of the small intestine has been seen in association with *Campylobacter* infection.[62*] Lymphoma in the gastrointestinal tract can present with abdominal pain and intestinal obstruction.[59*],[62*] Other causes of abdominal pain in HIV-positive patients[59*] include ileus, organomegaly, spontaneous aseptic peritonitis, toxic shock, herpes zoster, and Fitzhugh–Curtis syndrome (perihepatitis in association with tubal gonococcal or chlamydia infection).

Many antiretroviral agents are responsible for gastrointestinal symptoms but lactic acidosis, a rare but serious complication of some highly active antiretroviral therapy (HAART) regimens, can present with abdominal pain.[63*] Didanosine, zalcitabine, and stavudine can cause pancreatitis whereas patients taking indinavir are at increased risk for nephrolithiasis. Cholecystitis is a painful condition that may occur in HIV-infected patients as a result of opportunistic infection.[64*] Cytomegalovirus and *Cryptosporidium* are the most common infectious agents. Drug-induced hepatic toxicities as well as viral hepatitis as coinfection may lead to abdominal pain. Pancreatitis is an extremely painful condition often related to adverse effects of HIV-related therapies such as didanosine, stavudine and dideoxycytidine.[65*] Intravenous pentamidine is also associated with pancreatitis. Other causes of pancreatitis include CMV infection, MAI, cryptococcal lymphoma and Kaposi sarcoma.

Anorectal pain

Perirectal abscesses, CMV proctitis, fissure-in-ano, and human papillomavirus and HSV infection often cause painful anorectal syndromes.

Chest pain syndromes

Chest pain is a common complaint in patients with HIV disease, comprising approximately 13 percent of the pain syndromes encountered in a sample of ambulatory AIDS patients.[56*] The index of suspicion for coronary artery disease, even in young patients with no other risk factors, must be high if the patient is being treated with HAART. In immunosuppressed patients, infectious causes of chest pain should be considered, particularly in the presence of fever and some localizing sign such as dysphagia, dyspnea, or cough. Infectious causes of chest pain include *Pneumocystis* pneumonia, esophagitis (CMV, candidiasis), pleuritis/pericarditis, and PHN.

Opportunistic cancers, Kaposi's or lymphoma invading the esophagus, pericardium, chest wall, lung and pleura may also be sources of chest pain. Rarely, pulmonary embolus or bacterial endocarditis may be the cause of chest pain.

Neurological pain syndromes

Pain syndromes originating in the nervous system include headache, painful peripheral neuropathies, radiculopathies, and myelopathies. The human immunodeficiency virus is highly neurotropic, invading central and peripheral nervous system structures early in the course of HIV disease. Consequently, many complications of HIV/AIDS and opportunistic infections result in neurological pain, and many commonly used HIV/AIDS medications can also be implicated in neurological pain. Rarely cerebrovascular events (e.g. thalamic stroke) occurring in hypercoagulable states can result in central pain syndromes.

HEADACHE

Headache is extremely common in the HIV/AIDS patient and can pose a diagnostic dilemma for providers in that the underlying cause may range from benign stress and tension to life-threatening central nervous system infection.[59*] The differential diagnosis of headache in patients with HIV disease includes:

- HIV encephalitis and atypical aseptic meningitis
- Opportunistic infections of the nervous system
- AIDS-related central nervous system neoplasms
- Sinusitis
- Tension
- Migraine
- Headache induced by medication (particularly azathioprine [AZT])

Toxoplasmosis and cryptococcal meningitis are the two most commonly encountered opportunistic infections of the central nervous system that cause headaches in patients with HIV disease. More benign causes of headache in the patient with HIV disease include AZT-induced headache; tension headache; migraine with or without aura; and unclassifiable or idiopathic headache.[66*]

NEUROPATHIES

Neuropathic pain occurs in about 40 percent of AIDS patients.[54*,56*] The most common painful neuropathy seen is the predominantly sensory neuropathy (PSN) of AIDS. However, other potentially painful neuropathies in HIV/AIDS patients can have other viral and nonviral causes or may be caused by demyelination leading to Guillain–Barré syndrome, nutritional deficiencies, alcohol, and HIV therapies.[67*] Predominantly symmetrical sensory neuropathy of AIDS is the most frequently encountered neuropathy. This is typically a late manifestation, occurring most often in patients with an AIDS-defining illness.[68*] The prevalence of this neuropathy in hospice populations ranges from 19 percent to 26 percent.[69*,70*] The predominant symptom in about 60 percent of patients is pain in the soles of the feet. Paresthesia is frequent and usually involves the dorsum of the feet and soles. Most patients have signs of peripheral neuropathy and, although the signs progress, the symptoms often remain confined to the feet.[71*,72*] Although patients' complaints are predominantly sensory, electrophysiological studies demonstrate both sensory and motor involvement.

Rheumatological pain syndromes

In studies conducted by the Memorial Sloan–Kettering group, over 50 percent of pain syndromes were classified as rheumatological in nature including various forms of arthritis, arthropathy, arthralgias, myositis, and myalgias.[56*]

The most frequently reported arthritis is a reactive arthritis or Reiter's syndrome.[73*,74*,75*,76*,77*] Acute HIV infection may present with a polyarthralgia in association with a mononucleosis-like illness. There is also a syndrome of acute severe and intermittent articular pain, often referred to as HIV-associated painful articular syndrome, which commonly affects the large joints of the lower limbs and shoulders. Psoriasis and psoriatic arthritis have been reported in patients with HIV infection.[78*] Septic arthritis has been reported in patients with HIV disease, including arthritis due to bacterial infections and infections with *Cryptococcus neoformans* and *Sporothrix schenckii*.[73*,74*]

Key learning points

- Pain is the most common symptom for which palliative care specialists are consulted.

- Cancer pain is the most common pain encountered, but pain syndromes due to HIV/AIDS are on the rise in Africa and Asia.

- Pain is classified into nociceptive and neuropathic in broad terms, but the majority are mixed.

- Pain in cancer is caused by tumor, treatment, or as coexisting chronic pain.

- Tumor size may not correlate with pain intensity.

- There are well-defined pain syndromes described in the literature based on the cause and the location.

- Metastatic bone pain is often associated with neurological deficit due to close proximity between skull and cranial nerves, spinal cord and its roots with vertebral column.

- Not all bony metastatic sites hurt.

- Detailed history with emphasis on neurological examination will lead to early diagnosis of spinal cord compression.

- Suspect epidural disease with new onset neck, upper or lower back pain.

- Critical assessment of pain syndrome helps with optimal pain management, avoiding erroneous polypharmacy.

- A new pain or a sudden change in intensity of existing pain in cancer patient is invariably due to recurrence.

- Headache should always raise suspicion for base of skull metastasis or leptomeningeal disease.

- Exclude constipation as the cause of increased abdominal pain.

- Exclude infection as the cause of intractable pain, especially in head and neck cancers.

- Pain syndromes in HIV/AIDS often follow similar pattern as cancer. But neuropathic pain, rheumatic and musculoskeletal pain syndromes predominate, with high incidence of psychosomatic issues.

- Delirium can masquerade as pain.

- Generalized body pains may be a sign of somatization.

ACKNOWLEDGMENT

Thanks to Katja Sullivan for her help in the preparation of this manuscript.

REFERENCES

- 1   Twycross RG, Fairfield S. Pain in far-advanced cancer. *Pain* 1982; **14**: 303–10.
- 2   Daut RL, Cleeland CS, Dar R. Public attitudes toward cancer pain. *Cancer* 1985; **56**: 2337–9.
- 3   Portenoy RK. Cancer pain, epidemiology and syndromes. *Cancer* 1989; **63**: 2298–2307.
- 4   Cleeland CS. Pain control: public and physicians' attitudes. In: Hill CS, Fields WS, eds. *Advances in Pain Research and Therapy*. New York: Raven Press, 1989: 81–9.
- 5   Van Roenn JH, Cleeland CS, Gonin R, *et al*. Physician attitudes and practice in cancer pain management. A survey from the Eastern Cooperative Oncology Group. *Ann Intern Med* 1993; **119**: 121–6.
- 6   Cleeland CS. Undertreatment of cancer pain in elderly patients. *JAMA* 1998,17; **279**: 1877–82.
- 7   Cleeland CS, Gonin R, Hatfield AK, *et al*. Pain and its treatment in outpatients with metastatic cancer. *N Engl J Med* 1994; **330**: 592–6.
- 8   Foley KM. The treatment of cancer pain. *N Engl J Med* 1985; **313**: 84–95.
- 9   Weiner DK, Sakamoto S, Perera S, Breuer P. Chronic low back pain in older adults: prevalence, reliability, and validity of physical examination findings. *J Am Geriatr Soc* 2006; **54**: 11–20.
- 10 Pinals RS. Mechanisms of joint destruction, pain and disability in osteoarthritis. *Drugs* 1996; **52**(Suppl 3): 14–20.
- 11 Hardin JG. Complications of cervical arthritis. *Postgrad Med* 1992; **91**: 309–15, 318.
- 12 Yezierski RP. Spinal cord injury. A model of central neuropathic pain. *Neurosignals* 2005; **14**: 182–93.
- 13 Woolf CJ, Mannion RJ. Neuropathic pain: aetiology, symptoms, mechanisms, and management. *Lancet* 1999; **353**: 1959–64.
- 14 Dworkin RH, Backonja M, Rowbotham MC, *et al*. Advances in neuropathic pain: diagnosis, mechanisms, and treatment recommendations. *Arch Neurol* 2003; **60**: 1524–34.
- 15 Galasko CSB: Mechanisms of bone destruction in the development of skeletal metastasis. *Nature* 1976; **263**: 507.
- 16 Stambaugh J, Drew J. A double-blind parallel evaluation of the efficacy and safety of a single dose of ketoprofen in cancer pain. *J Clin Pharmacol* 1988; **Suppl 28**: S34.
- 17 Milne RJ, Foreman RD, Giesler GJ, *et al*. Converge of cutaneous and pelvic visceral nociceptive inputs onto primate spinothalamic neurons. *Pain* 1981; **11**: 163.
- 18 Payne R. Neuropathic pain syndromes, with special reference to causalgia and reflex sympathetic dystrophy. *Clin J Pain* 1989; **2**: 59.
- 19 Portenoy RK, Hagen NA. Breakthrough pain: definition, prevalence and characteristics. *Pain* 1990; 41:273–81.
- 20 Kelly JB, Payne R. Pain syndromes in the cancer patient. *Neurol Clin* 1991; **9**: 937–53.

● 21 Front D, Schneck SO, Frankel A. Bone metastasis and bone pain in breast cancer: Are they closely associated? *JAMA* 1979; **242**: 1747.

● 22 Levick S, Jacobos C, Loukas DF. Naproxen sodium in the treatment of bone pain due to metastatic cancer. *Pain* 1988; **35**: 253–8.

● 23 Greenberg HS, Deck MD, Vikram B *et al*: Metastasis to the base of the skull: clinical findings in 43 patients. *Neurology* 1981; **31**: 530.

✱ 24 Bryne TN, Waxman SG. *Epidural Spinal Cord Compression: Diagnosis and Treatment*. Contemporary Neurology Series. Vol. 33. Philadelphia: FA Davis, 1990.

✱ 25 Sundaresan N, DiGiacinto GV, Krol G, Hughes JEO. Spondylectomy for malignant of the spine. *J Clin Oncol* 1989; **7**: 1485–.

● 26 Kori SH, Foley KM, Posner JB. Brachial plexus lesions in patients with cancer: clinical findings in 100 cases. *Neurology* 1981; **31**: 45–50.

● 27 Blair DN, Rapoport S, Sostman HD, Blair OC. Normal brachial plexus: MR imaging. *Radiology* 1987; **165**: 763.

● 28 Payne R, Foley KM. Exploration of the brachial plexus in patients with cancer. *Neurology* 1986; **Suppl 36**: S329.

◆ 29 Kanner RM, Martini N, Foley KM. Incidence of pain and other clinical manifestations of superior pulmonary sulcus (Pancoast's tumors). In: Bonica JJ, Ventafridda V, eds. *Advances in Pain Research and Therapy*, Vol. 4. New York: Raven Press, 1982: 27.

✱ 30 Sundaresan N, Hilaris BS, Martini N. The combined neurosurgical-thoracic management of superior sulcus tumors. *J Clin Oncol* 1987; **5**: 1739.

● 31 Jaeckle K, Young DF, Foley KM. The natural history of lumbosacral plexopathy in cancer. *Neurology* 1985; **35**: 8–15.

● 32 Wasserstrom WR, Glass JP, Posner JB. Diagnosis and treatment of leptomeningeal metastases from solid tumors: experience with 90 patients. *Cancer* 1982; **49**: 759–72.

● 33 Watson CP, Evans RJ, Watt VR. The post-mastectomy pain syndrome and the effect of topical capsaicin. *Pain* 1989; **38**: 177–86.

● 34 Vecht CJ, Van De Brand HJ, Wajer OJM. Post-axillary dissection pain in breast cancer is due to a lesion of the intercostobrachila nerve. *Pain* 1989; **38**: 171–6.

◆ 35 Bradway JK, Malong JM, Racy J *et al*. Psychological adaptation to amputation: an overview. *Prosthet Orthot Int* 1984; **3**(8): 46–50.

● 36 Steinke NM, Ostgard SE, Jensen OM, *et al*. Interscapulothoracic amputation for sarcomas of the shoulder girdle. *Ugeskr Laeger* 1991; **153**: 2555–7.

● 37 Kroner K, Krebs B, Skov J, Jorgensen HS. Immediate and long-term phantom breast syndrome after mastectomy: incidence, clinical characteristics and relationship to pre-mastectomy breast pain. *Pain* 1989; **36**: 327–34.

● 38 Sugarbaker PH, Weiss CM, Davidson DD, Roth YF. Increasing phantom limb pain as a symptom of cancer recurrence. *Cancer* 1984; **54**: 373–5.

● 39 Boas RA, Schug SA, Acland RH. Perineal pain after rectal amputation: a five year follow-up. *Pain* 1993; **52**: 67–70.

◆ 40 Young DF, Postner JB. Nervous system toxicity of chemotherapeutic agents. In: Vinken PJ, Bruyn GW, eds. *Handbook of Clinical Neurology*. Amsterdam: North-Holland Publishing Company, 1969: 91.

◆ 41 Asbury AK, Bird SJ. Disorders of peripheral nerve. In: Asbury AK, McKhann GM, McDonald WI, eds. *Diseases of the Nervous System: Clinical Neurobiology*, 2nd ed. Vol 1. Philadelphia: WB Saunders Company, 1992.

● 42 Ihde DC, DeVita VT. Osteonecrosis of the femoral head in patients with lymphoma treated with intermittent combination chemotherapy (including corticosteroids). *Cancer* 1975; **36**: 1585–8.

◆ 43 Loeser JD. Herpes zoster and postherpetic neuralgia. *Pain* 1986; **25**: 149–64.

✱ 44 Thomas JE, Cascino TL, Earle JD. Differential diagnosis between radiation and tumor plexopathy of the pelvis. *Neurology* 1985; **35**: 1–7.

● 45 Aho I, Sainio K. Late irradiation induced lesions of the lumbosacral plexus. *Neurology* 1983; **33**: 953–5.

● 46 Jellinger K, Sturm KW. Delayed radiation myelopathy in man. *J Neurol Sci* 1971; **14**: 389–408.

◆ 47 Palmer JJ. Radiation myelopathy. *Brain* 1972; **95**: 109–22.

● 48 Foley KM, Woodruff JM, Ellis FT, *et al*. Radiation-induced malignant and atypical peripheral nerve sheath tumors. *Ann Neurol* 1980; **7**: 311–8.

● 49 Ducatman BS, Scheithauer BW. Postirradiation neurofibrosarcoma. *Cancer* 1983; **51**: 1028–33.

● 50 Thomas JE, Piepgras DG, Scheithauer B, *et al*. Neurogenic tumors of the sciatic nerve: a clinicopathologic study of 35 cases. *Mayo Clin Proc* 1983; **58**: 640–7.

● 51 Powers SK, Norman D, Edwards MSB. Computerized tomography of peripheral nerve lesions. *J Neurosurg* 1983; **59**: 131–6.

◆ 52 Penfold R, Clark AJM. Pain syndromes in HIV infection. *Can J Anaesth* 1992; **39**: 724–30.

◆ 53 Katz N. Neuropathic pain in cancer and AIDS. *Clin J Pain* 2000;**16**(2 Suppl): S41–8.

◆ 54 Wesselmann U. Pain syndromes in AIDS. *Anaesthesist* 1996; **45**: 1004–14.

● 55 Verma S, Estanislao L, Simpson D. HIV-associated neuropathic pain: epidemiology, pathophysiology and management. *CNS Drugs* 2005; **19**: 325–34.

● 56 Hewitt DJ, McDonald M, Portenoy RK, *et al*. Pain syndromes and etiologies in ambulatory AIDS patients. *Pain* 1997; **70**: 117–23.

● 57 Lebovits AH, Lefkowitz M, McCarthy D, *et al*. The prevalence and management of pain in patients with AIDS: a review of 134 cases. *Clin J Pain* 1989; **5**: 245–8.

● 58 Singer EJ, Zorilla C, Fahy-Chandon B, *et al*. Painful symptoms reported for ambulatory HIV-infected men in a longitudinal study. *Pain* 1993; **54**: 15–19.

◆ 59 Breckman B. Stoma management. In: Doyle D, Hanks GWC, MacDonald N, eds. *Oxford Textbook of Palliative Medicine*, 3rd ed. New York: Oxford University Press, 2004: 843–94.

● 60 Barone SE, Gunold BS, Nealson TF, *et al*. Abdominal pain in patients with acquired immune deficiency syndrome. *Ann Surg* 1986; **204**: 619–23.

● 61 Balthazar BJ, Reich CB, Pachter HL. The significance of small bowel intussusception in acquired immune deficiency. *Am J Gastroenterol* 1986; **1**: 1073–5.

● 62 Davidson T, Allen-Mersh TG, Miles AJG, *et al*. Emergency laparotomy in patients with AIDS. *Br J Surg* 1991; **789**: 924–6.

● 63 Cello JP. Acquired immune deficiency cholangiopathy: spectrum of disease. *Am J Med* 1989; **86**: 539–46.

● 64 Richman DD, Fischl MA, Grieco MH, *et al*. The toxicity of azidothymidine (AZT) in the treatment of patients with AIDS and AIDS-related complex. *N Engl J Med* 1987; **317**: 192–7.

● 65 Guo JJ, Jang R, Louder A, Cluxton RJ. Acute pancreatitis associated with different combination therapies in patients infected with human immunodeficiency virus. *Pharmacotherapy* 2005; **25**: 1044–54.

● 66 Evers S, Wibbeke B, Reichelt D, *et al.* The impact of HIV on primary headache. Unexpected findings from retrospective, cross-sectional, and prospective analyses. *Pain* 2000; **85**: 191–200.

◆ 67 Griffin JW, Wesselingh SL, Griffin DE, *et al.* Peripheral nerve disorders in HIV infection: Similarities and contrasts with CNS disorders. In: Price RW, Perry SW, eds. *HIV, AIDS and the Brain.* New York: Raven Press Ltd, 1994: 159–82.

● 68 Lange DJ, Britton CB, Younger DS, Hays AP. The neuromuscular manifestations of human immunodeficiency virus infections. *Arch Neurol* 1988; **45**: 1084–8.

● 69 Parry GJ. Peripheral neuropathies associated with human immunodeficiency virus infection. *Ann Neurol* 1988; **23** (Suppl): 349–53.

● 70 Dalakas MC, Pezeshkpour GA. Neuromuscular diseases associated with human immunodeficiency virus infection. *Ann Neurol* 1988; **23**(Suppl): S38–48.

● 71 Fuller GN, Jacobs JM, Guiloff RJ. Association of painful peripheral neuropathy in AIDS with cytomegalovirus infection. *Lancet* 1989; **334**: 937–41.

● 72 Harrison R, Soong S, Weiss H, *et al.* A mixed model for factors predictive of pain in AIDS patients with herpes zoster. *J Pain Symptom Manage* 1999; **17**: 410–17.

● 73 Espinoza LR, Aguilar JL, Berman A. Rheumatic manifestations associated with human immunodeficiency virus infection. *Arthritis Rheum* 1989; **32**: 1615–22.

● 74 Kaye BR. Rheumatologic manifestations of infection with human immunodeficiency virus. *Ann Intern Med* 1989; **111**: 158–67.

● 75 Rynes RI, Goldenberg DL, DiGiacomo R, *et al.* Acquired immunodeficiency syndrome-associated arthritis. *Am J Med* 1988; **84**: 810–16.

● 76 Dalakas MC, Pezeshkpour GH, Gravell M, Sever JL. Polymyositis associated with AIDS retrovirus. *JAMA* 1986; **256**: 2381–3.

● 77 Watts RA, Hoffbrand BI, Paton DF, Davie JC. Pyomyositis associated with human immunodeficiency virus infection. *Br Med J* 1987; **194**: 1524–5.

● 78 Johnson TM, Duvic M, Rapini RP, Rios A. AIDS exacerbates psoriasis. *N Engl J Med* 1986; **313**: 1415.

44

Opioid analgesics

PER SJØGREN, JØRGEN ERIKSEN

INTRODUCTION

Derivates of the opium poppy (*Papaver somniferum*) have a long history as pain-relieving agents. The main constituent, the alkaloid called morphine, was isolated by Sertürner in 1803, and was later shown to be almost completely responsible for the analgesic effects. Today morphine is still the most widely used opioid and remains the 'gold standard' when effects of other opioid analgesics are to be compared.

The concept of a specific opioid receptor was established in the middle of the twentieth century based on the stereospecificity and availability of selective antagonists to the analgesic actions.[1*,2*] In the 1970s, opioid receptors were recognized as specific biochemical structures and the evidence for the existence of multiple receptors was established.[3*,4,5*] Based on their activities *in vivo* opioids are now classified according to their sensitivity and selectivity in receptor-binding studies and it is now agreed that there are three main types of opioid receptor, μ (mu), δ (delta), and κ (kappa). In 1994, a fourth opioid receptor called the nociceptin/orphanin FQ (N/OFQ) receptor was discovered.[6*] Morphine as well as other opioids exert their analgesic action by a specific interaction with one or more subclasses of the three most important opioid receptors: μ, δ, and κ. Genes encoding for these receptors have been cloned. Based on their different pharmacology a number of subclasses have been described: μ_1 and μ_2, δ_1 and δ_2 and κ_{1-3}. Evidence for multiple μ-receptors came from binding studies, which showed biphasic binding properties of μ-agonists.[7*]

Clinically, differences were observed as patients who did not tolerate one μ-agonist could be switched to another, which was easily tolerated. Also incomplete cross-tolerance was observed in connection with 'rotation' from one μ-agonist to another: far lower doses than predicted of the new drug were necessary to control pain.[8,9*] Similar incomplete cross-tolerance has been confirmed in animal models.[10]

Most of the clinically relevant opioids are relatively selective for the μ-receptor, reflecting their similarity with morphine at least within normal dose ranges (Table 44.1). However, higher doses used to overcome development of tolerance may result in interaction with additional receptor subtypes and result in changes in their pharmacological profile.

Opioids act by inhibiting the ascending nociceptive signal transmission from the dorsal horn in the spinal cord. The periaqueductal gray region is a major anatomical locus for opioid activation of descending inhibitory pathways to the spinal cord and is thus an important site for μ-receptor mediated analgesia. Opioids do not excite descending fibers directly, but inhibit spontaneous γ-aminobutyric acid (GABA) release from GABAergic interneurons. Furthermore opioid receptors have also been demonstrated in inflamed tissue in terminals of peripheral nerves in animals as well as in humans.[11]

In this chapter the most widely used and clinically relevant opioid analgesics in palliative care are described.

MORPHINE

Morphine is the most thoroughly investigated opioid drug and it is recommended as a first-line opioid in the World Health Organization (WHO) Cancer Relief Guidelines.[12] Morphine is a pure opioid agonist with affinity primarily to the μ-receptors and to a lesser degree to the δ- and κ-receptors (see Table 44.1). Morphine can be administered by the oral, rectal, intravenous, intramuscular,

Table 44.1   *Primary receptor binding and pharmacologic data of important opioids in palliative medicine*

Opioid	Primary site of action	Bioavailability (average) (%)	Major metabolites	Major metabolic* and excretion† pathways	Safety in renal failure
Morphine	μ–receptor agonist	25	M6G+ M3G±	Hepatic* Renal†	Not safe
Methadone	μ–receptor agonist	80	Pyrrolidine− Pyrroline−	Hepatic* Fecal† Renal†	Safe
Oxycodone	μ–receptor agonist	60	Noroxycodone− Oxymorphone+	Hepatic* Renal†	Uncertain
Fentanyl	μ–receptor agonist	90	Phenylacetic acid− Norfentanyl− Hydroxyfentanyl	Hepatic* Renal†	Safe

+, active; −, inactive; ±, uncertain.

M6G, morphine-6-glucuronide; M3G, morphine-3-glucuronide.

subcutaneous, epidural, intrathecal, and intracerebroventricular routes.

Absorption

After oral administration morphine is almost completely absorbed from the gastrointestinal tract.[13] The rate of absorption from the gut depends on the pharmaceutical formulation. Immediate-release morphine tablets reach their maximum plasma concentrations within an average of 60–70 minutes and sustained-release morphine tablets designed for twice or thrice daily administration within an average of 140–200 minutes.[14,15**]

Pharmacokinetics

About 20–38 percent of morphine is bound to plasma proteins, primarily albumin.[16] The mean volume of distribution varies between 2.1 L/kg and 4.0 L/kg in cancer patients and healthy individuals, decreasing to half the value in elderly individuals.[17–19] In cancer patients and healthy individuals mean elimination half-life varies between 1.6 and 3.4 hours and mean systemic plasma clearance between 9 mL/kg and 33 mL/kg/min.[18,20]

Extensive first-pass metabolism after oral morphine administration results in a low and variable bioavailability between 19 percent and 47 percent[19,21] (see Table 44.1). The two most important metabolites quantitatively and qualitatively are morphine-3-glucuronide (M3G) and morphine-6-glucuronide (M6G) (see Table 44.1). Regardless of the route of administration approximately 44–55 percent of a morphine dose is converted into M3G, 9–10 percent to M6G and 8–10 percent is excreted in the urine unchanged.[19] The major pathway for morphine metabolism is conjugation with the co-substrate uridine-diphosphate

(UDP)-glucuronic acid. The process is catalyzed by UDP glucuronyltransferase (UDPGT) and takes place mainly in the liver, although a part takes place in the kidneys, gut, and brain[21,22] (see Table 44.1). Although the UDPGTs are a multienzyme family, it has been demonstrated that the human UGT2B7 is likely to be the major isoform responsible for morphine glucuronidation in humans, capable of catalyzing the glucuronidation process at the 3- as well as 6- positions.[23] A recent study indicated that during long-term treatment neither dose level nor treatment length influenced glucuronidation of morphine.[24]

Elimination

During the process of glucuronidation morphine is made more hydrophilic, and the enhanced water solubility eases its excretion via the kidneys (see Table 44.1). The role of the kidneys in the excretion process has been demonstrated in a study of patients with renal failure given intravenous morphine. Subsequent plasma concentrations of M3G and M6G were observed to be severalfold greater in these patients than in a control group with normal renal function.[25] The clearance of the metabolites is significantly correlated to the creatinine clearance.[26] As a consequence of the accumulation of M3G and M6G in patients with renal impairment toxic effects of morphine metabolites may be seen[27,28] (see Table 44.1).

Pharmacokinetics of M6G and M3G

In healthy volunteers the plasma protein binding of M3G and M6G has been found to be low, 15 percent and 11 percent, respectively. Formation of the metabolites takes time and T_{max} for M6G and M3G occur later than for morphine. After long-term administration of morphine to cancer patients the cerebrospinal fluid (CSF) and plasma ratios for M3G and M6G range between 0.08 and 0.18 and 0.07 and 0.15, respectively.[29,30]

M6G and analgesia

Animal studies demonstrated that, although M6G and morphine were almost equally potent after peripheral administration, the analgesic potency of M6G was >100-fold higher than morphine after intracerebroventricular injection. These pharmacological data suggest that the brain penetration of M6G is significantly attenuated relative to that of morphine.[31] A study using transcortical microdialysis in rat brain cells showed that systemically administered morphine entered brain cells, whereas M6G crossed the blood–brain barrier extremely slowly and was trapped in the extracellular fluid. A high concentration of M6G in this limited space in the brain may account for the durable availability of M6G to opioid receptors.[32] Another explanation for the prolonged analgesia elicited by systemically administered M6G compared with morphine was a threefold slower rate of elimination of M6G than morphine from the mouse brain.[33]

Intravenous M6G has analgesic effects in cancer patients; however, its potency compared with morphine has not been established in humans.[34] A critical clinical issue is the role and contribution of M6G to the analgesic action seen after long-term morphine administration. In this respect controversy exists as a few clinical studies have found evidence for M6G being a contributor to the analgesic action observed after morphine administration,[35,36] whereas other clinical studies have not been able to demonstrate this.[24,30,37,38] In general these studies are confounded by a multitude of other factors that influence patients' perception of pain, including psychological factors and varying responses to morphine administration due to different pain mechanisms and opioid receptor properties, concentration of opioids at the target sites, variability of nonspecific endogenous opioids and varying plasma sampling times for determining M6G/morphine.

M3G: antagonism of antinociception and neurotoxicity

M3G appears to have little or no μ-agonist properties and therefore to be devoid of analgesic activity. In some studies subcutaneous or intracerebroventricular administration of M3G prior to or after the administration of morphine or M6G has been shown to reduce the antinociceptive response of the two analgesic agents.[39,40] In contrast, other studies in rodents have not found any influence of M3G on morphine analgesia.[41,42] Apart from its possible role as an antianalgesic, M3G and high-dose morphine have also been associated with 'morphine-induced neurotoxicity' such as generalized hyperalgesia/allodynia and myoclonus.

Several studies in rodents have found that M3G and high-dose morphine administered by the intracerebroventricular[43,44] as well as the intrathecal routes produce symptoms of sensory and motor excitation.[45,46]

Clinically the symptoms of hyperalgesia, allodynia, and myoclonus have mostly been observed in cancer patients treated with high doses of morphine administered by several different routes,[47–49] although these side effects have also been associated with other opioids.[50,51] In several of the case reports describing these symptoms very high plasma levels of morphine and M3G as well as accumulation of M3G relative to morphine or M6G has been demonstrated.[47,49] A study has shown that although M3G does not cross the blood–brain barrier with the same ease as morphine, the mean steady state M3G concentration in the CSF is approximately twofold higher than the respective CSF morphine concentration following long-term morphine treatment.[52] Opioid switching or rotation, whereby a structurally dissimilar opioid (e.g. methadone (open-chain opioid analgesic) or fentanyl (anilinopiperidine opioid analgesic)) is substituted for a benzomorphan opioid, such as morphine (or hydromorphone) will also result in clearance of M3G from the brain tissue, giving a time-dependent resolution of the neuroexcitatory behaviors while maintaining analgesia with methadone or fentanyl.[49,53]

M3G has recently been given to healthy volunteers in small intravenous doses. In these doses, neurotoxicity did not occur.[54]

METHADONE

Methadone is increasingly being considered as a second-choice drug alternative to morphine in cancer pain treatment. It is a long-acting μ-receptor agonist with pharmacological properties qualitatively similar to those of morphine (see Table 44.1). Earlier reports of severe toxicity of methadone have given rise to misconceptions and render its effective use in cancer pain difficult.[55,56] With better understanding of the pharmacokinetics of methadone it has subsequently been found to be a safe, effective, and cheap alternative to other opioids when prescribed by physicians experienced in its use. Methadone is administered by the oral, rectal, and intravenous routes. Methadone is not suitable for subcutaneous administration because of the high frequency of local reactions.[57]

Absorption

Methadone is a synthetic opioid with an almost complete absorption when administered orally and rectally.[58]** Its oral bioavailability is generally high and considered to be higher than that of other oral opioids such as morphine; it is in the region of 80 percent and ranges from 41 percent to 99 percent[59,60] (see Table 44.1). It is a lipophilic drug and is subject to considerable tissue distribution.[61] The peripheral tissue reservoir sustains plasma concentrations during long-term treatment.[62] Methadone is extensively metabolized in the liver to inactive metabolites via N-demethylation[63] (see Table 44.1). In most countries methadone is used in a racemic mixture of S- and R-enantiomers, although the latter form has significantly longer elimination half-life, larger volume of distribution, slower clearance, and more analgesic potency.[64,65]

Pharmacokinetics

Methadone is characterized by a rapid and extensive distribution phase (half-life, 2–3 hours) followed by a slow elimination phase (β-half-life, 15–60 hours). After oral administration measurable concentrations appear in plasma after 30 minutes.[61] There is a large interindividual variation of the elimination phase, which can be the reason for accumulation and potential toxicity.[66]

Elimination

Methadone is mainly excreted by the fecal route and only a minor part is eliminated in the urine (see Table 44.1). Renal clearance is enhanced by lowering the urinary pH.[67***] As the elimination is primarily via feces significant accumulation is not likely in renal failure (see Table 44.1).

Clinical aspects

In recent years methadone has been used extensively for opioid switching or rotation.[68,69] In cancer patients, when switching for uncontrolled pain and opioid-induced toxicity, significant improvements have been reported in pain intensity and a number of toxicities.[70***] A major problem encountered when switching to methadone from another opioid is the huge interindividual variations in the equianalgesic ratio of methadone to other opioids. This equianalgesic dose ratio varies dramatically depending on the extent of previous exposure to opioids. Methadone becomes relatively more potent with increasing prior exposure to other opioids and can be up to 10 times more potent in patients given daily doses >500 mg of morphine than in patients given daily doses <100 mg of morphine.[71] Some mechanisms for the dynamic equipotency relations can be hypothesized: (i) incomplete cross-tolerance of opioid receptors, (ii) N-methyl-D-aspartate (NMDA) receptor antagonism, and (iii) elimination of active metabolites. In addition of course combinations of these mechanisms may be in play. Regarding the NMDA receptor antagonism methadone may possess a dual effect on opioid receptors and NMDA receptors, which clinically may be advantageous to other opioids in decreasing development of tolerance and increasing analgesia in neuropathic pain conditions. However, methadone has only been found to be a relatively potent NMDA inhibitor in *in vitro* studies.[72] A recent study in cancer patients comparing methadone with morphine orally did not indicate that methadone was advantageous in neuropathic pain conditions.[73**]

OXYCODONE

Oxycodone (14-hydroxy-7,8-dihydrocodeinone) has become the most commonly used opioid in the USA and can be administered by the oral, rectal, and intravenous routes. It is a μ-receptor agonist, but a part of its antinociceptive effects may be mediated by the κ-receptors (see Table 44.1).

Absorption

Oral bioavailability in humans is about 60 percent (range 50–87 percent)[74,75] (see Table 44.1). The mean lag time from oral administration to pharmacodynamic effect is 0.52 ± 0.33. Oxycodone is subject to extensive hepatic first-pass effects. Oxycodone is metabolized by the liver to the active metabolite, oxymorphone, and to the inactive, but quantitatively most prevalent metabolite, noroxycodone[76] (see Table 44.1).

Pharmacokinetics

T_{max} of oxycodone is approximately 1 hour, and the mean half-life after single-dose is 3.5–5.65 hours.[75,77] The half-life is not influenced by route of administration.[75] Oxycodone's physicochemical properties, liposolubility, and protein binding are similar to morphine.[77] Controlled-release oxycodone is absorbed in a bi-exponential fashion with a rapid mean half-life of 37 minutes and a slow phase of 6.2 hours. T_{max} is 3.2 ± 2.2 hours.[78]

Elimination

Oxycodone and its metabolites are mainly excreted via the kidneys. Oxycodone elimination is prolonged with renal failure and in end-stage liver disease[79,80] (see Table 44.1).

Clinical aspects

Oral equianalgesic ratios of oxycodone to morphine have varied from 1:1 to 1:2, 2:3, and 3:4 as a result of significant interindividual differences in oral bioavailability and unequal noncross-tolerance, and sex differences in the metabolism of oxycodone.[81**,82,83] Women seem to eliminate oxycodone 25 percent more slowly than men.[84]

FENTANYL

Fentanyl is a synthetic phenyl piperidine derivative and a chemical congener of the reversed ester of meperidine. It has selective high affinity for the μ-receptor, where it acts as a pure agonist[85] (see Table 44.1). Fentanyl has a short duration of action and is therefore administered continuously by the transdermal, subcutaneous, or spinal routes or used on demand by the intravenous and transmucosal routes. The transdermal therapeutic system (TTS) was designed to release fentanyl at a constant rate of 72 hours and has gained enormous popularity in Western countries for the treatment of cancer pain.

Absorption

A mean bioavailability of 92 percent (range 57–146 percent) has been reported for TTS fentanyl, although marked interindividual variation is apparent[86] (see Table 44.1). Although fentanyl has been detected in the blood 1–2 hours after initial application of TTS, considerable delays (17–48 hours) between patch application and occurrence of C_{max} were also apparent. The delay has been attributed to depot accumulation of the drug in the skin under the TTS before diffusion into the systemic circulation. Steady-state concentrations are achieved after application of the second patch.[87***]

Pharmacokinetics

Fentanyl is predominantly metabolized in the liver and produces phenylacetic acid, norfentanyl and small amounts of the active metabolite, p-hydroxy(phenethyl)fentanyl[87***] (see Table 44.1). It is highly lipid soluble, which facilitates rapid transfer across the blood–brain barrier and into the central nervous system (CNS). This is reflected in the half-life for equilibration between the plasma and CSF of approximately 5 minutes.[88]

Elimination

Renal elimination of fentanyl is prolonged after transdermal application compared with intravenous administration (see Table 44.1). Elimination half-life values of 13–25 hours have been reported after TTS.[87***]

Clinical aspects

The relative analgesic potency of intravenous fentanyl to morphine from single-dose studies is approximately 100:1 and the transdermal fentanyl to oral morphine during long-term administration is 150:1.[88,89] Two major difficulties have been identified with the transdermal route: a delay of

12–24 hours occurs in obtaining steady-state plasma concentrations and a prolonged period of continued fentanyl effect following removal of the patch.[90] In cancer patients the continuous subcutaneous route provides some advantages over the extensively described transdermal route in patients with unstable pain requiring rapid dose escalation or reduction. Furthermore on demand doses can be administered by the very same route for breakthrough pain.[88] Recently, oral transmucosal fentanyl citrate has been formulated as lollipops as well as intranasal sprays for breakthrough pain to achieve analgesic action within minutes.[91,92]

LONG-TERM CONSEQUENCES OF OPIOID TREATMENT

Apart from providing analgesia and other potentially desired effects opioids also induce side effects, which during long-term treatment often create substantial problems (see Chapter 45). However, long-term opioid treatment may also have other consequences that should be considered in palliative care.

Physical dependence

Physical dependence is a pharmacological phenomenon and the expected consequence of use of opioids. Physical dependence is defined by the appearance of withdrawal symptoms when the opioid dose is reduced or abruptly discontinued and may occur within few days of continuous use of opioids.[93,94] Withdrawal symptoms may include various physiological and psychological signs such as sweating, diarrhea, tremors and anxiety, irritability, and disturbed sleep. Also craving, pain or increased pain are common, often described as abdominal spasms, muscle pain, and bone pain.[94]

Intermittent withdrawal phenomena, breakthrough withdrawal symptoms, or on-off phenomena, which may appear as increased pain, are common in patients using short-acting opioids on demand.[95*] Hence, insufficient dosing may result in the so-called pseudo-addictive condition.[96]

Tolerance

Pharmacologically, tolerance may develop with the repeated use of opioids and is characterized by the necessity of increased doses in order to maintain the drug effects. A distinction, which may be due to the involvement of different neurotransmitter systems, could be made between associative (learned) tolerance and nonassociative (adaptive) tolerance.[97*] Associative tolerance involves environmental and psychological factors, whereas nonassociative tolerance is an adaptive process at the cellular level due to downregulation and/or desensitization of the opioid receptors.[98,99] In addition, changes in the metabolism, distribution or degradation of the drug may be of importance for the development of tolerance.[100,101]

Tolerance does not always occur in long-term opioid therapy, but when it does, it will often be described by the patient as increased pain.

Abnormal pain sensitivity

Increasing evidence not only in laboratory but also in clinical settings indicates that prolonged opioid treatment may lead to increased pain sensitivity. As described by Mao,[102***] the development of opioid-induced pain sensitivity is closely linked to the development of pharmacological tolerance. The two components of apparent opioid tolerance may involve opposing cellular mechanisms: a desensitization process (pharmacological tolerance) and a sensitization process (opioid-induced pain sensitivity). These mechanisms may be related to the development of opioid-induced neurotoxicity described in cancer patients treated with high doses.[47,49]

The NMDA receptor is involved in tolerance development, and this receptor has also been shown to be of importance for the cellular mechanisms engaged in opioid-induced pain sensitivity. Furthermore basic science studies and few clinical observations have suggested that the development of both pharmacological tolerance and opioid-induced pain sensitivity may be reduced or prevented by combination of an opioid with an NMDA receptor antagonist such as ketamine.[103–105]

Addiction and abuse

Addiction in the context of opioid therapy for pain constitutes a constellation of maladaptive behaviors including loss of control over use, preoccupation with opioid use despite adequate pain relief and continued use of the drugs despite apparent obvious adverse consequences due to their use.[106*] Other suggestive signs of addiction may be unwillingness to terminate opioid treatment even if other treatment possibilities are offered, preference for short-acting opioids used on demand, and not being interested in other treatment possibilities. Abuse refers to the condition in which the medication is used for a pain indication, but in a way that may cause harm to self or others. Abuse may or may not be associated with physical dependency or addiction.

Addiction is anticipated to have a complex etiology including genetic, psychologic, social, and cultural influences, and drug exposure. Neurobiologically, addiction is believed to related to dopaminergic phenomena in the limbic reward centers, which stimulate drug craving and compulsive use in vulnerable individuals.[107]

The factors that promote addiction in some people are not fully understood, although it is known that individuals with a family history of alcoholism or drug addiction or persons with a prior history of addiction have some increased risk of addiction or of relapse to addiction in association with therapeutic use of opioids.[108]

The immune system

Opioids have for years been known to influence the immune system, and recently several studies have shown that opioids may have detrimental immunomodulatory effects on nearly all measurable parts of the system. Opioids have been shown to suppress lymphocyte proliferation,[109*,110] trafficking,[111] natural killer cell activity,[112] antibody production,[113] and the overall number of circulating leukocytes.[114] Animal studies indicate that short-term opioid treatment has fewer adverse effects than long-term exposure, and that abrupt withdrawal may enhance the immunosuppression.[115] Also different opioids seem to act differently on the immune system, as exemplified through methadone, which may be less suppressive than morphine.[116,117]

Even if an enhanced sensitivity to bacterial infections is seen in drug abusers, the existing clinical data are inconclusive, and conclusions regarding the clinical relevance of opioid-induced immunosuppression cannot yet be made.

The reproductive system

Disturbance of libido, amenorrhea, and loss of potency have been described in connection with long-term opioid treatment especially with opioids administered intrathecally.[118,119] Abs et al.[120**] found among patients treated with opioids intrathecally decreased libido or impotence in almost all the men and significantly lowered serum testosterone levels. Decreased libido was present in about 70 percent of women receiving opioids and all premenopausal females developed amenorrhea or an irregular menstrual cycle. Serum luteinizing hormone, estradiol, and progesterone levels were significantly lower in the opioid-treated group than among the controls. Finch et al.[121] and Roberts et al.[122] have also found decreased libido and testosterone levels in men, and it can be concluded that opioids administered intrathecally may induce hypogonadotropic hypogonadism, which is of clinical importance for the majority of men and in premenopausal women. Even if it has been demonstrated that heroine addicts show a diminished semen quality with maintenance or a slightly reduced testosterone levels,[123,124] the clinical importance in patients receiving long-term oral opioid therapy has yet to be established.

SUMMARY

This chapter discussed the history and recent evidence regarding opioid receptors along with clinical observations of individual responses and incomplete cross-tolerance to different opioids. The up-to-date pharmacology of the four most commonly used strong opioids – morphine, methadone, oxycodone, and fentanyl was reviewed. Important clinical issues associated with long-term administration of these drugs were highlighted.

Key learning points

- Morphine is the most thoroughly investigated opioid drug, however, new and puzzling aspects of its metabolism are still unclear.

- Although M6G undoubtedly possesses analgesic effects its contribution to clinical analgesia is unknown. M3G may be involved in the development of antagonism of antinociception as well as opioid-induced neurotoxicity.

- Methadone is increasingly being considered as a second-choice drug alternative to morphine and has interesting properties when switching to it from other opioids. Methadone seems to become relatively more potent with increasing exposure to other opioids.

- Oxycodone has become the most commonly used opioid in the US, although its pharmacology at therapeutic dose levels seems to be closely related to that of morphine.

- The fentanyl patch is increasingly popular, however, in dynamic pain states titrating may be difficult.

- Long-term opioid treatment has other consequences than the 'classic' side effects and opioid-induced neurotoxicity. In palliative medicine physical dependence, tolerance, abnormal pain sensitivity and addiction should also be considered as they may be related to poor treatment outcomes.

- New knowledge concerning the potential influence of long-term administration of opioids on the immune and reproductive systems is emerging.

REFERENCES

● 1 Beckett AH, Casy AF. Synthetic analgesics: stereochemical considerations. *J Pharm Pharmacol* 1954; **6**: 986–1001.

● 2 Portoghese PS. Stereochemical factors and receptor interactions associated with narcotic analgesics. *J Pharm Sci* 1966; **55**: 865–87.

● 3 Terenius L. Specific uptake of narcotic analgesics by subcellular fractions of the guinea-pig ileum. *Acta Pharmacol Toxicol* 1972; **31**: 50–5.

4 Terenius L. Characteristics of the 'receptor' for narcotic analgesics in synaptic plasma membrane from rat brain. *Acta Pharmacol Toxicol* 1973; **33**: 377–84.

● 5 Martin WR, Eades CG, Thompson JA, et al. The effects of morphine and nalorphine-like drugs in the non-dependent and morphine-dependent chronic spinal dog. *J Pharmacol Exp Ther* 1976; **197**: 517–32.

● 6 Mollereau C, Parmentier M, Mailleux P, et al. ORL1, a novel member of the opioid receptor family. Cloning, functional expression and localization. *FEBS Lett* 1994; **341**: 33–8.

● 7 Pasternak GW. Pharmacological mechanisms of opioid analgesics. *Clin Neuropharmacol* 1993; **16**: 1–18.

8 Crews JC, Sweney NJ, Denson DD. Clinical efficacy of methadone in patients refractory to other mu-receptor agonist analgesics for management of terminal cancer pain. Case presentations and discussion of incomplete cross-tolerance among opioid agonist analgesics. *Cancer* 1993; **72**: 2266–72.

◆ 9 Mercadante S. Opioid rotation for cancer pain: rationale and clinical aspects. *Cancer* 1999; **86**: 1856–66.

● 10 Pasternak GW. Incomplete cross-tolerance and multiple mu peptide receptors. *Trends Pharmacol Sci* 2001; **22**: 67–70.

● 11 Stein C, Pflüger M, Yassouridis A, Hoelzl J, Lehrberger K, Welte C, Hasssan AHS. No tolerance to peripheral morphine analgesia in presence of opioid expression in inflamed synovia. *J Clin Invest* 1996; **98**: 793–9.

✳ 12 World Health Organization. *Cancer Pain Relief and Palliative Care*. Geneva; World Health Organization, 1996.

● 13 Brunk SF, Delle M. Morphine metabolism in man. *Clin Pharmacol Ther* 1974; **16**: 51–7.

14 Poulain P, Hoskin PJ, Hanks GW, et al. Relative bioavailability of controlled release morphine tablets (MST Continus) in cancer patients. *Br J Anaesth* 1988; **61**: 569–74.

15 Christrup LL, Sjogren P, Jensen N-H, et al. Steady-state kinetics and dynamics of morphine in cancer patients. Is sedation related to the absorption rate of morphine? *J Pain Symptom Manage* 1999; **18**: 164–73.

16 Olsen GD. Morphine binding to human plasma proteins. *Clin Pharmacol Ther* 1975; **17**: 31–5.

17 Owen JA, Sitar DS, Berger L, et al. Age-related morphine kinetics. *Clin Pharmacol Ther* 1983; **34**: 364–8.

● 18 Säwe J, Kager L, Svensson J-O, Rane A. Oral morphine in cancer patients: in vivo kinetics and in vitro hepatic glucuronidation. *Br J Clin Pharmac* 1985; **19**: 495–501.

● 19 Osborne R, Joel S, Trew D, Slevin M. Morphine and metabolite behavior after different routes of morphine administration: Demonstration of the importance of the active metabolite morphine-6-glucuronide. *Clin Pharmacol Ther* 1990; **47**: 12–19.

● 20 Crotty B, Watson KJR, Desmond PV, Mashford ML, Wood LJ, Colman J, Dudley FJ. Hepatic extraction of morphine is impaired in cirrhosis. *Eur J Clin Pharmacol* 1989; **36**: 501–6.

21 Wahlström A, Pacifici GM, Lindstrom B, Hammar L, Rane A. Human liver morphine UDP-glucuronyl transferase enantioselectivity and inhibition by opioid congeners and oxazepam. *Br J Pharmacol* 1988; **94**: 864–70.

● 22 King CD, Rios GR, Assouline JA, Tephly TR. Expression of UDP-glucuronosyltransferases (UGTs) 2B7 and 1A6 in the human brain and identification of 5-hydroxytryptamine as a substrate. *Arch Biochem Biophys* 1999; **365**: 156–62.

23 Coffman BL, Rios GR, King CD, Tephly TR. Human UGT2B7 catalyzes morphine glucuronidation. *Drug Met Disp* 1997; **25**: 1–4.

24 Andersen G, Sjogren P, Hansen SH, et al. Pharmacological consequences of long-term morphine treatment in patients with cancer and chronic non-malignant pain. *Eur J Pain* 2004; **8**: 263–71.

● 25 Osborne R, Joel S, Grebenik K, et al. The pharmacokinetics of morphine and morphine glucuronides in kidney failure. Clin Pharmacol Ther 1993; **54**: 158–67.

26 Klepstad P, Dale O, Kaasa S, et al. Influences on serum concentrations of morphine, M6G and M3G during routine clinical drug monitoring: A prospective survey in 300 adult cancer patients. Acta Anaesthesiol Scand 2003; **47**: 725–31.

27 Hasselström J, Berg U, Löfgren A, Säwe J. Long lasting respiratory depression induced by morphine-6-glucuronide? Br J Clin Pharmac 1989; **27**: 515–18.

28 Bodd E, Jacobsen D, Lund E, et al. Morphine-6-glucuronide might mediate the prolonged opioid effect of morphine in acute renal failure. Human Exp Toxicol 1990; **9**: 317–21.

29 Van Dongen RTM, Crul BJP, Koopman-Kimenai PM, Vree TB. Morphine and morphine-glucuronide concentrations in plasma and CSF during long-term administration of oral morphine. Br J Clin Pharmacol 1994; **38**: 271–3.

30 Goucke CR, Hackett LP, Ilett KF. Concentrations of morphine, morphine-6-glucuronide and morphine-3-glucuronide in serum and cerebrospinal fluid following morphine administration to patients with morphine-resistant pain. Pain 1994; **56**: 145–9.

● 31 Wu D, Kang YS, Bickel U, Pardrige WM. Blood-Brain Barrier permeability to morphine-6-glucuronide is markedly reduced compared with morphine. Drug Met Disp 1997; **25**: 768–71.

● 32 Stain-Texier F, Boschi G, Sandouk P, Scherrmann JM. Elevated concentrations of morphine 6-beta-D-glucuronide in brain extracellular fluid despite low blood-brain barrier permeability. Br J Pharmacol 1999; **128**: 917–24.

● 33 Frances B, Gout R, Monsarrat B, Cros J, Zajac J-M. Further evidence that morphine-6β-glucuronide is a more potent opioid agonist than morphine. J Pharmacol Exp Ther 1992; **262**: 25–31.

● 34 Osborne R, Thomsen P, Joel S, et al. The analgesic effect of morphine-6-glucuronide. Br J Clin Pharmacol 1992; **34**: 130–8.

35 Dennis GC, Soni D, Dehkordi O, et al. Analgesic responses to intrathecal morphine in relation to CSF concentrations of morphine-3β-glucuronide and morphine-6,beta-glucuronide. Life Sci 1999; **64**: 1725–36.

36 Klepstad P, Kaasa S, Borchgrevink PC. Start of oral morphine to cancer patients: effective serum morphine concentrations and contribution from morphine-6-glucuronide to the analgesia produced by morphine. Eur J Clin Pharmacol 2000; **55**: 713–19.

37 Quigley C, Joel S, Patel N, et al. Plasma concentrations of morphine, morphine-6-glucuronide and their relationship with analgesia and side effects in patients with cancer-related pain. Palliat Med 2003; **17**: 185–90.

38 Klepstad P, Borchgrevink PC, Dale O, et al. Routine drug monitoring of serum concentrations of morphine, morphine-3-glucuronide and morphine-6-glucuronide do not predict clinical observations in cancer patients. Palliat Med 2003; **17**: 679–87.

● 39 Smith MT, Watt JA, Cramond T. Morphine-3-glucuronide – a potent antagonist of morphine analgesia. Life Sci 1990; **47**: 579–85.

40 Gong Q-L, Hedner J, Björkman R, Hedner T. Morphine-3-glucuronide may functionally antagonize morphine-6-glucuronide induced antinociception and ventilatory depression in the rat. Pain 1992; **48**: 249–55.

41 Hewett K, Dickenson AH, McQuay HJ. Lack of effect of morphine-3-glucuronide on the spinal antinociceptive actions of morphine in the rat: an electrophysiological study. Pain 1993; **53**: 59–63.

42 Quellet DM-C, Pollack GM. Effect of prior morphine-3-glucuronide exposure on morphine disposition and antinociception. Biochem Pharmacol 1997; **53**: 1451–7.

● 43 Labella FS, Pinsky C, Havlicek V. Morphine derivatives with diminished opiate receptor potency show enhanced central excitatory activity. Brain Res 1979; **174**: 263–71.

44 Barlett SE, Cramond T, Smith MT. The excitatory effects of morphine-3-glucuronide are attenuated by LY274614, a competitive NMDA receptor antagonist, and by midazolam, an agonist at the benzodiazepine site on the GABA$_A$ receptor complex. Life Sci 1994; **54**: 687–94.

45 Yaksh TL, Harty GJ, Onofrio BM. High doses of spinal morphine produce a nonopiate receptor-mediated hyperesthesia: clinical and theoretic implications. Anesthesiology 1986; **64**: 590–7.

● 46 Yaksh TL, Harty GJ. Pharmacology of the allodynia in rats evoked by high dose intrathecal morphine. J Pharmacol Exp Ther 1988; **244**: 501–7.

47 Morley JS, Miles JB, Wells JC, Bowsher D. Paradoxical pain. Lancet 1992; **340**: 1045.

48 Rozan JP, Kahn CH, Warfield CA. Epidural and intravenous opioid-induced neuroexcitation. Anesthesiology 1995; **83**: 860–3.

49 Sjogren P, Thunedborg LP, Christrup L, et al. Is development of hyperalgesia, allodynia and myoclonus related to morphine metabolism during long-term administration? Acta Anaesthesiol Scand 1998; **42**: 1070–5.

50 Kaiko RF, Foley KM, Grabinski PY, et al. Central nervous system excitatory effects of mepiridine in cancer patients. Ann Neurol 1983; **13**: 180–5.

51 Bruera E, Pereira J. Acute neuropsychiatric findings in a patient receiving fentanyl for cancer pain. Pain 1997; **69**: 199–201.

52 Smith MT. Neuroexcitatory effects of morphine and hydromorphine: evidence implicating the 3-glucuronide metabolites. Clin Exp Pharmacol Physiol 2000; **27**: 524–8.

53 Sjogren P, Jensen N-H, Jensen TS. Disappearance of morphine-induced hyperalgesia after discontinuing or substituting morphine with other opioid agonists. Pain 1994; **59**: 313–16.

54 Penson TP, Joel SP, Clark S, et al. Limited phase 1 study of morphine-3-glucuronide. J Pharm Sci 2001; **90**: 1810–16.

55 Symonds P. Methadone and the elderly. Br Med J 1977; **1**: 512.

56 Hunt G, Bruera E. Respiratory depression in a patient receiving oral methadone for cancer pain. J Pain Symptom Manage 1995; **10**: 636–48.

57 Bruera E, Fainsinger R, Moore M, et al. Local toxicity with subcutaneous methadone. Experience of two centers. Pain 1991; **45**: 141–3.

58 Fainsinger R, Schoeller T, Bruera E. Methadone in the management of cancer pain: a review. Pain 1993; **52**: 137–47.

59 Nilsson MI, Meresaar U, Anggard E. Clinical pharmacokinetics of methadone. Acta Anaesthesiol Scand 1982; **74** (Suppl): S66–9.

60 Gourlay GK, Cherry DA, Cousins MJ. A comparative study of the efficacy and pharmacokinetics of oral methadone and

morphine in the treatment of severe pain in patients with cancer. *Pain* 1986; **25**: 297–312.

● 61 Säwe J. High-dose morphine and methadone in cancer patients. Clinical pharmacokinetic considerations of oral treatment. *Clin Pharmacokinet* 1986; **11**: 87–106.

62 Dole VP, Kreek MJ. Methadone plasma levels: sustained by a reservoir of drug in tissue. *Proc Natl Acad Sci USA* 1973; **70**: 10.

63 Inturrisi CE, Colbum WA, Kaiko RF, *et al*. Pharmacokinetics and pharmacodynamics of methadone in patients with chronic pain. *Clin Pharmacol Ther* 1987; **41**: 392–401.

● 64 Kristensen K, Christensen CB, Christrup L. The mu1, mu 2, delta, kappa opioid receptor binding profiles of methadone stereoisomers and morphine. *Life Sci* 1995; **56**: 45–50.

● 65 Kristensen K, Blemmer T, Angelo HR, *et al*. Stereoselective pharmacokinetics of methadone in chronic pain patients. *Ther Drug Monitor* 1996; **18**: 221–7.

66 Plummer JL, Gourlay GK, Cherry DA, Cousins MJ. Estimation of methadone clearance: application in management of cancer pain. *Pain* 1988; **33**: 313–22.

◆ 67 Ripamonti C, Zecca E, Bruera E. An update on the clinical use of methadone for cancer pain. *Pain* 1997; **70**: 109–15.

68 Mercadante S, Casuccio A, Calderone L. Rapid switching from morphine to methadone in cancer patients with poor response to morphine. *J Clin Oncol* 1999; **17**: 3307–12.

69 Mercadante S, Casuccio A, Groff L, *et al*. Switching from morphine to methadone to improve analgesia and tolerability in cancer patients. A prospective study. *J Clin Oncol* 2001; **19**: 2898–904.

◆ 70 Bruera E, Sweeney C. Methadone use in cancer patients with pain: a review. *J Palliat Med* 2002; **5**: 127–38.

71 Ripamonti C, De Conno F, Groff L, *et al*. Equianalgesic dose/ratio between methadone and other opioid agonists in cancer pain: comparison of two clinical experiences. *Ann Oncol* 1998; **9**: 79–83.

● 72 Ebert B, Andersen S, Krogsgaard-larsen P. Ketobemidone, methadone and pethidine are non-competitive N-methyl-D-aspartate (NMDA) antagonists in the rat cortex and spinal cord. *Neurosci Lett* 1995; **187**: 165–8.

73 Bruera E, Palmer LL, Bosjak S, *et al*. Methadone versus morphine as a first-line strong opioid for cancer pain: a randomised, double-blind study. *J Clin Oncol* 2004; **22**: 185–92.

74 Kalso E, Vainio A. Morphine and oxycodone hydrochloride in the management of cancer pain. *Clin Pharmacol Ther* 1990; **47**: 639–46.

75 Leow KP, Smith MT, Williams B, *et al*. Single-dose and steady-state pharmacokinetics and pharmacodynamics of oxycodone in patients with cancer. *Clin Pharmacol Ther* 1992; **52**: 487–95.

76 Heiskanen T, Olkkola KT, Kalso E. Effects of blocking CYP2D6 on the pharmacokinetics and pharmacodynamics of oxycodone. *Clin Pharmacol Ther* 1998; **64**: 603–11.

77 Poyhia R, Seppala R, Olkkola KT, Kalso E. The pharmacokinetics and metabolism of oxycodone after intramuscular and oral administration to healthy subjects. *Br J Clin Pharmacol* 1992; **33**: 617–21.

78 Mandema JW, Kaiko RF, Oshlak B, *et al*. Characterization and validation of a pharmacokinetic model or controlled-release oxycodone. *Br J Clin Pharmacol* 1996; **42**: 747–56.

79 Kirvela M, Lindgren L, Seppala T, Olkkola KT. The pharmacokinetics of oxycodone in uremic patients undergoing renal transplantation. *J Clin Anesth* 1996; **8**: 13–18.

80 Tallgren M, Olkkola KT, Seppala T, *et al*. Pharmacokinetics and ventilatory effects of oxycodone before and after liver transplantation. *Clin Pharmacol Ther* 1997; **61**: 655–61.

81 Heiskanen T, Kalso E. Controlled-release oxycodone and morphine in cancer related pain. *Pain* 1997; **73**: 37–45.

82 Zhukovsky DS, Walsh D, Doona M. The relative potency between high dose oral oxycodone and morphine: a case illustration. *J Pain Symptom Manage* 1999; **18**: 53–5.

✱ 83 Hanks GW, Conno F, Cherny N, *et al*. Expert Working Group of the Research Network of the European Association for Palliative Care. Morphine and alternative opioids in cancer pain: the EAPC recommendations. *Br J Cancer* 2001; **84**: 587–93.

84 Kaiko RF, Benziger DP, Fitzmartin RD, *et al*. Pharmacokinetic-pharmacodynamic relationship of controlled-release oxycodone. *Clin Pharmacol Ther* 1996; **59**: 52–61.

85 Villiger JW, Ray LJ, Taylor KM. Characteristics of fentanyl binding to the opiate receptor. *Neuropharmacology* 1983; **22**: 447–52.

86 Varvel JR, Sharfer SL, Hwang SS, *et al*. Absorption characteristics of transdermally administered fentanyl. *Anesthesiology* 1989; **70**: 928–34.

◆ 87 Jeal W, Benfield P. Transdermal fentanyl. *Drugs* 1997; **53**: 109–38.

88 Paix A, Cloeman A, Lees J, *et al*. Subcutaneous fentanyl and sufentanil infusion substitution for morphine intolerance in cancer pain management. *Pain* 1995; **63**: 263–9.

89 Sloan PA, Moulin DE, Hays H. A clinical evaluation of Transdermal Therapeutic System Fentanyl for the treatment of cancer pain. *J Pain Symptom Manage* 1998; **16**: 102–11.

● 90 Miser AW, Narang PK, Dothage JA, *et al*. Transdermal fentanyl for pain control in patients with cancer. *Pain* 1989; **37**: 15–21.

91 Zeppetella G. Nebulized and intranasal fentanyl in the management of cancer-related breakthrough pain. *Palliat Med* 2000; **14**: 57–8.

92 Streisand JB, Varvel JR, Stanski DR, *et al*. Absorption and bioavailability of transmucosal fentanylcitrate. *Anesthesiology* 1991; **75**: 223–9.

93 Way WL. Basic mechanisms in narcotic tolerance and physical dependence. *Ann N Y Acad Sci* 1978; **311**: 61–8.

94 Jaffe J. Opiates: Clinical aspects. In: Lowinson JH, Ruiz P, Millman RG, eds. *Substance Abuse. A Comprehensive Textbook*. Baltimore: Williams and Wilkens, 1992: 186–94.

● 95 Savage SR. Addiction in the treatment of pain: significance, recognition and treatment. *J Pain Symptom Manage* 1993; **8**: 265–78.

96 Weissman DE, Haddox JD. Opioid pseudoaddiction: an iatrogenic syndrome. *Pain* 1989; **36**: 363–6.

● 97 Mitchell JM, Basbaum AL, Fields HL. A locus and mechanism of action for associative morphine tolerance. *Nat Neurosci* 2000; **3**: 47–53.

98 Alvarez V, Arttamangkui S, Williams JT. A rave about opioid withdrawal. *Neuron* 2001; **32**: 761–3.

99 Finn AK, Whistletr JL. Endocytosis of the mu opioid receptor reduces tolerance and a cellular hallmark of tolerance to opioids. *Neuron* 2001; **32**: 829–39.

100 Portenoy RK, Payne R. Acute and chronic pain. In: Lowinson JH, Ruiz P, Millmann RG, Langrod JG, eds. *Substance Abuse. A Comprehensive Textbook.* Baltimore: Williams & Wilkins, 1997.

101 Collin E, Cesselin F. Neurobiological mechanisms of opioid tolerance and dependence. *Clin Neuropharmacol* 1991; **14**: 465–88.

● 102 Mao J. Opioid-induced abnormal pain sensitivity: implications in clinical opioid therapy. *Pain* 2002; **100**: 213–17.

103 Laulin JP, Maurette P, Corcuff JB, *et al.* The role of ketamine in preventing fentanyl-induced hyperalgesia and subsequent acute morphine tolerance. *Anesth Analg* 2002; **94**: 1263–9.

104 Sosnowski, M. Pain management: physiopathology, future research and endpoints. *Support Care Cancer* 1993; **1**: 79–88.

105 Mao J, Price DD, Mayer DJ. Mechanisms of hyperalgesia and opioid tolerance: a current view of their possible interactions. *Pain* 1995; **62**: 259–74.

● 106 American Society of Addiction Medicine, Public Policy Statement. *Definitions Related to the Use of Opioids for the Treatment of Chronic Pain.* Chevy Chase, MD: ASAM, 1997.

107 Gardner E. Brain rewarding mechanisms. In: Lowinson JH, Ruiz P, Millman RG, Langrod JG, eds. *Substance Abuse. A Comprehensive Textbook.* Baltimore: Williams and Wilkins, 1997.

108 Halikas J. Craving. In: Lowinson JH, Ruiz P, Millman RG, Langrod JG, eds. *Substance Abuse. A Comprehensive Textbook.* Baltimore: Williams and Wilkins, 1997; 85–90.

● 109 Bryant HU, Bernton EW, Holaday JW. Immunosuppressive effects of chronic morphine treatment in mice. *Life Sci* 1987; **41**: 1731–8.

110 Fecho K, Maslonek KA, Dykstra LA, Lysle DT. Mechanisms whereby macrophage-derived nitrous oxide is involved in morphine-induced suppression of splenic lymphocyte proliferation. *J Pharmacol Exp Ther* 1995; **272**: 477–83.

111 Flores LR, Wahl SM, Bayer BM. Mechanisms of morphine-induced immunosuppression: effect of acute morphine administration on lymphocyte trafficking. *J Pharmacol Exp Ther* 1995; **272**: 1246–51.

112 Yakota T, Uehara K, Nomota Y. Intrathecal morphine suppresses NK cell activity following abdominal surgery. *Can J Anaesth* 2000; **47**: 303–8.

113 Bussierre JL, Adler MW, Rogers TJ, Eisenstein TK. Cytokine reversal of morphine-induced suppression of the antibody response. *J Pharmacol Exp Ther* 1993; **264**: 591–7.

114 Fecho K, Lysle DT. Heroin-induced alterations in leukocyte numbers and apoptosis in the rat spleen. *Cell Immunol* 2000; **202**: 113–23.

115 Rahim RT, Adler MW, Meissler JJ Jr., *et al.* Abrupt or precipitated withdrawal from morphine induces immunosuppression. *J Neuroimmunol* 2002; **127**: 88–95.

116 Sacerdote P, Manfredi B, Mantegazza P, Panerai AE. Antinociceptive and immunosuppressive effects of opiate drugs: a structure related study. *Br J Pharmacol* 1997; **121**: 834–40.

117 De Waal EJ, Van Der Laan JW, Van Loveren H. Effects of prolonged exposure to morphine and methadone on in vivo parameters of immune function in rats. *Toxicology* 1998; **129**: 201–10.

118 Paice JA, Penn RD, Shott S. Intraspinal morphine for chronic pain: a retrospective multicenter study. *J Pain Symptom Manage* 1996; **11**: 71–80.

119 Gybels J, Erdine S, Maeyaert J. Neuromodulation of pain. A consensus statement of the European Federation of IASP Chapters (EFIC). *Eur J Pain* 1998; **2**: 2034–9.

◆ 120 Abs R, Verhelst J, Maeyaert J, *et al.* Endocrine consequences of long-term intrathecal administration of opioids. *J Clin Endocrinol Metab* 2000; **85**: 2215–22.

121 Finch PM, Roberts LJ, Price L, *et al.* Hypogonadism in patients treated with intrathecal morphine. *Clin J Pain* 2000; **16**: 251–4.

122 Roberts LJ, Finch PM, Bhagat CI, Price LM. Sex hormone suppression by intrathecal opioids: a prospective study. *Clin J Pain* 2002; **18**: 144–8.

123 Azizi F, Vagenakis A, Longcope C. Decreased serum testosterone concentration in male heroin and methadone addicts. *Steroids* 1973; **22**: 467–72.

124 Ragni G, De Lauretis L, Bestetti O. Gonadal function in male heroin and methadone addicts. *Int J Androl* 1988; **11**: 93–100.

45

Assessment and management of opioid side effects

CATHERINE SWEENEY, CATHRYN BOGAN

INTRODUCTION

Opioids have been used as analgesics since at least 4000 BC and common side effects such as sedation, nausea, and constipation have long since been recognized. Over the past 20 years opioid use for symptom relief has increased significantly in developed countries.[1] In many countries opioids are now being introduced at earlier stages and used in higher doses in palliative care.[1,2] This appropriate increase in the use of opioids, coupled with increased vigilance, has resulted in increased detection of a number of previously unidentified side effects. The spectrum of neurotoxic side effects is the most notable of these. The increased awareness and identification of opioid side effects has resulted in the development and improvement of management strategies for dealing with these unwanted effects.

In recent years with increased long-term use of opioids such as in the chronic nonmalignant pain situation, effects of prolonged use on the endocrine and immune system are increasingly being recognized and researched. The clinical importance of these effects for palliative care patients is not yet clear.

This chapter will discuss assessment and management of opioid side effects (Table 45.1) in palliative care. It is beyond the scope of this text to discuss the pathophysiology of opioid side effects in detail.

NAUSEA AND VOMITING

Nausea and vomiting are common after an opioid is commenced or the dose is increased. In most patients this

Table 45.1 *Opioid side effects*

Traditionally recognized	Recently recognized
Nausea/vomiting	Opioid-induced neurotoxicity:
Sedation	Severe sedation
Respiratory depression	Cognitive failure/delirium
Constipation	Hallucinations
Noncardiogenic pulmonary	Myoclonus/grand mal seizures
edema	Hyperalgesia/allodynia
Pruritus	Immune system effects
Urinary retention	Endocrine effects
Allergy	(hypopituitarism, hypogonadism)

responds well to antiemetic medication and disappears spontaneously within 3 or 4 days.[3] Occasionally patients experience chronic and severe nausea; this may be more likely in those receiving higher doses of opioids. Opioids can cause nausea by a number of mechanisms, including stimulation of the chemoreceptor trigger zone or the vomiting center,[4] gastroparesis, and constipation. Opioid-induced nausea and vomiting is discussed in detail in Chapter 59.

Assessment

There are many potential causes of nausea and vomiting in patients receiving palliative care, and frequently the etiology is multifactorial in an individual patient. Therefore assessment of these symptoms should take into account other potential contributors. Table 45.2 summarizes common contributors to nausea in patients with cancer. The presence of other symptoms such as constipation, abdominal pain,

Table 45.2 *Possible contributors to nausea in patients with advanced cancer*

Complications of cancer	Disease-modifying and symptom treatments	Other problems
Metabolic abnormalities (e.g. hypercalcemia)	Chemotherapy radiotherapy	Peptic ulcer disease
Bowel obstruction	Opioids	Anxiety
Constipation	Other drugs	
Uncontrolled symptoms (e.g. pain)		
Raised intracranial pressure		

and distension may give clues as to the underlying cause. Assessment and management of nausea in palliative care is discussed in detail in Chapter 59.

Management

Antiemetic medication should be available to patients commencing opioid therapy or who are having a significant dose increase. A number of different antiemetic medications can be used to effectively treat opioid-induced nausea and vomiting in palliative care patients. These include prokinetic agents such as metoclopramide[5,6] and drugs with central nervous system effects such as haloperidol,[7] levopromazine[4] and cyclizine.[8,9] Antiemetic agents which act centrally on the central nervous system (CNS) have the potential to cause side effects, such as sedation, which can add to opioid toxicity in some patients. Corticosteroids have antiemetic effects; there is evidence that the addition of corticosteroids may improve nausea and vomiting in patients who do not initially respond to prokinetic agents.[10**]

Other factors thought to be contributing to nausea and vomiting should if possible be corrected; constipation which frequently coexists in these patients should be treated, metabolic abnormalities corrected and other medications which might contribute should be reduced or discontinued if possible.

SEDATION

Sedation commonly occurs after initiation of opioids and may occur following significant dose increases.[11,12] In the majority of patients this settles after a few days of stable doses. In some patients with severe pain, somnolence during the first days of treatment or after an increase in dose may simply reflect increased comfort after days of pain-induced insomnia rather than true somnolence. In a small percentage of patients, the opioid dose needed for symptom control causes persistent sedation. Sedation is also a feature of opioid-induced neurotoxicity; this is discussed in greater detail below.

Assessment

There are many possible causes of sedation in patients with advanced cancer (Box 45.1). Assessment of sedation should

Box 45.1 Possible contributors to sedation in patients with advanced cancer

- Opioid medications and their metabolites
- Metabolic abnormalities (e.g. hypercalcemia, hyponatremia)
- Renal or hepatic impairment
- Dehydration
- CNS sedatives (e.g. tricyclic antidepressants, benzodiazepines, alcohol)
- Other medications (e.g. nonsteroidal anti-inflammatory drugs [NSAIDs]) causing renal impairment
- CNS involvement with cancer
- Infection

take into account these possible contributors; it is common for a number of factors to be present in an individual patient.

Management

If sedation is present and pain relief is good, it may be possible to reduce the opioid dose. Other potential contributors to sedation should be addressed where possible; metabolic abnormalities and dehydration should be corrected, infection treated, and the use of sedative medication minimized where appropriate. In patients where there is persistent sedation at opioid doses necessary to achieve pain control, adjuvant analgesic measures should be considered to allow reduction in the opioid dose. Such measures include pharmacological and nonpharmacological interventions. Pharmacological interventions include the use of NSAIDs, bisphosphonates, corticosteroids, tricyclic antidepressants, or anticonvulsants. Nonpharmacological measures include radiotherapy and nerve blocks. Alternative routes of administration of analgesics such as intrathecal and epidural administration may also be useful in allowing significant reductions in opioid doses.

If a patient who is obviously sedated continues to complain of pain it is important to consider the possibility that spiritual or psychological distress (somatization) is contributing to their expression of pain (see Chapter 55). In this situation further increases in the opioid dose will lead to increased side effects and will not relieve the patient's suffering. If somatization is suspected, the approach to management should include counseling, treatment of underlying anxiety or depression, and reduction in the opioid dose. The expression of psychosocial suffering as physical symptoms has been identified as an independent predictor of poor pain control in cancer patients.[13]

PSYCHOSTIMULANTS

In patients in whom the dose of opioid needed for analgesia results in persistent sedation, a trial of psychostimulant medication may be helpful. There is evidence that psychostimulants can improve cognitive function and reduce sedation in cancer patients receiving opioids.[14–17] In addition, the use of psychostimulants can allow increased opioid doses and improve analgesia in patients where sedation is limiting the dose of opioid that can be used.[15–18]

Psychostimulants have a number of potential adverse effects including neurotoxic side effects (such as hallucinations, delirium or psychosis), decreased appetite, tolerance and potential for addiction. Before prescribing psychostimulants, careful medical history must be taken to exclude any psychiatric disorder. This is important as stimulants are contraindicated in patients with a history of hallucinations, delirium or paranoid disorders. They are also relatively contraindicated with a history of substance abuse or hypertension.

The best type and dose of psychostimulant for the treatment of opioid-induced sedation has not been determined. Methylphenidate has been the most extensively studied of the group for this indication and is usually commenced at a dose of 5 mg twice daily. A beneficial effect is usually evident within 2 days of treatment and the dose can be increased to 10 mg twice daily. Morning and noon administration are recommended in an attempt to minimize potential sleep disturbance.

Recent preliminary research has highlighted a potential alternative to psychostimulants for the treatment of persistent opioid-induced sedation. Donepezil, a cholinesterase inhibitor used in the treatment of Alzheimer disease was found in an open label study in to reduce sedation and fatigue with cancer pain and opioid-induced sedation.[19] A retrospective study of 40 patients receiving opioids (mainly for cancer pain) also found a reduction in sedation with donepezil treatment.[20]

DRIVING AND OPIOIDS

Opioids have the potential to interfere with driving ability by impairing psychomotor skills and/or cognitive function.

A recent evidence-based review of driving-related skills in opioid-dependent/tolerant patients concluded that the majority of studies reviewed found no evidence of impaired driving-related skills.[21***] However, the review grouped three different populations of patients on opioids together: former addicts on maintenance programs, patients with chronic nonmalignant pain, and patients with chronic cancer pain. The majority of studies reviewed were carried out in the former population and there was some lack of consistency in the findings of studies in cancer patients.

In palliative care populations, the situation is more complicated. The underlying disease as well as other medications and treatments may contribute to impairment of skills that are considered to be important for driving. A number of studies looking at cognitive function and psychomotor abilities have been carried out in cancer patients receiving opioids.[22–26] In some studies, when compared with healthy controls, cancer patients receiving opioids have been found to have delayed continuous reaction times.[22,23] However, in studies comparing cancer patients receiving stable opioid doses with those not receiving opioids there appears to be some evidence that both populations are similar in terms of psychomotor and cognitive skills.[24*,25*] When both these groups were compared to healthy controls some deficits were found.[25] A study looking at the influence of opioid use, pain and performance status on neurophysiological function found that both pain and performance status appeared to affect neurophysiological tests; long-term use opioids did not in itself appear to negatively affect these tests.[26] Controlled studies of actual driving ability in cancer patients on opioids have not been carried out. Further research is needed in this area.

In general, cancer patients receiving opioids should be advised that their ability to drive may be compromised and that they should not drive if they feel drowsy or sedated. In addition, patients should be advised to avoid driving for 4–5 days after initiation of opioid medication or after a dose increase. They should also be informed that other medications used to treat symptoms can cause sedation and to check with their physician before driving if in doubt. Advising a patient to do a driving test may be appropriate if there is concern about a patient's driving ability and they are anxious to continue driving.

RESPIRATORY DEPRESSION

Respiratory depression is a potentially fatal side effect of opioids. It primarily occurs in opioid-naïve patients who are administered an excess dose of opioid. However it can occur in opioid-tolerant patients in a few situations. First, it may occur when there is a sudden reduction in opioid requirements, e.g. following a successful neurolytic block resulting in reduced pain. It is important to anticipate this possible situation and therefore consider reduction of opioid dose

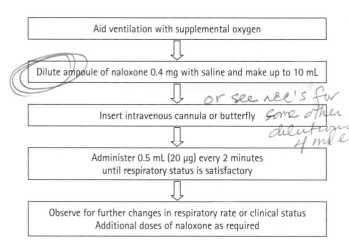

Handwritten note: *or see ref's for some other dilutions 4 ml etc*

Figure 45.1 *Guidelines for appropriate use of naloxone in opioid-induced respiratory depression based on recommendations of the American Pain Society.[31]*

following any intervention which may significantly reduce pain.[27] It may also occur following opioid rotation, in particular when rotating to methadone (see below).[28] Respiratory depression has also been described in a patient with renal impairment due to the build-up of morphine metabolites.[29]

Management involves reducing or omitting the next regular opioid dose or stopping an infusion temporarily to allow plasma levels to reduce and then recommencing the infusion at a lower dose. Opioid-induced sedation in the absence of respiratory depression is not an indication for using naloxone. Naloxone in these patients can result in opioid withdrawal syndrome and severe pain.[30] Naloxone is only indicated if there is significant respiratory depression, i.e. a respiratory rate of <8 breaths/minute, if the patient is barely rousable and/or cyanosed. Figure 45.1 summarizes the use of naloxone in opioid-induced respiratory depression. Naloxone has a shorter half-life than most opioids therefore it is important to observe patients carefully over a period of hours. Additional administration of naloxone may be required if the respiratory rate falls or clinical status changes.

CONSTIPATION

Opioids cause constipation by affecting the intestine by reducing gastrointestinal motility and secretions and increasing intestinal fluid absorption and blood flow.[32] Constipation is a common side effect of opioid therapy. It occurs in approximately 90 percent of patients treated with opioids.[33] Tolerance to constipation develops very slowly and most patients continue to require laxative therapy for the duration of opioid use. All opioids cause constipation although there is preliminary evidence to suggest that fentanyl may be less constipating than morphine,[34] and in a retrospective study of laxative use, laxative doses needed were found to be significantly lower with methadone than

with equianalgesic doses of morphine or hydromorphone.[35] Constipation is discussed in detail in Chapter 60 of this volume.

Assessment

Constipation should be suspected in all patients taking opioids. Frequently several other factors predisposing to constipation coexist in palliative care patients. Box 45.2 summarizes these factors.

Box 45.2 Factors contributing to constipation in palliative care patients

- Opioids
- Electrolyte disturbances (e.g. hypercalcemia, hypokalemia)
- Dehydration
- Other medication (e.g. tricyclic antidepressants)
- Reduced oral intake
- Abdominal surgery
- Abdominal involvement with cancer
- Immobility
- Autonomic failure

Assessment should include a history of the frequency and difficulty of defecation and consideration of other possible contributors. Physical examination should include palpation of the abdomen and a rectal examination. Occasionally an abdominal X-ray may be required if the history is unclear.[36,37]

Management

Prevention of constipation should be a priority when patients are starting opioid medication. Patients should be advised of the likelihood of developing constipation and have laxatives prescribed and the dose titrated until effective. Even patients with poor oral intake should be advised to use laxatives to prevent constipation. Patients should also be encouraged to take plenty of fluids.

Where a number of factors are thought to be contributing to constipation a multimodal approach to management will be required. Management can be divided into general and specific interventions. General interventions involve the elimination of medical factors that may be contributing to constipation (e.g. treatment of electrolyte abnormalities such as hypercalcemia, rehydration, discontinuation of all non-essential constipating drugs). Attention should be given to providing comfort and privacy to patients during defecation. Specific interventions involve the use of laxatives, suppositories and enemas, and manual disimpaction. Usually a combination of laxatives with different modes of action is used. However, treatment with a combination of laxatives is not sufficient for all patients; up to 40 percent of patients with advanced cancer also require other measures such as the use of enemas and/or manual disimpaction.[33] For most patients, enemas and rectal suppositories are only needed for short-term management of more severe episodes of constipation. Occasionally the use of long-term rectal laxatives or enemas is required.

There is evidence that the opioid antagonist naloxone (used orally)[38**] can be effective in the treatment of opioid-induced constipation in patients with advanced cancer. However, opioid withdrawal occurs in some patients treated with oral naloxone for constipation.[38–40] The first peripheral opioid receptor antagonist methylnaltrexone (used intravenously) has been found in a randomized controlled trial to be effective in treating opioid-induced constipation in subjects in a methadone maintenance program.[41**] Oral methylnaltrexone also offers a potential treatment option for this problem[42] Methylnaltrexone does not appear to cause problems with analgesia or withdrawal.[41,42] Other treatment options for patients with persistent troublesome constipation not responding to the usual measures include the use of prokinetic agents (e.g. metoclopramide, domperidone)[43] or to consider opioid rotation to methadone or fentanyl.

NONCARDIOGENIC PULMONARY EDEMA

Noncardiogenic pulmonary edema is a rare opioid side effect which has been mainly reported following illicit opioid use. It has recently been described in patients receiving treatment for cancer pain.[44] In this setting it has usually been reported following rapid escalation of opioid dose in the days prior to onset. Patients usually present with acute onset of tachypnea and cyanosis. The pathophysiology of opioid-induced noncardiogenic pulmonary edema is not clearly understood.

Assessment

Physical examination of the patient usually reveals bilateral rales (crepitations) in the absence of other signs of cardiac failure. Chest X-ray may show bilateral infiltrates. An electrocardiogram should be performed to rule out an acute cardiac cause for the symptoms. A high index of suspicion is necessary to make the diagnosis.

Management

In a palliative care setting with a conservative approach to management there appears to be high mortality associated with the development of this side effect. Evidence on the best management approach in this setting is lacking. Measures such as reduction in opioid dose and avoidance of possible precipitating factors such as overhydration, excessive oxygen therapy, and use of corticosteroids have been suggested.[44] One approach is to attempt to reduce the risk of development of noncardiogenic pulmonary edema by avoiding rapid escalation of opioid doses where possible. The use of adjuvant analgesics, epidural or intrathecal administration of analgesics, and opioid rotation are all measures that may be considered in circumstances where pain control is inadequate and opioid requirements have been rising rapidly.

URINARY RETENTION

Opioids can increase smooth muscle tone, resulting in increased sphincter tone. Urinary hesitancy and retention can therefore result from opioid use. These side effects are commoner in elderly patients and in those receiving opioids intrathecally.[45] In patients who develop hesitancy or retention while on opioid medication, other potential causes of these symptoms should also be considered such as concomitant use of tricyclic antidepressants, severe constipation, bladder outlet obstruction, and impending spinal cord compression. Approaches to management include changing the route of administration, changing the opioid, and the use of a urinary catheter.

PRURITUS

Pruritus (itch) is a relatively common side effect following intrathecal and epidural administration of opioids[46] and is less common after oral administration. It can be a very troublesome symptom for individual patients.[47] The pathophysiology of opioid-induced pruritus is not clearly understood; it does not appear to be related to histamine release.[48] Many conditions common in palliative patients can cause itch; Chapter 78 discusses pruritus in detail.

Treatment options for opioid-induced itch have mainly been researched in patients undergoing surgical procedures or cesarean sections under epidural or spinal anesthesia and several of these studies have looked at agents as prophylaxis rather than treatment.[49] There is evidence supporting the use of naloxone,[50**] droperidol,[51] butorphanol,[52] and ondansetron[53] to prevent opioid-induced pruritus in surgical and obstetric settings. Treatments that have been suggested in palliative care include opioid antagonists and ondansetron.[48] Use of opioid antagonists can result in antagonism of analgesia. A change to an alternative opioid has been reported to be very effective in individual case reports.[47,54]

ALLERGIC REACTIONS

Hypersensitivity reactions to opioids appear to be rare. Patients often consider side effects of a medication (e.g. nausea, sedation) to be an allergy; hence it is important to check what problems a specific medication has caused for an individual patient. In the case of opioid side effects reassurance, explanation, and appropriate treatment should be offered to patients.

OPIOID-INDUCED NEUROTOXICITY

Opioid-induced neurotoxicity (OIN) describes a syndrome of neuropsychiatric side effects seen with opioid therapy. This syndrome has been described only relatively recently.[55–57] Features of OIN are listed in Table 45.1. These features can exist singly or in combination. If any of these features are present in a patient taking opioid medication, OIN should be suspected.

Sedation

Sedation associated with OIN is persistent and frequently severe. It is often present with other features such as cognitive impairment and delirium. Sedation and its management have been discussed earlier in this chapter.

Cognitive impairment and delirium

Cognitive impairment and delirium are common features in patients with cancer.[58] While there are many potential causes (Box 45.3), opioid use is considered to be a major factor.[59,60]

Box 45.3 Causes of cognitive impairment/delirium

- Drug induced (e.g. opioids, antimuscarinics, corticosteroids)
- Biochemical (e.g. hypercalcemia, hyponatremia)
- Infection
- Dehydration
- Renal or hepatic failure
- Brain metastases
- Constipation
- General deterioration
- Withdrawal (e.g. alcohol, benzodiazepines, nicotine)

The extent to which various opioids contribute to delirium has not been well studied.[61]

Classically delirium is associated with an agitated hyperactive state, however, it must be remembered that delirium can also present with withdrawn, hypoactive features. This nonagitated delirium may be underrecognized by healthcare professionals. Occasionally, features of hyperactivity and hypoactivity may occur concurrently.[62,63]

Hallucinations

In OIN, hallucinations are typically visual in nature, although tactile hallucinations are not uncommon. Auditory hallucinations may also occur. The overall prevalence of hallucinations in the palliative care setting is unknown. The prevalence of visual hallucinations has been reported as 1 percent[64] while more recent work has reported the figure to be nearer 50 percent.[65] Patients are often reluctant to spontaneously admit to experiencing hallucinations. They may find them frightening and could fear that they have developed a psychiatric illness. While hallucinations are a known feature of OIN, they are also caused by other conditions and numerous medications, therefore one should look for other symptoms and signs of OIN. Hallucinations are commonly associated with cognitive impairment but are occasionally seen in patients who have not experienced cognitive impairment.[66] A sudden change in mood (anxiety or depression) may be the only indication of the presence of hallucinations.[67]

Myoclonus and seizures

Myoclonus is a sudden, shocklike involuntary movement caused by active muscular contractions which may involve a whole muscle or may be limited to a small number of muscle fibers.[63] It has been postulated that generalized myoclonus is a type of tonic-clonic seizure.[68] Myoclonus is one of the more frequently observed features of OIN and if present there should be a high index of suspicion for the diagnosis. It has been described following administration of morphine,[56,69] hydromorphone,[70,71] meperidine,[72,73] fentanyl,[74,75] and diamorphine.[76] It has been proposed that myoclonus results from accumulation of neurotoxic opioid metabolites.[77] Myoclonus may occur more commonly in those patients taking antidepressants, antipsychotics or NSAIDs.[78] Myoclonus may also occur with renal failure alone.

Hyperalgesia and allodynia

Abnormally heightened pain sensations can occur with opioids. These are characterized by a lowering of the pain threshold (hyperalgesia) and pain elicited by normally innocuous stimulation (allodynia).[79] Hyperalgesia may present as an exaggerated nociceptive response to a painful stimulus or as a worsening of the underlying pain syndrome, termed paradoxical pain.[80] This paradoxical pain may be misinterpreted by clinicians and the opioid dose increased further, resulting in worsening OIN. Morphine-3-glucuronide, normorphine, and hydromorphone have been shown to produce allodynia in rats after intrathecal administration; however, the exact mechanism is still unclear.[81,82]

Mechanism of opioid-induced neurotoxicity

It has been reported that several opioids and their active metabolites may contribute to OIN. Morphine, hydromorphone, and fentanyl have all been found to cause agitation, myoclonus, hyperalgesia, and tonic-clonic seizures in animals when administered systemically or intrathecally.[68,83–85] Morphine has been investigated extensively and is predominately metabolized to morphine-3-glucuronide (M3G) and morphine-6-glucuronide (M6G).[86,87] It has been postulated that M3G is responsible for some of the neuroexcitatory effects of morphine, while being devoid of analgesic properties.[88] Evidence for the role of M3G or similar metabolites is conflicting. More recent research reports that M3G failed to produce excitatory and antianalgesic effects in rats[89] and in a phase I healthy volunteer study M3G did not illicit any clinical effects when given alone nor did it antagonize the effects of morphine or M6G.[90] The possibility of interindividual variation in metabolism of opioids is but one of a number of possibilities for these conflicting findings. The precise mechanism of OIN remains unclear. Further research is required to gain a better understanding of the pathophysiology of OIN.

ASSESSMENT

Numerous risk factors predispose patients to the development of OIN. These are summarized in Box 45.4. Assessment includes an accurate history focusing particularly on symptoms of OIN. It is important to enquire specifically about hallucinations. Vivid dreams are sometimes a feature of OIN. A detailed medication history is important; information should be sought about the onset of features following commencement or dose increases of opioids, addition of psychoactive medications or drugs that may impair renal function.

Examination should look for signs of infection, dehydration and jerking movements should be noted. Cognitive function should be assessed as a matter of routine. A number of tools exist to assess cognitive function.[62] Although no gold standard tool has been identified, the Mini-Mental State Examination [91] has been widely used in this population.[92] Other tools include the Memorial Delirium Assessment Scale (MDAS)[93] and the Delirium Rating Scale (DRS).[94] Confusion and delirium assessment is covered in more detail in Chapter 72.

Box 45.4 Factors predisposing to OIN

- Large doses of opioids
- Extended period of treatment with opioids
- Dehydration
- Renal failure
- Infection
- Rapid opioid dose escalation (more likely to occur with): neuropathic pain; incident pain; tolerance; somatization/emotional pain; substance abuse
- Recent reduction in analgesic requirements (may follow): addition of nonopioid drugs (e.g. NSAIDs) or adjuvant analgesics (e.g. anticonvulsants, recent radiotherapy or chemotherapy or anesthetic intervention)
- Borderline cognitive impairment/delirium
- Use of other psychoactive drugs (e.g. benzodiazepines)
- Older age

If OIN is suspected, blood should be sent for biochemical and hematological analysis. An elevated white cell count may indicate the presence of infection, and the existence of renal failure or hypercalcemia must be excluded.

MANAGEMENT

Box 45.5 outlines the approaches to management of acute episodes of OIN. There are numerous reports detailing reduction in dose or discontinuation of opioids as successful treatment of OIN.[92,95,96] Dose reduction may not always be possible, especially if uncontrolled pain is a problem. In this situation the addition of nonopioid co-analgesics, adjuvant analgesics, and the use of specific antitumor therapies such as radiotherapy, chemotherapy, or anesthetic intervention to reduce opioid requirements should be considered.[97]

Opioid rotation, or opioid switching, is the term given to the practice of substituting one strong opioid with another to obtain better analgesic control and reduce opioid side effects. It requires knowledge of the approximate conversion ratios of the two different opioids. When switching it is common practice to use lower doses than predicted according to opioid dose conversion tables.[97,98] The situation with rotations involving methadone is more complex. The relation between increasing opioid doses and methadone dose is not linear; the higher the previous opioid dose the greater the relative potency of methadone.[99] It also should be remembered that methadone has complex pharmacokinetics resulting in a long and variable elimination half-life.

Box 45.5 Approaches to management of OIN

- Hydration (oral·or parenteral)

- Treat reversible causes (antibiotics for infection, bisphosphonates for hypercalcemia)

- Opioid reduction or in severe cases discontinuation of regular opioid

- Stop other contributing drugs (e.g. hypnotics)

- Maximize use of nonopioid analgesics (e.g. NSAIDs)

- Commence/titrate adjuvant analgesics (e.g. anticonvulsants, tricyclic antidepressants)

- Opioid rotation

- Symptomatic treatment (benzodiazepines for myoclonus, haloperidol for hallucinations)

- Reassurance and explanation

Box 45.6 Prevention of further episodes of neurotoxicity

- Identify and manage risk factors for OIN

- Carefully monitor for early signs of OIN

- Educate patient and family about risk factors and early signs of OIN

- Educate primary care physician about risk factors and early signs of OIN

- Careful monitoring post radiotherapy, chemotherapy or anesthetic intervention

---

Numerous conversion regimens exist[100–103] however, no gold standard has emerged. The most common error when opioid rotating to methadone is to underestimate its duration of action. Late toxicity may develop, possibly even 10 days following rotation. Extreme caution should be exercised when opioid rotating to methadone and one should be vigilant for signs of toxicity which may be subtle. Variations in analgesia or adverse effects following rotation are thought to result from a variety of mechanisms including receptor activity, asymmetry in cross-tolerance among different opioids, differing opioid efficacies, and accumulation of toxic metabolites.[98] Numerous studies have described the use of opioid rotation as a safe and effective method for reducing neurotoxicity while simultaneously retaining analgesia.[88,101,102,104–107] Although the success of opioid rotation has been extensively reported in the literature, these have been mainly case reports, retrospective studies or prospective uncontrolled studies. Despite the fact that opioid rotation is widely accepted in clinical practice, evidence to date is largely anecdotal or based on observational and uncontrolled trials.[108] Opioid rotation has, as yet, not been systematically studied in randomized controlled trials. Once OIN has been recognized and treated, steps must be taken to reduce the risk of further episodes (Box 45.6).

ENDOCRINE AND IMMUNE SYSTEM EFFECTS

Evidence is emerging that opioids have potential effects on the functioning of endocrine and immune systems. In one study patients with nonmalignant pain receiving long-term intrathecal opioid (n = 73) were compared with a group with similar pain syndromes; the opioid treatment group were found to be significantly more likely to have hypogonadic hypogonadism. Growth hormone deficiency and hypocorticism were also more likely in this group.[109] In intravenous drug users, opioids appear to affect the immune defense system and have been implicated in the pathogenesis of infection.[110]

The implications of these findings for palliative care patients and in particular for those with advanced disease are unknown and further research is required before evidence-based recommendations can be made on appropriate assessment and management.

PSYCHOLOGICAL DEPENDENCE AND SUBSTANCE ABUSE

Opioids are potential drugs of addiction. Psychological dependence is a key feature of addiction and involves compulsive behavior to obtain and take a drug for its psychological effects. Hence, psychological dependence involves substance misuse or abuse. Fear of addiction is common in patients and physicians and can lead to under-use of opioids in palliative care populations. Opiophobia should not prevent opioids being prescribed where they are needed. In clinical practice psychological dependence and opioid abuse are rare in patients who do not have a preexisting history of drug or alcohol abuse.[111,112] Physical dependence is often confused with psychological dependence. However, physical dependence (the appearance of withdrawal symptoms and signs when a drug is abruptly discontinued) is common when patients have been taking opioids for a period of time; this does not mean that a patient is addicted to an opioid. Abrupt discontinuation or dramatic reductions in opioid doses should be avoided. If a major dose reduction or discontinuation is desired, doses should be gradually reduced over several days. The management of pain in patients with drug and alcohol dependence is discussed in detail in Chapter 56.

Key learning points

- There are a number of common opioid side effects. It is important that these are identified as they can add significantly to symptom burden in palliative care patients; most are preventable or treatable with relatively simple measures.

- In palliative care patients there may be other contributors to common opioid side effects; these should be identified and corrected where possible.

- Nausea and vomiting are common after initiation or recent opioid dose increases. These symptoms often resolve spontaneously after a few days. Antiemetic medications such as metoclopramide, haloperidol or cyclizine are usually effective. Addition of corticosteroids can be helpful in resistant cases.

- Sedation is a common problem after initiation or recent opioid dose increases and usually resolves after 3–4 days. If it is a persistent problem the following measures can be considered: (i) reduction in opioid dose if pain control is good; (ii) reduce opioid requirements by treating pain with addition of nonopioid or adjuvant analgesic medications, alternative route of opioid delivery (epidural or intrathecal), radiotherapy or nerve blocks; (iii) if OIN is thought to be present it should be managed as described in text; (iv) psychostimulants or donepezil; (v) psychological or spiritual distress may be contributing to the patient's expression of pain. These issues should be explored and managed appropriately.

- Constipation is extremely common; the majority of patients require initiation of laxative treatment when opioids are started and continuation of this for the duration of treatment with opioids.

- Opioid-induced neurotoxicity is a relatively recently identified syndrome of opioid side effects. Features include severe sedation, cognitive failure, delirium, hallucinations, myoclonus, hyperalgesia, and allodynia, and one or more of these may be present. Treatment options include a combination of hydration, opioid dose reduction/opioid rotation, and correction of possible contributors such as infection and electrolyte abnormalities (see text).

REFERENCES

1   World Health Organization. *Cancer Pain Relief*, 2nd ed. Report of a WHO Expert Committee. Geneva: WHO, 1996.

2   Bruera E, Macmillan K, Hanson J, MacDonald RN. Palliative care in a cancer center: results in 1984 versus 1987. *J Pain Symptom Manage* 1990; **5**: 1–5.

3   Clarke RS. Nausea and vomiting. *Br J Anaesth* 1984; **56**: 19–27.

4   Twycross R, Barkby G, Hallwood P. The use of low dose levomepromazine in the management of nausea and vomiting. *Prog Palliat Care* 1997; **5**: 49–53.

5   Bruera E, Seifert L, Watanabe S, *et al.* Chronic nausea in advanced cancer patients: a retrospective assessment of a metoclopramide-based antiemetic regimen. *J Pain Symptom Manage* 1996; **11**: 147–53.

6   Bruera E, Belzile M, Neumann C, *et al.* A double-blind, crossover study of controlled-release metoclopramide and placebo for the chronic nausea and dyspepsia of advanced cancer. *J Pain Symptom Manage* 2000; **19**: 427–35.

7   Vella-Brincat J, Macleod AD. Haloperidol in palliative care. *Palliat Med* 2004; **18**:195–201.

8   Walder A, Aitkenhead A. A comparison of droperidol and cyclizine in the prevention of postoperative nausea and vomiting associated with patient-controlled analgesia. *Anaesthesia* 1995; **50**: 654–6.

9   Dundee J, Jones P. The prevention of analgesic-induced nausea and vomiting by cyclizine. *Br J Clin Pract* 1968; **22**: 379–82.

10   Bruera ED, Roca E, Cedaro L, *et al.* Improved control of chemotherapy-induced emesis by the addition of dexamethasone to metoclopramide in patients resistant to metoclopramide. *Cancer Treat Rep* 1983; **67**: 381–3.

11   Sjogren P, Banning AM, Christensen CB, Pedersen O. Continuous reaction time after single dose, long-term oral and epidural opioid administration. *Eur J Anaesth* 1994; **11**: 95–100.

12   Bruera E, Macmillan K, Hanson J, MacDonald RN. The cognitive effects of the administration of narcotic analgesics in patients with cancer pain. *Pain* 1989; **39**: 13–16.

13   Bruera E, Schoeller T, Wenk R, *et al.* A prospective multicenter assessment of the Edmonton staging system for cancer pain. *J Pain Symptom Manage* 1995; **10**: 348–55.

14   Bruera E, Miller MJ, Macmillan K, Kuehn N. Neuropsychological effects of methylphenidate in patients receiving a continuous infusion of narcotics for cancer pain. *Pain* 1992; **48**: 163–6.

15   Bruera E, Chadwick S, Brenneis C, *et al.* Methylphenidate associated with narcotics for the treatment of cancer pain. *Cancer Treat Rep* 1987; **71**: 67–70.

◆ 16   Rozans M, Dreisbach A, Lertora JJ, Kahn MJ. Palliative uses of methylphenidate in patients with cancer: a review. *J Clin Oncol* 2002; **20**: 335–9.

◆ 17   Dalal S, Melzack R. Potentiation of opioid analgesia by psychostimulant drugs: a review. *J Pain Symptom Manage* 1998; **16**: 245–53.

18   Bruera E, Fainsinger R, MacEachern T, Hanson J. The use of methylphenidate in patients with incident cancer pain receiving regular opiates. A preliminary report. *Pain* 1992; **50**: 75–7.

19   Bruera E, Strasser F, Shen L, *et al.* The effect of donepezil on sedation and other symptoms in patients receiving opioids for cancer pain: a pilot study. *J Pain Symptom Manage* 2003; **26**: 1049–54

20   Slatkin N, Rhiner M. Treatment of opioid-related sedation: utility of the cholinesterase inhibitors. *J Support Oncol* 2003; **1**: 53–63.

◆ 21   Fishbain DA, Cutler RB, Rosomoff HL, Rosomoff RS. Are opioid-dependent/tolerant patients impaired in driving-related skills?

A structured evidence-based review. *J Pain Symptom Manage* 2003; **25**: 559–77.

22 Sjogren P, Banning A. Pain, sedation and reaction time during long-term treatment of cancer patients with oral and epidural opioids. *Pain* 1989; **39**: 5–1.

23 Banning A, Sjogren P. Cerebral effects of long-term oral opioids in cancer patients measured by continuous reaction time. *Clin J Pain* 1990; **6**: 91–5.

24 Vainio A, Ollila J, Matikainen E, *et al.* Driving ability in cancer patients receiving long-term morphine analgesia. *Lancet* 1995; **346**: 667–70.

25 Clemons M, Regnard C, Appleton T. Alertness, cognition and morphine in patients with advanced cancer. *Cancer Treat Rev* 1996; **22**: 451–68.

26 Sjogren P, Olsen AK, Thomsen AB, Dalberg. Neuropsychological performance in cancer patients: the role of oral opioids, pain and performance status. *Pain* 2000: **86**: 237–45.

27 Hanks GW, Twycross RG, Lloyd JW. Unexpected complication of successful nerve block. Morphine induced respiratory depression precipitated by removal of severe pain. *Anaesthesia* 1981; **36**: 37–9.

28 Hunt G, Bruera E. Respiratory depression in a patient receiving oral methadone for cancer pain. *J Pain Symptom Manage* 1995; **10**: 401–4.

29 Osborne RJ, Joel SP, Slevin ML. Morphine intoxication in renal failure: the role of morphine-6-glucuronide. *Br Med J (Clin Res Ed)* 1986; **292**: 1548–9.

30 Manfredi PL, Ribeiro S, Chandler SW, Payne R. Inappropriate use of naloxone in cancer patients with pain. *J Pain Symptom Manage* 1996; **11**: 131–4.

✱ 31 Max MB and Payne R. *Principles of Analgesic Use in the Treatment of Acute Pain and Cancer Pain.* Skokie, IL: American Pain Society, 1992.

32 De Luca A, Coupar IM. Insights into opioid action in the intestinal tract. *Pharmacol Ther* 1996; **69**: 103–15.

33 Twycross RG, Lack SA, eds. *Control of Alimentary Symptoms in Far Advanced Cancer.* London: Churchill Livingstone, 1986: 166–207.

34 Hunt R, Fazekas B, Thorne D, Brooksbank M. A comparison of subcutaneous morphine and fentanyl in hospice cancer patients. *J Pain Symptom Manage* 1999; **18**: 111–19.

35 Mancini I, Hanson J, Neumann C, Bruera E. Opioid type and other clinical predictors of laxative dose in advanced cancer patients: A retrospective study. *J Palliat Med* 2000; **3**: 49–56.

36 Bruera E, Suarez-Almazor M, Velasco A, *et al.* The assessment of constipation in terminal cancer patients admitted to a palliative care unit: a retrospective review. *J Pain Symptom Manage* 1994; **9**: 515–19.

37 Starreveld JS, Pols MA, Van Wijk HJ, *et al.* The plain abdominal radiograph in the assessment of constipation. *Gastroenterology* 1990; **28**: 335–8.

38 Sykes NP. An investigation of the ability of oral naloxone to correct opioid-related constipation in patients with advanced cancer. *Palliat Med* 1996; **10**: 135–44.

39 Culpepper-Morgan JA, Inturrisi CE, Portenoy RK, *et al.* Treatment of opioid-induced constipation with oral naloxone: a pilot study. *Clin Pharmacol Ther* 1992; **52**: 90–5.

40 Meissner W, Schmidt U, Hartmann M, *et al.* Oral naloxone reverses opioid-associated constipation. *Pain* 2000; **84**: 105–9.

41 Yuan CS, Foss JF, O'Connor M, *et al.* Methylnaltrexone for reversal of constipation due to chronic methadone use: a randomized controlled trial. *JAMA* 2000; **283**: 367–72.

42 Yuan CS, Foss JF. Oral methylnaltrexone for opioid-induced constipation. *JAMA* 2000; **284**: 1383–4.

43 Bruera E, Brenneis C, Michaud M, MacDonald N. Continuous Sc infusion of metoclopramide for treatment of narcotic bowel syndrome. *Cancer Treat Rep* 1987; **71**:1121–2.

44 Bruera E, Miller MJ. Non-cardiogenic pulmonary edema after narcotic treatment for cancer pain. *Pain* 1989; **39**: 297–300.

◆ 45 Cousins MJ, Mather LE. Intrathecal and epidural administration of opioids. *Anesthesiology* 1984; **61**: 276–310.

46 Ballantyne JC, Loach AB, Carr DB. Itching after epidural and spinal opiates. *Pain* 1988; **33**: 149–60.

47 Katcher J, Walsh D. Opioid-induced itching: morphine sulfate and hydromorphone hydrochloride. *J Pain Symptom Manage* 1999; **17**: 70–2.

◆ 48 Twycross R, Greaves MW, Handwerker H, *et al.* Itch: scratching more than the surface. *Q J Med* 2003; **96**: 7–26.

◆ 49 Kjellberg F, Tramer MR. Pharmacological control of opioid-induced pruritus: a quantitative systematic review of randomized trials. *Eur J Anaesthesiol* 2001; **18**: 346–57.

50 Choi JH, Lee J, Choi JH, Bishop MJ. Epidural naloxone reduces pruritus and nausea without affecting analgesia by epidural morphine in bupivacaine. *Can J Anaesth* 2000; **47**:33–7.

51 Horta ML, Ramos L, Goncalves ZR. The inhibition of epidural morphine-induced pruritus by epidural droperidol. *Anesth Analg* 2000; **90**: 638–41.

52 Gunter JB, McAuliffe J, Gregg T, *et al.* Continuous epidural butorphanol relieves pruritus associated with epidural morphine infusions in children. *Paediatr Anaesth* 2000; **10**: 167–72.

53 Yeh HM, Chen LK, Lin CJ, *et al.* Prophylactic intravenous ondansetron reduces the incidence of intrathecal morphine-induced pruritus in patients undergoing cesarean delivery. *Anesth Analg* 2000; **91**: 172–5.

54 Mercadante S, Villari P, Fulfaro F. Rifampicin in opioid-induced itching. *Support Care Cancer* 2001; **9**: 467–8.

55 Sjogren P, Jonsson T, Jensen NH, *et al.* Hyperalgesia and myoclonus in terminal cancer patients treated with continuous intravenous morphine. *Pain* 1993; **55**: 93–7.

56 Sjogren P, Jensen NH, Jensen TS. Disappearance of morphine-induced hyperalgesia after discontinuing or substituting morphine with other opioid agonists. *Pain* 1994; **59**: 313–16.

57 Bruera E, Pereira J. Neuropsychiatric toxicity of opioids. In: Jensen TS, Turner JA, Wiesenfeld-Hallin Z, eds. *Proceedings of the 8th World Congress on Pain, Progress in Pain Research and Management,* Vol 8. Seattle: IASP Press, 1997: 717–37.

58 Bruera E, Miller L, McCallion J, *et al.* Cognitive failure in patients with terminal cancer: a prospective study. *J Pain Symptom Manage* 1992; **7**: 192–5.

59 Leipzig RM, Goodman H, Gray G, *et al.* Reversible, narcotic-associated mental status impairment in patients with metastatic cancer. *Pharmacology* 1987; **35**: 47–54.

60 Lawlor PG. The panorama of opioid-related dysfunction in patients with cancer: a critical literature appraisal. *Cancer* 2002; 94:1836–53.

◆ 61 McNicol E, Horowicz-Mehler N, Fisk RA, *et al.* Management of opioid side effects in cancer-related and chronic noncancer pain: a systematic review. *J Pain* 2003: **4**: 231–56.

◆ 62   Centeno C, Sanz A, Bruera E. Delirium in advanced cancer patients. *Palliat Med* 2004; **18**; 184–94.

63   Pereira J, Bruera E. Emerging neuropsychiatric toxicities of opioids. *J Pharm Care Pain Symptom Control* 1997; **5**: 3–29.

64   Regnard CL, Tempest S, ed. *Managing Opioid Adverse Effects. A guide to Symptom Relief in Advanced Disease*, 4th ed. Hale: Hochland and Hochland, 1998: 21.

65   Fountain A. Visual hallucinations: a prevalence study among hospice inpatients. *Palliat Med* 2001; **15**: 19–25.

66   Bruera E, Schoeller T, Montejo G. Organic hallucinosis in patients receiving high doses of opiates for cancer pain. *Pain* 1992; **48**: 397–9.

67   Lowe GR. The phenomenology of hallucinations as an aid to differential diagnosis. *Br J Psychiatry* 1973; **123**: 621–33.

68   Marsden CD, Hallet M, Fahn S. The nosology and patho- physiology of myoclonus. In: Marsden CD, Fahn S, eds. *Movement Disorders.* London: Butterworth, 1982: 196–248.

69   Sjogren P, Dragsted L, Christensen CB. Myoclonic spasms during treatment with high doses of intravenous morphine in renal failure. *Acta Anaesthesiol Scand* 1993; **37**: 780–2.

70   MacDonald N, Der L, Allan S, Champion P. Opioid hyper- excitability: the application of alternate opioid therapy. *Pain* 1993; **53**: 353–5.

71   Babul N, Darke AC. Putative role of hydromorphone metabolites in myoclonus. *Pain* 1992; **51**: 260–1.

72   Kaiko RF, Foley KM, Grabinski PY, *et al.* Central nervous system excitatory effects of meperidine in cancer patients. *Ann Neurol* 1983; **13**: 180–5.

73   Danziger LH, Martin SJ, Blum RA. Central nervous system toxicity associated with meperidine use in hepatic disease. *Pharmacotherapy* 1994; **14**: 235–8.

74   Rao TL, Mummaneni N, El Etr AA. Convulsions: an unusual response to intravenous fentanyl administration. *Anesth Analg* 1982; **61**: 1020–1.

75   Bowdle TA, Rooke GA. Postoperative myoclonus and rigidity after anesthesia with opioids. *Anesth Analg* 1994; **78**: 783–6.

76   Cartwright PD, Hesse C, Jackson AO. Myoclonic spasms following intrathecal diamorphine. *J Pain Symptom Manage* 1993; **8**: 492–5.

77   Mercandante S. Pathophysiology and treatment of opioid- related myoclonus in cancer patients. *Pain* 1998; **74**: 5–9.

78   Potter JM, Reid DB, Shaw RJ, *et al.* Myoclonus associated with treatment with high doses of morphine: the role of supplemental drugs. *BMJ* 1989; **299**: 150–3.

79   Mercadante S, Ferrera P, Villari P, Arcuri E. Hyperalgesia: An emerging iatrogenic syndrome. *J Pain Symptom Manage* 2003; **26**: 769–75.

80   Stillman MJ, Mouline DE, Foley K. Paradoxical pain following high-dose spinal morphine. *Pain* 1987; **4**(Suppl): S389.

81   Yaksh TL, Harty GJ. Pharmacology of the allodynia in rats evoked by high dose intrathecal morphine. *J Pharmacol Exp Ther* 1988; **244**: 501–7.

82   Yaksh TL, Harty GJ, Onofrio BM. High dose of spinal morphine produce a nonopiate receptor-mediated hyperesthesia: clinical and theoretic implications. *Anesthesiology* 1986; **64**: 590–7.

83   Shohami E, Evron S. Intrathecal morphine induces myoclonic seizures in the rat. *Acta Pharmacol Toxicol* 1985; **56**: 50–4.

84   Mao J, Price DD, Mayer DJ. Thermal hyperalgesia in association with the development of morphine tolerance in rats: roles of excitatory amino acid receptors and protein kinase C. *J Neurosci* 1994; **14**: 2301–12.

85   Borgbjerg FM, Frigast C. Segmental effects on motor function following different intrathecal receptor agonists and antagonists in rabbits. *Acta Anaesthesiol Scand* 1997; **41**: 586–94.

86   Hanna MH, Peat SJ, Woodham M, *et al.* Analgesic efficacy and CSF pharmacokinetics of intrathecal morphine-6- glucronate: comparison with morphine. *Br J Anaesth* 1990;**64**: 547–50.

87   Osborne R, Thompson P, Joel S, *et al.* The analgesic activity of morphine-6-glucronide. *Br J Clin Pharmacol* 1992;**34**: 130–8.

88   Smith MT. Neuroexcitatory effects of morphine and hydromorphone: evidence implicating the 3-glucuronate metabolites. *Clin Exp Pharmacol Physiol* 2000: **27**: 524–8.

89   Gong QL, Hedner J, Bjorkman R, Hedner T. Morphine -3- glucuronide may functionally antagonize morphine-6- glucronide induced antinociception and ventilatory depression in the rat. *Pain* 1992; **48**: 249–55.

90   Penson RT, Joel SP, Bakhshi K, *et al.* Randomised placebo- controlled trial pf activity of morphine glucuronides. *Clin Pharmacol Ther* 2000; **68**: 667–6.

● 91   Folstein MF, Folstein SE, McHugh PR. Mini-mental state. A practical method for grading the cognitive state of patients for the clinician. *J Psychiart Res* 1975; **12**: 189–98.

92   Lawlor P, Gagnon B, Mancini IL, *et al.* Occurrences, causes, and outcomes of delirium in patients with advanced cancer: a prospective study. *Arch Intern Med* 2000; **160**: 786–94.

93   Breibart W, Rosenfeld B, Roth A, *et al.* The Memorial Delirium Assessment Scale. *J Pain Symptom Manage* 1997; **13**: 128–37.

94   Trzepacz P, Baker R, Greenhouse J. A symptom rating scale for delirium. *Psychiatry Res* 1988; **23**: 89–97.

95   Krames ES, Gershow J, Glassberg A, *et al.* Continuous infusion of spinally administered narcotics for the relief of pain due to malignant disorders. *Cancer* 1985; **56**: 696–702.

96   Eisele JH, Grigsby EJ, Dea G. Clonazepan treatment of myoclonic contractions associated with high-dose opioids. *Pain* 1992; **49**: 231–2.

◆ 97   Cherny N, Ripamonti C, Pereira J, *et al.* Strategies to manage the adverse effects of oral morphine: an evidence-based report. *J Clin Oncol* 2001; **19**: 2542–54.

98   Mercadante S. Opioid rotation for cancer pain: rationale and clinical aspects. *Cancer* 1999; **86**: 1856–66.

◆ 99   Bruera E, Sweeney C. *Methadone Use in Cancer Patients With Pain: A Review.* J Palliat Med 2002; **5**: 127–38.

100   Morley JS, Makin MK. The use of methadone in cancer pain poorly responsive to other opioids. *Pain Rev* 1998; **5**: 51–8.

101   Bruera E, Pereira J, Watanabe S, *et al.* Opioid rotation in patients with cancer pain: a retrospective comparison of dose ratios between methadone, hydromorphone and morphine. *Cancer* 1996; **78**: 852–7.

102   Mercadante S, Casuccio A, Fulfaro F, *et al.* Switching from morphine to methadone to improve analgesia and tolerability in cancer patients: a prospective study. *J Clin Oncol* 2001;**19**: 2898–904.

103   Nauck, F, Ostgathe C, Dickerson ED, German model for methadone conversion. *Am J Hosp Palliat Care* 2001: **18**: 200–2.

104   de Stoutz ND, Bruera E, Suarez-Almazor M. Opioid rotation for toxicity reduction in terminal cancer patients. *J Pain Symptom Manage* 1995; **10**: 378–84.

105 Lawlor P, Walker P, Bruera E, Mitchell S. Severe opioid toxicity and somatization of psychosocial distress in a cancer patient with a background of chemical dependence. *J Pain Symptom Manage* 1997; **13**: 356–61.

106 Kloke M, Rapp M, Bosse B, Kloke O. Toxicity and/or insufficient analgesia by opioid therapy: risk factors and the impact of changing the opioid. A retrospective analysis of 273 patients observed at a single center. *Support Care Cancer* 2000; **8**: 479–86.

107 Moryl N, Santiago-Palma J, Kornick C, *et al.* Pitfalls of opioid rotation: substituting another opioid for methadone in patients with cancer pain. *Pain* 2002; **96**: 325–8.

◆ 108 Quigley C. Opioid switching to improve pain relief and drug tolerability. *Cochrane Database Syst Rev.* 2004: CD004847.

109 Abs R, Verhelst J, Maeyaert J, *et al.* Endocrine consequences of long-term intrathecal administration of opioids. *J Clin Endocrinol Metab* 2000; **85**: 2215–22.

◆ 110 Risdahl JM, Khanna KV, Peterson PK, Molitor TW. Opiates and infection. *J Neuroimmunol* 1998; **83**: 4–18.

111 Passik SD, Kirsh KI, McDonald MV, *et al.* A pilot survey of aberrant drug-taking attitudes and behaviors in samples of cancer and AIDS patients. *J Pain Symptom Manage* 2000; **19**: 274–86.

112 Porter J, Jick H. Addiction rare in patients treated with narcotics. *N Engl J Med* 1980; **302**: 123.

46

Adjuvant analgesic drugs

DAVID LUSSIER, RUSSELL K PORTENOY

INTRODUCTION

Pain due to cancer can be relieved by a simple opioid-based regimen in more than 70 percent of patients.[1,2**] Some patients are relatively less responsive to opioids, however, and require implementation of strategies to improve the balance between analgesia and adverse effects.[3***] Among these strategies is the use of adjuvant analgesics.

Adjuvant analgesics are drugs with a primary indication other than pain, but with analgesic properties in some painful conditions.[4] Although they can be used alone, they are usually coadministered with analgesics (acetaminophen, nonsteroidal anti-inflammatory drugs [NSAIDs], opioids) when treating cancer pain. They can be added to an opioid regimen to enhance pain relief provided by the opioid, address pain that has not or insufficiently responded, or allow the reduction of the opioid dose and hence reduce adverse effects (Box 46.1).[4] Numerous classes of drugs with diverse primary indications can be used as adjuvant analgesics. Some have been shown to have analgesic properties in diverse pain syndromes and warrant description as multipurpose adjuvant analgesics. Others are used for more specific indications, like neuropathic pain or bone pain (Table 46.1).

Box 46.1 Using adjuvant analgesics for pain management in the palliative care setting

1 Consider optimizing the opioid regimen before introducing an adjuvant analgesic

2 If appropriate, consider the use of other strategies for pain that is poorly responsive to an opioid, including opioid rotation, more aggressive adverse effects management, spinal drug administration, and trials of nonpharmacological approaches (e.g. nerve block, rehabilitative or psychological therapies)

3 Select the most appropriate adjuvant analgesic based on a comprehensive assessment of the patient (symptoms, comorbidities, goals of care) and the inference about the predominating type of pain.

4 When selecting an adjuvant analgesic, consider its pharmacological characteristics, actions, approved indications, unapproved indications accepted in medical practice, likely adverse effects, potential serious adverse effects, and interactions with other drugs

5 Administer the adjuvant analgesics with the best risk:benefit ratios as first-line treatment

6 Avoid initiating several adjuvant analgesics concurrently

7 In most cases, initiate treatment with low doses and titrate gradually according to analgesic response and adverse effects

8 Reassess the efficacy and tolerability of the therapeutic regimen on a regular basis, and taper or discontinue medications that do not provide additional pain relief

9 Consider combination therapy with multiple adjuvant analgesics in selected patients

---

Table 46.1 *Classification and dosing guidelines of adjuvant analgesics*

Drug	Starting dose	Usual effective dose	Drug	Starting dose	Usual effective dose
(I) Multipurpose adjuvant analgesics			Lidocaine topical	1–3 patches 12 hours/24	
Antidepressants					
Tricyclic antidepressants			*N*-methyl-D-aspartate receptor antagonists		
Amitriptyline	10–25 mg HS	50–150 mg HS	Ketamine	Different regimen (see text)	
Nortriptyline	10–25 mg HS	50–150 mg HS			
Desipramine	10–25 mg HS	50–150 mg HS	Dextromethorphan	15–20 mg tid	Unclear
Selective serotonin reuptake inhibitors (SSRIs)			Amantadine	100 mg qd	100–150 mg bid
Paroxetine	10–20 mg qd	20–40 mg qd	**(III) Adjuvant analgesics for bone pain**		
Citalopram	10–20 mg qd	20–40 mg qd	*Corticosteroids*		
Norepinephrine/serotonin reuptake inhibitors (NSRIs)			Calcitonin	1 IU/kg subcutaneous qd 200 IU intranasal qd	
Venlafaxine extended-release	37.5 mg qd	37.5–112.5 mg qd			
Duloxetine	20–30 mg qd	60 mg qd	*Bisphosphonates*		
Others			Pamidronate	60 mg IV q month[a]	60–90 mg IV q month[b]
Bupropion	50–75 mg bid	75–150 mg bid			
Corticosteroids			Ibandronate	6 mg IV q 3–4 weeks[a,b] 50 mg po qd	
Dexamethasone	1–2 mg qd or bid	Variable			
Prednisone	7.5–10 mg qd	Variable	Zoledronic acid	4 mg IV q 3 weeks[a]	
α_2-*Adrenergic agonists*			Radiopharmaceuticals		
Clonidine	0.1 mg po qd	Variable			
	½TTS-1 patch	0.3 mg transdermal/day	**(IV) Adjuvant analgesics for pain from bowel obstruction**		
Tizanidine	2 mg HS	Variable	Octreotide	0.2–0.3 mg/day SC infusion	
Neuroleptics					
Olanzapine	2.5 mg qd	Unclear efficacy	*Anticholinergics*		
Pimozide	1 mg qd	Unclear efficacy	Hyoscine (scopolamine)	40 mg/day SC infusion	60 mg/day SC infusion
(II) Adjuvant analgesics for neuropathic pain			Glycopyrrolate	0.1 mg SC or IV 3–4 times/day	Unclear
Anticonvulsants					
Gabapentin	100–300 mg HS	300–1200 mg tid	*Corticosteroids*		
Pregabalin	50–75 mg qd-bid	75–150 mg bid	Dexamethasone	4 mg bid	Variable
Lamotrigine	25 mg qd	100–200 mg bid	Methylprednisolone	10 mg tid	10–20 mg tid
Oxcarbazepine	75–150 mg bid	150–800 mg bid	**(V) Other adjuvant analgesics**		
Topiramate	25 mg qd	100–200 mg bid	Baclofen	5 mg tid	10–20 mg tid
Levetiracetam	250–500 mg bid	500–1500 mg bid			
Tiagabine	4 mg HS	4–12 mg bid	*Cannabinoids*		
Zonisamide	100 mg qd	100–200 mg bid	Dronabinol	2.5 mg bid	5–10 mg bid
Carbamazepine	100–200 mg qd-bid	300–800 mg bid	*Psychostimulants*		
Valproic acid	250 mg tid	500–1000 mg tid	Methylphenidate	2.5 mg q AM	Variable
Phenytoin	300 mg HS	100–150 mg tid	Modafinil	100 mg q AM	Variable
Local anesthetics					
Mexiletine	150 mg qd	100–300 mg tid			
Lidocaine intravenous	2 mg/kg over 30 min	2–5 mg/kg			

[a] Pamidronate should be infused over 2–4 hours, ibandronate over 1–2 hours and zoledronic acid over 15 minutes.
[b] High-dose IV ibandronate can also be used with 6 mg qd on three consecutive days, followed by q 4 weeks.
qd, once a day; bid, twice a day; tid, three times a day; HS, every night; q, every; IV, intravenous; SC, subcutaneous; IU, international units; AM, morning.

Few adjuvant analgesics have been studied in cancer populations. To a large extent, therefore, drug selection, dosing, and monitoring approaches are extrapolated from the literature on nonmalignant pain. Table 46.1 provides a list of the adjuvant analgesics for which there is some evidence of analgesic efficacy, along with dosing guidelines. Table 46.2 summarizes the postulated mechanisms of the analgesic activity of the main adjuvant analgesics.

MULTIPURPOSE ANALGESICS

Antidepressant drugs

TRICYCLIC ANTIDEPRESSANTS

The tricyclic antidepressants have been extensively studied, and there is compelling evidence for their analgesic properties in a variety of chronic nonmalignant pain conditions.[10,11**] Both the tertiary amines (amitriptyline, imipramine, doxepin, and clomipramine) and the secondary amines (nortriptyline and desipramine) are analgesic.[10,11**] Although few clinical trials have specifically evaluated these drugs for cancer pain, partially controlled[12–14**] and uncontrolled trials,[15*] as well as clinical experience, generally support their analgesic effects.

The use of the tricyclic antidepressants in medically ill or elderly patients may be limited by the frequent occurrence of adverse effects,[16] which include cardiotoxicity (arrhythmias), orthostatic hypotension, drug-induced delirium and precipitation of an acute glaucoma attack. The secondary amines, desipramine and nortriptyline, are less anticholinergic and, therefore, better tolerated than the tertiary amine drugs. Patients who are predisposed to adverse effects from tricyclics, or who have distressing adverse effects during a trial of a tertiary amine drug, should be considered for a trial of desipramine or nortriptyline.

The analgesic effect of tricyclic antidepressants is not dependent on their antidepressant activity. The usually effective analgesic dose is often lower than that required to treat depression, and the onset of analgesia typically occurs sooner, usually within a week.[10,11]

OTHER ANTIDEPRESSANTS

Although the evidence is far less than for tricyclics, randomized controlled trials suggest that other antidepressants are analgesic.[17**] The main advantage of the non-tricyclic antidepressants is their favorable side-effect profile, which makes them safer and better tolerated.

Among the selective serotonin reuptake inhibitors (SSRIs), the only ones for which controlled studies have suggested benefit are paroxetine[18**] and citalopram.[19**] No studies have been done in cancer pain. Venlafaxine, which inhibits the

Table 46.2 *Probable mechanisms of analgesic activity of adjuvant analgesics*[4]

Drug	Mechanism(s) of analgesic activity
Multipurpose adjuvant analgesics	
Antidepressants	
Tricyclics	Blockade of reuptake of norepinephrine and serotonin
Selective serotonin reuptake inhibitors	Blockade of serotonin reuptake
Venlafaxine	Low dose: blockade of serotonin reuptake
	High dose: blockade of norepinephrine reuptake
Bupropion	Blockade of reuptake of norepinephrine and dopamine
Corticosteroids	Decreased compression of pain-sensitive structures by reduction of peritumoral edema
	Shrinkage of steroid-sensitive tumor masses
	Decreased activation of nociceptors due to lower tissue concentrations of inflammatory mediators and lessened aberrant electrical activity in damaged nerves
α_2-Adrenergic agonists	Interaction with α-2 receptors in the spinal cord or brainstem activates endogenous systems that reduce nociceptive input to the central nervous system[5]?
Neuroleptics	Dopaminergic blockade[6]?
Adjuvant analgesics for neuropathic pain	
Anticonvulsants[7]	
Phenytoin, lamotrigine	Blockade of sodium channels
	Inhibition of presynaptic release of glutamate
Carbamazepine, oxcarbazepine	Blockade of sodium and calcium channels
Topiramate	Blockade of sodium channels
	Increase of inhibitory action of GABA
	Inhibition of excitatory action of glutamate
Gabapentin, pregabalin	Binding to the $\alpha 2\delta$ subunit of calcium channels blocks calcium influx and prevents presynaptic release of neurotransmitters[8]
Tiagabine	Direct agonist effect on GABA receptors
Levetiracetam	Unclear
Local anesthetics	Blockade of sodium channels
NMDA antagonists	Inhibition of the 'wind-up' phenomenon caused by activation of NMDA receptors by glutamate and aspartate[9]

GABA, γ-aminobutyric acid; NMDA, *N*-methyl-D-aspartate.

reuptake of both serotonin and norepinephrine, has been shown to provide good pain relief in nonmalignant painful polyneuropathy[20,21**] and pain following mastectomy for breast cancer;[22**] it also has reduced the incidence of postmastectomy pain if given prior to surgery.[23**] Duloxetine, another mixed reuptake inhibitor, is effective in treating painful symptoms associated with depression.[24**] Animal studies suggested that duloxetine might have a role in the treatment of neuropathic pain[25] and subsequent clinical trials led to approval by the US Food and Drug Administration as a treatment for painful diabetic polyneuropathy. The dual noradrenergic and dopaminergic compound bupropion can relieve nonmalignant neuropathic pain;[26,27**] its activating effects can be particularly helpful in hypoactive depressed, sedated or fatigued patients often encountered in the palliative care population.

Corticosteroids

Corticosteroids possess analgesic properties for a large variety of cancer pain syndromes, including bone pain, neuropathic pain from infiltration or compression of neural structures, headache due to increased intracranial pressure, arthralgia, and pain due to obstruction of a hollow viscus (e.g. bowel or ureter) or to organ capsule distension.[28***] They are also effective in the initial management of pain and symptoms from metastatic spinal cord compression[29,30**] while awaiting more definitive treatment (usually radiation therapy) if justified by the goals of care. Even though the risks and benefits of the various corticosteroids are unknown, dexamethasone is often selected because of its relatively low mineralocorticoid effects. Prednisone and methylprednisolone can also be used.

A high-dose regimen of corticosteroids is recommended for patients who experience spinal cord compression and can be helpful in an acute episode of severe pain that cannot be promptly reduced with opioids.[31***] There is a large experience in the administration of dexamethasone at an initial dose of 100 mg, followed by 96 mg/day in divided doses and a subsequent tapering over days or weeks after the initiation of other analgesic approaches (e.g. opioid therapy or radiation therapy). A low-dose corticosteroid regimen (e.g. dexamethasone 2–4 mg once or twice daily) can be used for patients with advanced cancer who continue to have pain despite optimal dosing of opioid drugs. Long-term usage of a corticosteroid in this dose range is associated with the possibility of adverse effects, including hypertension, hyperglycemia, fluid retention, gastrointestinal bleeding, skin fragility, and delirium. In patients with good prognoses for prolonged survival, repeated assessments are required to ensure that benefits are sustained. In all cases, the dose should be tapered to the lowest effective dose. The coadministration of a gastroprotective drug (usually a proton pump inhibitor) can be justified for patients

who present other risk factors for peptic ulcer disease, particularly the concomitant administration of an NSAID.

α₂-Adrenergic agonists

Although the α_2-adrenergic agonists may be considered multipurpose adjuvant analgesics, the limited supporting data and clinical experience, as well as the potential for adverse effects (mostly somnolence and hypotension) relegate these drugs to second-line use, after others have proved ineffective. Clonidine, administered either orally, transdermally or intraspinally, has been shown to be analgesic in nonmalignant neuropathic pain.[32–34***] Fewer than a quarter of patients who receive the drug systemically experience pain relief,[32] and adverse effects are a particular concern in frail palliative care patients. Intraspinal clonidine has been shown to reduce pain (especially neuropathic pain) in patients with severe intractable cancer pain partly responding to opioids.[35**] Tizanidine, which is more specific for the α_2-adrenergic receptor than clonidine, is approved as an antispasticity agent and is often better tolerated. Evidence of its analgesic efficacy is however limited to the nonmalignant syndromes of myofascial pain and chronic daily headache.[36***]

Neuroleptics

The second-generation 'atypical' neuroleptic, olanzapine, was reported to decrease pain intensity and opioid consumption, and improve cognitive function and anxiety in a case series of cancer patients.[37*] Nonetheless, the limited evidence of efficacy, combined with the potential for adverse effects, suggests a very limited role for neuroleptics as analgesics. They can be useful in the presence of a delirium or agitation, in which case the analgesic properties might provide better pain control and allow a decrease of opioid consumption, which might in turn be helpful in resolving the delirium.[38***]

ADJUVANT ANALGESICS SPECIFIC FOR NEUROPATHIC PAIN

The term 'neuropathic pain' is applied to those pain syndromes for which the sustaining mechanisms are presumed to be related to aberrant somatosensory processes in the peripheral nervous system, central nervous system (CNS), or both.[39] Surveys have reported that up to 40–50 percent of cancer pain syndromes can be categorized as exclusively or partly neuropathic.[40,41***]

Neuropathic pain may be relatively less responsive to opioid drugs that other types of pain. Adjuvant analgesics therefore play a very important role in the management of neuropathic pain. The use of opioid drugs as first-line analgesics should not, however, be abandoned when the pain is neuropathic, especially now that randomized controlled trials have established their potential efficacy in nonmalignant neuropathic pain syndromes.[17**] Addition of an adjuvant analgesic to the therapeutic regimen usually should follow the optimization of the opioid regimen.

Anticonvulsant drugs

There is good evidence that the anticonvulsant drugs are useful in the management of nonmalignant neuropathic pain.[7,42,43**] Gabapentin is recommended as a first-line agent for the treatment of nonmalignant neuropathic pain of diverse etiologies.[17] Randomized controlled trials have established its analgesic efficacy in several types of nonmalignant neuropathic pain.[44–47**] As an 'add on' therapy to patients whose neuropathic cancer-related pain is not controlled satisfactorily with an optimal dose of opioids, gabapentin 600–1800 mg daily reduces average pain and dysesthesias when compared with placebo.[48**] Gabapentin appears to be widely used to treat cancer-related neuropathic pain in palliative care units.[49*] It should be initiated at a daily dose of 100–300 mg at bedtime and can be increased every few days. The usual effective dose ranges between 900 mg and 3600 mg daily. An adequate trial should include 1–2 weeks at the maximum-tolerated dose. The most common adverse effects are somnolence, dizziness, and unsteadiness. If titrated carefully, gabapentin is usually well tolerated, but in frail palliative care patients, somnolence can be a limiting factor.[49] Since it is not metabolized by hepatic enzymes, gabapentin rarely has drug–drug interactions.

Although none of the other anticonvulsants have been studied in malignant neuropathic pain, there is evidence of analgesic efficacy in nonmalignant neuropathic pain. Lamotrigine was reported to be analgesic in several randomized trials.[50–53**] The risk of adverse effects (e.g. somnolence, dizziness, ataxia and cutaneous hypersensitivity syndromes including Stevens–Johnson syndrome) is lessened by slow dose titration. Pregabalin, a new anticonvulsant with a mechanism identical to that of gabapentin, now has a strong evidence of analgesic efficacy supported by randomized controlled trials.[54–56***] Oxcarbazepine, a metabolite of carbamazepine, has a similar spectrum of effects and better tolerability; it appears promising based on a few open-label trials.[57–60*] Topiramate,[61**] tiagabine,[62*] and zonisamide[63*] have some evidence of efficacy, and there is some favorable clinical experience with levetiracetam.[64,65*] Like gabapentin, pregabalin and levetiracetam lack any significant drug–drug interactions.

Among the older anticonvulsants, evidence of efficacy is best for carbamazepine and phenytoin. In cancer pain, phenytoin can provide mild to moderate analgesia and enhance opioid analgesia.[66**] An intravenous infusion of phenytoin has also been reported to be effective in reducing overall pain, as well as burning pain, shooting pain, sensitivity and numbness in acute flare-ups of nonmalignant neuropathic pain.[67**] Even though this effect is usually of short duration, it might be useful in refractory neuropathic pain. Valproate and clonazepam have been widely used but lack clear evidence of analgesic activity.

Oral and parenteral local anesthetics

Local anesthetics have analgesic properties in neuropathic pain.[4**] Due to their potential for serious side effects, they usually have been positioned as second-line therapies.[17,68]

A brief intravenous infusion of lidocaine has been shown to be effective in nonmalignant neuropathic pain.[69,70**] Although controlled trials in neuropathic cancer pain[71,72] have not demonstrated efficacy, clinical experience justifies a trial of intravenous lidocaine infusion in selected patients with severe refractory neuropathic pain. Brief infusions can be administered at varying doses within the range of 1–5 mg/kg infused over 20–30 minutes. In the medically frail patient often encountered in the palliative care population, it is prudent to start at the lower end of this range and provide repeated infusions at successively higher doses. A history of significant cardiac disease may relatively contraindicate this approach and should be evaluated before it is administered. An electrocardiogram should be done before starting the infusion or increasing the dose, and careful monitoring of vital signs is necessary during the period of the infusion and immediately thereafter.

Although prolonged relief of pain following a brief local anesthetic infusion may occur, relief usually is transitory. If lidocaine appears to be effective but pain recurs, long-term systemic local anesthetic therapy should be considered using an oral local anesthetic, such as mexiletine. For rare patients with refractory neuropathic cancer pain who respond only to intravenous lidocaine infusion, long-term subcutaneous administration has been reported to provide sustained relief.[73*]

There is no definitive evidence that an intravenous infusion of lidocaine predicts the response to an oral local anesthetic, the dose of which is slowly titrated. For this reason, an oral formulation, such as mexiletine, can be considered without a prior infusion and even those who do not respond to an infusion may be considered for a subsequent trial of an oral drug. Given the side-effect liability of these agents, they are typically positioned after trials of both anticonvulsants and antidepressants.

N-Methyl-D-aspartate receptor blockers

Interactions at the N-methyl-D-aspartate (NMDA) receptor are involved in the development of central nervous system changes that may underlie chronic pain and modulate opioid mechanisms, specifically tolerance.[74] Antagonists at the NMDA receptor may offer another novel approach to the treatment of neuropathic pain in cancer patients.

An intravenous infusion of ketamine can be effective in relieving cancer pain[75*,76**] and reducing opioid requirements,[77**] and may be therefore be considered in patients with refractory pain. The side-effect profile of ketamine, which includes hypertension, tachycardia, and serious psychotomimetic effects (such as a dissociative reaction), can be daunting, however, particularly in medically frail patients. Typically, ketamine therapy is initiated at low doses given subcutaneously or intravenously, such as 0.1–0.15 mg/kg by brief infusion or 0.1–0.15 mg/kg per hour by continuous infusion. The dose can be gradually escalated, with close monitoring of pain and adverse effects. For patients with refractory pain and limited life expectancy, long-term therapy can be maintained using continuous subcutaneous infusion or repeated subcutaneous injections.[78,79*] Oral administration also has been used, but experience is more limited.[80*] The ratio of doses needed to maintain effects when converting from parenteral to oral dosing is uncertain. Based on anecdotal data, some authors have suggested a 1:1 ratio,[81*] or an oral dose equivalent to 30–40 percent of the parenteral dose.[82*] It is also recommended to lower the opioid dose when starting ketamine.[82*]

The anti-tussive dextromethorphan is an NMDA-receptor antagonist. Following surgery for bone malignancy, dextromethorphan was shown to augment analgesia and lessen analgesic requirements.[83,84**] Other studies and clinical experience have yielded mixed results. If prescribed, a prudent starting dose is 45–60 mg/day, which can be gradually escalated until favorable effects occur, adverse effects supervene, or a conventional maximal dose of 1 g is achieved.

Amantadine is a noncompetitive NMDA antagonist, and limited data suggest that it might reduce pain, allodynia, and hyperalgesia in chronic neuropathic pain[85,86**] and surgical neuropathic cancer pain.[87**] Currently available data are, however, too meager to support recommending its use. Memantine is an NMDA antagonist approved for the treatment of Alzheimer disease. Although a preliminary study of analgesic effects was encouraging,[88] controlled trials have been disappointing thus far.[89,90] New NMDA receptor antagonists are in development and may ultimately prove useful for a variety of medical indications. Advances in this area have occurred rapidly, and it is likely that the role of these agents in the management of pain will be much better defined within a few years.

Other systemic drugs

BACLOFEN

Baclofen, an agonist at the γ-aminobutyric acid type B (GABA$_B$) receptor, has established efficacy in trigeminal neuralgia[91***] and is often considered for a trial in any type of neuropathic pain. The effective dose range is very wide (20 mg/day to >200 mg/day orally), and titration from a low initial dose is necessary. The possibility of a serious withdrawal syndrome on abrupt discontinuation must be avoided by a gradual dose taper.

CANNABINOIDS

Cannabinoids have antinociceptive effects in animal models and oral delta-9-tetrahydrocannabinol has been shown to be effective in cancer pain.[92**] Not all data are positive, however,[93] and more studies on the various cannabinoids are needed.

BENZODIAZEPINES

The evidence for analgesic effects from benzodiazepines is limited and conflicting, and overall provides little support for an analgesic activity of these drugs in neuropathic pain.[94,95]

PSYCHOSTIMULANTS

There is some evidence that psychostimulant drugs, including dextroamphetamine, methylphenidate and caffeine, have analgesic effects.[96***] Although pain is not considered a primary indication for these drugs, the potential for analgesic effects may influence the decision to institute a trial. In cancer patients, methylphenidate can also reduce opioid-induced somnolence, improve cognition, treat depression, and alleviate fatigue.[97**] The analgesic properties of the psychostimulants modafinil and atomoxetine have not yet been studied.

Topical analgesics

The development of a lidocaine 5 percent patch has facilitated the topical application of local anesthetics. This formulation has been shown to relieve pain from postherpetic neuralgia.[98**] Although never specifically studied in populations with advanced medical illness, clinical experience justifies a trial in diverse types of neuropathic pain and other types of focal pain problems. The patch is usually applied 12 hours per day, but a few studies indicate minimal systemic lidocaine absorption and a high level of safety with up to three patches for periods up to 24 hours.[99**] An adequate trial may require more than 1 week of applications. The most frequently reported adverse event is mild to moderate skin redness, rash, or irritation at the patch application site. EMLA®, an eutectic mixture of local anesthetics (prilocaine and lidocaine), can produce dense local cutaneous anesthesia but its use on large areas is limited by its fairly high cost. Topical lidocaine may be tried in various concentrations (up to a compounded formulation of 10 percent) as an alternative.

Capsaicin is the ingredient in chili pepper that produces its pungent taste. When applied topically, it causes the depolarization of C-fiber nociceptors and release of substance P. Regular use eventually leads to depletion of substance P from the terminals of these afferent C-fibers, potentially leading to decreased pain perception. In cancer patients, capsaicin cream was shown to be effective in reducing neuropathic postsurgical pain (such as postmastectomy pain).[100**] There are two commercially available concentrations (0.025 percent and 0.075 percent), and an initial trial usually involves application of the higher concentration three to four times daily. A trial of several weeks is needed to adequately judge effects. Many patients experience severe burning pain after the first applications (related to the initial release of substance P), which usually decreases gradually over a few days if the cream is applied regularly. Some patients tolerate the lower concentration cream better, or tolerate application only if preceded by a topical local anesthetic or ingestion of an analgesic.

Because of its presumed peripheral action at both opioid and sodium-potassium channels, topical ketamine (gel, ointment, cream) might provide local analgesia of neuropathic pain without any systemic absorption. Scientific evidence is limited to small open-label trials and case series.[101,102*] One small randomized controlled trial reported that ketamine cream applied for 2 days did not provide any analgesia; however, a 1-week application of a combination cream of ketamine and amitriptyline decreased local pain intensity.[103**] One anecdotal report suggests that ketamine oral rinse might provide effective analgesia for radiation-therapy induced mucositis.[104]

Numerous anti-inflammatory drugs have been investigated for topical use in populations with neuropathic pain, with mixed results from small controlled trials.[105,106] The analgesic effects of these formulations for musculoskeletal pain are also unclear.[107,108]

ADJUVANT ANALGESICS SPECIFIC FOR BONE PAIN

Bone pain is a common problem in the palliative care setting. Radiation therapy is usually considered when bone pain is focal and poorly controlled with an opioid, or is associated with a lesion that appears prone to fracture on radiographic examination. Multifocal bone pain may benefit from treatment with an NSAID or a corticosteroid. Other adjuvant analgesics that are potentially useful in this setting include calcitonin, bisphosphonate compounds, and selected radiopharmaceuticals.

Calcitonin

Calcitonin may have several pain-related indications in the palliative care setting, including pain from bone metastases.[109–111**] It can be administered subcutaneously or intranasally. If subcutaneous boluses are used, they should be preceded by skin testing with 1 IU to screen for hypersensitivity reactions. The optimal dose is not known. The intranasal formulation avoids the need for subcutaneous injections, facilitating the use of this drug in home care. Apart

from infrequent hypersensitivity reactions associated with subcutaneous injections, the main side effect is nausea. The likelihood and severity of this effect may be reduced by gradual escalation from a low starting dose. It usually subsides after a few days and is less frequent with the intranasal form.

Bisphosphonates

Bisphosphonates are analogs of inorganic pyrophosphate that inhibit osteoclast activity and, consequently, reduce bone resorption in a variety of illnesses. The analgesic efficacy of these compounds, particularly pamidronate, has been well established. Pamidronate has been extensively studied in populations with bone metastases.[112**] Its analgesic effects have been shown in breast cancer[113–115**] and multiple myeloma.[116**] The dose usually recommended is 60–90 mg intravenously (IV) (infused over 2–4 hours) every 3–4 weeks.[113] There are dose-dependent effects, and a poor response at 60 mg can be followed by a trial of 90 mg or 120 mg. The reduction of skeletal morbidity (pathological fractures, need for bone radiation or surgery, spinal cord compression, and hypercalcemia) is another incentive to use it as an adjuvant.[117,118**] Adverse effects, including hypocalcemia and a 'flulike syndrome, are dose related and typically transitory. Nephrotoxicity occurs rarely, usually following relatively rapid infusions, and typically is transitory; the drug can be used in those with impaired renal function, but renal function must be followed closely and the drug should be discontinued if deterioration occurs.

Zoledronic acid is a new bisphosphonate that is approximately two to three times more potent than pamidronate. It has been shown to reduce pain and the occurrence of skeletal-related events in breast cancer,[114,116,119**] prostate cancer,[120,121**] and multiple myeloma,[116**] as well as a variety of solid tumors, including lung cancer.[122**] It is as effective as pamidronate,[114,116**] and its use is more convenient, as it can be infused safely over 15 minutes at a dose of 4 mg every 3 weeks. The side effects are similar to those encountered with pamidronate, and the dose does not have to be adjusted in patients with mild-to-moderate renal failure.[123**]

Oral clodronate can reduce metastatic bone pain[124,125] but results are conflicting.[112] The main advantage of clodronate over pamidronate is its good oral bioavailability, which avoids the need for IV administration. An oral dose of 1600 mg daily seems to be optimal.[112] Clodronate is not available in the USA.

In a recent randomized controlled trial in patients with metastatic breast cancer, an intravenous infusion of 6 mg ibandronate every 3–4 weeks reduced bone pain, analgesic use and new bone events; the effects lasted for up to 2 years.[126**] Intravenous ibandronate administration of 6 mg for 3 consecutive days, repeated at 4-week intervals, provided relief from bone pain due to metastatic urological cancer.[127**] Oral ibandronate 50 mg daily decreased bone pain from metastatic breast cancer, starting at 6 weeks and persisting up to 2 years; it also had a positive effect on analgesic use and quality of life.[128**]

Radiopharmaceuticals

Radionuclides that are absorbed at areas of high bone turnover have been evaluated as potential therapies for metastatic bone disease. Strontium-89 and samarium-153, which are commercially available in the USA, may be effective as monotherapy or as an adjunct to conventional radiation therapy.[129–132**] Given the potential for myelosuppression associated with their use, these drugs usually are considered when pain is refractory to other modalities and no further cytotoxic chemotherapy is planned.

ADJUVANT ANALGESICS USED FOR PAIN CAUSED BY BOWEL OBSTRUCTION

The management of symptoms associated with malignant bowel obstruction may be challenging. If surgical decompression is not feasible, the need to control pain and other obstructive symptoms, including distension, nausea and vomiting, becomes paramount.

Octreotide

The somatostatin analog octreotide inhibits the secretion of gastric, pancreatic, and intestinal secretions, and reduces gastrointestinal motility. These actions, which can occur more rapidly than similar effects produced by anticholinergic drugs,[133**] probably underlie the analgesia and other favorable outcomes that have been reported in case series[134*] and one randomized trial[135**] in patients with bowel obstruction. Octreotide has a good safety profile, and its considerable expense may be offset in some situations by the avoidance of the necessity of gastrointestinal drainage procedures.

Anticholinergic drugs

Anticholinergic drugs could theoretically relieve the symptoms of bowel obstruction by reducing propulsive and nonpropulsive gut motility and decreasing intraluminal secretions. Two small series demonstrated that a continuous infusion of hyoscine butylbromide (scopolamine) at a dose of 60 mg daily can control symptoms from nonoperable malignant bowel obstruction, including pain.[134,136*] Glycopyrrolate has a pharmacological profile similar to that of hyoscine butylbromide, but may produce fewer adverse effects because of a relatively low penetration through the blood–brain barrier; this drug, however, has not been systematically evaluated in a population with symptomatic bowel obstruction.

Corticosteroids

The symptoms associated with bowel obstruction may improve with corticosteroid therapy. The mode of action is unclear, and the most effective drug, dose, and dosing regimen are unknown. Dexamethasone has been used in a dose range of 8–60 mg/day,[137*] and methylprednisolone has been administered in a dose range of 30–50 mg/day.[138*] The potential for complications during long-term therapy, including an increased risk of bowel perforation,[139,140] may limit this approach to patients with short life expectancies.

COMBINATIONS OF ADJUVANT ANALGESICS

When treating a complex pain pathology in palliative care patients, clinicians often use a combination of several analgesics (opioid and nonopioid) and adjuvant analgesics (e.g. an anticonvulsant, an antidepressant, and a lidocaine patch). This approach offers the advantage of acting on different pain mechanisms (Table 46.2) and minimizes the adverse effects associated with a specific drug by using a lower dose.[68] Scientific data on the additive analgesic effects obtained by combining several adjuvant analgesics are minimal. One small randomized controlled trial suggested that adding lamotrigine to phenytoin or carbamazepine was beneficial.[53**] For nonmalignant neuropathic pain, a combination of gabapentin and long-acting morphine has recently been shown to provide better pain relief with lower doses than each drug used separately.[141] An open-label trial suggested that the addition of levetiracetam in patients who responded only partially to gabapentin provided synergistic relief.[65*] Finally, a case series described 11 patients with multiple sclerosis and trigeminal neuralgia who did not respond satisfactorily to phenytoin or carbamazepine and for whom the addition of low dose gabapentin (300–1200 mg/day) provided good pain control.[142*]

Due to this lack of scientific evidence, the optimal sequences for the administration of drug combinations are unknown. Drug selection is a trial-and-error process based on the clinical situation and the clinician's experience.[143***] In all cases, careful attention should be given to potential interactions between the medications used.

DRUG INTERACTIONS

The risk for adverse drug–drug interactions is inherent in the use of drug combinations to optimize clinical effects. The common pharmacokinetic and pharmacodynamic interactions, which have been reviewed elsewhere recently,[143,144] must be appreciated to minimize risk when selecting drugs and adjusting doses.

CONCLUSIONS

The scientific evidence on the utility of adjuvant analgesics in the treatment of pain that responds only partly to the administration of opioid analgesics has evolved substantially in the past few years. The development of new molecules with a better adverse effect profile has greatly facilitated their use. Ongoing clinical and translational research should further improve our knowledge and offer new therapeutic options. The data on the use of adjuvant analgesics in cancer and palliative care patients are still relatively scarce, and the clinician must rely on studies of populations with nonmalignant pain and clinical experience. Hopefully, research in this area will continue to evolve.

Key learning points

- Adjuvant analgesics are drugs initially developed for an indication other than pain, but with analgesic properties in some painful conditions.

- Adjuvant analgesics can be classified as multipurpose nonspecific (e.g. antidepressants, ∴ α_2-adrenergic agonists, corticosteroids), specific for neuropathic pain (anticonvulsants, local anesthetics, NMDA antagonists), specific for bone pain (corticosteroids, calcitonin, bisphosphonates, radiopharmaceuticals) and specific for pain from bowel obstruction (octreotide, scopolamine, glycopyrrolate).

- In the treatment of pain in populations with advanced medical illness, adjuvant analgesics can be useful for pain that is only partly responsive to opioids and should usually be used in combination with an opioid regimen.

- The evidence on the use of most adjuvant analgesics for the treatment of pain due to advanced illness is often limited, and selection of the most appropriate adjuvant analgesic should be based on literature from nonmalignant pain and clinical experience.

- The adjuvant analgesics with the most favorable benefit:risk ratio should be used as first-line therapy.

REFERENCES

- ● 1 Grond S, Radbruch L, Meuser T et al. Assessment and treatment of neuropathic cancer pain following WHO guidelines. *Pain* 1999; **79**: 15–20.
- ◆ 2 Hanks GW, Justins DM. Cancer pain management. *Lancet* 1992; **339**: 1031–6.
- ◆ 3 Vielhaber A, Portenoy RK. Advances in cancer pain management. *Hematol Oncol Clin North Am* 2002; **16**: 527–41.
- ◆ 4 Lussier D, Portenoy RK. Adjuvant analgesics in pain management. In: Doyle D, Hanks G, Cherny N, Calman K, eds.

Oxford Textbook of Palliative Medicine, 3rd ed. Oxford: Oxford University Press, 2004: 349–77.
- 5 Puke MJ, Wiesenfeld-Hallin Z. The differential effects of morphine and the alpha 2-adrenoreceptor agonists clonidine and dexmedetomidine on the prevention and treatment of experimental neuropathic pain. *Anesth Analg* 1993; **77**: 104–9.
- 6 Kiritsky-Roy JA, Standish SM, Terry LC. Dopamine D-1 and D-2 receptor antagonists potentiate analgesic and motor effects of morphine. *Pharmacol Biochem Behav* 1989; **32**: 717–21.
- ◆ 7 Tremont-Lukats IW, Megeff C, Backonja MM. Anticonvulsants for neuropathic pain syndromes: mechanisms of action and place in therapy. *Drugs* 2000; **60**: 1029–52.
- 8 Field MJ, Hughes J, Singh L. Further evidence for the role of the alpha(2)delta subunit of voltage dependent calcium channels in models of neuropathic pain. *Br J Pharmacol* 2000; **131**: 282–6.
- 9 Fisher K, Coderre TJ, Hagen NA. Targeting the N-methyl-D-aspartate receptor for chronic pain management. Preclinical animal studies, recent clinical experience and future research directions. *J Pain Symptom Manage* 2000; **20**: 358–73.
- ◆ 10 Collins SL, Moore RA, McQuay HJ, Wiffen P. Antidepressants and anticonvulsants for diabetic neuropathy and postherpetic neuralgia: a quantitative systematic review. *J Pain Symptom Manage* 2000; **20**: 449–58.
- ◆ 11 Watson CP. The treatment of neuropathic pain: antidepressants and opioids. *Clin J Pain* 2000; **16**(2 Suppl): S49–5.
- 12 Breivik H, Rennemo F. Clinical evaluation of combined treatment with methadone and psychotropic drugs in cancer patients. *Acta Anaesth Scand* 1982; **74**: 135–40.
- 13 Ventafridda V, Bonezzi C, Caraceni A et al. Antidepressants for cancer pain and other painful syndromes with deafferentation component: comparison of amitriptyline and trazodone. *Ital J Neurol Sci* 1987; **8**: 579–87.
- 14 Walsh TD. Controlled study of imipramine and morphine in chronic pain due to advanced cancer. *Proc Am Soc Clin Oncol* 1986; **5**: 237.
- 15 Magni G, Arsie D, DeLeo D. Antidepressants in the treatment of cancer pain: a survey in Italy. *Pain* 1987; **29**: 347–53.
- 16 Preskorn SH, Irwin HA. Toxicity of tricyclic antidepressants – kinetics, mechanism, intervention: a review. *J Clin Psychiatry* 1982; **43**: 151–6.
- 17 Dworkin RH, Backonja M, Rowbotham MC et al. Advances in neuropathic pain: diagnosis, mechanisms and treatment recommendations. *Arch Neurol* 2003; **60**: 1524–34.
- 18 Sindrup SH, Gram LF, Brosen K, et al. The selective serotonin reuptake inhibitor paroxetine is effective in the treatment of diabetic neuropathy symptoms. *Pain* 1990; **42**: 135–44.
- 19 Sindrup SH, Bjerre U, Dejgaard A et al. The selective serotonin reuptake inhibitor citalopram relieves the symptoms of diabetic neuropathy. *Clin Pharmacol Ther* 1992; **52**: 547–52.
- ● 20 Rowbotham MC, Goli V, Kunz NR, Lei D. Venlafaxine extended release in the treatment of painful diabetic neuropathy: a double-blind, placebo-controlled study. *Pain* 2004; **110**: 697–706.
- 21 Sindrup SH, Bach FW, Madsen C, et al. Venlafaxine versus imipramine in painful polyneuropathy: A randomized, controlled trial. *Neurology* 2003; **60**: 1284–9.
- 22 Tasmuth T, Hartel B, Kalso E. Venlafaxine in neuropathic pain following treatment of breast cancer. *Eur J Pain* 2002; **6**: 17–24.
- ● 23 Reuben SS, Makari-Judson G, Lurie SD. Evaluation of efficacy of the perioperative administration of venlafaxine XR in the

prevention of postmastectomy pain syndrome. *J Pain Symptom Manage* 2004; **27**: 133–9.

24 Fava M, Mallinckrodt CH, Detke MJ, *et al*. The effect of duloxetine on painful physical symptoms in depressed patients: do improvements in these symptoms result in higher remission rates? *J Clin Psychiatry* 2004; **65**: 521–30.

25 Iyengar S, Webster AA, Hemrick-Luecke SK, Xu JY, Simmons RM. Efficacy of duloxetine, a potent and balanced serotonin-norepinephrine reuptake inhibitor in persistent pain models in rats. *J Pharmacol Exp Ther* 2004; **311**: 576–84.

26 Semenchuk MR, Davis B. Efficacy of sustained-release bupropion in neuropathic pain: an open-label study. *Clin J Pain* 2000; **16**: 6–11.

● 27 Semenchuk MR, Sherma S, Davis B. Double-blind, randomized trial of bupropion SR for the treatment of neuropathic pain. *Neurology* 2001; **57**: 1583–8.

28 Watanabe S, Bruera E. Corticosteroids as adjuvant analgesics. *J Pain Symptom Manage* 1994; **9**: 442–5.

29 Greenberg HS, Kim J, Posner JB. Epidural spinal cord compression from metastatic tumor: results with a new treatment protocol. *Ann Neurol* 1980; **8**: 361–6.

30 Vecht Ch.J, Haaxma-Reiche H, van Putten WLJ *et al*. Initial bolus of conventional versus high-dose dexamethasone in metastatic spinal cord compression. *Neurology* 1989; **39**: 1255–7.

31 Ettinger AB, Portenoy RK. The use of corticosteroids in the treatment of symptoms associated with cancer. *J Pain Symptom Manage* 1988; **3**: 99–103.

32 Byas-Smith MG, Max MB, Muir H, Kingman A. Transdermal clonidine compared to placebo in painful diabetic neuropathy using a two-staged 'enriched enrollment' design. *Pain* 1995; **60**: 267–74.

33 Rauck RL, Eisenach JC, Jackson K, *et al*. Epidural clonidine treatment for refractory reflex sympathetic dystrophy. *Anesthesiology* 1993; **79**: 1163–9.

34 Zeigler D, Lynch SA, Muir J, *et al*. Transdermal clonidine versus placebo in painful diabetic neuropathy. *Pain* 1992; **48**: 403–8.

35 Eisenach JC, Du Pen S, Dubois M, *et al*. Epidural clonidine analgesia for intractable cancer pain. *Pain* 1995; **61**: 391–400.

36 Chou R, Peterson K, Helfand M. Comparative efficacy and safety of skeletal muscle relaxants for spasticity and musculoskeletal conditions: a systematic review. *J Pain Symptom Manage* 2004; **28**: 140–75.

37 Khojainova N, Santiago-Palma J, Kornick C, *et al*. Olanzapine in the management of cancer pain. *J Pain Symptom Manage* 2002; **23**: 346–50.

38 Patt RB, Proper G, Reddy S. The neuroleptics as adjuvant analgesics. *J Pain Symptom Manage* 1994; **9**: 446–53.

◆ 39 Portenoy RK, Forbes K, Lussier D, Hanks G. Difficult pain problems: an integrated approach. In: Doyle D, Hanks G, Cherny N, Calman K, eds. *Oxford Textbook of Palliative Medicine*, 3rd ed. Oxford: Oxford University Press, 2004: 438–58.

● 40 Caraceni A, Portenoy RK, a working group of the IASP Task Force on Cancer Pain. An international survey of cancer pain characteristics and syndromes. *Pain* 1999; **82**: 263–74.

41 Manfredi PL, Gonzales GR, Sady R, *et al*. Neuropathic pain in patients with cancer. *J Palliat Care* 2003; **19**: 115–18.

◆ 42 Backonja MM. Anticonvulsants (antineuropathics) for neuropathic pain syndromes. *Clin J Pain* 2000; **16**: S67–72.

◆ 43 Backonja MM. Use of anticonvulsants for treatment of neuropathic pain. *Neurology* 2002; **59**(5 Suppl 2): S14–S17.

● 44 Backonja M, Beydoun A, Edwards KR *et al*. Gabapentin for the symptomatic treatment of painful neuropathy in patients with diabetes mellitus: a randomized controlled trial. *JAMA* 1998; **280**: 1831–6.

45 Backonja M, Glanzman RL. Gabapentin dosing for neuropathic pain: evidence from randomized, placebo-controlled clinical trials. *Clin Ther* 2003; **25**: 81–104.

46 Morello CM, Leckband SG, Stoner CP, *et al*. Randomized double-blind study comparing the efficacy of gabapentin with amitriptyline on diabetic peripheral neuropathy pain. *Arch Intern Med* 1999; **159**: 1931–7.

● 47 Rowbotham M, Harden N, Stacey B, *et al*. Gabapentin for the treatment of postherpetic neuralgia: a randomized controlled trial. *JAMA* 1998; **280**: 1837–42.

● 48 Caraceni A, Zecca E, Bonezzi C *et al*. Gabapentin for neuropathic cancer pain: a randomized controlled trial from the Gabapentin Cancer Pain Study Group. *J Clin Oncol* 2004; **22**: 2909–17.

49 Oneschuk D, al-Shahri MZ. The pattern of gabapentin use in a tertiary palliative care unit. *J Palliat Care* 2003; **19**: 185–7.

50 Simpson DM, McArthur JC, Olner D *et al*. Lamotrigine for HIV-associated painful sensory neuropathies: a placebo-controlled trial. *Neurology* 2003; **60**: 1508–14.

51 Simpson DM, Olney R, McArthur JC *et al*. A placebo-controlled trial of lamotrigine for painful HIV-associated neuropathy. *Neurology* 2000; **54**: 2115–19.

52 Vestergaard K, Andersen G, Gottrup H, *et al*. Lamotrigine for central poststroke pain: a randomized controlled trial. *Neurology* 2001; **56**: 184–90.

53 Zakrzewska JM, Chaudhry Z, Nurmikko TJ, *et al*. Lamotrigine (Lamictal) in refractory trigeminal neuralgia: results from a double-blind placebo controlled crossover trial. *Pain* 1997; **73**: 223–30.

● 54 Dworkin RH, Corbin AE, Young JP Jr *et al*. Pregabalin for the treatment of postherpetic neuralgia: A randomized, placebo-controlled trial. *Neurology* 2003; **60**: 1274–83.

● 55 Rosenstock J, Tuchman M, LaMoreaux L, Sharma U. Pregabalin for the treatment of painful diabetic peripheral neuropathy: a double-blind, placebo-controlled trial. *Pain* 2004; **110**: 628–38.

● 56 Sabatowski R, Galvez R, Cherry DA *et al*. Pregabalin reduces pain and improves sleep and mood disturbances in patients with post-herpetic neuralgia: results of a randomised, placebo-controlled clinical trial. *Pain* 2004; **109**: 26–35.

57 Beydoun A, Kobetz SA, Carrazana EJ. Efficacy of oxcarbazepine in the treatment of painful diabetic neuropathy. *Clin J Pain* 2004; **20**: 174–8.

58 Royal MA, Jenson M, Bhakta B *et al*. An open-label trial of oxcarbazepine in patients with complex regional pain syndrome refractory to gabapentin. *J Pain* 2002; 3(2 Suppl 1): 40 (abstract 756).

59 Ward S, Royal MA, Jenson M *et al*. An open-label trial of oxcarbazepine in patients with radiculopathy refractory to gabapentin. *J Pain* 2002; 3(2 Suppl 1): 42 (abstract 765).

60 Zakrzewska JM, Patsalos PN. Oxcarbazepine: a new drug in the management of intractable trigeminal neuralgia. *J Neurol Neurosurg Psychiatry* 1989; **52**: 472–6.

● 61 Raskin P, Donofrio PD, Rosenthal NR *et al*. Topiramate vs placebo in painful diabetic neuropathy: analgesic and metabolic effects. *Neurology* 2004; **63**: 865–73.

62 Jenson M, Ward S, Royal M *et al*. Tiagabine is an effective treatment of neuropathic pain: a prospective, open-label trial. *J Pain* 2002; 3(2 Suppl 1): 40 (abstract 757).

63 Takahashi Y, Hashimoto K, Tsuji S. Successful use of zonisamide for central poststroke pain. *J Pain* 2004; **5**: 192–4.

64 Price MM. Levetiracetam in the treatment of neuropathic pain: three case studies. *Clin J Pain* 2004; **20**: 33–6.

65 Ward S, Jenson M, Royal M *et al.* Gabapentin and levetiracetam in combination for the treatment of neuropathic pain. *J Pain* 2002; **3**(2 Suppl 1): 38 (abstract 750).

66 Yajnik S, Singh GP, Singh G, Kumar M. Phenytoin as a coanalgesic in cancer pain. *J Pain Symptom Manage* 1992; **7**: 209–13.

67 McCleane GJ. Intravenous infusion of phenytoin relieves neuropathic pain: a randomized, double-blinded, placebo-controlled, crossover study. *Anesth Analg* 1999; **89**: 985–8.

◆ 68 Namaka M, Gramlich CR, Ruhlen D *et al.* A treatment algorithm for neuropathic pain. *Clin Ther* 2004; **26**: 951–79.

69 Attal N, Gaudé V, Brasseur L *et al.* Intravenous lidocaine in central pain: a double-blind, placebo-controlled, psychophysical study. *Neurology* 2000; **54**: 564–74.

70 Rowbotham MC, Reisner-Keller LA, Fields HL. Both intravenous lidocaine and morphine reduce the pain of postherpetic neuralgia. *Neurology* 1991; **41**: 1024–8.

● 71 Bruera E, Ripamonti C, Brenneis C *et al.* A randomized double-blind crossover trial of intravenous lidocaine in the treatment of neuropathic cancer pain. *J Pain Symptom Manage* 1992; **7**: 138–40.

72 Ellemann K, Sjogren P, Banning AM *et al.* Trial of intravenous lidocaine on painful neuropathy in cancer patients. *Clin J Pain* 1989; **5**: 291–4.

73 Brose WG, Cousins MJ. Subcutaneous lidocaine for treatment of neuropathic cancer pain. *Pain* 1991; **45**: 145–8.

◆ 74 Parsons CG. NMDA receptors as targets for drug action in neuropathic pain. *Eur J Pharmacol* 2001; **429**: 71–8.

75 Jackson K, Ashby M, Martin P *et al.* 'Burst' ketamine for refractory cancer pain: an open-label audit of 39 patients. *J Pain Symptom Manage* 2001; **22**: 834–42.

76 Mercadante S, Arcuri E, Tirelli W, Casuccio A. Analgesic effect of intravenous ketamine in cancer patients on morphine therapy: a randomized, controlled, double-blind, crossover, double-dose study. *J Pain Symptom Manage* 2000; **20**: 246–52.

77 Lauretti GR, Lima ICPR, Reis MP, *et al.* Oral ketamine and transdermal nitroglycerin as analgesic adjuvants to oral morphine therapy for cancer pain management. *Anesthesiology* 1999; **90**: 1528–33.

78 Bell RF. Low-dose subcutaneous ketamine infusion and morphine tolerance. *Pain* 1999; **83**: 101–3.

79 Mercadante S, Lodi F, Sapio M, *et al.* Long-term ketamine subcutaneous continuous infusion in neuropathic cancer pain. *J Pain Symptom Manage* 1995; **10**: 564–8.

80 Kannan TR, Saxena A, Bhatnagar S, Bary A. Oral ketamine as an adjuvant to oral morphine for neuropathic pain in cancer patients. *J Pain Symptom Manage* 2002; **23**: 60–5.

81 Benitez-Rosario MA, Feria M, Salinas-Martin A. A retrospective comparison of the dose ratio between subcutaneous and oral ketamine. *J Pain Symptom Manage* 2003; **25**: 400–2.

82 Fitzgibbon EJ, Hall P, Schroder C, *et al.* Low dose ketamine as an analgesic adjuvant in difficult pain syndromes: A strategy for conversion from parenteral to oral ketamine. *J Pain Symptom Manage* 2002; **23**: 165–70.

83 Weinbroum AA, Bender B, Bickels J *et al.* Preoperative and postoperative dextromethorphan provides sustained reduction in postoperative pain and patient-controlled epidural analgesia requirement: A randomized, placebo-controlled double-blind study in lower-body bone malignancy-operated patients. *Cancer* 2003; **97**: 2334–9.

84 Weinbroum AA, Bender B, Nirkin A *et al.* Dextromethorphan-associated epidural patient-controlled analgesia provides better pain- and analgesics-sparing effects than dextromethorphan-associated intravenous patient-controlled analgesia after bone-malignancy resection: a randomized, placebo-controlled, double-blinded study. *Anesth Analg* 2004; **98**: 714–22.

85 Amin P, Sturrock ND. A pilot study of the beneficial effects of amantadine in the treatment of painful diabetic peripheral neuropathy. *Diabet Med* 2003; **20**: 114–18.

86 Eisenberg E, Pud D. Can patients with chronic neuropathic pain be cured by acute administration of the NMDA receptor antagonist amantadine? *Pain* 1998; **74**: 337–9.

87 Pud D, Eisenberg E, Spitzer A *et al.* The NMDA receptor antagonist amantadine reduces surgical neuropathic pain in cancer patients: a double blind, randomized, placebo-controlled trial. *Pain* 1998; **75**: 349–54.

88 Kirby LC, the Memantine Study Group. Memantine in the treatment of diabetics with painful peripheral neuropathy: a placebo-controlled phase IIB trial. *Pain Medicine* 2002; **3**: 182.

89 Maier C, Dertwinkel R, Mansourian N *et al.* Efficacy of the NMDA-receptor antagonist memantine in patients with chronic phantom limb pain—results of a randomized double-blinded, placebo-controlled trial. *Pain* 2003; **103**: 277–83.

90 Wiech K, Kiefer RT, Topfner S *et al.* A placebo-controlled randomized crossover trial of the N-methyl-D-aspartic acid receptor antagonist, memantine, in patients with chronic phantom limb pain. *Anesth Analg* 2004; **98**: 408–13.

91 Fromm GH. Baclofen as an adjuvant analgesic. *J Pain Symptom Manage* 1994; **9**: 500–9.

92 Noyes R, Brunk SF, Avery DAH, Canter AC. The analgesic properties of delta-9-tetrahydrocannabinol and codeine. *Clin Pharmacol Ther* 1975; **18**: 84–9.

93 Campbell FA, Tramer MR, Carroll D *et al.* Are cannabinoids an effective and safe treatment option in the management of pain? A qualitative systematic review. *BMJ* 2001; **323**: 13–6.

94 Dellemijn PLI, Fields HL. Do benzodiazepines have a role in chronic pain management. *Pain* 1994; **57**: 137–52.

95 Reddy S, Patt RB. The benzodiazepines as adjuvant analgesics. *J Pain Symptom Manage* 1994; **9**: 510–4.

◆ 96 Dalal S, Melzack R. Potentiation of opioid analgesia by psychostimulant drugs: a review. *J Pain Symptom Manage* 1998; **16**: 245–53.

97 Rozans M, Dreisbach A, Lertora JJ, Kahn MJ. Palliative uses of methylphenidate in patients with cancer: a review. *J Clin Oncol* 2002; **20**: 335–9.

● 98 Galer BS, Rowbotham MC, Perander J. Topical lidocaine patch relieves postherpetic neuralgia more effectively than a vehicle topical patch: results of an enriched enrollment study. *Pain* 1999; **80**: 533–8.

99 Gammaitoni AR, Davis MW. Pharmacokinetics and tolerability of lidocaine patch 5% with extended dosing. *Ann Pharmacother* 2002; **36**: 236–40.

● 100 Ellison N, Loprinzi CL, Kugler J *et al.* Phase III placebo-controlled trial of capsaicin cream in the management of surgical neuropathic pain in cancer patients. *J Clin Oncol* 1997; **15**: 2974–80.

101 Gammaitoni A, Gallagher RM, Welz-Bosna M. Topical ketamine gel: possible role in treating neuropathic pain. *Pain Med* 2000; **1**: 97–100.

102 Ushida T, Tani T, Kanbara T *et al.* Analgesic effects of ketamine ointment in patients with complex regional pain syndrome type 1. *Reg Anesth Pain Med* 2002; **27**: 524–8.

103 Lynch ME, Clark AJ, Sawynok J. A pilot study examining topical amitriptyline, ketamine, and a combination of both in the treatment of neuropathic pain. *Clin J Pain* 2003; **19**: 323–8.

104 Slatkin NE, Rhiner M. Topical ketamine in the treatment of mucositis pain. *Pain Med* 2003; **4**: 298–303.

105 DeBenedittis G, Besana F, Lorenzettit A. A new topical treatment for acute herpetic neuralgia and postherpetic neuralgia: the aspirin/diethyl ether mixture: An open-label study plus a double-blind controlled clinical trial. *Pain* 1992; **48**: 383–90.

106 McQuay HJ, Carroll D, Moxon A, *et al.* Benzydamine cream for the treatment of postherpetic neuralgia: minimum duration of treatment periods in a cross-over trial. *Pain* 1990; **40**: 131–5.

107 Lin J, Zhang W, Jones A, Doherty M. Efficacy of topical non-steroidal anti-inflammatory drugs in the treatment of osteoarthritis: meta-analysis of randomized controlled trials. *BMJ* 2004; **329**: 324–9.

108 Mason L, Moore RA, Edwards JE, *et al.* Topical NSAIDs for chronic musculoskeletal pain: systematic review and meta-analysis. *BMC Musculoskel Dis* 2004; **5**: 28–35.

109 Hindley AC, Hill AB, Leyland MJ, Wiles AE. A double-blind controlled trial of salmon calcitonin in pain due to malignancy. *Cancer Chemother Pharmacol* 1982; **9**: 71–4.

110 Roth A, Kolaric K. Analgesic activity of calcitonin in patient with painful osteolytic metastases of breast cancer: results of a controlled randomized study. *Oncology* 1986; **43**: 283–7.

111 Szanto J, Ady N, Jozsef S. Pain killing with calcitonin nasal spray in patients with malignant tumors. *Oncology* 1992; **49**: 180–2.

112 Fulfaro F, Casuccio A, Ticozzi C, Ripamonti C. The role of bisphosphonates in the treatment of painful metastatic bone disease: a review of phase III trials. *Pain* 1998; **78**: 157–69.

113 Glover D, Lipton A, Keller A *et al.* Intravenous pamidronate disodium treatment of bone metastases in patients with breast cancer. *Cancer* 1994; **74**: 2949–55.

● 114 Lipton A, Small E, Saad F *et al.* The new bisphosphonate, Zometa (zoledronic acid), decreases skeletal complications in both osteolytic and osteoblastic lesions: a comparison to pamidronate. *Cancer Investig* 2002; **20**(Suppl 20): 45–54.

115 Van Holten-Verzantvoort ATM, Kroon HM, Bijvoet OL *et al.* Palliative pamidronate treatment in patients with bone metastases from breast cancer. *J Clin Oncol* 1993; **11**: 491–8.

● 116 Rosen LS, Gordon D, Kaminski M *et al.* Zoledronic acid versus pamidronate in the treatment of skeletal metastases in patients with breast cancer or osteolytic lesions of multiple myeloma: a phase III, double-blind, comparative trial. *Cancer J* 2001; **7**: 377–87.

● 117 Berenson JR, Lichtenstein A, Porter L *et al.* Efficacy of pamidronate in reducing skeletal events in patients with advanced multiple myeloma. *N Engl J Med* 1996; **334**: 488–93.

● 118 Hortobagyi GN, Theriault RL, Porter L *et al.* Efficacy of pamidronate in reducing skeletal complications in patients with breast cancer and lytic bone metastases. *N Engl J Med* 1996; **335**: 1785–91.

119 Berenson JR, Rosen LS, Howell A *et al.* Zoledronic acid reduces skeletal-related events in patients with osteolytic metastases. *Cancer* 2001; **91**: 1191–200.

120 Saad F, Gleason DM, Murray R *et al.* A randomized, placebo-controlled trial of zoledronic acid in patients with hormone-refractory metastatic prostate carcinoma. *J Natl Cancer Inst* 2002; **94**: 1458–68.

● 121 Saad F, Gleason DM, Murray R *et al.* Long-term efficacy of zoledronic acid for the prevention of skeletal complications in patients with metastatic hormone-refractory prostate cancer. *J Natl Cancer Inst* 2004; **96**: 879–82.

122 Rosen LS. Efficacy and safety of zoledronic acid in the treatment of bone metastases associated with lung cancer and other solid tumors. *Semin Oncol* 2002; **29**(Suppl 21): 28–32.

123 Skerjanec A, Berenson J, Hsu C *et al.* The pharmacokinetics and pharmacodynamics of zoledronic acid in cancer patients with varying degrees of renal function. *J Clin Pharmacol* 2003; **43**: 154–62.

124 Lahtinen R, Laakso M, Palva I, *et al.* Randomised, placebo-controlled multicentre trial of clodronate in multiple myeloma. Finnish Leukaemia Group. *Lancet* 1992; **340**: 1049–52.

125 Robertson AG, Reed NS, Ralston SH. Effect of oral clodronate on metastatic bone pain: a double-blind, placebo-controlled study. *J Clin Oncol* 1995; **13**: 2427–30.

● 126 Body JJ, Diel IJ, Lichinitser MR *et al.* Intravenous ibandronate reduces the incidence of skeletal complications in patients with breast cancer and bone metastases. *Ann Oncol* 2003; **14**: 1399–405.

127 Heidenreich A, Ohlmann C, Olbert P, Hegele A. High-dose ibandronate is effective and well tolerated in the treatment of pain and hypercalcaemia due to metastatic urologic cancer. *Eur J Cancer* 2003; **1**(Suppl): S270 (abstract 897).

128 Pecherstorfer M, Diel IJ. Rapid administration of ibandronate does not affect renal functioning: evidence from clinical studies in metastatic bone disease and hypercalcaemia of malignancy. *Support Care Cancer* 2004; **12**: 877–81.

129 Anderson PM, Wiseman GA, Dispenzieri A *et al.* High-dose samarium-153 ethylene diamine tetramethylene phosphonate: low toxicity of skeletal irradiation in patients with osteosarcoma and bone metastases. *J Clin Oncol* 2002; **20**: 189–96.

130 Lewington VJ, McEwan AJ, Ackery DM *et al.* A prospective, randomised double-blind cross-over study to examine the efficacy of strontium-89 in pain palliation in patients with advanced prostate cancer metastatic to bone. *Eur J Cancer* 1991; **27**: 954–8.

131 Quilty PM, Kirk D, Bolger JJ *et al.* A comparison of the palliative effects of strontium-89 and external beam radiotherapy in metastatic prostate cancer. *Radiother Oncol* 1994; **31**: 33–40.

132   Serafini AN, Houston SJ, Resche I *et al.* Palliation of pain associated with metastatic bone cancer using samarium-153 lexidronam: a double-blind placebo-controlled clinical trial. *J Clin Oncol* 1998; **16**: 1574–81.

133   Mercadante S, Ripamonti C, Casuccio A, *et al.* Comparison of octreotide and hyoscine butylbromide in controlling gastrointestinal symptoms due to malignant inoperable bowel obstruction. *Support Care Cancer* 2000; **8**: 188–91.

134   Ripamonti C, Mercadante S, Groff L *et al.* Role of octreotide, scopolamine butylbromide, and hydration in symptom control of patients with inoperable bowel obstruction and nasogastric tubes: a prospective randomized trial. *J Pain Symptom Manage* 2000; **19**: 23–34.

135   Mystakidou K, Tsilika E, Kalaidopoulou O *et al.* Comparison of octreotide administration vs conservative treatment in the management of inoperable bowel obstruction in patients with far advanced cancer: a randomized, double-blind, controlled clinical trial. *Anticancer Res* 2002; **22**: 1187–92.

136   DeConno F, Caraceni A, Zecca E, *et al.* Continuous subcutaneous infusion of hyoscine butylbromide reduces secretions in patients with gastrointestinal obstruction. *J Pain Symptom Manage* 1991; **6**: 484–6.

137   Fainsinger RL, Spanchynski K, Hanson J, Bruera E. Symptom control in terminally ill patients with malignant bowel obstruction. *J Pain Symptom Manage* 1994; **9**: 12–18.

138   Farr WC. The use of corticosteroids for symptom management in terminally ill patients. *Am J Hospice Care* 1990; **7**: 41–6.

139   Fadul CE, Lemann W, Thaler HT, Posner JB. Perforation of the gastrointestinal tract in patients receiving steroids for neurologic disease. *Neurology* 1988; **38**: 348–52.

140   ReMine SG, McIlrath D. Bowel perforation in steroid-treated patients. *Ann Surg* 1980; **192**: 581–6.

141   Gilron I, Bailey JM, Tu D *et al.* Morphine, gabapentin, or their combination for neuropathic pain. *N Engl J Med* 2005; **352**: 1324–34.

142   Solaro C, Messmer Uccelli M, Uccelli A, *et al.* Low-dose gabapentin combined with either lamotrigine or carbamazepine can be useful therapies for trigeminal neuralgia in multiple sclerosis. *Eur Neurol* 2000; **44**: 45–8.

◆ 143   Lussier D, Huskey AG, Portenoy RK. Adjuvant analgesics in cancer pain management. *Oncologist* 2004; **9**: 571–91.

◆ 144   Bernard SA. The interaction of medications used in palliative care. *Hematol/Oncol Clin North Am* 2002; **16**: 641–55.

47

Alternative routes for systemic opioid delivery

CARLA RIPAMONTI, MAURO BIANCHI

INTRODUCTION

It is well recognized that oral administration of the opioid drugs is the mainstay of analgesic therapy in cancer patients. Indeed, it is safe, effective, and convenient. Moreover, the oral route for drugs makes home management more simple. However, in some clinical situations such as severe vomiting, bowel obstruction, severe dysphagia, or severe confusion, and in situations where rapid dose escalation is necessary, oral administration of opioids is impossible and an alternative route has to be implemented.

Recent data suggest that 53–70 percent of patients with cancer-related pain require an alternative route for opioid administration hours and months before death.[1,2*] In the last few years, a number of modes for opioid administration have been explored. Bruera suggested that our ability to deliver opioids safely using alternative routes is the single most important development in home management of cancer pain.[3] This chapter deals with the characteristics, the main aspects of pharmacokinetics, the clinical efficacy and indications of the following routes: rectal, sublingual, buccal (gingival, transmucosal), subcutaneous, intravenous, intranasal, and transdermal.

Table 47.1 shows the potential clinical applications of the above mentioned routes of opioid administration. Box 47.1 gives the recommendations of the European Association for Palliative Care (EAPC) regarding the different routes of opioid administration.[4]

Table 47.1 *Potential applications of alternative routes for systemic opioid administration*

Symptoms	Sublingual	Rectal	Continuous subcutaneous infusion	Intravenous	Transdermal fentanyl/ buprenorphine	Transmucosal
Vomiting	++	++	++	++	++	--
Bowel obstruction	++	++	++	++	++	--
Dysphagia	++	++	++	++	++	--
Cognitive failure	-	+	++	++	++	--
Diarrhea	++	-	++	++	++	
Hemorrhoids Anal fissures	++	-	++	++	++	--
Coagulation disorders	++	++	-	++	++	--
Severe immunosuppression	++	++	-	+	++	--
Generalized edema	++	++	-	++	-	--
Frequent dose changes	++	-	++[a]	++[a]	-	--
Titration	++	+	++[a]	++±[a]	-	--
Breakthrough pain	++	++	++[a]	++[a]	-	++

[a]Patient-controlled analgesia.
+, may be indicated; ++, indicated; -, contraindicated; --, not indicated.

Box 47.1 Opioid administration according to the EAPC recommendations[4]

- A small proportion of patients develop intolerable adverse effects with oral morphine (in conjunction with a nonopioid and adjuvant analgesic as appropriate) before achieving adequate pain relief. In such patients a change to an alternative opioid or a change in the route of administration should be considered.

- If patients are unable to take morphine orally the preferred alternative route is subcutaneous. There is generally no indication for giving morphine intramuscularly for chronic cancer pain because subcutaneous administration is simpler and less painful.

- The average relative potency ratio of oral morphine to subcutaneous morphine is between 1:2 and 1:3 (i.e. 20–30 mg of morphine by mouth is equianalgesic to 10 mg by subcutaneous injection).

- In patients requiring continuous parenteral morphine, the preferred method of administration is by subcutaneous infusion.

- Intravenous infusion of morphine may be preferred in patients:

   (a) who already have an indwelling intravenous line

   (b) with generalized edema

   (c) who develop erythema, soreness or sterile abscesses with subcutaneous administration

   (d) with coagulation disorders

   (e) with poor peripheral circulation.

- The average relative potency ratio of oral to intravenous morphine is between 1:2 and 1:3.

- Rectal administration may be preferred by some patients. The equianalgesic dose by oral and rectal routes is about 1:1.

- The buccal, sublingual, and nebulized routes of administration of morphine are not recommended because at the present time there is no evidence of clinical advantage over the conventional routes.

- Oral transmucosal fentanyl citrate (OTFC) is an effective treatment for 'breakthrough pain' in patients stabilized on regular oral morphine or an alternative step 3 opioid.

- Transdermal fentanyl is an effective alternative to oral morphine but is best reserved for patients whose opioid requirements are stable. It may have particular advantages for such patients if they are unable to take oral morphine, as an alternative to subcutaneous infusion.

- Spinal (epidural or intrathecal) administration of opioid analgesics in combination with local anesthetics or clonidine should be considered in patients who derive inadequate analgesia or suffer intolerable adverse effects despite the optimal use of systemic opioids and nonopioids.

RECTAL ROUTE

The surface area of the human rectum is small (200–400 cm^2) because of the absence of villi. Its fluid contents have a pH of 7–8. The main mechanism of absorption from the rectum is passive diffusion and is probably no different from that in the upper part of the gastrointestinal tract despite the fact that pH, surface area, and fluid content differs substantially.[5] The rectum is drained by the superior rectal vein into the portal system and by the middle and inferior rectal veins into the inferior cava vein. It is impossible to predict the quantity of drug that will bypass the hepatic filter, because there are several extensive anastomoses between the superior rectal vein that drains to the portal system and the median and inferior rectal veins that drain towards the systemic circulation.[5,6] Rectal drug vehicles may be liquid or solid.[5–7] The absorption of aqueous and alcoholic solutions may occur very rapidly but the absorption of suppositories is generally slower and very much dependent on the nature of the suppository base, the use of surfactants, and other factors such as the presence/absence/quantity of fecal mass and the total volume content inside the rectum. Although an almost complete absence of presystemic metabolism has been found for intrarectal lidocaine in humans, several other drugs have been found to metabolize equal to or more than orally when administered intrarectally.[5] Davis *et al.*[7] reviewed the clinical, pharmacologic, and therapeutic role of suppositories and rectal suspension of opioids and other analgesics.

Bioavailability studies have shown considerable interindividual variation.[5–7] Johnson et al.[8] found that after 24 hours of rectal and intravenous (IV) administration of 10 mg of morphine chloride in eight patients, the bioavailability of morphine after rectal administration was 53 ± 18 percent of the values obtained after IV administration. The authors conclude that probably first-passage elimination of morphine was partially avoided by the rectal administration since a previous study suggested that the bioavailability of oral morphine is 37 percent.[9] The bioavailability of free morphine and morphine-6-glucuronide (M6G) was found to be comparable after oral, sublabial and rectal administration of morphine in cancer patients.[10–12]

In a comparative study[13] between 10 mg of morphine sulphate in oral solution and rectal suppository carried out in 10 patients with cancer pain, a significantly higher mean concentration of free morphine was found after rectal administration at all evaluation times throughout a period of 4.5 hours, whereas there were no differences between the routes in mean morphine-3-glucuronide (M3G) concentrations. These data suggest the presence of some avoidance of first-pass metabolism. Moolenar et al.[14] studied the rectal absorption of morphine hydrochloride from different aqueous solutions with different pH values in seven volunteers. The rectal absorption of morphine appeared to be dependent on the pH of the solution: a significant improvement in the absorption was found with a rectal solution adjusted to pH 7–8. Kaiko et al.[15] carried out a randomized crossover multiple-dose study in 14 healthy men to compare the bioavailability of 30 mg of morphine sulfate tablets (MS Contin) administered orally and rectally. There was no significant difference in morphine absorption between the two methods of administration. At 24 hours the area under the curve for the rectal treatment group was 90 percent of that of the oral group. However, the rectally administered slow-release morphine tablet was associated with an attenuated maximum morphine concentration level. Furthermore, the highest plasma morphine concentrations occurred significantly later, delayed from 2.46 hours after oral ingestion to 5.38 hours after rectal administration. The results suggest that there is a slower rate of absorption for MS Contin administered rectally than when given orally. Rectal administration of drugs can be used to produce local or systemic effects. In some countries, preparations of opioids in the form of suppositories are not commercially available. To overcome this situation, microenemas made up of liquid opioid (the same used for parenteral administration) are prepared and then given rectally as a bolus using a needleless insulin-type syringe with the advantage of a rapid absorption.

Most of the cancer pain treatment studies are of the non-controlled type. Brumley[16] treated 30 patients with cancer pain who had good pain control on oral morphine tablets with an equianalgesic dose of the same tablets inserted rectally in two gelatin capsules. Up to six tablets were inserted into each gelatin capsule and several patients required the use of several gelatin capsules at the same time. The capsules were administered every 4 hours regularly. The authors report that 26 out of 30 patients required no further titration of dose for effective pain control. The highest dose was 330 mg every 4 hours in one patient. The homemade morphine sulfate suppositories were found to be much more economical and better tolerated by patients than the commercially prepared suppositories. Maloney et al.[17] reviewed the experience with 39 terminally ill patients who received slow-release morphine as a rectal suppository. All patients had terminal cancer and 38 patients were receiving oral slow-release morphine before starting the rectal administration. Good pain control was reported in all cases. In two patients the slow-release morphine tablets were administered into a colostomy and in one case a female patient with diarrhea received the tablets intravaginally. No local side effects using the standard commercial preparation of 30 mg tablets were reported. Patients were treated for an average of 11.5 days (range 1–30 days).

Long-term rectal administration of high-dose sustained-release morphine tablets was reported by Walsh et al.[18] Based on this case, the correct milligram relative potency conversion ratio for rectal to IV morphine during repeated dosing appears to be 3:1, which is similar to that for the conversion from oral to IV. For rectal to oral morphine dosing the conversion ratio seems to be 1.1. Table 47.2 presents the randomized controlled trials (RCTs) on rectal morphine compared with oral or subcutaneous morphine.[19–22]**

Few data are available on the analgesia and tolerability of rectally administered methadone. A study[23] was carried out to assess the pharmacokinetics and pharmacodynamics of 10 mg of methadone hydrochloride administered rectally (in the form of microenema) in six opioid-naïve cancer patients whose pain no longer responded to treatment with non-steroidal anti-inflammatory drugs (NSAIDs) given at fixed times. The pharmacokinetics of rectal methadone showed rapid and extensive distribution phases followed by a slow elimination phase. The plasma concentrations presented a great intraindividual variability, with no correlation between analgesia and plasma methadone concentration. Pain relief was statistically significant already after 30 minutes and continued more than 8 hours after administration. In five patients pain control lasted between 24 and 48 hours. Only one patient reported vomiting, confusion and vertigo after the administration of rectal methadone.

In a prospective, open study, Bruera et al.[24] demonstrated that custom-made capsules and suppositories of methadone were safe, effective, and low cost in 37 advanced cancer patients with poor pain control receiving high doses of subcutaneous hydromorphone. These patients had significant improvement in pain control with minimal toxicity, using doses higher than those reported in the literature. This study also demonstrated a large interindividual variation between methadone dosage and plasma level. Rectal methadone can be considered an effective, safe, and low cost therapy for

Table 47.2 *Randomized controlled trials on rectal morphine compared with oral or subcutaneous morphine*

Study	Study design	No. of patients	Route 1	Route 2	Results
Bruera et al.[19]	Double blind, crossover	23	CR morphine sulfate suppository every 12 hours	SC morphine Rectal/parenteral ratio 2.5:1	Comparable analgesia and side effects
Babul et al.[20]	Double blind, crossover	27	CR morphine suppository every 12 hours	CR morphine tablets every 12 hours Conversion rate 1:1	No difference in pain and sedation; small but significant difference in nausea in favor of rectal administration
De Conno et al.[21]	Double blind, double dummy, crossover, single dose study	34 opioid-naive	Rectal morphine prepared as microenema	Oral morphine Conversion rate 1:1	Rectal morphine had a faster onset of action and longer duration of analgesia than an acute dose of oral morphine. No significant difference in intensity of sedation, nausea, or number of vomiting episodes between the two routes
Bruera et al.[22]	Randomized, double blind crossover	126 evaluable	CR morphine sulfate suppository every 12 hours	CR morphine sulfate suppository every 24 hours	There was no significant difference between the q12h and q24h treatment groups in symptom (pain, nausea, sedation) intensity, adverse effects, patient choice

SC, subcutaneous; CSI, continuous subcutaneous infusion; CR, controlled release; IV, intravenous; q, every.

patients with cancer pain where oral and/or parenteral opioids are not indicated or available.

Oxycodone pectinate suppositories are available in countries such as the UK and need to be given every 8 hours. The single-dose pharmacokinetics and pharmacodynamics of oxycodone administered by intravenous and rectal routes were determined in 12 cancer patients. Intravenous oxycodone was associated with a rapid onset of analgesia (5–8 minutes) with respect to rectal route (0.5–1 hours) but with a shorter analgesic effect (4 hours via IV route compared with 8–12 hours via rectal route).[25] In a controlled clinical trial rectal administration of tramadol was as effective as oral tramadol in relieving cancer-related pain.[26**]

The colostomy administration route of opioids is not recommended. The results of the study of Hojsted et al.[27] comparing the pharmacokinetics of hydrochloride morphine administered via rectal and colostomic routes demonstrated that the bioavailability via colostomy showed a very wide variation, but the mean value as compared to rectal administration was 43 percent (range 0–127 percent). The authors suspect that the main reason for lower bioavailability may be poor vascularization of the colostomy, adsorption of morphine to feces, and the presence of first-passage elimination. Anecdotal reports of rectal administration of controlled-release morphine suggest

that these routes may be used for patients unable to take oral medications.

The rectal route of drug administration may present some disadvantages when used long term and when feces or diarrhea is present. This alternative route can be used successfully in patients with breakthrough pain (defined as transient flares of severe or excruciating pain in patients already managed with analgesics) and in some clinical situations as shown in Table 47.1. Compared with the subcutaneous and IV routes, the rectal route has the advantage of not requiring needles to be inserted or pumps to be carried. On the negative side, chronic and frequent rectal administration can lead to discomfort, and the presence of feces in the rectum, diarrhea, or normal peristalsis can reduce absorption.

There are some barriers to the development of rectally administered drugs. Sometimes physicians, caregivers, and patients find this route unappealing.

SUBLINGUAL AND BUCCAL ROUTES

The mouth has many areas with a potential for transmucosal administration: sublingual (beneath the tongue) and buccal (between the gingival edge of the upper molars and the cheek). The permeability is greatest in the sublingual area and lowest at the gingival level. The surface of the buccal and sublingual area is small ($200\,cm^2$) with a pH of 6.2–7.4. However, this region is rich in blood and lymphatic vessels and the possibility exists for rapid absorption with direct passage into the systemic circulation avoiding the hepatic first-pass metabolism.[5]

The conditions for the penetration of the drug improve with the smallness of molecules, a high concentration of nonionized drug, and a high degree of lipophilia. Thus, the amount of drug absorbed will depend on several factors including the pK_a, rate of partition of the nonionized form of the drug, the lipid/water partition coefficient, molecular weight of the drug, passive diffusion, and the pH of the solution in the mouth. Lipophilic drugs such as buprenorphine, fentanyl, and methadone are better absorbed than polar ones.[28] Studies on the buccal absorption of morphine report different results.[5,6]

The preferred preparation is the tablet form rather than liquids and pastes, which can spread all over the mouth and consequently increase the possibility of swallowing the drug. Saliva affects the absorption of the drug by dilution and by increasing the likelihood of the drug being swallowed before absorption.

Buprenorphine is the only commercial opioid formulated in a sublingual preparation. Single dose crossover studies have shown it to be 15 times as potent as morphine in terms of total analgesic effect.[29] The absorption half-life of sublingual buprenorphine is about 76 minutes, and peak plasma concentrations range from 20 to 360 minutes (mean 180 minutes) after administration, although there is a large intersubject variability.[30] A dose of 0.4 mg sublingually gives similar analgesia to 0.2–0.3 mg intramuscularly (IM), with an onset of analgesia within 30–60 minutes of administration and a duration of 6–9 hours.[31] The long duration of analgesia with buprenorphine may be related to its affinity for the μ-opioid receptor and an unusually slow dissociation constant for the drug-receptor complex.

Robbie[32] treated 141 cancer patients with sublingual buprenorphine in doses of 0.15–0.8 mg for an average of 12 weeks. This treatment was effective in most of the patients, particularly those with pain from head and neck cancer. Drowsiness was the most common side effect (seen in 22 patients maintained on sublingual buprenorphine), but dry mouth and nausea also occurred. De Conno et al.[33] found that patients previously treated with sublingual or IM buprenorphine required a dose of morphine significantly higher than those treated with other opioids (codeine, oxycodone, dextropropoxyphene, pentazocine) to obtain the same pain relief. Like the mixed agonist–antagonists, buprenorphine may precipitate withdrawal in patients who have received repeated doses of a morphine-like agonist and developed physical dependence. Naloxone is relatively ineffective in reversing serious respiratory depression caused by buprenorphine.[34]

There is still some controversy on the efficacy of sublingual morphine[35] because of the lack of controlled clinical studies. The few reports on the clinical effects of sublingual and buccal morphine are related to one-time dosage or anecdotal experience. Whitman et al.[36] report that 70–80 percent of 150 patients with cancer pain who were treated with sublingual morphine obtained 'adequate to good pain control'. Patients were treated with morphine sulfate tablets in a dose of 10–30 mg every 3–4 hours around the clock. The main side effects reported were intolerance to the taste of the drug and occasional confusion or unpleasant dreams. Pannuti et al.[12] treated 28 patients with cancer pain with sublingual drops of morphine hydrochloride every 4 hours. Patients were treated for an average of 5 weeks. Although the authors reported more rapid and significant pain remission for the sublingual route as compared to the rectal and oral route, no significant difference in the incidence or severity of side effects were reported. No patient required discontinuation of sublingual treatment because of toxicity.

The effects of sublingual fentanyl citrate (SLFC) were assessed in 11 hospice inpatients with cancer-related breakthrough pain.[37] SLFC was started at 25 μg (using parenteral formulation of 50 μg/mL) and the dose was progressively increased by 25 μg till pain was controlled. The maximum dose used was 150 μg as volumes greater than 3 mL were difficult to retain sublingually. Fifty-five percent of patients reported pain reduction after 10 minutes and 82 percent after 15 minutes. Ratings for SLFC were very good (18 percent), good (36 percent), moderate (28 percent), and bad (18 percent). Compared to the usual breakthrough medication (mostly normal release morphine), SLFC was better (46 percent), the same (36 percent), or worse (18 percent). No systemic adverse effects were reported. SLFC may be an option for patients unable to tolerate oral morphine in treating breakthrough pain.

Sublingual sufentanil at a dosage of 25 μg every 3 minutes × 3 doses, produced pain relief with minimal sedation in one patient previously treated with oral morphine and with sublingual fentanyl.[38] Sufentanil 25 μg is approximately equianalgesic to 70–100 mg sublingual morphine, whereas 50 μg sublingual fentanyl is equianalgesic to about 7–10 mg sublingual morphine.[39]

Oral transmucosal fentanyl citrate (OTFC) is a synthetic opioid agonist manufactured in a matrix of sucrose and liquid glucose base and fitted onto a radiopaque plastic handle. It is a drug delivery formulation used for management of breakthrough cancer pain. Doses are available in six different strengths (200 μg, 400 μg, 600 μg, 800 μg, 1200 μg, and 1600 μg). Absorption is via the oral mucosa. Administration of a drug through this route avoids the first-pass effect, and allows easy and rapid dose titration. From the pharmacokinetic point of view, OTFC is similar to IM and IV fentanyl, whereas the plasma concentrations are double in respect to oral fentanyl and are reached 86 minutes before.[40,41] Peak effect occurs in about 20 minutes. Approximately 25 percent of the dose of fentanyl goes directly into the bloodstream through mucosal absorption and accounts for 50 percent of the dose that reaches the plasma. Total bioavailability is approximately 50 percent as duration of action ranges from 2.5 to 5 hours. The onset of analgesic effect is obtained within 5 to 15 minutes,[42] in contrast to the 30–60 minutes with normal-release oral opioids. Seventy-six percent of patients with incident and breakthrough pain have experienced favorable results.[43]

In a multicenter, randomized, double-blind, placebo-controlled trial of OTFC for cancer-related breakthrough pain carried out by Farrar et al.,[44**] OTFC produced significantly larger changes in pain intensity and better pain relief than placebo. In another controlled dose titration study[45**] in cancer patients treated with OTFC, 74 percent of them were successfully titrated. Moreover, OTFC provided significantly greater analgesic effect at 15, 30, and 60 minutes, and a more rapid onset of effect, than the usual rescue drug. There was no relation between the total daily dose of the fixed schedule opioid regimen and the dose of OTFC required to manage breakthrough pain. As the optimal dose cannot be predicted, treatment should begin with a dose of 200 μg and increased at 15 minutes intervals. It emerged from controlled and uncontrolled studies that the adverse effects of the OTFC were similar to other opioids and very few adverse events were severe or serious.

In a double-blind, double-dummy, randomized, multiple crossover study, Coluzzi et al.[46**] compared OTFC and immediate-release morphine sulfate for management of breakthrough pain in 134 outpatients receiving a fixed scheduled opioid regimen equivalent to 60–1000 mg/day oral morphine or 50–300 μg/h transdermal fentanyl. Sixty-nine percent of patients (93/134) found a successful dose of OTFC and it was more effective than immediate-release oral morphine in treating breakthrough pain. In an open-label study,[47] OTFC was also shown to be safe and effective during long-term treatment of breakthrough pain in cancer patients cared for at home.

OTFC is approved the US Food and Drug Administration (FDA) solely for the management of breakthrough pain in opioid-tolerant cancer patients.[48] It is not recommended for treating acute and or postoperative pain. Future studies are required in order to establish the OTFC dose to be used as rescue dose in patients with breakthrough pain in respect to type and dose of opioid taken by the patient.

SUBCUTANEOUS ROUTE

The rate of absorption of a drug strongly depends on the blood flow to the site of absorption. In normal conditions, the perfusion of subcutaneous tissue is similar to that of muscles. However, the rate of absorption is slower. The main factors determining the subcutaneous absorption are the solubility of the drug, the site of the injection, the surface exposed, the blood pressure, the presence of cutaneous vaso-constriction, edema, or inflammatory processes.

Subcutaneous opioid administration can be intermittent or continuous. Intermittent injection may represent a valid option in some circumstances.[49] However, it can be associated with a 'bolus effect' characterized by acute toxicity and a brief analgesic effect. Moreover, because of the short duration of action of most opioids, injections need to be repeated frequently, usually at intervals of 4 hours or less. In palliative medicine, the results of this method are undesirable because it is painful for the patient, time consuming for the caregivers, and difficult to maintain in the home setting. Therefore, continuous subcutaneous infusion (CSI) is recommended. A recent review demonstrated that CSI is effective and safe for use in terminal illness.[50] Consistently with this evidence, it is gradually becoming a standard practice in palliative medicine.

The subcutaneous route can also be used for patient-controlled analgesia (PCA) using portable pumps.[51] PCA is a relatively new technique for managing pain in which patients are able to self-administer small doses of opioid analgesic when needed. This technique offers an alternative to traditional regimens and was developed in response to the under-treatment of pain in hospitalized patients. A number of uncontrolled and controlled trials have confirmed the safety and efficacy of PCA for postoperative pain in adults[51] as well as in children ranging from 5 to 15 years.[51] PCA is a very specific way of prescribing 'as needed' analgesics because all parameters such as route, drug concentration, dose, frequency, and maximum daily or hourly dose are actually prescribed by the physician, but the patient decides whether or not they should take a dose. The decision is not subject to external judgment and the administration is not slowed down by the intervention of the nurse or the doctor. A large variety of pumps are available for PCA. Most of them consist of a drug reservoir and an injection or infusion system, either manually or electronically operated. PCA devices permit the patient to choose an intermittent (demand) bolus, continuous infusion, or both intermittent, and continuous modes of administration. A continuous infusion plus an intermittent bolus dose allow patients to maintain a baseline level of opioid administration plus additional doses for breakthrough pain. The device can be used to deliver the drug through continuous intravenous, epidural, subcutaneous infusions. Whenever the patient feels that pain relief is necessary, he or she can activate the system by pressing a button. The unit dispenses an amount of analgesic that has been programmed by the physician. In some devices, unauthorized alteration of dose parameters is excluded by a number of safety factors. A lock-out time is available to prevent overdosage. Other simpler and less expensive devices do not contain a lock-out system. Although a lock-out system may be desirable for patients with confusion and/or a history of addiction, it is important to consider that oral prescriptions contain no lock-out mechanisms. The indications and contraindications for PCA are given in Box 47.2.

Box 47.2 Indications and contraindications for PCA

Indications

- Incident pain

- Circadian variation of pain intensity

- Patients with reduced 'therapeutic window'

- Renal failure

- Drugs with an unpredictable half-life (methadone)

- Patients who have a need to maintain control over their life (high locus of control)

- Patients who have an extreme fear of side effects

Contraindications

- Severe alcoholism

- History of drug addiction

- Cognitive failure

- Lack of knowledge and skill to use the technique safely and effectively

---

This is a well-known therapeutic strategy in analgesia. Many different portable pumps or nonportable devices are available for CSI, including a syringe pump, disposable plastic cylinder, and battery-operated computer-driven pumps. It is important to select the most suitable solution for each patient. The disadvantages of these devices are their cost and complexity. Simpler and less expensive devices should be developed in order to decrease the cost and increase the comfort of patients, families, and nurses. The most common problems that can occur with PCA systems are listed in Box 47.3. Subcutaneous PCA is particularly suitable also for the treatment of several types of postoperative pain.[52,53] This method is contraindicated in patients with coagulation disorders, cognitive failure or with a history of substance abuse.

Box 47.3 Most common problems with PCA

Operator errors

- Misprogramming of PCA device

- Failure to clamp or unclamp tubing

- Improper loading of syringe

- Failure to respond to safety alarm

- Misplacing pump key

Patient errors

- Poor understanding of PCA therapy

- Poor understanding of how to use PCA pump device

Mechanical problems

- Failure to deliver on demand

- Cracked drug vials or syringes

- Defective valves

- Faulty alarm system

- Malfunctions (e.g. lock-out feature)

Most studies of subcutaneous opioid administration have used morphine or hydromorphone. These drugs have short half-lives and hence reach the steady state rapidly. It has been reported that the blood levels of morphine during CSI are similar to those reached during continuous intravenous infusion.[54] Another study in healthy volunteers provided different results, indicating that the bioavailabilities of morphine and of its main metabolites (M6G and M3G) are significantly lower after subcutaneous than after IV administration. Despite this observation, the authors concluded that the subcutaneous route is an effective method for the systemic administration of morphine.[55] No clear differences seem to exist between subcutaneous morphine and hydromorphone from both the pharmacokinetic and the pharmacodynamic points of view.[56**,57**]

Drugs with longer half-lives, such as methadone, have also been evaluated. In most patients, CSI of methadone produced signs of local toxicity (specifically erythema and induration). Such a toxicity is manageable by changing the position of the needle and infusing dexamethasone concurrently with the methadone.[58,59] In general a 25 or 27 gauge butterfly needle inserted in the anterior chest or abdomen is recommended for infusion. The subcutaneous route, with special reference to SCI, should be considered as the standard alternative route for systemic opioid delivery.

INTRAVENOUS ROUTE

Intravenous administration of opioids permits complete systemic absorption, and produces rapid analgesia that is correlated to lipidic solubility (10–15 minutes for morphine, 2–5 minutes for methadone) but is of short duration. This makes it necessary to repeat infusions at least every 4 hours. Thus, this route of administration is painful for the patient, time-consuming for the nursing staff, and difficult to carry out in the home setting. Bolus administration can be substituted by continuous intravenous infusion (CIVI) using a pump. This is common among hospitalized cancer patients, above all in those with central venous catheters. Continuous intravenous infusion of opioids has been reported to be effective and safe in managing cancer pain in patients who are less responsive to analgesics administered at the maximum tolerated dose by other routes.[60,61] Patient-controlled analgesia is also possible by the IV route.[51]

The most frequently used drugs are short-acting opioid agonists such as morphine, hydromorphone, and fentanyl.[51,62**] Because these drugs have a short half-life, the risk of delayed toxicity due to gradually increasing their plasmatic levels will be less likely than with drugs having longer half-lives such as methadone or levorphanol. In the largest series reported to date, 117 consecutive cancer patients were treated with morphine (93 percent) or hydromorphone (7 percent) administered subcutaneously (87 percent) or IV (13 percent) with a PCA bolus set at 25 percent of the hourly infusion rate for breakthrough pain.[63] The mean duration of treatment was 23 days; 69 percent of patients were cared for at home, and the remaining patients were treated in an inpatient hospice. Most of the patients remained on PCA until death. After the initiation of PCA, 95 percent of patients achieved pain relief. Significant variability in opioid consumption was reported; the dose of morphine used ranged from 1 mg/h to 33 mg/h in the subcutaneous group and from 2 mg/h to 180 mg/h in the IV group. Complications developed in two patients (infection at the subcutaneous site in one patient and respiratory arrest within 24 hours of starting PCA in the other). The authors report that patients using the subcutaneous route who then required more than 40–50 mg/h were switched to the IV route. PCA has been successfully used in patients presenting severe oral pain due to mucositis who required systemically administered opioid medication.[51]

Over a certain period of time, some patients develop analgesic tolerance to this type of regimen, requiring frequent dose escalation. As noted above, if lower doses of opioid reduce psychological distress, one might rely on PCA alone during the day and a combination of PCA and continuous infusion during the night. Thus, these two modes of delivering PCA can be used together. Patient-controlled analgesia should be monitored by assessing the patient's respiratory rate and mental status with adequate modification of the opioid dosages if there is a decrease of the respiratory rate or hypoxemia or somnolence occur. Although morphine is the drug of choice, clinical experience has shown that other drugs, such as methadone, hydromorphone, and fentanyl, can also be used successfully.[61,64,65]

The choice of a drug for CIVI depends on the previous antalgic treatment and on the pharmacokinetic profile of the drug employed. A patient who reports good analgesia with a particular opioid but presents adverse effects to a bolus administration (plasma peak toxicity or pain during the reduction of the plasma concentration) is a suitable candidate for CIVI with the same drug. On the other hand, if the patient presents adverse effects at plasma peak and also reports poor or the absence of analgesia, the CIVI must be initiated with a different opioid. In choosing an analgesic drug, its half-life is by far the most important pharmacokinetic factor. For this reason morphine and hydromorphone, both having short half-lives, are the preferred infusion drugs. With the use of long half-life medication such as methadone, the delay to steady-state may result in the slow onset of analgesia when CIVI is increased or in the late appearance of toxicity developing after analgesia appears.

The opioid dosage at the beginning of treatment depends on the patient's pharmacological intake. Patients being treated with repeated parenteral doses can switch to CIVI with the same drug using the same daily dosage, whereas the administration of a different opioid would require a dosage reduction of between half to two-thirds.

Portenoy et al.[61] reviewed the clinical experience of 36 patients who received CIVI. Mean doses during CIVI were equivalent to maximum morphine initial doses of 17 mg/h (range 0.7–100), with maximum doses reaching 69 mg/h (range 4–480) and 52 mg/h (range 1–480) at the end of the treatment. Pain relief was acceptable in 28 CIVIs, unacceptable in 17, and unknown in one. The most important side effects, beginning or progressing during the CIVIs, were sedation, confusion, constipation and myoclonus. This review suggests that CIVI is safe, that analgesia may require rapid dose escalation, and that although not all the patients experienced acceptable analgesia, failure of CIVI with one medication because of incomplete cross-tolerance could be followed by effective analgesia obtained with a different opioid. In a case report[66] hydromorphone administered via CIVI and then orally was able to abolish itching present during IV morphine administration. Oral and IV oxycodone were compared in a single-dose study.[67] Although IV oxycodone produced a faster onset of pain relief, the duration of analgesia was about 4 hours with both routes of oxycodone administration; IV oxycodone produced significantly more adverse effects.

The pharmacokinetics of IV methadone showed rapid and extensive distribution phases followed by a slow elimination phase.[68] Manfredi et al.[69] described the dramatic beneficial effects of IV methadone in four patients in whom IV morphine and hydromorphone failed to produce adequate pain relief despite titration to dose-limiting side effects. All the patients had long-lasting pain relief without significant side effects at a methadone dose equal to 20 percent of the hydromorphone dose. Fitzgibbon et al.[70] described the successful use of large doses of IV methadone administered by PCA and continuous infusion for pain refractory to large doses of IV morphine. Morphine was stopped, and treatment with methadone via PCA was initiated (incremental dose 10 mg every 6 minutes) with a continuous infusion of methadone at a rate of 40 mg/h. On day 3, methadone was decreased to 200 mg with a good pain management and no adverse effects. The patient was discharged after 5 days with a dose of 220 mg/day (average daily methadone was approximately 1/10 that of morphine). After 6 weeks the dose was

Table 47.3 *Intravenous titration (dose finding) with morphine for severe cancer pain*

Study	Study design and patient population	Initial morphine dosage and route	Following dosage and route	Results
Radbruch et al.[73]	Prospective study 26 inpatients with uncontrolled pain, on step II opioids	IV PCA pump programmed for 24 h: 1 mg bolus, lock-out interval of 5 minutes. Maximum dose of 12 mg/h	Oral SR morphine q12h; dose on the basis of the previous IV requirements IV-PO conversion 1:2 BKP treated with IV PCA until stable analgesia was reached	Mean pain intensity (NRS 0–100): at entry: 67 after 5 h: 22 at day 7: 17 at day 14: 12 Mean morphine dosage (IV PCA) in the first 24 h: 32 mg (range 4–78) Mean daily morphine dosage (PO + IV PCA for BKP) at PCA termination (range 2–6 days): 139 mg (range 20–376) Mean morphine dosage (PO) at day 14: 154 mg (range 20–344) No significant adverse events
Mercadante et al.[74]	Prospective study 45 inpatients with severe (NRS $\geqslant$ 7) and prolonged pain At entry, 30 patients were on step II opioids, 15 were on step III opioids	IV bolus (2 mg every 2 minutes), repeated until analgesia or adverse effects were reported	Oral SR morphine; dose on the basis of the previous IV requirements IV-PO conversion: 1:3 for lower IV dosages, 1:2 for higher IV dosages The same IV dose was maintained for BKP in the first 24 hours	Mean pain intensity (NRS 0–10): At entry: 8.1 After 9.7 minutes: 3.0 with a mean IV morphine dosage of 8.5 mg Mean daily oral morphine dosage at time to discharge: 131 mg (107–156) + 10.8 mg (IV extra doses) No significant adverse events
Harris et al.[75]	Randomized controlled trial 62 strong opioid-naïve patients (pain intensity NRS $\geqslant$ 5) Patients were randomized to receive IV morphine (n = 31) or oral IR morphine (n = 31)	IV group: 1.5 mg bolus every 10 minutes until pain relief (or adverse effects) Oral group: IR morphine 5 mg every 4 h in opioid-naïve patients 10 mg in patients. on weak opioids. Rescue dose: the same dose every 1 h max.	IV group: Oral IR morphine q4h, on the basis of the previous IV requirements IV:PO conversion 1:1 Rescue dose: the same dose every 1 h max. Oral group: follow the same scheme	Percentage of patients achieving satisfactory pain relief: after 1 h: IV group, 84%; oral group, 25% (P < 0.001) after 12 h: IV group 97%; oral group 76% (P < 0.001) after 24 h: IV group and oral group similar IV group: Median morphine dosage (IV) to achieve pain relief: 4.5 mg (range 1.5–34.5). In the same group, mean morphine dosage (PO) after stabilization: 8.3 mg (range 2.5–30). Oral group: Median morphine dosage to achieve pain relief: 7.2 mg (2.5–15) No significant adverse events

IV, intravenous; PCA, patient-controlled analgesia; NRS, Numerical Rating Scale; step II, of the WHO analgesic ladder; BKP, breakthrough pain.

increased up to 400 mg/day with good pain control and no adverse effects.

Intravenous methadone administered by PCA was safe and effective in controlling cancer pain, sedation, and confusion in 18 patients previously treated with IV fentanyl. A conversion ratio of 25 μg/h of fentanyl to 0.1 mg/h of methadone was used to estimate the initial dose of methadone in all patients (0.25 ratio between fentanyl and

Table 47.4 *Intravenous titration (dose finding) with fentanyl for severe cancer pain*

Study	Study design and patient population	Initial morphine/ fentanyl dosage and route	Following dosage and route	Results
Soares et al.[76]	Prospective study 18 outpatients (pain intensity NRS ⩾ 7) on oral morphine therapy for at least 2 weeks Excluded patients with BKP and neuropathic pain	Repeated IV bolus in 4 steps, with 5 min intervals Evaluation of pain and side effects after each step Dosage: Oral morphine converted to IV morphine (dose ratio 1:3) and than to IV fentanyl (dose ratio 1:100) Steps 1 and 2: 10% of the total IV morphine taken in the previous 24 h Step 3 and 4: step 1 and 2 dosage increased by 50%	The protocol was not followed to find future doses of opioids The management of pain after the fast titration with fentanyl was 9 patients increased the previous morphine dose 3 patients switched the opioid 5 patients switched the route 5 patients received ketamine infusion	100% of patients achieving satisfactory pain relief Mean time to achieve pain relief: 11 minutes (range 5–25). Pain intensity less than 4 Mean previous oral morphine dosage 276 mg (range 180–600) Mean IV fentanyl required to achieve pain relief: 214 μg (range 60–525). No significant adverse events
Grond et al.[77]	Prospective study 50 GI or head and neck cancer patients with severe pain. Excluded patients with BKP and opioid unresponsive pain	Previous opioids were discontinued and PCA IV fentanyl started: demand dose 50 μg, lock-out time 5 min, hourly max dose 250 μg	On the second day TTS applied with a rate delivery calculated from the PCA dose[a] of the first 24 h + IV fentanyl for rescue doses during first and second day, there-after oral or SC morphine for rescue doses If pain intensity increased at the end of the 72-h period and an increase of the TTS-dose was ineffective, the systems were changed every 48 h	Patients were treated for 66 ± 101 days (3–535) Mean delivery rate was 5.9 ± 4.1 mg/day Mean pain intensity decreased from initially 45 ± 21 to 19 ± 15 in the titration phase and 15 ± 11 during long-term treatment 3 patients had moderate respiratory depression Moderate or severe constipation in 40% of the patients prior to study, in 18% during titration period and in 10% during long-term treatment

[a] PCAI V fentanyl (mg/day), 0.2–0.6, 0.6–1.0, 1.0–1.4, 1.4–1.8; TTS-fentanyl (mg/day), 0.6, 1.2, 1.8, 2.4.
IV, intravenous; NRS, Numerical Rating Scale; BKP, breakthrough pain; GI, gastrointestinal; TTS, transdermal therapeutic system; SC, subcutaneous.

methadone).[65] Self-administered bolus doses of IV methadone equal to 50–100 percent of the hourly infusion rate were allowed every 20 minutes and additional boluses of 100–200 percent of the hourly infusion rate every 60 minutes. To control pain, there was a 10 percent increase in the median hourly infusion dose of methadone from day 1 (64.45 mg) to day 2; after day 2 the median hourly infusion dose of methadone was the same and decreased to 54 mg on day 4.

Numerous medications prolong the rate-corrected QT (QTc) interval and induce arrhythmias by blocking ionic current through cardiac potassium channels composed of subunits expressed by the human ether-a-go-go-related gene (*HERG*). Recent reports suggest that high doses of methadone cause *torsades de pointes*.[71] Kornick et al.[72] found that methadone in combination with chlorobutanol (the preservative present in the formulation of parenteral methadone) is associated with QTc interval prolongation.

Even if the titration with strong opioids is routinely performed using immediate-release oral morphine every 4 hours, there are some clinical situation such as severe pain where pain relief has to be achieved as quickly as possible. Tables 47.3[73,74,75**] and 47.4[76,77] present the studies reporting 'fast titration' resulting in rapid pain relief of moderate to severe pain in cancer patients treated with bolus doses of intravenous morphine or fentanyl and then switched to oral morphine or transdermal fentanyl. These authors have shown that 'fast titration' with IV opioids is effective and safe.

At the Memorial Sloan–Kettering Cancer Center in New York the patients on transdermal fentanyl presenting severe episodes of pain are switched (transdermal therapeutic system [TTS] removed) to CIVI of fentanyl using a transdermal:IV conversion of 1:1.[78] PCA IV fentanyl is used to administer rescue on demand doses (50–100 percent of the CIVI rate). Relief of pain without serious adverse effects is reported.[78] Continuous parenteral (subcutaneous or intravenous) opioids have been shown to improve analgesia and tolerability in 71 percent of cancer patients previously treated with oral opioids (codeine, tramadol, morphine, methadone) or with transdermal fentanyl. On the basis of this study, parenteral opioids may be considered a good alternative to spinal opioids.[79]

Continuous intravenous infusion of opioids in cancer-related pain is specifically indicated in cases of generalized edema, coagulation disorders, increased frequency of subcutaneous local site infections, reduced peripheral circulation, when frequent IM or IV injections are required to maintain pain control, in the presence of prominent 'bolus effects' on repetitive injection and when rapid titration of drug doses is required to produce rapid pain relief.

Opioid administration through CIVI can be carried out via central venous catheters, however, these catheters are expensive and need to be surgically implanted and require considerable nursing expertise and/or teaching the patient's family. For these reasons CIVI should be considered only for patients with an implanted catheter and for patients who present bleeding diathesis or diminished muscle mass who develop intractable vomiting, bowel obstruction, or malabsorption.

INTRANASAL ROUTE

The nasal administration of opioids has been widely investigated in recent years. This route offers the advantage of more rapid drug absorption and onset of pain relief compared with oral dosing. This is due to the large surface area, porous endothelial membrane, high total blood flow, the avoidance of first-pass metabolism, and ready accessibility.[80] Pharmacokinetic data in volunteers are reported for fentanyl, alfentanil, sufentanil, butorphanol, oxycodone, morphine, diamorphine, hydromorphone, methadone, heroin, and buprenorphine.[80–85] From a clinical point of view, patient-controlled intranasal (PCIN) fentanyl has been compared with oral morphine for procedural wound care in patients with burns.[86**] It has been observed that PCIN fentanyl is similar in efficacy and safety to oral morphine. A rapid onset of analgesia and potential clinical utility for the treatment of postoperative pain have been suggested for a formulation of nasal fentanyl spray.[87]

Jackson et al.[88] reported the experience of the first seven applications of intranasal sufentanil via PCIN for breakthrough and incident pain in four cancer patients. The initial dose of 4.5 µg could be repeated at 10 minutes and 20 minutes until a maximum of three doses of 36 µg/daily. Very good pain relief was achieved within 30 minutes and lasted for around 2 hours. No serious adverse effects were reported. An open-label, uncontrolled study evaluated the pharmacokinetics, safety and efficacy of a single 40 mg dose of nasal morphine gluconate administered to 11 cancer patients in response to an episode of breakthrough pain.[89] This treatment was associated with effective plasma morphine concentrations, rapid onset of pain relief, and minor side effects (nasal irritation). Patient satisfaction ratings were high.

As morphine administered nasally has a bioavailability of the order of 10 percent compared with IV administration, a novel chitosan-morphine nasal formulation has been produced and tested in both healthy volunteers and in 14 cancer patients with breakthrough pain.[90,91] Morphine was rapidly absorbed (T_{max} of 15 minutes or less), with a bioavailability of nearly 60 percent. In clinical settings, encouraging results have been obtained in patients receiving 5–80 mg of nasal morphine-chitosan, with an onset of pain relief 5 minutes after dosing. Finally, it is interesting to note that transnasal butorphanol has proved to be effective in the treatment of opioid-induced pruritus unresponsive to 50 mg of IV dyphenhydramine.[92]

Inhalation route

In 1996 Lichtman et al.[93] demonstrated that the inhalation exposure to several opioids produced dose-dependent antinociception in mice, and suggested that the relative potency of morphine was greater when inhaled than when injected by IV route. Subsequently, variable results have been obtained using inhaled morphine in postoperative pain. More recently, promising results have been reported in patients with acute pain.[94,95] The pharmacokinetics of nebulized opioids needs to be studied in detail in order to design reliable clinical trials.

TRANSDERMAL ROUTE

Substances with high lipid solubility and molecular weight below 800–1000 kDa can pass through the skin. The absorption rate varies according to different factors such as the type of the vehicle, the skin characteristics (the thickness of stratum corneum) and conditions, the body surface. In general drugs that are successfully administered transdermally are those in which the daily dose is very low (no more than a few milligrams). Patient compliance with this route of administration is excellent, and skin reactions are rarely observed.

Among opioids, the potent synthetic drug fentanyl citrate is particularly suitable for transdermal administration, and its utility in pain therapy has been extensively evaluated. Transdermal fentanyl systems (TTS) are available in four release programs of 25, 50, 75, 100 µg/h depending on the patch size, and the drug is released continuously for 3 days. A substantial amount of fentanyl remains in used systems even after 3 days of application.[96] When a TTS is removed, fentanyl continues to be absorbed into the systemic circulation from the cutaneous depot. However, opioid withdrawal symptoms may occur after discontinuation of TTS administration, as well as after conversion from other opioids to TTS.[97,98] Moreover withdrawal symptoms were reported during chronic TTS administration and were managed with oral methadone.[99] Pharmacokinetic studies demonstrated that the rate of absorption of fentanyl from the transdermal delivery is constant beginning 4–8 hours after placement of the patches. Steady state is reached on the third day. However, a wide individual variability exists.[100] There is a lag period after patch application before plasma concentrations approach therapeutic levels. This lag period is highly variable, with a mean value of about 13 hours.[101] The TTS should be changed every third day. However, published data show that application intervals have to be shortened in about 25 percent of patients[102] at 48–60 hours because on the third day of each patch period the need for rescue doses of short-release oral morphine was more than on the first and second day.[101,102] In 11–43 percent of patients on long-term treatment, the patch had to be changed every 48 hours.[100]

The effectiveness of TTS fentanyl was first demonstrated in postoperative pain. Especially for the high incidence of respiratory depression, this use is now contraindicated. Conversely, in stable, chronic, cancer pain this formulation offers an interesting alternative to oral morphine.[101,103–105] In comparison with oral morphine TTS fentanyl seems to cause fewer gastrointestinal side effects, with special reference to constipation.[106,107] Its usefulness also in chronic, nonmalignant pain is strongly suggested by recently published papers.[108,109] Of course, this formulation is contraindicated during the titration phase, or to control breakthrough pain. The cost of TTS fentanyl is higher than that of other opioids. However, some pharmacoeconomic analyses suggest that its cost is closer to that for long-acting oral opioids when total medication costs are considered.[110–112]

The permeability coefficient for fentanyl is affected by temperature. A rise in body temperature to 40 °C may increase the absorption rate by about a third.[106] Acute toxicity related to increased absorption secondary to high temperature has been reported.[113] A recent study in volunteers demonstrated that the application of local heat to the transdermal patch significantly increased systemic delivery of fentanyl.[114]

Four cases of death due to the intravenous injection of fentanyl extracted from transdermal patches have been recently reported.[115] To minimize the problem of the 'dose dumping' due to membrane damage, and the risk of illegal diversion, a transdermal matrix patch formulation of fentanyl has been developed. Furthermore, a new system, called the electrotransport transdermal system has been developed, which allows the drug delivery rate to be varied electrophoretically. Further studies are necessary to verify the utility of this new formulation.

The partial agonist buprenorphine is another ideal candidate for delivery via a transdermal patch.[116] In the currently available formulation (buprenorphine transdermal delivery system) this drug is incorporated in a polymer adhesive matrix from which it is released through the skin. Transdermal buprenorphine has a bioavailability of about 50 percent, which is comparable with that observed after sublingual administration.[117] Buprenorphine patches are available in three dosage strengths. The patches are loaded with 20, 30, or 40 mg of buprenorphine and are designed to release the opioid at a controlled rate of 35, 52.5, and 70 µg/h, corresponding to a daily dose of 0.8, 1.2, and 1.6 mg, respectively. All of the patches are designed for a 72-hour application period. They should be applied to a flat and hairless area of noninflamed skin, preferably on the upper back, subclavicular region, or chest. Following their removal, buprenorphine plasma levels slowly decrease. The manufacturers suggest that additional opioids should not be administered within 24 hours of patch removal. Transdermal buprenorphine has been used and investigated less extensively than fentanyl TTS. The available data suggest that it may represent an effective analgesic against chronic pain.[118**]

Key learning points

- An alternative route for opioid administration should be considered when oral administration is not possible or in presence of poor pain control and/or adverse effects.

- The oral route is not suitable in clinical situations such as severe vomiting, bowel obstruction, dysphagia, severe confusion, and where rapid dose escalation is necessary.

- Each alternative route has indications or contraindications depending on the clinical history of the patient.

- Pharmacokinetic and pharmacodynamic characteristics of the different opioid analgesics should be carefully considered to individualize the therapy.

- The rectal route has the advantage of being simpler than the subcutaneous or IV routes; however chronic rectal administration can lead to patient discomfort.

- Sublingual and buccal routes may deserve special attention for the administration of highly lipophilic opioids such as methadone, fentanyl, and buprenorphine.

- Continuous SCI ± extra boluses (PCA), represents the standard alternative route for systemic opioid delivery.

- Intravenous administration is particularly indicated for 'fast titration' and dose finding in patients with severe pain and in those with an implanted central venous catheter.

- The intranasal route may offer some advantages; however further studies are needed in the palliative care setting.

- The transdermal route is a widely used and a comfortable way for opioid delivery. However, it should be reserved for patients whose opioid requirements are stable after the end of the 'titration phase'.

REFERENCES

1   Bruera E, MacMillan K, Hanson J. Palliative care in a cancer center: Results in 1984 versus 1987. *J Pain Symptom Manage* 1990; **5**: 1–5.

● 2   Cherny NJ, Chang V, Frager G, *et al.* Opioid pharmacotherapy in the management of cancer pain: a surwey of strategies used by pain physicians for the selection of analgesic drugs and routes of administration. *Cancer* 1995; **76**: 1283–93.

3   Bruera E. Alternative routes for home opioid therapy. *Pain Clin Updates* 1993; **1**: 1–7.

✱ 4   Hanks GW, De Conno F, Cherny N, *et al.* Expert Working Group of the Research Network of the European Association for Palliative Care. Morphine and alternative opioids in cancer pain: the EAPC recommendations. *Br J Cancer* 2001; **84**: 587–93.

◆ 5   Ripamonti C, Bruera E. Rectal, buccal, and sublingual narcotics for the management of cancer pain. *J Palliat Care* 1991; **7**: 30–5.

◆ 6   Cole L, Hanning CD. Review of the rectal use of opioids. *J Pain Symptom Manage* 1990; **5**: 118–26.

◆ 7   Davis MP, Walsh D, LeGrand SB, Naughton M. Symptom control in cancer patients: the clinical pharmacology and therapeutic role of suppositories and rectal suspension. *Support Care Cancer* 2002; **10**: 117–38.

● 8   Johnson T, Christensen CB, Jordening H, *et al.* The bioavailability of rectally administered morphine. *Pharmacol Toxicol* 1988; **62**: 203–5.

● 9   Sawe J, Dahlstrom B, Paalzow L, *et al.* Morphine kinetics in cancer patients. *Clin Pharmacol Ther* 1981; **30**: 629–35.

10   Breda M, Bianchi M, Ripamonti C, *et al.* Plasma morphine and morphine 6-glucuronide patterns in cancer patients after oral, subcutaneous, sublabial and rectal short-term administration. *J Clin Pharm Res* 1991; **11**: 93–7.

11   Osborne R, Joel S, Trew D. Morphine and metabolite behaviour after different route of morphine administration: demonstration of the importance of the active metabolite morphine 6-glucuronide. *Clin Pharmacol Ther* 1990; **47**: 12–19.

12   Pannuti F, Rossi AP, Iafelice G, *et al.* Control of chronic pain in very advanced cancer patients with morphine hydrochloride administered by oral, rectal, and sublingual route. *Pharmacol Res Commun* 1982; **14**: 369–81.

13   Ellison NM, Lewis GO. Plasma concentrations following single doses of morphine sulphate in oral solution and rectal suppository. *Clin Pharmacy* 1984; **3**: 614–17.

14   Moolenar F, Yska JP, Visser J, *et al.* Drastic improvement in the rectal absorption profile of morphine in man. *Clin Pharmacy* 1985; **29**: 119–21.

15   Kaiko RF, Healy N, Pav J, *et al.* The comparative bioavailability of MS Contin tablets (controlled-release oral morphine) following rectal and oral administration. In: Doyle D, ed. *The Edinburgh Symposium on Pain Control and Medical Education.* Royal Society of Medicine Serv Int'l Congresses and Symposium No 149. London: Royal Society of Medicine Services Ltd., 1989.

16   Brumley RD. Home made rectal morphine sulphate suppositories. *Hospice J* 1988; **4**: 95–100.

17   Maloney CM, Kesner RK, Klein G, *et al.* The rectal administration of MS Contin: Clinical implications of use in end-stage cancer. *Am J Hospice Care* 1989; **6**: 34–5.

18   Walsh D, Tropiano PS. Long-term rectal administration of high-dose sustained-release morphine tablets. *Support Care Cancer* 2002; **10**: 653–5.

● 19   Bruera E, Faisinger R, Spachinsky K, *et al.* Clinical efficacy and safety of a novel controlled-release morphine suppository and subcutaneous morphine in cancer pain: a randomized evaluation. *J Clin Oncol* 1995; **13**: 1520–7.

● 20   Babul N, Provencher L, Laberge F, *et al.* Comparative efficacy and safety of controlled-release morphine suppositories and tablets in cancer pain. *J Clin Pharmacol* 1998; **38**: 74–81.

● 21   De Conno F, Ripamonti C, Saita L, *et al.* Role of rectal route in treating cancer pain: a randomized cross-over clinical trial of oral vs rectal morphine administration in opioid-naive cancer patients with pain. *J Clin Oncol* 1995; **13**: 1004–8.

● 22   Bruera E, Belzile M, Neumann CM, *et al.* Twice-daily versus once-daily morphine sulphate controlled-release suppositories for the treatment of cancer pain. A randomized controlled trial. *Support Care Cancer* 1999; **7**: 280–3.

23   Ripamonti C, Zecca E, Brunelli C, *et al.* Rectal methadone in cancer patients with pain. A preliminary clinical and pharmacokinetic study. *Ann Oncol* 1995; **6**: 841–3.

24   Bruera E, Watanabe S, Faisinger R, *et al.* Custom-made capsules and suppositories of methadone for patients on high-dose opioids fo cancer pain. *Pain* 1995; **62**: 141–6.

25   Leow KP, Cramond T, Smith MT. Pharmacokinetics and pharmacodynamics of oxycodone when given intravenously and rectally to adults patients with cancer pain. *Anesth Analg* 1995; **80**: 296–302.

26   Mercadante S, Arcuri E, Fusco F, *et al.* Randomized double-blind, double-dummy crossover clinical trial of oral vs rectal tramadol administration in opioid-naive cancer patients with pain. *Support Cancer Care* 2005; **13**: 702–7.

27   Hojsted J, Rubeck K, Peterson H. Comparative bioavailability of a morphine suppository given rectally and in a colostomy. *Eur J Clin Pharmacol* 1990; **39**: 49–50.

● 28   Weinberg DS, Inturrisi CE, Reidewberg B, *et al.* Sublingual absorption of selected opioid analgesics. *Clin Pharmacol Ther* 1988; **44**: 335–42.

29   Wallenstein SL, Kaiko RF, Rogers AG, *et al.* Clinical analgesic assay of sublingual buprenorphine and intramuscular morphine. In: Cooper JR, Altman F, Brown BS, *et al.*, eds. *NIDA Research Monography Vol 41. Problems of Drug Dependence.* Rockville: USDHHS 1981: 288–93.

30   Bullingham RES, McQuay HJ, Dwyer D, *et al.* Sublingual buprenorphine used post-operatively: Clinical observations and preliminary pharmacokinetic analysis. *Br J Clin Pharmacol* 1981; **12**: 117–22.

31   Bullingham RES, McQuay HJ, Moore RA. Clinical pharmacokinetics of narcotic agonist-antagonist drug. *Clin Pharmacol* 1983; **8**: 332–43.

32   Robbie DS. A trial of sublingual buprenorphine in cancer pain. *Br J Clin Pharmacol* 1979; **7**: 315–17S.

33   De Conno F, Ripamonti C, Sbanotto A, Barletta L. A clinical note ob sublingual buprenorphine. *J Palliat Care* 1993; **9**: 44–6.

34   Gal T. Naloxone reversal of buprenorphine-induced respiratory depression. *Clin Pharmacol Ther* 1989; **45**: 66–71.

◆ 35   Coluzzi PH. Sublingual morphine: efficacy reviewed. *J Pain Symptom Manage* 1998; **16**: 184–92.

36   Whitman HH, Sublingual morphine: a novel route of narcotic administration. *Am J Nurs* 1984; **84**: 939–40.

37   Zeppetella G. Sublingual fentanyl citrate for cancer-related breakthrough pain: a pilot study. *Palliat Med* 2001; **15**: 323–8.

38   Kunz KM, Theisen JA, Schroeder ME. Severe episodic pain: management with sublingual sufentanyl. *J Pain Symptom Manage* 1993; **8**: 189–90.

39   Drug Information 1992. Bethesda: American Hospital Formulary Service, 1992: 1134, 1155.

40   Streisand JB, Varvel JR, Stanki DR, *et al*. Absorption and bioavailability of oral transmucosal fentanyl citrate. *Anesthesiology* 1991; **75**: 223–9.

41   Fine PG, Marcus M, De Boer AJ, *et al*. An open label study of oral transmucosal fentanyl citrate (OTFC) for the treatment of breakthrough cancer pain. *Pain* 1991; **45**: 149.

● 42   Streisand JB, Busch MA, Egan TD, *et al*. Dose proportionality and pharmacokinetics of oral transmucosal fentanyl citrate. *Anesthesiology* 1998; **88**: 305–9.

43   Christie JM, Simmonds M, Patt R, *et al*. Dose titration: A multicenter study of oral transmucosal fentanyl citrate for the treatment of breakthrough pain in cancer patients using transdermal fentanyl for persistent pain. *J Clin Oncol*, 1998; **16**: 3238–45.

44   Farrar JT, Clearly J, Rauck R, *et al*. Oral transmucosal fentanyl citrate: randomized, double-blinded, placebo-controlled trial for treatment of breakthrough pain in cancer patients. *J Natl Cancer Inst* 1998; **90**: 611–16.

● 45   Portenoy RK, Payne R, Coluzzi P, *et al*. Oral transmucosal fentanyl citrate (OTFC) for the treatment of breakthrough pain in cancer patients: a controlled dose titration study. *Pain* 1999; **79**: 303–12.

● 46   Coluzzi PH, Schwartzberg L, Conroy JD, *et al*. Breakthrough cancer pain: a randomized trial comparing oral transmucosal fen tanyl citrate (OTFC) and morphine sulphate immediate release (MSIR). *Pain* 2001; **91**: 123–30.

47   Payne R, Coluzzi P, Hart L, *et al*. Long-term safety of oral transmucosal fentanyl citrate for breakthrough cancer pain. *J Pain Symptom Manage* 2001; **22**: 575–83.

48   Lipman AG. New and alternative noninvasive opioid dosage forms and routes of administration. *Support Oncol Updates* 2000; **3**: 1–8.

49   Crane RA. Intermittent subcutaneous infusion of opioids in hospice home care; an effective, economical, manageable option. *Am J Hosp Palliat Care* 1994; **11**: 8–12.

◆ 50   Anderson SL, Shreve ST. Continuous subcutaneous infusion of opiates at the end-life. *Ann Pharmacother* 2004; **38**: 1015–23.

◆ 51   Ripamonti C, Bruera E. Current status of patient-controlled analgesia in cancer patients. *Oncology* 1997; **11**: 373–84.

52   Dawson L, Brockbank K, Carr EC, Barrett RF. Improving patients' postoperative sleep: a randomised control study comparing subcutaneous with intravenous patient-controlled analgesia. *J Adv Nurs* 1999; **30**: 875–81.

53   Keita H, Geachan N, Dahmani S, *et al*. Comparison between patient-controlled analgesia and subcutaneous morphine in elderly patients after total hip replacement. *Br J Anaesth* 2003; **90**: 53–7.

54   Waldmann C, Eason J, Ramboul E. Serum morphine levels: a comparison between continuous subcutaneous and intravenous infusion in postoperative patients. *Anaesth Analg* 1984; **39**: 768–73.

● 55   Stuart-Harris R, Joel SP, McDonald P, *et al*. The pharmacokinetics of morphine and morphine glucuronide metabolites after subcutaneous bolus injection and subcutaneous infusion of morphine. *Br J Clin Pharmacol* 2000; **49**: 207–14.

56   Moulin DE, Kreeft JH, Murray PN, Bouquillon AI. Comparison of continuous subcutaneous and intravenous hydromorphone infusions for management of cancer pain. *Lancet* 1991; **337**: 465–8.

57   Miller MG, McCarthy N, O'Boyle CA, Kearney M. Continuous subcutaneous infusion of morphine vs hydromorphone: a controlled trial. *J Pain Symptom Manage* 1999; **18**: 9–15.

58   Bruera E, Faisinger R, Moore M, *et al*. Local toxicity with subcutaneous methadone. Experience of two centers. *Pain* 1991; **45**: 141–3.

59   Mathew P, Storey P. Subcutaneous methadone in terminally ill patients: manageable local toxicity. *J Pain Symptom Manage* 1999; **18**: 49–52.

60   Citron ML, Johnson-Early A, Fassieck BE. Safety and efficacy of continuous intravenous morphine for severe cancer pain. *Am J Med* 1984; **17**: 199–204.

✱ 61   Portenoy RK, Moulin DE, Rogers A, *et al*. IV infusion of opioids for cancer pain: clinical review and guidelines for use. *Cancer Treat Rep* 1986; **70**: 575–81.

62   Bruera E, Brenneis C, Michaud M, *et al*. Patient-controlled subcutaneous hydromorphone vs continuous subcutaneous infusion for the treatment of cancer pain. *J Natl Cancer Inst* 1988; **80**: 1152–4.

63   Swanson G, Smith J, Bulich R, *et al*. Patient-controlled analgesia for chronic cancer pain in the ambulatory setting: a report of 117 patients. *J Clin Oncol* 1989; **7**: 1903–8.

✱ 64   Cherny N, Ripamonti C, Pereira J, *et al*. for the Expert Working Group of the EAPC network. Strategies to manage the adverse effects of oral morphine: an evidence-based report. *J Clin Oncol* 2001; **19**: 2542–54.

● 65   Santiago-Palma J, Khojainova N, Kornick C, *et al*. Intravenous methadone in the management of chronic cancer pain. Safe and effective starting doses when substituting methadone for fentanyl. *Cancer* 2001; **92**: 1919–25.

66   Catcher J, Walsh D. Opioid-induced itching: morphine sulphate and hydromorphone hydrochloride. *J Pain Symptom Manage* 1999; **17**: 70–2.

67   Leow K, Smith M, Williams B, Cramond T. Single-dose and steady-state pharmacokinetics and pharmacodynamics of oxycodone in patients with cancer. *Clin Pharmacol Ther* 1992; **52**: 487–95.

◆ 68   Ripamonti C, Bianchi M. The use of methadone for cancer pain. *Hematol Oncol Clin North Am* 2002; **16**: 543–55.

69   Manfredi PL, Borsook D, Chandler SW, Payne R. Intravenous methadone for cancer pain unrelieved by morphine and hydromorphone: clinical observations. *Pain* 1997; **70**: 99–101.

● 70 Fitzgibbon DR, Ready LB. Intravenous high-dose methadone administered by patient controlled analgesia and continuous infusion for the treatment of cancer pain refractory to high-dose morphine. *Pain* 1997; **73**: 259–61.

71 Walker PW, Klein D, Kasza L. High dose methadone and ventricular arrhythmias: a report of three cases. *Pain* 2003; **103**: 321–4.

72 Kornick CA, Kilborn MJ, Santiago-Palma J, *et al*. QTc interval prolongation associated with intravenous methadone. *Pain* 2003; **105**: 499–506.

● 73 Radbruch L, Loick G, Schulzeck S, *et al*. Intravenous titration with morphine for severe cancer pain: report of 28 cases. *Clin J Pain* 1999; **15**: 173–8.

● 74 Mercadante S, Villari P, Ferrera P, *et al*. Rapid titration with intravenous morphine for severe cancer pain and immediate oral conversion. *Cancer* 2002; **95**: 203–8.

● 75 Harris JT, Suresh Kumar K, Rajagopal MR. Intravenous morphine for rapid control of severe cancer pain. *Palliat Med* 2003; **17**: 248–56.

● 76 Soares LGL, Martins M, Uchoa R. Intravenous fentanyl for cancer pain: a 'fast titration' protocol for the emergency room. *J Pain Symptom Manage* 2003; **26**: 876–81.

● 77 Grond S, Zech D, Lehmann KA, *et al*. Transdermal fentanyl in the long-term treatment of cancer pain: a prospective study of 50 patients with advanced cancer of the gastro-intestinal tract ort he head and neck region. *Pain* 1997; **69**: 191–8.

78 Kornick CA, Santiago-Palma J, Schulman G, *et al*. A safe and effective method for converting patients from transdermal to intravenous fentanyl for the treatment of acute cancer-related pain. *Cancer* 2003; **97**: 3121–4.

79 Enting RH, Oldenmenger WH, van der Rijt C, *et al*. A prospective study evaluating the response of patients with unrelieved cancer pain to parenteral opioids. *Cancer* 2002; **94**: 3049–56.

80 Turker S, Onur E, Ozer Y. Nasal route and drug delivery systems. *Pharm World Sci* 2004; **26**: 137–42.

◆ 81 Dale O, Hjortkjaer R, Kharasch ED. Nasal administration of opioids for pain management in adults. *Acta Anaesth Scand* 2002; **46**: 759–70.

82 Takala A, Kaasalainen TA, Seppala T, *et al*. Pharmacokinetic comparison of intravenous and intranasal administration of oxycodone. *Acta Anaesth Scand* 1997; **41**: 309–12.

● 83 Kendall JM, Latter VS. Intranasal diamorphine as an alternative to intramuscular morphine: pharmacokinetic and pharmacodynamic aspects. *Clin Pharmacokinet* 2003; **42**: 501–13.

84 Dale O, Hoffer C, Sheffels P, Kharasch ED. Disposition of nasal, intravenous, and oral methadone in healthy volunteers. *Clin Pharmacol Ther* 2002; **72**: 536–45.

85 Coda BA, Rudy AC, Archer SM, Wermeling DP. Pharmaco-kinetics and bioavailability of single-dose intranasal hydromorphone hydrochloride in healthy volunteers. *Anesth Analg* 2003; **97**: 117–23.

86 Finn J, Wright J, Fong J, *et al*. A randomised crossover trial of patient controlled intranasal fentanyl and oral morphine for procedural wound care in adult patients with burns. *Burns* 2004; **30**: 262–8.

87 Paech MJ, Lim CB, Banks SL, *et al*. A new formulation of nasal fentanyl spray for postoperative analgesia: a pilot study. *Anaesthesia* 2003; **58**: 740–4.

88 Jackson K, Ashby M, Keech J. Pilot dose finding study of intranasal sufentanil for breakthrough and incident cancer-associated pain. *J Pain Symptom Manage* 2002; **23**: 450–2.

89 Fitzgibbon D, Morgan D, Dockter D, *et al*. Initial pharmacokinetic, safety and efficacy evaluation of nasal morphine gluconate for breakthrough pain in cancer patients. *Pain* 2003; **106**; 309–15.

● 90 Illum L, Watts P, Fisher AN, *et al*. Intranasal delivery of morphine. *J Pharmacol Exp Ther* 2002; **301**: 391–400.

91 Pavis H, Wilcock A, Edgecombe J, *et al*. Pilot study of nasal morphine-chitosan for the relief of breakthrough pain in patients with cancer. *J Pain Symptom Manage* 2002; **24**: 598–602.

92 Dunteman E, Karanikolas M, Filos KS. Transnasal butorphanol for the treatment of opioid-induced pruritus unresponsive to antihistamines. *J Pain Symptom Manage* 1996; **12**: 255–60.

93 Lichtman AH, Meng Y, Martin BR. Inhalation exposure to volatilized opioids produces antinociception in mice. *J Pharmacol Exp Ther* 1996; **279**: 69–76.

94 Thipphawong JB, Babul N, Morishige RJ, *et al*. Analgesic efficacy of inhaled morphine in patients after bunionectomy surgery. *Anesthesiology* 2003; **99**: 693–700.

95 Ballas SK, Viscusi ER, Epstein KR. Management of acute chest wall sickle cell pain with nebulized morphine. *Am J Hematol* 2004; **76**: 190–1.

96 Marquard KA, Tharratt RS, Musallam NA. Fentanyl remaining in a transdermal system following three days of continuous use. *Ann Pharmacother* 1995; **29**: 969–71.

97 Han PKJ, Arnold R, Bond G, *et al*. Myoclonus secondary to withdrawal from transdermal fentanyl: a case report and literature review. *J Pain Symptom Manage* 2002; **23**: 66–72.

98 Hunt R. Transdermal fentanyl and the opioid withdrawal syndrome. *Palliat Med* 1996; **10**: 347–8.

99 Ripamonti C, Campa T, De Conno F. Withdrawal symptoms during chronic transdermal fentanyl administration managed with oral methadone. *J Pain Symptom Manage* 2004; **27**: 191–4.

◆ 100 Grond S, Radbruch L, Lehmann KA. Clinical pharmacokinetics of transdermal opioids: focus on transdermal fentanyl. *Clin Pharmacokin* 2000; **38**: 59–89.

◆ 101 Gourlay GK. Treatment of cancer pain with transdermal fentanyl. *Lancet Oncology* 2001; **2**: 165–72.

102 Portenoy RK, Southam MA, Gupta SK, *et al*. Transdermal fentanyl for cancer pain. Repeated dose pharmacokinetics. *Anesthesiology* 1993; **78**: 36–43.

● 103 Mystakidou K, Parpa E, Tsilika E, *et al*. Pain management of cancer patients with transdermal fentanyl: a study of 1828 step I, II, & III transfers. *J Pain* 2004; **5**: 119–32.

104 Menten J, Desmedt M, Lossignol D, Mullie A. Longitudinal follow-up of TTS-fentanyl use in patients with cancer-related pain: results of compassionate-use study with special focus on elderly patients. *Curr Med Res Opin* 2002; **18**: 488–98.

● 105 Radbruch L, Elsner F. Clinical experience with transdermal fentanyl for the treatment of cancer pain in Germany. *Keio J Med* 2004; **53**: 23–9.

◆ 106 Muijsers RBR, Wagstaff AJ. Transdermal fentanyl. An updated review of its pharmacological properties and therapeutic efficacy in chronic cancer pain control. *Drugs* 2001; **61**: 2289–307.

107 Mystakidou K, Parpa E, Tsilika E, *et al.* Long-term management of noncancer patients with transdermal therapeutic system fentanyl. *J Pain* 2003; **4**: 298–306.

◆ 108 Kornick CA, Santiago-Palma J, Moryl N, *et al.* Benefit-risk assessment of transdermal fentanyl for the treatment of chronic pain. *Drug Saf* 2003; **26**: 951–73.

109 Menefee LA, Frank ED, Crerand C, *et al.* The effects of transdermal fentanyl on driving, cognitive performance, and balance in patients with chronic non-malignant pain conditions. *Pain Med* 2004; **5**: 42–9.

110 Guest J, Munrol V, Cookson R. Comparison of the cost of managing constipation in cancer patients receiving oral morphine or transdermal fentanyl. *Eur J Cancer* 1997; **33**: S19.

111 Neighbors DM, Bell TJ, Wilson J, Dodd SL. Economic evaluation of the fentanyl transdermal system for the treatment of chronic moderate to severe pain. *J Pain Symptom Manage* 2001; **21**: 129–43.

● 112 Frei A, Andersen S, Hole P, Jensen NH. A one year health economic model comparing transdermal fentanyl with sustained-release morphine in the treatment of chronic noncancer pain. *J Pain Palliat Care Pharmacother* 2003; **17**: 5–26.

113 Rose PG, Macfee MS, Boswell MV. Fentanyl transdermal system overdose secondary to cutaneous hyperthermia. *Anesth Analg* 1993; **77**: 390–1.

● 114 Ashburn MA, Ogden LL, Zhang J, *et al.* The pharmacokinetics of transdermal fentanyl delivered with and without controlled heat. *J Pain* 2003; **4**: 291–7.

115 Tharp AM, Winecker RE, Winston DC. Fatal intravenous fentanyl abuse: four cases involving extraction of fentanyl from transdermal patches. *Am J Forensic Med Pathol* 2004; **25**: 178–81.

116 Böhme K. Buprenorphine in a transdermal therapeutic system – a new option. *Clin Rheumatol* 2002; **Suppl 1**: S13–16.

◆ 117 Evans HC, Easthope SE. Transdermal buprenorphine. *Drugs* 2003; **63**: 1999–2010.

● 118 Sittl R, Griessinger N, Likar R. Analgesic efficacy, and tolerability of transdermal buprenorphine in patients with inadequately controlled chronic pain related to cancer and other disorders: a multicenter, randomised, double-blind, placebo-controlled trial. *Clin Ther* 2003; **25**: 150–68.

48

Epidural and intrathecal analgesia and neurosurgical techniques in the palliative setting

PHILLIP C PHAN, MADHURI ARE, SAMUEL J HASSENBUSCH III, ALLEN W BURTON

INTRODUCTION

According to the World Health Organization (WHO), an estimated 6.6 million people die from cancer every year, with cancer-related pain continuing to be a significant source of global health concern.[1] As cancer progresses, 65–85 percent of patients with advanced cancer will experience pain, with up to 80 percent of cancer patients describing their pain as having moderate to severe intensity.[2]

The WHO has established a three-step analgesic ladder that can be used to treat cancer pain.[1] The use of this analgesic ladder is described elsewhere in this book. Although effective in treating most cancer pain some 10–20 percent of patients with cancer fail to achieve adequate pain relief after use of the WHO analgesic ladder.[3] This failure of the WHO ladder approach arises either from pain that is refractory to opioids or the inability of the patient to tolerate the side effects of the opioids at higher doses.

It has been suggested that a fourth, 'interventional' step be added to the three-step WHO analgesic ladder[3,4] (Fig. 48.1). This step would encompass the vast armamentarium of interventional procedures to help alleviate pain not controlled with pharmacological treatment. One major class of interventions is neuraxial therapy, with the administration of epidural and intrathecal analgesics at the level of spinal cord.

INTRASPINAL ANALGESIA

Administration of neuraxial or spinal analgesics offers many advantages over irreversible neurodestructive procedures to

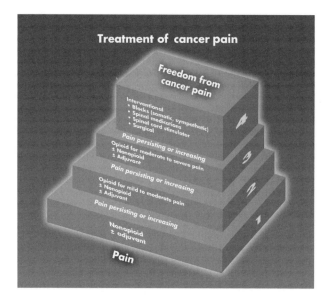

Figure 48.1 *The World Health Organization analgesic ladder with Step 4 'interventional management of pain' added. Adapted from Miguel[3] and Krames.[4]*

control pain, i.e. neurolytic blockade. It is very effective in patients with multiple pain sites, such as in those with advanced cancer with multiple sites of metastases.[5] An indwelling neuraxial catheter allows titration of opioid dosage and rotation of analgesic agents, if necessary. The use of intraspinal opioids is selective for the pain transmission pathway at the spinal level, without any discernable effect on the motor, sensory, or sympathetic systems. Further, for certain refractory syndromes, neurosurgical ablative procedures may have a favorable risk–benefit profile as described in the last section of this chapter.

Mechanism of action

The goal of intraspinal analgesics, including opioids, is local inhibition of nociceptive transmission at the spinal cord level. Intraspinally administered opioids modulate pain transmission by acting on receptors in the dorsal horn of the spinal cord where the primary sensory neuron synapses with the wide dynamic range interneurons and the second-order nociceptive neurons in the spinothalamic tract. Opioid receptors are concentrated in the dorsal horns in laminae I, II, V, and X of the spinal cord. Morphine was the first intraspinal opioid to be administered, and it is the standard for comparison of other intraspinally active analgesics.[6*,7] Opioids suppress postsynaptic excitability of second-order neurons at the level of spinal cord.[8–12]

Intraspinal analgesics

OPIOIDS

Many medications have been investigated for use as intraspinal analgesics, but data from controlled clinical studies are limited. Opioids as a class have been the most extensively studied.[13,14] Morphine is the only opioid approved for spinal administration by the US Federal Food and Drug Administration (FDA) although there is a growing body of literature supporting the use of other opioids, including hydromorphone, meperidine, fentanyl, alfentanil, sufentanil, and methadone.[15***]

The intraspinal analgesics target the receptor system within the spinal cord. Specifically for opioids, the target is the opioid μ receptors located within the dorsal horn. Many of the pharmacokinetic and pharmacodynamic properties of intraspinal opioids are related to their lipid solubility, specifically their ability to diffuse across the dura, spread within the cerebrospinal fluid (CSF), and diffuse into the dorsal horn. The oil–water coefficient of an analgesic agent is a good indicator of the hydrophilic or hydrophobic nature of that agent. Morphine, with an oil–water coefficient of 1.40, is a hydrophilic opioid. Thus, it will take longer to diffuse across the dura and to diffuse into the spinal cord. Furthermore this will result in slow receptor saturation, longer onset to peak action, and longer time to clearance from the spinal cord.[16] Slow clearance of hydrophilic morphine from spinal CSF accounts for delayed respiratory depression sometimes seen with intraspinally administered morphine. This is due to the rostral spread of morphine remaining within CSF and morphine's action on the respiratory centers in the brainstem.[17] This delayed effect, however, is rarely seen in opioid-tolerant patients.

Sufentanil, with an oil–water coefficient of about 1800, is the prototypical hydrophobic opioid. Once administered via either the epidural or the intrathecal route, this hydrophobic agent will quickly diffuse across the dura and be taken up into the spinal cord and vascular system. Receptor saturation of the spinal cord level corresponding to the catheter tip location is expected to be relatively rapid with rapid clearance from the CSF.[18]

OTHER INTRASPINAL AGENTS

Clonidine is a well-studied analgesic considered to be useful as an adjuvant in neuropathic pain states.[19] It acts on central α_2 adrenergic receptors, thereby modulating the spinal pain pathway. Clonidine binds to postsynaptic α_2 receptors within the dorsal horn and activates the descending noradrenergic inhibitory systems.[20,21] This spinal mechanism explains why clonidine is a poor analgesic when administered systematically.[22] Clonidine is hydrophobic, with an oil–water coefficient similar to fentanyl. It is quickly taken up in from the CSF and has a pronounced local effect at the spinal level.[23,24] Use of spinal clonidine has been investigated in both the postoperative pain control and in cancer pain management.[25**,26***] When clonidine is combined with an opioid, the intraspinal opioid requirement is less and tolerance takes longer to develop.[26***] The main side effect of intraspinally administered clonidine is postural hypotension.[27]

Spinally administered local anesthetics have a synergistic effect when combined with opioids. Bupivacaine, an amide local anesthetic, is commonly used in postoperative epidural infusions, but is also widely given by the intrathecal route in combination with opioids for cancer pain. Like clonidine, bupivacaine is more effective when used in combination with opioids than opioids alone in the treatment of neuropathic pain, however, bupivacaine is also used to treat nociceptive pain.[28***] The mechanism of action of local anesthetics involves blockade of voltage-sensitive sodium channels and preventing generation and conduction of nerve impulses across pain transmission pathways. As with other local anesthetics, bupivacaine dosing is limited by the occurrence of motor blockade at higher local anesthetic concentrations. Intrathecally administered, bupivacaine can cause a motor block at doses as low as 10 mg/day. However, with slow dose titration, bupivacaine doses up to 25–30 mg/day can be used without producing a motor blockade.

Ziconotide, a calcium channel blocker, produces its analgesic effect by selectively blocking neuronal N-type voltage-sensitive calcium channels. Calcium channel blockade prevents calcium ion influx and neurotransmitter release. This selectively inhibits transmission of primary afferents located in the dorsal horn of the spinal cord. Ziconotide is currently being evaluated in clinical studies for treatment of severe chronic pain in patients refractory to systemic opioid therapy.[29**] It was approved for intrathecal use by the FDA in December 2004. This is the first agent developed specifically for intraspinal administration in chronic pain states.

Its ultimate use will most likely be for those with pain states refractory to intraspinal opioids and severe neuropathic pain states.[15]

Neostigmine is another interesting nonopioid that may have a role as an intraspinal analgesic.[30,31] The drug is effective with minimal toxicity, but initial trials have seen some troublesome systemic dose-related side effects including nausea and vomiting and somnolence.[32]

A number of other α_2 adrenergic agonists, local anesthetics, and drugs from other classes (γ-aminobutyric acid [GABA] agonists such as baclofen, N-methyl-D-aspartate [NMDA] antagonists such as ketamine) have been delivered via the intraspinal route to treat intractable cancer pain, with varying degrees with success. According to a 2002 review, satisfactory analgesia has been reported with the use of these agents delivered intraspinally.[15] However, most of these agents are considered investigational at this time for intraspinal therapy. Clinical guidelines emerged in 2000 and have been recently revised in 2003. These form the basis for a treatment algorithm in intraspinal therapy to aid decision making (Fig. 48.2).[15]

Indications

As discussed earlier, intraspinal analgesics are effective in modulating pain pathways at the spinal level. The significant side effects from systemic high-dose opioid administration (including nausea, constipation, confusion, increased somnolence, or lethargy) can be minimized with intraspinal delivery of opioids. This therapy is effective in two broad groups of patients: those with refractory pain syndromes and those with intolerable opioid-related side effects. If the opioid is delivered to an epidural location, only 20–40 percent of the systemic dose is required to achieve analgesia equivalent to that achieved with systemic opioids. The intrathecal route is even more potent, requiring only 10 percent of the systemic dose for equianalgesia.[28,15] The ability to treat pain effectively while minimizing these side effects has a significant impact on the quality of life.[33]

Patient selection

When a comprehensive trial of pharmacological therapy fails to provide adequate analgesia or leads to unacceptable side effects, consideration should be given to alternative modalities. These modalities include parenteral opioid infusions, neuraxial medication infusion, neurolytic blockade, and other procedures such as vertebroplasty. Consultation with a pain specialist may help select patients most likely to benefit from one or another of these interventions. One advantage of intraspinal analgesia is that a trial therapy can be undertaken with minimal risk to the patient. If no benefit is seen with trial intraspinal therapy, a more permanent catheter or pump system need not be implanted. The trial is described below in more detail. With regard to placement of the permanent system, i.e. intrathecal pump, deciding which patients with cancer will benefit from such implantation is a complex process and involves multiple factors.

The role of interventional therapies must be placed in the proper context. In most cases, they cannot be employed as the sole treatment for cancer pain. Spinal analgesia should be used as part of a multimodality approach in treatment of cancer pain.[34***] As discussed previously, the causes of

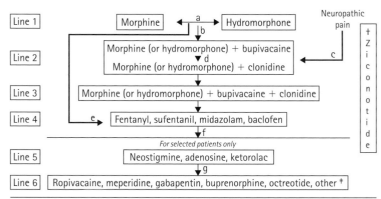

† The specific line to be determined after FDA review
‡ Potential spinal analgesics: methadone, oxymorphone, NMDA antagonists

a. If side effects occur, switch to other opioid.
b. If maximum dosage is reached without adequate analgesia, add adjuvant medication (Line 2).
c. If patient has neuropathic pain, consider starting with opioid monotherapy (morphine or hydromorphone) or, in selected patients with pure or predominant neuropathic pain, consider opioid plus adjuvant medication (bupivacaine or clonidine), (Line 2).
d. Some of the panel advocated the use of bupivacaine first because of concern about clonidine-induced hypotension.
e. If side effects or lack of analgesia on second first-line opioid, may switch to fentanyl (Line 4).
f. There are limited preclinical data and limited clinical experience, therefore, caution in the use of these agents should be considered.
g. There are insufficient preclinical data and limited clinical experience: therefore, extreme caution in the use of these agents should be considered.

Figure 48.2 *Treatment algorithm for intrathecal analgesia. Redrawn from reference 15.*

cancer pain are diverse, with nociception being one part of the constellation of symptoms experienced by the patients with cancer. Therefore, a comprehensive multidisciplinary approach to treatment of cancer pain is optimal. This would include appropriate palliative antineoplastic therapy, management of analgesics and adjuvant pain medications, behavioral and psychiatric support, and, finally, interventional therapies. Interventional pain procedures will not completely eliminate the need for pain medications, but should help significantly to minimize the nociceptive burden. The therapeutic goal of such procedures is to help alleviate cancer pain, reduce the overall analgesic need, and thereby minimize associated opioid-related side effects.

Communication

Prior to proceeding with any invasive pain procedure, communication between the pain physician and the relevant parties is absolutely essential. Effective communication with the patient entails a thorough discussion including outcomes of the procedure, duration of effectiveness, possible complications and their treatment, and the place of the interventional treatment in their overall treatment strategy. This discussion must be accomplished in terms the patient can understand and with involvement of the patient's family and/or caregivers. The patient and family must be given ample opportunity for questions, and, like the patient, the family must be also educated so that they have realistic expectations about the procedure.

Effective communication with other professional members of the care team is important for the optimal outcome. The team members include the patient's oncologist(s), primary care provider(s), and all the relevant consultant(s). As stated above, treatment of cancer is a multidisciplinary effort and the interventional procedure should be planned in coordination with the overall cancer treatment. For example, a patient with cancer may undergo chemotherapy with resultant thrombocytopenia. In such situations, an interventional procedure must be carried out prior to chemoinduction or afterward when the patient's platelet count has normalized. As a routine, other members of the patient's care team should be informed about the planned interventional procedure and given a chance to voice any input or concern.

Detailed history and physical examination

A thorough history and physical examination of the patient prior to the procedure is also critical. This entails a complete neurological evaluation. Interventional procedures for pain control generally involve placing needles and/or catheters near tissues such as nerves and other structures in central nervous system. The objective of intervention is to disrupt or modulate nociceptive pathways. Intrathecal infusion of opioids and local anesthetics will not only block pain transmission but at higher doses they may also reversibly block sensory and motor function. Consequently, it is important to have a thorough understanding of the patient's neurological and functional status before and after the procedure. Changes such as sensory and motor blockade are closely monitored after procedures, especially when high doses of local anesthetics are being used. Patients need to be fully informed about the use of high-dose local anesthetics as they may otherwise fear that they have become paralyzed if a motor block occurs.

Another important aspect of the pre-procedural evaluation is the assessment of overall symptom burden and psychological distress. If the overall symptom burden and/or magnitude of psychological distress is high, the result of the intervention aiming to decrease nociception may be disappointing in its seeming lack of overall effectiveness.

Delivery of intraspinal analgesics

Intraspinal delivery of opioids and other agents can be achieved by a variety of approaches, including epidural bolus, intermittent intrathecal injection, and continuous epidural and intrathecal infusions.[35] Continuous infusion via either the epidural or the intrathecal route requires the use of a catheter system and either external or implantable infusion pumps to deliver the analgesic medications. There is little consensus on when to use the intrathecal versus the epidural route of administration and when to use an implantable versus an external pump. With prolonged epidural infusions of greater than 6–9 months, complications such as catheter obstruction, fibrosis, and loss of analgesic efficacy have been observed, leading most clinicians to favor the intrathecal route for long-term intraspinal analgesic infusions.[36]

Many factors are considered in the decision whether to use an external pump system versus an implantable pump. Factors that are favorable of an external system include: a short life expectancy (<3 months), the need for frequent patient-controlled doses (such as with severe incident pain), the need for an epidural infusion (which generally requires infusion volumes which are too great for the implantable pump), the lack of reprogramming/refilling capabilities near the patient's home, payor constraints, as well as the ability of the patient and family to take care of an externalized catheter system.[37] We use a variety of catheters for our external systems including a tunneled Arrow Flex-Tip® catheter, the DuPen® epidural catheter, and Sims' Port-A-Cath® epidural system.

Factors that favor considering an implantable intrathecal pump include: a longer life expectancy (>3 months), access to pump refill/reprogramming capabilities, diffuse pain (e.g., widespread metastasis), and favorable response to an intrathecal trial. Our decision-making algorithm was recently published[37] and is also shown in Fig. 48.3. An economic analysis of an implantable versus externalized pump revealed the 3-month life expectancy to be the approximate

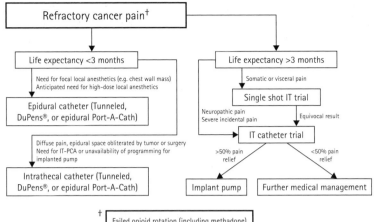

Figure 48.3 *Decision algorithm for intraspinal therapy. IT, intrathecal; PCA, patient-controlled analgesia. Redrawn from reference 38.*

'break-even' point for the implanted pump to become more cost effective than the externalized pump system.[38,39]

The rate of flow of implanted infusion pump systems can be fixed (factory preset at 0.5 mL or 1.0 mL/day) or programmable. All implantable pumps come with a refillable drug reservoir. In addition, they all have an access port and a side port system that allows for direct injection of a drug into the implanted catheter system. FDA-approved fixed infusion pump systems include Codman's model 400, Medtronic's Isomed® and Arrow's M-3000. Changing the dose in a fixed rate pump requires the medication concentration be changed, mandating a pump refill each time the dose is adjusted.

Medtronic Inc. (Minneapolis, MN) has the only programmable pump on the market today. Medtronic's Synchromed I and II pumps can hold up to 20 mL and 40 mL of medication, respectively. They can be programmed to deliver a single bolus, time-specific boluses, or a complex regimen of continuous infusion of intrathecal analgesic. A function exists for a patient-controlled 'demand dose' via a remote control, but this has not been approved for use in the USA as of the time of writing. Although these fixed rate and programmable pumps can be used to deliver either epidural or intrathecal medications, they are more suited to intrathecal delivery. Epidural infusions usually require a significantly higher daily volume and thus are typically managed with an external pump system.[36,37]

Intraspinal analgesic trial

Once intraspinal analgesia has been decided on, an intrathecal trial must be accomplished. This trial is to demonstrate efficacy of the intraspinal medication in improving pain control, level of functioning, and overall quality of life. There is no standard for neuraxial trials, although numerous approaches have been advocated.[36,37,40,41] We do not trial patients undergoing catheter–external pump systems, as the

trial procedure and catheter 'implant' procedure are virtually identical. For consideration of intrathecal catheter–pump implantation, our preference is a single shot (one subarachnoid opioid or opioid/local anesthetic injection) trial in most cases. If the analgesia is equivocal or the patient has a severe incidental pain syndrome, a tunneled intrathecal catheter trial is done, usually with opioid/local anesthetic or opioid/clonidine combination. Also in some cases when we anticipate the need for local anesthetic combination therapy, an intrathecal catheter trial is helpful in adjusting and achieving the right opioid and local anesthetic mix prior to pump implantation. Criteria for successful intraspinal opioid trial are variable, with some effective indicators being: reduction in pain scores, improvement in function, and decreased opioid requirement as well as reduction in opioid-related side effects.[37]

Pump implantation surgery

Prior to surgery, patients are again evaluated for any change in medical as well as neurological status since the last preoperative clinic visit. The procedure may be done under general anesthesia or monitored anesthetic care (sedation plus local anesthesia). The usual surgical aseptic precautions must be observed during the entire surgical procedure, with the use of preoperative prophylactic antibiotics to minimize the chance of perioperative infection. Under guidance of a fluoroscope, a spinal catheter is placed up to a specific level for optimal analgesia. The pump is implanted in the lower quadrant of the abdomen via an 8 cm incision, which is made to allow placement of the pump into the subcutaneous tissues with connection of the pump and catheter (Fig. 48.4). The patient is observed overnight and generally discharged the next morning with instructions regarding follow-up care, pump refill date, safety precautions, and routine postoperative wound care. The patient is also instructed to keep in touch with the

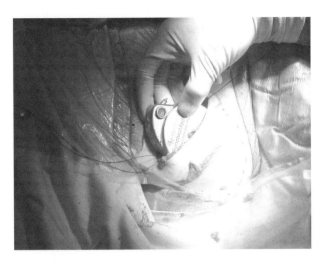

Figure 48.4 *Surgical placement of the intraspinal infusion pump into the left lower quadrant of the abdomen. Courtesy of A Burton.*

clinic in the coming week as we titrate the pump medication regimen for optimal pain control as needed.

Efficacy of intraspinal opioids in cancer pain

Intrathecal delivery of opioids has been shown to reduce pain levels in patients with intractable cancer pain.[37*,42*,43*,44*,45***,46*,47**] A recent review of literature found that use of intrathecal delivery of morphine by an implanted infusion pump provided 'good to excellent' pain relief, accompanied by increased activity and improved quality of life in patients with intractable pain.[45***] Furthermore, the results of three recent studies of intrathecal therapy have demonstrated the effectiveness of this therapy in management of severe cancer pain.[37*,46*,47**] Two of these studies examined the effectiveness of intrathecal drug delivery systems on the management of continuous severe cancer pain.[37*,47*] The third study examined the effectiveness of intrathecal therapy for episodic or breakthrough pain.[46*]

Our group at MD Anderson Cancer Center reported the results of use of intraspinal analgesia in 87 of 4107 evaluated patients using the previously mentioned algorithm.[37*] These patients were highly refractory to medical management with mean oral morphine doses of 588 mg/day and baseline mean pain scores of 7.9. Retrospective evaluation of 8-week follow-up revealed improved pain control, decreased oral opioid intake, and decreased drowsiness and mental clouding. This study analyzed the effectiveness of intraspinal analgesia on pain reduction by comparing pain scores, oral opioid intake, and self-reported symptoms before and after the intraspinal intervention. After administration of intraspinal analgesia either via epidural or intrathecal route, there was a significant reduction in the proportion of patients in severe pain (pain scores 7–10 on

a numerical rating scale [NRS]) from 86 percent to 17 percent ($P < 0.001$). The patients' NRS scores decrease significantly from a mean ($\pm$ SD) of 7.9 ± 1.6 to 4.1 ± 2.3 ($P < 0.001$). Oral opioid intake decreased from 588 mg/day MEDD to 294 mg/day ($P < 0.001$). Self-reported drowsiness and mental clouding (range 0–10) also significantly decreased from 6.2 ± 3.0 and 5.4 ± 3.4 to 3.2 ± 3.0 and 3.1 ± 3.0, respectively ($P < 0.001$).

In a prospective, randomized, multicenter clinical trial, the use of implanted intrathecal drug delivery system was shown to improve pain control, reduce toxicities, and improve survival in cancer patients with refractory pain.[47] At study entry, all patients (N = 202) had unrelieved cancer pain, as indicated by their visual analog pain scores of ≥ 5 on a 0–10 scale. Patients were randomized to receive either morphine via intrathecal delivery and comprehensive medical management according to the 1994 Agency for Health Care Policy and Research (AHCPR) cancer pain relief guidelines, or comprehensive medical management alone. At week 4 of follow-up, 60 of the 71 patients (84.5 percent) in the intrathecal delivery arm achieved clinical success, as indicated by ≥ 20 percent reduction in visual analog scale pain scores or ≥ 20 percent reduction in toxicity. In contrast, in the comprehensive medical management arm, only 51 of 72 patients (70.8 percent) achieved clinical success. Mean toxicity scores declined in the intrathecal delivery and comprehensive medical management only arm by 50 percent and 17 percent, respectively ($P = 0.004$). Further, the intrathecal delivery group had significant reduction in fatigue and depressed level of consciousness ($P < 0.05$). Moreover, slightly greater improvement in 6-month survival was seen in the intrathecal delivery group compared with the medical management only group (53.9 percent vs. 37.2 percent, $P = 0.06$).

In a third study, Rauck *et al.* evaluated intrathecal drug delivery systems in the management of episodic or breakthrough pain in a prospective, open label study.[46] In this study of 119 cancer patients with refractory cancer pain and/or uncontrollable side effects, better analgesia was achieved when the patients managed their pain with an implantable, patient-controlled intrathecal drug delivery system. Such a system allowed patients to self-administer a bolus dose of morphine sulfate on demand. The results showed that the mean numerical analog pain score significantly decreased from 6.1 to 4.2 at month 1 ($P < 0.01$, n = 99), and was maintained through month 7 ($P < 0.01$, n = 14) and month 13 ($P < 0.05$, n = 10). In addition, the morphine equivalent daily dose (MEDD) was significantly reduced throughout the study ($P < 0.01$). Overall success (≥ 50 percent reduction in numerical analog pain score, system opioid use, or severity of opioid side effects) was reported at month 1 at 83 percent and at month 4 at 91 percent of patients.

Clearly, in these three studies and many other studies, intraspinal administration of opioids and analgesics has been shown to play a significant role in controlling cancer pain, reducing opioid-related toxicities, and even improving survival outcomes. Intraspinal analgesic therapy is an effective mode of pain control in cancer patients with difficult-to-control refractory pain.

Complications

Complications fall into two broad categories: device and drug related. Device-related complications include wound infection, catheter breakage/migration, catheter tip granuloma. There is a growing body of literature on granulomas at the catheter tip, which are being increasingly reported. The consensus is that this is related to highly concentrated medications, especially morphine, and the index of suspicion should be high in patients with a new pain in their back prompting magnetic resonance imaging (MRI) evaluation and appropriate management as outlined elsewhere.[48] Drug-related complications include dosing/programming errors, misfiling, and the spectrum of opioid-related side effects including nausea, sedation, urinary retention, pruritus, and respiratory depression. These side effects are generally less pronounced than with systemic opioids.[47]

NEUROSURGICAL ABLATIVE TECHNIQUES IN THE MANAGEMENT OF CANCER PAIN

The relative roles of ablative procedures are still controversial in neurosurgical pain management. Many of these ablative procedures have been available for 40–50 years yet, in many situations, had been replaced by newer augmentative procedures over the past 10 years. Pain relief from ablative procedures may be of a shorter duration than that resulting from stimulation, and may be accompanied by deafferentation pain.[49] More recently, however, older techniques for intracranial ablative procedures have been updated. With the use of improved stereotactic equipment and guidance by computed tomography (CT) and MRI, the accuracy of intracranial procedures has improved and the need for ventriculography largely eliminated. The procedures can be carried out under local anesthesia with light sedation and require only a twist drill hole, rather than a burr hole or a craniotomy.

Patients generally must have severe pain that is not relieved adequately by systemic medications, neuraxial analgesics, or simple neurolytic procedures. Although some of the procedures, such as thalamotomy and cingulotomy often have been used for pain of noncancer causes, these operations are still quite beneficial for patients with cancer.[50–54] As with long-term spinal infusions of morphine, it remains unclear whether delayed recurrence of pain represents extension of the underlying tumor to new anatomical areas or late failure of the procedure.[55,56]

Neurosurgical procedures are used for both nociceptive and neuropathic pain, but it appears that, with the exception of thalamotomy, nociceptive pain responds better to intracranial procedures, which also cover larger body areas. Neuropathic pain often responds better to spinal procedures that have more limited areas of coverage. In addition to logistical issues, choice of a specific operation also needs to take into consideration the type of pain, severity, location, and the primary cause of the painful sensation.

Techniques

Though neurosurgical approaches to lesion placement are fairly standard, the requisite tools have changed as technology has progressed. Originally, ablations were placed using open surgical techniques.[57,58] Air or contrast ventriculography for intracranial lesions was the traditional, accurate method for placing lesions at coordinates defined by the anterior commissure–posterior commissure (AC–PC) line.[59,60] General anesthesia was often required to perform the procedure, which could not adjust for interpatient variability in anatomy. Now, however, closed operations using stereotaxis under ventriculogram, and CT or MRI guidance have become dominant.

The use of CT and MRI for stereotactic guidance eliminates the need for ventriculography and also increases the surgeon's ability to correct for individual patient variation in anatomy.[61,62] For example, using MRI, the actual trajectory for the electrode placement can be planned in relation to other brain structures. Special angled slices, which correspond to the trajectory for the electrode placement, can be taken allowing the target site and the actual trajectory through various brain structures to be found on these slices. Computed tomography has a high resolution and accuracy but also has a more limited level of resolution, thus making direct observation of the target difficult.[63] Magnetic resonance imaging is especially useful in the identification of relevant anatomy but does suffer from a somewhat lower accuracy because of magnetic field inhomogeneity.[64,65] Although there are statistically significant differences between CT and MRI-derived coordinates, the actual discrepancies are small enough that the MRI can be used alone for target localization.[63] Since neither method is entirely exact, a variety of intraoperative procedures are often used to confirm lesion placement.[63] Such techniques include the use of 'reversible' lesions, allowing intraoperative testing of the area without causing permanent damage; low-frequency stimulation that aids determination of the function of the region surrounding the target; and single-unit microelectrode recording to ensure preservation of critical structures in the area.[63]

Radiosurgery, for example using the gamma knife, is being increasingly employed to create ablative lesions for treatment of chronic pain and functional disorders. This method is particularly useful for sites found deep within the brain.[1] Targets in the thalamus and the anterior limb of the internal capsule have been frequently reported.[66–68]

The radiosurgical technique for these pain-relieving lesions uses a similar technique to that for focused radiation (radiosurgery) of a brain tumor. Although radiosurgery is noninvasive to the brain, it is unclear to what extent the lesions become smaller, and what degree of pain relief can be expected at various time points after the radiation exposure.

Specific procedures

The following procedures either are currently being practiced or, based upon past reports, offer significant efficacy of relief with minimal morbidity. As seen from the descriptions that follow, some of these procedures treat specific pain areas such as the head or legs whereas others treat more generalized areas of pain. The various approaches have been divided into ablative and augmentative techniques and described within each group, beginning with the most commonly used technique first.

INTRACRANIAL ABLATIVE TECHNIQUES

Hypophysectomy

The mechanism by which lesions of the pituitary gland bring pain relief is unclear, although it is generally agreed that neither the limbic system nor areas controlling affective responses are manipulated. Current research supports three theories for hormonal, hypothalamic, and neurotransmitter release mechanisms. A postulated hormonal mechanism involves changes in a humoral substance in the CSF or hormonal changes via a direct neural mechanism.[69,70] Contrary to this proposal, it has been noted that pain relief occurs almost immediately without any regard for tumor regression. Relief can also occur in the thalamic pain regions and hormonally unresponsive tumors on a scale that could not be inferred given the degree of pituitary ablation experienced.[71–75] Still, very small amounts of tumor regression cannot be discounted.[76]

Modalities used to perform a hypophysectomy lend credence to the hypothalamic mechanism theory. A possible relation to the pain relief properties of the posteromedial hypothalamus can be observed, although the morphological effects of hypophysectomy, regardless of the technique used to create the lesions, center in the anterior hypothalamus, specifically in the supraoptic and paraventricular nuclei.[76,77] Projections from the paraventricular nucleus to the periaqueductal gray, rostral ventral medulla, and lamina I of dorsal horn have been noted, linking the area to crucial elements in the descending antinociceptive system.[78–81] Information indicating the particularly strong impact that pituitary ablations have on the paraventricular nucleus coupled with knowledge of anatomical connections between this area and antinociceptive regions of the brain suggests the role of endogenous neurotransmitters. It has been observed, however, that naloxone does not reverse pain relief as it does with opioid-based relief. Although plasma concentrations of β-endorphin were elevated in one study, no changes have been found in CSF concentrations of met-enkephalin or β-endorphin.

Techniques for open surgery on the area include the transcranial hypophysectomy[82] and the open microsurgical hypophysectomy.[70,74,83,84] As technology has improved stereotactic methods, percutaneous stereotactic lesions are being created using radiofrequency thermal techniques, cryotherapy, or interstitial placement of radioactive seeds. The success of focused radiation therapy (e.g. gamma knife) on pituitary tumors has led to the use of this noninvasive modality to create similar lesions for pain relief.

Of these various techniques for hypophysectomy, stereotactic instillation of alcohol into the pituitary gland is one of the best-described and most common techniques at this time. Alcohol has been shown to pass to the floor of the third ventricle, hypophyseal portal vessels, and the hypothalamus.[76] The use of stereotaxy for chemical hypophysectomy enables an injection of alcohol volumes between 1 mL and 5 mL, a method first described in 1957.[85] Better results have been achieved using alcohol volumes extending to the upper volumes of this range that are clearly greater than the volume of the sella.[76]

After placing the patient under general anesthesia and securing the stereotactic frame, the surgeon locates the superoposterior part of the sella as the initial target. An 18 gauge, 15.24 cm (6 inch) spinal needle is introduced in a transnasal trajectory that passes through the floor of the sphenoid sinus. This needle is then replaced by a 20 gauge spinal needle directed through the sellar wall, with its progression observed by means of lateral X-ray fluoroscopy. Injection of 1–2 mL of alcohol in aliquots of 0.1 mL follows placement of the needle tip. After withdrawing the needle halfway to the floor of the sella, another 1–2 mL of alcohol is injected.[76] The needle is completely withdrawn after this last injection. Throughout the procedure, the eyes are monitored for compression of cranial nerves in the cavernous sinus as evidenced by changes in pupil size or movement of eyes from the midline. Other methods used to perform a hypophysectomy, such as stereotaxic radiofrequency hypophysectomy, stereotaxic cryohypophysectomy, and interstitial irradiation use standard stereotactic methods of intracranial operations.[54,73,86–88]

Hypophysectomy is generally recommended for patients with severe cancer pain such as metastatic breast or prostate carcinoma with diffuse areas of pain. It can also be effective for hormonally unresponsive tumors.[69,75,89–91] In two different series of greater than 100 patients each, chemical hypophysectomy appeared to provide significant pain relief. Excellent pain relief was reported in 45–65 percent of all patients and 75–85 percent of patients ceased using opioids. The mean postoperative survival time was 5 months, while the mean length of pain relief appeared to be 3 months. This length of pain relief was accomplished with one additional alcohol injection in 25–30 percent of patients and with two additional injections in another 3–9 percent.[69,76,92] Of the patients treated with alcohol injections, those with breast or prostate carcinoma (50–75 percent of patients) appeared to have slightly better pain relief than those with other types of tumors.[76] Approximately 25 percent of patients had at least one significant exacerbation of pain after the procedure whereas a third of these patients had more than one exacerbation.[76]

Common complications included hormonal deficiency, such as diabetes insipidus, in 5–20 percent of patients, CSF leak in 1–10 percent of patients, and ocular nerve palsy or temporal field visual loss in 2–10 percent of patients.[76,93] Most of these changes were temporary.[76] Other problems associated with the procedure on a far less frequent basis were meningitis in 0.5–1 percent of patients, hypothalamic changes, headaches, and carotid artery damage in approximately 0.5 percent of patients.[93] Despite a reported 2–5 percent mortality, it seems likely that these numbers have been significantly lowered with the adoption of newer percutaneous and stereotactic methods.[89,93]

Thalamotomy

The thalamus is the termination site of the spinothalamic tract (lateral nucleus and central lateral nucleus of the medial thalamus), the pathway responsible for transmitting information about pain and temperature from the body to higher areas in the brain.[49] The lateral thalamus seems to be principally involved with sensory discrimination aspects of pain, while the medial thalamic nuclei has more to do with affective responses.[49] In the late 1930s and early 1940s, there were increasing reports of the use of thalamotomy in the treatment of patients with Parkinson disease. In his attempt to create a means to preserve involuntary movements through an open pallidotomy, Russell Meyers also based his work on these ideas. Using the effectiveness of pallidal lesions as corroborating evidence, investigators reasoned that lesions of their thalamic projections in the ventrolateral nucleus of the thalamus would also be effective.[94] Advances in human stereotaxic procedures have led to a resurgence in use of the thalamotomy.

Despite its development for noncancer pain, thalamotomy can be highly effective for and has been reported in the treatment of cancer pain.[51,94] Thalamotomy is generally considered for intermittent shooting and hyperpathic or allodynic pain and not considered very effective for steady, burning, or dysesthetic components of central or de-afferentation pain.[94] The targets have been the basal thalamus, medial thalamus, and dorsomedian thalamus affecting extralemniscal fibers, and thalamic projections terminating in the intralaminar nucleus, centromedianus nucleus, and the frontal lobe.[95] One of the most effective sites appears to be the inferior posteromedial thalamus, containing the intralaminar, centromedianus, and parafascicularis nuclei, all of which might affect the paleospinothalamic tract.[96] More recent literature has proposed that the medial thalamus is related to the spinoreticular tract, the descending

passageway responsible for conducting impulses to many of the motor neurons.[49] Ablations of the lateral thalamus, particularly the ventrocaudal parvocellular nucleus, attempt to destroy the pain-receiving nucleus itself. Combination lesions, such as centromedianus and parafascicularis lesions with dorsomedial nucleus or the thalamic pulvinar lesions, might provide better long-term results.[96] Although lesion size is an important component of this type of operation, a standard does not truly exist because many surgeons have personal preferences. Specific cases may dictate a particular lesion size so as not to inflict damage on the surrounding areas.[94]

Currently, a thalamotomy includes the use of stereotactic methods, frame imaging, referencing, target location(s) selection, and careful introduction of the probe so that sensitive motor structures remain intact.[94] These operative steps are followed by physiological testing to confirm the site.[94] The interactive nature of these tests requires the use of local anesthesia to ensure patient cooperation. The testing site according to Tasker[94] should be approximately in the 15 mm sagittal plane or the tactile representation of the contralateral manual digits. A 5 cm (2 inch) diameter head shave and prep is made for the entry point.

Two types of physiological testing can be used to determine target accuracy. Macrostimulation requires nominal instrumentation with quick progression and total identification of the brain and the spectrum of structures at variable distances from the probe. The process can be executed simultaneously with deep brain recording using the same electrode. The microelectrode recording technique is capable of identifying a limited group of structures. Located on the arc of the stereotactic frame, the microelectrode extends from its protective tubing with the aid of a hydraulic microdrive.[94] Actual stimulation with the microelectrode occurs every 1.0 mm at 300 Hz, 100 mA, 0.1 ms, until responses occur below about 15 mA.[94] A bipolar concentric electrode, 1.1 mm in diameter with a 0.5 mm tip separated by a 0.5 mm ring, monitors the stimulation. In the medial thalamus, neurons that fire spontaneously in a burst fashion provide clear hallmarks of the region, whereas an absence of touch-responsive neurons signals the proximity to the ventrocaudal parvocellular nucleus in the lateral thalamus.[49] Both types of stimulation effect are used in order to minimize damage, procedural failure, and any morbidity resulting when a lesion is made in a position other than the anticipated anatomical target. A documented example of this can be seen in Nashold's work where he implanted electrodes as a testing method prior to performing a thalamotomy.[88] The implanted electrodes permitted an accurate direction for the placement of the thalamotomy electrode tip during the actual operation.[88]

Complications often depend on the problem necessitating the operation and include paresis, cognitive disorders, infection and mortality (although rare in nociceptive pain cases), seizures, speech disturbance, and other matters related to specific areas of disease. Both medial and lateral lesions of the thalamus are moderately effective (approximately 60 percent pain relief) in dealing with cancer pain, but lateral thalamotomy carries with it higher rates of complication, nearly 32 percent.[49] In treatment of nociceptive pain, thalamotomy has been reported to produce transient loss of all contralateral sensory modalities after the operation and also pseudoparesis in many of the cases studied by Tasker; patients seemed to lose the appreciation of position and vibration sense due to the lesions in the ventrocaudal nucleus.[94] Though lesions do not seem to affect cognitive ability, studies have shown that left-sided lesions affect language and the dominance of the right ear in listening exercises (right ear advantage).[49] Enthusiasm for the use of thalamotomy, however, has waned over the past few years because of concerns of pain recurrence after 6–12 months. Due to this decreased efficacy and the significant risks, more recent reports have suggested that thalamic stimulation should be carried out before considering the creation of a lesion.[94]

Cingulotomy

Dating back to 1948, the method calling for the creation of lesions in the cingulate gyrus originated when Hugh Cairns at Oxford removed a portion of the anterior cingulate gyrus in an open operation.[58] The use of the open cingulotomy in the 1940s and 1950s produced significant improvements in psychiatric symptoms in most patients.[57] In 1962, Foltz first described the application of stereotaxy to bilateral anterior cingulate lesions for pain relief while Ballantine began to use ventriculogram-guided stereotaxy to create smaller lesions in the anterior cingulate gyrus. Although cingulotomy has most often has been applied to patients with affective disorders, there are numerous reports of its use for severe pain control.[50–52,97–100] The procedure has been quite successful in patients with cancer suffering from diffuse or multiply-located pain, but it has not been fully adopted because of neurosurgical stereotactic techniques required to perform the operation.[64,65,101]

With the availability of technology capable of guiding closed procedures, there is not any present role for open surgical techniques for cingulotomy. The specific target is the cingulate gyrus, 20–30 mm posterior to the anterior tip of the lateral ventricles. The target is 1.5 mm lateral to midline and 15 mm superior to the roof of the lateral ventricles.[102,103] The radiofrequency method is used more commonly, with each lesion being created at 75°C for 60–90 seconds. The result is a cylindrical lesion approximately 10–20 mm long and 5–7 mm in diameter, centered in each cingulate gyrus.

Although its exact role in pain transmission is unclear, the anterior cingulate cortex incorporates motor, affective, memory, and nociceptive functions, accounting for the various pathways connecting this area with the basal ganglia, frontal subsytems, and lateral frontal and parietal regions.[101,104] The involvement of the cingulate gyrus in emotional processes has led to the suggestion that the anterior cingulate cortex is most notable for its role in human response to pain rather than sensitivity to pain stimuli.[104] Still, studies of cingulate gyrus lesions in laboratory animals have shown a reduction contralaterally in the response to pain, particularly noxious thermal stimuli.[101,105] The anterior cingulate cortex, particularly the posterior side of this region, has been shown to be particularly responsive to nociceptive signals from the thalamus.[105] A recent study indicates that the anterior section of this region is activated by attention-demanding tasks. Some patients studied a year after cingulotomy were seen to have executive and attentional deficits, particularly in the areas of focused and sustained attention.[104]

As many as 30 percent of patients were treated for severe chronic pain in the many reports of patients undergoing cingulotomy. Approximately 51 percent of these patients who were treated with intractable cancer pain had moderate, marked, or complete pain relief 3 months after the procedure. Like many ablative procedures, cingulotomy is more effective for patients with a shorter survival time.[64,65] The main complications resulting from cingulotomy using ventriculogram-guidance (in the treatment of psychiatric or pain symptoms) have been controllable seizures (9 percent incidence), transient mania (6 percent incidence), decreased memory (3 percent incidence), hemiplegia from intracerebral hematoma (0.3 percent incidence), and a low, but measurable, mortality (0.9 percent).[102,103,106] In neuropsychiatric examination, the only abnormalities noted were occasional difficulties in copying complex figures, performing two tapping tests, and successfully completing memory components of an organized serial learning test.[97,107,108] Present evidence suggests that changes in attention due to cingulate gyrus lesions do not significantly affect daily functioning and social behavior for patients with severe cancer pain.

Trigeminal tractotomy

The discovery that lesions in the descending trigeminal tract affected pain and temperature without diminishing touch sensation led to the study of this area and the adjacent nucleate caudalis as a target site for the ablative treatment of trigeminal neuralgia.[109] The caudalis nucleate lies on the surface of the medulla posterior to the dorsal spinocerebellar tract, lateral to the fasciculus cuneatus, and inferior to the restiform body.[110] It appears to act as a relay station for pain and temperature transmission from cranial nerves II, V, IX, and X so that destruction of its oral pole decreases neuron hyperexcitability and severs the ascending multisynaptic pathways for pain.[111]

Trigeminal tractotomy is used primarily for treatment of patients with head and neck cancer and with intractable pain in the distribution of the trigeminal nerve. For those patients whose pain is more diffuse in the head and neck, mesencephalotomy often is a more effective choice.[112] Although trigeminal tractotomy was originally used to treat trigeminal neuralgia and postherpetic neuralgia, it is not frequently used for these conditions because of the availability of other percutaneous and open operations. Newer research indicates that, because the trigeminal, glosso-pharyngeal, and vagal nerves all meet at the spinobulbar juncture, ablative therapy in this region can also be used to treat vagoglossopharyngeal and geniculate neuralgias.[111] Other treatment options have higher rates of morbidity and mortality as well as more extreme complications.[111]

Both percutaneous and open surgical techniques have been described for this operation. A percutaneous technique has been reported with needle penetration at the C1–fora-men magnum area under stereotactic guidance.[113,114] Use of CT technology in particular allows direct visualization of the target and generates measurements of the spinal cord that are patient specific.[111] An electrode with a 0.5–0.6 mm diam-eter is angled 30° cephalad and placed in the spinal cord, 6 mm lateral to the midline, to a depth of 4 mm. Under local anesthesia, electrical stimulation at 50 Hz should provide facial response to low voltage. Stimulation will be felt in con-tralateral body areas via the spinothalamic tract if placement is too ventral, whereas placement that is too dorsal will be felt in ipsilateral areas via the fasciculus cuneatus.

Based on the procedures described by Sjoqvist,[109] the open operation uses a prone position to remove bone uni-laterally from the occiput and C1. After opening the dura, a lesion is created on the nucleus caudalis, 3–5 mm below the surface of the cervicomedullary junction, using a transverse knife. Located 4–8 mm inferior to the obex, the incision extends medially from the fasciculus cuneatus to the rootlets of the spinal accessory nerve. An oblique incision that is angled from superior to inferior as it is made from posterior to anterior minimizes the chance of accidentally injuring the restiform body. Extension of the lesion to include part of both the spinothalamic tract and the fasci-culus is recommended for mouth coverage. The tractotomy is often combined with other nerve and/or root sections in the same area.

Limited published reports of the results of this proce-dure, either with open or percutaneous techniques, suggest that about 75–85 percent of patients with head and neck cancer have good pain relief. Postoperative sensory changes in the area of the pain accompanied by limited relief have been documented as well. Duration of efficacy appears to be months rather than years after the procedure.[110] In some cases, pain associated with the percutaneous operation may result in termination of the procedure before completion. Temporary complications consist of changes in ipsilateral arm coordination, contralateral leg sensation, and ipsilateral arm (rarely leg) proprioception. Less frequent complications include Horner syndrome, dysarthria, gait changes, and hic-cups. Overall mortality has been estimated at 5–10 percent in patients with advanced cancer.

Mesencephalotomy

Mesencephalic tractotomy (mesencephalotomy), the surgical production of lesions in the midbrain, has been reported to provide significant pain relief in greater than 80 percent of cancer patients on both short-term and long-term (2–4 years) follow-ups.[49] The longest duration of pain relief in cancer patients is in the extremities whereas pain in the chest and abdomen does not respond adequately.[115] The procedure is particularly effective in the treatment of head and neck can-cer. A common target site is found by locating the spinothal-amic tract (STT) and the spinoreticular tract (SRT), which are found 7–9 mm lateral to the midline and 4–7 mm lateral of the midline, respectively (carefully avoiding the medial lemniscus which is 9–12 mm lateral of the mid-line).[49] By disrupting the junction of the STT and the SRT, the lesions on the mesencephalon disrupt two nociceptive pathways.[49]

The target has been at the superior colliculus or inferior colliculus level although it appears that the inferior collicu-lus target provides a lower incidence of ocular problems but perhaps with lesser success (50–70 percent). In the studies carried out by Bosch, the target was identified based on intraoperative ventriculography with water-soluble medium using the frontal burr-hole route.[115] The usual stereotactic techniques are performed under general anesthesia to fur-ther standardize the procedure. The area of evoked pain is limited to a very small range (about 2–3 mm of target) and requires the use of a bipolar concentric electrode for extremely precise localized stimulation. Stimulation of the STT results in thermal or noxious sensation contralaterally, while stimulation of the media lemniscus results in tempo-rary paresthesias of the contralateral side.[49]

The accuracy of the stereotactic trajectory to the rostral midbrain also reduces morbidity and other risks.[116] Because of neuropathic side effects, the operation should be limited to patients with short life expectancy and lateralized nociceptive pain. With a well-defined target, the operation can produce pain relief comparable to other pain relief operations like open anterior cordotomy, midline myelo-tomy, and dorsal root entry zone (DREZ) lesions.[115] The major side effect appear to be difficulties with ocular move-ment and binocular vision with mortality varying from 1 percent to 7 percent.[88,117] Postoperative dysesthesia has been reported in studies of the medial lemniscus after large mesencephalic lesions in patients with different types of pain.[116,118] These side effects have been reduced by using a smaller electrode, neural recording, and more precise elec-trical stimulation.[116]

The results of this operation vary due to the nature of the particular diseases. Although nociceptive pain is often sensitive to opioids, mesencephalic surgery is a successful and viable alternative.

Pulvinotomy

Pulvinotomy appears to be ideally suited to treatment of intractable cancer pain whose symptoms are similar to those indicated for cingulotomy, particularly in patients with survival times up to 18 months.[119] Kudo et al. first described lesions in the pulvinar of the thalamus for pain relief in 1966,[120] and by 1975, 30 patients had undergone this treatment. Exact mechanisms for pain relief have not yet been ascertained, but research indicates that the oral and medial parts of the pulvinar are involved in pain appreciation.[121] Electrophysiological studies in cats have demonstrated that the pulvinar is involved in an indirect route for afferent stimuli.[82] From the pulvinar, afferent transmission connections have been traced to the temporal lobe and, from there, to the posterior sensory cortex.[122]

Typically, lesion placement has occurred only in the medial area or in both the medial and lateral areas of pulvinar. Concentration of the lesions in the hemisphere contralateral to the site of pain appears to be less effective than lesions positioned bilaterally.[86,96,118] The coordinates for pulvinar lesions have been 4 mm superior to the AP–PC line, 5 mm posterior to the posterior commissure, and lateral to the AP–PC line by either 10–11 mm for a medial target or 15–16 mm for a lateral target.[119] Lesions are created using ultrasonic probes, with a setting of 75 W and 2.5 megacycles for 30 seconds, at two to six separate sites, resulting in lesions 5–6 mm in diameter.[119] Currently, MRI-guided stereotaxis and radiofrequency thermal tools are also used to generate lesions in the pulvinar.

Moderate to excellent pain relief has been reported in as many as 25 percent of patients for periods ranging from 1 to 2.5 years.[119,122] When the lesions are extended backward to involve the pulvinar, the lesions, especially in the anterior pulvinar, have been found to be more effective than the centromedianus thalamotomy.[122] Extension of the lesions to a more posterior region of the pulvinar, particularly when coupled with thalamotomy lesions in the centromedianus and parafascicularis provides an increase in pain relief.[123] Preexisting pain is most affected by this operation and there is no reported loss of somatic sensation after the procedure.[96] Analysis of patients after pulvinotomy has shown no apparent changes in cognitive functions, although temporary changes in behavior, such as tendencies toward childishness, excessive excitability and euphoria, have all been observed.[124]

Hypothalamotomy

Lesions of the hypothalamus were reported initially for control of cancer pain in 1971, with 28 patients reported to have received the procedure for pain control between 1971 and 1982.[125,126] β-Endorphin concentrations in ventricular cerebrospinal fluid, believed to increase in response to nociceptive stimuli, elevate as a result of electrical stimulation of the target prior to actual ablation of the area and remain at a higher level for at least 2 days after the hypothalamotomy.[127] A postoperative degeneration of axon fibers occurs in regions found ipsilateral to the hypothalamus, including the nucleus ventrocaudalis parvocellularis of Hassler (Vcpc), nucleus parafascicularis, somatosensory cortices, pallidum, and the reticular formation but not in the dorsomedial nucleus of the thalamus.[128] Patients with cancer suffering from diffuse pain, particularly when an emotional or visceral component is present, are good candidates for the operation.[129]

Target sites had previously been localized 2 mm below the midpoint and 2 mm lateral to the lateral wall of the third ventricle, but more recent reports have suggested that a more posterior placement may provide greater pain control.[128] In one series, 15 of 21 hypothalamotomy procedures were bilateral with 'good' results reported in 62 percent of patients.[127,129] Hypothalamotomy does not seem to result in any significant complications; however, published reports are limited.

Combined procedures

As technology enables intracranial procedures to be performed with much more ease, combinations of these techniques should be increasingly used, with particular attention paid to those combinations already used to treat affective disorders. For instance, the use of cingulotomy and anterior capsulotomy, in which lesions are created in both the cingulate gyrus and the anterior limb of the internal capsule, is well reported within the realm of affective disorders. The same combination also has proved useful in the area of severe cancer-related pain, yielding better pain relief, including neuropathic pain, than cingulotomy alone.[130] Targets for thalamotomy also include the pulvinar as an additional target because of the increase in pain relief that this combination brings.[123] As experience and technological advances improve and become more accessible, it is hoped that interest in the research of combination therapy will result in more modalities that provide better long-term efficacy in pain control.

SPINAL ABLATIVE TECHNIQUES

Cordotomy

Until recently, intraspinal ablative procedures have been favored despite the variety of intracranial procedures available as the older spinal methods are 'rediscovered' by using newer percutaneous techniques and CT-guidance. Although its use appears to be decreasing as technological innovations focus more and more attention on intracranial ablative and intraspinal augmentative procedure, the most acknowledged intraspinal ablative procedure, cordotomy, is still a standard option. The aim of the operation is to disrupt the spinothalamic tract as it enters the medulla. However, the mechanism of action for this procedure has been suggested to affect more than just C-fibers because pain relief coincides with a lessened sensation of pinching skin and temperature cooling.[131]

In the percutaneous method, X-ray fluoroscopy is used to position a radiofrequency electrode needle at the level of the C1–2 interspace in the lateral spinothalamic tract as determined by the area of pain.[132] CT-guidance allows for better visualization and more accurate insertion of the electrodes into the spine. A cordotomy needle puncture is made in the side of the neck contralateral to the site of pain with the aid of a questioning stimulation in which the patient is asked about sensory changes and twitching. The open surgical technique for cordotomy is similar to the percutaneous method except that it is often carried out with the patient seated in an upright position. In this procedure, the anterolateral surface of the spinal cord is viewed and an avascular area is found for the incision. The blade projects 6 mm through the cervical area and 4–5 mm in the thoracic area, and then cuts ventrally in order to transect the ventral quadrant but spare the medial funiculus. The open operation is currently considered the less effective surgical option because of the greater risks it entails in comparison with the percutaneous operation.

A patient's case must be exactly suited to the procedure for pain relief to be successfully achieved. Proper preoperative respiratory/pulmonary function is critical because mortality is almost always related to respiratory problems. The main complication during and after surgery is the possible loss of the sensation of temperature. Possible side effects of the percutaneous operation include contralateral limb weakness from lesioning too deep, transient Horner syndrome, respiratory problems, and burning postcordotomy dysesthetic syndromes. Postlesional dysesthesias and new pain either in the contralateral limb or above the level of the previous pain have been reported. Some patients also have been reported to experience low levels of analgesia due to the failure of the surgery or lack of adequate anatomical localization of target sites during the operation. A small group experienced new pain formation in a similar and/or different location, whereas others did not experience relief at all. In other words, the operation is fairly successful in achieving pain relief although many small impediments may hinder success along the way.

In the large series of Tasker,[133] long-term success with no pain was found in 33 percent of patients, and partial pain relief in 12 percent. Persistent pain was noted in 6 percent and a dysesthetic pain in 34 percent, whereas 2.6 percent required a repeat cordotomy for continued pain relief. Others, however, have found that absolute pain relief has decreased through postoperative time with only 37 percent having satisfactory analgesia even after 5–10 years.[134] Complications in the Tasker series included persistent paresis (2 percent), bladder dysfunction (2 percent), temporary respiratory failure (0.5 percent), and death (0.5 percent).

Midline myelotomy

First conceived by Armour in 1927 as a way of treating a patient with tabetic abdominal pain,[135] the midline myelotomy was first performed by Putnam in 1934.[136] Since its first use, the procedure has undergone many mechanical and functional adjustments for new applications. The procedure for midline myelotomy also has undergone adjustments as technologies have changed; it can now be performed with mechanical ablation, radiofrequency techniques, or carbon dioxide laser[137] to section midline fibers posterior to the central canal of the spinal cord.

The lesions are usually created at the lower thoracic spinal cord level although Gildenberg and Hirshberg[138] and others also have reported lesions at C1. The percentage of patients reporting moderate to marked pain relief has been approximately 70 percent with only rare complications or side effects noted. This procedure is particularly effective for visceral lower body pain in patients with cancer in whom other procedures are inapplicable or unsuccessful. There is evidence for a tract in the anterior part of the medial borders of the posterior columns mediating both pelvic and more proximal epigastric visceral pain.[139–142] Research conducted with laboratory animals has shown that lesions in the dorsal column reduce responses to noxious colorectal pain stimulation by 60–80 percent, compared with the 20 percent reduction that results from lesioning the ventral posterolateral nucleus of the thalamus.[143] Orthograde and retrograde tracers have shown the presence of a postsynaptic pathway (separate from the spinothalamic tract) that ascends in the gray matter around the central canal to the nucleus gracilis.[144] From there, nociceptive stimuli are relayed to the ventral posterolateral nucleus of the thalamus using the medial lemniscus.[144] A study of cancer patients with visceral pain has confirmed that punctate midline myelotomy of the mid-thoracic spinal cord can reduce visceral pain and use of narcotics without changes in sensation or motor function.[144] In general, analgesia from hyperpathia and background pain has been obtained without sensory loss but with preserved ability to localize and discriminate between sharp and dull stimuli.[145]

A commissural myelotomy on the spinal cord aims to interrupt all decussating second-order spinothalamic fibers that are contributing to pain perception on both sides of the body through the posterior commissure of the spinal cord. Two methods are presently available: open and closed. The open operation requires an incision in the spinal cord down the exact midline between the two gracilis tracts and ventrally configured down until completely divided. This transection disconnects the two sides of the posterior half of the spinal cord so that they are now independent of each other and can no longer communicate dorsally. The closed operation involves placement of a radiofrequency electrode between the two gracilis tracts using CT guidance.

Although many different methods have been described over many decades, there continues to be a lack of knowledge about the myelotomy, particularly the mechanism of pain relief. Since the use of this procedure has been diminishing over the last 15 years, there have only been about 425 total cases reported throughout neurosurgical journals.[137,138,145–156]

AUGMENTATIVE PROCEDURES

Intraventricular infusion of opioids

Intraventricular infusion of opioids is one of the best-known intracranial augmentative procedures. The mechanism by which it regulates pain appears to involve supraspinal pathways for analgesia. This treatment option is normally among the last resort options for a patient's treatment.[157]

The opioid can be delivered by an implanted infusion pump placed subcutaneously in the anterior abdominal wall and connected by subcutaneous tubing to an implanted ventricular catheter. The length of action of the intraventricular injections appears to be significantly longer than with intraspinal delivery. Patients may be able to receive adequate relief with an implanted ventricular catheter connected to a subcutaneous Ommaya reservoir-type device with one to two injections per day.[158] Morphine sulfate is the usual agent and appears to provide a marked increase in potency as compared to intrathecal or epidural infusions, with daily morphine doses for intraventricular delivery ranging from 50 μg/day to 700 μg/day.[159–161]

Recent studies using sheep indicated that certain drugs, particularly lipophilic morphine-type drugs, have problems diffusing through the CSF pathways to reach distant receptors. Thus, the type of opioid must be carefully considered. Payne et al. used drugs like hydromorphone, morphine, methadone, naloxone, and then sucrose to test the spread of specific opioids in cerebrospinal fluid (CSF).[154] Morphine, hydromorphone, and sucrose were identified at approximately 90 minutes in the lumbar CSF after an intracerebroventricular (ICV) injection. Hydromorphone was located after 50 minutes. Methadone was never found in the CSF due to the fact that the ICV and intrathecal dosage of lipophilic opioids creates distinctly different CSF distributions from hydrophilic drugs, like morphine.[162]

Most significantly, it has been shown that there is a rapid spread of hydrophilic compounds in CSF after lumbar intrathecal injections. The hydrophilic nature of these compounds, however, does make it more difficult for them to attach to the desired receptors. The lipophilicity of the opioid determines the extent of diffusion and concentration in the brain after ICV administration.[162] Brain concentrations of the morphine persist for a few hours after injection although the drug is unevenly dispersed in the tissue. Since morphine is hydrophilic, the movement of the drug through the ventricles of the brain is more like passive diffusion than active transport. Fentanyl, sufentanil, and etorphine, the lipophilic opioids, are cleared in the CSF after one hour as they bind better to lipophilic receptors.[162]

This procedure appears to be best suited for head and neck cancer pain. Occasionally, it is used for patients with limited survival time (1–3 months) who develop a tolerance to intraspinal infusion of opioids despite an good initial response to the treatment. Several factors must be weighed for effective treatment with intraventricular morphine delivery via an Ommaya reservoir, such as the location of the pain, age of the patient and the history of opioid usage. The lower limbs benefit from lumbar subarachnoid administration of morphine, whereas craniofacial or diffuse pain was shown to be more responsive to the analgesic effect of ICV delivery.[163]

Seiwald and Kofler[164] have described in detail their experience with 20 patients (18 patients had cancer) treated with ICV morphine injections between 1990 and 1993.

Administration of morphine into the ventricle through a catheter-reservoir system was nondestructive and effectively relieved nociceptive pain.[164] They also found that lower doses were slower to bring about pain relief. Somatogenic pain was ameliorated in 95 percent of the patients; however, minimal effects were seen in the management of neurogenic pain.[164] The safety and side effects of the intraventricular injections or infusions are similar to intraspinal infusions with the exception of the increased risk of respiratory depression noted in the first 3 days of the intraventricular delivery.[158,160]

Deep brain stimulation

Interest in stimulation swelled in the late 1960s and early 1970s as the severe morbidity rates and limited scope of some early ablative procedures came to light.[165] In 1972, the first stimulation of periventricular and periaqueductal gray matter were performed in humans.[165] Particularly effective in those with chronic pain that activates the paleospinothalamic tract, deep brain stimulation is currently the most useful technique for central pain caused by spinal cord lesions as well as pain that is inadequately relieved with spinal cord or peripheral nerve stimulation.[165] The use of deep brain stimulation has also been reported in the relief of chronic pain of noncancer etiology.[166]

During this procedure, an electrode is implanted by placing the patient under local anesthesia while a burr hole is made 3 cm from the midline in the coronal structure. These burr holes are made easily with CT and MRI-guided stereotaxis because the technology enables accurate placement of the stimulating electrodes.[166] For this operation, the initial targets are either the periventricular gray/periaqueductal gray (PVG/PAG) area, the ventral posterior lateral thalamus, or the internal capsule.[166] To implant an electrode in the PVG/PAG, the exploring electrode tip is placed 10 mm posterior to the midpoint of the AC–PC line at a depth of 4–5 mm.[165] The internal capsule can be found using the atlas of Tasker and Emmers and test stimulation performed at the junction of the thalamus and internal capsule.[165]

In the PVG/PAG, stimulation sets off an endogenous opioid system, mediated primarily by β-endorphins, which inhibits noxious pain impulses.[165] Judging from failed trials with naloxone, the system in the thalamus and internal capsule does not involve opioids, although the mechanism of action is not precisely known.[165] The type of pain being experienced and the severity of the situation help in determining which target site will provide sufficient analgesia. Stimulation of the PVG/PAG is best suited to nociceptive pain, while stimulation of areas in and around the thalamus is thought to work better for neuropathic pain.[167] The small size of thalamic targets as well as the numbness that may result from implantation have led some surgeons to prefer the internal capsule to the lateral thalamus.[165] Many surgeons place electrodes temporarily in both areas and allow the patient to choose the location that best alleviates pain; others rely on intraoperative stimulation to determine placement. After 4 days, routine tests of the apparatus determine the frequencies that generate pain relief. Several days to 3 months after implantation, a radiofrequency-receiving device can be attached so that the patient can freely use the device.[165]

In cancer pain, deep brain stimulation can accommodate patients with pain refractory to ablative procedures. This includes pain from diffuse bone metastases, midline or bilateral pain (especially of the lower body), brachial or lumbosacral plexopathy, and recurrent pain from head and neck cancer.[168] In a series of 31 patients with cancer pain who were treated with deep brain stimulation, 87 percent of the patients experienced satisfactory relief with 55 percent of these experiencing lasting relief until death.[168] In a trial of 68 patients over 15 years, 78 percent underwent internalization of their devices and 79 percent reported long-term relief.[167]

Complications are unavoidable because they are greatly influenced by the placement of the deep brain stimulator electrode. They occur less frequently when the electrode is placed in the PVG region than when it is placed in the PAG. The most reported complication in the Kumar study resulted from hardware malfunction, although 20–25 percent of patients involved in the study reported the development of migraine-type headaches.[167] One complication specific to PVG/PAG is the development of tolerance. It has been suggested that ramp stimulation (intermittent stimulation) and administration of L-tryptophan for a period of 2–3 weeks can diminish this occurrence.[165] Although individual variations can reduce the chance for successful analgesia as a result of deep brain stimulation, the possibility of effective pain relief is both promising and realistic for most patients.[166]

information is still not complete concerning the best application of many of these procedures. Most certainly, it should be emphasized that these techniques are applied only to patients with severe pain since many of the noninterventional options will suffice for pain that is minimal or mild in severity.

- Selection of a specific technique can be based upon expected survival time of the patient with cancer, pain location, and/or preference toward ablative or augmentative options.

- Despite the praise heaped by different clinical groups upon individual methods, information regarding the best modalities of treatment for specific pain syndromes is still lacking. This might be an indication that technology has outpaced our knowledge of the most effective application for each procedure.

- In the modern era, palliative care can and should make use of these modalities to become both 'high-touch' and 'high-tech', which need not be mutually exclusive concepts in the care of patients with cancer.

REFERENCES

1 World Health Organization. *Cancer Pain Relief and Palliative Care*, 2nd ed. Geneva: World Health Organization, 1996: 12–15.

2 Lesage P, Portenoy RK. Trends in cancer pain management. *Cancer Control* 1999; **6**: 136–45.

3 Miguel R. Interventional treatment of cancer pain: the fourth step in the WHO analgesic ladder? *Cancer Control* 2000; **7**: 149–56.

4 Krames E. Interventional pain management: appropriate when less invasive therapies fail to provide adequate analgesia. *Med Clin North Am* 1999; **83**: 787–808.

5 Waldman SD. The role of spinal opioids in management of cancer pain. *J Pain Symptom Manage* 1990; **5**: 163.

6 Ventafidda V, Spoldi E, Caraceni A, *et al.* Intraspinal morphine for cancer pain. *Acta Anaesthesiol Scand Suppl* 1987; **85**: 47–53.

7 Chaney MA. Side effects of intraspinal and epidural opioids. *Can J Anaesth* 1995; **42**: 891–903.

8 Saek S, Yaksh T. Suppression of nociceptive responses by spinal mu agonists: effects of stimulus intensity and agonist efficacy. *Anesth Analg* 1993; **77**: 265.

9 Yaksh TL. Spinal opiates: a review of their effect on spinal function with an emphasis on pain processing. *Acta Anaesthesiol Scand* 1987; **31**: 25.

10 Sanowski M, Yaksh TL. Spinal administration of receptor-selective drugs as analgesics: new horizons. *J Pain Symptom Manage* 1990; **5**: 204.

11 Yaksh TL, Noueihed R. The physiology and pharmacology of spinal opioids. *Annu Rev Pharmacol Toxicol* 1985; **25**: 433.

12 Zieglgansberger W. Opiate actions on mammalian spinal neurons. *Int Rev Neurobiol* 1984; **25**: 243.

13 Coda BA, Brown MC, Schaffer R, *et al.* Pharmacology of epidural fentanyl, alfentanil, and sulfentanil in volunteers. *Anesthesiology* 1994; **81**: 1149–61.

Key learning points

- The management of cancer pain is a complicated challenge, requiring a thorough understanding of the cancer disease process, the pain diagnosis, and the treatment modalities available to treat the painful condition.

- In addition to pain, the patient with cancer often presents with a constellation of symptoms arising from the cancer and the oncological treatment. Full utilization of all available treatment modalities should help to optimize the patient's pain control and quality of life.

- In selected patients, neuraxial intervention via epidural or intrathecal delivery system can help the physician and patient to achieve effective control of cancer pain, minimize opioid-related side effects, and thereby optimize quality of life.

- Over the past decade, the technology for and use of spinal procedures has remained fairly constant and as a result,

14 Jacobson L, Chabal C, Brody MC, et al. Intrathecal methadone: a dose-response study and comparison with intrathecal morphine. Pain 1990; 43: 141–8.

● 15 Hassenbusch SJ, Portenoy RK, Cousins M, et al. Polyanalgesic Consensus Conference 2003: An update on the management of pain by intraspinal drug delivery – report of an expert panel. J Pain Symptom Manage 2004; 27: 540–63.

16 Max MB, Inturrisi CE, Kaido RF, et al. Epidural and intrathecal opiates: CSF and plasma profiles in patients with chronic cancer pain. Clin Pharmacol Ther 1985; 38: 631.

17 Gourley RF, Cherry BA, Cousins MJ. Cephalad migration of morphine in CSF following lumbar epidural administration in patients with cancer pain. Pain 1985; 23: 317.

18 Miguel R, Barlow I, Morrell M, et al. A prospective, randomized double-blinded comparison of epidural and intravenous sulfentanil infusions. Anesthesiology 1994; 81: 346–52.

19 Sullivan AF, Dashwood MR, Dickenson AN. Alpha-2 adrenoreceptor modulation of nociceptor in rat spinal cord: location, effects, and interactions with morphine. Eur J Pharmacol 1987; 138: 169–77.

20 Yaksh TL. Pharmacology of spinal adrenergic systems which modulate spinal nociceptive processing. Pharmacol Biochem Behav 1985; 22: 845–58.

21 Ono H, Mishima A, Ono S, et al. Inhibitory effects of clonidine and tizanidine on release of substance P from slices of rat spinal cord and antagonism by alpha-adrenergic receptor antagonists. Neuropharmacology 1991; 30: 585–9.

22 Segal IS, Jarvis DI, Duncan SR, et al. Clinical efficacy of oral-transdermal clonidine combinations during the perioperative period. Anesthesiology 1991; 74: 220–5.

23 Surrott B, Conway EL, Macarrone C, et al. Clonidine: understanding its disposition, sites, and mechanism of action. Clin Exp Pharmacol Physiol 1987; 14: 471–9.

24 Fibs KS, Goudas LC, Palran O, et al. Hemodynamic and analgesic profile after intrathecal clonidine in humans. A dose-response study. Anesthesiology 1994; 81: 591–601.

● 25 Eisenach SC, DuPen S, Dubois M, et al. Epidural clonidine analgesia for intractable cancer pain. Pain 1995; 61: 391–9.

26 Coombs DW, Saunder RL, Fratkin SD, et al. Continuous intrathecal hydromorphone and clonidine for intractable cancer pain. J Neurosurg 1986; 64: 890–4.

27 Eisenach SC, Tong CY. Site of hemodynamic effects of intrathecal alpha 2-adrenergic agonists. Anesthesiology 1991; 74: 766–71.

● 28 Walker SM, Goudas LC, Cousins MJ, Carr DB. Combination spinal analgesic chemotherapy: a systematic review. Anesth Analg 2002; 95: 674–715.

● 29 Staats PS, Yearwood T, Chapapata SG, et al. Intrathecal ziconotide in treatment of refractory pain in patients with cancer or AIDS: a randomized controlled trial. JAMA 2004; 291: 63–70.

30 Almeida RA, Lauretti GR, Mattis AL. Antinociceptive effect of low-dose intrathecal neostigmine combined with intrathecal morphine following gynecologic surgery. Anesthesiology 2003: 495–8.

31 Naguib M, Yaksh TL. Antinociceptive effects of spinal cholinesterase inhibition and isobolographic analysis of the interaction with mu and alpha 2 receptor systems. Anesthesiology 1994; 80: 1338–48.

32 Hood DD, Eisenach SC, Tuttle R. Phase I safety assessment of intrathecal neostigmine methylsulfate in humans. Anesthesiology 1995; 82: 331–45.

33 Gallagher RM. Epidural and intrathecal cancer pain management: prescriptive care for quality of life. Pain Med 2004; 5: 235.

● 34 Ferrante FM, Bedder M, Caplan KA, et al. Practice guidelines for cancer pain management. Anesthesiology 1996; 94: 1243–57.

35 Dupen SL, Williams AR. Spinal and peripheral drug delivery systems. Pain Digest 1995; 5: 307–17.

36 Kedlaya D, Reynolds L, Waldman S. Epidural and intrathecal analgesia for cancer pain. Best Pract Res Clin Anaesthesiol 2002; 16: 651–5.

● 37 Burton AW, Rajagopal A, Shah HN, et al. Epidural and intrathecal analgesia is effective in treating refractory cancer pain. Pain Med 2004; 5: 238–46.

38 Bedder MD, Burchiel JK, Larson A. Cost analysis of two narcotic delivery systems. J Pain Symptom Manage 1991; 6: 397–409.

39 Hassenbusch SJ. Cost modeling for alternative routes of administration of opioids for cancer pain. Oncology 1999; 13: 63–7.

40 Burton AW, Hassenbusch SJ. The double catheter technique for intrathecal medication trial: A brief clinical note and report of five cases. Pain Med 2001; 2: 352–354.

41 Krames ES. Intraspinal opioid therapy for chronic nonmalignant pain: current practice and clinical guidelines. J Pain Symptom Manage 1996; 11: 333–52.

42 Hassenbusch SJ, Pillay PK, Magdinec M, et al. Constant infusion of morphine for intractable cancer pain using implanted pump. J Neurosurg 1990; 73: 405–9.

43 Kanoff RB. Intraspinal delivery of opiates by an implantable, programmable pump in patients with chronic, intractable pain of nonmalignant origin. J Am Osteopath Assoc 1994; 94: 487–93.

44 Krames ES. Continuous infusion of spinally administered narcotics for the relief of pain due to malignant disorders. Cancer 1985; 56: 696–702.

● 45 Gilmer-Hill HS, Boggan JE, Smith KA, et al. Intrathecal morphine delivered via subcutaneous pump for intractable cancer pain: a review of the literature. Surg Neurol 1999; 51: 12–15.

● 46 Rauck RL, Cherry D, Boyer MF, et al. Long-term intrathecal opioid therapy with a patient-activated implanted delivery system for the treatment of refractory cancer pain. J Pain 2003; 4: 441–7.

● 47 Smith TJ, Staats P, Deer T, et al. Randomized clinical trial of an implantable drug delivery system compared with comprehensive medical management for refractory cancer pain: impact on pain, drug-related toxicity, and survival. J Clin Oncol 2002; 20: 4040–9.

● 48 Bennett G, Burchiel K, Buchser E, et al. Clinical guidelines for intraspinal infusion: report of an expert panel. J Pain Symptom Manage 2000; 20: 537–43.

49 Davis KD, Lozano Am, Tasker RR, Dostrovsky JO. Brain targets for pain control. Stereotact Funct Neurosurg 1998; 71: 173–9.

50 Foltz EL, White LE. Pain 'relief' by frontal cingulumotomy. J Neurosurg 1962; 19: 89–100.

51 Hurt RW, Ballantine HT. Stereotactic anterior cingulate lesions for persistent pain: a report on 68 cases. Clin Neurosurg 1974; 21: 334–51.

52 Mempel E, Dietrich RZ. Favorable effect of cingulotomy on gastric crisis pain. Neurol Neurochir Pol 1977; 11: 611–13.

53 Sano K. Neurosurgical treatments of pain – a general survey. Acta Neurochir Suppl 1987; 38: 86–96.

54 Santo JL, Arias LM, Barolat G, *et al.* Bilateral cingulumotomy in the treatment of reflex sympathetic dystrophy. *Pain* 1988; **41**: 55–9.

55 Coombs DW. Intraspinal analgesic infusion by implanted pump. *Ann N Y Acad Sci* 1988; **531**: 108–22.

56 Yaksh TL, Onofrio B. Retrospective consideration of the doses of morphine given intrathecally by chronic infusion in 163 patients by 19 physicians. *Pain* 1987; **31**: 211–23.

57 Lewin W. Observations on selective leucotomy. *J Neurol Neurosurg Psychiatry* 1961; **24**: 37–44.

58 Lewin W. Selective leucotomy: a review. In: Laitinen LV, Livingston KE, eds. *Surgical Approaches in Psychiatry.* Baltimore: University Park Press, 1972:69–73.

59 Spiegel EA, Wycis HT, Marks M, *et al.* Stereotaxic apparatus for operations on the human brain. *Science* 1947; **106**: 349–50.

60 Spiegel EA. *Guided Brain Operations.* Basel: S. Karger, 1982.

61 Hadley MN, Shetter AG, Amos MR. Use of the Brown-Roberts-WElls stereotactic frame for functional neurosurgery. *Appl Neurophysiol* 1985; **48**: 61–8.

62 Hassenbusch SJ, Pillay P. Ablative intracranial neurosurgery for cancer pain: three-year experience and modification of techniques [abstract]. *J Neurosurg* 1992; **76**: 396A.

63 Holsheimer J, Demeulemeester H, Nuttin B, de Sutter P. Identification of the target neuronal elements in electrical deep brain stimulation. *Eur J Neurosci* 2000; **12**: 4573–7.

64 Hassenbusch SJ, Pillay P. *Cingulotomy for Treatment of Cancer-related Pain.* Mt Kisco, NY: Futura, 1993: 297–312.

65 Pillay PK, Hassenbusch SJ. Cingulotomy for cancer pain: two year experience. *Stereotactic Funct Neurosurg* 1992; **59**: 33–8.

66 Leksell L. Cerebral radiosurgery. Gammathalamotomy in two cases of intractable pain. *Acta Chir Scand* 1968; **134**: 585–95.

67 Steiner L, Forster D, Leksell L, Gammathalamotomy in intractable pain. *Acta Neurochir* 1980; **52**: 173–84.

68 Lindquist C, Kilstrom L, Hellstrand E. Functional neurosurgery: a future for the gamma knife? *Stereotactic Funct Neurosurg* 1991; **57**: 72–81.

69 Miles J. Chemical hypophysectomy. *Adv Pain Res Ther* 1979; **2**: 373–80.

70 Tindall GT, Payne NS, Nixon DW. Transsphenoidal hypophysectomy for disseminated carcinoma of the prostate gland. *J Neurosurg* 1979; **50**: 275–82.

71 Kapur TR, Dalton GA. Trans-sphenoidal hypophysectomy for metastatic carcinoma of the breast. *Br J Surg* 1969; **56**: 332–7.

72 Zervas NT. Stereotaxic radiofrequency surgery of the normal and abnormal pituitary gland. *N Engl J Med* 1969; **280**: 429–37.

73 Maddy JA, Winternitz WW, Norrell H. Cryohypophysectomy in the management of advanced prostatic cancer. *Cancer* 1971; **28**: 322–8.

74 Silverberg GD. Hypophysectomy in the treatment of disseminated prostate carcinoma. *Cancer* 1977; **39**: 1727–31.

75 Levin AB, Ramirez LF, Katz J. The use of stereotaxic chemical hypophysectomy in the treatment of thalamic pain syndrome. *J Neurosurg* 1983; **59**: 1002–6.

76 Levin AB. Hypophysectomy in the treatment of cancer pain. In: Arbit E. *Management of Cancer-Related Pain.* Mt. Kisco, NY: Futura Publishing Company, Inc., 1993: 281–95.

77 Daniel PM. The human hypothalamus and pituitary stalk after hypophysectomy of pituitary stalk section. *Brain* 1972; **95**: 813–24.

78 Nilaver G, Zimmerman EA, Wilkins J, *et al.* Magnocellular hypothalamic projections to the lower brain stem and spinal cord of the rat: immunocytochemical evidence for predominance of the oxytocin-neurophysin system compared to a vasopressin-neurophysin system. *Neuroendocrinology* 1980; **30**: 150–8.

79 Sofroniew MV. Projections from vasopressin, oxytocin, and neurophysin neurons to neural targets in the rat and human. *J Histochem Cytochem* 1980; **28**: 475–8.

80 Swanson LW, Sawchenko PE. Paraventricular nucleus: a site for the integration of neuroendocrine and autonomic mechanism. *Neuroendocrinology* 1980; **31**: 410–17.

81 Silverman AJ, Zimmerman EA. Magnocellular neurosecretory system. *Annu Rev Neurosci* 1983; **6**: 357–380.

82 Kudo T, Toshii N, Shimizu S, *et al.* Stereotactic thalamotomy for pain relief. *Tohoku J Exp Med* 1968; **96**: 219–23.

83 Gros C, Frerebeau P, Privat JM, *et al.* Place of hypophysectomy in the neurosurgical treatment of pain. *Adv Neurosurg* 1975; **3**: 264–72.

84 Tindall GT, Ambrose SS, Christy JH. Hypophysectomy in the treatment of disseminated carcinoma of the breast and prostate gland. *South Med J* 1976; **69**: 579–83.

85 Greco T, Sbaragli F, Cammilli L. L'alcolizzazione della ipofisi per via transfenoidal nella terapia di particoloari tumori maligni. *Settim Med* 1957; **45**: 355–6.

86 Yoshii N, Fukuda S, Effects of unilateral and bilateral invasion of thalamic pulvinar for pain relief. *Tohoku J Exp Med* 1979; **127**: 81–4.

87 Lipton S. Percutaneous cervical cordotomy and pituitary injection of alcohol. In: Swerdlow M, ed. *Relief of Intractable Pain.* Amsterdam: Elsevier, 1983: 269–304.

88 Shieff C, Nashold B. Stereotactic mesencephalic tractotomy for thalamic pain. *Neurol Res* 1987; **9**: 101–4.

89 Perrault M, LeBeau J, Klotz B, *et al.* L'hypophysectomie totale dans le traitment du cancer sein: premier cas francais: avenir de la methode. *Therapie* 1952; **7**: 290–300.

90 Katz S, Levin AB. Treatment of diffuse metastatic pain by instillation of alcohol in to the sella turcia. *Anesthesiology* 1977; **46**: 115–21.

91 Williams NE, Miles JB, Lipton S, *et al.* Pain relief and pituitary function following injection of alcohol into the pituitary fossa. *Ann R Coll Surg Engl* 1980; **62**: 203–7.

92 Madrid JL. Chemical hypophysectomy. *Adv Pain Res Ther* 1979; **2**: 381–91.

93 Tasker R. Neurosurgical and neuroaugmentative intervention. In: Patt RB, ed. *Cancer Pain.* Philadelphia: JB Lippincott Company, 1993: 471–500.

94 Tasker RR. Thalamotomy. *Neurosurg Clin North Am* 1990; **1**: 841–66.

95 Gildenberg PL, Lin PM, Polakoff PP, *et al.* Anterior percutaneous cervical cordotomy. Determination of target point and calculations of angle of insertion. Technical note. *J Neurosurg* 1968; **28**: 173–7.

96 Sweet WH. Central mechanisms of chronic pain (neuralgias and certain other neurogenic pain). *Res Publ Assoc Res Nerv Ment Dis* 1980; **58**: 287–303.

97 Faillace LA, Allen RP, McQueen JD, Northrup B. Cognitive deficits from bilateral cingulotomy for intractable pain in man. *Dis Nerv Sys* 1981; **32**: 171–75.

98 Ortiz A. The role of the limbic lobe in central pain mechanisms: an hypothesis relating to the gate control theory of pain. In: Laitinen LV, Livingston KE, eds. *Surgical*

Approaches in Psychiatry. Baltimore: University Park Press, 1972: 59–64.

99 Sharma T. Absence of cognitive deficits from bilateral cingulotomy for intractable pain in humans. *Tex Med* 1973; **69**: 79–82.

100 Sharma T. Abolition of opiate hunger in humans following bilateral anterior cingulotomy. *Tex Med* 1974; **70**: 49–52.

101 Wong ET, Gunes S, Gaughan E, *et al.* Palliation of intractable cancer pain by MRI-guided cingulotomy. *Clin J Pain* 1997; **13**: 260–3.

102 Ballantine HT. A critical assessment of psychiatric surgery: Past, present, and future. In: Berger PA, Brodie HKH, eds. *American Handbook of Psychiatry*, Vol. 8. New York: Basic Books, 1986: 1029–45.

103 Ballantine HT, Bouckoms AJ, Thomas EK, *et al.* Treatment of psychiatric illness by stereotactic cingulotomy. *Biol Psychiatry* 1987; **22**: 807–817.

104 Cohen RA. Impairments of attention after cingulotomy. *Neurology* 1999; **53**: 819–24.

105 Davis KD, Taub E, Duffner F, *et al.* Activation of the anterior cingulate cortex by thalamic stimulation in patients with chronic pain: a positron emission tomography study. *J Neurosurg* 2000; **92**: 64–9.

106 Jenike MA, Baer L, Ballantine T, et al, Cingulotomy for refractory obsessive-compulsive disorder. *Arch Gen Psychiatry* 1991; **48**: 548–55.

107 Allen RP, Faillace LA. A clinical test for detecting defects of cingulate lesions in man. *J Clin Psychol* 1972; **28**: 63–5.

108 Corkin S, Twitchell TE, Sullivan EV. Safety and efficacy of cingulotomy for pain and psychiatric disorder. In: Hitchcock ER, Ballantine HT, Myerson BA, eds. *Modern Concepts in Psychiatric Surgery*. New York: Elsevier North-Holland, 1979: 253–72.

109 Sjoqvist O. Studies on pain conduction in trigeminal nerve: a contribution to the surgical treatment of facial pain. *Acta Psychiatr Neurol Suppl* 1938: 1–139.

110 White JC, Sweet WH. *Pain and the Neurosurgeon: a Forty-year Experience*. Springfield, IL: Charles C Thomas, 1969: 232–51, 314–20.

111 Kanpolat Y, Saras A, *et al.* CT-guided trigeminal trachotomy-nucleotomy in the management of vagoglossopharyngeal and geniculate neuralgias. *Neurosurgery* 1998; **43**: 484–8.

112 Spiegel EA, Wycis HT. Mesencephalotomy in the treatment of 'intractable' facial pain. *Arch Neurol* 1953; **69**: 1.

113 Nashold BS Jr, Crue BL. Stereotaxic mesencephalotomy and trigeminal tractotomy. In: Youmans JR, ed. *Neurological Surgery*, 2nd ed. Philadelphia: WB Saunders, 1982: 3702–16.

114 Schvarcz JR. Spinal cord stereotactic techniques re trigeminal nucleotomy and extralemniscal myelotomy. *Appl Neurophysiol* 1978; **41**: 99–112.

115 Harris B. Dorsal rhizotomy. In: Wilkins RS, ed. *Neurosurgery*. New York: McGraw-Hill, 1985: 2430–7.

116 Amano K, Kitamura K, Tatsuya T, *et al.* Stereotactic mesencephalotomy for pain relief. *Stereotact Funct Neurosurg* 1992; **59**: 25–32.

117 Frank F, Fabrizi AP, Gaist G. Stereotactic mesencephalic tractotomy in the treatment of chronic pain. *Acta Neurochir (Wein)* 1989; **99**: 38–40.

118 Shieff C, Nashold B. Stereotactic mesencephalotomy. *Neurosurg Clin North Am* 1990; **1**: 825–39.

119 Yoshii N, Mizokami T, Ushikubo Y, *et al.* Comparative study between size of lesioned area and operative effects after pulvinotomy. *Appl Neurophysiol* 1982; **45**: 492–7.

120 Kudo T, Toshii N, Shimizu S, *et al.* Effects of stereotactic thalamotomy to intractable pain and numbness. *Keio J Med* 1966; **15**: 191–4.

121 Strenge H. The functional significance of the pulvinar thalami. *Fortschr Neurol Psychiatr* 1978; **46**: 491–507.

122 Laitinen LV. Anterior pulvinotomy in the treatment of intractable pain. In: Sweet WH, Obrador S, Martin Rodriguez JG, eds. *Neurosurgical Treatment in Psychiatry, Pain, and Epilepsy*. Baltimore, University Park Press, 1977: 669–672.

123 Mayanagi Y, Bouchard G. Evaluation of stereotactic thalamotomies for pain relief with reference to pulvinar intervention. *Appl Neurophysiol* 1976; **39**: 154–7.

124 Yoshii N, Fukuda S. Several clinical aspects of thalamic pulvinotomy. *Appl Neurophysiol* 1977; **39**: 162–4.

125 Sano K. Sedative neurosurgery with reference to posteromedial hypothalamotomy. *Neurol Medicochir* 1962; **4**: 112–42.

126 Fairman D. Hypothalamotomy as a new perspective for alleviation of intractable pain and regression of metastatic malignant tumors. In: Fusek K, ed. *Present Limits of Neurosurgery*. Prague, Avicenum Czechoslovakian Medical Press, 1971: 525–8.

127 Mayanagi Y, Sano K, Suzuki I, *et al.* Stimulation and coagulation of the posteromedial hypothalamus for intractable pain, with reference to beta-endorphins. *Appl Neurophysiol* 1982; **45**: 136–42.

128 Sano K, Sekino H, Hashimoto I, *et al.* Posteromedial hypothalamotomy in the treatment of intractable pain. *Confinia Neurol* 1975; **37**: 285–90.

129 Amano K, Kitamura K, Sano K, *et al.* Relief of intractable pain from neurosurgical point of view with reference to present limits and clinical indications: a review of 100 consecutive cases. *Neurol Med Chir (Tokyo)* 1976; **16**: 141–53.

130 Hassenbusch SJ, Pillay P. Cingulotomy for intractable pain using stereotaxis guided by magnetic resonance imaging. In: Rengachary SS, Wilkins RH, eds. *Neurosurgical Operative Atlas*. Baltimore: Williams & Wilkins, 1992; **1**: 449–58.

131 Lahuerta I, Bowsher D, Campbell J. Clinical and instrumental evaluation of sensory function before and after percutaneous anterolateral cordotomy at cervical level in man. *Pain* 1990; **42**: 23–30.

132 Faillace LA, Allen RP, McQueen JD, Northrup B. Cognitive deficits from bilateral cingulotomy for intractable pain in man. *Dis Nerv Sys* 1981; **32**: 171–175.

133 Tasker R. Neurosurgical and neuroaugmentative intervention. In: *Cancer Pain*. Philadelphia: Lippincott, 1990: 471–500.

134 Rosomoff HL, Papo I, Loeser JD. Neurosurgical operations on the spinal cord. In: Bonica JJ, ed. *The Management of Pain*. Philadelphia: Lea & Febiger 1990: 2067–81.

135 Armour D. Surgery of the spinal cord and its membranes. *Lancet* 1927; **1**: 691–7.

136 Putnam TJ. Myelotomy of the commissure. *Arch Neurol Psychiatry* 1934; **32**: 1189–93.

137 Fink RA. Neurosurgical treatment of non-malignant intractable rectal pain: microsurgical commissural myelotomy with the carbon dioxide laser. *Neurosurgery* 1984; **14**: 64–5.

138 Gildenberg PL, Hirshberg RM. Limited myelotomy for the treatment of intractable cancer pain. *J Neurol Neurosurg Psychiatry* 1984; **47**: 94–6.

139 Hirshberg RM, Al-Chaer NM, Lawand NB, *et al.* Is there a pathway in the posterior funiculus that signals visceral pain? *Pain* 1996; **67**: 291–305.

140 Al-Chaer ED, Lawand NB, Westlund KN, Willis WD. Pelvic visceral input into the nucleus gracilis is largely mediated by the postsynaptic dorsal column pathway. *J Neurophysiol* 1996; **76**: 2675–90.

141 Al-Chaer ED, Lawand NB, Westlund KN, Willis WD. Visceral nociceptive input into the ventral posterolateral nucleus of the thalamus: A new function for the dorsal column pathway. *J Neurophysiol* 1996; **76**: 2661–74.

142 Feng Y, Cui ML, Al-Chaer ED, *et al.* Epigastric pain relief by cervical dorsal column lesion in rats. *Anesthesiology* 1998; **89**: 411–20.

143 Willis WD, Al-Chaer ED, Quast MJ, Westlund KN. A visceral pathway in the dorsal column of the spinal cord. *Proc Natl Acad Sci U S A* 1999; **96**: 7675–9.

144 Nauta JW, Soukup VM, Fabian RH, *et al.* Punctate midline myelotomy for relief of visceral cancer pain. *J Neurosurg* 2000; **92**: 125–30.

145 Schvarcz JR. Stereotactic extralemniscal myelotomy. *J Neural Neurosurg Psychiatry* 1976; **39**: 53–7.

146 Sunder-Plassmann M, Grunert V. Commissural myelotomy for drug resistant pain. In: Koos WT, Spetzler RF ed. *Clinical Neurosurgery*. Stuttgart: Georg Thieme Verlag, 1976: 165–70.

147 Hitchcock ER, Tsukamoto Y. Distal and proximal sensory responses during stereotactic spinal tractotomy in man. *Ann Clin Res* 1973; **5**: 68–73.

148 Schvarcz JR. Stereotactic high cervical extralemniscal myelotomy for pelvic cancer pain. *Acta Neurochir* 1984; (Suppl 33): 431–5.

149 Broager B. Commissural myelotomy. *Surg Neurol* 1974; **2**: 71.

150 Cook AW. Commissural myelotomy. *J Neurosurg* 1977; **47**: 1.

151 Lippert RG, Hosobuchi Y, Nielsen SL. Spinal commissurotomy. *Surg Neurol* 1974; **2**: 373.

152 Papo I, Luongo A. High cervical commissural myelotomy in the treatment of pain. *J Neurol Neurosurg Psychiatry* 1976; **39**: 105.

153 King RB. Anterior commissurotomy for intractable pain. *J Neurosurg* 1977; **47**: 7–1.

154 Payne NS. Dorsal longitudinal myelotomy for the control of perineal and lower body pain [abstract]. *Pain* 1984; (Suppl2): S320.

155 Sweet WH, Poletti CE. Operations in the brain stem and spinal canal, with an appendix on open cordotomy. In: Wall PD, Melzack R, eds. *Textbook of Pain*. Edinburgh, UK: Churchill Livingstone, 1984:615–31.

156 Adams JE, Lippert R, Hosobuchi Y. Commissural myelotomy. In: Schmidek HH, Sweet WH, eds. *Current Techniques in Operative Neurosurgery*. New York: Grune & Stratton, 1988: 1185–9.

157 Siegfried]. Intracerebral neurosurgery in the treatment of chronic pain. *Schweiz Rundsch Med Prax* 1998; 87: 314–17.

158 Brazenor GA Long-term intrathecal administration of morphine: a comparison of bolus injection via reservoir with continuous infusion by implanted pump. *Neurosurgery* 1987; **21**:, 484–91.

159 Tseng LF, Fujimoto JM. Differential actions of intrathecal naloxone on blocking the tail flick inhibition induced by intraventricular beta-endorphin and morphine in rats. *J Pharmacol Exp Ther* 1985; **232**: 74–9.

160 Dennis GC, DeWitty RL. Long-term intraventricular infusion of morphine for intractable pain in cancer of the head and neck. *Neurosurgery* 1990; **26**: 404–8.

161 Lazorthes Y. Intracerebroventricular administration of morphine for control of irreducible cancer pain. *Ann N Y Acad Sci* 1988; **531**: 123–32.

162 Payne R, Inturris C. Cerebrospinal fluid distribution of opioids after intraventricular and lumbar subarachnoid administration in sheep. *Life Sci* 1996; **59**: 1307–21.

163 Karavelis A, Foroglou G, Selviaridis P, Fountzilas G. Intraventricular administration of morphine for control of intractable cancer pain in 90 patients. *Neurosurgery* 1996; **39**: 57–62.

164 Seiwald M, Kofler A. Intraventricular morphine administration as a treatment possibility for patients with intractable pain. *Wien Klin Wochenschr* 1996; **108**: 5–8.

165 Richardson DE. Deep brain stimulation for pain relief. In: Wilkins RH, Rengachary SS, eds. *Neurosurgery*. New York: McGraw-Hill, 1985: 2421–6.

166 Goodman RR. Surgical management of pain. *Neurosurg Clin North Am* 1990; **1**: 701–17.

167 Kumar K, Wyant CM, Nath R. Deep brain stimulation for control of intractable pain in humans, present and future: A ten-year follow-up. *Neurosurgery* 1990; **26**: 774–82.

168 Laitinen RF. Clinical experience with radiofrequency and laser DREZ lesions. *J Neurosurg* 1990; **72**: 715–20.

49

Topical administration of analgesics

ANDREAS KOPF, STEFFEN SCHMIDT, CHRISTOPH STEIN

INTRODUCTION

Systemic application of analgesics is the preferred route of drug administration to achieve pain control in malignant as well as nonmalignant pain. However, recent findings suggest a role for topical administration of analgesics as well as the use of local receptor systems. This can be achieved by a variety of application forms, e.g. creams, lotions, gels, patches, aerosols, and occlusion systems. They allow high local drug concentrations at the site of pain with low or absent adverse drug effects due to low systemic drug levels. By definition, topical analgesia targets a site immediately at the location of drug delivery whereas transdermal analgesia uses the skin merely as an alternative delivery route to achieve systemically active drug levels. Tissue affected by cancer may be more responsive to topical analgesia due to injury of skin or membrane integrity. Peripheral pain signaling is influenced by a number of excitatory and inhibitory mediators released by local tissue injury and inflammation. Neurotransmitter receptors are expressed and/or upregulated on sensory nerve endings, which may be targeted by topical analgesics. Inhibitory receptors which may be useful clinically include μ-, λ- and δ-opioid and cannabinoid receptors. An extensive review of this topic has been published recently.[1] A number of different drug classes have been administered topically (Table 49.1).

DRUG CLASSES

Opioids

Opioids are mostly used orally or parenterally. Lately the transdermal route has gained popularity for patients with and without cancer. Less frequently, opioids are administered

Table 49.1 *Drug classes which have been used for topical administration*

Drug class	Target
Opioids	μ-, κ- and δ-opioid receptors
Nonsteroidal anti-inflammatory drugs	Cyclooxygenase
Local anesthetics	Na channel
Menthol	TRPM8 receptor
Capsaicin	TRPV-1 receptor
Tetrahydrocannabinol	CB$_2$ receptor
Clonidine	α_2 receptor
Ketamine	NMDA receptor
Tricyclic antidepressants	Na channel, adenosine receptor

intranasally or intraorally to achieve high and reliable systemic drug concentrations, mostly in postoperative[2*] but also in cancer pain.[3*] Still, in some patients systemic side effects of opioids limit their use. Therefore using topical effects of opioids may help achieve analgesia and at the same time reduce systemic blood levels and side effects.

Opioid receptors have been identified outside the central nervous system in animals[4] and in humans.[5] They are expressed in the neuronal cell bodies in the dorsal root ganglia and then transported intraaxonally to peripheral sensory nerve terminals of C- and A-fibers.[6*] The presence of local inflammation and secretory stimulants (e.g. interleukin [IL]-1, corticotrophin-releasing hormone [CRH]) determines the migration of opioid-producing cells and opioid peptide release.[7] In certain pain situations where affected tissue may be approached externally (e.g. skin ulcers or oral mucositis) local opioid receptors may be used to achieve analgesia. μ-Agonists like morphine seem to be the most potent at producing peripheral analgesia. Patients with ulcerating cancers may benefit not only from local analgesia but also from the local anti-inflammatory effects of opioids.[8,9]

While the therapeutic concept of local opioid analgesia is regularly used and well documented in the case of intraarticular application of morphine for perioperative analgesia,[10] there is scarce literature on local opioid analgesia in other locations like skin, bladder, or nerve plexus.[11*,12*,13] Only few studies have examined the effects of local opioid analgesia in cancer patients. Oral mucositis is a frequent complication of cytoreductive radio- or chemotherapy.[14] In particular, pain from oral mucositis remains a therapeutic challenge in patients with bone marrow transplantation.[15***] Ulcerations of the oral cavity are a consequence of the direct toxic effects to the epithelial layer, enhanced by cytokines[16] and local superinfections,[17] resulting in damage to the epithelial integrity.[18] The majority of patients with oral mucositis will depend on the World Health Organization (WHO) step III systemic analgesics to achieve pain reduction,[19**] usually for 10–20 days. Patient-controlled intravenous opioid analgesia is the first choice.[20] In radiochemotherapy-induced oral mucositis it has been shown that the topical administration of 15 mL of 0.2 percent morphine reduced pain intensity and duration, which might be interpreted as a local analgesic and/or anti-inflammatory opioid effect.[21**] In a similar study that used repeated applications of 200 μg fentanyl sufficient analgesia could not be achieved or a healing tendency of the oral mucosa.[22] To achieve local opioid analgesia and to avoid systemic uptake a less lipophilic substance like morphine may be more suitable. For example, it has been shown that less than 20 percent of (5 mg) morphine after being in the oral cavity for 10 minutes was absorbed systemically.[23]

Apart from intraoral local opioid analgesia there is a growing body of experimental and clinical evidence that opioids are also useful when applied topically to cutaneous ulcers. A number of case reports and case studies describe profound and long-acting analgesia with minimal adverse effects.[11,12*,24–28] In most cases morphine was used locally, usually in a commercially available gel formulation, and in some instances with an occlusion tape. One study evaluated the ability of morphine to penetrate intact skin and its subsequent systemic uptake.[29] The maximum calculated systemic bioavailability for morphine after topical application was 20 percent. In most patients absorption was negligible. It was concluded that topical morphine has local analgesic effects without considerable systemic absorption, with the possible exception of ulcers with a large surface. However, it has yet to be determined systematically how specific formulations and application techniques influence bioavailability and systemic uptake, which drugs are optimal and what is the potential for cutaneous side effects.

Nonsteroidal anti-inflammatory drugs

Nonsteroidal anti-inflammatory drugs are an integral part of the World Health Organization (WHO) analgesic ladder.

Due to their gastroenterological and renal toxicity they are often used with caution in the management of pain in palliative care patients. Selective inhibitors of cyclooxygenase (COX)-2 have the advantage of longer dosing intervals and do not need to be combined with gastroprotective agents. Nevertheless in many instances topical NSAID preparations would be welcome, since plasma concentrations following topical application are 15 percent lower than those after systemic application.[30***] Whether the possible increase in cardiovascular morbidity and mortality with COX-2 inhibitors is a real concern in the palliative care patient population is questionable, since only patients with long-term treatment seem to be at risk.[31**] Topical NSAIDs are typical over-the-counter medications which are widely advertised and used for acute and chronic pain, but usually not for cancer pain. A large number of formulations (cream, gel, ointment) are commercially available with varying drug delivery to the skin.[32,33***] Most studies examined patients with acute pain due to sports injuries or chronic pain in osteoarthritis.[34**] In contrast to the general belief that NSAID concentrations in tissues below the dermis are low, two meta-analyses concluded that topical NSAIDs are effective for a limited period of time in acute painful conditions[35***,36] and chronic conditions.[37,38***] The long-term use of topical NSAIDs in the treatment of osteoarthritis did not support efficacy.[39***] For the palliative care situation specific indications for topical NSAIDs are unknown. However, there are some situations when their application might be justified, e.g. to alleviate pain and inflammation at sites of cannulation,[40*] to reduce pain and discomfort from topical treatments in actinic keratoses[41*] or to control pain in acute herpetic neuralgia,[42**] a painful complication frequently seen in cancer patients. In the latter study 30 mL of ethyl-ether added to 1500 mg acetylsalicylic acid were applied locally onto the affected dermatome with beneficial effects on pain. No active drug concentrations could be detected in plasma after topical administration.[43] In a more recent study this effect could be reproduced using a topical aspirin-moisturizer solution.[44**]

Local anesthetics

Topical formulations of local anesthetics produce analgesia by blockade of sodium channels in cutaneous primary afferent neurons. Sodium channel blockade reduces impulse generation both in normal sensory neurons and in damaged sensory neurons with ectopic repetitive firing. Therefore, topical local anesthetics are effective in acute pain states as well as in chronic neuropathic pain states. Remarkably, in neuropathic pain states with altered expression, distribution and function of sodium channels along axons, pain relief is achieved with local anesthetic tissue concentrations far below those which totally block impulse conduction. Therefore, pain reduction in neuropathic pain states is possible without achieving anesthesia of the skin.[45]

Most evidence for pain relief through topical local anesthetics exists for lidocaine either as a eutectic mixture with prilocaine (EMLA®)[46***] or as a patch.

EMLA is used for alleviating pain resulting from invasive procedures. A variety of controlled studies have demonstrated analgesic effectiveness for procedures such as venipuncture,[47**,48,49] central venous port access[50*] or lumbar puncture,[51] especially in children with cancer. A minimal application time of 60 minutes with occlusion is necessary for optimal results. Invasive procedures therefore have to be prearranged. A new formulation with liposomal lidocaine seems to have a faster onset and could therefore be advantageous.[52] For the palliative care patient there is good evidence for efficacy of EMLA in reducing pain in venous leg ulcers.[53***] There is one case report of pain control with EMLA in a patient with rectal pain caused by a malignant mass.[54] Side effects are rare and include erythema or pruritus. Prilocaine-induced methemoglobinemia has been described primarily in infants but there are case reports of occurrence in adults.[55] Due to its short duration of action (2–4 hours) EMLA is normally not suitable for treatment of chronic pain conditions.

Lidocaine patches have been reported to be effective in the treatment of chronic neuropathic pain and are a valuable alternative or supplement to systemic neuropathic pain therapy. The coated lidocaine patch contains 5 percent lidocaine and is easy to apply. It has to be attached for 12 hours per day at the site of pain. Controlled studies showed pain reduction in patients with longstanding postherpetic neuralgia and mechanical allodynia.[56**,57*,58**] However, reduction of allodynia seems to be at least in part due to patch protection of the allodynic skin. Also, in patients with painful diabetic polyneuropathy,[59] complex regional pain syndrome (CRPS), postmastectomy syndrome or postthoracotomy syndrome[60] pain relief can be achieved with the lidocaine patch. A recent controlled study reported significant reduction in pain and allodynia in patients with focal nonherpetic neuropathies.[61*] There have been no reports of serious side effects,[62] but local skin irritation can occur. In certain situations gel formulations of lidocaine may be useful without systemic adverse effects, e.g. in a 5 percent concentration for the treatment of postherpetic neuralgia[63**] or oral mucositis.[64]

Some years ago the local anesthetic n-butyl-p-aminobenzoate (BAB), also known as butamben, a highly lipid-soluble congener of benzocaine, was reintroduced into clinical practice for end-stage cancer patients. It was shown that (repeated) injections in the epidural space, at peripheral nerves, and at the celiac plexus resulted in a prolonged and profound analgesia without impairment of motor function.[65*,66*,67*] The prolonged period of effect was achieved without pathomorphological changes of nerve structures. More recently the ability of butamben to penetrate skin when applied locally was tested in an animal study.[68] In this study butamben was superior to lidocaine and displayed synergistic interactions with morphine.

Phytotherapeutics

Peppermint oil containing 10 percent menthol (the active ingredient) has been used successfully in a patient with neuropathic pain.[69] Also, itching may be relieved with menthol through its possible interaction with the TRPM8 receptor.[70,71] Arnica gel (combined with salicylate) may also be useful.[72,73*]

An interesting observation regarding traditional herbal medicine in India is the analgesic and anti-inflammatory effect of topical gall extract of *Quercus infectoria* Olivier (Fagaceae).[74] Commonly used externally for pain control and internally for its supposed anticancer potential but with only anecdotal evidence is noni (*Morinda citrifolia*), a traditional Polynesian medicinal plant.[75]

CAPSAICIN

Capsaicin is the active pungent ingredient in hot red chili pepper. Topically applied capsaicin interacts with nociceptive neurons in the skin via the vanilloid receptor (TRPV-1).[76] It causes an initial activation of neurons with release of substance P. This is perceived as burning or itching sensation with a flare response. After repeated application desensitization and hypalgesia occurs, probably due to depletion of substance P both peripherally and centrally.[77] Another potential mechanism for hypalgesia after repeated application is a direct neurotoxic effect on small diameter sensory afferents, resulting in degeneration of those fibers.[78]

Topical capsaicin was shown to achieve significant pain relief in the treatment of postherpetic neuralgia when used as a 0.075 percent cream three to four times daily for 8 weeks.[79**] A small controlled study reported pain reduction in postmastectomy syndrome.[80] A recently published systematic review[36] pooled data from six double blind, placebo controlled trials with analysis of capsaicin application for neuropathic pain. It revealed a moderate to poor efficacy of topically applied capsaicin 0.075 percent, and the NNT (number needed to treat) was 5.7. A different treatment approach using concentrations up to 10 percent was successfully tested in CRPS.[81] To tolerate this treatment, patients needed regional anesthesia, since pretreatment with topical EMLA failed to control pain induced by capsaicin above a concentration of 1 percent.[82*] In conclusion, topical capsaicin may be a valuable supplement for the treatment of neuropathic pain in a small number of patients unresponsive to or intolerant to other therapeutic approaches.

TETRAHYDROCANNABINOL

The effects of systemic tetrahydrocannabinol (THC) tend to be overestimated in palliative care.[83] Comparative levels of analgesia may be achieved with 'weak' opioids like 60 mg codeine.[84] Furthermore the antiemetic effect of ondansetron is superior to THC[85] and anorexia may be treated more effectively with megestrol.[86,87**] Intractable pruritus secondary to cholestatic liver disease may be a new indication for THC.[88] Side effects such as sedation and vertigo limit the doses of THC used in clinical practice. The analgesic activity of cannabinoids is generally believed to be mediated via CB_1 and CB_2 receptors.[89,90] Interestingly, for certain situations in palliative care where injury of epidermis or mucosa is present, CB_2 receptors may play a particularly prominent role in the periphery.[91,92] In animals a local effect[93] and interaction with topical morphine antinociception[94] could be demonstrated. Local peripheral formulations of cannabinoid derivatives have not been tested yet.

Clonidine

α_2-Adrenergic agonists such as clonidine cause antinociception due to the inhibition of postsynaptic spinothalamic neurons and presynaptic primary sensory nerve terminals and due to a generalized attenuation of sympathetic efferent activity. Systemic, spinal, and supraspinal analgesic effects of clonidine have been reported.[95] Therapeutic utility for general pain management is confined to mild pain because of dose-limiting central side effects, e.g. sedation and hypotension.[96] Topical administration may be an alternative since α_2 receptors are expressed by nociceptive sensory neurons and are mediators of sympathetic afferent coupling.[97–100] Peripheral antinoceptive effects devoid of central side effects could be demonstrated in animals[101*] and in a human case report with clonidine ointment.[102] Clonidine is available as a patch for transdermal administration, but relief of symptoms has been ascribed to systemic action.[103**] Local intraarticular clonidine may enhance the effects of local anaesthetics[104] and opioids[105] when inflammation is present.

Ketamine

The analgesic and dissociative properties have made ketamine, the most prominent N-methyl-D-aspartate (NMDA) receptor antagonist with combined activity at opioid receptors, a frequently used anesthetic for minor surgery. However, its undesired psychomimetic effects do limit its use. Ketamine binds noncompetitively to NMDA receptors and to opioid receptors. NMDA receptors are seen to play a key role in spinal processing of neuroplasticity mainly by inhibiting the effects of excitatory amino acids like glutamate. The clinical use of NMDA receptor antagonists in palliative care remains anecdotal since clinical studies are rare and mostly case reports. Ketamine oral rinse was tested with some success in mucositis in one cancer patient.[106] Case reports on the efficacy of ketamine administered topically for pain in the palliative care setting[107] and different neuropathic pain states[108,109] have been published. Apart from the NMDA receptor antagonism other actions and interactions from ketamine may contribute to local analgesia.[110–112] The value of NMDA receptors in cancer pain remains to be defined.

Tricyclic antidepressants

Tricyclic antidepressants (TCAs) are the mainstay of treatment for neuropathic pain. In a variety of neuropathies of different origin systemically administered TCAs have the lowest NNT to produce pain relief. Their efficacy is only partial and can be limited by the occurrence of troublesome side effects.[113***] To limit side effects the topical application of amitriptyline and desipramine was studied in a rat model, demonstrating antinoceceptive properties.[114] According to studies with doxepin 5 percent[115] and 3.3 percent[116**] either a cream or gel formulation may be useful in both inflammatory and neuropathic pain. Additionally TCAs have been tested as a mouthwash in oral mucositis due to cancer or cancer therapy.[117]

Other approaches

Other approaches to topical analgesia have been tried, but without major practical significance for cancer pain and the palliative care situation. Experimental research has demonstrated modulatory effects on pain of the endogenous nucleoside adenosine and its analogs.[118,119] This is probably due to the activation of the antinociceptive adenosine A_1 receptor. Peripheral adenosine kinase inhibitors might produce a direct effect on pain by adenosine actions on the sensory nerve terminal via A_1 receptors and through effects on the inflammatory process via A_2 receptors. In rodents local application caused neurogenic edema.[120,121]

Since γ-aminobutyric acid A ($GABA_A$) receptors are present on afferent axons, peripherally acting GABA agonists may inhibit pain.[122] A recent study evaluated the analgesic potency of a mouthwash with clonazepam, which possesses a high affinity for the $GABA_A$ receptor.[123**] Without considerable systemic blood levels patients with clonazepam achieved significant pain reduction, an effect which might be used in cancer-related mucositis as well.

Neuraxial administration of cholinesterase inhibitors like neostigmine has been studied in different patient populations,[124] but there are no reports of topical administration, although peripheral muscarinic receptor activation results in sensory neuron desensitization.[125] The findings of a clinical study[126*] with iontophoretically applied topical vincristine in postherpetic neuralgia could not demonstrate a reduction in neuropathic pain in comparison with placebo.

Neuropeptide FF is an octapeptide present in the central nervous system with specific receptors in the human spinal cord. It is believed to modulate morphine-induced analgesia. A recent study[127] in rats reported the effects of an analog of neuropeptide FF on hyperalgesia and morphine-induced analgesia. Unfortunately these effects were weakest in neuropathic pain states. Peripheral modulatory influences of neuropeptides on pain signaling have been postulated but are poorly understood at present.

Table 49.2 *Possible useful indications for topical analgesics*

Topical analgesic	Possible useful indication
Morphine, fentanyl	Oral mucositis, ulcerating skin cancer
Acetylsalicylic acid	Skin lesions in (acute) herpes zoster
EMLA, 5% lidocaine, butamben	Skin ulcers, postherpetic neuralgia with allodynia
Menthol 10%	Itching with hyperbilirubinemia
Capsaicin $\geq$ 0.075%	Peripheral neuropathic pain, e.g., in HIV/AIDS
Ketamine	Oral mucositis, peripheral neuropathic pain
Doxepin 5%	Peripheral neuropathic pain, urethral hyperesthesia

Possible useful indications for topical analgesics are shown in Table 49.2.

Key learning points

- Topical analgesia targets local (e.g. cutaneous or subcutaneous) receptors and neurotransmitters to inhibit pain signaling.

- Due to reduced or absent systemic uptake side effects of analgesic substances are reduced.

- Local anesthetics and capsaicin are currently the most widely used topical analgesics.

- Especially opioids but also ketamine and cannabinoids are promising drugs for clinical studies and practice.

- Increasing understanding of the peripheral mechanisms of pain signaling holds the promise of future advancement of topical analgesia.

- Postherpetic neuralgia, regional allodynia, oral mucositis and exulcerating cancer are the current indications for topical analgesia with most satisfying results.

- Topical analgesia should be part of a multimodal approach to palliative symptom control whereever possible.

REFERENCES

◆ 1 Sawynok J. Topical and peripherally acting analgesics. *Pharmacol Rev* 2003; **55**: 1–20.

2 Striebel HW, Oelmann T, Spies C, *et al.* Patient-controlled intranasal analgesia: a method for noninvasive postoperative pain management. *Anesth Analg* 1996; **83**: 548–51.

3 Pavis H, Wilcock A, Edgecombe J, *et al.* Pilot study of nasal morphine-chitosan for the relief of breakthrough pain in patients with cancer. *J Pain Symptom Manage* 2002; **24**: 598–602.

4 Hassan AH, Ableitner A, Stein C, Herz A. Inflammation of the rat paw enhances axonal transport of opioid receptors in the sciatic nerve and increases their density in the inflamed tissue. *Neuroscience* 1993; **55**: 185–95.

◆ 5 Stein C. The control of pain in peripheral tissue by opioids. *N Engl J Med* 1995; **332**: 1685–90.

6 Stein C, Pfluger M, Yassouridis A, *et al.* No tolerance to peripheral morphine analgesia in presence of opioid expression in inflamed synovia. *J Clin Invest* 1996; **98**: 793–9.

◆ 7 Stein C, Schäfer M, Machelska H. Attacking pain at its source: New perspectives on opioids. *Nat Med* 2003; **9**: 1003–8.

◆ 8 Barber A, Gottschlich R. Opioid agonists and antagonists: an evaluation of their peripheral actions in inflammation. *Med Res Rev* 1992; **12**: 525–62.

9 Yaksh TL. Substance P release from knee joint afferent terminals: modulation by opioids. *Brain Res* 1988; **458**: 319–24.

◆ 10 Kalso E, Smith L, McQuay HJ, Andrew Moore R. No pain, no gain: clinical excellence and scientific rigour – lessons learned from IA morphine. *Pain* 2002; **98**: 269–75.

11 Krajnik M, Zylicz Z, Finlay I, *et al.* Potential uses of topical opioids in palliative care – report of 6 cases. *Pain* 1999; **80**: 121–5.

12 Twillman RK, Long TD, Cathers TA, Mueller DW. Treatment of painful skin ulcers with topical opioids. *J Pain Symptom Manage* 1999; **17**: 288–92.

◆ 13 Picard PR, Tramèr MR, McQuay HJ, Moore RA. Analgesic efficacy of peripheral opioids (all except intra-articular): a qualitative systematic review of randomised controlled trials. *Pain* 1997; **72**: 309–18.

14 Barasch A, Peterson DE. Risk factors for ulcerative oral mucositis in cancer patients: unanswered questions. *Oral Oncol* 2003; **39**: 91–100.

15 Epstein JB, Schubert MM. Management of orofacial pain in cancer patients. *Eur J Cancer B Oral Oncol* 1993; **29**: 243–50.

16 Sonis ST. Mucositis as a biological process: a new hypothesis for the development of chemotherapy-induced stomatotoxicity. *Oral Oncol* 1998; **34**: 39–43.

17 Epstein JB, Schubert MM. Oral mucositis in myelosuppressive cancer therapy. *Oral Surg Oral Med Oral Pathol Oral Radiol Endod* 1999; **88**: 273–6.

◆ 18 Duncan M, Grant G. Oral and intestinal mucositis – causes and possible treatments. *Aliment Pharmacol Ther* 2003; **18**: 853–74.

19 Pillitteri LC, Clark RE. Comparison of a patient-controlled analgesia system with continuous infusion for administration of diamorphine for mucositis. *Bone Marrow Transplant* 1998; **22**: 495–8.

◆ 20 Worthington HV, Clarkson JE, Eden OB. Interventions for treating oral mucositis for patients with cancer receiving treatment. *Cochrane Database Syst Rev* 2004: CD001973.

21 Cerchietti LC, Navigante AH, Korte MW, *et al.* Potential utility of the peripheral analgesic properties of morphine in stomatitis-related pain: a pilot study. *Pain* 2003; **105**: 265–73.

22 Shaiova L, Lapin J, Manco LS, *et al.* Tolerability and effects of two formulations of oral transmucosal fentanyl citrate (OTFC; ACTIQ) in patients with radiation-induced oral mucositis. *Support Care Cancer* 2004; **12**: 268–73.

◆ 23 Weinberg DS, Inturrisi CE, Reidenberg B, *et al.* Sublingual absorption of selected opioid analgesics. *Clin Pharmacol Ther* 1988; **44**: 335–42.

24 Back IN, Finlay I. Analgesic effect of topical opioids on painful skin ulcers. *J Pain Symptom Manage* 1995; **10**: 493.

25 Krajnik M, Zylicz Z. Topical morphine for cutaneous cancer pain. *Palliat Med* 1997; **11**: 325.

26 Flock P, Gibbs L, Sykes N. Diamorphine-metronidazole gel effective for treatment of painful infected leg ulcers. *J Pain Symptom Manage* 2000; **20**: 396–7.

27 Zeppetella G, Paul J, Ribeiro MD. Analgesic efficacy of morphine applied topically to painful ulcers. *J Pain Symptom Manage* 2003; **25**: 555–8.

28 Ballas SK. Treatment of painful sickle cell leg ulcers with topical opioids. *Blood* 2002; **99**: 1096.

29 Ribeiro MD, Joel SP, Zeppetella G. The bioavailability of morphine applied topically to cutaneous ulcers. *J Pain Symptom Manage* 2004; **27**: 434–9.

30 Heyneman CA, Lawless-Liday C, Wall GC. Oral versus topical NSAIDs in rheumatic diseases: a comparison. *Drugs* 2000; **60**: 555–74.

31 Bombardier C, Laine L, Reicin A, *et al.* VIGOR Study Group. Comparison of upper gastrointestinal toxicity of rofecoxib and naproxen in patients with rheumatoid arthritis. VIGOR Study Group. *N Engl J Med* 2000; **343**: 1520–8.

32 Gallagher SJ, Trottet L, Heard CM. Ketoprofen: Release from, permeation across and rheology of simple gel formulations that simulate increasing dryness. *Int J Pharmaceutics* 2003; **268**: 37–45.

33 Tramèr MR, Williams JE, Carroll D, *et al.* Comparing analgesic efficacy of non-steroidal anti-inflammatory drugs given by different routes in acute and chronic pain: A qualitative systematic review. *Acta Anaesthesiol Scand* 1998; **42**: 71–9.

34 Trnavsky K, Fischer M, Vogtle-Junkert U, Schreyer F. Efficacy and safety of 5% ibuprofen cream treatment in knee osteoarthritis. Results of a randomized, double-blind, placebo-controlled study. *J Rheumatol* 2004; **31**: 565–72.

35 Mason L, Moore RA, Edwards JE, *et al.* Topical NSAIDs for acute pain: a meta-analysis. *BMC Fam Pract* 2004; **5**: 10–19.

◆ 36 Mason L, Moore RA, Derry S, *et al.* Systematic review of topical capsaicin for the treatment of chronic pain. *BMJ* 2004; **328**: 991–5.

37 Moore RA. Topical nonsteroidal antiinflammatory drugs are effective in osteoarthritis of the knee. *J Rheumatol* 2004; **31**: 1893–5.

38 Mason L, Moore RA, Edwards JE, *et al.* Topical NSAIDs for chronic musculoskeletal pain: systematic review and meta-analysis. *BMC Musculoskelet Disord* 2004; **19**: 28–31.

39 Lin J, Zhang W, Jones A, Doherty M. Efficacy of topical non-steroidal anti-inflammatory drugs in the treatment of osteoarthritis: Meta-analysis of randomised controlled trials. *BMJ* 2004; **329**: 324–34.

40 Dutta A, Puri GD, Wig J. Piroxicam gel, compared to EMLA cream is associated with less pain after venous cannulation in volunteers. *Can J Anaesth* 2003; **50**: 775–8.

41 Rivers JK, McLean DI. An open study to assess the efficacy and safety of topical 3% diclofenac in a 2.5% hyaluronic acid gel for the treatment of actinic keratoses. *Arch Dermatol* 1997; **133**: 1239–42.

42 De Benedittis G, Lorenzetti A. Topical aspirin/diethyl ether mixture versus indomethacin and diclofenac/diethyl ether mixtures for acute herpetic neuralgia and postherpetic neuralgia: a double-blind crossover placebo-controlled study. *Pain* 1996; **65**: 45–51.

43 Bareggi SR, Pirola R, DeBenedittis G. Skin and plasma levels of acetylsalicylic acid: a comparison between topical aspirin/diethyl ether mixture and oral aspirin in acute herpes zoster and postherpetic neuralgia. *Eur J Clin Pharmacol* 1998; **54**: 231–5.

44 Balakrishnan S, Bhushan K, Bhargava VK, Pandhi P. A randomized parallel trial of topical aspirin-moisturizer solution vs. oral aspirin for acute herpetic neuralgia. *Int J Dermatol* 2001; **40**: 535–8.

45 Tanelian DL, MacIver MB. Analgesic concentrations of lidocaine suppress tonic A-delta and C fiber discharges produced by acute injury. *Anesthesiology* 1991; **74**:934–6.

◆ 46 Gajraj NM, Pernant JR, Watcha MR. Eutectic mixture of local anesthetics (EMLA) cream. *Anesth Analg* 1994; **78**: 558–74.

47 Cooper CM, Gerrish SP, Hardwick M, Kay R. EMLA reduces the pain of venipuncture in children. *Eur J Anesthesiology.* 1987; **4**: 441–8.

48 Robieux I, Eliopoulos C, Hwang P, *et al.* Pain perception and effectiveness of the eutectic mixture of local anesthetics in children undergoing venipuncture. *Pediatr Res* 1992; **32**: 520–3.

49 Vaghadia H, al Ahdal OA, Nevin K. EMLA patch for intra-venous cannulation in adult surgical outpatients. *Can J Anaesth* 1997; **44**: 798–802.

50 Miser AW, Goh TS, Dose AM. Trial of a topically administered local anesthetic (EMLA cream) for pain relief during central venous port accesses in children with cancer. *J Pain Symptom Manage* 1994; **9**: 259–64.

51 Halperin DL, Koren G, Attias D, *et al.* Topical skin anesthesia for venous, subcutaneous drug reservoir and lumbar punctures in children. *Pediatrics* 1989; **84**: 281–4.

52 Goldman RD. ELA-max: A new topical lidocaine formulation. *Ann Pharmacother* 2004; **38**: 892–4.

◆ 53 Briggs M, Nelson EA. Topical agents or dressings for pain in venous leg ulcers (Cochrane Review). *Cochrane Library*, Issue 3, 2004.

54 Stegman MB, Stoukides CA. Resolution of tumor pain with EMLA cream. *Pharmacotherapy* 1996; **16**: 694–7.

55 Hahn IH, Hoffman RS, Nelson LS. EMLA-induced methemoglobinemia and systemic topical anesthetic toxicity. *J Emerg Med* 2004; **26**: 85–8.

56 Rowbotham MC, Davies PS, Verkempinck C, Galer BS. Lidocaine patch: Double-blind controlled study of a new treatment method for post-herpetic neuralgia. *Pain* 1996; **65**: 39–44.

57 Galer BS, Rowbotham MC, Perander J, Friedman E. Topical lidocaine patch relieves postherpetic neuralgia more effectively than a vehicle topical patch: results of an enriched enrollment study. *Pain* 1999; **80**: 533–8.

58 Galer BS, Jensen MP, Ma T, *et al.* The lidocaine patch 5% effectively treats all neuropathic pain qualities: results of a randomized, double-blind, vehicle-controlled, 3-week efficacy study with use of the neuropathic pain scale. Clin *J Pain* 2002; **18**: 297–301.

59 Barbano RL, Herrmann DN, Hart-Gouleau S, *et al.* Effectiveness, tolerability, and impact on quality of life of the 5% lidocaine patch in diabetic polyneuropathy. *Arch Neurol* 2004; **61**: 914–18.

60 Devers A, Galer BS. Topical lidocaine patch relieves a variety of neuropathic pain conditions: an open-label study. *Clin J Pain* 2000; **16**: 205–8.

61   Meier T, Faust M, Huppe M, Schmucker P. Reduction of chronic pain for non-postherpetic peripheral neuropathies after topical treatment with a lidocaine patch. *Schmerz* 2004; **18**: 172–8.

62   Gammaitoni AR, Davis MW. Pharmacokinetics and tolerability of lidocaine patch 5% with extended dosing. *Ann Pharmacother* 2002; **36**: 236–40.

63   Rowbotham MC, Davies PS, Fields HL. Topical lidocaine gel relieves postherpetic neuralgia. *Ann Neurol* 1995; **37**: 246–53.

64   Yamashita S, Sato S, Kakiuchi Y, *et al*. Lidocaine toxicity during frequent viscous lidocaine use for painful tongue ulcer. *J Pain Symptom Manage* 2002; **24**: 543–5.

65   Shulman M, Lubenow TR, Nath HA, *et al*. Nerve blocks with 5% butamben suspension for the treatment of chronic pain syndromes. *Reg Anesth Pain Med* 1998; **23**: 395–401.

66   Korsten HH, Ackerman EW, Grouls RJ, *et al*. Long-lasting epidural sensory blockade by n-butyl-p-aminobenzoate in the terminally ill intractable cancer pain patient. *Anesthesiology* 1991; **75**: 950–60.

67   Shulman M, Harris JE, Lubenow TR, *et al*. Comparison of epidural butamben to celiac plexus neurolytic block for the treatment of the pain of pancreatic cancer. *Clin J Pain* 2000; **16**: 304–9.

68   Kolesnikov YA, Cristea M, Pasternak GW. Analgesic synergy between topical morphine and butamben in mice. *Anesth Analg* 2003; **97**: 1103–7.

69   Davies SJ, Harding LM, Baranowski AP. A novel treatment of postherpetic neuralgia using peppermint oil. *Clin J Pain* 2002; **18**: 200–2.

70   Peier AM, Moqrich A, Hergarden AC, *et al*. A TRP channel that senses cold stimuli and menthol. *Cell* 2002; **108**: 705–15.

71   Anand P. Capsaicin and menthol in the treatment of itch and pain: Recently cloned receptors provide the key. *Gut* 2003; **52**: 1233–5.

72   Kucera M, Horacek O, Kalal J, *et al*. Synergetic analgesic effect of the combination of arnica and hydroxyethyl salicylate in ethanolic solution following cutaneous application by transcutaneous electrostimulation. *Arzneimittelforschung* 2003; **53**: 850–6.

73   Knüsel O, Weber M, Suter A. Arnica montana gel in osteoarthritis of the knee: an open, multicenter clinical trial. *Adv Ther* 2002; **19**: 209–18.

74   Kaur G, Hamid H, Ali A, *et al*. Antiinflammatory evaluation of alcoholic extract of galls of Quercus infectoria. *J Ethnopharmacol* 2003; **90**: 285–92.

75   McClatchey W. From Polynesian healers to health food stores: changing perspectives of *Morinda citrifolia* (Rubiaceae). *Integr Cancer Ther* 2002; **1**: 110–20.

◆ 76   Caterina MJ, Schumacher MA, Tominga M, *et al*. The capsaicin receptor: a heat-activated ion channel in the pain pathway. *Nature (Lond)* 1997; **389**: 816–24.

77   Winter J, Bevan S, Campbell EA. Capsaicin and pain mechanisms. *Br J Anaesth* 1995; **75**: 157–68.

78   Nolano M, Simone DA, Wendelschafer-Crabb G, *et al*. Topical capsaicin in humans: Parallel loss of epidermal nerve fibres and pain sensation. *Pain* 1999; **81**: 35–45.

79   Watson CP, Tyler KL, Bickers DR, *et al*. A randomized vehicle-controlled trial of topical capsaicin in the treatment of postherpetic neuralgia. *Clin Ther* 1993; **15**: 510–16.

80   Watson CP, Evans RJ. The postmastectomy pain syndrome and topical capsaicin: A randomized trial. *Pain* 1992; **51**: 375–9.

81   Robbins WR, Staats PS, Levine J, *et al*. Treatment of intractable pain with topical large-dose capsaicin: preliminary report. *Anesth Analg* 1998; **86**: 579–83.

82   Fuchs PN, Pappagallo M, Meyer RA. Topical EMLA pretreatment fails to decrease the pain induced by 1% topical capsaicin. *Pain* 1999; **80**: 637–42.

◆ 83   Campbell FA, Tramer MR, Carroll D, *et al*. Are cannabinoids an effective and safe treatment option in the management of pain? A qualitative systematic review. *BMJ* 2001; **323**: 13–16.

84   Gill A, Williams AC. Preliminary study of chronic pain patients' concerns about cannabinoids as analgesics. *Clin J Pain* 2001; **17**: 245–8.

85   Tramer MR, Carroll D, Campbell FA, *et al*. Cannabinoids for control of chemotherapy induced nausea and vomiting: quantitative systematic review. *BMJ* 2001; **323**: 16–21.

86   Soderpalm AH, Schuster A, de Wit H. Antiemetic efficacy of smoked marijuana: subjective and behavioral effects on nausea induced by syrup of ipecac. *Pharmacol Biochem Behav* 2001; **69**: 343–50.

87   Jatoi A, Windschitl HE, Loprinzi CL, *et al*. Dronabinol versus megestrol acetate versus combination therapy for cancer-associated anorexia: a North Central Cancer Treatment Group study. *J Clin Oncol* 2002; **20**: 567–73.

88   Neff GW, O'Brien CB, Reddy KR, *et al*. Preliminary observation with dronabinol in patients with intractable pruritus secondary to cholestatic liver disease. *Am J Gastroenterol* 2002; **97**: 2117–19.

89   Richardson JD, Kilo S, Hargreaves KM. Cannabinoids reduce hyperalgesia and inflammation via interaction with peripheral CB1 receptors. *Pain* 1998; **75**: 111–19.

◆ 90   Iversen L, Chapman V. Cannabinoids: a real prospect for pain relief? *Curr Opin Pharmacol* 2002; **2**: 50–5.

91   Rice AS, Farquhar-Smith WP, Nagy I. Endocannabinoids and pain: spinal and peripheral analgesia in inflammation and neuropathy. *Prostaglandins Leukot Essent Fatty Acids* 2002; **66**: 243–56.

92   Walker JM, Huang SM. Cannabinoid analgesia. *Pharmacol Ther* 2002; **95**: 127–35.

93   Dogrul A, Gul H, Akar A, *et al*. Topical cannabinoid antinociception: synergy with spinal sites. *Pain* 2003; **105**: 11–16.

94   Yesilyurt O, Dogrul A, Gul H, *et al*. Topical cannabinoid enhances topical morphine antinociception. *Pain* 2003; **105**: 303–8.

95   Asano T, Dohi S, Ohta S, *et al*. Antinociception by epidural and systemic alpha(2)-adrenoceptor agonists and their binding affinity in rat spinal cord and brain. *Anesth Analg* 2000; **90**: 400–7.

96   Puskas F, Camporesi EM, O'Leary CE, *et al*. Intrathecal clonidine and severe hypotension after cardiopulmonary bypass. *Anesth Analg* 2003; **97**: 1251–3.

97   Kawasaki Y, Kumamoto E, Furue H, Yoshimura M. Alpha 2 adrenoceptor-mediated presynaptic inhibition of primary afferent glutamatergic transmission in rat substantia gelatinosa neurons. *Anesthesiology* 2003; **98**: 682–9.

98   Koltzenburg M, Habler HJ, Janig W. Functional reinnervation of the vasculature of the adult cat paw pad by axons originally innervating vessels in hairy skin. *Neuroscience* 1995; **67**: 245–52.

99   Arnold JM, Teasell RW, MacLeod AP, *et al*. Increased venous alpha-adrenoceptor responsiveness in patients with reflex sympathetic dystrophy. *Ann Intern Med* 1993; **118**: 619–21.

100 Chen Y, Michaelis M, Janig W, Devor M. Adrenoreceptor subtype mediating sympathetic-sensory coupling in injured sensory neurons. *J Neurophysiol* 1996; **76**: 3721-30.

101 Dogrul A, Uzbay IT. Topical clonidine antinociception. *Pain* 2004; **111**: 385-91.

102 Hagihara R, Meno A, Arita H, Hanaoka K. A case of effective treatment with clonidine ointment for herpetic neuralgia after bone marrow transplantation in a child. *Masui* 2002; **51**: 777-9.

103 Byas-Smith MG, Max MB, Muir J, Kingman A. Transdermal clonidine compared to placebo in painful diabetic neuropathy using a two-stage 'enriched enrollment' design. *Pain* 1995; **60**: 267-74.

104 Joshi W, Reuben SS, Kilaru PR, *et al*. Postoperative analgesia for outpatient arthroscopic knee surgery with intraarticular clonidine and/or morphine. *Anesth Analg* 2000; **90**: 1102-6.

105 Buerkle H, Schapsmeier M, Bantel C, *et al*. Thermal and mechanical antinociceptive action of spinal vs peripherally administered clonidine in the rat inflamed knee joint model. *Br J Anaesth* 1999; **83**: 436-41.

106 Slatkin-NE, Rhiner M. Topical ketamine in the treatment of mucositis pain. *Pain Med* 2003; **4**: 298-303.

107 Wood RM. Ketamine for pain in hospice patients. *Int J Pharmaceutical Compounding* 2000; **4**: 253-4.

108 Gammaitoni A, Gallagher RM, Welz-Bosna M. Topical ketamine gel: possible role in treating neuropathic pain. *Pain Med* 2000; **1**: 97-100.

109 Crowley KL, Flores JA, Hughes CN Iacono RP. Clinical application of ketamine ointment in the treatment of sympathetically maintained pain. *Int J Pharmaceutical Compounding* 1998; **2**: 122-7.

110 Hirota K, Lambert DG. Ketamine: its mechanism(s) of action and unusual clinical uses. *Br J Anaesth* 1996; **77**: 441-4.

111 Meller ST. Ketamine: relief from chronic pain through actions at the NMDA receptor? *Pain* 1996; **68**: 435-6.

112 Sawynok J, Reid A. Modulation of formalin-induced behaviors and edema by local and systemic administration of dextromethorphan, memantine and ketamine. *Eur J Pharmacol* 2002; **450**: 153-62.

113 McQuay HJ, Tramér M, Nye BA, *et al*. A systematic review of antidepressants in neuropathic pain. *Pain* 1996; **68**: 217-7.

114 Sawynok J, Esser MJ, Reid AR. Peripheral antinociceptive actions of desipramine and fluoxetine in an inflammatory and neuropathic pain test in the rat. *Pain* 1999; **82**: 49-58.

115 McCleane G. Topical application of doxepin hydrochloride can reduce the symptoms of complex regional pain syndrome: a case report. *Injury* 2002; **33**: 88-9.

116 McCleane G. Topical application of doxepin hydrochloride, capsaicin and a combination of both produces analgesia in chronic human neuropathic pain: a randomized, double-blind, placebo-controlled study. *Br J Clin Pharmacol* 2000; **49**: 574-9.

117 Epstein JB, Truelove EL, Oien H, *et al*. Oral topical doxepin rinse: analgesic effect in patients with oral mucosal pain due to cancer or cancer therapy. *Oral Oncol* 2001; **37**: 632-7.

118 Pöyhiä R, Xu M, Kontinen VK, *et al*. Systemic physostigmine shows antiallodynic effects in neuropathic rats. *Anesth Analg* 1999; **89**: 428-33.

119 Gomes JA, Li X, Pan HL, Eisenach JC. Intrathecal adenosine interacts with a spinal noradrenergic system to produce antinociception in nerve-injured rats. *Anesthesiology* 1999; **91**: 1072-9.

120 Sawynok J, Reid A, Liu XJ. Involvement of mast cells, sensory afferents and sympathetic mechanisms in paw oedema induced by adenosine A(1) and A(2B/3) receptor agonists. *Eur J Pharmacol* 2000; **395**: 47-50.

121 Esquisatto LC, Costa SK, Camargo EA, *et al*. The plasma protein extravasation induced by adenosine and its analogues in the rat dorsal skin: evidence for the involvement of capsaicin sensitive primary afferent neurones and mast cells. *Br J Pharmacol* 2001; **134**: 108-15.

122 Carlton SM, Zhou S, Coggeshall RE. Peripheral GABA(A) receptors: evidence for peripheral primary afferent depolarization. *Neuroscience* 1999; **93**: 713-22.

123 Gremeau-Richard C, Woda A, Navez ML, *et al*. Topical clonazepam in stomatodynia: a randomised placebo-controlled study. *Pain* 2004; **108**: 51-7.

124 Roelants F, Rizzo M, Lavand'homme P. The effect of epidural neostigmine combined with ropivacaine and sufentanil on neuraxial analgesia during labor. *Anesth Analg* 2003; **96**: 1161-6.

125 Bernardini N, Sauer SK, Haberberger R, *et al*. Excitatory nicotinic and desensitizing muscarinic (M2) effects on C-nociceptors in isolated rat skin. *J Neurosci* 2001; **21**: 3295-02.

126 Dowd NP, Day F, Timon D, *et al*. Iontophoretic vincristine in the treatment of postherpetic neuralgia: a double-blind, randomized, controlled trial. *J Pain Symptom Manage* 1999; **17**: 175-9.

127 Courteix C, Coudoré-Civiale M-A, Privat A-M, *et al*. Spinal effect of a neuropeptide FF analogue on hyperalgesia and morphine-induced analgesia in mononeuropathic and diabetic rats. *Br J Pharmacol* 1999; **127**: 1454-62.

50

Pain and opioids in children

RICHARD D W HAIN, MARY DEVINS, ANGELA MISER

INTRODUCTION

The management of pain in the palliative care of children is somewhat different from that of adults. It also differs in approach from management of other types of acute and chronic pain in childhood. Where once opioids were thought to be highly dangerous drugs, often unsuitable for use in children, they have now taken their place as the mainstay of provision of good analgesia in the palliative phase.

The verb 'to palliate' means to relieve without curing. Palliative medicine was first recognized as a medical specialty in the UK in 1987. It has been defined as 'the study and management of patients with active progressive, far advanced disease for whom the prognosis is limited and the focus of care is on the quality of life'.[1] The World Health Organization (WHO) further elaborated on the multidimensional care inherent in this ideal, summarizing palliative care as 'the active total care of patients whose disease is not responsive to curative treatment. Control of pain, of other symptoms and of psychologic, social and spiritual problems is paramount. The goal of palliative care is the achievement of the best quality of life for patients and their families'.[2]

Palliative medicine in children was initially defined in 1997 by the Royal College of Paediatrics and Child Health working with the Association of Children with Life-limiting or Threatening conditions and their families (ACT).[3,4] The basic principle remains the same as for adults; palliative care for children and young people with life-limiting conditions is described as 'an active and total approach to care embracing physical, emotional, social and spiritual elements. It focuses on enhancement of quality of life for the child and support for the family, and includes the management of distressing symptoms, provision of respite care through death and bereavement'. Life-limiting conditions are those for which there is no hope of cure and from which children will eventually die, though often years or even decades after diagnosis. For many the progress of the disease is such that they become increasingly dependent on others. Because an end to life is imminent or anticipated in the foreseeable future, care and interventions may sometimes differ from those chosen in acute care, where therapy is aimed at reversing a disease process. They may even differ from chronic care, where optimal management of long-term conditions is the goal.

Opioids often play a central role in analgesic management in palliative care. They are commonly divided into weak and strong opioids, and they have no 'ceiling effect'. The dose can be escalated as required to achieve adequate analgesia. Occasionally this is limited by increasing toxicity, in which case an alternative may be equally effective with fewer adverse effects. Such a limitation is more likely with weak opioids. Strong opioids are the predominant analgesics used in palliative care, and this chapter is limited to aspects of their use in treating pain in children with life-limiting conditions. Their use in neonates, and in management of acute postoperative pain or for sickle crisis, will not be addressed here. The interested reader is referred to the extensive published literature on these topics.

Historically, the approach taken by physicians to using major opioids in their patients has been an illustration of the human tendency to place more faith in myth than in evidence. We are particularly prone to believe myths that appear to carry the authority of scientific research. For decades it was believed that opioids were highly addictive drugs whose therapeutic potential was trivial compared with their threat to society. The fear of prescribing morphine, now often termed 'morphophobia', has been and perhaps remains the single greatest threat to the comfort of patients with moderate to severe pain.

Children are especially vulnerable to undertreatment of their pain. In caring for a child, the instinct of adults may be to adopt a precautionary approach. The belief that morphine is a highly dangerous drug, however ill supported by evidence, is enough to cause many pediatricians to hesitate before prescribing it. Other myths have developed to justify such an approach. These include the traditional notion that children are physiologically less capable of feeling pain,[5] or that they can and should 'tolerate discomfort well'.[6] Provided that basic prescribing principles are observed throughout, morphine and other strong opioids are very safe in the management of moderate to severe pain. The risks of adverse effects and addiction in adult palliative care are small[7] and there is no evidence that children differ in this regard.[8]

MAJOR OPIOIDS IN PALLIATIVE MEDICINE IN CHILDREN

Measuring pain in children

Pain is one of the most prevalent and distressing symptoms experienced by children with life-limiting conditions, and is rightly given high priority by the WHO.[9] For the dying child, accurate assessment of pain is often difficult and it is frequently necessary to review the effectiveness of therapy. Furthermore, many children with life-limiting illnesses are unable to verbalize their symptoms and will instead communicate their discomfort nonverbally. A great deal of work on the development of age-appropriate scales for measuring pain has been published.[10,11] Choosing a pain assessment scale suitable for day-to-day clinical use is important. However, it can be problematic. There are multiple tools available and this reflects the fact that none is ideal. Also, the measurement of pain in cognitively impaired children remains a challenge.[12] Whatever tool is chosen, it must remain part of the cycle of assessment, intervention, and review or reassessment.

The place of morphine in pain control

In attempting to address misunderstandings about opioids, the WHO developed an analgesic ladder[2,9,13] (Fig. 50.1). This provides a rational, simple, stepwise approach to pain, in which simple analgesics comprise the first rung, weak (minor) opioids such as codeine the second, and strong (major) opioids such as morphine the third. Analgesia on a higher rung of the ladder is introduced only if the previous one becomes ineffective.

This 3-step approach has to be taken in conjunction with a number of other principles. First, at each stage, adjuvant analgesics appropriate to the nature of pain should be

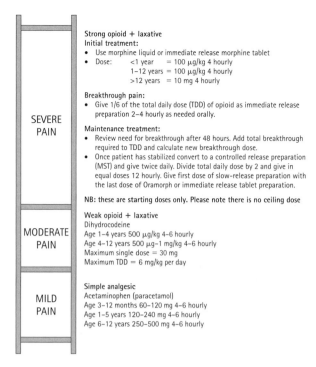

Figure 50.1 *An example of the World Health Organization pain ladder approach to pain relief. At each 'rung' appropriate analgesics should be considered (for example, radiation for metastatic bone pain, nonsteroidal anti-inflammatory drugs for musculoskeletal pain, antidepressants or anticonvulsants for neuropathic pain).*

introduced. It is particularly important to identify features of neuropathic or bone pain. Second, there is no place for strong opioids to be given only *pro re nata*; if a strong opioid is required it should always be given on a regular schedule by the clock. The prescription of a regular dose of strong opioid should always be accompanied by a breakthrough dose that should be a fixed fraction of the total daily requirement. The total dose should be reviewed every 48 hours, with increases in the regular dose being indicated if more than two breakthrough doses per day have been required during any 48-hour period. Third, the oral route is always preferred unless there is a contraindication (for example, cytotoxic-induced mucositis).

Notwithstanding these general principles, a child suddenly presenting with severe pain may need a strong opioid from the outset, often parenterally and in frequent doses, until pain control is achieved.

PHARMACOKINETICS OF MORPHINE IN CHILDREN

Morphine remains the most frequently prescribed strong opioid in children and is the one about which most is known. It is the archetype strong opioid. Here we will consider opioids in children by examining the characteristics of morphine first, and then other strong opioids insofar as they differ in indication or in pharmacology from morphine itself.

Morphine appears to be well absorbed from the child's gastrointestinal tract.[14,15] The oral to parenteral potency is approximately 50 percent; in other words, to achieve the same effect, an oral dose of morphine should be twice that given intravenously or subcutaneously. There is extensive biotransformation in the liver to a number of compounds, of which the two most important are morphine-3-glucuronide (M3G) and morphine-6-glucuronide (M6G).[15,16] Both are more soluble in water than the parent compound. Morphine-3-glucuronide is quantitatively the most important but has little or no affinity for the μ-opioid receptor and no analgesic activity.[17,18] There is some evidence to suggest that it may contribute to some of the adverse effects of morphine, particularly neuroexcitability[18] though this is hard to explain. The 6-glucuronide on the other hand, has a high affinity for μ-opioid receptors[19] and is a powerful analgesic[20,21] with an effectiveness that exceeds that of morphine. The capacity to form both glucuronides is present from an early stage in fetal development[22] and there is some evidence that it increases over the first 12 months of life.[23,24]

The distribution of morphine and M6G seems to be similar in children and adults.[15,16] Clearance of the glucuronides is almost entirely renal and much of the parent compound is also excreted in the urine. The clearance of morphine and M6G in children appears to exceed that in adults.[15,16,23,25] This may be due to both better renal clearance and faster glucuronidation in children. To have a therapeutic effect, morphine and M6G must cross the blood–brain barrier to have access to receptors in the brain. Both morphine and M6G can penetrate into the cerebrospinal fluid of children. There is no evidence to suggest that outside infancy this happens more easily in children than in adults,[16] making it unlikely that children are any more sensitive to centrally mediated effects of opioids, such as respiratory depression.[26,27]

Morphine is the only major opioid whose pharmacokinetics have been extensively studied in children. The results have often been inconsistent. Some studies suggest that the volume of distribution per kilogram in children is much the same as adults, but that clearance and half-life are shorter.[15,16] The ratio of glucuronides to morphine may be higher in children than in adults.[15] Kinetics in the infant under 12 months of age is very different, with rather lower clearance particularly in neonates under 2 weeks of age.[28–30] One study, which concluded that clearance appeared to reach adult levels by 2 years of age,[25] did not exclude the possibility that it may then improve further before declining to adult levels at puberty.

There is anecdotal evidence to support the use in children of a smaller opioid dosage interval than in adults, particularly in the use of slow-release morphine and fentanyl patches. The slow-release formulations of morphine seem to result in a less sustained serum concentration in children than in adults and it is common in practice for children to require slow-release preparations of morphine to be given 8 hourly, rather than the recommended 12 hourly. Such a difference has not been shown in immediate release preparations of morphine, but this may be because when the appropriate breakthrough-dosing interval of 2–4 hours is used the difference does not have time to manifest.

CLINICAL USE AND ADVERSE EFFECTS OF MORPHINE IN CHILDREN

Typical guidelines for management of pediatric pain are shown in Figure 50.1. The adverse effect profile in children may be slightly different from that in adults. It is distinctly unusual in clinical practice for a child to complain of nausea as a result of opioid therapy, and prophylactic antiemetics are not usually indicated. On the other hand, constipation is very common, and laxatives should always be started at the time as prescribing a strong opioid. The mechanism of opioid-induced constipation is a reduction in bowel motility. To overcome this requires a stimulant laxative such as senna. Lactulose, which enjoys a prominent role in the management of constipation in children in the UK, is not an appropriate laxative for opioid-induced constipation. It is not primarily a stimulant. Furthermore, the breakdown products of lactulose cause flatulence, abdominal distension, and colic.[31,32] Where a softener is required, magnesium hydroxide is effective. Co-danthrusate, a combination of sodium docusate and dantron conveniently combines a softener and a stimulant laxative. It is currently licensed only for use in palliative care.[31,32]

Another adverse effect that seems to occur more commonly in children is urinary retention. The mechanism is not clear; it could be due to direct stimulation of opioid receptors in the smooth muscle of the internal sphincter, or else antimuscarinic activity. This uncomfortable complication is an indication to consider an alternative major opioid.

Alternative major opioids in children

Alternative opioids (Table 50.1) should probably only be considered in children when there is a good reason to abandon morphine. There are several potential reasons, and it is helpful to consider the alternative opioids that are available in terms of the advantages they confer over morphine. Of all the steps in the WHO pain ladder, the final major opioid step offers the greatest variety to choose from. Large numbers of opioids and synthetic or semisynthetic opioids are available. Many offer dubious advantage over morphine itself and do not have the benefit of its long track record and predictable clinical effectiveness.[35*,36*] Others, however, offer real benefits to the individual patient who has specific difficulties using morphine.

DIAMORPHINE

Diamorphine is currently thought to act in precisely the same way as morphine itself. The major difference is simply that it is more easily soluble in water. It has a role where a child requires a parenteral dose of morphine that cannot be dissolved in a convenient volume of fluid. Many units

Table 50.1 *Dose equivalents of major opioids commonly used in children, and their potential advantages over morphine*

Opioid	Advantage over morphine	Relative potency compared with oral morphine (approx)
Diamorphine (PO)	More soluble (when given parenterally)	1.5
Fentanyl (patch)	Patch formulation Less constipation[33] Less itch* Less retention*	100
Methadone (PO)	Anti-neuropathic activity[34]	Variable
Hydromorphone (PO)	None	5
Pethidine (PO)	None	0.125
Tramadol (PO)	None	0.25
Oxycodone (PO)	None	1.5–2

*Anecdotal information not based on trial.
PO, per oral.

have made diamorphine their standard parenteral opioid while retaining morphine as their standard oral opioid. Diamorphine is slightly more potent than morphine, approximately two-thirds of the dose is needed to give the same effect. To have the same effect as an oral dose of morphine, a parenteral dose of diamorphine should therefore be one-third of the dose.

FENTANYL

Fentanyl is a synthetic opioid which may offer a number of advantages over morphine itself for some children.[35*,36*] It does not appear to accumulate to the same degree when renal clearance is impaired,[37,38] it may cause less constipation than morphine,[33*] and does not seem to cause urinary retention. Perhaps most importantly from the child's perspective is that it is available as a transdermal patch, which can avoid the need for a subcutaneous or intravenous syringe driver in children needing prolonged major opioid therapy at home. The smallest patch size currently available, which delivers 25 µg/h of fentanyl, is rather too high a starting dose for many children. Fentanyl, being a completely different molecule from morphine, may also be effective when tolerance has developed to morphine or diamorphine. Fentanyl is often used in children as second-line strong opioid after morphine or diamorphine.[39]

HYDROMORPHONE

Hydromorphone is approximately five times more potent than morphine[40,41] and can therefore offer an alternative solution to the problem of solubility of large parenteral doses of opioid. It is metabolized in a similar way to morphine[42] and probably confers little advantage over diamorphine where the latter is available. Its main role is in

countries where diamorphine is not yet freely available for prescription, usually because of unfounded fears of heroin addiction.

METHADONE

Despite anecdotal reports of its safe use even in outpatients, there is little published experience of methadone in children.[43,44] This is a pity; potentially methadone has an important role in the management of pediatric pain. Methadone combines the effects of an opioid with those of an NMDA (*N*-methyl-D-aspartate) antagonist.[34] This gives it a potentially major role in the management of neuropathic pain, such as when following thoracotomy, amputation, or nerve damage due to compression by a tumor.[45–49] More research is required into the use of methadone in children before it can be recommended. It has an unusual distribution curve which can result in toxicity many hours or even days after the drug is commenced.[50,51]

OTHER OPIOIDS

Buprenorphine

There is anecdotal evidence that buprenorphine is effective and well tolerated in children, but this has yet to be substantiated in clinical trials. Potentially it has a valuable role in managing pain in pediatric palliative medicine, as it has the advantage over morphine of a transdermal matrix formulation that can be divided to enable small doses to be given. Evidence in adults also suggests constipation is relatively rare.[52*,53*] It may therefore have a particular role in children with neurological disorders such as cerebral palsy or metabolic conditions, where long-term weak opioid therapy is often needed but patients are susceptible to constipation and the enteral route for medications may be difficult. Clinical experience suggests that in children buprenorphine may be more nauseating than other opioids, but again this has yet to be confirmed in studies.

Pethidine

Nowadays, pethidine has little role in pediatric pain relief. It is considerably less potent than morphine (see Table 50.1). Enteral absorption is erratic.[54,55] The major toxicities of pethidine are in the brain, where accumulation of its metabolites causes convulsions.[56–59] Its one advantage over morphine is that it causes less constriction of the sphincter of Oddi, and proved biliary colic is perhaps its only – rare – indication in children.

Oxycodone

Although oxycodone is a κ as well as a μ agonist, its properties are similar to those of morphine.[60,61] Its oral bioavailability is about 75 percent and like morphine it is biotransformed in the liver to a potent analgesic metabolite (oxymorphone). Again like morphine, the onset of action for oral oxycodone is 20–30 minutes and its duration of action is around 4–6 hours. Its clearance is impaired in renal failure. There is little experience of the use of oxycodone in pediatric palliative medicine, but it appears safe and effective in acute pain.[62] The risk of ventilatory depression may be higher than with morphine.[63] In general, there is little evidence that oxycodone offers significant advantage over morphine in children. Its role in pediatric palliative care, if any, remains unclear. It seems little different from morphine.

Tramadol

Tramadol is a weak opioid but its analgesic strength is augmented by an additional effect in inhibiting monoamine neurotransmitter reuptake.[64] Nevertheless its potency is only one-fifth to one-tenth that of morphine and it is probably best considered a weak or intermediate opioid. Its bioavailability is about 75 percent, and its onset and duration of action are similar to morphine. Its clearance is significantly impaired in liver dysfunction. Tramadol has a potency intermediate between codeine and morphine. It is more nauseating than oxycodone[65] and, like pethidine, can induce seizures.[66,67] Most research in children has been in the perioperative or postoperative context rather than the palliative. Like morphine, any effects on respiratory depression appear clinically insignificant.[68]

EPISODIC AND BREAKTHROUGH PAIN

Breakthrough pain has been defined as 'a transitory exacerbation of pain superimposed on a background of persistent but usually well controlled pain'.[69] The difficulty in managing episodic pain is that a dose of analgesic adequate for pain at its worst is often toxic when pain is at its least. Extra doses of morphine may be ineffective for severe episodic pain, since the time taken for it to reach effective serum levels means the pain has often subsided before it can work.

Pain may be episodic for three reasons. The dose of regular medication may be too small, resulting in intermittent breakthrough pain. The solution is to review the regular medication. The cause for pain may be episodic. For example, pain from a dislocated hip in cerebral palsy, or from bony metastasis in cancer can be provoked by movement (incident pain). Identifying, anticipating and where possible avoiding the provoking factors are the mainstays of treatment. Finally, the pain may simply be of an episodic nature, for example intestinal colic or muscle spasm. This is a situation in which adjuvant therapy such as anticholinergics or muscle relaxants may be helpful.

Because these causes for breakthrough pain are closely related, the definitions are often confused and incidence is therefore difficult to estimate.[70] The prevalence and characteristics of episodic and breakthrough pains have been evaluated. Patients report a wide variety of types of pain that can break through their regular analgesia, and similarly variable events that could precipitate it.[71] See also Chapter 54 (Episodic pain).

CHOOSING THE MOST APPROPRIATE ROUTE

The oral route is usually best for children. However, not all patients are able to swallow tablets or capsules. This is particularly true of children with neurodegenerative conditions, though many may have alternative enteral routes such as gastrostomy. Patients who are experiencing nausea and vomiting may simply be unable to tolerate oral medication. A range of alternative routes is available.

Transdermal patch

Fentanyl and buprenorphine are available as a self-adhesive patch.[35,36] The usual interval between changes of patch is 72 hours but a significant minority of patients may need the patch to be changed every 48 hours. It is important that adequate breakthrough medication continues to be made available, usually as immediate-release oral morphine or transmucosal fentanyl.[72]

Subcutaneous infusion

The subcutaneous route is often overlooked in the management of children. Portable syringe drivers, which are battery operated, are a convenient method for administering many drugs through subcutaneous infusion (CSCI). This approach combines the advantages of intravenous infusion (consistent delivery, easy titration, and potential for simultaneous administration of multiple drugs) with simplicity. Subcutaneous syringe drivers can be sited by nurses and can be managed at home with little medical or nursing input. Adverse effects can include local irritation at the site but this is usually easily managed by rotation through different sites.

Patient-controlled analgesia

Patient-controlled analgesia is an effective means of delivering postoperative pain relief. A modification of patient-controlled analgesia in children is nurse-controlled analgesia. This approach requires interpretation by an adult of a child's pain experience and risks delays to drug administration or even overruling of a child's reports of pain.

Continuous intravenous infusion

Where a child already has an indwelling central line, the intravenous route may be preferred.[73] This again permits constant plasma concentration, although this advantage is sometimes offset by difficulties maintaining the line. Multiple peripheral cannulation for intravenous infusion is not usually appropriate in the palliative phase since the subcutaneous route is at least equally effective and much easier to set up and maintain at home or in the hospice.

Rectal route

Many children will find rectal administration of medications unacceptable and this route should probably be discouraged nowadays, although it can provide rapid absorption and avoids the need for injection. The rectal route is contraindicated in children with neutropenia or thrombocytopenia. Relatively few strong opioids are available in rectal formulations. They include oxycodone, morphine,[74] and hydromorphone.

Transmucosal routes

Many strong opioids can be absorbed directly from the nasal or oral mucosa and can therefore be given via the buccal or intranasal route. This approach is particularly widespread among those working in children's hospices, where facilities for immediate intravenous or subcutaneous infusion may not immediately be available. The transmucosal route avoids first-pass metabolism, which may influence the effectiveness of opioids that are extensively metabolized in the liver.

OPIOID ROTATION OR SUBSTITUTION

It is likely that in some children tolerance to strong opioid analgesia can occur even in a therapeutic setting. The solution to this is usually simply to increase the dose of the major opioid. Rarely, such increases are constrained by dose-limiting toxicity such as neuroexcitability. One solution is to change to an alternative strong opioid of a different class.[39,75] A patient who has developed tolerance to the analgesic effects of morphine may well be less tolerant to those of fentanyl, for example. This phenomenon is termed 'incomplete cross-tolerance'. When substituting one opioid for another, the dose can and should be reduced, because tolerance to the analgesic effect of the new opioid will be incomplete. A corresponding reduction in toxicity will occur. The dose reduction is conventionally 25 percent.

Thus, a child who is toxic but not pain free on 1000 mg oral morphine per day can receive instead a fentanyl dose equivalent to only 750 mg oral morphine, and yet enjoy better analgesia and less toxicity. This is further helped by the fact that tolerance to the adverse effects of opioids often occurs more rapidly than tolerance to the beneficial effects. It is probable that there is little advantage in changing drugs within a class, for example substituting diamorphine for morphine, since cross-tolerance is not likely to be incomplete.

CONCLUSION

Clinical evidence is accumulating that strong opioids can be used safely and effectively in children with moderate to severe pain. They should be used as part of a rational approach to the diagnosis, assessment, and management of pain (Box 50.1, Fig. 50.2). The WHO pain ladder gives a straightforward structure to such an approach and is recommended to all those who wish to approach the management of a child with pain.

The evolution of clinical expertise and experience has been paralleled and supported by an expansion of the

---

Box 50.1 Using opioids effectively: principles of good pain management in children

Do not be afraid of strong opioids in children – the risks of serious toxicity or addiction are vanishingly small when they are used therapeutically and rationally. Always:

- use a rational approach to diagnose pain and its cause
- use a rational approach to manage pain (use pain ladder)
- balance benefit of any diagnostic or therapeutic approach with burden to patient or family
- use the simplest approach that is effective (e.g. oral route where possible)
- use appropriate adjuvants at each 'rung'
- prescribe stimulant laxatives when major opioid is started

Avoid:

- intramuscular route
- strong opioids 'prn' except as breakthrough
- novel opioids unless they are a genuine improvement on morphine

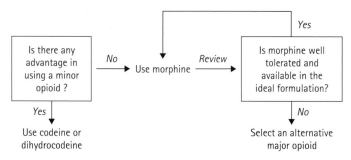

Figure 50.2 *A logical approach to the use of opioids in children. Until and unless evidence accumulates to suggest that another major opioid is more effective, less toxic, or cheaper (or ideally all of these), oral morphine should usually remain first line.*

research evidence base. This seems to show that, where children differ from adults in their handling of morphine, the result is that morphine is cleared more rapidly. It is plausible that this may make them more resilient than adults to its effects. More research is needed, as in so many other areas of pediatric clinical pharmacology. Important research areas include the clinical use of methadone and buprenorphine in children, and clarifying the dose–response relation of this important but often ill-understood class of analgesics in children.

Key learning points

- Children differ from adults in the pathophysiology and the pharmacology of pain management.

- Children experience pain at least as intensely as adults, but may not be able to express or quantify it verbally.

- After the first year of life, children may require higher doses of opioids than adults (relative to size) to obtain the same degree of analgesia. This may be because they clear some opioids more quickly. More research is needed.

- Pharmacokinetics in the neonatal period is very different from other periods in childhood, and in particular renal clearance is slower.

- The range of causes for pain in pediatric palliative medicine is wide, reflecting a great variety of life-limiting conditions other than cancer.

- Despite these differences, basic principles of pain management in adults can often be extrapolated to children, albeit with caution.

- Management of pain in children requires a combination of expertise in pediatrics and in symptom control. Where specialist pediatric palliative medicine is not available, close cooperation between pediatric and palliative medicine teams is essential.

ACKNOWLEDGMENTS

This chapter has been adapted with permission from RD Hain, A Miser, M Devins, WHB Wallace. Strong opioids in pediatric palliative medicine. *Pediatric Drugs* 2005; **7**(1): 1–9.

The authors gratefully acknowledge the contributions of Dr A Miser and Dr WHB Wallace.

REFERENCES

1 Doyle D, Hanks GW, Macdonald N. Introduction. In: Doyle D, Hanks GW, Macdonald N, eds. *Oxford Textbook of Palliative Medicine*, 2nd ed. Oxford: Oxford University Press, 1998: 1–8.

✱ 2 World Health Organization. *Cancer as a Global Problem.* Geneva: WHO, 1984.

◆ 3 Baum D, Curtis H, Elston S, *et al. A Guide to the Development of Children's Palliative Care Services.* 1st ed. Bristol: ACT/RCPCH, 1997.

◆ 4 Association of Children with Life-limiting or Threatening conditions and their families/Royal College of Paediatrics and Child Health. *A Guide to the Development of Children's Palliative Care Services – Second Edition, September 2003. Updated Report.* Bristol: ACT/RCPCH, 2003.

5 McGraw MB. Neural maturation as exemplified in the changing reactions of the infant to pin prick. *Child Dev* 1941; **12**: 31–42.

6 Swafford, A. Pain relief in the pediatric patient. *Med Clin North Am* 1968; **52**: 131–6.

7 Schug SA, Zech D, Grond S, *et al.* A long-term survey of morphine in cancer pain patients. *J Pain Symptom Manage* 1992; **7**: 259–66.

8 Desparmet J, Guelen P, Brasseur L. Opioids for the management of severe pain in children and infants. *Clin Drug Investig* 1997;14(Suppl 1): 15–21.

✱ 9 World Health Organization. Guidelines for analgesic drug therapy. In: *Cancer Pain Relief and Palliative Care in Children.* Geneva: WHO/IASP, 1998: 24–8.

◆ 10 Franck LS, Greenberg CS, Stevens B. Pain assessment in infants and children. *Pediatr Clin North Am* 2000; **47**: 487–512.

◆ 11   Hain RD. Pain scales in children: a review. *Palliat Med* 1997; **11**: 341–50.

12   Hunt A, Goldman A, Seers K, *et al.* Clinical validation of the paediatric pain profile. *Dev Med Child Neurol* 2004; **46**: 9–18.

13   Ventafridda V, Tamburini M, Caraceni A, *et al.* A validation study of the WHO method for cancer pain relief. *Cancer* 1987; **59**: 850–6.

14   Hunt TL, Kaiko RF. Comparison of the pharmacokinetic profiles of two oral controlled- release morphine formulations in healthy young adults. *Clin Ther* 1991; **13**: 482–8.

● 15   Hunt A, Joel S, Dick G, Goldman A. Population pharmacokinetics of oral morphine and its glucuronides in children receiving morphine as immediate-release liquid or sustained- release tablets for cancer pain. *J Pediatr* 1999; **135**: 47–55.

● 16   Hain RD, Hardcastle A, Pinkerton CR, Aherne GW. Morphine and morphine-6-glucuronide in the plasma and cerebrospinal fluid of children. *Br J Clin Pharmacol* 1999; **48**: 37–42.

17   Woods L. Distribution and fate of morphine in nontolerant and tolerant dogs and rats. *J Pharmacol Exp Ther* 1954; **112**: 158–75.

18   Bartlett S, Dodd P, Smith M. Pharmacology of morphine and morphine-3-glucuronide at opioid, excitatory amino acid, GABA and glycine binding sites. *Pharmacol Toxicol* 1994; **74**: 1–9.

● 19   Paul D, Standifer KM, Inturrisi CE, Pasternak GW. Pharmacological characterization of morphine-6-beta glucuronide, a very potent morphine metabolite. *J Pharmacol Exp Ther* 1989; **251**: 477–83.

20   Hoskin PJ, Hanks GW, Heron CW, *et al.* M6G and its analgesic action in chronic use. *Clin J Pain* 1989; **5**: 199–200.

21   Hanks GW, Hoskin PJ, Aherne GW, *et al.* Explanation for potency of repeated oral doses of morphine. *Lancet* 1987; **2**: 723–6.

22   Pacifici GM, Söwe J, Kager L, Rane A. Morphine glucuronidation in human fetal and adult liver. *Eur J Clin Pharmacol* 1982; **22**: 553–8.

23   Lynn A, Nespeca MK, Bratton SL, *et al.* Clearance of morphine in postoperative infants during intravenous infusion: the influence of age and surgery. *Anesth Analg* 1998; **86**: 958–63.

24   Hartley R, Green M, Quinn M, Levene MI. Pharmacokinetics of morphine infusion in premature neonates. *Arch Dis Child* 1993; 69(1 Spec No): 55–8.

25   McRorie TI, Lynn AM, Nespeca MK, *et al.* The maturation of morphine clearance and metabolism. *Am J Dis Child* 1992; **146**: 972–6.

26   Lloyd-Thomas A. Assessment and control of pain in children. *Anaesthesia* 1995; **50**: 753–5.

27   Lloyd-Thomas AR, Howard RF. A pain service for children. *Paediatr Anaesth* 1994; **4**: 3–15.

28   Choonara I, Lawrence A, Michalkiewicz A, *et al.* Morphine metabolism in neonates and infants. *Br J Clin Pharmacol* 1992; **34**: 434–7.

29   Choonara I, McKay P, Hain RDW, Rane A. Morphine metabolism in children. *Br J Clin Pharmacol* 1989; **28**: 599–604.

30   Lynn AM, Slattery JT. Morphine pharmacokinetics in early infancy. *Anesthesiology* 1987; **66**: 136–9.

31   Twycross R, Wilcock A, Thorp S. *Palliative Care Formulary.* Oxford: Radcliffe Medical Press, 1998: 20.

32   Hammer HF, Petritsch W, Pristautz H, Krejs GJ. Evaluation of the pathogenesis of flatulence and abdominal cramps in patients with lactose malabsorption. *Wien Klin Wochenschr* 1996; **108**: 175–9.

33   Ahmedzai S, Brooks D. Transdermal fentanyl versus sustained-release oral morphine in cancer pain: preference, efficacy, and quality of life. *J Pain Symptom Manage* 1997; **13**: 254–61.

◆ 34   Sang CN. NMDA-receptor antagonists in neuropathic pain: experimental methods to clinical trials. *J Pain Symptom Manage* 2000; **19**(1 Suppl): S21–S25.

● 35   Collins JJ, Dunkel IJ, Gupta SK, *et al.* Transdermal fentanyl in children with cancer pain: feasibility, tolerability, and pharmacokinetic correlates. *J Pediatr* 1999; **134**: 319–23.

36   Hunt AM, Goldman A, Devine T, Phillips M. Transdermal fentanyl for pain relief in a paediatric palliative care population. *Palliat Med* 2001; **15**: 405–12.

37   Koren G, Crean P, Goresky GV, *et al.* Pharmacokinetics of fentanyl in children with renal disease. *Res Commun Chem Pathol Pharmacol* 1984; **46**: 371–9.

38   Koehntop DE, Rodman JH. Fentanyl pharmacokinetics in patients undergoing renal transplantation. *Pharmacotherapy* 1997; **17**: 746–52.

39   Noyes M, Irving H. The use of transdermal fentanyl in pediatric oncology palliative care. *Am J Hosp Palliat Care* 2001; **18**: 411–16.

40   Lawlor P, Turner K, Hanson J, Bruera E. Dose ratio between morphine and hydromorphone in patients with cancer pain: a retrospective study. *Pain* 1997; **72**: 79–85.

● 41   Collins JJ, Geake J, Grier HE, *et al.* Patient-controlled analgesia for mucositis pain in children: a three-period crossover study comparing morphine and hydromorphone. *J Pediatr* 1996; **129**: 722–8.

42   Babul N, Darke AC, Hain R. Hydromorphone and metabolite pharmacokinetics in children. *J Pain Symptom Manage* 1995; **10**: 335–7.

43   Miser AW, Miser JS. The use of oral methadone to control moderate and severe pain in children and young adults with malignancy. *Clin J Pain* 1986; **1**: 243–8.

44   Shir Y, Shenkman Z, Shavelson V, *et al.* Oral methadone for the treatment of severe pain in hospitalized children: a report of five cases. *Clin J Pain* 1998; **14**: 350–3.

45   Gourlay GK, Cherry DA, Cousins MJ. A comparative study of the efficacy and pharmacokinetics of oral methadone and morphine in the treatment of severe pain in patients with cancer. *Pain* 1986; **25**: 297–312.

46   Bruera E, Neumann CM. Role of methadone in the management of pain in cancer patients. *Oncology (Huntingt)* 1999; **13**: 1275–82; discussion 1285–8, 1291.

47   De Conno F, Groff L, Brunelli C, *et al.* Clinical experience with oral methadone administration in the treatment of pain in 196 advanced cancer patients. *J Clin Oncol* 1996; **14**: 2836–42.

48   Mercadante S, Casuccio A, Fulfaro F, *et al.* Switching from morphine to methadone to improve analgesia and tolerability in cancer patients: a prospective study. *J Clin Oncol* 2001; **19**: 2898–904.

49   Bruera E, Sweeney C. Methadone use in cancer patients with pain: a review. *J Palliat Med* 2002; **5**: 127–38.

● 50   Inturrisi CE, Colburn WA, Kaiko RF, *et al.* Pharmacokinetics and pharmacodynamics of methadone in patients with chronic pain. *Clin Pharmacol Ther* 1987; **41**: 392–401.

51   Fainsinger R, Schoeller T, Bruera E. Methadone in the management of cancer pain: a review. *Pain* 1993; **52**: 137–47.

52   Muriel C, Failde I, Mico JA, *et al.* Effectiveness and tolerability of the buprenorphine transdermal system in patients with moderate to severe chronic pain: A multicenter, open-label, uncontrolled, prospective, observational clinical study. *Clin Ther* 2005; **27**: 451–62.

53   Ray R, Pal H, Kumar R, *et al.* Post marketing surveillance of buprenorphine. *Pharmacoepidemiol Drug Saf* 2004; **13**: 615.

54   Pokela ML, Olkkola KT, Koivisto M, Ryhanen P. Pharmacokinetics and pharmacodynamics of intravenous meperidine in neonates and infants. *Clin Pharmacol Ther* 1992; **52**: 342–9.

55   Hamunen K, Maunuksela EL, Seppala T, Olkkola KT. Pharmacokinetics of i.v. and rectal pethidine in children undergoing ophthalmic surgery. *Br J Anaesth* 1993; **71**: 823–6.

56   Kussman BD, Sethna NF. Pethidine-associated seizure in a healthy adolescent receiving pethidine for postoperative pain control. *Paediatr Anaesth* 1998; **8**: 349–52.

57   Pryle BJ, Grech H, Stoddart PA, *et al.* Toxicity of norpethidine in sickle cell crisis. *BMJ* 1992; **304**: 1478–9.

58   Kyff JV, Rice TL. Meperidine-associated seizures in a child. *Clin Pharm* 1990; **9**: 337–8.

59   Waterhouse RG. Epileptiform convulsions in children following premedication with Pamergan SP100. *Br J Anaesth* 1967; **39**: 268–70.

60   Heiskanen TE, Ruismaki PM, Seppala TA, Kalso EA. Morphine or oxycodone in cancer pain? *Acta Oncol* 2000; **39**: 941–7.

◆ 61   Rischitelli DG, Karbowicz SH. Safety and efficacy of controlled-release oxycodone: a systematic literature review. *Pharmacotherapy* 2002; **22**: 898–904.

62   Sharar SR, Carrougher GJ, Selzer K, *et al.* A comparison of oral transmucosal fentanyl citrate and oral oxycodone for pediatric outpatient wound care. *J Burn Care Rehabil* 2002; **23**: 27–31.

63   Olkkola KT, Hamunen K, Seppala T, Maunuksela EL. Pharmacokinetics and ventilatory effects of intravenous oxycodone in postoperative children. *Br J Clin Pharmacol* 1994; **38**: 71–6.

◆ 64   Lee CR, McTavish D, Sorkin EM. Tramadol. A preliminary review of its pharmacodynamic and pharmacokinetic properties, and therapeutic potential in acute and chronic pain states. *Drugs* 1993; **46**: 313–40.

65   Silvasti M, Tarkkila P, Tuominen M, *et al.* Efficacy and side effects of tramadol versus oxycodone for patient-controlled analgesia after maxillofacial surgery. *Eur J Anaesthesiol* 1999; **16**: 834–9.

66   Tobias JD. Seizure after overdose of tramadol. *South Med J* 1997; **90**: 826–7.

67   Spiller HA, Gorman SE, Villalobos D, *et al.* Prospective multicenter evaluation of tramadol exposure. *J Toxicol Clin Toxicol* 1997; **35**: 361–4.

68   Finkel JC, Rose JB, Schmitz ML, *et al.* An evaluation of the efficacy and tolerability of oral tramadol hydrochloride tablets for the treatment of postsurgical pain in children. *Anesth Analg* 2002; **94**: 1469–73.

69   Gomez-Batiste X, Madrid F, Moreno F, *et al.* Breakthrough cancer pain: prevalence and characteristics in patients in Catalonia, Spain. *J Pain Symptom Manage* 2002; **24**: 45–52.

◆ 70   Mercadante S, Radbruch L, Caraceni A, *et al.* Episodic (breakthrough) pain: consensus conference of an expert working group of the European Association for Palliative Care. *Cancer* 2002; **94**: 832–9.

71   Portenoy RK, Payne D, Jacobsen P. Breakthrough pain: characteristics and impact in patients with cancer pain. *Pain* 1999; **81**: 129–34.

72   Rees E. The role of oral transmucosal fentanyl citrate in the management of breakthrough cancer pain. *Int J Palliat Nurs* 2002; **8**: 304–8.

73   Sirkia K, Hovi L, Pouttu J, Saarinen-Pihkala UM. Pain medication during terminal care of children with cancer. *J Pain Symptom Manage* 1998; **15**: 220–6.

74   Lundeberg S, Beck O, Olsson GL, Boreus LO. Rectal administration of morphine in children. Pharmacokinetic evaluation after a single-dose. *Acta Anaesthesiol Scand* 1996; **40**: 445–51.

75   Cherny N, Ripamonti C, Pereira J, *et al.* Strategies to manage the adverse effects of oral morphine: an evidence-based report. *J Clin Oncol* 2001; **19**: 2542–54.

51

Pain in older people

WENDY M STEIN

INTRODUCTION

Young patients fear new or increasing pain as a sign of impending death, whereas their older counterparts most fear that pain will reflect declining functional status and a loss of independence. In older patients where pain is often chronic, pain loses its diagnostic significance and degenerates instead into chronic depression as their world begins to revolve solely around unremitting pain. In advanced disease, unrelieved pain may actually shorten life,[1] and certainly limits the time spent in activities consistent with quality of life. Despite advances in understanding of the mechanisms of pain, improvements in drug delivery systems and increasing educational requirements of physicians already in practice as well as those in training, a substantial number of patients are in pain, particularly those from special populations like older people. These people remain vastly underrepresented in drug studies, when often they are the very population ultimately targeted for the product's use. Insurance carriers are more apt to fund high-tech surgical or anesthesia interventions as opposed to ongoing medication or physical therapy. Older patients often do not volunteer pain as a problem at an outpatient visit when presenting with multiple other medical problems, feeling that pain is a natural part of aging. Older patients have a greater potential for drug–drug and drug–disease interactions due to changes in pharmacokinetics with aging and thus present a greater treatment challenge.

Despite these obstacles, pain can be successfully assessed and treated in the older patient, and when done so successfully fulfills the mission of geriatric care to improve function as the patient defines it. The purpose then of this chapter is to outline those issues unique to pain assessment and treatment in the older person. As this textbook is quite comprehensive in nature, this chapter will not review information already presented, but rather seek to supply the practitioner with a framework with which to competently approach the older person in pain.

DEFINITION AND EPIDEMIOLOGY

The International Association for the Study of Pain defines pain as an 'unpleasant sensory and emotional experience'.[2] Sensation and transmission is mitigated against the backdrop of previous pain experiences which are often far richer than for their younger counterparts. The multifactorial nature of pain separates it from many of the other syndromes commonly observed in geriatric medicine. Like dementia and incontinence, pain occurs with increasing prevalence as an individual ages, but should never be considered a normal or necessary part of the aging process. As many patients consider pain a natural sequela of aging, they will not volunteer clinical information unless specifically queried.

Exact estimates of pain in older cohorts are not known, particularly in those community dwelling elders over age 75. In most studies significant pain is defined as pain severe enough to prompt a patient to take medication several times a week or daily or to impair functional status. Studies have suggested that the prevalence of significant pain in community-dwelling elders may range from 25 percent to 56 percent,[3] and in nursing home residents from 45 percent to 80 percent.[4] The most common causes are related to musculoskeletal sources such as arthritis or chronic back pain. A Harris poll in 1997 found that 18 percent of older persons surveyed took analgesic medication several times a week or daily, and of this group, more than 70 percent each self-reported taking prescription and over-the-counter medications for their pain.[5] This finding is of particular concern as anti-inflammatory related complications are one of the most common reasons why older persons are admitted to acute care hospitals. As these medications can be purchased without prescription, they are often not reported to physicians at office or home visits. It is not unusual for an older person to have explored every option available to him or her before reaching the physician's office with a pain complaint.

Pain should be classified by physiological mechanism thus allowing the clinician to focus treatment interventions appropriately. Nociceptive pain arises from stimulation from nociceptors and is divided between somatic and visceral sources of pain. Somatic pain such as tendonitis commonly arises from injury to a specific tissue, joint or tendon. Pain can be localized to the injured area and is often described as aching pain. This type of pain responds well to common analgesic medications and topical interventions as well as physical therapy. Visceral pain arising from an organ may be dull, constant or sharp but may be referred to a site distant from the involved organ. Visceral pain may require surgical intervention depending on the cause and may require analgesics for moderate to severe pain. Neuropathic pain such as postherpetic neuralgia or diabetic neuropathy is generated from aberrant nerve signals in the periphery or central nervous system. Neuropathic pain is distinctly different from the nociceptive sources of pain; although traditional analgesics may 'take the edge off' the pain, adjuvant medications or invasive interventions are often needed to effectively treat these syndromes. Patients will often describe this type of pain as burning, shooting, electric, or shocklike. The patient's self-description will often lead the clinician to the most appropriate intervention more quickly than diagnostic testing, and without the waiting time required to obtain test results so that relief can be initiated almost immediately.

PAIN ASSESSMENT

The Joint Commission on Accreditation of Hospitals (JCAHO) now stipulates that pain assessment should be initiated upon admission to every healthcare setting, but wisely leaves it to that setting to determine how that should be best accomplished. In the acute care hospital, this provides the opportunity to identify pain and order any necessary consultations or studies prior to discharge, thus minimizing lengthy trips back and forth to the hospital. Subsequent pain assessments should be performed in the outpatient office setting and upon initial admission to the assisted living, nursing home, or subacute care unit after acute illness, with each change in level of care or with each pain intervention, and finally as part of the Minimum Data Set (MDS). The greatest challenge at each of these step points is transfer of key information and treatment plans.

Pain assessment may present unique challenges in the older person. The population of older persons living in some kind of community care setting is rising rapidly. The long-term care environment may pose difficulties in obtaining diagnostic testing and evaluation. In-house laboratories, radiology or other resources for the accurate and timely evaluation of patients are uncommon. Expert consultants from neurology, palliative medicine, anesthesia, physiatry, and psychiatry are usually unwilling to travel from the acute care environment. This often results in residents being transported to distant facilities for evaluation of active problems and for scheduled state-of-the-art diagnostic evaluations. From the older person's perspective this means missed meals and medications as well as hours waiting at the diagnostic center for studies, and the potential for iatrogenic illness (complications due to invasive diagnostic requirements such as radiographic dye), or increased musculoskeletal discomfort incurred while lying on hard surfaces without premedication for prolonged time periods in order to procure diagnostic information. The key question in geriatric palliative medicine, or geriatric primary care for that matter, is always will the findings change the plan of care enough to make the burden of procuring the information worthwhile?

A second significant challenge is the meaning of pain to an older person. It is uncommon for older people to have only one pain complaint, and since musculoskeletal sources of pain (arthritis) are prevalent in this population along with other pain types occurring with high prevalence (vasculitis, neuropathy, etc.), often pain goes unreported as it is assumed to be a natural part of aging. Although like dementia and incontinence, pain increases in prevalence with aging it should never be assumed to be a natural or requisite part of aging. In addition, the provider should listen carefully for terms other than pain which may be suggestive such as discomfort, or indications of depression which may be related to chronic unremitting pain.[6]

Initial pain assessments for the older person should always start with complete histories and physical examinations, including careful neurological and musculoskeletal assessments, and include history of trauma and previously used pharmacological and nonpharmacological approaches as well as indications of their success or failure (see Fig. 51.1).[7] Information concerning the length of time a particular intervention was used is as important as information regarding what specific interventions were used as often drugs have not been given adequate clinical trials or at adequate dose levels.

If medication review is done on an outpatient visit asking the patient to 'brown bag' anything she or he puts in

NAME: _____   AGE: _____

PRIMARY DIAGNOSES: _____   _____   _____

_____   _____   _____

MEDICATIONS & SCHEDULE: _____   _____   _____

_____   _____   _____

_____   _____   _____

NON-PHARMACOLOGIC PAIN
TREATMENTS: _____

_____

SUCCESS OF ABOVE: _____

_____

PAIN INTENSITY: NOW: 0   1   2   3   4   5
                               NONE   MODERATE   SEVERE

WORST IN 24 HOURS: 0   1   2   3   4   5
                               NONE   MODERATE   SEVERE

PAIN LOCATION:

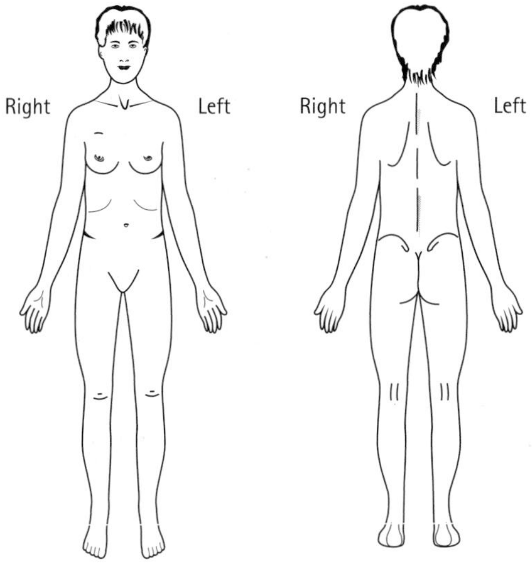

Right   Left   Right   Left

PAIN DESCRIPTORS: _____

_____

MANEUVERS THAT EXACERBATE: _____

_____

MANEUVERS THAT ALLEVIATE: _____

VISUAL ANALOG SCALE (PLACE AN X ON SCALE TO INDICATE PAIN SEVERITY)

|———|

EFFECTS OF PAIN ON: MOOD: _____   SLEEP: _____

ADLs/IADLs: _____

MMSE SCORE: _____   DEPRESSION SCALE SCORE: _____

GAIT & BALANCE ASSESSMENT: _____

Figure 51.1 *The initial geriatric pain assessment form. Redrawn from Stein WM. Pain in the nursing home.* Clin Geriatr Med *2001; 17: 585*[7] *with permission from Elsevier.*

their mouth or on their body for symptoms, illness, or discomfort is helpful as often older patients are apt not to count anything not prescribed by a provider as medicine. If this is done at a home visit asking the patient to 'show me the pills' until the patient runs out of places is helpful. It is not uncommon to find medications from several physicians as well as medications which are many years outdated, some of which could be toxic if taken, especially outdated antibiotics. Older patients will commonly hold on to unused portions of prescriptions because of the cost and in some cases the sacrifices they may have had to make to purchase a prescription. This exercise is a wonderful opportunity to discuss appropriate storage and use of medications, as well as finding out about other treating physicians. In addition, older patients are often unaware of the potential for interactions among prescriptions and over-the-counter medications or alternative/complementary therapies.

Common medication side effects such as nausea or sedation in the first 48–72 hours with an opioid need to be carefully separated from allergies likely to lead to anaphylaxis which are obviously a true medical concern. All major active diagnoses should be outlined and addressed to ensure that all chronic and currently symptomatic problems will be treated appropriately. Any diagnoses which are no longer active should be removed, allowing the clinician to streamline the medication list and decrease the potential for drug–drug interactions.

In addition, the assessment of the older person should also include some measure of mental status such as the Folstein Mini-Mental State Examination (MMSE),[8] a screen for depression such as the Geriatric Depression Scale (GDS), and a review of activities of daily living (ADLs) and instrumental activities of daily living (IADLs),[9] as well as the impact of pain on daily function. Although some research with limited numbers of subjects has not disclosed statistically significant relations between pain intensity and standard geriatric measures of function, this should not deter the use of these instruments with individual patients as a measurement of progress or worsening of underlying burden of disease. Pain often interferes with what patients perceive as overall function, however the usual geriatric measures of function may not be sensitive or specific enough to identify fine changes. Improving function means less assistance required with ADLs and thus less staff or caregiver involvement over time. Also, a patient delirious with pain, or sleep deprived secondary to pain is unlikely to score well on a MMSE but should improve significantly with effective pain management. Many of these measures are routinely collected on long-term care residents at the time of admission and subsequently updated at monthly, quarterly and annual physician visits, and therefore readily available. Care plans need to be developed for any abnormalities found on screening with scheduled visits at intervals to check on progress or new symptoms such as increased constipation. Functional status may also assist in providing an outcome measure for improvement of pain in follow-up visits.

Due to the high rate of dementing illness in this population, particularly in those over age 80, it is important on the initial assessment to identify significant others or caregivers. Unfortunately many older persons may be living in the community without close family and may be relying on close friends as 'the keepers of the med box', to refill prescriptions, fill out pain diaries, and get them to physician appointments. This fact is important to identify as often the 'caregiver' is as functionally impaired as the patient, and without this individual the patient may be unable to remain independently in the community.

There are many standardized pain assessment tools, both unidimensional and multidimensional. The key to pain assessment tools is which tool works best for a particular individual, and can be used with multiple providers of varying skill levels on different occasions with reliable results. The 'gold standard' of the multidimensional tools is the McGill Pain Questionnaire.[10–12] However, as with most multidimensional scales it is extremely burdensome for the older person in pain and not apt to be completed at multiple visits in a reliable fashion. Additionally, this tool is not easily adaptable to ill or incapacitated individuals and has been used primarily in the outpatient setting as the standard against which newer tools have been tested. The Geriatric Pain Measure is one such tool which includes multiple domains, consists of 24 items, and showed significant validity and reliability in older persons with multiple medical problems.[13] Unidimensional tools consist of a single item which gauges pain intensity.[14–16] If different pain scales are attempted upon admission to determine which may be best used with that patient, information concerning the most successful scale with *that patient* should be documented clearly in the record, and communicated to each member of the interdisciplinary team for continuity. The Initial Geriatric Pain Assessment Form (see Fig. 51.1)[7] as first developed and published includes gait and balance; bowel function should be added as well. It is imperative to pick up any potential problems in these key areas before adding any medications which could result in, or exacerbate, complications such as impactions or falls and fractures.

Key components of the pain evaluation should be performed initially and repeated on a consistent and continual basis, and include pain location, intensity using both a numerical scale and a patient-generated list of descriptors, and a review of alleviating and exacerbating factors. Often patients have extremely useful nonpharmacologic interventions which in an institutional environment (hospital, SNF) require a physician's order. Potential influences on sleep and mood need to be elicited. There are changes which occur in sleep patterns with 'normal' aging such as increased sleep latency and decreased REM sleep, which often prompt older patients to use medications inappropriately such as sleeping medications or diphenhydramine, both of which carry with them increased risk of falls. When these changes are coupled with unrelieved pain, sleep is often vastly disturbed by the time a patient reaches their provider.

These items can be incorporated into a pain diary, the patient record, kept at the bedside or with the nursing medication administration record (MAR) for easy acquisition. Entries should be accompanied by dates and times in order to assist in correlating pain entries with administration times of medications or nonpharmacologic interventions. Assessments should be obtained as often as needed while patients continue to require aggressive titration of medications, and at least once every shift in an acute or long-term care setting. Although more frequent assessments may be desirable, it is often difficult to obtain assessments more than once per nursing shift in a long-term care facility.

Chronic pain may present very differently in the older person than their younger counterpart. Acute pain commonly presents with autonomic discharge leading to elevations in pulse, temperature, blood pressure, or respiratory rate. Patients may have changes in facial expression, fidgeting, or changes in posture or mood. Patients with chronic pain may not exhibit any of these signs or symptoms, and thus the assessment of pain is all the more challenging.

Depression and pain are often inextricably bound together and so depression when present needs to be identified and treated aggressively in order to successfully manage the patient's total pain. Cohen-Mansfield and Marx[17] performed a study of 408 nursing home residents and demonstrated that depressed residents were more likely to have pain regardless of the presence of cognitive impairment.[17] Parmalee et al.'s 1991 study of 598 nursing home and congregate housing residents also showed a significant association of pain with depression.[18] Those meeting Diagnostic and Statistical Manual (DSM)-IIIR criteria for major depression reported both more intense pain and a greater number of localized pain complaints than did those with minor or no depression in this study. Although no causal mechanisms were established, the authors suggested that older patients with significant depression might be more sensitive to pain caused by a preexisting physical disorder.[18]

PAIN IN THE COGNITIVELY IMPAIRED

This section will address the most challenging assessment problems clinicians face which include alterations of cognitive status such as delirium and dementia, and vision and hearing impairments which may further complicate the assessment of pain in the cognitively impaired. Although delirium has been specifically identified in a large number of patients with cancer,[19] these challenges predominantly involve older people; therefore, this section will focus primarily on research and clinical suggestions developed for this rapidly growing section of the population.

Cognitive impairment or altered mental state has been defined as 'a change in the patient's usual premorbid state of mind'.[8] This may include delirium and dementia as well as alterations in emotions and behaviors. The most critical task is to establish the patient's premorbid mental status, and the nature and association of any clinical changes which may have occurred. Changes in mental status may occur in as many as 20–30 percent of medical inpatients and 50–90 percent of nursing home residents,[20] and significantly impact upon an individual's ability to participate actively in symptom assessment.

Delirium

Delirium has also been called 'acute confusional state' and clinicians have often colloquially referred to this state as 'temporary brain failure'. Delirium is best defined as 'an organic mental syndrome featuring global cognitive impairment, disturbances of attention, reduced level of consciousness, increased or reduced psycho-motor activity, and disorganized sleep–wake cycle'.[21] Symptoms include restlessness, anxiety, difficulty in thinking coherently, insomnia, disturbing dreams as well as fleeting hallucinations. Age greater than 65, chronic cerebral disease and brain damage are the main predisposing factors for delirium. Psychological stress, sleep loss and sensory deprivation and overload can all facilitate and maintain delirium. DELIRIUMS is a mnemonic offered as a way to remember the causes of delirium.[20]

D – alludes to drugs which can include a number of drugs, especially those with anticholinergic properties, as well as drug overdose or withdrawal

E – stands for emotional causes such as agitated depression or mania

L – includes low oxygenation as is found in cardiac ischemia, chronic pulmonary disease, congestive heart failure or pulmonary embolism

I – represents infection of any sort, and typically in hospitalized older patients includes pneumonia or urosepsis

R – refers to retention of urine or feces

I – represents ictal states

U – stands for undernutrition as well as dehydration which occur commonly in community-dwelling as well as institutionalized older people

M – includes metabolic causes such as organ failure or specifically, hypo- or hyperthyroidism

S – raises the possibilities of stroke or subdural hematoma.

All of these possible causes need to be considered when entertaining the diagnosis of delirium.

The aging of America

The population over the age of 60 in the USA is expected to increase by 69 percent by the year 2020, and those over 85 represent the most rapidly growing subsegment of this population.[22] There have been substantial scientific and technological breakthroughs in the field of medicine, all of which have contributed to the growth of an older, chronically ill population. Prevalence rates of dementia, and specifically Alzheimer disease, rise exponentially after age 65. Rates of Alzheimer disease have ranged as high as 50 percent in those over the age of 90.[22]

Dementia

Dementia has been defined as 'a syndrome characterized by a decline in multiple cognitive functions occurring in clear consciousness'.[23] Dementia has been documented in 10–15 percent of older surgical patients, one-third of older medical inpatients, and more than 50 percent of nursing home residents.[23] The more than 50 causes of dementia include primary dementia with no other signs, dementia with signs of vascular disease, dementia with evidence of chronic infection, secondary dementia with signs of an underlying neurological condition such as is seen in neoplasm and movement disorders as well as motor neuron disease or multiple sclerosis. Dementia may also follow diffuse brain trauma as well as occur with endocrine disorders and vitamin deficiencies, toxic disorders, psychiatric disorders such as chronic schizophrenia or pseudodementia, as well as other conditions largely affecting adolescents or young adults such as Wilson disease, tuberous sclerosis, progressive myoclonic epilepsy, and the metabolic storage diseases.

For convenience, dementia may be divided up into cortical causes such as Alzheimer disease, Jakob–Creutzfeldt disease, Pick disease, and stroke, and subcortical causes. Cortical causes feature prominent amnesia, aphasia, apraxia, agnosia, and in Alzheimer disease specifically, preservation of fine motor movement until late in the illness.[23] Subcortical causes include Parkinson disease, Huntington disease, and hydrocephalus. The latter characteristically exhibit amnesia, slowness of thought, apathy and lack of initiative in all aspects of cognitive function, and early disorders of movement.[23]

The issue of potentially reversible dementias has received much attention in the medical literature. These include drugs, depression, hypothyroidism, B_{12} deficiency, sensory impairment, normal pressure hydrocephalus, tumor, subdural hematoma, infection, and anemia.[20] The chief concern in identifying these phenomena is in limiting further deleterious consequences, not in the potential to reverse the cognitive impairment that has already occurred.

Delirium versus dementia

It is vital to differentiate between delirium and dementia. Both conditions may also occur simultaneously. Rates of delirium have ranged as high as 50 percent in hospitalized patients with previously diagnosed dementia.[20] Delirium favors an acute onset lasting days to weeks in its subacute phase, fluctuating over time leading to disrupted sleep–wake cycle and waxing and waning level of consciousness. Ability to attend to task is impaired as well as orientation. Autonomic changes are common and electroencephalograms (EEGs) show diffuse slow waves. Language may be incoherent and the patient may be fearful and agitated.

Dementia is usually insidious in onset, excluding vascular dementia which follows a stepwise connection. Symptoms tend to be persistent and stable over time with a normalized sleep–wake cycle and normal level of consciousness in a particular patient. Ability to attend to task is not affected, but orientation is impaired and aphasia and apathy are quite common. Autonomic changes are unusual and EEGs, if anything, will show a mild slowing.

The impact of sensory impairment

Uncompensated sensory impairment can impact upon functional decline, social isolation, depression, falls, and accidents, leading to increased patient frustration and resentment. Visual and auditory impairments are the two sensory losses which most often complicate both symptom assessment and management.

Senile miosis, decreased amplitudes of accommodation of the lens (presbyopia), and age-related changes in color vision occur with normal aging. Cataracts, glaucoma, age-related macular degeneration and diabetic retinopathy represent the four most common causes of blindness in older persons and affect 9 percent of adults 65–74 years old. The incidence rises to greater than 50 percent in those over 75 years old.[24]

Hearing loss is the third most commonly reported chronic problem in those over age 65.[25] In nursing homes, prevalence statistics for hearing loss range between 50 and 100 percent with prevalence rising with advancing age.[26] In the Framingham Heart Study cohorts, although 41 percent of those over age 65 had some level of hearing impairment, only 10 percent of these individuals had tried hearing aids.[26] This is a significant problem among older people which can seriously impede the clinician's ability to conduct meaningful symptom assessment. Hearing impairment can be broken down into the conductive type (cerumen impaction, middle ear disease and otosclerosis), sensorineural disease (cranial nerve VIII damage from noise, cochlear damage, ototoxic drugs such as gentamicin, presbycusis, trauma, infection, and acoustic neuroma), mixed and central hearing loss which itself affects 50 percent of those aged 51–91 years.[26]

Studies of pain in the cognitively impaired

Of all the symptoms seen in individuals at the end of life, pain is the single symptom which has been most well studied in the cognitively impaired. In a study designed to assess physicians' detection of pain among geriatric nursing home residents, Sengstaken and King[27] found that 66 percent of those able to communicate were identified as having pain by chart review as well as patient interview. Only 34 percent of these patients, however, had pain identified by their treating physicians. When the noncommunicative residents were compared to those able to communicate, the physicians were found to have identified pain less frequently in those who were noncommunicative. There were no differences between these groups in regard to demographic or medical diagnoses other than dementia, so one might expect that they would be equally likely to suffer pain, although the treating physicians identified chronic pain more than twice as frequently in those who were able to communicate. Parmalee et al.[28] studied self-reported pain in 758 nursing home and congregate housing older people with mild to moderate levels of cognitive impairment as defined by the Blessed Memory Information Concentration Test. This study showed that, in general, pain complaints decreased with increasing levels of cognitive impairment. Markedly impaired subjects reported less intense pain, and a smaller number of pain complaints than those who had intact cognition or mild impairment. However, when cognitively impaired individuals reported pain, their pain complaints were no less valid.

Ferrell et al.[29] examined the problem of pain in nursing homes and explored the usefulness of currently existing pain scales for cognitively impaired residents utilizing a patient base drawn from 10 different community nursing homes. Their study population consisted of patients with moderate to severe degrees of cognitive impairment (mean 12.1 ± 7.9 on the MMSE) and scales included the McGill Present Pain Intensity Subscale (0 to 5 with word anchors) the Rand Coop Chart (cartoon figures with word anchors), the Memorial Pain Card Subscale, and a verbal 0 to 10 scale in enlarged format and with adequate amounts of light and hearing augmentation. Although only 32 percent of patients could complete all five scales presented, 83 percent of these individuals with significant degrees of cognitive impairment could complete at least one of the existing scales presented. This finding validated the utility of attempting to utilize established pain assessment tools in communicative, cognitively impaired older people. The study participants were quite good at communicating how intense their pain was at a particular moment, but were unable to convey the intensity of pain at a past point in time.

Studies of pain in noncommunicative cognitively impaired

Multiple attempts have been and are being made to use pediatric instruments, and specifically those developed for neonates, with noncommunicative cognitively impaired older people. There are some fundamental issues to address when using pediatric assessment tools in older patients. First, pediatric tools have been developed to measure acute, and often specifically procedure-related pain; in cognitively impaired older patients clinicians are often evaluating chronic, or acute on chronic pain, which might be expected

to present differently. In acute pain, the observer might expect to see changes in facial expression, vocalization, increased muscle tension and autonomic discharge resulting in alterations of heart rate, blood pressure and respiratory rate. Although in chronic pain states such as arthritis, which is highly prevalent in both community-dwelling and institutionalized older people, clinicians may witness vocalizations and increased muscle tension, chronic pain may more likely present as primary depression or change in baseline mental status. Second, infants have no wealth of pain memory to influence their pain interpretation, and so existing knowledge cannot attach any meaning to induced pain. It is currently unknown whether cognitively impaired older people retain this ability.

There are fewer studies published on pain assessment in noncommunicative cognitively impaired older people; those that currently exist include relatively small numbers of subjects. Marzinski[30] reviewed 60 patients living in a dementia unit, 43 percent of whom had potentially painful conditions on the basis of chart review. Only three of these patients received routinely scheduled analgesics. However, one of the most interesting findings of this study was the nursing staff could quickly identify what amounted to normative behavior for a particular patient. Once deviations were identified, they were noted and acted upon.

The Assessment of Discomfort in Dementia (ADD) Protocol was designed by Kovach et al.[31] to more accurately assess discomfort, more accurately treat pain, and decrease use of psychotropic medications. This program focused first on educating the nursing staff who best knew the patients to identify even subtle changes in behavior which may represent abnormal versus normal behaviors for a particular patient, to perform basic physical examination and chart review looking for new findings. They were then taught a protocol of nondrug soothing interventions once abnormal behaviors were identified. Only last did this protocol go on to physician ordered as needed analgesics and if successful, the physician was notified and medication for pain ordered on a routine basis. A convenience sample of 104 residents with dementia were drawn from the 32 participating facilities. Utilization of the ADD protocol resulted in increased use of scheduled analgesics and nonpharmacological soothing interventions. Difficulties in this setting involved limited time, challenges getting staff sufficiently educated, and resistance to change. Staff reported that the main benefits were increased sense of residents' discomfort and improved pain and physical assessments.

The Pain Assessment in Advanced Dementia (PAINAD) Scale developed by Warden et al.[32] is a 0–10 scale that allows a caregiver or proxy to rate a patient's pain from 0 to 2 in terms of breathing, negative vocalization, facial expression, body language, and consolability, and was found to be reliable and valid in the nonverbal cognitively impaired population. This tool is also particularly useful for professionals using 0–10 scales with their verbal patients as it simplifies intensity; however, we do not know whether increasing scores are associated with higher levels of pain as this tool is a compilation of scores in five separate areas and thus cannot be directly compared to VAS-type intensity scores.

RECOMMENDATIONS FOR PAIN ASSESSMENT AND MANAGEMENT

In order to accommodate for sight and hearing impairment, it is recommended that extra time be given for the patient to assimilate questions. Large print visual cues, adequate ambient light, and ensuring that hearing aids or pocket amplification devices and refractive lenses are in place are vital. Limited attention span may necessitate performing symptom assessments in portions over time. Subjective responses or descriptions must carry equal weight with fixed answers to standardized tools. In the case of pain, multiple tools should be presented upon initial assessment if standardized instruments are being utilized. Whichever tool is most clinically useful with a particular patient should be carefully recorded in the chart and this information communicated to other members of the interdisciplinary team. This procedure will ensure that each subsequent assessment is performed exactly the same regardless of the team member involved. As cognitively impaired older people are often able to report on pain at the time of but not previous to pain assessment, pain assessment should be conducted more frequently than would be necessary with a cognitively intact patient.[33]

In the case of the noncommunicative cognitively impaired the single most important sign is deviation from what is baseline or 'normal' behavior for that particular individual. When this occurs, a careful bedside examination should be undertaken with laboratory studies consistent with the patient and family's wishes. Examination should focus particularly on occult sources or atypical presentations of infection in older people such as pneumonia or urinary tract infections. The aid of nursing staff should be enlisted to exclude alterations in sleeping, eating or elimination as the source of change in behavior. Chart review should exclude medication changes as an etiology. After all of these have been carefully undertaken, there may be a role for a well defined empirical trial of short acting pain medication with consistent and continual reassessment.[33]

PAIN TREATMENT

Pain treatment may present several unique challenges in the older population. The World Health Organization (WHO) three-step ladder approach to pain based on pain intensity[34,35] is as applicable in the older population as in the young with certain caveats. The ladder assumes that the patient will enter the protocol based on their current pain, i.e. a patient with severe pain does not have to go through steps 1 and 2 first. Pain relief should be provided even while the patient is in the diagnostic phase of their work-up. Finally, if pain ratchets up from mild to severe the step 2 medications can be skipped. Or if it is recognized that the patient is presenting with advanced disease, it makes more sense to go from step 1 drugs to low-dose step 3 drugs with appropriate adjuvants along the way.

Aging is associated with an increased fat to lean body mass combined with decreased hepatic and renal clearance of medications that may lead to slower breakdown of medications in general, and specifically of potentially harmful metabolites. For example, meperidine and propoxyphene both have potentially harmful active metabolites which may accumulate and cause central nervous system hyperexcitability.[36]

Almost every over-the-counter pharmaceutical product available is compounded with acetaminophen or aspirin. The step 2 medications most commonly ordered for pain also contain these common ingredients. Although there are general guidelines for the acute use (7–14 days) of acetaminophen of no more than 4 g/day in a younger patient and no more than 3 g/day in an older patient, no chronic dosing guidelines have ever been released. The prevalence of both drug–drug and drug–disease interactions are higher in this population and may result in worsened cognitive status, orthostatic hypotension, and the potential for falls. It is important to remember that older patients are often already at increased risk of constipation secondary to decreased activity, decreased fluid intake, and multiple concomitant medications, and so should be started on an aggressive bowel regimen as soon as any potentially constipating medications (opioids, tricyclics, anticholinergics) are started. The high prevalence of laxative dependence in this age group may require starting with the patient's daily laxative requirement and titrating over this amount to effect as needed. Side effects should be anticipated and appropriate measures taken to avoid them, particularly constipation, with thorough follow-up on subsequent visits. And finally, nonsteroidal anti-inflammatory drug (NSAID) use is more problematic because of increased frequencies of gastric and renal toxicities in this age group.[37] The frail older person over 85 years has the highest risk of both silent bleeds and fatal bleeds.[38] The newer cyclooxygenase 2 (COX-2) agents, although specifically formulated to decrease the risk of gastrointestinal side effects, may still carry some risk of gastric irritation, as well as the usual renal and central nervous system toxicities, and did not turn out to be the anticipated panacea. General recommendations remain regarding the cautious use of NSAIDs in this population and then coupled with misoprostol[39] or proton pump inhibitors. However, as there are no generally accepted published guidelines for clinical follow-up in this population, the usual advice to start low, go slow, and use only for as long as absolutely necessary pertains.

Older people may be more sensitive to the analgesic effects of opioids with a higher peak effect and longer duration of action secondary to decreased elimination.[40,41] This does not mean, however, that pain in older patients should not be as aggressively treated as in younger patients. In fact, unlike acetaminophen and NSAIDs, opioids are the only drugs which can be taken for years with no threat of end-organ toxicity. Patients and their caregivers need to be educated regarding the expected side effects of nausea and sedation associated with opioids in the first 24–72 hours so that the patient continues to take the medication and not assume she or he has developed a drug allergy. Education regarding the concept of dependence which occurs with chronic opioid use, as it does with β blockers, needs to be separated from the concepts of tolerance and addiction.

The clinician should anticipate a higher peak effect and longer drug half-life because of slower clearance and dose accordingly. For these reasons, drugs like meperidine and propoxyphene should be avoided; extremely extended duration and particularly potent drugs like levorphanol, methadone and sustained release fentanyl should be considered only in special circumstances and for opioid-tolerant patients only. Methadone has gained increased attention as it is inexpensive and is the only opioid to date that has also demonstrated N-methyl-D-aspartate receptor activity which is often helpful in recalcitrant nerve pain. However, methadone is extremely long-acting and thus difficult to titrate, particularly in the institutional setting. Nonpharmacological and pharmacological measures should be used concomitantly to act synergistically and to decrease the incidence of drug–drug interactions and side effects.

Neuropathic pain is often the most challenging pain to treat in older persons. Traditionally tricyclics were used, however in a multiarm study Max and colleagues found no greater benefit in less anticholinergic drugs such as desipramine than with amitriptyline.[42] It is most likely that tricyclics work through the norepinephrine-mediated downward inhibitory pain pathway. The serotonin-mediated antidepressants have not been found to be beneficial adjuvants in neuropathic pain. Gabapentin was used in two large multicenter, randomized, double blind, placebo controlled clinical trials and found to be effective in the treatment of diabetic neuropathy and postherpetic neuralgia.[43,44] The main side effect was sedation necessitating low initial doses and very gradual dose increases to a therapeutic range of 1000–1600 mg/day. Other drugs for neuropathic pain have included valproic acid and intravenous lidocaine.

ROUTES OF ADMINISTRATION AND DELIVERY

Whenever possible the least invasive route of medication delivery should be employed to maximize patient and caregiver independence and limit risk. Because of the increased risk of side effects, short acting medications should be started first, titrated to comfort and then converted to long acting medications with an appropriate amount of medication prescribed for breakthrough pain. Whenever possible, only one drug should be titrated at a time in order to more

accurately identify side effects and limit stopping whole regimens. Pharmacokinetic realities should be respected, i.e. medications which should reasonably last 4–6 hours and may in this population last 6–8 hours should be ordered that way to avoid overshooting the mark and risking oversedation or worse. Unfortunately clinicians need to keep medication costs uppermost in their minds when prescribing. Older patients are often unable to pay for needed medications on fixed incomes. Insurers are more apt to cover an invasive procedure or medication pump rental costing thousands of dollars than medications or physical therapy if needed on an ongoing basis. And finally, there may indeed be a role for consultation with an anesthesiologist who is trained in the special needs and anatomical concerns of older people.[45]

TOPICALS AND ADJUVANTS

Topical therapy has attracted significant attention due to patient acceptability, increased sense of control, and limited untoward side effects. Capsaicin is extracted from hot chili peppers, and when applied faithfully multiple times every day depletes the supply of substance P from the terminus of unmyelinated C fibers.[46] The patient needs to adhere to a treatment regimen and endure the initial skin irritation and burning before the onset of anesthesia which must then be maintained. Breaks in treatment regimen require restarting capsaicin and waiting for therapeutic effect. This product has best been used as an adjuvant to drug therapy and rarely as sole therapy.

EMLA® (Eutectic Mixture of Lidocaine and Prilocaine anesthetics) was initially developed for temporary analgesia in pediatric patients. The cream is applied thickly to a specific area 1–1.5 hours before a scheduled procedure such as a planned dose of ceftriaxone (Rocephin), venepuncture or intravenous stick, covered with a plastic membrane to keep it in place, then the area is prepped as usual. Analgesia is effective but temporary necessitating additional applications for longer pain relief. Although intended for procedure-related analgesia, some clinicians have evolved protocols involving EMLA or lidocaine gel with morphine for various pain problems to decrease dose-related side effects of pain medications or in some cases as sole therapy.

In response to the early success with EMLA, researchers developed the 5 percent lidocaine patch. Rowbotham et al.[47] studied 35 adults (mean age 75 years) with a diagnosis of postherpetic neuralgia in a four session, random order, double blind, vehicle controlled study. Up to three patches were applied to the patient's most painful area, 12 hours on, 12 hours off. The lidocaine patch was superior to both no-treatment and vehicle patches, without systemic side effects, and was well tolerated. New roles for this product continue to be developed, with varying application schedules, and in different pain presentations. Originally developed as an adjuvant to medications as a strategy to cut down dose, it is now used in patients who wish to avoid any oral medications, or as an adjunct in patients with either inadequate response to customary treatment, or in whom higher doses would inflict intolerable side-effects.

Older patients often benefit greatly from the use of non-pharmacological interventions. The use of heat, cold, massage, distraction and relaxation techniques can be routinely integrated with appropriately prescribed medicines, and while waiting for doses of breakthrough medications to take effect. These augment, not replace, medication and can help give the patient and caregivers a sense of participation in the therapeutic process. Often patients have been using some of these techniques successfully prior to admission to acute care hospitals or long-term care facilities, and integrating these with the total care plan after admission can improve outcome; however, it is vital that these be listed on the initial assessment as in institutional settings these nonpharmacological interventions require physicians' orders. Alternatively, techniques which might have been difficult for an older person to utilize alone at home on an ongoing basis can be provided in the long-term care facility with assistance from nursing and restorative personnel. Physical therapy, restorative services and activities personnel, all of whom are available in the long-term care, can be part of the plan of care to integrate nonpharmacological therapies. Restorative nursing assistants after an initial assessment by a physical therapist can continue helpful therapies without extending limited resources under Medicare Part B in the USA. These therapies can strengthen deconditioned and sore muscles, helping to decrease overall fall risk, improve pain related to problems affecting posture and gait, decrease muscle spasm from overcompensation from pain associated with compression fracture, and use helpful modalities such as ultrasound, hydrotherapy or paraffin.

Older patients have historically been less interested in cognitive modalities. Cognitive interventions are made all the more complex by sensory or cognitive impairments. Many older patients have been socialized by traditional Western medicine into thinking about pills as the only solution to medical conditions or problems, and so are more likely to welcome what they perceive as a 'quick fix' approach. Many cognitive modalities require instruction and reinforcement by an expert, and finally are usually not reimbursed by insurers. Acupuncture and chiropractic have become increasingly more accepted practices and in some cases even covered by insurers. In their review of alternative medicine in older Americans, Foster et al.[48] questioned 2055 adults, of whom 311 were aged 65 and older about their use of 20 alternative medicine therapies in the previous 12 months. Thirty percent of people aged 65 and older used at least one alternative treatment in the last year compared with 46 percent of those less than 65. The two most commonly used modalities were chiropractic and herbs.

Alternative and complementary therapies hold great promise as adjuvants in pain management in older persons.

They have become increasingly acceptable, increase patient and caregiver autonomy, decrease side effect profiles by potentially working synergistically with traditionally pharmaceutical agents, and often have multisymptom use. These therapies may require a special practitioner, however, are limited or uncovered by most insurance carriers, and require a prescription in an institutional setting. Finally, some of these therapies may be positively or negatively affected by sensory or cognitive impairments. There currently are few studies involving these therapies, partly because of difficulties creating 'sham' control arms, and specifically few if any in older people especially those over age 75. More research needs to be done in this necessary area to answer these basic questions.

PAIN IN THE LONG-TERM CARE ENVIRONMENT

The assessment and treatment of pain in the long-term care environment continues to present several unique and challenging problems. Increasingly, studies are focusing on the large number of older people with important pain problems in long-term care.[49–51] The inclusion of pain as an area of clinical research interest in the minimum data set (MDS) has generated interest in this problem and will provide an ongoing data stream for continued study. Researchers are attempting to establish reliability and validity data of standardized assessment tools previously validated in younger populations, and utilizing both traditional and novel assessment tools in the cognitively impaired. Assessment strategies in the noncommunicative cognitively impaired resident are being developed in tandem with unique clinical protocols focusing on the role of the primary care nurse who best knows that patient to decipher 'normal' from 'abnormal' behavior.

The application of available pharmacological interventions poses greater challenges because of the higher incidence of drug–drug and drug–disease interactions as well as side effects in older people; this picture is in turn complicated by the decreased hepatic metabolism and renal clearance present in many older patients. The long-term care environment has limited resources which can present logistical concerns for both diagnosis and treatment, but can also positively limit overly invasive or extensive modalities which may not in the end positively alter treatment and may pose iatrogenic concerns of their own. This section will explore these issues and offer suggestions for the appropriate assessment and management of pain in the resident in long-term care.

ISSUES RELATIVE TO CARE IN THE LONG-TERM CARE ENVIRONMENT

A significant proportion of individuals over the age of 65 now make their home in some part of the long-term care community, whether these individuals are recovering from acute illness and able to return home, admitted for long stays, or in the last 6 months of life.[20] By the year 2030, it is anticipated that in the USA, the number of persons over 65 will double to over 60 million, with the greatest increase in those frail elders over age 85.[20] Nursing home beds are expected to double over the next 30 years to keep up with this boom, and may exceed 5 million by the year 2040.[20]

Long-term care is growing rapidly, and the quality of care provided in a nursing home affects a significant proportion of our older population. By necessity, the older person is looking for more diverse choices, and there is often a considerable range in available finances to spend for care. To that end, the term long-term care now also includes a variety of different care settings such as senior apartments, RCFEs (residential care facilities for the elderly) or in some areas of the USA board and care, and assisted living homes, as well as specialized units within each of these care settings for individuals with dementia.

As the acuity level of the acute care hospital has risen with the boom in technology, patients are apt to be released to long-term care with much higher care needs. Traditional rehabilitation units require the patient to be able to tolerate at least 3 hours per day of therapy to qualify for admission. Many older patients after an acute event cannot meet this requirement but can make therapeutic gains and thus began the development of subacute care units or transitional care units. The older stroke patient who would have remained in the hospital a decade ago, now is sent out to subacute care in a nursing home. The typical nursing home resident of the 1960s would today more likely be placed in an assisted living or residential care facility. Nursing homes are less and less composed of homogeneous populations; most nursing homes have populations of residents admitted near end of life, those with lengths of stay ranging from 6 months to years, patients admitted for rehabilitation after an acute hospital stay, and those in their last years of life lacking adequate community or family support to remain at home.[20] With tighter budgets and higher enforced federal and state requirements, it becomes an even greater challenge to provide individualized resident-focused care to all of these individuals.

One of the first successful legal cases involving inadequate pain management involved a nursing home resident with end-stage prostate cancer whose plan of care clearly delineated an adequate pain treatment plan, but whose plan of care was not followed.[52] Including pain within the scope of the MDS and as a quality indicator, and the initiation of JCAHO guidelines to have pain assessed in every healthcare site including long-term care, have also resulted in more appropriate recognition of, and treatment for, pain in long-term residents. Under or untreated pain is no longer acceptable regardless of the setting.

PAIN PREVALENCE IN LONG-TERM CARE

Estimates of pain prevalence specifically among nursing home residents vary widely with some estimates as high as 45–80 percent,[4] whereas in the community-dwelling older population estimates range between 25 percent and 50 percent.[5] The occurrence of concomitant sensory impairments, dementia and disability make assessing and managing pain a challenge in the long-term setting.

One of the earliest studies in the long-term care population involved 97 patients from a 311-bed long-term care multilevel facility.[51] Existence of pain problems and their management in addition to functional status, depression, and cognitive impairment were obtained from chart review and patient interview. Seventy-one percent of these patients had at least one pain complaint, of which 34 percent described continuous pain. Of the 43 subjects with intermittent pain, 51 percent had pain on a daily basis. Types of pain varied widely, although the majority involved musculoskeletal sources. The most striking finding was that only 15 percent had received pain medications within the previous 24 hours despite the fact that 84 percent had physician orders for pain medications. There were moderately strong correlations between pain and activity attendance. There was little statistical correlation between pain and depression scale, MMSE, and ADL scales although individuals often reported functional impairments with pain. Of greatest clinical significance was that the subjects reported substantial impairments in both their activities of daily living and quality of life due to pain. If we are to believe the patient report as the single best measure of the intensity and impact of pain,[14,53–55] then perhaps the patient's report of the effect of pain on their life is the most vital measure of all.

Arthritis is the single most common musculoskeletal source of pain in those over age 65. The prevalence of arthritis alone in nursing homes has been identified as between 23 percent and 24 percent.[56] In a study of 629 nursing home residents in the greater Boston area,[56] 23.3 percent had some form of arthritis. Even controlling for age, the residents with arthritis more often reported requiring assistance at least some of the time for six of eight functional task items, and using more assistive devices. The implication is that these residents would also likely need greater assistance from caregivers. Those with arthritis had higher visual analog scale scores (76.25 ± 31.75) than those without arthritis (51.93 ± 30.67).

In addition to the pains which likewise affect younger patients, there are also a number of problems occurring with higher prevalence in older patients such as polymyalgia rheumatica, angina, atherosclerotic vascular disease, temporal arteritis, cancer, herpes zoster, and peripheral neuropathies; and it is likely for an older patient to have two or more sources of pain. Therefore, it is vital that the provider assess each pain separately and continue to do so on an ongoing basis in order to treat the older person's total pain problem adequately. Pain in the older long-term care resident can significantly impact healthcare and quality of life concerns.

Pain occurs with approximately a 75 percent prevalence rate in cancer patients,[57] and undertreatment particularly of older patients has been fairly well described in various settings;[58–60] many of these patients may at some point in the disease trajectory require long-term care. As the incidence of most cancers increases with advancing age with rare exceptions, this amounts to a significant number of older individuals experiencing cancer pain. Despite the inclusion of other nonmalignant end-stage conditions such as renal failure, dementia, congestive heart failure and others, the majority of patients requiring hospice care continue to be admitted with cancer diagnoses.[61] Many hospice patients either are admitted already in long-term care or ultimately require nursing home admission as their illness worsens either temporarily or long term; in some areas hospices are establishing inpatient hospice units within or adjoining to existing nursing homes. Some long-term care facilities are even acquiring their own licenses for inpatient hospice care. Previously the hospice advised the nursing home in the area of pain assessment and management. With the advent of JCAHO, AMDA (American Medical Directors' Association), AGS (American Geriatrics Society), and other guidelines on pain and its management, and the increasing use of long-term care as a core clinical training site, long-term care facilities now have the potential to demonstrate clinical expertise in this area. The establishment of multiple guidelines which include the assessment and treatment of nonmalignant as well as malignant pain has led to a greater acceptance of the imperative to treat regardless of the pain etiology.[14,34,53–55]

CHALLENGES TO OVERCOME IN THE NURSING HOME

Although pain management in general has improved significantly over the last decade, there are many concerns unique to the long-term care environment that make pain assessment and management particularly challenging. These include systems barriers intrinsic to the nursing home care setting, physiological barriers to pain management in older persons, and research and educational barriers which interfere with effective clinical care.

Nursing homes lack the extensive diagnostic, nursing, and pharmacy resources present in higher acuity settings. Until the advent of the recent JCAHO, AGS, AMDA guidelines, the institution-wide commitment to pain assessment and management was not a long-term care priority. Whereas patients or caregivers can administer 'as needed' or prn doses in the home environment, the ability to respond to this request is severely hampered in long-term care by the significant number of planned medications required for each patient. Nursing home residents have on average seven to nine or more routine medications; in most states, regulations require that the medication be distributed within 1 hour before or 1 hour after the scheduled time period to get that medication to a resident, observed and properly recorded. It is therefore not unusual for patients to sometimes ask family

members to provide acetaminophen or other pain relievers handy for self dosing in lieu of requesting 'as needed' medications, resulting in potentially harmful situations. A useful exercise when making a home visit to a long-term care resident is asking permission to look in the bedside stand. It is not unusual to find almost any prescription or over-the-counter medication. In addition, interventions such as hot or cold packs which family members may have provided at home with good effect, require physician orders in long-term care. Each medication or laboratory test ordered also requires an accompanying diagnosis; medications in the five quality indicator categories (sedatives, anxiolytics, 'others' including mood stabilizers, antidepressants, and antipsychotics) also require the terminology 'AEB' (as exhibited by) with appropriate symptoms which the nursing staff can then flowsheet and track. The intent of this requirement is to have staff use a nondrug intervention and gauge its effectiveness before a medication in these categories is given. Pain adjuvants (valproate, gabapentin, tricyclics, etc.) given specifically for this purpose should be so labeled and would not require psychiatric tracking language.

Often long-term care residents have multiple medical problems and many potential sources of pain. Memory and sensory impairments, and increased sensitivity to adverse drug reactions are among the physiological barriers often encountered in the older population. Lack of family understanding of the goals of treatment, the difference between physical dependence and addiction, and often family inability to be present and involved during physician rounds in the nursing home may hinder communication and thus the provision of optimal pain management.

Educational and attitudinal barriers may exist among staff, families and patients as well. There are still misconceptions about changes in pain tolerance with aging, or that medications suitable for young patients cannot be used safely in older people, despite available evidence to the contrary even in cognitively impaired populations. And finally, many regulatory and policy barriers also exist, including the use of increasingly restricted formularies, and difficulty in obtaining opioid drugs in states where multiple copy prescriptions are required. The identification of potential barriers to pain management is an integral component of improving pain management in long-term care. With improved institutional commitment to optimal pain relief many of these barriers can be reduced or eliminated.

NURSING HOMES AS UNIQUE ENVIRONMENTS

Nursing homes are unique as evidenced by their interdisciplinary approach to care planning and provision. Team-based care is not only encouraged but required by state and federal and where applicable JCAHO rules and regulations, and is at least, therefore, indirectly reimbursed. Each resident's

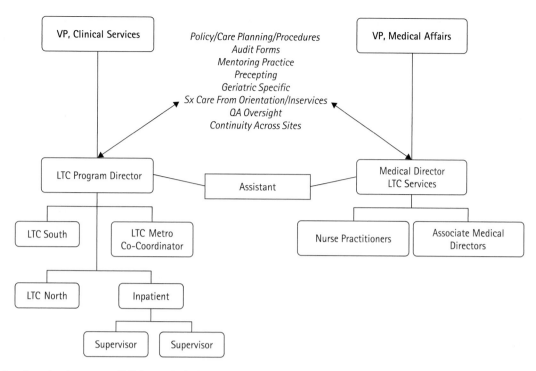

Figure 51.2 *Organization, responsibilities, and relationships between the interdisciplinary team members and nursing home residents with pain problems. LTC, long-term care; QA, quality assurance. Redrawn from Stein WM. Pain in the nursing home.* Clin Geriatr Med 2001; *17:* 582[7] *with permission from Elsevier.*

plan of care is required to be reviewed by an interdisciplinary team composed of nursing, social service, appropriate therapies, dietary, medical, and pharmacy services. Care plans are developed using a problem-oriented approach and revised every 30–90 days depending on the patient's acuity level. Pain management, like most areas of palliative care, is best accomplished by an interdisciplinary approach and thus adapts particularly well to the nursing home milieu. Figure 51.2 illustrates the organization, responsibilities, and relationships between the interdisciplinary team members and nursing home residents with pain problems. In community nursing homes, the administrator and nursing home board of directors/owner(s) have the ultimate responsibility for establishing and maintaining the function of the interdisciplinary team. Moreover, it is the administrator and ownership who are ultimately responsible for compliance with state and federal guidelines, regulatory issues, and the total quality of care provided in the facility. The individual healthcare team members each provide their particular expertise and share responsibility for pain management. They develop living care plans and work toward a common goal of pain management for individual patients based on the frequent and appropriate assessment of the resident's pain. Using this framework the team is usually successful in assisting the resident in reaching important goals including restoration and maintenance of function as the resident defines it, preservation of autonomy, delaying

the progression of chronic medical problems, and ensuring quality of life.

QUALITY OF LIFE AND OUTCOME MEASURES

Quality of life involves many dimensions. Some of the domains of quality of life frequently cited by investigators include physical concerns, functional ability, family well being, spirituality, social functioning, treatment satisfaction, financial concerns, future orientation, sexuality, intimacy, and occupational functioning. Most patients and clinicians agree that pain and its management substantially improve quality of life. An individual incapacitated by pain will not participate in rehabilitative or restorative therapy because of increased pain with movement, resulting in further deconditioning and isolation which limit the individual's ability to participate in social activities and interpersonal relationships. Patients with chronic pain may lose their sense of purpose and hope for the future when all they experience is unremitting pain and often present with chronic depression. Life stops focusing around activities and people that bring joy and meaning to their life and instead revolves around unremitting pain. Residents who have entered some part of the long-term care trajectory have already experienced multiple losses associated with aging and chronic disease. Unremitting pain only worsens this sense of loss.

Several investigators have developed instruments for the assessment of quality of life as an outcome measure for pain management but the role of these instruments in clinical practice remains uncertain. For example, it has been observed that although pain may improve dramatically, it may be overshadowed by other issues confounding the assessment of overall quality of life. In an era of ever increasing quantity of life, the quality of that life should demand equal attention.

Key learning points

- Pain assessment and treatment in the older person continues to offer considerable challenges. Multiple studies indicate a high prevalence of pain which is often poorly managed in both the cognitively intact and cognitively impaired.

- A variety of barriers to pain management have been identified that can be overcome with appropriate educational interventions and correction of common misconceptions concerning pain in this population.

- Clearly to date, no research has definitively shown changes in pain perception with the aging process.[62–65] Additional research still remains to be done to more accurately identify and treat pain in this population, particularly in the case of the cognitively impaired resident.

- The validity and reliability of standard pain assessment tools need to be better defined, and new pain tools developed which are specific to this population.

- Drugs with milder side effect profiles are desperately needed, and as new drugs are developed more studies need to be done in every segment of the older population particularly in those over 80 years of age.

- Nonpharmacological strategies including exercise programs, and physical methods of pain control need to be scientifically evaluated in this population.

- These challenges will require practical clinical solutions that take into account the physiological barriers to pain management in long-term care residents, the pharmacokinetic changes which occur with normal aging, as well as the limited resources and logistical issues often encountered in various care settings where older persons often reside.

REFERENCES

1 Loeser JD, Melzack R. Pain: an overview. *Lancet* 1999; **353**: 1607–9.
2 Max MB, Payne R, eds. *Principles of Analgesic Use in Treatment of Acute Pain and Cancer Pain*. 4th ed. Glenview, IL: American Pain Society, 1999.
3 Helm RD, Gibson SJ. Epidemiology of pain in elderly people. *Clin Geriatr Med* 2001; **17**: 417–31.
4 Ferrell BA. Pain evaluation and management in the nursing home. *Ann Intern Med* 1995; **123**: 681–7.
5 Cooner E, Amorosi S. *The Study of Pain and Older Americans*. New York: Louis Harris and Associates, 1997.
6 Parmalee PA, Smith B, Katz, IR. Pain complaints and cognitive status among elderly institution residents. *J Am Geriatr Soc* 1993; **41**: 517–22.
7 Stein WM. Pain in the nursing home. *Clin Geriatr Med* 2001; **17**: 575–94.
8 Folstein MF, Folstein SE, McHugh PR. Mini Mental State: a practical method for grading the cognitive state of patients for the clinician. *J Psychiatr Res* 1975; **12**: 89–198.
9 Katz, S, Downs TD, Cash, HR, Grotz RC. Progress in development of the Index of ADL. *Gerontologist.* 1970; **10**: 20–30.
10 Melzack R, Katz J. The McGill Pain Questionnaire: appraisal and current status. In Turk D, Melzack R, eds. *Handbook of Pain Assessment*. New York. Guilford Press 1992: 152–68.
11 Melzack R. The McGill Pain Questionnaire: major properties and scoring methods. *Pain* 1975; **1**: 277–99.
12 Melzack R. The Short-Form McGill Pain Questionnaire. *Pain* 1987; **30**: 191–7.
13 Ferrell BA, Stein WM, Beck JC. The Geriatric Pain Measure: validity, reliability and factor analysis. *J Am Geriatr Soc* 2000; **48**: 1669–73.
14 AGS Panel on Chronic Pain in Older Persons. The management of chronic pain in older persons. *J Am Geriatr Soc* 1998; **46**: 635–51.
15 Gloth FM III, Scheve AA, Stober CV, *et al*. The Functional Pain Scale: reliability, validity and responsiveness in an elderly population. *J Am Dir Assoc* 2001; **2**: 110–14.
16 Herr KA, Garand L. Assessment and measurement of pain in older adults. *Clin Geriatr Med* 2001; **17**: 457–78.
17 Cohen-Mansfield J, Marx MS. Pain and depression in the nursing home: corroborating results. *J Gerontol* 1993; **48**: 96–97.
18 Parmalee PA, Katz IR, Lawton MP. The relation of pain to depression among institutionalized aged. *J Gerontol* 1991; **46**: 15–21.
19 Derogatis LR, Morrow GR, Fetting J, *et al*. The prevalence of psychiatric disorders among cancer patients. *JAMA* 1983; **249**: 751–7.
20 Ouslander JG, Osterweil D, Morley J, eds. *Medical Care in the Nursing Home*. New York: McGraw-Hill. 1997.
21 Lipowski ZJ. Delirium. In: Hazzard WB, Bierman EL, Blass JP, *et al*., eds. *Principles of Geriatric Medicine and Gerontology*. New York: McGraw-Hill, Inc., 1994: 1021–6.
22 Mittlemark MB. The epidemiology of aging. In: Hazzard WB, Bierman EL, Blass JP, *et al*., eds. *Principles of Geriatric Medicine and Gerontology*. New York: McGraw-Hill, Inc., 1994: 221–8.
23 Folstein MF, Folstein SE. Syndromes of altered mental state. In: Hazzard WB, Bierman EL, Blass JP, *et al*., eds. *Principles of Geriatric Medicine and Gerontology*. New York: McGraw-Hill, Inc., 1994: 1197–204.
24 Michaels DD. The eye. In: Hazzard WB, Bierman EL, Blass JP, *et al*., eds. *Principles of Geriatric Medicine and Gerontology*. New York: McGraw-Hill, Inc., 1994: 441–56.
25 Rees TS, Duckert LG, Milczuk HA. Auditory and vestibular dysfunction. In: Hazzard WB, Bierman EL, Blass JP, *et al*., eds. *Principles of Geriatric Medicine and Gerontology*. New York: McGraw-Hill, Inc., 1994: 457–72.

26 Mangione CM. Vision and hearing: screening and treatment efficacy. Lecture. *Proceedings of the Intensive Course in Geriatric Medicine*. UCLA Multicampus Program in Geriatrics and Gerontology, 1997: 267–76.

27 Sengstaken EA, King SA. The problem of pain and its detection among geriatric nursing home residents. *J Am Geriatr Soc* 1993; **41**: 541–4.

28 Parmalee PA. Pain in cognitively impaired older persons. *Clin Geriatr Med* 1996; **12**: 473–87.

29 Ferrell BA, Ferrell BR, Rivera L. Pain in cognitively impaired nursing home patients. *J Pain Symptom Manage* 1995; **10**: 591–8.

30 Marzinski LR. The tragedy of dementia: clinically assessing pain in the confused, nonverbal elderly. *J Gerontol Nurs* 1991; **17**: 25–8.

31 Kovach CR, Weissman DE, Griffie J, *et al*. Assessment and treatment of discomfort for people with late-stage dementia. *J Pain Symptom Manage* 1999; **18**: 412–19.

32 Warden V, Hurley AC, Volicer L. Development and psychometric evaluation of the Pain Assessment in Advanced Dementia (PAINAD) Scale. *J Am Med Dir Assoc* 2003; **4**: 9–15.

33 Stein WM. Assessment of symptoms in the cognitively impaired. In: Bruera E, Portenoy RK, eds. *Topics in Palliative Care*. New York: Oxford University Press, 2001: 123–33.

34 Jacox A, Carr DB, Payne R, *et al*. *Management of Cancer Pain. Clinical Practice Guideline 9*. AHCPR Publication 94-0592. Rockville MD: Agency for Health Care Policy and Research, US Department of Health and Human Services, Public Health Service, 1994.

35 Forman WB. Opioid analgesic drugs in the elderly. *Clin Geriatr Med* 1996; **12**: 489–500.

36 Beers MH. Explicit criteria for determining potentially inappropriate medication use by the elderly. *Arch Intern Med* 1997; **157**: 1531–6.

37 Gurwitz JH, Avorn J, Ross-Degnan D, Sipsitz LA. Nonsteroidal anti-inflammatory drug associated azotemia in the very old. *JAMA* 1990; **264**: 471–5.

38 Griffin MR, Piper JM, Daugherty JR, *et al*. Nonsteroidal anti-inflammatory drug use and increased risk for peptic ulcer disease in elderly persons. *Ann Intern Med* 1991; **114**: 257–63.

39 Silverstein FE, Graham DY, Senior JR, *et al*. Misoprostol reduces serious gastrointestinal complications in patients with rheumatoid arthritis receiving nonsteroidal anti-inflammatory drugs. *Ann Intern Med* 1995; **123**: 241–9.

40 Kaiko RF. Age and morphine analgesia in cancer patients with postoperative pain. *Clin Pharmacol Ther* 1980; **28**: 823–6.

41 Kaiko RF, Wallenstein SL, Rogers AG, *et al*. Narcotics in the elderly. *Med Clin North Am* 1982; **66**: 1079–89.

42 Max MB, Lynch SA, Muir J, *et al*. Effects of desipramine, amitriptyline, and fluoxetine on pain in diabetic neuropathy. *N Engl J Med* 1992; **326**: 1250–6.

43 Backonja M, Beydoun A, Edwards KR, et al, for the Gabapentin Diabetic Neuropathy Study Group. Gabapentin for the symptomatic treatment of painful neuropathy in patients with diabetes mellitus: a randomized controlled trial. *JAMA* 1998; **280**: 1831–6.

44 Rowbotham M, Harden N, Stacey B, et al for the Gabapentin Postherpetic Neuralgia Study Group. Gabapentin for the treatment of postherpetic neuralgia: a randomized controlled trial. *JAMA* 1998; **280**: 1837–42.

45 Prager JP. Invasive modalities for the diagnosis and treatment of pain in the elderly. *Clin Geriatr Med* 1996; **12**: 549–61.

46 Watson CP. Topical capsaicin as an adjuvant analgesic. *J Pain Symptom Manage* 1994; **9**: 425–33.

47 Rowbotham MC, Davies PS, Verkempinck C, Galer BS. Lidocaine patch: a double-blinded controlled study of a new treatment method for postherpetic neuralgia. *Pain* 1996; **65**: 39–44.

48 Foster DF, Phillips RS, Hamel MB, Eisenberg DM. Alternative medicine use in older americans. *J Am Geriatr Soc* 2000; **48**: 1560–5.

49 Miller SC, Mor V, Teno J. Hospice enrollment and pain assessment and management in nursing homes. *J Pain Symptom Manage* 2003; **26**: 791–9.

50 Ferrell BA. Pain management in elderly people. *J Am Geriatr Soc* 1991; **39**: 64–73.

51 Ferrell BA, Ferrell BR, Osterweil D. Pain in the nursing home. *J Am Geriatr Soc* 1990; **38**: 409–14.

52 Shapiro RS. Liability issues in the management of pain. *J Pain Symptom Manage* 1994; **9**: 146–52.

53 Acute Pain Management Guideline Panel. *Acute Pain Management: Post-operative or Medical Procedures and Trauma. Clinical Practice Guideline. #1*. AHCPR Publication 92-0032. Rockville, MD: Agency for Health Care Policy and Research, Public Health Service, US Department of Health and Human Services, 1993.

54 APS Task Force on Pain, Symptoms, and End of Life Care. Treatment at the End of Life: A Position Statement from the American Pain Society. *APS Bull* 1997; **7**: 11.

55 American Medical Directors' Association. *Chronic Pain Management in the Long-Term Care Setting. Clinical Practice Guideline*. Columbia, MD: AMDA, 1999.

56 Guccione AA, Meenan RF, Anderson JJ. Arthritis in nursing home residents. *Arthritis Rheum* 1989; **32**: 1546–53.

57 Stein WM. Cancer pain in the elderly. In: Ferrell BR, Ferrell BA, eds. *Pain in the Elderly*. Seattle: IASP Press, 1996: 69–80.

58 Bernabei R, Gambassi G, Lapane K, *et al*. Management of pain in elderly patients with cancer. *JAMA* 1998; **279**: 1877–82.

59 Cleeland CS, Gonin R, Hatfield AK, *et al*. Pain and its treatment in outpatients with metastatic cancer. *N Engl J Med* 1994; **330**: 592–6.

60 Von Roenn JH, Cleelan CS, Gonin R, *et al*. Physician attitudes and practice in cancer pain management. A survey from the eastern cooperative oncology group. *Ann Intern Med* 1993; **119**: 121–6.

61 Stein WM, Miech RP. Cancer pain in the elderly hospice patient. *J Pain Symptom Manage* 1993; **8**: 474–82.

62 Gibson SJ, Helme RD. Age differences in pain perception and report: a review of physiological psychological, laboratory and clinical studies. *Pain Rev* 1995; **2**: 111–37.

63 Gibson SJ, Helme RD. Age related differences in pain perception and report. *Clin Geriatr Med* 2001; **17**: 433–56.

64 Harkins SW. Pain perceptions in the old. *Clin Geriatr Med* 1996; **12**: 435–59.

65 Porter FL, Malhotra KM, Wolf CM, *et al*. Dementia and response to pain in the elderly. *Pain* 1996; **68**: 413–21.

52

Neuropathic pain

MARCO LACERENZA, FABIO FORMAGLIO, LIA TELONI, PAOLO MARCHETTINI

INTRODUCTION

Diagnosing and treating neuropathic pain remains a major challenge for neurologists, oncologists, and pain specialists. Major advances in clinical and experimental research in the past decade(s) have shed light on the multiple types of neuropathic pain; it is now recognized that the same clinical condition may have diverse pathophysiological mechanisms.[1] The International Association for the Study of Pain[2] defines neurogenic pain as 'Pain initiated or caused by a primary lesion or dysfunction or transitory perturbation in the peripheral or central nervous system'. Neuropathic pain is a subentity where 'transitory perturbation' is omitted. The inclusion of 'dysfunction' in the definition of neuropathic pain raises confusion, because it allows improper labeling of nociceptive and psychogenic conditions as neurogenic/neuropathic. To clarify and simplify the definition of neuropathic pain, we proposed[3] amending the definition to 'pain due to primary lesion of the peripheral or central nervous system', a concept now approved by recognized pain experts.[4,5]

Neuropathic pain originates from diseases or trauma to the peripheral or central nervous system, and exhibits an acute or chronic temporal profile, the latter being by far more common and disabling. Pain and related neuropathic symptoms and signs may fluctuate according to the temporal evolution of the painful disease, mood and anxiety of the patient, and even weather conditions (trigeminal neuralgia).

Neuropathic pain can be spontaneous (stimulus-independent pain) with an episodic or continuous temporal profile. Episodic paroxysms are typical of trigeminal and glossopharyngeal neuralgias, but other pains in neuropathy may appear as isolated attacks or attacks of increasing intensity superimposed on continuous pain. Spontaneous symptoms are described as uncommon tactile and thermal sensations associated with numbness, tingling, pins and needles, burning, shooting, or electric shocklike sensation. In addition, the common aching pain, attributable to the nociceptive component, may be part of the clinical picture of painful peripheral neuropathies and a frequent complaint in patients with central pain due to multiple sclerosis[6] and syringomyelia.[7]

Neuropathic pain may also be evoked. The evoking stimulus may cause massive activation of ectopic sensory discharges by acting on mechanosensitive neural pathways. The maneuvers evoking the latter are improperly called clinical signs and classically referred to by their eponyms (Lhermitte, Lasègue, and Spurling are widely known). Pain may also be evoked by direct stimulation of cutaneous nerve endings (stimulus-dependent pain) unchaining a sequence of spontaneous attacks, such as trigger point activation of tic douloureux, or remaining time locked within the original stimulus, however, with exaggeratedly intense or distorted quality. Dysesthesia, hyperalgesia, and allodynia are the terms applied to define aberrant evoked sensory phenomena. Such aberrant sensations appear following a lesion in the peripheral or central nervous system; obviously similar symptoms originating from anatomically different sites and causes are likely to have different pathophysiology. Sensitization of nociceptors, ectopic activity, and multiplication of impulses are probable peripheral mechanisms of dysesthesia and hyperalgesia.[8] Disinhibition of the spinothalamic pathway and, again, ectopic activity, are likely central mechanisms, although the evidence in humans is still weak. It is at least recognized that central pain and pain evoked by central stimuli require abnormal spinothalamic function.[9*,10*] Allodynia is a more complex condition. By definition the term implies a painful perception evoked by stimuli (mechanical or thermal) of intensity below nociceptor threshold. Therefore allodynia is widely viewed as the clinical 'sign' of central sensitization.[1] However, nociceptor threshold is remarkably lower than pain threshold, the pain perception requiring temporal and spatial summation of nociceptive impulses to overcome the endogenous inhibitory state. Thus, what common experience would reasonably define as stimulus of painless intensity might be sufficient to activate nociceptors.[11] Hyperactivity and multiplication of discharges in peripheral nociceptive afferents may well give rise to allodynia. Novel recordings from nociceptors in patients with allodynia due to painful neuropathies provide objective evidence for this peripheral explanation.[12]

When considering the somato-topical organization of the peripheral and central nervous systems, all neuropathic pains are perceived to occur within the innervation territory of the damaged structure. A thorough exploration of the neuroanatomical distribution of pain and sensory alteration using a pain drawing completed by the patient aids the diagnosis[3] that otherwise relies on the medical history and bedside examination. The evaluation aims at correlating sensory, motor, and autonomic signs with the anatomical localization of the lesion based on a careful history.

Autonomic signs may be a direct consequence of the nerve injury or a consequence of spinal/supraspinal reflex to nociceptive input, and care should be taken to distinguish between these phenomena.[13] Clinical neurophysiological tests such as electromyography, nerve conduction studies, evoked potentials, infrared telethermography, and quantitative mechanical and thermal threshold tests supplement the clinical diagnosis allowing definition of nerve fibers or central sensory pathways involved.

NEUROPATHIC PAIN SYNDROMES IN PATIENTS WITH CANCER

In the final stages of the disease 80 percent of cancer patients complain of pain,[14] and a neurological complication is frequently heralded by pain.[15*] Direct activity of the tumor causes nerve trunk, nerve plexus or radiculospinal compression; among the indirect consequences are paraneoplastic polyneuropathies, ischemic mononeuropathy, and postherpetic neuralgia. In the early clinical phase, compression or invasion of the peripheral or central nervous system by tumor generates a nociceptive pain due to stimulation of the perineurium or the meninges. This nerve-trunk pain[16] or meningeal pain, responds well to drugs effective against nociceptive pain, such as nonsteroidal anti-inflammatory drugs (NSAIDs) or opioids. In the following phase, when the axonal membranes get damaged, typical neuropathic symptoms enter the clinical picture. Two clinical studies tried identifying the different types of pain in cancer patients and found that 5 percent and 10 percent had pure neuropathic pain, 64 percent and 49 percent had nociceptive pain, 31 percent and 41 percent had mixed pain. Overall, 36 percent of pains in one study[17*] and 51 percent in the other study[18**] had a neuropathic component. A multicenter survey of IASP Task Force on

Cancer Pain reporting in 1999, found neuropathic mechanisms in 39.7 percent of 1095 patients from 24 countries.[19*]

Neuropathic pain syndromes due to direct or indirect activity of the tumor

Classic trigeminal neuralgia is among the presenting symptoms of malignancies of middle and posterior cranial fossae.[20*] Most commonly, bone or meningeal invasion causes constant deep aching pain overlapping with paroxysmal electric shocklike trigeminal pain. With the progression of the illness, neuropathic pain becomes continuous. Spontaneous deep burning sensation combined with sensory loss and other focal neurological signs appear following axonal loss. A progressively worsening pain in the territory of the trigeminal or other cranial sensory nerves, coupled with evolving neurological signs or symptoms is almost pathognomonic of head/neck tumors.

The intercostal nerve syndrome, caused by metastatic spread into a rib, is a common example of syndromes caused by peripheral nerve compression and infiltration by the evolving cancer. A period of deep aching pain in the chest precedes the appearance of a continuous burning pain with superimposed episodes of segmentally distributed, shooting pain. Later, positive and negative sensory symptoms combine and worsen progressively, culminating in the fracture of the rib.

Plexopathies

Nerve plexus lesions in cancer frequently lead to pain with a neuropathic component. The nerve injury can be caused by direct invasion by the primary tumor, dissemination via lymph nodes, postradiation therapy or surgery. Cervical plexus involvement is witnessed in primary or metastatic head or neck tumors, resulting from invasion or compression from the growing mass or from surgical and/or radiation treatment. The neuropathic pain syndrome reflects the anatomical distribution of the damaged nerve fibers. Pain and sensory symptoms can arise from the lesser and greater occipital nerves territories in the occipital region, the preauricular area supplied by the greater auricular nerve, and the anterior part of the neck and shoulder innervated by the transverse cutaneous and supraclavicular nerves, and may also project to the jaw.[21*] A combination of nociceptive and neuropathic pains with positive and negative sensory symptoms in multiple nerves territories is the rule in patients with postsurgery and postradiation syndromes.

Brachial plexopathy is a frequent neurological complication in patient with cancer and occurs in lymphoma and breast and lung carcinoma. Pain usually precedes focal neurological signs, even up to 9 months; it is the most common symptom in 85 percent of patients.[22*] Lower plexus invasion is by far the most common, as in Pancoast syndrome due to apical lung cancer. An aching pain in the shoulder, subscapular area and upper back may appear some months before a burning pain in the armpit. Clinical examination usually reveals sensory loss in the intercostobrachial nerve territory, of which patients are frequently unaware. In the early phase, an X-ray of the chest often has normal findings and only computed tomography (CT) or magnetic resonance imaging (MRI) of the chest reveals the neoplasm.[23] The advanced clinical picture includes Horner syndrome (Fig. 52.1) and focal weakness, atrophy, sensory loss in the hand and severe electromyographic-electroneurographic abnormalities in the C7, C8, and T1 root distribution. Involvement of the upper plexus (C4, C5, C6 roots) by metastatic breast carcinoma and lymphoma is less frequent. Pain is localized in the shoulder girdle, worsened by neck movement, and projected to the radial side of the hand with tingling, sensory loss, burning and shooting sensations. The combination of Lhermitte sign, Horner syndrome, and pan-plexopathy strongly suggests epidural extension, which can be occur even in the absence of bony erosion in patients with lymphoma.[22*]

Painful lumbosacral plexopathy (LSP), and its complications, is a most disabling condition in cancer. Pelvic tumors and metastatic malignancies almost always cause pain in the buttocks and/or legs following lumbosacral plexus invasion.[24*] The insidious onset of an aching and cramping nociceptive pain, provoked by perineural invasion and activation of nociceptors in the nervi nervorum, typically precedes neuropathic pain. In Jaeckle and coworkers' series of 85 patients with proved LSP, causalgic pain was present in 8 percent. They described three types of pain: local pain (85 percent), radicular pain (85 percent) and referred pain (44 percent), which was associated with an upper plexopathy (L1–L4) in about a third of the cases, a lower plexopathy (L4–S1) in half of the cases, and a pan-plexopathy in less than a fifth. The anatomical distribution of weakness and sensory symptoms and signs, usually appearing after the pain, does not always correlate with CT imaging – the examination usually reveals wider invasion.[24*] Presence of pain and neurological signs of LSP with normal findings on CT of the abdomen and pelvis calls for a differential diagnosis of meningeal carcinomatosis, epidural cord compression, and cauda equina compression.

Radiculopathies and myelopathies

Painful radiculopathies in patients with cancer are usually related to direct compression or invasion of nerve roots by vertebral and paraspinal cancers or leptomeningeal metastases. There can be nociceptive focal and neuropathic pain projected along the distribution of the damaged root. When multifocal radiculopathies are associated with headache and changes in mental status, the clinical picture is highly suggestive of leptomeningeal metastases.[25] The clinical picture of myelopathy is often preceded by local nociceptive pain due to invasion of vertebral body or epidural space and

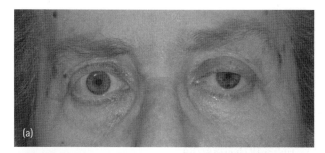

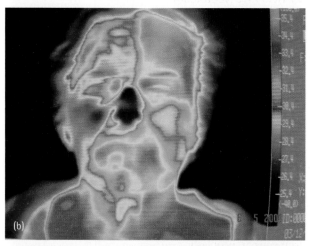

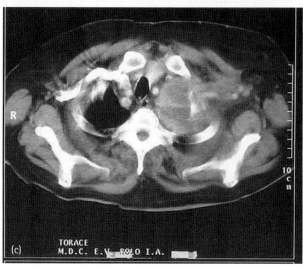

Figure 52.1 *(a) This 72-year-old woman developed aching pain in the left shoulder followed by projected burning pain in the left upper limb 4 months prior to examination. The neurological evaluation revealed Horner syndrome and signs of left lower brachial plexus involvement. (b) Telethermography revealed straightforward thermal asymmetry of the face, the left side warmer being than the right due to sympathetic denervation. (c) Computed tomography of the pulmonary apex disclosed a Pancoast tumor on the left side.*

then neuropathic pain of radicular origin. When the compression extends to the dorsal column of the spinal cord, generating focal demyelination, the presence of Lhermitte sign confirms the onset of clinical myelopathy.

Rarely, in case of advanced myelopathy, neuropathic pain originates from compression/invasion of spinothalamic pathways. The pain is usually unilateral, a few myelomeres below the affected level – extended down to the foot or with a patchy distribution, associated with tingling and allodynias, mainly due to cold and spontaneous thermal sensations.

POSTHERPETIC NEURALGIA

Postherpetic neuralgia is a painful radiculopathy following herpes zoster infection usually in the mid-thoracic dermatomes and in the ophthalmic branch of the trigeminal nerve. It is more common in altered immune states, e.g. in older people and in patients with cancer (mainly leukemia and lymphomas), and it has been shown that the site of the primary tumor correlates with the site of subsequent herpes zoster infection.[26*] Neuropathic pain can be spontaneous with deep aching, burning and shooting components, or stimulus dependent with allodynia and/or hyperalgesia.[27]

Polyneuropathies

Peripheral paraneoplastic neuropathies, due to either indirect cancer activity or the immune reaction against the cancer, may be painful. Altogether, these are a rare complication of cancer and an accurate diagnosis is crucial: sometimes it may uncover the tumor. Paraneoplastic sensory neuronopathy is a disabling condition presenting with neuropathic pain and progressive sensory loss in the limbs, trunk, and face. Burning pain and shooting sensations are present and associated with asymmetrically distributed numbness and tingling. Symptoms usually appear before, by weeks or months, the diagnosis of tumor, which most frequently is a small-cell lung cancer or less frequently a breast carcinoma. Given the high specificity (99.8 percent) and sensitivity (82 percent) of anti-Hu antibodies,[28] in patients with no evidence of cancer a CT study of the chest should be done.

Although paraneoplastic sensory neuropathy is related to an inflammatory, probably immune-mediated lesion of sensory neurons, usually it does not respond to plasma exchange, intravenous immunoglobulin, or immunosuppressants but to early treatment of the tumor.[29] Early symptomatic treatment of neuropathic pain is mandatory. Among other painful paraneoplastic disorders affecting the peripheral nervous system is the Guillain–Barré syndrome, which sometimes can be heralded by radicular pains, and a nonsystemic vasculitic neuropathy. This subacute and progressive condition can be associated with small-cell lung cancer and lymphomas and involves sensory and motor fibers in a symmetric or asymmetric fashion. Early diagnosis of paraneoplastic vasculitis encourages combined treatment with steroids and cyclophosphamide, with better results than steroids alone.[30] Severe local pain can be related to the inflammatory biochemical cascade that leads to activation/sensitization of nervi nervorum, followed by ischemia and consequent axonal damage and neuropathic pain along the anatomical distribution of the damaged nerve.

Table 52.1 summarizes the neuropathic pain syndromes in the patient with cancer along with their etiology.

IATROGENIC NEUROPATHIC PAIN IN CANCER

Bleuler in 1924 introduced the term 'iatrogenic' to define any disorder 'generated or caused by medicine or medical doctors'. Longer survival times and more aggressive surgical and medical treatment of cancer have led to an increase in iatrogenic painful conditions. Iatrogenic neuropathic pain in cancer patients may arise as a consequence of radiotherapy, chemotherapy, or surgical nerve lesions.[31] Pain in malignancies is often associated with cancer recurrence. The appearance of a novel painful condition deserves extensive examination aimed at early diagnosis of the cause of the pain. Informing the patient that the pain is iatrogenic and not a direct consequence of the tumor reduces their anxiety and results in a favorable response to specific treatment.

Neuropathic pain as a consequence of radiotherapy

Radiation may provoke painful myelopathy or peripheral nerve lesions. High-dose radiotherapy close to the spine causes transient or, less frequently, delayed progressive myelopathy that occasionally has the features of a central pain syndrome.[32*,33*] Sometimes the presenting complaint of a post-radiation myeloradiculopathy is the Lhermitte sign.[34*] Painful brachial plexopathy is the most common post radiotherapy syndrome. The nerve injury may be direct or indirect, i.e. infarction of the brachial plexus due to thrombosis of the subclavian artery and its branches.[35*] High-voltage radiation may cause acute painful but reversible brachial plexopathy.[36*] A delayed, but usually not painful, brachial plexopathy due to radiation fibrosis may develop several months after radiotherapy, with tingling and large fiber sensory loss within the upper plexus distribution.[37] In contrast, recurrent cancer with invasion of the peripheral nerves is often severely painful with neuropathic and nociceptive pains. Electromyographic studies help in differentiating the two conditions, with radiation being associated with myokymias more often than tumor invasion.[38]

Lumbosacral plexopathy, which is rarely painful, may also follow radiotherapy as a late delayed complication.[39] However, pelvic pain and lower extremity paralysis are described as an acute complication, occurring up to 10 weeks following completion of radiation therapy for cervical cancer.[40*]

Table 52.1 *Neuropathic pain in patients with cancer*

	Clinical syndrome	Etiology
Nerve compression/invasion	Trigeminal neuralgia	Middle and posterior cranial fossa tumors, base of skull metastases
	Glossopharyngeal neuralgia	Jugular foramen invasion, leptomeningeal metastases
	Intercostal neuralgia	Primary or metastatic lung, pleural, rib cancer
Direct effects of cancer		
Cervical compression/invasion plexopathies	Postauricular neuralgia	Primary head and neck cancer and cervical lymph node metastases
	Preauricular neuralgia	
	Anterior part of the neck neuralgia	
Brachial compression/invasion plexopathies	Upper brachial plexus neuralgia	Lymphoma and cervical lymph node metastases from breast and lung cancer
	Pancoast syndrome	Breast metastases and lung cancer
Lumbosacral compression/invasion plexopathies	Upper lumbar (L1–L4) neuralgia	Primary cancer: colorectal, genitourinary and sarcoma, lymphoma
	Lower lumbar (L5–S1) neuralgia	Metastatic cancer: colorectal, breast, lymphoma, genitourinary, melanoma, lung, gastric
	Sacrococcygeal neuralgia	
Compression/invasion of nerve root	Unilateral pain in the cervical and lumbosacral radicular territories	Vertebral cancer
	Frequently bilateral distribution in the thoracic dermatomes	Paraspinal invasion
		Epidural invasion
		Leptomeningeal dissemination
Compression/invasion of spinal cord	Rarely, central pain with Brown–Séquard syndrome	Primary and metastatic cancer
Compression/invasion of thalamocortical projections	Rarely, central pain with thalamic syndrome	Primary and metastatic cancer
Indirect effects of cancer		
Paraneoplastic neuropathies	Sensory ganglionopathy	Small cell lung, ovary, colon, and breast carcinomas
	Guillain–Barré syndrome	
	Nonsystemic vasculitis	Small cell lung cancer, lymphoma
	Brachial plexopathy	
Acute herpes zoster	Frequently in the thoracic dermatomes, ophthalmic branch of the trigeminal nerve and in previously irradiated dermatomes	Leukemia, lymphomas, post irradiation
Postherpetic neuralgia		
Nerve entrapment due to lymphedema	Brachial plexopathy	Post mastectomy
Ischemic neuropathy/ies	Painful mono/multiple neuropathy	Thrombosis, compression/invasion of small arteries
Cerebral hemorrhage	Central pain with thalamic syndrome	Primary and metastatic cancer
Iatrogenic neuropathic pain in cancer		
Postsurgical nerve lesion	Post neck surgery syndrome	Neck dissection
	Intercostobrachial neuralgia	Mastectomy
	Intercostal neuralgia	Thoracotomy
	Post-thoracotomy pain	Thoracotomy
	Phantom pain	Limb, breast, rectal amputation
	Stump pain	
Postradiation neuropathies	Painful brachial plexopathy acute and delayed, rarely painful lumbosacral plexopathy	Radiotherapy
Postradiation myelopathy	Central pain with Brown–Séquard syndrome	
Painful polyneuropathy associated with chemotherapy	Distal ascending pain and sensory symptoms	Platinum compounds, vincristine, taxanes, and their combination

Neuropathic pain as a consequence of chemotherapy

Peripheral polyneuropathy is a common complication of chemotherapy. Neuropathic pain and sensory symptoms are often the limiting factor in chemotherapy with cisplatin, vincristine, and the taxanes. The severity of nerve damage is directly proportional to drug dosage.[41–43] Patients with preexisting neuropathy due to diabetes mellitus, alcohol, hereditary neuropathies, paraneoplastic neuropathy, or earlier treatment with neurotoxic chemotherapy are thought to be more vulnerable to developing chemotherapy-induced peripheral neuropathy.[44] Ascending distal paresthesias and dysesthesias together with burning pain and allodynia to cold or mechanical stimuli in a glove and stocking distribution often appear after chemotherapy. The mechanisms producing the nerve injury, and in particular neuropathic pain and sensory symptoms, are not clear.

A common mechanism has been proposed for the toxicity of cisplatin, vincristine, and taxol.[45] Vincristine therapy provokes a predominantly sensory, sometimes autonomic subacute neuropathy in almost all patients. Cisplatinum neuropathy becomes clinically evident with cumulative dosages of the drug, nerve deterioration continuing months after drug withdrawal.[46*] The widely used paclitaxel is known to provoke neuropathic pain and sensory dysfunctions that mostly affect the hands and feet, and is related to a myelinated fiber neuropathy preferentially affecting the largest fibers (with sparing of C fibers).[45]

Brachial and lumbosacral plexopathy may also be related to chemotherapy. Chemotherapy administration through the subclavian or iliac artery may cause an acute painful brachial or lumbosacral plexopathy, which is sometimes irreversible. This is probably due to direct damage to small vessels and thrombosis, which leads to infarction of the nerve plexus.[47*]

Postsurgical neuropathies

Postinjury neuralgia is a relatively rare event compared with the large number of nerve injuries provoked by surgical trauma, perioperative ischemia, compression, and delayed scar entrapment. Although reliable clinical data are lacking, the incidence of painful neuralgia following peripheral nerve injury seems to be about 2.5–5 percent of the injuries.[48]

Post-neck surgery syndrome

Neck and nuchal pain may arise as a consequence of cutaneous nerve lesions provoked by surgical interventions for primary or metastatic head or neck tumor. Pain affects almost 50 percent of patients, sometimes weeks after neck dissection.[49*] According to the aggressiveness of tumor and the timing and location of the surgery, the pain may have nociceptive and neuropathic components. In half of the patients the pain subsides in a few months, whereas in the other half it lasts for years.[49*] In studies reporting on pain following neck surgery, 8 percent of patients complained of shoulder and arm pain, increasing to around 30 percent after a 1-year period.[49*,50,51] Only 2 percent of the patients reported this pain as 'severe',[49*] but most of them judged it to be debilitating.[51] Shoulder pain and disability were shown to be proportional to the surgical extension; they seem to be reduced in modified radical neck dissection and selective neck dissection compared with standard radical neck dissection.[52*] Therefore it is likely that the surgical technique influences the pain occurrence.

Pain following breast cancer surgery

More than 50 percent of patients have chronic pain syndromes after breast cancer surgery.[53] Acute postoperative pain has both nociceptive and neuropathic components, whereas persistent pain has predominantly a neuropathic origin. A recent, validated classification of neuropathic pain following breast cancer surgery has identified four classes: phantom breast pain, intercostobrachial neuralgia, neuroma pain, and other nerve injury pain.[53] In another study pain occurrence correlated significantly with the surgical extension: infrequent in lumpectomy but involving up to 72 percent of patients who underwent axillary lymph node dissection.[54*] In these cases, pain appearance was positively associated with the number of lymph nodes removed.[54*] Pain seems to be less frequent when careful surgical techniques are used, or when surgeons perform more interventions, as in hospitals experienced in breast surgery.[55*]

Post-thoracotomy pain

One year after thoracic surgery up to 61 percent of the patients report post-thoracotomy pain. Chronic pain development is directly related to the degree of postoperative pain severity.[56*] This pain may be due to intercostal nerve lesions, or to brachial plexus traction. Transaxillary rib resection is one of the causes of brachial plexopathy.[57] Persistent chest pain may also be due to complete intercostal nerve transection, sometimes followed by painful neuroma. Seventy percent of patients undergoing thoracotomy report severe pain (usually subsiding after 2 months time) with a neuropathic component. Progressive pain, worsening over weeks or months, and recurrence of chest pain following a pain-free period are significant negative prognostic symptoms, suspicious for cancer recurrence.[58*]

THERAPY

Treatment for neuropathic pain at the end of life differs from the management of chronic nonmalignant pain. In palliative care relief of pain is the priority while preservation of functionality becomes a secondary issue. Therefore, the overall side effects, and in particular the sedative effects of opioids and adjuvant drugs may become acceptable, providing the drugs offer adequate pain control. The current recommendation of care is to follow the World Health Organization (WHO) ladder, choosing an analgesic regimen on the basis of pain intensity, and adding adjuvant drugs in selected pain syndromes.[17*,59*] Adjuvants analgesic mechanisms are often complementary to opioids. Well-established guidelines recommend a combination of opioids and adjuvant drug to improve the analgesic regimen of patients with neuropathic cancer pain.[17*,60]

Nerve trunk pain, i.e. the nociceptive component of neuropathic pain syndromes caused by compression, invasion or acute nerve ischemia, is treatable with NSAIDs, steroids, and eventually opioids.[14] Conversely, in the experience of most clinicians, neuropathic pain of the deafferentation type responds poorly to NSAIDs.

For a long time opioids were considered barely effective in neuropathic pain. However, in the past few years several retrospective reports on long-term therapy for neuropathic pain related to nonmalignant diseases and cancer have supported opioid efficacy and low risk of addiction and tolerance.[18*,61*] Since then, several clinical studies have supported the use of opioids in the treatment of peripheral neuropathic pain.[61,62**,63**,64**,65**] However, the evidence for their efficacy with regard to central pain is weak.[66**] Some opioids are potentially more effective than others in neuropathic pain due to their pharmacological properties: methadone[67,68**] and propoxyphene have weak N-methyl-D-aspartate (NMDA) receptor antagonism, and tramadol[69**] has noradrenergic/serotonergic activity. However, comparative studies of opioids in neuropathic pain syndromes are still lacking.

Anticonvulsants, other channel blockers, and antidepressants, commonly referred to as adjuvant drugs, are considered effective treatment for neuropathic pain.[70***,71***,72***] Gabapentin is an anticonvulsant structurally related to γ-aminobutyric acid (GABA) and binds the $α_2δ$ subunits of voltage-gated calcium channels with well-documented efficacy in peripheral neuropathic pain related to diabetic neuropathy and postherpetic neuralgia.[73**,74**,75**] Gabapentin added to opioids in cancer patients with neuropathic pain reduced pain in one study,[76*] but it had a limited effect in a larger patient population investigated by the same group.[77**] Pregabalin modulates the $α_2δ$ subunits of voltage-gated calcium channels with better kinetics properties compared to gabapentin; its efficacy in neuropathic pain due diabetic polyneuropathy and postherpetic neuralgia is also well documented.[78**,79**] Carbamazepine is an old anticonvulsant that unselectively blocks sodium channels. It is still considered the gold standard treatment for trigeminal neuralgia.[80**] In older clinical studies proved efficacy of carbamazepine was shown in painful diabetic neuropathy[81**] although with a higher incidence of side effects

compared with the newer anticonvulsants. Its analog oxcarbazepine is also effective in trigeminal neuralgia[82*] and in painful diabetic polyneuropathy, with a better tolerability profile.[83**] Lamotrigine is an antiepileptic agent that stabilizes the neural membrane, blocking voltage-sensitive sodium channels and inhibiting presynaptic release of glutamate. Its analgesic efficacy has been shown in trigeminal neuralgia,[84**] post-stroke central pain[85**] and human immunodeficiency virus (HIV)-related polyneuropathy.[86**]

Tricyclic antidepressants (TCAs) were the mainstay of neuropathic pain therapy before the introduction of the new anticonvulsants.[87***] Among these drugs, amitriptyline and imipramine are the most commonly prescribed TCAs in neuropathic pain. Amitriptyline reduces pain in diabetic neuropathy[88**] and central post-stroke pain.[89**] Randomized trials of selective serotonin reuptake inhibitors have shown inconstant efficacy in neuropathic pain.[72***] The noradrenergic/serotonergic reuptake inhibitor venlafaxine seems a promising drug, because at high doses it has shown analgesic efficacy in peripheral neuropathic pain.[90**,91**] Bupropion, a second-generation non-TCA antidepressant, has demonstrated efficacy and good tolerability in a single double-blind randomized trial on different types of peripheral neuropathic pain.[92**] A lidocaine patch decreases pain and allodynia in postherpetic neuralgia.[93**] Intravenous lidocaine[62**] and parenteral ketamine[94**] quickly, although only transiently, reduce pain and may help control episodic neuropathic pain unresponsive to conventional analgesics.

Neuromodulation with spinal drug delivery is a recognized treatment for patients with severe refractory pain and life expectancy of at least 6 months.[95,96*] The most commonly used drugs in neuraxial analgesia are morphine, bupivacaine, clonidine, and ketamine. Recently intrathecal ziconotide, an N-type calcium-channel blocker derived from a sea-snail peptide, has shown statistically significant analgesic efficacy in advanced cancer and acquired immune deficiency syndrome (AIDS) patients with intractable pain.[97**] On the other hand, a lack of cost–benefit efficacy and concomitant poor long-term prognosis precludes electrical spinal cord stimulation.[98]

As a general rule, for treating the neuropathic component of a pain, the initial approach could be based on gabapentin or pregabalin (particularly for peripheral pain), alternatively on amitriptyline or lamotrigine (also effective in central pain), given 'round the clock' in a regular fashion with an appropriate titration dose. Other anticonvulsants or antidepressants might be considered as second step in poorly responsive patients. Opioids, and sometimes NSAIDs and steroids, may be used as rescue medication for treating episodes of incident or worsening pain, or may be available on an 'as needed' basis, or added at regular times in the presence of pain of mixed origin or severe intensity. Figure 52.2 summarizes our standard approach to treating neuropathic pain in palliative care patients.

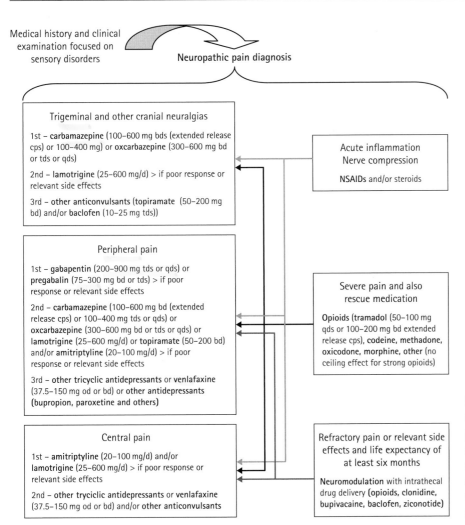

Medical history and clinical examination focused on sensory disorders → Neuropathic pain diagnosis

Trigeminal and other cranial neuralgias

1st – **carbamazepine** (100–600 mg bds (extended release cps) or 100–400 mg) or **oxcarbazepine** (300–600 mg bd or tds or qds)

2nd – **lamotrigine** (25–600 mg/d) > if poor response or relevant side effects

3rd – **other anticonvulsants** (topiramate (50–200 mg bd) and/or **baclofen** (10–25 mg tds))

Peripheral pain

1st – **gabapentin** (200–900 mg tds or qds) or **pregabalin** (75–300 mg bd or tds) > if poor response or relevant side effects

2nd – **carbamazepine** (100–600 mg bd (extended release cps) or 100–400 mg tds or qds) or **oxcarbazepine** (300–600 mg bd or tds or qds) or **lamotrigine** (25–600 mg/d) or **topiramate** (50–200 bd) and/or **amitriptyline** (20–100 mg/d) > if poor response or relevant side effects

3rd – **other tricyclic antidepressants or venlafaxine** (37.5–150 mg od or bd) or other antidepressants (bupropion, paroxetine and others)

Central pain

1st – **amitriptyline** (20–100 mg/d) and/or **lamotrigine** (25–600 mg/d) > if poor response or relevant side effects

2nd – **other tryciclic antidepressants or venlafaxine** (37.5–150 mg od or bd) and/or other anticonvulsants

Acute inflammation Nerve compression

NSAIDs and/or steroids

Severe pain and also rescue medication

Opioids (tramadol (50–100 mg qds or 100–200 mg bd extended release cps), **codeine, methadone, oxicodone, morphine, other** (no ceiling effect for strong opioids)

Refractory pain or relevant side effects and life expectancy of at least six months

Neuromodulation with intrathecal drug delivery (opioids, clonidine, bupivacaine, baclofen, ziconotide)

Figure 52.2 *Management of neuropathic pain in palliative care patients. *Based on the clinical practice at the authors' center. This management protocol is not fully supported by randomized clinical trials. bds, twice daily; tds, thrice daily; qds four times daily, od, once daily; d, day.*

In conclusion, we emphasize the need to identify the cause of the pain, unravel its neuropathic nature and possibly hypothesize or search for the mechanisms. A thorough investigation might lead to a more specific treatment, which even in the palliative stages could be relevant for improving the patient's autonomy, cognition, and dignity.

Key learning points

- Neuropathic pain is not a single entity but encompasses a variety of different, complex clinical pictures with diverse pathophysiological mechanisms.

- Neuropathic pain is frequently present in cancer patients either in isolation or combined with nociceptive pain (mixed pain).

- Direct and indirect activity of cancer cause different neuropathic pain syndromes depending on the anatomy and the pathophysiology of the injured part of the nervous system.

- The number of cancer patients with neuropathic pain of iatrogenic origin is increasing due to longer survival times and the more aggressive surgical and medical treatment.

- Radiotherapy, chemotherapy, and surgery may cause multiple painful neuropathic syndromes.

- A thorough evaluation of the patient's pain informs the most appropriate treatment and enhances the patient's ability to cope.

- Treatment of neuropathic pain is moving out of the empirical era to an evidence-based scientific approach. Novel adjuvant compounds have become available for neuropathic pain, supported by clinical studies on their efficacy and tolerability.

- Improved understanding of neuropathic pain pathophysiology is steering clinical research and patient management.

REFERENCES

◆ 1 Woolf CJ, Mannion RJ. Neuropathic pain: aetiology, symptoms, mechanisms, and management. *Lancet* 1999; **5**: 1959–64.

◆ 2 Merskey H, Bogduk N. *Classification of Chronic Pain: Descriptions of Chronic Pain Syndromes and Definitions of Pain Terms.* Seattle: IASP Press, 1994: 222.

◆ 3 Hansson PT, Lacerenza M, Marchettini P. Aspects of clinical and experimental neuropathic pain: the clinical perspective. In: Hansson PT, Fields HL, Hill RG, Marchettini P, eds. *Neuropathic Pain: Pathophysiology and Treatment.* Progress in Pain Research and Management Vol 21. Seattle: IASP Press, 2001: 1–18.

4 Max MB. Clarifying the definition of neuropathic pain. *Pain* 2002; **96**: 406–7.

5 Backonja MM. Defining neuropathic pain. *Anesth Analg* 2003; **97**: 785–90.

6 Osterberg A, Boivie J, Holmgren H, *et al.* The clinical characteristics and sensory abnormalities of patients with central pain caused by multiple sclerosis. In: Gebhart GF, Hammond DL, Jensen TS, eds. *Proceedings of the 7th World Congress on Pain.* Progress in Pain Research and Management, Vol. 2. Seattle: IASP Press 1994: 789–96.

◆ 7 Boivie J. Central pain. In: Wall PD, Melzack R, eds. *Textbook of Pain.* Edinburgh: Churchill Livingstone 1999: 879–914.

8 Ochoa JL, Serra J, Campero M. Pathophysiology of human nociceptor function. In: Belmonte C, Cervero F, eds. *Neurobiology of Nociceptors.* Oxford: Oxford University Press, 1996; 489–516.

● ◆ 9 Beric A. Central pain: 'new' syndromes and their evaluation. *Muscle Nerve* 1993; **16**: 1017–24.

● 10 Leijon G, Boivie J, Johansson I. Central post-stroke pain – neurological symptoms and pain characteristics. *Pain* 1989; **36**: 13–25.

● 11 Marchettini P, Simone D, Caputi G, Ochoa J. Pain from excitation of identified muscle nociceptors in humans. *Brain Res* 1996; **740**: 109–16.

● 12 Ochoa J, Campero M, Serra J, Bostock H. Hyperexcitable polymodal and insensitive nociceptors in painful human neuropathy. *Muscle Nerve* 2005; **32**: 459–72.

13 Bennett GJ, Ochoa JL. Thermographic observations on rats with experimental neuropathic pain. *Pain* 1991; **45**: 61–7.

◆ 14 Vecht CJ. Cancer pain: a neurological perspective. *Curr Opin Neurol.* 2000; **13**: 649–53.

15 Gilbert MR, Grossman SA. Incidence and nature of neurologic problems in patients with solid tumors. *Am J Med* 1986; **81**: 951–4.

● 16 Asbury AK, Fields HL. Pain due to peripheral nerve damage: an hypothesis. *Neurology* 1984; **34**: 1587–90.

● * 17 Grond S, Radbruch L, Meuser T, *et al.* Assessment and treatment of neuropathic cancer pain following WHO guidelines. *Pain* 1999; **79**: 15–20.

● 18 Cherny NI, Thaler HT, Friedlander-Klar H *et al.* Opioid responsiveness of cancer pain syndromes caused by neuropathic or nociceptive mechanisms: a combined analysis of controlled, single-dose studies. *Neurology* 1994; **44**: 857–61.

● 19 Caraceni A, Portenoy RK. An international survey of cancer pain characteristics and syndromes. IASP Task Force on Cancer Pain. International Association for the Study of Pain. *Pain* 1999; **82**: 263–74.

20 Cheng TM, Cascino TL, Onofrio BM. Comprehensive study of diagnosis and treatment of trigeminal neuralgia secondary to tumors. *Neurology* 1993; **43**: 2298–302.

● ◆ 21 Vecht CJ, Hoff AM, Kansen PJ, *et al.* Types and causes of pain in cancer of the head and neck. *Cancer* 1992; **70**: 178–84.

● 22 Kori SH, Foley KM, Posner JB. Brachial plexus lesions in patients with cancer: 100 cases. *Neurology* 1981; **31**: 45–50.

23 Marangoni C, Lacerenza M, Formaglio F, *et al.* Sensory disorder of the chest as presenting symptom of lung cancer. *J Neurol Neurosurg Psychiatry* 1993; **56**: 1033–4.

● 24 Jaeckle KA, Young DF, Foley KM. The natural history of lumbosacral plexopathy in cancer. *Neurology* 1985; **35**: 8–15.

◆ 25 Elliott K, Foley KM. Neurological pain syndromes in patients with cancer. *Neurol Clin* 1989; **7**: 333–60.

26 Rusthoven JJ, Ahlgren P, Elhakim T, *et al.* Varicella-zoster infection in adult cancer patients. A population study. *Arch Intern Med* 1988; **148**: 1561–6.

● 27 Fields HL, Rowbotham M, Baron R. Postherpetic neuralgia: irritable nociceptors and deafferentation. *Neurobiol Dis* 1998; **5**: 209–27.

28 Molinuevo JL, Graus F, Serrano C, *et al.* Utility of anti-Hu antibodies in the diagnosis of paraneoplastic sensory neuropathy. *Ann Neurol* 1998; **44**: 976–80.

◆ 29 Rudnicki SA, Dalmau J. Paraneoplastic syndromes of the spinal cord, nerve, and muscle. *Muscle Nerve* 2000; **23**: 1800–18.

30 Oh SJ. Paraneoplastic vasculitis of the peripheral nervous system. *Neurol Clin* 1997; **15**: 849–63.

31 Marchettini P, Formaglio F, Lacerenza M. Iatrogenic painful neuropathic complications of surgery in cancer. *Acta Anaesthesiol Scand* 2001; **45**: 1090–4.

32 Marcus RB Jr, Million RR. The incidence of myelitis after irradiation of the cervical spinal cord. *Int J Radiat Oncol Biol Phys* 1990; **19**: 3–8.

33 Jellinger K, Sturm KW. Delayed radiation myelopathy in man. *J Neurol Sci* 1971; **14**: 389–408.

34 Lewanski CR, Sinclair JA, Stewart JS. Lhermitte's sign following head and neck radiotherapy. *Clin Oncol* 2000; **12**: 98–103.

35 Gerard JM, Franck N, Moussa Z, Hildebrand J. Acute ischemic brachial plexus neuropathy following radiation therapy. *Neurology* 1989; **39**: 450–1.

36 Malow BA, Dawson DM. Neuralgic amyotrophy in association with radiation therapy for Hodgkin's disease. *Neurology* 1991; **41**: 440–1.

◆ 37 Foley KM. Pain syndromes in patients with cancer. In: Bonica JJ, Ventafridda V, eds. *Advances in Pain Research and Therapy.* New York: Raven Press, 1979; 59–78.

38 Lederman RJ, Wilbourn AJ. Brachial plexopathy: recurrent cancer or radiation? *Neurology* 1984; **34**: 1331–5.

● 39 Thomas JE, Cascino TL, Earle JD. Differential diagnosis between radiation and tumor plexopathy of the pelvis. *Neurology* 1985; **35**: 1–7.

40 Abu-Rustum NR, Rajbdhandari D, Glusman S, Massad LS. Acute lower extremity paralysis following radiation therapy for cervical cancer. *Gynecol Oncol* 1999; **75**: 152–4.

41 Alberts DS, Noel JK. Cisplatin-associated neurotoxicity: can it be prevented? *Anticancer Drugs* 1995; **6**: 369–83.

● 42 Casey EB, Jellife AM, Le Quesne PM, Millett YL. Vincristine neuropathy. Clinical and electrophysiological observations. *Brain* 1973; **96**: 69–86.

43 Kaplan JG, Einzig AI, Schaumburg HH. Taxol causes permanent large fiber peripheral nerve dysfunction: a lesson for preventative strategies. *J Neurooncol* 1993; **16**: 105–7.

◆ 44 Verstappen CC, Heimans JJ, Hoekman K, Postma TJ. Neurotoxic complications of chemotherapy in patients with cancer: clinical signs and optimal management. *Drugs* 2003; **63**: 1549–63.

45 Dougherty PM, Cata JP, Cordella JV, *et al.* Taxol-induced sensory disturbance is characterized by preferential impairment of myelinated fiber function in cancer patients. *Pain* 2004; **109**: 132–42.

46 Siegal T, Haim N. Cisplatin-induced peripheral neuropathy: frequent off-therapy deterioration, demyelinating syndromes and muscle cramps. *Cancer* 1990; **66**: 1117–23.

47 Castellanos AM, Glass JP, Young KWA *et al.* Regional nerve injury after intra-arterial chemotherapy. *Neurology* 1987; **37**: 834–837.

48 Kline DG, Hudson AR, eds. *Nerve Injuries.* Philadelphia: WB Saunders Company, 1995.

49 Chaplin JM, Morton RP. A prospective, longitudinal study of pain in head and neck cancer patients. *Head Neck* 1999; **21**: 531–7.

50 Krause HR. Shoulder-arm-syndrome after radical neck dissection: its relation with the innervation of trapezius muscle. *Int J Oral Maxillofacial Surg* 1992; **21**: 276–9.

51 Shone GR, Yardley MP. An audit into the incidence of handicap after unilateral radical neck dissection. *J Laryngol Otol* 1991; **105**: 760–2.

52 Kuntz AL, Weymuller EA Jr. Impact of neck dissection on quality of life. *Laryngoscope* 1999; **109**: 1334–8.

● ◆ 53 Jung BF, Ahrendt GM, Oaklander AL, Dworkin RH. Neuropathic pain following breast cancer surgery: proposed classification and research update. *Pain* 2003; **104**: 1–13.

54 Hack TF, Cohen L, Katz J, *et al.* Physical and psychological morbidity after axillary lymph nodes dissection for breast cancer. *J Clin Oncol* 1999; **1**: 143–9.

● 55 Tasmuth T, Blomqvist C, Kalso E. Chronic post-treatment symptoms in patients with breast cancer operated in different surgical units. *Eur J Surg Oncol* 1999; **25**: 38–43.

56 Perttunen K, Tasmuth T, Kalso E. Chronic pain after thoracic surgery: a follow up study. *Acta Anesth Scand* 1999; **43**: 563–7.

57 Horowitz SH. Brachial plexus injury with causalgia resulting from transaxillary rib resection. *Arch Surg* 1985; **120**: 1189–91.

58 Kanner RM, Martini N, Foley KM. Nature and incidence of post-thoracotomy pain. *Proc Am Soc Clin Oncol* 1982; **1**: 152.

● 59 Stute P, Soukup J, Menzel M, *et al.* Analysis and treatment of different types of neuropathic cancer pain. *J Pain Symptom Manage* 2003; **26**: 1123–31.

✱ 60 Agency for Health Care Policy and Research, US Department of Health and Human Service. *Management of Cancer Pain.* Clinical Practice Guideline No. 9. Rockville MD: AHCPR Publication N94-0592, 1994.

● 61 Portenoy RK, Foley KM, Inturrisi CE. The nature of opioid responsiveness and its implications for neuropathic pain: new hypotheses derived from studies of opioid infusions. *Pain* 1990; **43**: 273–86.

● 62 Rowbotham MC, Reisner-Keller LA, Fields HL Both intravenous lidocaine and morphine reduce the pain of postherpetic neuralgia *Neurology* 1991; **41**: 1024–8.

● 63 Dellemijn PL, Vanneste JA. Randomised double-blind active-placebo-controlled crossover trial of intravenous fentanyl in neuropathic pain. *Lancet* 1997; **349**: 753–8.

● 64 Watson CP, Babul N. Efficacy of oxycodone in neuropathic pain: a randomized trial in postherpetic neuralgia. *Neurology* 1998; **50**: 1837–41.

● 65 Rowbotham MC, Twilling L, Davies PS, *et al.* Oral opioid therapy for chronic peripheral and central neuropathic pain. *N Engl J Med* 2003; **348**: 1223–32.

66 Attal N, Guirimand F, Brasseur L, *et al.* Effects of IV morphine in central pain: a randomized placebo-controlled study. *Neurology* 2002; **58**: 554–63.

67 Foley KM. Opioids and chronic neuropathic pain. *N Engl J Med* 2003; **348**: 1279–81.

68 Morley JS, Bridson J, Nash TP, *et al.* Low-dose methadone has an analgesic effect in neuropathic pain: a double-blind randomized controlled crossover trial. *Palliat Med* 2003; **17**: 576–87.

69 Sindrup SH, Andersen G, Madsen C, *et al.* Tramadol relieves pain and allodynia in polyneuropathy: a randomised, double-blind, controlled trial. *Pain* 1999; **83**: 85–90.

● ◆ 70 McQuay H, Carrol D, Jadad AR, *et al.* Anticonvulsant drugs for management of pain: a systematic review. *BMJ* 1995; **311**: 1047–52.

● ◆ 71 McQuay H, Tramer MR, Nye BA, *et al.* A systematic review of antidepressants in neuropathic pain. *Pain* 1996; **68**: 217–27.

● ◆ 72 Sindrup SH, Jensen TS. Efficacy of pharmacological treatments of neuropathic pain: an update and effect related to mechanism of drug action. *Pain* 1999; **83**: 389–400.

● 73 Backonja M, Beydoun A, Edwards KR, *et al.* Gabapentin for the symptomatic treatment of painful neuropathy in patients with diabetes mellitus. *JAMA* 1998; **280**:1831–6.

● 74 Rowbotham M, Harden N, Stacey B, *et al.* Gabapentin for the treatment of postherpetic neuralgia. *JAMA* 1998; **280**: 1837–42.

75 Serpell MG, Neuropathic Pain Study Group. Gabapentin in neuropathic pain syndromes: a randomized, double-blind, placebo-controlled trial. *Pain* 2002; **99**: 557–66.

● 76 Caraceni A, Zecca E, Martini C, De Conno F Gabapentin as an adjuvant to opioid analgesia for neuropathic cancer pain. *J Pain Symptom Manage* 1999; **17**: 441–5.

77 Caraceni A, Zecca E, Bonezzi C, *et al.* Gabapentin for neuropathic cancer pain: a randomized controlled trial from the Gabapentin Cancer Pain Study Group. *J Clin Oncol* 2004; **22**: 2909–17.

78 Sabatowski R, Gálvez R, Cherry DA, *et al.* Pregabalin reduces pain and improves sleep and mood disturbances in patients with post-herpetic neuralgia: results of a randomised, placebo-controlled clinical trial *Pain* 2004; **109**: 26–35.

79 Richter RW, Portenoy R, Sharma U, *et al.* Relief of painful diabetic peripheral neuropathy with pregabalin: a

randomized, placebo-controlled trial. *J Pain* 2005; **6**: 253–60.

● 80   Campbell FG, Graham JG, Zilkha KJ. Clinical trial of carbazepine (Tegretol) in trigeminal neuralgia. *J Neurol Neurosurg Psychiatry* 1966; **29**: 265–7.

● 81   Rull JA, Quibrera R, Gonzalez-Millan H, *et al.* Symptomatic treatment of peripheral diabetic neuropathy with carbamazepine (Tegretol): double blind crossover trial. *Diabetologia* 1969; **5**: 215–18.

82   Zakrzewska JM, Patsalos PN Long-term cohort study comparing medical (oxcarbazepine) and surgical management of intractable trigeminal neuralgia. *Pain* 2002; **95**: 259–66.

83   Dogra S, Beydoun S, Mazzola J, *et al.* Oxcarbazepine in painful diabetic neuropathy: a randomized, placebo-controlled study *Eur J Pain* 2005; **9**: 543–54.

84   Zakrzewska JM, Chaudhry Z, Nurmikko TJ, *et al.* Lamotrigine (Lamictal) in refractory trigeminal neuralgia: results for a double blind placebo controlled crossover trial. *Pain* 1997; **73**: 223–30.

85   Vestergaard K, Andersen G, Gottrup H *et al.* Lamotrigine for central poststroke pain; a randomized controlled trial. *Neurology* 2001; **56**: 184–90.

86   Simpson DM, McArthur JC, Olney R, *et al.* Lamotrigine for HIV-associated painful sensory neuropathies. *Neurology* 2003; **60**: 1508–14.

◆ 87   Collins SL, Moore RA, McQuay HJ, Wiffen P. Antidepressants and anticonvulsants for diabetic neuropathy and postherpetic neuralgia: a quantitative systematic review. *J Pain Symptom Manage* 2000; **20**: 449–58.

● 88   Max MB, Culnane M, Schafer S, *et al.* Amitriptyline relieves diabetic neuropathy pain in patients with normal or depressed mood. *Neurology* 1987; **37**: 589–96.

89   Leijon G. Boivie J. Central post-stroke pain – a controlled trial of amitriptyline and carbamazepine. *Pain* 1989; **36**: 27–36.

90   Tasmuth T, Hartel B, Kalso E. Venlafaxine in neuropathic pain following treatment of breast cancer. *Eur J Pain* 2002; **6**: 17–24.

91   Rowbotham MC, Goli V, Kunz NR, Lei D. Venlafaxine extended release in the treatment of painful diabetic neuropathy: a double-blind, placebo-controlled study. *Pain* 2004; **110**: 697–706; erratum in: *Pain* 2005; **113**: 248.

92   Semenchuk MR, Sherman S, Davis B. Double-blind, randomized trial of bupropion SR for the treatment of neuropathic pain. *Neurology* 2001; **57**: 1583–8.

93   Galer BS, Rowbotham MC, Perander J, Friedman E. Topical lidocaine patch relieves postherpetic neuralgia more effectively than a vehicle topical patch: results of an enriched enrollment. *Pain* 1999; **80**: 533–8.

94   Mercadante S, Arcuri E, Tirelli W, *et al.* Analgesic effect of intravenous ketamine in cancer patients on morphine therapy: A randomized controlled, double-blind, cross-over, double dose study. *J Pain Symptom Manage* 2000; **20**: 246–62.

◆ ✱ 95   Hassenbusch SJ, Portenoy RK, Cousins M, *et al.* Polyanalgesic Consensus Conference 2003: an update on the management of pain by intraspinal drug delivery-report of an expert panel. *J Pain Symptom Manage* 2004; **27**: 540–63.

● 96   Burton AW, Rajagopal A, Shah HN, *et al.* Epidural and intrathecal analgesia is effective in treating refractory cancer pain. *Pain Med* 2004; **5**: 239–47.

● 97   Staats PS, Yearwood T, Charapata SG, *et al.* Intrathecal ziconotide in the treatment of refractory pain in patients with cancer or AIDS: a randomized controlled trial. *JAMA* 2004; **291**: 63–70.

✱ 98   Gybels J, Erdine S, Maeyaert J, *et al.* Neuromodulation of pain a consensus statement prepared in Brussels, 16–18 January 1998, by the following task force of the European Federation of IASP chapters (EFIC). *Eur J Pain* 1998; **2**: 203–9.

Bone pain

YOKO TARUMI

INTRODUCTION

The disease-related event that has the most significant impact on quality of life for patients with malignant disease is cancer-induced pain.[1] Bone metastases are most commonly associated with cancers of the breast, prostate, lung, kidney, and with multiple myeloma (Table 53.1). Approximately 40–70 percent of patients with bone metastases will develop skeletal complications (skeletal-related events [SRE]) at some point during the course of their disease, most commonly bone pain, pathological fractures, hypercalcemia and spinal cord compression.[11,**12**,13] Malignant bone pain is the most common source of pain in patients with malignant disease.[14,15*] At its onset, malignant bone pain can be intermittent, but it progresses rapidly into continuous pain (background pain) that is exacerbated by episodes of spontaneous aggravation of pain or movement-induced (incident) pain. Patients with established chronic malignant bone pain syndrome who show perception of severe pain to normally nonpainful activity or stimulation such as coughing, turning in bed, gentle touching, or gentle limb movements have developed mechanical allodynia and hyperalgesia.[16–18] Pain management in this population is particularly important to maintain function, especially in patients with primary malignancy of breast and prostate, and multiple myeloma whose may have a long life expectancy after the diagnosis of metastatic bone disease.

PATHOPHYSIOLOGY OF MALIGNANT BONE PAIN: WHY IS TUMOR-INDUCED BONE DESTRUCTION PAINFUL?

Not all the bone metastases are painful. Although the most common presenting symptom of metastatic disease to the bone is pain, 30–50 percent of patients have asymptomatic bone metastases found during staging studies for primary tumors.[19] On the other hand, in the animal model of bone cancer, pain-related behavior is present before any significant bone destruction is evident.[20]

Animal model of malignant bone pain

In the past, malignant bone pain was understood to be due to vascular occlusion, compression of the bone or peripheral nerve, or mechanical instability. Since 1999, an animal model of malignant bone disease has been established, which shares key features with human malignant bone pain with

Table 53.1 *Incidence of bone metastases and life expectancy after diagnosis*

Type of cancer	Frequency	Life expectancy
Prostate cancer	75–100%[2,4]	53 months without visceral metastases and 30 months with visceral metastases[3]
Breast cancer	80%[2]	34 (1–90) months[2,5]
Multiple myeloma	95–100%[2]	20 months[2]
Nonsmall and small cell lung cancer	30–40%[2]	<1 year[6**]
Renal cell cancer	35%[7]	1–2 years[8***]
Bladder cancer	22%[9*]	1–2 years[10]

progressive bone destruction leading to a pathological fracture, accompanying progressive limping, guarding, spontaneous flinching and vocalization on palpation, reduced movement secondary to hyperalgesia, and allodynia, while, at the same time, the animal remains well with good weight gain.[16,21,22] The level of pain behaviors observed correlated with the extent of disease-induced osteolysis.[17,18] The response to systemic opioids in the mouse model was similar to that found in humans, which showed reduced attenuation with morphine compared with the model with inflammatory pain.[23]

Neurochemical alterations

In the animal malignant bone pain model, three significant and specific neurochemical alterations in the spinal cord are observed:

1 Expression of the prohyperalgesic peptide dynorphin (an opioid family relating to maintenance of chronic pain.[24]
2 Increased neuronal activity.
3 Increased number of astrocytes (the most numerous type of glial cell in the central nervous system).[16]

These neurochemical findings were correlated with the degree of bone destruction.[16–18,20] In the neurochemical studies measures of pain have been compared in mice or rats with inflammatory pain, neuropathic pain, and malignant bone pain; the findings indicated that bone pain results in a unique neurochemical pain state: a condition that differs clearly from inflammatory pain or neuropathic pain.[18,25]

Tumor–nociceptor interface

In malignant bone pain expression, multiple types of tumor-associated cells including immune-system cells such as macrophages, neutrophils and T cells, secrete factors such as prostaglandins, multiple cytokines, and endothelin (a peptide activating nociceptors, inflammation, and angiogenesis). These factors are thought to play an important role in exciting or sensitizing the peripheral and central nervous system through continuous nociceptive activation, resulting in the release of neurotransmitters such as calcitonin gene-related peptide (CGRP), glutamine, histamine, and substance P (a neurotransmitter, synthesized and transported to the C-fiber after painful stimuli, potential mediator of hyperalgesia).[26] Bone has rich sensory and sympathetic fiber innervations involving mineralized bone and periosteum.[27,28] The stimulation of sensory afferent nerves endings located in the bone cortex, periosteum, and surrounding soft tissue are ultimately involved in pain transmission.[28]

Osteoclast and malignant bone pain

Although the mechanisms of malignant pain are largely unknown, data from clinical trials with bisphosphonates

and analysis of bone metabolism in patients with bone metastases suggest that cancer-induced bone resorption is linked to malignant bone pain.[2,3,11,29,30**,31**,32**] It is now understood that the osteoclast plays the major role in the resorption of bone instead of the cancer cell itself. Cancer cells produce and secrete a variety of cytokines and growth factors such as transforming growth factor β (TGFβ and parathyroid hormone-related protein (PTHrP) that recruit osteoclast precursors and activate mature osteoclasts[33] (Fig. 53.1). Osteoclasts are derived from myelo-monocytic precursors and destroy bone by forming an acidic extracellular compartment at sites of bone resorption.[16,34] Many primary afferent neurons that innervate the periosteum have been shown to express acid-sensing ion channels.[35]

Osteoprotegerin as bone resorption 'regulator'

Macrophage colony-stimulating factor and the receptor activator of nuclear factor κB-ligand (RANKL) and its receptor system are important components of osteoclastogenesis.[34] RANKL is produced by osteoblasts and stromal cells, and osteoclast precursors express RANK. RANKL stimulates recruitment, differentiation, and activation of osteoclasts.[34] Osteoprotegerin (OPG) is a 'decoy' receptor that competes with RANK for RANKL, and thus modulates the effects of RANKL.[36,37] Although OPG has been shown to decrease pain behaviors in animal models of malignant bone pain, it is still being developed for use in cancer patients.[17,20,26]Although an animal model of malignant bone pain treated with OPG halted progression and stabilized bone destruction, the pain behavior or neuromechanical measure of pain did not improve.[17,20] Osteoprotegerin has also been shown to increase bone mineral density and bone volume, which are associated with a decrease in active osteoclast number in women with osteoporosis and patients with multiple myeloma.[38**,39]

ASSESSMENT

Diagnosis of malignant bone pain can usually be made by history and physical examination. The clinician should enquire about the onset, quality, intensity, location, radiation of the pain, factors that exacerbate or alleviate the pain, and other systemic symptoms such as bowel and urinary problems, and functional problems. Malignant bone pain syndrome consists of a triad of background pain, spontaneous pain, and movement-induced (incident) pain[15,40] (Table 53.2). Patients often describe a sudden flare of their pain which keeps them from moving freely, resulting in disability (see Chapter 54, page 505).

Besides the general physical examination, a musculoskeletal and neurological examination should be completed focusing on palpable tenderness in the skeletal system and neurological deficits/alterations. Patients who have back

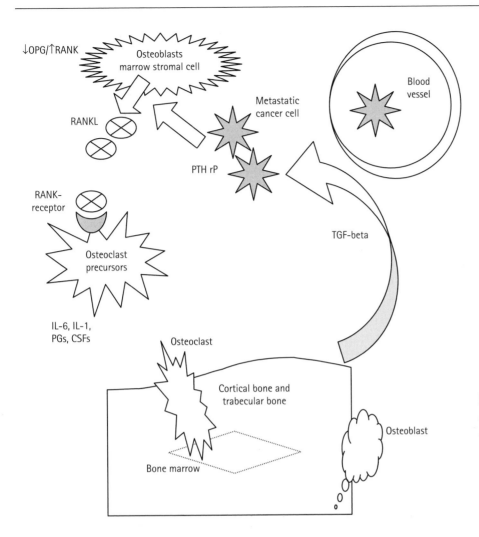

Figure 53.1 *Osteoclast and bone metastases. OPG, osteoprotegerin; RANKL, receptor activator of nuclear factor κ B-ligand; PTHrP, parathyroid hormone related protein; TGFβ, transforming growth factor β; IL, interleukin; PG, prostaglandin; CSF, colony stimulating factor.*

Table 53.2 *Triad of clinical signs of malignant bone pain*

Sign	Characteristic features
Background pain	Constant dull ache Increase in intensity over time
Spontaneous pain	Intermittent episodes of intense pain without trigger
Movement-induced (incident) pain	Intermittent episodes of intense pain upon movement/weight bearing

pain with or without weakness of the limbs, paresthesias, sensory change, or bladder or bowel impairment should be carefully assessed for potential spinal cord compression and cauda equina syndrome (see Chapter 88, page 817). The differential diagnosis of bone pain includes degenerative disease due to osteoporosis in older women with a history of malignancy (such as breast cancer) who may present with acute back pain due to collapsed vertebrae, or Paget disease of bone in older men with a history of prostate cancer with sclerotic radiographic changes in the pelvis. In all cases, it is important to emphasize that the imaging tests should be interpreted in conjunction with the clinical picture, information from measurement of biochemical markers of bone metabolism and serum tumor markers when appropriate. Tables 53.3 and 53.4 provide summaries of the use of diagnostic modalities.

Bone consists of 85 percent dense cortical bone composed of minerals, and 15 percent porous and spongy trabecular bone composed of collagens which encompasses the marrow component. Most of the red marrow is located in axial bones, such as vertebrae, pelvis, proximal femora, while fat marrow is located in appendicular bones.

Plain radiography

On X-rays, bone metastases may appear as areas of absent density or absent trabecular structure which represents osteolytic lesions. Osteoblastic lesions may appear as increased density and sclerotic lesions or rims. X-ray is specific to confirm symptomatic lesions or suspicious lesions on bone scintigraphy (bone scan). It is also useful for

Table 53.3   *Comparison of bone structure and various bone imaging modalities*

	Cortical bone	Trabecular bone	Bone marrow	Tumors	Bone metabolism	Tumor glucose metabolism
X-ray (plain radiography)	√	√				
Computed tomography	√	√	√	√		
Magnetic resonance imaging			√√	√√		
Bone scan					√	
Positron emission tomography						√

Table 53.4   *Comparison of diagnostic sensitivity/specificity and advantages/disadvantages*

	Sensitivity	Specificity	Advantages	Disadvantage
X-ray (plain radiography)	Low	Not available	Assessment of risk for pathologic fracture Less expensive Detects structural changes	Delayed appearance
Computed tomography	High	High	Evaluates cortical and trabecular bone	Relatively expensive
Magnetic resonance imaging	High	High	Evaluates spinal cord compression and soft tissue	Expensive
Bone scan	Varies	Low	Detects new lesions Reasonable screening tool	Low specificity
Positron emission tomography	Varies	High	Detects new marrow lesions	Very expensive

assessing patients at high risk for pathological fractures, for example, persistent pain on weight bearing, which may guide planning for prophylactic management surgically or nonsurgically. However, because 30–75 percent of normal bone mineral content must be lost before osteolytic lesions in the vertebrae become apparent on X-ray, metastatic lesions may not appear on X-ray for several months.[41] A recent systematic review suggests that the diagnostic sensitivity of X-ray is 44–50 percent, which is less sensitive than bone scan for detecting initial bone metastases.[42***]

X-ray may be used as the primary investigation for bone malignancies with pure lytic disease such as multiple myeloma in which bone scintigraphy (bone scan) is falsely negative in up to 50 percent of lesions.[43*,44] Pure lytic disease can also occur in other tumor types when there are rapidly growing lytic lesions.[44]

Bone scan

Bone scan, unlike X-ray, is highly sensitive for the detection of bone metastasis but lacks specificity.[45] In their systematic review, Hamaoka *et al.* reported that its diagnostic sensitivity ranges from 62 percent to 100 percent and specificity from 78 percent to 100 percent.[42***] A bone scan commonly shows abnormality where there is osteoblastic activity; it may be negative in purely lytic lesions, such as in multiple myeloma, or in rapidly progressive disease which allows little chance for new bone formation (cold spots).[44] However, it may be positive in osteoarthritis, infections, trauma, and

Paget disease.[45] Therefore, the advantage of bone scan is not for diagnosis but rather for screening, as it is widely available and can produce rapid whole-body images at a reasonable cost.[42***] Despite the usefulness of bone scan, other imaging modalities such as X-ray, CT (computed tomography), or MRI (magnetic resonance imaging) may be performed to characterize lesions further.

The 'flare' phenomenon, which may be misinterpreted as disease progression, has been reported in prostate cancer or breast cancer patients who show escalation of activity or new lesions on bone scan due to their repair process during the first 3 months of treatment. However, after 6 months, the activity associated with the flare gradually decreases.[41,46] It is important to note that determining the final response of bone metastases to oncological treatment solely on the basis of changes in bone scan is not appropriate.[42***]

Computed tomography or magnetic resonance imaging

Computed tomography with bone window setting offers superior skeletal detail, including bone marrow, because of its ability to distinguish among materials of different densities.[41,46] A systematic review suggests that its diagnostic sensitivity of bone metastases ranges from 71 percent to 100 percent.[42***] Metastases in the marrow can be detected on CT before bone destruction becomes evident.[47]

Magnetic resonance imaging can provide detailed information of the bone and bone marrow, and has better contrast resolution than CT for visualizing soft tissue and spinal cord, especially when spinal cord involvement is suspected.[46] The diagnostic sensitivity and specificity of skeletal MRI have been reported as 82–100 percent and 73–100 percent, respectively, in a systemic review.[42***] In one retrospective survey of 100 patients, 47 percent had therapy changes associated with MRI findings.[48*] In this survey, 40 out of 78 patients who had symptoms such as back pain, weakness, paresthesia, or sphincter dysfunction had MRI-associated change in further therapy, whereas 7 out 22 patients without spinal symptoms detected on bone scintigraphy had a change in further therapy.[48*] MRI results influenced the addition or modification of radiation therapy treatment in 33 percent of the patients suspected of metastatic disease to the spine.[48*] Clinically asymptomatic presentations of spinal cord compression are not uncommon. A poor correlation between the site of vertebral body metastases and extent of epidural disease has been emphasized.[49*]

Occasionally, despite the presence of pain, no abnormalities are detected in X-ray or bone scan,[50*] and MRI may have a role in this setting. In a survey of 734 vertebral lesions, 255 were of an intertrabecular pattern; these intertrabecular lesions were detected by only 7.1 percent of radiographs and 4.5 percent of bone scans, but were demonstrated by all MRI scans.[51*]

Positron emission tomography

Positron emission tomography (PET), which visualizes the uptake of a positron-emitting radioactive form of biochemicals by tissues to trace the metabolism of the natural form of that chemical through imaging, may have role in early detection of soft tissue or bone metastases. Although high in sensitivity and specificity, its high cost, relative lack of availability, and additional time required for scanning are disadvantages.[42***] In the palliative care setting, the significance of this modality would be limited.

Biochemical markers

Markers of bone remodeling in metastatic bone disease may be useful tools when considering the cost of repeated imaging studies and possible radiation exposures. Markers of bone resorption could play a variety of roles in the management of metastatic bone disease.[41] For example, they could be indicated to identify patients at risk of developing skeletal complications or patients who may or may not benefit from bisphosphonate therapy.[41,52,53*,54] Some studies suggest that markers may predict the rate of bone loss, the risk of disease progression, and the potential for fracture in patients with lytic bone disease.[41,55*] It also has been suggested that the newer bone-specific markers may be sensitive enough to provide early diagnosis of bone metastases. However, the currently available evidence does not allow

final conclusions in regard to the accuracy and clinical validity of any of these indices in the primary diagnosis of bone metastases. As regards the monitoring of anticancer therapy, markers of bone resorption such as the pyridinium crosslinks, N- and C-terminal crosslinked telopeptide of type I collagen, react promptly and profoundly to bisphosphonate, hormonal, or chemical treatments. However, there have been no controlled studies on the usefulness of bone markers in monitoring of clinical symptoms of malignant bone disease.[56]

CURRENT THERAPEUTIC OPTIONS FOR MANAGEMENT OF MALIGNANT BONE PAIN

Goal of management

Once the etiology of pain has been determined, it is important that the patient and care-providers, including family members, have shared expectations and goals of the management of pain. The treatment modalities may be influenced by the individual situation, such as life expectancy, function prior to the pain experience, disease status, comorbidities, and availability of the modalities.

Table 53.5 shows the available therapies for management of malignant bone pain.

Opioid analgesics and episodic pain

Opioid analgesics are widely available and often effective; therefore they should be commenced and optimized as promptly as possible, before any other modalities are considered. Clinicians should be aware that patients may experience multifocal malignant bone pain besides other types of pain such as visceral or neuropathic pain.[15,57] Goals for the management of pain should include immediate relief of pain, restoration and maintenance of function, and prevention of complications.[58]

There is no single opioid analgesic that is preferable for malignant bone pain. The dosage should be individualized accordingly (see Chapters 44 and 45, pages 380 and 390, respectively). One of the challenges in the management of malignant bone pain with opioid analgesics is the management of spontaneous flares of pain and movement-induced (incident) pain, which may be categorized as episodic pain.[59] Because background pain can often easily be controlled by opioid analgesics, higher dosing of opioids to manage primarily the incidental component may lead to opioid toxicity. Anticipatory rescue (breakthrough) analgesics may be used prior to the activity for movement-induced pain (see Chapter 54, page 505). Newer, highly liposoluble opioids such as transmucosal fentanyl were developed particularly for management of episodic pain;[60*,61**,62*] however, this preparation is not widely available worldwide at present.

Table 53.5 *Therapies available for management of malignant bone pain*

Therapy (cost)	Mechanism	Effect	Onset	Adverse events
Opioids (relatively low cost)	μ-Opioid receptor agonism	Analgesia	Immediate	Side effects through multiple opioid receptors (See Chapter 45)
NSAIDs (relatively low cost)	COX-1 + 2 synthesis inhibitor	Analgesia + anti-inflammatory	Immediate to days	GI ulceration, interstitial nephritis, bleeding, etc.
Corticosteroids (low cost)	Inhibit eicosanoids, cytokines and substance P release	Analgesia + anti-inflammatory	Immediate to days	Psychosis, infection, proximal myopathy, edema
Bisphosphonates (high cost)	Inhibit osteoclasts activity; induce apoptosis of osteoclasts	Suppression of osteoclasts + some analgesia	Days to weeks	GI toxicity, 'flulike symptoms, electrolyte imbalances
Radiation (very high cost)	Cause apoptosis of osteoclasts + control release of cytokines	Tumor shrinkage + analgesia	Weeks	Fatigue, variety of local adverse effects (nausea, diarrhea, skin reaction, etc.)
Systemic radioisotope (very high cost)	Destruction of tumor cells	Tumor shrinkage + analgesia	Weeks	Leukocytopenia, thrombocytopenia
Surgery (very high cost)	Stabilization of unstable skeletal system	Prevention of further fracture	Immediate to days	Postsurgical complications

COX, cyclooxygenase; GI, gastrointestinal; NSAIDs, nonsteroidal anti-inflammatory drugs.

Nonsteroidal anti-inflammatory drugs

A recently reported systematic review found that the efficacy of nonsteroidal anti-inflammatory drugs (NSAIDs) in cancer pain control, especially for bone pain management, is inconclusive. Analysis is limited due to the short duration and the heterogeneity of studies.[63***] Overall, the long-term advantage/efficacy and safety of NSAIDs in bone pain management with or without opioid analgesics have not been established. Prostaglandins, which are released by tumor cells as well as through nociceptor activation from peripheral terminals of sensory fibers, are involved in the sensitization and/or direct excitation of nociceptors.[64,65] Cyclooxygenase 2 (COX-2) enzyme, which is one of two isomers involved in prostaglandin synthesis, is expressed only under inflammatory conditions, and is also expressed by cancer cells and tumor-associated macrophages. COX-2 has also been associated with angiogenesis and tumor growth.[66] Newer and more selective COX-2 inhibitors than celecoxib or rofecoxib showed efficacy in both background and movement-induced malignant bone pain in an animal model, in addition to reducing tumor burden and inducing osteoclast destruction.[67,68]

Corticosteroids

Corticosteroids play an extensive role as an adjuvant analgesic in malignant bone pain. However, there is little evidence to indicate the ideal type of corticosteroid and treatment regimen (dose, duration, etc.). Corticosteroids,

as inhibitors of adrenal androgen synthesis, are used as third-line hormonal therapy in prostate cancer in combination with mitoxantrone. Corticosteroids attenuate bone pain by inhibiting synthesis of eicosanoids, cytokines, substance P, and sprouting of sensory nerve fibres.[69,70**,71**,72] In multiple myeloma without prior treatment, high-dose dexamethasone alone or combined with thalidomide seemed to improve lytic bone lesions; however, analgesic effect was not included in the endpoint of these studies.[73**,74**,75**] Dexamethasone is commonly used due to its long-acting efficacy and absent mineralocorticoid effect. As breast cancer, prostate cancer, and multiple myeloma patients' life expectancies are relatively long, an extended period of high-dose corticosteroids should be avoided, in view of adverse effects such as proximal myopathy, which aggravates immobility, immunosuppression, and avascular necrosis.[76] Although little supporting evidence exists, the use of a nonfluorinated steroids such as methyl prednisone may delay the development of proximal myopathy.[77]

Calcitonin

Calcitonin is a hormone produced in the thyroid gland. It has a hypocalcemic action that is due primarily to the inhibition of osteoclastic bone resorption, and secondarily by action on the kidneys that results in increased urinary excretion of calcium and phosphorus. A recent systematic review suggested a nonsignificant effect of calcitonin on analgesia, reduction of analgesic consumption, control of skeletal complications, and improvement in quality of life or survival in the malignant bone pain setting. Although statistically nonsignificant, a greater number of adverse effects (facial brushing, subcutaneous pain) were observed in the calcitonin group.[78***]

Bisphosphonates

Bisphosphonates have been recognized as an effective treatment option for hypercalcemia of malignancy due to their strong affinity for the hydroxyapatite crystal of the bone. Preclinical research has recognized that bisphosphonates inhibit the formation of osteoclasts, interfere with signaling between osteoclasts and osteoblasts (see Fig. 53.1), induce apoptosis (programmed cell death) in osteoclasts, and show disease-modifying and antinociceptive effects.[21,79,80] Newer bisphosphonates such as ibandronate and zoledronic acid show 10 000 to 100 000-fold greater potency in inhibiting osteoclast-mediated bone resorption than older agents such as clodronate or pamidronate.[81]

A systematic review supports the efficacy of bisphosphonates in providing some pain relief for bone metastases.[82***] In a total of 3682 subjects included, the number needed to treat to achieve 50 percent pain relief at 4 weeks was 11, falling to 7 at 12 weeks.[82***] However the superiority in analgesic efficacy of one agent for different primary neoplasms cannot be established due to lack of direct comparisons between bisphosphonates. Another important finding is that there is insufficient evidence to recommend bisphosphonates for immediate pain relief or as first-line therapy. Thus, bisphosphonates should be considered where analgesics and/or radiotherapy are inadequate for the management of painful bone metastases.[82***]

A number of large controlled, longitudinal, disease-specific studies have been reported since the last systematic review, primarily for breast cancer,[83**,84**,85**] prostate cancer,[86**,87**,88**,89**,90**] and multiple myeloma,[91**,92**] regarding the efficacy of different bisphosphonates for reducing SRE. However, there are still unanswered questions, such as in which primary disease, which bisphosphonate, when to start and stop therapy, especially in longer survivors, and what is the role of the therapy in the absence of symptoms.

External beam radiation therapy

External beam radiotherapy continues to be a mainstay in the palliative treatment of malignant bone pain of all primary types. A systematic review supported the efficacy in pain relief by radiotherapeutic intervention in both localized or multifocal bone metastases, with 25 percent of patients experiencing complete pain relief at one month, and 41 percent of patients experiencing at least 50 percent pain relief.[93***] Single or multiple fractions did not produce different outcomes in pain management, and the number needed to treat to achieve complete relief at 1 month (compared with an assumed natural history of 1 in 100 patients

whose pain resolved without treatment) was 4.2.[93***] Although one of the largest studies suggested that complete pain relief was achieved within 4 weeks and lasted for 12 weeks (median), no pooled estimates of the speed of onset of relief or its duration could be obtained.[93***] The description of adverse effects was poor over all.[93***]

Another systematic review suggested no difference between single-fraction and multifraction radiotherapy arms in overall rates of partial pain relief (60 percent and 59 percent, respectively) and complete pain relief in patients with any primary site, but mainly prostate, breast, and lung.[94***] A higher re-treatment rate was seen in the single-fraction arm than the multifraction arm (odds ratio 3.44).[94***] Three percent of patients in the single-fraction arm developed pathological fractures compared with 1.6 percent patients in multifraction arm (odds ratio 1.82).[94***] The incidence of spinal compression was similar for both arms.[94***] Single-fraction radiotherapy may have a significant role in the palliative setting.

The mechanism of action of radiotherapy in the relief of pain is not well-defined. The speed of onset and pain relief over the first 14 days appears to be independent of tumor type when based on retrospective subgroup analysis.[95*] Roughly 50 percent of patients record an improvement within 2 weeks, and another 10–20 percent within 4 weeks, although those with lung cancer appear to have a lower prospect of pain relief.[95*,96*] These observations led to the hypothesis that tumor shrinkage may not be an essential requirement for pain relief.[97*] This may indicate the possibility that radiosensitive host cells, including macrophages and osteoclasts, which respond to low doses of ionizing radiation by apoptosis, may be therapeutic targets. Recent data suggest that the response to radiotherapy may reduce osteoclast activity.[98*]

For treatment of generalized bone pain, hemibody irradiation may alleviate pain, although serious adverse effects such as bone marrow suppression and radiation pneumonitis limit its application.

Radioisotopes

Radioisotopes, which concentrate in sites of bone metabolism due to malignant tumor activity, produce similar analgesic results to external-beam radiotherapy for management of multifocal malignant bone pain.[93***] Strontium-89, samarium-153, phosphorus-32 and lexidronam (Quadramet) have been found to be effective and are widely available.[99**,100*,101**] There is no evidence suggesting that one particular kind of radioisotope is more effective than the others in management of malignant bone pain.[102] A systemic review suggested a small effect of radioisotopes on pain control for 1–6-month period without available evidence for long-term effects (12 months) in management of metastatic bone pain.[103***] A high incidence of leukocytopenia (relative risk 4.56) in association with radioisotope therapy was found.[103]*** A recently evaluated 'bone consolidation approach', which is the combination of a systemic chemotherapy regimen (doxorubicin) followed by Metastron (strontium-89), seemed promising for reduction of SRE as well as survival benefit in patients with metastatic prostate cancer.[104]

Radioisotopes may have a role in recurrent pain sites after maximum dose of external beam radiotherapy. However, the timing of administration with respect to chemotherapy and radiotherapy is important. A rapid fall in leukocyte or platelet count may be contraindications. The presence of disseminated intravascular coagulation is also a contraindication for this therapy.[105]* Radioisotopes should not be considered as an alternative option to external beam radiotherapy for an existing or impending pathological fracture and spinal cord compression since it would not provide sufficient radiation to soft tissues.[106]

Orthopedic surgery

Pathological fractures of bones will generally not heal by themselves because of excessive osteolytic activity in the area of the metastasis. These fractures may contribute to the development of pneumonia, pressure ulcers, urinary tract infections, thromboembolism, and caregiver burden due to extremely limited functional status. In fractured bone, internal fixation or endoprosthetic reconstruction provides superior relief of pain and restoration of function, compared with nonoperative treatment of most pathological fractures.[107] An expected survival of only weeks to months is not necessarily a contraindication to surgery.[108]

In painful bone metastases without fracture, the first prospective, consecutive series of pilot studies to evaluate surgical treatment did not find a clear benefit to quality of life for patients with advanced skeletal metastases.[109]* The complications associated with these procedures include spinal cord compression, urinary retention, ileus, intractable pain, and pulmonary compromise due to osteolytic fractures.[110]*,[111]* Postoperative radiotherapy generally is recommended after surgical fixation of pathological fractures, stabilization of impending fractures, decompression of the spinal cord, or stabilization of the spine. Postoperative therapy has been associated with a decrease in the need for second surgical procedures and improved functional status in patients with previously unirradiated long bone and acetabular lesions.[112]* Treatment generally is started within 2–4 weeks of surgery.

Kyphoplasty

Kyphoplasty is a new technique evolving from vertebroplasty, which combines injection of polymethylmethacrylate to strengthen a vertebra with balloon angioplasty.[113]* This technique was developed after vertebroplasty, which showed a high incidence of complications especially epidural leakage of cement outside of vertebral bodies. This procedure may lead to early and sustained clinical improvement in pain and function through timely intervention of effective skeletal reconstruction for those suffering from ongoing osteolytic destruction of vertebral bodies with minimum complication.[114],[115]* Further controlled study will be warranted for clinical implication in the setting of metastatic bone disease.

Percutaneous image–guided radiofrequency ablation

A small study of consecutive patients examining the efficacy of percutaneous image-guided radiofrequency ablation using multiple needles for patients with painful osteolytic metastasis suggests that this therapy may have a role in reducing malignant bone pain, reducing the amount of opioid requirement, and preventing the painful consequence of disease progression.[116]* The possible mechanisms of action include destroying tumor cells and decreasing the production of cytokines and tumor factors involved in bone nerve sensitization and osteoclastic activity.[116]*

CONCLUSION

Identification of the multiple mechanisms responsible for production of distinct pain syndromes and their molecular components as well as identification of clinical malignant bone pain syndrome has been a major contribution in further advancement in management of malignant bone pain. Mechanism-based therapies are under development that target specific components of bone cancer pain. However, there are still unanswered questions regarding currently available treatment modalities, such as: How should we integrate the use of each treatment modality with our understanding of the heterogeneity of malignancies and individual factors?, and How should we determine the cost-benefit consequences?

Key learning points

- Recent evidence from the basic sciences supports that malignant bone pain is a distinctive pain state compared with inflammatory or neuropathic pain.

- Diagnosis of malignant bone pain should include a thorough history and physical examination, particularly musculoskeletal and neurological examination, in conjunction with information from imaging tests.

- Bone pain accompanied by progressive neurological symptoms or signs of pathological fracture may need to be assessed and treated urgently.

- Opioid analgesics, possibly in conjunction with NSAIDs or corticosteroids, may be considered as first-line therapy for malignant bone pain management because of their rapid onset of action.

- Limited evidence supports the analgesic efficacy of currently available treatment modalities, such as bisphosphonates and external beam radiotherapy for malignant bone pain.

- Further research into new mechanism-based therapy in malignant bone pain and integration of currently available treatment modalities is warranted.

REFERENCES

- 1   Clohisy D, Mantyh P. Bone cancer pain. *Cancer* 2003; **97**(3 Suppl): 866–73.
   2   Coleman RE. How can we improve the treatment of bone metastases further? Curr Opin Radiol 1998; **10** (Suppl 1): S7–S13.
- 3   Coleman RE. Skeletal complications of malignancy. *Cancer* 1997; **80**: 1588–94.
   4   Carlin BI, Andriole GL. The natural history; skeletal complications and management of bone metastases in patients with prostate carcinoma. *Cancer* 2000; **88**: 2989–94.
   5   Koendersm PG, Beex LV, Kloppenborg PWC, *et al.* Human breast cancer: survival from metastases. *Breast Res Treat* 1992; **21**: 173–80.
   6   Thongprasert S, Sanguanmitra P, Juthapan W. Relationship between quality of life and clinical outcomes in advanced non-small cell lung cancer: best supportive care (BSC) versus BSC plus chemotherapy. *Lung Cancer* 1999; **24**: 17–24.
   7   Koga S, Tsuda S, Nishikido M, *et al.* The diagnostic value of bone scan in patients with renal cell carcinoma. *J Urol* 2001; **166**: 2126–8.
   8   Coppin C, Porzsolt F, Kumpf J, *et al.* Immunotherapy for advanced renal cell cancer. (Cochrane Review). In: *Cochrane Library*, Chichester, UK: John Wiley & Sons, Ltd, 2004(3).
   9   Wallmeroth A. Wagner U, Moch H, *et al.* Pattern of metastases in muscle-invasive bladder cancer (pT2–4): an autopsy study on 367 patients. *Urol Int* 1999; **62**: 69–75.
  10   von der Maasse H. Current and future perspectives in advanced bladder cancer: is there a new standard? *Semin Oncol* 2002; **29**: 3–14.
  11   Hortobagyi GN, Theriault RL, Porter L, *et al.* Efficacy of pamidronate in reducing skeletal complications in patients with breast cancer and lytic bone mets. *N Engl J Med* 1996; **335**: 1836–7.
  12   Theriault RL, Lipton A, Hortobagyi GN, *et al.* Pamidronate reduces skeletal morbidity in women with advanced breast cancer and lytic bone lesions: a randomised, placebo-controlled trial Protocol 18 Aredia Breast Cancer Study Group. *J Clin Oncol* 1999; **17**: 846–54.
  13   Lote K, Walloe A, Bjersand A. Bone metastases: prognosis diagnosis and treatment. *Acta Radiol Oncol* 1986; **25**: 227–32.
- 14   Portenoy RK, P. L. Management of cancer pain. *Lancet* 1999; **353**: 1695–700.

  15   Portenoy RK, Payne D, Jacobson P. Breakthrough pain: characteristics and impact in patients with cancer pain. *Pain* 1999; **81**: 129–34.
  16   Schwei MJ, Honore P, Rogers SD, *et al.* Neurochemical and cellular recognition of the spinal cord in a murine model of bone cancer pain. *J Neurosci* 1999; **19**: 10886–97.
  17   Honore P, Luger NM, Sabino MA, *et al.* Osteoprotegerin blocks bone cancer-induced skeletal destruction, skeletal pain and pain-related neurochemical reorganization of the spinal cord. *Nat Med* 2000; **6**: 521–8.
  18   Honore P, Rogers SD, Schwei MJ, *et al.* Murine models of inflammatory, neuropathic, and cancer pain each generates a unique set of neurochemical changes in the spinal cord and sensory neurons. *Neuroscience* 2000; **98**: 585–98.
  19   Galasko C. Diagnosis of skeletal metastases and assessment of response to treatment. *Clin Orthop* 1995; **312**: 64–75.
  20   Luger NM, Honore P, Sabino MA, *et al.* Osteoprotegerin diminishes advanced bone cancer pain. *Cancer Res* 2001; **61**: 4038–47.
  21   Medhurst SJ, Walker K, Bowes M, *et al.* A rat model of bone cancer pain. *Pain* 2002; **96**: 129–40.
  22   Wacnik PW, Kehl LJ, Trempe TM, *et al.* Tumor implantation in mouse humerus evokes by intramuscular carrageenan. *Pain* 2003; **101**: 175–86.
  23   Luger NM, Sabino MA, Schwei MJ, *et al.* Efficacy of systemic morphine suggests a fundamental difference in the mechanisms that generate bone cancer vs inflammatory pain. *Pain* 2002; **99**: 397–406.
  24   Vanderah TW, Ossipov MH, Lai J, *et al.* Mechanisms of opioid-induced pain and antinociceptive tolerance: descending facilitation and spinal dynorphin. *Pain* 2001; **92**: 5–9.
  25   Urch CE, Donovan-Rodriguez T, Dickenson AH. Alteration in dorsal horn neurones in a rat model of cancer-induced bone pain. *Pain* 2003; **106**: 347–56.
  26   Mantyh PW, Clohisy DR, Koltzenburg M, *et al.* Molecular mechanisms of cancer pain. *Nat Rev Caner* 2002; **2**: 201–9.
  27   Bjurholm A, Kreicbergs A, Bordin E, Schultzberg M. Substance P- and CGRP-immunoreactive nerves in bone. *Peptides* 1988; **9**: 165–71.
  28   Mach DB, Rogers SD, Sabino MC, *et al.* Origins of skeletal pain: sensory and sympathetic innervation of the mouse femur. *Neuroscience* 2002; **113**: 155–66.
  29   Berruti A, Dogliotti L, Gorzegno G, *et al.* Differential patterns of bone turnover in relation to bone pain and disease extent in bone in cancer patients with skeletal metastases. *Clin Chem* 1999; **45**: 1240–7.
  30   Lipton A, Theriault RL, Hortobagyi GN, *et al.* Pamidronate prevents skeletal complications and is effective palliative treatment in women with breast carcinoma and osteolytic bone metastases: long-term follow-up of two randomised, placebo-controlled trials. *Cancer* 2000; **88**: 1082–90.
  31   Pelger RC, Hamdy NA, Zwinderman AH, *et al.* Effects of the bisphosphonate olpadronate in patients with carcinoma of the prostate metastatic to the skeleton. *Bone* 1998; **22**: 403–8.
  32   Hortobagyi GN, Theriault RL, Lipton A, *et al.* Long-term prevention of skeletal complications of metastatic breast cancer with pamidronate. For the Protcol 19 Aredia Breast Cancer Study Group. *J Clin Oncol* 1998; **16**: 2038–44.
- 33   Hortobagyi GN. Novel approaches to the management of bone metastases. *Semin Oncol* 2003; **30**(5 suppl 16): 161–6.

◆ 34 Mundy GR. Mechanisms of bone metastases. *Cancer* 1997; **80**: 1546–56.

35 Olson TH, Rield MS, Vulchanova XR, Elde R. An acid sensing ion channel (ASIC) localizes to small primary afferent neurons in rats. *Neuroreport* 1998; **9**: 1109–13.

36 Simonet WS, Lacey DL, Dunstan CR, *et al.* Osteoprotegerin: a novel secreted protein involved in the regulation of bone density. *Cell* 1997; **89**: 309–19.

37 Lacey DL, Timms E, Tan HL, *et al.* Osteoprotegerin ligand is a cytokine that regulates osteoclast differentiation and activation. *Cell* 1998; **93**: 165–76.

38 Bekker PJ, Holloway D, Nakanishi A, *et al.* The effect of a single dose of osteoprotegerin in postmenopausal women. *J Bone Miner Res* 2001; **16**: 348–60.

39 Standal T, Seidel C, Hjertner O, *et al.* Osteoprotegerin is bound, internalized, and degrated by multiple myeloma cells. *Blood* 2002; **100**: 3002–7.

● 40 Mercadante S, Arcuri E. Breakthrough pain in cancer patients: pathophysiology and treatment. *Cancer Treat Rev* 1998; **24**: 425–32.

◆ 41 Vinholes J, Coleman R, Eastell R. Effects of bone metastases on bone metabolism: implications for diagnosis, imaging and assessment of response to cancer treatment. *Cancer Treat Res* 1996; **22**: 289–331.

42 Hamaoka T, Madewell JE, Podoloff DA, *et al.* Bone imaging in metastatic breast cancer. *J Clin Oncol* 2004; **22**: 2942–53.

43 Corcoran RJ, Thrall JH, Kyle RW, *et al.* Solitary abnormalities in bone scans of patients with extraosseous malignancies. *Radiology* 1976; **121**: 663–7.

44 Coleman RE, Rubens RD. Bone metastasis. In: Abeloff MD, Armitage JO, Niederhuber JE, *et al.*, eds. *Clinical Oncology*. Philadelphia: Elsevier, Churchill Livingstone, 2004: 1091–129.

45 Peter JE. Skeletal imaging in metastatic disease. *Curr Opin Radiol* 1991; **3**: 791–0.

46 Tryciecky EW, Cottschalk A, Ludema K. Oncologic imaging: interactions of nuclear medicine with CT and MRI using the bone scan as a midel. *Semin Nucl Med* 1997; **27**: 142–51.

◆ 47 Rybak LD, Rosenthal DI. Radiological imaging for the diagnosis of bone metastases. *Q J Nucl Med* 2001; **45**: 53–64.

48 Colletti PM, Siegel HR, Woo MY, *et al.* The impact on treatment planning of MRI of the spine in patients suspected if vertebral metastasis: an efficacy study. *Comput Med Imaging Graph* 1996; **20**: 159–62.

49 Pigott KH, Baddeley H, Maher EJ. Pattern of disease in spinal cord compression on MRI scan and implications for treatment. *Clin Oncol* 1994; **6**: 7–10.

50 Kattapuram SV, Khurana JS, Scott JA, Khourygy E. Negative scintigraphy with positive magnetic resonance imaging in bone metastases. *Skeletal Radiol* 1990; **19**: 113–16.

51 Yamaguchi T, Tamai K, Yamato M, *et al.* Intertrabecular pattern of tumors metastatic to bone. *Cancer* 1996; **78**: 1288–394.

◆ 52 Souberbielle JC, Cormier C, Kindermans C. Bone markers in clinical practice. *Curr Opin Rheumatol* 1999; **11**: 312–19.

53 Lipton A, Demers L, Curley E, Chinchilli V, *et al.* Markers of bone resorption in patients treated with pamidronate for metastatic bone disease. *Ann Oncol* 1998; **8**: 1243–50.

◆ 54 Woitge HW, Pecherstorfer M, Li Y, *et al.* Novel serum markers of bone resorption: clinical assessment and comparison with established urinary indices. *J Bone Miner Res* 1999; **14**: 792–801.

55 Miura H, Yamamoto I, Takada M, *et al.* Diagnostic validity of bone metabolic markers for bone metastases. *Endocr J* 1997; **44**: 751–7.

◆ 56 Fohr B, Dunstan CR, Seibel MJ. Clinical Review 165: Markers of bone remodeling in metastatic bone disease. *J Clin Endocrinol Metab* 2003; **88**: 5059–75.

57 Twycross R. Cancer pain classification. *Aca Anaesthesiol Scand* 1997; **41**: 141–5.

58 Cheville AL. Pain management in cancer rehabilitation. *Arch Phys Med Rehabil* 2001; **82**(Suppl 1): S84–7.

◆ 59 Mercadante S, Radbruch L, Caraceni A, *et al.* Episodic (breakthrough) pain: consensus conference of an expert working group of the European Association for Palliative Care. *Cancer* 2002; **94**: 832–9.

60 Coluzzi PH, Schwartzberg L, Conroy JD, *et al.* Breakthrough cancer pain: a randomised trial comparing oral transmucosal fentanyl citrate (OTFC) and morphine sulphate immediate. *Pain* 2001; **91**: 123–30.

61 Portenoy RK, Payne R, Coluzzi P, *et al.* Oral transmucosal fentanyl citrate (OTFC) for the treatment of breakthough pain in cancer patients: a controlled dose titration study. *Pain* 1999; **79**: 303–12.

62 Payne R, Coluzzi P, Hart L, *et al.* Long-term safety or oral transmucosal fentanyl citrate for breakthough cancer pain. *J Pain Symptom Manage* 2001; **22**: 575–83.

63 McNicol E, Strassels S, Goudas L, *et al.* Nonsteroidal anti-inflamatory drugs, alone or combined with opioids, for cancer pain: a systematic review. *J Clin Oncol* 2004; **22**: 1975–92.

64 Lembeck F, Gamse R. Substance P in peripheral sensory processes. *Ciba Found Symp* 1982; **91**: 35–54.

65 Vasko M. Prostaglandin-induced neuropeptide release from spinal cord. *Prog Brain Res* 1995; **104**: 367–80.

66 Moore BC, Simmons DL. COX-2 inhibition, apoptosis, and chemoprevention by nonsteroidal anti-inflammatory drugs. *Curr Med Chem* 2000; **7**: 1131–44.

67 Sabino MA, Ghilardi JR, Jongen JL, *et al.* Simultaneous reduction in cancer pain, bone destruction, and tumor growth by selective inhibition of cyclooxygenase-2. *Cancer Res* 2002; **62**: 7343–49.

68 Fox A, Medhurst SJ, Courade J, *et al.* Anti-hyperalgesic activity of the cox-2 inhibitor lumiraxoxib in a model of bone cancer pain in the rat. *Pain* 2004; **107**: 33–40.

69 Small EJ, Vogelzang NJ. Second-line hormonal therapy for advanced prostate cancer: a shifting paradigm. *J Clin Oncol* 1997; **15**: 382–8.

70 Tannock IF, Osoba D, Stockler MR, *et al.* Chemotherapy with mitoxantrone plus prednisone or prednisone alone for symptomatic hormone-resistant prostate cancer: a Canadian randomised trial with palliative end point. *J Clin Oncol* 1996; **14**: 1756–64.

71 Kantoff PW, Halabi S, Conaway M, *et al.* Hydrocortisone with or without mitoxantrone in men with hormone-refractory prostate cancer: results of the Cancer and Leukemia Group B 9182 study. *J Clin Oncol* 1999; **18**: 2506–13.

72 Kingrery WS, Castellote JM, Maze M. Methylprednisolone prevents the development of autotomy and neuropathic edema in rats, but has no effect on nociceptive thresholds. *Pain* 1999; **80**: 555–66.

73 Weber D, Rankin K, Gavino M, *et al.* Thalidomide alone or with dexamethasone for previously untreated multiple myeloma. *J Clin Oncol* 2003; **21**: 16–19.

74 Rajkumar SV, Hayman S, Gertz MA, *et al.* Combination therapy with thalidomide plus dexamethasone for newly diagnosed myeloma. *J Clin Oncol* 2002; **20**: 4319–23.

75 Alexanian R, Dimopoulos MA, Delasalle K, Barlogie B. Primary dexamethasone treatment of multiple myeloma. *Blood* 1992; **80**: 887–90.

76 Twycross R. The risks and benefits of corticosteroids in advanced cancer. *Drug Saf* 1994; **11**: 163–78.

77 Dropcho EJ, Twycross R, Truenman T. Steroid-induced weakness in patients with primary brain tumors. *Postgrad Med* 1983; **59**: 702–6.

78 Martinez MJ, Roque M, Alonso-Coello P, *et al.* Calcitonin for metastatic bone pain (Cochrane Review). In: *Cochrane Library.* Chichester, UK: John Wiley & Sons, Ltd, 2004(3).

● 79 Green J. Anti-tumor effects of bisphosphonates. *Cancer* 2003; **97**(Suppl 3): 840–7.

80 Walker K, Medhurst SJ, Kidd BL, *et al.* Disease modifying and anti-nociceptive effects of the bisphosphonate, zolendronic acid in a model of bone cancer pain. *Pain* 2002; **100**: 219–29.

81 Green JR, Rogers MJ. Pharmacologic profile of zoledronic acid: a highly potent inhibitor of bone resorption. *Drug Dev Res* 2002; **55**: 210–24.

82 Wong R, Wiffen PJ. Bisphosphonates for the relief of pain secondary to bone metastases (Cochrane Review). In: *Cochrane Library.* Chichester, UK: John Wiley & Sons, Ltd, 2004(3).

83 Rosen LS, Gordon D, Kaminski M, *et al.* Long-term efficacy and safety of zoledronic acid compared with pamidronate disodium in the treatment of skeletal complications in patients with advanced multiple myeloma or breast cancer. *Cancer* 2003; **98**: 1735–44.

84 Body JJ, Diel IJ, Lichinitzer M, *et al.* Oral ibandronate reduces the risk of skeletal complications in breast cancer patients with metastatic bone disease: results from two randomised, placebo-controlled phase III studies. *Br J Cancer* 2004; **90**: 1133–7.

85 Diel IJ, Body JJ, Lichinitser MR, *et al.* Improved quality of life after long-term treatment with the bisphosphonate ibandronate in patients with metastatic bone disease due to breast cancer. *Eur J Cancer* 2004; **40**: 1704–12.

86 Dearnaley DP, Sydes MR, Mason MD, *et al.* A double-blind, placebo-controlled, randomised trial of oral sodium clodronate for metastatic prostate cancer (MRC PR05 Trial). *J Natl Cancer Inst* 2003; **95**: 1300–11.

87 Ernst DS, Tannock IF, Winquist EW, *et al.* Randomised, double-blind, controlled trial of mitoxantrone/prednisone and clodronate versus mitoxantrone/prednisone and placebo in patients with hormone-refractory prostate cancer and pain. *J Clin Oncol* 2003; **21**: 3335–42.

88 Gleason DM, Saad F, Goas A, Zheng M. Continuing benefit of zoledronic acid in preventing skeletal complications after the first occurence in patients with prostate cancer and bone metastases [abstract 1522]. Program and Proceedings of the American Society of Clinical Oncology 39th annual meeting, Chicago, IL Alexandria (Virginia), 2003: 379.

89 Saad F, Gleason DM, Murray R, *et al.* A randomised, placebo-controlled trial of zoledronic acid in patients with hormone-refractory metastatic prostate cancer. *J Natl Cancer Inst* 2002; **94**: 1458–68.

90 Small EJ, Smith MR, Seaman JJ, Petrone S, Kowalsaki MO. Combined analysis of two multicentre, randomised, placebo-controlled studies of pamidronate disodium for the palliative of bone pain in men with metastatic prostate cancer. *J Clin Oncol* 2003; **21**: 4277–84.

91 Menssen HD, Sakalova A, Fontana A, *et al.* Effects of long-term intravenous ibandronate therapy on skeletal-related events, survival, and bone resorption markers in patients with advanced multiple myeloma. *J Clin Oncol* 2002; **20**: 2353–9.

92 Musto P, Falcone A, Sanpaolo G, *et al.* Pamidronate reduces skeletal events but does not improve progression-free survival in early-stage untreated myeloma: results of a randomized trial. *Leuk Lymphoma* 2003; **44**: 1545–8.

93 McQuay HJ, Collins SL, Carroll D, Moore RA. Radiotherapy for the palliation of painful bone metastases (Cochrane Review). In: *Cochrane Library.* Chichester, UK: John Wiley & Sons, Ltd, 2002(4).

94 Sze WM, Shelley M, Held I, Mason M. Palliation of metastatic bone pain: single fraction versus multifraction radiotherapy (Cochrane Review). In: *Cochrane Library.* Chichester, UK: John Wiley & Sons, Ltd, 2004(3).

95 Price P, Hoskin PJ, Easton D, *et al.* Prospective randomised trial of single and multifraction radiotherapy schedules in the treatment of painful bony metastases. *Radiother Oncol* 1986; **6**: 247–55.

96 Hoskin PJ, Price P, Easton D, *et al.* A prospective randomised trial of 4 Gy or 8Gy single doses in the treatment of metastatic bone pain. *Radiother Oncol* 1992; **23**: 74–8.

97 Bone Pain Trial Working Party. 8 Gy single fraction radiotherapy for the treatment of metastatic skeletal pain: randomised comparison with a multifraction schedule over 12 months of patient follow-up. *Radiother Oncol* 1999; **52**: 111–21.

98 Papatheofani FJ. Serum PICP as a bone formation marker in 89Sr and external beam radiotherapy of bone metastasis. *Br J Radiol* 1997; **70**: 584–8.

99 Lewington VJ, McEwan AJB, Ackery DM, *et al.* A prospective, randomised double-blind crossover study to examine the efficacy of strontium-89 in pain palliation in patients with advanced prostate cancer metastatic to bone. *Eur J Cancer* 1991; **27**: 954–8.

100 Quilty PM, Kirk D, Bolger JJ, *et al.* A comparison of the palliative effects of strontium-89 and external beam radiotherapy in metastatic prostate cancer. *Radiother Oncol* 1994; **31**: 33–40.

101 Serafini AN, Houston SJ, Resche I, *et al.* Palliation of pain associated with metastatic bone cancer using samarium-153 lexidronam: a double-blind placebo-controlled clinical trial. *J Clin Oncol* 1998; **16**: 1574–81.

● 102 Mertens WC, Filipczak LA, Ben-Josef E, *et al.* Systemic bone-seeking radionuclides for palliation of painful osseous metastases: current concepts. *CA Cancer J Clin* 1998; **48**: 361–74.

103 Raqué M, Martinez MJ, Alonso-Coello P, *et al.* Radioisotopes for metastatic bone pain (Cochrane Review). In: *Cochrane Library.* Chichester, UK: John Wiley & Sons, Ltd, 2004(3).

104 Tu SM, Millikan RE, Mengistu B, *et al.* Bone-targeted therapy for advanced androgen-independent carcinoma of the prostate: a randomized Phase II trial. *Lancet* 2001; **357**: 336–41.

105 Leong C, Mckenzie MR, Coupland DB, *et al.* Disseminated intravascular coagulation in patients with metastatic

prostate cancer: fatal outcome following strontium-89 therapy. *J Nucl Med* 1994; **35**: 1662–4.

◆ 106 Silberstein EB, Eugene M, Saenger SR. Painful osteoblastic metastases: the role of nuclear medicine. *Oncology* 2001; **15**: 157–63.

◆ 107 Harrington KD. Orthopedic surgical management of skeletal complications of malignancy. *Cancer* 1997; **80**(8 Suppl): 1614–27.

● 108 Frassica FJ, Frassica DA, Lietman SA, *et al.* Surgical palliation of malignant bone pain. In: Portenoy R Bruera E, eds. *Topics in Palliative Care*. Vol. 3. New York: Oxford; **1998**: 139–62.

109 Clohisy DR, Le CT, Cheng EY, *et al.* Evaluation of the feasibility of and results of measuring health-status changes in patients undergoing surgical treatment for skeletal metastases. *J Orthop Res* 2000; **18**: 1–9.

110 Cortet B, Cotten A, Boutry N, *et al.* Percutaneous vertebroplasty in patients with osteolytic metastases or multiple myeloma. *Rev Rheum Engl Ed* 1997; **64**: 145–6.

111 Cetton A, Dewatre F, Cortet B, *et al.* Percutaneous vertebroplasty for osteolytic metastases and myeloma: effects of the percentage of lesion filling and the leakage of methylmethacrylate at clinical follow up. *Radiology* 1996; **200**: 525–30.

112 Townsend PW, Rosenthal HG, Smalley SR, *et al.* Impact of postoperative radiation therapy and other perioperative factors on outcome after orthopaedic stabilization of impending or pathologic fractures due to metastatic disease. *J Clin Oncol* 1994; **12**: 2345–50.

113 Dudeney S, Lieberman I, Reinhardt MK, Hussein M. Kyphoplasty in the treatment of osteolytic vertebral compression fractures as a result of multiple myeloma. *J Clin Oncol.* 2002: 2382–7.

● 114 Lieberman I, Reinhhardt MK. Vertebroplasty and kyphoplasty for osteolytic vertebral collapse. *Clin Orthop Relat Res* 2003; **415**: 176–86.

115 Lane JM, Hong R, Koob J, *et al.* Kyphoplasty enhances function and structural alignment in multiple myeloma. *Clin Orthop Relat Res* 2004; **426**: 49–53.

116 Goetz MP, Callstrom MR, Charboneau W, *et al.* Percutaneous image-guided radiofrequency ablation of painful metastases involving bone: a multicenter study. *J Clin Oncol* 2004; **22**: 300–6.

Episodic pain

SHIRLEY H BUSH

INTRODUCTION

The intensity of cancer pain commonly fluctuates over time and challenges usual cancer pain management using the World Health Organization (WHO) analgesic 'ladder'. It is an important clinical problem, often significantly impacting on a patient's quality of life, and can be difficult to assess and predict. A bewildering array of terminology and definitions has been used to describe this heterogeneous phenomenon but the lack of a standardized worldwide definition has led to difficulty in comparisons of reported prevalence and management.

Background to terminology and definitions

In 1989, the Edmonton staging system for cancer pain defined 'incidental pain' as 'pain aggravated suddenly as a result of movements, swallowing, defecation or urination'.[1] Portenoy and Hagen developed a working definition for 'breakthrough pain' in 1990, for a prospective survey of cancer pain patients.[2] Breakthrough pain was defined as 'a transitory increase in pain to greater than moderate intensity, which occurred on a baseline pain of moderate intensity or less'. Opioid use was not included in the working definition, but evaluated patients had been on relatively stable doses of opioids for two consecutive days. Breakthrough pain required controlled background pain for this definition.[3] It has been felt that breakthrough pain cannot be assessed in patients with uncontrolled pain.[4] Breakthrough pain has also been defined as pain that 'breaks through' the regular doses of an analgesic schedule.[5] This includes 'end-of-dose failure', where pain worsens before the next scheduled dose of opioid.

The term 'incident pain' is frequently used to describe pain induced by movement.[6] The definition is often broadened to define pain due to, or exacerbated by a specific inducing event (action) or activity.[7,8] McQuay and Jadad classified 'incident pain' into two subtypes. The first was pain on movement that included walking, turning, lifting, coughing, and deep breathing. The other subtype was intermittent pain not related to activity or movement.[9] 'Incident pain' has also been used to represent pain with a volitional precipitant, i.e. induced by the patient's voluntary actions, which should be predictable.[2,10]

Other terms that have been used include 'pain in motion'[11*] and 'transitory pain'.[12] In an international survey of 58 clinicians from 24 countries, where breakthrough pain was defined as an episode of 'pain flare', there was a large variation in the rates of breakthrough pain identification, suggesting that the concept of breakthrough pain varies geographically.[13]

'Episodic pain' is the term agreed on by an expert working group of the European Association for Palliative Care, in December 2000, as it translates better into different languages.[14] 'Episodic pain' is a transitory exacerbation of pain that changes with time. It can occur with controlled or uncontrolled baseline pain (Fig. 54.1). In the absence of significant baseline pain, it can be further differentiated into movement-related (incident) episodic pain, which is usually due to bone metastases, and nonmovement-related episodic pain. The working group also recognized pains which are volitional and not induced by a specific movement, e.g. swallowing in presence of mucositis or touch if hyperesthesia, and nonvolitional pains, e.g. sneezing, coughing, laughing or myoclonus. Spontaneous pains are independent of movement or volition, e.g. neuropathic pain.

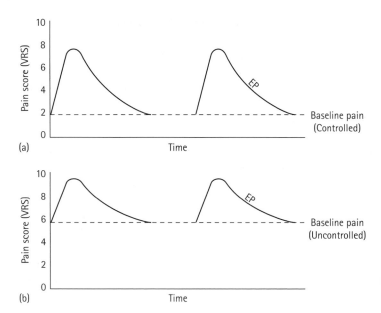

Figure 54.1   *(a,b) Episodic pain (EP) crescendos. VRS, verbal rating scale.*

From these assorted definitions, episodic pain can be more usefully classified into three subtypes: activity and movement-related, spontaneous and end-of-dose failure.

ETIOLOGY OF EPISODIC PAIN

As with cancer pain etiology, episodic pain may be caused by the cancer or by the cancer treatment. Episodic pain may also be related to the cancer or debility, or be due to a concurrent disorder.

EPISODIC PAIN MECHANISMS

Episodic pain, like cancer pain, is categorized according to different anatomical and pathophysiological pain mechanisms.[15] The mechanistic categories are: nociceptive, comprising superficial somatic, deep somatic and visceral pains, and neuropathic pains. Episodic pain may have a different pathophysiology to the baseline pain.

PREVALENCE AND CHARACTERISTICS OF EPISODIC PAIN

The prevalence of episodic pain differs enormously depending on the definition and survey instrument used and the population sampled. Reported prevalence has been as low as 19 percent[16*] to around 90 percent.[17–19] Many studies report prevalence in the range of 40–70 percent.[2,3,12,20,21*] Internationally, prevalence has been found to vary according to region with a reported prevalence of 80.1 percent from English-speaking countries, 69.4 percent from North

and Western Europe, 54.8 percent from South America, and only 45.9 percent from Asia.[22]

Episodic pain commonly occurs a median 4–6 times/day, although the range can markedly vary, as in the reported case of a patient with a rib fracture and cough experiencing episodic pain every minute.[2] Box 54.1 gives the mean time for pain to peak and the mean duration, although the upper limit of the range can be as long as 2 or even 4 hours. Most cases of episodic pain are exacerbations of the baseline pain, but they can be a worsening of a different pain. A minority of patients experience more than one type of episodic pain.

Box 54.1 Features of typical episodic pain

- Mean time to peak – 3 minutes

- Mean duration – 15–30 minutes

The onset of episodic pain is often unpredictable, despite 20–40 percent being movement-related and 13–30 percent classified as end-of-dose failure.[3,18,21*] Neuropathic episodic pain is significantly briefer and more frequent than nociceptive episodic pain.[12,18]

REGARDING THE IMPACT OF EPISODIC PAIN

Patients with episodic pain tend to have higher pain scores and more intense baseline pain than patients without episodic pain. The presence of episodic pain significantly impacts on walking and causes functional interference on the Brief Pain Inventory, manifesting as increased levels of depression and anxiety.[3,21*,22] Episodic pain often interferes with sleep and impairs quality of life by restricting social and general activities. Cancer patients with episodic pain are more likely to have endured increased medical costs, due to pain-related hospitalization and physician visits.[23]

Movement-related episodic pain, which is commonly due to metastatic bone disease, is relatively resistant to treatment with analgesics.[21*,24*] The presence of bone metastases had a significant impact for patients attending a multidisciplinary pain clinic in Denmark as only 6 percent of these patients became pain free 'in motion' after pain treatment.[11*] In a prospective multicenter assessment of the Edmonton clinical staging system, patients with 'incidental pain' were less likely to respond well to any analgesic treatment.[25]

MANAGEMENT OF EPISODIC PAIN

For the appropriate management of episodic pain, a multimodality approach is needed while maintaining a holistic framework. Ongoing explanation with the patient and family is essential for professional care.

Assessment of episodic pain

A detailed assessment of the patient and the episodic pain(s) experienced should include episodic pain characteristics and mechanisms, in addition to those of the baseline pain, and a psychosocial evaluation. The Breakthrough Pain Questionnaire was designed to characterize breakthrough pain.[2] It should be noted that the assessment algorithm used in the 1999 survey had not been validated.[3]

Primary therapies to treat the underlying cause

Oncological interventions may be appropriate, depending on the patient's condition and anticipated prognosis. Radiotherapy is effective at reducing pain from painful bone metastases (see Chaper 91). Single and multiple fractionation schedules have been used with similar efficacy.[26***] For extensive bone metastatic disease causing pain, hemibody irradiation has been used. There is some evidence that radioisotopes, e.g. strontium-89, relieve pain over 1–6 months, but with a risk of leukopenia and thrombocytopenia.[27***] Bisphosphonates have been shown to be effective in reducing pain due to bone metastases (see Chapter 53).[28***]

There may be a role for chemotherapy or hormone therapy in responsive disease. Surgery may also be used palliatively after an assessment of benefits and attendant risks, e.g. stabilization of a pathological fracture, or prophylactically for a femur at risk of fracture. Percutaneous vertebroplasty has been shown to reduce pain and improve mobility in patients with fractured spinal metastases, who have failed radiation.[29*] Some cases of bowel obstruction may be remediable with surgery, thus eliminating episodic pain due to colic.

Optimizing the analgesic regimen

Implementation of the principles of the WHO 'ladder' should optimize the treatment of baseline pain. Episodic pain regularly improves as often baseline pain has been poorly controlled. However, it is important not to over-sedate the patient by increasing baseline opioid analgesia levels excessively in pursuit of around-the-clock control of episodic pain crescendos, as the pain signal will often diminish with rest or time (Fig. 54.2a). If opioid side effects are excessive, then opioid substitution or 'switching' should be considered (see Chapter 45). Another strategy to decrease sedation from opioids is the addition of methylphenidate.[16*] Increasing the opioid dose or reducing the interval between opioid doses can manage end-of-dose failure. For example, a few patients require 12-hourly modified release morphine to be given every 8 hours or transdermal fentanyl patches changed every 48 hours, rather than the usual 72 hours.

Depending on the pain mechanism, the use of non-opioid analgesic regimens may also improve baseline analgesia. Anti-inflammatory agents, such as nonsteroidal anti-inflammatory drugs (NSAIDs) and short-term use of steroids like dexamethasone, are indicated for pain due to bone metastases, mucosal or skin lesions. They also provide relief for pain originating from organ capsules, such as liver capsule inflammation, and from mesothelial membranes (pleura and peritoneum). Steroids also have an analgesic effect on neuropathic pain by reducing edema around peripheral nerves. The regular use of adjuvants for neuropathic pain, including tricyclic antidepressants, anticonvulsants and antiarrhythmics, should diminish episodic pain from this mechanism. Patients with either multiple bone metastases and severe movement-related episodic pain, mucositis or neuropathic pain have responded to ketamine, an N-methyl-D-aspartate (NMDA) receptor antagonist, given as a 'burst' subcutaneous infusion for 3–5 days.[30*]

Other drugs used for episodic pain include antispasmodics, e.g. hyoscine butylbromide for bowel spasm, oxybutynin for bladder spasm, and diazepam or baclofen for muscle spasm.

Using 'rescue' analgesia for episodic pain

A 'rescue' dose of analgesia should be administered when needed to 'top-up' baseline analgesia, either in anticipation of a predicted episodic pain or at the onset of an episodic pain. Frequently, a patient will have concluded that their prescribed oral 'rescue' dose is pointless, as their episodic pain will have resolved long before the onset of the extra pain relief. Often an opioid is used, but sometimes an NSAID is prescribed. Properties of an ideal 'rescue' analgesic include:

- quick absorption with rapid onset of analgesia and early peak effect

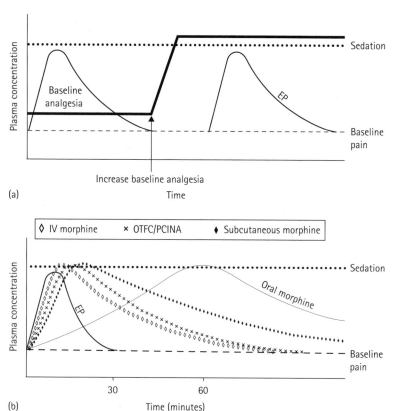

(a)

Increase baseline analgesia

Time

(b)

Time (minutes)

| ◊ IV morphine   × OTFC/PCINA   ♦ Subcutaneous morphine |

Figure 54.2 *Drug management of episodic pain (EP). (a) Increasing the baseline analgesia to meet the peaks of episodic pain, leading to oversedation. (b) Rescue doses of analgesia – schematic representation. OTFC, oral transmucosal fentanyl citrate; PCINA, patient-controlled intranasal analgesia.*

- a short duration of action, but long enough to treat the episodic pain event
- minimal side effects
- a good safety profile.

The drug should target the implicated pain mechanism. The ideal 'rescue' analgesic would be responsive to the peaks and troughs of episodic pain with a rapid on/off effect to counter a fluctuating pain trajectory over a short period of time, analogous to the current 'gold standard' of intravenous patient controlled analgesia (PCA). It should also be easy to self-administer, available for both inpatients and those in the community and should not be expensive. The choice of drug for the 'rescue' dose and the route used will also be influenced by the accessibility of opioids and their formulations in different countries.

Routes of administration of opioid 'rescue' analgesia for episodic pain

See Table 54.1 and Figure 54.2b.

ORAL ROUTE

For patients on an oral regularly scheduled morphine regimen for baseline pain, it has been recommended that the 'rescue' dose be equivalent to the 4-hourly dose of morphine, i.e. 16 percent of the 24-hour dose.[31] Other clinicians suggest 5–10 percent. More recent studies suggest that an individual's 'rescue' dose should be found by titration.[32*]

Table 54.1 *Comparing the efficacy of different routes of administration of opioids*

Route	Average time for onset of analgesia	Average duration of analgesic effect
Intravenous, e.g. morphine	5 minutes	1–2 hours
Oral transmucosal/ intranasal, e.g. fentanyl series	5–15 minutes	1–2 hours
Subcutaneous, e.g. morphine	10–15 minutes	3–4 hours
Oral, as immediate (normal) release, e.g. morphine	30 minutes	4 hours

The immediate (normal) release formulation of morphine has a mean T_{max} (time at which maximum concentration is reached) of 1 hour.[33***] Analgesia then lasts about 4 hours, indicating that the time taken for onset of analgesia and its duration are usually too prolonged for the majority of episodic pain events.

INTRAVENOUS ROUTE

Pain relief should begin within 5 minutes of intravenous (IV) administration, and last for 1–2 hours.[34] On using a fixed ratio of IV morphine, given by bolus injection, pain intensity of episodic pain has been reported to be reduced by more than 50 percent within a mean of 16.6 minutes.[35*] Patients have had their uncontrolled bone pain successfully and safely managed at home by skilled and accessible staff, using a PCA pump and either the IV or subcutaneous route.[36*]

SUBCUTANEOUS ROUTE

Following a subcutaneous injection of opioid, analgesia begins within 10–15 minutes and lasts for 3–4 hours.[34] Mean time to pain relief with subcutaneous morphine for episodic pain is 17 minutes.[20]

ORAL AND NASAL TRANSMUCOSAL ROUTES

These routes have the advantage of bypassing the first-pass effect of the liver. The nasal and oral mucosae are highly vascular areas enabling rapid absorption and superior bioavailability for those drugs with suitable physicochemical properties.[37,38] Drugs meeting these requirements are lipophilic, with a high permeability coefficient, and potent. The properties of the fentanyl series of drugs make them the best of the available opioids for transmucosal administration. Sublingual administration of fentanyl citrate,[39] sufentanil[40] and alfentanil[41] have been reported. Volumes of fluid greater than 1–2 mL have been found to be problematic, due to reflex swallowing. Buprenorphine can be given sublingually, but sublingual absorption of morphine is poor due to low lipid solubility and over 90 percent ionization.[42]

There are a multitude of published studies on oral transmucosal fentanyl citrate (OTFC). OTFC is a compressed, sweetened lozenge with an artificial berry flavor, attached to a plastic applicator. It is available in six dose strengths but is relatively expensive. A unit should be consumed slowly over 15 minutes by rubbing it across the oral, particularly buccal, mucosa. The units must be kept out of the reach of children and correctly discarded. Randomized, double blinded trials have shown significantly better pain relief compared with placebo or immediate (normal) release morphine.[32*,43**] In an open label study of OTFC, the average time for onset of pain relief was 9.5 minutes.[44*] The T_{max} of a 15 µg/kg dose is 22 minutes with the effect lasting 1–2 hours. The overall bioavailability of OTFC is 50 percent, with 25 percent from rapid oromucosal absorption and 25 percent from slower gastrointestinal absorption, after swallowing the remaining dose.[45] It has been found that there is no fixed relationship between the total daily dose of scheduled opioid and dose of OTFC required for the episodic pain,[46*,32*] so individual dose titration of this formulation is mandatory. Common adverse effects are somnolence, nausea, and dizziness.

The fentanyl series of drugs have also been administered by intranasal spray.[40,47*,48*] The T_{max} for their intranasal single dose administration in healthy volunteers is 5–10 minutes, with bioavailabilities of 65–78 percent.[37] The maximum volume for one nostril in a single administration is 150–200 µL. The use of a patient-controlled intranasal analgesia (PCINA) device mimics the efficacy of IV PCA.[48*] Morphine has been administered intranasally using chitosan to enhance penetration.[49*] In a pediatric population with clinical fractures, a nasal diamorphine spray provided a quicker onset of pain relief compared with intramuscular morphine.[50**] Adverse effects of nasal administration are mainly related to the opioid used, as opposed to the route itself.

Other drugs used for episodic pain

Intermittent subcutaneous midazolam has been used for the temporary sedation of patients with pathological hip fractures and severe episodic pain.[51] Subanesthetic ketamine, in a subcutaneous bolus dose of 20–40 mg, is often used before predictable movement-related episodic pain, such as difficult dressing changes or repositioning of a patient with a fractured long bone. It may be combined with a bolus injection of midazolam.[52] The utilization of intranasal ketamine for episodic pain appears promising following evidence from a recent placebo controlled, crossover trial in 20 patients with chronic pain.[53**]

Nonpharmacological approaches

There are a variety of contributing pain-relieving factors, including rest, repositioning, movement, heat, massage, relaxation, or diversion.[12,19] Referral to physiotherapy and occupational therapy is beneficial for patients with movement-related episodic pain. Orthotic devices, bracing or aids may be necessary, in addition to lifestyle modification.

Interventional approaches

For patients with resistant episodic pain, anesthetic or neurosurgical intervention may be required. Techniques used include: peripheral nerve or neurolytic blocks, spinal (intrathecal or epidural) analgesia, and percutaneous or open cordotomy.

FUTURE DIRECTIONS

Uniform worldwide and precise definitions of episodic pain are needed for consistency in characterization and to enable direct comparisons of trial data and management. Validated instruments to measure pain intensity over short periods of time are warranted. Further studies should investigate the appropriate dosing and titration of 'rescue' analgesia. 'Flexible' drugs are needed as 'rescue' analgesics, being responsive to changes in the pain intensity/time profile.

Studies should examine and refine the most appropriate management of the different episodic pain mechanisms.

Key learning points

- Episodic pain challenges the WHO 'ladder' for pain management.

- Current terminology and definitions are confusing.

- Prevalence is in the range of 40–70 percent.

- It is typically characterized by both rapid onset and brief duration.

- The parenteral and transmucosal routes are the most efficacious for 'rescue' analgesia, for drugs with appropriate pharmacodynamic properties.

REFERENCES

1 Bruera E, MacMillan K, Hanson J, MacDonald RN. The Edmonton staging system for cancer pain: preliminary report. *Pain* 1989; **37**: 203–9.

- 2 Portenoy RK, Hagen NA. Breakthrough pain: definition, prevalence and characteristics. *Pain* 1990; **41**: 273–81.

- 3 Portenoy RK, Payne D, Jacobsen P. Breakthrough pain: characteristics and impact in patients with cancer pain. *Pain* 1999; **81**: 129–34.

4 Cleary JF. Pharmacokinetic and pharmacodynamic issues in the treatment of breakthrough pain. *Semin Oncol* 1997; **24** (5 Suppl 16): 13–19.

◆ 5 Caraceni A, Weinstein SM. Classification of cancer pain syndromes. *Oncology* 2001; **15**: 1627–40, 1642.

6 Portenoy RK. Treatment of temporal variations in chronic cancer pain. *Semin Oncol* 1997; **24** (5 Suppl 16): 7–12.

7 Reddy SK, Nguyen P. Breakthrough pain in cancer patients: new therapeutic approaches to an old challenge. *Curr Rev Pain* 2000; **4**: 242–7.

8 Harlos M. Palliative care incident pain and incident dyspnea protocol. Available at: http://palliative.info/IncidentPain.htm (accessed July 22, 2004).

- 9 McQuay HJ, Jadad AR. Incident pain. *Cancer Surv* 1994; **21**: 17–24.

10 Sykes J, Johnson R, Hanks GW. ABC of palliative care: Difficult pain problems. *BMJ* 1997; **315**: 867–9.

11 Banning A, Sjogren P, Henriksen H. Treatment outcome in a multidisciplinary cancer pain clinic. *Pain* 1991; **47**: 129–34.

12 Petzke F, Radbruch L, Zech D, *et al.* Temporal presentation of chronic cancer pain: transitory pains on admission to a multidisciplinary pain clinic. *J Pain Symptom Manage* 1999; **17**: 391–401.

13 Caraceni A, Portenoy RK. An international survey of cancer pain characteristics and syndromes. IASP Task Force on Cancer Pain. International Association for the Study of Pain. *Pain* 1999; **82**: 263–74.

- 14 Mercadante S, Radbruch L, Caraceni A, *et al.* Episodic (breakthrough) pain: consensus conference of an expert working group of the European Association for Palliative Care. *Cancer* 2002; **94**: 832–9.

- 15 Ashby MA, Fleming BG, Brooksbank M, *et al.* Description of a mechanistic approach to pain management in advanced cancer. Preliminary report. *Pain* 1992; **51**: 153–61.

16 Bruera E, Fainsinger R, MacEachern T, Hanson J. The use of methylphenidate in patients with incident cancer pain receiving regular opiates. A preliminary report. *Pain* 1992; **50**: 75–7.

17 Fine PG, Busch MA. Characterization of breakthrough pain by hospice patients and their caregivers. *J Pain Symptom Manage* 1998; **16**: 179–83.

18 Zeppetella G, O'Doherty CA, Collins S. Prevalence and characteristics of breakthrough pain in cancer patients admitted to a hospice. *J Pain Symptom Manage* 2000; **20**: 87–92.

19 Swanwick M, Haworth M, Lennard RF. The prevalence of episodic pain in cancer: a survey of hospice patients on admission. *Palliat Med* 2001; **15**: 9–18.

20 Gomez-Batiste X, Madrid F, Moreno F, *et al.* Breakthrough cancer pain: prevalence and characteristics in patients in Catalonia, Spain. *J Pain Symptom Manage* 2002; **24**: 45–52.

21 Hwang SS, Chang VT, Kasimis B. Cancer breakthrough pain characteristics and responses to treatment at a VA medical center. *Pain* 2003; **101**: 55–64.

22 Caraceni A, Martini C, Zecca E, *et al.* Breakthrough pain characteristics and syndromes in patients with cancer pain. An international survey. *Palliat Med* 2004; **18**: 177–83.

23 Fortner BV, Okon TA, Portenoy RK. A survey of pain-related hospitalizations, emergency department visits, and physician office visits reported by cancer patients with and without history of breakthrough pain. *J Pain* 2002; **3**: 38–44.

24 Mercadante S, Maddaloni S, Roccella S, Salvaggio L. Predictive factors in advanced cancer pain treated only by analgesics. *Pain* 1992; **50**: 151–5.

25 Bruera E, Schoeller T, Wenk R, *et al.* A prospective multicenter assessment of the Edmonton staging system for cancer pain. *J Pain Symptom Manage* 1995; **10**: 348–55.

26 McQuay HJ, Collins SL, Carroll D, Moore RA. Radiotherapy for the palliation of painful bone metastases (Cochrane Review). In: *Cochrane Library*, Issue 3, 2004 (accessed September 29, 2004).

27 Roque M, Martinez MJ, Alonso-Coello P, *et al.* Radioisotopes for metastatic bone pain (Cochrane Review). In: *Cochrane Library*, Issue 3, 2004 (accessed September 29, 2004).

28 Wong R, Wiffen PJ. Bisphosphonates for the relief of pain secondary to bone metastases (Cochrane Review). In: *Cochrane Library*, Issue 3, 2004 (accessed September 29, 2004).

29 Chow E, Holden L, Danjoux C, *et al.* Successful salvage using percutaneous vertebroplasty in cancer patients with painful spinal metastases or osteoporotic compression fractures. *Radiother Oncol* 2004; **70**: 265–7.

30 Jackson K, Ashby M, Martin P, *et al.* 'Burst' ketamine for refractory cancer pain: an open-label audit of 39 patients. *J Pain Symptom Manage* 2001; **22**: 834–42.

◆ 31 Expert Working Group of the Research Network of the European Association for Palliative Care. Morphine and alternative opioids in cancer pain: the EAPC recommendations. *Br J Cancer* 2001; **84**: 587–93.

32 Coluzzi PH, Schwartzberg L, Conroy JD, *et al.* Breakthrough cancer pain: a randomized trial comparing oral transmucosal fentanyl citrate (OTFC) and morphine sulfate immediate release (MSIR). *Pain* 2001; **91**: 123–30.

33 Collins SL, Faura CC, Moore A, McQuay HJ. Peak plasma concentrations after oral morphine: a systematic review. *J Pain Symptom Manage* 1998; **16**: 388–402.

◆ 34 Levy MH. Drug therapy: Pharmacologic treatment of cancer pain. *N Engl J Med* 1996; **335**: 1124–32.

35 Mercadante S, Villari P, Ferrera P, *et al.* Safety and effectiveness of intravenous morphine for episodic (breakthrough) pain using a fixed ratio with the oral daily morphine dose. *J Pain Symptom Manage* 2004; **27**: 352–9.

36 Swanson G, Smith J, Bulich R, *et al.* Patient-controlled analgesia for chronic cancer pain in the ambulatory setting: a report of 117 patients. *J Clin Oncol* 1989; **7**: 1903–8.

◆ 37 Dale O, Hjortkjaer R, Kharasch ED. Nasal administration of opioids for pain management in adults. *Acta Anaesthesiol Scand* 2002; **46**: 759–70.

◆ 38 Zhang H, Zhang J, Streisand JB. Oral mucosal drug delivery: clinical pharmacokinetics and therapeutic applications. *Clin Pharmacokinet* 2002; **41**: 661–80.

39 Zeppetella G. Sublingual fentanyl citrate for cancer-related breakthrough pain: a pilot study. *Palliat Med* 2001; **15**: 323–8.

40 Gardner-Nix J. Oral transmucosal fentanyl and sufentanil for incident pain. *J Pain Symptom Manage* 2001; **22**: 627–30.

41 Duncan A. The use of fentanyl and alfentanil sprays for episodic pain. *Palliat Med* 2002; **16**: 550.

42 Coluzzi PH. Sublingual morphine: efficacy reviewed. *J Pain Symptom Manage* 1998; **16**: 184–92.

43 Farrar JT, Cleary J, Rauck R, *et al.* Oral transmucosal fentanyl citrate: randomized, double-blinded, placebo-controlled trial for treatment of breakthrough pain in cancer patients. *J Natl Cancer Inst* 1998; **90**: 611–16.

44 Fine PG, Marcus M, De Boer AJ, Van der Oord B. An open label study of oral transmucosal fentanyl citrate (OTFC) for the treatment of breakthrough cancer pain. *Pain* 1991; **45**: 149–53.

45 Streisand JB, Varvel JR, Stanski DR, *et al.* Absorption and bioavailability of oral transmucosal fentanyl citrate. *Anesthesiology* 1991; **75**: 223–9.

46 Portenoy RK, Payne R, Coluzzi P, *et al.* Oral transmucosal fentanyl citrate (OTFC) for the treatment of breakthrough pain in cancer patients: a controlled dose titration study. *Pain* 1999; **79**: 303–12.

47 Zeppetella G. An assessment of the safety, efficacy, and acceptability of intranasal fentanyl citrate in the management of cancer-related breakthrough pain: a pilot study. *J Pain Symptom Manage* 2000; **20**: 253–8.

48 Jackson K, Ashby M, Keech J. Pilot dose finding study of intranasal sufentanil for breakthrough and incident cancer-associated pain. *J Pain Symptom Manage* 2002; **23**: 450–2.

49 Pavis H, Wilcock A, Edgecombe J, *et al.* Pilot study of nasal morphine-chitosan for the relief of breakthrough pain in patients with cancer. *J Pain Symptom Manage* 2002; **24**: 598–602.

50 Kendall JM, Reeves BC, Latter VS, on behalf of the Nasal Diamorphine Trial Group. Multicentre randomised controlled trial of nasal diamorphine for analgesia in children and teenagers with clinical fractures. *BMJ* 2001; **322**: 261–5.

51 Benitez del Rosario MA, Martin AS, Ortega JJM, Feria M. Temporary sedation with midazolam for control of severe incident pain. *J Pain Symptom Manage* 2001; **21**: 439–42.

52 Kotlinska-Lemieszek A, Luczak J. Subanesthetic ketamine: an essential adjuvant for intractable cancer pain. *J Pain Symptom Manage* 2004; **28**: 100–2.

53 Carr DB, Goudas LC, Denman WT, *et al.* Safety and efficacy of intranasal ketamine for the treatment of breakthrough pain in patients with chronic pain: a randomized, double-blind, placebo-controlled, crossover study. *Pain* 2004; **108**: 17–27.

55

Somatization and pain expression

MARILU P BERRY, DIANE M NOVY

INTRODUCTION

In most clinical settings, the term somatization is loosely thought to be the presence of any physical complaints without a recognized organic basis. If a patient has a physical symptom or symptoms that have no apparent physiological cause, this may be viewed as the conversion of mental distress into physical symptoms. However, this clinical impression does not meet all of the strictly formulated inclusion criteria of a true somatization disorder.

DIFFERENTIAL DIAGNOSES OF SOMATIZATION

Somatization disorder is one of a group of disorders known as somatoform disorders. The Diagnostic and Statistic Manual of Mental Disorders (DSM)-IV[1] defines somatoform disorders as a group of specific disorders or problems characterized by persistent bodily symptoms or concerns that cannot be fully accounted for by a diagnosable disease. Hypochondriasis, for example, is the persistent, unfounded worry or conviction, despite adequate medical assurance to the contrary, that one has a serious medical illness. Body dysmorphic disorder involves preoccupation with an imagined or exaggerated physical defect. Conversion disorder is characterized by medically unexplained deficits or alterations of motor or sensory function. Somatization is a chronic condition consisting of multiple and specific categories of medically unexplained physical complaints that occur over a prolonged period of time. Pain disorder involves the persistence of medically unexplained pain symptoms. In each of these somatoform disorders, the physical symptoms are not under voluntary control and often coexist with anxiety or depression or both.[1,2*,3*] Somatoform disorders are widespread and largely unsolved problems that involve physical and psychological components.[4]

Somatoform disorders are distinguished from factitious disorder and malingering by the intentional production of symptoms in the latter two. Factitious disorder, as defined by the DSM-IV, is the *intentional* production or feigning of symptoms to assume the sick role. In malingering, the motivation for producing the symptoms is an external incentive such as economic gain or avoiding legal responsibility. This intentional 'faking' for secondary gain differs from somatization and its typically unconscious nature. Alternatively, some patients may consciously amplify their existing symptoms as a 'cry for help', and this not uncommon amplification of symptoms may accompany somatization and/or other psychiatric diagnoses.

In the medical literature, the term functional somatic syndrome refers to several syndromes in which the symptoms and subsequent suffering and disability are not fully explained by demonstrable tissue abnormality.[5] These syndromes include irritable bowel syndrome, fibromyalgia, chronic fatigue syndrome, multiple chemical sensitivity, chronic whiplash, and tension headache. These patients express symptoms such as gastrointestinal symptoms and fatigue in addition to pain. Individuals with functional somatic syndromes have higher rates of somatization, somatoform disorders, anxiety, and depression.[5]

PREVALENCE OF SOMATIZATION

In actuality, most patients in medical settings, including pain clinics and centers, do not meet the strict criteria of somatization as defined by the DSM-IV. However, when the overarching group of somatoform disorders is loosely defined as a medically unexplained symptom or symptoms, prevalence rates are quite high. For example, the prevalence is as high as 80 percent in primary care settings.[6*] In a secondary care orthopedic clinic, more than 50 percent of patients seen with chronic low-back pain had multiple unexplained symptoms, and 34 percent had pain diagrams that were believed to be incompatible with an organic cause.[7*] Among patients with chronic noncancer pain, the prevalence of multiple medically unexplained symptoms ranges from 0 percent to 53 percent.[8] In a recent comparison study on patients with chronic noncancer pain and patients with cancer pain, prevalence rates for having at least one somatic symptom that was in excess or unrelated to disease or side effects of medication were as high as 80 percent in both groups.[9*,10*] Some of the commonly reported symptoms of those patients with noncancer and cancer pain that could not be fully explained by existing medical information and physical examination include pain in arms and legs, fatigue, backache, pain in multiple sites, tingling or numbness, weakness of body, pain in joints, and sleep problems.

Because these comparison studies[9*,10*] had the patients' physicians rate the degree to which they thought the patient-reported symptoms were medically unexplainable, a broader understanding of patients' somatic symptoms was possible. Physicians noted that many patient-reported somatic symptoms could not be clearly differentiated between medically explainable and unexplainable. Hence, these symptoms were considered indeterminate. The overall findings from these studies were of complex profiles of somatic symptoms that are mostly medically explainable or indeterminate and only partially medically unexplainable. Therefore, the authors concluded that it would be difficult to assign a specific somatoform disorder diagnosis to most of the patients in these studies. Further, the authors noted that even those somatic symptoms that were rated as highly unexplained medically could not automatically be considered to be of psychological origin.[11*] They also pointed out that patients in pain are likely to be sleep-deprived and depleted of energy, which influences their experience and reporting of symptoms.[12*,13]

DEFINING MEDICALLY UNEXPLAINED SYMPTOMS

The pain literature provides other competing explanations for medically unexplained symptoms. Explanations with inconsistent and weak support include: the 'pain-prone personality' perspective; the pain as a variant of an affective disorder perspective; and the functional relation between secondary gain and disability in patients with chronic pain.[8] A more tenable explanation is that unexplained or indeterminate somatic symptoms among patients with pain may

be related to a sensitizing effect to physiological events that heighten bodily awareness.[14] Several researchers have found that patients with chronic pain blur certain experiences, including affective distress, and interpret them in terms of pain.[15] Another viable explanation is that cultural factors and medical and social institutions that focus on physical symptoms rather than the accompanying psychological distress may also be responsible for heightening the perception of physical problems.[15] Finally, work by Geisser and colleagues[16*] supports Field's neurobiological model of pain in which the patient's tendency to focus on somatic symptoms activates pain facilitation neurons. These neurons, in turn, are believed to sharpen the perception of the stimulus. The current theory for the majority of patients with chronic pain is that unexplained somatic symptoms are related to both pain and negative mood states.[17]

Indeed, pain and negative mood states are considered part of the multidimensional nature of chronic pain syndromes. Other relevant dimensions are behavioral and cognitive. There is wide acceptance that individuals with chronic pain may exhibit symptoms including negative mood states (depression, anxiety, anger), behavioral changes (inactivity, pain behaviors), and maladaptive beliefs and thoughts about pain, in addition to the somatic pain complaints. This multifaceted expression of pain is supported by clinical evidence for a multiplicity of treatments for chronic pain.[18]

Several possible reasons have been offered to explain the connection between negative mood states and somatic complaints. One possibility is that negative mood may contribute directly to bodily dysfunction and symptoms or more indirectly by causing changes in habit patterns and behavior, thus increasing vulnerability. Another possibility is that negative mood state may be associated with bodily arousal that then may be appraised as symptoms of various kinds. Third, negative mood state may affect the interpretation of physical changes as symptoms.[19*]

RELATION BETWEEN SOMATIC SYMPTOMS AND MOOD

Empirical evidence supports the relationship between somatic symptoms, which definitely include pain, and negative mood states in patients with pain. For example, with chronic cancer pain, data reported by Berry and Novy and colleagues[9*,10*] show scores on anxiety, depression, and somatization, as rated on the Brief Symptom Inventory (BSI)-18, approximately one standard deviation above the norm for the BSI oncology normative sample.[20] Using these illness-specific norms, the anxiety, depression, and somatic symptoms of patients with cancer seem to be greater among those who have pain. The difference may be because the participants in the normative sample were not being treated for pain, *per se*, and pain is known to be associated with greater psychological dysfunction.[3*,12*] In Zimmerman's[21*] study of cancer patients with and without pain, the data showed that somatization, hostility, anxiety, and depression were more problematic for patients with pain.

The relation between somatic symptoms and negative mood states has also been demonstrated in patients with chronic noncancer pain. In Berry and Novy and colleagues'[9*,10*] studies, the sample of patients with chronic noncancer pain had *t* score means approximately one standard deviation above the community norms for anxiety, depression, and somatization.[10*] This increase over community norms may be related to patients' experience of pain which is known to impact many different emotions, all of them negative.[22,23] Berry *et al.* and Novy *et al.* also found strong relations between their somatic symptom checklist and negative mood states among their sample of patients with cancer and noncancer pain.[9*,10*] Taken together, the conclusion of these studies is a rejection of a reductionist explanation (real body pain versus a psychological problem) of somatic and negative mood states, particularly for most of patients who have complex profiles of medical problems, pain, and negative mood states.

It appears that many somatic symptoms cannot be fully explained by the extent of organic pathology alone. The frequency of this occurrence and physician endorsement of the indeterminate basis of somatic symptoms in the Berry and Novy and colleagues' studies[9*,10*] should lessen the negative connotations that often are associated with somatoform symptoms and the possibility of any one of the somatoform disorder diagnoses.

SIGNIFICANCE OF SOMATIC SYMPTOMS

As the data presented here suggest, and as most healthcare professionals who work with patients with chronic noncancer or cancer pain know, unexplained symptoms do not necessarily indicate a psychiatric or somatoform diagnosis. The presence of unexplainable somatic symptoms is common in this population. To the frustration of physicians and patients alike, diagnostic and radiographic studies do not always reveal the cause of all of the underlying problems. Once healthcare providers give patients a somatoform disorder or other psychiatric diagnosis, that label often serves to invalidate patients' physical symptoms and prevent them from having credibility in the future.

However, there still is the tendency of some physicians to question the credibility of patients' reports of somatic symptoms when medical evidence does not support their presence. At those times, some physicians may think that negative mood states or other psychological symptoms are the cause of the unexplained somatic symptoms. Regretfully, those physicians have little appreciation for the potential interaction among sensory/physical, affective, behavioral, and cognitive components of patients' problems. Another regrettable situation is created by failure to gather patients'

extensive medical and psychosocial histories and repeatedly pursuing organic causes of unexplained somatic symptoms by tests, procedures, medications, and operations. In such cases, the dollar cost of strictly organic work-ups and treatments are exceeded only by the potential for iatrogenic harm in patients with and without chronic pain.[24,25**]

Patients with a somatic focus typically have a history of repeated hospitalizations and surgeries, see many physicians for consultation and work-up, take many medications, and resist psychological explanations for their symptoms. Because of this overutilization of the healthcare system, one important aspect of management is to have a heightened threshold for instituting aggressive diagnostic and treatment procedures.[26] It is important to note that the physician must rule out treatable medical problems but balance this with caution to avoid repeating unnecessary tests and procedures that reinforce the focus on the symptoms, cause added expense, and may be damaging to the patient in other ways. Taking the suggestions of Barsky and Borus[5] and Purcell[27*] together, we present management guidelines in Box 55.1. When working with this type of patient, it is important to avoid statements such as 'It is all in your head' and 'The symptom does not exist' that could harm the working relationship and cause the patient to feel defensive.

Box 55.1 Management guidelines for somatization

- Rule out diagnosable medical disease
- Assess for psychiatric disorders
- Build a collaborative relationship with the patient
- Establish that improved function is the goal for treatment
- Provide limited reassurance
- Refer for cognitive behavioral therapy
- Provide a caring physician attitude
- Refer patient to a support system such as a support group

Detection rates for anxiety, depression, and other psychological distress and appropriateness of referral to support services tend to be different across noncancer and cancer pain groups. The literature reports evidence of low detection and referral for psychological problems in oncology settings.[28*,29*] Although patients with chronic nonmalignant pain often are referred for multidisciplinary assessment and treatment, those with cancer pain are not. The findings of Berry *et al.* and Novy *et al.* highlight the importance of routine screening for psychological distress in cancer pain groups so that there will be improved detection and more appropriate referrals.[9*,29*]

SUMMARY

In summary, prevalence rates for a medically unexplained symptom or symptoms in pain populations range from 0 percent to 80 percent, and unexplainable somatic symptoms remain a frustrating phenomenon for many healthcare providers and patients alike. Research supports a connection between number of somatic symptoms experienced and negative mood states, although many patients with a complex presentation of somatic symptoms are mistakenly written off as having purely psychogenic pain. Improved assessment and management of these complex cases is needed so as not to err on the sides of over- or underutilization of healthcare services. Both medical and psychological screening and treatment are needed with this patient group, and various nonpharmacological techniques are suggested for the management of this type of patient. Further research is needed in somatoform disorders to better understand the mind–body connection.

Key learning points

- Somatization is loosely, and incorrectly, thought to be the mere presence of a medically unexplained symptom or symptoms.

- Prevalence rates for an unexplained symptom or symptoms in pain populations range from 0 percent to 80 percent.

- Research supports a connection between somatization and negative mood states.

- In both patients with cancer pain and with noncancer pain, somatization, anxiety, and depression were higher than in patients without pain.

- Unexplained symptoms do not necessarily indicate a psychiatric or somatoform diagnosis.

- Physicians should rule out diagnosable medical disease but with caution to avoid unnecessary testing and procedures.

- Management should include assessment for psychological problems and appropriate referral as needed for cognitive behavioral treatment.

REFERENCES

1 American Psychiatric Association. *Diagnostic and Statistical Manual of Mental Disorders*, 4th ed. Washington DC: American Psychiatric Association, 1994: 445–52.

2 Escobar JI, Burnam A, Karno M, *et al.* Somatization in the community. *Arch Gen Psychiatry* 1987; **44**: 713–18.

3 Simon G, Gater R, Kisely S, *et al.* Somatic symptoms of distress: An international primary care study. *Psychosom Med* 1996; **58**: 481–8.

◆ 4 Lipowski AJ. Somatization: The concept and its clinical application. *Am J Psychiatry* 1988; **145**: 1358–68.

◆ 5 Barsky, AJ Borus, JF. Functional somatic syndromes. *Ann Intern Med* 1999; **130**: 910–21.

6 Kroenke K, Spitzer RL, Williams JBW, *et al.* Physical symptoms in primary care: Predictors of psychiatric disorders and functional impairment. *Arch Fam Med* 1994; **3**: 774–9.

7 Sikorski JM, Stampfer HG, Cole RM *et al.* Psychological aspects of chronic low back pain. *Aust N Z J Surg* 1996; **66**: 294–7.

8 Dworkin RH, Caligor E. Psychiatric diagnoses and chronic pain: DSM-IIIR and beyond. *J Pain Symptom Manage* 1988; **3**: 87–98.

9 Berry, MP, Palmer, JL, Bruera, E, Novy, DM. Predictors of unexplained somatic symptoms in cancer and noncancer pain. *Proceedings of the American Psychological Association Annual Meeting*, July 2004.

10 Novy DM, Berry MP, Palmer, JL, *et al.* Somatic symptoms in patients with chronic noncancer and cancer pain. *J Pain Symptom Manage* 2005; **29**: 603–12.

● 11 Portenory R, Thaler HT, Kornblith AB, *et al.* The Memorial Symptom Assessment Scale: An instrument for the evaluation of symptom prevalence, characteristics and distress. *Eur J Cancer* 1994; **30**: 1326–36.

12 Swartz M, Blazer D, George L, *et al.* Somatization disorder in a community population. *Am J Psychiatry* 1986; **134**: 1403–8.

13 Syrjala KL, Abrams J. Cancer pain. In Gatchel RJ, Turk DC, eds. *Psychosocial Factors in Pain: Critical Perspectives.* New York: Guilford Press, 1999: 301–14.

14 Barsky AJ, Goodson DJ, Lane RS. The amplification of somatic symptoms. *Psychosom Med* 1988; **50**: 510–19.

15 Dworkin SF, Wilson L, Masson DL. Somatizing as a risk factor for chronic pain. In: Grzesiak RC, Ciccone DS, eds. *Psychological Vulnerability to Chronic Pain.* New York: Springer, 1994, 28–54.

● 16 Geisser ME, Gaskin ME, Robinson ME, *et al.* The relationship of depression and somatic focus to experimental and clinical pain in chronic pain patients. *Psychol Health* 1993; **8**: 415–20.

17 Robinson ME, Riley JL. The role of emotion in pain. In: Gatchel RJ, Turk DC, eds. *Psychosocial Factors in Pain: Critical Perspectives.* New York: Guilford Press, 1999: 74–88.

◆ 18 Novy DM, Nelson, DV, Francis, DJ, Turk, DC. Perspectives of chronic pain: An evaluative comparison of restrictive and comprehensive models. *Psychol Bull* 1995; **118**: 238–47.

19 Mechanic D. The experience and reporting of common physical complaints. *J Health Soc Behav* 1980; **21**: 146–55.

20 Derogatis LR. *Brief Symptom Inventory-18.* Minneapolis, MN: National Computer Systems, Inc., 2000.

21 Zimmerman, L, Story KT, Gaston-Johansson, F, Rowles, JR. Psychological variables and cancer pain. *Cancer Nurs* 1996; **19**: 44–53.

22 Fernandez E, Turk DC. The scope and significance of anger in the experience of chronic pain. *Pain* 1995; **61**: 165–75.

23   Rudy TE, Kerns RD, Turk DC. Chronic pain and depression: Toward a cognitive-behavioral meditation model. *Pain* 1988; **35**: 129–40.

◆ 24   Quill TE. Somatization disorder: One of medicine's blind spots. *JAMA* 1985; **254**: 3075–79.

● 25   Chaturvedi SK, Maguire GP. Persistent somatization in cancer: A controlled follow-up study. *J Psychosomatic Res* 1998; **45**: 249–56.

26   Ketterer, MW, Buckholtz, CD. Somatization disorder. *J Am Osteopath Assoc* 1989; **89**: 489–90, 495–99.

27   Purcell, TB. The somatic patient. *Emerg Med Clin North Am* 1991; **9**: 137–59.

28   Cull A, Stewart M, Altmann DG. Assessment of and intervention for psychosocial problems in routine oncology practice. *Br J Cancer* 1995; **72**: 229–35.

29   Ford S, Fallowfield L, Lewis S. Can oncologists detect distress in their out-patients and how satisfied are they with their performance during bad news consultations. *Br J Cancer* 1994; **70**: 767–70.

56

Pain in patients with alcohol and drug dependence

STEVEN D PASSIK, KENNETH L KIRSH

INTRODUCTION

Substance abuse and addiction are difficult problems both theoretically and clinically in the arena of pain management and palliative care.[1***] Patients with histories of alcohol and substance dependence are seen often by palliative care specialists, as well as those with the less obvious aberrant drug-taking behaviors sometimes in evidence in the treatment of patients without formal psychiatric histories of substance use disorders. An example of this is when a patient with advanced disease and pain is unilaterally escalating drug doses, using medications to treat other symptoms or when prescriptions are being mishandled. The clinician therefore is challenged to understand such happenings and plan interventions accordingly. Once these aberrant behaviors are identified the clinician must decide on a course of action that is fair and in the best interests of the patient as well as his or her own career. Thus, the problem of alcoholism, chemical dependence and drug abuse spans a continuum from formal psychiatric disorders to problematic behaviors in the absence of these disorders.

PREVALENCE

Nearly one-third of the US population has used illicit drugs and an estimated 6–15 percent have a substance use disorder of some type.[2–4*] As a result of this high prevalence, and the association between drug abuse and life-threatening diseases, problems related to abuse and addiction are encountered commonly in palliative care settings.[5*] In diverse patient populations with progressive life-threatening diseases, a remote or current history of drug abuse presents a constellation of physical and psychosocial issues that carry a stigma that can both complicate the management of the underlying disease and undermine palliative therapies. Clearly, the interface between the therapeutic use of potentially abusable drugs and the abuse of these drugs is complex and must be understood to optimize palliative care.

Substance abuse appears to be less frequent among palliative care patients than the prevalence of substance use disorders in society at large, in general medical populations, and in emergency medical departments.[2–4*,6] This relatively low prevalence was also reported in the Psychiatric Collaborative Oncology Group study, which assessed psychiatric diagnoses in ambulatory cancer patients from several tertiary care hospitals.[7*] Following structured clinical interviews, less than 5 percent of 215 cancer patients met the Diagnostic and Statistical Manual for Mental Disorders (DSM)-III criteria for a substance use disorder.[8*] Thus, the problem reflects a minority of patients, but one that can only be adequately and successfully treated when their addiction problems are noted by staff and the patient's special needs can be addressed.[9,10*]

CURRENT DEFINITIONS OF ABUSE AND ADDICTION

The pharmacological phenomena of tolerance and physical dependence are commonly confused with abuse and addiction. All the definitions applied to medical patients have been developed from addict populations without medical illness, as well as sociocultural considerations, which may lead to mixed messages in the clinical setting. The clarification of this terminology is an essential step in improving the diagnosis and management of substance abuse in the palliative care setting.

Tolerance, a pharmacological property defined by the need for increasing doses to maintain effects, has been a particular concern during opioid therapy.[11,12] Clinicians and patients both commonly express concerns that tolerance to analgesic effects may compromise the benefits of therapy and lead to the requirement for progressively higher, and ultimately unsustainable, doses. Additionally, the development of tolerance to the reinforcing effects of opioids, and the consequent need to increase doses to regain these effects, has been speculated to be an important element in the pathogenesis of addiction.[13]

Notwithstanding these concerns, extensive clinical experience with opioid drugs in the medical context has not confirmed that tolerance causes substantial problems.[14–16] Although tolerance to a variety of opioid effects can be reliably observed in animal models,[17**] and tolerance to nonanalgesic effects, such as respiratory depression and cognitive impairment,[9*] occurs routinely in the clinical setting, analgesic tolerance does not appear to routinely interfere with the clinical efficacy of opioid drugs. Most patients can attain stable doses associated with a favorable balance between analgesia and side effects for prolonged periods. Dose escalation, when it is required, usually heralds the appearance of a progressive painful lesion.[18–24*] Unlike tolerance to the side effects of the opioids, clinically meaningful analgesic tolerance appears to be a rare phenomenon, and is rarely the cause for dose escalation.

Physical dependence is defined solely by the occurrence of a withdrawal syndrome following abrupt dose reduction or administration of an antagonist.[11,12,25*] Neither the dose nor duration of administration required to produce clinically significant physical dependence in humans is known. Most practitioners assume that the potential for withdrawal exists after opioids have been administered repeatedly for only a few days.

There is great confusion among clinicians about the differences between physical dependence and addiction. Physical dependence, like tolerance, has been suggested to be a component of addiction, and the avoidance of withdrawal has been postulated to create behavioral contingencies that reinforce drug-seeking behavior.[13,26–28] These speculations, however, are not supported by experience acquired during opioid therapy for chronic pain. Physical dependence does not preclude the uncomplicated discontinuation of opioids during multidisciplinary pain management of nonmalignant pain, and opioid therapy is routinely stopped without difficulty in the cancer patients whose pain disappears following effective antineoplastic therapy.[29] Indirect evidence for a fundamental distinction between physical dependence and addiction is even provided by animal models of opioid self-administration, which have demonstrated that persistent drug-taking behavior can be maintained in the absence of physical dependence.[30**]

CONCERNS OVER CURRENT DEFINITIONS

These definitions of tolerance and physical dependence highlight deficiencies in the nomenclature applied to substance abuse. The terms 'addiction' and 'addict' are particularly troublesome and are often inappropriately applied to describe both aberrant drug use and phenomena related to tolerance or physical dependence. Clinicians and patients may use the word 'addicted' to describe compulsive drug taking in one patient and nothing more than the possibility for withdrawal in another. It is not surprising, therefore, that patients, families and staff become very concerned about the outcome of opioid treatment when this term is applied, and which often leads to misperceptions of this mode of therapy for all involved.[31]

The accurate assessment of drug-related behaviors in patients with advanced medical disease usually requires detailed information about the role of the drug in the patient's life. The existence of mild mental clouding or the time spent out of bed may be less meaningful than other outcomes, such as noncompliance with primary therapy related to drug use, or behaviors that jeopardize relationships with physicians, other healthcare providers or family members.

AN ALTERNATIVE APPROACH FOR DEFINING ABUSE AND ADDICTION IN THE MEDICALLY ILL

Previous definitions that include phenomena related to physical dependence or tolerance cannot be the model terminology for medically ill populations who receive potentially abusable drugs for legitimate medical purposes. A more appropriate model definition of addiction notes that it is a chronic disorder characterized by 'the compulsive use of a substance resulting in physical, psychological or social harm to the user and continued use despite that harm'.[32] This definition appropriately emphasizes that addiction is, fundamentally, a psychological and behavioral syndrome. Any appropriate definition of addiction must include the concepts of loss of control over drug use, compulsive drug use, and continued use despite harm.

The spectrum of aberrant drug-taking behavior

If drug-taking behavior in a medical patient can be characterized as aberrant, a differential diagnosis for this behavior can be explored. A true addiction is only one of several possible explanations. Of the behaviors likely to represent true addiction, some recent research suggests that multiple unsanctioned dose escalations and obtaining opioids from multiple prescribers may have some specific relevance.[33] If the problem is not addiction, the challenging diagnosis of pseudo-addiction must be considered if the patient is reporting distress associated with unrelieved symptoms. Behaviors such as aggressively complaining about the need for higher doses, or occasional unilateral drug escalations may be signs that the patient's pain is under-medicated. Also, impulsive drug and alcohol use may indicate the existence of another psychiatric disorder, which may have therapeutic implications. For example, patients with borderline personality disorder can express fear and rage through aberrant drug taking and behave impulsively and self destructively during pain therapy.[34] Similarly, patients who self-medicate psychiatric conditions such as anxiety, panic, depression or even periodic dysphoria and loneliness can present as aberrant drug takers. In such instances careful diagnosis and treatment of these additional problems can at times obviate the need for such self-medication.[35] Other rule-outs for addiction include mild encephalopathy and criminal intent through diversion or sale of medications.

In assessing the differential diagnosis for drug-related behavior, it is useful to consider the degree of aberrancy. The less aberrant behaviors (such as aggressively complaining about the need for medications) are more likely to reflect untreated distress of some type, rather than addiction-related concerns. Conversely, the more aberrant behaviors (such as injection of an oral formulation) are more likely to reflect true addiction. Although empirical studies are needed to validate this conceptualization, it may be a useful model when evaluating aberrant behaviors.

Empirical validation of the aberrant drug-taking concept

The spectrum of aberrant drug-taking has been used as a heuristic to guide the assessment of problematic drug-taking in several recent studies. The studies performed to date all involve small samples, though they have shown the utility of the spectrum concept as an assessment tool yielding important implications for clinicians.

The first study examined the relationship between aberrant drug-taking behaviors and compliance in patients with a history of substance abuse receiving chronic opioid therapy for nonmalignant pain. Dunbar and Katz examined outcomes and drug-taking in a sample of 20 patients with diverse histories of drug abuse during a year of chronic opioid therapy.[36] During the study, 11 patients were compliant with the drug regimen and 9 were not. The authors examined patient characteristics and aberrant drug-taking behaviors that differentiated the two groups. The patients who did not abuse the therapy were current abusers of alcohol only (or had remote histories of polysubstance

abuse), were in a solid drug-free recovery as evidenced by participation in 12-step programs, and had good social support. The patients who abused the therapy were polysubstance abusers, were not participating in 12-step programs and had poor social support. The specific behaviors that were recorded more frequently by those who abused the therapy were unscheduled visits and multiple phone calls to the clinic, unsanctioned dose escalations and obtaining opioids from more than one source.

A second study examined the relationship between aberrant drug-taking and the presence or absence of a psychiatric diagnosis of substance use disorder in pain patients. Compton and colleagues studied 56 patients seeking pain treatment in a multidisciplinary pain program who were referred for 'problematic drug-taking.'[37*] The patients all underwent structured psychiatric interviews and the sample was divided between those qualifying and not qualifying for psychiatric diagnoses of substance use disorders. The authors then examined the subjects' reports of aberrant drug-taking behaviors on a structured interview assessment. Those with a substance use disorder were more likely to have engaged in unsanctioned dose escalations, received opioids from multiple sources and had lost of control of their prescribed medications.

Passik and researchers examined the self-reports of aberrant drug-taking attitudes and behaviors in samples of cancer (n = 52) and acquired immune deficiency syndrome (AIDS) (n = 111) patients with a questionnaire designed for the purposes of the study.[31*] Reports of past drug use and abuse were more frequent than present reports in both groups. Current aberrant drug-related behaviors were seldom reported. Attitude items, however, revealed that patients would consider engaging in aberrant behaviors, or would possibly excuse them in others, if pain or symptom management were inadequate. Overall, patients greatly overestimated the risk of addiction in pain treatment. Experience with this questionnaire suggests that patients with both cancer and AIDS respond in a forthcoming fashion to drug-taking behavior questions and describe attitudes and behaviors which may be highly relevant to the diagnosis and management of substance use disorders.

Such studies will help us to better understand the particular diagnostic meanings of the various behaviors so that clinicians may recognize which are the true 'red flags' in a given population. Far too often anecdotal accounts shape the way clinicians view these behaviors. Some behaviors are regarded almost universally as aberrant despite limited systematic data to suggest that this is the case. Consider for example the patient who requests a specific pain medication, or a specific route or dose. Such behavior often reflects a patient who is knowledgeable about what works for him or her but is almost always greeted with suspicion on the part of practitioners. Other behaviors may be found to be common in nonaddicts, and although they seem aberrant based upon their face value, they may have little predictive value for true addiction.

ADDICTION IN PATIENTS WITH DRUG ABUSE HISTORY VERSUS THOSE WITHOUT

It is interesting to explore the differences inherent in populations of patients with and without histories of drug abuse or addiction. The following discussion highlights the known differences while also highlighting the fact that we have a long way to go regarding true understanding of the effects of prior abuse and addiction on current treatments for oncology patients.

Abuse and addiction in patients without prior drug abuse

An extensive worldwide experience in the long-term management of cancer pain with opioid drugs has demonstrated that opioid administration in cancer patients with no prior history of substance abuse is only rarely associated with the development of significant abuse or addiction.[26,38–49*] Indeed, concerns about addiction in this population are now characterized by an interesting paradox: Although the lay public and inexperienced clinicians still fear the development of addiction when opioids are used to treat cancer pain, specialists in cancer pain and palliative care widely believe that the major problem related to addiction is not the phenomenon itself, but rather the persistent undertreatment of pain driven by inappropriate fear that it will occur.

The traditional view of long-term opioid therapy is negative and early surveys of addicts, which noted that a relatively large proportion began their addiction as medical patients administered opioid drugs for pain, provided some indirect support for this perspective.[50–52*] The most influential of these surveys recorded a history of medical opioid use for pain in 27 percent of white male addicts and 1.2 percent of black male addicts.[52*]

Surveys of addict populations, however, do not provide a valid measure of the addiction liability associated with chronic opioid therapy in populations without known abuse. Prospective patient surveys are needed to define this risk accurately. One project evaluated 11 882 inpatients who had no prior history of addiction and were administered an opioid while hospitalized; only four cases of addiction could be identified subsequently.[53*] A national survey of burn centers could find no cases of addiction in a sample of more than 10 000 patients without prior drug abuse history who were administered opioids for pain, and a survey of a large headache clinic identified opioid abuse in only three of 2369 patients admitted for treatment, most of whom had access to opioids.[54–55*]

Other data suggest that the typical patient with chronic pain is sufficiently different from the addict without painful disease that the risk of addiction during therapy for pain is likely to be low. For example, surveys of cancer patients and postoperative patients indicate that euphoria, a phenomenon believed to be common during the abuse of opioids, is extremely uncommon following administration of an opioid for pain; dysphoria is observed more typically, especially in those who receive meperidine.[56*] Although the psychiatric comorbidity identified in addict populations could be an effect, rather than a cause, of the aberrant drug-taking, the association suggests the existence of psychological risk factors for addiction. The likelihood of genetically determined risk factors for addiction also has been suggested by a twin study that demonstrated a significant concordance rate for aberrant drug-related behaviors.[57*]

Favorable surveys of pain patients are not definitive, of course, and there are conflicting data collected by multidisciplinary pain management programs that suggest a high prevalence of abuse behaviors among the patients referred to this setting.[58–66*] The latter surveys, however, are subject to an important selection bias, and this bias, combined with other methodological concerns, limit the generalizability of these data to the large and heterogeneous populations with chronic nonmalignant pain.[67*]

The inaccurate perception that opioid therapy inherently yields a relatively high likelihood of addiction has encouraged assumptions that are not supportable in populations without a prior history of substance abuse. For example, agonist–antagonist opioid analgesics are less likely to be abused by addicts than pure μ agonist opioids, and, consequently, some clinicians view the agonist–antagonist drugs as safer in terms of addiction liability. There is no evidence for this conclusion in populations without drug abuse histories, and the extensive experience with long-term opioid therapy for cancer pain and chronic nonmalignant pain has relied on the pure μ agonists.[22–24*,68–70*] Similarly, there is a common perception that short-acting oral opioids and opioids delivered by the parenteral route carry a relatively greater risk of addiction because of the rapid delivery of the drug. Again, these perceptions derive from observations in the healthy addict population and are not relevant to the treatment of pain in medical patients with no prior history of substance abuse.

Risk of abuse and addiction in populations with current or remote drug abuse

There is very little information about the risk of abuse or addiction during, or after, the therapeutic administration of a potentially abusable drug to patients with a current or remote history of abuse or addiction. Anecdotal reports suggest that successful long-term opioid therapy in patients with cancer pain or chronic nonmalignant pain is possible, particularly if the history of abuse or addiction is remote.[36*,71*,72*] Indeed, one study showed that patients with AIDS-related pain were able to be successfully treated with morphine whether or not they were substance users or nonusers. In fact, the major difference found was that substance users required considerably more morphine to reach stable pain control.[73*] However, a modicum of caution should be employed. For example, although there is no empirical evidence that the use of short-acting drugs or the parenteral route is more likely to lead to problematic drug-related behaviors than other therapeutic approaches, it may be prudent to avoid such therapies in patients with histories of substance abuse.

CLINICAL MANAGEMENT

Out-of-control aberrant drug-taking among palliative care patients (with or without a prior history of substance abuse) represents a serious and complex clinical occurrence. Perhaps the more difficult situations involve the patient who is actively abusing illicit or prescription drugs or alcohol concomitantly with medical therapies. The following guidelines can be useful whether the patient is an active drug abuser, has a history of substance abuse, or is not complying with the therapeutic regimen.

Multidisciplinary approach

A multidisciplinary team approach is recommended for the management of substance abuse in the palliative care setting. Mental health professionals with specialization in the addiction field can be instrumental helping palliative care team members develop strategies for management and patient treatment compliance, though often such professionals are not readily available. Providing care to these patients can lead to feelings of anger and frustration among staff. Such feelings can unintentionally compromise the level of patient care surrounding the patient's pain management and contribute to feelings of isolation and alienation by the patient. A structured multidisciplinary approach can be effective in helping the staff better understand the patient's needs and develop effective strategies for controlling pain and aberrant drug use simultaneously. Staff meetings can be helpful in establishing treatment goals, facilitating compliance, and coordinating the multidisciplinary team.

Assessment

The first member of the medical team to suspect problematic drug taking or a history of drug abuse should alert the patient's palliative care team, thus beginning the multidisciplinary assessment and management process.[74***] A physician should assess the potential of withdrawal or other pressing concerns and begin involving other staff (i.e. social work and/or psychiatry) to begin planning management strategies. Obtaining as detailed as possible a history of duration, frequency, and desired effect of drug use is crucial. Frequently, clinicians avoid asking patients about substance abuse out of fear that they will anger the patient or that they are incorrect in their suspicion of abuse. However, such approaches will likely contribute to continued problems with treatment compliance and frustration among staff. Empathic and truthful communication is always the best approach. The use of a careful, graduated interview approach can be instrumental in slowly introducing the assessment of drug use. This approach entails starting the assessment interview with broad questions about the role of drugs (e.g. nicotine, caffeine) in the patient's life and gradually becoming more specific in focus to include illicit drugs. Such an approach is helpful in reducing the denial and resistance that the patient may express. This interviewing style also assists in the detection of coexisting psychiatric disorders that may be present. Comorbid psychiatric disorders can significantly contribute to aberrant drug-taking behavior. Anxiety, personality disorders, and mood disorders are the most commonly encountered.[75–76] The assessment and treatment of comorbid psychiatric disorders can greatly enhance management strategies and reduce the risk of relapse. The patient's desired effects from illicit drugs can often be a clue to comorbid psychiatric disorders (i.e. drinking to quell panic symptoms).

Development of a multidisciplinary treatment plan

Drug abuse is often a chronic, progressive disorder. Therefore, the development of clear treatment goals is essential for the management of drug abuse. Team members should not expect a complete remission of the patient's substance use problems. The distress of coping with a life-threatening illness and the availability of prescription drugs for symptom control can make complete abstinence an unrealistic goal.[77] Rather, a harm reduction approach should be employed that aims to enhance social support, maximize treatment compliance, and contain harm done through episodic relapse. The following guidelines are recommended for the management of patients with a substance disorder.

1 The clinician should first establish a relationship based on empathic listening and accept the patient's report of distress.
2 It is important to utilize nonopioid and behavioral interventions when possible, but not as substitutes for appropriate pain management.
3 The team should consider tolerance, route of administration and duration of action when prescribing medications for pain and symptom management. Preexisting tolerance should be taken into account for patients who are actively abusing drugs or are being maintained on methadone maintenance programs. Failure to realize any existing tolerance can result in undermedication and contribute to the patient's attempts to self-medicate.
4 The team should consider using longer-acting drugs (e.g. fentanyl patch, and sustained-release opioids).

The longer duration and slow onset may help to reduce aberrant drug-taking behaviors when compared to the rapid onset and increased frequency of dosage associated with short-acting drugs. Finally, the team should make plans to frequently reassess the adequacy of pain and symptom control, as well as compliance via use of urine drug screens and any other forms of monitoring.[78*]

Patients in recovery

Pain management with patients in recovery presents a unique challenge. Depending on the structure of the recovery program (e.g. Alcoholics Anonymous, methadone maintenance programs), a patient may fear ostracism from the program's members or may have an increased fear regarding susceptibility to re-addiction. The first choice should be to explore nonopioid therapies with these patients, which may require referral to a pain center.[79] Alternative therapies may include the use of nonsteroidal anti-inflammatory drugs, anticonvulsants (for neuropathic components), bio-feedback, electrical stimulation, neuroblative techniques, acupuncture, or behavioral management. If the pain condition is so severe that opioids are required, care must be taken to structure their use with opioid management contracts, random urine toxicology screens, and occasional pill counts. If possible, attempts should be made to include the patient's recovery program sponsor to garner their cooperation and aid in successful monitoring of the condition.

The patient with advanced disease

Managing addiction problems in patients with advanced cancer is labor intensive and can be extremely time-consuming. This begs the question as to why a clinician should even bother to address such a complex health concern in the patient with advanced disease. In fact, many clinicians might opt to overlook a patient's use of illicit substances or alcohol entirely, viewing these behaviors as a last source of pleasure for the patient. However, addiction has a deleterious impact on palliative care efforts. Proper addiction management plays an important part in the success of palliative efforts to reduce suffering and increase quality of life. Complete abstinence may not be a realistic outcome, but reduction in use can certainly have positive effects for the patient.[80]

CONCLUSION

Although the most prudent actions on the part of clinicians cannot obviate the risk of all aberrant drug-related behavior, clinicians must recognize that virtually any drug that acts on the central nervous system can be abused. The effective management of patients with pain who engage in aberrant drug-related behavior necessitates a comprehensive approach that recognizes the biologic, chemical, social, and psychiatric aspects of substance abuse and addiction, and provides practical means to manage risk, treat pain effectively and assure patient safety. An accepted nomenclature for abuse and addiction, and an operational approach to the assessment of patients with medical illness, are prerequisite to an accurate definition of risk in populations with and without histories of substance abuse.

Key learning points

- Substance abuse and addiction are difficult challenges in practice and theory when addressing pain management issues in palliative care patients.

- Traditional definitions for defining addiction (i.e. those focusing on tolerance and physical dependence) are subpar for application in the medically ill population. Rather, a focus on use despite harm is a better approach for identifying patients at risk.

- It is important to embrace an understanding of aberrant drug taking as a spectrum of behaviors that can be viewed as potentially problematic by prescribers.

- The use of opioid analgesics in patients without a history of addiction is very unlikely to create a problem unless the patient has genetic, social, and familial vulnerabilities, and a predisposition toward addiction. In essence, we do not 'create addicts' simply by prescribing opioids.

- Managing patients with known alcohol or other drug dependence creates a complex clinical management challenge that is best addressed through a multi-disciplinary team approach.

REFERENCES

1 Kirsh KL, Whitcomb LA, Donaghy K, Passik SD. Abuse and addiction issues in medically ill patients with pain: attempts at clarification of terms and empirical study. *Clin J Pain* 2002; **4**(Suppl): S52–60.

2 Colliver JD, Kopstein AN. Trends in cocaine abuse reflected in emergency room episodes reported to DAWN. *Publ Health Rep* 1991; **106**: 59–68.

3 Groerer J, Brodsky M. The incidence of illicit drug use in the United States, 1962–1989. *Br J Addict* 1992; **87**: 1345–51.

4 Regier DA, Meyers JK, Dramer M, *et al.* The NIMH epidemiologic catchment area program. *Arch Gen Psychiatry* 1984; **41**: 934–7.

5 Wells KB, Golding JM, Burnam MA. Chronic medical conditions in a sample of the general population with anxiety, affective, and substance use disorders. *Am J Psychiatry* 1989; **146**: 1440–5.

6 Burton RW, Lyons JS, Devens M, Larson DB. Psychiatric consults for psychoactive substance disorders in the general hospital. *Gen Hosp Psychiatry* 1991; **13**: 83–7.

● 7 Derogatis LR, Morrow GR, Fetting J, *et al.* The prevalence of psychiatric disorders among cancer patients. *JAMA* 1983; **249**: 751–8.

8   American Psychiatric Association. *Diagnostic and Statistical Manual for Mental Disorders–III.* Washington, D.C: American Psychiatric Association, 1983.

9   Bruera E, Macmillan K, Hanson JA, MacDonald RN. The cognitive effects of the administration of narcotic analgesics in patients with cancer pain. *Pain* 1989; **39**: 13–17.

10 Bruera E, Moyano J, Seifert L, *et al.* The frequency of alcoholism among patients with pain due to terminal cancer. *J Pain Symptom Manage* 1995; **10**: 599–606.

11 Dole VP. Narcotic addiction, physical dependence and relapse. *N Engl J Med* 1972; **286**: 988–94.

● 12 Martin WR, Jasinski DR. Physiological parameters of morphine dependence in man – tolerance, early abstinence, protracted abstinence. *J Psychiatr Res* 1969; **7**: 9–13.

13 Wikler A. *Opioid Dependence: Mechanisms and Treatment.* New York: Plenum Press, 1980.

14 Portenoy RK. Opioid therapy for chronic nonmalignant pain: current status. In: Fields HL, Liebeskind JC, eds. Progress in pain research and management, Vol 1. *Pharmacological Approaches to the Treatment of Chronic Pain: New Concepts and Critical Issues.* Seattle: IASP Publications, 1994: 247–9.

15 Portenoy RK. Opioid tolerance and efficacy: basic research and clinical observations. In: Gebhardt G, Hammond D, Jensen T, eds. *Proceedings of the VII World Congress on Pain.* Progress in Pain Research and Management, Vol. 2. Seattle: IASP Press, 1994: 595–7.

16 Foley KM. Clinical tolerance to opioids. In: Basbaum AI, Besson J-M, eds. *Towards a New Pharmacotherapy of Pain.* Chichester: John Wiley & Sons, 1991: 181–6.

● 17 Ling GSF, Paul D, Simantov R, Pasternak GW. Differential development of acute tolerance to analgesia, respiratory depression, gastrointestinal transit and hormone release in a morphine infusion model. *Life Sci* 1989; **45**: 1627–33.

18 Twycross RG. Clinical experience with diamorphine in advanced malignant disease. *Int J Clin Pharmacol Ther Toxicol* 1974; **9**: 184–8.

19 Kanner RM, Foley KM. Patterns of narcotic drug use in a cancer pain clinic. *Ann N Y Acad Sci* 1981; **362**: 161–7.

20 Chapman CR, Hill HF. Prolonged morphine self-administration and addiction liability: evaluation of two theories in a bone marrow transplant unit. *Cancer* 1989; **63**: 1636–9.

21 France RD, Urban BJ, Keefe FJ. Longterm use of narcotic analgesics in chronic pain. *Soc Sci Med* 1984; **19**: 1379–85.

22 Portenoy RK, Foley KM. Chronic use of opioid analgesics in nonmalignant pain: report of 38 cases. *Pain* 1986; **25**: 171–5.

23 Urban BJ, France RD, Steinberger DL, *et al.* Longterm use of narcotic antidepressant medication in the management of phantom limb pain. *Pain* 1986; **24**: 191–6.

24 Zenz M, Strumpf M, Tryba M. Long-term opioid therapy in patients with chronic nonmalignant pain. *J Pain Symptom Manage* 1992; **7**: 69–75.

25 Redmond DE, Krystal JH. Multiple mechanisms of withdrawal from opioid drugs. *Annu Rev Neurosci* 1984; **7**: 443–78.

26 World Health Organization. *Cancer Pain Relief and Palliative Care,* Geneva: World Health Organization, 1990.

27 World Health Organization. *Technical Report No. 516, Youth And Drugs.* Geneva: World Health Organization, 1973.

28 American Psychiatric Association. *Diagnostic and Statistical Manual for Mental Disorders–IV.* Washington, DC: American Psychiatric Association, 1994.

29 Halpern LM, Robinson J. Prescribing practices for pain in drug dependence: a lesson in ignorance. *Adv Alcohol Subst Abuse* 1985; **5**: 184–7.

30 Dai S, Corrigal WA, Coen KM, Kalant H. Heroin self-administration by rats: influence of dose and physical dependence. *Pharmacol Biochem Behav* 1989; **32**: 1009–12.

31 Passik S, Kirsh, KL, McDonald M, *et al.* A pilot survey of aberrant drug-taking attitudes and behaviors in samples of cancer and AIDS patients. *J Pain Symptom Manage* 2000; **19**: 274–286.

32 Rinaldi RC, Steindler EM, Wilford BB, Goodwin D. Clarification and standardization of substance abuse terminology. *JAMA* 1988; **259**: 555.

33 Passik SD, Kirsh KL, Whitcomb LA, *et al.* A new tool to assess and document pain outcomes in chronic pain patients receiving opioid therapy. *Clin Ther* 2004; **26**: 552–61.

34 Hay JL, Passik SD. The cancer patient with borderline personality disorder: suggestions for symptom-focused management in the medical setting. *Psychooncology.* 2000; **9**: 91–100.

35 Khantzian EJ, Treece C. DSM-III psychiatric diagnosis of narcotic addicts. *Arch Gen Psychiatry* 1985; **42**: 1067–71.

36 Dunbar SA, Katz NP. Chronic opioid therapy for nonmalignant pain in patients with a history of substance abuse: report of 20 cases. *J Pain Symptom Manage* 1996; **11**: 163–70.

37 Compton P, Darakjian J, Miotto K. Screening for addiction in patients with chronic pain with 'problematic' substance use: evaluation of a pilot assessment tool. *J Pain Symptom Manage* 1998: **16**: 355–63.

38 Jorgensen L, Mortensen M-J, Jensen N-H, Eriksen J. Treatment of cancer pain patients in a multidisciplinary pain clinic. *Pain Clin* 1990; **3**: 83–7.

39 Moulin DE, Foley KM. Review of a hospital-based pain service. In: Foley KM, Bonica JJ, Ventafridda V, eds. *Advances in Pain Research and Therapy,* Vol 16. Second International Congress on Cancer Pain. New York: Raven Press 1990:413–20.

✱ 40 Schug SA, Zech D, Dorr U. Cancer pain management according to WHO analgesic guidelines, *J Pain Symptom Manage* 1990; **5**: 27–33.

41 Schug SA, Zech D, Grond S, *et al.* A long-term survey of morphine in cancer pain patients. *J Pain Symptom Manage* 1992; **7**: 259–65.

42 Ventafridda V, Tamburini M, DeConno F. Comprehensive treatment in cancer pain. In: Fields HL, Dubner R, Cervero F, eds. *Advances in Pain Research and Therapy,* Vol 9. Proceedings of the Fourth World Congress on Pain. New York: Raven Press 1985: 617–21.

43 Ventafridda V, Tamburini M, Caraceni A, *et al.* A validation study of the WHO method for cancer pain relief. *Cancer* 1990; **59**: 850–4.

44 Walker VA, Hoskin PJ, Hanks GW, White ID. Evaluation of WHO analgesic guidelines for cancer pain in a hospital-based palliative care unit. *J Pain Symptom Manage* 1988; **3**: 145–53.

45 Health and Public Policy Committee, American College of Physicians. Drug therapy for severe chronic pain in terminal illness. *Ann Intern Med* 1983; **99**: 870–6.

46 Ad Hoc Committee on Cancer Pain, American Society of Clinical Oncology: Cancer pain assessment and treatment curriculum guidelines. *J Clin Oncol* 1992; **10**: 1976–84.

47 Agency for Health Care Policy and Research, US Department of Health and Human Services: *Clinical Practice Guideline Number 9: Management of Cancer Pain.* Washington, DC: US Department of Health and Human Services, 1994.

48   American Pain Society. *Principles of Analgesic Use in the Treatment of Acute Pain and Cancer Pain*. Skokie, IL: American Pain Society, 1992.

49   Zech DFJ, Grond S, Lynch J, *et al.* Validation of the World Health Organization Guidelines for cancer pain relief: a 10 year prospective study. *Pain* 1995; **63**: 65–8.

50   Kolb L. Types and characteristics of drug addicts. *Ment Hyg* 1925; **9**: 300–6.

51   Pescor MJ. The Kolb classification of drug addicts. Washington, DC: *Public Health Rep Suppl* 155, 1939–42.

52   Rayport M. Experience in the management of patients medically addicted to narcotics. *JAMA* 1954; **156**: 684–91.

53   Porter J, Jick H. Addiction rare in patients treated with narcotics. *N Engl J Med* 1980; **302**: 123–4.

54   Perry S, Heidrich G. Management of pain during debridement: a survey of US burn units. *Pain* 1982; **13**: 267–72.

55   Medina JL, Diamond S. Drug dependency in patients with chronic headache. *Headache* 1977; **17**: 12–16.

56   Kaiko RF, Foley KM, Grabinski PY, *et al.* Central nervous system excitatory effects of meperidine in cancer patients. *Ann Neurol* 1983; **13**: 180–7.

57   Grove WM, Eckert ED, Heston L, *et al.* Heritability of substance abuse and antisocial behavior: a study of monozygotic twins reared apart. *Biol Psychiatry* 1990; **27**: 1293–7.

58   Buckley FP, Sizemore WA, Charlton JE. Medication management in patients with chronic non-malignant pain. a review of the use of a drug withdrawal protocol. *Pain* 1986; **26**: 153–8.

59   Finlayson RD, Maruta T, Morse BR. Substance dependence and chronic pain: profile of 50 patients treated in an alcohol and drug dependence unit. *Pain* 1986; **26**: 167–74.

60   Finlayson RD, Maruta T, Morse BR, Martin MA. Substance dependence and chronic pain: experience with treatment and follow-up results. *Pain* 1986; **26**: 178–82.

61   Maruta T. Prescription drug-induced organic brain syndrome. *Am J Psychiatry* 1978; **135**: 376–83.

62   Maruta T, Swanson DW, Finlayson RE. Drug abuse and dependency in patients with chronic pain. *Mayo Clin Proc* 1979; **54**: 241–8.

63   Maruta T, Swanson DW. Problems with the use of oxycodone compound in patients with chronic pain. *Pain* 1981; **11**: 389–97.

64   McNairy SL, Maruta T, Ivnik RJ, *et al.* Prescription medication dependence and neuropsychologic function. *Pain* 1984; **18**: 169–74.

65   Ready LB, Sarkis E, Turner JA. Self-reported vs. actual use of medications in chronic pain patients. *Pain* 1982; **12**: 285–91.

66   Turner JA, Calsyn DA, Fordyce WE, Ready LB. Drug utilization pattern in chronic pain patients. *Pain* 1982; **12**: 357–64.

67   Fishbain DA, Rosomoff HL, Rosomoff RS. Drug abuse, dependence, and addiction in chronic pain patients. *Clin J Pain* 1992; **8**: 77–84.

68   Gardner-Nix JS. Oral methadone for managing chronic nonmalignant pain. *J Pain Symptom Manage* 1996; **11**: 321–8.

69   Tennant FS, Uelman GF. Narcotic maintenance for chronic pain: medical and legal guidelines. *Postgrad Med* 1983; 73–6.

70   Taub A. Opioid analgesics in the treatment of chronic intractable pain of nonneoplastic origin. In: Kitahata LM, Collins D, eds. *Narcotic Analgesics in Anesthesiology*. Baltimore: Williams & Wilkins, 1982: 199–215.

71   Macaluso C, Weinberg D, Foley KM. Opioid abuse and misuse in a cancer pain population [abstract]. *J Pain Symptom Manage* 1988; **3**: S24–25.

72   Gonzales GR, Coyle N. Treatment of cancer pain in a former opioid abuser: fears of the patient and staff and their influence on care. *J Pain Symptom Manage* 1992; **7**: 246–9.

73   Kaplan R, Slywka J, Slagle S, et al: A titrated analgesic regimen comparing substance users and non-users with AIDS-related pain. *J Pain Symptom Manage* 2000; **19**: 265–71.

◆ 74   Lundberg JC, Passik SD. Alcohol and cancer: A review for psycho-oncologists. *Psychooncology* 1997; **6**: 253–66.

75   Regier DA, Farmer ME, Rae, DS, *et al.* Comorbidity of mental disorders with alcohol and other drug abuse. *JAMA* 1985; **264**: 2511–18.

76   Penick E, Powell B, Nickel E, *et al.* Comorbidity of lifetime psychiatric disorders among male alcoholics. *Alcohol Clin Exp Res* 1994; **18**: 1289–93.

77   Passik SD, Portenoy RK. Substance abuse issues in palliative care. In: Berger A, Portenoy R, Weissman D, eds. *Principles and Practice of Supportive Oncology*. Philadephia: Lippincott Raven Publishers, 1998.

78   Passik S, Schreiber J, Kirsh *et al.* A chart review of the ordering and documentation of urine toxicology screens in a cancer center: do they influence patient management? *J Pain Symptom Manage* 2000; **19**: 40–44.

79   Parrino M. State methadone treatment guidelines. *TIPS 1 DHHS Publication No. (SMA) 93–1991*. Washington, DC.

80   Passik S, Theobald D. Managing addiction in advanced cancer patients: why bother? *J Pain Symptom Manage* 2000; **19**: 229–34.

PART 9

Gastrointestinal systems

57

Pathophysiology of cachexia/anorexia syndrome

EGIDIO DEL FABBRO, EDUARDO BRUERA

INTRODUCTION

The cachexia/anorexia syndrome is a common, debilitating condition characterized by involuntary weight loss, weakness, and poor appetite in up to 80 percent[1] of patients with advanced cancer. Cachexia is commonly found in patients with chronic illnesses such as acquired immune deficiency syndrome (AIDS), chronic obstructive pulmonary disease (COPD), congestive heart failure (CHF), renal failure, liver failure, rheumatological disorders, tuberculosis (TB), and malaria. The pathophysiology of cachexia and even the response to treatment modalities may be quite similar in these seemingly disparate illnesses. The syndrome is distressing for both patients and families.[2] It decreases the quality of life, compromises the sense of body integrity, self-confidence, and attractiveness,[3] and is a marker for poor prognosis.[4**] This chapter describes the interactions between the disease and host, which may lead to increased resting energy expenditure, the loss of both lean muscle mass and fat through lipolysis and proteolysis, and the neurohormonal dysregulation of compensatory mechanisms such as appetite.

Certain tumors, such as pancreatic (83 percent) and gastric (83 percent) cancers, are more likely to cause weight loss,[5**] whereas others, such as lung (57–61 percent), colon (54 percent), prostate (56 percent) and breast (36 percent) cancers, are less likely to cause weight loss. Hematological tumors other than unfavorable non-Hodgkin (36 percent) are unlikely to produce cachexia. Although there is limited evidence of an association between weight loss and the extent of the cancer, some studies have demonstrated an increased weight loss in those patients with more than one organ involved. The metabolic effects of tumor factors produced by the genetic expression of the individual cancer are more important than the extent of metastases or the size of the primary tumor.

PRIMARY VERSUS SECONDARY CACHEXIA

In patients with advanced cancer primary metabolic cachexia should be distinguished from secondary cachexia or starvation. Secondary cachexia occurs when there is impaired oral intake, impaired gastrointestinal absorption, or loss of nutrients. This may be due to taste abnormalities, dysphagia, delirium, dementia, mucositis, constipation, diarrhea, chronic nausea, clinical depression, or bowel obstruction. Patients with advanced cancer typically have early satiety due to decreased gastric motility, an enlarged liver or spleen, an intraabdominal mass, or severe constipation. The pathophysiology and treatment of primary and secondary cachexia are different, yet both may be present in a particular patient (Fig. 57.1). However, there is evidence of some shared mechanisms for primary cachexia and secondary cachexia. Cytokines not only play a significant role in primary cachexia, but they also appear to affect gastric motility[6] and small bowel absorption.[7]

DEFINITION

Cancer cachexia has been defined as 'a wasting syndrome involving muscle and fat directly caused by tumor factors, or indirectly caused by an aberrant host response to tumor presence'.[8] Cachexia is characterized by involuntary weight loss. As little as 5 percent weight loss over a 4–6-month period is associated with increased mortality in patients with human immunodeficiency virus (HIV) infection.[9,10**] Lung cancer patients with a pretreatment weight loss of >5 percent have a poorer prognosis[11**] and a greater risk for treatment toxicity.[12**] Measurement of body mass index (BMI) may not be useful as the prevalence of obesity has

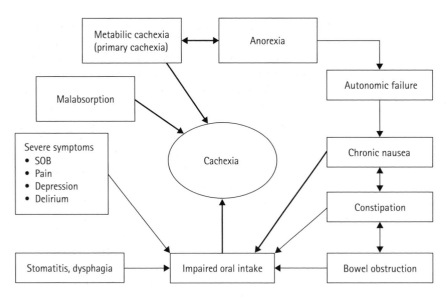

Figure 57.1 *Causes of cachexia in cancer, SOB, shortness of breath.*

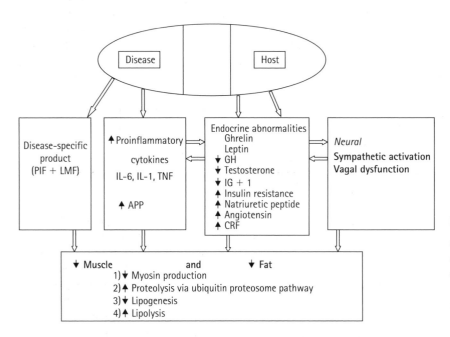

Figure 57.2 *Metabolic abnormalities in primary cachexia. APP, acute phase proteins; TNF, tumor necrosis factor; PIF, proteolysis inducing factor; CRF, corticotropin releasing factor; LMF, lipid mobilizing factor; GH, growth hormone; IL, interleukin.*

increased and patients are now more likely to have a much higher pre-illness weight. Fluid retention (ascites, pleural effusions) may also mask significant weight loss. The severity of anorexia, which often accompanies cachexia, can be measured by a numerical scale (usually >3/10), however, there is no specific threshold or duration of loss of appetite to define anorexia.

Other parameters which are consistent with the diagnosis are increased resting energy expenditure as measured by indirect calorimetry, decreased lean muscle mass and fat as demonstrated by anthropometric testing and bioelectrical impedance. Commonly available laboratory tests such as albumin, and C-reactive protein (CRP) may provide correlation with weight loss and also prognosis.[13**]

MECHANISMS OF CACHEXIA (FIG. 57.2)

Nutrition and metabolic abnormalities

Patients with chronic illnesses such as rheumatoid arthritis, COPD, CHF, and advanced cancer often experience weight loss despite an intact gastrointestinal tract and 'sufficient' nutritional intake. These patients may still benefit from nutrition support if there is a significant starvation or secondary cachexia component. In contrast with starvation where the patient undergoes adaptation to reduce energy expenditure, conserve protein, and use fatty acids and ketones as an energy source, in primary cachexia there is

Table 57.1 *Metabolic alterations in primary and secondary cachexia*

	Secondary cachexia (starvation)	Primary cachexia (metabolic)
Protein synthesis	⇑	⇓
Muscle proteins	⇓	⇓
Acute phase proteins	⇑	⇔
Lipogenesis	⇓	⇓
Proteolysis	⇑⇑⇑	⇔
Lipolysis	⇑	⇑⇑⇑
Glucose turnover	⇑	⇓

Note: Clinically both forms of cachexia are identical.

accelerated catabolism despite declining energy intake, as well as normal or increased resting energy expenditure, mobilization of protein and lipid stores and augmented gluconeogenesis (Table 57.1).

Primary cachexia is not simply a nutrition deficit caused by the combination of increased energy consumption by the tumor and decreased caloric intake due to the action of tumor-related factors on the satiety center. Past attempts at increasing nutrition intake with aggressive nutritional therapies failed to reverse the cachexia/anorexia syndrome and did not improve clinical outcomes such as survival or tumor response.[14***] Performance status or symptom control did not improve[15**] with dietary counseling, and invasive artificial nutrition had a negative impact on quality of life[16] and a higher rate of complications[17**] compared with oral intake. High caloric oral nutritional therapy was also unsuccessful in COPD[18*] patients with cachexia and relative anorexia. Despite the general poor response, the support of food intake should not be neglected as shown in one prospective randomized trial[19**] which added nutritional intervention to existing pharmacological treatment and found significant benefit in weight gain, function, and survival.

In contrast with starvation, where more than 75 percent of weight loss is from body fat, studies of cancer patients have found approximately equal losses of fat and body-cell mass, particularly skeletal muscle.[20,21*] With the introduction of retroviral therapy, patients with HIV rarely experience the catastrophic weight loss which was common in the past, however, the loss of lean body mass is still common.[22*] Investigation of changes in body composition on longitudinal follow-up of up to 5 years[23*] reveals that weight loss in cancer patients on anti-inflammatories appears to be predominantly from loss of body fat, primarily from the trunk and then leg tissue and arm tissue, respectively. Lean mass is predominantly lost from arm tissue. There may be a gender difference in cancer cachexia, with increased muscle loss in males.[24*] In patients with moderate-to-severe COPD[25] fat free mass is an independent predictor of mortality irrespective of fat mass.

Metabolic abnormalities include increased resting energy expenditure (with reduced physical activity level and total energy expenditure) and are more likely to be found in certain tumor types[26] and even in some tumors without evidence of[27] metastatic disease. Similar abnormalities are found in CHF, rheumatoid arthritis,[28] and kidney failure.[29] The increased resting energy expenditure may represent an increase in futile metabolic cycles such as the Cori cycle (which converts the large amount of lactate produced by the tumor back into glucose in the liver) or may be due to an increased expression and activity of mitochondrial uncoupling proteins,[30] which are involved in the control of energy metabolism and cause increased thermogenesis and blood flow of brown adipose tissue in cachectic states. Tumor necrosis factor (TNF) is able to increase gene expression[31] of uncoupling proteins and can also induce uncoupling in the mitochondria[32] of rats, however, muscle samples from cachectic pancreatic cancer patients demonstrated increased mRNA for ubiquitin but not uncoupling proteins.[33] Inhibition of fatty acid synthase (and therefore fatty acids) has been shown to decrease food intake in mice by decreased expression of neuropeptide Y, which is probably mediated by increased levels of malonyl coenzyme A (proposed to act as a signal of the availability of physiological fuels).[34] Progressive cachexia is also associated with other metabolic abnormalities including relative glucose intolerance, insulin resistance and gluconeogenesis.[35]

Tumor and host factors

CYTOKINES

Cytokines may be produced by the tumor or by the host and include TNF-α, interleukin (IL)-1, IL-6, and interferon-γ. Cytokines are also elevated in other conditions characterized by a chronic inflammatory response, such as TB, malaria,[36] rheumatoid arthritis, and COPD. Patients with CHF and cachexia have significantly elevated levels of cytokines (TNF-α, IL-6, soluble TNF-receptor-1) compared with noncachectic patients.[37**] Proinflammatory cytokines such as TNF-α, IL-6 and IL-1β promote weight loss, anorexia, and protein and fat breakdown. They increase the levels of cortisone and glucagon, and increase insulin resistance and decrease insulin levels. Furthermore, cytokines increase the resting energy expenditure in humans and animals and promote the acute phase response by the liver (characterized by the synthesis of acute phase proteins, such as CRP, fibrinogen, and α_1-antitrypsin).

TNF-α modulates the activity of glucose-sensitive neurons in the hypothalamus[38] and stimulates prostaglandin E_2 (PGE$_2$) synthesis, which induces the release of anorectic corticotropin releasing factor (CRF).[39] Administration of a TNF inhibitor to anorectic rats results in improved food intake and body weight.[40] In COPD patients hypoxemia appears to be associated with activation of TNF-α and may be a contributing factor to weight loss.[41] However, in humans with cancer cachexia, serum levels of TNF-α do not appear to correlate directly with appetite and weight loss[42] and some animal experiments suggest that administration of cytokines may induce an acute phase response without causing weight loss. By itself, TNF may not be able to cause muscle wasting and would require the synergistic effect of a combination of cytokines.[43] In myotubes and mouse muscle, the combination of TNF-α and interferon-γ strongly reduces myosin expression through an RNA-dependent mechanism[44] via the transcription factor nuclear factor kappa B (NF-κB).[45] In addition, loss of myosin was found to be caused by a second mechanism, the activation of the ubiquitin-dependent proteasome pathway. Ultimately, the preferential loss of the myosin-heavy chain protein relative to actin, tropomyosin and troponin may alter the ratio between thick and thin filaments, possibly inducing atrophy to restore balance in the formation of a functional contractile lattice.[46]

Proteasomal degradation of intracellular skeletal muscle proteins via the ubiquitin–proteasome pathway involves enzymes which bind (E3) to the protein substrate, and conjugate (E1) and transfer (E2) ubiquitin. Activation of this pathway is important in the mediation of muscle atrophy in a number of disease models including renal failure,[47] diabetes, and heart failure. Experimentally, the genetic deletion[48] of muscle-specific E3 ligases protects against muscle[49] atrophy following denervation and disuse. The expression of ubiquitin ligase E3 alpha-II is increased by proinflammatory cytokines and accelerates ubiquitin conjugation to endogenous cellular proteins.[50] Ubiquitin–proteasome-dependent proteolysis is probably the predominant mechanism of muscle protein loss, but there is evidence that several other regulatory mechanisms may be important as well.[51]

The role of NF-κB in the activation of the transcription of genes is well established, and it also functions in promoting cell growth. It is activated by TNF, muscle disuse[52] and IL-1, and leads to the production of a host of related proteins including cytokines and acute phase response proteins as well as regulators of apoptosis. Activation of the NF-κB pathway of skeletal muscle in mice induces serious skeletal muscle atrophy[53] and is characterized by increased catabolism via the ubiquitin–proteasome pathway. Genetic inactivation of NF-κB has been shown to prevent atrophy whereas a pharmacological blocker sodium salicylate partially suppressed the atrophy. Although activation of NF-κB in skeletal muscle may be an appropriate response during periods of starvation, providing amino acids for energy, in pathological conditions, such as cancer, it may have catastrophic consequences. Activation of NF-κB has been demonstrated in the skeletal muscle of COPD patients with low body weight,[54] adding support for the role of NF-κB as a potential molecular mechanism leading to cachexia.

Another important proinflammatory cytokine, IL-6, does not consistently induce weight loss when administered alone to animals, but a review of trials using monoclonal antibody to IL-6 showed a decrease in CRP and cachexia.[55] High mobility group box 1 is a ubiquitous protein present in the nuclei and cytoplasm of nearly all cell types and causes anorexia and weight loss when administered to normal animals.[56] Other growth factors which have been demonstrated to produce cachexia in animal models include ciliary neurotrophic factor and leukemia inhibitory factor. Their importance in human cachexia is yet to be determined. Some cytokines, in contrast, may have an anabolic effect. Myosin heavy chain accretion in human skeletal myogenic cultures has been shown to be stimulated by IL-15,[57] and when administered to tumor-bearing rats, IL-15 partly inhibits skeletal muscle wasting.[58]

PROTEOLYSIS–INDUCING FACTOR

Proteolysis-inducing factor (PIF) is a sulfated glycoprotein, tumor-derived product whose biological effect is mediated by its sulfated oligosaccharide chains.[30] It is detectable in the urine of 80 percent of patients with pancreatic cancer, and these patients have a significantly greater rate of weight loss than those in whom PIF is undetectable.[59] A longitudinal study also demonstrated that over time patients who were positive for PIF experienced weight loss whereas those with a negative test gained weight.[60] A correlation has also been reported between PIF expression in gastrointestinal tumors, its detection in urine, and weight loss.[61] Human melanoma cells produce PIF and induce cachexia and depletion of lean muscle mass in nude mice.[62] Mouse skeletal muscle and in vitro murine myotubes show an increased activity and expression of the ubiquitin–proteasome proteolytic pathway when treated with PIF.[63] Proteasome inhibitors attenuated the enhanced degradation of myofibrillar proteins. The expression of the ubiquitin–proteasome pathway in skeletal muscle and PIF-induced proteolysis appears to be mediated via NF-κB,[64] therefore agents capable of inhibiting NF-κB activation may be able to prevent muscle degradation; PIF activates NFκB, resulting in increased IL-6 and IL-8 production and to a lesser degree CRP, as well as inducing the signal transducers and activators of transcription pathway (STAT3),[65] which are involved in the induction of acute phase protein response. Recently, tumor xenografts engineered to overexpress human PIF did not induce cachexia in mice.[66] The reason for this unexpected result is not clear.

Lipolytic factors

Cancer patients with weight loss show urinary excretion of a lipid-mobilizing factor (LMF),[67] which is characterized by its ability to stimulate lipolysis in isolated murine epididymal adipocytes. This bioactivity was not detected in the urine of patients without weight loss. When LMF or Zn-α_2-glycoprotein (ZAG) is administered to mice or to human adipocytes, lipid is mobilized and glycerol and 3-hydroxybutyrate is increased.[68] When LMF is administered to murine myoblasts there appears to be an increase in protein synthesis and a decrease in protein catabolism.[69] More recent work has demonstrated that ZAG/LMF is produced locally by adipocytes and is upregulated in cachexia.[70] ZAG also induces uncoupling protein expression in skeletal muscle and adipose tissue.[71] Eicosapentaenoic acid (EPA) attenuates body weight loss in mice and downregulates ZAG expression in adipose tissue, whereas dexamethasone-stimulated lipolysis is attenuated by anti-ZAG antibody; EPA may preserve adipose tissue in cachectic mice by downregulation of ZAG expression through interference with glucocorticoid signaling.[72] Natriuretic peptides, known to play a key role in blood pressure and volume homeostasis, have been found to promote lipolysis in human fat cells[73] and lipid mobilization, and therefore may have a potential role in cardiac cachexia.

NEUROHORMONAL MECHANISMS

Neurohormonal mechanisms are an important compensatory means by which caloric intake is increased in response to hormonal signals of energy balance. Before examining the abnormalities documented in the cachectic/anorexic state, a summary of the normal physiology may be helpful to understand the process.

PHYSIOLOGY

Evidence suggests that reciprocal circadian rhythms in two peripheral hormones, anorexigenic leptin from adipocytes and orexigenic ghrelin from the stomach, are major afferent signals for the activation of the appetite regulating network in the hypothalamus.[74] Another hormone, cholecystokinin, released from the proximal small intestine, signals postprandial satiety and has been shown to inhibit the orexigenic effect of peripheral ghrelin[75] while mobilizing gastric leptin and increasing plasma leptin levels.[76] However, the recent discovery that the precursor preproghrelin produces obestatin in addition to ghrelin in rats is further demonstration of the complexity of the 'gut–brain' axis. Obestatin[77] appears to decrease food intake, weight gain, gastric emptying, and jejunal motility. The hypothalamic melanocortin system is also an important regulator of caloric intake via proopiomelanocortin neurons that produce and release α-melanocyte-stimulating hormone (MSH) which binds to melanocortin receptors (MC3-R and MC4-R) resulting in decreased food intake. Leptin may increase the potency of the anorexigenic effects of α-MSH by enzymatic N-acetylation.[78] In mice, leptin has been shown to play an inhibiting role in an alternative orexigenic pathway involving the endocannabinoid receptor CB-1 and the endogenous agonists anandamide and 2-arachidonyl-glycerol.[79]

Agouti-related peptide (AgRP) is an endogenous antagonist which binds to MC3-R and MC4-R thereby inhibiting the effect of anorexigenic melanocortin peptides. The expression of AgRP is stimulated by fasting and inhibited by leptin and cytokines. Other hormones which increase feeding include melanin concentrating hormone (MCH), opioid peptides, orexin, and galanin. Those peptides that decrease food intake include corticotropin releasing factor (CRF), urocortin, bombesin, glucagons and cocaine and amphetamine-regulated transcript. When there is reduced energy intake there is an increase in the number and amplitude of episodic ghrelin discharges. Leptin is secreted in a pulsatile manner similar to ghrelin, but in contrast decreased caloric intake diminishes the amplitude of the pulse.[80] Gastric ghrelin crossing the blood–brain barrier and locally produced hypothalamic ghrelin causes a release of orexigenic neuropeptide Y, AgRP, and increased appetite.[81] Another hormone which may play a role is peptide YY (PYY), which is secreted in the ileum and crosses the blood–brain barrier to reduce food intake by binding to the inhibitory neuropeptide Y2 receptor (NPY Y2) in the hypothalamus.[82,83]

Metabolism of sugars and fats has an established role in regulating feeding. The infusion of glucose[84] or ketones[85] inhibits feeding via vagal afferent signaling, and the inhibition of glucose or fatty acid oxidation stimulates caloric intake.

PATHOPHYSIOLOGY (FIG. 57.3)

Patients with cachexia and lung cancer have elevated plasma levels of ghrelin.[86] Compared with cancer patients without cachexia, those who have cancer-induced cachexia have significantly higher active ghrelin levels and the active to total ghrelin ratio is also increased. Because appetite is not increased in patients with cachexia despite high ghrelin levels, cachexia may be a state of ghrelin resistance.[87] In a long-term follow-up of cancer patients, survival and body fat were predicted by insulin, ghrelin, and leptin levels.[88] In patients with CHF, the plasma levels of ghrelin are significantly higher in cachectic than in noncachectic patients, possibly as a compensatory mechanism for the catabolic state.[89] Ghrelin appears to counteract the elevated sympathetic activity and high norepinephrine levels in COPD patients with cachexia[90] and probably has a similar role in CHF.

In uremia-associated cachexia and in children with renal failure leptin levels are elevated. Uremia-associated cachexia is attenuated mice deficient in leptin receptor and in MC-4R-deficient mice or those who had the antagonist AgRP administered.[91] This suggests a major role for the leptin–melanocortin pathway in this form of cachexia. In patients with COPD, leptin and ghrelin levels are lower[92] than in healthy controls but leptin appears to increase significantly in patients experiencing acute exacerbations.[93] In experimental models leptin does not appear to play a significant role in cancer cachexia, and in humans with cancer the leptin levels are low and inversely proportional to cytokines such as IL-6. In patients with TB and HIV plasma leptin concentrations are not associated with loss of appetite or wasting.[94] In HIV-negative TB patients there was no significant difference in leptin (corrected for energy balance) and muscle mass at baseline and after 1 month and 6 months of treatment.[95]

Despite the decreased fat stores in cancer patients, the levels of leptin may be inappropriately low, possibly due to inhibition by chronically high growth hormone levels and low insulin levels.[96] Some studies have found no significant

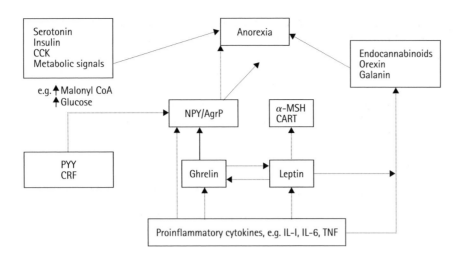

Figure 57.3 *Mechanisms of anoexia (via blood and neural signalling). .... inhibition; _____ stimulation, PVY, peptide YY, AgRP, Agouti-related protein (hypothalamus); CCK, cholecystokinin; TNF, tumor necrosis factor; CART, cocaine and amphetamine regulated transcript; NPY, neuropeptide Y (hypothalamus); MSH, melanocyte-stimulating hormone; IL, interleukin.*

difference in terms of insulin resistance in patients with cachectic or noncachectic cancer,[97] but increased peripheral resistance to insulin mediated by TNF-α[98] has been implicated in the development of cachexia in CHF and rheumatoid arthritis. When human oral squamous cell carcinoma cells are inoculated into mice, they produce weight loss but no compensatory hyperphagia. Corticotropin-releasing hormone mRNA is increased[99] in these mice and this is thought to inhibit NPY-induced feeding. Peptide YY levels have been found to be similar in patients with cachexia and those without, suggesting that it is unlikely to play an important role in cancer-induced cachexia.[87] The hormone orexin reverses cholecystokinin-induced loss of appetite in mice,[100] but its role in humans is unclear.

Proinflammatory cytokines are known to have anorexic effects and may interact with the neurohormonal system to cause decreased caloric intake. Proinflammatory cytokines (IL-1, IL-6, TNF-α) are believed to activate the melanocortin system by an unknown mechanism that leads to anorexia.[101] The mechanism of action of IL-1 may include the stimulation of leptin receptors, which decrease NPY[102] production and increase MSH, thereby reducing appetite. Interleukin-1 also increases hypothalamic levels of CRH[103] and serotonin.[104] Serotonin is found to be elevated in cachectic rats compared with controls.[105] In addition, IL-1 increases cholecystokinin levels and delays gastric emptying. However, in an experiment, an IL-1 receptor antagonist was not able to reverse the cachexia syndrome in animals.[106]

It seems likely that the failure of compensatory mechanisms to increase appetite is due to elevated levels of cytokines and disease products, which either decrease sensitivity to orexigenic hormones or inhibit hunger by direct stimulation of or increased sensitivity to anorexigenic peptides.

Anabolic hormone abnormalities

Cachexia has been associated with low testosterone levels in patients with pancreatic[107] cancer and in patients with lung cancer.[108] Long-term treatment with opioids may be

another important factor which produces hypogonadism[109] in patients with cancer. Up to one third of COPD patients have hypogonadism (which may be aggravated by corticosteroids[110]), however this is not necessarily associated with weight loss or muscle weakness when compared to eugonadal COPD patients.[111] When compared to normal controls, hypogonadic nonsteroid-using COPD patients with normal arterial oxygen have decreased quadriceps muscle strength.[112] Also, patients with COPD and reduced mid thigh muscle cross-sectional area have significantly lower levels of dihydroepiandrosterone sulfate (DHEAS) when compared to healthy subjects.[113] Decreased testosterone is present in up to 50 percent of HIV patients and is highly correlated with loss of lean muscle mass, increased GH levels and decreased Insulin-like growth factor (IGF-I).[114] This suggests that a combination of GH resistance and androgen deficiency may play a role in the weight loss. Hypoandrogenemia is also found in HIV-infected women[115] and is associated with advanced disease state and weight loss. IGF-I induces hypertrophy of human myotubes in vitro and an increase in myosin heavy chain content,[116] and it is decreased in cachectic colorectal patients probably as a result of GH resistance.[117] There is also evidence that angiotensin II downregulates IGF-I in skeletal muscle, leading to proteolysis and wasting.[118] In CHF, local IGF-I expression is reduced in the presence of normal serum levels of IGF-I (this correlates with decreased muscle fiber cross-sectional area and inversely with local expression of IL-1beta.).[119]

Autonomic nervous system

Clinical manifestations of autonomic dysfunction are well described in patients with advanced cancer,[120*] rheumatoid arthritis, HIV disease, CHF, and COPD.[121] Whether the gastrointestinal (chronic nausea, early satiety, anorexia, pseudo-bowel obstruction) and cardiovascular (postural hypotension, fixed heart rate) manifestations represent the same underlying mechanism is unknown. In the patient with advanced cancer and autonomic neuropathy, vagal nerve dysfunction may not only result in gastroparesis but may also lead to dysregulation of neurohormonal feeding signals and immune homeostasis, thereby contributing to the anorexia/cachexia syndrome.

Humoral and neural signals for satiety and hunger can be conveyed via the vagus nerve and may be the major pathway conveying ghrelin's starvation signals to the brain.[122] Ghrelin appears to suppress vagal afferent discharges when administered intravenously[123] to rats, whereas cholecystokinin and another anorectic peptide, PYY,[124] increase discharges and transmit a satiety signal to the nucleus tractus solitarius. Conversely, the electrical activity of efferent fibers of the vagus nerve is stimulated by ghrelin resulting in increased gastric acid secretion and motility. Ghrelin contributes to an anabolic state by stimulating growth hormone release via vagal afferents[125] (the growth hormone-releasing effect of ghrelin appears to be more potent than that of the growth hormone-releasing hormone[126]) and it also decreases fat utilization through growth hormone-independent mechanisms.[127] Decreased sensitivity to ghrelin and dysfunctional signaling by other peptides may cause abnormal regulation of satiety/hunger by the vagus. Abnormalities of the autonomic nervous system may be linked to a loss of circadian variation of leptin levels[83] in cachectic COPD patients, which in turn may lead to alteration of the afferent signaling to the hypothalamus.

In humans, stimulation of the vagus nerve may be associated with marked peripheral increases in pro and anti-inflammatory cytokines.[128] Efferent signals in the vagus nerve in response to peripheral inflammation provide a direct mechanism for neural regulation of the immune response that is reflexive and rapid. Proinflammatory cytokines are decreased,[129] as is NF-κB[130] via the release of acetylcholine in the vicinity of macrophages.[131] In rats with cancer anorexia, vagotomy markedly attenuates tumor-induced declines in food intake, suggesting that afferent neural signals also play an important role.[132]

Autonomic remodeling of the host by HIV has been proposed as a contributor to the immunodeficiency and cachexia in these patients.[133] Patients with cardiac cachexia exhibit severely impaired autonomic reflex control compared with noncachectic patients[134] and have higher norepinephrine and epinephrine levels. Experiments in rats indicate that angiotensin II stimulates lipolysis in subcutaneous and visceral adipocytes by sympathetic activation and β-adrenergic receptor stimulation. The nonselective blockade of β-adrenergic and angiotensin II receptors markedly attenuated the rise of norepinephrine.[135]

CONCLUSION

The cachexia/anorexia syndrome is a cascade of events that is initiated by the interaction between host and disease, and is caused by multiple interrelated mechanisms, which include the secretion of tumor products and cytokines, neuroendocrine abnormalities, autonomic failure, diminished calorie intake, muscle proteolysis, lipolysis, and the inability to accrue lean muscle mass or fat. This complex syndrome is not likely to be managed by a single treatment modality, but rather by the simultaneous institution of several nonpharmacological and pharmacological therapies.

Key learning points

- Inflammation, sympathetic activation, and hormonal abnormalities are mechanisms of cachexia that are common to a variety of diseases.

- Primary cachexia is characterized by increased proteolysis and increased acute phase protein production.

- Secondary cachexia or starvation is characterized by insufficient calories and utilization of fat as an energy source in order to conserve protein.

- Cytokines are important mediators of proteolysis, lipolysis, neurohormonal activation and anorexia.

- Dysregulation of hypothalamic hormones (e.g. neuropeptide Y, the melanocortin system) and peripherally secreted hormones (e.g. ghrelin, leptin, cholecystokinin, insulin) contribute to loss of appetite.

- Degradation of protein via the ubiquitin–proteasome pathway and decreased expression of myosin result in the loss of lean muscle.

- Successful management of cachexia/anorexia will require treatments targeted at multiple pathways.

REFERENCES

◆ 1   Bruera E, MacDonald RN. Nutrition in cancer patients: an update and review of our experience. Issues in symptom control. part 3. *J Pain Symptom Manage* 1988; **3**: 133–40.

2   Hockley JM, Dunlop R, Davies RJ. Survey of distressing symptoms in dying patients and their families in hospital and the response to a symptom control team. *BMJ* 1988; **296**: 1715–17.

3   Vigano A, Watanabe S, Bruera E. Anorexia and cachexia in advanced cancer patients. *Cancer Surv* 1994; **21**: 99–115.

● 4   Reuben DB, Mor V, Hiris J. Clinical symptoms and length of survival in patients with terminal cancer. *Arch Intern Med* 1988; **148**: 1586–91.

● 5   Dewys WD, Begg C, Lavin PT, *et al*. Prognostic effect of weight loss prior to chemotherapy in cancer patients. Eastern Cooperative Oncology group. *Am J Med* 1980; **69**: 491–7.

6   McCarthy DO. TNF alpha and IL-6 have differential effects on food intake and gastric emptying in fasted rats. *Res Nurs Health* 2000; **23**: 222–8.

7   Suzuki S, Goncalves CG, Meguid MM. Catabolic outcome from non-gastrointestinal malignancy-related malabsorption leading to malnutrition and weight loss. *Curr Opin Nutr Metab Care* 2005; **8**: 419–27.

8   MacDonald N, Easson A, Mazurak V, *et al.* Understanding and managing cancer cachexia. *J Am Coll Surg* 2003;143–61.

9   Wheeler DA, Gilbert CL, Launer CA, *et al.* Weight loss as a predictor of survival and disease progression in HIV. *J Acquire Immun Defic Syndr Hum Retrovirol* 1998; **18**: 80–5.

● 10 Tang AM, Jacobson DL, Spiegelman D, *et al.* Increasing risk of 5% or greater unintentional weight loss in a cohort of HIV-infected patients, 1995–2003. *J Acquire Immun Defic Syndr* 2005; **40**: 70–6.

11 Jeremic B, Shibamoto Y. Pre-treatment prognostic factors in patients with stage III NSCLC treated with hyperfractionated radiation therapy with or without concurrent chemotherapy. *Lung Cancer* 1995; **13**: 21–30.

12 Socinski MA, Zhang C, Herndon JE, *et al.* Combined modality trials of the cancer and leukemia Group B in stage III NSCLC: analysis of factors influencing survival and toxicity. *Ann Oncol* 2004; **15**: 1033–41.

13 Elahi MM, McMillan DC, McArdle CS, *et al.* Score based on hypoalbuminemia and elevated C-reactive protein predicts survival in patients with advanced gastrointestinal cancer. *Nutr Cancer* 2004; **48**: 171–3.

◆ 14 Klein S, Kinney J, Jeejeebhoy K, *et al.* Nutrition support in clinical practice: review of published data and recommendations for future directions. *Am J Clin Nutr* 1997; **66**: 683–706.

● 15 Ovesen L, Allingstrup L, Hannibal J, *et al.* Effect of dietary counseling on food intake, body weight, response rate, survival, and quality of life in cancer patients undergoing chemotherapy: a prospective randomized study. *J Chem Oncol* 1993; **11**: 2043–9.

● 16 Torelli GF, Campos AC, Meguid MM. Use of TPN in terminally ill patients. *Nutrition* 1999; **15**: 665–7.

17 Hyltander A, Bosaeus I, Svedlund J, *et al.* Supportive nutrition on recovery of metabolism, nutritional state, health related quality of life, and exercise capacity after major surgery: a randomized study. *Clin Gastroenterol Hepatol* 2005; **3**: 466–74.

18 Creutzberg EC, Schols AM, Weling-Scheepers CA, *et al.* Characterization of nonresponse to high caloric oral nutritional therapy in depleted patients with COPD. *Am J Respir Crit Care Med* 2000; **161**: 745–52.

19 Lundholm K, Daneryd P, Bosaeus I, *et al.* Palliative nutritional intervention in addition to cyclooxygenase and erythropoietin treatment for patients with malignant disease: effects on survival, metabolism, and function. A randomized prospective study. *Cancer* 2004; **100**: 1967–77.

20 Segal RJ, Reid RD, Courneya KS, *et al.* Resistance exercise in men receiving androgen deprivation therapy for prostate cancer. *J Clin Oncol* 2003; **21**: 1653–59.

21 MacFie J, Burkinshaw L. Body composition in malignant disease. *Metabolism* 1987; **36**: 290–4.

22 Roubenoff R, Greenspoon N, Skolnik PR, *et al.* Role of cytokines and testosterone in regulating lean body mass and resting energy expenditure in HIV-infected men. *Am J Physiol Endocrinol Metab* 2002; **283**: E138–145.

23 Fouladian M, Korner U, Bosaeus I, *et al.* Body composition and time course changes in regional distribution of fat and lean tissue in unselected cancer patients on palliative care-correlations with food intake, metabolism, exercise capacity, and hormones. *Cancer* 2005; **103**: 189–98.

24 Sarhill N, Mahmoud F, Walsh D, *et al.* Evaluation of nutritional status in advanced metastatic cancer. *Support Care Cancer* 2003; **10**: 652–9.

25 Schols AM, Broekhuizen R, Weling-Scheepers CA, *et al.* Body composition and mortality in COPD. *Am J Clin Nutr* 2005; **82**: 53–9.

● 26 Fredrix EN, Soeters PB, Wouters EF, *et al.* Effect of different tumor types on resting energy expenditure. *Cancer Res* 1991; **51**: 6138–41.

27 Jatoi A, Daly BD, Hughes VA, *et al.* Do patients with non-metastatic non-small cell lung cancer demonstrate altered resting energy expenditure? *Ann Thorac Surg* 2001; **72**: 348–51.

28 Rall LC, Roubenoff RR. Rheumatoid Cachexia: Metabolic abnormalities, mechanisms and interventions. *Rheumatology* 2004; **43**: 1219–23.

29 Wang AY, Sea MM, Tang N, *et al.* Resting energy expenditure and subsequent mortality risk in peritoneal dialysis patients. *J Am Soc Nephrol* 2004; **15**: 3134–43.

◆ 30 Tisdale M. Molecular pathways leading to cancer cachexia. *Physiology* 2005; **20**: 340–8.

31 Busqets S, Sanchis D, Alvarez B, *et al.* In the rat TNF administration results in an increase in both UCP2 and UCP3 mRNA's in skeletal muscle: a possible mechanism for cytokine induced thermogenesis? *FEBS Lett* 1998; **440**: 348–50.

32 Busqets S, Aranda X, Ribas-Carbo M, *et al.* Tumor necrosis factor-alpha uncouples respiration in isolated rat mitochondria. *Cytokine* 2003; **22**: 1–4.

33 De Jong CH, Busqets S, Moses AG, *et al.* Systemic inflammation correlates with increased expression of skeletal muscle ubiquitin but not uncoupling proteins in cancer cachexia. *Oncol Rep* 2005; **14**: 257–63.

● 34 Loftus TM, Jaworsky DE, Frehywot GL, *et al.* Reduced food intake and body weight in mice treated with fatty acid synthase inhibitors. *Science* 2000; **288**: 2299–300.

35 Tayek JA. A review of cancer cachexia and abnormal glucose metabolism in humans with cancer. *J Am Coll Nutr* 1992; **11**: 445–56.

36 Onwuamaegbu ME, Henein M, Coats AJ. Cachexia in malaria and heart failure: therapeutic considerations in clinical practice. *Postgrad Med J* 2004; **80**: 642–9.

● 37 Anker SD, Ponikowski PP, Clark AL, *et al.* Cytokines and neurohormones relating to body composition alterations in the wasting syndrome of chronic heart failure. *Eur Heart J* 1999; **20**: 683–93.

● 38 Plata-Salaman CR, Oomura Y, Kai Y. Tumor necrosis factor and interleukin -1 beta: suppression of food intake by direct action in the central nervous system. *Brain Res* 1988; **448**: 106–14.

39 Uehara A, Sekiya C, Takasugi M, *et al.* Anorexia induced by interleukin-1:involvement of corticotropin releasing factor. *Am J Physiol* 1989; **257**: R613–R617.

40 Torelli GF, Meguid MM, Moldawer LL, *et al.* Use of recombinant human soluble TNF receptor in anorectic tumor-bearing rats. *Am J Physiol* 1999; **277**: R850–855.

41 Takabatake N, Nakamura H, Abe S, *et al.* The Relationship between chronic hypoxemia and activation of the tumor necrosis factor-alpha system in patients with COPD. *Am J Respir Crit Care Med* 2000; **161**: 1179–84.

42 Maltoni M, Fabbri L Nanni O, et al. Serum levels of tumor necrosis factor alpha and other cytokines do not correlate with weight loss and anorexia in cancer patients. *Support Care Cancer* 1997; **5**: 130–5.

43 Argiles JM, Lopez-Soriano FJ. The role of cytokines in cancer cachexia. *Med Res Rev* 1999; **19**: 223–48.

● 44 Acharyya S, Ladner K, Nelsen L, et al. Cancer cachexia is regulated by selective targeting of skeletal muscle gene products. *J Clin Invest* 2004; **114**: 370–8.

45 Guttridge DC, Mayo MW, Madrid LV, et al. NFkB induced loss of Myo-D m-RNA: possible role in muscle decay and cachexia. *Science* 2000; **289**: 2293–4.

◆ 46 Chamberlain J. Cancer in cachexia – zeroing in on myosin. *N Engl J Med* 2004; **351**: 2124–5.

47 Schulze PC, Spate U. Insulin-like growth factor-1 and muscle wasting in chronic heart failure. *Int J Biochem Cell Biol* 2005; **37**: 2023–5.

48 Bodine SC, Latres E, Baumheuter S, et al. Identification of ubiquitin ligases required for skeletal muscle atrophy. *Science* 2001; **294**: 1704–8.

49 Glass DJ. Signalling pathways that mediate skeletal muscle hypertrophy and atrophy. *Nat Cell Biol* 2003; **5**: 87–90.

50 Kwak K, Zhou X, Solomon V, et al. Regulation of protein catabolism by muscle-specific and cytokine-inducible ubiquitin ligase E3alpha-II during cancer cachexia. *Cancer Res* 2004; 8193–8.

51 Hasselgren PO, Wray C, Mammen J. Molecular regulation of muscle cachexia: it may be more than the protesome. *Biochem Biophys Res Commun* 2002; **290**: 1–10.

52 Hunter RB, Stevenson E, Koncarevic A, et al. Activation of an alternative NF kB pathway in skeletal muscle during disuse atrophy. *FASEB J* 2002; **16**: 529–38.

● 53 Cai D, Frantz JD, Tawa NE, et al. IKKbeta/NFkB Activation causes severe muscle wasting in mice. *Cell* 2004; **119**: 285–98.

54 Agusti A, Morla M, Sauleda J, et al. NFkB activation and iNOS upregulation in skeletal muscle of patients with COPD and low body weight. *Thorax* 2004; **59**: 483–7.

55 Trikha M, Corringham R, Klein B, et al. Targeted anti-interleukin-6 antibody therapy for cancer: a review of the rationale and clinical evidence. *Clin Cancer Res* 2003; **9**: 4653–65.

56 Yang H, Wang H, Czura CJ. The cytokine activity of HMGB1. *J Leukoc Biol* 2005; **78**: 1–8.

57 Furmanczyk PS, Quinn LS. Interleukin-15 increases myosin accretion in human skeletal myogenic cultures. *Cell Biol Int* 2003; **27**: 845–51.

58 Carbo N, Lopez-Soriano J, Costelli P, et al. Interleukin-15 antagonizes muscle protein waste in tumor-bearing rats. *Br J Cancer* 2000; **83**: 526–31.

● 59 Wigmore FJ, Todorov PT, Barber MD, et al. Characteristics of patients with pancreatic cancer expressing a novel cancer cachectic factor. *Br J Surg* 2000; **87**: 53–5.

60 Williams ML, Torres-Duarte A, Brant LJ, et al. The relationship between a urinary cachectic factor and weight loss in advanced cancer patients. *Cancer Invest* 2004; **22**: 866–70.

61 Cabal-Manzano R, Bhargava P, Torres-Duarte A, et al. Proteolysis inducing factor is expressed in tumors of patients with gastrointestinal cancers and correlates with weight loss. *Br J Cancer* 2001; **84**: 1599–602.

62 Todorov PT, Field WN, Tisdale MJ. Role of proteolysis inducing factor (PIF) in cachexia induced by a human melanoma (G361). *Br J Cancer* 1999; **80**: 1734–7.

63 Lorite MJ, Smith HJ, Arnold AJ, et al. Activation of ATP-ubiquitin-dependent proteolysis in skeletal muscle in vivo and murine myoblasts in vitro by a proteolysis-inducing factor (PIF). *Br J Cancer* 2001; **85**: 297–302.

64 Wyke SM, Tisdale MJ. NFkappaB mediates proteolysis inducing factor induced protein degradation and expression of the ubiquitin proteasome system in skeletal muscle. *Br J Cancer* 2005; **92**: 711–721.

65 Watchorn TM, Waddell ID, Dowidar N, et al. Proteolysis inducing factor regulates hepatic gene expression via the transcription factors NFkappaB and STAT3. *FASEB J* 2001; **15**: 562–64.

66 Monitto CL, Dong SM, Jen J, Sidransky D. Characterization of a human homologue of proteolysis-inducing factor and its role in cancer cachexia. *Clin Cancer Res* 2004; **10**: 5862–9.

● 67 Todorov PT, McDevitt TM, Meyer DJ, et al. Purification and characterization of a tumor lipid mobilizing factor. *Cancer Res* 1998; **58**: 2353–8.

68 Hirai K, Hussey HJ, Barber MD, et al. Biological evaluation of a lipid mobilizing factor isolated from the urine of cancer patients. *Cancer Res* 1998; **58**: 2359–65.

69 Islam-Ali BS, Tisdale MJ. Effect of a tumor-produced lipid-mobilizing factor on protein synthesis and degradation. *Br J Cancer* 2001; **84**: 1648–55.

70 Bing C, Bao Y, Jenkins J, et al. Zinc-alpha2-glycoprotein, a lipid mobilizing factor, is expressed in adipocytes and is upregulated in mice with cancer cachexia. *Proc Natl Acad Sci U S A* 2004; **101**: 2500–5.

71 Sanders PM, Tisdale MJ, Effect of ZAG on expression of uncoupling proteins in skeletal muscle and adipose tissue. *Cancer Lett* 2004; **212**: 71–81.

72 Russel ST, Tisdale MJ. Effect of EPA on expression of a lipid mobilizing factor in adipose tissue in cancer cachexia. *Prostaglandins Leukot Essent Fatty Acids* 2005; **72**: 409–14.

73 Lafontan M, Moro C, Sengenes C, et al. An unsuspected metabolic role for atrial natriuretic peptides: the control of lipolysis, lipid mobilization, and systemic nonesterified fatty acid levels in humans. *Arterioscler Thromb Vasc Biol* 2005; **25**: 2032–42.

74 Kalra S, Ueno N, Kalra P. Stimulation of appetite by ghrelin is regulated by leptin restraint: peripheral and central sites of action. *J Nutr* 2005; **135**: 1331–5.

75 Kobelt P, Tebbe J, Tjandra I, et al. CCK inhibits the orexigenic effect of peripheral ghrelin. *Am J Physiol Regul Integr Comp Physiol* 2005; **288**: R751–R758.

76 Bado A, Levasseur S, Attoub S, et al. The stomach is a source of leptin. *Nature* 1998; **394**: 790–3.

● 77 Zhang J, Ren PG, Avsian-Kretchmer O, et al. Obestatin, a peptide encoded by the ghrelin gene, opposes ghrelin's effects on food intake. *Science* 2005; **5750**: 996–9.

78 Guo L, Munzberg H, Stuart RC, et al. N-acetylation of hypothalamic alpha-melanocyte-stimulating-hormone and regulation by leptin. *Proc Natl Acad Sci U S A* 2004; **101**: 11797–802.

79 Di Marzo V, Goparaju S, Wang L, et al. Leptin regulated endocannabinoids are involved in maintaining food intake. *Nature* 2001; **410**: 822–5.

80 Bagnasco M, Kalra P, Kalra S. Ghrelin and leptin pulse discharge in fed and fasted rats. *Endocrinology* 2002; **143**: 726–9.

● 81 Nakazato M, Murakami N, Date Y, et al. A role for ghrelin in the central regulation of feeding. *Nature* 2001; **409**: 194–8.

82 Batterham RL, Cowley MA, Small CJ, et al. Gut hormone PYY physiologically inhibits food intake. Nature 2002; **418**: 650–4.

83 Takabatake N, Nakamura H, Minamihaba O, et al. A novel pathophysiologic phenomenon in cachexic patients with chronic obstructive pulmonary disease. Am J Respir Care Med 2001; **163**: 1314–19.

84 Niijima A. Glucose sensitive afferent fibres in the liver and their role in food intake and blood glucose regulation. J Autonom Nerv Syst 1983; **9**: 207–20.

85 Langhans W, Egli G, Scharrer E. Selective hepatic vagotomy eliminates the hypophagic effect of different metabolites. J Autonom Nerv Syst 1985; **13**: 255–62.

86 Shimizu Y, Nagaya N, Isobe T, et al. Increased plasma ghrelin level in lung cancer cachexia. Clin Cancer Res 2003; **9**: 774–8.

87 Garcia J, Garcia-Touza M, Hijazi R, et al. Active ghrelin levels and active to total ghrelin ratio in cancer-induced cachexia. J Clin Endocrinol Metab 2005; **90**: 2920–6.

88 Fouladiun M, Korner U, Bosaeus I, et al. Body composition and time course changes in regional distribution of fat and lean tissue in unselected cancer patients on palliative care-correlations with food intake, metabolism, exercise capacity, and hormones. Cancer 2005; **103**: 189–98.

89 Nagaya N, Kangawa K. Ghrelin improves left ventricular dysfunction and cardiac cachexia in heart failure. Curr Opin Pharmacol 2003; **3**: 146–51.

● 90 Nagaya N, Ito T, Murakami S, et al. Treatment of cachexia with ghrelin in patients with COPD. Chest 2005; **128**: 1187–93.

91 Cheung W, Yu P, Little B, et al. Role of leptin and melanocortin signaling in uremia associated cachexia. J Clin Invest 2005; **6**: 1476–8.

92 Luo FM, Liu XJ, Li SQ, et al. Circulating ghrelin in patients with COPD. Nutrition 2005; **21**: 793–8.

93 Calikoglu M, Sahin G, Unlu A, et al. Leptin and TNF alpha levels in patients with COPD and their relationship to nutritional parameters. Respiration 2004; **71**: 45–50.

94 van Lettow M, van der Meer JW, West CE, et al. IL-6 and HIV load, but not plasma leptin concentration predict anorexia and wasting in adults with pulmonary tuberculosis in Malawi. J Clin Endocrinol Metab 2005; **90**: 4771–6.

95 Schwenk A, Hodgson L, Rayner CF, et al. Leptin and energy metabolism in pulmonary tuberculosis. Am J Clin Nutr 2003; **77**: 392–8.

96 Huang Q, Zhang X, Jiang ZW, et al. Hypoleptinemia in gastric cancer patients: relation to body fat mass, insulin and growth hormone. J Parent Enteral Nutr 2005; **29**: 229–35.

97 Dulger H, Alici S, Sekeroglu MR, et al. Serum levels of leptin and proinflammatory cytokines in patients with gastrointestinal cancer. Int J Clin Pract 2004; **58**: 545–9.

◆ 98 Argiles JM, Lopez-Soriano FJ. Catabolic proinflammatory cytokines. Curr Opin Clin Nutr Metab Care 1998; **1**: 245–51.

99 Lee JH, Cha MJ, Choi SH, et al. Neuropeptide Y immuno-reactivity and corticotrophin-releasing hormone mRNA level are increased in the hypothalamus of mouse bearing a human oral squamous cell carcinoma. Neuropeptides 2004; **38**: 345–50.

100 Asakawa A, Inui A, Inui T, et al. Orexin reverses cholecystokinin-induced reduction in feeding. Diabetes Obes Metabolism 2002; **4**: 399–401.

◆ 101 Wisse B, Schwatrz MW, Cummings DE. Melanocortin signaling and anorexia in chronic disease states. Ann N Y Acad Sci 2003; **994**: 275–81.

102 Plata-Salman CR. Central nervous mechanisms contributing to the cachexia-anorexia syndrome. Nutrition 2000; **16**: 1009–12.

103 Sapolsky R, Rivier C, Yamamoto G, et al. Interkeukin-1 stimulates the secretion of hypothalamic corticotrophin releasing factor. Science 1987; **238**: 522–4.

104 Shintani F, Kanba S, Nakaki T, et al. Interleukin-1 beta augments release of norepinephrine, dopamine and serotonin in the rat anterior hypothalamus. J Neurosci 1993; **13**: 3574–81.

105 Blaha V, Yang ZJ, Meguid MM, et al. Ventromedial nucleus of hypothalamus is related to the development of cancer-induced cachexia: in vivo microdialysis study. Acta Med 1998; **41**: 3–11.

106 Costelli P, Llovera M, Carbo N, et al. Interleukin-1 receptor antagonist is unable to reverse cachexia in rats bearing an ascites hepatoma. Cancer Lett 1995; **95**: 33–8.

107 Todd BD. Pancreatic carcinoma and low serum testosterone; a correlation secondary to cancer cachexia? Eur J Surg Oncol 1988; **14**: 199–202.

108 Simons JP, Schols AM, Buurman WA, et al. Weight loss and low body cell mass in males with lung cancer: relationship with systemic inflammation, acute phase response, resting energy expenditure, and catabolic and anabolic hormones. Clin Sci (Lond)1999; **97**: 215–23.

● 109 Rajagopal A, Vassilopoulou-Sellin R, Palmer JL, et al. Symptomatic hypogonadism in male survivors of cancer with chronic exposure to opioids. Cancer 2004; **100**: 851–8.

110 Kamischke A, Kemper DE, Castel MA, et al. Testosterone levels in men with COPD with or without glucocorticoid therapy. Eur Respir J 1998; **11**: 41–5.

111 Laghi F, Langbein WE, Antonescu-Turcu A, et al. Respiratory and skeletal muscles in hypogonadal men with COPD. Am J Respir Crit Care Med 2005; **171**: 598–605.

112 Van Vliet M, Spruit MA, Verleden G, et al. Hypogonadism, quadriceps weakness, and exercise intolerance in COPD. Am J Respir Crit Care Med 2005; **172**: 1105–11.

113 Debigare R, Marquis K, Cote CH, et al. Catabolic/anabolic balance and muscle wasting in patients with COPD. Chest 2003; **124**: 83–9.

114 Grinspoon S, Corcoran C, Lee K, et al. Loss of lean body and muscle mass correlates with androgen levels in hypogonadal men with AIDS and wasting. J Clin Endocrinol Metab 1996; **81**: 4051–8.

115 Huang JS, Wilkie SJ, Dolan S, et al. Reduced testosterone levels in HIV-infected women with weight loss and low weight. Clin Infect Dis 2003; **36**: 499–506.

116 Jacquemin V, Furling D, Bigot A, et al. IGF-1 induces human myotube hypertrophy by increasing cell recruitment. Exp Cell Res 2004; **299**: 148–58.

117 Huang Q, Nai YJ, Jiang ZW, Li JS. Change of the Growth hormone–insulin-like growth factor-1 axis in patients with gastrointestinal cancer: related to tumor type and nutritional status. Br J Nutr 2005; **93**: 853–8.

118 Song YH, LI Y, Du J, et al. Muscle specific expression of IGF-1 blocks angiotensin II-induced skeletal muscle wasting. J Clin Invest 2005; **115**: 451–8.

119 Schulze PC, Gielen S, Adams V, *et al.* Muscular levels of proinflammatory cytokines correlate with a reduced expression of insulin-like growth factor-I in chronic heart failure. *Basic Res Cardiol* 2003; **98**: 267–74.

● 120 Bruera E, Chadwick S, Fox R, *et al.* Study of cardiovascular autonomic insufficiency in advanced cancer patients. *Cancer Treat Rep* 1986; **70**: 1383–7.

121 Tug T, Terzi SM, Yoldas TK. Relationship between the frequency of autonomic dysfunction and the severity of COPD. *Acta Neurol Scand* 2005; **112**: 183–8.

122 Ueno H, Yamaguchi H, Kangawa K, Nakazato M. Ghrelin: a gastric peptide that regulates food intake and energy homeostasis. *Regul Pept* 2005; **126**: 11–19.

123 Date Y, Toshinai K, Koda S, *et al.* Peripheral interaction of ghrelin with cholecystokinin on feeding regulation. *Endocrinology* 2005; **146**: 3518–25.

124 Koda S, Date Y, Murakami N, *et al.* The role of the vagal nerve in peripheral PYY induced feeding reduction in rats. *Endocrinology* 2005; **146**: 2369–75.

● 125 Date Y, Murakami N, Toshinai K, *et al.* The role of the gastric afferent vagal nerve in ghrelin-induced feeding and growth hormone secretion in rats. *Gastroenterology* 2002; **123**: 1120–8.

● 126 Takaya K, Ariyasu H, Kanamoto N, *et al.* Ghrelin strongly stimulates growth hormone release in humans. *J Clin Endocrinol Metab* 2000; **85**: 4908–11.

127 Tachop M, Smiley DL, Helman ML. Ghrelin induces adiposity in rodents. *Nature* 2000; **407**: 908–13.

128 Corcoran C, Connor TJ, O'Keane V, Garland MR. The effects of vagus nerve stimulation on pro- and anti-inflammatory cytokines in humans: a preliminary report. *Neuroimmunomodulation* 2005; **12**: 307–9.

129 Czura CJ, Friedman SG, Tracy KJ. Neural inhibition of inflammation: the cholinergic anti-inflammatory pathway. *J Endotoxin Res* 2003; **9**: 409–13.

130 Guarini S, Altavilla D, Cainazzo MM, *et al.* Efferent vagal fibre stimulation blunts NFkB activation and protects against hypovolemic hemorrhagic shock. *Circulation* 2003; **107**: 1189–94.

◆ 131 Czura CJ, Tracey KJ. Autonomic neural regulation of immunity. *J Intern Med* 2005; **257**: 156–66.

132 Bernstein IL. Neural mediation of food aversions and anorexia induced by tumor necrosis factor and tumors. *Neurosci Biobehav Rev* 1996; **20**: 177–81.

133 Yun A, Lee P, Bazar K. Modulation of Host immunity by HIV may be partly achieved through usurping host autonomic functions. *Med Hypotheses* 2004; **63**: 362–6.

134 Ponikowski P, Piepolo M, Chua TP, *et al.* The impact of cachexia on cardiorespiratory reflex control in chronic heart failure. *Eur Heart J* 1999; **20**: 1667–75.

135 Cabassi A, Coghi P, Govoni P, *et al.* Sympathetic modulation by carvedilol and losartan reduces Angiotensin II mediated lipolysis in subcutaneous and visceral fat. *J Clin Endocrinol Metab* 2005; **90**: 2888–97.

58

Overview of the management of the anorexia/weight loss syndrome

CARA BONDLY, AMINAH JATOI

OVERVIEW AND DEFINITIONS

The anorexia/weight loss syndrome occurs in patients with a variety of illnesses, including cancer, acquired immune deficiency syndrome (AIDS), and congestive heart failure. The cancer anorexia/weight loss syndrome is particularly devastating and is characterized by loss of appetite and weight, and functional decline, which occurs as a result of tissue wasting, in particular, muscle wasting. This syndrome affects approximately two-thirds of patients who die from advanced cancer.[1]

Weight loss of 10 percent is a well-accepted diagnostic criterion for severe malnutrition. However, among patients with cancer, previous studies have clearly shown that the anorexia/weight loss syndrome can be invoked if an involuntary weight loss of even 6 percent has occurred. This degree of weight loss has been observed in conjunction with incurable cancer, progressive debility, and a decline in performance status.[2]

From a clinical standpoint, the assessment of nutritional status is often viewed as multifaceted, if not cumbersome. A variety of approaches are utilized, and these span anything from a quick hands-off assessment shortly after entering a patient's room to a detailed modeling of nutritional parameters into a single risk assessment to an elaborate assessment of body composition that includes measurement of total body potassium, ingestion and sampling of tritiated water, and dual X-ray absorptiometry. All these approaches have their merits. However, we believe that the most clinically useful, practical, and validated measurement is patient-reported weight loss. As discussed above, weight loss of 6 percent or greater over the preceding 6 months predicts a

poor prognosis among cancer patients, and everyone will agree that it is relatively simple to acquire.

The anorexia/weight loss syndrome is distressing to patients and their families; in their eyes, the patient is 'starving'. Walsh et al. interviewed 1000 patients with advanced cancer referred to a palliative care program. Anorexia was tied for third, superseded only by pain and fatigue, as the most prevalent and bothersome symptom experienced by these patients.[3] Some of the distress associated with this symptom may be derived specifically from loss of appetite, but, at the same time, this decline in oral intake brings with it tremendous turmoil for the patient and family. This fear of 'starvation', as noted above, provides an extra emotional burden in the setting of an incurable, refractory malignancy.

Although these patients are not starving (Table 58.1), the anorexia/weight loss syndrome does portend an unfavorable prognosis in patients with cancer as well as in patients with human immunodeficiency virus (HIV) infection and congestive heart failure. In the cancer setting, Dewys et al. formally analyzed the impact of weight loss on prognosis. They retrospectively evaluated 3047 patients from 12 different Eastern Cooperative Oncology Group clinical trials.

Table 58.1 *Cancer anorexia/weight loss versus starvation*

Cancer anorexia/weight loss	Starvation
Loss of fat and lean tissue	Loss of fat
No hunger	Hunger
Resting energy expenditure sometimes increased	Drop in resting energy expenditure
Specific mediators have been implicated	Specific mediators not as well implicated

Patient-reported weight loss of more than 5 percent over the preceding 6 months predicted early mortality independently of tumor stage, histology, and patient performance status. This weight loss was also associated with a trend toward lower chemotherapy response rates.[4] Similarly, Anker et al. demonstrated a much worse prognosis among congestive heart failure patients who had lost weight compared with those who had maintained their weight. Both groups of patients had similar degrees of left ventricular dysfunction.[5] Finally, in HIV-infected patients, weight loss has been associated with increased mortality,[6–12] accelerated disease progression,[12] and impairment of strength and functional status.[13] Thus, in several disease states, involuntary weight loss clearly predicts a shortened survival (Fig. 58.1).

There are multiple readily observable clinical factors that contribute to involuntary weight loss in patients with chronic diseases such as cancer, HIV, or congestive heart failure. In cancer patients, the systemic and local effects of the tumor and side effects from anticancer treatments all contribute, whereas fatigue, anxiety, depression, and pain appear also to contribute to the weight loss. These patients face many challenges in maintaining adequate caloric intake, including difficulty swallowing due to obstructing tumors or nerve compromise, mucositis, dry mouth, odor sensitivity, taste changes, diarrhea, constipation, and nausea and vomiting. Changes in the capacity to recognize and taste sweetness in foods occur in over a third of cancer patients. Bitterness, sourness, and saltiness are less frequently affected.[14,15] Multiple theories have been proposed regarding this change in taste, including zinc deficiency, alterations in brain neuropeptides, and opioid peptides.[16–18] Alterations have also been described in the gastrointestinal tract of weight-losing patients, and these almost certainly play a role in the weight loss of these patients. Early satiety is seen in weight-losing cancer patients even without direct tumor involvement of the gastrointestinal tract. Proinflammatory cytokines such

as interleukin (IL)-1β and central corticotropin-releasing factor have been implicated in early satiety.[19,20] Central corticotropin-releasing factor may also induce delayed gastric emptying and gastric stasis, ultimately resulting in early satiety.[18,21,22]

PATHOPHYSIOLOGY

The anorexia/weight loss syndrome is a complex metabolic derangement that includes anorexia, early satiety, weakness, and anemia, as well as weight loss. Patients experience inadequate energy intake, possibly increased resting energy expenditure, and abnormalities induced by proinflammatory cytokines.[23] Bruera et al. demonstrated that weight-losing cancer patients consumed 3200 kJ (800 calories) per day less than patients without weight loss.[24] This observation is important because it shows that weight loss occurs not only as a result of inappropriately spent energy sources but also as a result of diminished energy intake. At the same time, however, multiple studies have shown that provision of increased energy through increased oral nutritional support does not result in weight gain.[25,26] In the anorexia/weight loss syndrome, unlike starvation, loss of skeletal muscle in relation to adipose tissue is accelerated. In contrast, starvation results in preferential consumption of fat rather than glucose as the primary fuel, perhaps in an effort to spare lean body mass.[27]

The exact pathophysiology of the cancer anorexia/weight loss syndrome has not yet been clearly defined, but the development of this syndrome is associated with multiple hormonal and metabolic alterations. Leptin is a hormone secreted by adipose tissue in response to changes in weight. Levels of circulating leptin decline as weight loss occurs and, through complex feedback mechanisms, stimulates food intake in healthy people.[2] In weight-losing cancer patients, however, the leptin system appears to be dysregulated; studies are inconsistent on whether weight loss is truly associated with a drop in serum leptin.[28] In addition to leptin, several cytokines have also been implicated as mediators of weight loss and anorexia. These include tumor necrosis factor α (TNFα), IL-1, IL-6, and interferon γ (IFNγ). High levels of serum TNFα, IL-1β, and IL-6 have been found in some patients with cancer. When elevated levels of these cytokines are present they seem to correlate with the progression of the tumor.[29–31] However, a recent North Central Cancer Group study has questioned the role of serum cytokines and hypothesized instead that cytokines in the peripheral blood mononuclear cells may be more reflective of what occurs at the tissue level.[32] Several studies have also shown that administration of these cytokines to healthy patients reduces food intake and reproduces the features of anorexia/weight loss syndrome.[17,27–33] Hypermetabolism, which is defined as an elevation in the resting energy expenditure, is sometimes a feature of this syndrome. Some studies suggest that this

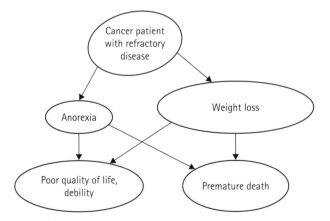

Figure 58.1 *The anorexia/weight loss syndrome is associated with diminished survival and quality of life.*

occasional phenomenon may be caused by induction of the mitochondrial uncoupling protein in muscle and adipose tissue. The induction of this protein may be due to cytokine activation. Ultimately, these mechanisms lead to increased heat production and muscle wasting.[17,34]

A variety of changes in nutrient metabolism have also been described in weight-losing patients (Box 58.1). Glucose metabolism is altered in weight-losing cancer patients. Lactate is produced in excess quantities by many solid tumors and is converted back to glucose via the Cori cycle in the liver.[35,36] This cycle of producing glucose from lactate uses ATP in a highly inefficient manner. Possibly this process contributes to the increased resting energy expenditure mentioned above. In one study, a 40 percent increase in hepatic glucose production was observed in weight-losing cancer patients.[35–37] Changes in lipid metabolism have also been described in patients with the cancer anorexia/weight loss syndrome. These include increased lipid mobilization, decreased lipogenesis, and decreased activity of lipoprotein lipase, which is responsible for clearance of triglyceride from plasma.[18,35,36] A lipid mobilizing factor has also been isolated.[27,36,38,39] Studies in animal models have suggested that lipid mobilizing factor may contribute to loss of body fat and increased resting energy expenditure.[39]

Box 58.1 Mediators of the cancer anorexia/weight loss syndrome

- TNFα
- IL-1β
- IL-6
- 'Cancer cachectic factor'
- Lipid-mobilizing factor
- Leptin (possibly)
- IFNγ

Along with the changes in glucose and lipid metabolism, changes in protein metabolism have also been documented in weight-losing cancer patients. During starvation, glucose utilization by the brain is replaced by use of ketone bodies derived from fat. This process decreases the amino acid driven gluconeogenesis by the liver. In weight-losing cancer patients, however, amino acids are not spared and lean body mass is depleted.[2] Skeletal muscle biopsies from patients with cancer have demonstrated both increased rates of protein synthesis and increased rates of protein degradation.[40,41] The cancer cachectic factor is a 24 kDa proteoglycan that has recently been implicated as a mediator in cancer-associated weight loss. Utilizing a rodent model, Todorov et al.[42] found that direct injection of this 'cancer cachectic factor' into the body results in weight loss. In contrast, if an antibody to the 'cancer cachectic factor' is administered 24 hours before the injection, this same wasting effect is not observed. Providing provocative clinical data, these investigators found that this proteoglycan is highly specific for weight loss in patients with cancer as opposed to weight loss from trauma or sepsis or the mere presence of cancer with no weight loss.

In general, the pathophysiology of the cancer anorexia/weight loss syndrome continues to be studied, and much of what is described above still requires further investigation. Nonetheless, the available data clearly point to pathophysiological mechanisms that are markedly different from those observed in classic starvation. Thus, the most important point of the above discussion is that caloric repletion is not the answer to managing this syndrome and that other approaches, such as counseling patients on prognosis and, on occasion, pharmacological manipulation of the appetite, should be considered.

THERAPEUTIC OPTIONS

Treatment of the anorexia/weight loss syndrome has led to only modest improvements in clinical outcome. In the cancer anorexia/weight loss syndrome treating the underlying malignancy appears to reverse at least some aspects of the syndrome. Geels et al. examined 300 patients who were receiving chemotherapy for breast cancer, a relatively chemotherapy-sensitive solid tumor. Patients completed questionnaires that included an assessment of appetite, and a direct relation between tumor response and improvement in appetite was observed. Specifically, 82 percent of patients with a complete or partial response to chemotherapy also reported an improvement in appetite.[43] To our knowledge, no major studies have examined weight or body composition in cancer survivors or in patients whose cancer responds dramatically to cancer therapy to assess what sort of changes in weight or eating patterns occur in these settings. However, the above data suggest that at least some aspects of the cancer anorexia/weight loss syndrome can be reversed with chemotherapy.

Caloric supplementation

Intuitively, and at a first glance, caloric supplementation seems to be the ideal approach for managing weight loss in patients with the cancer anorexia/weight loss syndrome. This strategy, however, has shown to be beneficial in only a few, specific situations, particularly in the cancer setting. Indeed, it is our contention that, by definition, patients who benefit from nutritional supplementation do not truly have the cancer anorexia/weight loss syndrome. Cancer patients who do sometimes benefit from nutritional support include those with perioperative cancer, those who have undergone stem cell or bone marrow transplantation, and those who are receiving radiation for head and neck cancer. The unifying theme behind all these situations is that these patients all appear to have potentially curable malignancies or a high likelihood of long-term tumor response.

In contrast, in patients with advanced, incurable, metastatic disease, no benefit has been derived from parenteral or enteral nutritional support. McGeer et al. published a meta-analysis showing no benefit with parenteral nutrition in cancer patients receiving chemotherapy. In fact in this meta-analysis, patients receiving parenteral nutrition experienced higher rates of infectious complications compared with patients receiving no parenteral nutrition.[44] Similarly, Ovesen et al. found that among cancer patients receiving chemotherapy, dietary counseling did lead to increased caloric intake but that this increased caloric intake did not result in improved survival, tumor response rates, or quality of life.[26] With regard to patients with congestive heart failure, there have been no large controlled studies of nutritional strategies in the management of cardiac-associated anorexia/weight loss. However, in patients with clinically stable congestive heart failure and no evidence of severe malnutrition, nutritional support alone has not been shown to carry a significant effect on clinical status.[45]

Unlike studies in cancer and congestive heart failure patients, studies of total parenteral nutrition in HIV-infected patients with severe wasting have shown significant improvement in weight. The patients receiving total parenteral nutrition experienced an 8 kg weight increase compared with a 3 kg weight loss in patients receiving no parenteral nutrition.[46] The effects of total parenteral nutrition on lean body mass were greatest in HIV-infected patients with documented malabsorption compared with patients with active secondary infections.[47]

Is there ever a situation among patients with incurable, metastatic cancer where nutritional support, such as total parenteral nutrition, appears to benefit patients? As emphasized above, we believe that this approach is outside the standard of care for most patients with cancer. However, case reports and small series suggest that occasionally these patients may benefit from total parenteral nutrition. Certainly, selection bias may result in publication of the most favorable outcomes. Recently, the Mayo Clinic published a report on a 20-year retrospective experience with total parenteral nutrition in this group of patients.[48] Overall, the use of total parenteral nutrition at this institution was quite conservative; only 52 patients with incurable cancer, or 15 percent of all patients treated at home received this intervention. Although most patients did poorly, 16 did live for one year or longer, presumably as a result of the total parenteral nutrition. In an attempt to tease out predictive factors in order to provide guidance on who might benefit from total parenteral nutrition from a practice perspective, no such predictive factor emerged. Thus the conclusion of this study was that clinical discretion – in the setting of a multidisciplinary approach and after indepth

discussions with the patient and family members – should guide management when this nonstandard approach is considered.

In cancer, the limited role of increased caloric intake emphasizes the need to discuss goals and realistic expectations of any intervention for patients suffering from the anorexia/weight loss syndrome. First, the healthcare provider should determine who actually is most bothered by the decreased oral intake and weight loss. Is it the patient or the family? Often, family members, and not the patient, are more distressed by these signs and symptoms. Family members often feel tremendous guilt over their inability to convince their loved ones to increase their oral intake and thereby presumably stop ongoing weight loss. Their attempts to encourage oral intake can become a source of frustrating disagreement between patients and their families. Second, frank discussions with patients and their family members regarding the fact that simple increased oral intake of food is unlikely to prolong life or improve quality of life in terminally ill cancer patients often relieves this source of anxiety. Studies of patients near the end of life indicate that they usually do not feel hunger and dehydration even in the absence of nutritional or fluid supplementation.[49] These findings should be explicitly conveyed to family members. Therefore, patients should base the use of pharmacological measures to improve appetite, as discussed below, on their own wishes for appetite improvement rather than on the guilt and frustration of family members. Third, it is important to point out to patients and family members symptoms such as loss of appetite and weight often occur at the end of life. The major role of dietary counseling in this setting is to provide education that the cancer anorexia/weight loss syndrome is common, out of the patient's control, and not representative of lack of volition on the part of the patient.

Pharmacological interventions

When the decision is made to initiate pharmacological treatment for the cancer anorexia/weight loss syndrome, progestational agents or glucocorticoids are reasonable options. These two classes of agents are the only ones that have been shown in multiple, placebo controlled, randomized trials to stimulate appetite.

PROGESTATIONAL AGENTS

Progestational agents used in the management of this syndrome include megestrol acetate and medroxyprogesterone acetate. Megestrol acetate is a synthetic, orally active derivative of naturally occurring progesterone. Medroxyprogesterone acetate is also be available as an injectable, depot formulation, although, to our knowledge, the depot formulation has not been used extensively for appetite stimulation. Multiple studies suggest that progestational agents improve appetite in patients with advanced cancer and anorexia. Some have speculated that this effect is exerted partially by downregulation of IL-6, although some studies refute this mechanism of action. Approximately 15 published, placebo controlled trials in cancer patients have evaluated the appetite-stimulating effects of megestrol acetate. Thirteen of these studies demonstrated that megestrol acetate improved appetite.[50] For example, in a North Central Cancer Treatment Group trial, Loprinzi et al. examined 133 cancer patients in a placebo controlled trial and found that those who received megestrol acetate at 800 mg/day manifested both an increase in appetite and an increase in nonfluid weight.[51]

A recent meta-analysis by Pascual Lopez et al. included 26 studies published between 1990 and 1999 investigating the effectiveness of megestrol acetate in the treatment of anorexia/weight loss syndrome in comparison with placebo and other drugs used in the treatment of cachexia. All together, 3368 patients were included in the meta-analysis. Eighty-six percent of patients had cancer, 11 percent had HIV, and 2 percent had other illnesses (failure to round up apparently precluded summing to 100%), including cystic fibrosis in 12 children and a wide range of other diseases in the geriatric population. In general, the study revealed an increase in appetite and weight gain with megestrol acetate. Results regarding quality of life were somewhat less clear cut. However, when the Karnofsky performance index was used as surrogate marker for quality of life the overall results were in favor of megestrol.[52]

Megestrol acetate has been shown to have a dose-related benefit starting at doses of 160 mg. The optimal dosage is generally considered 800 mg/day, and increasing the dose beyond this level provides no further benefit.[53] It is generally recommended that patients start at 160 mg/day and titrate upward according to clinical response.[2] However, the clinician may choose to start at 800 mg/day if a rapid clinical decline is anticipated, and the option of gradual titration is thought to be unavailable.

Progestational agents are reasonably well tolerated for the most part. However, adverse effects of both megestrol acetate and medroxyprogesterone include thromboembolic phenomena, breakthrough uterine bleeding, peripheral edema, hyperglycemia, hypertension, adrenal suppression, and adrenal insufficiency.[2] The risk of thromboembolic events with the use of megestrol acetate is minimal. In Pascual Lopez et al.'s meta-analysis, the only statistically significant adverse effect observed in patients receiving megestrol acetate versus placebo was edema with a relative risk of 1.67.[52] However, a history of thromboembolism remains a definite contraindication to initiating megestrol acetate for the anorexia/weight loss syndrome, as the risk: benefit ratio is too great. Whereas use of progestational agents for the anorexia/weight loss syndrome in cancer or HIV patients may provide benefit, their use in weight-losing congestive heart failure has not been extensively studied. Progestational agents promote fluid retention and may therefore lead to deleterious side effects in this particular patient group. In general, their use in congestive heart failure patients is not routinely recommended.

GLUCOCORTICOIDS

In addition to progestational agents, corticosteroids have been extensively studied as a treatment approach for the anorexia/weight loss syndrome. These agents are thought to exert their effects through suppression of inflammatory mediators and possibly through a direct effect on appetite centers in the hypothalamus.[54] Moertel et al. published the first placebo controlled trial investigating the effectiveness of corticosteroids in the cancer anorexia/weight loss syndrome. This study included 116 patients with advanced gastrointestinal malignancies. At 4 weeks, 55 percent of patients in the corticosteroid group reported an improvement in appetite compared with 26 percent in the placebo group.[55] Multiple subsequent studies have demonstrated similar results with corticosteroids in the treatment of cancer-associated anorexia.

Which are better: corticosteroids or progestational agents? In a North Central Cancer Treatment Group study, Loprinzi et al. answered this question by a randomized controlled trial in 475 weight-losing and/or anorexic cancer patients. Patients were randomly assigned to receive megestrol acetate 800 mg daily versus dexamethasone 0.75 mg four times daily versus the androgen fluoxymesterone. Fluoxymesterone did not provide favorable results. However, the key point of this trial was that, at the doses studied, megestrol acetate and dexamethasone provided equivalent orexigenic effects. Toxicity was different in these two effective arms. Myopathy was more frequent in the dexamethasone group: 6 percent and 18 percent in the megestrol acetate and dexamethasone groups, respectively. Other adverse effects that were seen more commonly in the dexamethasone group included cushingoid changes (1 percent vs. 6 percent) and peptic ulcer disease (0 percent vs. 3 percent). Twenty-five percent of megestrol acetate-treated patients and 36 percent of dexamethasone-treated patients discontinued therapy because of either their wishes and/or toxicity.[56]

Based on these findings, corticosteroids are generally reserved for patients in whom megestrol acetate is contraindicated, such as in those with thromboembolism. Patients with a limited life expectancy and therefore likely to receive only short-term benefits may prefer corticosteroids.[54] For other patients who do not fall into these categories, progestational agents may be viewed as a more favorable choice.

INEFFECTIVE OR RELATIVELY INEFFECTIVE AGENTS

Other pharmacological agents have been proposed as possible treatments for the cancer anorexia/weight loss syndrome. The list of agents that have not proved as effective in large randomized, comparative trials is extensive (see Box 58.2) and includes fluoxymesterone (as discussed above).

Box 58.2 What does not work

- Dronabinol
- Cyproheptadine
- Pentoxifylline
- Hydrazine sulfate
- Dietary counseling as a single intervention
- Eicosapentaenoic acid

OTHER PROMISING AGENTS

Other agents appear more promising and merit further study (Box 58.3). First, in cancer patients, melatonin appears promising. This is a pineal gland hormone that has been demonstrated to decrease the level of circulating TNFα. In one study, the addition of melatonin to chemotherapy for lung cancer resulted in improved response and survival rates and a reduced incidence of myelosuppression, neuropathy, and weight loss in the group treated with melatonin compared with the control group.[57] Although promising, this finding needs to be confirmed in larger trials. Second, thalidomide is another promising agent that may work in the treatment of cancer anorexia/weight loss syndrome by means of TNFα inhibition. Bruera et al. observed in their study that the majority of cancer patients who were at the end of life, reported an overall improved sense of wellbeing with this agent.[58] Third, phase III testing of the androgen

---

Box 58.3 Some of the agents that merit further study

- Ghrelin
- Neuropeptide Y
- TNF inhibitors
- Oxandrolone
- Thalidomide
- Adenosine triphosphate
- Melatonin
- Creatine

---

oxandrolone has been recently completed following promising pilot data. The results of this larger trial are eagerly awaited. Finally, the North Central Cancer Treatment Group is currently testing other agents including TNFα inhibitors (etanercept and infliximab) and creatine. Preliminary results are anticipated in 2007.

In AIDS patients, modest doses of thalidomide have been associated with a significant improvement in well-being and weight gain.[59] There is now accumulating evidence that the combination of aggressive nutritional counseling, appetite stimulants, progressive strength training, and anabolic hormones can reverse weight loss and increase lean body mass. This approach requires further study, but at this point appears promising. The first goals of therapy for these patients should be treatment of any secondary infections and optimization of antiretroviral therapy.[60] Nutritional strategies employed in these patients with some success include total parenteral nutrition, β-hydroxy-β-methylbutyrate, and high-quality oral proteins including whey protein supplements. Improvement in weight has been shown with the use of megestrol acetate. Physiological testosterone administration in hypogonadal men with AIDS wasting has been shown to result in sustained improvement in lean body mass. Another agent associated with improvement in lean body mass in HIV patients is growth hormone.[61] Again, further study of all these approaches appears to be indicated.

Multiple drugs have been investigated as potential treatments for the anorexia/weight loss syndrome in the setting of congestive heart failure. Freeman et al. suggested that fish oil supplementation reduces circulating levels of IL-1 and improves cachexia in dogs.[61] Specific anticytokine therapies have been tested in this patient population. Etanercept, an anti-TNFα antibody, was studied in a large scale trial. Unfortunately, the trial was stopped early based on unfavorable preliminary results.[62] There are preliminary data that the angiotensin inhibitor enalapril can prevent development of weight loss in congestive heart failure patients although definitive evidence is lacking.[63] Hryniewicz et al. reported promising results with the use of β blocker therapy in patients with anorexia/weight loss and congestive heart failure. In this study, 27 patients with baseline anorexia/weight loss were treated with carvedilol or long-acting metoprolol. Compared with a similar control group, the patients treated with β blocker therapy demonstrated a significantly greater weight gain.[64] Anecdotal evidence has been reported supporting the use of short-term, high-dose growth hormone therapy in cardiac anorexia/weight loss patients. Two case reports of three 'cachectic' patients stated that there were profound increases in muscle mass and strength without significant side effects.[65,66] The use of anabolic steroids has also been proposed as a treatment option for patients with cardiac anorexia/weight loss, but the side effects of these medications often limit their usefulness in this patient population. Interestingly, treatment with left ventricular assist devices provides little benefit with regard to weight gain in this patient population.[67]

Key learning points

- Anorexia and weight loss are devastating aspects of a syndrome that complicates several chronic diseases.

- When present, the anorexia/weight loss syndrome is not only psychologically difficult for patients and their families but portends a worse outcome.

- The goals of nutritional/pharmacological management of this syndrome vary for individual patients depending on their underlying disease, but the approach is primarily palliative in nature.

- Aggressive nutritional support, particularly with total parenteral nutrition, is beneficial in only a few well-defined circumstances.

- Pharmacological interventions that are considered reasonable, particularly in patients with advanced cancer or HIV, include progestational agents or corticosteroids.

- Management of the cancer anorexia/weight loss syndrome is challenging because this syndrome represents a set of complex metabolic aberrations, but the exact pathophysiology remains unclear.

- Certainly, the most pressing issues surrounding this syndrome center around its etiology and finding effective means to palliate associated symptoms, improve quality of life, and prolong survival.

- Future research should focus on gaining a better grasp on pathophysiology for purposes of eventually developing better therapies.

REFERENCES

1 Splinter TA. Cachexia and cancer: a clinicians view. *Ann Oncol* 1992; **3**: 25–7.

2 Inui A. Cancer anorexia-cachexia syndrome: current issues in research and management. *Cancer J Clin* 2002; **52**: 72–91.

3 Walsh D, Donnelly S, Rybicki L. The symptoms of advanced cancer: relationship to age, gender and performance status in 1000 patients. *Support Care Cancer* 2000; **8**: 175–9.

4 Dewys WD, Begg C, Lavin PT, et al. Prognostic effect of weight loss prior to chemotherapy in cancer patients. Eastern Cooperative Oncology Group. *Am J Med* 1980; **69**: 491–7.

5 Anker S, Ponikowski P, Varney S, et al. Wasting as an independent risk factor for mortality in chronic heart failure. *Lancet* 1997; **349**: 1050–3.

6 Kotler D, Tierney AR, Wang J, Pierson RN Jr. Magnitude of body-cell-mass depletion and the timing of death from wasting in AIDS. *Am J Clin Nutr* 1989; **50**: 444–7.

7 Chlebowski R, Grosvenor MB, Bernhard NH, et al. Nutritional status, gastrointestinal dysfunction and survival in patients with AIDS. *Am J Gastroenterol* 1989; **84**: 1288–93.

8 Guenter P, Muurahainen N, Simons G, et al. Relationships among nutritional status, disease progression, and survival in HIV infection. *J Acquir Immune Defic Syndr* 1993; **6**: 1130–8.

9 Palenicek J, Graham NM, He YD, et al. Weight loss prior to clinical AIDS as a predictor of survival. *J Acquir Immune Defic Syndr* 1995; **10**: 366–73.

10 Semba R, Caiaffa WT, Graham NM, et al. Vitamin A deficiency and wasting as predictors of mortality in human immunodeficiency virus-infected injection drug users. *J Acquir Immune Defic Syndr* 1995; **171**: 1196–202.

11 Suttmann U, Ockenga J, Selberg O, et al. Incidence and prognostic value of malnutrition and wasting in human immunodeficiency virus-infected outpatients. *J Acquir Immune Defic Syndr* 1995; **8**: 239–46.

12 Wheeler D, Gibert CL, Launer CA, et al. Weight loss as a predictor of survival and disease progression in HIV Infection. *J Acquir Immune Defic Syndr* 1998; **18**: 80–5.

13 Grinspoon S, Corcoran C, Rosenthal D, et al. Quantitative assessment of cross-sectional muscle area, functional status and muscle strength in men with AIDS wasting syndrome. *J Clin Endocrinol Metab* 1999; **84**: 201–6.

14 Dewys WD. Anorexia as a general effect of cancer. *Cancer* 1979; **41**: 2013–19.

15 Dewys WD, Walters K. Abnormalities of taste sensation in cancer patients. *Cancer* 1975; **36**: 1888–96.

16 Glass MJ, Billington CJ, Levine AS. Opioids and food intake: distributed functional neural pathways? *Neuropeptides* 1999; **33**: 360–8.

17 Inui A. Cancer anorexia-cachexia syndrome: are neuropeptides the key? *Cancer Res* 1999; **59**: 4493–501.

18 Nelson KA, Walsh D, Sheehan FA. The cancer anorexia-cachexia syndrome. *J Clin Oncol* 1994; **12**: 213–25.

19 Fujimiya M, Inui A. Peptidergic Regulation of gastrointestinal motility in rodents. *Peptides* 2000; **21**: 1565–82.

20 Tache Y, Garrick T, Raybould H. Central nervous system action of peptides to influence gastrointestinal motor function. *Gastroenterology* 1990; **98**: 517–28.

21 Inui A, Okano H, Miyamoto M, et al. Delayed gastric emptying in bulimic patients. *Lancet* 1995; **346**: 1240.

22 Okano H, Inui A, Ueno N, et al. EM523L, a nonpeptide motilin agonist, stimulates gastric emptying and pancreatic polypeptide secretion. *Peptides* 1996; **17**: 895–900.

23 Capra S, Ferguson M, Ried K. Cancer: impact of nutrition intervention outcome – nutrition issues for patients. *Nutrition* 2001; **17**: 769–72.

24 Bruera E, Carraro S, Roca E, et al. Association between malnutrition and caloric intake, emesis, psychological depression, glucose taste and tumour mass. *Cancer Treat Rep* 1984; **68**: 873.

25 Evans WK, Nixon DW, Daly JM, et al. A randomized study of oral nutritional support versus ad lib nutritional intake during chemotherapy for advanced colorectal and non-small cell lung cancer. *J Clin Oncol* 1987; **5**: 113.

26 Ovesen L, Allingstrup L, Hannibal J, et al. Effect of dietary counseling on food intake, body weight, response rate, survival and quality of life in cancer patients undergoing chemotherapy: a prospective, randomized study. *J Clin Oncol* 1993; **11**: 2043.

27 Tisdale MJ. Biology of cachexia – a review. *J Natl Cancer Inst* 1997; **89**: 1763.

28 Jatoi A, Loprinzi CL, Sloan JA, et al. Neuropeptide y, leptin, and cholecystokinin 8 in patients with advanced cancer and

anorexia. A North Central Cancer Treatment Group exploratory investigation. *Cancer* 2001; **92**:629–33.

29 Moldawer LL, Rogy MA, Lowry SF. The role of cytokines in cancer cachexia. *J Parent Enteral Nutr* 1992; **16**: 43–9.

30 Noguchi Y, Yoshikawa T, Matsumoto A, *et al.* Are cytokines possible mediators of cancer cachexia? *Surg Today* 1996; **26**: 467–75.

31 Matthys P, Billiau A. Cytokines and cachexia. *Nutrition* 1997; **13**: 763–70.

32 Jatoi A, Egner J, Loprinzi CL, *et al.* Investigating the utility of serum cytokine measurements in a multi-institutional cancer anorexia/weight loss study. *Support Care Cancer* 2004; **12**: 640–4.

33 Gelin J, Moldawer LL, Lonnroth C, *et al.* Role of endogenous tumor necrosis factor alpha and interleukin 1 for experimental tumor growth and the development of cancer cachexia. *Cancer Res* 1991; **51**: 415–21.

34 Bessesen DH, Faggioni, R. Recently identified peptides involved in the regulation of body weight. *Semin Oncol* 1998; **25**: 28–32.

35 Barber MD, Ross JA, Fearon KC. Cancer cachexia. *Surg Oncol* 1999; **8**: 133–41.

36 Tisdale MJ. Metabolic abnormalities in cachexia and anorexia. *Nutrition* 2000; **16**: 1013–14.

37 Tayek JA. A review of cancer cachexia and abnormal glucose metabolism in humans with cancer. *J Am Coll Nutr* 1992; **11**: 445–56.

38 Hirai K, Hussey HJ, Barber MD, *et al.* Biological evaluation of a lipid-mobilizing factor isolated from the urine of cancer patients. *Cancer Res* 1998; **58**: 2359–65.

39 Tisdale MJ. Cancer anorexia and cachexia. *Nutrition* 2001; **17**: 438–42.

40 Baracos VE. Regulation of skeletal muscle protein turnover in cancer associated cachexia. *Nutrition* 2000; **16**: 1015–18.

41 Lundholm K, Bylund AC, Holm J, Schersten T. Skeletal muscle metabolism in patients with malignant tumor. *Eur J Cancer* 1976; **12**: 465–73.

42 Todorov P, Variuk P, McDevitt T, *et al.* Characterization of a cancer cachectic factor. *Nature* 1996; **379**: 739–42.

43 Geels P, Eisenhauer E, Bezjak A, *et al.* Palliative effect of chemotherapy: objective tumor response is associated with symptom improvement in patients with metastatic breast cancer. *J Clin Oncol* 2000; **18**: 2395–405.

44 McGeer AJ, Detsky AS, O'Rourke, K. Parenteral nutrition in cancer patients undergoing chemotherapy: a meta-analysis. *Nutrition* 1990; **6**: 233.

45 Broqvist M, Arnqvist H, Dahlstrom U, *et al.* Nutritional assessment and muscle energy metabolism in severe chronic congestive heart failure – effects of long-term dietary supplementation. *Eur Heart J* 1994; **15**: 1641–50.

46 Kotler D, Tierney AR, Ferraro R, *et al.* Enteral alimentation and repletion of body cell mass in malnourished patients with acquired immunodeficiency syndrome. *Am J Clin Nutr* 1991; **53**: 149–54.

47 Kotler D, Tierney AR, Culpepper-Morgan JA, *et al.* Effect of home total parenteral nutrition on body composition in patients with acquired immunodeficiency syndrome. *J Parent Enteral Nutr* 1990; **14**: 454–8.

48 Hoda D, Jatoi A, Burnes J, *et al.* Should patients with advanced, incurable cancers ever be sent home with total parenteral nutrition? *Cancer* 2005; **103**:863–8.

49 Vullo-Navich K, Smith S, Andrews M, *et al.* Comfort and incidence of abnormal serum sodium, bun, creatinine, and osmolality in dehydration of terminal Illness. *Am J Hosp Palliat Care* 1993; **15**: 77–84.

50 Jatoi A, Kumar S, Sloan JA, Nguyen PL. On appetite and its loss. *J Clin Oncol* 2000; **59**: 166.

51 Loprinzi CL, Ellison NM, Schaid DJ, *et al.* Controlled trial of megestrol acetate for the treatment of cancer anorexia and cachexia. *J Natl Cancer Inst* 1990; **82**: 1127–32.

52 Pascual Lopez A, Roque i Figuls M, Urrutia Cuchi G, *et al.* Systematic review of megestrol acetate in the treatment of anorexia-cachexia syndrome. *J Pain Symptom Manage* 2004; **27**: 360–9.

53 Loprinzi, CL, Michalak JC, Schaid DJ, *et al.* Phase III evaluation of four doses of megestrol acetate as therapy for patients with cancer anorexia and/or cachexia. *J Clin Oncol* 1993; **11**: 762–7.

54 Jatoi A, Loprinzi CL. Drug therapy for cancer-associated anorexia. In: Ripamonti C, Bruera E (eds). *Gastrointestinal symptoms in advanced cancer patients*. New York: Oxford University Press, 2002: pp. 361–72.

55 Moertel CG, Schutt AJ, Reitemeier RJ, Hahn RG. Corticosteroid therapy of preterminal gastrointestinal cancer. *Cancer* 1974; **33**: 1607.

56 Loprinzi CL, Kugler JW, Sloan JA, *et al.* Randomized comparison of megestrol acetate versus dexamethasone versus fluoxymesterone for the treatment of cancer anorexia/cachexia. *J Clin Oncol* 1999; **17**: 3299.

57 Lissoni P, Paolorossi F, Ardizzoia A, *et al.* A randomized study of chemotherapy with cisplatin plus etoposide versus chemoendocrine therapy with cisplatin, etoposide and the pineal hormone melatonin as a first-line treatment of advanced non-small cell lung cancer patients in poor clinical state. *J Pineal Res* 1997; **23**: 15–19.

58 Bruera E, Neumann CM, Pituskin E, *et al.* Thalidomide in patients with cachexia due to terminal cancer: preliminary report. *Ann Oncol* 1999; **10**: 857–9.

59 Klausner JD, Makonkawkeyoon S, Akarasewi P, *et al.* The effect of thalidomide on the pathogenesis of human immunodeficiency virus type 1 and M. tuberculosis infection. *J Acquir Immune Defic Syndr* 1996; **11**: 247–57.

60 Grinspoon S, Mulligan K, Department of Health and Human Services Working Group on the Prevention and Treatment of Wasting and Weight Loss. Weight loss and wasting in patients infected with human immunodeficiency virus. *Clin Infect Dis* 2003; **36**: S69–78.

61 Freeman L, Rush JE, Kehayias JJ, *et al.* Nutritional alterations and the effect of fish oil supplementation in dogs with heart failure. *J Vet Intern Med* 1998; **12**: 440–8.

62 Johnston C. IHFS: Etanercept no benefit in treating heart failure – international study stopped prematurely. July 2001. Available at: www.pslgroup.com/dg/2001D6.htm (accessed October 17, 2005).

63 Anker S. Weight loss in chronic heart failure and the impact of treatment with ACE inhibitors – results from the SOLVD treatment trial. *Circulation* 1999; **100**: I-78.

64 Hryniewicz K, Androne AS, Hudaihed A, Katz SD. Partial reversal of cachexia by beta adrenergic receptor blocker therapy in patients with chronic heart failure. *J Card Fail* 2003; **9**: 464–8.

65 Cuneo RC, Wilmshurst P, Lowy C, *et al.* Cardiac failure responding to growth hormone. *Lancet* 1989; **1**: 838–9.

66 O'Driscoll JG, Green DJ, Ireland M, *et al.* Treatment of end-stage cardiac failure with growth hormone. *Lancet* 1997; **34**: 1068.

67 Clark AL, Loebe M, Potapov EV, *et al.* Ventricular assist device in severe heart failure: effects on cytokines, complement and body weight. *Eur Heart J* 2001; **22**: 2275–83.

59

Nausea/vomiting

SEBASTIANO MERCADANTE

INTRODUCTION

Nausea and vomiting are demeaning, reduce patients' quality of life, and affect compliance with therapy. Nausea occurs both at an early stage and in the advanced stage of cancer disease. The frequency reported in literature varies according to the setting: primary tumor, concurrent treatment, stage and life expectancy, different evaluation tools or study design, and sex. For example, nausea and vomiting occur more frequently in women, probably due to cancer type and increased sensitivity to drugs.[1]

Thus it is reasonable to distinguish two forms of nausea and vomiting: that associated with chemotherapy and other oncological treatments, and the chronic multifactorial nausea and vomiting, commonly observed in advanced cancer or associated with progressive diseases. Other than in cancer patients, patients with progressive neurological diseases such as central nervous diseases, peripheral nervous diseases, dysfunction of neuromuscular junction, and muscle diseases, may also develop nausea and vomiting with different mechanisms.[2]

DEFINITIONS

Accurate use of terminology and an understanding of the symptom experience are essential for reliable, valid assessment and measurement. Three components of vomiting are recognized: nausea, retching, and emesis. Nausea is an unpleasant sensation of the need to vomit and is associated with autonomic symptoms, including pallor, cold sweats, tachycardia, and diarrhea. It may occur without retching or vomiting. It is not clear if nausea and vomiting represent

different points along the spectrum of outputs from the vomiting center, or if they are related, but independent, phenomena. Nausea, differently from vomiting and retching, which are objective and definitive signs, arises from subjective components and dimensions unique to the individual.

While nausea is an expression of autonomic stimulation, characterized by a decrease in gastric tone and peristalsis and associated with an increase in the tone of duodenum, retching and vomiting are mediated by somatic nerves. Retching is an attempt to vomit without bringing anything up. It is characterized by a spasmodic movement of the diaphragm and abdominal musculature with the glottis closed, and denotes the labored rhythmic respiratory activity that frequently precedes emesis. The vomiting act involves forceful contraction of the abdominal wall musculature, contraction of pylorus and antrum, a raised gastric cardia, diminished lower esophageal sphincter pressure, and esophageal dilatation. Intestinal contents are commonly present in vomited material, implying a possible reverse peristalsis. Hypersalivation and cardiac rhythm disturbances are frequent associated phenomena.[3] Although the neural pathways that mediate nausea are not known, evidence suggests that they are the same pathways that mediate vomiting.[4] It may be that mild activation leads to nausea, whereas more intense activation leads to retching or vomiting.

PATHOPHYSIOLOGY AND CAUSES OF NAUSEA AND VOMITING

The distress resulting from these symptoms may escalate over time with the continuing symptom experience, regardless of the frequency, duration, and severity. Although people may experience seemingly identical symptoms, the cause of the symptoms and each person's response to the symptoms may vary, so that an accurate assessment of the individual's symptoms and recognition of the possible causes forms the basis for customized treatments.

Vomiting involves a complex set of activities that suggests a central neurological control by a vomiting center. Stimulation of the dorsal portion of the lateral reticular formation in the vicinity of the fasciculus solitarius produces vomiting. This vomiting center is anatomically adjacent to the medullary centers that control respiration and salivation. The emetic pattern generator is in the third ventricle, close to the area postrema, but lying fully within the blood–brain barrier. It contains D_2-receptors, histaminic (H_1) receptors, muscarinic-cholinergic receptors, serotonin (5-hydroxytryptamine [5-HT] 2 and 3) receptors, which are emetogenic, and μ_2-opioid receptors, which are antiemetic at this location. Intracranial lesions are an important cause of nausea and vomiting. The increased intracranial pressure compresses and stimulates the emetic center on the floor of the fourth ventricle. Circumscribed lesions – vascular lesions, neoplasm, or local inflammatory lesions of the brain – may directly affect the emetic center or its afferent pathways. The emetic center may also be stimulated through ventricular dilatation without increased intracranial pressure, as in low-pressure hydrocephalus. Infectious diseases of the central nervous system may also produce vomiting.[2]

Psychological or emotional factors may also contribute to the generation of nausea at this level, where there is a group of motor nuclei, including the nucleus ambiguous, ventral and dorsal respiratory groups, and the dorsal motor nucleus of the vagus.

A chemoreceptor trigger zone (CTZ), sensitive to chemical stimuli, lies in the floor of the fourth ventricle in the brain stem and is able to stimulate the vomiting center. This area is outside the blood–brain barrier and is bathed in the systemic circulation. The CTZ contains emetic receptors for dopamine (D_2), serotonin (5-HT_3), acetylcholine (ACHr), and opioids (μ_2), which when stimulated provide input for the vomiting center sited in the third ventricle. High plasma concentrations of emetogenic substances, such as calcium ions, urea, morphine, and digoxin may stimulate dopamine receptors in this area. Anorexia, dehydration, weight loss, abnormal metabolites, and toxins produced by associated infections may also contribute. Moreover, it also receives input from the vestibular apparatus and the vagus (see Box 59.1). The deeper layers of the area postrema are partly formed of the nucleus tractus solitarius, which predominantly contains 5-HT receptors and is considered the main central connection of the vagus. Visceral afferent impulses arising from the gastrointestinal tract may reach the medullary vomiting center by way of the vagus, without traversing the CTZ.[1,5]

Vomiting is an integrated somatovisceral process. The central emetic pattern generator coordinates emetic processes, receiving and integrating input from various sources. The efferent pathways are mainly somatic, involving the vagus

---

Box 59.1 Factors stimulating the CTZ

- Glycosides
- Opioids
- Ergot derivatives
- Chemotherapeutic agents, enterotoxins, salicylates
- Metabolic abnormalities: uremia, hypercalcemia, hyponatremia, diabetic ketoacidosis
- Hypoxia
- Radiation sickness

---

nerve, the phrenic nerves, and the spinal nerves. Changes in tone and mobility of the stomach during vomiting are likely mediated by visceral efferent neurons. Once the vomiting center has been sufficiently stimulated, the vomiting reflex is initiated. The person takes a deep breath which is held, the glottis closes to avoid aspiration of vomitus, the soft palate elevates to close off the nasal passage, and finally the diaphragm and abdominal muscles contract. As a consequence intraabdominal pressure squeezes the stomach between the two sets of muscles, and the gastrointestinal sphincter relaxes, allowing the expulsion of gastric contents.[3]

RECEPTORS AND NEUROTRANSMITTERS

Different neuromediators are implicated in the genesis of gastrointestinal symptoms, including dopamine, serotonin (via 5-HT_3 receptors), histamine, norepinephrine, GABA, acetylcholine, and enkephalin.[6] The CTZ is also implicated in delaying the reflex of gastric emptying, and production of taste aversion, which could contribute to vomiting. Acoustic neuroma, bone metastases at the base of the skull, brain tumors, or metastases affecting the vestibular apparatus are possible other causes of vestibular stimulation of H_1 receptors and muscarinic cholinergic receptors. In addition to the direct afferent pathways from the gastrointestinal tract to the vomiting center, the anatomical region of the area postrema receives emetic impulses from the pharynx, heart, peritoneum, mesenteric vasculature, and bile ducts. Impulses from these peripheral receptors are also transmitted directly to the vomiting center.

Drugs, particularly aspirin and opioids, directly stimulate the vestibular apparatus, which in turn provides input to the vomiting centre. Receptors in the gastrointestinal tract play an equally important part in the pathogenesis and treatment of nausea and vomiting, particularly 5-HT_3, 5-HT_4, and D_2 receptors. Activation of D_2 receptors produces gastroparesis. Vagus receptors include 5-HT_3 receptors, which are emetogenic, and 5-HT_4 receptors, which enhance

Table 59.1 *Receptor site affinities of principal antiemetics*

	Dopamine D$_2$ antagonist	Histamine H$_1$ antagonist	Acetylcholine antagonist	5-HT$_2$ antagonist	5-HT$_3$ antagonist	5-HT$_4$ agonist
Metoclopramide	++				+	++
Domperidone	++					
Ondansetron					+++	
Cyclizine		++	++			
Hyoscine			+++			
Haloperidol	+++					
Prochlorperazine	++	+				
Chlorpromazine	++	++	+			
Levomepromazine	++	+++	++	+++		

5-HT, 5-hydroxytryptamine.

the propulsion, resulting in a prokinetic effect. This effect is mediated by the cholinergic myenteric plexus, so that it could be inhibited by anticholinergics. Various stimuli, notably bowel distension and inflammation, may produce massive release of 5-HT from enterochromaffin cells contained in the bowel wall. Slowed gastric emptying and constipation, frequently observed in patients progressively immobilized and anorectic, may activate the same process. The activation of these peripheral receptors leads to the stimulation of the vomiting center via vagal and sympathetic afferents. There are also corticobulbar afferents to the vomiting center that mediate vomiting in response to some smells, sights, and tastes, and may play a role in psychogenic vomiting. Stress, anxiety, and nausea from any cause induce delayed gastric emptying via peripheral dopaminergic receptors on the myenteric plexus interneurons. Therefore, nausea and vomiting are influenced by a complex network of central and peripheral factors which interact with each other. The receptor site affinities of principal antiemetics are listed in Table 59.1.

SPECIFIC CONDITIONS ASSOCIATED WITH VOMITING

Chemotherapy-induced nausea and vomiting

Although chemotherapy and radiation may no longer be indicated for curative reasons in patients with advanced disease, they may provide symptom palliation. Chemotherapy-induced nausea and vomiting is one the most feared effects of cancer treatment. There are five levels of emetic potential of chemotherapeutic agents, and preemptive treatment with antiemetics is mandatory for the highest levels.[7] Neurotransmitters, such as dopamine, acetylcholine, histamine, and serotonin are involved in the emetogenic pathways stimulated by chemotherapy and radiation. It has been suggested that chemotherapy causes release of serotonin from enterochromaffin cells of the gastrointestinal tract, which then stimulate emesis via both the vagus and greater splanchnic

nerve as well as stimulating the area postrema of the brain, which is rich in serotonin receptors. Thus, serotonin receptors, both central and peripheral, are particularly important in the pathophysiology of acute emesis and drugs that inhibit this group of receptors are the cornerstone of the prevention and treatment of chemotherapy-related nausea and vomiting. Contributing factors include emetogenic potential of the chemotherapy drug combination, dosages, route, time of day, and length of administration, other therapies, anxiety, previous episodes, sex, and age.[8]

Anticipatory nausea and vomiting

This phenomenon occurs on the day or some hours before the expected chemotherapy, and often symptoms present in particular conditions, such as talking or thinking about the treatment. It affects a third of patients attending for chemotherapy. A psychological mechanism of association is probable, and is strongly related to the intensity of adverse effects associated with the previous chemotherapy, and the number of treatments received. Younger age, expectation, and motion sickness are well recognized risk factors for developing anticipatory nausea and vomiting, probably due to the higher doses used and anxiety.[9]

Disorders affecting the central nervous system

Different neurological diseases may produce a disturbance in central control of gut motility, resulting in gastrointestinal syndromes, such as vomiting or intestinal pseudo-obstruction with or without gastric stasis (Table 59.2).

Lesions of various origin of the spinal cord, above T5, may isolate the spinal sympathetic control from the influence of high centers. This results in a delayed gastric emptying and delay in duodenal progression. In the early period, severe gastric stasis and dilatation, and ileus are commonly present. In cases of long-term loss of function, patients who develop

Table 59.2 *Nervous system diseases associated with nausea and vomiting[2]*

Disease group	Mechanisms
Central nervous system	
Cerebral and brainstem disorders	
Multiple sclerosis	Gastroparesis
Parkinson disease	Gastrointestinal dysmotility
Cerebral masses	Compression of vomiting center
Spinal cord disorders	
Amyotrophic lateral sclerosis	Gastric atony, ileus
Poliomyelitis	Gastric atony, ileus
Autonomic dysfunction, gastric atony	Esophageal dysfunction
Peripheral nervous system	
Alcohol-related gastroparesis	Gastritis (acute), neuropathy – impaired esophageal peristalsis
Myenteric plexus dysfunction (Chagas disease, Hirschsprung disease, achalasia, ganglioneuromatosis)	Pseudo-obstruction
Neuromuscular junction	
Myasthenia gravis	Oropharyngeal incoordination
Muscle disease	
Myotonic dystrophy	Dysphagia, gastric atony, pseudo-obstruction
Dermatomiositis-polymyositis	Dysphagia, gastric atony, pseudo-obstruction
Oculopharyngeal muscular dystrophy	Dysphagia
Duchenne muscular dystrophy	Dysphagia, pseudo-obstruction
Familiar visceral neuropathy	Dysphagia, pseudo-obstruction

quadriplegia are more likely to have gut complications than those with paraplegia. The incidence of gastroesophageal reflux is increased and gastric emptying impaired. Chronic constipation may worsen the clinical picture possibly facilitating the development of nausea and vomiting. Neuropathies are frequently encountered in patients with cancer.[2]

Autonomic failure

Autonomic failure is more common in patients with poor performance status often associated with anorexia-cachexia syndrome. The mechanisms remain unclear and appear to be multifactorial – tumor invasion of nervous tissue, malnutrition, damage from chemotherapy or radiotherapy, drugs, preexisting disease – and could be considered a sort of paraneoplastic syndrome, producing gastroparesis.[10]

Other disorders may affect the extrinsic gastrointestinal innervation. There is evidence that vagal autonomic neuropathy may be responsible for gastric motor disturbances in diabetic patients with gastroparesis. It is well known that the motility disorder involves not only the stomach, but also the upper small bowel. This has been commonly attributed to gastric motor dysfunction with delayed gastric emptying. Peripheral neuropathy, manifestations of autonomic neuropathy, with bladder dysfunction, sweat disorder, orthostatic hypotension, impotence, nephropathy, and retinopathy are frequently found, as gastroparesis is commonly reported in patients with longstanding, insulin-dependent poorly controlled diabetes.[11] Neurological diseases, such as dystrophia

myotonica and progressive muscular dystrophy, amyloidosis, collagen vascular diseases, and autoimmune neurological diseases may affect parietal structures of the gastrointestinal tract, inducing motility dysfunction, which can precipitate nausea and vomiting.[2] Radiation injury is another important cause of gastrointestinal dysmotility. Early vomiting is probably due to direct mucosal injury, whereas late vomiting and gastrointestinal stasis may be related to radiation-induced inflammation or strictures.[3,11]

Metabolic disorders

Significant gastrointestinal disturbances may be associated with thyroid and parathyroid disorders. Intestinal pseudo-obstruction may develop both in hyperthyroidism and hypothyroidism. The role of gastrointestinal hormones in disorders of upper intestinal motility remains unclear.[5]

Drug-induced nausea and vomiting

Many drugs commonly cause nausea and vomiting. Adrenergic agents, such as β agonists, generally delay gastric emptying, whereas β blockers enhance gastric emptying. Clonidine, an α_2 agonist, may induce nausea and vomiting. Anticholinergic agents, such as some tricyclic antidepressants, inhibit contractile activity and delay gastric emptying.

Dopamine agonists, opioids, digitalis, and chemotherapeutic agents such as cisplatin remain the major offenders.

Opioids have central and peripheral actions. Centrally, they may stimulate the emetic center via D_2 receptors of the CTZ, richly distributed in the area prostrema. In addition, they induce a relevant delay in gastric emptying and a delay in intestinal transit. The narcotic bowel syndrome is characterized by a picture similar to pseudo-obstruction. Non-steroidal anti-inflammatory drugs (NSAIDs) may induce nausea and vomiting by damaging gastric mucosa and activating peripheral ascending impulses. A central effect of alcohol on the CTZ has been recognized, other than the well known consequence of damage to the gastric mucosa.

ASSESSMENT AND DIAGNOSIS

Like pain, nausea is a subjective experience and presents all of the problems inherent in measuring pain. Nausea is usually assessed by visual analog or numerical scales.[12] Vomiting can be objectively recorded as events in a manner reminiscent of the methodology used to study antiemesis related to chemotherapy.

Many factors should be considered when choosing antiemetic treatment. History, examination, and review of the ongoing drug regimen are generally helpful in finding the cause of gastrointestinal symptoms in the neurological population. A multitude of medications, including opioids, digoxin, antibiotics, imidazoles, and cytotoxics can cause nausea and vomiting by acting on the CTZ, whereas NSAIDs, iron supplements, antibiotics, and tranexamic acid may damage gastric mucosa. Opioids, tricyclics, phenothiazines, and anticholinergics induce gastric stasis. Finally, selective serotonin reuptake inhibitors and cytotoxic drugs may induce $5-HT_3$ receptor stimulation. Uncontrolled pain *per se* may be a cause of nausea and vomiting.

In patients with neurological diseases such as diabetic neuropathy, or with advanced cancer, autonomic failure occurs with gastroparesis, nausea, vomiting, and constipation. Movement-related nausea with vomiting suggests either vestibular dysfunction or mesenteric traction. Nausea increasing with head motion, with tinnitus, decreased hearing, or skull tenderness is suggestive of vestibular involvement due to drug toxicity and local lesions. Presence of vertigo may be helpful in distinguishing the two conditions. Candidal infection may produce pharyngeal irritation, activating the afferent arm of the vomiting circuit via the vagus nerve and should be suspected in patients taking steroids.

Emesis produced with cough occurs at the end or during a coughing paroxysm and is associated with chronic pulmonary disease, esophageal fistulas, and brain metastases. Morning vomiting, sometime projectile, associated with cognitive changes or neurological deficits may be due to brain tumors or secondaries. Papilledema may be a possible associated sign. Neck stiffness and headache may be signs of underlying meningitis. Computed tomography (CT) or magnetic resonance imaging (MRI) can confirm the diagnosis. Nausea produced by hyperglycemia or hypercalcemia is associated with polyuria and polydipsia. Patients treated for prolonged periods with steroids for chronic neurological disease may develop Addison disease after abrupt suspension of medication.

Vomiting that occurs in relation to meals is frequently of diagnostic importance. Patients with gastric outlet obstruction or gastric atony often will complain of vomiting several hours after eating. In contrast, patients who vomit as a result of viral gastroenteritis or psychogenic causes are usually symptomatic in the immediate postprandial period. Appropriate screening tests include a biochemistry profile consisting of electrolytes, blood urea nitrogen, creatinine, glucose, albumin and calcium. In patients taking digoxin or anticonvulsants the plasma drug levels should be considered. A pattern of infrequent large-volume vomitus which relieves nausea suggests a partial bowel obstruction. Abdominal examination and an abdominal X-ray are helpful to screen for situations involving sub-obstruction. Abdominal CT and ultrasound may be required to complete the investigation. Emotional experience may trigger psychogenic vomiting.

TREATMENT

Long periods or repeated episodes of vomiting can lead to dehydration. To avoid this, it is important to replace fluids lost through vomiting. In some circumstances it is necessary to administer fluids and drugs by the parenteral route, either subcutaneously or intravenously. Treating any identifiable cause of nausea and vomiting is the first step. Reversible causes include hypercalcemia, hyperglycemia, hypocortisolism, hyponatremia, uremia, obstipation, and increased intracranial pressure. Bisphosphonates for hypercalcemia and dexamethasone for intracranial tumors are the first-line treatments in these specific conditions. Identifiable offending drugs should be stopped. A calm and reassuring environment may be useful, avoiding exposure to foods precipitating nausea. Control of malodor from decubitus ulcers is mandatory. Behavioral techniques, relaxation exercises, and benzodiazepines may be helpful for anticipatory nausea.

Generally, widely accepted management guidelines are not available, except for the treatment of nausea and vomiting associated with chemotherapy. The use of the modern antiemetic regimens based on combinations of drugs has dramatically reduced the incidence, which was reported to be about 80 percent in the past decades. The fact that different agents cause nausea and vomiting by different mechanisms prompted researchers to develop regimens with multiple drug with different mechanisms of action.[13***] Although the mechanism considered to play the predominant role in the induction of nausea and vomiting is the activation of the CTZ, gastrointestinal stimulation or damage, vestibular and cortical mechanisms, or alterations of taste and smell, may equally contribute in different ways in producing these symptoms. As discussed earlier in the chapter chemotherapeutic agents interact with the CTZ to release various transmitters, such as dopamine, histamine, serotonin, and neurokinin, largely represented in this area.

The pharmacological treatment of nausea and vomiting in the palliative care setting usually involves established drugs. Many classes of medication have been used as antiemetics. If vomiting prevents drug absorption a nonoral route should be used at first. Patients should be reevaluated at regular intervals to optimize the dose or to switch drugs. The choice of medication depends upon drug receptor selectivity and drug interactions, as patients are frequently receiving several medications that potentially interact with or antagonize the antiemetics. The afferent pathway involved and the group of antiemetics that antagonize the involved neuroreceptors are key factors that influence the choice of the first drug, i.e. a mechanistic approach should be the basis for choosing first-line antiemetic drugs. The sites and possible receptor mechanisms of the principal antiemetic drugs are listed in Table 59.1.

An important principle is to use combinations of antiemetics with different modes of action,[14,15] primarily based on starting with a metoclopramide regimen.[10] On the other hand, antiemetics may have specific adverse effects in patients with neurological diseases. Moreover, anticholinergic medications may antagonize the prokinetic effects of drugs acting via the cholinergic system in the myenteric plexus.[1,6,16,17]

In a recent systematic review of the efficacy of antiemetics in the treatment of nausea in patients with terminal cancer, uncontrolled studies had high response rates (75–93 percent) to standard regimens, whereas randomized controlled trials reported much lower response rates (23–36 percent for nausea, 18–52 percent for vomiting), regardless of an empirical or a more selective clinical approach.[18***]

Metoclopramide

Metoclopramide, in addition to its recognized dopamine antagonist action, also acts as a weak serotonin antagonist and can stimulate gastrointestinal motility by increasing acetylcholine release, which explains the potential for central adverse effects, such as extrapyramidal reactions. Metoclopramide, usually combined with steroids, appears to be as effective as the 'setrons' (see below) in preventing delayed emesis, and is cheaper than specific antiserotonin agents.

Metoclopramide enhances the transit of the contents of the gastrointestinal tract as far as the jejunum, speeding gastric emptying, and decreasing small intestinal transit time, probably by increasing cholinergic activity through the activation of $5\text{-}HT_4$ receptors. In high doses metoclopramide also has $5\text{-}HT_3$ receptor antagonist activity. Domperidone,

a D_2 antagonist that poorly crosses the blood–brain barrier, acts primarily on gastric D_2 receptors and D_2 receptors in the CTZ, which are outside the blood–brain barrier, facilitating gastric motor activity and emptying.[1,4] Although in same studies the efficacy was similar to that observed with placebo,[19**] metoclopramide in doses of 60 mg daily was quite effective in a cancer population with chronic nausea. Three percent of patients required other antiemetics because of extrapyramidal side effects.[20*] Controlled-release metoclopramide 40 mg every 12 hours, significantly reduced nausea without producing the pertinent adverse effects in patients with a history of cancer-associated dyspepsia syndrome.[21**] Metoclopramide use confers an increased risk for the initiation of treatment generally reserved for the management of Parkinson disease in patients with drug-induced parkinsonian symptoms.[22*]

Setron family

As mentioned above, serotonin receptors, both central and peripheral, are particularly important in the pathophysiology of acute emesis and drugs that target this group of receptors underpin the prevention and treatment of chemotherapy-related nausea and vomiting. The role of the $5\text{-}HT_3$ receptor was recognized during the evaluation of the mechanism of high-dose metoclopramide, which unlike other D_2 receptor antagonists, has a good capacity to reduce the emesis induced by cisplatin administration.

Several $5\text{-}HT_3$ antagonists are commercially available, including ondansetron, granisetron, tropisetron, and dolasetron. Many randomized controlled trials have demonstrated that these agents have equivalent antiemetic activity and safety at the recommended doses, despite differences in structure and pharmacokinetic profiles,[3] both orally and intravenously, due to their good bioavailability following oral administration. These drugs are well tolerated, and central adverse effects are not commonly observed with serotonin antagonists. The effect of the setrons on the serotonin-mediated emetic pathways may lend itself to the management of chronic nausea. Ondansetron, a selective $5\text{-}HT_3$ antagonist, has been used in palliative care setting in patients not responding to conventional treatments. In 9 of 16 patients with advanced human immunodeficiency disease, the treatment was effective and well tolerated.[23*] However, in a controlled study the efficacy of ondansetron at relatively large doses was similar to that reported with placebo.[19**] Tropisetron-containing combinations or tropisetron as a single agent are much more effective in the control of emesis in patients with advanced cancer than the conventional antiemetic combination of chlorpromazine plus dexamethasone.[24**] Not being antidopaminergic, setrons are potentially useful when the risk of extrapyramidal reactions is high, such as in children or elderly people who have neurological diseases with an extrapyramidal component. They appear to have no effect on motion sickness.[1]

Phenothiazines and butyrophenones

Phenothiazines and butyrophenones belong to the class of D_2 antagonists. Haloperidol has a relatively narrow spectrum and is a potent D_2 antagonist with negligible anticholinergic activity, so that it produces less sedation than phenothiazines but greater extrapyramidal reactions.[1,16]

Phenothiazines, including prochlorpromazine, promethazine, and chlorpromazine, possess a broader spectrum of activity with dopaminergic, cholinergic, and histamine receptor antagonism. Hypotension, sedation, decreased salivary flow are the main adverse effects. Central and hemo-dynamic adverse effects are more likely with major tranquilizers. Levomepromazine is a phenothiazine closely related chemically to chlorpromazine. Its proved analgesic properties make it unique among the phenothiazines. It is efficacious and generally nonsedative in doses of 5–12.5 mg/day. It is a potent antagonist at 5-HT$_2$, H$_1$, D$_2$, and α_1-receptors.[25*]

Anticholinergics

Hyoscine is a naturally occurring compound which competitively inhibits the action of acetylcholine and other muscarinic agonists. The primary indication of hyoscine is motor sickness and labyrinthic disturbances. It is also indicated for reducing intestinal secretions in patients with inoperable bowel obstruction. Unlike the other antimuscarinic agents, hyoscine produces central nervous system depression in therapeutic doses – manifesting as drowsiness, euphoria, amnesia, disorientation, restlessness, and hallucinations.[1]

Antihistamines

Cyclizine is effective in nausea associated with motion sickness, pharyngeal stimulation, bowel obstruction, and increased intracranial pressure. Drowsiness and antimuscarinic effects are the main adverse effects.[1,5,16]

Neurokinin-1 receptor antagonists

These substances inhibit the effects of substance P on the nucleus tractus solitarius. In early clinical trials, the neurokinin-1 receptor antagonist aprepitant was shown to improve the protection provided by the best available therapy, including a 5-HT$_3$ receptor antagonist and dexamethasone, against chemotherapy-induced nausea and vomiting over multiple cycles of cisplatin-based chemotherapy.[26**]

Cisapride

This drug acts on acetylcholine receptors in the myenteric plexus of the gut, improving gastroduodenal and pyloroduodenal coordination. It also affects colonic transit. As it is not a dopamine antagonist, and has no central nervous system penetration, it does not cause the central adverse effects of many other antiemetic drugs and can be extremely useful in most neurological patients with gastrointestinal disorders resulting in nausea vomiting. Its prokinetic effect is not limited to the upper bowel but extends throughout the gastrointestinal tract. The enhancement of gastric motor activity by prokinetics may reduce afferent activity in the vagus nerve and so diminish the stimulus to nausea and vomiting from visceral sensation (for example, distension).[1,3]

Steroids

Dexamethasone has synergistic or additive antiemetic effects combined with setrons, metoclopramide, or phenothiazines. The mechanism remains unknown. The antiemetic actions of dexamethasone are not well characterized, except for use in the treatment of nausea and vomiting due to increased intracranial pressure. Adverse effects include glucose intolerance, myopathy, osteopenia, and infections.[1,5]

Dronabinol

Cannabinoids appear to be of low antiemetic efficacy and adverse effects may occur. The mechanism of the antiemetic effect of cannabinoids is unknown. It has been hypothesized that an indirect inhibition of the vomiting center in the medulla occurs as a result of binding to opioid receptors in the forebrain. Dronabinol has been used in diffuse metastatic disease in the gastrointestinal tract mucosa for intractable nausea and vomiting unresponsive to conventional antiemetics.[27*]

Olanzapine

Olanzapine, an atypical antipsychotic, possesses a unique neurotransmitter binding profile that is similar to methotrimeprazine. It has been shown to relieve nausea in some patients with advanced cancer who fail to respond to the usual antiemetics.[28*] Olanzapine has been also used to reduce the incidence of delayed emesis in patients receiving moderate to highly emetogenic chemotherapy and is well tolerated.[29*,30*]

Key learning points

- Nausea and vomiting are frequent symptoms reported by cancer patients. Several causes are recognized, including curative and symptomatic treatments, as well as disease itself.

- Different and complex systems are involved in the mechanisms producing these symptoms.

- Except for chemotherapy-induced vomiting, no clear guidelines have been produced for the remaining conditions, particularly in advanced-stage disease, when multiple factors may play a role in producing or exacerbating nausea and vomiting.

- Different classes of antiemetics or their combinations are usually chosen according to the supposed mechanism with variable efficacy.

- The need for controlled studies is justified by the finding that uncontrolled studies show high response rates whereas randomized controlled studies have shown lower response rates.

REFERENCES

◆ 1 Twycross R, Back I. Nausea and vomiting in advanced cancer. *Eur J Palliat Care* 1998; **5**: 39–45.

◆ 2 Mercadante S. Nausea and vomiting. In: Voltz R, Bernat JL, Borasio GD, eds. *Palliative Care in Neurology*. Oxford: Oxford University Press, 2004.

◆ 3 Nailor R, Rudd JA. Emesis and anti-emesis. In: Hanks GW, ed. *Cancer Surveys, Vol. 21. Palliative Medicine: Problem Areas in Pain and Symptom Management*. New York: Cold Spring Harbor Laboratory Press, 1994: 117–35.

◆ 4 Allan SG. Nausea and vomiting. In: Doyle D, Hanks GW, MacDonald N, eds. *Oxford Textbook of Palliative Medicine*. Oxford: Oxford Medical Press, 1993: 282–90.

◆ 5 Fallon B. Nausea and vomiting unrelated to cancer treatment. In: Berger AM, Portenoy RK, Weissman DE, eds. *Principles and Practice of Supportive Oncology*. Philadelphia: Lippincott Williams and Wilkins, 1998: 179–90.

◆ 6 Peroutka SJ, Snyder SH. Antiemetics: neurotransmitter receptor binding predicts therapeutic actions. *Lancet* 1982; **i**: 658–9.

◆ 7 Roila F, Ballatori E, Tonato M, et al. 5-HT3 receptor antagonists: differences and similarities. *Eur J Cancer* 1997; **33**: 1364.

◆ 8 Rhodes V, McDaniel R. Nausea, vomiting, and retching: complex problems in palliative care. *Ca Cancer J Clin* 2001; **51**: 232–48.

◆ 9 Morrow GR, Dobkin PL. Anticipatory nausea and vomiting in cancer patients undergoing chemotherapy treatment: prevalence, etiology, and behavioral interventions. *Clin Psychol Rev* 1988; **8**: 517.

✱ 10 Bruera E, Sweeney C. Chronic nausea and vomiting. In: Berger AM, Portenoy RK, Weissman DE, eds. *Principles and Practice of Supportive Oncology*, 2nd ed. Philadelphia: Lippincott Williams and Wilkins, 2002:222–32.

◆ 11 Lee M, Feldman M. Nausea and vomiting. In: Slesinger MH, Fordtran JS. *Gastrointestinal Disease*. Philadelphia: WB Saunders Co, 1993: 509–23.

● 12 Melzack R. Measurement of nausea. *J Pain Symptom Manage* 1989; **4**: 157–60.

✱ 13 Gralla RJ, Osoba D, Kris MG, et al. Recommendations for the use of antiemetics: evidence-based clinical practice guidelines. *J Clin Oncol* 1999; **17**: 2971.

✱ 14 Bentley A, Boyd K. Use of clinical pictures in the management of nausea and vomiting: a prospective audit. *Palliat Med* 2001; **15**: 247–53.

◆ 15 Herndon CM, Jackson KC, Hallin PA. Management of opioid-induced gastrointestinal effects in patients receiving palliative care. *Pharmacotherapy* 2002; **22**: 240–50.

✱ 16 Regnard C, Comiskey M. Nausea and vomiting in advanced cancer – a flow diagram. *Palliat Med* 1992; **6**: 146–51.

◆ 17 Lichter I. Which antiemetic? *J Palliat Care* 1993; **9**: 42–50.

◆ 18 Glare P, Pereira G, Kristjanson LJ, et al. Systematic review of the efficacy of antiemetic in the treatment of nausea in patients with far-advanced cancer. *Support Care Cancer* 2004; **12**: 432–40.

● 19 Hardy J, Daly S, McQuade B, et al. A double-blind, randomised parallel group, multi-national, multi-centre study comparing ondansetron 24 mg p.o. with placebo and metoclopramide 10 mg tds p.o. in the treatment of opioid induced nausea and emesis in cancer patients. *Support Care Cancer* 2002; **10**: 231–6.

● 20 Bruera E, Seifert L, Watanabe S, et al. Chronic nausea in advanced cancer patients: a retrospective assessment of a metoclopramide-based antiemetic regimen. *J Pain Symptom Manage* 1996; **11**: 147–53.

● 21 Bruera E, Balzile M, Neumann C, et al. A double-blind, crossover study of controlled-release metoclopramide and placebo for the chronic nausea and dyspepsia of advanced cancer. *J Pain Symptom Manage* 2000; **19**: 427–35.

● 22 Avorn J, Gurwitz JH, Bohn RL, et al. Increased incidence of levodopa therapy following metoclopramide use. *JAMA* 1995; **274**: 1780–2.

● 23 Currow DC, Coughlan M, Fardell B, Cooney NJ. Use of ondansetron in palliative medicine. *J Pain Symptom Manage* 1997; **13**: 302–7.

● 24 Mystakidou K, Befon S, Liossi C, Vlachos L. Comparison of tropisetron and chlorpromazine combinations in the control of nausea and vomiting in patients with advanced cancer. *J Pain Symptom Manage* 1998; **15**: 176–84.

● 25 Twycross RG, Barkby GD, Hallwood PM. The use of low dose levomepromazine in the management of nausea and vomiting. *Prog Palliat Care* 1997; **5**: 49–53.

● 26 de Wit R, Herrstedt J, Rapoport B, et al. The oral NK(1) antagonist, aprepitant, given with standard antiemetics provides protection against nausea and vomiting over multiple cycles of cisplatin-based chemotherapy. a combined analysis of two randomised, placebo-controlled phase III clinical trials. *Eur J Cancer* 2004; **40**: 403–10.

● 27 Gonzales-Rosales F, Walsh D. Intractable nausea and vomiting due to gastrointestinal mucosal metastases relieved by tetrahydrocannabinol. *J Pain Symptom Manage* 1997; **14**: 311–14.

● 28 Passik SD, Kirsh KL, Theobald DE, et al. A retrospective chart review of the use of olanzapine for the prevention of delayed emesis in cancer patients. *J Pain Symptom Manage* 2003; **25**: 485–8.

● 29 Srivastava M, Brito-Dellan N, Davis MP, et al. Olanzapine as an antiemetic in refractory nausea and vomiting in advanced cancer. *J Palliat Med* 2003; **6**: 251–5.

● 30 Brown J. A retrospective chart review of the use of olanzapine for the prevention of delayed emesis in cancer patients. *J Pain Symptom Manage* 2003; **25**: 485–8.

60

Constipation and diarrhea

EDUARDO BRUERA, NADA FADUL

INTRODUCTION

Constipation and diarrhea are common and distressing symptoms in palliative care patients. In some patients these symptoms occur together, and others alternate between episodes of diarrhea and constipation. However, in the majority of cases, the patient presents with one manifestation or the other according to the clinical situation. During the trajectory of illness of patients with cancer or acquired immunodeficiency syndrome (AIDS), there will be episodes of chronic constipation related to opioid medications, decreased oral intake, immobility or autonomic failure; and episodes of diarrhea related to antibiotic therapy and chemotherapy-induced mucositis. For educational purposes, this chapter discusses the assessment and management of constipation and diarrhea independently. However, in clinical practice, the syndromes frequently occur in a less independent fashion.

CONSTIPATION

Definition

Constipation is a common symptom in the palliative care population. It affects more than 50 percent of the patients in a palliative care unit or hospice. This might actually underestimate the problem since many of these patients are already on stool softeners and/or laxatives. Constipation is a clinical syndrome, rather than a symptom. It is defined as infrequent or difficult defecation with reduced number of bowel movements, which may or may not be abnormally hard, with increased difficulty or discomfort.[1] Because of the variability of normal bowel movement pattern from one patient to another, it is difficult to find an objective measure of constipation. The Rome criteria are often used to define constipation (Box 60.1).[2] Constipation is inadequately assessed and is underdiagnosed in the palliative care settings, even though it has been found to cause greater distress than pain in this patient population.[3**] Untreated constipation may progress to obstipation, which may potentially lead to life threatening complications associated with bowel obstruction.[4**]

Box 60.1 Definition of constipation according to the Rome criteria

The presence of two or more of the following symptoms for a period of at least three months:

- Straining at least 25 percent of the time
- Hard stools at least 25 percent of the time
- Incomplete evacuation at least 25 percent of the time
- Two or fewer bowel movements per week

Pathophysiology

Normal bowel function requires the coordination of motility, mucosal transport, and defecation reflexes. Motility of the small intestine, colon, and sphincteric regions is controlled by myogenic characteristics, central nervous system mechanisms, the activity of the peripheral autonomic nervous system (sympathetic and parasympathetic systems, and circulating gastrointestinal hormones [Fig. 60.1]).[2]

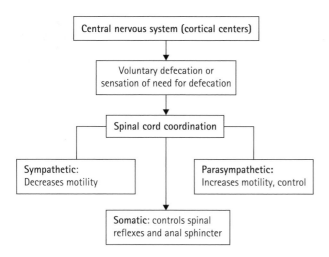

Figure 60.1 *Neurological control of bowel motility.*

Gut smooth muscle is innervated by extrinsic nerves that relay information to and from the extraintestinal ganglia, the spinal cord, and the central nervous system, and by intrinsic nerves within the intestinal wall. The vagus nerve provides parasympathetic supply to the ascending colon and proximal half of the transverse colon, and the reminder of the large intestine is supplied by parasympathetic fibers from the second, third, and fourth sacral segments.[5] The external anal sphincter and pelvic floor muscles receive sacral spinal input from the pudendal nerves. Sympathetic fibers innervate the proximal part of the large intestine though the superior mesenteric plexus, and the distal part of the large intestine through the inferior mesenteric and superior hypogastric plexuses. Sympathetic innervation generally inhibits excitatory cholinergic transmission in the myenteric plexus of both the small intestine and colon.[6,7] The functional significance of these pathways is exemplified by the long inhibitory intestinal reflexes that decrease motility through neural arcs involving the prevertebral ganglia. Conversely, sympathectomy either has no effect on bowel function or may unmask colonic propulsion.

Colonic propulsion and defecation appear to be coordinated by a spinal center that is modulated by excitatory and inhibitory influences from the brain.[8] Patients with neurological lesions involving the cauda equina or lower spinal cord have all the neurological abnormalities observed after section of the pelvic nerves, but in addition the external anal sphincter contractions are weak or absent and may not occur in response to rectal distension, increase intra-abdominal pressure, and anal stimulation.[8] These types of lesion produce constipation associated with hypomotility, colonic dilation, decreased rectal tone and sensation, stasis of the distal colon, and impaired defecation.[9,10] Patients with lesions involving the high spinal cord are often constipated, probably because they are unable to perceive the presence of feces in the rectum. However, colonic reflexes are intact and sphincter pressure is often normal and defecation

can often be triggered by digital stimulation of the anal canal.[11] Although the motor response of the sigmoid colon after a meal is reduced in persons with high spinal injuries, responses to pharmacological stimuli are normal. Colonic motility can also be abnormal in patients with pontine, hypothalamic, or cortical lesions.[8] The myenteric plexus provides the major intrinsic innervation to the small intestine and colon, although the submucous plexus may play a minor role in some reflexes. These two groups of nerve cells integrate the motor and secretory activities of the gastrointestinal tract.[12] The number of intrinsic neurons greatly exceeds the number of vagal, pelvic, or splanchnic fibers. The human enteric nervous system contains 10–100 million neurons versus 2000 efferent fibers in the vagus; thus, intrinsic nerves direct most motor activities, whereas extrinsic innervation provides a modulatory function.

A number of neurotransmitters participate in extrinsic neural control of small intestinal and colonic motor function. Peptidergic fibers containing somatostatin, substance P, cholecystokinin (CCK), neuropeptide Y (NPY), encephalin, and other transmitters are present in the vagus and splanchnic nerves.

Assessment

HISTORY

Because of interindividual variability of the normal elimination pattern, constipation in an individual patient should be defined according to that patient's experience. It is helpful to use the patient's prior stool pattern and regularity as a basis for comparison. It is also important to determine when was the last time the patient had a bowel movement and what were the characteristics of the bowel movement, whether straining was necessary or whether there was pain on defecation. If the patient has an urge to move the bowel but is unable to, this might suggest rectal obstruction or impaction of stool. In contrast, if the patient has lost the urge to move the bowel, this suggests a spinal cord problem causing neurogenic bowel dysfunction. Patients with impaired mobility are predisposed to constipation partly because of difficulty accessing the toilet or commode.

It is also important to determine whether there are other associated symptoms, because these might indicate development of complications or they could be atypical presentation of constipation (Box 60.2). Severely constipated patients can complain of diarrhea and continue to pass fecal material.[13] Patient can also complain of variable abdominal or rectal pain, which is colicky in nature. Unexplained nausea or vomiting should prompt investigations to rule out constipation.[14] Fecal impaction is well-recognized cause of urinary retention in elderly patients. Certain medications can predispose to constipation (Box 60.3) and it is essential to obtain a thorough history of prescription as well as over-the-counter medications and whether the patient is using laxatives along with these medications.[1]

Box 60.2 Symptoms associated with constipation

- Flatulence
- Abdominal pain
- Nausea and/or vomiting
- Pseudodiarrhea (see section on diarrhea)
- Urinary retention
- Abdominal distension
- Anorexia
- Mental status change and delirium

Box 60.3 Drugs commonly associated with constipation in palliative care patients

- Opioids
- Anticholinergic (antispasmodics, antidepressants and phenothiazines)
- Haloperidol
- Anticonvulsants
- Iron
- Calcium-channel blockers
- Vinca alkaloids
- Aluminum (antacids)
- Calcium
- Barium sulfate
- Ganglionic blockers
- 5-Hydroxytryptamine (5-HT$_3$) blockers
- Diuretics
- Antihypertensives

PHYSICAL EXAMINATION

Abdominal examination may reveal distension, tenderness, firmness, or the presence of fecal mass, particularly in the descending colon. Several features can help distinguish between a fecal mass and a tumor. Fecal masses usually indent with deep palpation and can have a crepituslike feeling because of the presence of entrapped gas. Over time the fecal mass will move.[9] Auscultation can detect high-pitched, hyperactive sounds, which are characteristic of intestinal obstruction, or loss of bowel sounds, which signifies ileus.

Digital rectal examination is essential in the assessment of constipation. It may reveal stenosis, fissure, scarring,

rectal tumor, hemorrhoids, or rectal prolapse. It can aid in the diagnosis and management of fecal impaction by removal of the impacted feces to facilitate bowel movement. An empty rectal vault may indicate proximal impaction or obstruction. Perineal sensation should be assessed, and reflex contraction of the anal canal after pinprick of the perianal area (anal wink) also can be used to test neurological function of the perineal areas.[10] The actual stool can be examined: small hard pellets suggest slow colonic transit time; ribbonlike stool suggests bowel stenosis or the presence of hemorrhoids. The presence of blood or mucus is suggestive of hemorrhoids, tumor, or inflammation.

DIAGNOSTIC TESTS

An important laboratory test in patients with constipation is serum calcium, since hypercalcemia is an easily reversible cause of constipation. Serum potassium level can also be helpful since hypokalemia can cause constipation. Thyroid hormone studies to rule out hypothyroidism can be helpful in patients with other signs and symptoms of this disorder.

A plain abdominal radiograph can be extremely useful in the assessment of constipation. Diagnosis of constipation by history and physical examination alone has been shown to be unreliable, inaccurate, and often omitted by healthcare professionals.[11**] The diagnosis can be greatly improved by obtaining an abdominal radiograph, a noninvasive and inexpensive test that is more appropriate to the palliative care population than other more sophisticated tests, such as defecography and colonic transit time studies. The abdominal radiograph can provide an objective assessment of fecal load by obtaining a constipation score. A constipation scoring system has been proposed based on the amount of stool in each quadrant (ascending, transverse, descending colon, and rectum). Each quadrant is assigned a score from 0 to 3 where:

- 0 = no stool
- 1 = stool occupies less than 50 percent
- 2 = stool occupies >50 percent but <100 percent
- 3 = stool occupies 100 percent of the lumen.

A score greater than or equal to 7/12 is considered to reflect severe constipation.[15**]

Etiology

In the palliative care population the causes of constipation can be related to the primary illness or secondary associated factors (Fig. 60.2). Chronic illnesses often lead to physical and mental impairments that can produce or exaggerate constipation. This condition may be further exacerbated by inactivity or physical immobility, which can lead to fecal retention. A bedridden patient may be unable to respond to defecatory signals because of inadequate toileting arrangements; as a result, fecal retention may lead to

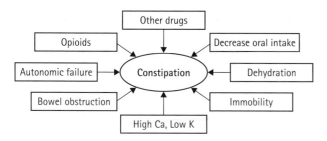

Figure 60.2 *Common causes of constipation in palliative care patients.*

megarectum, diminished rectal sensation, and fecal impaction. Other factors that may contribute to constipation in the bedridden patient include underlying illness, medications such as opioids, low fluid intake, low-fiber diet, sedation, and depression.[2,16] A survey conducted by Twycross suggested the importance of these factors: in a hospice population, 50 percent of the patients not receiving opioids required regular laxatives.[28]

Diseases associated with constipation include structural disorders that lead to mechanical obstruction (intra- or extraluminal), metabolic and endocrine disorders, and those neurogenic disorders that affect the gastrointestinal tract. Structural disorders include both intracolonic and extracolonic mass lesions, either primary or metastatic, radiation fibrosis and other anorectal pathology including painful anal fissures, hemorrhoids, or perianal abscess. Metabolic disorders that predispose to constipation include dehydration (due to poor oral intake, vomiting, fever, polyuria or diuretics), hypercalcemia, hypokalemia, and uremia.[16] Other systemic endocrine disorders that can cause constipation may also coexist in these patients such as diabetes and hypothyroidism.[17,18] Because colonic and anorectal motor functions are coordinated by both the enteric nerves and the extrinsic innervation of the sympathetic and parasympathetic nerves, diseases of the central and peripheral nervous systems are often associated with constipation.[19] Constipation can be caused by epidural metastasis leading to compression of the spinal cord, conus medullaris or cauda equina. Other neurological disorders that can cause constipation include peripheral neuropathy and local sacral plexus disease. In addition patient with advance cancer frequently develop autonomic failure that leads to abnormal gastrointestinal motility and symptoms such as chronic nausea, anorexia, and constipation. This abnormality is more frequent in patients with the anorexia/cachexia syndrome.

Several medications induce constipation (see Box 60.3). Opioid analgesics are the most common offending agents. In a large retrospective study, Skyes showed that opioids accounted for about a quarter of constipation found in terminally ill cancer patients in a hospice.[20*] Opioids affect the intestine by one of three mechanisms: reduction in motility (propulsive peristalsis), reduction in secretions (pancreatic, biliary, fluid, and electrolyte abnormalities), and increase in intestinal absorption and blood flow.[21,22] Opioids also increase transit time in the colon and ileum. Morphine can lead to constipation partly by local accumulation in the intestinal tissue.[23] Opioid receptors are present on the gut smooth level and at all levels of the nervous input to the intestine. Tolerance to the constipation effect of opioids develops slowly and many patients require laxatives as long as they take the medication. The effect on the bowel varies between the different opioids and there is also wide interindividual variability. Research suggests that methadone and transdermal fentanyl cause less constipation than other opioids.[24*,25**] In a report of four cases, Daeninck and Bruera found reduction of laxative requirements after opioid rotation to methadone.[24*] Other medications that are commonly used in palliative care patients have prominent constipating effect, including those with anticholinergic action (antispasmodics, antidepressants, phenothiazines, antacids, and haloperidol), some anticonvulsants or anti-hypertensive drugs, antiemetics (ondansetron), and diuretics.[2] Chemotherapeutic agents that can cause peripheral neuropathy such as vinca alkaloids can also lead to constipation.

Complications

Chronic constipation may lead to pudendal nerve damage and fecal incontinence in middle-aged and older women.[10] In more advanced cases, rectal prolapse may result. Stercorous ulcers with bleeding or perforation constitute a hazard in patients with fecal impaction. Constipation has also been determined to be a risk factor for patients receiving corticosteroids for intracranial lesions.[1,2]

Management

Management of constipation can be divided into preventive measures and therapeutic measures. Preventive measures include prophylaxis with laxatives when initiating opioids.[26] Nonpharmacological interventions are appropriate in some patients, such as increase in dietary fiber and fluid intake. It is important to ensure adequate fluid intake when increasing dietary fiber, since fiber can be problematic in some patients and can lead to paradoxical worsening of constipation. Patients with partial obstruction should not be given fiber because of the risk of increased obstructive symptoms.[2] Anorectic patients should be given fiber cautiously since the satiety produced by a high-fiber diet worsens malnutrition. Patients should be encouraged to increase physical activity to avoid decrease in colonic motility caused by inactivity.[27] It is also important to educate the patient, family and healthcare providers about the myth of the relation between regularity of bowel movement and food intake. Palliative care professionals should emphasize the fact that stool content is comprised mostly of sloughed intestinal endothelial cells and microorganisms rather than digested food.

Table 60.1 *Classification, dosages, and pharmacological properties of laxatives*

Laxative	Onset of action (h)	Mechanism	Usual adult dose	Comments
Bulk forming agents	12–24	Hold water in stool and cause distension		Patients should be able to increase fluid intake, otherwise fluid impaction might occur
Natural (psyllium)			7 g/day	
Synthetic (methylcellulose)			4–6 g/day	
Saline laxatives	0.5–3	Draw fluid into the intestine		Avoid in patients with renal or heart failure
Magnesium hydroxide			30 mL	
Magnesium citrate			200 mL	
Hyperosmolar agents	Variable, generally 24–48	Increase stool osmolarity leading to accumulation of fluid in the colon		Might cause flatulence and distension
Polyethylene glycol			8–25 g/day	
Lactulose			15–30 mL	
Sorbitol			15–30 mL	
Contact cathartics	6–10	Stimulate peristalsis by direct action on the myenteric plexus. Reduce net absorption of water and electrolytes		Additive risk of hepatotoxicity when docusate is used in combination with other contact cathartics
Anthraquinones *Senna*			Variable	
Diphenylmethane *Bisacodyl*			65–130 mg	
Castor oil	2–6		15–60 mL	
Docusate	24–72		100–800 mg	
Emollient laxatives	6–8	Lubricant and stool softener	15–45 mL/day	Might lead to serious lipoid pneumonia if aspiration occurs
Mineral oil				
Prokinetic agents	Variable	Decrease transit time through intestine		For refractory constipation. Might be useful in colonic inertia secondary to spinal cord injury
Metoclopramide			40–120 mg/day	
Domperidone			30–80 mg/day	

Therapeutic modalities to treat existing constipation can be divided into general interventions and pharmacological treatment. The nonpharmacological measures used in prevention can also be incorporated in treatment of constipation. Other measures include treatment of underlying medical factors that can lead to constipation (discontinuation of offending drugs, treatment of electrolyte and metabolic abnormalities) and the availability of comfort, privacy, and convenience during defecation. Therapeutic interventions for the routine management of constipation could be administered orally or rectally.[1,2,9,16] For most patients, the use of enemas and rectal suppositories is limited for the acute short-term management of more severe episodes.[1] Surveys of hospice populations suggest that more than 40 percent of

these patients use rectally administered laxative therapy on a regular basis.[28] Oral laxatives include bulk forming agents, osmotic (saline) agents, hyperosmolar agents, contact cathartics, agents for colonic lavage, lubricants, prokinetic drugs, and opioid antagonists (Table 60.1).[1]

Bulk-forming laxatives comprise natural (psyllium) or synthetic polysaccharides or cellulose derivatives that act in a manner similar to fiber that is naturally contained in the diet. Because fluid intake should be increased with these preparations,[29**] they should be used cautiously in patients who are unable to maintain good oral intake, otherwise a viscous mass may form and aggravate a partial bowel obstruction. These products are typically effective after 2–4 days of regular use and they are generally unsuitable for palliative care patients and/or for relief of severe constipation.

Saline laxatives including magnesium salts (magnesium hydroxide and magnesium citrate) and sodium salts (sodium phosphate) contain relatively nonabsorbable cations and anions that exert an osmotic effect to increase intraluminal water content. Magnesium increases intestinal motor activity; because an appreciable amount of magnesium may be absorbed, these agents should be avoided in patients with renal insufficiency because of the danger of magnesium toxicity. Saline laxatives can also be administered by enemas or suppositories.

Hyperosmolar agents include polyethylene glycol and nonabsorbable sugars such as lactulose and sorbitol. Sorbitol and lactulose are degraded by colonic bacteria to low-molecular-weight acids that increase stool acidity and osmolarity and lead to accumulation of fluid in the colon. The use of these substances may cause flatulence in about 20 percent of patients and their sweet taste is sickly to some. Doses should be adjusted to reduce abdominal bloating and flatulence and to modulate defecation.

Contact cathartics are the most commonly prescribed agents for opioid-induced constipation.[1] This group comprises the anthraquinones (cascara sagrada, senna, casanthranol, and danthron), diphenylmethanes (phenolphthalein and bisacodyl, and oxyphenisatin), the docusates, and castor oil. Although there is some difference in action in different classes, all of these drugs stimulate peristalsis by direct stimulation of the myenteric plexus and reducing net absorption of water and electrolytes from the intraluminal content.[30*,31,32] Anthraquinone derivatives increase fluid and electrolyte accumulation in the distal ileum and colon through incompletely understood actions. They act primarily on the colon, and colonic electromyography following administration of senna in humans shows an increase in myoelectrical activity of the type seen in diarrhea. Pathological changes in the colon produced by long-term anthraquinone use include melanosis coli, a benign and reversible condition. Although smooth muscle atrophy and damage to the myenteric plexus were suggested in earlier studies, there is no evidence that anthraquinones given in clinically relevant doses cause enteric damage in experimental animals or humans.[33**] These laxatives are generally effective within 12–24 hours. The diphenylmethane derivatives (phenolphthalein and bisacodyl, and oxyphenisatin) also act primarily on the colon and produce effects similar to those of anthraquinone derivatives. Allergy to these substances has been reported. In 1997, the phenolphthaleins were voluntarily withdrawn from the market after the US Food and Drug Administration (FDA) reclassified the drugs as 'not generally recognized as safe and effective' after a study in rodents found an increased incidence of nongastrointestinal neoplasms. This has not been proved to be the case in humans.[34*,35*,36*] Bisacodyl is structurally similar to phenolphthalein and exhibits similar actions on small intestine fluid accumulation and colonic motor activity.[37] Because the drug is a gastric irritant, tablets

are enteric coated and should not be broken or chewed. Docusate salts are anionic surfactants that lower the surface tension of stool to allow mixing of aqueous and fatty substances. This action softens stool to permit easier defecation. These agents also stimulate intestinal fluid and electrolyte secretion by increasing mucosal cyclic adenosine monophosphate.[38] Although not absorbed, they alter intestinal mucosal permeability and increase the absorption of other laxatives, such as mineral oil, phenolphthalein, and danthron. Docusate salts are often added to other laxatives as a stool softener. This is reasonable although there are no controlled studies establishing the efficacy of such a combination. There is an additive risk of hepatotoxicity when used in combination with other contact cathartics, and liver function should be evaluated periodically.[39*] Castor oil is hydrolyzed by gut microflora to ricinoleic acid, which acts on small intestine producing abundant mucosal secretions. Castor oil may have a rapid onset of action and can cause considerable cramping. With chronic use, malabsorption of nutrients may occur. This drug should be reserved only for the management of acute constipation.

Agents for colonic lavage such as polyethylene glycol electrolyte solutions are most often given for bowel cleansing before colonoscopy or before institution of bowel programs. Consumption of small quantities (25–500 mL) can be used to reverse chronic constipation in patients who are refractory to other laxatives.[2,40**] Lubricant laxatives (mineral oil) lubricate the stool surface and soften the stool, allowing easier elimination. These substances are generally recommended for the management of acute transient constipation and are not suitable for chronic laxative use. Long-term use is limited by perianal irritation, malabsorption of fat-soluble vitamins and the serious potential for lipoid pneumonia should aspiration occur. Mineral oil should not be used in obtunded or demented patients.[1,2]

Prokinetic agents (bethanechol, metoclopramide, or domperidone) are drugs that stimulate gastrointestinal motor activity to enhance transit of intraluminal contents. These drugs enhance intestinal motility by one of two mechanisms; they mediate the effect of a local transmitter that enhances motility such as acetylcholine or by antagonizing the effect of an inhibitory transmitter such as dopamine.[41,42] These agents could be considered for the treatment of constipation that does not respond to conventional measures. Cholinergic agents such as bethanechol have been used with little success and exhibit moderate side effects, including abdominal cramps, diarrhea, salivation, flushing, bradycardia, and blurred vision. Cisapride appeared to enhance transit through the proximal colon and has been shown to stimulate colonic motility and improve rectal sensation in chronically constipated patients. Although some studies suggest that clinical improvement occurs with the drug,[43**] others report highly variable and often disappointing results in patients with severe idiopathic constipation. Cisapride had been withdrawn by the FDA because of the risk of cardiac toxicity. Metoclopramide enhances gastrointestinal motility through three distinct mechanisms: central antidopamine effect, peripheral antidopamine effect, and both direct and indirect stimulation of cholinergic receptors.[44] Basic studies have shown the effect of metoclopramide on colonic activity,[45,46] but clinical studies have failed to demonstrate effectiveness in treatment of constipated patients.[47] Domperidone is a benzimidazole derivative that acts as a specific antagonist to the inhibitory effects of dopamine on the upper intestinal tract and causes dose-dependent antroduodenal coordination.[48,49] It has no cholinergic activity and diffuses poorly into the central nervous system causing less extrapyramidal side effects than metoclopramide.

It has been shown that the opioid receptor antagonist naloxone can reverse certain cases of constipation. Scintigraphic techniques have shown that naloxone accelerates transit in various parts of the colon in normal volunteers.[50] Presumably this is because opioid receptors are involved in normal control of gut motility. Preliminary studies suggest that oral naloxone, compared with placebo, may increase stool volumes in elderly constipated persons.[51]** Such agents have been used successfully to treat constipation associated with long-term use of narcotic agents.[52] In a study by Skyes, the daily oral administration of naloxone at 20 percent or more of the prevailing 24-hour morphine dose was capable of providing a clinical effect without antagonizing the analgesic effect of opioid.[53]** However, opioid withdrawal was observed and it is suggested that initial naloxone administration dose should not exceed 5 mg. Methylnaltrexone is a quaternary ammonium opioid receptor antagonist, which does not cross the blood–brain barrier in humans. Intravenous or oral methylnaltrexone has been shown to reverse chronic opioid-induced constipation in patients in methadone maintenance programs without causing adverse effects such as withdrawal or abdominal cramps.[54,55] The dose of methylnaltrexone ranged from 0.3 mg/kg to 3 mg/kg with an effect that was significantly dose dependent.

The use of rectally administered agents including enemas and rectal suppositories should generally be limited to the acute short-term management of severe and intractable constipation. The occasional patient who cannot tolerate oral laxatives may be able to use long-term rectal laxatives or enemas effectively. These are usually administered two to three times per week. Surveys of hospice population suggest that more than 40 percent of this population uses rectally administered laxative therapy on a regular basis.[28] These agents are contraindicated in patients with thrombocytopenia. Rectal suppositories may be inert or active. Inert suppositories are usually fashioned from glycerin alone. They draw fluid into the rectum and act as a stimulus to defecation. Active suppositories contain a cathartic agent. Enemas are used to treat constipation unrelieved by suppositories. Enema may consist of small volume (microenemas) or large volume. Various commercially prepared formulations are available, based on a variety of laxative substances. Sodium phosphate enemas may cause fluid and electrolyte imbalance particularly in dehydrated patients. Large volume enemas can use tap water, soap suds, or saline. These can lead to mucosal irritation and can potentially cause fluid overload if a significant amount of water is absorbed.[1,2]

Future trends

There has been intense interest in the pharmacological actions of serotonin (5-HT) agonists on gastrointestinal motility; 5-HT$_4$ agonists stimulate intestinal motility, in part by facilitating enteric cholinergic transmission.[56,57] Clinical trials indicate that several 5-HT$_4$ receptor agonists accelerate colonic transit time and improve symptoms in patients with constipation. Tegaserod, a partial 5-HT$_4$ receptor agonist, reduces symptoms in patients with constipation-predominant irritable bowel syndrome. Tegaserod has also been shown to accelerate gastric emptying and small bowel transit. It is being evaluated for gastroparesis.[58]

The preliminary study on donepezil found that this drug could help constipation. Bruera et al. found that bowel movement per week (bm/week) did not increase among nonconstipated patients, but did increase from 2.9 to 5.5 bm/week in the eight constipated patients after 1 week of donepezil 5 mg/day. This centrally acting cholinergic drug has diarrhea as its main side effect and therefore it would be appropriate to consider clinical trials of its potential usefulness in constipation in patients requiring it for sedation or fatigue.[59]

DIARRHEA

Definition

Diarrhea is loosely defined as passage of abnormally liquid or unformed stools at an increased frequency. For adults on a typical Western diet, stool weight >200 g/day can generally be considered diarrheal. Because of the fundamental importance of duration to diagnostic considerations, diarrhea may be further defined as acute if <2 weeks, persistent if 2–4 weeks, and chronic if >4 weeks in duration.[13] Pseudodiarrhea and fecal incontinence are caused by anorectal problems or neuromuscular problems, respectively. These disorders are associated with passage of less than 200 g of stool and must be distinguished from diarrhea.[60–62] Diarrhea can also be an atypical presentation of constipation. Stool consistency probably best defines diarrhea, but it cannot be easily measured. Consistency is best defined as the ratio of fecal water to the water-holding capacity of insoluble solids.[63] Infectious agents cause more than 90 percent of cases of acute diarrhea; these cases are often accompanied by vomiting, fever, and abdominal pain. The remaining 10 percent or so are caused by medications, toxic ingestions, ischemia, and other conditions. Infectious diarrhea is one of the most frequent categories of nosocomial infections in many hospitals and long-term

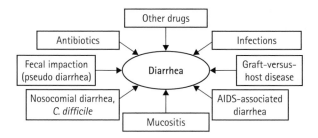

Figure 60.3 *Common causes of diarrhea in palliative care patients.*

care facilities; the causes include a variety of microorganisms but most commonly *Clostridium difficile* (Fig. 60.3). Special categories of diarrhea including graft-versus-host disease (GVHD) and diarrhea in HIV patients will be discussed separately.

Pathophysiology

Most of the diarrheal conditions that have been studied have shown alterations of both intestinal fluid and electrolyte transport and the induction of propagative forms of intestinal motility. Diarrhée motrice is diarrhea caused by autonomic dysfunction in patients with hexosaminidase B deficiency (Sandhoff disease). It is thought to be caused specifically and only by abnormal motility. Deranged motility may reduce the contact time between the intestinal epithelium and luminal content. This commonly occurs in patient with postsurgical disorders (such as post-gastrectomy dumping syndrome, post-vagotomy, iliocecal valve resection) or neoplastic and chronic disease (such as malignant carcinoid syndrome, medullary carcinoma of the thyroid, and diabetes). Diarrhea in diabetic patients is a complication of diabetic neuropathy leading to sympathetic denervation of the bowel with prevalence of unopposed cholinergic innervation.

During each 24 hours, about 8–10 L of fluid enters the duodenum. This fluid contains 800 mmol sodium (Na^+), 700 mmol chloride (Cl^-), and 100 mmol potassium (K^+). Two liters of this duodenal load is derived from the diet; the remainder comes from secretions of the salivary glands, stomach, liver, pancreas, and the duodenum itself. Generally 1.5 L is absorbed in the small intestine and the remainder is presented to the colon. The absorptive capacity of the small intestine is undefined, but the capacity of the normal adult human colon is 4–5 L/24 h.[64]

Theoretically, diarrhea can result from decreased absorption by either the small intestine or the colon. If either deranged epithelial transport mechanisms or the presence of nonabsorbable solutes in the intestinal lumen reduce the absorptive capacity of the small intestine by 50 percent, the daily volume of fluid then presented to the normal colon (approximately 5 L) would exceed its absorptive capacity.

In recent decades it has been shown that intestinal secretions contribute greatly to the development of diarrhea. It was initially thought that bacterial enterotoxins cause secretion only by a direct effect on enterocyte receptors, but it has now been shown that 50 percent or more of the intestinal secretion initiated by bacterial enterotoxins *in vivo* comes about from stimulation of receptors on enterochromaffin cells that release hormones that activate the enteric nervous system, secondarily stimulating the enterocyte.[65,66] Inflammatory mediators also play a role. Phagocytes such as eosinophils, macrophages, and neutrophils and mesenchymal cells (myofibroblasts, endothelium, and smooth muscle) in the lamina propria and submucosa are also capable of initiating intestinal secretion. These mediators may directly stimulate the enterocyte and may also activate the enteric nervous system.

Chronic diarrhea is divided into three general categories: malabsorption (osmotic diarrheas), secretory diarrheas, and inflammatory diarrheas.

OSMOTIC DIARRHEA

This is caused by the ingestion of poorly absorbable solutes such polyethylene glycol and lactulose. The proximal small bowel is highly permeable to water and sodium, and water influx across the duodenum rapidly adjusts the osmolarity of the luminal content toward that of plasma. The mucosa of the ileum and colon is not readily permeable to sodium and solutes. However, there is an efficient active ion transport mechanism that allows the reabsorption of electrolytes and water even against electrochemical gradients.[67] Colonic bacteria play a major protective role by fermenting dietary proteins and carbohydrates into short chain fatty acids and gas. Anaerobic colonic flora is necessary for the fermentation of fiber into short chain fatty acids and constitutes the bulk of the fecal mass. Lactulose, an unabsorbable sugar in the small intestine, when ingested in large amount, leads to loss of this protective mechanism of colonic flora and diarrhea will occur. Osmotic diarrhea due to carbohydrate malabsorption is characterized by low pH due to short chain fatty acids, a high carbohydrate content, high stool osmolality, and flatulence. In osmotic diarrhea caused by poorly absorbable salts such as magnesium and sulfate, the pH is normal. Osmotic diarrhea commonly subsides by fasting or discontinuation of the poorly absorbable solute laxatives. With ingestion of either unabsorbable solute (i.e. Mg^{2+} or polyethyleneglycol) or unabsorbed carbohydrate (i.e. lactulose[68] or, in some persons, lactose),[69] a considerable amount of the osmolality of stool results from the nonabsorbed solute, so there is a significant difference, or gap, between stool osmolality and the sum of the electrolytes in the stool.[70]

Secretory diarrhea is rarely present as a sole mechanism and is often associated with other mechanisms. An abnormal ion transport in the intestinal epithelial cells, with a reduction in absorptive function or increase in increase in the secretion of the epithelial cells, is observed in secretory diarrhea. In contrast to osmotic diarrhea, the anionic gap is usually small and the diarrhea does resolve by fasting. As is the case with osmotic causes of diarrhea, the stimuli causing secretory diarrhea may be of exogenous origin or they may be endogenous. The detergent stool softener dioctyl sodium sulfosuccinate and the cathartic ricinoleic acid (castor oil)[71] are examples of exogenous long-chain fatty acids that stimulate colonic secretion.

INFLAMMATORY DIARRHEA

Inflammatory diarrhea is characterized by enterocyte damage and death, villus atrophy, and crypt hyperplasia. In cases of severe inflammation, immune-mediated vascular damage or ulceration allows protein to exudate from capillaries and lymphatics and contribute to the diarrhea. Activation of lymphocytes, phagocytes, and fibroblasts releases various inflammatory mediators that induce intestinal chloride secretion.[72] Release of mediators such as prostaglandins, leukotrienes, platelet-activating factor, and hydrogen peroxide from phagocytes induces intestinal secretion by acting on the enterocyte and also by activating enteric nerves.[65,66,73] There are four general categories of inflammatory diarrhea: infection, hypersensitivity, cytostatic (anticancer) agents, and idiopathic (possibly autoimmune) diseases.

ACUTE DIARRHEA

Acute diarrhea is defined as diarrhea of less than 2–3 weeks' duration and, at most, 6–8 weeks' duration. The most common causes are infectious, medications, and chemicals. Acute infectious diarrhea is a major cause of death in developing countries. Death rates from diarrhea in the USA are probably underestimated, but they may be as high as 5000/year from food-borne infections alone.[74] Preliminary data from the US Centers for Disease Control and Prevention (CDC) indicate that the rates of *Salmonella*, *Shigella*, *Listeria*, *Escherichia coli*, and *Yersinia* (but not *Vibrio*) infections have declined by 20–30 percent, most likely as the result of increased attention to food safety.

Assessment

Experienced clinicians[75,76] suggest that 75–80 percent of chronic diarrheas can be diagnosed by an expert history and physical examination, coupled with certain screening and focused laboratory examinations.

HISTORY

Frequency, amount, and consistency of the stool should be carefully obtained. Stools that are large in volume, light in color, watery or greasy, and contain undigested food particles are associated with small bowel and proximal colon etiology. Stools that are small in volume, dark, often contain mucus or blood, and are frequent are associated with left colonic or rectal etiologies. Diarrhea associated with flatus and mushy stool is associated with carbohydrate malabsorption. Intermittent diarrhea and constipation is frequent in diabetic neuropathy. Fecal impaction can cause apparent diarrhea because only liquids pass through a partial obstruction. The association of heat intolerance, palpitations and weight loss suggest hyperthyroidism. Dietary habits, alcohol consumption, or food intolerances should be investigated. Medications should be reviewed including prescription medications and antibiotic use in the preceding few months. Impact of diarrhea on quality of life should also be elucidated from history.

PHYSICAL EXAMINATION

A complete physical examination may reveal important clues to the etiology of diarrhea, including abdominal mass, abdominal tenderness or distension, ascites, fever, lymphadenopathy, and postural hypotension. Rectal examination should be performed to rule out fecal impaction or rectal mass, perianal fistula or abscess, loss of anal sphincter tone and to exclude intestinal obstruction. Rectal involvement is suggested by presence of little or no stool with a sense of rectal urgency, commonly named tenesmus.

INVESTIGATIONS

The diagnostic evaluation must be rationally directed by a careful history and physical examination, and simple triage tests are often warranted before complex investigations are launched. If feasible, collected stool should be sent for chemical and microbiological analysis. Peripheral blood counts may reveal leukocytosis that suggests inflammation; anemia that reflects blood loss or nutritional deficiencies; or eosinophilia that may occur with parasitoses, neoplasia, collagen-vascular disease, allergy, or eosinophilic gastroenteritis. Blood chemistries may demonstrate electrolyte, hepatic, or other metabolic disturbances. Quantitative stool collection and analyses can yield important objective data that may establish a diagnosis or characterize the type of diarrhea as a triage for focused additional studies. If stool weight is >20 g/day, additional stool analyses should be performed that might include electrolyte concentration, pH, occult blood testing, leukocyte inspection (or leukocyte protein assay), fat quantitation, and laxative screens.[77] Microbiological studies should be done including fecal bacterial cultures (including media for *Aeromonas* and *Plesiomonas*), inspection for ova and parasites, and *Giardia* antigen assay (the most sensitive test for giardiasis). This should be guided by suggestive history and physical examination. Gram stain of the stool can reveal the presence of *Staphylococcus*, *Campylobacter*, or *Candida* infection. The presence of microorganisms in the stool is diagnostic. Fecal occult blood testing should also be performed. Positive fecal occult blood or stool leukocyte test would suggest an exudative mechanism, such as radiation colitis, colonic neoplasm, or infectious diarrhea. Fecal leukocyte tests have poor sensitivity for ruling out inflammatory diarrheas.[78–80]

Stool analysis for *C. difficile* toxins A and B is an essential element of work-up of nosocomial diarrhea.

Abdominal radiography may reveal the presence of fecal impaction, intestinal obstruction or mass. Routine contrast radiographs of the gastrointestinal tract are not usually helpful in the diagnosis of watery diarrheas, unless they show a previous vagotomy, extensive small bowel resection or cholecystectomy, the presence of a tumor (carcinoid or villous adenoma), or a bowel filled with fluid (endocrine tumor). Contrast radiography may show diagnostic evidence of inflammatory bowel disease or changes suggestive of eosinophilic gastroenteritis or radiation enterocolitis.[81] Endoscopy and other invasive tests are rarely needed to establish the diagnosis of diarrhea.

Management

Treatment of chronic diarrhea depends on the specific etiology and may be curative, suppressive, or empirical. If the cause can be eradicated, treatment is curative as with resection of a colorectal cancer, antibiotic administration for Whipple disease, or discontinuation of an offending drug. For many chronic conditions, diarrhea can be controlled by suppression of the underlying mechanism.

In the majority of cases oral dietary therapy may provide effective symptom management. A gluten-free diet can reduce abdominal cramping and bowel movement frequency in the presence of intestinal fermentation with bowel distension, Binders of osmotically active substances (kaolin-pectin) give a thicker consistency to the stool, but their antidiarrheal effectiveness is unclear. Oral hydration solutions are rich in glucose and electrolytes, which takes advantage of the presence of the intestinal glucose–sodium cotransporter to promote increased sodium and water absorption. Dietary sugar beet fiber may ameliorate the diarrhea caused by abdominal irradiation.[82]

Because death in acute diarrhea is caused by dehydration, an important principle is to assess the degree of dehydration and replace fluid and electrolyte deficits. Severely dehydrated individuals should be rehydrated with intravenous Ringer lactate or saline solutions to which additional K^+ and $NaHCO_3^-$ may be added as necessary. Alert patients should be given oral rehydration solutions. Intravenous hydration is also indicated in presence of clinical signs of dehydration in patients with nausea and vomiting, in whom oral therapy is ineffective.

Antidiarrheal agents are of two types: agents useful for mild-to-moderate diarrheas and agents helpful in secretory and other severe diarrheas. The bulk-forming agents (kaolin-pectin, psyllium, and methylcellulose) increase the consistency of stool and have no antisecretory activity. Pectin has been shown to have proabsorptive activity. Other antidiarrheal agents have only mild proabsorptive or antisecretory action, and most have antidiarrheal activity by altering the intestinal motility. Bismuth salicylates, opioids, loperamide, clonidine, phenothiazine,

and somatostatin have mild antisecretory activity but also cause dilation of the small intestine and colon and decrease peristalsis.

Opioids increase anal sphincter tone leading to fluid entrapment within the intestine and put it in contact with the mucosa for a greater period of time, allowing more complete absorption. Opioids may be symptomatically useful in mild diarrheas. Opioid receptors are present at different sites, including smooth muscle, the myenteric plexus, the spinal cord, and the brain. Paregorics, deodorized tincture of opium, codeine, and diphenoxylate with atropine largely have been supplanted by loperamide. Loperamide does not pass the blood–brain barrier and has a high first-pass metabolism in the liver; it has a high therapeutic-to-toxic ratio and is essentially devoid of addiction potential. It is safe in adults, even in total doses of 24 mg/day. The usual dose is 2–4 mg two to four times daily. The dosage should be titrated against the effect, and higher doses, 2 mg every 2 hours, have been recommended in conjunction with chemotherapeutic agents associated with high incidence of diarrhea.[83] When giving opioids, stool output is not a reliable gauge for replacing fluid losses because the antimotility effects of opioids cause fluid to sequester in the bowel lumen (third space).

Sucralfate has been shown to mitigate diarrhea after pelvic radiation therapy. However, recent controlled studies were not able to demonstrate significant benefit.[84] Cholestyramine has been favorably used in radiation-induced diarrhea. In the same way aspirin has been reported effective in post radiotherapy diarrhea. It reduced prostaglandin synthesis, thereby increasing water and electrolyte secretion, which has a role in many types of diarrhea due to an inflammatory process.[85] Corticosteroids may exert a positive effect in treatment of radiation-induced diarrhea. Steroids can also decrease intestinal tract edema in cases of pseudoobstruction and exert a proabsorptive effect on the intestine that is demonstrable by 5 hours after administration. Budesonide, a topical active steroid is effective in treatment of diarrhea induced by 5-fluorouracil and irinotecan-induced diarrhea after failure of loperamide treatment.[86] Bismuth subsalicylate (Pepto-Bismol) is safe and efficacious in bacterial infectious diarrheas. Because of the possibility of worsening the colonization or invasion of infectious organisms by paralyzing intestinal motility, and because of evidence that the use of motility-altering drugs may prolong microorganism excretion time, neither opioids nor anticholinergic drugs are recommended for infectious diarrheas. Racecadotril, an intestinal enkephalinase inhibitor that is antisecretory but does not paralyze intestinal motility, is effective in the treatment of acute diarrhea in children and adults.[87]

Certain infectious diarrheas should be treated with antibiotics: shigellosis, cholera, traveler's diarrhea, pseudomembranous enterocolitis, parasitic infestations, and sexually transmitted diseases. Antibiotics are not usually indicated in viral diarrhea and cryptosporidiosis because they are not effective. Treatment of *E. coli* serotype O157:H7 infection is not recommended at present because current antibiotics do not seem to be helpful, and the incidence of complications (hemolytic uremic syndrome) may be greater after antibiotic therapy. Regardless of the cause of infectious diarrhea, patients should be treated if they are immunosuppressed; have valvular, vascular, or orthopedic prostheses; have congenital hemolytic anemias or if they are elderly.

Refractory diarrhea that does not respond to specific therapy may present a challenging and serious clinical problem. Octreotide, a somatostatin analog with a more favorable pharmacokinetic profile, exerts a wide range of physiological effects on the gastrointestinal tract.[88] Several clinical trials suggest that this antisecretory agent may be useful in the symptomatic management of refractory diarrhea. The mechanisms by which octreotide produces these effects are probably multifactorial. It suppresses the secretion on many of the gut peptides implicated in the control of secretory and motor activity. Furthermore, it reduces splanchnic blood flow, inhibits exocrine secretion from the stomach, pancreas and small intestine, thus impairing gastrointestinal motility and facilitating absorption of water and electrolytes.[89,90] Octreotide may not be helpful in the diarrhea of medullary carcinoma of the thyroid, and it is of only limited usefulness in short bowel syndrome, and the refractory diarrhea of AIDS. Octreotide has been found to be effective in the management of chemotherapy-induced diarrhea[91] and diarrhea induced by celiac-plexus block, as well as diabetic diarrhea.[92,93] The newer long-acting preparations, Sandostatin-LAR (Novartis) and Lanreotide-PR (Ipsen-Biotech), for monthly subcutaneous administration have made therapy with this drug more convenient for the patient.

Agents such as phenothiazine, calcium-channel blockers, or clonidine can have serious side effects but may be tried if octreotide fails. Clonidine can be useful in the diarrhea of opioid withdrawal and occasionally in patients with diabetic diarrhea. Indometacin, a cyclooxygenase blocker that inhibits prostaglandin production, occasionally may be useful in neuroendocrine tumors, irritable bowel syndrome, and food allergy and is most useful in patients with diarrhea caused by acute radiation, AIDS, and villous adenomas of the rectum or colon. Cyclooxygenase blockers may be harmful in inflammatory bowel disease.

Diarrhea associated with special situations

NOSOCOMIAL DIARRHEA

Diarrhea is either the first or the second most common nosocomial illness among hospitalized patients and residents in long-term care facilities. Fecal impaction, medication and infections (*E. coli* and *C. difficile*) are common causes. Often this is a hidden problem, known only to the nurse's aide who changes the bed sheets. In the intensive care setting, it occurs in 30–50 percent of patients. Fecal impaction is thought to be one of the most common causes of diarrhea in hospitalized or institutionalized patients. Such paradoxical diarrhea and incontinence appear to be most common in patients with dementia or psychosis.[61] Any of a patient's medications may

initiate diarrhea. However, certain medications are more apt to cause diarrhea than others[62] (Box 60.4). Antibiotic-associated diarrhea is certainly the most common manifestation of drug-related diarrhea. Liquid formulations of any medication may cause diarrhea (elixir diarrhea) because of the high content of sorbitol used to sweeten the elixir. Patients prescribed liquid medications through feeding tubes may receive more than 20 g of sorbitol daily. An important but poorly understood cause of diarrhea is enteral (tube) feeding, particularly in critically ill patients, who often develop diarrhea. Dysmotility, increased intestinal permeability, and low sodium content in enteral formulas may be contributing factors. The incidence of acute, mild diarrhea with cancer chemotherapy or radiation therapy is high, approaching 100 percent with some agents, such as amsacrine, azacitidine, cytarabine, dactinomycin, daunorubicin, doxorubicin, floxuridine, 5-fluorouracil, 6-mercaptopurine, methotrexate, plicamycin, and irinotecan (CPT-11). Interleukin-2 therapy and the combination of 5-fluorouracil plus leucovorin are frequent causes of severe watery diarrhea.

Box 60.4 Drugs commonly associated with diarrhea in palliative care patients

Osmotic diarrhea

- Laxatives
- Antacid (containing magnesium)
- Olestra, orlistat (lipase inhibitor)
- Colchicine
- Cholestyramine
- Neomycin
- Methyldopa
- Paraaminosalicylic acid
- Biguanides

Secretory diarrhea

- Laxatives
- Diuretics (furosemide, thiazides)
- Theophylline
- Thyroxine
- Metformin
- Cholinergic drugs (glaucoma eye drops)
- Cholinesterase inhibitors
- Quinidine and quinine
- Metoclopramide
- Chemotherapy
- Misoprostol
- Gold
- Nonsteroidal anti-inflammatory drugs (NSAIDs)

DIARRHEA ASSOCIATED WITH GRAFT-VERSUS-HOST DISEASE

Graft-versus-host disease (GVHD) occurs when genetically disparate lymphocytes are transferred into an immunologically compromised recipient incapable of rejecting the donor graft. Acute GVHD involves primarily three organ systems: the skin, the gastrointestinal tract, and the liver. Risk factors for the development of acute GVHD include the degree of the human leukocyte antigen (HLA) match, a sex mismatch with the donor, a prior history of donor parity, an increased dose of total body irradiation (TBI), and the type of acute GVHD prophylaxis used.[94,95] The CD34-positive cell dose is an independent risk factor for acute GVHD after peripheral blood stem cell transplantation.[96] The severity of the intestinal condition generally parallels that of the skin and liver involvement, although profound gastrointestinal symptoms can occur without any gross skin or liver changes. Gastrointestinal GVHD involves the small and large intestines, which may result in diarrhea, nausea or vomiting, crampy abdominal pain, intestinal bleeding, and ileus. The onset or continuance of profuse, watery diarrhea 3 weeks following bone marrow transplantation is indicative of intestinal acute GVHD.

The clinical picture, when severe, includes anorexia, vomiting, buccal mucositis, abdominal pain, intestinal bleeding, protein loss, and secondary infection. High-volume diarrhea may occur, and the amount of fluid generated is an index of the extent and severity of disease activity. Extensive disease may be associated with up to 10 L of diarrheal fluid loss per day. The large stool volume may lead to distension and pain. Distension of the bowel may be exacerbated by opioid analgesics, which should be used with caution. Features that distinguish acute GVHD from the enteritis associated with the induction protocol and opportunistic intestinal infection include an erythematous, maculopapular skin rash over the palms, soles, and trunk, as well as liver test abnormalities, including hyperbilirubinemia. The patient who presents with gastrointestinal symptoms but without jaundice or skin rash represents a much more difficult diagnostic challenge.

Stool analysis and barium radiography might help the diagnosis. The stool usually contains large amounts of cellular debris and red and white blood cells. Protein loss in the stool may be sufficiently severe to lead to profound hypoalbuminemia. The absence of pathogens in the stool is important but does not necessarily rule out an infection of the gastrointestinal tract. Barium roentgenography may be helpful in the differential diagnosis and in establishing extent of disease. Widespread changes may occur, including mucosal and submucosal edema, pneumatosis cystoides intestinalis, and mucosal ulcerations.

Management of intestinal acute GVHD consists of nutritional support, maintenance of fluid and electrolyte balance, steroid and immunosuppressive treatment, and vigilance for secondary infectious complications. Common opportunistic pathogens include astrovirus, C. difficile, and adenovirus.[97] For patients with severe high-volume diarrhea, subcutaneous administration of octreotide may provide relief.[98] To improve long-term survival, doses ranging up to 2 mg/kg of prednisone, for up to 1–2 weeks, may be used. Ciclosporin may be used in combination with specific anti-T-cell monoclonal antibodies and inhibition of tumor necrosis factor α (TNF-α) is promising.[99,100]

AIDS-ASSOCIATED DIARRHEA

Acute or chronic diarrhea is a frequent complication of AIDS and may be caused by medications, opportunistic infections, or common causes occurring in the general population such as viral gastroenteritis or irritable bowel syndrome. The antiretroviral agents that most commonly cause diarrhea are lopinavir, nelfinavir, didanosine, and saquinavir. Treatment with bacterial agents may be complicated by C. difficile-associated diarrhea or colitis, but the frequency and severity do not appear to be increased by immunosuppression. Infections of the small and large intestine leading to diarrhea, abdominal pain, and occasionally fever are among the most significant gastrointestinal problems in HIV-infected patients. They include infections with bacteria, protozoa, and viruses. Among the bacteria may be those responsible for secondary infections of the gastrointestinal tract. Infections with enteric pathogens such as Salmonella, Shigella, and Campylobacter are more common in homosexual men and are often more severe and more apt to relapse in patients with HIV infection. Patients with untreated HIV have approximately a 20-fold increased risk of infection with S. typhimurium. With CD4 counts less than 200/mm^3 especially if less than 50/mm^3, acute diarrhea may represent the early stages of enteric infection caused by pathogens more commonly associated with chronic diarrhea. Common opportunistic pathogens that cause chronic diarrhea with CD4 counts less than 200/mm^3 are typically referred to as the 'big four', which are Cryptosporidium parvum, microsporidia (Enterocytozoon bieneusi and Encephalitozoon intestinalis), M. avium, and cytomegalovirus (CMV); less common is Isospora belli. Fungal infections may also be a cause of diarrhea in patients with HIV infection. Histoplasmosis, coccidioidomycosis, and penicilliosis have all been identified as a cause of fever and diarrhea in patients with HIV infection. Peritonitis has been seen with C. immitis.

In addition to disease caused by specific secondary infections, patients with HIV infection may also experience a chronic diarrheal syndrome for which no etiological agent other than HIV can be identified. This entity is referred to as AIDS enteropathy or HIV enteropathy. It is most likely a direct result of HIV infection in the gastrointestinal tract. The diagnostic evaluation is dictated by the symptoms and CD4 count. Standard screening tests for HIV-infected patients who have diarrhea that is severe, chronic, and not medication-associated includes a stool culture for enteric pathogens, ova and parasite exam times two with acid-fast stain (to detect cryptosporidia, isospora, and cyclospora), stool stain, and microscopy for microsporidia (×1000 magnification with trichrome stain), *C. difficile* toxin assay (especially with recent antibiotic use), and stool analysis for fecal leukocytes and red blood cells. Approximately 50 percent of the time this work-up will demonstrate infection with pathogenic bacteria, mycobacteria, or protozoa. Endoscopy is usually reserved for patients with severe or persistent symptoms and a negative evaluation using noninvasive studies. Endoscopy is often necessary to establish the diagnosis of CMV colitis or enteritis.

Treatment of chronic infectious diarrhea in the HIV-infected patient is determined by the severity of symptoms and pathogen. With chronic cryptosporidiosis and most cases of CMV colitis and microsporidiosis, the only intervention that is likely to be effective is immune reconstitution with antiretroviral agents. Nonspecific interventions that are commonly used and are effective include antiperistaltic agents such as loperamide and diet modification including small, frequent, bland feedings without caffeine, fat, milk, or milk products. Octreotide is often used in symptomatic treatment of diarrhea associated with HIV, however clinical evidence of its efficacy in controlling diarrhea is not conclusive.[101,102] Antimicrobial agents are used to treat specific pathogens. Cryptosporidiosis is commonly treated with paromomycin, but evidence of benefit by this or other antimicrobials is sparse. *E. intestinalis* responds to albendazole, but *E. bieneusi* causes 80 percent of microsporidia cases and cannot be treated with antimicrobials. Cytomegalovirus is usually treated with intravenous ganciclovir or oral valganciclovir, but response is modest and recurrence rates are high. *M. avium* usually responds to standard treatment, but therapy must be lifelong unless there is immune reconstitution.

MUCOSITIS-ASSOCIATED DIARRHEA

Mucositis pertains to pharyngeal-esophago-gastrointestinal inflammation that manifests as red, burnlike sores or ulcerations throughout the mouth. Stomatitis is an inflammation of the oral tissues, which can present with or without sores, and is made worse by poor dental hygiene. Gastrointestinal mucositis increases mortality and morbidity and contributes to rising healthcare costs. Mucositis is common among oncology patients. Early estimates proposed that mucositis occurred in over 40 percent of patients who receive cancer chemotherapy or irradiation. Other recent data indicate that oral and gastrointestinal mucositis can affect up to 100 percent of patients undergoing high-dose chemotherapy and hematopoietic stem cell transplantation, 80 percent of patients with malignancies of the head and neck receiving radiotherapy, and over 50 percent of patients receiving chemotherapy.[103] The pathophysiology of mucositis in the alimentary tract beyond the oral cavity is a collective consequence of a number of concurrent and sequential biological processes. After radiotherapy or chemotherapy, mucositis is heralded by an initiation phase that is characterized by injury to tissues of the submucosa.

After the upregulation of a series of early-response genes, changes are observed in the endothelium, connective tissue, and extracellular matrix that are mediated by reactive oxygen species (ROS), the ceramide pathway, and a number of transcription factors, including nuclear factor kappa B (NF-κB). Diarrhea is frequently associated with gastrointestinal mucositis secondary to chemotherapy, hematopoietic stem cell transplant (HSCT), radiation therapy and GVHD. Chemotherapy-induced mucositis and diarrhea is a common clinical problem associated with certain drugs used to treat colon cancer and other solid tumors (5-fluorouracil, irinotecan) and with high-dose chemotherapy coupled with HSCT. Irinotecan-induced diarrhea occurs in two phases: an acute syndrome (within the first 24 hours), which is mediated by acetylcholine and blocked by atropine, followed by a delayed phase, which is inflammatory.

Prevention of radiation and chemotherapy-induced mucositis and diarrhea was outlined in the clinical practice guidelines for the prevention and treatment of cancer therapy-induced oral and gastrointestinal mucositis.[104] The panel suggests the use of 500 mg of sulfasalazine orally twice daily to help reduce the incidence and severity of radiation-induced enteropathy in patients receiving external-beam radiotherapy to the pelvis. Radiation-induced enteropathy with abdominal pain and diarrhea occurs in 75–90 percent of patients receiving external-beam radiotherapy for such common pelvic malignancies as prostate, rectal, or cervical cancer and typically begins in the second or third week of treatment.[105] Oral sucralfate does not prevent acute diarrhea in patients with pelvic malignancies who are undergoing external-beam radiotherapy. Compared with placebo, sucralfate was found to be associated with increased gastrointestinal side effects, including rectal bleeding.[84,106] 5-Aminosalycylic acid (ASA) and the related compounds mesalazine and olsalazine are not generally recommended for the prevention of gastrointestinal mucositis. In randomized clinical studies it has been found that 5-ASA, mesalazine, and olsalazine were of no benefit or caused more diarrhea than placebo in patients receiving pelvic radiotherapy.[107–109]

Loperamide can be used to treat mucositis associated-diarrhea. When loperamide fails to control diarrhea induced by standard-dose or high-dose chemotherapy associated with HSCT recipients, the panel recommends octreotide at a dose of at least 100 μg administered subcutaneously twice daily. Octreotide administration during radiation and for 2 weeks after radiation was complete was associated with a reduction in both acute and subsequent chronic intestinal toxicity.[110,111]

SUMMARY

Constipation is a multidimensional clinical syndrome that requires thorough assessment and high degree of clinical suspicion. The etiology of constipation is multifactorial and involves derangement in neurological as well as endocrine factors that ultimately affect the bowel motility and function. Assessment of the patient who presents with constipation requires thorough history, including medications, associated symptoms and underlying comorbid conditions. The management of constipation involves eradicating any precipitation factors and treatment of reversible causes. Several medication classes can be used to treat constipation in the palliative care patient, and clinical judgment should be used in individualizing the appropriate treatment algorithm. Novel agents include opioid antagonists such as methylnaltrexone, the 5-HT$_4$ receptor agonist tegaserod, and donepezil.

Diarrhea is also a multidimensional and common clinical syndrome in the palliative care population. Diarrhea is generally divided into acute or chronic, secretory or osmotic diarrhea. Common causes of diarrhea include medications, infections, mucositis, GVHD and AIDS. Assessment of diarrhea requires a thorough history and physical examination as well as targeted laboratory test and radiological investigations. Treatment of diarrhea should focus initially on rehydration and correction of electrolyte abnormalities. Further management should be individualized to treat the underlying etiology of diarrhea as well as general measures such as antidiarrheal agents. Octreotide might be helpful in treatment of refractory diarrhea associated with mucositis, GVHD, and AIDS.

Key learning points

Constipation

- Common and multidimensional problem.
- Can present as atypical symptoms and frequently coexists with diarrhea.
- Requires high degree of clinical suspicion, especially in the delirious patient.
- Needs thorough assessment to determine the underlying cause.
- Multiple laxatives forms and preparations are available.
- Rectally administered medications should be preserved for short-term use only.

Diarrhea

- Common and distressing symptom.
- Diarrhea is a multifactorial and multidimensional syndrome.
- Careful history and examination along with targeted investigations are needed.
- Treatment is divided into general measures such as hydration and antidiarrheal agents and specific treatment for the underlying cause.

REFERENCES

1 Mancini I, Bruera E. Constipation. In: Ripamonti C, Bruera E, eds. *Gastrointestinal Symptoms in Advanced Cancer Patients.* New York: Oxford University Press, 2002: 193–206.

2 Derby S, Portenoy RK. Assessment and management of opioid induced constipation. In: Portenoy RK, Bruera E, eds. *Topics in Palliative Care.* New York: Oxford University Press, 1997: 95–112.

● 3 Holmes S. Use of a modified symptom distress scale in assessment of the cancer patient. *Int J Nurs Stud* 1989; **26**: 69–79.

4 Drossman *et al.* Identification of sub-groups of functional gastrointestinal disorders. *Gastroenterol Int* 1990; **3**: 159–72.

5 Collman PI, Grundy D, Scratcherd T. Vagal control of colonic motility in the anaesthetized ferret: evidence for a non-cholinergic excitatory innervation. *J Physiol (Lond)* 1984; **348**: 35.

6 Kosterlitz HW, Lees GM. Pharmacological analysis of intrinsic intestinal reflexes. *Pharmacol Rev* 1964; **16**: 301.

7 Crema A, Frigo GM, Lecchini S. Pharmacological analysis of the peristaltic reflex in the isolated colon of the guinea-pig or cat. *Br J Pharmacol* 1970; **39**: 334.

8 Read NW, Timms JM. Defecation and the pathophysiology of constipation. *Clin Gastroenterol* 1986; **15**: 937–65.

9 Wald A. Constipation. In: Yamada T, Alpers DH, Laine L, *et al.*, eds. *Textbook of Gastroenterology.* Philadelphia: Lippincott Williams & Wilkins 2003: 895–907.

10 Bruera E, Suarez-Almazor M, Velasco A, *et al.* The assessment of constipation in terminal cancer patients admitted to a palliative care unit: a retrospective review. *J Pain Symptom Manage* 1994; **9**: 515–19.

● 11 Starreveld JS, Pols MA, van Wijk HJ, *et al.* The plain abdominal radiograph in the assessment of constipation. *Gastroenterology* 1990; **28**: 335–8.

12 Kutchai HC. Gastrointestinal system. In: Berne RM, Levy MN, eds. *Principles of Physiology.* St Louis: Mosby, 1990: 352–414.

13 Goldfinger SE. Constipation and diarrhea. In: Wilson ID, Braunwald E, Isselbacher KJ, eds. *Harrison's Principles of Internal Medicine.* Toronto: Mcgraw-Hill, 1991: 256–9.

14 Pereira J, Bruera E. Chronic nausea. In: Bruera E, Higginson I, eds. *Cachexia-Anorexia in Cancer Patients.* Oxford: Oxford University Press, 1996: 23–37.

15 Skyes NP. Constipation and diarrhea. In: Doyle D, Hanks GWC, MacDonald N, eds. *Palliative Medicine.* Oxford: Oxford University Press, 1993: 299–310.

◆ 16 Portenoy RK. Constipation in the cancer patient: causes and management. *Med Clin North Am* 1987; **71**: 303–11.

17 Feldman M, Schiller LR. Disorders of gastrointestinal motility associated with diabetes mellitus. *Ann Intern Med* 1983; **98**: 378.

18 Solano FX, Starling RC, Levey GS. Myxedema megacolon. *Arch Intern Med* 1985; **145**: 231.

19 Devroede G, Lamarche J. Functional importance of extrinsic parasympathetic innervation to the distal colon and rectum in man. *Gastroenterology* 1974; **66**: 273.

20 Skyes NP, The relationship between opioid use and laxatives use in terminally ill cancer patients. *Palliat Med* 1998; **12**: 375–82.

21 De Luca A, Couper IM. Insights into opioid action in the intestinal tract. *Pharmacol Ther* 1996; **69**: 103–15.

22 Manara L, Bianchetti A. The central and peripheral influences of opioids on gastrointestinal propulsion. *Annu Rev Pharmacol Toxicol* 1985; **25**: 249–73.

23 Bianchi G, Ferretti P, Recchia M, *et al.* Morphine tissue levels and reduction of gastrointestinal transit time in rats. Correlation supports primary action site in the gut. *Gastroenterology* 1983; **85**: 852–8.

24 Daeninck PJ, Bruera E. Reduction in constipation and laxative requirements following opioid rotation to methadone: a report of four cases. *J Pain Symptom Manage* 1999; **18**: 303–9.

25 Radbruch L, Sabatowski R, Loick G, *et al.* Constipation and the use of laxatives: a comparison between transdermal fentanyl and oral morphine. *Palliat Med* 2000; **14**: 11–19.

26 Walch TD, Prevention of opioid side effects. *J Pain Symptom Manage* 1990; **5**: 363–7.

27 Rader MC, Vaughen MD. Management of the frail deconditioned patient. *South Med J* 1994; **87**: S61–S65.

28 Twycross RG, Lack SA. *Control of Alimentary Symptoms in Far Advanced Cancer.* London: Churchill Livingstone, 1986: 166–207.

29 Anti M, Pignataro G, Armuzzi A, *et al.* Water supplementation enhances the effect of high fiber diet on stool frequency and laxative consumption in adult patients with functional constipation. *Hepatogastroenterology* 1998; **45**: 727.

30 Sonnenberg A, Koch TR. Physician visits in the United States for constipation: 1958–1986. *Dig Dis Sci* 1989; **34**: 606.

◆ 31 Gaginella TS, Bris P. Laxatives: an update on the mechanism of action. *Life Sci* 1978; **23**: 1001–10.

32 Hardcastle JD, Wilkins JL. The action of sennosides and related compounds on human colon and rectum. *Gut* 1970; **11**: 1038–42.

33 Reicken EO, Zeitz M, Emde C, *et al.* The effect of an anthraquinone laxative on colonic nerve tissue: a controlled trial in constipated women. *Z Gastroenterol* 1990; **28**: 660.

34 Coogan PF, Rosenberg L, Palmer JR, *et al.* Phenolphthalein laxatives and risk of cancer. *J Natl Cancer Inst* 2000; **92**: 1943.

35 Seigers C-P, von Hertzberg E, Otte M, Schneider B. Anthranoid laxative abuse: a risk for colorectal cancer. *Gut* 1993; **34**: 1099.

36 Van Gorkom BAP, DeVries EGE, Karrenbeld A, Kleibeulier JH. Anthranoid laxatives and their potential carcinogenic effects. *Aliment Pharmacol Ther* 1999; **13**: 443.

37 Preston DM, Lennard-Jones JE. Pelvic motility and response to intraluminal bisacodyl in slow-transit constipation. *Dig Dis Sci* 1985; **30**: 289.

38 Donowitz M, Binder HJ. Effect of dioctyl sodium sulfosuccinate on colonic fluid and electrolyte movement. *Gastroenterology* 1975; **69**: 941.

39 Tolman KG, Hammer S, Sannilla JJ. Possible hepatotoxicity of Doxidan. *Ann Intern Med* 1976; **84**: 290–2.

● 40 Androsky RI, Goldner F. Colonic lavage solution (polyethylene glycol electrolyte lavage solution) as a treatment for chronic constipation: a double blind, placebo-controlled study. *Am J Gastroeneterol* 1990; **85**: 261–5.

◆ 41 Reynolds JC. Prokinetic agents: a key in the future of gastroenterology. *Gastroenterol Clin North Am* 1989; **18**: 437–57.

42 Reynolds JC, Putnam PE. Prokinetic agents. *Gastroenterol Clin North Am* 1992; **21**: 567–96.

43 Krevsky B, Maurer AH, Malmud LS, Fisher RS. Cisapride accelerates colonic transit in constipated patients with colonic inertia. *Am J Gastroenterol* 1989; **84**: 882–7.

44 Jacoby HI, Brodic DA. Gastrointestinal actions of metoclopramide. An experimental study. *Gastroenterology* 1967; **52**: 676–84.

45 Harrington RA, Hamilton CW, Brodgen RN, *et al.* Metoclopramide an updated review of its pharmacological properties and clinical use. *Drugs* 1983; **25**: 451–4.

46 Eisner M. Gastrointestinal effect of metoclopramide in man. In vitro experiment with human smooth muscle preparation. *Br Med J* 1968; **4**: 679–80.

47 Wald A. Constipation. *Med Clin North Am* 2000; **84**: 1231.

48 Brodgen RN, Carmine AA, Hecl RC, *et al.* Domperidone: a review of its pharmacological activity, pharmacokinetics and therapeutic efficacy in the symptomatic treatment of chronic dyspepsia and as an antiemetic. *Drugs* 1982; **24**: 360–400.

49 Schuurkes JAJ, Van Nueten JM. Domperidone improves myogenically transmitted antroduodenal coordination by blocking dopaminergic receptor sites. *Scand J Gastroenterol* 1984; **19**: 101–10.

50 Kaufman PN, Krevsky B, Malmud LS, *et al.* Role of opiate receptors in the regulation of colonic transit. *Gastroenterology* 1988; **94**: 1351.

● 51 Kreek MJ, Paris P, Bartol MA, Mueller D. Effects of short-term oral administration of the specific opioid antagonist naloxone on fecal evacuation in geriatric patients. *Gastroenterology* 1984; **86**: 1144.

52 Kreek MJ, Schaffer RA, Hahn EF, Fishman J. Naloxone, a specific opioid antagonist, reverses chronic idiopathic constipation. *Lancet* 1983; **1**: 261.

53 Skyes NP. An investigation of the ability of oral naloxone to correct opioid-related constipation in patients with advanced cancer. *Palliat Med* 1996; **10**: 135–44.

● 54 Yuan CS, Foss JF, O'Connor M. Methylnaltrexone for reversal of constipation due to chronic methadone use. *JAMA* 2000; **283**: 367–72.

55 Yuan CS, Foss JF. Oral methylnaltrexone for opioid induced constipation. *JAMA* 2000; **284**: 1383–4.

56 Tally NJ. 5-Hydroxytryptamine agonists and antagonists in the modulation of gastrointestinal motility and sensation: clinical implications. *Aliment Pharmacol Ther* 1992; **6**: 273.

57 Foxx-Orenstein AE, Jin J-G, Grider JR. 5HT4 receptor agonists and δ-opioid receptor antagonists act synergistically to stimulate colonic propulsion. *Am J Physiol* 1998; **275**: G979.

58 Degen L, Petrig C, Studer D, *et al.* Effect of tegaserod on gut transit in male and female subjects. *Neurogastroenterol Motil* 2005; **17**: 821–6.

59 Bruera E, Strasser F, Shen L, *et al.* The effect of donepezil on sedation and other symptoms in patients receiving opioids for cancer pain: a pilot study. *J Pain Symptom Manage* 2003; **26**: 1049–54.

60 Soffer EE, Hull T. Fecal incontinence: a practical approach to evaluation and treatment. *Am J Gastroenterol* 2000; **95**: 1873.

61 Bliss DZ, Johnson S, Savik K, *et al.* Fecal incontinence in hospitalized patients who are acutely ill. *Nurs Res* 2000; **49**: 101.

62 Johanson JF, Irizarry F, Doughty A. Risk factors for fecal incontinence in a nursing home population. *J Clin Gastroenterol* 1997; **24**: 156.

63 Wenzl HH, Fine KD, Schiller LR, Fordtran JS. Determinants of decreased fecal consistency in patients with diarrhea. *Gastroenterology* 1995; **108**: 1729.

64 Phillips S, Giller J. The contributions of the colon to electrolyte and water conservation in man. *J Lab Clin Med* 1973; **81**: 733.

65   Turvill JL, Connor P, Farthing MJ. Neurokinin 1 and 2 receptors mediate cholera toxin secretion in rat jejunum. *Gastroenterology* 2000; **119**: 1037.

66   Crowe SE, Powell DW. Fluid and electrolyte transport during enteric infections. In: Blaser MJ, Smith PD, Ravdin JI, et al, eds. *Infections of the Gastrointestinal Tract*. New York: Raven Press, 1994: 107.

67   Fine KD, Krejs GJ, Fordtran JS. Diarrhea. In: Sleisenger MH, Fordtran JS, eds. *Gastrointestinal Disease*. Philadelphia: Saunders, 1993: 1043–72.

68   Hammer HF, Santa Ana CA, Schiller LR, Fordtran JS. Studies of osmotic diarrhea induced in normal subjects by ingestion of polyethylene glycol and lactulose. *J Clin Invest* 1989; **84**: 1056.

69   Christopher NL, Bayless TM. Role of the small bowel and colon in lactose-induced diarrhea. *Gastroenterology* 1971; **60**: 845.

● 70   Shiau YF, Feldman GM, Resnick MA, Coff PM. Stool electrolyte and osmolality measurements in the evaluation of diarrheal disorders. *Ann Intern Med* 1985; **102**: 773.

71   Gaginella TS, Chadwick VS, Debongnie JC, et al. Perfusion of rabbit colon with ricinoleic acid: dose-related mucosal injury, fluid secretion, and increased permeability. *Gastroenterology* 1977; **73**: 95.

72   Blaser MJ, Smith PD, Ravdin JI, et al, eds. *Infections of the Gastrointestinal Tract*. New York: Raven Press, 1994.

73   Sartor RB, Powell DW. Mechanisms of diarrhea in intestinal inflammation and hypersensitivity. In: Field M, ed. *Diarrheal Diseases*. New York: Elsevier, 1991: 75.

74   Mead PS, Slutsker L, Dietz V, et al. Food-related illness and death in the United States. *Emerg Infect Dis* 1999; **5**: 607.

◆ 75   Fine KD, Schiller LR. AGA technical review on the evaluation and management of chronic diarrhea. *Gastroenterology* 1999; **116**: 1464.

76   Schiller LR. Diarrhea. *Med Clin North Am* 2000; **84**: 1259.

77   Rhoads JM, Powell DW. Diarrhea. In: Walker WA, Durie PR, Hamilton JR, eds. *Pediatric Gastrointestinal Disease*. Toronto: BC Decker.

● 78   Harris JC, DuPont HL, Hornick RB. Fecal leukocytes in diarrheal illness. *Ann Intern Med* 1972; **76**: 697.

79   Savola KL, Baron EJ, Tompkins LS, Passaro DJ. Fecal leukocyte stain has diagnostic value for outpatients but not inpatients. *J Clin Microbiol* 2001; **39**: 266.

80   Herbert ME. Medical myth: Measuring white blood cells in the stools is useful in the management of acute diarrhea. *West J Med* 2000; **172**: 414.

81   Horton KM, Corl FM, Fishman EK. CT evaluation of the colon: inflammatory disease. *Radiographics* 2000; **20**: 399.

82   Ishizuka S, Ito S, Kasai T, Hara H. Dietary sugar beet fiber ameliorates diarrhea as an acute gamma-radiation injury in rats. *Radiat Res* 2000; **154**: 261–7.

● 83   Cascinu S, Bichisao E, Amadori D, et al. High dose loperamide in the treatment of 5-fluorouracil-induced diarrhea in colorectal cancer patients. *Support Care Cancer* 2000; **8**: 65–7.

84   Martenson JA, Bollinger JW, Sloan JA, et al. Sucralfate in the prevention of treatment induced diarrhea in patients receiving pelvic radiation therapy: a North Central Cancer Treatment Group Phase III double blind placebo-controlled trial. *J Clin Oncol* 2000; **18**: 1239–45.

85   Earnest DL, Trier JS. Radiation enteritis and colitis. In: Sleisenger MH, Fordtran JS, eds. *Gastrointestinal Disease*. Philadelphia: Saunders, 1993: 1257–69.

86   Lenfers BH, Loeffler TM, Droege CM, Hausamen TU. Substantial activity of budesonide in patients with irinotecan (CPT-11) and 5-fluorouracil induced diarrhea and failure of loperamide treatment. *Ann Oncol* 1999; **10**: 1251–3.

87   Vetel JM, Berard H, Fretault N, Lecomte JM. Comparison of racecadotril and loperamide in adults with acute diarrhea. *Aliment Pharmacol Ther* 1999; **13**: 21–6.

88   Fried M. Octreotide in the management of refractory diarrhea. *Digestion* 1999; **60**(suppl. 2): 42–6.

89   Harris AG. Octreotide in the treatment of disorders of gastrointestinal tract. *Drugs* 1992; **4**(suppl 3): 1–54.

● 90   Simon DM, Cello JP, Valenzuela J, et al. Multicenter trial of octreotide in patients with refractory acquired immunodeficiency syndrome-associated diarrhea. *Gastroenterology* 1995; **108**: 1753.

91   Pirelli NJ, Rodriguez-Bias M, Frustum Y, et al. Bowel rest, intravenous hydration, and continuous high dose infusion of octreotide acetate for the treatment of chemotherapy-induced diarrhea in patients with colorectal carcinoma. *Cancer* 1993; **72**: 1543–6.

92   Dean AP, Reed WD. Diarrhea, an unrecognized hazard of celiac plexus block. *Aust N Z J Med* 1991; **21**: 47–8.

◆ 93   Mercadante S. The role of octreotide in palliative care. *J Pain Symptom Manage* 1994; **9**: 406–11.

94   Nash RA, Peep MS, Sorb R, et al. Acute graft-versus-host disease: analysis of risk factors after allogeneic marrow transplantation and prophylaxis with cyclosporine and methotrexate. *Blood* 1992; **80**: 1838–45.

95   Weider D, Hake R, Blazer B, et al. Risk factors for acute graft-versus-host disease in histocompatible donor bone marrow transplantation. *Transplantation* 1991; **51**: 1197–203.

96   Przepiorka D, Smith TL, Folloder J, et al. Risk factors for acute graft-versus-host disease after allogeneic blood stem cell transplantation. *Blood* 1999; **94**: 1465–70.

97   Cox GJ, Matsui SM, Lo RS, et al. Etiology and outcome of diarrhea after marrow transplantation: a prospective study. *Gastroenterology* 1994; **17**: 1398.

98   Ippoliti C, Champlin R, Bugazia N. Use of octreotide in the symptomatic management of diarrhea induced by graft-versus-host disease in patients with hematological malignancies. *J Clin Oncol* 1997; **15**: 3350–4.

99   Brown GR, Lindberg G, Meddings J, et al. Tumor necrosis factor inhibitor ameliorates murine intestinal graft-versus-host disease. *Gastroenterology* 1999; **116**: 593.

● 100   Kornblau S, Benson AB, Catalano R, et al. Management of cancer treatment-related diarrhea. Issues and therapeutic strategies. *J Pain Symptom Manage* 2000; **19**: 118–29.

101   Kotler DP. Octreotide therapy for human immunodeficiency virus–associated diarrhea: pitfalls in drug development. *Gastroenterology* 1995; **108**: 1939.

● 102   Cello JP, Grendell JH, Bausk P, et al. Effect of octreotide in refractory AIDS-associated diarrhea: a prospective, multicenter clinical trial. *Ann Intern Med* 1991; **115**: 705–10.

● 103   Pico JL, Avila-Garavito A, Naccache P. Mucositis: its occurrence, consequences, and treatment in the oncology setting. *Oncologist* 1998; **3**: 446–51.

✱ 104   Rubenstein EB, Peterson DE, Schubert M, et al. Clinical practice guidelines for the prevention and treatment of cancer therapy-induced oral and gastrointestinal mucositis. *Cancer* 2004; **100**: 2026–46.

● 105   Kilic D, Egehan I, Ozenirler S, Dursun A. Double-blinded, randomized, placebo-controlled study to evaluate the effectiveness of sulphasalazine in preventing acute gastrointestinal complications due to radiotherapy. *Radiother Oncol* 2000; **57**: 125–1.

106   Kneebone A, Mameghan H, Bolin T, *et al.* The effect of oral sucralfate on the acute proctitis associated with prostate radiotherapy: a double-blind, randomized trial. *Int J Radiat Oncol Biol Phys* 2001; **51**: 628–35.

107   Baughan CA, Canney PA, Buchanan RB, Pickering RM. A randomized trial to assess the efficacy of 5-aminosalicylic acid for the prevention of radiation enteritis. *Clin Oncol (R Coll Radiol)* 1993; **5**: 19–24.

108   Resbeut M, Marteau P, Cowen D, *et al.* A randomized double blind placebo controlled multicenter study of mesalazine for the prevention of acute radiation enteritis. *Radiother Oncol* 1997; **44**: 59–63.

109   Martenson JA Jr., Hyland G, Moertel CG, *et al.* Olsalazine is contraindicated during pelvic radiation therapy: results of a double-blind, randomized clinical trial. *Int J Radiat Oncol Biol Phys* 1996; **35**: 299–303.

110   Gebbia V, Carreca I, Testa A, *et al.* Subcutaneous octreotide versus oral loperamide in the treatment of diarrhea following chemotherapy. *Anticancer Drugs* 1993; **4**: 443–5.

111   Wang J, Zheng H, Sung CC, Hauer-Jensen M. The synthetic somatostatin analogue, octreotide, ameliorates acute and delayed intestinal radiation injury. *Int J Radiat Oncol Biol Phys* 1999; **45**: 1289–96.

Malignant ascites

JEREMY KEEN

INTRODUCTION

A survey of Canadian physicians and their management of malignant ascites produced comments such as 'generally impossible to manage', 'it is a frustrating clinical situation', and 'a practical and effective solution is needed'.[1]

This chapter will aim to review briefly the pathophysiology of ascites formation in malignant disease and then to examine the prevalence, associated symptoms and, in more detail, the reported methods of clinical management. The main frustrations in the management of ascites relate to questions such as the role of diuretic therapy, imaging and the method of paracentesis, each of which remain poorly tested in formal trials. However, new work in the pathophysiology of ascites formation may lead to more individualized and novel methods of management.

INCIDENCE/PREVALENCE

Problems related to the presence of malignant ascites are present in 3.6–6 percent of patients admitted to palliative care units.[2,3] Malignant ascites is most frequently associated with a primary diagnosis of ovarian carcinoma and less frequently with endometrial, breast, colonic, gastric, pancreatic, or unknown primary carcinoma.[4–6] The presence of ascites is usually an indicator of advanced disease and, unfortunately, is detectable at the time of initial diagnosis in over half of the patients in whom it develops.[7] Patients with ovarian cancer, however, do have a longer mean survival from the time of development of ascites compared with those with other malignancies.[6] This may relate to ascites being a complication of relatively early stage ovarian cancer

and its relative sensitivity to cytotoxic chemotherapy. However, in one study of patients with stage III and IV disease receiving chemotherapy, the presence of ascites at the start of treatment reduced 5-year survival from 46 percent to 5 percent.[8] In another study of debulking surgery for patients with stage IV disease the presence of ascites was the only independent predictive factor for early tumor progression.[9] Control of ascites often requires repeated inpatient episodes that, in one recent series of patients with ovarian cancer, showed a rapid increase in frequency over the last year of life to a median of seven admissions in the last 3 months.[10]

SYMPTOMS

Symptoms requiring palliation relate to increased intra-abdominal pressure; discomfort of the abdominal wall, dyspnea, anorexia, early satiety, nausea and vomiting, esophageal reflux, poor mobility, insomnia related to general discomfort, pain in the groins and subcostal regions, and lower limb edema (Table 61.1). Abdominal compartment syndrome with resultant multisystem failure has also been recently

Table 61.1 *Malignant ascites in 1000 consecutive admissions to St Columba's Hospice (January 1, 1997 to October 16, 1999)*

No of admissions with ascites	36 (3.6% of all admissions)
With visceral pain	15 (42% of those with ascites)
With nausea	13 (36%)
With dyspnea	9 (25%)
With pain, nausea, and dyspnea	3 (8%)

reported.[11] Easily overlooked can be the significant negative effect of abdominal distension on body image.

PATHOPHYSIOLOGY

The accumulation of ascites is a result of an imbalance in the normal state of influx and efflux of fluid from the peritoneal cavity. The absorption of radiolabeled serum albumin after intraperitoneal injection has been measured in humans to be 4–5 mL/h.[12] Drainage of peritoneal fluid occurs via the lymphatic system with the open-ended diaphragmatic lymphatics probably providing the major pathway.

A decreased rate of fluid efflux may occur as a result of blockage of the lymphatic system by tumor and this has been shown histologically in association with malignant ascites in animal models.[13] In human subjects, one study demonstrated that 32 of 38 patients with malignant ascites showed no lymphatic absorption of radiolabeled sulfur colloid that had been injected into the peritoneum.[14] Conversely 13 of 14 control subjects with either no ascites or nonmalignant ascites did demonstrate lymphatic uptake of the colloid. It is unlikely that a reduced rate of fluid efflux alone is sufficient to cause the accumulation of massive amounts of ascitic fluid. Indeed, the rate of efflux has been shown to increase as ascites accumulates and intra abdominal pressure increases, possibly up to rates approaching 80 mL/h.[15]

The rate of fluid influx into the peritoneal space may be increased in malignancy as a result of two distinct mechanisms. Each mechanism will result in ascitic fluid of different biochemical properties and may respond to different modes of treatment.

1 Increased hepatic venous pressure, as an anatomical consequence of multiple hepatic metastases, or single large (sometimes benign) tumors causing a Budd–Chiari syndrome.[16] An increase in venous pressure results in both fluid leakage into the peritoneum from the sinusoids and, via an increase in plasma renin concentration, to the retention of salt and water by the kidneys. The ascitic fluid resulting from this mechanism is similar to that seen as a result of cirrhosis and has the properties of a transudate.

2 An exudate of relatively high protein concentration may be produced as a result of increased vascular permeability. Tumor neovasculature is thought to be intrinsically leaky, allowing extravasation of fluid, and from peritoneal tumor deposits would contribute to ascites formation. However it has long been recognized that ascitic fluid also arises from areas of peritoneum unaffected by tumor.[15] Beecham and colleagues observed marked neovascularization of the parietal peritoneum in patients with malignant ascites and ovarian carcinoma.[17]

In rats there appears to be an increase in permeability of peritoneal capillaries after cell-free malignant ascitic fluid is infused intraperitoneally.[7] The permeability of normal microvessels, such as those which line the peritoneal cavity, can be increased by a variety of cytokines including transforming growth factors α and β, epidermal growth factor and vascular endothelial growth factor (VEGF).[18] Cytokines may be secreted by tumor cells and/or inflammatory monocytes and macrophages.

VEGF is expressed by the normal ovary during phases of follicular development and corpora lutea formation[19] and, in one series, the degree of tumor expression was related to patient survival.[20] VEGF not only increases capillary permeability but also stimulates angiogenesis, facilitating tumor growth and also, potentially, the observed neovascularization of normal peritoneum. Animal experiments have demonstrated a significant relation between the degree of tumor cell expression of VEGF and observed levels of angiogenesis and ascites production.[21,22] VEGF has been detected in high concentrations in malignant as opposed to nonmalignant ascites and associated with metastases from a variety of primary sites.[23–25] The exception has been the observation of high levels of VEGF in ovarian hyperstimulation syndrome, also associated with ascites formation.[26] The potential for therapeutic interventions that target the production or actions of VEGF will be discussed below.

In an individual patient, the relative contribution of these two principal mechanisms of ascitic fluid production can be estimated from the calculation of the serum–ascites albumin gradient. The serum–ascites gradient is calculated by subtracting the albumin concentration of the ascitic fluid from that within a serum specimen obtained on the same day. The gradient correlates with the portal venous pressure and a value of ≥11 g/L is indicative of a transudate and the presence of portal hypertension.[27] This may be of importance in assessing the likelihood of response to diuretic therapy with an aldosterone antagonist.

The formation of chylous ascites is a complication of retroperitoneal tumor spread or its treatment and arises either from damage to lymphatic vessels or through obstruction of lymphatic flow through lymph nodes or the pancreas.

DIAGNOSIS

The diagnosis of the presence of ascites in an individual is usually straightforward, relying on relevant clinical history and examination.[28] Where there is doubt, usually with typical symptoms present in a patient with an obese abdomen or with potential bowel obstruction, ultrasound examination can detect as little as 100 mL of free fluid in the peritoneum.[29] Computed tomography is equally as accurate but not always as easily available as ultrasound. Plain abdominal X-rays may be helpful not only in excluding signs suggestive of bowel obstruction but also positive signs of ascites such as a 'ground glass' appearance, loss of psoas shadows and organ definition, and increased spacing of intestinal loops. Clearly the presence of ascites in a patient with known malignancy cannot always be assumed to be secondary to the presence of intraabdominal tumor, and other causes, such as cirrhosis, congestive heart failure, nephrotic syndrome, tuberculosis, and pancreatitis which necessitate specific modalities of treatment, must be excluded.

Several tests have been proposed to differentiate malignant from other forms of ascites such as fluid levels of sialic acid,[30] telomerase,[31] β-human chorionic gonadotrophin (β-hCG),[32] fibronectin[33] or, in one study, a combination of total protein, lactate dehydrogenase, tumor necrosis factor α (TNFα), C4, and haptoglobin.[34] Such diagnostic tests may, of course, be helpful in terms of prognosis and possibly decisions regarding antitumor therapy but not as an aid to decisions about other forms of palliative treatment.

MANAGEMENT

The palliation of all symptoms related to malignant disease follows the same broad principles of totally individualized care based on the best evidence available from larger populations. Guidelines and treatment algorithms for management of problems such as ascites have been developed and are helpful[18,35,36] but the temptation is to manipulate every patient into particular protocols or guidelines and lose sight of the individual risk-benefit analyses for certain management plans.

Antitumor therapy

For the relief of symptoms resulting from complications, such as ascites, which reflect tumor activity, specific antitumor therapy should always be considered particularly for patients with ovarian or breast carcinoma. The development of ascites often complicates ovarian carcinoma relatively early in the course of the disease and is, in fact, a presenting feature in a third of all cases.[37] Malik et al.[38*] demonstrated complete clearance or significant reduction of ascites in 46 percent of patients with ovarian cancer treated with systemic cytotoxic chemotherapy. Significant response in ovarian cancer can be observed with second- and even third-line chemotherapy, so should always be considered.

Cytotoxic agents have been given intraperitoneally from as early as the 1950s.[39] There has been a resurgence of interest with the development of a hyperthermic intraperitoneal technique that appears to allow greater tissue penetration and lowers levels of drug resistance.[40] This technique has been particularly used in combination with aggressive cytoreductive surgery.[41*,42*] Chylous ascites, when associated with retroperitoneal lymphoma and a consequent disruption of normal lymphatic drainage pathways, may be expected to show some response to chemotherapy if it be first- or second-line treatment. Radiotherapy may also have a role in the relief of symptoms of lymphoma.

The success of the intracavitary instillation of a variety of agents in the control of malignant pleural effusions has encouraged a similar approach to the treatment of malignant ascites. There have been numerous small trials and case series reporting the use of radioisotopes, cytotoxics,

and more recently, biological agents and response modifiers to reduce ascitic fluid formation (Box 61.1). A recently reported phase II study found that intraperitoneal instillation of the corticosteroid triamcinolone hexacetonide resulted in a significant slowing of ascites accumulation.[43*] The effect was noted particularly in patients with an albumin serum–ascites gradient of <11 g/L. The authors postulated the effect to have been mediated through a steroid-induced reduction of the secretion of VEGF.

Box 61.1 Agents employed for intra-peritoneal instillation in the management of peritoneal malignancy and ascites

^{198}Au

^{32}CrPO$_4$

Thiotepa

Fluorouracil

Mustine

Bleomycin

Cisplatinum

Carboplatin

Etoposide

Mitomycin C

Adriamycin

Docetaxel

Mitoxantrone

Interferon α

Interferon β

Tumor necrosis factor

Interleukin-2

Radiolabeled monoclonal antibodies

Metalloproteinase inhibitors

Corticosteroids

Corynebacterium parvum

OK-432 (extract from *Streptococcus pyogenes*)

Other approaches

Initial preclinical trials with anti-VEGF antibodies, anti-VEGF receptor antibodies, and an inhibitor of VEGF receptor tyrosine kinase activity[44] have been reported to show a reduction in ascites formation in animal models. Transfection of a mutated gene controlling production of VEGF has decreased ascites production in mice.[45] Tumor necrosis factor has been found to block reaccumulation of ascites in an animal model by inhibiting the expression of VEGF mRNA[46] and an early clinical study suggested benefit from the administration of recombinant TNFα.[47*] Interestingly, a recent report of the use of the anti-TNF agent infliximab showed a reduction in levels of VEGF and angiogenesis in the synovia of patients with psoriatic arthritis.[48*] VEGF expression and associated angiogenesis has also been shown to be reduced by ketoprofen,[49] green tea,[50] and angiotensin-converting enzyme inhibitors.[51]

Matrix metalloproteinases are a group of enzymes that, after loss of normal inhibitory control during tumor development, potentiate tumor invasion and metastases. Early clinical trials of metalloproteinase inhibitors have been reported to have benefit.[52*] Octreotide, the somatostatin analog, has been suggested to have therapeutic potential for a myriad of different disorders and indeed, there has been a small case series demonstrating a reduction in malignant ascites in two of three patients treated.[53*] The physiological mechanism remains unclear although one other report does suggest a benefit to patients with hepatic cirrhosis and ascites.[54]

DIURETIC THERAPY

Diuretic therapy remains the mainstay of the treatment of patients with ascites of nonmalignant origin but the role of diuretics in the management of malignant ascites remains controversial. A recent Canadian survey of the management of malignant ascites reported that whereas 98 percent of physicians used paracentesis, only 61 percent prescribed diuretics and of these a quarter felt them to be ineffective.[1] The rates of response to diuretics in reported studies range from 38 percent[55*] to 86 percent.[56*] Theoretically, it would be expected that those patients who demonstrate raised plasma renin activity and hence increased sodium and water retention would have a greater likelihood of response to diuretics. These patients are those who tend to demonstrate a serum–ascites albumin gradient of ≥11 g/L where ascites is formed exclusively or principally as a result of intrahepatic metastases. A small study of the use of diuretics in patients with ascites and either massive hepatic metastases, 'peritoneal carcinomatosis' or chylous ascites only demonstrated a reduction in estimated ascitic volume in the group with hepatic metastases.[57] Each of the three patients in the group with hepatic metastases had raised plasma renin levels, a high serum–ascites albumin gradient and responded to the aldosterone antagonist spironolactone. In another small series 13 of 15 patients with malignant ascites responded to spironolactone therapy.[56*] Plasma renin levels were measured in only five patients but were raised in each case. There is a significant body of evidence relating to the optimum use of diuretics in ascites secondary to cirrhosis where 90 percent of patients would be expected to respond to treatment.[27] The majority of trials report the use of spironolactone, but given the long half-life of the parent drug and its active metabolites there is often a delay of up to 2 weeks before the onset of a significant diuresis. The alternative potassium-sparing diuretic amiloride has a much faster onset of action. Although amiloride is not a classical mineralocorticoid receptor antagonist it appears to interfere with aldosterone effects in model systems.[58] Interestingly, both amiloride and spironolactone interfere with the effect of aldosterone on endothelial cells. Amiloride with a faster onset of action may be a more appropriate choice for patients with relatively short prognoses or in whom early prevention of reaccumulation of ascites after paracentesis is desired. The use of a loading dose of spironolactone has not been reported and the usual regimen comprises a starting dose of 100 mg as a single daily dose increasing at 2- to 3-day intervals to 400 mg if needed and tolerated. Regular girth measurement may be a more appropriate method of monitoring response to treatment than daily weights and accurate fluid balance recordings. The response to diuretics is thought to occur, in part, as a result of a redistribution of fluid within body compartments rather than being wholly dependent on a diuresis.[59] The addition of a loop diuretic may improve the speed of response, with one study reporting a rapid initial response to the use of an intravenous infusion of furosemide during the accumulation period of spironolactone therapy.[60]

The initiation of spironolactone therapy is not infrequently associated with nausea unrelated to electrolyte imbalance. The most debilitating side effects however relate to intravascular volume depletion and include postural hypotension, uremia and, in some cases, renal failure. A proportion of patients will have a concurrent paraneoplastic autonomic neuropathy and resultant postural hypotension[61] that will be augmented by aggressive diuretic therapy. Hepatic encephalopathy is an additional potential complication of aggressive diuresis in patients with limited residual hepatic function. It is important to monitor the response to diuretics and titrate the dose to a maintenance level to lessen the chance of side effects.

PARACENTESIS

Abdominal paracentesis remains the most commonly employed modality of treatment for malignant ascites.[1] It affords quick symptomatic relief in a population that often has a relatively short prognosis and for whom diuretic therapy, if effective, may include a significant lag period and be associated with postural hypotension. The reported techniques and equipment used for the procedure are numerous and particularly amongst palliative care physicians appear to allow full expression of their creativity. The most significant differences in approach relate to the cannula or catheter used for puncturing the peritoneum, the rate of ascitic fluid drainage and the necessity or not of maintenance of intravascular volume with albumin, colloid, or crystalloid infusions.

The large experience of the potential problems associated with paracentesis in patients with hepatic cirrhosis, particularly hypotension and renal impairment, has colored the approach of many to the procedure in malignant ascites. It is likely that, in the absence of a serum–ascites gradient of $\geqslant 11\,g/L$, these complications of paracentesis are rare in patients with malignant ascites and fluid may be drained off relatively rapidly with no need to routinely administer intravenous colloid or albumin.[36] Indeed, the use of vacuum bottles allowing several liters to be removed in a matter of minutes, with apparently few complications, has been reported to be particularly useful in the outpatient clinic or even the patient's home.[62]

A study of 35 patients with ascites and ovarian cancer demonstrated a direct correlation between the measured value of intraperitoneal pressure and the severity of symptoms reported.[63*] Another recent study helps to confirm that raised intraabdominal pressure and related symptoms can be significantly relieved after drainage of just a 'few liters' over 2 hours.[64*] The group of patients reported had a mean of 5.3 L drained over 24 hours but no significant improvement in symptom relief (of those assessed) after 24 hours than that noted after only 2 hours of drainage. Indeed only dyspnea (and not discomfort, nausea, or vomiting) was improved significantly more at 72 hours than at 2 hours of ascitic drainage. It would be of interest if perception of body image had been factored into these studies.

Since symptoms can often be relieved by the removal of relatively small volumes of ascites over a short time period this is to be recommended particularly in the very frail with a limited prognosis. One to two liters of fluid can be removed simply over 30 minutes via a plastic intravenous cannula. The insertion of the cannula is simple and, if used in conjunction with local infiltration of local anesthetic, is a relatively comfortable procedure. The removal of such a modest volume is unlikely to cause symptomatic hypovolemia and the use of a small cannula for a short time is highly unlikely to cause local complications.

Clearly, however, ascites is likely to reaccumulate and should a prognosis be more than a few days then frequent recurrent small volume paracenteses will be required. Two case series and two case reports suggest that this can be achieved by a permanent indwelling catheter that allows frequent small volume drainage without the risks of large volume fluid shifts and repeated peritoneal puncture.[65–68] However, most clinicians in this situation would give consideration to the less frequent drainage of larger volumes of ascites through some form of temporary catheter. Peritoneal dialysis, suprapubic urinary bladder and self-retaining nephrostomy catheters have all been described as useful drainage devices.

Stephenson and Gilbert reported the successful introduction of guidelines for paracentesis into an oncology unit that resulted in reductions in the use of ultrasound to mark sites for drainage, the mean duration of drainage and length of inpatient stay.[36] Catheters were left in for no more than 6 hours with up to 5 L being drained and intravenous fluids only considered if patients were hypotensive, dehydrated, or known to have severe renal impairment. Patients without

peripheral edema may be particularly prone to hypovolemia. It is prudent to monitor blood pressure during the procedure with intravascular volume replenished by intravenous infusion of either colloid or plasma protein solution should hypotension develop. A low threshold for the administration of intravenous fluid should be present for patients with high serum–ascitic albumin gradient who do not respond to diuretics and are treated by paracentesis.

After withdrawal of the drain there is a tendency for a continued leakage of fluid from the drain site. This can be lessened by the use of a 'Z-technique' when introducing the catheter through the skin and then the peritoneal wall. Some operators tie a purse-string suture around the site, others place a stoma bag over the site until leakage stops, and one group has suggested the application of enbucrilate adhesive to seal the skin.[69]

Complications of paracentesis relate mainly to the potential for a relatively rapid shift of fluid between body compartments. One study reported two deaths from hypotension in a series of 109 consecutive paracenteses performed on 43 patients.[70] More likely in malignant ascites are procedural complications including bowel perforation, peritonitis, and localized cellulitis surrounding the drain site. One study reported two deaths from peritonitis in a series of 127 paracenteses in 100 patients.[12] Infection was a particular problem in a reported case series of patients with permanent implanted drains.[66] A recent series of 10 patients treated with tunneled Pleurx catheters recorded no catheter-related infections with a mean catheter survival of 70 days.[71] In this series serial serum albumin measurements demonstrated a progressive decline. However, one case report of the use of an implanted peritoneal dialysis catheter reported only one superficial infection in 17 months during which time the patient drained 1000–1500 mL of ascites twice a week.[67] Interestingly, this same patient maintained serum albumin levels despite such prolonged and frequent drainage. However, anecdotal experience would suggest that many patients feel extremely tired for several days following paracentesis and both hyponatremia and a progressive fall in plasma albumin concentration with repeated paracenteses has been recorded in some series. Patients with severely compromised hepatic function are at particular risk of hepatic failure and encephalopathy over the first 24 hours after ascitic drainage.

PERITONEOVENOUS SHUNTING

Potential problems of repeated paracentesis such as intravascular hypovolemia, hypoalbuminemia, infection, and visceral damage, and the expense, discomfort, and inconvenience of repeated hospital admissions have prompted the development of alternative drainage procedures. Peritoneovenous shunting was established in the mid-1970s[72] and remains the most common procedure performed. Shunting of ascitic fluid into the stomach[73] and urinary bladder[74] have also been reported but have presented too many technical difficulties to be useful at present. There have, however, been no randomized controlled trials to date comparing peritoneovenous shunting with repeated abdominal paracentesis.

Two forms of shunt are commonly used, the original Le Veen and the Denver shunt. Both are designed to allow drainage of ascites into the central venous system, usually via the internal jugular or femoral veins. They may be placed surgically, laparoscopically, or percutaneously with a recent study reporting no difference in performance or complication rate on direct comparison of these methods.[75*] The most common reason for shunt failure is lumen occlusion, which appears to occur more frequently during drainage of malignant ascites than cirrhotic ascites (for the control of which these shunts were first described). The Denver shunt has the theoretical advantage of a manual pumping mechanism to facilitate ascitic flow and clearance of debris. However, no statistical difference in the performance of the two shunts could be found in one comparative study.[76*]

Successful resolution of ascites and symptom relief with the use of peritoneovenous shunts has been reported in between 62 and 87 percent of patients.[55,77–80] One noncontrolled study showed, in addition, a maintenance of serum albumin levels in comparison to a progressive decrease in patients treated with repeated paracentesis.[55*] This same study measured 'quality of life' by a single question and visual analog scale and found a nonsignificant trend to an improvement with either paracenteses or shunts and no difference between the two methods of drainage. In the previously quoted survey of physicians' practice only 12 of 44 respondents had used peritoneovenous shunts and seven found them to be useful.[1] The apparent reluctance to use this method is probably a result of the significant complication rate of both the operative procedure and the ongoing operation of the shunt. There is a significant operative mortality in patients with malignant ascites quoted as 13 percent in one of the larger studies,[77] although this is less than that associated with the procedure for ascites associated with cirrhosis. Whereas this high mortality rate is in part to be expected in a frail population undergoing a general anesthetic or even local anesthetic and sedation, specific procedure-related mortality is more commonly a result of pulmonary edema. This complication of a sudden increase in fluid volume within the central venous system can be avoided, in part, by removing a proportion of the ascites (50–70 percent quoted in one study[81]) at operation to reduce pressure and hence flow through the shunt. Many centers would still advocate 'intensive' monitoring with central venous pressure lines for the first 24 hours after surgery.

Overall, complication rates of peritoneovenous shunts of between 25 percent and 50 percent are reported.[55,77,78] The most common complication is shunt occlusion, either, more commonly, from thrombosis of the venous terminal or alternatively from debris in the peritoneal end. Two studies reported alterations in laboratory measurements of coagulation parameters (increased concentration of fibrinogen degradation products) consistent with subclinical disseminated intervascular coagulation (DIC) in all patients with patent shunts.[82*,76*] Indeed, while such findings may be used as surrogate evidence of shunt patency, frank DIC remains a rare complication. The incidence of DIC is greater in patients with shunts and cirrhotic ascites possibly as a result of a higher concentration of plasminogen-activator-inhibitor in malignant ascites with consequently less potential for fibrinolytic activity.[83] The incidence of postoperative DIC can be reduced by removal of a significant proportion of the ascitic volume intraoperatively.[82] Other complications include thromboembolism, vena caval thrombosis, hepatic encephalopathy, peritonitis, and tumor seeding to the subcutaneous tissues of the anterior abdominal wall.

The potential effects of the introduction of tumor cells from the peritoneal cavity into the circulation via the shunt has been examined in a small series of postmortem examinations.[84] The study reported a variety of observations but concluded that metastases, although occurring in some patients as a direct result of shunt placement, are not clinically significant and do not alter prognosis. This is likely to be related to the short prognosis of the majority of patients who develop malignant ascites. Peritoneovenous shunts are clearly unsuitable for patients with loculated ascites and are not advised if the ascites is hemorrhagic or chylous or the patient has poor cardiac or renal function or a tendency to hepatic encephalopathy. Patients with elevated bilirubin levels have an increased risk of intravascular coagulation with shunting.[85*] Portal hypertension, massive pleural effusion, and coagulation disorders are relative contraindications.[86,87] The presence of malignant cells in ascitic fluid, if no antitumor treatment is to be given, correlates with a poor prognosis (median survival of 26 days compared with 140 days if cytology is negative) and is thus also a relative contraindication.[88] A recently reported series of patients with ascites and nongynecological primary tumors showed the best outcomes of peritoneovenous shunts to occur in patients with normal renal function and tumors of non-gastrointestinal primary origin.[89] The relatively long survival of patients with ascites and gynecological malignancies and the potential savings in terms of repeated hospitalizations for paracentesis makes peritoneovenous shunting an option to be considered in all cases.

SUMMARY

The burden of ascites as a complication of malignancy remains highly significant, particularly for the individual patient but also in terms of the healthcare resources consumed in clinical management. Despite numerous small studies of the intraperitoneal administration of various cytotoxic agents, radioisotopes, and immune/biological response modifiers, management continues to rely upon the use of diuretics, abdominal paracentesis, and peritoneovenous shunts.

There has been recent interest in hyperthermic intra-peritoneal chemotherapy. However, it is from recent studies into the pathophysiology of ascites production in intra-abdominal malignancy that new and specific ways to slow or halt ascitic fluid production are likely to emerge. In particular, the present interest in the role of VEGF in tumor angiogenesis along with the realization of the role of peritoneal neovascularization in ascites production has highlighted a possible new, specific, target for therapy. One would hope, given the high frequency of occurrence of this complication of malignancy, that there would be good levels of recruitment to large, multicenter, trials. However, surprisingly, such trials have not been a feature of research into ascites management to date.

Key learning points

Diuretics

- Most effective if serum–ascites albumin gradient is ≥11 g/L.

- Spironolactone requires high doses and does have a significant lag-time. Amiloride, a faster acting diuretic that interferes with the effects of aldosterone, is potentially useful but has not been assessed in formal trials.

Paracentesis

- Most widely used method of managing malignant ascites.

- Symptomatic relief is often afforded with the removal of a relatively small volume of ascites. For patients with a prognosis measured in days consider using an intravenous cannula to drain ascitic fluid for minimal discomfort.

- For patients with a longer prognosis, larger volumes of ascites may be drained relatively quickly without the necessity of intravenous fluid replacement in all individuals.

- Consider the use of implanted/tunneled catheters with regular drainage performed by the patient at home.

Peritoneovenous shunts

- Associated with significant morbidity but potentially useful if ascites is rapidly recurrent after paracentesis and is diuretic-resistant.

- Most useful for patients with gynecological (principally ovarian) and nongastrointestinal primary tumors and normal renal function.

- Complications can be significantly reduced if the majority of the ascitic volume is removed at the time of shunt insertion.

REFERENCES

1 Lee CW, Bociek G, Faught W. A survey of practice in management of malignant ascites. *J Pain Symptom Manage* 1998; **16**: 96–101.

2 Keen J, Fallon M. Malignant ascites. In: Ripamonti C, Bruera E, eds. *Gastrointestinal Symptoms in Advanced Cancer Patients.* Oxford: Oxford University Press, 2002: 279–90.

3 Preston N. New strategies for the management of malignant ascites. *Eur J Cancer Care (Engl)* 1995; **4**: 178–83.

4 Ringenberg QS, Doll DC, Loy TS, Yarbro JW. Malignant ascites of unknown origin. *Cancer* 1989; **64**: 753–5.

5 Malik I, Abubakar S, Rizwana I, *et al.* Clinical features and management of malignant ascites. *J Pak Med Assoc* 1991; **41**: 38–40.

6 Parsons SL, Lang MW, Steele RJ. Malignant ascites: a 2-year review from a teaching hospital. *Eur J Surg Oncol* 1996; **22**: 237–39.

7 Garrison RN, Kaelin LD, Galloway RH, Heuser LS. Malignant ascites. Clinical and experimental observations. *Ann Surg* 1986; **203**: 644–51.

8 Puls LE, Duniho T, Hunter JE, *et al.* The prognostic implication of ascites in advanced-stage ovarian cancer. *Gynecol Oncol* 1996; **61**: 109–12.

9 Zang RY, Zhang ZY, Cai SM, *et al.* Cytoreductive surgery for stage IV epithelial ovarian cancer. *J Exp Clin Cancer Res* 1999; **18**: 449–54.

10 von Gruenigen VE, Frasure HE, Reidy AM, Gil KM. Clinical disease course during the last year in ovarian cancer. *Gynecol Oncol* 2003; **90**: 619–24.

11 Etzion Y, Barski L, Almog Y. Malignant ascites presenting as abdominal compartment syndrome. *Am J Emerg Med* 2004; **22**: 430–1.

12 Parsons SL, Watson SA, Steele RJ. Malignant ascites. *Br J Surg* 1996; **83**: 6–14.

13 Feldman GB, Knapp RC, Order SE, Hellman S. The role of lymphatic obstruction in the formation of ascites in a murine ovarian carcinoma. *Cancer Res.* 1972; **32**: 1663–6.

14 Coates G, Bush RS, Aspin N. A study of ascites using lymphoscintography with 99m Tc-sulphur colloid. *Radiology* 1973; **107**: 577–83.

15 Hirabayashi KI, Graham J. Genesis of ascites in ovarian cancer. *Am J Obstet Gynecol* 1970; **106**: 492–7.

16 Sebastian S, Tuite D, Crotty P, *et al.* Painful ascites. *Gut* 2004; **53**: 1344, 1355.

17 Beecham JB, Kucera P, Helmkamp BF, Bonfiglio TA. Peritoneal angiogenesis in patients with ascites. *Gynecol Oncol* 1983; **15**: 142.

18 De Simone GG. Treatment of malignant ascites. *Prog Palliat Care* 1999; **7**: 10–16.

19 Yamamoto S, Konishi I, Tsuruta Y, *et al.* Expression of vascular endothelial growth factor (VEGF) during folliculogenesis and corpus luteum formation in the human ovary. *Gynecol Endocrinol* 1997; **11**: 371–81.

20 Yamamoto S, Konishi I, Mandai M, *et al.* Expression of vascular endothelial growth factor (VEGF) in epithelial ovarian neoplasms: correlation with clinicopathology and patient survival, and analysis of serum VEGF levels. *Br J Cancer* 1997; **76**: 1221–7.

21 Yoneda J, Kuniyasu H, Crispens MA, *et al.* Expression of angiogenesis-related genes and progression of human ovarian carcinomas in nude mice. *J Natl Cancer Inst* 1998; **90**: 447–54.

22 Zhang L, Yang N, Garcia JR, *et al.* Generation of a syngeneic mouse model to study the effects of vascular endothelial growth factor in ovarian carcinoma. *Am J Pathol* 2002; **161**: 2295–309.

23 Zebrowski BK, Liu W, Ramirez K, *et al.* Markedly elevated levels of vascular endothelial growth factor in malignant ascites. *Ann Surg Oncol* 1999; **6**: 373–8.

24 Verheul HM, Hoekman K, Jorna AS, *et al.* Targeting vascular endothelial growth factor blockade: ascites and pleural effusion formation. *Oncologist* 2000; **5**(Suppl 1): 45–50.

● 25 Kraft A, Weindel K, Ochs A, *et al.* Vascular endothelial growth factor in the sera and effusions of patients with malignant and nonmalignant disease. *Cancer* 1999; **85**: 178–87.

26 Gomez R, Simon C, Remohi J, Pellicer A. Administration of moderate and high doses of gonadotropins to female rats increases ovarian vascular endothelial growth factor (VEGF) and VEGF receptor-2 expression that is associated to vascular hyperpermeability. *Biol Reprod* 2003; **68**: 2164–71.

27 Runyon BA. Care of patients with ascites. *N Engl J Med* 1994; **330**: 337–42.

28 Williams JW, Jr., Simel DL. The rational clinical examination. Does this patient have ascites? How to divine fluid in the abdomen. *JAMA* 1992; **267**: 2645–8.

● 29 Goldberg BB, Goodman GA, Clearfield HR. Evaluation of ascites by ultrasound. *Radiology* 1970; **96**: 15–22.

30 Colli A, Buccino G, Cocciolo M, *et al.* Diagnostic accuracy of sialic acid in the diagnosis of malignant ascites. *Cancer* 1989; **63**: 912–16.

31 Tangkijvanich P, Tresukosol D, Sampatanukul P, *et al.* Telomerase assay for differentiating between malignancy-related and nonmalignant ascites. *Clin Cancer Res* 1999; **5**: 2470–5.

32 Gerbes AL, Hoermann R, Mann K, Jungst D. Human chorionic gonadotropin-beta in the differentiation of malignancy-related and nonmalignant ascites. *Digestion* 1996; **57**: 113–17.

33 Colli A, Buccino G, Cocciolo M, *et al.* Diagnostic accuracy of fibronectin in the differential diagnosis of ascites. *Cancer* 1986; **58**: 2489–93.

34 Alexandrakis MG, Moschandrea J, Kyriakou DS, *et al.* Use of a variety of biological parameters in distinguishing cirrhotic from malignant ascites. *Int J Biol Markers* 2001; **16**: 45–9.

✱ 35 Regnard C, Mannix K. Management of ascites in advanced cancer – a flow diagram. *Palliat Med* 1989; **4**: 45–47.

36 Stephenson J, Gilbert J. The development of clinical guidelines on paracentesis for ascites related to malignancy. *Palliat Med* 2002; **16**: 213–18.

37 Lifshitz S. Ascites, pathophysiology and control measures. *Int J Radiat Oncol Biol Phys* 1982; **8**: 1423–6.

38 Malik I, Abubakar S, Rizwana I, *et al.* Clinical features and management of malignant ascites. *J Pak Med Assoc* 1991; **41**: 38–40.

● 39 Weisberger AS, Levine B, Storaasli JP. Use of nitrogen mustard in treatment of serous effusions of neoplastic origin. *JAMA* 1955; **159**: 1704–7.

◆ 40 Witkamp AJ, de Bree E, Van Goethem R, Zoetmulder FA. Rationale and techniques of intra-operative hyperthermic intraperitoneal chemotherapy. *Cancer Treat Rev* 2001; **27**: 365–74.

41 de Bree E, Romanos J, Michalakis J, *et al.* Intraoperative hyperthermic intraperitoneal chemotherapy with docetaxel as second-line treatment for peritoneal carcinomatosis of gynaecological origin. *Anticancer Res* 2003; **23**: 3019–27.

42 Loggie BW, Perini M, Fleming RA, *et al.* Treatment and prevention of malignant ascites associated with disseminated intraperitoneal malignancies by aggressive combined-modality therapy. *Am Surg* 1997; **63**: 137–43.

43 Mackey JR, Wood L, Nabholtz J, *et al.* A phase II trial of triamcinolone hexacetanide for symptomatic recurrent malignant ascites. *J Pain Symptom Manage* 2000; **19**: 193–9.

44 Xu L, Yoneda J, Herrera C, *et al.* Inhibition of malignant ascites and growth of human ovarian carcinoma by oral administration of a potent inhibitor of the vascular endothelial growth factor receptor tyrosine kinases. *Int J Oncol* 2000; **16**: 445–54.

45 Huang S, Robinson JB, Deguzman A, *et al.* Blockade of nuclear factor-kappaB signaling inhibits angiogenesis and tumorigenicity of human ovarian cancer cells by suppressing expression of vascular endothelial growth factor and interleukin 8. *Cancer Res* 2000; **60**: 5334–9.

46 Stoelcker B, Echtenacher B, Weich HA, *et al.* VEGF/Flk-1 interaction, a requirement for malignant ascites recurrence. *J Interferon Cytokine Res* 2000; **20**: 511–17.

47 Rath U, Kaufmann M, Schmid H, *et al.* Effect of intraperitoneal recombinant human tumour necrosis factor alpha on malignant ascites. *Eur J Cancer* 1991; **27**: 121–5.

48 Canete JD, Pablos JL, Sanmarti R, *et al.* Antiangiogenic effects of anti-tumor necrosis factor alpha therapy with infliximab in psoriatic arthritis. *Arthritis Rheum* 2004; **50**: 1636–41.

49 Sakayama K, Kidani T, Miyazaki T, *et al.* Effect of ketoprofen in topical formulation on vascular endothelial growth factor expression and tumor growth in nude mice with osteosarcoma. *J Orthop Res* 2004; **22**: 1168–74.

50 Kojima-Yuasa A, Hua JJ, Kennedy DO, Matsui-Yuasa I. Green tea extract inhibits angiogenesis of human umbilical vein endothelial cells through reduction of expression of VEGF receptors. *Life Sci* 2003; **73**: 1299–313.

51 Yoshiji H, Kuriyama S, Noguchi R, Fukui H. Angiotensin-I converting enzyme inhibitors as potential anti-angiogenic agents for cancer therapy. *Curr Cancer Drug Targets* 2004; **4**: 555–67.

52 Beattie GJ, Smyth JF. Phase I study of intraperitoneal metalloproteinase inhibitor BB94 in patients with malignant ascites. *Clin Cancer Res* 1998; **4**: 1899–902.

53 Cairns W, Malone R. Octreotide as an agent for the relief of malignant ascites in palliative care patients. *Palliat Med* 1999; **13**: 429–30.

54 McCormick PA, Chin J, Greenslade L, Karatapanis S. Cardiovascular effects of octreotide in patients with hepatic cirrhosis. *Hepatology* 1995; **21**: 1255–60.

◆ 55 Gough IR, Balderson GA. Malignant ascites. A comparison of peritoneovenous shunting and nonoperative management. *Cancer* 1993; **71**: 2377–82.

56 Greenway B, Johnson PJ, Williams R. Control of malignant ascites with spironolactone. *Br J Surg* 1982; **69**: 441–2.

57 Pockros PJ, Esrason KT, Nguyen C, *et al.* Mobilization of malignant ascites with diuretics is dependent on ascitic fluid characteristics. *Gastroenterology* 1992; **103**: 1302–6.

58   Oberleithner H, Ludwig T, Riethmuller C, *et al*. Human endothelium: target for aldosterone. *Hypertension* 2004; **43**: 952–6.

59   Twycross RG, Lack SA. Ascites. *Control of Alimentary Symptoms in Far Advanced Cancer*. Edinburgh: Churchill Livingstone, 1986: 282–99.

60   Amiel SA, Blackburn AM, Rubens RD. Intravenous infusion of frusemide as treatment for ascites in malignant disease. *Br Med J* 1984; **288**: 1041.

● 61   Bruera E, Chadwick S, Fox R, *et al*. Study of cardiovascular autonomic insufficiency in advanced cancer patients. *Cancer Treat Rep* 1986; **70**: 1383–7.

✱ 62   Moorsom D. Paracentesis in a home care setting. *Palliat Med* 2001; **15**: 169–70.

63   Gotleib WH, Feldman B, Feldman-Moran O, *et al*. Intraperitoneal pressures and clinical parameters of total paracentesis for palliation of symptomatic ascites in ovarian cancer. *Gynecol Oncol* 1998; **71**: 381–5.

64   McNamara P. Paracentesis – an effective method of symptom control in the palliative care setting? *Palliat Med* 2000; **14**: 62–4.

65   Lee A, Lau TN, Yeong KY. Indwelling catheters for the management of malignant ascites. *Support Care Cancer* 2000; **8**: 493–9.

66   Belfort MA, Stevens PJ, DeHaek K, *et al*. A new approach to the management of malignant ascites; a permanently implanted abdominal drain. *Eur J Surg Oncol* 1990; **16**: 47–53.

67   Bui CDH, Martin CJ, Currow DC. Effective community palliation of intractable malignant ascites with a permanently implanted abdominal drain. *J Palliat Med* 1999; **2**: 319–21.

● 68   Sabatelli FW, Glassman ML, Kerns SR, Hawkins IF, Jr. Permanent indwelling peritoneal access device for the management of malignant ascites. *Cardiovasc Intervent Radiol* 1994; **17**: 292–4.

69   Blackwell N, Burrows M. A sticky tip. *Palliat Med* 1994; **8**: 256–7.

70   Ross GJ, Kessler HB, Clair MR, *et al*. Sonographically guided paracentesis for palliation of symptomatic malignant ascites. *AJR Am J Roentgenol* 1989; **153**: 1309–11.

71   Richard HM, III, Coldwell DM, Boyd-Kranis RL, *et al*. Pleurx tunneled catheter in the management of malignant ascites. *J Vasc Interv Radiol* 2001; **12**: 373–5.

● 72   Le Veen HH, Christoudias G, Moon IP, Luft R, Falk G, Grosberg S. Peritoneovenous shunting for ascites. *Ann Surg* 1974; **180**: 580–90.

73   Lorentzen T, Sengelov L, Nolsoe CP, *et al*. Ultrasonically guided insertion of a peritoneo-gastric shunt in patients with malignant ascites. *Acta Radiol* 1995; **36**: 481–4.

74   Stehman FB, Ehrlich CE. Peritoneo-cystic shunt for malignant ascites. *Gynecol Oncol* 1984; **18**: 402–7.

75   Clara R, Righi D, Bortolini M, *et al*. Role of different techniques for the placement of Denver peritoneovenous shunt (PVS) in malignant ascites. *Surg Laparosc Endosc Percutan Tech* 2004; **14**: 222–5.

76   Edney JA, Hill A, Armstrong D. Peritoneovenous shunts palliate malignant ascites. *Am J Surg* 1989; **158**: 598–601.

77   Schumacher DL, Saclarides TJ, Staren ED. Peritoneovenous shunts for palliation of the patient with malignant ascites. *Ann Surg Oncol* 1994; **1**: 378–81.

78   Helzberg JH, Greenberger NJ. Peritoneovenous shunts in malignant ascites. *Dig Dis Sci* 1985; **30**: 1104–7.

◆ 79   Adam RA, Adam YG. Malignant ascites: past, present, and future. *J Am Coll Surg* 2004; **198**: 999–1011.

◆ 80   Zanon C, Grosso M, Apra F, *et al*. Palliative treatment of malignant refractory ascites by positioning of Denver peritoneovenous shunt. *Tumori* 2002; **88**: 123–7.

81   Holm A, Halpern NB, Aldrete JS. Peritoneovenous shunt for intractable ascites of hepatic, nephrogenic, and malignant causes. *Am J Surg* 1989; **158**: 162–6.

82   Reinhold RB, Lokich JJ, Tomashefski J, Costello P. Management of malignant ascites with peritoneovenous shunting. *Am J Surg* 1983; **145**: 455–7.

83   Scott-Coombes DM, Whawell SA, Vipond MN, *et al*. Fibrinolytic activity of ascites caused by alcoholic cirrhosis and peritoneal malignancy. *Gut* 1993; **34**: 1120–2.

● 84   Tarin D, Price JE, Kettlewell MG, *et al*. Mechanisms of human tumor metastasis studied in patients with peritoneovenous shunts. *Cancer Res* 1984; **44**: 3584–92.

85   Schwartz ML, Swaim WR, Vogel SB. Coagulopathy following peritoneovenous shunting. *Surgery* 1979; **85**: 671–6.

86   Markey W, Payne JA, Straus A. Hemorrhage from esophageal varices after placement of the LeVeen shunt. *Gastroenterology* 1979; **77**: 341–3.

87   Qazi R, Savlov ED. Peritoneovenous shunt for palliation of malignant ascites. *Cancer* 1982; **49**: 600–2.

88   Cheung DK, Raaf JH. Selection of patients with malignant ascites for a peritoneovenous shunt. *Cancer* 1982; **50**: 1204–9.

89   Bieligk SC, Calvo BF, Coit DG. Peritoneovenous shunting for nongynecologic malignant ascites. *Cancer* 2001; **91**: 1247–55.

Jaundice

NATHAN I CHERNY

INTRODUCTION

In the West, jaundice in patients with terminal illness is most commonly encountered in advanced malignancy. In this setting it is generally caused by obstruction of biliary drainage, extensive hepatocellular failure due to liver infiltration by metastases, or a combination of both. Indeed, cancer-related jaundice is one of the most common causes of severe jaundice. In a recent series from Sweden it accounted for 58 of 173 sequential cases.[1] Uncommonly it may be due to comorbid conditions such as infectious or drug-induced hepatitis.

GENERALIZED HEPATIC DYSFUNCTION

Jaundice is a common feature of generalized hepatic dysfunction. Intrahepatic cholestasis involves either diffuse injury to small bile ducts or metabolic derangements in the bile secretory apparatus at the level of the hepatocyte and canaliculus. Intrahepatic cholestasis is typically not associated with ductal dilatation and is not amenable to mechanical interventions.

Cancer

Jaundice caused by primary liver cancer or intrahepatic metastases is a sign of extensive dysfunction and it is usually accompanied by other features of liver failure. Patients commonly display signs of incipient encephalopathy, ascites and have evidence of hypoalbuminemia, and laboratory findings of coagulopathy. Ultrasonic or computed tomography (CT) of the liver usually demonstrates extensive involvement of

the liver by metastases. Gastrointestinal malignancies are especially prone to spread to the liver because of its portal venous drainage. Extraabdominal tumors such as bronchogenic carcinoma, breast cancer, and malignant melanoma often spread hematogenously to the liver. Irrespective of the site of origin of the tumor, jaundice associated with extensive tumor infiltration of the liver is a sign of far advanced disease and is an adverse prognostic factor associated with a relatively short anticipated survival.[2–7] The role of antitumor therapies in this setting depends on the likelihood of anticipated response, the performance status of the patient and the goals of care. Among patients with tumors that are sensitive to systemic therapies (chemotherapy, hormonal therapy, tyrosine kinase inhibitors, or immunotherapy) occasionally patients will achieve a remission with adequate restoration of liver function to facilitate resolution of jaundice. In patients with unresponsive disease, liver failure ensues with progression until death.

AIDS cholangiopathy

Acquired immune deficiency syndrome (AIDS) may be associated with a number of biliary tract abnormalities.[8] Patients with advanced immunodeficiency may develop acalculous cholecystitis, focal distal biliary stenosis at the ampulla of Vater, or multifocal stenoses of the biliary tree which resembles primary biliary cirrhosis. AIDS cholangiopathy is strongly associated with colonization of bile with cryptosporidia or microsporidia. Patients typically describe right upper quadrant abdominal pain and often have abnormal liver test results, particularly that of alkaline phosphatase. The diagnosis may be warranted when an ultrasound examination of the gallbladder reveals edema of the wall;

endoscopic retrograde cholangiopancreatography (ERCP) demonstrates strictures and delayed emptying and may permit direct sampling of bile for pathogens. These syndromes are late complications of AIDS which, although rarely fatal of itself, indicate a poor prognosis.

Chronic graft–versus–host disease

After bone marrow transplantation chronic graft-versus-host disease may be associated with an intrahepatic cholestasis syndrome.[9] Liver involvement is characterized by mononuclear infiltration of portal tracts with obliteration of small bile ductules, similar to that seen in primary biliary cirrhosis. Intensive immunosuppression may control the graft-versus-host reaction, and if this fails, ursodeoxycholic acid may improve cholestasis; however, the cholestasis often progresses to biliary cirrhosis.

BILIARY OBSTRUCTION

Tumors may obstruct biliary flow within the liver parenchyma, at the porta hepatis or at any point along the common bile duct until the ampulla of Vater. High obstruction at the ductal confluence may be caused by cholangiocarcinoma, gallbladder carcinoma, intrabiliary metastases or adenopathy in the porta hepatis secondary to a variety of metastases.[10,11] Rarely sarcoid reaction in hilar lymph nodes has been associated with obstructive jaundice in cases of cholangiocarcinoma.[12]

Obstruction of the common bile duct is most commonly caused by cancer of the head of pancreas, ampullary carcinoma, or less commonly cholangiocarcinoma or gallbladder carcinoma.[13–15] Among patients with hepatocellular carcinoma, bile duct thrombosis is one of the main causes for obstructive jaundice, and the reported incidence is 1.2–9 percent.[16] Thrombi can be benign (clots, pus, or sludge), malignant, or a combination of both. Rarely, rupture of hepatocellular carcinoma into the common bile duct may cause a fluctuating obstruction by floating tumor debris.[17] Extensive tumor metastases within the liver may produce intrahepatic cholestasis by obstructing smaller intrahepatic ducts. Diffuse infiltration of malignant cells along hepatic sinusoids with consequent cholestasis also may occur, especially in small cell carcinoma of the lung and in lymphoma.

CLINICAL PRESENTATION

Patients with advanced cholestatic jaundice experience generalized malaise, weakness, easy fatigability, nausea, anorexia, and pruritus. Introduction of bacteria into bile above an obstructing lesion can cause ascending cholangitis; purulent infection of the biliary tree and liver. Contributing factors include high biliary pressure and stasis. In the absence of infection, however, cholestasis may be well tolerated for long periods of time. Chronic biliary obstruction, regardless of cause, eventually leads to cirrhosis with all its complications. The mechanism by which increased bile secretory pressure leads to cirrhosis has not as yet been established, but it can occur with either extrahepatic or intrahepatic obstruction.

INVESTIGATION

Clinical evaluation often yields substantial information in the assessment of the cancer patient who presents with jaundice. It is important to ascertain the tumor type and history to date, if known. The presence of pale stools is strongly suggestive of cholestasis. The abdomen is examined for evidence of hepatomegaly, ascites, and features of portal hypertension. Patients should undergo a brief mental status examination and neurological examination for evidence of asterixis.

Diagnostic evaluation

BLOOD TESTS

The diagnosis of jaundice is confirmed by the finding of hyperbilirubinemia. Serum bilirubin concentration in normal adults is less than 1–1.5 mg/dL and varies directly with bilirubin production and inversely with hepatic bilirubin clearance. A serum bilirubin value of 3 mg/dL is usually required for jaundice or scleral icterus to be clinically evident.

Other initial studies should include a complete blood cell count as well as liver function tests including activities of alkaline phosphatase and alanine and aspartate aminotransferases, albumin and prothrombin time. Both γ-glutamyl transpeptidase and alkaline phosphatase are typically elevated in patients with cholestasis; the combination of an elevated alkaline phosphatase and normal γ-glutamyl transpeptidase suggests that the alkaline phosphatase is from bone. Conversely, an isolated elevation of γ-glutamyl transpeptidase may result from certain drugs (e.g. phenytoin) or alcohol even in the absence of liver disease.

IMAGING STUDIES

Imaging studies help identify the presence or absence of intrahepatic metastases, the presence of intrahepatic or extrahepatic cholestasis and the site of obstruction if present.

Ultrasound

External ultrasound is a noninvasive test that can identify the presence or absence of metastases and determine whether the intrahepatic and/or extrahepatic biliary system is dilated. The sensitivity of abdominal ultrasonography for the detection of biliary obstruction in jaundiced patients ranges from 55 percent to 91 percent, and the specificity ranges from 82 percent to 95 percent.

Computed tomography

Computed tomography (CT) may be preferred when precise definition of anatomical structure and information about the level of obstruction are desired. Both CT and ultrasound may occasionally fail to identify dilated ducts in obstructed patients with cirrhosis and poorly compliant hepatic parenchyma or in patients with primary sclerosing cholangitis. Conversely, the presence of dilated ducts in a patient who has previously undergone cholecystectomy does not necessarily signify obstruction. To maximize lesion detection CT images should be routinely evaluated by two different window levels. A soft-tissue window (width of 300–500 Hounsfield Units [HU]) is used for the initial examination of the liver; this allows for evaluation of adjacent abdominal architecture. A second setting with a narrow window and a lower width (100–150 HU) is then used to evaluate the liver, since this setting increases contrast differences between the normal liver parenchyma and abnormalities.

Endoscopic retrograde cholangiopancreatography

Endoscopic retrograde cholangiopancreatography (ERCP) is highly accurate in the diagnosis of biliary obstruction, with a sensitivity of 89 percent to 98 percent and specificity of 89 percent to 100 percent. If dilated ducts are identified, it is generally appropriate to visualize the biliary tree directly by ERCP. The procedure involves passing an endoscope into the duodenum, introducing a catheter into the ampulla of Vater, and injecting contrast medium into the distal common bile duct and/or pancreatic duct. Choledochoscopy and bile duct brushing cytology are potentially useful techniques in the differentiating obstructions due to intraluminal mass, infiltrating ductal lesions or extrinsic mass compression applicable before and after duct exploration. Furthermore, if a focal cause for biliary obstruction is identified (e.g. choledocholithiasis, biliary stricture), therapeutic maneuvers to relieve obstruction (e.g. sphincterotomy, stone extraction, dilation, stent placement) can be performed during the procedure. It is not a benign procedure and significant adverse events occur in 0.5–2 percent of patients. Risks include respiratory depression, aspiration, bleeding, perforation, cholangitis, and pancreatitis.

Percutaneous transhepatic cholangiography

Percutaneous transhepatic cholangiography (PTC) involves percutaneous passage of a needle through the hepatic parenchyma and injection of contrast medium into the proximal biliary tree through a peripheral bile duct. It is often preferred when the level of biliary obstruction is proximal to the common hepatic duct or when altered anatomy precludes ERCP. When, however, bile ducts are not dilated, this approach may be technically difficult and it may be unsuccessful in up to 25 percent of attempts. As with ERCP, interventional procedures, such as balloon dilation and stent placement can be performed at the time of PTC.

Magnetic resonance cholangiopancreatography

Magnetic resonance cholangiopancreatography (MRCP) is a technical refinement of standard magnetic resonance imaging that permits rapid clear-cut delineation of the biliary tree without the requirement of intravenous contrast agents. This approach is superior to ERCP in interpreting the cause and depicting the anatomical extent of the perihilar obstructive jaundice, and is particularly distinctive in cases associated with tight biliary stenosis and along segmental biliary stricture.[18,19] Its greatest usefulness may be in circumstances in which the patient is thought to be at high risk for complications from ERCP or PTC. In patients with hilar tumor MRCP can be used to determine the dominant ductal drainage for the liver segments for subsequent stent placement.[20]

Endoscopic ultrasonography

Endoscopic ultrasound is a valuable imaging test for diagnosing and staging pancreatic cancer. In skilled hands it is more accurate than spiral CT scanning[21,22] or MRCP.[23] This approach is particularly useful when no visible mass is observed on routine imaging studies. In this setting it has both a high positive and negative predictive value.[21] It is also particularly useful in the diagnosis of cancer of papilla of Vater.[22]

MANAGEMENT OF BILIARY OBSTRUCTION

Symptomatic management

Biliary obstruction that is asymptomatic in a patient who has a short life expectancy does not require intervention. In many cases, however, jaundice is associated with symptoms of itch, anorexia, and fatigue. Indeed studies that have evaluated the quality of life of patients before and after relief of biliary obstruction highlight improvements in itch, anorexia, fatigue, and global wellbeing.[24]

Surgical management

Historically, the approach to obstructive jaundice has been biliary bypass surgery. In an extensive review of the literature from 1965 to 1980, Sarr and Cameron explored the role of surgical palliation for patients with unresectable pancreas cancer.[25*] In this collected series of over 8000 patients, in comparison with those who underwent abdominal exploration alone, patients who underwent biliary bypass had a lower operative mortality (19 percent vs. 26 percent) and longer survival (5.4 months vs. 3.5 months). Whether these results reflect therapeutic benefit or simply selection of better-risk patients for the bigger operation remains speculative. Nonetheless, in this review, 56–85 percent of patients who underwent biliary bypass surgery had some degree of clinical benefit; most notably relief of pruritus, improvement in hepatic function, and return of appetite. In modern studies, the mortality associated with bypass surgery is approximately 1–3 percent.[26–30]

The preferred surgical bypass procedure remains a matter of debate. Bypass procedures include cholecystojejunostomy, choledochoduodenostomy, and a choledocho/hepaticoduodenostomy with jejunal Roux-en-Y reconstruction. Some surgeons have advocated cholecystoenterostomy because it can be performed quickly, however, recurrent jaundice is more common due to obstruction at the cystic duct. A major retrospective cohort study of 1919 patients confirmed that patients who initially had a gallbladder bypass were more likely to require further surgery and that this approach was associated with a shorter median survival was longer following bile duct bypass.[31**]

Whereas surgery of this sort had previously required extensive laparotomy, in some centers bypass surgery can be achieved with minimally invasive laparoscopic techniques.[30,32]

PERCUTANEOUS DRAINAGE

Percutaneous drainage can be achieved with an internal–external catheter that can drain either externally or internally.[33–35] These transhepatic catheters are designed with side-holes both above and below the level of obstruction in the biliary tree; the tip of the catheter resides within the bowel, so that bile drains through the catheter across the obstruction and out of the side-holes into the duodenum. Even when biliary obstruction is complete, in many instances an interventional radiologist can negotiate through a stricture with a combination of guidewires and catheters under fluoroscopic guidance. With placement of an internally draining catheter, nutrition is improved, and metabolic imbalance no longer becomes an issue. Transhepatic catheters are associated with complications of obstruction, leakage, and infection.[36] Usually transhepatic biliary catheters are routinely changed every 2 months to avoid any chance of obstruction.

Recently, some authors have suggested that there may be benefit in bile replacement following external drainage. They hypothesize that impaired intestinal barrier function does not recover by external drainage without bile replacement. In a pilot experience with 25 patients bile replacement through a nasoduodenal tube was able to restore the intestinal barrier and that this was primarily due to repair of physical damage to the intestinal mucosa.[37]

PERCUTANEOUS BILIARY STENT

The percutaneous approach to biliary cannulation can be used to inset expandable metallic stents. A comparison of direct stent insertion with an approach of delayed stenting after initial drainage and dilatation demonstrated substantially less morbidity with the more direct approach.[38] In a recent series of 224 patients, there were no procedure-related

deaths and the clinical success rate within the first 30 days was 88 percent.[39]

ENDOSCOPIC BILIARY STENT

Endoscopic placement of biliary endoprostheses overcomes the stigma and care requirement of an external drain. A 1990 review of the extensive literature describing the results of this technique found that stent placement was successful in 91 percent of attempts.[40] Procedure-related mortality was 1.3 percent, and the overall incidence of cholangitis, fever, or hemorrhage was 20 percent. Median time before occlusion was 4.6 months. Median survival of patients with stents was 4.9 months. Percutaneous insertion can be employed successfully in the majority of the 10–15 percent of patients who fail attempts at endoscopic stenting.

There are data to suggest that this is a safer approach than the percutaneous route. In a small, randomized trial which included patients with distal as well as proximal malignant biliary obstruction, endoscopic stent insertion was associated with a lower frequency of complications than percutaneous insertion.[41] Although both techniques resulted in cholangitis in approximately 20 percent of patients, the percutaneous technique was associated with a higher 30-day mortality, attributed to complications resulting from hemorrhage or leakage of bile into peritoneal cavity or pleural space. In addition, the percutaneous technique resulted in discomfort at the insertion site, not experienced by the patients who had endoscopic insertion. In a study comparing the course, costs and outcome of surgical bypass and metallic stents in patients with unresectable pancreatic cancer, both procedures had high rates of procedural success and there was no difference in survival.[42***] Biliary bypass without gastric bypass was sometimes complicated by delayed duodenal obstruction. Metallic stent insertion was associated with shorter hospitalization and lower cost, but a higher prevalence of late complications. In particular, stent occlusion tended to occur in patients with uncovered metallic stents. This study concluded that insertion of covered metallic stents is preferable to surgical bypass, but, in patients with a relatively long expected prognosis, or in those with existing duodenal obstruction, biliary bypass with gastrojejunostomy may provide an advantage.[42]

Combined percutaneous-endoscopic procedures have been described for patients in whom endoscopic insertion is unsuccessful.[43–45] In this approach, a guidewire and fine-bore catheter is introduced percutaneously, and the biliary tree is decompressed. The guidewire is advanced through the obstruction, and into the duodenum. An endoscopist then introduces a stent over the guidewire. Once adequate internal drainage has been achieved, the percutaneously placed guidewire and catheter may be withdrawn.

Multiple prospective controlled trials have compared endoscopic polyethylene or Teflon stent placement with surgical bypass in patients with malignant extrahepatic biliary obstruction.[46***] The overwhelming majority of patients in the three trials had pancreas cancer, although some included patients with bile duct cancer as well. The results of all three studies are quite consistent. The two methods were equally successful in alleviating jaundice, and there was no difference in overall survival. Patients who underwent endoscopic stent placement had a shorter initial hospital stay, but a greater frequency of late complications. Occlusion of plastic endoprostheses generally is managed with repeat endoscopy and stent replacement. Exchange of endoprostheses may be done as long as duodenal intubation with an adequate endoscope remains possible, but does require a second endoscopy. Early prophylactic stent exchange at 3–6 months has been advocated, but an optimal time has not been defined. In patients whose stents have occluded but who are not candidates for endoscopic replacement, percutaneous stenting may be palliative.

Stent blockage is a major problem with Teflon catheters. Obstruction has been attributed to adherence of bacteria to the wall of the stent, resulting in the production of a biofilm that traps debris and ultimately occludes the lumen.[47] Self-expanding metal prostheses were introduced to overcome the problem of occlusion. The most commonly used device, the Wallstent®, consists of a stainless steel mesh that is mounted on a 9 Fr delivery catheter. These metal stents have a larger diameter (8–10 mm) and are not removable. They are introduced into the bile duct enclosed in a sheath which is then retracted, enabling the stent to expand against the wall of the bile duct. However, metal stents also are permanent, and much more expensive than plastic.

There have been four prospective trials in which patients with biliary obstruction were randomized to stenting with either polyethylene or metal stents[47–49,50***] and one trial in which patients were randomized to percutaneous transhepatic stenting with either plastic or metal stents.[51***] The results are quite consistent. Successful stent placement is seen in at least 95 percent of patients, and is independent of stent material. There is no impact of type of stent on survival, but the duration of patency is greater for metal stents, resulting in fewer episodes of cholangitis, and fewer total days in the hospital. In contrast to plastic stents, when metal stents become occluded, the occlusion is usually the result of tumor growth invading into the lumen around the wire that makes up the wall of the stent. These occlusions are best managed by insertion of a plastic stent through the occluded metal stent.[52]

Special case: obstruction at the bifurcation of the hepatic ducts

Patients with biliary obstruction at the bifurcation of the hepatic ducts present a difficult challenge and there is much controversy as to the importance of establishing drainage of both liver lobes in malignant hilar obstruction. Data from a retrospective review of 141 patients indicated that the longest survival was achieved with bilateral drainage, and the worst survival in those with obstruction of both lobes but drainage of only one.[53*]

Recently one group has described an approach using MRCP to determine the dominant ductal drainage for the liver segments, thus directing stent placement. In a series of 35 patients who underwent MRCP with subsequent unilateral stent deployment at ERCP jaundice resolved in 86 percent.[20]

SYMPTOMATIC MANAGEMENT OF CHOLESTATIC PRURITUS

Pruritus is the major symptom of obstructive jaundice.[54,55] It may occur with any type of liver disease but is primarily associated with acute or chronic cholestasis. It has been estimated to occur in 20–50 percent of jaundiced patients. The intensity of the pruritus varies from mild to severe. It can be persistent or intermittent and it may be generalized or localized to specific parts of the body: commonly the soles of the feet and palms of the hands.

The pathogenesis of cholestatic jaundice is complex and multifactorial.[56] Indirect evidence suggests that it may be caused, at least in part by dermal itch receptor stimulation by a bile acid, a bile acid derivative, or some other substance that undergoes enterohepatic circulation. A central mechanism, associated with altered neurotransmission in the brain has also been imputed based on observations that opioid and serotonin antagonists reduce scratching activity in cholestatic patients.

The management of pruritus in this setting is often difficult and it should involve specific antipruritic therapies along with general supportive measures.

Anion exchange resins

Anion exchange resins, which are given by mouth, bind bile acids and other anionic compounds in the intestine, resulting in increased fecal excretion of bound substances. Thus they decrease the enterohepatic circulation of bile acids. The most widely administered treatment for the pruritus of cholestasis has been the basic anion exchange resin cholestyramine but other resins, colestipol and colesevelam, are also available.[56*] The maximum recommended dose of cholestyramine is 16 g/24 h. The resins should be taken at least 2 hours apart from other medications to ensure adequate absorption of the latter. Cholestyramine is not very palatable. The most common side effects of resin treatment are bloating and constipation. It is prudent to monitor the prothrombin time during prolonged administration of these agents, because treatment may result in malabsorption of fat-soluble vitamins.

Antihistamines

Despite common application in this setting, antihistamines are rarely effective in this setting.[56]

Phenobarbital

Phenobarbital may relieve pruritus in individual patients, but its utility has not been supported in controlled trials.[57] It has sedative effects as well as effects on the liver. This drug nonspecifically increases the activity of the hepatic microsomal enzyme system by enzyme induction and it is hypothesized that it may act by enhancing the excretion of pruritogens.

Rifampicin

Rifampicin is another microsomal enzyme inducer. There are conflicting data regarding the efficacy of rifampicin. When effective, the onset of effect is relatively rapid. The usual dose is 300–600 mg/day in divided oral doses.[58–60] In a double blind, crossover, randomized short-term study that included nine patients with primary biliary cirrhosis, rifampicin therapy at doses of 150 mg orally twice a day or 150 mg three times a day in patients with serum bilirubin less than or higher than 3 mg/dL, respectively, was reported to be associated with amelioration of the pruritus of cholestasis as assessed by a visual analog scale of the perception of pruritus.[61***] The long-term administration of rifampicin for refractory pruritus is associated with occasional hepatotoxicity.[60]

Opioid antagonists

The observation that intravenous naloxone can reduce cholestatic pruritus[62,63] prompted trials of therapy with orally administered antagonists nalmefene and naltrexone. In an open label study of nalmefene 2 mg orally twice was associated with a significant subjective amelioration of pruritus, as measured by a visual analog scale of pruritus, and a significant decrease in scratching activity.[64***] Naltrexone at doses of 50 mg per day has been studied in a placebo controlled study of patients with the pruritus of cholestasis without apparent toxicity and with subjective relief of their pruritus as assessed subjectively.[65***] In a small study, some patients achieved relief with buprenorphine.[66]

5–Hydroxytryptamine 3 antagonists

Very limited data from two small placebo-controlled studies support a trial of the 5-HT$_3$ antagonist ondansetron in the management of cholestatic pruritis.[67,68]

Propofol

Propofol, at subhypnotic doses of 15 mg, was reported to ameliorate the cholestatic pruritus in a small placebo-controlled trial.[69,70]

Other measures

In addition to these specific therapies, simple measures have been recommended. Such measures include the use of emollients and mild fragrance-free soaps (e.g. fragrance-free Dove, Basis, Aveeno), less frequent bathing, wearing light clothing, and frequent cutting of fingernails.

Key learning points

- Jaundice in patients with terminal illness is most commonly encountered in the setting of advanced malignancy.

- Jaundice caused by primary liver cancer or intrahepatic metastases is a sign of extensive dysfunction and it is usually accompanied by other features of liver failure.

- Imaging studies help identify the presence or absence of intrahepatic metastases, the presence of intrahepatic or extrahepatic cholestasis and the site of obstruction if present.

- Management of biliary obstruction may be symptomatic or surgical.

- Several treatment options exist for the symptomatic management of cholestatic juandice.

REFERENCES

1 Bjornsson E, Ismael S, Nejdet S, Kilander A. Severe jaundice in Sweden in the new millennium: causes, investigations, treatment and prognosis. *Scand J Gastroenterol* 2003; **38**: 86–94.

2 Fischerman K, Petersen CF, Jensen SL, *et al.* Survival among patients with liver metastases from cancer of the colon and rectum. *Scand J Gastroenterol Suppl* 1976; **37**: 111–15.

3 Bengmark S, Domellof L, Hafstrom L. The natural history of primary and secondary malignant tumours of the liver. 3. The prognosis for patients with hepatic metastases from pancreatic carcinoma verified by laparotomy. *Digestion* 1970; **3**: 56–61.

4 O'Reilly SM, Richards MA, Rubens RD. Liver metastases from breast cancer: the relationship between clinical, biochemical and pathological features and survival. *Eur J Cancer* 1990; **26**: 574–7.

5 Hoe AL, Royle GT, Taylor I. Breast liver metastases – incidence, diagnosis and outcome [see comments]. *J R Soc Med* 1991; **84**: 714–16.

6 Hogan BA, Thornton FJ, Brannigan M, *et al.* Hepatic metastases from an unknown primary neoplasm (UPN): survival, prognostic indicators and value of extensive investigations. *Clin Radiol* 2002; **57**: 1073–7.

7 Polee MB, Hop WC, Kok TC, *et al.* Prognostic factors for survival in patients with advanced oesophageal cancer treated with cisplatin-based combination chemotherapy. *Br J Cancer* 2003; **89**: 2045–50.

◆ 8   Yusuf TE, Baron TH. AIDS Cholangiopathy. *Curr Treat Options Gastroenterol* 2004; **7**: 111–17.

9   Arai S, Lee LA, Vogelsang GB. A systematic approach to hepatic complications in hematopoietic stem cell transplantation. *J Hematother Stem Cell Res* 2002; **11**: 215–29.

10   Koea J, Holden A, Chau K, McCall J. Differential diagnosis of stenosing lesions at the hepatic hilus. *World J Surg* 2004; **28**: 466–70.

11   Takamatsu S, Teramoto K, Kawamura T, *et al.* Liver metastasis from rectal cancer with prominent intrabile duct growth. *Pathol Int* 2004; **54**: 440–5.

12   Onitsuka A, Katagiri Y, Kiyama S, *et al.* Hilar cholangiocarcinoma associated with sarcoid reaction in the regional lymph nodes. *J Hepatobiliary Pancreat Surg* 2003; **10**: 316–20.

13   Holzinger F, Schilling M, Z'Graggen K, *et al.* Carcinoma of the cystic duct leading to obstructive jaundice. A case report and review of the literature [see comments]. *Dig Surg* 1998; **15**: 273–8.

14   Hu J, Pi Z, Yu MY, *et al.* Obstructive jaundice caused by tumor emboli from hepatocellular carcinoma. *Am Surg* 1999; **65**: 406–10.

◆ 15   NIH state-of-the-science statement on endoscopic retrograde cholangiopancreatography (ERCP) for diagnosis and therapy. *NIH Consens State Sci Statements* 2002; **19**: 1–26.

16   Qin LX, Tang ZY. Hepatocellular carcinoma with obstructive jaundice: diagnosis, treatment and prognosis. *World J Gastroenterol* 2003; **9**: 385–91.

17   Chen MF, Jan YY, Jeng LB, *et al.* Obstructive jaundice secondary to ruptured hepatocellular carcinoma into the common bile duct. Surgical experiences of 20 cases. *Cancer* 1994; **73**: 1335–40.

◆ 18   Kaltenthaler E, Vergel YB, Chilcott J, *et al.* A systematic review and economic evaluation of magnetic resonance cholangiopancreatography compared with diagnostic endoscopic retrograde cholangiopancreatography. *Health Technol Assess* 2004; **8**: iii, 1–89.

19   Romagnuolo J, Bardou M, Rahme E, *et al.* Magnetic resonance cholangiopancreatography: a meta-analysis of test performance in suspected biliary disease. *Ann Intern Med* 2003; **139**: 547–57.

20   Hintze RE, Abou-Rebyeh H, Adler A, *et al.* Magnetic resonance cholangiopancreatography-guided unilateral endoscopic stent placement for Klatskin tumors. *Gastrointest Endosc* 2001; **53**: 40–6.

21   Agarwal B, Abu-Hamda E, Molke KL, *et al.* Endoscopic ultrasound-guided fine needle aspiration and multidetector spiral CT in the diagnosis of pancreatic cancer. *Am J Gastroenterol* 2004; **99**: 844–50.

22   Maluf-Filho F, Sakai P, Cunha JE, *et al.* Radial endoscopic ultrasound and spiral computed tomography in the diagnosis and staging of periampullary tumors. *Pancreatology* 2004; **4**: 122–8.

23   Ainsworth AP, Rafaelsen SR, Wamberg PA, *et al.* Is there a difference in diagnostic accuracy and clinical impact between endoscopic ultrasonography and magnetic resonance cholangiopancreatography? *Endoscopy* 2003; **35**: 1029–32.

24   Luman W, Cull A, Palmer KR. Quality of life in patients stented for malignant biliary obstructions. *Eur J Gastroenterol Hepatol* 1997; **9**: 481–4.

25   Sarr MG, Cameron JL. Surgical management of unresectable carcinoma of the pancreas. *Surgery* 1982; **91**: 123–33.

26   Proposito D, Santoro R, Mancini B, *et al.* [Palliative procedures in the treatment of non-resectable pancreatic tumors. Retrospective study of 294 cases and review of the literature]. *Ann Ital Chir* 1998; **69**: 185–93.

27   van Wagensveld BA, Coene PP, van Gulik TM, *et al.* Outcome of palliative biliary and gastric bypass surgery for pancreatic head carcinoma in 126 patients. *Br J Surg* 1997; **84**: 1402–6.

28   Shirahatti RG, Alphonso N, Joshi RM, *et al.* Palliative surgery in malignant obstructive jaundice: prognostic indicators of early mortality. *J R Coll Surg Edinb* 1997; **42**: 238–43.

◆ 29   Lillemoe KD. Palliative therapy for pancreatic cancer. *Surg Oncol Clin North Am* 1998; **7**: 199–216.

30   Kuriansky J, Saenz A, Astudillo E, *et al.* Simultaneous laparoscopic biliary and retrocolic gastric bypass in patients with unresectable carcinoma of the pancreas. *Surg Endosc* 2000; **14**: 179–81.

31   Urbach DR, Bell CM, Swanstrom LL, Hansen PD. Cohort study of surgical bypass to the gallbladder or bile duct for the palliation of jaundice due to pancreatic cancer. *Ann Surg* 2003; **237**: 86–93.

32   Ali AS, Ammori BJ. Concomitant laparoscopic gastric and biliary bypass and bilateral thoracoscopic splanchnotomy: the full package of minimally invasive palliation for pancreatic cancer. *Surg Endosc* 2003; **17**: 2028–31.

33   Born P, Rosch T, Triptrap A, *et al.* Long-term results of percutaneous transhepatic biliary drainage for benign and malignant bile duct strictures. *Scand J Gastroenterol* 1998; **33**: 544–9.

34   Tipaldi L. A simplified percutaneous hepatogastric drainage technique for malignant biliary obstruction. *Cardiovasc Intervent Radiol* 1995; **18**: 333–6.

35   Gunther RW, Schild H, Thelen M. Percutaneous transhepatic biliary drainage: experience with 311 procedures. *Cardiovasc Intervent Radiol* 1988; **11**: 65–71.

36   Nomura T, Shirai Y, Hatakeyama K. Bacteribilia and cholangitis after percutaneous transhepatic biliary drainage for malignant biliary obstruction. *Dig Dis Sci* 1999; **44**: 542–6.

37   Kamiya S, Nagino M, Kanazawa H, *et al.* The value of bile replacement during external biliary drainage: an analysis of intestinal permeability, integrity, and microflora. *Ann Surg* 2004; **239**: 510–7.

38   Inal M, Aksungur E, Akgul E, *et al.* Percutaneous placement of metallic stents in malignant biliary obstruction: one-stage or two-stage procedure? Pre-dilate or not? *Cardiovasc Intervent Radiol* 2003; **26**: 40–5.

39   Inal M, Akgul E, Aksungur E, *et al.* Percutaneous self-expandable uncovered metallic stents in malignant biliary obstruction. Complications, follow-up and reintervention in 154 patients. *Acta Radiol* 2003; **44**: 139–46.

40   Naggar E, Krag E, Matzen P. Endoscopically inserted biliary endoprosthesis in malignant obstructive jaundice. A survey of the literature. *Liver* 1990; **10**: 321–4.

41   Speer AG, Cotton PB, Russell RC, *et al.* Randomised trial of endoscopic versus percutaneous stent insertion in malignant obstructive jaundice. *Lancet* 1987; **2**: 57–62.

42   Maosheng D, Ohtsuka T, Ohuchida J, *et al.* Surgical bypass versus metallic stent for unresectable pancreatic cancer. *J Hepatobiliary Pancreat Surg* 2001; **8**: 367–73.

43 Hall RI, Denyer ME, Chapman AH. Percutaneous-endoscopic placement of endoprostheses for relief of jaundice caused by inoperable bile duct strictures. *Surgery* 1990; **107**: 224–7.

44 Tsang TK, Crampton AR, Bernstein JR, *et al.* Percutaneous-endoscopic biliary stent placement. A preliminary report. *Ann Intern Med* 1987; **106**: 389–92.

45 Wayman J, Mansfield JC, Matthewson K, *et al.* Combined percutaneous and endoscopic procedures for bile duct obstruction: simultaneous and delayed techniques compared. *Hepatogastroenterology* 2003; **50**: 915–8.

46 Taylor MC, McLeod RS, Langer B. Biliary stenting versus bypass surgery for the palliation of malignant distal bile duct obstruction: a meta-analysis. Liver Transpl 2000; **6**: 302–8.

47 Huibregtse K, Carr-Locke DL, Cremer M, Domschke W, Fockens P, Foerster E, *et al.* Biliary stent occlusion – a problem solved with self-expanding metal stents? European Wallstent Study Group. *Endoscopy* 1992; **24**: 391–4.

48 Prat F, Chapat O, Ducot B, *et al.* A randomized trial of endoscopic drainage methods for inoperable malignant strictures of the common bile duct. *Gastrointest Endosc* 1998; **47**: 1–7.

49 Knyrim K, Wagner HJ, Pausch J, Vakil N. A prospective, randomized, controlled trial of metal stents for malignant obstruction of the common bile duct. *Endoscopy* 1993; **25**: 207–12.

50 Davids PH, Groen AK, Rauws EA, *et al.* Randomised trial of self-expanding metal stents versus polyethylene stents for distal malignant biliary obstruction. *Lancet* 1992; **340**: 1488–92.

51 Lammer J, Hausegger KA, Fluckiger F, *et al.* Common bile duct obstruction due to malignancy: treatment with plastic versus metal stents. *Radiology* 1996; **201**: 167–72.

52 Kaskarelis IS, Papadaki MG, Papageorgiou GN, *et al.* Long-term follow-up in patients with malignant biliary obstruction after percutaneous placement of uncovered Wallstent endoprostheses. *Acta Radiol* 1999; **40**: 528–33.

53 Chang WH, Kortan P, Haber GB. Outcome in patients with bifurcation tumors who undergo unilateral versus bilateral hepatic duct drainage. *Gastrointest Endosc* 1998; **47**: 354–62.

◆ 54 Mela M, Mancuso A, Burroughs AK. Review article: pruritus in cholestatic and other liver diseases. *Aliment Pharmacol Ther* 2003; **17**: 857–70.

55 Bosonnet L. Pruritis: scratching the surface. *Eur J Cancer Care* (Engl) 2003; **12**: 162–5.

◆ 56 Bergasa NV. Pruritus in chronic liver disease: mechanisms and treatment. *Curr Gastroenterol Rep* 2004; **6**: 10–16.

57 Laatikainen T. Effect of cholestyramine and phenobarbital on pruritus and serum bile acid levels in cholestasis of pregnancy. *Am J Obstet Gynecol* 1978; **132**: 501–6.

58 Price TJ, Patterson WK, Olver IN. Rifampicin as treatment for pruritus in malignant cholestasis. *Support Care Cancer* 1998; **6**: 533–5.

59 Yerushalmi B, Sokol RJ, Narkewicz MR, *et al.* Use of rifampin for severe pruritus in children with chronic cholestasis. *J Pediatr Gastroenterol Nutr* 1999; **29**: 442–7.

60 Talwalkar JA, Souto E, Jorgensen RA, Lindor KD. Natural history of pruritus in primary biliary cirrhosis. *Clin Gastroenterol Hepatol* 2003; **1**: 297–302.

61 Ghent CN, Carruthers SG. Treatment of pruritus in primary biliary cirrhosis with rifampin. Results of a double-blind, crossover, randomized trial. *Gastroenterology* 1988; **94**: 488–93.

62 Terra SG, Tsunoda SM. Opioid antagonists in the treatment of pruritus from cholestatic liver disease. *Ann Pharmacother* 1998; **32**: 1228–30.

63 Bergasa NV, Talbot TL, Alling DW, *et al.* A controlled trial of naloxone infusions for the pruritus of chronic cholestasis. *Gastroenterology* 1992; **102**: 544–9.

64 Bergasa NV, Schmitt JM, Talbot TL, *et al.* Open-label trial of oral nalmefene therapy for the pruritus of cholestasis. *Hepatology* 1998; **27**: 679–84.

65 Wolfhagen FH, Sternieri E, Hop WC, *et al.* Oral naltrexone treatment for cholestatic pruritus: a double-blind, placebo-controlled study. *Gastroenterology* 1997; **113**: 1264–9.

66 Juby LD, Wong VS, Losowsky MS. Buprenorphine and hepatic pruritus. *Br J Clin Pract* 1994; **48**: 331.

67 Schworer H, Hartmann H, Ramadori G. Relief of cholestatic pruritus by a novel class of drugs: 5-hydroxytryptamine type 3 (5-HT3) receptor antagonists: effectiveness of ondansetron. *Pain* 1995; **61**: 33–7.

68 Muller C, Pongratz S, Pidlich J, *et al.* Treatment of pruritus in chronic liver disease with the 5-hydroxytryptamine receptor type 3 antagonist ondansetron: a randomized, placebo-controlled, double-blind cross-over trial. *Eur J Gastroenterol Hepatol* 1998; **10**: 865–70.

69 Borgeat A, Wilder-Smith OH, Mentha G. Subhypnotic doses of propofol relieve pruritus associated with liver disease. *Gastroenterology* 1993; **104**: 244–7.

70 Borgeat A, Wilder-Smith O, Mentha G, Huber O. Propofol and cholestatic pruritus. *Am J Gastroenterol* 1992; **87**: 672–4.

63

Bowel obstruction

CARLA RIPAMONTI

FREQUENCY AND PATHOPHYSIOLOGY OF BOWEL OBSTRUCTION

Bowel obstruction is defined as any process preventing the movement of bowel contents. Bowel obstruction may be a mode of presentation of intraabdominal and pelvic malignancy or a feature of recurrent disease following anticancer therapy. Malignant bowel obstruction (MBO) is well recognized in gynecological patients with advanced cancer. Retrospective and autopsy studies found the frequency of MBO to be approximately 5–51 percent of patients with gynecological malignancy.[1–5,6***] It is particularly frequent in patients with ovarian cancer where it is the most frequent cause of death.[3,4,6***] Patients with stage III and IV ovarian cancer and those with high-grade lesions are at higher risk for MBO as compared with patients with lower stage or low-grade tumors.[7,8] The reported frequency of bowel obstruction ranges from 4 percent to 24 percent in colorectal cancer.

Bowel obstruction can be partial or complete, single or multiple. Benign causes are reported in nearly half the patients with colorectal cancer and in approximately 6 percent of patients with gynecological cancer. The small bowel is more commonly involved than the large bowel (61 percent vs. 33 percent, respectively) and both are involved in over 20 percent of the patients.[1–5]

Several pathophysiological mechanisms may be involved in the onset of bowel obstruction and there is variability in both presentation and etiology (Box 63.1). Any mechanism limiting or preventing the propulsion of the intestinal content from passing distally induces a cascade of events producing definitive bowel obstruction (Fig. 63.1).

Box 63.1 Pathophysiological mechanisms of MBO

Mechanical obstruction is caused by:

- extrinsic occlusion of the lumen due to an enlargement of the primary tumor or recurrence, mesenteric and omental masses, abdominal or pelvic adhesions (caused either by the tumor or secondary to surgery), postirradiation fibrosis

- intraluminal occlusion of the lumen due to neoplastic mass or annular tumoral dissemination

- intramural occlusion of the lumen due to intestinal linitis plastica

Functional obstruction (or adynamic ileus) is caused by intestinal motility disorders consequent to:

- tumor infiltration of the mesentery or bowel muscle and nerves (carcinomatosis), malignant involvement of the coeliac plexus

- paraneoplastic neuropathy in patients with lung cancer

- chronic intestinal pseudoobstruction (CIP) mainly due to diabetes mellitus, previous gastric surgery and other neurological disorders. These factors may affect extrinsic neural control to viscera. Vagal dysfunction is confirmed in a majority of patients with CIP associated with diabetes or neurological disorders

- paraneoplastic pseudoobstruction

Other causes such as inflammatory edema, fecal impaction, constipating drugs (such as opioids, anticholinergics, etc.), and dehydration, are likely to contribute to the development of bowel obstruction or to worsen the clinical picture.

At least three factors occur in bowel obstruction

1 Accumulation of gastric, pancreatic, and biliary secretions that are a potent stimulus for further intestinal secretions
2 Decreased absorption of water and sodium from the intestinal lumen.
3 Increased secretion of water and sodium into the lumen as distension increases[9] (see Fig. 63.1).

As a result of the breakdown of the sequence and reabsorption in the gastrointestinal tract, there is a loss of fluids and electrolytes. The pancreatic, biliary, and gastrointestinal secretions accumulate in the bowel above the obstruction,

and the volume of secretions tends to increase following intestinal distension and the consequent increase in the surface area, thus producing a vicious circle of secretion-distension-secretion.[9] Depletion of water and salt in the lumen is considered the most important 'toxic factor' in bowel obstruction.

SIGNS AND SYMPTOMS: ASSESSMENT AND DIFFERENTIAL DIAGNOSIS

In patients with cancer, compression of the bowel lumen develops slowly and often remains partial. The initial symptoms are frequently abdominal cramps, nausea, vomiting, and abdominal distension, which usually present periodically and resolve spontaneously. These episodes are frequently followed by passage of gas or loose stools. Gastrointestinal symptoms caused by the sequence of distension-secretion-motor activity of the obstructed bowel (Fig. 63.1) occur in different combinations and intensity depending on the site

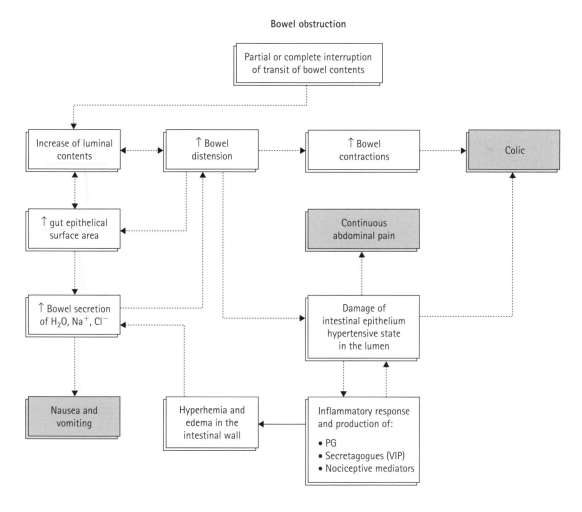

Figure 63.1 *Bowel obstruction. Distension-secretion-motor activity causing gastrointestinal symptoms. PG, prostaglandins; VIP, vasoactive intestinal polypeptide.*

Table 63.1 *Common symptoms in cancer patients with malignant bowel obstruction*

Symptom		
Vomiting	Intermittent or continuous	Develops early and in large amounts in gastric, duodenum and small bowel obstruction and develops later in large bowel obstruction	Biliary vomiting is almost odorless and indicates an obstruction in the upper part of the abdomen. The presence of bad smelling and fecaloid vomiting can be the first sign of an ileal or colic obstruction
Nausea	Intermittent or continuous		
Colicky pain	Variable intensity and localization due to distension proximal to the obstruction; secondary to gas and fluid accumulation, most of which are produced by the gut	If it is intense, periumbilical and occurring at brief intervals, may be an indication of an obstruction at the jejunum–ileal level. In large bowel obstruction the pain is less intense, deeper, occurring at longer intervals and spreads toward the colon wall	An overall acute pain which begins intensely and becomes stronger, or a pain which is specifically localized, may be a symptom of a perforation or an ileal or colic strangulation. A pain which increases with palpation may be due to peritoneal irritation or the beginning of a perforation
Continuous pain	Variable intensity and localization	It is due to abdominal distension, tumor mass, tumor mass growth compressing the intestine, intestinal distension and/or hepatomegaly	
Dry mouth		It is due to severe dehydration, metabolic alterations but above all it is due to the use of drugs with anticholinergic properties	
Constipation	Intermittent or complete	In case of complete obstruction there is no evacuation of feces and no flatus	In case of partial obstruction the symptom is intermittent
Overflow (paradoxical) diarrhea		It is the result of bacterial liquefaction of the fecal material blocked in the sigma or rectum	

Table 63.2 *Radiologic investigations*

Plain radiography	Abdominal radiography taken in supine and standing position to document the dilated loops of bowel, air–fluid interfaces or both
Contrast radiography	Helps to evaluate dysmotility, partial obstruction and to define the site and extent of obstruction
	Barium can interfere with subsequent endoscopic studies or cause severe impaction or aspiration pneumonia
	Gastrografin (diatrizoate meglumine) is useful in such cases; moreover, it often provides excellent visualization of proximal obstructions and can reduce luminal edema and help resolve partial obstructions. Contrast studies of the stomach, gastric outlet and small bowel can distinguish obstructions from metastases, radiation injury or adhesions
	The diagnosis of a motility disorder is revealed by the slow passage of barium through undilated bowel with no demonstrable point of obstruction
	Retrograde, transrectal contrast studies (barium or water-soluble medium enema) can rule out and diagnose isolated or concomitant obstruction of the large bowel
Computed tomography	Abdominal CT is useful to evaluate the global extent of disease, to perform staging and to assist in the choice of surgical, endoscopic or simple pharmacological palliative intervention for the management of the obstruction
Endoscopy	Once a site of obstruction is identified in either the gastric outlet or colon, endoscopic studies may be helpful to evaluate the exact cause of the obstruction. This is particularly important when endoscopic treatment approaches, such as stent placement, are considered

of obstruction and tend to worsen (Table 63.1). Vomiting can be assessed in terms of numbers, volume, and overall duration. Other symptoms such as nausea, pain (both colicky and/or continuous), xerostomia, somnolence, dyspnea, even sensation of hunger can be present and can be evaluated with visual analog, numerical, or verbal scales. The assessment of patients with suspected MBO should consider:

- Other causes of nausea, vomiting and constipation
- Metabolic abnormalities
- Type and dosages of drugs
- Nutritional and hydration status
- Bowel movements and the presence of overflow diarrhea
- Presence of abdominal fecal masses, distension to all the abdomen or above the obstacle, ascites as well as painful sites
- Presence of feces in the rectal ampulla (rectal exploration)

From the metabolic point of view, dehydration, electrolyte losses and disorders of acid–base balance are frequently associated with bowel obstruction. The hypovolemic state may induce a functional renal failure due to a decrease of the renal flow and, as a consequence, of the glomerular filtration. Different respiratory patterns may be observed, depending on the level of obstruction. Whereas the level is high, metabolic alkalosis, hypochloremia and hypokalemia, due to a prevalent loss of gastric secretions, determine hypoventilation. If the level of obstruction is distal, the secondary deficit is global including chlorum, sodium, potassium, bicarbonates owning to intestinal stasis of biliary, pancreatic, intestinal as well as gastric secretions. The dehydration

reflects the accumulation of fluids and electrolytes in the third space. With a low level of obstruction, including ileum or colon, acidosis prevails due to ischemic lesions or septic complications.

The diagnosis of intestinal obstruction is established or suspected on clinical grounds and usually confirmed with abdominal radiographs demonstrating air–fluid levels. Table 63.2 shows the possible radiological investigations that might be performed in patients with symptoms and signs of bowel obstruction. However, there is no point in proceeding with any of these if the patient is too ill or has declined surgery.

MANAGEMENT OF BOWEL OBSTRUCTION: THERAPEUTIC APPROACHES

The management of patients with malignant bowel obstruction is one of the greatest challenges for physicians who care for patients with cancer. This management has to be highly individualized according to the stage of the illness, the prognosis, the possibility of further antineoplastic therapies, and the general status and choices of the patients.

In the face of a clearly incurable situation, significant patient discomfort and suffering must be balanced with the need to simplify the care of those patients with a short time to live. A multidisciplinary working group of the European Association for Palliative Care reviewed issues regarding bowel obstruction, and published clinical practice recommendations for the management of MBO in patients with end-stage cancer.[5]

Surgery

Surgery remains the primary treatment in these patients. Palliative surgery is usually considered when relief from symptoms due to bowel obstruction is not obtained within 48–72 hours after decompression with a nasogastric tube has been implemented.[4] In advanced cancer patients, however, guidelines for conservative vs. surgical treatment are still unresolved. Published data show that, in advanced cancer, the operative mortality is 30–40 percent and complication rates vary from 27 percent to 90 percent. The type of obstruction (partial vs. complete) and the method of surgical treatment (bypass vs. resection and reanastomosis) has no significant effect on the outcome. As recently published results are no better than those published in the past, improvements in surgical techniques and perioperative care appear not to influence the outcome. Not all patients are fit for surgery. According to different authors, the rate of inoperable patients ranges from 6.2 percent to 50 percent.[1–5]

Several authors have emphasized that prognostic criteria are needed to help doctors select patients who are likely to benefit from surgical intervention. The available data suggesting the poor prognostic factors are shown in Box 63.2.[1–5] Surgical palliation in advanced cancer patients is a complex issue, and the decision to proceed with surgery must be carefully evaluated for each individual patient.

Box 63.2 Prognostic indicators of low likelihood of clinical benefit from surgery of MBO

- Obstruction secondary to cancer
- Intestinal motility problems due to diffuse intraperitoneal carcinomatosis*
- Widespread tumor†
- Patients over 63 years in association with cachexia†
- Ascites requiring frequent paracentesis*
- Low serum albumin level and low serum prealbumin level
- Previous radiotherapy of the abdomen or pelvis†
- Poor nutritional status†
- Diffuse palpable intraabdominal masses*
- Liver metastases, distant metastases, pleural effusion or pulmonary metastases producing dyspnea†
- Multiple partial bowel obstruction with prolonged passage time on radiograph examination*
- Elevated blood urea nitrogen levels, elevated alkaline phosphatase levels, advanced tumor stage, short diagnosis to obstruction interval†
- Poor performance status†
- A recent laparotomy which demonstrated that further corrective surgery was not possible*
- Previous abdominal surgery which showed diffuse metastatic cancer*
- Involvement of proximal stomach*
- Extraabdominal metastases producing symptoms difficult to control (e.g. dyspnea)†

Data from retrospective studies. * Absolute and † relative contraindications to surgery

Modified from Ripamonti *et al.* Clinical-practice recommendations for the management of bowel obstruction in patients with end-stage cancer. *Support Care Cancer* 2001; **19**: 23–34.[5]

Venting procedures

In inoperable patients, the usual treatment consists of drainage using a **nasogastric suction associated with parenteral hydration**. This treatment decompresses the stomach and/or intestine, and corrects fluid and electrolyte imbalance before surgery, or while a decision is being made. The tube often becomes occluded and requires flushing and/or replacement. During long-term drainage, a nasogastric tube can interfere with coughing for clearing pulmonary secretions and may be associated with nasal cartilage erosion, otitis media, aspiration pneumonia, esophagitis, and bleeding. This treatment can also create discomfort in patients who are already distressed by previous anticancer and surgical therapies. Long-term use of nasogastric tube should only be considered when pharmacological therapy for symptom control is ineffective or when gastrostomy cannot be carried out.[1–3]

The **percutaneous endoscopically placed gastrostomy (PEG) tube**, initially developed for enteral feeding, has been recently used effectively for intractable vomiting due to obstruction of the upper gastrointestinal tract.[10,11] In PEG, a tube is inserted at the stomach, through the abdominal wall, under endoscopic, ultrasonographic, or fluoroscopic guidance.[11,12] This procedure can easily conducted under mild sedation and local anesthetics. Gastrostomy drainage allows for nausea and vomiting control in 83–93 percent of patients.[13–16] It is a much more acceptable method for longer term decompression of an obstructed gastrointestinal tract than a nasogastric tube. Intermittent decompression allows patients to continue to eat and drink small quantities and to maintain an active lifestyle without the physical and psychological distress associated with the presence of the nasogastric tube. A decompressive gastrostomy must be avoided in patients with portal hypertension, large volume of ascites, and those at risk for systemic bleeding. Relative contraindications include previous multiple abdominal surgeries, carcinomatosis, adhesions, colostomies, and abdominal ulcers that are open and infected. Occasionally a decompressive gastrostomy can end up being useful for feeding if the patient is able to resume intestinal transit.[17] Decompressive tube esophagostomy is an under-utilized, minimally invasive alternative in patients with complete, irreversible upper gastrointestinal tract obstruction.[18]

Self-expanding metallic stents

In recent years there has been a growing experience in the use of expandable metallic stents in the management of bowel obstructions in the gastric outlet, proximal small bowel and colon. The goal is to convert an emergent procedure to a safer, elective operation and one that can be curative.[19]

These stents may be useful in the management of patients with advanced metastatic disease, who are at poor surgical risk or in those presenting with large bowel obstruction in which decompression by a stent allows treatment of coexisting medical complications to enable surgery to be carried out at a later date, after staging of the disease and optimal colonic preparation.[20] This technique can be palliative or can serve as an adjunct to curative resection.

Malignant duodenal obstruction is most commonly secondary to neoplastic invasion but more frequently due to extrinsic compression from carcinoma of the head of the pancreas or from compression by lymphadenopathy. In patients unfit for general anesthesia and/or surgery or in patients unfit for laparoscopic drainage procedure such as gastroenterostomy because of ascites and/or peritoneal metastases, internal stenting of the lesion may be indicated. Flexible, self-expanding metallic stents may be inserted using radiological or endoscopic techniques. The major limiting factor using the endoscopic technique is the inability to pass the endoscope through the stricture. Several authors report relief of malignant gastric and/or duodenal obstruction in the majority of patients treated by peroral[21–23] or percutaneous insertion of a metal stent.[24–26] Most patients had an immediate benefit and were able to eat small amounts of food without vomiting. No recurrence of gastric outlet obstruction was noted in the follow-up period of 1–5 months.[23–25]

As with any procedure, complications are possible. The major complications reported were gastric ulceration, bowel perforation after balloon dilatation of the stent and stent migration. Contraindications for the position of self-expanding stent are the presence of multiple stenoses, peritoneal carcinomatosis located distally in the small bowel that may be undiagnosed at the preprocedural opacification because of the severity of the duodenal stenosis. Failure to relieve the obstruction may be secondary to an inability to cross the stricture, incomplete opening of the stent or stent malposition that fails to traverse the entire stricture. In this case it is necessary to apply additional stents across the remaining obstruction.

Seventy percent of colon and rectal cancers are left sided and are considered accessible to stent placement.[19] Positive results have been reported by various authors after insertion of colonic stents in colorectal obstruction.[19,20,27–29] Complications, which potentially include perforation, bleeding and stent migration, have been reported in less than 3 percent of cases[19, 27–29] and only in few patients treated with self-expanding mesh stents was there a recurrent obstruction due to tumor ingrowth.[30] Temporary incontinence may be observed.[30]

Normal bowel contractions could cause stent migration especially if the stent diameter is too small, if the stent length is too short, or if the stent is placed too distal in the lesion. The migration into the rectal ampulla can result in obstruction and in painful spasm. Canon et al.[31] stated that before a patient is selected as a candidate for having an expandable metal stent placed in the colon, three factors were determined:

- location of the lesion within the colon
- length of the tumor
- presence or absence of a synchronous carcinoma.

Thus, meticulous evaluation of the digestive tract downstream is mandatory to avoid pointless stent placement. The usefulness of metallic stents in patients with end-stage cancer has not yet been formally evaluated. Further studies are necessary to identify those patients with advanced and terminal cancer and MBO who may have some benefit in terms of symptom control and quality of life after these procedures.

Pharmacological management

The pharmacological management of bowel obstruction due to advanced cancer focuses on the treatment of nausea, vomiting, pain and other symptoms without the use of a nasogastric tube. If a central venous catheter has been previously inserted, this can be used to administer drugs for symptom control. Continuous subcutaneous infusion of drugs using a portable syringe driver allows the parenteral administration of different drug combinations, produces minimal discomfort for the patient, and is easy to use in a home setting.

Drug therapy comprising analgesics, antisecretory drugs, and antiemetics, without using a nasogastric tube, was first described by Baines et al.[32] Several authors have confirmed the efficacy of this approach.[1–5] Medications should be tailored to each patient regarding both the drugs to be administered, the dosages, the drug associations and the route of their administration (Fig. 63.2).[5] In most patients with bowel obstruction, oral administration is not suitable and

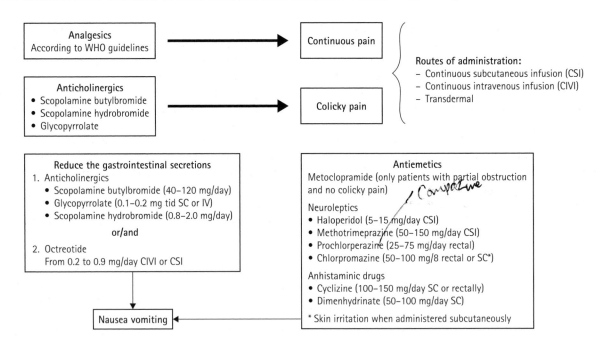

Figure 63.2 *Symptomatic pharmacological approach. CIVI, continuous intravenous infusion; CSI, continuous subcutaneous infusion; SC, subcutaneous; tid, three times daily; IV, intravenous.*

alternatives routes have to be considered. Most of the recommended drugs can be administered in association via parenteral continuous infusion.

To relieve continuous abdominal pain, opioid analgesics via continuous subcutaneous or intravenous infusion are necessary in most of the patients. The dosage has to be titrated for each patient until pain relief is achieved. Anticholinergics may be administered in association with opioids to control colicky pain[5] (Fig. 63.2).

Vomiting can be managed using two different pharmacological approaches and reduced to an acceptable level for the patient (e.g. one to two times per day):

1 Drugs such as anticholinergics (scopolamine butylbromide, glycopyrrolate) or/and octreotide, which reduce gastrointestinal secretions.
2 Antiemetics acting on the central nervous system, alone or in association with drugs to reduce gastrointestinal secretions (Fig. 63.2).

Several authors recommend the use of corticosteroids for the symptoms due to bowel obstruction because it can reduce peritumoral inflammatory edema, thus improving intestinal motility. No controlled clinical trials have been carried out and administration routes and dosing of these drugs have not been standardized as yet. The role of corticosteroids in treating bowel obstruction is still controversial.[33***]

SCOPOLAMINE BUTYLBROMIDE

Scopolamine butylbromide is a frequently used drug for both vomiting and colicky pain by some palliative care

centers.[32,34–36] This drug differs from both atropine and scopolamine hydrobromide in having a low lipid solubility. It does not penetrate the blood–brain barrier as well as these other drugs and, consequently, may produce fewer side effects, such as somnolence and hallucinations, when administered in combination with opioids. The anticholinergic activity of scopolamine butylbromide decreases the tonus and peristalsis in smooth muscle and decreases the secretions in the gastrointestinal tract. The antiemetic, antisecretory as well as the analgesic role of scopolamine butylbromide administered subcutaneously by a syringe driver has been well documented by different authors. Dry mouth is reported to be the most significant side effect, but patients tolerated it by sucking ice cubes and drinking small sips of water. Also anticholinergic agents such as scopolamine hydrobromide or butylbromide and glycopyrrolate, reduce colicky pain and the volume of intestinal secretions. Glycopyrrolate, which is used as an antisecretory drug in the USA, is more potent than scopolamine hydrobromide and may be effective in some patients who fail to respond to scopolamine.[37] It has little central nervous system penetration and is unlikely to cause the delirium that has been associated with tertiary amine anticholinergics.

OCTREOTIDE

This is a synthetic analog of somatostatin that has a more potent biological activity and a longer half-life has also been used to manage the symptoms of bowel obstruction. Somatostatin and its analogs have been shown to inhibit the release and activity of gastrointestinal hormones, modulate gastrointestinal function by reducing gastric acid secretion, slow intestinal motility, decrease bile flow, increase mucus production, and reduce splanchnic blood flow. It reduces gastrointestinal contents and increases absorption of water and electrolytes at intracellular level, via cAMP and calcium regulation. Submucosal somatostatin-containing neurons, activated by octreotide, inhibit excitatory nerves, mainly by an inhibition of acetylcholine output. As a result muscle relaxation can occur, ameliorating the spastic activity responsible for colicky pain. These effects may be due to vasoactive intestinal polypeptide (VIP) inhibition, which is increased in experimental bowel obstruction and is known to have adverse effects on intestinal secretions, splanchnic flow and peristalsis.[38]

The inhibitory effect of octreotide on both peristalsis and gastrointestinal secretions reduces bowel distension and the secretion of water and sodium by the intestinal epithelium, thereby reducing vomiting and pain. The drug may therefore break the vicious circle represented by secretion, distension, and contractile hyperactivity. Octreotide has been shown to have a potent anti-VIP effect resulting in the inhibition of intestinal secretions.[39,40] Also in the *in vitro* experiments on rabbit ileum, somatostatin was able to stimulate water and sodium chloride absorption and inhibit bicarbonate secretion and to inhibit water secretion in the jejunum.[9, 41]

Experimental studies suggest that the principal mechanism of fluid secretion in bowel obstruction depends on VIP-induced inflammatory events.[38,42] Another inhibitory mechanism of hormonal release occurs through the activation of a G-protein which, on stimulating the potassium channels, determines the hyperpolarization of the cell, with the consequent blockage of the flux of calcium to the cell.[43] Octreotide may be administered by subcutaneous bolus or continuous subcutaneous or intravenous infusion. Its half-life is about 1.5 hours after intravenous or subcutaneous administration, and its kinetics are linear. The recommended starting dose is 0.3 mg/day subcutaneously. The dose can be titrated upward until symptom control is achieved, in general 0.6–0.9 mg/day. Octreotide is an expensive drug and its cost–benefit ratio should be carefully considered, especially for prolonged treatment. However, the cost of the drug should be interpreted in the widest possible sense, that is if the use of a drug results in a more rapid improvement of gastrointestinal symptoms which potentially limits the bed stay or the admission to an inpatient unit in addition to a better quality of life of the patient.[9,44]

Many experimental studies have evaluated the efficacy of somatostatin and octreotide in respect to placebo on intestinal distension, electrolyte losses, and ischemia.[9]

Efficacy of octreotide before surgery for bowel obstruction

Surgical gastrointestinal complications are common and postoperative outcome is poor in patients with advanced cancer. As luminal contents accumulate proximal to the obstruction, the bowel becomes distended and the increase in intraluminal pressure stimulates intestinal fluid secretion, which further stretches the bowel wall. The consequent pathological findings are accumulation of fluids and gases above the obstruction with altered motility producing distension, wall edema, vessel congestion, necrosis and perforation of the bowel above the obstruction and the presence of peritoneal fluids. Patients with obstruction are hypovolemic, tachycardiac, and frequently hypotensive as a result of fluids and electrolytes sequestered in the gut wall and in its lumen. Successful surgery may be compromised by these alterations and higher morbidity and mortality are expected.[45]

Octreotide at a daily dose of 0.3 μg has been preoperatively administered in patients undergoing surgery for bowel obstruction due to cancer. The patients were managed by an intravenous replacement of fluids and electrolytes, nasogastric tube and antibiotics. Diameter of the bowel above the obstruction was normal and no local gross pathological findings due to the accumulation of fluids in the lumen, such as edema, vessel congestion, or necrosis of the bowel above the obstruction, commonly observed in this situation, were observed. Samples of intestine above and below the obstruction revealed a normal anatomical and biochemical pattern. Intestinal anastomosis after resection was successful.[46] These preliminary results were confirmed in a randomized, double blind clinical trial carried out on 54 consecutive patients with mechanical bowel obstruction. Patients who received octreotide preoperatively required surgery less often than patients who did not receive the drug. Moreover, severe dilatation and necrosis of the bowel proximal to the area of obstruction was significantly less frequent as compared with those patients who did not receive the drug preoperatively.[47]

EFFICACY OF OCTREOTIDE IN PATIENTS WITH GASTROINTESTINAL SYMPTOMS DUE TO INOPERABLE MALIGNANT BOWEL OBSTRUCTION

Table 63.3 shows the efficacy of octreotide administration in the control of gastrointestinal symptoms due to bowel obstruction.[48–53] All the authors were able to show the efficacy on emesis in cancer patients with intractable continual vomiting due to small/large bowel obstruction that was unresponsive to conventional therapy (prochlorperazine, metoclopramide, cyclizine and dexamethasone). Octreotide was administered subcutaneously in association or not with opioid analgesics and with antiemetics.

Symptom control was maintained until death. No adverse effects were attributable to the drugs. The nasogastric tube was removed in most patients. In the presence of marked and diffuse bowel distension the administration of octreotide may reduce gastrointestinal secretions and thus allow an appropriate site for PEG placement to be obtained.[54]

Table 63.3 *Role of octreotide (OCT) in malignant bowel obstruction*

Author(s)	No. of patients	Site of cancer(s) Site of obstruction	Symptom(s)	OCT dose/route other drugs	Results
Khoo et al.[48a]	5	Various intraabdominal Small bowel	Intractable vomiting unresponsive to conventional therapy	0.1–0.5 mg/day SCb at start then CSI	Vomiting stopped within 1 hour of start of treatment The only patient with a NGT presented a reduction in aspirate from 2000 mL/day to under 300 mL/day No important toxicity was reported
Mercadante et al.[49a]	2	Intraabdominal Small and/or large bowel carcinomatosis	Abdominal pain and vomiting (1°) Colic pain and vomiting despite the use of NGT and haloperidol (2°)	0.3–0.2 mg/day Buprenorphine CSI 0.9 mg/day + 3 mg haloperidol	Pain and vomiting disappeared within 24 hours NGT was removed. No adverse effects were reported Within 24 hours NGT secretions decreased from 2600 mL/day to 350 mL/day and vomiting disappeared NGT was removed. No further need for analgesics or IV fluids. No adverse effects were reported
Mercadante et al.[50]	14	Various intraabdominal Small and/or large bowel	Nausea, vomiting unresponsive to haloperidol or chlorpromazine	0.3–0.6 mg/day SCb or CSI +haloperidol +analgesics	Vomiting was controlled in 12 patients and reduced in 2 In 2 out of 3 patients NGT was removed and the symptoms controlled No important toxicity was reported
Riley et al.[51]	24	Various intraabdominal Small and/or large bowel	Intractable vomiting not responsive to a combination of antiemetics, steroids and/or NGT drainage for 24 hours	0.1–1.2 mg/day SCb or CSI	14 patients had no further vomiting and 4 patients showed some improvements with a dose 0.1–0.6 mg/day There was a reduction of aspirate in all 5 patients with NGT 6 patients did not respond despite dosages of 0.6–1.2 mg/day no adverse effects were reported also at higher dosages
Mangili et al.[52]	13	Ovary Small and/or large bowel	Vomiting not responsive to metoclopramide and haloperidol	0.3–0.6 mg/day SCb or CSI ± analgesics	Vomiting was controlled in all cases within 3 days (range 1–6). In 8 patients with a NGT there was a reduction of secretions and NGT was removed No adverse effects were reported
Steadman et al.[53a]	1	Pancreas Small bowel	Vomiting and drowsiness with diamorphine, cyclizine, hyoscine	0.2 mg/day + diamorphine	Good symptom relief without causing unwanted uncomfortable drowsiness

[a] Case reports.
SCb, subcutaneous bolus; CSI, continuous subcutaneous infusion; IV, intravenous; NGT, naso-gastric tube.

These studies, although uncontrolled, support the use of octreotide in the management of gastrointestinal symptoms due to inoperable MBO. Reported effective doses range from 0.1 mg/day to 0.6 mg/day either as a continuous parenteral infusion or as intermittent subcutaneous or intravenous boluses. Octreotide, administered in association respectively with morphine or hyoscine butylbromide or haloperidol (0.5–1.2 mg/mL) does not show visual precipitation when mixed in the syringe.[5]

COMPARATIVE STUDIES BETWEEN OCTREOTIDE AND SCOPOLAMINE BUTYLBROMIDE

Two randomized prospective studies were carried out to compare the antisecretory effects of octreotide (0.3 mg/day) and scopolamine butylbromide (SB) (60 mg/day) administered by continuous subcutaneous infusion for 3 days in 17 patients with inoperable bowel obstruction having a nasogastric tube[55**] and in 15 patients without a nasogastric tube.[56**] In both studies 50 percent of the patients were cared for at home and the rest were hospitalized in surgical wards. In both studies the hospitalized patients received significantly more parenteral hydration (2000 mL vs. 500 mL daily) compared with the patients cared for at home.

Ripamonti et al.[55] showed that octreotide significantly reduced the amount of gastrointestinal secretions already 2 days after baseline ($P = 0.016$) and 3 days after baseline ($P = 0.020$). The nasogastric tube could be removed in all 10 homecare patients and in 3 hospitalized patients without changing the dosage of the drug. In three patients, it was possible to remove the nasogastric tube when the octreotide was added to SB (1 patient) or when the SB dose was doubled and parenteral hydration was reduced (1 patient). Also in these patients, octreotide showed a trend toward better efficacy than SB. It can be hypothesized that in the hospitalized patients the major difficulty in removing the nasogastric tube was associated with the higher amount of parenteral hydration.

In the second study[56**] octreotide treatment induced a significantly rapid reduction in the number of daily episodes of vomiting and intensity of nausea when compared to SB-treated patients, examined at the different time intervals. The association of the two drugs (octreotide and SB) may reduce gastrointestinal secretions and vomiting whenever one drug alone is ineffective.[55**,57]

In a recent study of 68 terminally ill cancer patients randomly receiving continuous subcutaneous administration of chlorpromazine 15–25 mg/day, combined with hyoscine butylbromide 60–80 mg/day or octreotide 600–800 μg/day, significant favorable differences in vomiting and nausea, fatigue and anorexia were reported in patients receiving octreotide.[58**]

PARTIAL OR REVERSIBLE BOWEL OBSTRUCTION

Other than reducing the gastrointestinal symptoms in definitive bowel obstruction, octreotide may be useful in reversing clinical conditions of subobstruction, as it can reduce the hypertensive state in the lumen, producing the sequence distension-secretion, which proceeds to definitive obstruction if not treated.[46,59] The most important mechanism in these circumstances is functional and can be reversible, if an aggressive treatment is initiated early before fecal impaction and edema render MBO irreversible. An early and intensive pharmacological treatment may not only reduce gastrointestinal symptoms but also reverse malignant bowel obstruction, in clinical conditions commonly considered definitive.[59] Octreotide, combined with metoclopramide, dexamethasone and an initial bolus of amidotrizoate, allowed the recovery of intestinal transit within 1–5 days in most advanced cancer patients, who continued this treatment without presenting symptoms of bowel obstruction until death.[60]

HYDRATION AND TOTAL PARENTERAL NUTRITION

In patients with inoperable bowel obstruction the amount of fluid administered should be assessed carefully. High levels of intravenous fluids may result in more bowel secretions, thus it is necessary to keep a balance between the efficacy of the treatment and the side effects such as increased vomiting, abdominal distension, and pain. The intensity of dry mouth and thirst are independent of the quantity of both intravenous or oral hydration.[55,56] However the intensity of nausea is significantly lower in patients treated with more than 1 L/day of parenteral fluids. Intravenous hydration can be difficult and uncomfortable for patients with end-stage cancer, so it should be reserved for patients who have a central venous catheter. Hypodermoclysis is a simple technique for rehydration that offers many advantages over the intravenous route.[61] The role of total parenteral nutrition (TPN) in the management of patients with inoperable bowel obstruction is controversial. No data are available on the survival rates or quality of life in advanced cancer patients treated with this modality. Depending on the context a patient provides, TPN may be considered a futile treatment or an acceptable means of maintaining patient autonomy.[5,62,63]

CONCLUSIONS

The optimal treatment of bowel obstruction in patients with advanced cancer is still an open and widely debated issue. Patient are usually considered suitable candidates for surgery when survival is expected to be more than 2 months. Studies of prognostic indicators of survival in advanced cancer patients are necessary to assist doctors in making appropriate therapeutic decisions, together with the patient and family members. Medical treatment by continuous subcutaneous or intravenous administration of opioids, corticosteroids, anticholinergic drugs, octreotide, and antiemetic drugs can be an effective approach for controlling pain, nausea and vomiting in patients with inoperable gastrointestinal obstruction. Nasogastric suction or percutaneous gastrostomy may be considered for patients with refractory symptoms and/or upper bowel obstruction who do not respond satisfactorily to pharmacological measures alone. The efforts of the doctor/nurse team must be aimed at both symptom control and other aspects of the patient's suffering, including psychological distress and spiritual concerns.

Key learning points

- Bowel obstruction is a distressing outcome above all in patients with abdominal and pelvic cancer in the advanced and terminal stage of disease.

- Surgery should not routinely be undertaken in patients with poor prognostic criteria such as intraabdominal carcinomatosis, poor performance status and massive ascites.

- Medical measures such as analgesics, antisecretory drugs and antiemetics administered alone or in combination should be used to relieve symptoms.

- A nasogastric tube should be used only as a temporary measure and a venting gastrostomy should be considered if drugs fail in reducing vomiting to an acceptable level.

- TPN should be considered only for patients who may die for starvation rather than from tumor spread.

- Parenteral hydration is sometimes indicated to correct nausea and regular mouth care is the treatment of choice for dry mouth.

- A collaborative approach by surgeons and physicians can offer patients an individualized and appropriate symptom management plan.

Results of the Consensus Conference on malignant bowel obstruction: from Ripamonti *et al*. Clinical-practice recommendations for the management of bowel obstruction in patients with end-stage cancer. *Support Care Cancer* 2001; **19**: 23–34.[5]

REFERENCES

◆ 1 Baines M. The pathophysiology and management of malignant intestinal obstruction. In: Doyle D, Hanks GWC, MacDonald N, eds. *Oxford Textbook of Palliative Medicine*, 2nd ed. Oxford: Oxford University Press, 1998: 526.

◆ 2 Ripamonti C. Malignant bowel obstruction. In: Ripamonti C, Bruera E, eds. *Gastrointestinal Symptoms in Advanced Cancer Patients*. Oxford: Oxford University Press 2002: 235.

◆ 3 Ripamonti C, Mercadante S. Pathophysiology and management of malignant bowel obstruction. In: Doyle D, Hanks G, Cherny NI, Calman K, eds. *Oxford Textbook of Palliative Medicine*, 3rd ed. New York: Oxford University Press, 2004: 496–506.

● 4 Krebs HB, Goplerud DR. Mechanical intestinal obstruction in patients with gynecologic disease: a review of 368 patients. *Am J Obstet Gynecol* 1987; **157**: 577–9.

✱ 5 Ripamonti C, Twycross R, Baines M, *et al*. Clinical-practice recommendations for the management of bowel obstruction in patients with end-stage cancer. *Support Care Cancer* 2001; **19**: 23–34.

◆ 6 Feuer DJ, Broadley KE, Shepherd JH, Barton DPJ. Systematic review of surgery in malignant bowel obstruction in advanced gynecological and gastrointestinal cancer. *Gynecol Oncol* 1999; **75**: 313–22.

● 7 Tunca JC, Buchler DA, Mack EA, *et al*. The management of ovarian-cancer-caused bowel obstruction. *Gynecol Oncol* 1981; **12**: 186–92.

● 8 Krebs HB, Goplerud DR. Surgical management of bowel obstruction in advanced ovarian carcinoma. *Obstet Gynecol* 1983; **61**: 327–30.

◆ 9 Ripamonti C, Panzeri C, Groff L, *et al*. The role of somatostatin and octreotide in bowel obstruction: pre-clinical and clinical results. *Tumori* 2001; **87**: 1–9.

10 Pictus D, Marx MV, Weyman PJ. Chronic intestinal obstruction: value of percutaneous gastrostomy tube placement. *Am J Radiol* 1988; **150**: 295–7.

11 George J, Crawford D, Lewis T, *et al*. Percutaneous endoscopic gastrostomy: a two year experience. *Med J Aust* 1990; **152**: 17–20.

12 Malone JM, Koonce T, Larson DM, *et al*. Palliation of small bowel obstructon by percutaneous gastrostomy in patients with progressive ovarian carcinoma. *Obstet Gynecol* 1986; **68**: 431–3.

13 Herman LL, Hoskins WJ, Shike M. Percutaneous endoscopic gastrostomy for decompression of the stomach and small bowel. *Gastrointest Endosc* 1992; **38**: 314–18.

14 Cunningham MJ, Bromberg C, Kredentser DC, *et al*. Percutaneous gastrostomy for decompression in patients with advanced gynecologic malignancirs. *Gynecol Oncol* 1995; **59**: 273–6.

15 Campagnutta E, Cannizzaro R, Gallo A, *et al*. Palliative treatment of upper intestinal obstruction by gynecological malignancy: the usefulness of percutaneous endoscopic gastrostomy. *Gynecol Oncol* 1996; **62**: 103–5.

16 Forgas I, Macpherson A, Tibbs C. Percutaneous endoscopic gastrostomy. The end of the line for nasogastric feeding? *BMJ* 1992; **304**: 1395–6.

● 17 Gemlo B, Rayner AA, Lewis B. Home support of patients with end-stage malignant bowel obstruction using hydration and venting gastrostomy. *Am J Surg* 1986; **152**: 100–4.

18 Mack LA, Pereira J, Temple WJ. Decompressive tube esophagostomy: a forgotten palliative procedure? *J Palliat Med* 2004; **7**: 265–7.

19 Mainar A, Tejero E, Maynar M, *et al*. Colorectal obstruction: treatment with metallic stents. *Radiology* 1996; 198; 761–4.

20 Wallis F, Campbell KL, Eremin O, Hussey JK. Self-expanding metal stents in the management of colorectal carcinoma-a preliminary report. *Clin Radiol* 1998; **53**: 251–4.

21 Scott-Mackie P, Morgan R, Farrugia M, *et al.* The role of metallic stents in malignant duodenal obstruction. *Br J Radiol* 1997; **70**: 252–5.

22 Pinto IT. Malignant gastric and duodenal stenosis: palliation by peroral implantation of a self-expanding metallic stent. *Cardiovasc Intervent Radiol* 1997; **20**: 431–4.

23 Park HS, Do YS, Suh SW, *et al.* Upper gastrointestinal tract malignant obstruction: initial results of palliation with a flexible covered stent. *Radiology* 1999; **210**: 865–70.

24 Feretis C, Benakis P, Dimopoulos C, *et al.* Duodenal obstruction caused by pancreatic head carcinoma: palliation with self-expandable endoprostheses. *Gastrointest Endosc* 1997; **46**: 161–5.

25 de Baere T, Harry G, Ducreux M, *et al.* Self-expanding metallic stents as palliative treatment of malignant gastroduodenal stenosis. *AJR Am J Roentgenol* 1997; **169**: 1079–83.

26 Sebastian JJ, Zaragozano R, Vicente J, *et al.* Duodenal obstruction secondary to a metastasis from an adenocarcinoma of the cecum: a case report. *Am J Gastroenterol* 1997; **92**: 1051–2.

27 Arnell T, Stamos MJ, Takahashi P, *et al.* Colonic stents in colorectal obstruction. *Am Surg* 1998; **64**: 986–8.

28 Tejero E, Fernandez-Lobato R, Mainar A *et al.* Initial results of a new procedure for treatment of malignant obstruction of the left colon. *Dis Colon Rectum* 1997; **40**: 432–6.

29 Saida Y, Sumiyama Y, Nagao J, Takase M. Stent endoprosthesis for obstructing colorectal cancers. *Dis Colon Rectum* 1996; **39**: 552–5.

30 Dohmoto M, Hunerbein M, Schlag PM. Application of rectal stents for palliation of obstructing rectosigmoid cancer. *Surg Endosc* 1997; **11**: 758–61.

31 Canon CL, Baron TH, Morgan DE, *et al.* Treatment of colonic obstruction with expandable metal stents: radiologic features. *AJR Am J Roentgenol* 1997; **168**: 199–205.

● 32 Baines M, Oliver DJ, Carter RL. Medical management of intestinal obstruction in patients with advanced malignant disease: a clinical and pathological study. *Lancet* 1985; **2**: 990–3.

◆ 33 Feuer DJ, Broadley KE, Members of the Systematic Review Steering Committee. Systematic review and meta-analysis of corticosteroids for the resolution of malignant bowel obstruction in advanced gynaecological and gastrointestinal cancers. *Ann Oncol* 1999; **10**: 1035–41.

34 Ventafridda V, Ripamonti C, Caraceni A, *et al.* The management of inoperable gastrointestinal obstruction in terminal cancer patients. *Tumori* 1990; **76**: 389–93.

35 Fainsinger RL, Spachynski K, Hanson J, *et al.* Symptom control in terminally ill patients with malignant bowel obstruction. *J Pain Symptom Manage* 1994; **9**:12–18.

36 De Conno F, Caraceni A, Zecca E, *et al.* Continuous subcutaneous infusion of hyoscine butylbromide reduces secretions in patients with gastrointestinal obstruction. *J Pain Symptom Manage* 1991; **6**: 484–6.

37 Davis MP, Furste A. Glycopyrrolate: a useful drug in the palliation of mechanical bowel obstruction. *J Pain Symptom Manage* 1999; **18**: 153–4.

38 Basson MD, Fielding LP, Bilchik AJ, *et al.* Does vasoactive intestinal polypeptide mediate the pathophysiology of bowel obstruction? *Am J Surg* 1989; **157**: 109–15.

39 Nellgard P, Bojo L, Cassuto J. Importance of vasoactive intestinal peptide and somatostatin for fluid losses in small-bowel obstruction. *Scand J Gastroenterol* 1995; **30**: 464–9.

40 Neville R, Fielding P, Cambria RP, Modlin I. Vascular responsiveness in obstructed gut. *Dis Colon Rectum* 1991; **34**: 229–35.

41 Dharmsathaphorn K, Binder HJ, Dobbins WJ. Somatostatin stimulates sodium and chloride absorption in the rabbit ileum. *Gastroenterology* 1980; **78**: 1559–65.

42 Nellgard P, Cassuto J. Inflammation as a major cause of fluid losses in small-bowel obstruction. *Scand J Gastroenterol* 1993; **28**: 1035–41.

43 Yatani A, Birnbaumer L, Brown AM. Direct coupling of the somatostatin receptor to potassium channels by a G protein. *Metabolism* 1990; **39**(9 Suppl): 91–5.

44 Ripamonti C, Mercadante S. How to use octreotide for malignant bowel obstruction. *J Support Oncol* 2004; **2**: 357–64.

45 Yamaner S, Bugra D, Muslumanoglu M, *et al.* Effects of octreotide on healing of intestinal anastomosis following small bowel obstruction in rats. *Dis Colon Rectum* 1995; **38**: 308–12.

● 46 Mercadante S, Avola G, Maddaloni S, *et al.* Octreotide prevents the pathological alterations of bowel obstruction in cancer patients. *Support Care Cancer* 1996; **4**: 393–4.

47 Sun X, Li X, Li H. Management of intestinal obstruction in advanced ovarian cancer: an analysis of 57 cases. *Chung Hua Chung Liu Tsa Chih* 1995; **17**: 39–42.

48 Khoo D, Riley J, Waxman J. Control of emesis in bowel obstruction in terminally ill patients. *Lancet* 1992; **339**:, 375–6.

● 49 Mercadante S, Maddaloni S. Octreotide in the management of inoperable gastrointestinal obstruction in terminal cancer patients. *J Pain Symptom Manage* 1992; **7**: 496–8.

50 Mercadante S, Spoldi E, Caraceni A, *et al.* Octreotide in relieving gastrointestinal symptoms due to bowel obstruction. *Palliat Med* 1993; **7**: 295–9.

51 Riley J, Fallon MT. Octreotide in terminal malignant obstruction of the gastrointestinal tract. *Eur J Palliat Care* 1994; **1**: 23–8.

52 Mangili G, Franchi M, Mariani A, *et al.* Octreotide in the management of bowel obstruction in terminal ovarian cancer. *Gynecol Oncol* 1996; **61**: 345–8.

53 Steadman K, Franks A. A woman with malignant bowel obstruction who did not want to die with tubes. *Lancet* 1996; **347**: 944.

54 Sartori S, Trevisani L, Nielsen I, *et al.* Identification of a safe site for percutaneous endoscopic gastrostomy placement in patients with marked bowel distension: may octreotide have a role? *Endoscopy* 1994; **26**: 710–11.

55 Ripamonti C, Mercadante S, Groff L, *et al.* Role of octreotide, scopolamine butylbromide and hydration in symptom control of patients with inoperable bowel obstruction having a nasogastric tube. A prospective, randomized clinical trial. *J Pain Symptom Manage* 2000; **19**: 23–34.

56 Mercadante S, Ripamonti C, Casuccio A, *et al.* Comparison of octreotide and hyoscine butylbromide in controlling gastrointestinal symptoms due to malignant inoperable bowel obstruction. *Support Care Cancer* 2000; **8**: 188–91.

57 Mercadante S. Scopolamine butylbromide plus octreotide in unresponsive bowel obstruction. *J Pain Symptom Manage* 1998; **16**: 278–9.

58 Mystakidou K, Tsilika E, Kalaidopoulou O, *et al.* Comparison of octreotide administration vs conservative treatment in the management of inoperable bowel obstruction in patients with far advanced cancer: a randomized, double- blind, controlled clinical trial. *Anticancer Res* 2002; **22**: 1187–92.

● 59 Mercadante S, Kargar J, Nicolosi G. Octreotide may prevent definitive intestinal obstruction. *J Pain Symptom Manage* 1997; **13**: 352–5.

60 Mercadante S, Ferrera P, Villari P, Marrazzo A. Aggressive pharmacological treatment for reversing bowel obstruction. *J Pain Symptom Manage* 2004; **28**: 412–16.

61 Fainsinger RL, MacEachern T, Miller MJ *et al.* The use of hypodermoclysis for rehydration in terminally ill cancer patients. *J Pain Symptom Manage* 1994; **9**: 298–302.

✱ 62 Bozzetti F, Amadori D, Bruera E, *et al.* Guidelines on artificial nutrition versus hydration in terminal cancer patients. *Nutrition* 1996; **12**: 163–7.

63 Cozzaglio L, Balzala F, Casentino F, *et al.* Outcome of cancer patients receiving home parenteral nutrition. *JPEN J Parenter Enteral Nutr* 1997; **21**: 339–42.

64

Endoscopic treatment of gastrointestinal symptoms

PASQUALE SPINELLI

INTRODUCTION

Most tumors, and 99 percent of the digestive ones, are *endo*cavitary and thus *endo*scopy is the most suitable approach for them, for diagnostic as well as for therapeutic purposes. Endocavitary treatment of cancer may lead to the cure of superficial, locally extending, nonmetastatic lesions or palliation of noncurable tumors. Digestive cancers form about 20 percent of all diagnosed cancers; when these are advanced, most of them are poorly responsive to curative treatments; consequently, patients not responding to curative treatment will need symptomatic, palliative treatment.

Palliative care has appropriately been receiving increased attention in recent years. Palliation, by itself, can be defined as the treatment of the symptoms of a disease. Palliative treatment is planned when it is impossible to treat a disease for cure. Palliation would be better defined by dividing it into:

- Palliative care – which includes the treatments required during the course of patients with advanced tumors from a stage of specific disease status to the stage of terminal events.
- Control of symptoms – which concerns an earlier stage in the natural history of the disease, when there is an acceptable disease-related quality of life.[1]

In view of these distinctions, palliative treatments to control symptoms should start as soon as the disease is classified as being incurable.[2] It could happen at the time of the diagnosis if conditions preventing curative treatments already exist. Palliation must be undertaken if anticancer treatments are not considered advisable because of general or local reasons, such as in cases where anticancer treatments would waste the time and resources that could be used for a more tolerable and profitable symptomatic approach.

Diagnosis of a solid cancer must be followed by the staging, as therapeutic options and prognosis are strictly related to the stage. Staging procedures are based on sophisticated and precise diagnostic tools, so that the oncologist should be able to separate localized from diffused and curable from noncurable diseases in the majority of cases. In fact, all suitable diagnostic possibilities must be considered to identify patients with noncurable disease as early as possible, and thus avoid giving them inefficacious, sometime toxic and always costly anticancer treatments, instead managing their symptoms appropriately.[3] Before deciding on palliative care to treat only the symptoms and waiving the possibility of directly treating the disease, the following points should be considered:

- the different curative potentials of surgery, radiotherapy, chemotherapy, immunotherapy, and any other kind of certified treatments
- risk factors in a particular patient
- side effects of a treatment
- quality of the remaining life of the patient
- weighing up the real impact of the therapeutic procedures with regard to the expected benefits.[4*]

With the availability of a variety of new prognostic indicators in the form of molecular, clinical, and pathological testing, the possibility that they could be used also for selecting potentially curable from noncurable patients has emerged. Analysis of gene expression patterns may be useful in the future for predicting the response to an anticancer treatment.[4,5*]

PALLIATIVE TREATMENTS: GENERAL CONCEPTS

Surgery

Surgery can be indicated in various contexts and is generally the first option to be considered.[6**] From the surgeon's standpoint, therapy is considered palliative when resection of all known tumor sites is no longer possible or advisable. Since a cure, as it is commonly defined, is not possible, the success of the therapy is determined by the alleviation of the suffering. A part of the gastrointestinal tract may be resected in presence of painful obstructive symptoms with the aim of relieving pain, restoring the lumen and reducing bleeding by removing a tumor. Bypass operations, indicated in cases of nonresectable tumor masses, may be performed through traditional laparotomy and also through laparoscopic access, achieving the double goal of minimum trauma and quick recovery. The appropriate use of surgery in these settings can improve the quality of life of patients with cancer.

Radiotherapy

In presence of unresectable tumors, radiotherapy reduces the tumor volume. It does seem to be of benefit in selected cases with large cancers because it may reduce the mass and make it resectable. Under specific circumstances, it can be given together with endoscopic treatments, thus combining endoluminal with the extraluminal benefits of mass reduction. In some cancers causing local symptoms, reduction of the size of the tumor and of the extravisceral extension of the tumor with radiation therapy results in partial control of pain. This treatment can be used alone or in combination with other anticancer treatments.[7] Among the different radiotherapeutic options, brachytherapy can better localize radiation dose with limited side effects; this is important when treating previously irradiated areas.[8]

Chemotherapy

Chemotherapy using multiagent regimens has an advantage for palliation of unresectable or metastatic cancer in cases of medium survival, but there is no confirmed advantage in cases of long-term survival. Chemotherapy is used to reduce the size of masses and to alleviate symptoms. Furthermore, in patients who have locally advanced, unresectable disease and in patients in whom tumors are resected with positive margins the duration of survival can be increased with palliative chemotherapy and irradiation.[9] Along with chemotherapy, endoscopic treatments aimed at immediately relieving obstruction of an occluded cavity may be strongly advisable in selected cases, allowing for functional recovery.[10]

PALLIATIVE CARE FOR GASTROINTESTINAL SYMPTOMS

From the endoscopic point of view, both primary digestive cancers as well as their metastases can compromise esophageal, tracheobronchial, biliary, and urinary functions, depending on their location. In consideration of these concepts, palliative care should not be limited to the patients with preterminal disease, but greatly expanded, starting with the control of symptoms as soon as the disease is classified as incurable and avoiding unnecessary anticancer treatments. As stated earlier in this chapter, when a solid cancer is diagnosed, the disease must be staged, as therapeutic options and prognosis are related to the stage. Since the disease is staged through precise diagnostic procedures, one should be able to separate localized from diffused and curable from noncurable cancers in most cases.

The continuing increase of the lifespan that has happened in recent years entails a constant increase in the incidence of age-related malignant neoplasms; advanced age, together with related risk factors, reduces the possibility of performing radical treatments and opens the doors to palliative treatments. In current clinical practice, however, most patients are treated with curative intent, even when palliation of symptoms would have been the right choice. Furthermore, the majority of clinical trials currently in progress are evaluating the response to treatments in terms of decrease in the volume of the tumor mass and global survival, but neglecting the evaluation of the impact of the treatment toxicity, of the general side effects on the quality of life and on the relationships of the patients with the people around them.

Although the primary purpose of a palliative procedure is not to increase survival, the treatment of severe symptoms (nutritional, respiratory, or metabolic) as in tumors resulting in stenosis of the esophagus, trachea, or intestinal, biliary, or urinary tracts, very often results in an effective extension of the survival time. Consequently, palliation becomes, in many cases, not just the simple treatment of symptoms, but it offers to the patient a wide range of therapeutic opportunities during the entire course of the disease.

Endoscopic palliative treatments aim to obtain the best possible quality of life with immediate and durable benefits with negligible trauma, side effects and incidence of complications related to the proposed advantages. Although these objectives seem to be obvious, it often happens that these simple principles – essential to the correct approach to the oncological patient – are not adopted and patients are submitted to treatments that are not suited to their requirements and their health status. In everyday practice it frequently happens that patients who only need control of symptoms related to the size and site of the tumor masses and to their relations with the surrounding anatomical structures, are over treated.

Palliative treatment of an oncological patient under these conditions must be tailored so that the quality of life offered by the treatment is more consistent with their lifestyle and, when possible, it should be planned in agreement with the patient. This is because there are different ways to achieve relief from one symptom. The physician must be able to inform the patient about the different methods available so that they can choose the one that fits better with their preferred lifestyle. For example, esophageal stenosis can be relieved by a nasogastric tube, by a laser treatment, by a gastrostomy, or by a palliative radiochemotherapy: patients must be informed about these options so that they can decide which one is the most suitable for their way of life.

In the field of clinical research, human resources are insufficient and dedicated researchers are spread out among numerous – and partly curative – projects and not focused on specific palliation research. This is of concern also to endoscopic palliative treatments, as these are less widely known and used than they should be, considering the palliative opportunities they offer to oncological patients. Methodologically appropriate research is needed to bring into focus the indications of these methods and disseminate awareness about them.

Gastrointestinal symptoms may be produced by digestive or extradigestive tumors. Most of these tumors affect the digestive cavities and grow into them, occupying the spaces required for the digestive functions. The gastrointestinal tract has cavities that function as 'containers' or as 'canals' (stomach, esophagus, intestine, biliary, and pancreatic tract). Tumors reduce the space available and impair the functions of containing and flowing; moreover, tumors that infiltrate and ulcerate the walls of these cavities generate symptoms, in particular, they cause hemorrhage, obstruction, perforation and fistula formation. The most important symptoms of digestive tumors are: dysphagia, salivation, vomiting, jaundice, pain, and hemorrhage. All these symptoms can be treated by endoscopic modalities.

Dysphagia

Dysphagia is the most severe symptom of pharyngo-esophageal tumors. Malignant dysphagia can be in relation to the presence of a primary or secondary esophageal tumor or it can be consequent to a surgical treatment or to a radiotherapy or chemotherapy. Dysphagia can be defined as an abnormal swallowing, characterized by difficulty in transferring solid or liquid food from the mouth to the stomach; it is the initial symptom of an esophageal cancer in 90 percent of cases, but it also may be caused by compression or infiltration by thyroid or lung tumors, mediastinal lymphomas or by metastatic involvement of the mediastinum, mainly by breast cancer. Dysphagia can be associated with pain (odynophagia) and aspiration of food and saliva into the trachea and bronchi and with chronic cough, asthma, laryngitis, and, eventually, pneumonia.

Beyond the most common causes, in oncological patients dysphagia may be due to:

- neurological reasons, e.g. cricopharyngeal dysphagia because of recurrent nerve palsy due to perineural and neural infiltration by tumor tissue; neurological dysphagia may be also due to vagal or sympathetic tumoral infiltration, with involvement of the skull base or due to brain metastases.
- mucositis related to candidosis, bacterial infection, herpes, radiotherapy, chemotherapy.
- asthenia/cachexia.

From the mechanical viewpoint, a patient becomes dysphagic when the diameter of the esophageal lumen is less than 14 mm, but an uncertain feeling of trouble in swallowing is generally complained of some weeks or months before the diagnosis of esophageal cancer.

Esophagoscopy is indicated when a patient complains of dysphagia; its performance can be indicated in the various phases of diagnosis, staging and treatment. It allows the surgeon to characterize and exactly locate a tumor, to measure its length and appreciate the circular extent and the size of the residual esophageal lumen, and to obtain histological confirmation of the clinical diagnosis. Echoendoscopy is extremely useful for determining the level of infiltration of the lesion across the esophageal wall, the involvement of neighboring anatomical structures and the eventual presence of metastatic lymph nodes. Infiltration of the wall interrupts the progression of peristaltic contraction and stops, temporarily or definitively, the progression of food; this interruption is related to the extent of the obstruction and it causes a variety of symptoms, depending on whether it is partial or total. Partial obstruction can stop solid food, but allows passage of liquids; total obstruction, which stops the flow of liquids too, causes liquids to collect above the site of the obstruction, between the obstruction and the upper esophageal sphincter.

Regurgitation, salivation, odynophagia

Longstanding stenoses can cause incompetence – permanent or episodic – of the upper esophageal sphincter and the regurgitation of undigested material together with the possibility of inhalation; the amount of this collection is related to the level of the obstruction, being much larger when the lesion is close to the cardia; moreover, total obstruction stops the passage of saliva and causes the onset of another invalidating symptom, that is, salivation.

The patient complaining of salivation is obliged to spit or dribble continuously and walks around with a bag full of handkerchiefs – deprived of a social life. Dysphagia can be associated with odynophagia, generally caused by inflammation of the esophageal wall or by candidiasis or herpesvirus; odynophagia too may cause salivation. Salivation and regurgitation often cause coughing as patients attempt to swallow and may simulate an esophagorespiratory fistula. This false diagnosis can be confirmed by a bronchogram due to the regurgitation of contrast medium when performing an esophagogram; it may be further confirmed by the fact that, after insertion of a stent into a stenotic esophagus, cough on swallowing disappears not because the inexistent fistula has been closed, but because, after opening of the esophageal transit, there is no more esophagorespiratory regurgitation. Consequently, the diagnosis of esophagorespiratory fistula must be confirmed by a tracheobronchoscopy, although nasal regurgitation is suggestive of the presence of a tracheoesophageal or bronchoesophageal fistula. When dealing with an oncological patient for palliative purposes, one should learn to give the patient the opportunity to fully explain the symptoms of the disease. A combination of an accurate clinical history and the results of the investigations often allows planning of treatment with a reduced number and frequency of traumatic and time-consuming examinations in these patients with a limited survival time.

Palliative endoscopic options for dysphagia

NASOGASTRIC TUBE

The objective of esophagoscopic treatment of dysphagia and its sequelae is based on crossing the obstacle that prevents the passage of food: this can be achieved by a nasogastric tube, by restoring the esophageal lumen by dilation, laser treatment, photodynamic treatment, or prostheses insertion, or performing a gastrostomy. These different options have specific indications.[10] The purpose of inserting a nasogastric tube is feeding liquid food, and it is an alternative to a gastrostomy. The indication is restricted to cases in which the stenotic obstacle cannot be dilated more than 4–5 mm; this mainly happens when there is postoperative or postradiotherapy fibrotic stenosis that makes forced dilation dangerous as there is a possibility of perforation.

There are several different disadvantages of the nasogastric tube:

- esthetic – the patient is obliged to live with the tube coming out of his or her nose
- functional – the external surface of the tube adheres strictly to the inner surface of the stenotic tract and this prevents saliva being swallowed leading to salivation
- sensuous – with food introduced through the tube, the patient is unable to enjoy its taste, one of the few pleasant sensations remaining at this stage of the life.

These disadvantages have to be considered also when planning to perform a gastrostomy, because, except for the presence of the nasal tube, patients complain of these symptoms after the creation of a gastrostomy.

DILATION

Dilation can be performed by pneumatic balloon dilators or by plastic bougies: both can slide along a guidewire and enlarge the esophageal lumen up to 20 mm. There are also balloons that can be introduced through the operative channel of the endoscope and guided into the stenotic tract under direct vision; the drawback of the dilation is that the stenosis will recur in 1–3 weeks and dilations must be frequently repeated.

LASER TREATMENT

This aims to reopen the esophageal lumen through the thermal coagulation-destruction of the cancer tissue: power laser radiation increases the local temperature of the irradiated tissues and causes the tissue water to evaporate. The neodymium:yttrium aluminum garnet (Nd:YAG) laser is the most frequently used due to the depth of penetration of its radiation into the cancer tissue. The treatment is precise and safe in appropriate hands and the esophageal lumen can be fully restored so as to obtain a satisfactory eating function; the mean duration of the patency of the lumen is estimated to be 4–8 weeks.[11]

PHOTODYNAMIC THERAPY

Photodynamic therapy (PDT) uses photosensitizing drugs from the group of porphyrins that are selectively fixed by the tumor. The photosensitizer, activated by light, produces singlet oxygen that is toxic for biological tissues and causes a necrotic effect; unlike the procedures discussed above which are performed to allow the passage of food, the necrotic effect of PDT needs 4–8 days to become apparent and the relief from obstruction lasts for 5–10 weeks.[12] However, patients submitted to PDT have to avoid direct sunlight for 4–6 weeks because of the skin photosensitization.[13]

PROSTHESES

The fate of all these procedures is the recurrence of the obstruction due to the regrowth of the tumor, unless a prosthesis is inserted after dilation of the stenotic tract.[14] Both disposal plastic as well as metallic prostheses are available. The plastic ones require full dilation of the lumen (17 mm to insert a 15 mm prosthesis), unlike the metallic ones, that, being expandable, can be introduced through a narrow (7–9 mm) passage, to reach, at the end of the expansion, an internal diameter of 20–22 mm, allowing an optimal and immediate transit for any kind of food.[15] The insertion of an expandable prosthesis is no more traumatic than a flexible esophagoscopy.

The differences between plastic and expandable prostheses are: the plastic ones have a narrower lumen and give rise to a larger number of complications (migration, perforation, obstruction by solid food) whereas the expandable ones are much more expensive, cannot be removed and, being woven as meshes, cannot be used to close fistulas. Recently, covered stents to be used in cases with fistulas have been manufactured, but the possibility of migration is higher than with noncovered stents, particularly when inserted through the cardia. Prostheses can be obstructed by large morsels or by regrowth of the tumor. The best results are obtained when the prosthesis does not interfere with the mechanism of a sphincter (the pharyngo-esophageal or the cardiac sphincter).[16] When the cardiac sphincter is infiltrated by the tumor, and the prosthesis keeps it open, the valvular antireflux mechanism is impaired and the gastric content flows back into the esophagus. The acid gastric secretion can be responsible for supra-prosthetic esophagitis and this condition causes dysphagia even though the esophagus is patent. However, in patients submitted to gastrectomy or operated on with techniques including vagotomy, in which the gastric environment is alkaline, the reflux through the prosthesis may give rise to an alkaline esophagitis. While in the first group of patients drugs that increase the pH, such as proton pump inhibitors, are indicated, in the second group, with alkaline esophagitis, these drugs worsen the dysphagic symptoms. Therefore special attention must be paid to the medical treatment of patients with patent prosthesis complaining of resistant dysphagia. Special prostheses with antireflux mechanisms have been recently manufactured, but definite results of their use are not yet available.[17,18] When the pharyngo-esophageal sphincter is involved and the insertion of the prosthesis keeps it open, the patient must adapt the swallowing mechanism to this new condition and that may need some days or weeks to be perfected.

In patients predicted to have a long survival, the evolution of the cancer through the esophageal wall can be in the form of the development of a fistula, connecting the esophageal lumen with the skin of the neck, the trachea, a bronchus, the mediastinum or the pleural space. Prostheses are equally used in these patients to bypass the fistula, allowing immediate passage of the oral intake. Fistulas can be consequent to tumor infiltration or previous surgery or radiotherapy. Insertion of a prosthesis to bypass a fistula allows immediate restoration of oral feeding and curing of concomitant dermatitis (in cervical fistulas), bronchopneumonia (in tracheo- and broncho-esophageal fistulas), mediastinitis (in mediastinal fistulas) and pleural effusions (in esophago-pleural fistulas). Obviously, only plastic stents or covered mesh stents can be used in the indication of closing a fistulous passage, because a simple mesh stent would allow the filtration of liquids through the mesh.[19] Covered stents have a tendency to migrate and their application must be carefully evaluated, because an eventual removal may be extremely difficult. The new self-expanding plastic stents have been used in the treatment of thoracic leaks after esophagectomy for cancer; these stents can be easily removed after the fistula repair and their application reduces leak-related morbidity and mortality and can be considered as a cost-effective alternative to surgery and to the other endoscopic treatments.[20]

If an esophago-tracheal or an esophago-bronchial fistula cannot be treated by inserting a stent into the esophagus (no concomitant stenosis to avoid migration of the stent), the prosthesis can be inserted into the respiratory tract to close the tracheal or the bronchial opening to avoid aspiration pneumonia, a frequent cause of death in these patients. Generally, plastic stents are used. The most widely marketed are the Dumon stents, introduced with a rigid tracheobronchoscope under general anesthesia. These stents have the advantage that they can be easily repositioned in case of migration or removed if the fistula closes, as it can happen in postsurgical cases.

PERCUTANEOUS GASTROSTOMY

Percutaneous gastrostomy is considered only when there is no possibility to carry out one of the previously described procedures. Percutaneous endoscopic gastrostomy (PEG) consists of the insertion of a feeding/venting tube into the stomach, through the abdominal wall under direct endoscopic control, to choose the best position to access the gastric cavity. Such a tube can be advanced to reach the jejunum, thus becoming a jejunostomy and it can be used also for decompressing an obstructed intestine.

Bleeding and vomiting

Endoscopic treatment can be beneficial for bleeding and vomiting, when these symptoms result mainly from intragastric or pancreatic tumors infiltrating the gastric wall. Polypoid or ulcerated, they may be endoscopically treated because they produce symptoms linked to the bleeding or to the food progression. This second group of symptoms is generally linked to the compression of the gastric antrum. Malignant ulcerations bleed and produce anemic conditions speeding up the progression toward cachexia. Decisions concerning the management of a bleeding gastrointestinal cancer need to consider the general clinical condition of the patient and the burden and the extent of the disease.

PALLIATIVE ENDOSCOPIC OPTIONS FOR BLEEDING AND VOMITING

To stop bleeding, endoscopic laser photocoagulation, unipolar or multipolar electrocoagulation, cryotherapy, injection of sclerosing drugs can be used for cytoreductive as well as for hemostatic purposes. These treatments are effective, but the duration of the effect is limited and the recurrence of the bleeding is a rule. The progression of the infiltration of the gastric wall and the presence of polypoid intragastric masses, mainly in the antrum, obstructs the gastric passage and causes gastric distension, nausea and, finally, vomiting. Because all these symptoms are produced by gastric obstruction, they disappear when the obstruction is relieved after an endoscopic treatment performed through administration of thermal energy (electrocoagulation, laser [argon beam] coagulation) or positioning a stent. Duodenal obstructions, as well as the gastric ones, can also be treated by performing a translaparoscopic bypass between the gastric body and the first jejunal loop, although expandable prostheses are also used to bypass duodenal and gastric compressive and stenosing lesions. Duodenum and gastric antrum can be obstructed by primary or metastatic tumors. Malignant lymph nodes, pancreatic and ampullary cancers are the most frequent causes of duodenal obstruction. Together with biliary tumors, these conditions are responsible for biliary obstruction and cause malignant jaundice.

Malignant jaundice

After the first cannulation of the papilla of Vater performed by Classen and Demling in 1972[21] and the consequent operative procedures, jaundice became one of the most important fields of application of the endoscopic techniques.

Biliary obstruction causes malignant jaundice. The obstruction can be caused by biliary, pancreatic, or metastatic cancer or by lymphomas, obstructing the common bile duct or the hepatic ducts. It is generally concomitant with whitish stools, brown urine and diffuse itching. Pancreatic cancer is the most common cause of malignant biliary obstruction, followed by cholangiocarcinoma, carcinoma of the papilla of Vater, and metastatic tumors. When biliary obstruction and the consequent jaundice occurs, the patient has advanced stage disease and palliation of the jaundice is the real purpose of the treatment.

PALLIATIVE ENDOSCOPIC OPTIONS FOR MALIGNANT JAUNDICE

An endoscopic approach[22] by inserting biliary endoprostheses through the transpapillary route has become the palliative treatment of choice, particularly for distal stenoses located at the choledochal level. When the obstruction is located into the hepatic hilum, the endoscopic approach is more difficult. However, palliative treatments that are alternatives to the endoscopic ones (surgical and percutaneous) have higher costs and complications and a lower success rate. They are indicated in case of failure of the endoscopic procedure.[23] Moreover the endoscopic approach allows a careful inspection of the alimentary tract and particularly of the antro-pyloric and duodenal area: this inspection is useful because of the frequent association of biliary and duodenal obstruction.

Insertion of gastroduodenal prostheses can relieve a concomitant obstruction of the gastric outlet and of the gastroduodenal passage. To obtain endoscopic biliary drainage, the obstructed biliary tract must be crossed with a guidewire introduced through the papilla under endoscopic guidance; a guide catheter is then passed over it and, lastly, a plastic prosthesis is pushed through the stenotic tract and allows bile to flow. These plastic stents present a main late complication consisting of the occlusion with biliary sludge; in this case they must be removed and replaced with new ones, it generally happens within 6 months after the stent is introduced. Metallic expandable prostheses, similar to those used in the coronary vessels, in the urethra and in the tracheobronchial tree, have been proposed for the biliary tract. They have a low occlusion and complication rate, are easy to place and can be considered as a permanent procedure in the malignant jaundice.

The main advantages of the endoscopic approach are the low rate of trauma and the immediate effect. In fact, whitish stools become well-stained in the 24–48 hours after the procedure, the urine loses progressively its intensive brown color and itchiness disappears. When endoscopic drainage is impossible, percutaneous, video-laparoscopic or open surgical routes can be used: the first one allows the insertion of a transhepatic tube, whereas the second and third allow wide exploration of the peritoneal cavity and the performance of a bilio-digestive bypass.[22]

Constipation

Constipation is a very frequent symptom; more than 50 percent of advanced cancer patients need to be treated for the infrequent passage of hard stool. The cause should be clarified. When caused by anticancer chemotherapeutic drugs (mainly vincristine), opioids, metabolic problems like hypokalemia or global electrolyte imbalances, it is mostly of the type of adynamic ileus and is frequently accompanied by generalized abdominal pain. Intestinal obstruction by endoluminal masses or by extraintestinal compressions is more frequently accompanied by colicky pain.

PALLIATIVE ENDOSCOPIC OPTIONS FOR CONSTIPATION

Longstanding constipation resistant to common treatments must be managed in an effective way, but the safety of the treatment is compulsory. Endoscopy can help in the purpose of perfecting the diagnosis as well as in treating the distension. These patients are generally submitted to nasogastric intubation or other venting procedures for gastroduodenal decompression. A transanal approach can be necessary, so that, after cleaning enemas have been performed at low pressure, colonoscopy with large channel endoscopes allows gas and liquid aspiration and distension of the bowel wall. It must be performed carefully, injecting small quantities of warm water to clean the lumen, considering that the bowel wall is often very fragile because of concomitant ischemic lesions.

PALLIATIVE OPTIONS FOR OBSTRUCTION

A cancer growing into the intestinal lumen will obstruct the progression of intestinal content. Obstruction can also occur due to metastatic involvement of the mesenteric lymph nodes or diffuse peritoneal nodular metastases, e.g. in papillary carcinomas, mainly, ovarian and pancreatic. About 10 percent of intestinal obstructions are caused by malignancies; up to 30 percent of obstructions result in resolution. More than 60 percent of malignant obstructions are caused by recurrent cancers.

The plan of investigations and the treatment in each case is tailored to the individual patient. If a patient, already treated for an intestinal tumor, presents with abdominal distension, vomiting, constipation and crampy pain, and plain X-ray of the abdomen shows air–fluid levels and bowel distension, the first choice is endoscopy. This is to locate precisely the cause of the obstruction and to perform, when possible, the first palliative treatment by dilation, laser, or stenting.

Surgery

Surgery is indicated consequent to endoscopic examination and to re-staging examinations. Surgical procedures can be classified as bowel resections, preparing ostomy or bypass operations; the kind of procedure is related to the position of the stenosing lesion and to the type of previous surgery. Providing optimal palliative care for the patient with advanced colorectal cancer is a complex and challenging process and may be a departure from the traditional surgical satisfaction derived from the complete excision of a malignancy. However, surgeons aspiring excellence in palliative care will likely find this a rewarding endeavor.[23]

Considering the pros and the cons of the different surgical procedures, on the one hand bypass operations and diverting stomas do not remove the tumor and consequently do not interfere with symptoms related to its presence, such as bleeding and pain due to infiltration of anatomical structures (peritoneum in intraabdominal cancers or periosteum in the pelvic localizations) although they alleviate symptoms due to obstruction. On the other hand surgical removal, when possible, alleviates all the tumor-related symptoms, but morbidity and mortality rates are higher in patients who undergo palliative versus curative surgery.

When only palliation of symptoms is possible, the purpose of surgery is to bypass the stenotic tract, removing the malignancy. Before surgery, some points must be noted, such as the location of the lesion, whether it is single or multiple, the degree of the stenosis, the viability of the bowel wall, the real and ultimate cause of symptoms (malignancy, adherences, bands), and the likelihood of spontaneous resolution. Persistence of bowel obstruction has a strong influence on prognostic outcome and in a multivariate analysis it was the only symptom that had an independent effect. Consequently, it must be managed, and possibly interrupted as soon as possible. Conventional medical treatment has to be established with nasogastric or nasojejunal intubation, and supply of intravenous fluids and electrolytes. The patient must be monitored with serial physical examinations

performed by the same physician, enemas should be performed to clean the colon and a colonoscopy should be done with the purpose of localizing and possibly treating the obstructing lesion. This type of examination must be performed carefully by an experienced endoscopist because of the fragility of the patient and of the intestinal wall, of the hypersensitivity to pain, and the risk of perforation.

Endoscopic options

Endoscopic procedures to be considered in case of obstruction are dilation, electrocoagulation, laser coagulation, cryotherapy and, lastly, endoprostheses, all of them with low mortality and morbidity.[24] Any treatment has to be performed only in patients presenting symptoms (obstruction, pain, bleeding) clearly attributable to the tumor and must be directed to bypass the symptom. In asymptomatic patients any palliative treatment must be deferred. Patients to be submitted to palliation are those with very advanced and nonremovable cancers. They generally present with cachexia and weight loss and surgical operations carry a high mortality, about 10 percent, and a survival rate of around 5 percent at 5 years.

There are different endoscopic possibilities of treatment, related to the kind of the obstructing lesion and in particular to its shape and to the tumor bulk, growing into the lumen or infiltrating the bowel wall. In the first case – the presence of an obstructing mass – the mass has to be removed to reopen the intestinal lumen; this can be done through an endoscopic laser treatment. In the second case – lesion infiltrating the bowel wall – introduce under endoscopic visual guidance a trans-stenotic guidewire and slide a dilator on it; once dilation has been achieved, the fecal transit can been reestablished and the emergency problem overcome and the bowel cleaned. If the tumor is operable, the lesion can be resected or a bypass operation performed through a surgical laparotomy or a laparoscopic procedure which is planned for the following days; if the patient is inoperable because of high risk conditions or because the lesion is not removable, the endoscopic alternative is the only feasible option. To keep open the intestinal lumen and maintain the bowel functions, an expandable prosthesis must be inserted in these cases to obtain a durable effect.[25] The results of the endoscopic treatments can be summarized as follows:

- Dilation with inflatable balloons has a high rate of success (~90 percent), but stenosis recurs in 1–2 weeks
- Similar rate of success is obtained with Nd:YAG laser but the duration of the dilation is longer
- Insertion of a prosthesis with a correct technique and indication allows the patency of the large bowel to be maintained in more than 80 percent of treated patients. We started to insert stents in primary rectal tumors and in recurrences in rectal anastomoses with a success rate of more than 90 percent. In most of our cases patency of the stent lasts until death.[26]

CONCLUSION

The features of endoscopic palliation are: (i) achievement of an immediate result in the control of symptoms and in the restoration of a normal function, whereas other options of palliation, like radiotherapy and chemotherapy and surgery are generally more risky, and need incomparably longer times to become effective; (ii) absence of contraindications and side effects; and (iii) the possible combination of endoscopic treatments with any other form of treatment.

Palliative treatments, in each case, should be tailored to the individual patient, and some clinical benefit, subject to the patient's capacity to undergo the treatments, consisting of a decrease or disappearance of symptoms and of improvement of performance status, should be the primary endpoint.

Key learning points

- Palliative treatments should start to control the symptoms as soon as the disease is classified as incurable.

- Digestive cancers form about 20 percent of all diagnosed cancers and most of them, when advanced, are poorly responsive to curative treatments; consequently, patients not responding to curative treatment will need symptomatic, palliative treatments.

- Before deciding to treat only symptoms, we should consider the different curative options offered by surgery, radiotherapy, chemotherapy, immunotherapy, through a multidisciplinary approach.

- Gastrointestinal symptoms may be produced by digestive or extradigestive tumors. Most of them affect the digestive cavities and grow into them, occupying spaces required for digestive functions.

- Tumors reduce the spaces and impair the functions of containing and flowing, and they infiltrate and lead to ulceration the walls of these cavities thus producing symptoms; in particular, they cause hemorrhages, obstructions, perforations and fistulas.

- More than 95 percent of the digestive tumors are *endo*cavitary and *endo*scopy is the most suitable approach for precise and selective treatment.

REFERENCES

◆ 1 Nelson KA. The cancer anorexia-cachexia syndrome. *Semin Oncol* 2000; **27**: 64.

◆ 2 Baines MJ. Symptom control in advanced gastrointestinal cancer. *Eur J Gastroenterol Hepatol* 2000; **12**: 375–9.

◆ 3 Ikeda M. Significant host and tumor-related factors for predicting prognosis in patients with esophageal carcinoma. *Ann Surg* 2003; **238**: 197–202.

◆ 4 Brown JM, Wouters BG. Apoptosis, p53, and tumor cell sensitivity to anticancer agents. *Cancer Res* 1999; **59**: 1391–9.

5 Jernvall P, Makinen MJ, Karttunen TJ, *et al.* Loss of heterozygosity at 18q21 is indicative of recurrence and therefore poor prognosis in a subset of colorectal cancers. *Br J Cancer* 1999; **79**: 903–8.

● 6 Silberman AW. Surgical debulking of tumors. *Surg Gynecol Obstet* 1982; **155**: 577–85.

✱ 7 Morris DE. Clinical experience with retreatment for palliation. *Semin Radiation Oncol* 2000; **10**: 210–21.

● 8 De Vita VT, Schein PS. The use of drugs in combination for the treatment of cancer. *N Engl J Med* 1973; **288**: 998.

9 Lipsky MH, Chu MY, Yee LK, *et al.* Predictive sensitivity of human cancer cells to anticancer agents in vivo. *Proc Am Assoc Cancer Res* 1994; **35**: 371.

◆ 10 Goodwin WJ, Byers PM. Nutritional management of the head and neck cancer patients. *Med Clin North Am* 1993; **77**: 597–610.

11 Spinelli P, Dal Fante M, Mancini A. Endoscopic palliation of malignancies of the upper gastrointestinal tract using Nd:YAG laser: results and survival in 308 treated patients. *Lasers Surg Med* 1991; **11**: 550–5.

12 Lightdale CJ, Heier SK, Marcon NE, *et al.* Photodynamic therapy with porfimer sodium versus thermal ablation therapy with Nd: YAG laser for palliation of esophageal cancer: a multicenter randomized trial. *Gastrointest Endosc* 1995; **42**: 507–12.

◆ 13 Lightdale CJ. Role of photodynamic therapy in the management of advanced esophageal cancer. *Gastrointest Endosc Clin North Am* 2000; **10**: 397–408.

✱ 14 Spinelli P, Cerrai FG, Meroni E. Pharingo-esophageal prostheses in malignancies of the cervical esophagus. *Endoscopy* 1991; **23**: 213–14.

◆ 15 Boyce HW Jr. Stents for palliation of dysphagia due to esophageal cancer [editorial]. *N Engl J Med*.1993; **329**: 1345–6.

✱ 16 Decker P, Lippler J, Decker D, Hirner A. Use of the Polyflex stent in the palliative therapy of esophageal carcinoma: results in 14 cases and review of the literature. *Surg Endosc* 2001; **15**: 1444–7.

17 Dormann AJ, Eisendrath P, Wigginghaus B, *et al.* Palliation of esophageal carcinoma with a new self-expanding plastic stent. *Endoscopy* 2003; **35**: 207–11.

18 O'Donnell CA, Fullarton GM, Murray GD, *et al.* A comparison of the effectiveness of metallic stents and plastic endoprostheses in the palliation of oesophageal cancer: A pilot randomised controlled trial. *Br J Surg* 2002; **89**: 985.

◆ 19 Boyce HW Jr. Palliation of dysphagia of esophageal cancer by endoscopic lumen restoration techniques. *Cancer Control* 1999; **6**: 73–83.

✱ 20 Hünerbein M, Stroszczynski C, Moesta KT, Schlag PM. Treatment of thoracic anastomotic leaks after esophagectomy with self-expanding plastic stents. *Ann Surg* 2004; **240**: 801.

● 21 Classen M, Koch H, Demling L. Diagnostische Bedeutung des endoscopischen Kontrastdarstellung des Pankreasgangsystems. *Leber Magen Darm* 1972; **2**: 79–81.

◆ 22   Costamagna G. Therapeutic biliary endoscopy. *Endoscopy*
       2000; **32**: 209.

● 23   Bismuth H, Casting D, Traynor O. Resection or palliation:
       priority of surgery in the treatment of hilar cancer. *World J
       Surg* 1988; **12**: 39–47.

✱ 24   Matthew R, Dixon A, Michael J, Stamos B. Strategies for
       palliative care in advanced colorectal cancer. *Dig Surg* 2004;
       21: 344–51.

◆ 25   Spinelli P, Mancini A, Dal Fante M. Endoscopic treatment of
       gastrointestinal tumors: indications and results of laser
       photocoagulation and photodynamic therapy. *Semin Surg
       Oncol* 1995; **11**: 307–18.

  26   Spinelli P, Mancini A. Use of self-expanding metal stents for
       palliation of rectosigmoid cancer. *Gastrointest Endosc* 2001;
       53: 203–6.

PART 10

Fatigue

65

Pathophysiology of fatigue

CLAUDIA GAMONDI, HANS NEUENSCHWANDER

INTRODUCTION

Fatigue is the most frequent symptom in patients with advanced cancer.[1] It is reported as a symptom that heavily interferes with daily life. The prevalence is estimated, depending on the studies, to be between 60 percent and 90 percent among advanced cancer patients.[2–6**] In many malignant and nonmalignant diseases, fatigue becomes a leading, nonspecific symptom that accompanies patients from diagnosis to death. Fatigue can be one of the symptoms that leads to diagnosis; it may first occur during chemotherapy and radiotherapy and may remain one of the major complaints of the patient during the recovery after treatment.

Fatigue commonly has a major impact on function. Descriptive studies show an inverse relation between fatigue and various indicators of quality of life.[7–13*] Some studies have explored the gender difference in fatigue: data suggest that there is no gender difference, even if there are some indications that women generally report higher rates of symptoms than men.[14–19] Fatigue may easily interfere with social and physical activities, may influence the patient's decision making and may lead a patient to refuse a potentially curative treatment. For all these reasons, during the past few years, there has been an increasing awareness of the importance of this symptom in palliative care and oncology.

The basic mechanisms by which fatigue is caused are not well understood. Occasionally one predominant abnormality is present and appears to be the main contributor to the symptom, but in most cases several abnormalities and many symptoms coexist and may contribute to the genesis of fatigue. There are, however, three main types of mechanism causing asthenia: direct tumor effects, tumor-induced products, and tumor-accompanying factors.

DIRECT TUMOR EFFECTS AND TUMOR-INDUCED PRODUCTS

On the one hand, cancer by itself is able to release a number of substances, termed 'asthenine', able to interfere with host metabolism. On the other hand cancer can induce host macrophages and lymphocytes to produce a number of inflammatory cytokines such as tumor necrosis factor α (TNFα), interleukin (IL)-1, IL-6, and IL-2, which are active in the muscle tissue and in the central nervous system (Fig. 65.1).

Muscle is a main target tissue of cancer fatigue: histologically, there is an atrophy of type II muscle fibres, which are responsible for anaerobic performance.[1] Muscles of cancer-bearing animals show alterations in the activity of various enzymes, distribution of isoenzymes and synthesis and breakdown of myofibrillar and sarcoplastic proteins.[20,21] In humans there is an evidence of excessive lactate production in tumor-free muscle tissue: this represents an expression of both weakness and pathophysiological mechanism.[22,23]

Patients with chronic heart failure may show profound metabolic abnormalities leading to a catabolic state with progressive loss of muscle bulk: indeed a significant correlation between muscular fatigability and reduced electromyographic activity was found in patients with chronic heart failure.[24] A reduction in skeletal muscle protein stores may result from endogenous TNF or from TNF administered as antineoplastic therapy.[25] Thorud et al., in a study conducted on rats with congestive heart failure, observed that elevated circulatory concentrations of TNFα and monocyte chemoattractant protein-1 is a frequent finding. These molecules are supposed to stimulate matrix metalloproteinase activity and thereby contribute to distort the normal contractile muscle function, increasing skeletal muscle fatigue.[26] Prolonged bed rest and immobility leads to loss

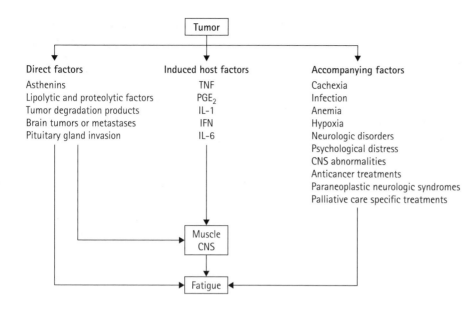

Figure 65.1 *Fatigue generating mechanisms. TNF, tumor necrosis factor; IFN, interferon; IL, interleukin; PGE, prostaglandine E; CNS, central nervous system.*

of muscle mass and reduced cardiac output. This deconditioning results in reduced endurance for exercise and activities of daily living and may be compounded by other muscle abnormalities in patients with cancer.[27,28]

Franssen *et al.* pointed out the contribution of starvation, deconditioning, and aging to alterations of peripheral skeletal muscle in chronic organ diseases, such as chronic obstructive pulmonary disease, chronic heart, and renal failure.[29] Studies have demonstrated that endurance training can reduce fatigue and improve physical performance in cancer patients while they are receiving chemotherapy and bone marrow or autologous stem cell transplantation.[30–35]

Aerobic training and combination of exercise modalities in patients with heart failure are shown to be effective in decreasing global rating of symptoms, including fatigue.[36]

TUMOR-ACCOMPANYING FACTORS

Fatigue and cachexia

The relationship between fatigue and cachexia is complex. In the main, there is agreement that these two conditions are strongly associated or at least coexist.[1] Malnutrition, muscle mass loss, and progressive cachexia are valid reasons for fatigue and they are strongly related one to the other. Cancer patients present a catabolic metabolism: they show increased rate of metabolism and energy expenditure compared with control groups with similar weight loss; in addition they show an increased need for amino acids, which leads to protein breakdown.[37–39]

Cachexia in cancer is characterized by severe muscle wasting: reactive oxygen and nitrogen species have been proposed as underlying mechanisms. The inefficiency of the antioxidant enzymes may be responsible for the development

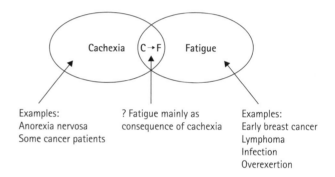

Figure 65.2 *Possible relation between cachexia and fatigue.*

of both oxidative and nitrosative stress in cancer-induced cachexia.[40] These muscle abnormalities, such as reduced skeletal muscle and impaired skeletal muscle quality, are common in a variety of chronic conditions. In patients with chronic heart failure, cardiac cachexia is common: some authors observed raised plasma levels of norepinephrine, epinephrine, and cortisol, with high plasma renin activity and increased plasma aldosterone levels. There is increasing evidence that neurohormonal and immune abnormalities may play a crucial role.[41] However, in a number of conditions this relationship is not as close as expected: patients with breast cancer or lymphomas might complain of profound fatigue, but they have low incidence of cachexia.[42] Furthermore, patients with chronic fatigue syndrome or major depression show no malnutrition but high incidence of fatigue. On the other hand, in diseases such as anorexia nervosa there is severe malnutrition without fatigue.[1]

In conclusion, cachexia and fatigue may be part of an expression of major metabolic abnormalities, rather than simply expression of malnutrition *per se* (Fig. 65.2).[1]

Anemia

Anemia is a common finding in patients with malignant disease. It can be caused by the cancer itself or it can be cancer-induced or due to correlated factors such as bleeding, hemolysis, nutritional deficiencies, iron deficiency, antineoplastic treatment such as chemotherapy or radiotherapy, or by cancer independent factors. Hemoglobin levels below 8 g/dL are associated with profound fatigue.[1]

In some circumstances anemia may be a major factor in cancer-related fatigue and impairment of quality of life in cancer patients.[5,43,44] For individual patients, it is difficult to discern the real impact of anemia from that of other competing contributing factors to fatigue. The impact of anemia varies depending on factors such as the rapidity of onset, patient's age, plasma volume status, and the number and severity of co-morbidities.[45]

In patients with mean levels of hemoglobin between 9 g/dL and 11 g/dL receiving chemotherapy, the correction of anemia is shown to be effective in ameliorating quality of life, activity levels, and energy levels.[43] In our experience, even though anemia is a major contributor to asthenia, the correction of anemia is not always followed by an improvement in fatigue. The difficulty is correlating hemoglobin levels with degree of fatigue and its potential alterability.

In a study conducted among women undergoing pelvic radiotherapy for uterine cancer, Ahlberg et al. observed an increase in fatigue during treatment and no significant correlation between general fatigue and hemoglobin levels after 3 weeks of therapy.[46] Combined data from three randomized, placebo controlled trials on epoetin alfa, the recombinant form of human erythropoietin, revealed an association between increased hematocrit and an improvement in overall quality of life.[47] Patients with an increase in hematocrit of >6 percent had significant improvement in energy level and daily activities. Three large, prospective, nonrandomized, multicenter, community trials similarly observed that epoetin alfa-treated patients who experienced a rise in hemoglobin reported significant improvements in energy level, activity level, functional status, and overall quality of life.[43,44,48,49]

Since none of these studies had fatigue as a primary endpoint caution in interpreting these findings remains mandatory. All the studies refer to fatigue and chemotherapy; no controlled trials have been published so far on the correlation between fatigue and anemia in a palliative care population.

Infection

Correlation between fatigue and infection is well documented. Fatigue can be a prodromal symptom and it can outlast the infection for weeks and months.[50,51] In cancer patients, because of the immunodepression, acute and chronic infections are very common, and one of the underlying mechanisms of pathophysiology is the production of some mediators of inflammatory response, such as TNFα.[52] The production of some cytokines (TNFα, IL-1, IL-2, IL-6, interferon [IFN]) and the consequent activation of the inflammatory reaction can, in some cases, be considered the main mechanism leading to the cachexia-anorexia syndrome.[20,53,54] It can be assumed that there is a similar underlying mechanism in the genesis of infection-induced fatigue.

Metabolic and endocrine disorders

In many abnormalities of the metabolism and the endocrine system, e.g. diabetes mellitus, Addison disease, or electrolytic disorders, fatigue is a leading symptom. Dysfunction of the hypothalamic–pituitary–adrenal (HPA) axis is a field of research. Abnormalities of the HPA axis have been postulated as possible additional factors in the chronic fatigue syndrome.[1]

There is also evidence suggesting that IFNα initiates a cytokine cascade that affects the HPA and hypothalamic–pituitary–gonadal axis, thus affecting regulation of glucocorticoid and sex steroid hormone secretion. However the clinical significance of these observations has not yet been established.[55] There is clear evidence that hormonal deficiency syndromes, such as hypothyroidism, occur in a relatively large portion of patients receiving systemic IFNα therapy.

Some authors, after acknowledging the limitations of current clinical data, have concluded that adrenal and gonadal axis dysfunction also must be considered in patients with IFNα-induced fatigue.[56] The possibility of hypothyroidism must be considered. However, diagnosis of hypothyroidism in cancer patients might be complicated by the occurrence of the 'sick euthyroid syndrome' (ESS). This syndrome is defined as the decrease of serum free triiodothyronine with normal free L-thyroxin and thyrotropin.[57] Recent reports have shown that IL-6 plays a key role in the pathogenesis of ESS: some authors have demonstrated that IL-6 can suppress the thyroid function.[58–60]

Kumar et al. conducted a prospective observational study on 198 consecutive breast cancer patients receiving adjuvant chemotherapy.[61] Changes in anthropometric data, fatigue, nutritional intake, physical activity, thyroid and steroid hormones were monitored from start to end of the chemotherapy and 6 months after therapy. They concluded that cytotoxic agents may influence thyroid function in this population, contributing to and progressively worsening symptoms such as weight gain, amenorrhea, fatigue and lowered physical activity. They suggested to screen breast cancer patients for thyroid function at diagnosis or at the beginning of the adjuvant treatment.[61]

The role of testosterone has also been studied: age-associated hypogonadism occurs in 30 percent of men after the age of 55. It is associated with decreased muscle mass, bone mineral density, and libido, hemoglobin levels and with anorexia, fatigue, and irritability.[62] Even if some of these symptoms overlap with those of depression, the association between the two disorders is unclear. There is some evidence that there is an increased incidence of depressive illness and a shorter time to diagnosis of depression in hypogonadal men.[63] In male patients with cancer, hypogonadism is correlated with fatigue, and androgen insufficiency can be caused by anorexia-cachexia syndrome.

Profound hypogonadism with low levels of serum testosterone or estrogen coupled with low levels of pituitary gonadotropins has been noted in male and female patients receiving intrathecal opioids.[64,65] Hormone levels are related to the opioid consumed, dosage and dosage form, nonopioid medication use, and several personal characteristics.[66] A recent study demonstrated that cancer survivors who were chronic opioids consumers experienced symptomatic hypogonadism with significantly higher levels of depression, fatigue, and sexual dysfunction.[67] The reduction in opioid consumption can dramatically increase libido and sexual function with a possible mechanism involving opioid-related effects on the HPA axis.[68*]

The determination of testosterone in men under opioid treatment who are experiencing fatigue might therefore be worthwhile, since there might be some therapeutic consequences. Hormonal ablative therapy in prostate cancer patients can double the incidence of fatigue and the replacement therapy in hypogonadic and testosterone depleted HIV patients results in an improvement of energy, libido and hemoglobin levels.[1]

Psychological distress

The prevalence of depression in cancer patients varies: major depression has a prevalence of 0–38 percent, depression spectrum syndromes from 0 percent to 58 percent. In palliative care, the reported prevalence of depression varies from 17 percent to 42 percent.[69] In psychiatric patients, fatigue is a common somatic symptom of clinical depression and it is included in the diagnostic criteria for major depressive disorders, bipolar disorders, and dysthymic disorders. Anderson *et al.* conclude that patients with cancer report significantly more severe fatigue and fatigue-related interference in their daily life activities than the community-dwelling subjects. Furthermore, patients with depressive disorders reported more severe fatigue and more interference with their daily lives due to fatigue than either cancer or community individuals.[70]

Several investigators have suggested that depression and fatigue may have overlapping but not equivalent physiopathological mechanisms: this could explain why patients with clinical depression who respond to antidepressant medication may continue to experience residual fatigue.[71] In a large representative sample of cancer patients where the most frequently reported problem was fatigue, 37.8 percent met criteria for general distress in the clinical range.[72] This

finding supports the view of the chronic stress condition mentioned above. In addition a recent study supports the evidence that in treating depression with sustained released (SR) bupropion there can be a reduction of the symptom fatigue experienced by cancer patients.[73]

Central nervous system abnormalities

The relation between central nervous system (CNS) and fatigue is poorly studied. Abnormalities of the CNS can themselves be a cause of fatigue, and, at the same time, the brain is also the area where fatigue is perceived.[1] Primary or secondary CNS tumors may cause endocrine abnormalities and, as a consequence, fatigue. Patients with acute lymphoblastic leukemia receiving cranial radiotherapy experience fatigue, depression and sleepiness.[74] Chronic pain stimulates the reticular activating system, which seems to be responsible for the experience of fatigue. All these findings should stimulate research in this field.

Anticancer treatments

Anticancer treatments have a high impact on energy levels: most of the patients complain of fatigue while receiving chemotherapeutic agents.[75–78] Several studies have shown a correlation between fatigue and different types of oncological treatment: it has been observed that 65–100 percent of patients undergoing radiotherapy and up to 82–96 percent of those receiving chemotherapy suffer from fatigue during treatment.[79] In supportive care, drugs used to control nausea and vomiting are themselves contributors to fatigue. However, it may be difficult, in the individual patient, to demonstrate if fatigue is more related to treatment or to the underlying disease.

In a multivariate analysis, 43 percent of the variance in fatigue was ascribed to disease-related symptoms and 35 percent to toxicity of treatment.[79] Radiotherapy and chemotherapy can result in anemia, diarrhea, anorexia and weight loss, all contributors to fatigue. For example, treatment with dexamethasone may be beneficial to reduce postchemotherapy symptoms induced by irinotecan, specifically anorexia and fatigue.[80**] In patients treated with biological response modifiers such as IFNα, fatigue is an important dose-limiting side effect.

Autoimmune thyroid disease, another contributor to fatigue, is a well-recognized consequence of IFNα therapy and may be mediated by the induction of IFNγ production by lymphocytes.[56] Recent data suggest that IFNα depression may be composed of two overlapping syndromes: a depression-specific syndrome characterized by mood, anxiety, and cognitive complaints, and a neurovegetative syndrome characterized by fatigue, anorexia, and psychomotor slowing.[81]

Fann *et al.* in a study conducted on delirium episodes in patients undergoing hematopoietic stem cell transplantation observed that affective distress and fatigue were common and appeared to be associated most with psychosis-behavioral delirium symptoms.[82] The new emerging feature called 'chemobrain' should stimulate further research in the possible relation between delirium and fatigue.[83]

Paraneoplastic neurological syndromes

Even though quite rare, these neurological complications of cancer are probably underestimated. Sometimes these symptoms can precede the outbreak of the malignant disease by months or even more, or may lead to the diagnosis of cancer. Box 65.1 shows some of the syndromes associated with fatigue. Lung cancer has the highest incidence of paraneoplastic syndrome.[84]

Box 65.1 Paraneoplastic neurological syndromes associated with fatigue

- Progressive multifocal leukoencephalopathy
- Peripheral paraneoplastic neurological syndrome
- Paraneoplastic encephalomyelitis
- Ascending acute polyneuropathy
- Amyotrophic lateral sclerosis
- Neuromuscular paraneoplastic syndromes: dermatomyositis; polymyositis; Eaton–Lambert syndrome; myasthenia gravis
- Subacute motor neuropathy
- Subacute necrotic myelopathy

Symptom control oriented treatments

OPIOIDS

Nearly 90 percent of patients with advanced cancer receive opioids;[1] these drugs are known to act on the reticular system and cause sedation and drowsiness, which can be perceived by patients as a dimension of fatigue. Opioids may interfere with concentration and can contribute to mental fatigue. On the other hand, their effect in relieving pain may contribute to a less sleep deprivation and possibly to less fatigue.

ANTIDEPRESSANTS

Common side effects of antidepressants are weight gain, sexual dysfunction, sleep disturbances, fatigue, apathy, and cognitive impairment. Selective serotonin reuptake inhibitors and atypical antidepressants (e.g. venlafaxine, bupropion, and nefazodone) show relatively favorable short-term as

well as long-term tolerability compared with older drugs (e.g. tricyclics and monoamine oxidase inhibitors).[85]

ANXIOLYTICS

All central actions of the benzodiazepines are based on a common molecular mechanism. Reactions that are CNS depressant, such as sedation, fatigue, ataxia, impairment of motor coordination, and intellectual functions including memory are most frequent, especially in the elderly.[86]

ANTIEMETICS

There is clear evidence that almost all antiemetics might cause fatigue. In an anecdotal report, however, five female patients with chronic fatigue syndrome were eligible to receive oral granisetron for one month: the treatment with granisetron resulted in significant improvement in fatigue and functional impairment. Activity level showed no significant increase.[87] The significance of this finding has still to be assessed.

STEROIDS

On the one hand steroids can be a cause of fatigue by inducing myopathy, and on the other hand they can be part of the treatment of asthenia and their withdrawal can contribute to a worsening of the symptom.

Other symptoms as contributors to fatigue

Uncontrolled pain or dyspnea exacerbate fatigue. Poorly controlled symptoms may lead to insomnia, depression and anxiety, all contributors to fatigue.[1] Autonomic dysfunction, a common finding in patients with advanced cancer, characterized in others by postural hypotension, fixed heart rate, gastroparesis, is in many cases an important contributor to fatigue.

Sleep disturbance, defined as insomnia or hypersomnia occurring nearly every day, may appear as a self-standing symptom or as an epiphenomenon of depression. Among cancer patients it has received limited attention in clinical studies: it is estimated to range from 23 percent to over 50 percent.[70] There is a correlation between sleep patterns and fatigue: most patients with chronic fatigue syndrome complain of unrefreshing sleep. It can be supposed that the perceived sleep quality is of greater importance than the sleep characteristics. There is some evidence that sleep disturbance is associated with patient's fatigue level: a recent study, conducted in patients undergoing radiotherapy, found a correlation between improvement in sleep patterns and decrease in fatigue.[88] The relation between sleep disturbance and fatigue in cancer patients may be related to disease and treatment-induced abnormalities in cytokine levels. Many cytokines involved in cancer and cancer treatments have been associated with fatigue and sleep disorders. For example, injection of TNFα or IL-1 induces non-REM sleep and IFNα reduces the amount of both slow-wave and REM sleep.[89] Anderson *et al.* indicate that symptoms of sleep disturbance are highly prevalent among cancer patients and that sleep disturbance is a significant predictor of severe fatigue in these patients.[70]

Key learning points

- Fatigue is the most prevalent finding in patients with malignant disease. In the mean time it is the most underestimated condition that impairs function and quality of life. It has unfortunately still to be considered a mostly silent symptom, because it is not reported by the patient, not perceived and therefore not investigated by the physician.

- Even though quite often fatigue, or at least a part of it, might be attributed to other findings (symptoms, therapy side effects) therefore considered as an epiphenomenon, there is now enough evidence that fatigue is a self-standing symptom complex. In this sense, it deserves to be considered as a syndrome.

- Fatigue is almost always a multifactorial symptom. However in several cases one of the contributing factors may be apparently predominant. For this reason it is worth investigating the different possible causes, with respect to important therapeutic consequences.

- A lot of research in the field of fatigue is needed. In the past few years some contributing factors, such as cachexia and anemia have been investigated much more than others. Unfortunately the choice of research fields is sometimes also influenced by the pharmaceutical companies, which identify a potentially huge market for their products. There are two sides to the coin: on the one hand this helps to recognize fatigue as a major problem with major impact on quality of life and stimulates research. On the other hand fields of research that might also be important are overlooked. We feel that beside clinical interest and research on anemia and cachexia, clinical researchers should also have an interest in the study of sleep disturbances, endocrinological dysfunction, psychiatric conditions and the therapeutic balance between utility and futility of physical training and rest.

REFERENCES

1   Sweeney C, Neuenschwander H, Bruera E. Fatigue and asthenia. In: Doyle D, Hanks G, Cherny NI, Calman K, eds. *Oxford Textbook of Palliative Medicine*, 3rd ed. Oxford: Oxford University Press, 2004: 560–8.

● 2   Bruera E. Research into symptoms other than pain. In: Doyle D, Hanks G, MacDonald N, eds. *Oxford Textbook of Palliative Medicine*, 2nd ed. Oxford: Oxford University Press, 1998: 179–85.

3   Coyle N, Adelhardt J, Foley KM, *et al.* Character of terminal illness in the advanced cancer patient: Pain and other symptoms during the last 4 weeks of life. *J Pain Symptom Manage* 1990; **5**: 83–93.

4   Cella DF, Tulsky DS, Gray G, *et al.* The functional assessment of cancer therapy scale: Development and validation and of the general measure. *J Clin Oncol* 1993; **11**: 570–9.

● 5   Vogelzang NJ, Breitbart W, Cella D, *et al.* Patient, caregiver and oncologist perception of cancer related – fatigue: result of a tripart assessment survey. The Fatigue Coalition. *Semin Hematol* 1997; **34**: 4–12.

6   Portenoy RK, Thaler HT, Kornblith AB, *et al.* Symptom prevalence, characteristics and distress in a cancer population. *Qual Life Res* 1994; **3**: 183–9.

7   Dodd MJ, Miaskowski C, Paul SM. Symptom cluster and their effect on the functional status of patients with cancer. *Oncol Nurs Forum* 2001; **28**: 465–70.

8   Schwartz AL. Fatigue mediates the effects of exercise on quality of life. *Qual Life Res* 1999; **8**: 529–38.

9   Ferrell BR, Grant M, Dean GE, *et al.* 'Bone tired': the experience of fatigue and its impact on quality of life. *Oncol Nurs Forum* 1996; **23**: 1539–47.

10   Servaes P, van der Werf S, Prins J, *et al.* Fatigue in disease-free cancer patients compared with fatigue in patients with chronic fatigue syndrome. *Support Care Cancer* 2001; **9**: 11–17.

11   Hickok JT, Morrow GR, McDonald S, *et al.* Frequency and correlates of fatigue in lung cancer patients receiving radiation therapy: implications for management. *J Pain Symptom Manage* 1996; **11**: 370–7.

12   Akechi T, Kugaya A, Okamura H, *et al.* Fatigue and its associated factors in ambulatory cancer patients: a preliminary study. *J Pain Symptom Manage* 1999; **17**: 42–8.

13   Stone P, Hardy J, Broadley K, *et al.* Fatigue in advanced cancer: a prospective controlled cross- sectional study. *Br J Cancer* 1999; **79**: 1479–86.

14   Heinonen H, Volin L, Uutela A, *et al.* Gender associated differences in the quality of life after allogenic BMT. *Bone Marrow Transplant* 2001; **28**: 503–9.

● 15   Pater JL, Zee B, Palmer M, *et al.* Fatigue in patients with cancer: results with the National Cancer Institute of Canada Clinical Trials Group studies employing the EORT QLQ-C30. *Support Care Cancer* 1997; **5**: 410–13.

16   Walsh D, Donnelly S, Rybicki L. The symptoms of advanced cancer: relationship to age, gender and performance status in 1000 patients. *Support Care Cancer* 2000; **8**: 175–9.

● 17   Kronke K, Wood Rd, Mangelsdrorff AD, *et al.* Chronic fatigue in primary care. Prevalence, patient characteristics, and outcome. *JAMA* 1998; **260**: 929–34.

18   Van Wijk CM, Kolk AM. Sex differences in physical symptoms: the contribution of symptom perception theory. *Soc Sci Med* 1997; **45**: 231–46.

19   Verbrugge LM. Gender and health: an update on hypotheses and evidence. *J Health Soc Behav* 1985; **26**: 156–82.

20   Theologides A. Anorexins, asthennins, and cachectins in cancer. *Am J Med* 1986; **81**: 696–8.

21   Nelson KA, Walsh D, Sheehan FA. The cancer anorexia-cachexia syndrome. *J Clin Oncol* 1994; **12**: 213–25.

22   Bruera E, Brenneis C, Michaud M, *et al.* Association between involuntary muscle function and asthenia, nutritional status, lean body mass, psychometrical assessment and tumour mass in patient with advanced breast cancer. *Proc Am Soc Clin Oncol* 1987; **6**: 261.

23 Holroyde CP, Axelrod RS, Skutches CL, *et al.* Lactate metabolism in patient with metastatic colorectal cancer. *Cancer Res* 1979; **39**: 4900–4.

24 Schulze PC, Linke A, Schoene N, *et al.* Functional and morphological skeletal muscle abnormalities correlate with reduced electromyographic activity in chronic heart failure. *Eur J Cardiovasc Prev Rehabil* 2004; **11**: 155–61.

25 St Pierre BA, Kasper CE, Lindsey AM. Fatigue mechanisms in patients with cancer: effects of tumour necrosis factor and exercise on skeletal muscle. *Oncol Nurs Forum.* 1992; **19**: 419–25.

26 Thorud HM, Stranda A, Birkeland JA, et. al. Enhanced matrix metalloproteinase activity in skeletal muscles of rats with congestive heart failure. *Am J Physiol Regul Integr Comp Physiol* 2005; **289**: R389–R394.

27 Germain P, Guell A, Marini JF. Muscles strength during bed-rest with and without muscle exercise as a countermeasure. *Eur J Appl Physiol Occup Physiol* 1995; 71: 342–8.

28 Levine BD, Zuckerman JH, Pawelczyk JA. Cardiac atrophy after bed-rest deconditioning: a nonneural mechanism for orthostatic intolerance. *Circulation* 1997; **96**: 517–25.

29 Franssen FM, Wouters EF, Schols AM. The contribution of starvation, deconditioning and ageing to the observed alterations in peripheral skeletal muscle in chronic organ diseases. *Clin Nutr* 2002; **21**: 1–14.

30 Dimeo FC, Stieglitz RD, Novelli-Fischer U, *et al.* Effects of physical activity on the fatigue and psychologic status of cancer patients during chemotherapy. *Cancer* 1999; **85**: 2273–7.

31 Dimeo F, Fetscher S, Lange W, *et al.* Effects of aerobic exercise on the physical performance and incidence of treatment related complications after high dose chemotherapy. *Blood* 1997; **90**: 3390–4.

32 Dimeo F, Bertz H, Finke J, *et al.* An aerobic exercise program for patients with haematological malignancies after Bone Marrow Transplantation. *Bone Marrow Transplant* 1996; **18**: 1157–60.

33 Dimeo FC. Effects of exercise on cancer-related fatigue. *Cancer* 2001; **92**(6 Suppl): 1689–93.

34 Dimeo F, Schwartz S, Fietz T, *et al.* Effects of endurance training on the physical performance of patients with hematological malignancies during chemotherapy. *Support Care Cancer* 2003; **11**: 623–8.

35 Crevenna R, Zielinski C, Keilani MY, *et al.* Aerobic endurance training for cancer patients. *Wien Med Wochenschr* 2003; **153**: 212–16.

36 Corvera-Tindel T, Doering LV, Woo MA, *et al.* Effects of a home walking exercise program on functional status and symptoms in heart failure. *Am Heart J* 2004; **147**: 339–46.

37 Argiles JM, Moore-Carrasco R, Busquets S, *et al.* Catabolic mediators as targets for cancer cachexia. *Drug Discov Today* 2003; **15**: 838–44.

38 Legaspi A, Jeevanadam M, Stanes HF, *et al.* Whole body lipid and energy metabolism in the cancer patient. *Metabolism* 1987; **10**: 958–63.

39 Nelson KA, Walsh D, Shehan FA. The cancer anorexia-cachexia syndrome. *J Clin Oncol* 1994; **12**: 213–25.

40 Barreiro E, de la Puente B, Busquets S, *et al.* Both oxidative and nitrosative stress are associated with muscle wasting in tumour-bearing rats. *FEBS Lett* 2005; **579**: 1646–52.

41 Anker SD, Sharma R. The syndrome of cardiac cachexia. *Int J Cardiol* 2002; **85**: 51–66.

42 Bruera E, Brenneis C, Michaud M, *et al.* Association between asthenia and nutritional status, lean body mass, anaemia, psychological status, and tumour mass in patients in advanced breast cancer. *J Pain Symptom Manage* 1989; **4**: 59–63.

43 Glaspy J, Bukowski R, Steinberg D *et al.* Impact of therapy with epoetin alfa on clinical outcomes in patients with nonmyeloid malignancies during cancer chemotherapy in community oncology practice. Procrit Study Group. *J Clin Oncol* 1997; **15**: 1218–34.

44 Demetri GD, Kris M, Wade J, *et al.* Quality-of-life benefit in chemotherapy patients treated with epoetin alfa is independent of disease response or tumour type: results from a prospective oncology study. Procrit Study Group. *J Clin Oncol* 1998; **16**: 3412–25.

45 Johnston E, Crawford J. The haematological support of the cancer patient. In: Berger A, Portenoy RK, Weissman DE, eds. *Principles and Practice of Supportive Oncology*. Philadelphia: Lippincott-Raven Publishers, 1998: 549–69.

46 Ahlberg K, Ekman T, Gaston-Johansson F. Levels of fatigue compared to levels of cytokines and haemoglobin during pelvic radiotherapy: a pilot study. *Biol Res Nurs* 2004; **5**: 203–10.

47 Abels RI. Recombinant human erythropoietin in the treatment of the anaemia of cancer. *Acta Haematol* 1992; **1**(87 suppl): 4–11.

48 Glaspy J. The impact of epoetin alfa on quality of life during cancer chemotherapy: a fresh look at an old problem. *Semin Hematol* 1997; **34**(3 suppl 2): 20–6.

49 Gabrilove J. Overview: erythropoiesis, anaemia, and the impact of erythropoietin. *Semin Hematol* 2000; **37**(4 suppl 6): 1–3.

50 Jones JF, Ray CG, Minnich LL, *et al.* Evidence for active Epstein-Barr virus infection in patients with persistent, unexplained illnesses: elevated anti-early antigen antibodies. *Ann Intern Med* 1985; **102**: 1–7.

51 Straus SE, Tosato G, Armstrong G, *et al.* Persisting illness and fatigue in adults with evidence of Epstein-Barr virus infection. *Ann Intern Med* 1985; **102**: 7–16.

52 Neuenschwander H, Bruera E. Pathophysiology of cancer asthenia. In: Portenoy RK, Bruera E, eds. *Topics in Palliative Care*, Vol. 2. Oxford: Oxford University Press, 1998.

53 Beutler B, Cerami A. Cachetin: more than a tumour necrosis factor. *N Engl J Med* 1987; **316**: 379–85.

54 Tisdale MJ. New cachexie factors. *Curr Opin Clin Nutr Metab Care* 1998; **1**: 253–6.

55 Gisslinger H, Svoboda T, Clodi M, *et al.* Interferon-alpha stimulates the hypothalamic-pituitary-adrenal axis in vivo and in vitro. *Neuroendocrinology* 1993; **57**: 489–95.

56 Jones TH, Wadler S, Hupart KH. Endocrine-mediated mechanism of fatigue during treatment with interferon-alpha. *Semin Oncol* 1998; **25**(1 suppl 1): 54–63.

57 Vexiau P, Perez-Castiglioni P, Socie G, *et al.* The 'euthyroid sick syndrome': incidence, risk factors and prognostic value soon after allogeneic Bone Marrow Transplantation. *Br J Haematol* 1993; **85**: 778–82.

58 Kimura T, Kanda T, Kotajima N, *et al.* Involvement of circulating interleukin-6 and its receptor in the development of euthyroid sick syndrome in patients with acute myocardial infarction. *Eur J Endocrinol* 2000; **143**: 179–84.

59 Kotajima N, Kanda T, Kimura T, *et al.* Studies on circulating interleukin-6 and thyroid functions in acute myocardial infarction. *Rinsho Byori* 2000; **48**: 276–81.

60 Davies PH, Black EG, Sheppard MC, *et al.* Relation between serum interleukin-6 and thyroid hormone concentrations in 270 hospital in-patients with non-thyroidal illness. *Clin Endocrinol (Oxford)* 1996; **44**: 199–205.

61 Kumar N, Allen KA, Riccardi D, *et al.* Fatigue, weight gain, lethargy and amenorrhea in breast cancer patients on chemotherapy: is subclinical hypothyroidism the culprit? *Breast Cancer Res Treat* 2004; **83**: 149–59.

62 Cavallini G, Caracciolo S, Vitali G, *et al.* Carnitine versus androgen administration in the treatment of sexual dysfunction, depressed mood, and fatigue associated with male aging. *Urology* 2004; **63**: 641–6.

63 Shores MM, Sloan KL, Matsumoto AM, *et al.* Increased incidence of diagnosed depressive illness in hypogonadal older men. *Arch Gen Psychiatry* 2004; **61**: 162–7.

64 Finch PM, Roberts LJ, Price L, *et al.* Hypogonadism in patients treated with intrathecal morphine. *Clin J Pain* 2000; **16**: 251–4.

65 Roberts LJ, Finch PM, Pullan PT, *et al.* Sex hormone suppression by intrathecal opioids: a prospective study. *Clin J Pain* 2002; **18**: 144–8.

66 Daniell HW. Hypogonadism in men consuming sustained-action oral opioids. *J Pain* 2002; **3**: 377–84.

67 Rajagopal A, Vassilopoulou-Sellin R, Palmer JL, *et al.* Symptomatic hypogonadism in male survivors of cancer with chronic exposure to opioids. *Cancer* 2004; **100**: 851–8.

68 Rajagopal A, Bruera E. Improvement in sexual function after reduction of chronic high-dose opioid medication in a cancer survivor. *Pain Med* 2003; **4**: 379–83.

69 Massie MJ. Prevalence of depression in patients with cancer. *J Natl Cancer Inst Monogr* 2004: 57–7.

● 70 Anderson KO, Getto CJ, Mendoza TR, *et al.* Fatigue and sleep disturbance in patients with cancer, patients with clinical depression, and community-dwelling adults. *J Pain Symptom Manage* 2003; **25**: 307–18.

71 Menza MA, Kaufmann KR, Castellanos A. Modafinil augmentation of antidepressant treatment in depression. *J Clin Psychiatry* 2000; **61**: 378–81.

72 Carlson LE, Angen M, Cullum J, *et al.* High levels of untreated distress and fatigue in cancer patients. *Br J Cancer* 2004; **90**: 2297–304.

73 Cullum JL, Wojciechowski AE, Pelletier G, *et al.* Bupropion sustained release treatment reduces fatigue in cancer patients. *Can J Psychiatry* 2004; **49**: 139–44.

74 Proctor SJ, Kernaham J, Taylor P. Depression as component of postcranial irradiation somnolence syndrome. *Lancet* 1981; **1**: 1215–16.

75 Greene D, Nail LM, Fieler VK, *et al.* A comparison of patient reported side effects among three chemotherapy regimens for breast cancer. *Cancer Pract* 1994; **2**: 57–62.

76 Stone P, Richards M, A'Hern R, *et al.* Fatigue in patients with cancers of the breast or prostate undergoing radical radiotherapy. *J Pain Symptom Manage* 2001; **22**: 1007–15.

77 Irvine D, Vincent L, Graydon JE, *et al.* The prevalence and correlates of fatigue in patients receiving treatment with chemotherapy and radiotherapy. A comparison with fatigue experience by healthy individuals. *Cancer Nurs* 1994; **17**: 367–78.

78 Blesch KS, Paice JA, Wickham R, *et al.* Correlates of fatigue in people with breast or lung cancer. *Oncol Nurs Forum* 1991; **18**: 81–7.

79 Donald P, Lawrence, Kupelnick B, *et al.* Report on the Occurrence, Assessment, and Treatment of Fatigue in Cancer Patients. *J Natl Cancer Inst Monographs* 2004: 40–50.

80 Inoue A, Yamada Y, Matsumura Y, *et al.* Randomized study of dexamethasone treatment for delayed emesis, anorexia and fatigue induced by irinotecan. *Support Care Cancer* 2003; **11**: 528–32.

81 Raison CL, Demetrashvili M, Capuron L, *et al.* Neuropsychiatric adverse effects of interferon-alpha: recognition and management. *CNS Drugs* 2005; **19**: 105–23.

82 Fann JR, Alfano CM, Burington BE, *et al.* Clinical presentation of delirium in patients undergoing hematopoietic stem cell transplantation. *Cancer* 2005; **15**: 810–20.

83 Wefel JS, Lenzi R, Theriault R, *et al.* 'Chemobrain' in breast carcinoma?: a prologue. *Cancer* 2004; **101**: 466–75.

84 Jurado Gamez B, Garcia de Lucas MD, Gudin Rodriguez M. Lung cancer and paraneoplastic syndromes. *An Med Interna* 2001; **18**: 440–6.

85 Cassano P, Fava M. Tolerability issues during long-term treatment with antidepressants. *Ann Clin Psychiatry* 2004; **16**: 15–25.

86 Klotz U. Effects and side effects of benzodiazepines. *Anasth Intensivster Notfallmed* 1988; **23**: 122–6.

87 Prins J, Bleijenberg G, van der Meer JW. The effect of granisetron, a 5-HT3 receptor antagonist, in the treatment of chronic fatigue syndrome patients – a pilot study. *Neth J Med* 2003; **61**: 285–9.

88 Sharpley A, Clements A, Hawton K, *et al.* Do patients with 'pure' chronic fatigue syndrome (neuroasthenia) have abnormal sleep? *Psychosom Med* 1997; **59**: 592–6.

89 Kubota T, Majde JA, Brown RA, *et al.* Tumour necrosis factor receptor fragment attenuates interferon-gamma-induced non-REM sleep in rabbits. *J Neuroimmunol* 2001; **119**: 192–8.

66

Assessment of fatigue in palliative care

JON H LOGE

WHAT IS FATIGUE?

Fatigue is an ambiguous phenomenon commonly described by patients as a sensation of tiredness, lack of energy, or exhaustion. In accordance with this, fatigue is often defined as a nonspecific and subjective feeling of tiredness, physically and/or mentally. However, no common agreed upon definition exists.[1,2] Fatigue may therefore represent different phenomena.

First, fatigue may be a physical symptom commonly defined as a perception, feeling or belief about the state of the body.[3] Physical symptoms are most commonly associated with pathological processes. Still, there is not a direct association between the pathological processes and the accompanying physical symptoms. Physical symptoms are influenced by the individual's perceptions, such as stated in the current definition of pain.[4] Second, fatigue may be a psychophysical symptom. These symptoms are commonly associated with mental health such as in the chronic fatigue syndrome (CFS) and in other psychosomatic conditions dominated by medically unexplained symptoms.[3] Psychophysical symptoms are not clearly physical or psychological in origin. Third, fatigue may be an emotional symptom. Fatigue is commonly observed in depressive conditions, and it is included as a depressive symptom in the current diagnostic criteria for depression.[3,5] However, it has been suggested that fatigue should be excluded as a depressive symptom in somatically ill patients due to the similarities between fatigue and the expressions of the disease processes (i.e. fatigue is a physical symptom).[3,5]

Thus there are different types of fatigue, but at present we are not able to clearly distinguish between them.[6] Fatigue is often categorized in various dimensions, but experts do not agree into which dimensions it should be categorized.[2,7] The multidimensionality of fatigue is grounded on theory and empirical data from different populations including cancer patients,[8–10] patients with nonmalignant diseases,[11,12] and disease-free cancer survivors.[13–15] Qualitative studies have suggested that cancer-related fatigue implies at least three distinct dimensions: a physical sensation (decreased capacity for physical work), affective sensations (reduced energy level, low mood), and cognitive sensations (lack of concentration, impaired memory).[8] However, it is unresolved whether these dimensions are stable and reproduced in more general settings.

FATIGUE IS A FINAL COMMON ENDPOINT

Several factors may cause fatigue, but specific biological mechanisms are at present relatively poorly understood.[7,16] The majority of the studies on fatigue have been cross-sectional which limits the possibility to explore causality. Although several proposed mechanisms are theoretically sound, a simple mechanistic approach (one cause – one symptom) is too simplistic in most clinical and scientific settings. The latter view is supported by the fact that most physical diseases are accompanied by fatigue.[7] Further, in cancer and palliative patients, many common symptoms such as pain, dyspnea, cachexia, and sleep disturbances correlate significantly with fatigue.[17–19] Additionally, correlates of fatigue also differ between populations. Stone et al. demonstrated that among palliative care inpatients, fatigue severity was significantly associated with pain and dyspnea scores. In healthy controls fatigue severity was significantly associated with anxiety and depression.[20] Finally, fatigue characteristics do not differentiate between fatigue of physical or mental origin.[21] The predictive value of fatigue as a symptom is consequently low, and fatigue is probably best seen as a final common pathway to which many factors contribute.[22] The pathways may differ between populations. In palliative patients, fatigue is strongly related to physical aspects of the disease as opposed to healthy persons. In the latter, fatigue is most strongly related to psychological distress.[20]

FATIGUE: A SIMPLE SYMPTOM OR PART OF ILLNESS BEHAVIOR?

The individual patient will probably experience fatigue as a symptom comparable to other subjective symptoms such as nausea, pain or dyspnea. As stated, there is never a direct relationship between a pathological process and a symptom, and this is important to be aware of in assessments of fatigue.[23] Symptoms are more or less influenced by psychological and social factors.[24] The distinction between the pathological process (the disease) and the subjective experience of disease (the illness) is therefore of special relevance in relation to fatigue.[23] For some symptoms such as nausea and pain there are specific neuronal pathways, which convey the message from the affected part of the body to the brain where the information is processed and eventually expressed. In clinical settings we can therefore assume that a subjective sensation of pain reflects an underlying pathological process (for example skeletal metastases) that has activated the neuronal pathway. No specific neuronal pathway has been demonstrated for fatigue, and the specificity of fatigue as a symptom is low, i.e. most known diseases and many different pathological processes are accompanied by fatigue. Fatigue is therefore a common part of being ill.

Fatigue in patients with cancer correlates with increased symptom distress, decreased quality of life and even shortened survival.[25] Approaching fatigue as a 'simple' symptom that can be alleviated through one single intervention is therefore an oversimplification. Fatigue must be assessed and understood as part of the illness experience in most situations. Thus, patients with terminal cancer and other severe diseases probably have to experience fatigue at some level. Fatiguelike behavior can also be observed in other mammals, and from an evolutionary viewpoint one may argue that the 'fatiguelike' behavior must have been selected for some reason, for example improved protection from predators.

These points illustrate the complexity of the fatigue phenomenon in research and in practice. Instead of asking if a patient experiences fatigue, one should ask how much fatigue she or he experiences. Ideally one should anchor the level of fatigue to other criteria such as an expected level or a relevant comparison group. Comparison groups must be adjusted or matched for age and gender since these variables have an effect upon fatigue.[26]

HOW PREVALENT IS FATIGUE?

Fatigue is reported to be prevalent in most studied populations including patients with cancer and palliative care patients.[7,9] Prevalence estimates above 75 percent among cancer patients are commonly cited.[9,16,22,27,28] All palliative care patients will experience fatigue during their disease trajectory.[20,29]

Still, the prevalence of fatigue is strongly related to how fatigue is measured. The prevalence of 'severe' fatigue (defined as fatigue above a certain cut-point originally defined in the validation study of the Fatigue Questionnaire [the FQ][30]) in the general Norwegian population was 22 percent.[26] When a time-criterion was included (6 months or longer duration), the prevalence dropped to 11 percent.[26] This also illustrates the importance of the distinction between acute and chronic fatigue (usually defined by duration $\geqslant 6$ months[31]).

Figure 66.1 illustrates the distribution of fatigue scores measured by the FQ in the general Norwegian population. Fatigue is close to normally distributed, and this has consequences for measurement and their interpretation.[19] Based upon such a distribution researchers on the CFS have proposed that severe fatigue as seen in CFS is the extreme part of a normally distributed phenomenon.[7] Another way of interpreting the distribution is to apply an analogy with blood pressure. Blood pressure is normally distributed, and a high level is defined by the consequences such as renal failure or cardiovascular diseases. An elevated level of blood pressure is defined on the basis of empirical data on acute and late morbidity (cardiovascular disease or renal failure). Further, an elevated blood pressure does not indicate anything about the possible underlying mechanisms (i.e. renal, endocrinologic, essential, etc.). Consequently, assessments of fatigue without referring to clinical consequences,

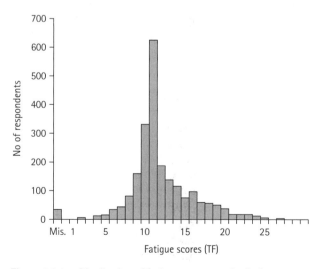

Figure 66.1 *Distribution of fatigue-scores on the Fatigue Questionnaire in the Norwegian general population (possible range: 0–33). Mis., missing data; TF, total fatigue.*

comparison groups or other external criteria are often of limited value.

MEASUREMENT OF FATIGUE: SOME GENERAL ASPECTS

A prerequisite for including fatigue as a study endpoint are valid and reliable measurement techniques. Several different measurement techniques have been used. These include observation, self-rating scales and objective tests.[7,27,28,32,33] There is a lack of consensus on how to define fatigue, but there is agreement on the subjective nature of the phenomenon.[34] Consequently, measurement by self-report is the preferred method.[2] Most of the early studies on fatigue used single-item self-rating measures. The validity of such measures is questionable because the wording so strongly influences the answers. For example, 'feeling tired' is reported 10 times more often than 'feeling weak'.[7] Studies in the general populations report prevalences of fatigue in the range of 11–50 percent.[7,26] This large difference is most probably explained by the use of different questions/questionnaires.

Efforts have been made to measure fatigue objectively by for example counting movements by an electronic device and using the number of movements as an expression for fatigue.[33] This is simple from a technical point of view, but the number of movements (i.e. the validity) corresponds poorly with the subjective experience of fatigue.[33]

An expert panel recently pointed to the need for systematic assessment of subjective symptoms including fatigue in cancer care.[35] In spite of the challenges related to definitions, operationalizations, and measurement of fatigue, a nihilistic approach which has been common among physicians partly related to these challenges[1] is not in line with the burden fatigue represents for the patients. In practical clinical work the choice of a measure will often be a compromise between optimal psychometric properties, brevity, simplicity, and the purpose of the assessment. It is better to measure fatigue by a single item with a verbal/numerical rating scale as response alternatives than not measuring it at all. Still, the single items have limited reliability which restricts their use in studies. A simple question combined with a numerical rating scale such as in the Edmonton Symptom Assessment Scale is found to be a useful clinical tool.[36]

FATIGUE INSTRUMENTS

At present, measurement by self-rating multi-item instruments is the preferred method for studies of fatigue. Several self-rating fatigue instruments are available and relatively recent publications present data on the instruments' content and psychometric properties.[2,37] The instruments can be grouped within the terminology of health-related quality-of-life (HRQOL) instruments. These are commonly divided into generic (i.e. not specific to any population or disease such as the Medical Outcome Survey Short Form 36 (SF-36)[38]), disease-specific (such as EORTC QLQ-C30[39] for use in cancer patients) and domain-specific instruments, which generally include measures for psychological distress, pain, fatigue or other symptoms. Most recent generic and disease-specific HRQOL instruments include fatigue and measure fatigue in one dimension.[40] By inspection, the items on fatigue within these instruments measure physical fatigue. The psychometric properties of these instruments are generally the best documented.

Domain-specific fatigue instruments have become relatively numerous during the last 10 years, and some of the most commonly used instruments are presented in Table 66.1. Some instruments measure fatigue as a one-dimensional phenomenon, others measure it as a multidimensional phenomenon. This reflects the lack of consensus on definition and measurement of fatigue.[2] Most of the publications on the instruments are from patients with cancer in general, and the optimal instrument for palliative care is at present not agreed-upon. Still, there are some points that relate specifically to palliative patients. First, the length of the instrument is of special concern in palliative care.

Table 66.1 *Some fatigue-specific instruments applied in cancer patients*

Instruments	Characteristics	Reference
Unidimensional instruments		
Rhoten Fatigue Scale	Single item + visual analog scale	41
Visual Analog Fatigue Scale	Single item + visual analog scale	42
Brief Fatigue Inventory	9 items on numerical rating scales	43
FACIT-F	13 items, 5 response categories	44
Multidimensional instruments		
Fatigue Symptom Inventory	14 items, 4 subscales	45
Revised Piper Fatigue Scale	22 items, 4 subscales	46
Fatigue Questionnaire	11 items, 2 subscales	30
Multidimensional Fatigue Inventory	20 items, 5 subscales	10

Table 66.2 *The Fatigue Questionnaire (FQ)[30] versus the Multidimensional Fatigue Inventory (MFI-20)[10]*

	FQ	MFI-20
Number of items	11	20
Number of subscales	2	5
Number of response categories	4	5
Caseness-score	Yes	No
Intercorrelations[a]	0.55	0.30–0.86
Reliability[b]	0.79 and 0.89	0.79–0.93
Correlations with HADS-depression[c]	0.39 and 0.46	0.61–0.77
Percentage of max/min scores	0/0	3.7–15.7/9.2–33.6
Percentage of complete questionnaires	87	89

[a] Correlations between subscales.
[b] Assessed by Cronbach α.
[c] Correlation with the depression subscale of the Hospital Anxiety and Depression Scale (HADS).[51]

This was found to be of special relevance to the measurement of pain, and is probably as relevant in relation to measurement of fatigue.[47] Long instruments are too demanding to fill in, resulting in missing forms and increasing the possibility for introducing a selection bias. Second, physical fatigue, which is the feeling of being exhausted physically, is probably the most relevant type of fatigue in palliative care as opposed to, for example, mental fatigue or affective fatigue.[48] Third, including functional limitations due to fatigue (interference) is disputable since the majority of palliative patients experience several symptoms at the same time, and most of them have functional consequences. It is questionable whether it is possible to differentiate between, for example, functional limitations due to fatigue, dyspnea, nausea, or pain. Fourth, some measures presuppose fatigue, and these are inappropriate to use in individuals not experiencing fatigue. Fifth, the time frame covered by the instrument should be considered as this may vary significantly. If the purpose is to assess the level of fatigue before and after an intervention a shorter time frame is preferable. On the other hand if the purpose is to assess fatigue in cancer survivors, minor fluctuations are of lesser relevance and a longer time frame is preferable.

Generally, recent instruments have acceptable internal consistency (Cronbach $\alpha > 0.70$).[2,32] Few measures have been tested for their responsiveness to change, and the instruments' capacity to detect changes during interventions is consequently uncertain. The content of each instrument should be carefully evaluated to see if it is appropriate. This might be a challenge, and a similar challenge has been reported in relation to measurement of pain.[49] Furthermore, few instruments have been validated in palliative patients. One study compared a fatigue-specific instrument to a cancer-specific HRQOL instrument.[48] Thus, the documentation on the strengths of the instruments' validity and reliability should always be considered carefully.

The possibility to perform external validation of fatigue instruments is restricted because of the lack of a 'gold standard', and validation must consequently be indirect. However, the construct validity of fatigue-specific instruments is generally not very well documented. It is therefore not known to what degree the instruments measure the same or different phenomena. The convergent validity, which means the degree to which instruments supposed to measure the same phenomenon actually do so, has not been documented for most of the instruments. The divergent validity, which means the degree to which a measure assesses a phenomenon as distinct from similar but different phenomena, has to our knowledge not been addressed for the majority of the instruments.

Some data from the validation studies of the Multidimensional Fatigue Inventory (MFI-20)[2] and data on the FQ[30] from studies of Hodgkin disease survivors[15,50] illustrate these points and are presented in Table 66.2. The table demonstrates that the FQ and the MFI-20 differ substantially in their psychometric properties. However, the examples are from different samples and therefore definite conclusions cannot be drawn. In the study of Smets *et al.* the correlations between physical and mental fatigue and HADS depression were 0.67 and 0.61, respectively.[52] The same dimensions of the FQ correlated 0.46 and 0.39 with Hospital Anxiety Depression Scale – depression.[50] The correlation between the two dimensions (mental and physical fatigue) in the FQ was 0.55.[50] Except for low to moderate correlations between the Mental Fatigue subscale and the other subscales, all the other subscales in the MFI-20 correlated in the range of 0.66–0.86.[52] These correlations indicate that the postulated dimensions of the MFI-20 are questionable, and that the MFI-20 measures depression to a higher degree than the FQ. Studies comparing different fatigue instruments are therefore needed. A recent study which compared three fatigue instruments concluded that single questions about lack of energy or fatigue severity may provide a simple and acceptable way to assess fatigue.[53]

INTERPRETING MEASUREMENTS OF FATIGUE

Most studies of fatigue in patients with cancer have been performed in convenience samples by cross-sectional designs and without use of comparison groups.[19,28] Our present knowledge of fatigue in cancer patients may therefore consist of arbitrary snapshots of a phenomenon that fluctuates over time. The cross-sectional studies of fatigue in convenience samples can generate hypotheses, but do not give opportunities for generalizations. Further, without knowing the natural course, it is also difficult to assess the need for interventions. For example, fatigue may be a self-limiting process as demonstrated by Greenberg et al., who measured fatigue during radiotherapy after lumpectomy in women with breast cancer (stages I and II).[54] The level of fatigue increased during the first part of the radiotherapy, then reached a plateau and dropped to the pretreatment level after termination of the radiotherapy.[54]

The choice of comparison groups in studies of fatigue may strongly affect the results and thereby the interpretation of the findings. This is illustrated by an example from a survey on fatigue in a representative sample of the Norwegian general population.[26] The respondents were asked if they had any of five different target diseases or nine different current health problems as used in the International Quality of Life Assessment project.[55] Based upon the answers, the sample was divided into four groups (no disease or current health problem, past or current disease only, current health problem only, both past or current disease and current health problem).[26] Fatigue is reported as cases (i.e. fatigue of a substantial level for 6 months or longer).[56] As presented in Figure 66.2, there were few patients with fatigue in the group not reporting diseases or health problems. The percentage of patients was fairly equally distributed in the groups only reporting diseases or current health problems. The highest proportion of cases was found in the group reporting both health problems and past or current diseases. Due to the normal distribution of fatigue in the general population, comparing cancer patients with subjects without health problems will boost up the differences. Such differences might be of lesser clinical significance. In the worst case, such comparisons may result in type I errors.

In general, several possibilities for interpretation of fatigue measurements exist.[57] The use of general population norms (norm-based comparisons) has some advantages and is of special relevance in cross-sectional studies. One advantage is that the level in the patient group is anchored to the population as a whole. The clinical significance of the findings may therefore be addressed without the tautological deduction from statistical significance to clinical significance. The norms are the best estimate for an expected value in the general population. Other comparison groups might be more or less representative, and it is generally a challenge to decide the representativity of a comparison group. The selection of an appropriate control

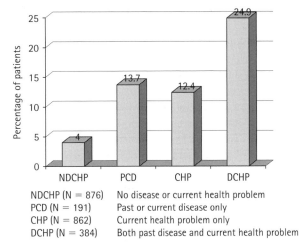

NDCHP (N = 876)   No disease or current health problem
PCD (N = 191)   Past or current disease only
CHP (N = 862)   Current health problem only
DCHP (N = 384)   Both past disease and current health problem

Figure 66.2 *Fatigue cases in the Norwegian general population grouped by health condition. NDCHP, no disease or current health problem; PCD, past or current disease only; CHP, current health problem only; DCHP, both past or current disease and current health problem.*

group is the main difficulty with the case–control study.[58] Population norms might be used several times, and subgroups of the norms can be matched with the patient group on age, gender, and other variables known to impact upon fatigue or these variables can be controlled for.[26] Further, the norms may be used for estimation of effect sizes by calculating standardized deviations from the norms (subtracting the norm mean score from the patients' mean score and dividing by the standard deviation of the norm).[57] Effect sizes calculated in this way compare well with evidence-based effect sizes.[59] Effect sizes can be used to interpret both cross-sectional and longitudinal group-based differences.[60] Additionally, clinical meaningful effect sizes are also necessary for performing power calculations in the planning phase of a study.

ASSESSMENT OF FATIGUE IN CLINICAL PRACTICE

Assessment of fatigue in palliative practice might be a challenge, and fatigue is probably often neglected or overlooked.[61] Physicians' neglect of fatigue might have historical reasons,[1] but it is also probably related to the nonspecificity of fatigue as a symptom. By asking, the physician might fear ending up in a long consultation, taking several tests, not finding any treatment options and ending up with presenting general advice. For these reasons, physicians probably omit to address fatigue, and the lack of documentation on treatment alternatives might further support such a nihilistic or avoidant approach. The physicians' beliefs about fatigue are therefore of relevance.[62]

However, the prevalence of fatigue, the overall aim of palliative care to prioritize the patients' quality of life and the burden fatigue imposes on the patients and their families both psychologically and functionally do not support an avoidant approach. In fact, many patients are relieved just by being asked, they feel assured by adequate information tailored to their level of knowledge, and many are well aware of the limited possibilities for documented treatment alternatives. The aims for assessment of a patient with a possible CFS can be modified for use in palliative care:[62]

- to establish a working relationship with the patient
- to elaborate on the symptom with a biopsychosocial assessment
- to address possible medical explanations
- to consider possible psychiatric explanations
- create an initial management plan.

The clinical assessment of fatigue as a symptom should follow general guidelines for symptom assessment in palliative care.[63] The assessment should include characterizing the severity, temporal features (onset, duration, course and daily pattern), exacerbating and relieving factors, associated distress and if possible impact on daily life.[22,61] To measure fatigue severity, a simple verbal rating scale or a numerical rating scale such as the item on fatigue in the Edmonton Symptom Assessment Scale might be useful both for the physician and the patient.[22,36] It is not documented that multi-item instruments have advantages compared to single-item measures in individual assessments of fatigue in palliative care. This is because the multi-item measures are designed for group assessments. However, one should be aware of the effect of the wordings in the single-item measures.

Illness beliefs are found to be of particular relevance in assessment of chronic fatigue in settings other than palliative care,[62] but might be relevant in palliative care as well. In general, addressing illness beliefs open-mindedly and in respect of the patient's beliefs strengthens the physician–patient relationship.[62] Assessment of illness beliefs is also of practical use because it might help to clear up misconceptions and also indicate possibilities for successful treatment. For example, a patient with a strong belief of fatigue being a direct consequence of a specific physiological disturbance might need more information and prompting to start physical training than a patient who believes fatigue to be the consequence of all the stressors affecting her or him. Further, assessment of previous experiences with health personnel in relation to fatigue is often productive. Many fatigued patients report that previous complaints about fatigue have not been taken seriously, and this might have been experienced as a rejection. Such 'illness disconfirmation' from health personnel might negatively affect the working alliance with the patient, and airing previous negative experiences might be a good starting point for a constructive therapeutic alliance.[62] Fatigue is for most patients a personnel experience and often accompanied by feelings of personnel insufficiency.[34] For example, lack of

energy might limit the possibility to take part in the family's life, and lowered self-efficacy and self-esteem and in the worst case feelings of guilt and personal failure might be the result. An inability to participate in ordinary life due to fatigue can be experienced as a serious loss and might further add to the stress of having a life-threatening disease.[34] The patient's way of coping with their fatigue might therefore be as relevant to assess as the functional consequences *per se.*

Finally, specific factors potentially contributing to fatigue should be assessed. These should include pain, mood, sleep disturbances, immobility and lack of exercise, medications and comorbid conditions.[61] This part of the assessment should focus on possible correctable causes. The list of possible 'causes' is long and includes direct effects of the underlying disease, effects of treatments, intercurrent systemic disorders such as anemia or infections, medications such as opioids, and psychiatric conditions such as depression.[22,61] In practical clinical work the distinction towards depression is best assessed by asking about mood. The simple question 'Are you depressed?' is a good screening tool for depression in palliative patients.[64] The question might easily be supplemented with questions about mood during the day, about what brings pleasure and about loss of interest in things or persons that usually bring pleasure. If a patient does not feel depressed, experiences normal mood during the day and experiences pleasure as expected, a depression is not the likely cause for the fatigue. It is also noteworthy that the standard criteria for depression are not fully valid in somatically ill people, and the correlation between fatigue and depression is probably much weaker in palliative care patients than in other cancer patients.[20,65]

An ordinary physical examination should always be done. Signs of infection, anemia, weight loss, and respiratory distress should be looked for. Since fatigue has so many possible etiologies, a number of laboratory tests can be relevant. Such tests should be guided by the clinical picture. A management algorithm for cancer-related fatigue has been suggested, but its usefulness in clinical practice in general and in palliative clinical practice in particular has not been documented.[22]

Diagnostically the proposed criteria for cancer-related fatigue might be of some use although they have not yet become 'official' and are not fully validated.[66] An interview guide to facilitate and standardize the diagnostic process has also been tested out.[67] The diagnostic criteria have been tested out in a mixed population of cancer survivors.[68] At the moment it is uncertain whether there is any gain in using them in clinical settings. However, the criteria might be of greater value in relation to research, similar to the criteria for CFS which were developed for use in research.[31]

CONCLUDING REMARKS

Fatigue is fascinating, complex and hard to explore. In the beginning of the last century, it was proposed to ban the identical phenomenon, asthenia, from science.[69] Our present technology makes research on fatigue possible, but the complexity of the phenomenon should be reflected in the research questions, study designs, measurements, and interpretation of results. Clinical experience tells us that fatigue is of great concern for palliative patients. Therefore the lack of knowledge on specific mechanisms and effective treatment options should not keep us from addressing the issue in clinical settings.

Key learning points

- Fatigue is a subjective phenomenon with multi-causal etiology.

- Fatigue is assessed by reports from the patients (i.e. by questionnaires).

- Many questionnaires are available, but few have been compared.

- The dimensionality of fatigue is unresolved but physical fatigue is most relevant in palliative care.

- A comparison group is warranted in most assessments and population norms have some major advantages.

- In clinical settings the most important assessment is to ask the patients about their fatigue, how it affects them and how they handle it.

- Assessment of possible underlying mechanisms in clinical settings should be guided by the possibility to base treatment decisions on the findings.

REFERENCES

◆ 1 Wessely S. The epidemiology of chronic fatigue syndrome [review]. *Epidemiol Rev* 1995; **17**: 139–51.

◆ 2 Jacobsen PB. Assessment of fatigue in cancer patients. *J Natl Cancer Inst Monogr* 2004; **32**: 93–97.

3 Wilson IB, Cleary PD. Linking clinical variables with health-related quality of life. A conceptual model of patient outcomes. *JAMA* 1995; **273**: 59–65.

4 Pain terms: a list with definitions and notes on usage. Recommended by the IASP Subcommittee on Taxonomy. *Pain* 1979; **6**: 249.

5 American Psychiatric Association. *Diagnostic and Statistical Manual of Mental Disorders*, 4th ed. Washington DC: APA, 1994.

6 Shapiro CM. Fatigue: how many types and how common? *J Psychosom Res* 1998; **45**(1 Spec No): 1–3.

◆ 7 Lewis G, Wessely S. The epidemiology of fatigue: more questions than answers [review]. *J Epidemiol Comm Health* 1992; **46**: 92–7.

● 8 Glaus A, Crow R, Hammond S. A qualitative study to explore the concept of fatigue/tiredness in cancer patients and in healthy individuals. *Support Care Cancer* 1996; **4**: 82–96.

◆ 9 Smets EM, Garssen B, Schuster-Uitterhoeve AL, de Haes JC. Fatigue in cancer patients [review]. *Br J Cancer* 1993; **68**: 220–4.

10 Smets EM, Garssen B, Bonke B, de Haes JC. The Multidimensional Fatigue Inventory (MFI) psychometric qualities of an instrument to assess fatigue. *J Psychosom Res* 1995; **39**: 315–25.

11 Ford H, Trigwell P, Johnson M. The nature of fatigue in multiple sclerosis [see comments]. *J Psychosom Res* 1998; **45**(1 Spec No): 33–8.

12 Wysenbeek AJ, Leibovici L, Weinberger A, Guedj D. Fatigue in systemic lupus erythematosus. Prevalence and relation to disease expression. *Br J Rheumatol* 1993; **32**: 633–5.

13 Bloom JR, Fobair P, Gritz E, *et al.* Psychosocial outcomes of cancer: a comparative analysis of Hodgkin's disease and testicular cancer. *J Clin Oncol* 1993; **11**: 979–88.

14 Joly F, Henry-Amar M, Arveux P, *et al.* Late psychosocial sequelae in Hodgkin's disease survivors: a French population-based case-control study. *J Clin Oncol* 1996; **14**: 2444–53.

15 Loge JH, Abrahamsen AF, Ekeberg O, Kaasa S. Hodgkin's disease survivors more fatigued than the general population. *J Clin Oncol* 1999; **17**: 253–61.

◆ 16 Morrow GR, Andrews PL, Hickok JT, *et al.* Fatigue associated with cancer and its treatment. *Support Care Cancer* 2002; **10**: 389–98.

● 17 Stone P, Richards M, A'Hern R, Hardy J. A study to investigate the prevalence, severity and correlates of fatigue among patients with cancer in comparison with a control group of volunteers without cancer. *Ann Oncol* 2000; **11**: 561–7.

18 Ancoli-Israel S, Moore PJ, Jones V. The relationship between fatigue and sleep in cancer patients: a review. *Eur J Cancer Care (Engl)* 2001; **10**: 245–55.

● 19 Hotopf M. Definitions, epidemiology, and models of fatigue in the general population and in cancer. In: Armes J, Krishnasamy M, Higginson IJ, eds. *Fatigue in Cancer*. Oxford: Oxford University Press, 2004.

● 20 Stone P, Hardy J, Broadley K, Tookman AJ, *et al.* Fatigue in advanced cancer: a prospective controlled cross-sectional study. *Br J Cancer* 1999; **79**: 1479–86.

21 Katerndahl DA. Differentiation of physical and psychological fatigue. *Fam Pract Res J* 1993; **13**: 81–91.

✱ 22 Portenoy RK, Itri LM. Cancer-related fatigue: guidelines for evaluation and management. *Oncologist* 1999; **4**: 1–10.

23 Aronowitz RA. When do symptoms become a disease? *Ann Intern Med* 2001; **134**(9 Pt 2): 803–8.

24 Kroenke K, Harris L. Symptoms research: a fertile field. *Ann Intern Med* 2001; **134**(9 Pt 2): 801–2.

● 25 Hwang SS, Chang VT, Cogswell J, Kasimis BS. Clinical relevance of fatigue levels in cancer patients at a Veterans Administration Medical Center. *Cancer* 2002; **94**: 2481–9.

26 Loge JH, Ekeberg O, Kaasa S. Fatigue in the general Norwegian population: normative data and associations. *J Psychosom Res* 1998; **45** (1 Spec No): 53–65.

27 Richardson A. Fatigue in cancer patients: a review of the literature [review]. *Eur J Cancer Care (Engl)* 1995; **4**: 20–32.

◆ 28   Stone P, Richards M, Hardy J. Fatigue in patients with cancer. *Eur J Cancer* 1998; **34**: 1670–6.

29   Coyle N, Adelhardt J, Foley KM, Portenoy RK. Character of terminal illness in the advanced cancer patient: pain and other symptoms during the last four weeks of life. *J Pain Symptom Manage* 1990; **5**: 83–93.

30   Chalder T, Berelowitz G, Pawlikowska T, *et al*. Development of a fatigue scale. *J Psychosom Res* 1993; **37**: 147–53.

31   Holmes GP, Kaplan JE, Gantz NM, *et al*. Chronic fatigue syndrome: a working case definition. *Ann Intern Med* 1988; **108**: 387–9.

32   Loge JH, Kaasa S. Fatigue and cancer – prevalence, correlates and measurement. *Prog Palliat Care* 1998; **6**: 43–7.

◆ 33   Swain M. Fatigue in chronic disease. *Clin Sci* 2000; **99**: 1–8.

34   Armes J. The experience of cancer – related fatigue. In: Armes J, Krishnasamy M, Higginson IJ, eds. *Fatigue in Cancer*. Oxford: Oxford University Press, 2004.

35   Wang L. Cancer care should include symptom management, panel says. *J Natl Cancer Inst* 2002; **94**: 1123–4.

36   Bruera E, Kuehn N, Miller MJ, *et al*. The Edmonton Symptom Assessment System (ESAS): a simple method for the assessment of palliative care patients. *J Palliat Care* 1991; **7**: 6–9.

37   Wu HS, McSweeney M. Measurement of fatigue in people with cancer. *Oncol Nurs Forum* 2001; **28**: 1371–84.

38   Ware JE, Jr., Sherbourne CD. The MOS 36-item short-form health survey (SF-36). I. Conceptual framework and item selection. *Med Care* 1992; **30**: 473–83.

39   Aaronson NK, Ahmedzai S, Bergman B, *et al*. The European Organization for Research and Treatment of Cancer QLQ-C30: a quality-of-life instrument for use in international clinical trials in oncology. *J Natl Cancer Inst* 1993; **85**: 365–76.

40   Ware JE, Jr. The status of health assessment 1994 [review]. *Annu Rev Public Health* 1995; **16**: 327–54.

41   Blesch KS, Paice JA, Wickham R, *et al*. Correlates of fatigue in people with breast or lung cancer. *Oncol Nurs Forum* 1991; **18**: 81–7.

42   Glaus A. Assessment of fatigue in cancer and non-cancer patients and in healthy individuals. *Support Care Cancer* 1993; **1**: 305–15.

43   Mendoza TR, Wang XS, Cleeland CS, *et al*. The rapid assessment of fatigue severity in cancer patients: use of the Brief Fatigue Inventory. *Cancer* 1999; **85**: 1186–96.

44   Yellen SB, Cella DF, Webster K, *et al*. Measuring fatigue and other anemia-related symptoms with the Functional Assessment of Cancer Therapy (FACT) measurement system. *J Pain Symptom Manage* 1997; **13**: 63–74.

45   Hann DM, Jacobsen PB, Azzarello LM, *et al*. Measurement of fatigue in cancer patients: development and validation of the Fatigue Symptom Inventory. *Qual Life Res* 1998; **7**: 301–10.

46   Piper BF, Dibble SL, Dodd MJ, *et al*. The revised Piper Fatigue Scale: psychometric evaluation in women with breast cancer. *Oncol Nurs Forum* 1998; **25**: 677–84.

47   Caraceni A, Cherny N, Fainsinger R, *et al*. Pain measurement tools and methods in clinical research in palliative care: recommendations of an Expert Working Group of the European Association of Palliative Care. *J Pain Symptom Manage* 2002; **23**: 239–55.

48   Knobel H, Loge JH, Brenne E, *et al*. The validity of EORTC QLQ-C30 fatigue scale in advanced cancer patients and cancer survivors. *Palliat Med* 2003; **17**: 664–72.

◆ 49   Jensen MP. The validity and reliability of pain measures in adults with cancer. *J Pain* 2003; **4**: 2–21.

50   Loge JH, Abrahamsen AF, Ekeberg, Kaasa S. Fatigue and psychiatric morbidity among Hodgkin's disease survivors. *J Pain Symptom Manage* 2000; **19**: 91–9.

51   Zigmond AS, Snaith RP. The hospital anxiety and depression scale. *Acta Psychiatr Scand* 1983; **67**: 361–70.

52   Smets EM, Garssen B, Cull A, de Haes JC. Application of the multidimensional fatigue inventory (MFI-20) in cancer patients receiving radiotherapy. *Br J Cancer* 1996; **73**: 241–5.

● 53   Hwang SS, Chang VT, Kasimis BS. A comparison of three fatigue measures in veterans with cancer. *Cancer Invest* 2003; **21**: 363–73.

54   Greenberg DB, Sawicka J, Eisenthal S, Ross D. Fatigue syndrome due to localized radiation. *J Pain Symptom Manage* 1992; **7**: 38–45.

55   Gandek B, Ware JE, Jr. Methods for validating and norming translations of health status questionnaires: the IQOLA Project approach. International Quality of Life Assessment. *J Clin Epidemiol* 1998; **51**: 953–9.

56   Fukuda K, Straus SE, Hickie I, *et al*. The chronic fatigue syndrome: a comprehensive approach to its definition and study. International Chronic Fatigue Syndrome Study Group. *Ann Intern Med* 1994; **121**: 953–9.

57   Osoba D, King M. Meaningful differences. In: Fayers P, Hays R, eds. *Assessing Quality of Life in Clinical Trials*. Oxford: Oxford University Press, 2005.

58   Altman DG. *Practical Statistics for Medical Research*, 1st ed. London: Chapman and Hall, 1991.

● 59   Osoba D, Rodrigues G, Myles J, *et al*. Interpreting the significance of changes in health-related quality-of-life scores. *J Clin Oncol* 1998; **16**: 139–44.

60   Cohen J. *Statistical Power Analysis for the Behavioural Sciences*. Hillsdale, NJ: Lawrence Erlbaum Associates, 1988.

◆ 61   Barnes EA, Bruera E. Fatigue in patients with advanced cancer: a review. *Int J Gynecol Cancer* 2002; **12**: 424–8.

62   Wessely S, Hotopf M, Sharpe M. *Chronic Fatigue and Its Syndromes*. Oxford: Oxford University Press, 1999.

63   Ingham J, Portenoy RK. The measurement of pain and other symptoms. In: Doyle D, Hanks GWC, Cherny N, Calman K, eds. *Oxford Textbook of Palliative Medicine*. Oxford: Oxford University Press, 2004: 167–84.

64   Chochinov HM, Wilson KG, Enns M, Lander S. 'Are you depressed?' Screening for depression in the terminally ill [see comments]. *Am J Psychiatry* 1997; **154**: 674–6.

65   Jacobsen P, Weitzner MA. Fatigue and depression in cancer patients: conceptual and clinical issues. In: Armes J, Krishnasamy M, Higginson IJ, eds. *Fatigue in Cancer*. Oxford: Oxford University Press, 2004.

◆ 66   Cella D, Peterman A, Passik S, *et al*. Progress toward guidelines for the management of fatigue [review]. *Oncology (Huntingt)* 1998; **12**: 369–77.

✳ 67   Sadler IJ, Jacobsen PB, Booth-Jones M, *et al*. Preliminary evaluation of a clinical syndrome approach to assessing cancer-related fatigue. *J Pain Symptom Manage* 2002; **23**: 406–16.

68   Cella D, Davis K, Breitbart W, Curt G. Cancer-related fatigue: prevalence of proposed diagnostic criteria in a United States sample of cancer survivors. *J Clin Oncol* 2001; **19**: 3385–91.

69   Muscio B. Is a fatigue test possible? *Br J Psychol* 1921; **12**: 31–46.

67

Exercise, physical function, and fatigue in palliative care

KERRY S COURNEYA, JEFFREY K H VALLANCE, MARGARET L McNEELY, CAROLYN J PEDDLE

INTRODUCTION

Cancer-related fatigue (CRF) is defined as a common, persistent, and subjective sense of tiredness related to cancer and/or its treatments that interferes with usual functioning.[1***] This is distinguishable from normal fatigue in that CRF symptoms are severe, distressing, and persist regardless of adequate amounts of sleep and rest.[2] Whereas approximately 20–30 percent of the general population report frequent tiredness,[3] between 60 percent and 90 percent of cancer survivors report CRF.[2] The etiology of CRF is unclear but multiple factors are likely involved. It may be caused by tumor-related and/or treatment-related factors such as decreases in the availability of metabolic substrates, hormonal changes, increase in proinflammatory cytokines, cachexia, neurophysiological changes in skeletal muscle, muscle wasting, decreased ventilatory ability, anemia, and altered sleep patterns.[4–7]

Cancer-related fatigue has proved to be a difficult symptom to manage.[2] One pharmacological intervention that has been found to be effective is correction of anemia by erythropoietin.[8***] Most nonpharmacological interventions can be categorized as energy conserving (i.e. a passive response to the fatigue). These interventions include rest, sleep, pacing oneself, relaxation training, and group psychotherapy. Interestingly, these approaches to managing fatigue have had limited success.[8***] For example, a meta-analysis of 15 randomized controlled trials found that relaxation training in cancer survivors showed significant

improvements in blood pressure, pulse rate, nausea, pain, depression, tension, anxiety, mood, and hostility, but not fatigue.[9***] Similarly, a randomized controlled trial of group psychotherapy in 235 women with metastatic breast cancer showed improvements in depression, anxiety, anger, and confusion but not fatigue or vigor.[10**] Despite these data, however, energy conserving strategies are still commonly recommended to cancer survivors with CRF. For example, one survey reported that when cancer survivors asked their physicians what they recommended to reduce fatigue, 40 percent said nothing, 37 percent said rest or relaxation, and only 5 percent said exercise.[11] In the present chapter, we review the growing literature examining exercise as a therapy for managing CRF.

POSSIBLE MECHANISMS FOR HOW EXERCISE MIGHT REDUCE CANCER-RELATED FATIGUE

Exercise may reduce fatigue in cancer survivors by alterations in physical functioning, behavioral functioning, psychological functioning, and/or social functioning (Fig. 67.1). In the present chapter, we focus on the physical functioning category. Exercise training has the potential to attenuate fatigue by means of optimizing physical efficiency and performance.[12] The ability to resist physical fatigue is determined, in part, by both muscular and cardiopulmonary fitness.[13] With repeated bouts of appropriately prescribed exercise the various body systems undergo a progressive adaptation to the imposed stress. These adaptations result in improved physical functioning[14] and an enhancement of energy capacity.[15]

Muscular fatigue may be defined as a reversible decrease in contractile strength that occurs after repeated muscle activity.[16] Local muscle fatigue may occur due to disturbances in the contractile mechanism of the muscle itself because of a decrease in energy stores, insufficient oxygen, and/or a build-up of lactic acid.[16] Endurance muscle fibers, or oxidative muscle fibers, are used in everyday activity both at work and in the home. These slow-twitch muscle fibers do not produce much force but are highly aerobic and therefore can sustain low levels of work for long periods of time. Disuse or deconditioning due to a period of significantly reduced activity or bed rest results in muscle atrophy and a decrease in the population of efficient, oxidative muscle fibers.[17***] Functional limitations from impaired muscular endurance can lead to significant fatigue when simply performing instrumental activities of daily living (e.g. housework or yard work).

Muscular endurance is improved by performing repeated contractions against a mild resistance.[16,18] Endurance training results in cells with increased mitochondrial size, number, and enzymatic activity.[15,16] Increased enzymatic activity in the cells allows the muscle to better use the oxygen delivered. Muscles trained for endurance also exhibit increased local glycogen fuel storage.[15,16] In addition to improving fuel stores, the endurance-trained muscle also increases fatty acid use and decreases the use of glycogen as a fuel.[15,16] Furthermore, endurance muscle training enhances the oxygen delivery system by increasing the local capillary network, producing more capillaries per muscle fiber.[16] These changes improve efficiency of the muscular system and thus allow more exercise to be performed before muscular fatigue occurs.

Cardiopulmonary endurance is determined by the ability of the cardiopulmonary system to consume, extract, deliver, and use oxygen, and to remove waste products from the body tissues. Cardiopulmonary endurance is necessary to be able to perform activities for extended periods of time without becoming short of breath.[16] Although cardiopulmonary endurance also requires muscular endurance, activities requiring muscular endurance do not always require high levels of cardiopulmonary endurance.

Cardiopulmonary endurance is improved by activities such as walking, swimming and cycling. These activities use large muscle groups, are maintained for a prolonged period of time, and are rhythmic and aerobic in nature. Cardiopulmonary endurance training produces significant changes in both cardiovascular and pulmonary systems.[15] These changes include increases in stroke volume and cardiac output and an increase in the weight and volume of the heart.[16] Blood volume is expanded along with increases in plasma volume, total hemoglobin concentration, and peripheral capillary formation. Increased breathing volumes accompany improvements in fitness and exercise training results in a significant increase in the quantity of oxygen extracted from the circulating blood.[15] Oxygen use is improved with increases in aerobic enzyme and muscle myoglobin levels, while substrate use is enhanced with increases in fat-mobilizing enzymes and free fatty acid delivery to muscle. Regular exercise also reduces resting and submaximal heart rate, systolic and diastolic blood pressure, and can alter body composition by decreasing body fat.[16] As a result, a prescribed submaximal activity can be carried out more readily and with less subjective perception of effort.[16] Furthermore, a higher peak rate of working becomes possible, and the rate of recovery of physiological variables after physical activity is enhanced.[14]

While typical day-to-day activities primarily require adequate muscular and cardiopulmonary endurance, many work and recreational activities require muscular strength and power. As the force requirement for work increases,

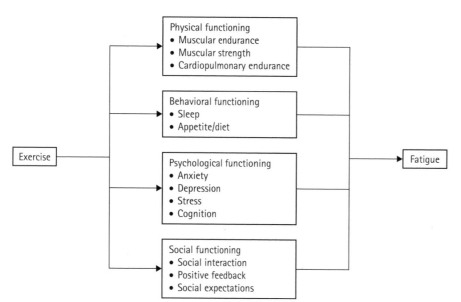

Figure 67.1 *Model of exercise and fatigue in cancer survivors.*

intermediate (oxidative-glycolytic) and fast-twitch (glycolytic) muscle fibers are recruited by the central nervous system.[18] Fast twitch muscle fibers are able to generate energy rapidly for quick forceful contractions; however, they do so with greater reliance on anaerobic pathways, resulting in earlier fatigue.[18]

Muscular strength is best enhanced by progressive resistance exercise training performed with high intensity (resistance) but fewer repetitions.[16] As the strength of a muscle increases, the cardiovascular response of the muscle improves so that muscular endurance and power also increase.[19] Increase in muscle cross-sectional area, as well as energy sources (creatine phosphate, ATP, myokinase, and phosphofructokinase) result from appropriately prescribed progressive resistance exercise training.[16] Neural adaptations to exercise include increases in neural activation and in the muscle's ability to produce torque.[16] Progressive resistance exercise training can also increase the maximum tensile strength of connective tissues such as tendon and ligaments, and can maintain or improve bone density.[16] Long-term performance of resistance training also benefits the cardiovascular system as evidenced by a decrease in heart rate and improvements in blood pressure and maximum oxygen consumption.[16] Muscular strength

training is particularly important to attenuate both sarcopenia and disease-related declines in muscle mass.[17]***

EXERCISE AND FATIGUE IN CANCER SURVIVORS

A literature review of all studies examining exercise and fatigue in cancer survivors was conducted in July 2004 using the CD-ROM databases CancerLit, CINAHL, HERACLES, MEDLINE, PsycINFO, and SPORT Discus. Key words that related to cancer (i.e. cancer, oncology, tumor, neoplasm, carcinoma), the postdiagnosis time period (i.e. rehabilitation, therapy, adjuvant therapy, treatment, intervention, palliation), and exercise (i.e. exercise, physical activity, physical therapy, sport, weight training) were combined and searched. Relevant articles were then hand searched for further pertinent references. To be included in the review, a study had to be published in a peer-reviewed journal and examine aerobic or resistance exercise. Studies also had to include fatigue as an endpoint. We found 28 studies that examined exercise and fatigue in cancer survivors. Details of the studies are reported in Tables 67.1 (observational studies) and 67.2 (intervention studies) and we briefly summarize them here.

Table 67.1 *Summary of observational studies examining the association between exercise and fatigue in cancer survivors*

Author(s)	Sample	Design	Exercise measurement	Fatigue measure(s)	Fatigue results
Dimeo et al., 1997[27]*	78 cancer survivors (34 breast, 21 non-Hodgkin lymphoma, 11 testicular, 12 other) admitted for chemotherapy and bone marrow transplantation	Cross-sectional	Maximal performance assessed by treadmill test	POMS	Higher maximal exercise significantly associated with lower fatigue
Berger, 1998[21]*	72 breast cancer survivors	Prospective	Wrist actigraphs to quantify participants movement	Piper Fatigue Scale	Higher activity levels during treatment associated with lower fatigue
Courneya et al., 2000[26]*	25 cancer survivors (8 breast, 7 multiple myeloma, 7 non-Hodgkin lymphoma, 3 other) who had just completed chemotherapy and bone marrow transplantation	Prospective	Self-reported stationary cycling during hospital stay	FACT-F	Higher cycling duration per day associated with lower fatigue at discharge
Pinto and Trunzo, 2004[22]*	119 breast cancer survivors	Prospective	Self-reported exercise (7-day recall), Rockport 1-Mile Walk Test	POMS	Exercisers reported less fatigue than non exercisers

(Continued)

Table 67.1 (*Continued*)

Author(s)	Sample	Design	Exercise measurement	Fatigue measure(s)	Fatigue results
Jones et al., 2004[23]*	88 multiple myeloma survivors	Retrospective	Self-reported exercise during treatment and off-treatment	FACT-F	Higher strenuous and total exercise associated with lower fatigue both during and off treatment
Vallance et al., 2005[24]*	438 non-Hodgkin lymphoma survivors	Retrospective	Self-reported exercise during treatment and off-treatment	FACT-F	Survivors meeting public health exercise guidelines reported less fatigue than survivors not meeting guidelines both during and off treatment
Courneya et al., 2005[25]*	386 endometrial cancer survivors	Retrospective	Self-reported exercise during the past month	FACT-F	Survivors meeting public health exercise guidelines reported less fatigue than survivors not meeting guidelines

FACT-F, Functional Assessment of Cancer Therapy – Fatigue; POMS, Profile of Mood States.

Table 67.2 *Summary of intervention studies examining the effects of exercise on fatigue in cancer survivors*

Author(s)	Sample	Design	Exercise intervention	Fatigue measure(s)	Fatigue results
MacVicar and Winningham, 1986[28]*	10 breast cancer survivors receiving treatment, 6 healthy controls	Nonrandomized controlled trial	Laboratory-based cycle ergometer, 3/week at 60–80% HR max. for 10 weeks	POMS	Exercise group and control group both decreased in fatigue
Mock et al., 1994[29]**	14 breast cancer survivor receiving treatment	Randomized controlled trial	Home-based walking, 4–5/week for 30 minutes + social support group for 6 weeks	Visual analog scale	Exercise group reported less fatigue than control 1 month post chemotherapy
Dimeo et al., 1997[20]*	32 cancer survivors (17 breast, 12 non-Hodgkin lymphoma, 3 other) who underwent high-dose chemotherapy and autologous peripheral blood stem cell transplantation	Nonrandomized controlled trial	Supervised treadmill walking 5/week, 15–30 minutes at 80% HR max. using interval training for 6 weeks	Not specified	0% of exercise group and 25% of controls reported fatigue with usual daily activities
Mock et al., 1997[30]**	46 breast cancer survivors receiving treatment	Randomized controlled trial	Home-based, self-paced walking, 4–5/week for 20–30 minutes at 'brisk' intensity for duration of radiation therapy for 6 weeks	Visual analog scale, Piper Fatigue Scale	Exercise group reported less fatigue at posttest compared to controls
Dimeo et al., 1998[31]*	5 cancer survivors who reported fatigue	Uncontrolled trial	Daily supervised treadmill walking, 15–30 minutes at 80% HR max. for 6 weeks	Clinical observation of fatigue	Clear decrease in fatigue

Table 67.2 *(Continued)*

Author(s)	Sample	Design	Exercise intervention	Fatigue measure(s)	Fatigue results
Dimeo et al., 1999[32]*	59 cancer survivors (31 breast, 28 other) who had just completed high-dose chemotherapy and bone marrow transplantation	Nonrandomized controlled trial	Daily supervised bed ergometer biking during hospitalization (about 2 weeks) for 30 minutes at 50% HR reserve.	POMS	Exercise group reported no change in fatigue. Control group reported increased fatigue
Schwartz, 1999[33]*	27 breast cancer survivors starting chemotherapy	Uncontrolled trial	Home-based aerobic exercise, 3–4 times/week, 15–30/minutes, at low-to-moderate intensity for 8 weeks	POMS, Schwartz Cancer Fatigue Scale	Exercise adherers reported lower fatigue than nonadherers
Porock et al., 2000[34]*	9 advanced cancer patients (4 bowel, 2 pancreas, 1 breast, 1 oral, 1 melanoma)	Uncontrolled trial	Home-based individualized program (walking and stretching) of daily activity for 28 days	Multidimensional Fatigue inventory	No change in fatigue
Schwartz, 2000[35]*	27 breast cancer survivors receiving treatment	Uncontrolled Trial	Home-based walking or patient choice, 3–4 times/week for 30 minutes for 8 weeks	Visual analog scale	Exercise reduced the levels of average and worst fatigue. Exercise adherers reported fewer days of high fatigue levels and more days of low fatigue levels
Mock et al., 2001[36]**	50 breast cancer survivors receiving treatment	Randomized controlled trial ('as treated' analysis performed)	Home-based walking, 4–5/week for 30 minutes for the duration of chemotherapy (approximately 4–6 months)	Piper Fatigue Scale	Survivors who exercised at least 90 minutes per week on 3 or more days reported significantly less fatigue than survivors who were less active during treatment
Schwartz et al., 2001[37]*	61 breast cancer survivors receiving treatment	Uncontrolled Trial	Home-based walking or patient choice, 3–4 times/week for 30 minutes for 8 weeks	Visual analog scale	Exercise significantly reduced fatigue
Burnham and Wilcox, 2002[38]**	18 cancer survivors (15 breast, 3 colon) posttreatment	Randomized controlled trial	Supervised low intensity (25–35% HR reserve) or moderate intensity (40–50% HR reserve) aerobic exercise program, 3 times/week for 10 weeks	Visual analog scale	Exercise group reported significantly lower fatigue compared with controls
Schwartz et al., 2002[39]*	12 melanoma patients prescribed methylphenidate and 6 usual care historical controls with melanoma	Nonrandomized controlled trial	Aerobic exercise 15–30 minutes, 4/week for 4 months	Schwartz Cancer Fatigue Scale	Exercise + methylphenidate group reported reduced fatigue compared with historical controls who only took methylphenidate

(Continued)

Table 67.2   (*Continued*)

Author(s)	Sample	Design	Exercise intervention	Fatigue measure(s)	Fatigue results
Coleman *et al.*, 2003[47**]	16 multiple myeloma cancer survivors receiving high-dose chemotherapy and bone marrow transplant	Randomized controlled trial	Home-based combined aerobic and upper and lower strength training program, 3/week for 30–60 minutes, walking or preferred exercise for 6 months	POMS	Exercise group reported less fatigue than control group
Courneya *et al.*, 2003[40**]	108 cancer survivors (44 breast, 10 colon, 54 other)	Randomized controlled trial	Home-based, moderate-intensity walking program for 20–30 minutes, 3–5/week at 65–75% estimated HR max. for approximately 10 weeks	FACT-F	Exercise + group psychotherapy reported less fatigue than group psychotherapy alone
Courneya *et al.*, 2003[41**]	93 postsurgical colorectal cancer survivors, 66% were receiving adjuvant therapy	Randomized controlled trial	Home-based exercise program, 3–5/week, moderate intensity for 20–30 minutes for 16 weeks	FACT-F	Intention-to-treat analysis revealed no significant differences. 'As treated' analysis revealed that survivors who had ↑ fitness reported less fatigue that survivors who had ↓ finess levels
Courneya *et al.*, 2003[42**]	52 breast cancer survivors	Randomized controlled trial	Supervised cycle ergometer, 3 times/week for 15–35 minutes for 15 weeks	FACT-F	Exercise group reported less fatigue than the control group
Galantino *et al.*, 2003[43**]	11 breast cancer survivors reporting CRF	Randomized controlled trial	3 × 60 minute sessions of tai chi vs. home walking program 3/week minimum for 6 weeks	Brief Fatigue Inventory	Both the walking and tai chi groups reported a trend toward lower fatigue
Oldervoll *et al.*, 2003[44*]	9 posttreatment Hodgkin cancer survivors reporting fatigue	Uncontrolled trial	Home-based aerobic exercise training program 3/week, 40–60 minutes at 65–80% intensity for 20 weeks	Fatigue Questionnaire	Exercise reduced fatigue
Segal *et al.*, 2003[45**]	155 men with prostate cancer receiving androgen deprivation	Randomized controlled trial	Supervised resistance exercise, 2 sets of 8–12 reps at 60–70% 1 RM, 3/week for 12 weeks	FACT-F	Exercise group reported lower fatigue compared with controls
Windsor et al., 2004[46**]	66 men with localized prostate carcinoma receiving radiation	Randomized controlled trial	Home-based, moderate intensity, continuous walking for 30 minutes, 3/week at 60–70% of HR max. for the duration of their radiation treatments	Brief Fatigue Inventory	Exercise group reported no significant increase in fatigue. Control group reported significant increase in fatigue

FACT-F, Functional Assessment of Cancer Therapy – Fatigue; POMS, Profile of Mood States; HR, heart rate.

SUMMARY OF STUDIES EXAMINING EXERCISE AND FATIGUE IN CANCER SURVIVORS

Seven observational studies have examined the association between exercise and fatigue in cancer survivors.[21*,22*,23*,24*,25*,26*,27*] Overall, the results showed that all seven observational studies reported a significant negative association between exercise/fitness and fatigue. That is, higher levels of exercise/fitness were associated with lower levels of fatigue. The primary limitation of these studies, of course, is that the causal association between exercise and fatigue cannot be established. It is certainly possible that fatigue causes reductions in exercise activity or that some third variable (e.g. depression) causes both higher levels of fatigue and lower levels of exercise.

A total of 21 intervention studies have examined the effects of exercise on fatigue in cancer survivors.[20*,28**,29**,30*,31*,32*,33*,34*,35*,36**,37*,38**,39*,40**,41**,42**,43**,44*,45**,46**,47**] With the exception of one study,[34*] all of the intervention studies showed positive effects of exercise on fatigue. Generally speaking, the intervention studies examining exercise and fatigue in cancer survivors were of good quality, consisting of randomized controlled trial designs, supervised exercise sessions, an appropriate exercise stimulus, objective fitness indicators, and validated fatigue scales. The primary methodological limitations of these studies include :

- failure to describe the methodology in sufficient detail (e.g. enrolment, randomization, blinding, loss to follow-up, and analytical plan)
- recruitment of small convenience samples
- relatively short exercise interventions
- limited follow-up
- unidimensional measures of fatigue.

Moreover, it is important to note that few studies:

- explicitly focused on cancer survivors with CRF
- included cancer survivors with metastatic or advanced disease
- attempted to identify the mechanisms for the exercise effect.

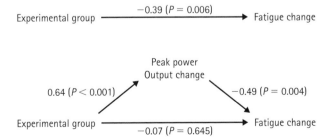

Figure 67.2 *Mediation of fatigue by peak power output. Data from Courneya et al.[40]*

Although the focus of this chapter is on cancer, the supportive role of exercise in other chronic and progressive populations has also been documented. In particular, exercise is an important component of symptomatic and supportive treatment(s) for patients with multiple sclerosis,[48***] chronic heart failure,[49***] chronic obstructive pulmonary disease,[50***] and human immunodeficiency virus (HIV)/ acquired immune deficiency syndrome (AIDS).[51***]

STUDIES OF MECHANISMS OF REDUCED FATIGUE FROM EXERCISE IN CANCER SURVIVORS

Only one study has examined the potential mechanisms for the effects of exercise on fatigue in cancer survivors. Courneya et al.[40**] conducted a randomized controlled trial to determine the effects of a 15-week exercise training program in 52 postmenopausal breast cancer survivors who had completed adjuvant therapy with or without current hormone therapy use. The authors reported significant effects of the intervention on various fitness indices including peak oxygen consumption and peak power output, and various psychosocial measures including fatigue. Multiple regression analyses were used to provide a statistical test of the possible mediating role of physical fitness. The researchers found evidence that the reduction in fatigue that occurred with the exercise intervention was largely mediated by a change in peak power output (Fig. 67.2). These data suggest that fitness changes may mediate the effects of exercise on fatigue in cancer survivors.

FUTURE RESEARCH DIRECTIONS

Although there are almost 30 studies that have examined exercise and fatigue in cancer survivors a significant amount of research remains to be done. The primary limitation of our current knowledge is that few studies have focused on fatigue as the primary endpoint in cancer survivors with CRF. Consequently, there is good evidence that exercise reduces fatigue in the general population of cancer survivors but limited evidence that exercise can reduce fatigue in cancer survivors with CRF, especially severe CRF. It is not at all obvious that exercise will prove therapeutic for cancer survivors with severe CRF, therefore, randomized controlled trials of exercise interventions that explicitly target cancer survivors with various levels of CRF are needed.

Studies focusing on cancer survivors with metastatic or advanced disease are also needed. Most of what is known about exercise and fatigue in cancer survivors is based on studies of early-stage breast cancer survivors. Research should also examine all dimensions of CRF including physical, emotional, and cognitive to determine if exercise will be particularly effective for one dimension of fatigue (e.g. physical) or will be equally effective for all dimensions of fatigue. It will also be important to elucidate the mechanisms by which exercise may reduce fatigue. For example, is it really necessary to improve physical fitness in order to reduce CRF? Finally, it will be important to determine the optimal type (e.g. aerobic versus resistance training), volume (i.e. frequency, intensity, and duration), progression, and context (e.g. center-based versus home-based, individual versus group format) of exercise for fatigued cancer survivors. Moreover, this research will need to overcome the methodological limitations of previous research including the use of rigorous randomized controlled trials, randomly selected samples, and longer interventions with longer follow-up.

CLINICAL IMPLICATIONS

Convincing evidence suggests that exercise reduces fatigue in cancer survivors although few studies have focused on cancer survivors with CRF. Nevertheless, exercise is now recommended as a therapy for cancer survivors with CRF.[36***,52***] For example in the USA, the National Comprehensive Cancer Network (NCCN) recommends that clinicians encourage cancer survivors with CRF to at least maintain current levels of physical activity. Furthermore, the NCCN suggests that most cancer survivors could experience benefits from a moderate exercise program implemented throughout the duration of their treatment regimen.[36***,52***] In all patients a thorough screening for comorbidities is required. Such screening should identify contraindications to exercise or a need for a referral of specialized services such as physiotherapy or rehabilitation services. Cancer survivors suffering from high levels of fatigue should be prescribed exercise on an individual basis[52***] including information from functional tests.

Tests of functional capacity are used extensively in research and clinical settings to evaluate patients suffering from heart and lung diseases (i.e. chronic obstructive pulmonary disease, heart failure, peripheral arterial disease, surgical candidates, pediatric cystic fibrosis).[53***] The tests used most often are the 6-minute walk test (6MWT), 2-minute walk test (2MWT), 12-minute walk test (12MWT), self-paced walk test (SPWT), and the shuttle walk test (SWT).[53***] The most widely researched of these is the 6MWT, which is considered easy to administer and is generally well tolerated. This test also tends to be most reflective of activities of daily living and is often used to assess response to medical interventions in patients with mild, moderate, or severe heart and lung disease.[53] The 6MWT has been indicated for use as a tool in evaluating functional status, as well as for the prediction of morbidity and mortality.[54] The 2MWT has also been proposed for populations who are not able to ambulate for 6 minutes.[55] This test has been shown to be sensitive to change following surgery, but

has not been extensively validated.[55] The shuttle walk test has also been proposed for use in patients with a wide range of disease and functional status. The SWT has preliminary evidence of sensitivity to change following a rehabilitation intervention, but has not been extensively tested. Overall, the 6MWT is the most widely researched and established functional walk test used in clinical and research settings.[53***]

Programming must make considerations for various factors such as age, current level of physical activity, type of cancer, stage of cancer, as well as the type of cancer treatment.[52***] These factors will impact the type, frequency, intensity, and duration of the exercise prescribed. Exercise should begin at low levels of intensity and duration. Modification and gradual increase of exercise is dependent upon individual ability and tolerance.[52***] Survivors with metastasis to bone, immunosuppression, anemia, neutropenia, thrombocytopenia, or fever require special attention in prescription and delivery of exercise programs.[52***] Moreover, the NCCN notes that survivors suffering from immunosuppression or neutropenia should exercise only in environments where risk of infection is a minimized (i.e. swimming pools are contraindicated by the NCCN).[36***,52***] It may be that exercise will be most appropriate for cancer survivors with chronic mild-to-moderate CRF or in the prevention of CRF. Pharmacological and energy conserving strategies may be more appropriate for cancer survivors with acute and/or severe CRF.

Exercise may also be beneficial to manage symptoms and optimize quality of life in patients with advanced stages of illness. An exercise regimen can be developed to help maintain and/or attenuate declines in physical functioning, within the context of the patient's health status, level of function and personal goals. Determining the optimal regimen may be best accomplished by an interdisciplinary team that includes physician, nurse, physical and occupational therapists, dietician, respiratory therapist, and the exercise specialist.

Cardiorespiratory exercise may be performed by 'biking' with a bed ergometer.[20*] Arm ergometry is an alternative option for those who are able to sit but unable to use their lower extremities. The primary focus of resistance exercise for the bedridden patient should be on strengthening of the extensor muscle groups (e.g. quadriceps, triceps) which are most affected by bed rest. Resistance exercise may be performed using resistance exercise bands/tubing, free weights and/or devices such as the horizontal leg press training device.[56*] Stretching and range of motion exercises may also be prescribed to maintain range of motion of a joint, improve muscle capability for circulation and oxygen exchange, provide a stimulus for bone and joint tissue integrity and reduce muscle tension (promote relaxation).[16,19] Active range of motion exercise is used when there is no contraindication to active movement and no inflammation. Active-assisted and passive range of motion exercises are beneficial when support of the body segment allows for movement without pain or when a patient is unable to actively move a segment.[19]

Exercise regimens, in general, will need to be performed at a lower intensity, shorter duration, and with longer rest periods. Therefore, exercise sessions may need to occur more frequently during the day (two to five sessions per day) to obtain benefit and yet avoid exacerbating fatigue.[16] Furthermore, to enhance a sense of well-being, exercise may be incorporated into self-care and/or functional activities that are in line with the patient's goals.

SUMMARY AND CONCLUSIONS

Compelling evidence suggests that exercise may play an important role in reducing fatigue in cancer survivors although few studies have focused explicitly on cancer survivors with CRF. Nevertheless, there are plausible physiological mechanisms by which exercise may reduce CRF. Future research is needed, however, to delineate the role of exercise in the management of CRF. Until then, exercise may be recommended for CRF on an individual basis. It may be that exercise will be an effective therapy for the prevention and management of chronic mild-to-moderate CRF but that pharmacological and energy-conserving strategies are indicated in cases of acute and/or severe CRF.

Key learning points

- Cancer-related fatigue (CRF) has proved to be a difficult symptom to manage.

- Energy conserving interventions (e.g. rest, sleep, relaxation training) have had modest success.

- The ability to resist physical fatigue is partly determined by muscular and cardiopulmonary fitness.

- Exercise may reduce fatigue in cancer survivors by alterations in physical functioning.

- Seven observational studies and 21 intervention studies have demonstrated that exercise training can reduce fatigue in various cancer survivor populations including during and after adjuvant therapies.

- Future exercise trials should explicitly target cancer survivors with high levels of CRF.

- The NCCN encourages cancer survivors with CRF to maintain current levels of physical activity and to adopt a moderate intensity exercise program if feasible.

- Exercise may be most appropriate for cancer survivors with mild-to-moderate CRF or in the prevention of CRF.

ACKNOWLEDGMENT

KSC is supported by the Canada Research Chairs Program and a Research Team Grant from the National Cancer Institute of Canada (NCIC) with funds from the Canadian Cancer Society (CCS) and the CCS/NCIC Sociobehavioral Cancer Research Network. JKHV is supported by a Canada Graduate Scholarship from the Canadian Institutes for Health Research and a Doctoral Incentive Award from the Alberta Heritage Foundation for Medical Research (AHFMR). MLM and CJP are supported by Health Research Studentships from AHFMR.

REFERENCES

1 Mock V, Atkinson A, Barsevick A, et al. NCCN Practice guidelines for cancer-related fatigue. Oncology (Huntingt) 2000; 14: 151–61.
2 Cella D, Davis K, Breitbart W, Curt G. Cancer-related fatigue: prevalence of proposed diagnostic criteria in a United States sample of cancer survivors. J Clin Oncol 2001; 19: 3385–91.
3 Hjermstad MJ, Fayers PM, Bjordal K, Kaasa S. Using reference data on quality of life – the importance of adjusting for age and gender, exemplified by the EORTC QLQ-C30 (+3). Eur J Cancer 1998; 34: 1381–9.
4 Baracos VE. Management of muscle wasting in cancer-associated cachexia: understanding gained from experimental studies. Cancer 2001; 92(6 Suppl): 1669–77.
5 Gutstein HB. The biologic basis of fatigue. Cancer 2001; 92(6 Suppl): 1678–83.
6 Kurzrock R. The role of cytokines in cancer-related fatigue. Cancer 2001; 92(6 Suppl): 1684–8.
7 Stasi R, Abriani L, Beccaglia P, et al. Cancer-related fatigue: evolving concepts in evaluation and treatment. Cancer 2003; 98: 1786–801.
8 Mock V. Evidence-based treatment for cancer-related fatigue. J Natl Cancer Inst Monogr 2004: 112–18.
9 Luebbert K, Dahme B, Hasenbring M. The effectiveness of relaxation training in reducing treatment-related symptoms and improving emotional adjustment in acute non-surgical cancer treatment: a meta-analytical review. Psychooncology 2001; 10: 490–502.
10 Goodwin PJ, Leszcz M, Ennis M, et al. The effect of group psychosocial support on survival in metastatic breast cancer. N Engl J Med 2001; 345: 1719–26.
11 Curt GA. The impact of fatigue on patients with cancer: Overview of FATIGUE 1 and 2. Oncologist 2000; 5(Suppl 2): 9–12.
12 Winningham ML. Strategies for managing cancer-related fatigue syndrome. Cancer 2001; Suppl 92: 988–97.
13 Wilmore JH, Costill D. Physiology of Sport and Exercise, 3rd ed. Champaign, IL: Human Kinetics, 2004.
14 Hasson SM. Clinical Exercise Physiology. Salem: Mosby, 1994.
15 McArdle WD, Katch FI, Katch VL. Exercise Physiology. 5th ed. Philadelphia: Lippincott, Williams & Wilkins, 2001.
16 Hall CM, Brody LT. Therapeutic Exercise: Moving Towards Function. Philadelphia: Lippincott, Williams & Wilkins, 1999.
17 Lucia A, Earnest C, Perez M. Cancer-related fatigue: can exercise physiology assist oncologists? Lancet 2003; 4: 616–25.

18 Bacharach DW. Review of exercise physiology. In: Lemura LM, ed. *Clinical Exercise Physiology*. Philadelphia: Lippincott Williams & Wilkins, 2004: 3–14.

19 Kisner C, Colby LA. *Therapeutic Exercise: Foundations and Techniques*. 4th ed. Philadelphia: FA Davis Co., 2002.

● 20 Dimeo FC, Tilmann MH, Bertz H, *et al.* Aerobic exercise in the rehabilitation of cancer patients after high dose chemotherapy and autologous peripheral stem cell transplantation. *Cancer* 1997; **79**: 1717–22.

21 Berger AM. Patterns of fatigue and activity and rest during adjuvant breast cancer chemotherapy. *Oncol Nurs Forum* 1998; **25**: 51–62.

22 Pinto BM, Trunzo JJ. Body esteem and mood among sedentary and active breast cancer survivors. *Mayo Clin Proc* 2004; **79**: 181–6.

23 Jones LW, Courneya KS, Vallance JKH, *et al.* Association between exercise and quality of life in multiple myeloma cancer survivors. *Support Care Cancer* 2004; **12**: 780–8.

24 Vallance JKH, Courneya KS, Jones LW, Reiman T. Differences in quality of life between non-Hodgkin's lymphoma survivors meeting and not meeting public health exercise guidelines. *Psychooncology* 2005; **14**: 979–991.

25 Courneya KS, Karvinen TH, Campbell KL, *et al.* Associations among exercise, body weight, and quality of life in endometrial cancer survivors: a population-based survey. *Gynecol Oncol* 2005; **97**: 422–430.

26 Courneya KS, Keats MR, Turner AR. Physical exercise and quality of life in cancer patients following high dose chemotherapy and autologous bone marrow transplantation. *Psychooncology* 2000; **9**: 127–36.

27 Dimeo F, Stieglitz RD, Novelli-Fischer U, *et al.* Correlation between physical performance and fatigue in cancer patients. *Ann Oncol* 1997; **8**: 1251–5.

● 28 MacVicar MG, Winningham ML. Promoting the functional capacity of cancer patients. *Cancer Bull* 1986; **38**: 235–9.

● 29 Mock V, Burke MB, Sheehan P, *et al.* A nursing rehabilitation program for women with breast cancer receiving adjuvant chemotherapy. *Oncol Nurs Forum* 1994; **21**: 899–907; discussion 908.

● 30 Mock V, Dow KH, Meares CJ, *et al.* Effects of exercise on fatigue, physical functioning, and emotional distress during radiation therapy for breast cancer. *Oncol Nurs Forum* 1997; **24**: 991–1000.

● 31 Dimeo F, Rumberger BG, Keul J. Aerobic exercise as therapy for cancer fatigue. *Med Sci Sports Exerc* 1998; **30**: 475–8.

● 32 Dimeo FC, Stieglitz RD, Novelli-Fischer U, *et al.* Effects of physical activity on the fatigue and psychologic status of cancer patients during chemotherapy. *Cancer* 1999; **85**: 2273–7.

33 Schwartz AL. Fatigue mediates the effects of exercise on quality of life. *Qual Life Res* 1999; **8**: 529–38.

34 Porock D, Kristjanson LJ, Tinnelly K, *et al.* An exercise intervention for advanced cancer patients experiencing fatigue: a pilot study. *J Palliat Care* 2000; **16**: 30–6.

35 Schwartz AL. Daily fatigue patterns and effect of exercise in women with breast cancer. *Cancer Pract* 2000; **8**: 16–24.

✱ 36 Mock V. Fatigue management. Evidence and guidelines for practice. *Cancer* 2001; **92**: 1699–707.

● 37 Schwartz AL, Mori M, Gao R, *et al.* Exercise reduces daily fatigue in women with breast cancer receiving chemotherapy. *Med Sci Sports Exerc* 2001; **33**: 718–23.

38 Burnham TR, Wilcox A. Effects of exercise on physiological and psychological variables in cancer survivors. *Med Sci Sports Exerc* 2002; **34**: 1863–7.

39 Schwartz AL, Thompson JA, Masood N. Interferon-induced fatigue in patients with melanoma: a pilot study of exercise and methylphenidate. *Oncol Nurs Forum* 2002; **29**: E85–90.

40 Courneya KS, Mackey JR, Bell GJ, *et al.* Randomized controlled trial of exercise training in postmenopausal breast cancer survivors: cardiopulmonary and quality of life outcomes. *J Clin Oncol* 2003; **21**: 1660–8.

● 41 Courneya KS, Friedenreich CM, Quinney HA, *et al.* A randomized trial of exercise and quality of life in colorectal cancer survivors. *Eur J Cancer Care (Engl)* 2003; **12**: 347–57.

● 42 Courneya KS, Friedenreich CM, Sela RA, *et al.* The group psychotherapy and home-based physical exercise (group-hope) trial in cancer survivors: physical fitness and quality of life outcomes. *Psychooncology* 2003; **12**: 357–74.

43 Galantino ML, Capito L, Kane RJ, *et al.* The effects of tai chi and walking on fatigue and body mass index in women living with breast cancer: a pilot study. *Rehabil Oncol* 2003; **21**: 17–22.

44 Oldervoll LM, Kaasa S, Knobel H, Loge JH. Exercise reduces fatigue in chronic fatigued Hodgkins disease survivors – results from a pilot study. *Eur J Cancer* 2003; **39**: 57–63.

● 45 Segal RJ, Reid RD, Courneya KS, *et al.* Resistance exercise in men receiving androgen deprivation therapy for prostate cancer. *J Clin Oncol* 2003; **21**: 1653–9.

46 Windsor PM, Nicol KF, Potter J. A randomized, controlled trial of aerobic exercise for treatment-related fatigue in men receiving radical external beam radiotherapy for localized prostate carcinoma. *Cancer* 2004; **101**: 550–7.

47 Coleman EA, Coon S, Hall-Barrow J, *et al.* Feasibility of exercise during treatment for multiple myeloma. *Cancer Nurs* 2003; **26**: 410–19.

48 Rietberg M, Brooks D, Uitdehaag B, Kwakkel G. Exercise therapy for multiple sclerosis. *Cochrane Database Syst Rev* 2005; **328**: CD003980.

49 Piepoli MF, Davos C, Francis DP, Coats AJ. Exercise training meta-analysis of trials in patients with chronic heart failure (ExTraMATCH). *BMJ* 2004; **328**(7433):189.

50 Lacasse Y, Brosseau L, Milne S, *et al.* Pulmonary rehabilitation for chronic obstructive pulmonary disease. *Cochrane Database Syst Rev* 2002: CD003793.

51 O'Brien K, Nixon S, Tynan AM, Glazier RH. Effectiveness of aerobic exercise in adults living with HIV/AIDS: systematic review. *Med Sci Sports Exerc* 2004; **36**: 1659–66.

✱ 52 Clinical Practice Guidelines in Oncology, Cancer-Related Fatigue Version 1. At www.nccn.org/professionals/physician_gls/PDF/fatigue.pdf (accessed September 20, 2005), National Comprehensive Cancer Network, 2004.

53 Solway S, Brooks D, Lacasse Y, Thomas S. A qualitative systematic overview of the measurement properties of functional walk tests used in cardiorespiratory domain. *Chest* 2001; **119**: 256–70.

54 American Thoracic Society Statement: Guidelines for the six-minute walk test. *Am J Respir Crit Care Med* 2003; **167**: 1287.

55 Brooks D, Parsons J, Tran D, *et al.* The two-minute walk test as a measure of functional capacity in cardiac surgery patients. *Arch Phys Med Rehabil* 2004; **85**: 1525–9.

56 Akima H, Kubo K, Imai M, *et al.* Inactivity and muscle: effect of resistance training during bed rest on muscle size in the lower limb. *Acta Physiol Scand* 2001; **172**: 269–78.

68

Treatment of fatigue in palliative care

JEANETTE A BOOHENE, EDUARDO BRUERA

INTRODUCTION

Fatigue has been defined as tiring easily with decreased capacity to maintain adequate performance.[1–3] It is one of the most common symptoms in palliative care. This is because most patients seen in palliative care have advanced disease, such as acquired immune deficiency syndrome (AIDS), end-stage congestive heart failure, and most common of all, cancer. All of these diseases in their advanced stage have a high degree of fatigue, for instance fatigue is present in 60–90 percent of all patients with advanced cancer.[4–6,7*,8*,9**] Assessment and treatment of this common symptom however, is difficult as it is subjective and often underreported.

The pathophysiology and assessment of fatigue has already been discussed in the previous chapters and it is clear that fatigue is usually multifactorial. To this end, when considering how to treat fatigue, a multidimensional approach is the best. It is important to determine whether the etiology is reversible and treating these reversible causes as best as possible. However, despite treating reversible causes fatigue often persists in this patient population and treatment then needs to be symptomatic, based on the presumed mechanism.

In this chapter, we will discuss the treatment of reversible and irreversible causes of fatigue using both pharmacological and nonpharmacological modalities. To be able to manage fatigue adequately, the contributing factors, often multiple, need to be determined (Fig. 68.1), some of which may be irreversible. Detailed assessment is required to be able to target therapy and this has been discussed elsewhere in this book. Once appropriate assessment is completed, the therapeutic approach to fatigue can be divided into treating underlying causes and symptomatic treatment (Fig. 68.2).

TREATING THE UNDERLYING CAUSES OF FATIGUE

Cancer treatment

The complex association between cancer and fatigue has not been completely defined. There is little doubt however, that most patients with cancer at some time in their illness develop fatigue, and especially in the terminal phase this is thought to be as a direct result of the cancer.[6,10*,11] In a cross-sectional follow-up study of 459 Hodgkin disease patients, fatigue was significantly higher than in controls from the general population. Follow-up was by mail, and a fatigue questionnaire measuring physical and mental fatigue as well as total fatigue score was used.[12*] In patients with cancer, there is a complex interaction occurring between tumor and host, which is not well understood but is thought to result in fatigue in several ways. Tumors produce proteolytic and lipolytic factors which can interfere with host metabolism. These factors are thought to play a role in the development of cancer cachexia with which there is complex overlap and interplay with fatigue[13] as discussed in other chapters in this book and also below. Moreover, there may be other substances induced or released directly by the tumor which can also lead to fatigue.[14,15] Tumors can also act by direct invasion of brain tissue, particularly the pituitary gland, and cause fatigue by both direct (disturbance in cognition) or indirect (endocrine disturbances via the pituitary axis) mechanisms.[2,16] Management in this case is essentially treating the cancer. The successful treatment of the malignancy can result in significant and sustained improvement in fatigue.[17***] The patient and caregivers must be educated about how common fatigue is as a complication of cancer and its treatment.

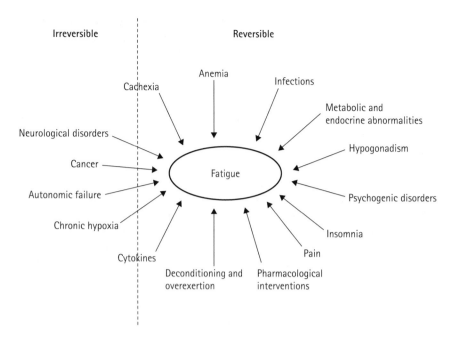

Figure 68.1 *Contributors to fatigue.*

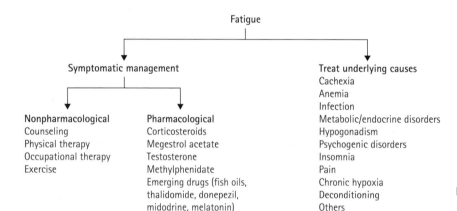

Figure 68.2 *Therapeutic approaches to the management of fatigue.*

They must also be counseled and educated about what to anticipate during and after therapy is completed with regards fatigue and mechanisms by which this common symptom can be managed such as vigilance with structured exercise and energy conservation.

Many of the cancer therapies and symptomatic treatment of other effects of the cancer such as pain, can themselves result in transient and/or prolonged fatigue and management of this is discussed below.

Therapies and medications

CHEMOTHERAPY AND RADIOTHERAPY

These treatment modalities in patients with cancer cause a specific fatigue syndrome. In isolation they both can cause

fatigue but this is augmented further when both modalities are given concurrently. Fatigue associated with chemotherapy tends to have a cyclical pattern. It occurs within the first few days of starting therapy, gets to a peak at about the time the white blood cell count is at its lowest level then improves in the week or so thereafter. The cycle is repeated with each cycle of chemotherapy and worsens with subsequent cycles, suggestive of a cumulative dose-related toxic effect.[3] Multiple chemotherapeutic agents have been studied in fatigue either in isolation or in combination with most generating some degree of fatigue. Different types of cancer have also been studied with specific chemotherapeutic regimens with varying degrees of fatigue noted depending on the cancer and the regimen.[18,19*,20**,21*,22*,23*,24*,25*,27*] A longitudinal prospective controlled study assessed 104 women with breast cancer receiving adjuvant chemotherapy and 102 controls. Tools used included the Functional Assessment of Cancer Treatment-General Quality of Life questionnaire, with subscales for fatigue and endocrine symptoms and the High Sensitivity Cognitive Screen. Ninety-one and 83 patients, and 81 controls were assessable at the end of 1 and 2 years, respectively. Differences between patients and controls were significant for both scales. It showed that fatigue, menopausal symptoms and cognitive dysfunction were important adverse effects of chemotherapy that improved in most patients with time.[28*]

Radiotherapy causes a different pattern of fatigue when given alone. It tends to start more abruptly soon after treatment and diminishes soon thereafter but may get progressively worse as therapy continues. A prospective study of 15 women with stage I or II breast cancer having radiation treatment revealed fatigue that did not increase linearly with cumulative radiation dose over time. There was a decrease in fatigue from the first to second week then increase in the third week. Cumulative effects reached a plateau in the fourth week then were maintained for the remaining treatment course. Fatigue diminished within 3 weeks after treatment.[29*] Fatigue has been noted to diminish but not completely resolve when short breaks in therapy occur, for example at weekends.[30]

BIOLOGICAL THERAPY

Biological response modifying agents such as interferon-α cause fatigue in 70 percent of patients who receive this therapy.[31] Fatigue is one of the most important dose limiting side effects of this type of therapy. The mechanism here is unknown though some investigators have postulated diffuse encephalopathy may occur.[32*,33*]

Management of fatigue in these situations is essentially symptomatic and nonpharmacological. Patients and their caregivers need to be counseled and educated prior to commencing therapy about the anticipated fatigue associated with the different treatment modalities. Exercise, without overexertion as well as physical and occupational therapy during treatment can help minimize the sometimes overwhelming fatigue and prevent deconditioning. One common side effect of chemotherapy which may impact fatigue and has been associated with symptom improvement if treated early is anemia. This will be discussed later in this chapter.

OPIOIDS

A large proportion of cancer patients experiencing pain are on opioids. This group of medications has significant effects on the reticular system and can cause sedation, cognitive changes, and fatigue in some but not all patients. The central acting effects would explain the mental fatigue but it is more likely that the drowsiness or somnolence is what is perceived as fatigue by some patients. Most patients develop tolerance over time to the drowsiness and may as such perceive improvement in fatigue.[1,2] A trial of dose reduction if pain is well controlled and fatigue is becoming the predominant symptom can be effective. Psychostimulants such as methylphenidate and donepezil have been used to improve opioid-induced fatigue.[34**,35*,36*]

Cytokine modulation

Circulating cytokines and inflammatory proteins are thought to be associated with many of the symptoms exhibited in patients with advanced cancer such as fatigue, pain, depression, cachexia, and sleep disorders.[37,38*,39*] These products have also been associated with infections, the effects of cancer treatments including chemotherapy and radiation therapy, and with the presence of the cancer itself. One of the mechanisms shown in laboratory studies by which cytokines mediate symptoms is via a number of signals through the hypothalamic–pituitary–adrenal axis.[40*] Since fatigue is one of the most common symptoms in advanced cancer, researchers have proposed that one possible explanation for fatigue in this patient population is the increased secretion of proinflammatory cytokines, such as interleukin (IL)-2, IL-6, interferon α (INFα) and tumor necrosis factor α (TNFα), in response to both the disease and its treatment.[41,42*] Several lines of evidence support cytokines in the pathophysiology of fatigue. These include:

- The occurrence of fatigue as a major side effect of cytokines used in the treatment of cancer patients.[2,43*,44*]
- The increased levels of cytokines in nononcological conditions characterized by fatigue, such as chronic fatigue syndrome.[3,45*,46*]
- The elevation of cytokine levels seen in chemotherapy treatments for cancer.[4,47*]
- The upregulation of proinflammatory cytokines seen in several malignancies and their correlation with fatigue.[42,48,49*]

Treatment in this case can be challenging and depends to some extent on the mechanism. Evidence to date strongly supports a role for cytokine modulation with agents such as corticosteroids, cyclooxygenase (COX) 1 and 2 inhibitors (nonsteroidal anti-inflammatory drugs, nabumetone) thalidomide, monoclonal antibodies (anti-TNF, infliximab), and specific soluble receptor antagonists, some of which are currently being studied to modulate the effects of cytokines on the brain and other sites.[50,51***]

Treatment of cachexia

Cachexia has been covered in detail elsewhere in this book but there are a number of important points to note with cachexia in association with fatigue.[2] There is a complex overlap between cachexia and fatigue especially in advanced cancer. Cachexia can be reversible when due to malnutrition or starvation or in catabolic states such as acute or chronic infections. However, when due to underlying illness usually in the terminal phase such as cancer, AIDS, end-stage cardiac disease, or chronic obstructive airways disease, it is often more difficult to reverse.[52] The significant loss of muscle mass in cachexia could explain the profound weakness and fatigue with which it is associated. Of note though is that fatigue can be present in the absence of significant weight loss and vice versa where profound cachexia and malnutrition may exist without fatigue.[2]

Treatment for cachexia secondary to malnutrition or starvation involves nutritional support. Though there is no evidence that aggressive nutritional therapy improves the quality of life in advanced cancer patients or that parenteral feeding has much impact on fatigue,[53,54] in patients where cachexia is deemed to be secondary to malnutrition these are exactly the measures that should be employed. In such patients aggressive nutritional support can result in reversing the cachexia and associated fatigue.[55*] The majority of cachexia in palliative care patients is unfortunately irreversible and treatment is often symptomatic. In addition to established agents in use including progestins (megestrol acetate), corticosteroids, and prokinetics (metoclopramide), many newer agents are being studied such as thalidomide, cannabinoids and omega 3 fatty acids found in fish oils.[56***]

Management of autonomic failure

Autonomic failure is a common outcome of advanced cancer,[57*] but can also occur in other noncancer diseases encountered in palliative care such as Parkinson disease. Symptoms associated with autonomic failure include postural hypotension with or without intermittent episodes of syncope, gastrointestinal symptoms such as nausea, vomiting, diarrhea or constipation, and anorexia.[57,58] Some of these symptoms may contribute directly or indirectly to fatigue such as postural hypotension, anorexia, and persistent diarrhea. A subset of chronic fatigue syndrome has been associated with autonomic dysfunction,[59] but this association has not been studied much in advanced diseases encountered in palliative care.

Autonomic failure is usually irreversible and can be difficult to treat in the setting of fatigue. Midodrine, a specific α_1 sympathomimetic agent, has been used to manage autonomic failure in other conditions such as diabetes and might have a therapeutic role in autonomic failure in the palliative care population. In a double-blind randomized crossover study with midodrine and ephedrine, eight patients with refractory orthostatic hypotension secondary to autonomic failure were assessed. Midodrine produced a significant increase in both systolic and diastolic blood pressure with associated improved ability to stand as compared with ephedrine and placebo.[60**] Another double-blind, placebo controlled, four way crossover trial looked at 25 patients with neurogenic orthostatic hypotension. Patients were randomized to receive either placebo or three different doses of midodrine (2.5, 10, or 20 mg) on successive days. Supine and standing blood pressures were measured sequentially and midodrine was shown to significantly increase standing systolic blood pressure (peaking at 1 hour after dosing) with mean score of global improvement of symptoms being significantly higher for midodrine at doses of 10 mg and 20 mg compared with placebo.[61**] Other measures, including discontinuing all possible contributing medications, plasma volume expansion with increased salt intake and use of fludrocortisone, wearing pressure stockings and rising up in stages and slowly for patients with postural hypotension used in other causes of autonomic failure might also be applicable in this patient population.[62***]

Neurological disorders

A number of neurological disorders are associated with fatigue, some of which may be the primary disease such as amyotrophic lateral sclerosis, myasthenia gravis, Parkinson disease, multiple sclerosis, and other demyelinating diseases.[2] On the other hand, some neurological disorders occur as a result of the terminal disease and may sometimes precede the disease by quite a long time, such as the paraneoplastic syndromes including Eaton–Lambert syndrome and dermatomyositis/polymyositis (Table 68.1).[63] Treatment here is disease specific though most of these diseases are progressive despite treatment and both the disease and associated fatigue become irreversible, at which point symptomatic therapies both pharmacological and nonpharmacological are introduced (see Fig. 68.1).

Treating anemia

The patient group in which mild to moderate levels of anemia may exacerbate fatigue for which there is evidence that treating less severe anemia improves energy levels and quality of life includes those receiving chemotherapy. In an open label study 2342 patients from community-based hospitals, with malignancies undergoing chemotherapy, were treated with epoetin alfa. A total of 1047 patients completed the full 4 months of epoetin therapy and showed significant increase in mean self-rated scores of energy level, activity level, and overall quality of life. These improvements correlated with the magnitude of the hemoglobin increase.[64*] Another prospective community-based study with 2289 patients with nonmyeloid malignancies receiving chemotherapy received epoetin for 16 weeks. Patients reported improvement in quality of life parameters which correlated with significant increases in hemoglobin levels independent of tumor response.[65*] Some authors, however, believe that the improvement noted in treating this level of anemia may be secondary to improvement in exertional dyspnea rather than fatigue *per se*. In a retrospective cohort study of 355 patients receiving chemotherapy, both palliative and potential curative, 19 percent received blood transfusion (18 percent for anemia, 1 percent for bleeding). The chemotherapy caused reduced hemoglobin in all groups of

Table 68.1   *Paraneoplastic neurological syndromes associated with fatigue*

Syndrome	Association
Progressive multifocal leukoencephalopathy	Lymphoma, leukemia
Paraneoplastic encephalomyelitis	70% lung, 30% other malignancies,
Subacute motor neuropathy	e.g. after irradiation in lymphoma
Subacute necrotic myelopathy	Lung cancer
Peripheral paraneoplastic neuropathy	Often precedes the primary
Ascending acute polyneuropathy (GBS)	Lymphoma
Dermatomyositis/polymyositis	Associated with malignancy in 50%
Eaton–Lambert syndrome	Small cell lung cancer
Myasthenia gravis	Lymphoma, thymoma (30%)
Amyotrophic lateral sclerosis	Primary disorder with fatigue

GBS, Guillain–Barré syndrome.

cancer studied but of note was that lung cancer patients required transfusion at much higher hemoglobin levels. This was thought to be due to underlying lung disease causing more symptoms associated with anemia particularly dyspnea. Factors significantly associated with transfusion were lung cancer, leukemia, and low baseline hemoglobin ($<$8 g/dL).[66*]

In patients with advanced disease and in the palliative care patient population, anemia is probably overdiagnosed as a cause for fatigue. Fatigue measured on a scale of 0–10 in a retrospective study of 147 patients seen in palliative care consultation with a median hemoglobin level of 11.6 g/dL did not show significant correlation between fatigue and hemoglobin level though there was a trend ($P = 0.09$).[67*] There is little doubt that anemia is prevalent in such disease states, especially advanced cancer, but it is unclear at what hemoglobin level the treatment of anemia either with blood transfusions or epoeitin impacts fatigue. A retrospective cohort study on 31 patients who received transfusions of packed red blood cells in a palliative care unit in the presence of a low hemoglobin ($\leqslant$8 g/dL) with or without severe fatigue or dyspnea showed some subjective improvement in wellbeing which was not related to the severity of dyspnea or fatigue. Pretransfusion hemoglobin level did not differ significantly in patients who benefited and did not benefit from transfusion.[68*] This lack of significant benefit from transfusion alone for severe anemia in this patient population further confirms the multifactorial etiology of fatigue where other more overwhelming factors such as cachexia, depression, pain, and overall debilitation may become more predominant in the terminal phase of disease.

In managing fatigue thought to be associated with anemia, assessment of the underlying cause as well as the acuity of anemia becomes important as this may influence the choice of treatment. The two mainstays of treatment here are blood transfusions, often indicated in severe anemia (hemoglobin $<$ 8 g/dL) or synthetic erythropoietin. The goals of care need to be determined on an individual basis as well as overall prognosis since transfusions would give almost immediate results and erythropoietin could take up

to 4 weeks to show response. Moreover, erythropoietin is administered by subcutaneous injection either weekly or in the case of darbepoetin sometimes less often (every 2 weeks).[64,65*,69*,70***] Iron deficiency can also be fairly easily corrected with iron supplements but again this takes weeks to produce significant effect and may not be practical in palliative care patients with short life expectancies.[71**]

Infection

Patients with advanced cancer and other advanced disease states seen in palliative care are at increased risk of infection due to relative and sometimes profound immunosuppression. Fatigue is often associated with infections, especially when the course is protracted or when infections are recurrent. Prolonged viral infections are especially notorious for producing longlasting episodes of fatigue.[72*,73*,74] Fatigue may occur as a prodromal symptom and persist sometimes long after the infection has resolved. Chronic infection and cancer induce the same cytokine mediators for cachexia such as TNFα,[15] so it is possible that they share similar mediators for fatigue as well due to the overlap between cachexia and fatigue described earlier. Vigilance in avoiding recurrent infections is important here and having a low threshold for using appropriate antimicrobial therapy can minimize some of these infections.

Treating psychogenic disorders

Depression and anxiety are discussed in more detail elsewhere in this book but a few key points are worth mentioning here due to the strong correlation between these disorders and fatigue. The diagnosis of psychological distress makes up approximately 75 percent of patients without cancer presenting with fatigue.[3,75] Symptoms of psychological distress and adjustment disorders with depressive or anxious moods are much more common in this patient population than major psychiatric disorders. The incidence of depression in this group tends to be overestimated.

Self-reported scales suggest a prevalence as high as 25 percent, but in fact only 6 percent of cancer patients are estimated to have major depression and 2 percent have anxiety disorders.[76,77*] Fatigue can be the prevalent symptom in any of these disorders. It is sometimes difficult to tease out cause and effect as depression for instance may be the cause of or occur as a result of fatigue. Some groups have found significant association between fatigue and psychological distress but again this is by no means the only variable causing fatigue, reiterating the multifactorial contributors to fatigue.[78*]

Treatment here is by and large symptomatic with good expressive supportive counseling though antidepressants may sometimes be indicated especially when depressive mood makes up a large component of the adjustment disorder. Mirtazapine, an antidepressant which enhances norepinephrine and serotonin release and inhibits 5-hydroxytryptamine $(5\text{-}HT)_2$ and $5\text{-}HT_3$ receptors, has been shown in pilot studies with fibromyalgia syndrome to improve multiple symptoms including depression, fatigue, pain and sleep disturbance.[79] It will be interesting to see if this can be confirmed with double-blind, placebo controlled studies and also shown to be effective in the palliative care patient population.

Insomnia

Lack of sleep occurs for multiple reasons which themselves may be indirectly causing fatigue. Sleep may be disturbed because of uncontrolled symptoms such as pain, depression or anxiety, mild delirium with sleep cycle inversion, drugs and suboptimal conditions causing poor sleep hygiene. Insomnia is less likely therefore to be an independent variable in the etiology of fatigue and though it can cause fatigue does not cause physical weakness.[4,80*]

Appropriately assessing the patient and treating the underlying contributing factors such as pain and psychogenic disorders, as well as teaching good sleep hygiene, can improve the insomnia and may sometimes be more effective in the long run than using hypnotics and sedatives which sometimes may be indicated for short-term use.[81,82]

Metabolic and endocrine abnormalities

These are often very reversible causes of fatigue, which can be easy to treat. It is therefore important when a patient presents with fatigue to run a simple chemistry panel as part of the work-up. Abnormalities such as hyponatremia, hypokalemia, hypomagnesemia, hypercalcemia, and hyper or hypoglycemia can be readily diagnosed and corrected with simple measures such as hydration and replacement therapy. A lot of these electrolyte disturbances cause physical/muscle weakness, which can cause significant fatigue. Endocrine disorders are easily missed but can also often be readily reversible or treatable causes of fatigue. Addison disease for instance causes significant fatigue and although this is now uncommon in

Western society, hypoadrenalism *per se* is still fairly common. Many drugs can cause secondary hypoadrenalism, which has identical symptoms to the primary disorder, e.g. steroids (when discontinued abruptly). Other common endocrine disorders such as diabetes and hypothyroidism should also be excluded and if diagnosed treated promptly with appropriate replacement therapies.[1,2]

Hypogonadism

This condition deserves a separate mention from the other endocrine disorders due to recent research interest in this as a cause of fatigue with associated loss of muscle mass. Low testosterone results in loss of muscle mass, fatigue, reduced libido, and reduced hemoglobin.[83] Two large patient groups encountered in palliative care, namely cancer patients and patients with AIDS, have been found to have testosterone deficiency which in males can often be easily reversible by replacement therapy with testosterone. Some antineoplastic therapies as well as both systemic and intrathecal opioids have been shown to cause hypogonadotropic hypogonadism[84*,85*,86*,87*] and a low threshold for measuring testosterone levels and offering replacement therapy is key in managing fatigue in this patient population. Hormonal ablative therapy has been shown to double the incidence of fatigue in men with prostate cancer[88*] but of note is that this is one patient population in which testosterone replacement therapy is contraindicated.[89***]

Chronic hypoxia

The association here with fatigue is probably best studied in chronic airways disease where oxygen therapy has been shown to improve quality of life in patients with fatigue as one of the symptoms. In a prospective longitudinal study of 43 consecutive chronic obstructive pulmonary disease (COPD) patients fulfilling criteria for long-term oxygen therapy and 25 patients not fulfilling criteria, there was significant improvement noted in health-related quality of life in patients on long-term oxygen therapy. This improvement in symptoms included fatigue, emotional, and mental function and was sustained over a 6-month period.[90*]

The use of supplemental oxygen in decreasing dyspnea and fatigue or improving exercise tolerance has not been shown to be beneficial in cancer patients with mild hypoxemia. A double-blind, randomized controlled crossover trial with 31 lung cancer patients without severe hypoxemia (O_2 saturation level $\geqslant$ 90 percent) assessed whether or not oxygen is more effective than air in decreasing dyspnea and fatigue and increasing physical performance. There was no significant difference observed between treatment and control groups in dyspnea, fatigue, or physical performance.[91**] Earlier studies showed that patients with cancer who had hypoxemia and dyspnea at rest benefit from oxygen therapy, but further studies are required to determine whether oxygen therapy could improve fatigue or exercise tolerance in hypoxia patients with advanced disease.[92**,93**]

Pain

Some authors have found a strong correlation between pain intensity/severity and fatigue in patients with cancer.[94***,95*] Others however, found no association between the two symptoms.[78] It is more likely that there is an indirect correlation with chronic uncontrolled pain causing psychological distress, insomnia, etc. thus impacting fatigue. Moreover, as mentioned above, some of the treatment modalities of pain can cause fatigue, for example opioids. As such, detailed assessment and targeting treatment toward the associated factors and symptoms, as well as achieving good pain control, would be the most appropriate management here.

SYMPTOMATIC MANAGEMENT OF FATIGUE

This can be divided into pharmacological and nonpharmacological management.

Pharmacological management

Pharmacological management can be further divided into established and emerging agents (Box 68.1).

Box 68.1 Pharmacological agents for fatigue

Established agents

- Corticosteroids

- Megestrol acetate

- Psychostimulants, e.g. methylphenidate, modafinil, dextroamphetamine

- Testosterone

Emerging agents

- Agents that inhibit cytokine action, e.g. thalidomide, COX-1 and COX-2 inhibitors (NSAIDs), selective COX-2 inhibitors, omega 3 fatty acids, α-melanocyte stimulating hormone

- Agents that block cytokine release, e.g. pentoxifylline, bradykinin antagonists

- Donepezil

- Monoclonal antibodies, e.g. infliximab, soluble receptor antagonists

- L-Carnitine

ESTABLISHED AGENTS

Unfortunately there is no single agent that can be used to treat fatigue in advanced diseases effectively. This is probably because of the multifactorial etiologies contributing to fatigue. However, a number of agents have been studied and shown to be effective in treating fatigue, often in combination with other modalities including nonpharmacological ones.

Corticosteroids

Studies have been done on steroids, dexamethasone, and methylprednisone and have shown improvement in fatigue. One group showed a significant improvement in appetite and strength following 2 weeks of dexamethasone. In a double-blind controlled study with 116 patients with advanced gastrointestinal cancer, dexamethasone given at a dose of 0.75 mg and 1.5 mg four times daily showed improvement in appetite and sense of wellbeing. There was however, no associated weight gain or improvement in performance status. There was also initial symptomatic improvement in the placebo group but after 4 weeks this disappeared and at this point, dexamethasone showed a statistically significant advantage over placebo.[96**] Other groups found methylprednisolone caused improvement in activity level quite rapidly but this was not sustained over a 3-week period. Forty terminally ill cancer patients were studied in a 14-day randomized double-blind, crossover trial comparing methylprednisolone with placebo. The daily dose was 32 mg and endpoints studied were pain, appetite, nutritional status, psychiatric status, daily activity, and performance. Appetite and daily activity increased in 77 percent and 21 percent of patients, respectively, with 71 percent and 57 percent reduction in depression and analgesic use, respectively.[97**] Corticosteroids to treat fatigue are probably best used on a short-term basis, as long-term use can cause myopathy and other side effects which could make fatigue worse. Moreover, studies have shown that the beneficial effects generally last between 2 and 4 weeks. Recommended doses based on studies are a dose equivalent of prednisone 40 mg daily.[2] Other beneficial effects of steroids that may impact fatigue include the effect on nausea, appetite, and pain. The mechanism of action of corticosteroids on fatigue is not known though there is evidence that they inhibit cytokines and may also have inhibitory effects directly on tumor.[98**,99*,100] The central euphoric effects of steroids are also another potential mechanism.[97]

Megestrol acetate

A number of studies in terminally ill patients given megestrol acetate have shown a rapid improvement within 1 week to 10 days, in a number of symptoms including fatigue, appetite, calorie intake, and nutritional status. Doses used range from 160 to 480 mg per day. In a randomized, double-blind crossover study with 53 evaluable patients with advanced solid tumors not responsive to hormone therapy, megestrol acetate given at a dose of 160 mg three times daily for 10 days reported a significant improvement in appetite, activity, and wellbeing. There was also significant improvement in overall fatigue score. There was no significant change in nausea, nutrition, or energy intake.[101**] Another double-blind crossover trial to assess effects of megestrol acetate on cancer-induced cachexia looked at 40 consecutive malnourished patients with advanced non-hormone responsive tumors receiving no antineoplastic treatment. The dose used here was 480 mg daily for 7 days with crossover on days 8–15. Pain, nausea, depression, appetite, energy level, and wellbeing were assessed on a visual analog scale. Among the 31 evaluable patients, there was significant improvement in appetite, energy, and wellbeing. Caloric intake was also increased.[102**] The mechanism of action of megestrol acetate is unclear and may be due to the glucocorticoid or anabolic activity or due to effects on cytokine release or a combination.

Psychostimulants

Methylphenidate at doses of 5–10 mg in the morning and 5 mg at noon has been shown in pilot studies to be useful in treating patients with advanced cancer. In a prospective open study with 31 patients with advanced cancer and fatigue, methylphenidate at a dose of 5 mg every 2 hours as needed was given for a total of 7 days. The daily maximum dose was 20 mg. The primary endpoint was fatigue (though multiple other symptoms were also assessed daily) measured on a 0–10 scale and Functional Assessment for Chronic Illness Therapy – Fatigue (FACIT-F) was performed at baseline, and days 7 and 28. Thirty patients were evaluable and showed significantly improved fatigue between baseline and day 7. Anxiety, pain, appetite, nausea, depression, and drowsiness also improved significantly.[103*] A phase II study enrolled 37 patients with a history of breast cancer and absence of disease for >6 months but <5 years, hemoglobin level >12 g/dL, less than moderate depression and a score of ≥4 on the Brief Fatigue Inventory (BFI) scale. Patients received methylphenidate 5 mg orally twice daily for 6 weeks. Response was defined as a decrease in BFI score of at least 2 points. On weeks 4 and 6, 54 percent had a response though 19 percent withdrew due to adverse events.[104*] There is also evidence that methylphenidate results in significant improvement in activity level in patients on large doses of opioids. In a randomized double-blind crossover study, 28 patients with chronic pain due to advanced cancer (on opioids) were treated with methylphenidate (10 mg with breakfast and 5 mg with lunch) for 3 days. Activity improved and drowsiness decreased on methylphenidate. The intensity of pain and number of extra doses of analgesics also decreased.[34**] The effect of methylphenidate in this patient population may therefore be an indirect effect by improving opioid-induced sedation as well as improving pain. Also of note are the rapid onset antidepressant effects of psychostimulants such as methylphenidate, which may indirectly impact fatigue.

Subsequent studies have not shown methylphenidate to be any more effective than placebo in the management of fatigue. Larger studies are currently under way to clarify the role of methylphenidate in fatigue. A double-blind, randomized controlled study as a follow-up to a preliminary pilot study, which showed methylphenidate to be effective for treatment of cancer-related fatigue, revealed that patient-controlled methylphenidate was not significantly superior to placebo after 1 week. This study looked at 105 evaluable patients (52 patients and 53 patients in placebo arm) randomized to patient-controlled methylphenidate taking 5 mg of methylphenidate every 2 hours as needed by mouth (maximum daily dose 20 mg) for 7 days.[105**] Currently there is insufficient evidence to use psychostimulants for the management of fatigue in cancer patients without opioid-related sedation.

Other psychostimulants studied in noncancer palliative groups include modafinil and amantadine in multiple sclerosis,[106,107] and modafinil in human immunodeficiency virus (HIV) and amyotrophic lateral sclerosis (ALS). A pilot study and a 4-week open-label trial was conducted on 30 HIV-positive patients with clinically significant fatigue on antiretroviral medications without any treatable medical conditions known to cause fatigue. After 4 weeks on modafinil, the 24 responders showed statistically significant improvement on all measures of fatigue, depressive symptoms, and executive function. The most common side effects included headache, irritability and feeling hyperactive.[108*] In an open-label trial of modafinil looking at effect on fatigue in ALS, 15 patients with ALS were treated with 200 mg or 400 mg of modafinil. After treatment for 2 weeks, fatigue and drowsiness were assessed on the Fatigue Severity Scale (FSS) and Epsworth Sleepiness Scale (ESS). There was significant reduction in scores on both scales after modafinil use.[109*] The use of modafinil in the cancer population is currently being studied.[110] Dextroamphetamine has also been studied in HIV patients with some improvement in fatigue. Wagner and Rabkin[111] have shown initially in an open-label pilot study, and later in a small double-blind, placebo controlled trial, that dextroamphetamine in this patient population is a potentially effective antidepressant treatment for both depression and debilitating fatigue. The pilot study looked at 19 men with DSM-III-R criteria for a depressive disorder with debilitating low energy, CD4 count of <200 cells/mm^3 and no history of drug dependence. There was a treatment period of 6 weeks with indefinite follow-up. Ninety-five percent of the patients reported substantial improvement in mood and energy level at a median dosage of 10 mg/day of dextroamphetamine.[111*] In the placebo-controlled trial, the inclusion criteria were essentially the same with a 2-week randomized placebo controlled trial period and blinding maintained until week 8 for responders followed by open treatment to completion of 6 months. Seventy-three percent of patients randomly assigned to dextroamphetamine reported significant improvement in mood and energy compared with 25 percent of the placebo patients. There was no evidence of development of tolerance, abuse, or dependence on taking dextroamphetamine for the trial duration.[112]**

Testosterone

This has been discussed earlier with the treatment of hypogonadism as a cause of fatigue. The use of testosterone and its derivatives and other androgenic anabolic steroids have been shown, predominantly in patients with hypogonadism due to HIV disease, to increase muscle mass, improve energy and libido and increase hemoglobin levels. In a prospective longitudinal study over a 3-year period, 18 hypogonadal men who had never been treated were given transdermal testosterone. The mean testosterone level reached the normal range by 3 months of treatment and remained normal for the duration of treatment. Outcomes measured were bone mineral density, fat free mass, prostate volume, erythropoiesis, energy, and sexual function. The full effect on bone mineral density took 24 months but the full effects on the other tissues and energy levels took 3–6 months.[113]* A randomized, double-blind, placebo controlled study in a group of hypogonadal men with AIDS wasting looked at the effect of testosterone administration on the depression score. Fifty-two hypogonadal males with AIDS demonstrated significantly higher scores on the BDI than matched eugonadal men also with AIDS. The hypogonadal men were then treated with testosterone and there was a significant decrease noted in the BDI score for the 39 patients who completed the study.[114]** The correlation between depression and fatigue has been made earlier and hence by improving depression in this way, fatigue could potentially improve. Testosterone deficiency has also been shown to occur as a result of cancer therapy including radiation and chemotherapy as well as in the hormonal treatment of certain cancers such as prostate cancer (where testosterone replacement is not possible). The use of testosterone replacement therapy either transdermally or parenterally in patients who are hypogonadic is now on the increase.

EMERGING PHARMACOLOGICAL AGENTS

Fatigue, as stated earlier in this chapter, is the most common symptom in palliative patients and yet is probably one of the most difficult symptoms to treat. Multiple agents have been studied and found not to be effective in the treatment of fatigue, such as mazindol.[115]** With regards the established agents, results are often short term or they are associated with unacceptable side effects, e.g. corticosteroids with myopathy in long-term use or megestrol acetate with associated thrombotic risk. This often makes them unsuitable for many in this patient population. Moreover because of the multifactorial complex etiology of fatigue, it has been challenging to find a single effective pharmacological

agent to treat fatigue. Currently a number of agents are under investigation for the treatment of fatigue (see Box 68.1), some of which are discussed below.

Thalidomide

Thalidomide has been shown to be of potential benefit in the management of cachexia and may have some beneficial effect on fatigue due to the complex overlap between these two symptoms as mentioned earlier. Cytokines are thought to play a key role in this complex interaction and thalidomide is thought to act by inhibiting TNFα and modulating interleukins. It has been shown to improve the overall sensation of wellbeing in patients with cancer cachexia.[38]* A randomized controlled trial with patients with advanced pancreatic cancer and cachexia showed a statistically significant improvement in physical function associated with weight gain. Fifty patients with advanced pancreatic cancer and at least 10 percent of body weight loss were randomized to receive either 200 mg of thalidomide daily or placebo for a total of 24 weeks in a single center, double-blind, randomized controlled trial. The primary outcome was nutritional status and change in weight and there was a positive correlation between weight gain and improvement in physical function.[116]** Thalidomide was found to preserve performance status in a randomized placebo-controlled study in patients with advanced HIV disease and cachexia. Twenty-eight adult patients with advanced HIV disease on antiretroviral therapy for at least 6 months without any active opportunistic infection and who had 10 percent weight loss in the previous 6 months were randomized to receive 100 mg of thalidomide four times daily or placebo for 12 weeks. The primary outcomes measured were weight gain or no progression of wasting and secondary outcomes were Karnofsky performance status, HIV viral burden and CD4 cell count. The Karnofsky index was significantly higher in the thalidomide group by the end of the study period.[117]**

Omega 3 fatty acids

Omega 3 fatty acids (fish oil) has been shown to improve performance status in pancreatic cancer patients with cachexia after 3 weeks of treatment. Twenty patients with unresectable pancreatic adenocarcinoma consumed two cans of a fish oil-enriched nutritional supplement per day in addition to their usual dietary daily intake. At the end of 3 weeks and again at 7 weeks, patients showed a significant weight gain with improvement in performance status and appetite.[118]* The mechanism here is thought to be similar to thalidomide acting on cytokines and studies have mainly been in cachexia.[119]*** Other studies however, have not found any significant difference between fish oil and placebo in influencing fatigue, nutritional status, or function in patients with advanced cancer. In a randomized double-blind, placebo-controlled study of 60 patients with advanced cancer randomly assigned to take fish oil capsules or placebo, there was no significant improvement in appetite, fatigue, nutritional status, caloric intake, wellbeing, or functional status after 2 weeks.[120**]

Donepezil

Medications which enhance intracerebral cholinergic activity may offer an alternative approach to psychostimulants such as methylphenidate for treating opioid-induced sedation and fatigue with less side effects. Pilot studies have shown donepezil, a centrally acting acetylcholine esterase inhibitor, to be effective in the treatment of opioid-induced sedation and related symptoms (fatigue, anxiety, depression, anorexia, insomnia and wellbeing) in patients with cancer pain. In a retrospective study in which 40 patients (37 of whom had cancer) receiving long-term opioid therapy (on a stable dose for at least 2 weeks) were also taking donepezil at a dose of on average 9 mg/day for an average of 21 days, 73 percent of the evaluable 19 patients experienced improvement on the Epworth Sleepiness Scale and Clinical Global Improvement Scale. The morphine equivalent daily dose in these patients was on average 844 mg.[35*] A pilot study assessed 27 patients receiving strong opioids for pain related to cancer and reporting sedation. They were given 5 mg donepezil every morning for 7 days and symptoms including pain, sedation, and fatigue were assessed using the Edmonton Symptom Assessment Scale. Fatigue was also measured with the FACIT-F scale. Twenty evaluable patients reported significant improvement in multiple symptoms including fatigue and sedation.[36*] Randomized controlled trials are currently under way to study this effect further.

L-Carnitine

Nutritional deficiencies are among the postulated causes of fatigue in cancer patients. Deficiency in the micronutrient carnitine has been postulated to play a role here by reducing energy production through fatty acid oxidation. Some early studies have found that a number of cancer patients are deficient in carnitine and have shown some improvement in fatigue scores after supplementation with L-carnitine. An open-label dose-finding study assessed 18 cancer patients for carnitine deficiency and found 83 percent to be deficient. Preliminary data analysis of 13 patients revealed an increase in carnitine levels following supplementation with L-carnitine for 1 week. Outcome measures included fatigue, depression, sleep disruption, and performance status. With the exception of performance status, there was improvement in all the other symptoms.[121*] More well-conducted (randomized, double-blind, placebo-controlled) studies are needed to further clarify the role of L-carnitine in fatigue.

Other emerging and proposed agents for targeting the treatment of fatigue in palliative care include α-melanocyte-stimulating hormone, monoclonal antibodies against TNFα

such as infliximab, COX-1 and COX-2 inhibitors, to name a few. Herbal remedies are often used by patients with cancer-related fatigue. Ginkgo biloba for example has some activity against TNF and the potential benefits of natural products in fatigue should also be explored with good clinical studies.[51***]

Nonpharmacological management

EDUCATION

Educating the patient and caregivers about the possible causes of fatigue and informing them of how frequent a symptom it is at this stage in their disease may help them have more realistic expectations. Also providing them with information about the different modalities of treatment, some of which can be self-implemented, such as education about sleep hygiene and progressive limitation in physical activity can help empower the patient.

COUNSELING

There is some overlap here with education. Counseling a patient about what symptoms to expect, including fatigue, with disease progression or with cancer treatment helps to better prepare them for the symptom when it occurs. Studies have shown that only a small percentage of patients expect fatigue from their therapy whereas up to 89 percent of them experience it.[122*] Counseling for coping with other symptoms, such as adjustment disorder with depressed mood and anxiety, which may impact fatigue could also help with improving fatigue.

EXERCISE (OVEREXERTION/DECONDITIONING)

This has been discussed in detail in other chapters of this book. It is important however, to mention this again briefly here as it does impact the management of fatigue. Impaired muscle function may be one of the underlying mechanisms in fatigue (at least the physical component to fatigue). There are a number of studies showing muscle alterations in cancer patients and the association between reduced muscle mass in cachexia and fatigue.[123*] Prolonged bed rest or immobility has been shown to cause deconditioning with associated loss of muscle mass and decreased cardiac output. This state results in reduced endurance both for normal activities of daily living and exercise. Normal exercise has been shown to have a beneficial effect on muscle and cardiovascular fitness, however, overexertion is a frequent cause of fatigue in noncancer patients. This is an important problem to recognize in younger cancer patients who are trying to maintain their social and professional lives while receiving aggressive antineoplastic therapies such as chemotherapy and radiotherapy.[3]

Exercise is recommended as part of the therapy for fatigue in cancer patients,[124*,125] and physiotherapists and occupational therapists can suggest suitable exercises and help achieve increased activity. The precaution here however, is that the level of exercise is appropriate for the patient and does not result in overexertion and subsequent worsening of the fatigue.[126**]

CONCLUSION

Fatigue is a multifactorial symptom which is extremely common in advanced cancer and other advanced disease states. Approach to the management of this complex symptom must therefore be multidimensional to be effective. Detailed assessment is key to appropriate management and as noted here there is still a lot of research to be done to offer adequate therapy to this patient population for such a common symptom.

Key learning points

- Fatigue is a common yet complex multifactorial symptom in palliative care.

- To offer appropriate treatment a detailed assessment is important.

- Treat reversible causes then add in symptomatic treatment if indicated – pharmacological as well as nonpharmacological.

- Multiple agents are emerging with constant research, but it will be difficult to find a single agent to manage this complex symptom.

REFERENCES

1 Cleary JF. The reversible causes of asthenia in cancer patients. In: Portenoy R, Bruera E, eds. *Topics in Palliative Care* Vol 2. New York: Oxford University Press, 1998: 183–202.

2 Sweeney C, Neuenschwander H, Bruera E. Fatigue and asthenia. In: Doyle D, Hanks G, Cherny N, Calman K, eds. *Oxford Textbook of Palliative Medicine*. Oxford: Oxford University Press, 2004: 560–8.

3 Bruera E. Fatigue and dyspnea. In: Pazdur R, Coia LR, Hoskins WJ, Wagman LD, eds. *Cancer Management: A Multidisciplinary Approach*. CMP United Business Media, 2005–2006: 919–28.

4 Neuenschwander H. Fatigue. In: Fisch MJ, Bruera E, eds. *Handbook of Advanced Cancer*. Cambridge: Cambridge University Press, 2003: 374–81.

5 Bruera E. Research into symptoms other than pain. In: Doyle D, Hanks G, MacDonald N, eds. *Oxford Textbook of Palliative Medicine*. Oxford: Oxford University Press, 1998: 179–85.

6 Coyle N, Adelhardt J, Foley KM, Portenoy RK. Character of terminal illness in the advanced cancer patient: pain and other symptoms during the last four weeks of life. *J Pain Symptom Manage* 1990; **5**: 83–93.

● 7 Cella DF, Tulsky DS, Gray G, *et al.* The functional assessment of cancer therapy scale: development and validation of the general measure. *J Clin Oncol* 1993; **11**: 570–9.

8 Vogelzang NJ, Breitbart W, Cella D, *et al.* Patient, caregiver and oncologist perceptions of cancer-related fatigue: results of a tripart assessment survey. The Fatigue Coalition. *Semin Hematol* 1997; **34**: 4–12.

9 Portenoy RK, Thaler HT, Kornblith AB, *et al.* Symptom prevalence, characteristics and distress in a cancer population. *Qual Life Res* 1994; **3**: 183–9.

10 Donnelly S, Walsh D, Rybicki L. The symptoms of advanced cancer: identification of clinical and research priorities by assessment of prevalence and severity. *J Palliat Care* 1995; **11**: 27–32.

11 Bruera E, MacDonald RN. Overwhelming fatigue in advanced cancer. *Am J Nurs* 1988; **88**: 99–100.

12 Loge JH, Abrahamsen AF, Ekeberg O, Kaasa S. Hodgkin's disease survivors more fatigued than the general population. *J Clin Oncol* 1999; **17**: 253–61.

♦ 13 Tisdale MJ. New cachexic factors. *Curr Opin Clin Nutr Metab Care* 1998; **1**: 253–6.

♦ 14 Theologides A. Anorexins, asthenins and cachectins in cancer. *Am J Med* 1986; **81**: 696–8.

♦ 15 Beutler B, Cerami A. Cachectin: more than a tumor necrosis factor. *N Engl J Med* 1987; **316**: 379–85.

♦ 16 Valentine AD, Meyers CA. Cognitive and mood disturbance as causes and symptoms of fatigue in cancer patients. *Cancer* 2001; **92**: 1694–8.

17 Barnes EA, Bruera E. Fatigue in patients with advanced cancer: a review. *Int J Gynecol Cancer* 2002; **12**: 424–8.

18 Dahlgren S, Holm G, Svanborg N. Clinical and morphological side effects of busulfan. *Acta Med Scand* 1972; **192**: 129–35.

19 Jabboury K, Frye D, Holmes FA, *et al.* Phase II evaluation of gallium nitrate by continuous infusion in breast cancer. *Invest New Drugs* 1989; **7**: 225–9.

20 Moertel CG, Fleming TR, Macdonald JS, *et al.* Levamisole and fluorouracil for adjuvant therapy of resected colon carcinoma. *N Engl J Med* 1990; **322**: 352–8.

21 Catimel G, Verweij J, Mattijssen V, *et al.* Docetaxel (Taxotere): an active drug for the treatment of patients with advanced squamous cell carcinoma of the head and neck. *Ann Oncol* 1994; **5**: 533–7.

22 Catimel G, Coquard R, Guastalla JP, *et al.* Phase I study of RP 48532A, a new protein-synthesis inhibitor, in patients with advanced refractory solid tumors. *Cancer Chemother Pharmacol* 1995; **35**: 246–8.

23 Christman K, Kelsen D, Saltz L, Tarassoff PG. Phase II trial of gemcitabine in patients with advanced gastric cancer. *Cancer* 1994; **73**: 5–7.

24 Poplin EA, Corbett T, Flaherty L, *et al.* Diflourodeoxycytidine (dFdC)-gemcitabine: a phase I study. *Invest New Drugs* 1992; **10**: 165–70.

25 Berlin J, Tutsch KD, Hutson P, *et al.* Phase I clinical and pharmacokinetic study of oral carboxyamidotriazole, a signal transduction inhibitor. *J Clin Oncol* 1997; **15**: 781–9.

26 Jamar S. Fatigue in women receiving chemotherapy for ovarian cancer. In: Funk SG, *et al*, eds. *Key Aspects of Comfort: Management of Pain, Fatigue and Nausea*. New York: Springer-Verlag, 1989: 224–8.

27 Nail LM, Jones LS, Greene D, *et al.* Use and perceived efficacy of self-care activities in patients receiving chemotherapy. *Oncol Nurs Forum* 1991; **18**: 883–7.

28 Fan HG, Houede-Tchen N, Yi QL, *et al.* Fatigue, menopausal symptoms and cognitive function in women following adjuvant chemotherapy for breast cancer: One and two year follow-up of a prospective controlled study. *J Clin Oncol* 2005; **23**: 8025–32.

29 Greenberg DB, Sawicka J, Eisenthal S, Ross D. Fatigue syndrome due to localized radiation. *J Pain Symptom Manage* 1992; **7**: 38–45.

30 Kobashi-Schoot JA, Hanewald GJ, van Dam FS, Bruning PF. Assessment of malaise in cancer patients treated with radiotherapy. *Cancer Nurs* 1985; **8**: 306–13.

◆ 31 Jones TH, Wadler S, Hupart KH. Endocrine-mediated mechanisms of fatigue during treatment with interferon-alpha. *Semin Oncol* 1998; **25**: 54–63.

32 Jones GJ, Itri LM. Safety and tolerance of recombinant interferon alfa-2a (Roferon (R)-A) in cancer patients. *Cancer* 1986; **57**(Suppl): 1709–15.

33 Adams F, Quesada J, Gutterman J. Neuropsychiatric manifestations of human leucocyte interferon therapy in patients with cancer. *JAMA* 1984; **7**: 938–41.

34 Bruera E, Chadwick S, Brennies C. Methylphenidate associated with narcotics for the treatment of cancer pain. *Cancer Treat Rep* 1987; **71**: 120–7.

35 Slatkin NE, Rhiner M. Treatment of opioid-related sedation: utility of the cholinesterase inhibitors. *J Support Oncol* 2003; **1**: 53–63.

36 Bruera E, Strasser F, Shen L, *et al.* The effect of donepezil on sedation and other symptoms in patients receiving opioids for cancer pain: a pilot study. *J Pain Symptom Manage* 2003; **26**: 1049–54.

◆ 37 Kurzrock R. The role of cytokines in cancer-related fatigue. *Cancer* 2001; **92**: 1684–8.

38 Bruera E, Neumann CM, Pituskin E, *et al.* Thalidomide in patients with cachexia due to terminal cancer. Preliminary report. *Ann Oncol* 1999; **10**: 857–9.

39 Haack M, Pollmacher T, Mullington J. Diurnal and sleep-wake dependent variations of soluble TNF- and IL-2 receptors in healthy volunteers. *Brain Behav Immun* 2004; **18**: 361–7.

40 Sephton SE, Sapolsky RM, Kraemer HC, Spiegel D. Diurnal cortisol rhythm as a predictor of breast cancer survival. *J Natl Cancer Inst* 2000; **92**: 994–1000.

◆ 41 Ahlberg K, Ekman T, Gaston-Johansson F, Mock V. Assessment and management of cancer-related fatigue in adults. *Lancet* 2003; **362**: 640–50.

42 Greenberg DB, Gray JL, Mannix CM, *et al.* Treatment-related fatigue and serum interleukin-1 levels in patients during external beam irradiation for prostate cancer. *J Pain Symptom Manage* 1993; **8**: 196–200.

43 Eskander ED, Harvey HA, Givant E, Lipton A. Phase 1 study combining tumor necrosis factor with interferon alpha and interleukin-2. *Am J Clin Oncol* 1997; **20**: 511–14.

44 Veldhuis G, Willemse PH, Sleijfer DT, *et al.* Toxicity and efficacy of escalating dosages of recombinant human interleukin-6 after chemotherapy in patients with breast cancer or non-small cell lung cancer. *J Clin Oncol* 1995; **13**: 2585–93.

45 Gupta S, Aggarwal S, See D, Starr A. Cytokine production by adherent and nonadherent mononuclear cells in chronic fatigue syndrome. *J Psychiatr Res* 1997; **31**: 149–56.

46 Moss RB, Mercandetti A, Vojdani A. TNF-alpha and chronic fatigue syndrome. *J Clin Immunol* 1999; **19**: 314–16.

47 Pusztai L, Mendoza TR, Reuben JM, *et al.* Changes in plasma levels of inflammatory cytokines in response to paclitaxel chemotherapy. *Cytokine* 2004; **25**: 94–102.

48 Rigas JR, Hoopes PJ, Meyer LA, *et al.* Fatigue linked to plasma cytokines in patients with lung cancer undergoing combined modality therapy [abstract]. *Proc A S C O* 1998; **17**: 68a.

49 Adler HL, McCurdy MA, Kattan MW, *et al.* Elevated levels of circulating interleukin-6 and transforming growth factor-B1 in patients with metastatic prostatic carcinoma. *J Urol* 1999; **161**: 182–7.

50 Webster JI, Tonelli L, Sternberg EM. Neuroendocrine regulation of immunity. *Annu Rev Immunol* 2002; **20**: 125–63.

◆ 51 Burks TF. New agents for the treatment of cancer-related fatigue. *Cancer* 2001; **15**(Suppl 6): 1714–8.

52 Strasser F. Pathophysiology of the anorexia/cachexia syndrome. In: Doyle D, Hanks G, Cherny N, Calman K, eds. *Oxford Textbook of Palliative Medicine.* Oxford: Oxford University Press, 2004: 520–33.

◆ 53 Nelson KA, Walsh D, Sheehan FA. The cancer anorexia-cachexia syndrome. *J Clin Oncol* 1994; **12**: 213–25.

54 Bruera E, Fainsinger RL. Clinical management of cachexia and anorexia. In: Doyle D, Hanks G, MacDonald N, eds. *Oxford Textbook of Palliative Medicine.* New York: Oxford University Press, 1993: 330–7.

55 De Cicco M, Panarello G, Fantin D, *et al.* Parenteral nutrition in cancer patients receiving chemotherapy: effects on toxicity and nutritional status. *J Parenter Enteral Nutr* 1993; **17**: 513–18.

56 Finley JP. Management of cancer cachexia. *AACN Clin Issues* 2000; **11**: 590–603.

57 Bruera E, Chadwick S, Fox R, *et al.* Study of cardiovascular autonomic insufficiency in advanced cancer patients. *Cancer Treat Rep* 1986; **70**: 1383–7.

58 Henrich WL. Autonomic insufficiency. *Arch Intern Med* 1982; **142**: 339–44.

59 Calkins H, Rowe PC. Relationship between chronic fatigue syndrome and neurally mediated hypotension. *Cardiol Rev* 1998; **6**: 125–34.

60 Fouad-Tarazi FM, Okabe M, Goren H. Alpha sympathomimetic treatment of autonomic insufficiency with orthostatic hypotension. *Am J Med* 1995; **99**: 604–10.

61 Wright RA, Kaufmann HC, Perera R, *et al.* A double-blind, dose-response study of midodrine in neurogenic orthostatic hypotension. *Neurology* 1998; **51**: 120–4.

62 Stumpf JL, Mitrzyk B. Management of orthostatic hypotension. *Am J Hosp Pharm* 1994; **51**: 648–60.

63 Warenius HM. Paraneoplastic neurological syndromes. In: Tallis R, ed. *Clinical Neurology of Old Age.* New York: John Wiley and Sons, 1989: 323–34.

64 Glaspy J, Bukowski R, Steinberg D, *et al.* Impact of therapy with epoetin alfa on clinical outcomes in patients with nonmyeloid malignancies during cancer chemotherapy in community oncology practice. Procrit Study Group. *J Clin Oncol* 1997; **15**: 1218–34.

65 Demetri GD, Kris M, Wade J, *et al.* Quality-of-life benefit inchemotherapy patients treated with epoetin alfa is independent of disease response or tumor type: results from a prospective community oncology study. Procrit Study Group. *J Clin Oncol* 1998; **16**: 3412–25.

66 Skillings JR, Sridhar FG, Wong C, Paddock L. The frequency of red cell transfusion for anemia in patients receiving chemotherapy: a retrospective cohort study. *J Clin Oncol* 1993; **16**: 22–5.

67 Munch TN, Zhang T, Willey J, *et al*. The association between anemia and fatigue in patients with advanced cancer receiving palliative care. *J Palliat Med* 2005; **8**: 1144–9.

68 Monti M, Castellani L, Berlusconi A, Cunietti E. Use of red blood cell transfusions in terminally ill cancer patients admitted to a palliative care unit. *J Pain Symptom Manage* 1996; **12**: 18–22.

69 Gabrilove JL, Cleeland CS, Livingston RB, *et al*. Clinical evaluation of once-weekly dosing of epoetin alfa in chemotherapy patients: improvements in hemoglobin and quality of life are similar to three times weekly dosing. *J Clin Oncol* 2001; **19**: 2875–82.

70 Seidenfeld J, Piper M, Flamm C, *et al*. Epoetin treatment of anemia associated with cancer therapy: a systematic review and meta-analysis of controlled clinical trials. *J Natl Cancer Inst* 2001; **93**: 1204–14.

71 Candelaria M, Cetina L, Duenas-Gonzalez A. Anemia in cervical cancer patients: implications for iron supplementation therapy. *Med Oncol* 2005; **22**: 161–8.

72 Jones JF, Ray CG, Minnich LL, *et al*. Evidence for active Epstein-Barr virus infection in patients with persistent, unexplained illnesses: elevated anti-early antigen antibodies. *Ann Intern Med* 1985; **102**: 1–7.

73 Strauss E, Tosato G, Armstrong G, *et al*. Persisting illness and fatigue in adults with evidence of Epstein-Barr virus infection. *Ann Intern Med* 1985; **102**: 7–16.

74 Schooley RT. Epstein-Barr virus infections, including infectious mononucleosis. In: Isselbacher KJ, Braunwald E, Wilson JD, *et al*, eds. *Harrison's Principles of Internal Medicine*. New York: McGraw Hill, 1994: 790–3.

75 Adams R. Anxiety, depression, asthenia and personality disorders. In: Petersdorf R, Adams R, Brawnnald E, eds. *Harrison's Principles of Internal Medicine*. New York: McGraw-Hill, 1993: 68–75.

◆ 76 Massie MJ, Gagnon P, Holland JC. Depression and suicide in patients with cancer. *J Pain Symptom Manage* 1994; **9**: 346–50.

77 Derogatis LR, Morrow GR, Fetting J, *et al*. The prevalence of psychiatric disorders among cancer patients. *JAMA* 1983; **249**: 751–7.

78 Bruera E, Brenneis C, Michaud M, *et al*. Association between asthenia and nutritional status, lean body mass, anemia, psychological status and tumor mass in patients with advanced breast cancer. *J Pain Symptom Manage* 1989; **4**: 59–63.

79 Samborski W, Lezanska-Szpera M, Rybakowski JK. Open trial of mirtazapine in patients with fibromyalgia. *Pharmacopsychiatry* 2004; **37**: 168–70.

80 Dorrepaal KL, Aaronson NK, van Dam FS. Pain experience and pain management among hospitalized cancer patients. A clinical study. *Cancer* 1989; **63**: 593–8.

◆ 81 O'Donnell JF. Insomnia in cancer patients. *Clin Cornerstone* 2004; **6**(Suppl 1D): S6–14.

◆ 82 Portenoy RK, Itri LM. Cancer related fatigue – guidelines for evaluation and management. *Oncologist* 1999; **4**: 1–10.

◆ 83 Basaria S, Wahlstrom JT, Dobs AS. Clinical review 138: Anabolic-androgenic steroid therapy in the treatment of chronic diseases. *J Clin Endocrinol Metab* 2001; **86**: 5108–17.

84 Rajagopal A, Vassilopoulou-Sellin R, Palmer JL, *et al*. Symptomatic hypogonadism in male survivors of cancer with chronic exposure to opioids. *Cancer* 2004; **100**: 851–8.

85 Rajagopal A, Vassilopoulou-Sellin R, Palmer JL, *et al*. Hypogonadism and sexual dysfunction in male cancer survivors receiving chronic opioid therapy. *J Pain Symptom Manage* 2003; **26**: 1055–61.

86 Finch PM, Roberts LJ, Price L, *et al*. Hypogonadism in patients treated with intrathecal morphine. *Clin J Pain* 2000; **16**: 251–4.

87 Strasser F, Degracia B, Palmer JL, *et al*. Hypogonadism in patients with advanced cancer: Impact on fatigue, anxiety and depression, hemoglobin and sexual desire. *J Clin Oncol* 2004; **22**(14 Suppl): Abstract 8112.

88 Stone P, Hardy J, Huddart R, *et al*. Fatigue in patients with prostate cancer receiving hormone therapy. *Eur J Cancer* 2000; **36**: 1134–41.

◆ 89 Gould DC, Kirby RS. Testosterone replacement therapy for late onset hypogonadism: what is the risk of inducing prostate cancer? *Prostate Cancer Prostatic Dis* 2005; November 1 [Epub ahead of print].

90 Eaton T, Lewis C, Young P, *et al*. Long term oxygen therapy improves health related quality of life. *Respir Med* 2004; **98**: 285–93.

91 Bruera E, Sweeney C, Willey J, *et al*. A randomized controlled trial of supplemental oxygen versus air in cancer patients with dyspnea. *Palliat Med* 2003; **17**: 659–63.

92 Bruera E, de Stoutz N, Velasco-Leiva A, *et al*. Effects of oxygen on dyspnoea in hypoxaemic terminal-cancer patients. *Lancet* 1993; **342**: 13–14.

93 Bruera E, Schoeller T, MacEachern T. Symptomatic benefit of supplemental oxygen in hypoxemic patients with terminal cancer: the use of N of 1 randomized controlled trial. *J Pain Symptom Manage* 1992; **7**: 365–8.

94 Fishbain DA, Cole B, Cutler RB, *et al*. Is pain fatiguing? A structured evidence-based review. *Pain Med* 2003; **4**: 51–62.

95 Stone P, Richards M, A'Hern R, Hardy J. A study to investigate the prevalence, severity and correlates of fatigue among patients with cancer in comparison with a control group of volunteers without cancer. *Ann Oncol* 2000; **11**: 561–7.

96 Moertel C, Schutt AJ, Reitemeier RJ, Hahn RG. Corticosteroid therapy of preterminal gastrointestinal cancer. *Cancer* 1974; **33**: 1607–9.

97 Bruera E, Roca E, Cedaro L, *et al*. Action of oral methylprednisolone in terminal cancer patients: a prospective randomized double-blind study. *Cancer Treat Rep* 1985; **69**: 751–4.

98 Ettinger AB, Portenoy RK. The use of corticosteroids in the treatment of symptoms associated with cancer. *J Pain Symptom Manage* 1988; **3**: 99–103.

99 Hardy JR, Rees E, Ling J, *et al*. A prospective survey of the use of dexamethasone on a palliative care unit. *Palliat Med* 2001; **15**: 3–8.

◆ 100 McEwen BS, Biron CA, Brunson KW, *et al*. The role of adenocorticoids as modulators in immune function in health and disease: neural, endocrine and immune interactions. *Brain Res Brain Res Rev* 1997; **23**: 79–133.

101 Bruera E, Ernst S, Hagen N, *et al*. Effectiveness of megestrol acetate in patients with advanced cancer: a randomized, double-blind, crossover study. *Cancer Prev Control* 1998; **2**: 74–8.

102 Bruera E, Macmillan K, Kuehn N, *et al.* A controlled study of megestrol acetate on appetite, caloric intake, nutritional status and other symptoms in patients with advanced cancer. *Cancer* 1990; **66**: 1279–82.

103 Bruera E, Driver L, Barnes EA, *et al.* Patient controlled methylphenidate for the management of fatigue in patients with advanced cancer: A preliminary report. *J Clin Oncol* 2003; **21**: 4439–43.

104 Hanna A, Sledge G, Mayer ML, *et al.* A phase II study of methylphenidate for the treatment of fatigue. *Support Care Cancer* 2005; August 12 [Epub ahead of print].

105 Bruera E, Driver L, Valero V, *et al.* Patient controlled methylphenidate for cancer-related fatigue: A randomized controlled trial [abstract]. *ASCO Annual Meeting Proceedings* 2005.

◆ 106 Zifko UA. Management of fatigue in patients with multiple sclerosis. *Drugs* 2004; **12**: 1295–304.

◆ 107 MacAllister WS, Krupp LB. Multiple sclerosis-related fatigue. *Phys Med Rehabil Clin North Am* 2005; **16**: 483–502.

108 Rabkin JG, McElhiney MC, Rabkin R, Ferrando SJ. Modafinil treatment for fatigue in HIV+ patients: a pilot study. *J Clin Psychiatry* 2004; **65**: 1688–95.

109 Carter GT, Weiss MD, Lou JS, Jensen MP, *et al.* Modafinil to treat fatigue in amyotrophic lateral sclerosis: an open label pilot study. *Am J Hosp Palliat Care* 2005; **22**: 55–9.

◆ 110 Morrow GR, Shelke AR, Roscoe JA, *et al.* Management of cancer-related fatigue. *Cancer Invest* 2005; **23**: 229–39.

111 Wagner GJ, Rabkin JG, Rabkin R. Dextroamphetamine as a treatment for depression and low energy in AIDS patients: a pilot study. *J Psychosomatic Res* 1997; **42**: 407–11.

112 Wagner GJ, Rabkin R. Effects of dextroamphetamine on depression and fatigue in men with HIV: a double-blind, placebo-controlled trial. *J Clin Psychiatry* 2000; **61**: 436–40.

113 Snyder PJ, Peachey H, Berlin JA, *et al.* Effects of testosterone replacement in hypogonodal men. *J Clin Endocrinol Metab* 2000; **85**: 2670–7.

114 Grinspoon S, Corcoran C, Askari H, *et al.* Effects of androgen administration in men with the AIDS wasting syndrome. A randomized, double-blind, placebo-controlled trial. *Ann Intern Med* 1998; **129**: 18–26.

115 Bruera E, Carraro S, Roca E, *et al.* Double-blind evaluation of the effects of mazindol on pain, depression, anxiety, appetite and activity in terminal cancer patients. *Cancer Treat Rep* 1986; **70**: 295–8.

116 Gordon JN, Trebble TM, Ellis RD, *et al.* Thalidomide in the treatment of cancer cachexia: a randomized placebo controlled trial. *Gut* 2005; **54**: 447–8.

117 Reyes-Teran G, Sierra-Madero JG, Martinez del Cerro V, *et al.* Effects of thalidomide on HIV-associated wasting syndrome: a randomized, double-blind, placebo-controlled clinical trial. *AIDS* 1996; **10**: 1501–7.

118 Barber MD, Ross JA, Voss AC, *et al.* The effects of oral nutritional supplement enriched with fish oil on weight-loss in patients with pancreatic cancer. *Br J Cancer* 1999; **81**: 80–6.

119 Peuckmann V, Fisch M, Bruera E. Potential novel uses of thalidomide: focus on palliative care. *Drugs* 2000; **60**: 273–92.

120 Bruera E, Strasser F, Palmer JL, *et al.* Effect of fish oil on appetite and other symptoms in patients with advanced cancer and anorexia/cachexia: a double-blind, placebo-controlled study. *J Clin Oncol* 2003; **21**: 129–34.

121 Cruciani RA, Dvorkin E, Homel P, *et al.* L-carnitine supplementation for the treatment of fatigue and depressed mood in cancer patients with carnitine deficiency: a preliminary analysis. *Ann N Y Acad Sci* 2004; **1033**: 168–76.

122 Love RR, Leventhal H, Easterling DV, Nerenz DR. Side effects and emotional distress during cancer chemotherapy. *Cancer* 1989; **63**: 604–12.

123 Smith KL, Tisdale MJ. Mechanism of muscle protein degradation in cancer cachexia. *Br J Cancer* 1993; **68**: 314–18.

∗ 124 Mock V. Fatigue management. Evidence and guidelines of practice. *Cancer* 2001; **92**: 1699–707.

125 Clinical Practice Guidelines in Oncology, Cancer-Related Fatigue Version 2. In: National Comprehensive Cancer Network 2005. www.nccn.org/professionals/physician_gls/PDF/fatigue.pdf.

126 Dimeo F, Stieglitz R, Novelli-Fischer U, *et al.* Effects of physical activity on the fatigue and psychological status of cancer patients during chemotherapy. *Cancer* 1999; **85**: 2273–7.

PART 11

Respiratory systems

69

Dyspnea

JAY R THOMAS, CHARLES F VON GUNTEN

DEFINITION/SCOPE

Dyspnea is a highly prevalent source of suffering for palliative care patients. Many patients, caregivers, and practitioners use the synonymous term breathlessness to refer to dyspnea. It is most simply defined as an uncomfortable sensation or awareness of breathing. This definition highlights the subjective nature of dyspnea. Furthermore, it supports the concept that psychological, social, and spiritual/existential issues can amplify the suffering a person experiences with dyspnea. This concept is similar to the concept of total pain or total suffering.

Dyspnea in palliative medicine must be approached within the context of a patient's goals of care. Dependent on these goals, investigations to identify and interventions to reverse sources of dyspnea may be warranted. While waiting for underlying etiologies to be reversed, palliation of dyspnea should still be pursued. Sometimes sources of dyspnea are irreversible or their reversal is incapable of restoring a patient to a subjectively defined state of quality of life. In these cases symptomatic relief of dyspnea may be the goal.

We will first present the epidemiology and what is known about the pathophysiology of dyspnea. Then we will briefly discuss the identification and treatment of the reversible causes of dyspnea. Other sources for more indepth coverage of treatment for specific causes will be indicated. The management of congestive heart failure (CHF) and chronic obstructive pulmonary disease (COPD) are presented in Chapters 97 (page 918) and 99 (page 935), respectively. The primary focus of this chapter will be to present the evidence base for the symptomatic relief of dyspnea.

EPIDEMIOLOGY

Dyspnea is a common complaint in both cancer and noncancer diagnoses. In a representative population sample of 988 Americans living at home identified by their physicians as being terminally ill with a prognosis of less than 6 months, 71 percent had shortness of breath.[1] Depending on the stage of cancer, the prevalence of dyspnea ranges from 21 percent to 90 percent.[2-4] When there is primary or metastatic involvement of the lung, dyspnea is understandable; however, it is also a common complaint of patients with no direct lung involvement. In one study, 24 percent of cancer patients had dyspnea but no known cardiopulmonary pathology.[4] Moreover, cancer is often diagnosed in patients who have significant underlying cardiopulmonary problems, such as COPD and CHF, the two most common noncancer causes of chronic progressive dyspnea.

Worldwide, there are no good estimates of the incidence and prevalence of noncancer conditions that cause dyspnea. In 2002, the prevalence of COPD and CHF in the USA was estimated at 11.2 million and 5 million, respectively. The World Health Organization (WHO) estimates deaths in 2002 from noncancer conditions that are likely to be associated with dyspnea as follows: cardiovascular disease ~8 million, lower respiratory infections ~3.9 million, COPD ~2.7 million, asthma ~0.24 million, and iron deficiency anemia ~0.14 million.[5]

PATHOPHYSIOLOGY OF DYSPNEA

With the advent of functional brain imaging using positron emission tomography (PET) and functional magnetic resonance imaging (fMRI), researchers may be identifying cortical areas involved in the perception of dyspnea.[6–11] One area implicated in all studies to date is the anterior insula, a part of the limbic system. Animal studies have identified neural connections between the medullary respiratory center and the cortex, including the anterior insula.[12] These connections support the hypothesis that the respiratory center may send signals concomitantly to activate respiratory muscles as well as to the cortex leading to conscious perceptions of breathing. Interestingly, the anterior insula has also been implicated in the perception of pain, hunger, and thirst.[13–19] Thus, it is intriguing to speculate that there may be some commonality to the perception of unpleasant sensations or suffering.

What signals are transmitted to the brain that trigger dyspnea? Although incompletely understood, most studies indicate three types of signal:[20,21]

- the work of breathing
- chemoreception of oxygen and carbon dioxide levels
- neuromechanical dissociation.

The respiratory center in the medulla and pons coordinates the activity of the diaphragm, the intercostal muscles, and the accessory muscles of respiration (Fig. 69.1). It

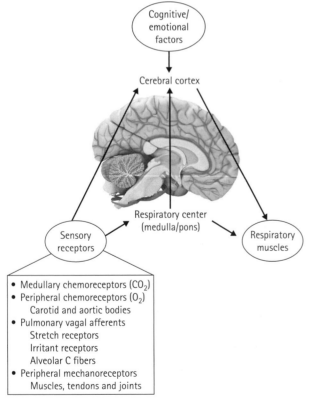

Figure 69.1 *Scheme of the flow of information between the peripheral and central components involved in the perception of breathing and breathlessness.*

receives sensory information from multiple sources. Peripheral mechanoreceptors in muscles, tendons, and joints send information regarding lung expansion and contractile force. The increased effort required for breathing against increased resistance (e.g. COPD) or breathing with weakened muscles (e.g. neuromuscular disease or cachexia) is sensed as dyspnea. This sense of effort probably comes not only from the increased work of ventilation relayed by mechanoreceptors but also from the increased strength of central nervous system efferent signals required to activate the muscles of breathing. As mentioned previously, these efferent signals appear to be sent concomitantly to the cortex where they presumably trigger dyspnea.

There are also pulmonary vagal afferents. These include:

- pulmonary stretch receptors, which are activated by lung inflation
- pulmonary irritant receptors triggered by certain chemicals, airflow, and smooth muscle tone
- alveolar C fibers that respond to pulmonary interstitial and capillary pressure.

These afferents may also send information directly to the cerebral cortex. An example of the role vagal afferents may play was elucidated by an experiment comparing dyspnea induced by bronchoconstriction to that induced by an external increase in breathing load.[22] The work of breathing was similar in both cases, but bronchoconstriction induced more dyspnea. Moreover, inhaled lidocaine blocked dyspnea from bronchoconstriction whereas dyspnea from external resistance was unchanged. This result implies pulmonary afferents are involved in some causes of dyspnea.

There are central and peripheral chemoreceptors sensitive to oxygen and carbon dioxide levels. Medullary chemoreceptors predominantly sense hypercapnia. Carotid and aortic body chemoreceptors predominantly sense hypoxemia. These sensations can lead to dyspnea in a way that is independent of increased respiratory effort.[23,24] Despite common belief, hypoxemia appears to play a less significant role in dyspnea. First, it takes moderately severe levels of hypoxemia to trigger the peripheral chemoreceptors.[25] Second, the compensatory increase in ventilation triggered by hypoxemia drives down the carbon dioxide level, which then partially negates the effect of the hypoxemia.

Finally, the concept of neuromechanical dissociation proposes that when there is a mismatch between what the brain desires for respiration and the sensory feedback it receives, dyspnea is enhanced.[26] For example, when researchers limit the inspiratory flow rate at which a subject is allowed to breathe, dyspnea results despite there being no change in respiratory work or chemical status.[27] Therefore, there are multiple independent and potentially synergistic mechanisms that can trigger dyspnea. Although these mechanisms all lead to dyspnea, individual mechanisms may trigger different perceptions in the type of dyspnea. Questionnaires have identified different words used by patients to describe dyspnea that may have mechanistic implications. For example, the bronchospasm of asthma is often characterized as 'tightness'; whereas hypercapnia is often described as 'air hunger'.[23,28,29] Further study is needed to determine if treatment can reliably be based on this 'language of dyspnea'.

ASSESSMENT AND IDENTIFICATION OF CAUSES OF DYSPNEA

Box 69.1 lists the important elements of a thorough assessment. The degree of assessment is determined by the burdens

and benefits of interventions in the context of a patient's goals of care.

Patient self-report is the only accurate measure of dyspnea. Although objective measures such as respiratory rate or arterial blood gas determinations may imply dyspnea and possibly help identify the causes, they do not directly measure dyspnea. For example, patients may be hypoxic, tachypneic, and 'look dyspneic', but when they are well palliated they report no sense of dyspnea. Validated scales such as a visual analog scale[30] or the Borg scale[31] are clinically useful to quantify dyspnea.

After thorough assessment, it may be possible to identify and treat underlying causes of dyspnea. Box 69.2 lists common causes for dyspnea associated with malignant and nonmalignant processes.

Box 69.1 Assessment of dyspnea

History

- Characterization of dyspnea (onset, description, quantification, associated symptoms, exacerbators and relievers)
- Past medical history (including smoking history, occupational history, prior radiation or chemotherapy)
- Psychosocial/spiritual history

Physical

- Observation (cachexia, cyanosis, clubbing, breathing pattern)
- Vital signs
- Cardiac examination (rhythm, adventitious sounds, murmurs, jugular venous distention, paradoxical pulse)
- Pulmonary examination (hyperinflation, stridor, adventitious sounds)
- Ascites
- Peripheral edema

Additional studies

- Laboratory studies (complete blood count, arterial blood gas, B-type natriuretic peptide)
- Pulse oximetry
- Pulmonary function tests
- Electrocardiogram
- Echocardiogram
- Angiography
- Imaging studies (chest X-ray, computed tomography, MRI, PET, ventilation–perfusion scan)

Box 69.2 Causes of dyspnea

- Infection
- Anemia
- Deconditioning
- Hypoxia
- Hypercapnia
- Metabolic acidosis
- Bronchospasm
- Pulmonary edema
- Pleural effusion
- Restrictive processes (chest wall restriction, decreased lung compliance)
- Pneumothorax
- Pulmonary embolus
- Muscle weakness (neuromuscular diseases, cachexia, steroid myopathy, phrenic nerve paralysis)
- Airway mechanical obstruction
- Lymphangitic carcinomatosis
- Pulmonary hypertension
- Pericardial effusion
- Ascites
- Psychosocial/spiritual issues

SYMPTOMATIC MANAGEMENT OF DYSPNEA

Opioids

Opioids are the first-line therapy for the symptomatic relief of dyspnea. Unfortunately, the mechanism is not well understood. Endogenous opioids have been implicated in the control of dyspnea by the following experiment:[32] opioid-naïve normal volunteers were exercised to the point of dyspnea. When given intravenous naloxone, a systemically acting opioid antagonist, dyspnea was enhanced. This finding implies antagonism of endogenous opioids which were working to dampen dyspnea.

Opioid receptors are located throughout the peripheral and central nervous systems. They are also located throughout the lung with the highest concentration in the alveoli.[33] As previously noted, fMRI has identified loci in the brain believed to be involved in the perception of dyspnea, such as the anterior insula, that also seems to be involved in perceiving other types of suffering, such as pain. Thus, it is possible that opioids alter the perception of dyspnea in a manner similar to that of pain.

There is evidence that opioids can be safe and effective in controlling dyspnea in several clinical populations. In a placebo-controlled crossover study in cancer patients, Bruera et al. demonstrated that opioids relieved dyspnea without a decrease in respiratory rate or oxygen saturation.[34] In this study at baseline, patients were dyspneic at rest despite opioids being used for pain with tolerable pain control. Thus additional opioids were effective for dyspnea even on this background of opioid use for pain. In opioid-naïve patients, as little as 5 mg of subcutaneous morphine sulfate was shown to be effective in controlling dyspnea.[35] The effect lasted for 4 hours, which is consistent with morphine's known half-life and its effects for pain relief. Allard et al. showed that a 25 percent increase in the baseline opioid dose for cancer pain provided relief of dyspnea for up to 4 hours.[36] Extrapolating from these results and by analogy with the treatment of pain, a reasonable regimen to control chronic dyspnea would include both a sustained-release opioid for baseline control and an immediate-release opioid for breakthrough dyspnea (Box 69.3).

Box 69.3 Opioid dosing recommendations for opioid-naïve patients

1   Start with oral morphine or equivalent 2.5–5 mg

2   Based on response at the time of maximum serum concentration (~1 hour per oral, ~30 minutes for subcutaneus/intramuscular, ~6 minutes for intravenous), the dose may be repeated or titrated up (for continued mild to moderate dyspnea, the dose can be titrated up 25–50 percent; for moderate to severe dyspnea, the dose can be titrated up 50–100 percent)

3   Calculate 24-hour opioid requirements and provide equivalent as long-acting opioid

4   Allow 5–15 percent of the 24-hour opioid dose for breakthrough dyspnea every hour orally as needed

---

Three small randomized, double-blind, placebo-controlled studies have investigated the effect of opioids in relief of dyspnea in opioid-naïve CHF patients. Chua et al. studied patients with an average ejection fraction of 21.3 percent who were New York Heart Association (NYHA) class II or III despite a good medical regimen.[37] Compared with placebo, patients who received a single oral dose of dihydrocodeine (1 mg/kg) had better exercise tolerance with less dyspnea 1 hour after dosing. Williams et al. also studied bolus dosing just before exercise using intravenous diamorphine (1 or 2 mg) versus placebo.[38] In these CHF patients with an average ejection fraction of 35.5 percent, diamorphine yielded a significant improvement in aerobic exercise capacity without suppressing respirations. Using a crossover design, Johnson et al. treated stable NYHA class III or IV patients on a good medical regimen with either placebo or morphine 5 mg orally four times a day over 4 days.[39] At steady state, morphine led to a significant reduction in breathlessness on a visual analog scale without evidence of respiratory depression. Several patients were noted to remain on opioids long term with good effects.

The effects of opioids on patients with COPD have also been examined. In one single-dose study, opioid-naïve COPD patients with an average FEV_1 (forced expiratory volume in 1 second) of 0.99 L, $PaCO_2 < 46$ mmHg, and $PaO_2 > 55$ mmHg were given an oral morphine dose of 0.8 mg/kg prior to exercise.[40] At this dosing, a patient weighing 70 kg would have received 56 mg of oral morphine, which is many times greater than a typically effective starting dose of 2.5–5 mg for an opioid-naïve COPD patient. Although there was an increase in $PaCO_2$ and decrease in PaO_2, respirations were not suppressed in a life-threatening way. In fact, dyspnea and exercise tolerance improved. Abernethy et al. performed a randomized, double-blind, placebo-controlled crossover trial of oral morphine in a group of patients who were dyspneic at rest despite maximal medical therapy.[41] The majority of the patients (88 percent) had COPD. These opioid-naïve patients received either 20 mg of sustained-release morphine per day or placebo over 4 days. At steady state, morphine significantly decreased visual analog scores of dyspnea, again without suppressing respirations.

Unfortunately, most studies have included small numbers of patients. To overcome this problem, one systematic meta-analysis was performed.[42] The authors identified double-blind, randomized, placebo-controlled studies that had assessed the efficacy of opioids in the treatment of dyspnea from any cause at the time of analysis: nine studies using oral or parenteral opioids (n = 7 for COPD, n = 1 for cancer, and n = 1 for CHF) and nine studies using nebulized opioids (n = 7 for COPD, n = 1 for cancer, and n = 1 for interstitial lung disease). The meta-analysis demonstrated a statistically significant overall subjective improvement in dyspnea. A subgroup analysis of the COPD studies also demonstrated benefits of the opioids. Importantly, no deaths were attributed to the opioids. Patients did experience opioid side effects such as nausea, lethargy, and constipation. Typically, tolerance develops to these effects with the exception of constipation, but their presence highlights the need to treat these predictable side effects proactively when chronic opioids are prescribed. Despite known opioid receptors in lung and anecdotal reports that nebulized opioids improve dyspnea, a subgroup analysis failed to show any benefit from nebulized opioids. Opioid antagonists that are only peripherally acting may help further define the role of opioid receptors outside the central nervous system (CNS), such as those present in lung. Because such agents will not cross the blood–brain barrier, it should be possible to block lung opioid receptors without affecting those in the CNS. Thus, the potential contribution of lung opioid receptors in the control of dyspnea could be assessed. Methylnaltrexone is one such agent currently undergoing clinical trials for opioid-induced constipation.

Further research is needed to define the benefits and burdens of opioids in specific diseases and individuals. However, given what is currently known, a trial of a low-dose opioid such as 2.5–5 mg of oral morphine or equivalent for an opioid-naïve patient is warranted. Oral opioid peak serum levels are reached in about 1 hour. If patients remain symptomatic, an appropriate dose of opioid can be safely given again. Patients can be monitored for any adverse event. The half-life of short-acting opioids ensures that any adverse event is equally short lived. In the rare event of a severe opioid adverse event, specific antagonists exist that are highly effective.

Anxiolytics

Benzodiazepines are frequently prescribed for anxiety that often coexists with dyspnea. Overall, however, the data indicate benzodiazepines alone should not be first line therapy for dyspnea. One placebo-controlled, single-blind study of four patients with COPD demonstrated that moderate doses of diazepam improved dyspnea.[43] However, subsequent double-blind studies on healthy subjects or COPD patients with diazepam or alprazolam failed to show any benefit over placebo.[44**,45**,46**] Dudgeon and Lertzman[47] found anxiety to be correlated with dyspnea; but in their multivariate model, it was sufficient to explain only 10 percent of the variance of dyspnea. Opioids, by removing the perception of dyspnea, may be sufficient to relieve anxiety in many cases. Nevertheless, some patients may continue

to have anxiety despite appropriate opioid dosing or may have an underlying anxiety disorder. In these patients, it is rational and safe to prescribe benzodiazepines in conjunction with opioids. As long as dosing guidelines are followed, there is no fear of respiratory depression.

Other psychoactive agents have also been studied. Buspirone, a nonbenzodiazepine anxiolytic, has yielded conflicting results in two studies.[48,49] The major tranquilizer chlorpromazine was tested in a small randomized, double-blind trial in healthy volunteers.[50**] Chlorpromazine 25 mg orally was able to significantly reduce dyspnea compared with placebo without increasing sedation. Larger studies will be needed to clarify its role in the symptomatic treatment of dyspnea. However, in dyspneic patients with a component of delirium/psychosis, it may be a reasonable choice.

Oxygen

Many clinicians use oxygen for dyspnea independent of etiology, whether or not hypoxemia is present. Often, patients report improved dyspnea with oxygen when they are not hypoxemic or when they remain hypoxemic despite oxygen. A partial explanation for this observation may be that oxygen has a placebo effect, potentially due to the medical symbolism inherent in its use. However, another explanation comes from studies that have demonstrated that stimulation of the trigeminal nerve (V2 branch) dampens dyspnea.[51**,52**,53**] Subjects who are made experimentally dyspneic report less dyspnea or have a decreased ventilatory response to provocation when cool, moving air is directed at the cheek or nasal mucosa. This result is consistent with the observed improvement in dyspnea seen simply by having a fan blow air across a patient's face.

Thus, if patients are hypoxemic and symptomatic, it is rational to attempt to reverse the hypoxemia and dyspnea with oxygen. If palliation of dyspnea is unsuccessful, oxygen does not need to be continued simply because of the hypoxemia. The use of oxygen must be individualized. In COPD patients with hypoxemia, oxygen may decrease mortality without significantly affecting quality of life. However, oxygen also has burdens that must be included in the decision about its use. Oxygen is costly, explosive, restricts mobility, affects self-image, and may cause CO_2 retention in some patients. If these burdens outweigh its benefits, it should not be used. However, independent of dyspnea etiology, one can consider a fan that provides cool, moving air across the trigeminal nerve distribution.

Lidocaine

As previously cited, inhaled lidocaine decreased dyspnea experimentally induced by bronchoconstriction.[22] However, small studies of patients with interstitial lung disease[54] and cancer[55] failed to show lidocaine to be better than saline. Larger studies need to be conducted to determine what, if any, subset of dyspnea is responsive to inhaled lidocaine.

NONPHARMACOLOGICAL THERAPIES

Cognitive/behavioral interventions

Dyspnea occurs in a whole person. In palliative care, there is a firm belief that to treat dyspnea and other symptoms optimally, psychological, social, and spiritual/existential issues must also be addressed. This includes assisting patients and families with education, practical care issues, interpersonal relationships, coping with fears, redefining meaning and hope, and attaining a self-defined sense of peace despite an illness. This task is best accomplished with an interdisciplinary team. This concept is beginning to gain support from clinical studies.

Bredin et al. conducted a multicenter, randomized controlled study that evaluated the effect of a nurse-run dyspnea clinic for patients with lung cancer.[56**] This approach is similar to pulmonary rehabilitation clinics for COPD, which have also been shown to improve quality of life and function.[57] The intervention consisted of teaching breathing control, activity pacing, relaxation techniques, and psychosocial support. Relative to controls, the patients who underwent the intervention showed improvement in dyspnea scores, performance status, and emotional states. Such nonpharmacological approaches include:

- A healthcare provider employing a calm demeanor to deescalate the anxiety a patient may be feeling.
- Educating patients and their caregivers about the underlying causes of dyspnea and proactive techniques to treat dyspnea in order to reestablish some sense of control of their lives.
- Simple repositioning to improve ventilation and perfusion matching when a disease process affects the lungs asymmetrically.
- Leaning forward while sitting or standing and supporting the thorax by bracing the arms against a chair or a patient's knees has been shown to increase ventilatory capacity.
- Use of devices such as a wheelchair to reduce metabolic demands.
- Education on the optimal preemptive use of medications such as opioids or bronchodilators before known exertional triggers to improve exercise tolerance.
- Pursed lip breathing to increase end-expiratory pressure, which in turn prevents alveolar collapse and thus improves oxygenation.
- Keeping a room well ventilated, with a fan gently blowing cool air across a patient's face (trigeminal nerve stimulation as discussed previously), while maintaining a line of sight to the outside.

Integrative therapies

Pan et al. performed a systematic review of integrative therapies (formerly known as complementary and alternative

medicine) for several symptoms including dyspnea.[58] In single-blind, randomized controlled trials of COPD patients, acupuncture[59] and acupressure[60] significantly relieved dyspnea compared with sham interventions. The role acupuncture and other integrative therapies will play in the control of dyspnea awaits more study.

NONINVASIVE POSITIVE PRESSURE VENTILATION

Noninvasive positive pressure ventilation (NIPPV) employing facemasks, nasal masks, or helmets has been used in several scenarios of respiratory failure, including neuromuscular disease,[61–63] COPD,[64] and cancer.[65] Both lung failure (primarily hypoxia) and respiratory pump failure (primarily hypercapnia) have been treated using NIPPV. Gas under pressure inflates the lungs, and exhalation occurs by passive recoil of the respiratory system. Often, pressure support ventilation is used together with continuous positive airway pressure (CPAP). A patient triggers an inspiration and the ventilator assists the breath with a preset pressure. When flow rate decreases to a certain point, the ventilator cycles down, and expiration is allowed to occur.

When CPAP is used, end-expiratory alveolar collapse is reduced enhancing oxygenation and reducing right-to-left shunting. In certain stages of a chronic condition such as amyotrophic lateral sclerosis and in some acute, reversible clinical situations such as a COPD exacerbation or pneumonia in a patients with cancer, there may be some utility to the use of NIPPV. Patients may be restored to some level of quality of life or enabled to achieve some short-term goal. This benefit must be carefully weighed against the burdens of the intervention for each individual. The role NIPPV will play in palliative care remains to be elucidated.

REFRACTORY DYSPNEA

Rarely, some patients may have dyspnea that is refractory to interventions. In these cases, palliative sedation is an ethical and legal option with patient or surrogate informed consent. The reader is referred to Chapter 103 (page 976) for further details of palliative sedation.

Key learning points

- The physiological basis of dyspnea is still being elucidated but is likely related to chemical signals (O_2, CO_2), the work of breathing, and/or neuromechanical dissociation.

- Dyspnea is a subjective phenomenon that can only be quantified by asking a patient.

- When consistent with a patient's goals of care, an attempt to identify and reverse the underlying causes of dyspnea is reasonable. While waiting for an etiology to be reversed, effective palliation is still indicated.

- When interventions to reverse the causes of dyspnea are not possible or when these interventions are not consistent with a patient's goals of care, opioids are the best therapy for the symptomatic relief of dyspnea.

- Benzodiazepines are not a first-line therapy for dyspnea but can be safely used as an adjunct to opioid therapy.

- For symptomatic relief, oxygen can be rationally tried if hypoxia is present but does not need to be continued if symptoms remain unabated. Stimulation of the trigeminal nerve distribution with cool, moving air is reasonable for symptomatic relief of dyspnea independent of cause.

- Dyspnea must also be understood in the context of a whole person, and all sources of suffering must be addressed for optimal symptom control.

REFERENCES

1 Emanuel EJ, Fairclough DL, Slutsman J, Emanuel LL. Understanding economic and other burdens of terminal illness: the experience of patients and their caregivers. *Ann Intern Med* 2000; **132**: 451–9.

2 Muers MF, Round CE. Palliation of symptoms in non-small cell lung cancer: a study by the Yorkshire Regional Cancer Organisation Thoracic Group. *Thorax* 1993; **48**: 339–43.

3 Higginson I, McCarthy M. Measuring symptoms in terminal cancer: are pain and dyspnoea controlled? *J R Soc Med* 1989; **82**: 264–7.

4 Reuben DB, Mor V. Dyspnea in terminally ill cancer patients. *Chest* 1986; **89**: 234–6.

5 World Health Organization. Beaglehole R, Irwin A, Prentice T. *The World Health Report 2004: Changing History*. Geneva: World Health Organization, 2004.

● 6 Evans KC, Banzett RB, Adams L, et al. BOLD fMRI identifies limbic, paralimbic, and cerebellar activation during air hunger. *J Neurophysiol* 2002; **88**: 1500–11.

7 Banzett RB, Mulnier HE, Murphy K, et al. Breathlessness in humans activates insular cortex. *Neuroreport* 2000; **11**: 2117–20.

8 Brannan S, Liotti M, Egan G, et al. Neuroimaging of cerebral activations and deactivations associated with hypercapnia and hunger for air. *Proc Natl Acad Sci U S A* 2001; **98**: 2029–34.

9 Liotti M, Brannan S, Egan G, et al. Brain responses associated with consciousness of breathlessness (air hunger). *Proc Natl Acad Sci U S A* 2001; **98**: 2035–40.

10 Parsons LM, Egan G, Liotti M, et al. Neuroimaging evidence implicating cerebellum in the experience of hypercapnia and hunger for air. *Proc Natl Acad Sci U S A* 2001; **98**: 2041–6.

11 Peiffer C, Poline JB, Thivard L, et al. Neural substrates for the perception of acutely induced dyspnea. *Am J Respir Crit Care Med* 2001; **163**: 951–7.

12 Gaytan SP, Pasaro R. Connections of the rostral ventral respiratory neuronal cell group: an anterograde and retrograde tracing study in the rat. *Brain Res Bull* 1998; **47**: 625–42.

13 Baciu MV, Bonaz BL, Papillon E, et al. Central processing of rectal pain: a functional MR imaging study. *AJNR Am J Neuroradiol* 1999; **20**: 1920–4.

14 Binkofski F, Schnitzler A, Enck P, et al. Somatic and limbic cortex activation in esophageal distention: a functional magnetic resonance imaging study. *Ann Neurol* 1998; **44**: 811–15.

15 Derbyshire SW, Jones AK, Gyulai F, et al. Pain processing during three levels of noxious stimulation produces differential patterns of central activity. *Pain* 1997; **73**: 431–45.

16 Iadarola MJ, Berman KF, Zeffiro TA, et al. Neural activation during acute capsaicin-evoked pain and allodynia assessed with PET. *Brain* 1998; **121**(Pt 5): 931–47.

17 Peyron R, Garcia-Larrea L, Gregoire MC, et al. Haemodynamic brain responses to acute pain in humans: sensory and attentional networks. *Brain* 1999; **122**(Pt 9): 1765–80.

18 Denton D, Shade R, Zamarippa F, et al. Correlation of regional cerebral blood flow and change of plasma sodium concentration during genesis and satiation of thirst. *Proc Natl Acad Sci U S A* 1999; **96**: 2532–7.

19 Tataranni PA, Gautier JF, Chen K, et al. Neuroanatomical correlates of hunger and satiation in humans using positron emission tomography. *Proc Natl Acad Sci U S A* 1999; **96**: 4569–74.

◆ 20 Manning HL, Schwartzstein RM. Pathophysiology of dyspnea. *N Engl J Med* 1995; **333**: 1547–53.

21 American Thoracic Society. Dyspnea. Mechanisms, assessment, and management: a consensus statement. *Am J Respir Crit Care Med* 1999; **159**: 321–40.

22 Taguchi O, Kikuchi Y, Hida W, et al. Effects of bronchoconstriction and external resistive loading on the sensation of dyspnea. *J Appl Physiol* 1991; **71**: 2183–90.

23 Banzett RB, Lansing RW, Reid MB, et al. 'Air hunger' arising from increased PCO_2 in mechanically ventilated quadriplegics. *Respir Physiol* 1989; **76**: 53–67.

24 Lane R, Cockcroft A, Adams L, Guz A. Arterial oxygen saturation and breathlessness in patients with chronic obstructive airways disease. *Clin Sci (Lond)* 1987; **72**: 693–8.

25 Eyzaguirre C, Zapata P. Perspectives in carotid body research. *J Appl Physiol* 1984; **57**: 931–57.

26 O'Donnell DE, Webb KA. Exertional breathlessness in patients with chronic airflow limitation. The role of lung hyperinflation. *Am Rev Respir Dis* 1993; **148**: 1351–7.

27 Manning HL, Molinary EJ, Leiter JC. Effect of inspiratory flow rate on respiratory sensation and pattern of breathing. *Am J Respir Crit Care Med* 1995; **151**(3 Pt 1): 751–7.

28 Simon PM, Schwartzstein RM, Weiss JW, et al. Distinguishable types of dyspnea in patients with shortness of breath. *Am Rev Respir Dis* 1990; **142**: 1009–14.

29 Binks AP, Moosavi SH, Banzett RB, Schwartzstein RM. 'Tightness' sensation of asthma does not arise from the work of breathing. *Am J Respir Crit Care Med* 2002; **165**: 78–82.

30 Adams L, Chronos N, Lane R, Guz A. The measurement of breathlessness induced in normal subjects: validity of two scaling techniques. *Clin Sci (Lond)* 1985; **69**: 7–16.

31 Borg GA. Psychophysical bases of perceived exertion. *Med Sci Sports Exerc* 1982; **14**: 377–81.

32 Akiyama Y, Nishimura M, Kobayashi S, et al. Effects of naloxone on the sensation of dyspnea during acute respiratory stress in normal adults. *J Appl Physiol* 1993; **74**: 590–5.

33 Zebraski SE, Kochenash SM, Raffa RB. Lung opioid receptors: pharmacology and possible target for nebulized morphine in dyspnea. *Life Sci* 2000; **66**: 2221–31.

● 34 Bruera E, MacEachern T, Ripamonti C, Hanson J. Subcutaneous morphine for dyspnea in cancer patients. *Ann Intern Med* 1993; **119**: 906–7.

35 Mazzocato C, Buclin T, Rapin CH. The effects of morphine on dyspnea and ventilatory function in elderly patients with advanced cancer: a randomized double-blind controlled trial. *Ann Oncol* 1999; **10**: 1511–14.

36 Allard P, Lamontagne C, Bernard P, Tremblay C. How effective are supplementary doses of opioids for dyspnea in terminally ill cancer patients? A randomized continuous sequential clinical trial. *J Pain Symptom Manage* 1999; **17**: 256–65.

● 37 Chua TP, Harrington D, Ponikowski P, et al. Effects of dihydrocodeine on chemosensitivity and exercise tolerance in patients with chronic heart failure. *J Am Coll Cardiol* 1997; **29**: 147–52.

38 Williams SG, Wright DJ, Marshall P, et al. Safety and potential benefits of low dose diamorphine during exercise in patients with chronic heart failure. *Heart* 2003; **89**: 1085–6.

39 Johnson MJ, McDonagh TA, Harkness A, et al. Morphine for the relief of breathlessness in patients with chronic heart failure – a pilot study. *Eur J Heart Fail* 2002; **4**: 753–6.

● 40 Light RW, Muro JR, Sato RI, et al. Effects of oral morphine on breathlessness and exercise tolerance in patients with chronic obstructive pulmonary disease. *Am Rev Respir Dis* 1989; **139**: 126–33.

41 Abernethy AP, Currow DC, Frith P, et al. Randomised, double blind, placebo controlled crossover trial of sustained release morphine for the management of refractory dyspnoea. *BMJ* 2003; **327**: 523–8.

◆ 42 Jennings AL, Davies AN, Higgins JP, et al. A systematic review of the use of opioids in the management of dyspnoea. *Thorax* 2002; **57**: 939–44.

43 Mitchell-Heggs P, Murphy K, Minty K, et al. Diazepam in the treatment of dyspnoea in the 'Pink Puffer' syndrome. *Q J Med* 1980; **49**: 9–20.

44 Stark RD, Gambles SA, Lewis JA. Methods to assess breathlessness in healthy subjects: a critical evaluation and application to analyse the acute effects of diazepam and promethazine on breathlessness induced by exercise or by exposure to raised levels of carbon dioxide. *Clin Sci (Lond)* 1981; **61**: 429–39.

45 Woodcock AA, Gross ER, Geddes DM. Drug treatment of breathlessness: contrasting effects of diazepam and promethazine in pink puffers. *Br Med J (Clin Res Ed)* 1981; **283**: 343–6.

46 Man GC, Hsu K, Sproule BJ. Effect of alprazolam on exercise and dyspnea in patients with chronic obstructive pulmonary disease. *Chest* 1986; **90**: 832–6.

47 Dudgeon DJ, Lertzman M. Dyspnea in the advanced cancer patient. *J Pain Symptom Manage* 1998; **16**: 212–19.

48 Argyropoulou P, Patakas D, Koukou A, et al. Buspirone effect on breathlessness and exercise performance in patients with chronic obstructive pulmonary disease. *Respiration* 1993; **60**: 216–20.

49 Singh NP, Despars JA, Stansbury DW, et al. Effects of buspirone on anxiety levels and exercise tolerance in patients with chronic airflow obstruction and mild anxiety. *Chest* 1993; **103**: 800–4.

50 O'Neill PA, Morton PB, Stark RD. Chlorpromazine – a specific effect on breathlessness? *Br J Clin Pharmacol* 1985; **19**: 793–7.

● 51 Schwartzstein RM, Lahive K, Pope A, et al. Cold facial stimulation reduces breathlessness induced in normal subjects. *Am Rev Respir Dis* 1987; **136**: 58–61.

52 Liss HP, Grant BJ. The effect of nasal flow on breathlessness in patients with chronic obstructive pulmonary disease. *Am Rev Respir Dis* 1988; **137**: 1285–8.

53 Burgess KR, Whitelaw WA. Effects of nasal cold receptors on pattern of breathing. *J Appl Physiol* 1988; **64**: 371–6.

54 Winning AJ, Hamilton RD, Guz A. Ventilation and breathlessness on maximal exercise in patients with interstitial lung disease after local anaesthetic aerosol inhalation. *Clin Sci (Lond)* 1988; **74**: 275–81.

55 Wilcock A, Corcoran R, Tattersfield AE. Safety and efficacy of nebulized lignocaine in patients with cancer and breathlessness. *Palliat Med* 1994; **8**: 35–8.

● 56 Bredin M, Corner J, Krishnasamy M, et al. Multicentre randomised controlled trial of nursing intervention for breathlessness in patients with lung cancer. *BMJ* 1999; **318**: 901–4.

57 Pulmonary rehabilitation – 1999. American Thoracic Society. *Am J Respir Crit Care Med* 1999; **159**(5 Pt 1): 1666–82.

◆ 58 Pan CX, Morrison RS, Ness J, et al. Complementary and alternative medicine in the management of pain, dyspnea, and nausea and vomiting near the end of life. A systematic review. *J Pain Symptom Manage* 2000; **20**: 374–87.

59 Jobst K, Chen JH, McPherson K, et al. Controlled trial of acupuncture for disabling breathlessness. *Lancet* 1986; **2**: 1416–19.

60 Maa SH, Gauthier D, Turner M. Acupressure as an adjunct to a pulmonary rehabilitation program. *J Cardiopulm Rehabil* 1997; **17**: 268–76.

61 Voltz R, Borasio GD. Palliative therapy in the terminal stage of neurological disease. *J Neurol* 1997; **244**(Suppl 4): S2–S10.

62 Borasio GD, Voltz R. Palliative care in amyotrophic lateral sclerosis. *J Neurol* 1997; **244**(Suppl 4): S11–S17.

63 Polkey MI, Lyall RA, Davidson AC, et al. Ethical and clinical issues in the use of home non-invasive mechanical ventilation for the palliation of breathlessness in motor neurone disease. *Thorax* 1999; **54**: 367–71.

64 Lightowler JV, Wedzicha JA, Elliott MW, Ram FS. Non-invasive positive pressure ventilation to treat respiratory failure resulting from exacerbations of chronic obstructive pulmonary disease: Cochrane systematic review and meta-analysis. *BMJ* 2003; **326**: 185.

65 Nava S, Cuomo AM. Acute respiratory failure in the cancer patient: the role of non-invasive mechanical ventilation. *Crit Rev Oncol Hematol* 2004; **51**: 91–103.

70

Other respiratory symptoms (cough, hiccup, and secretions)

TABITHA THOMAS, ROSEMARY WADE, SARA BOOTH

INTRODUCTION

The aim of this chapter is to outline the management of cough, hiccup, and excessive respiratory secretions in the palliative care setting. The majority of research into chronic cough and hiccup has been carried out in patients with non-malignant disease, and this provides the bulk of evidence for their management in palliative care. Evidence for the management of excessive bronchial secretions and death rattle is lacking because of the difficulties in undertaking research in these areas. For this reason, some therapies are included in this chapter based on general consensus within the specialty, despite there being very little evidence for their efficacy.

COUGH

Cough is common in the general population and is generally self-limiting or can be managed by treating the precipitating cause.[1] Where this cannot be achieved, however, cough can become a persistent and distressing symptom. Approximately 65 percent of patients with lung cancer complain of cough at presentation, and its incidence and severity remain the same throughout the disease course, indicating that it is generally not well palliated.[2] Cough is also a common symptom in patients with any type of advanced cancer. In one survey, 37 percent of patients with advanced cancer complained of cough, and of these, 38 percent of these rated it as moderate or severe.[3,4]

Relentless coughing can have a profound impact on quality of life. It leads to exhaustion, breathlessness, musculoskeletal pain, vomiting, and incontinence. Disturbed sleep affects both patients and partners with consequent strain on family and social relationships.

Physiology

Cough serves as a reflex defense mechanism to remove either inhaled foreign material, or excess endogenous inflammatory products. The reflex begins with either mechanical or chemical stimulation of irritant receptors in the epithelium of the respiratory tract. Impulses are then transmitted via vagal afferents to the medulla oblongata where a cough response is coordinated. The efferent pathways are anatomically distinct from those involved in spontaneous respiration and travel via the phrenic and spinal motor nerves to the respiratory musculature, and via the recurrent laryngeal nerve to the larynx. Bronchial smooth muscle constriction is also necessary for cough production and is under vagal control.

Cough involves the initial inspiration of air followed by glottis closure and the development of high intrapleural pressure. The greater the volume of inspired air, the better the length tension ratio of the expiratory muscles, and the greater the intrathoracic pressure. When the glottis opens, a biphasic turbulent blast of air is produced as a result of the high pressure and the dynamic compression of the central airways. At high airflow velocities, the surface of the mucus is sheared off and droplets are propelled into the airway lumen.[5]

Pathogenesis

An effective cough, resulting in mucus displacement, depends upon:

- the velocity of the airstream

- the tenacity of the mucus
- a functioning mucociliary transport system.

Thus weak respiratory and abdominal muscles, for example in paraplegic patients, reduce the ability to produce a high expiratory pressure and therefore reduce the velocity of airflow and produce an ineffective cough. Mucus tenacity increases when the water content of mucus decreases, which leads to ineffective clearance. Finally, a functioning mucociliary apparatus is required to move mucus from the periphery to the more central airways from where it can be expelled by coughing.

Causes

Any form of malignant lung disease can cause an inflammatory or mechanical stimulus to cough. It may be the direct result of the tumor itself, or a consequence of consolidation associated with bronchial obstruction, aspiration or tracheoesophageal fistulae. In addition, the combination of pain and cachexia diminishes cough effectiveness and increases susceptibility to infection. Some tumors, particularly bronchoalveolar carcinoma, actively secrete mucus and therefore continuously stimulate the cough reflex. Occasionally, cough associated with increasing breathlessness is the result of an interstitial pneumonitis associated with radiotherapy.

There are many nonmalignant causes of chronic cough, which may nevertheless be relevant in palliative care. Smoking is a prime cause in adults and induces both airway inflammation and mucus hypersecretion. Because the mucociliary apparatus is also damaged, there is constant stimulation of the cough reflex. Lung damage due to smoke or persistent infection leads to chronic bronchitis and bronchiectasis, conditions characterized by chronic cough and excessive sputum production. Management is usually directed at treating the underlying cause, i.e. treating infection and increasing cough clearance, rather than cough suppression.

In nonsmoking, immunocompetent patients with a normal chest radiograph, who are not taking an angiotensin-converting enzyme (ACE) inhibitor and who do not have exposure to irritants, the most common causes of cough are postnasal drip syndrome, asthma, and gastroesophageal reflux disease. In 20 percent of patients cough is due to more than one cause.[1]

Assessment

Cough may make an important contribution to symptoms such as pain, nausea, insomnia and breathlessness, and its treatment can therefore have considerable benefits. As well as looking for an underlying cause, care should be taken to determine whether cough frequency or difficulty with expectoration is most troublesome. Once this is established

it helps make the decision as to whether therapy should be curative, protussive, or antitussive. The patient's prognosis should also be taken into account when deciding on management: if cough is severe and the prognosis short, there may be no time to treat infection or reflux, and a powerful opioid antitussive might be more appropriate.

Management strategies

SUPPORTIVE

The severity of a cough may be used as a gauge of disease progression by some patients, particularly if it was the presenting symptom of their cancer. Paroxysms of coughing are distressing to experience, alarming to watch and can lead to a fear that death will occur during an attack. Discussion, reassurance, and the establishment of a management plan to use during a coughing fit are helpful for both patients and carers.

STOP COUGH CAUSING MEDICATIONS

Among approximately 10 percent of users, ACE inhibitors cause a dry cough, which tends to be a class effect and is not dose related. There may be no correlation between the timing of drug usage and the onset of cough. It is important to note that cough of any cause can be aggravated by ACE inhibitors and this effect can take up to 4 weeks to resolve once the drug is stopped.[6**]

PHARMACOLOGIC

Pharmacological therapy can be used to treat an underlying cause or to modify the cough, in which case it is either protussive or antitussive. Protussive therapy makes the cough more effective and therefore less distressing, and is also useful if the cough is providing a useful physiological function, for example clearing a treatable infection. Antitussive therapy involves nonspecific cough suppression.

Treatment of the underlying cause

DECONGESTANTS AND ANTIHISTAMINES

Postnasal drip syndrome is the most common cause of chronic cough. Secretions from the nose or sinuses drip into the hypopharynx and stimulate the cough reflex. Symptoms of nasal congestion or discharge or a history of a recent cold are relatively sensitive but not necessarily specific[5] and ultimately a diagnosis of postnasal drip syndrome is made if cough shows a response to therapy. Sedative antihistamines and decongestants have been shown to be beneficial for both acute[7**] and chronic cough[8*] caused by postnasal drip but the effect is gradual and can take up to 2 weeks.

BRONCHODILATORS

In those with asthma or airway hyperresponsiveness, cough will respond transiently to bronchodilator therapy with

β_2 agonists,[9*] and in the long term has been shown to respond to sodium necrodomil,[10**] antileukotriene agents,[11*] and corticosteroids.[12*] In addition, the bronchodilator ipratropium bromide has been found to be useful as an antitussive in patients with chronic obstructive pulmonary disease by decreasing both sputum production and cough.[13**]

The use of bronchodilators to aid expectoration in chronic lung disease is controversial. They may reduce cough effectiveness because the increase in bronchial compliance causes the airways to collapse during the dynamic compression phase of the cough.[5] However, in one study nebulized terbutaline significantly enhanced the effects of physiotherapy on cough clearance for patients with bronchiectasis.[13*] This may have been because of enhanced ciliary beating and increased mucus hydration.

PROTON PUMP INHIBITORS/ANTACIDS

Cough due to gastroesophageal reflux can take a number of weeks to resolve in healthy subjects treated with antacids.[14] Because cough may aggravate reflux and reflux may then further aggravate cough, treatment with prokinetics and antacids may be worth considering in the palliative care setting for people with particularly troublesome symptoms.

CORTICOSTEROIDS

A dry cough associated with increasing dyspnea in those who have recently received radiotherapy to the lung should raise the suspicion of radiation pneumonitis.[15] Interstitial pneumonitis is also a rare complication of some chemotherapeutic agents.[16,17] If appropriate, radiological imaging should be carried out to confirm the diagnosis, as both are likely to respond to steroids.

RADIOTHERAPY

Radiotherapy can improve cough in nonsmall cell lung cancer in about 50 percent of patients,[18*] and seems to be related to the degree of shrinkage of the tumor. Re-treatment can be beneficial for those with cough who have previously received radiotherapy (palliation lasted for more than 50 percent of their remaining lifespan in one study).[19,20*] Intraluminal brachytherapy for endobronchial lesions improved cough at 6 weeks in 62 percent of patients.[21*]

CHEMOTHERAPY

Patients receiving single agent gemcitabine[22**] or carboplatin and etoposide[23**] for inoperable nonsmall cell lung cancer reported a greater improvement in cough and required less radiotherapy for symptom control than those receiving 'best supportive care'. However, the total number of patients who experienced any palliation of their cough was small and 'best supportive care' was loosely defined and did not necessarily include specialist palliative care.

BRONCHOSCOPIC THERAPIES

These include endobronchial laser therapy, electrocautery, argon plasma coagulation, cryotherapy, with or without intraluminal stent insertion. Their main indication in palliative care is for the relief of malignant central airway obstruction and in the case of the first three, management of hemoptysis. No studies have specifically investigated their use in the palliation of intractable cough. Indeed retention of secretions and cough are known complications of intraluminal stent insertion.[24–26]

Protussive cough enhancers (mucoactive agents)

EXPECTORANTS

Expectorants improve cough effectiveness by increasing airway water or the volume of airway secretions. Simple hydration has not been shown to improve cough and may be detrimental, since overhydration has been shown to decrease airway clearance in some patients with chronic cough.[27*]

HYPERTONIC SALINE

Nebulized hypertonic saline has been shown to enhance mucociliary clearance both *in vitro* and *in vivo*. As well as stimulating mucociliary transport, it is postulated that hypertonic saline breaks the ionic bonds within mucus gel and therefore lowers viscosity and elasticity.[28] It may also induce an osmotic flow of water into the mucus layer and thereby alter the mucus rheology. The effect appears to be concentration dependent: patients with cystic fibrosis were found to have better cough clearance with increasing concentrations of nebulized hypertonic saline.[29*] Therefore more evidence exists for the use of nebulized hypertonic saline as opposed to normal saline, which tends to be administered routinely.

GUAIFENESIN

This expectorant is found in many over-the-counter preparations, although few studies have evaluated its efficacy. One placebo controlled trial showed that patients treated with guaifenesin maintained steady levels of sputum production compared with the decline in sputum volume found with those taking placebo.[30**] In addition, guaifenesin has recently been shown to decrease cough reflex sensitivity in patients with upper respiratory tract infection.[31]

MUCOLYTIC AGENTS

Mucolytic medications increase the expectoration of sputum by depolymerizing either the mucin network (classic mucolytics) or the DNA-actin polymer network (peptide mucolytics), thereby reducing its viscosity and aiding cough clearance.[32]

Classic mucolytics, e.g. *N*-acetylcysteine, carbocysteine

These mucolytics hydrolyze the disulfide bonds that link mucin monomers within sputum. Classic mucolytics are widely used in parts of Europe and Asia for chronic bronchitis. Although they have some benefit in reducing the number and length of exacerbations,[33***] their relevance for patients with advanced cancer is unclear. Oral preparations are gastric irritants while nebulized *N*-acetylcysteine has a sulfurous odor and can cause bronchospasm, making it unsuitable for symptom palliation.

Peptide mucolytics

Recombinant DNAase is approved for use in patients with cystic fibrosis. It reduces the size of DNA molecules within mucus, thereby reducing sputum viscosity and aiding clearance. It has been shown to improve forced expiratory volume in one second (FEV_1), reduce exacerbations and improve quality of life in cystic fibrosis patients, but has shown no benefit for patients with chronic bronchitis and is not generally used for symptom control in other conditions.[32]

CHEST PHYSIOTHERAPY

Advice from a physiotherapist on cough technique is important. 'Huffing', a technique that involves forcible exhalation with the glottis open from a medium-to-low lung volume, can be helpful for weak, breathless patients with extensive disease.

Cough suppression

HOME REMEDIES/OVER-THE-COUNTER PREPARATIONS

Any sweet thickened drink will help relieve cough and many popular 'cough medicines' and herbal remedies rely on the presence of demulcents such as sugars and gum arabic which absorb fluid and produce a soothing covering in the throat. They are probably most useful if the cough is due to receptor irritation in the oropharynx.[34]

ANTITUSSIVES

Relatively little is known about how antitussive drugs act to inhibit cough.[35] Some have a predominantly central mode of action, for example opioids, whereas others are thought to work peripherally. The concept of 'opioid-resistant cough' appears in the literature as a distinct entity,[36–38] and may be due to either peripheral or central sensitization of the cough reflex. Various drugs have been suggested to be beneficial in this situation and are discussed below.

OPIOIDS AND RELATED COMPOUNDS

The antitussive activity of opioids is distinct from their analgesic effect and some opioid-related antitussives have no analgesic effect at all. For palliative care patients, it is often necessary to treat both cough and pain, in which case a strong opioid analgesic is appropriate. If cough persists while a patient is taking a strong opioid for pain relief, it is not currently clear whether it is beneficial to use a separate opioid, that has greater antitussive activity, for cough. If, however, predominantly the antitussive activity is required, codeine or one of its nonanalgesic derivatives can be used.

Codeine

Codeine's antitussive activity is much greater than its analgesic action and has been extensively studied both clinically and experimentally.[39***] A 4-hourly dose of 30–60 mg is known to be effective, but has all the typical opioid side effects such as nausea, drowsiness, and constipation.

Hydrocodone

Hydrocodone is one of the metabolites of codeine and has analgesic and antitussive activity. It was used in a phase II open label study in cancer patients with cough as an alternative to codeine because it had been found to be better tolerated.[40*] A median dose of 10 mg a day was associated with the best response (most patients achieved >50 percent improvement in cough frequency). Most patients were using other opioids for analgesia.

Methadone

The dextroisomer of methadone is particularly active and is a more potent antitussive than codeine or morphine.[39*] Methadone linctus can be given at a dose of 1–2 mg every 4–6 hours, reducing to twice daily with prolonged use. Because of its long half life and potential to accumulate, it should be used with caution and under specialist supervision.

OPIOID-RELATED ANTITUSSIVES WITH NO ANALGESIC ACTIVITY

Pholcodine

This is structurally related to codeine and possibly has greater antitussive activity, but no analgesic action. It has few side effects and does not give rise to tolerance or dependence.[39**] It can be used at a dose of 5–10 mg three to four times per day.

Dextromethorphan

Dextromethorphan is a non-narcotic codeine analog and is the active ingredient in many over-the-counter preparations. It is the most commonly used antitussive in the USA and compares favorably to codeine in patients with chronic cough. In one comparative study, both were effective in reducing cough frequency at a dose of 20 mg, but dextromethorphan was preferred by the majority of patients and had fewer side effects.[41**]

Dimemorfan

Dimemorfan is widely used in Japan. Although an opioid derivative, dimemorfan is thought to have a central antitussive activity which is independent of the narcotic antitussive mechanism. Its action is not affected by levallorphan, an opioid receptor antagonist. In animal experiments its antitussive activity is greater than codeine and it has a stimulant rather than a depressant effect on the respiratory center. It shows marked or moderate efficacy in about 50 percent of patients treated at doses of 20 mg three times daily. It does not cause dependence and has no analgesic action.[42**]

NONOPIOID ANTITUSSIVE DRUGS

Benzonatate

Benzonatate is chemically related to para-aminobenzoic acid anesthetics and is thought to act peripherally by anesthetizing stretch receptors. It has been described in a case series as useful for opioid-resistant cough in cancer patients at a dose of 100 mg three times daily and has few side effects.[38*]

Levodropropizine

Levodropropizine is also thought to have a peripheral mechanism of action involving modulation of C fiber sensitivity. It is a phenylpiperazinopropane derivative which has been shown to be as effective as dihydrocodeine in patients with malignant involvement of the lung at a dose of 75 mg three times daily. Although adverse effects were low in both groups, there was significantly less somnolence reported in the levodropropizine group.[43**] The side effect profile of levodropropizine was also significantly better when it was compared to dextromethorphan in patients with moderate nonproductive cough, although both had similar antitussive activity.[44**]

Moguisteine

Moguisteine is a peripherally acting non-narcotic antitussive drug. It has been shown to produce a significant reduction in cough when compared with placebo (42 percent vs. 14 percent, respectively). Patients with chronic respiratory disorders and chronic cough, some of whom had lung cancer, were randomized to receive moguisteine syrup, 200 mg three times daily, or placebo over a period of 4 days.[45**] In a separate study a dose of 100 mg three times daily was found to be equally as effective as codeine 15 mg and 30 mg.[46**]

Glaucine

This centrally acting antitussive is mainly available in eastern European countries and should not be confused with a β blocker, metipranolol, which is marketed in Europe under the same name.[5] Antitussive effects and side effect profile were significantly better than codeine in one randomized controlled trial.[47**] Both drugs were taken at a dose of 30 mg three times daily.

Sodium cromoglycate

Sodium cromoglycate may suppress unmyelinated C fibers involved in the afferent pathway of the cough reflex. A trial in patients with neoplastic, irritative cough which had been unresponsive to conventional treatment found there was a significant reduction in cough amongst those receiving inhaled sodium cromoglycate when compared with placebo.[37**]

LOCAL ANESTHETICS

Experimentally, local anesthetics delivered either intravenously or by inhalation have been shown to inhibit the cough response to a variety of stimuli.[35] Nebulized bupivacaine has been used for persistent cough in the palliative care setting, although evidence exists in case reports only.[48*] Its use is limited by its unpleasant taste, risk of aspiration, risk of bronchospasm, and short duration of action and patients also frequently develop tachyphylaxis.

SEROTONIN SELECTIVE REUPTAKE INHIBITORS

It has been postulated that serotonin selective reuptake inhibitors may be beneficial in opioid resistant dry cough based on observations that increased serotonin levels depress the cough reflex in cats.[49] One case series reported paroxetine to be effective for cancer patients with cough for whom codeine had been ineffective.[36*] However, there is known to be a powerful placebo effect with all cough treatment, and therefore, any study which has no placebo control is difficult to interpret.[50]

HICCUP

Chronic hiccup is an infrequent but distressing problem. Whether it occurs in patients with advanced cancer or those who are otherwise healthy, it leads to fatigue, insomnia, depression, and weight loss and can have a significant effect on quality of life.

Physiology

Hiccup may exist as an exercise to coordinate respiratory muscles in the fetus, but serves no known physiological purpose in the adult.[51] The reflex arc consists of:

1 afferent input via the phrenic and vagus nerves and the thoracic sympathetic chain
2 a central mediator thought to be in the cervical spine and brainstem
3 an efferent limb via motor fibers of the phrenic nerve.

The pathophysiology of chronic hiccup is poorly understood but probably results from persistent disturbance of one of the components of the reflex arc. Conditions associated with hiccup can be grouped into three main categories:

- physical causes within the anatomical distribution of the phrenic and vagus nerve
- neurological conditions thought to interfere with central control mechanisms
- metabolic/toxic and drug-induced causes: steroids in particular have been linked with the onset of hiccups and are thought to lower the threshold for synaptic transmission in the midbrain.[52]

Clinical management

It is important to consider the probable etiology (Box 70.1): removal of an underlying cause is more likely to be successful than medication. However, in most cases the cause is untreatable or cannot be found.

Box 70.1 Conditions associated with intractable hiccup

Physical causes within the anatomical distribution of the phrenic and vagus nerve

- Gastritis
- Gastric distension
- Bowel obstruction
- Gastroesophageal reflux
- Subphrenic and hepatic disease
- Foreign body in external auditory meatus
- Pleural effusion
- Lateral myocardial infarction
- Mediastinal disease
- Thoracic aortic aneurysm

Neurological conditions – structural or functional disorders of the brainstem

- Brainstem infarction
- Multiple sclerosis
- Brainstem tumors
- Tuberculoma
- Sarcoidosis

Metabolic/toxic and drug-induced

- Hyponatremia
- Uremia
- Hypocalcemia
- Addison disease
- Hypocapnia
- Alcohol
- Corticosteroids
- Midazolam

Treatment strategies

Hiccup often occurs in short episodes requiring no specific treatment. As with all symptoms an assessment of the extent and impact of the symptom on the patient and family should be documented to establish the benefit of any treatments. There are many 'traditional' remedies for hiccups which often involve some form of pharyngeal stimulation or diaphragmatic interruption/splinting:

- Cold key on the back of the neck
- Drinking water from the wrong side of a cup
- Sucking on a spoon of sugar
- Stimulation of the soft palate

These may be more effective for an acute bout of hiccups rather than the chronic, intractable form but may be tried as they are unlikely to cause any harm.

Phrenic nerve crush, cervical phrenic nerve block, and phrenic nerve stimulation have all been used to treat chronic hiccup in an attempt to disrupt the reflex arc. A number of papers have been published on the use of acupuncture and this is worth considering if drug side effects are intolerable.

Pharmacological management

Rare and self-limiting symptoms, such as hiccup, are particularly difficult to research and there are few published trials. Treatments discussed here (Table 70.1) are those for which there is a small amount of evidence, or those which have found their way into general use.

SECRETIONS

Salivary or bronchial secretions can be problematic either because of excessive production (e.g. bronchorrhea) or because of defective clearance (e.g. an ineffective cough or swallow reflex). The volume of bronchial secretions is partly under parasympathetic control: an increase in vagal activity increases the volume of secretions. However adrenergic nerves, cough receptor stimulation, and inflammatory changes also influence secretory output.

Rattle

Prospective studies of terminally ill cancer patients have reported the incidence of death rattle to be between 41 percent and 56 percent.[63–66] Rates in smaller observational studies vary widely.

PATHOPHYSIOLOGY

Noisy, rattly breathing is caused by an accumulation of secretions in a patient who is either weak or tired, has lost their cough and swallowing reflexes, is semi-conscious, unconscious or poorly positioned. The noise occurs when secretions bubble with respiration. It is has been postulated that there may be two types of rattle: type 1, a consequence of pooled salivary secretions that accumulate when the patient is close to death; and type 2, caused mainly by bronchial secretions when the patient has been deteriorating over a few days.[67] Among cancer patients it seems that

Table 70.1 *Drugs used for control of hiccup*

Drug	Evidence	Common side effects
Metoclopramide	Used with success in a case series of 14 patients with a variety of conditions[53*]	Few side effects and not sedative so reasonable to use first line
Haloperidol 3–5 mg nocte (oral or subcutaneous)	Licensed for use in intractable hiccup but evidence for efficacy in case reports only Commonly used in palliative care	Extrapyramidal side effects and sedation (usually at higher doses)
Chlorpromazine 25 mg tds (orally)	Licensed for use in intractable hiccup but scant evidence for efficacy	Hypotension and sedation
Baclofen 5 mg tds (orally), increasing each dose by 5 mg every 3 days until effective	A number of case series and an extremely small randomized controlled trial support its use[54–57*]	Sedation – particularly in renal failure
Gabapentin starting dose 100–300 mg tds	May be beneficial when central cause most likely (e.g., brainstem ischemia/inflammation) Reported to be effective in this situation in a number of case series[58–61*]	Drowsiness, dizziness and ataxia
Nifedipine 30–60 mg/day (orally)	4 patients in a series of 7 gained complete relief and the fifth felt improvement with nifedipine[62*]	Headache, vasodilation, peripheral edema

tds, three times daily.

cerebral tumors and malignant lung involvement predispose to death rattle.[64,67] It is possible that some cases of refractory rattle associated with cerebral tumors are due to neurogenic pulmonary edema. This is described in the literature in association with a variety of neurological conditions and is unresponsive to anticholinergic agents.[68]

MANAGEMENT STRATEGIES

Reassure patient and carers

Good terminal care often implies 'dying peacefully'. Controlling 'death rattle' can be an important component of this but is probably only effective about a third to a half of treated patients.[64,69] Making extreme efforts to control death rattle may not be necessary for patient comfort but it can be very distressing for relatives spending long periods of time at the patient's bedside. It is absolutely vital that time is spent giving explanation and reassurance to relatives, and it is important that nursing staff feel confident to do this.[70]

Positioning

Repositioning the patient to a lateral or more upright position to promote drainage of secretions is often recommended. In one study, nursing interventions such as repositioning and suction improved symptoms in 31 percent of patients.[65*]

Suctioning

This can be appropriate if secretions have accumulated in the pharynx and are easily reachable, but can cause significant distress in some patients.[66*] Assessment should be made on an individual basis according to the extent to which excessive secretions are preventing peace and dignity.

Pharmacological management

Pharmacological management involves reduction of salivary and bronchial secretions and dilatation of airways to allow a more laminar flow. Anticholinergic medications are more effective at reducing saliva secretion and dilating bronchial smooth muscle than reducing bronchial secretions.[67] They have no effect upon secretions which have already accumulated and are therefore more effective in preventing rattle if used early.

Clinical guidelines have been published giving guidance for doses of anticholinergic drugs (see Table 70.2) in death rattle based on one-off doses in healthy volunteers.[71] The choice of drug is less clear from the literature and therefore depends upon knowledge of the side effect profile, cost, and availability. All can cause dry mouth and urinary retention and those that cross the blood–brain barrier are more sedative and antiemetic. Although this can be beneficial they may also cause confusion and agitation, particularly in the elderly.

Bronchorrhea

Bronchorrhea is arbitrarily defined as the production of >100 mL of sputum per day. Excessive sputum production is seen in chronic, benign lung diseases such as bronchiectasis and chronic bronchitis. However, massive bronchorrhea, in which liters of clear frothy sputum are generated, is usually associated with malignancy, and can lead to severe fluid and electrolyte depletion in addition to respiratory distress. It is most commonly associated with bronchoalveolar carcinoma, but has been described in metastatic pancreatic, colonic and cervical adenocarcinoma.[72–74] The mechanism of massive

Table 70.2 *Anticholinergic drugs for death rattle*

	Cross blood–brain barrier[a]	Stat dose (SC)	Continuous SC infusion in 24 hours	Comments
Atropine	Yes	300–600 μg	1.2–2.4 mg	No evidence to support its use, but could be considered if no alternative available
Hyoscine hydrobromide	Yes	400 μg	1.2–2 mg	Available in transdermal patches in doses 0.5–1.5 mg for use over 24–72 hours, multiple patches can be used
Hyoscine butylbromide	No	20 mg	400 mg	Poor oral absorption
Glycopyrrolate	No	400 μg	1.2–2 mg	

[a] Sedation, antiemetic, confusion.
SC, subcutaneous.

MANAGEMENT

Bronchorrhea caused by an underlying malignancy will diminish if the tumor responds to therapy. Most cases, however, are due to bronchoalveolar carcinoma which is not very chemoresponsive.

There are a few case reports, in the literature, of the successful treatment of bronchorrhea using indometacin, erythromycin, and furosemide. However, in one randomized, placebo controlled trial, nebulized indometacin at a dose of 2 mL three times daily (1.2 μg/mL) was used to treat bronchorrhea associated with chronic bronchitis, diffuse panbronchiolitis, and bronchiectasis. Sputum production was significantly reduced and breathlessness improved.[75**] Subsequently nebulized indometacin has been reported to have been used successfully to treat bronchorrhea in two patients with bronchioalveolar carcinoma.[76]

Based on evidence that erythromycin inhibits bronchial hypersecretion *in vivo* and from epithelial cells *in vitro*, there are case reports of its successful use in benign and malignant causes of bronchorrhea.[77,78]

SUMMARY

Cough, hiccup, and respiratory secretions are common problems that cause great distress both to patients with advanced disease and to their families and carers. There are few effective evidence-based treatments available for these conditions at present, hence the wide variety of management strategies cited here.

The patient's aims and priorities must guide the treatments used and their prognosis and clinical state will impose limitations on the options available and appropriate. It is important that the patient (and family) understand that it may take time and several therapeutic interventions to improve symptom control and that treatment may involve pharmacological and nonpharmacological approaches.

There is an urgent need for a better evidence base on which to base our treatment decisions.

Key learning points

Cough

- Cough is common but generally not well palliated.

- It is important to decide: if there is a treatable underlying cause; if difficulty with expectoration is the main issue; and if there is associated pain and breathlessness.

- If no analgesia is required, the choice of antitussive depends upon drug availability and side effect profile.

- Some opioids have more antitussive activity than others and can be used in addition to a regular opioid analgesic.

Hiccup

- Establish site of underlying cause (central or peripheral) and treat if possible.

- Nonpharmacological remedies involving vagal or phrenic stimulation can be tried but may be of more use for acute rather than chronic hiccup.

- Metoclopramide is an appropriate first-line drug, particularly if gastric stasis or distension is implicated.

- More sedative drugs have a role, particularly if there is associated distress or insomnia.

- Consider gabapentin if a central cause is most likely.

Rattle

- Secretions can be salivary or bronchial in origin.
- Anticholinergic medications affect saliva production more than bronchial mucus production.
- Pharmacological management of rattle should be instituted early, before secretions have accumulated.
- Reassurance and support for relatives is vital.

REFERENCES

1 Harding SM. Chronic cough: practical considerations. *Chest* 2003; **123**: 659–60.

2 Muers MF, Round CE. Palliation of symptoms in non-small cell lung cancer: a study by the Yorkshire Regional Cancer Organisation Thoracic Group. *Thorax* 1993; **48**: 339–43.

3 Donnelly S, Walsh D. The symptoms of advanced cancer. *Semin Oncol* 1995; **22**: 67–72.

4 Donnelly S, Walsh D, Rybicki L. The symptoms of advanced cancer: identification of clinical and research priorities by assessment of prevalence and severity. *J Palliat Care* 1995; **11**: 27–32.

◆ 5 Irwin SI, Boulet L-P, Cloutier MM, *et al.* Managing cough as a defence mechanism and as a symptom: a consensus panel report of the American College of Chest Physicians. *Chest* 1998; **114**: S133–S181.

6 Lacourciere Y, Brunner H, Irwin R, *et al.* Effects of modulators of the renin-angiotensin-aldosterone system on cough. Losartan Cough Study Group. *J Hypertens* 1994; **12**: 1387–93.

7 Curley FJ, Irwin RS, Pratter MR, *et al.* Cough and the common cold. *Am Rev Respir Dis* 1988; **138**: 305–11.

8 Pratter MR, Bartter T, Akers S, DuBois J. An algorithmic approach to chronic cough. *Ann Intern Med* 1993; **119**: 977–83.

9 de Benedictis FM, Canny GJ, Levison H. Methacholine inhalational challenge in the evaluation of chronic cough in children. *J Asthma* 1986; **23**: 303–8.

10 A double-blind multicenter group comparative study of the efficacy and safety of nedocromil sodium in the management of asthma. North American Tilade Study Group. *Chest* 1990; **97**: 1299–306.

11 Spector SL, Tan RA. Effectiveness of montelukast in the treatment of cough variant asthma. *Ann Allergy Asthma Immunol* 2004; **93**: 232–6.

12 Cheriyan S, Greenberger PA, Patterson R. Outcome of cough variant asthma treated with inhaled steroids. *Ann Allergy* 1994; **73**: 478–80.

13 Sutton PP, Gemmell HG, Innes N, *et al.* Use of nebulised saline and nebulised terbutaline as an adjunct to chest physiotherapy. *Thorax* 1988; **43**: 57–60.

◆ 14 Harding SM, Richter JE. The role of gastroesophageal reflux in chronic cough and asthma. *Chest* 1997; **111**: 1389–402.

15 Abratt RP, Morgan GW, Silvestri G, Willcox P. Pulmonary complications of radiation therapy. *Clin Chest Med* 2004; **25**: 167–77.

16 Kudrik FJ, Rivera MP, Molina PL, *et al.* Hypersensitivity pneumonitis in advanced non-small-cell lung cancer patients receiving gemcitabine and paclitaxel: report of two cases and a review of the literature. *Clin Lung Cancer* 2002; **4**: 52–6.

17 Fassas A, Gojo I, Rapoport A, *et al.* Pulmonary toxicity syndrome following CDEP (cyclophosphamide, dexamethasone, etoposide, cisplatin) chemotherapy. *Bone Marrow Transplant* 2001; **28**: 399–403.

18 Langendijk JA, ten Velde GP, Aaronson NK, *et al.* Quality of life after palliative radiotherapy in non-small cell lung cancer: a prospective study. *Int J Radiat Oncol Biol Phys* 2000; **47**: 149–55.

19 Kramer GW, Gans S, Ullmann E, *et al.* Hypofractionated external beam radiotherapy as retreatment for symptomatic non-small-cell lung carcinoma: an effective treatment? *Int J Radiat Oncol Biol Phys* 2004; **58**: 1388–93.

20 Gressen EL, Werner-Wasik M, Cohn J, *et al.* Thoracic reirradiation for symptomatic relief after prior radiotherapeutic management for lung cancer. *Am J Clin Oncol* 2000; **23**: 160–3.

21 Gollins SW, Burt PA, Barber PV, Stout R. High dose rate intraluminal radiotherapy for carcinoma of the bronchus: outcome of treatment of 406 patients. *Radiother Oncol* 1994; **33**: 31–40.

22 Anderson H, Hopwood P, Stephens RJ, Thatcher N, *et al.* Gemcitabine plus best supportive care (BSC) vs BSC in inoperable non-small cell lung cancer – a randomized trial with quality of life as the primary outcome. UK NSCLC Gemcitabine Group. Non-Small Cell Lung Cancer. *Br J Cancer* 2000; **83**: 447–53.

23 Helsing M, Bergman B, Thaning L, Hero U. Quality of life and survival in patients with advanced non-small cell lung cancer receiving supportive care plus chemotherapy with carboplatin and etoposide or supportive care only. A multicentre randomised phase III trial. Joint Lung Cancer Study Group. *Eur J Cancer* 1998; **34**: 1036–44.

24 Freitag L, Tekolf E, Steveling H, *et al.* Management of malignant esophagotracheal fistulas with airway stenting and double stenting. *Chest* 1996; **110**: 1155–60.

25 Witt C, Dinges S, Schmidt B, *et al.* Temporary tracheobronchial stenting in malignant stenoses. *Eur J Cancer* 1997; **33**: 204–8.

26 Wood DE, Liu YH, Vallieres E, *et al.* Airway stenting for malignant and benign tracheobronchial stenosis. *Ann Thorac Surg* 2003; **76**: 167–72.

27 Shim C, King M, Williams MH, Jr. Lack of effect of hydration on sputum production in chronic bronchitis. *Chest* 1987; **92**: 679–82.

28 King M, Rubin BK. Pharmacological approaches to discovery and development of new mucolytic agents. *Adv Drug Deliv Rev* 2002; **54**: 1475–90.

29 Robinson M, Hemming AL, Regnis JA, *et al.* Effect of increasing doses of hypertonic saline on mucociliary clearance in patients with cystic fibrosis. *Thorax* 1997; **52**: 900–3.

30 Parvez L, Vaidya M, Sakhardande A, *et al.* Evaluation of antitussive agents in man. *Pulm Pharmacol* 1996; **9**: 299–308.

31 Dicpinigaitis PV, Gayle YE. Effect of guaifenesin on cough reflex sensitivity. *Chest* 2003; **124**: 2178–81.

32 Rubin BK. The pharmacologic approach to airway clearance: mucoactive agents. *Respir Care* 2002; **47**: 818–22.

◆ 33 Poole PJ, Black PN. Oral mucolytic drugs for exacerbations of chronic obstructive pulmonary disease: systematic review. *BMJ* 2001; **322**: 1271–4.

34 Ziment I. Herbal antitussives. *Pulm Pharmacol Ther* 2002; **15**: 327–33.

35 Bolser DC. Mechanisms of action of central and peripheral antitussive drugs. *Pulm Pharmacol* 1996; **9**: 357–64.

36 Zylicz Z, Krajnik M. What has dry cough in common with pruritus? Treatment of dry cough with paroxetine. *J Pain Symptom Manage* 2004; **27**: 180–4.

37 Moroni M, Porta C, Gualtieri G, *et al.* Inhaled sodium cromoglycate to treat cough in advanced lung cancer patients. *Br J Cancer* 1996; **74**: 309–11.

38 Doona M, Walsh D. Benzonatate for opioid-resistant cough in advanced cancer. *Palliat Med* 1998; **12**: 55–8.

39 Eddy NB, Friebel H, Hahn KJ, Halbach H. Codeine and its alternates for pain and cough relief. 4. Potential alternates for cough relief. *Bull World Health Organ* 1969; **40**: 639–719.

40 Homsi J, Walsh D, Nelson KA, *et al.* A phase II study of hydro-codone for cough in advanced cancer. *Am J Hosp Palliat Care* 2002; **19**: 49–56.

41 Matthys H, Bleicher B, Bleicher U. Dextromethorphan and codeine: objective assessment of antitussive activity in patients with chronic cough. *J Int Med Res* 1983; **11**: 92–100.

42 Ida H. The nonnarcotic antitussive drug dimemorfan: a review. *Clin Ther* 1997; **19**: 215–31.

43 Luporini G, Barni S, Marchi E, Daffonchio L. Efficacy and safety of levodropropizine and dihydrocodeine on nonproductive cough in primary and metastatic lung cancer. *Eur Respir J* 1998; **12**: 97–101.

44 Catena E, Daffonchio L. Efficacy and tolerability of levo-dropropizine in adult patients with non-productive cough. Comparison with dextromethorphan. *Pulm Pharmacol Ther* 1997; **10**: 89–96.

45 Aversa C, Cazzola M, Clini V, *et al.* Clinical trial of the efficacy and safety of moguisteine in patients with cough associated with chronic respiratory diseases. *Drugs Exp Clin Res* 1993; **19**: 273–9.

46 Barnabe R, Berni F, Clini V, *et al.* The efficacy and safety of moguisteine in comparison with codeine phosphate in patients with chronic cough. *Monaldi Arch Chest Dis* 1995; **50**: 93–7.

47 Gastpar H, Criscuolo D, Dieterich HA. Efficacy and tolerability of glaucine as an antitussive agent. *Curr Med Res Opin* 1984; **9**: 21–7.

48 Howard P, Cayton RM, Brennan SR, Anderson PB. Lignocaine aerosol and persistent cough. *Br J Dis Chest* 1977; **71**: 19–24.

49 Kamei J. Role of opioidergic and serotonergic mechanisms in cough and antitussives. *Pulm Pharmacol* 1996; **9**: 349–56.

50 Eccles R. The powerful placebo in cough studies? *Pulm Pharmacol Ther* 2002; **15**: 303–8.

51 Orr CF, Rowe DB. *Helicobacter pylori* hiccup. *Intern Med J* 2003; **33**: 133–4.

52 Dickerman RD, Jaikumar S. The hiccup reflex arc and persistent hiccups with high-dose anabolic steroids: is the brainstem the steroid-responsive locus? *Clin Neuropharmacol* 2001; **24**: 62–4.

53 Madanagopolan N. Metoclopramide in hiccup. *Curr Med Res Opin* 1975; **3**: 371–4.

54 Walker P, Watanabe S, Bruera E. Baclofen, a treatment for chronic hiccup. *J Pain Symptom Manage* 1998; **16**: 125–32.

55 Petroianu G, Hein G, Petroianu A, *et al.* Idiopathic chronic hiccup: combination therapy with cisapride, omeprazole, and baclofen. *Clin Ther* 1997; **19**: 1031–8.

56 Guelaud C, Similowski T, Bizec JL, *et al.* Baclofen therapy for chronic hiccup. *Eur Respir J* 1995; **8**: 235–7.

57 Ramirez FC, Graham DY. Treatment of intractable hiccup with baclofen: results of a double-blind randomized, controlled, cross-over study. *Am J Gastroenterol* 1992; **87**: 1789–91.

58 Hernandez JL, Pajaron M, Garcia-Regata O, *et al.* Gabapentin for intractable hiccup. *Am J Med* 2004; **117**: 279–81.

59 Moretti R, Torre P, Antonello RM, *et al.* Gabapentin as a drug therapy of intractable hiccup because of vascular lesion: a three-year follow up. *Neurologist* 2004; **10**: 102–6.

60 Porzio G, Aielli F, Narducci F, *et al.* Hiccup in patients with advanced cancer successfully treated with gabapentin: report of three cases. *N Z Med J* 2003; **116**: U605.

61 Petroianu G, Hein G, Stegmeier-Petroianu A, *et al.* Gabapentin 'add-on therapy' for idiopathic chronic hiccup (ICH). *J Clin Gastroenterol* 2000; **30**: 321–4.

62 Lipps DC, Jabbari B, Mitchell MH, Daigh JD, Jr. Nifedipine for intractable hiccups. *Neurology* 1990; **40**: 531–2.

63 Back IN, Jenkins K, Blower A, Beckhelling J. A study comparing hyoscine hydrobromide and glycopyrrolate in the treatment of death rattle. *Palliat Med* 2001; **15**: 329–36.

64 Morita T, Tsunoda J, Inoue S, Chihara S. Risk factors for death rattle in terminally ill cancer patients: a prospective exploratory study. *Palliat Med* 2000; **14**: 19–23.

65 Lichter I, Hunt E. The last 48 hours of life. *J Palliat Care* 1990; **6**: 7–15.

66 Morita T, Hyodo I, Yoshimi T, *et al.* Incidence and underlying etiologies of bronchial secretion in terminally ill cancer patients: a multicenter, prospective, observational study. *J Pain Symptom Manage* 2004; **27**: 533–9.

67 Bennett MI. Death rattle: an audit of hyoscine (scopamine) use and review of management. *J Pain Symptom Manage* 1996; **12**: 229–33.

68 Macleod AD. Neurogenic pulmonary edema in palliative care. *J Pain Symptom Manage* 2002; **23**: 154–6.

● 69 Hughes A, Wilcock A, Corcoran R, *et al.* Audit of three anti-muscarinic drugs for managing retained secretions. *Palliat Med* 2000; **14**: 221–2.

70 Watts T, Jenkins K. Palliative care nurses' feelings about death rattle. *J Clin Nurs* 1999; **8**: 615–16.

✳ 71 Bennett M, Lucas V, Brennan M, *et al.* Using anti-muscarinic drugs in the management of death rattle: evidence-based guidelines for palliative care. *Palliat Med* 2002; **16**: 369–74.

72 Lembo T, Donnelly TJ. A case of pancreatic carcinoma causing massive bronchial fluid production and electrolyte abnormalities. *Chest* 1995; **108**: 1161–3.

73 Shimura S, Takishima T. Bronchorrhea from diffuse lymphangitic metastasis of colon carcinoma to the lung. *Chest* 1994; **105**: 308–10.

74 Epaulard O, Moro D, Langin T, *et al.* Bronchorrhea revealing cervix adenocarcinoma metastatic to the lung. *Lung Cancer* 2001; **3131**: 331–4.

75 Tamaoki J, Chiyotani A, Kobayashi K, *et al.* Effect of indomethacin on bronchorrhea in patients with chronic bronchitis, diffuse panbronchiolitis, or bronchiectasis. *Am Rev Respir Dis* 1992; **145**: 548–52.

76 Homma S, Kawabata M, Kishi K, *et al.* Successful treatment of refractory bronchorrhea by inhaled indomethacin in two patients with bronchioloalveolar carcinoma. *Chest* 1999; **115**: 1465–8.

77 Suga T, Sugiyama Y, Fujii T, Kitamura S. Bronchioloalveolar carcinoma with bronchorrhoea treated with erythromycin. *Eur Respir J* 1994; **7**: 2249–51.

78 Marom ZM, Goswami SK. Respiratory mucus hypersecretion (bronchorrhea): a case discussion – possible mechanisms(s) and treatment. *J Allergy Clin Immunol* 1991; **87**: 1050–5.

PART 12

Neuropsychiatric

71

Depression/anxiety

MICHAEL J FISCH

INTRODUCTION

The length and quality of life of patients with serious chronic illnesses such as cancer are influenced not only by their malignant disease but also by comorbid medical and psychological conditions, such as depression. The complexity of care for these patients makes it particularly challenging to ascertain whether a patient is struggling with serious depression. Moreover, compared with the statistics on the overall population of general medical patients, there are fewer data to draw upon that would help clinicians determine what treatments are effective for depression in the advanced cancer or other advanced disease settings. This chapter will examine the assessment and treatment of depression in general medical patients and in patients with cancer. Cancer will be used as a paradigm for a serious chronic illness that benefits from good palliative care, and from which available data could be generalized to many other serious chronic diseases. Some of the unique aspects of managing depression in the end-of-life setting will be examined, and the diagnosis and management of anxiety will be distinguished from depression as well.

PREVALENCE, EFFECT, AND ASSESSMENT OF DEPRESSION

General medical patients

To better understand how to recognize and treat depression in patients with cancer, it is useful to first review the existing paradigms for finding and treating depression in the primary care setting. Depression is estimated to affect more than 120 million people worldwide.[1] Large prospective studies have shown that the prevalence of major depression in the outpatient primary care setting is 6–14 percent, and the lifetime incidence of major depression is approximately 15 percent.[2**] The point prevalence of depression in preadolescent children is in the 1–3 percent range, and it is about three times higher in adolescents.[3] Depression is two to three times more common in hospitalized patients and patients with chronic illnesses.[4] Physicians recognize psychological distress in about two-thirds of the general medical patient population and prescribe antidepressants for about half of those distressed patients.[2] Major depressive disorder can cause severe functional impairment and increase the risk of suicide.[5**] Depressive symptoms are associated with a higher-than-normal risk of physical decline and with long-term mortality in older adults;[6*,7*,8*,9*] depression is also a risk factor for coronary heart disease and stroke,[10,11] and it is associated with greater use of healthcare services.[12,13]

The standard paradigm for identifying depression in the primary care setting is to view depression as a syndromal diagnosis made on the basis of patient history and the exclusion of competing diagnoses, using criteria from the Diagnostic and Statistical Manual of Mental Disorders (DSM)-IV.[14] Major depression is defined as depressed mood or anhedonia (loss of interest in pleasurable activities) that lasts for at least 2 weeks plus the presence of three or four other specific psychological or somatic symptoms. If two to four rather than more than five symptoms are present, then the patient may be defined as having minor depression, an unofficial research diagnosis in the DSM-IV.[15] A recent review of case-finding instruments used in primary care showed that at least 11 questionnaires, ranging in length from 1 to 30 questions and ranging in time of administration from 1 to 5 minutes, show reasonable performance characteristics when compared with a semi-structured interview applying standard diagnostic criteria.[15] The US Preventive Services Task Force recommends depression screening in clinical practices that have systems in place to ensure accurate diagnosis and effective treatment and follow-up.[16] Unfortunately, such systems are not available in most primary care practices or oncology/hematology subspecialty practices.

The decision regarding whether to treat a patient for depression in the primary care setting is not always made on the basis of rigid diagnostic criteria; it often arises from clinical judgment about the severity and duration of symptoms and the likelihood of spontaneous recovery within a supportive environment.[17] Between 50 percent and 60 percent of cases of major depression respond to initial therapy with antidepressants, psychotherapy, or both.[17***] Minor depression and dysthymia have similar response rates to antidepressants or psychotherapy over placebo.[18] Depression may be treated by a patient's primary care physician, who can use either a collaborative care model that involves augmentation with one or more visits with a mental healthcare provider or a stepped-care approach in which patients whose depression does not respond to initial therapy are referred to a mental healthcare provider.[4] Physicians and patients show considerable variability in how they think depression should be treated. This variability arises from not only physician, patient, and spouse or caregiver preferences but also health system variables, such as the availability of mental healthcare providers and reimbursement for mental healthcare.[4] Unfortunately, the vast majority of depressed patients who receive antidepressants are not prescribed an adequate dose for a long enough time.[2] Likewise, the duration of psychotherapy is often too brief; effective therapy requires 6–16 visits.[17*] These data underscore the basis of the US Preventive Services Task Force emphasis on having appropriate systems in place so that patients who have depression detected by screening achieve the best possible outcomes.

Depression is associated with significant morbidity, and the estimated economic impact of depression in the USA alone is more than US$40 billion annually.[19*] Fortunately, depression is treatable, and thus cost effective interventions to improve the detection and treatment of depression are important. A randomized trial to determine the cost effectiveness of a specific quality improvement program in 46 primary care clinics and six community-based managed care organizations found that the cost per quality-adjusted life year (QALY) associated with the specific quality improvement program was US$15 000–35 000, comparable with that of other accepted medical interventions.[20] Moreover, employment retention for depressed patients improved over a 1-year period without an overall increase in medical visits.[21]

Cancer: a paradigm for serious chronic illness

In a comprehensive, evidence-based review of the literature of depression in cancer, Pirl[22] reported that despite standardized criteria for diagnosing major depressive disorder in cancer patients, it remains difficult to draw firm conclusions about the prevalence of major depression in this population because of the wide range of reported rates. There were 11 cross-sectional studies of major depression in cancer published between 1983 and 2000, drawing upon nearly 2000 patients.[23–33] The best estimate is that major depression has a point prevalence of 10–25 percent in cancer patients. This prevalence is similar to that seen in patients with other chronic medical illnesses, such as diabetes and heart disease, and slightly lower than that observed for patients with debilitating chronic neurological diseases, such as multiple sclerosis or Parkinson disease.[1]

Although some comprehensive cancer centers have adequate behavioral healthcare resources, most hospitals and oncology clinics rely on general psychiatry and psychology staff and resources. Limited funding for mental healthcare resources is a serious problem, and care is often fragmented among private practitioners, for-profit and not-for-profit clinics, and community mental health centers.[34*] Limited resources in standard areas of care also affect the research environment.

Even though it may be ideal to use a two-stage strategy that combines an assessment of severity with an assessment of the number of depressive symptoms, it is far more common to perform only a short instrument to assess symptom severity in the typical environment where time and resources are limited. Numerous symptom scales have been used to assess depression symptom severity at a specific time or over time. The most commonly reported instruments are shown in Box 71.1.

Box 71.1 Self-report measures used to assess depressive symptoms in cancer patients

- Hospital and Anxiety Depression Scale (HADS)
- Zung Self-Rating Depression Scale (ZSRDS)
- Brief version, Zung Self-Rating Depression Scale (BZSDRS)
- Beck Depression Inventory (BDI)
- Beck Depression Inventory, Short Form (BDI-SF)
- Center for Epidemiologic Studies Depression Scale (CES-D)
- Brief Symptom Inventory (BSI)
- Rotterdam Symptom Checklist (RSCL)
- Geriatric Depression Scale (GDS)
- Profile of Mood States (POMS)
- General Health Questionnaire (GHQ)

The instrument that has been investigated most extensively is the HADS. Since its original publication in 1983 by

Zigmond and Snaith,[35] this instrument has been translated into more than 20 languages and has become one of the most often cited articles in the medical literature. There have been no fewer than 14 published studies of cancer patients assessed with the HADS since 1989, and six of those studies included more than 200 patients each. One of the largest validation studies of the HADS included 514 patients from four sites and found that, using the DSM-III, as the reference standard, the HADS had a sensitivity of 80 percent, a specificity of 76 percent, and a positive predictive value of 41 percent in outpatients with various cancers.[36] In a large primary care population, the HADS had a positive likelihood ratio of 7.0 (95 percent CI 2.9 to 11.2) and a negative likelihood ratio of 0.3 (95 percent CI 0.3 to 0.4).[37] When symptom scales are used, the prevalence of depression is usually found to be in the 15–35 percent range, which is slightly higher than the prevalence of major depression assessed by a diagnostic interview.

Challenges in the assessment of depression in cancer patients

Patients, family members, and healthcare providers sometimes believe that feeling down, depressed, or hopeless is perfectly natural and understandable in the context of living with cancer. Clinicians are encouraged to acknowledge the difficulty and disappointment that often confront cancer patients and their families,[38] but depression and hopelessness are not accepted by expert clinicians as an inevitable consequence of living with cancer. In addition, cancer patients often have physical symptoms of depression (so-called neurovegetative symptoms), such as sleep disturbance, psychomotor retardation, appetite disturbance, poor concentration, and low energy, as a consequence of their underlying illness or treatment, thus confounding the diagnosis of depression. Indeed, depression is just one of many symptoms that clinicians must recognize and manage in inpatients and outpatients with cancer. For example, roughly two-thirds of outpatients with cancer experience pain, and more than a third report significant disruption in daily function associated with the pain.[39**] For patients with advanced cancer, the median number of symptoms (e.g. pain, trouble sleeping, fatigue, and anhedonia) expressed by self-report is generally five or more.[40*,41*,42*] It may be that the problem of concurrent symptoms is the most relevant difference between depression in the general medical setting and in the cancer care setting. Relatively few cancer care providers have sufficient knowledge and skill to assess and treat depression in this context, and it is often difficult to decide whether the depressive symptoms should be the primary focus of treatment or whether these symptoms may improve if other problems are better managed. Clinicians sometimes use verbal or nonverbal cues to focus on symptoms for which they have a broader comfort zone for assessing and treating. Currently, many cancer providers

are most comfortable treating somatic symptoms, such as pain, nausea, constipation, or dyspnea.

The large number of instruments and techniques used to assess cancer patients for depression does not seem to translate into an overall improvement in the assessment of depression in this complex population of patients. A 'Don't ask, don't tell' policy appears to be in place all too often.[34] A list of nine of the most significant barriers to the assessment of depression is presented in Box 71.2. With a growing appreciation for the need to simplify the starting point in assessing depression, the use of 1- or 2-item screening techniques has become popular (Box 71.3). Chochinov et al.[43] have studied a simple 1-item survey and found it to have acceptable psychometric properties in patients with advanced cancer. Akizuki et al.[44] have described a clever 1-item survey that was tested in 275 patients and was found to correlate well with both the HADS ($r = 0.66$) and the Distress Thermometer ($r = 0.71$). At optimal cutoffs, the sensitivity (80 percent) and specificity (61 percent) for diagnosing major depression and adjustment disorders for this 1-item survey were similar to those of the HADS and Distress Thermometer. Finally, Whooley and colleagues[45] have used 2-item screening in medically ill patients who did not have cancer with an approach that targeted depressed mood and anhedonia. This 2-item screening approach has been endorsed by the US Preventive Health Task Force for use in primary care settings.[16,46] Once again, this simple approach appears to be about as effective as the more complex instruments for decision-making purposes,

---

Box 71.2 Common barriers to the assessment of depression in patients with cancer

- Time constraints in busy oncology settings

- Cost constraints limiting access to professionals with behavioral health training

- Overlap of physical symptoms of depression and symptoms of cancer or its treatment

- Stigma concerning mental illness or weakness perceived by the patient/family

- Patient/family fear that revealing depression will lead to undertreatment of the cancer

- Clinician underrecognition of hopelessness, feelings of worthlessness, or suicidal ideation

- Clinician uncertainty about how to interpret screening instrument cut-offs

- Poor continuity of care over the trajectory of illness

- Limited understanding by cancer professionals regarding which patients are most at risk

---

Box 71.3 Examples of 1- or 2-question screening methods for depression

One question

- 'Are you depressed?' (Chochinov et al.[43])

- 'Please grade your mood during the past week by assigning it a score from 0 to 100, with a score of 100 representing your usual relaxed mood. A score of 60 is considered a passing grade.' (Akizuki et al.[44])

Two questions

- 'Have you often been bothered by feeling down, depressed, or hopeless?'

- 'Have you often been bothered by having a lack of interest or pleasure in doing things?' (Whooley et al.[45])

---

and this 2-item screening approach has also been used in cancer patients.[47*]

In addition to brief screening approaches specific to depression, a more global approach to distress screening has been developed by Holland[48,49] and endorsed by the National Comprehensive Cancer Network. This approach involves a thermometer with a numerical scale ranging from 0 to 10 for the patient to indicate 'How much distress you have been experiencing in the past week, including today?' This is coupled with a 34-item checklist organized into practical areas, family issues, emotional issues, spiritual/religious issues, and physical symptoms. This approach embeds depression screening in a broad context that can be less stigmatizing to some patients. The drawback of this approach is that it is not easy to use in face-to-face discussions between the physician and patient. Rather, it is well suited to a practice setting in which other providers are available to do the screening and initiate an appropriate response to the patient on the basis of the information provided. In general, the distress screening approach works best in a resource-rich environment. In the USA, support for psychosocial services is expected to be hindered even more by reduced payments for oncology care through the Medicare Prescription Drug, Improvement, and Modernization Act of 2003.

TREATMENT OF DEPRESSION

General medical patients

Antidepressant therapy and psychotherapy seem to be equally effective for treating mild-to-moderate depression in the general medical population.[4,50*] For treating severe depression, antidepressant therapy combined with psychotherapy may be better than psychotherapy alone.[51**] Antidepressants are also effective for treating depression in patients with concomitant physical illnesses. In 1998, a systematic review of randomized trials comparing antidepressants with placebo to treat depression in physically ill patients was published; the review comprised 18 studies including more than 800 patients with a variety of chronic diseases.[52***] Depression treated with antidepressants was significantly more likely to improve than that treated with placebo (odds ratio = 0.37; 95 percent CI 0.27 to 0.51). However, the study also showed that approximately four patients would need to be treated to produce one recovery that would not have occurred with placebo alone (number needed to treat = 4.2; 95 percent CI 3.2 to 6.4). Approximately 10 cases of depression needed to be treated with antidepressants to cause one treatment dropout relative to placebo.[52***]

Interestingly, the response rates to both antidepressants and placebo are substantial, having increased considerably over the past 20 years.[53*] This may reflect a 'stage migration' effect, wherein the study cohorts at inception have tended to have less severe depressive symptoms over time. Evidence suggests that severe depression is less likely than mild or moderate depression to respond to placebo.[54,55] Of note, the widely used herbal remedy St John's wort (*Hypericum perforatum*) has not been found to be effective compared with placebo for treating moderately severe depression.[56]

More than 24 antidepressants that work by at least seven distinct mechanisms of action are available.[57] However, no single drug or category of drugs has proved most effective for relieving depressive symptoms or treating the syndrome of major depression (see Box 71.4 for summary of antidepressant agents).[17,58] In the USA, many adults take medications to improve their health and wellbeing; in any given week, most American adults take at least one medication, and 7 percent take five or more.[59] This growing affinity for taking medication also is manifested in a national trend in the outpatient treatment of depression. Specifically, the proportion of depressed patients receiving antidepressant medications nearly doubled between 1987 and 1997 (from 37.3 percent to 74.5 percent), whereas the proportion of depressed patients receiving psychotherapy declined (71.1 percent to 60.2 percent).[60*]

Cancer patients

CHOOSING PATIENTS FOR TREATMENT

The largest barrier to the effective treatment of depression in patients with cancer is the difficulty recognizing which patients are depressed and need treatment. The factors associated with increased risk of depression in cancer patients are shown in Box 71.5. Because of the complexity of assessing patients in modern cancer care environments, many cases of depression are missed, and the patients with more severe

Box 71.4 Commonly used antidepressants grouped by mechanism of action

Selective serotonin reuptake inhibitors (SSRIs)

- Fluoxetine
- Paroxetine
- Sertraline *Zoloft also panic disorder*
- Citalopram
- Escitalopram

Comment: These agents have few anticholinergic or cardiovascular side effects, and they are not fatal in overdose. Sexual dysfunction, insomnia, headache, or nausea may occur with any of these agents.

SSRI and presynaptic α_2-receptor antagonist

- Mirtazapine

Comment: This agent may cause sedation and weight gain. For this reason, it can be dosed at night to improve sleep and given to patients who have poor appetite. It can cause constipation, edema, hypertension, or orthostatic hypotension.

SSRI and norepinephrine reuptake inhibitor

- Venlafaxine *Effexor*

Comment: In addition to its effect on depression, this agent has been used to decrease the frequency and intensity of hot flashes in cancer patients. Dose-related sustained hypertension is an important possible side effect to monitor. May cause sexual dysfunction, insomnia, headache, constipation, or nausea.

Dopamine and norepinephrine reuptake inhibitor

- Bupropion

Comment: This agent is also indicated to improve rates of successful smoking cessation. Sometimes used to avoid the sexual dysfunction seen with other agents. Does not treat anxiety. Known to lower the seizure threshold. May cause insomnia, agitation, confusion, headache, or weight loss.

Psychostimulants

- Methylphenidate
- Dextroamphetamine

Comment: These agents are known for the rapid onset of action in terms of antidepressant efficacy. They are activating agents also used to counteract opioid-induced sedation. Generally given in the waking hours (morning and early afternoon). Should be avoided in patients with unstable ischemia or cardiac arrhythmias. Drug tolerance, abuse, and dependence can occur. May cause nervousness, agitation, or insomnia.

Tricyclic antidepressants

- Nortriptyline
- Amitriptyline
- Doxepin
- Desipramine

Comment: These agents can cause cardiac arrhythmias, and overdoses are lethal. Baseline electrocardiography is recommended. Often used as adjuvant analgesics at doses subtherapeutic for depression. May cause sexual dysfunction, weight gain, anticholinergic effects (dry mouth, sedation, or constipation), or orthostatic hypotension.

symptoms, ironically, are more easily overlooked. Investigators in Indiana, USA, working in the community setting[61] evaluated 1109 outpatients with cancer and found that physicians were most accurate at correctly identifying the absence of depression. However, when depression was severe, only 13 percent of affected patients were correctly classified by their oncologists. In general, oncologists and oncology nurses appear to be most responsive to sad, tearful patients with minor depression rather than patients with a flat affect, feelings of pervasive guilt or worthlessness, or suicidal thoughts. In a sense, sicker patients may create thicker smokescreens that impede easy recognition of the underlying problem. These patients are particularly vulnerable, and their inability to advocate for themselves may be part of the illness.[34]

Box 71.5 Risk factors for depression in cancer

Social factors

- Recent losses
- Financial stressors
- Poor social support
- Sexual and/or physical abuse
- Childhood trauma or parental loss
- History of substance abuse

Genetic factors

- Family history of depressive disorder

Cancer-related factors

- Advanced stage of disease
- Poor performance status
- Poor pain control
- Pancreatic cancer

Cancer treatment factors

- Corticosteroids
- Interferon alfa
- Interleukin-2
- Amphotericin-B
- Procarbazine
- L-Asparaginase

Symptom research is an emerging interest within the discipline of academic general medicine.[61–63] Within this new paradigm, symptoms are conceptualized in terms of a functional disturbance of the nervous system. There is a growing appreciation for the physical changes in the nervous system associated with depression and its treatment.[64,65] Understanding depressive symptoms in the context of symptom science rather than solely within the standard psychiatric paradigm is being explored in the context of cancer care to try to overcome some of the barriers to recognition and management of depression in this population.

TREATMENT OPTIONS

Drugs used to treat depression in cancer patients are quite similar to those used in the primary care setting; these include tricyclic antidepressants, SSRIs, newer antidepressants, and psychostimulants. Specific examples of commonly used antidepressants grouped by mechanism of action are presented in Box 71.4. The National Institutes of Health consensus statement regarding symptom management in cancer states that 'depression related to cancer is not substantially different from depression in other medical conditions, but treatments may need to be adapted or refined for cancer patients'.[66] One refinement for patients with cancer, particularly in the palliative care setting, is the growing interest in the use of psychostimulants to treat depression.[67*,68*,69*,70*] This interest is driven by the potential of these agents to rapidly produce clinical effects and to alleviate concomitant symptoms, such as fatigue, sedation, and poor concentration. Another refinement that is often important to cancer patients is being mindful of potentially important drug interactions that can occur with antidepressants that are metabolized using the cytochrome P450 (CYP) enzyme system of the liver. In particular, agents such as fluoxetine and nefazodone that inhibit the CYP 3A4 enzyme system may increase the effects of some commonly used chemotherapeutic agents. Moreover, because many patients with cancer are older adults with complex medical problems, other coadministered drugs may be influenced by the antidepressants. Although the clinical relevance of these potential interactions is not well described or understood, it is useful for clinicians to be aware of this issue. Selected CYP interaction possibilities are summarized in Table 71.1.

Psychological therapies include psychoeducational interventions, cognitive behavioral therapy, interpersonal therapy, and problem-solving therapy. Although these therapies are often used to treat depression in patients with cancer, there is a barrier to their use: the sheer complexity of patient care (multiple providers, laboratory and radiographic tests, and scheduled treatments such as radiation or infusions) makes scheduling psychological interventions difficult. Electroconvulsive therapy, an invasive modality known to be effective for severe depression, is rarely used and has not been studied for depression in the context of cancer care.

Difficult issues in designing interventions for cancer-related depression include identifying an acceptable standard for depression treatment in cancer, choosing an appropriate duration of therapy, and finding a feasible strategy to assess compliance with the intervention. In addition, assessment of outcomes is particularly challenging because the researcher must choose feasible numbers and types of outcome measures and decide the importance of depression-specific outcomes relative to secondary outcomes, such as quality of life. Other difficulties in researching depression in cancer patients include the lack of a standard primary endpoint; the high frequency of missing data; the clash of expectations and paradigms inherent to interdisciplinary review of depression

Table 71.1 *Selected cytochrome P450 drug interactions*

Agents	2C9	2C19	2D6	3A4
Substrates	Fluoxetine	Tricyclic antidepressants	Tricyclic antidepressants	Benzodiazepines
	Celecoxib	Benzodiazepines	Venlafaxine	Theophylline
	Warfarin		Fluoxetine	Methadone
	Trimethoprim/sulfameth		Haloperidol	Cyclosporine
	Oxazole		Phenothiazines	Tacrolimus
	Cyclophosphamide		Oxycodone	Tamoxifen
			Hydrocodone	Etoposide
			β Blockers	Vinca alkaloids
			Ondansetron	Paclitaxel
			Tamoxifen	Gefinitib
				Imatinib
				Calcium channel blockers
Inhibitors	Paroxetine	Fluoxetine	Fluoxetine	Nefazodone
	Sertraline	Paroxetine	Paroxetine	Fluoxetine
	Fluconazole	Omeprazole	Sertraline	Quinolones
	Amiodarone		Methadone	Macrolide antibiotics
			Doxorubicin	Ketoconazole
			Vinblastine	Amiodarone
				Grapefruit juice
				HIV protease inhibitors
Inducers		Corticosteroids		St John's wort
				Barbiturates
				Phenytoin
				Corticosteroids
				Rifampin

Note: This table highlights some of the most serious known P450 drug interactions. Appropriate, updated reference material should be consulted to establish the presence or absence of important P450 interactions before prescribing.

research proposals; the shortage of patient access to behavioral health specialists; and the relative aversion of patients, family members, and some healthcare providers to placebo controlled study designs.

RANDOMIZED TRIALS

With all of these challenges in mind, it is not surprising that data from controlled trials regarding the efficacy of treatment of depression in cancer patients is sparse. Only eight published placebo controlled randomized trials have compared an antidepressant drug (a tricyclic antidepressant or serotonin reuptake inhibitor) with a placebo in cancer patients (Table 71.2). Fewer than 1000 patients were included; none of these studies included children, and three of the studies[71**,72**,73**] included women only. The trend in these studies was in favor of the treatment arm, but the small sample size of the individual trials, short follow-up duration, and heterogeneity of outcome measures limit the conclusions that can be made from this body of research.

The handful of other randomized, controlled trials involving patients with cancer and assessment of depression outcomes are equally difficult to interpret. Three randomized,

placebo controlled trials assessed depression outcomes but studied drugs (methylprednisolone, thioridazine, and mazindol) that are not typically used to treat depression.[78**,79**,80**] These studies included a total of 116 patients. There are also three published double-blind, randomized trials comparing two interventions without a placebo control.[81–83] These trials compared alprazolam versus muscle relaxation,[81] fluoxetine versus desipramine,[82] and trazadone versus clorazepate[83] in a total of 211 patients. Overall, research related to drug therapy for depression in patients with cancer spans 30 years. Unfortunately, these studies include a myriad of different endpoints, and most of the trials had small sample sizes and short durations of follow-up. The trend in these trials suggested that antidepressants alleviate depression in cancer patients much as in other medically ill patients. Further research is needed to better define the magnitude and duration of the treatment effect and to improve the precision of the estimate of this effect. In addition, the toxicities and costs of drug therapy for cancer patients who have depressive symptoms have not been adequately studied.

Psychological therapies are most often applied in addition to drug treatments for depressed patients, but this kind of

Table 71.2 *Clinical trials comparing antidepressant with placebo in patients with cancer*

Author(s)	Intervention (No. of subjects)	Patient description	Inclusion criteria for depression	Outcome measures	Measures improved compared with placebo
Purohit et al., 1978[74]	Imipramine (39)	Hospitalized patients receiving radiation therapy	Not stated	HDRS	No statistical evaluation
Costa et al., 1985[73]	Mianserin (73)	Adult women with cancer	Major depression: HDRS ⩾ 16 ZSDRS ⩾ 41	CGI, HDRS, ZSDRS	CGI (77% vs. 50%), HDRS at days 7, 21, and 28, ZSDRS at days 7 and 28
Eija et al., 1996[72]	Amitriptyline (15)	Patients with breast cancer and neuropathic pain	None	2 questions about depression on a 4-point scale	No statistical evaluation
Van Heeringen and Zivkov, 1996[71]	Mianserin (55)	Adult women with early-stage breast cancer treated with radiation	DSM-III depressive disorder	HDRS	HDRS at 4 weeks and 7 weeks
Razavi et al., 1996[75]	Fluoxetine (91)	Adults with depression or adjustment disorder in relation to cancer	DSM-III depression or adjustment disorder, HADS ⩾ 13	HADS, MADRS, SCL-90-R, HAS, SQOLI	SCL-90-R at 5 weeks
Musselman et al., 2001[76]	Paroxetine (40)	Adults beginning high-dose interferon alpha for melanoma	None	HDRS, HAS, DSM-IV criteria	HDRS and HAS at 8 and 12 weeks, major depression (11% vs. 45%)
Fisch et al., 2003[47]	Fluoxetine (163)	Adults with advanced solid tumors and expected survival of 3–24 months	Depressed mood and/or anhedonia revealed by 2-question survey	FACT-SP, Brief ZSRDS	FACT-G, Brief ZSRDS (12-week study)
Morrow et al., 2003[77]	Paroxetine (479)	Adults with cancer beginning chemotherapy	None	CES-D, POMS D/D	CES-D and POMS D/D at 12 weeks, POMS D/D at 9 weeks

Brief ZSRDS' Brief version of the ZSDRS; HAS, Hamilton Anxiety Scale; CES-D, Center for Epidemiological Studies–Depression; HDRS, Hamilton Depression Rating Scale; CGI, Clinical Global Impression scale; MADRS, Montgomery–Åsberg Depression Rating scale; DSM, Diagnostic and Statistical Manual of Mental Disorders; POMS D/D = Profile of Mood States Depression-Dejection scale; SCL-90-R; Revised Symptom Checklist; FACT-G, Functional Assessment of Cancer Treatment; SQOLI, Spitzer Quality of Life Index; FACT-SP, FACT-G plus spiritual wellbeing subscale; ZSRDS, Zung Self-Rating Depression scale; HADS, Hospital Anxiety Depression Scale.

therapy can also be used alone to treat moderate to severe depression.[4] There are no data regarding the added value of psychological therapies plus antidepressants compared with antidepressants alone specifically in cancer patients. In fact, there are very few studies in the medically ill in which the effect of psychotherapy has been described with sufficient methodological detail.[84] There are several published meta-analyses of controlled trials of psychological interventions for decreasing psychological distress in cancer patients. Sheard and Maguire[85] reported the results of two meta-analyses and found 20 trials with sufficient data to show a combined effect size of 0.36 (95 percent CI 0.06 to 0.66; 1101 patients). This study did not reveal a difference in the efficacy of group therapy compared with individual therapy in patients with cancer. A recent systematic review of psychological therapies for cancer patients was completed by the New South Wales Cancer Council Cancer Education Research Program.[86***] This review evaluated 627 eligible papers published since 1954, and 129 trials were identified that involved psychosocial outcomes. The data from this systematic review regarding depression are summarized in Table 71.3. Only 21 percent of the 114 studies showed an advantage for the therapies in terms of the endpoint of depression. Similar to the situation with antidepressant trials, the data regarding the efficacy of psychological interventions for the treatment of depressive symptoms in cancer patients remain equivocal.

It is useful to note that application of unwanted (but received) support or counseling has been uniquely associated with poor psychosocial adjustment.[87*] As such, clinicians would do well to make counseling and support available to cancer patients but to respect the boundaries that some patients set regarding such services.

Table 71.3 *Psychological intervention trials with depression as an endpoint*

Description of intervention	Significant benefit found/ total trials
Individual therapy	2/18
Therapist-delivered	4/24
Significant-other involvement	1/5
Information and education	4/13
Unstructured counseling	1/5
Structured counseling	2/5
Relaxation training	3/15
Cognitive–behavioral therapy	3/10
Communication/expression training	2/7
Guided imagery/visualization	0/3
Self-practice	1/6
Improving self-esteem/self-image	1/3
Total	24/114 (21%)

Reproduced with permission from Fisch, MJ. Treatment of depression in cancer. *J Natl Cancer Inst Monogr* 2004; **32**: 109. Data from[86].

UNIQUE ISSUES IN END-OF-LIFE CARE

The prevalence of significant depression in palliative care settings is similar to those described for cancer settings above, as most palliative care cohorts are dominated by patients with advanced cancer. Ambiguity surrounding the definition of end-of-life care makes this particular literature difficult to interpret and apply. The 1-item screening question 'Are you depressed?' explored by Chochinov involved a cohort of 197 palliative care inpatients and had perfect sensitivity and specificity of 1.0 in this single study.[43] However, in a palliative care cohort of 74 patients in the UK receiving only palliative and supportive day care, Lloyd-Williams and colleagues found that 27 percent of patients had depression by semi-structured interview criteria, and the single-item screening question had a sensitivity of 55 percent, a specificity of 74 percent, a positive predictive value of 44 percent, and a negative predictive value of 82 percent.[88] Nevertheless, even use of the 14-item HADS had significant limitations in another UK study in a hospice population, as the positive predictive value of this instrument using a cut-off threshold of 20 was only 48 percent with a sensitivity of 77 percent and specificity of 89 percent.[89] Overall, there are insufficient data in end-of-life patient populations to distinguish the assessment issues from those that have been described for cancer patients in general. It should be noted, however, that the occurrence of counter-transference of hopelessness on the part of families and clinicians may discourage dying patients from seeking assessment and treatment for depression.[90]

Regarding the treatment of patients with depression toward the end of life, several consensus statements have been published.[90–92] These statements are limited by the paucity of evidence, but several themes emerge across these statements. First, there should be a low threshold for treating patients with suspected depression using short-term therapeutic trials of carefully selected interventions.[84***,92] In addition, the rapid onset of action of psychostimulants make this class of drugs particularly appealing in patients toward the very end of life. Moreover, psychotherapeutic interventions focused on issues related to meaning and/or dignity[93,94] have shown promising results in the terminally ill.

Finally, one of the more dreaded issues in managing patients with serious illness toward the end of life is the problem of patients who express desire for death. Desire for death statements may indicate that a patient is depressed or suicidal, but may also be a way of coping or expressing suffering.[95*] The prevalence of desire for death statements in terminally ill patients varies widely, ranging from less than 2 percent to 30 percent, depending on the patient population and how patients are identified.[96*,97*,98*] Depressive disorders and delirium are clearly the most common underlying cause of suicidal ideation in patients with potentially fatal illnesses.[99*,100*,101*,102*] However, the presence of a potentially fatal illness, by itself, only carries a modest two- to fourfold increased risk for suicide.[103*] Challenging aspects of assessing patients with desire for death include evaluation and treatment of depression and delirium, assessing the adequacy of palliative care overall, and dealing with broader issues such as personality, family dynamics, as well as important ethnic and cultural issues.[104,105***] It is important to understand that most patients appreciate being asked about their mood in depth, including questions about desire for death or suicide.[106]

MANAGING ANXIETY

It is the rare patient living with cancer or a serious chronic illness who does not confront anxiety. Most patients adapt readily with reassurance from friends, family, and providers. However, some patients have comorbid psychiatric conditions that may manifest with anxiety such as depressive disorders, delirium, or underlying anxiety disorders. Moreover, there may be other underlying causes of anxiety that need to be explored and treated. The common causes of anxiety in palliative care are outlined in Box 71.6.

Symptoms that are uniquely attributable to anxiety include physical symptoms such as tremor, sweating, tachycardia, hyperventilation, and restlessness. Psychological symptoms of anxiety include worry, rumination, and fear.[107] These symptoms may cause patients to flee their environment or display avoidant behaviors. Anxiety symptoms often co-exist with depression and delirium.[108] It is important to consider the diagnosis of delirium in anxious patients, for use of benzodiazepine therapy in patients with subtle manifestations of disordered attention and confusion may lead to an exacerbation of the delirium. Assessment tools that are used to screen for delirium in patients with anxiety who are also at risk for cognitive disturbance are described in Chapter 74.

Box 71.6 Common causes of anxiety symptoms in palliative care

Situational

- Recent diagnosis of serious illness
- Impending surgery or chemotherapy
- Impending diagnostic imaging
- Perceived risk for receiving bad news
- Fear of death/existential anxiety

Symptom-related

- Pain
- Dyspnea
- Palpitations
- Nausea

Metabolic disturbances

- Hypercalcemia
- Hypoglycemia
- Carcinoid syndrome

Drug-associated

- Akathisia due to phenothiazines
- Thyroid replacement
- Allergic reactions

Psychiatric disorders

- Delirium
- Depressive disorders
- Panic disorder
- Posttraumatic stress disorder
- Phobias
- Generalized anxiety disorder

For patients with pervasive worry and autonomic hyperreactivity, pharmacotherapy may be indicated. The categories of medications used to treat anxiety are listed in Box 71.7. Unfortunately, there is an overall lack of evidence on the role of benzodiazepines and most other anxiolytics in palliative care patients.[109] Benzodiazepines are the most commonly prescribed agents and they are effective first-line agents. These medications may cause significant sedation or trigger delirium in patients who are on other psychoactive medications (including opioids) or who are particularly frail. These drugs should be used cautiously and, when feasible, should be discontinued. The short-acting benzodiazepines

lorazepam and alprazolam are used most frequently. For patients with panic disorder, alprazolam is effective as are several antidepressants (imipramine, sertraline, paroxetine). For patients with coexisting delirium or possible opioid toxicity, haloperidol or other neuroleptic agents are useful for management of symptoms while the underlying problem is addressed. In particular, the newer antidepressants are being explored with increasing frequency to treat patients who have complex symptoms including anxiety.[110] Antihistamines and other sedative hypnotic agents can also provide useful anxiolysis, particularly at night when insomnia is an issue. Finally, counseling is effective for treatment of anxiety and it generally involves substitution of more adaptive behaviors and problem-solving approaches for expression of anxiety (which is less adaptive). Counseling may be psychoeducational, behavioral, cognitive – behavioral, or group oriented.

Box 71.7 Drug therapy of anxiety

Benzodiazepines

- Clonazepam
- Alprazolam
- Diazepam
- Lorazepam

Antidepressant agents

- SSRI and newer antidepressants
- Tricyclic antidepressants

Neuroleptic agents

- Haloperidol
- Atypical antipsychotics

Other drug therapies

- Buspirone
- β blockers (for autonomic symptom relief)
- Sedative hypnotics (for relief of insomnia)

Key learning points

- Depression and anxiety are common in patients with serious illness.

- Despite a body of research that spans several decades and includes hundreds of clinical trials, one can make no strong recommendations about the effectiveness of antidepressants or psychological interventions at improving depression or anxiety outcomes for patients with cancer and other serious chronic illnesses.

- Simple, direct questions to explore issues about mood, anxiety, or desire for death are important and appreciated by patients.

- An awareness of the potential for drug interactions with antidepressants and some other drugs commonly used in palliative care is important.

- Patients with serious chronic illnesses would benefit from multidisciplinary care that includes access to specialists in behavioral health when needed.

REFERENCES

◆ 1 Massie MJ. Prevalence of depression in patients with cancer. *J Natl Cancer Inst Monogr* 2004; **32**: 57–71.

◆ 2 Hirschfeld RM, Keller MB, Panico S, *et al.* The National Depressive and Manic-Depressive Association consensus statement on the undertreatment of depression. *JAMA* 1997; **277**: 333–40.

3 Waslick BD, Kander R, Kakouros A. Depression in children and adolescents: an overview. In: Shaffer D, Waslick D, eds. *The Many Faces of Depression in Children and Adolescents.* Washington, DC: American Psychiatric Publishing; 2002.

4 Kroenke K. A 75-year-old man with depression. *JAMA* 2002; **287**: 1568–76.

● 5 Wells KB, Stewart A, Hays RD, *et al.* The funcitoning and well-being of depressed patients: results from the Medical Outcomes Study. *JAMA* 1989; **262**: 914–19.

6 Penninx BW, Guralnik JM, Ferrucci L, *et al.* Depressive symptoms and physical decline in community-dwelling older persons. *JAMA* 1998; **279**: 1720–6.

● 7 Covinsky KE, Fortinsky RH, Palmer RM, *et al.* Relation between symptoms of depression and health status outcomes in acutely ill hospitalized older persons. *Ann Intern Med* 1997; **126**: 417–25.

● 8 Covinsky KE, Kahana E, Chin MH, *et al.* Depressive symptoms and 3-year mortality in older hospitalized medical patients. *Ann Intern Med* 1999; **130**: 563–9.

● 9 Callahan CM, Wolinsky FD, Stump TE, *et al.* Mortality, symptoms, and functional impairment in late-life depression. *J Gen Intern Med* 1998; **13**: 746–52.

10 Ford DE, Mead LA, Chang PP, *et al.* Depression is a risk factor for coronary artery disease in men: the precursors study. *Arch Intern Med* 1998; **158**: 1422–6.

11 Everson SA, Roberts RE, Goldberg DE, Kaplan GA. Depressive symptoms and increased risk of stroke mortality over a 29-year period. *Arch Intern Med* 1998; **158**: 1133–8.

● 12 Wagner HR, Burns BJ, Broadhead WE, *et al.* Minor depression in family practice: functional morbidity, co-morbidity, service utilization and outcomes. *Psychol Med* 2000; **30**: 1377–90.

● 13 Callahan CM, Kesterson JG, Tierney WM. Association of symptoms of depression with diagnostic test charges among older adults. *Ann Intern Med* 1997; **126**: 426–32.

14 American Psychiatric Association. *Diagnostic and Statistical Manual of Mental Disorders*, 4th ed. Washington, DC: American Psychiatric Association, 1994.

◆ 15 Williams JW Jr, Noel PH, Cordes JA, *et al.* Is this patient clinically depressed? *JAMA* 2002; **287**: 1160–70.

✱ 16 US Preventive Services Task Force. Screening for depression: recommendations and rationale. *Ann Intern Med* 2002; **136**: 760–4.

◆ 17 Whooley MA, Simon GE. Managing depression in medical outpatients. *N Engl J Med* 2000; **343**: 1942–50.

18 Williams JW Jr, Barrett J, Oxman T, *et al.* Treatment of dysthymia and minor depression in primary care: A randomized controlled trial in older adults. *JAMA* 2000; **284**: 1519–26.

19 Nease DE, Malouin JM. Depression screening: a practical strategy. *J Fam Pract* 2003; **52**: 118–24.

20 Schoenbaum M, Unutzer J, Sherbourne C, *et al.* Cost-effectiveness of practice-initiated quality improvement for depression: results of a randomized controlled trial. *JAMA* 2001; **286**: 1325–30.

21 Wells KB, Sherbourne C, Schoenbaum M, *et al.* Impact of disseminating quality improvement programs for depression in managed primary care: a randomized controlled trial. *JAMA* 2000; **283**: 212–20.

◆ 22 Pirl WF. Evidence report on the occurrence, assessment, and treatment of depression in cancer patients. *J Natl Cancer Instit Monogr* 2004; **32**: 32–9.

23 Alexander PJ, Dinesh N, Vidyasagar MS. Psychiatric morbidity among cancer patients and its relationship with awareness of illness and expectations about treatment outcome. *Acta Oncol* 1993; **32**: 623–6.

● 24 Berard RM, Boermeester F, Viljoen G. Depressive disorders in an outpatient oncology setting: prevalence, assessment, and management. *Psychooncology* 1998; **7**: 112–20.

● 25 Breitbart W, Rosenfeld B, Pessin H, *et al.* Depression, hopelessness, and desire for hastened death in terminally ill patients with cancer. *JAMA* 2000; **284**: 2907–11.

● 26 Bukberg J, Penman D, Holland JC. Depression in hospitalized cancer patients. *Psychosom Med* 1984;199–212.

27 Colon EA, Callies AL, Popkin MK, McGlare PB. Depressed mood and other variables related to bone marrow transplantation survival in acute leukemia. *Psychosomatics* 1991; **32**: 420–5.

● 28 Derogatis L, Morrow G, Fetting J, *et al.* The prevalence of psychiatric disorders among cancer patients. *JAMA* 1983; **249**: 751–7.

29 Evans DL, McCartney CF, Nemeroff CB, *et al.* Depression in women treated for gynecological cancer: clinical and neuroendocrine assessment. *Am J Psychiatry* 1986; **143**: 447–52.

30 Golden RN, McCartney CF, Haggerty JJ, *et al.* The detection of depression by self-report in women with gynecological cancer. *Int J Psychiatry Med* 1991; **21**: 17–27.

31 Grandi S, Fava GA, Cunsolo A, *et al.* Major depression associated with mastectomy. *Med Sci Res* 1987; **15**: 283–4.

32 Morton RP, Davies AD, Baker J, *et al.* Quality of life in treated head and neck cancer patients: a preliminary report. *Clin Otolaryngol* 1984; **9**: 181–5.

33 Sneeuw KC, Aaronson NK, van Wouwe MC, *et al.* Prevalence and screening of psychiatric disorder in patients with early stage breast cancer. *Qual Life Res* 1993; **2**: 50–1.

34 Greenberg DB. Barriers to the treatment of depression in cancer. *J Natl Cancer Instit Monogr* 2004; **32**: 127–35.

35 Zigmond AS, Snaith RP. The hospital anxiety and depression scale. *Acta Psychiatr Scand* 1983; **67**: 361–70.

36 Ibbotson T, Maguire P, Selby P, *et al.* Screening for anxiety and depression in cancer patients: the effects of disease and treatment. *Eur J Cancer* 1994; 30A: 37–40.

37 Spitzer R, Williams J, Kroenke K, *et al.* Utility of a new procedure for diagnosing mental disorders in primary care: The Prime-MD 1000 Study. *JAMA* 1994; **272**: 1749–56.

38 Quill TE, Arnold RM, Platt F. 'I wish things were different': expressing wishes in response to loss, futility, and unrealistic hopes. *Ann Intern Med* 2001; **135**: 551–5.

39 Cleeland CS, Gonin R, Hatfield AK, *et al.* Pain and its treatment in outpatients with metastatic cancer. *N Engl J Med* 1994; **330**: 592–6.

40 Walsh D, Donnelly S, Rybicki L. The symptoms of advanced cancer: relationship to age, gender, and performance status in 1,000 patients. *Support Care Cancer* 2000; **8**: 175–9.

41 Portenoy RK, Thaler HT, Kornblith AB. Symptom prevalence, characteristic and distress in a cancer population. *Qual Life Res* 1994; **3**: 183–9.

42 Schuit KW, Sleijfer DT, Meijler WJ, *et al.* Symptoms and functional status of patients with disseminated cancer visiting outpatient departments. *J Pain Symptom Manage* 1998; **16**: 290–7.

43 Chochinov H, Wilson K, Enns M, Lander S. 'Are you depressed?' Screening for depression in the terminally ill. *Am J Psychiatry* 1997; **154**: 674–6.

44 Akizuki N, Akechi T, Nakanishi T, *et al.* Development of a brief screening interview for adjustment disorders and major depression in patients with cancer. *Cancer* 2003; **97**: 2005–13.

45 Whooley M, Avins A, Miranda J, Browner W. Case-finding instruments for depression: two questions are as good as many. *J Gen Intern Med* 1997; **12**: 439–45.

46 Pignone MP, Gaynes BN, Rushton JL, *et al.* Screening for depression in adults: a summary of the evidence for the U.S. Preventive Services Task Force. *Ann Intern Med* 2002; **136**: 765–6.

47 Fisch MJ, Loehrer PJ, Kristeller J, *et al.* Fluoxetine versus placebo in advanced cancer outpatients: a double-blinded trial of the Hoosier Oncology Group. *J Clin Oncol* 2003; **21**: 1937–43.

48 Holland JC. Preliminary guidelines for the treatment of distress. *Oncology* 1997; **11**: 109–14; discussion 115–17.

49 Holland JC. NCCN Practice guidelines for the management of psychosocial distress. *Oncology* 1999; **13**: 113–48.

50 Coulehan JL, Schulberg HC, Block MR, *et al.* Treating depressed primary care patients improves their physical, mental, and social functioning. *Arch Intern Med* 1997; **157**: 1113–20.

51 Keller MB, McCullough JP, Klein DN, *et al.* A comparison of nefazodone, the cognitive behavioral-analysis system of psychotherapy, and their combination for the treatment of chronic depression. *N Engl J Med* 2000; **342**: 1462–70.

52 Gill D, Hatcher S. A systematic review of the treatment of depression with antidepressant drugs in patients who also have a physical illness. *Cochrane Database Syst Rev* 1999; 2.

53 Walsh BT, Seidman SN, Sysko R, Gould M. Placebo response in studies of major depression: variable, substantial, and growing. *JAMA* 2002; **287**: 1840–7.

54 Charney DS, Nemeroff CB, Lewis L, *et al.* National Depressive and Manic-Depressive Association consensus statement on the use of placebo in clinical trials of mood disorders. *Arch Gen Psychiatry* 2002; **59**: 262–70.

55 Khan A, Leventhal RM, Khan SR, Brown WA. Severity of depression and response to antidepressants and placebo: an analysis of the Food and Drug Administration database. *J Clin Psychopharmacol* 2002; **22**: 40–5.

56 Hypericum Depression Trial Study Group. Effect of *Hypericum perforatum* (St. John's Wort) in major depressive disorder: a randomized controlled trial. *JAMA* 2002; **287**: 1807–14.

57 Stahl SM. Basic psychopharmacology of antidepressants, part 1: Antidepressants have seven distinct mechanisms of action. *J Clin Psychiatry* 1998; **59**(Suppl 4): 5–14.

58 Kroenke K, West SL, Swindle R, *et al.* Similar effectiveness of paroxetine, fluoxetine, and sertraline in primary care: a randomized trial. *JAMA* 2001; **286**: 2947–55.

59 Kaufman DW, Kelly JP, Rosenberg L, *et al.* Recent patterns of medication use in the ambulatory adult population of the United States: The Slone Survey. *JAMA* 2002; **287**: 337–44.

60 Olfson M, Marcus SC, Druss B, *et al.* National trends in the outpatient treatment of depression. *JAMA* 2002; **287**: 203–9.

61 Aronowitz RA. When do symptoms become a disease? *Ann Intern Med* 2001; **134**(9 Part 2 Suppl S): 803–8.

62 Kroenke K, Harris L. Symptoms research: A fertile field. *Ann Intern Med* 2001; **134**(9 Part 2 Suppl S): 801–2.

63 Kroenke K. Studying symptoms: Sampling and measurement issues. *Ann Intern Med* 2001; **134**(9 Part 2 Suppl S): 844–53.

64 Holden C. Neuroscience. Drugs and placebos look alike in the brain. *Science* 2002; **295**: 947.

65 Vastag B. Decade of work shows depression is physical. *JAMA* 2002; **287**: 1787–8.

66 National Institutes of Health State-of-the-Science Conference Statement: symptom management in cancer: pain, depression, and fatigue, July 15–17, 2002. *J Natl Cancer Inst Monogr* 2004; **32**: 9–16.

67 Homsi J, Nelson KA, Sarhill N, *et al.* A phase II study of methylphenidate for depression in advanced cancer. *Am J Hosp Palliat Care* 2001; **18**: 403–7.

68 Rozans M, Dreisbach A, Lertora JJ, Kahn MJ. Palliative uses of methylphenidate in patients with cancer: a review. *J Clin Oncol* 2002; **20**: 335–9.

69 Meyers CA, Weitzner MA, Valentine AD, Levin VA. Methylphenidate therapy improves cognition, mood, and function of brain tumor patients. *J Clin Oncol* 1998; **16**: 2522–7.

70 Bruera E, Fainsinger R, MacEachern T, Hanson J. The use of methylphenidate in patients with incident cancer pain receiving regular opiates. A preliminary report. *Pain* 1992; **50**: 75–7.

71 van Heeringen K, Zivkov M. Pharmacological treatment of depression in cancer patients. A placebo-controlled study of mianserin. *Br J Psychiatry* 1996; **169**: 440–3.

72 Eija K, Tiina T, Pertti NJ. Amitriptyline effectively relieves neuropathic pain following treatment of breast cancer. *Pain* 1996; **64**: 293–302.

73 Costa D, Mogos I, Toma T. Efficacy and safety of mianserin in the treatment of depression of women with cancer. *Acta Psychiatr Scand* 1985; **72**: 85–92.

74 Purohit DR, Navlakha PL, Modi RS, Eshpumiyani R. The role antidepressants in hospitalised cancer patients. (A pilot study). *J Assoc Physicians India* 1978; **26**: 245–8.

● 75 Razavi D, Allilaire JF, Smith M, *et al.* The effect of fluoxetine on anxiety and depression symptoms in cancer patients. *Acta Psychiat Scand* 1996; **94**: 205–10.

● 76 Musselman DL, Lawson DH, Gumnick JF, *et al.* Paroxetine for the prevention of depression induced by high-dose interferon alfa. *N Engl J Med* 2001; **344**: 961–6.

77 Morrow GR, Hickok JT, Roscoe JA, *et al.* University of Rochester Cancer Center Community Clinical Oncology Program. Differential effects of paroxetine on fatigue and depression: a randomized, double-blind trial from the University of Rochester Cancer Center Community Clinical Oncology Program. *J Clin Oncol* 2003; **21**: 4635–41.

78 Johnston B. Relief of mixed anxiety-depression in terminal cancer patients. Effect of thioridazine. *N Y State J Med* 1972; **72**: 2315–17.

● 79 Bruera E, Roca E, Cedaro L, *et al.* Action of oral methyl-prednisolone in terminal cancer patients: a prospective randomized double-blind study. *Cancer Treat Rep* 1985; **69**: 751–4.

● 80 Bruera E, Carraro S, Roca E, *et al.* Double-blind evaluation of the effects of mazindol on pain, depression, anxiety, appetite, and activity in terminal cancer patients. *Cancer Treat Rep* 1986; **70**: 295–8.

● 81 Holland JC, Morrow GR, Schmale A, *et al.* A randomized clinical trial of alprazolam versus progressive muscle relaxation in cancer patients with anxiety and depressive symptoms. *J Clin Oncol* 1991; **9**: 1004–11.

● 82 Holland JC, Romano SJ, Heiligenstein JH, *et al.* A controlled trial of fluoxetine and desipramine in depressed women with advanced cancer. *Psychooncology* 1998; **7**: 291–300.

● 83 Razavi D, Kormoss N, Collard A, *et al.* Comparative study of the efficacy and safety of trazodone versus clorazepate in the treatment of adjustment disorders in cancer patients: a pilot study. *J Int Med Res* 1999; **27**: 264–72.

◆ 84 Stiefel F, Die Trill M, Berney A, *et al.* Depression in palliative care: a pragmatic report from the Expert Working Group of the European Association for Palliative Care. *Support Care Cancer* 2001; **9**: 477–88.

● 85 Sheard T, Maguire P. The effect of psychological interventions on anxiety and depression in cancer patients: results of two meta-analyses. *Br J Cancer* 1999; **80**: 1770–80.

◆ 86 Newell SA, Sanson-Fisher RW, Savolainen NJ. Systematic review of psychological therapies for cancer patients: overview and recommendations for the future. *J Natl Cancer Inst* 2002; **94**: 558–84.

87 Reynolds JS, Perrin NA. Mismatches in social support and psychological adjustment to breast cancer. *Health Psychol* 2004; **23**: 425–30.

● 88 Lloyd-Williams M, Dennis M, Taylor F, Baker I. Is asking patients in palliative care, 'Are you depressed?' appropriate? Prospective study. *BMJ* 2003; **327**: 372–3.

● 89 Le Fevre P, Devereux J, Smith S, *et al.* Screening for psychiatric illness in the palliative care inpatient setting: a comparison between the Hospital Anxiety and Depression Scale and the General Health Questionnaire-12. *Palliat Med* 1999; **12**: 399–407.

✱ 90 APM's Ad Hoc Committee on End-of-Life Care. Psychiatric aspects of excellent end-of-life care: A position statement

of the Academy of Psychosomatic Medicine. *J Palliat Med* 1998; **1**: 113–15.

✱ 91 Stiefel R, Die Trill M, Berney A, *et al.* Depression in palliative care: a pragmatic report from the Expert Working Group of the European Association for Palliative Care. *Support Care Cancer* 2001; **9**: 477–88.

◆ 92 Block SD. Assessing and managing depression in the terminally ill patient. *Ann Intern Med* 2000; **132**: 209–18.

93 Chochinov HM, Hack T, Hassard T, *et al.* Dignity and psychotherapeutic considerations in end-of-life care. *J Palliat Care* 2004; **20**: 134–42.

94 Breitbart W. Reframing hope: meaning-centered care for patients near the end of life. Interview by Karen S. Heller. *J Palliat Med* 2003; **6**: 979–88.

95 Van Loon RA. Desire to die in terminally ill people: a framework for assessment and intervention. *Health Soc Work* 1999; **24**: 260–8.

● 96 Akechi T, Okuyama T, Sugawara Y, *et al.* Suicidality in terminally ill Japanese patients with cancer. *Cancer* 2004; **100**: 183–91.

● 97 Tiernan E, Casey P, O'Boyle C, *et al.* Relations between desire for early death, depressive symptoms and antidepressant prescribing in terminally ill patients with cancer. *J R Soc Med* 2002; **95**: 386–90.

● 98 Lloyd-Williams M. How common are thoughts of self-harm in a UK palliative care population? *Support Care Cancer* 2002; **10**: 422–4.

● 99 Chochinov HM, Wilson KG, Enns M, *et al.* Desire for death in the terminally ill. *Am J Psychiatry* 1995; **152**: 1185–91.

● 100 Wilson KG, Scott JF, Graham ID, *et al.* Attitudes of the terminally ill toward euthanasia and physician-assisted suicide. *Arch Intern Med* 2000; **160**: 2454–60.

● 101 Akechi T, Kugaya A, Okamura H, *et al.* Suicidal thoughts in cancer patients: clinical experience in psycho-oncology. *Psychiatry Clin Neurosci* 1999; **53**: 569–73.

● 102 Akechi T. Desire or early death in cancer patients and clinical oncology. *Japanese J Clin Oncol* 1999; **29**: 616.

● 103 Henriksson MM, Isometsa ET, Hietanen PS, *et al.* Mental disorders in cancer suicides. *J Affect Disord* 1995; **36**: 11–20.

104 Cohen LM, Steinberg MD, Hails KC, *et al.* Psychiatric evaluation of death-hastening requests. Lessons from dialysis discontinuation. *Psychosomatics* 2000; **41**: 195–203.

◆ 105 Mann JJ. A current perspective on suicide and attempted suicide. *Ann Intern Med* 2002; **136**: 302–11.

106 Meyer HA, Sinnott C, Seed PT. Depressive symptoms in advanced cancer. Part 1. Assessing depression: the Mood Evaluation Questionnaire. *Palliat Med* 003; **17**: 596–603.

◆ 107 Stiefel F, Razavi D. Common psychiatric disorders in cancer patients. II. Anxiety and acute confusional states. *Support Care Cancer* 1994; **2**: 233–7.

◆ 108 Roth AJ, Modi R. Psychiatric issues in older cancer patients. *Crit Rev Oncol Hematol* 2003; **48**: 185–97.

● 109 Jackson KC, Lipman AG. Drug therapy for anxiety in palliative care. *Cochrane Database Syst Rev* 2004; 1.

◆ 110 Fisch MJ, Kim HF. Use of atypical antipsychotic agents for symptom control in patients with advanced cancer. *J Support Oncol* 2004; **2**: 447–452.

72

Confusion/delirium

WILLIAM BREITBART, MIRIAM FRIEDLANDER

INTRODUCTION

Cognitive failure is unfortunately all too common in patients with advanced illness. The Diagnostic and Statistical Manual of Mental Disorders (DSM)-IV[1] divides cognitive disorders into the subcategories of:

- Delirium, dementia, amnesic and other cognitive disorders
- Mental disorders due to a general medical condition (including mood disorder, anxiety disorder and personality change due to a general medical condition)
- Substance-related disorders.

While virtually all of these mental syndromes can be seen in the patient with advanced disease, the most common include delirium, dementia, and mood and anxiety disorders due to a general medical condition. Lipowski categorized organic mental disorders into those that were characterized by general cognitive impairment, (i.e. delirium and dementia) and those where cognitive impairment was rather selective or limited (i.e. amnesic disorder, organic hallucinosis, organic mood disorder, etc.).[2] With organic mental disorders where cognitive impairment is selective, limited, or relatively intact, the more prominent symptoms tend to consist of either anxiety, mood disturbance, delusions, hallucinations or personality change. For instance, the patient with mood disturbance meeting criteria for major depression, who is severely hypothyroid or on high-dose corticosteroids is most accurately diagnosed as having a mood disorder due to a general medical condition or substance-induced mood disorder, respectively (particularly if organic factors are judged to be the primary etiology related to the mood disturbance). Similarly, the patient with hyponatremia, or the patient on aciclovir for central nervous system (CNS) herpes who is experiencing visual hallucinations but has an intact sensorium with minimal cognitive deficits, is more accurately diagnosed as having a psychotic disorder due to a general medical condition or a substance-induced psychotic disorder, respectively.

In spite of very little being known about the neuropathogenesis of delirium, its symptoms suggest that it is a dysfunction of multiple regions of the brain.[3] Delirium has been characterized as an etiologically nonspecific, global, cerebral dysfunction characterized by concurrent disturbances of level of consciousness, attention, thinking, perception, memory, psychomotor behavior, emotion, and the sleep–wake cycle. Disorientation, fluctuation, or waxing and waning of these symptoms, as well as an acute or abrupt onset of such disturbances are other critical features of delirium. Delirium, in contrast with dementia, is conceptualized as a *reversible* process. Reversibility of the process of delirium is often possible even in the patient with advanced illness; however it may *not* be reversible in the last 24–48 hours of life. This is most likely due to the fact that irreversible processes such as multiple organ failure are occurring in the final hours of life. Delirium occurring in these last days of life is often referred to as terminal restlessness or terminal agitation in the palliative care literature.

At times it is difficult to differentiate delirium from dementia since they frequently share such common clinical features as impaired memory, thinking, and judgment, and disorientation. Dementia appears in relatively alert individuals with little or no clouding of consciousness. The temporal onset of symptoms in dementia is more subacute or chronically progressive, and the sleep–wake cycle seems less impaired. Most prominent in dementia are difficulties in short-term and long-term memory, impaired judgment, and abstract thinking as well as disturbed higher cortical functions (such as aphasia and apraxia). Occasionally, delirium superimposed on an underlying dementia is encountered such as in the case of an older patient, a patient with acquired immune deficiency syndrome (AIDS), or a patient with a paraneoplastic syndrome. Clinically, a number of scales or instruments aid clinicians in the diagnosis of delirium, dementia, or cognitive failure.

DELIRIUM IN THE TERMINALLY ILL PATIENT

Prevalence of delirium

Delirium is the most common and serious neuropsychiatric complication in the patient with advanced illness. Cognitive disorders and delirium in particular, have enormous relevance to symptom control and palliative care. Delirium is highly prevalent in cancer and AIDS patients with advanced disease, particularly in the last weeks of life, with prevalence rates ranging from 25 percent to 85 percent.[4–11] Delirium is one of the most common mental disorders encountered in general hospital practice. Knight and Folstein estimated that 33 percent of hospitalized medically ill patients have serious cognitive impairments.[12] Massie and coworkers found delirium in 25 percent of 334 hospitalized cancer patients seen in psychiatric consultation and in 85 percent (11 of 13) of terminal cancer patients.[5] Pereira and coworkers found the prevalence of cognitive impairment in cancer inpatients to be 44 percent, and just prior to death, the prevalence rose to 62.1 percent.[13] Delirium also occurs in up to 51 percent of post-operative patients.[14,15] The incidence of delirium is currently increasing, which reflects the growing numbers of older patients, who are particularly susceptible.[14] Studies of older patients admitted to medical wards estimate that between 30 and 50 percent of patients age 70 years or more showed symptoms of delirium at some point during hospitalization.[16–20] Older patients who develop delirium during hospitalization have been estimated to have a 22–76 percent chance of dying during that hospitalization.[21]

Delirium is associated with increased morbidity in the terminally ill, causing distress in patients, family members, and staff.[22–24] In a recent study of the 'Delirium Experience' of terminally ill cancer patients, Breitbart and colleagues found that 54 percent of patients recalled their delirium experience after recovery from delirium.[22] Factors predicting delirium recall included the degree of short-term memory impairment, delirium severity, and the presence of perceptual disturbances (the more severe the less likely recall). Distress related to the episode of delirium was rated by patients, spouses/caregivers, and nurses on a 0–4 numerical rating scale (with 4 being most severe). Patients scored an average rating of 3.2, spouses 3.75, and nurses 3.2. The most significant factor predicting distress for patients was the presence of delusions. Patients with hypoactive delirium were just as distressed as patients with hyperactive delirium. Predictors of spouse distress included the patients' Karnofsky Performance Status (the lower the Karnofsky, the worse the spouse distress), and nurse distress included delirium

severity and perceptual disturbances. Delirium can interfere dramatically with the recognition and control of other physical and psychological symptoms such as pain in later stages of illness.[23,25,26]

A recent retrospective study of 284 hospice patients sought to identify factors that contribute to impairment of communication capacity in terminally ill cancer patients.[27] The study demonstrated that communication capacity was frequently impaired in terminally ill cancer patients and the degree of impairment was significantly associated with higher doses of opioids. Patients who did not require high doses of opioids were able to retain complex and simple communication capacity longer than those who required high doses of opioids prior to death. Delirium was present in 20 percent of patients in this study which emphasized the importance of further investigations to explore new strategies for maintaining communication capacity in this population.

Often a preterminal event, delirium is a sign of significant physiological disturbance, usually involving multiple medical causes, including infection, organ failure, medication side effects (including opioids), as well as extremely rare paraneoplastic syndromes.[11,28–31] Lawlor and colleagues recently reported on their experience in the management of delirium in advanced cancer patients in a palliative care unit.[32] Whereas 42 percent of patients had delirium upon admission to their palliative care unit, terminal delirium occurred in 88 percent of the deaths. Unfortunately, delirium is often underrecognized or misdiagnosed and inappropriately treated or untreated in terminally ill patients. Impediments to progress in the recognition and treatment of delirium have included confusion regarding terminology and lack of consistency in the use of diagnostic classification systems. In addition, the signs and symptoms of delirium can be diverse and are sometimes mistaken for other psychiatric disorders such as mood or anxiety disorders. Practitioners caring for patients with life-threatening illnesses must be able to diagnose delirium accurately, undertake appropriate assessment of the etiologies, and be knowledgeable about the benefits and risks of the pharmacological and nonpharmacological interventions currently available in managing delirium among the terminally ill.

Diagnosing delirium

The clinical features of delirium are quite numerous and include a variety of neuropsychiatric symptoms that are also common to other psychiatric disorders such as depression, dementia, and psychosis.[33] Clinical features of delirium include prodromal symptoms (restlessness, anxiety, sleep disturbance, and irritability); rapidly fluctuating course; reduced attention (easily distractible); altered arousal; increased or decreased psychomotor activity; disturbance of sleep–wake cycle; affective symptoms (emotional lability, sadness, anger, and euphoria); altered perceptions (misperceptions, illusions, delusions, and hallucinations);

disorganized thinking and incoherent speech; disorientation to time, place, or person; and memory impairment (cannot register new material). Neurological abnormalities can also be present during delirium, including cortical abnormalities (dysgraphia, constructional apraxia, dysnomia, aphasia); motor abnormalities (tremor, asterixis, myoclonus, and reflex and tone changes); and electroencephalographic (EEG) abnormalities (usually global slowing). It is this protean nature of delirious symptoms, the variability and fluctuation of clinical findings, and the unclear and often contradictory definitions of the syndrome that have made delirium so difficult to diagnose and treat.

Box 72.1 lists the DSM-IV[1] criteria for delirium. The essential defining features of delirium, based on DSM-IV criteria, have shifted from the extensive list of typical symptoms and abnormalities described above, to a focus on the two essential concepts of disordered attention (arousal) and cognition while continuing to recognize the importance of acute onset and organic etiology. Associated phenomena such as psychomotor behavioral changes, perceptual disturbances, hallucinations or delusions are no longer viewed as essential to the diagnosis of delirium. Delirium is now conceptualized primarily as 'a disorder of arousal and cognition'[3] in contrast with dementia, which is a disorder of cognition without an arousal disturbance. It is this disorder of the arousal system, with consequent disturbances in level of consciousness and attention that is pathognomonic of delirium and is, in part, the basis for classifying delirium into several subtypes.

Box 72.1 DSM-IV criteria for delirium

Delirium due to a general medical condition:

A   Disturbance of consciousness (that is, reduced clarity of awareness of the environment) with reduced ability to focus, sustain, or shift attention.

B   Change in cognition (such as memory deficit, disorientation, language disturbance, or perceptual disturbance) that is not better accounted for by a preexisting, established, or evolving dementia.

C   The disturbance develops over a short period of time (usually hours to days) and tends to fluctuate during the course of the day.

D   There is evidence from the history, physical examination, or laboratory findings of a general medical condition judged to be etiologically related to the disturbance.

SUBTYPES OF DELIRIUM

Three clinical subtypes of delirium, based on arousal disturbance and psychomotor behavior, have been described. These subtypes included the 'hyperactive' (hyperaroused, hyperalert, or agitated) subtype, the 'hypoactive' (hypoaroused, hypoalert, or lethargic) subtype, and a 'mixed' subtype with alternating features of hyperactive and hypoactive delirium.[2,3] Research suggests that the hyperactive form is most often characterized by hallucinations, delusions, agitation, and disorientation, while the hypoactive form is characterized by confusion and sedation, but is rarely accompanied by hallucinations, delusions, or illusions.[34] In addition, there is evidence suggesting that specific delirium subtypes may be related to specific etiologies of delirium, may have unique pathophysiologies, and differential responses to treatment.[35,36] It is estimated that approximately two-thirds of deliria are either of the hypoactive or mixed subtype, hence, the prototypically agitated delirious patient most familiar to clinicians is actually a minority of the deliria which occur.[2,34,37]

DIFFERENTIAL DIAGNOSIS

Many of the clinical features and symptoms of delirium can be also be associated with other psychiatric disorders such as depression, mania, psychosis, and dementia. For instance, delirious patients, not uncommonly, exhibit mood disturbances such as anxiety, fear, depression, irritability, anger, euphoria, apathy, or lability. Delirium, particularly the 'hypoactive' subtype, is often initially misdiagnosed as depression. Symptoms of major depression, including altered level of activity (hypoactivity), insomnia, reduced ability to concentrate, depressed mood, and even suicidal ideation, can overlap with symptoms of delirium making an accurate diagnosis more difficult. In distinguishing delirium from depression, particularly in the context of advanced disease, an evaluation of the onset and temporal sequencing of depressive and cognitive symptoms is particularly helpful. Importantly, the degree of cognitive impairment in delirium is much more severe and pervasive than in depression, with a more abrupt temporal onset. Also, in delirium the characteristic disturbance in arousal or consciousness is present, while it is usually not a feature of depression. Similarly, a manic episode may share some features of delirium, particularly a 'hyperactive' or 'mixed' subtype of delirium. Again, the temporal onset and course of symptoms, the presence of a disturbance of consciousness (arousal) as well as of cognition, and the identification of a presumed medical etiology for delirium are helpful in differentiating these disorders. Delirium that is characterized by vivid hallucinations and delusions must be distinguished from a variety of psychotic disorders. In delirium, such psychotic symptoms occur in the context of a disturbance in consciousness or arousal, as well as memory impairment and disorientation, which is not the case in other psychotic disorders. Delusions in delirium tend to be poorly organized and of abrupt onset, and hallucinations are predominantly visual or tactile rather than auditory as is typical of schizophrenia. Finally, the development of these psychotic symptoms in the context of advanced medical illness makes delirium a more likely diagnosis.

The most common differential diagnostic issue is whether the patient has delirium, or dementia, or a delirium superimposed upon a preexisting dementia. Both delirium and dementia are cognitive impairment disorders and so share such common clinical features as impaired memory, thinking, judgment, and disorientation. The patient with dementia is alert and does not have the disturbance of consciousness or arousal that is characteristic of delirium. The temporal onset of symptoms in dementia is more subacute and chronically progressive, and the sleep–wake cycle is less impaired. Most prominent in dementia are difficulties in short-term and long-term memory, impaired judgment, and abstract thinking as well as disturbed higher cortical functions (such as aphasia and apraxia). Occasionally, delirium superimposed on an underlying dementia is encountered such as in the case of an older patient, an AIDS patient, or a patient with a paraneoplastic syndrome. Delirium, in contrast with dementia, is conceptualized as a reversible process. Reversibility of the process of delirium is often possible even in the patient with advanced illness. However, delirium may not be reversible in the last 24–48 hours of life. This is most likely due to the fact that irreversible processes such as multiple organ failure are occurring in the final hours of life. Delirium occurring in these last days of life is sometimes referred to as 'terminal delirium' in the palliative care literature.

DELIRIUM SCREENING/DIAGNOSTIC SCALES

A number of scales or instruments have been developed which can aid the clinician in rapidly screening for cognitive impairment disorders (dementia or delirium), or in establishing a diagnosis of delirium[38–46] (see Box 72.2). Such scales have been described and their relative strengths and weaknesses reviewed elsewhere.[43,47] Perhaps most helpful to clinicians are the Mini-Mental State Examination (a cognitive impairment screening tool) and several delirium diagnostic and rating scales, including the Delirium Rating Scale, the Delirium Rating Scale–Revised–98, the Confusion Assessment Method, the Abbreviated Cognitive Test for Delirium, and the Memorial Delirium Assessment Scale. These tools are described briefly below.

Box 72.2   Assessment methods for delirium in cancer patients

Diagnostic classification systems

- DSM-IV
- Internation Classification of Diseases (ICD)-9, ICD-10

Diagnostic interviews/instruments

- Delirium Symptom Interview (DSI)
- Confusion Assessment Method (CAM)

Delirium rating scales

- Delirium Rating Scale (DRS)
- Delirium Rating Scale–Revised–98 (DRS-R-98)
- Confusion Rating Scale (CRS)
- Saskatoon Delirium Checklist (SDC)
- Memorial Delirium Assessment Scale (MDAS)
- Abbreviated Cognitive Test for Delirium (CTD)

Cognitive impairment screening instruments

- Mini-Mental State Examination (MMSE)
- Short Portable Mental Status Questionnaire (SPMSQ)
- Cognitive Capacity Screening Examination (CCSE)
- Blessed Orientation Memory Concentration Test (BOMC)

Mini-Mental State Examination

The MMSE is useful in screening for cognitive failure, but does not distinguish between delirium and dementia.[45] The MMSE provides a quantitative assessment of the cognitive performance and capacity of a patient, and is a measure of severity of cognitive impairment. It is also most sensitive to cortical dementias such as Alzheimer disease, and less sensitive in detecting subcortical deficits such as those found in AIDS dementia. The MMSE assesses five general cognitive areas including orientation, registration, attention and calculation, recall, and language. Although a score of 23 or less has generally been considered the cut-off score for cognitive impairment, a three tiered system is now often used suggesting that a score of 24–30 indicates no impairment, 18–23 indicates mild impairment, and 0–17 indicates severe impairment.

Delirium Rating Scale

The DRS, developed by Trzepacz and colleagues is a 10-item clinician-rated symptom rating scale for diagnosing delirium.[47] The scale is based on DSM-III-R diagnostic criteria for delirium and is designed to be used by the clinician to identify delirium and distinguish it reliably from dementia and other neuropsychiatric disorders. Each item is scored by choosing the appropriate rating which carries a numerical weight selected to distinguish the phenomenological characteristics of delirium. A score of 12 or greater is diagnostic of delirium.

Delirium Rating Scale-Revised-98

The DRS-R-98 is a revision of the DRS. The DRS-R-98 has 13 severity and three diagnostic items with descriptive anchors for each rating level. It includes more items than the DRS and was designed for phenomenological and treatment research although it may be used clinically. The DRS-R-98 is a valid, sensitive, and reliable instrument for rating delirium severity. It has advantages over the original DRS for repeated measures and phenomenological studies due to its enhanced breadth of symptoms and separation into severity and diagnostic subscales.[48]

Confusion Assessment Method

The CAM is a 9-item delirium diagnostic scale that uses the DSM-III-R criteria for delirium, and can be administered quickly by a trained clinician.[49] A unique and helpful feature of the CAM is that it has been simplified into a diagnostic algorithm that includes only four items of the CAM designed for rapid identification of delirium by nonpsychiatrists. The 4-item algorithm requires the presence of: (i) acute onset and fluctuating course, (ii) inattention, and either (iii) disorganized thinking or (iv) altered level of consciousness.

Abbreviated Cognitive Test for Delirium

The abbreviated CTD was developed as a tool to help identify delirium in patients in the intensive care unit setting who have limited ability to communicate verbally.[50] This brief tool uses visualization span and recognition memory for pictures as two of nine content scores that produces a total score that reliably identifies delirium and discriminates delirium from dementia, depression, and schizophrenia.

Memorial Delirium Assessment Scale

The MDAS is a 10-item delirium assessment tool (see Box 72.3), validated in hospitalized inpatients with advanced cancer and AIDS.[38] The MDAS is both a good delirium diagnostic screening tool as well as a reliable tool for assessing delirium severity among patients with advanced disease. A cut-off score of 13 is diagnostic of delirium. The

MDAS has advantages over other delirium tools in that it is both a diagnostic as well as a severity measure that is ideal for repeated assessments and for use in treatment intervention trials. Recently, Lawlor and colleagues further examined the clinical utility and validation of the MDAS in a population of advanced cancer patients in a palliative care unit.[51] These investigators found the MDAS to be useful in this population, and found that a cut-off score of 7 out of 30 yielded the highest sensitivity (98 percent) and specificity (76 percent) for a delirium diagnosis in this palliative care population.

MANAGEMENT OF DELIRIUM IN THE TERMINALLY ILL PATIENT

The standard approach to the managing delirium in the medically ill, and even in those with advanced disease, includes a search for underlying causes, correction of those factors and management of the symptoms of delirium. The desired and often achievable outcome is a patient who is awake, alert, calm, cognitively intact, not psychotic, and communicating coherently with family and staff. In the terminally ill patient who develops delirium in the last days of life ('terminal' delirium), the management of delirium is unique, presenting a number of dilemmas, and the desired clinical outcome may be significantly altered by the dying process (see Fig. 72.1).

Assessment of etiologies of delirium

When confronted with delirium in the terminally ill or dying patient, a differential diagnosis should always be formulated as to the likely etiology or etiologies. There is an ongoing debate as to the appropriate extent of diagnostic evaluation that should be pursued in a dying patient with a terminal delirium.[52,53] Most palliative care clinicians would undertake diagnostic studies only when a clinically suspected etiology can be identified easily, with minimal use of invasive procedures, and treated effectively with simple

---

> **Box 72.3 Items from the Memorial Delirium Assessment Scale (MDAS)**
>
> 1   Reduced level of consciousness (awareness)
>
> 2   Disorientation
>
> 3   Short-term memory impairment
>
> 4   Impaired digit span
>
> 5   Reduced ability to maintain and shift attention
>
> 6   Disorganized thinking
>
> 7   Perceptual disturbance
>
> 8   Delusions
>
> 9   Decreased or increased psychomotor
>
> 10   Sleep–wake cycle disturbance (disorder of arousal)

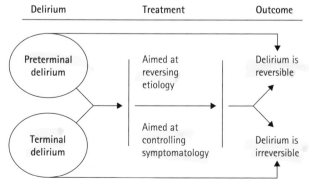

Figure 72.1 *Overview of delirium management.*

interventions that carry minimal burden or risk of causing further distress. Diagnostic workup in pursuit of an etiology for delirium may be limited by either practical constraints such as the setting (home, hospice) or the focus on patient comfort, so that unpleasant or painful diagnostics may be avoided. Most often, however, the etiology of terminal delirium is multifactorial or may not be determined. Bruera and colleagues report that an etiology is discovered in less than 50 percent of terminally ill patients with delirium.[6] When a distinct cause is found for delirium in the terminally ill, it is often irreversible or difficult to treat. Studies, however, in patients with earlier stages of advanced cancer have demonstrated the potential utility of a thorough diagnostic assessment.[6,25] When such diagnostic information is available, specific therapy may be able to reverse delirium. One study found that improvement could be achieved in 68 percent of delirious cancer patients, despite a 30-day mortality of 31 percent.[54] Another found that a third of the episodes of cognitive failure improved following evaluation that yielded a cause for these episodes in 43 percent.[6]

In a recent prospective study of delirium in patients on a palliative care unit, investigators reported that the etiology of delirium was multifactorial in the great majority of cases.[32] Even though delirium occurred in 88 percent of dying patients in the last week of life, delirium was reversible in approximately 50 percent of episodes. Causes of delirium that were most associated with reversibility included dehydration and psychoactive or opioid medications. Hypoxic and metabolic encephalopathies were less likely to be reversed in terminal delirium.

The diagnostic evaluation includes an assessment of potentially reversible causes of delirium. A full physical examination should assess for evidence of sepsis, dehydration, or major organ failure. Medications that could contribute to delirium should be reviewed. A screen of laboratory parameters will allow assessment of the possible role of metabolic abnormalities, such as hypercalcemia, and other problems, such as hypoxia or disseminated intravascular coagulation. Imaging studies of the brain and assessment of the cerebrospinal fluid may be appropriate in some instances.

Delirium can have multiple potential etiologies (see Box 72.4). In patients with advanced cancer, for instance, delirium can be due either to the direct effects of cancer on the CNS, or to indirect CNS effects of the disease or treatments (medications, electrolyte imbalance, failure of a vital organ or system, infection, vascular complications and preexisting cognitive impairment or dementia).[6,32] Given the large numbers of drugs cancer patients require, and the fragile state of their physiological functioning, even routinely ordered hypnotics are enough to tip patients over into a delirium. Narcotic analgesics such as levorphanol, morphine sulfate, and meperidine, are common causes of confusional states, particularly in older patients and the terminally ill. Chemotherapeutic agents known to cause delirium include methotrexate, fluorouracil, vincristine, vinblastine, bleomycin, BCNU, cis-platinum, asparaginase,

---

> **Box 72.4 Causes of delirium in patients with advanced disease**
>
> **Direct CNS causes**
>
> - Primary brain tumor
> - Metastatic spread to CNS
> - Seizures
>
> **Indirect causes**
>
> - Metabolic encephalopathy due to organ failure
> - Electrolyte imbalance
> - Treatment side effects from chemotherapeutic agents: steroids; radiation; narcotics; anticholinergics; antiemetics; antivirals
> - Infection
> - Hematological abnormalities
> - Nutritional deficiencies
> - Paraneoplastic syndromes

procarbazine, and corticosteroids.[7,11,28,55–60] Most patients receiving chemotherapeutics will not develop prominent CNS effects unless dexamethasone or prednisone is included in the regimen. The spectrum of mental disturbances related to steroids includes minor mood lability, affective disorders (mania or depression), cognitive impairment (reversible dementia), and delirium (steroid psychosis). The incidence of these disorders ranges from 3 percent to 57 percent in the noncancer populations, and they occur most commonly on higher doses.[25] Symptoms usually develop within the first two weeks on steroids, but in fact can occur at any time, on any dose, even during the tapering phase.[25] These disorders are often rapidly reversible upon dose reduction or discontinuation.[25]

Nonpharmacological interventions

In addition to seeking out and potentially correcting underlying causes of delirium, symptomatic and supportive therapies are important.[8,24,26,52] In fact, in the dying patient they may be the only steps taken. Fluid and electrolyte balance, nutrition, vitamins, measures to help reduce anxiety and disorientation, interactions with and education of family members may be useful. Measures to help reduce anxiety and disorientation (i.e. structure and familiarity) may include a quiet, well-lit room with familiar objects, a visible clock or calendar, and the presence of family. Judicious use of physical restraints, along with one-to-one nursing observation may also be necessary and useful.

Recently, Inouye and colleagues reported on a successful multicomponent intervention program to prevent delirium in hospitalized older patients.[61] They focus on a set of risk factors that were highly predictive of delirium in older patients which included: preexisting cognitive impairment, visual impairment, hearing impairment, sleep deprivation, immobility, dehydration and severe illness. Interventions directed at constant reorientation, correction of hearing and visual impairment, reversal of dehydration and early mobilization appeared to significantly reduce the number and duration of episodes of delirium in hospitalized older patients. The applicability of these interventions and the likelihood that they would prevent delirium in the terminally ill, particularly in the last days of life, is likely minimal.

Pharmacological interventions in delirium

Supportive techniques alone are often not effective in controlling the symptoms of delirium, and symptomatic treatment with neuroleptics or sedative medications are necessary (see Table 72.1). Neuroleptic drugs (dopamine-blocking drugs) such as haloperidol, are utilized frequently as antiemetics in the medical setting, however, only 0.5 percent to 2 percent of hospitalized cancer patients, for instance, receive haloperidol for the management of the symptoms of delirium.[62,63] Among terminally ill patients, only 17 percent receive an antipsychotic for agitation or psychological distress, despite an estimated prevalence of delirium ranging from 25 percent in the hospitalized cancer patient to 85 percent in the terminally ill.[64,65]

NEUROLEPTICS

Haloperidol, a neuroleptic drug that is a potent dopamine blocker, is often the drug of choice in the treatment of delirium in patients with advanced disease.[65–73] Haloperidol in low doses, 1–3 mg/day, is usually effective in targeting agitation, paranoia, and fear. Typically 0.5–1.0 mg haloperidol (per oral [PO], intravenous [IV], intramuscular [IM], subcutaneous [SC]) is administered, with repeat doses every 45–60 minutes titrated against target symptoms.[53,74] An IV route can facilitate rapid onset of medication effects. If IV access is unavailable, start with IM or SC administration and switch to the oral route when possible. The majority of delirious patients can be managed with oral haloperidol. Parenteral doses are approximately twice as potent as oral doses. Haloperidol is administered by the SC route by many palliative care practitioners.[6,75] Low doses of neuroleptic medication are usually sufficient in treating delirium in elderly terminally ill patients. In general, doses need not exceed 20 mg of haloperidol in a 24-hour period. However, a few clinicians have advocated high doses (up to 250 mg/24-hour of haloperidol intravenously) in selected cases.[73]

A common strategy in the management of symptoms related to delirium is to add parenteral lorazepam to a regimen of haloperidol.[76,77] Lorazepam (0.5 mg to 1.0 mg every 1–2 hours PO or IV) along with haloperidol may be more effective in rapidly sedating the agitated delirious patient and may minimize extrapyramidal side effects associated with haloperidol.[77] An alternative strategy is to switch from haloperidol to a more sedating neuroleptic such as chlorpromazine (see Fig. 72.2 later). In a double blind, randomized

Table 72.1 *Medications used in the management of delirium in patients with advanced disease*

Generic name	Approximate daily dosage range	Route
Neuroleptics		
Haloperidol	0.5–5 mg every 2–12 hours	PO, IV, SC, IM
Thioridazine	10–75 mg every 4–8 hours	PO
Chlorpromazine	12.5–50 mg every 4–12 hours	PO, IV, IM
Methotrimeprazine	12.5–50 mg every 4–8 hours	IV, SC, PO
Molindone	10–50 mg every 8–12 hours	PO
Droperidol	0.625–2.5 mg every 4–8 hours	IV, IM
Atypical neuroleptics		
Olanzapine	2.5–20 mg every 12–24 hours	PO
Risperidone	0.5–3 mg every 12–24 hours	PO
Quetiapine	12.5–200 mg every 12–24 hours	PO
Ziprasidone (note max IM daily dose 40 mg)	10–80 mg every 12–24 hours	PO, IM
Benzodiazepines		
Lorazepam	0.5–2.0 mg every 1–4 hours	PO, IV, IM
Midazolam	30–100 mg every 24 hours	IV, SC
Anesthetics		
Propofol	10–70 mg every hour Up to 200–400 mg/h	IV

PO, per oral; IM, intramuscular; IV, intravenous; SC, subcutaneous.

comparison trial of haloperidol versus chlorpromazine versus lorazepam, Breitbart and colleagues demonstrated that lorazepam alone, in doses up to 8 mg in a 12-hour period, was ineffective in the treatment of delirium and contributed to worsening delirium and cognitive impairment.[4**] Both neuroleptic drugs however, in low doses (approximately 2 mg of haloperidol equivalent/per 24 hours), were highly effective in controlling the symptoms of delirium (dramatic improvement in DRS scores) and improving cognitive function (dramatic improvement in MMSE scores). In addition, both haloperidol and chlorpromazine were demonstrated to significantly improve the symptoms of delirium in both the 'hypoactive' as well as the 'hyperactive' subtypes of delirium.[4**] Methotrimeprazine, a phenothiazine neuroleptic with properties similar to chlorpromazine, is often used parenterally (IV or by SC infusion) to control confusion and agitation in terminal delirium.[78*] Dosages range from 12.5 mg to 50 mg every 4–8 hours up to 300 mg per 24 hours for most patients, including the elderly where doses at the lower end of the range are preferable. Hypotension and excessive sedation are potential limitations of this drug; however, methotrimeprazine has the advantage of also being an analgesic, equipotent to morphine, through nonopioid mechanisms.[78]

ATYPICAL NEUROLEPTICS

Several new, atypical, antipsychotic agents with less or more specific dopamine-blocking effects (less risk of extrapyramidal side effects or tardive dyskinesia) are now available and include such agents as risperidone, olanzapine, quetiapine, and ziprasidone.[79–83] Risperidone has been useful in the treatment of dementia and psychosis in AIDS patients at doses of 1–6 mg daily, suggesting safe use in patients with delirium.[82] Until recently, there have been only a limited number of published studies of the use of these agents in the treatment of delirium.[80–83] Schwartz and Massand's review of the use of atypical antipsychotics in delirium in 2002 included mostly case reports and retrospective studies.[84] In the interval, a number of additional studies have been published.

A retrospective analysis of 77 patients who received either haloperidol or risperidone for delirium indicated that both were effective in reducing symptoms of delirium and suggested that risperidone reduced the need for prescribing anticholinergic agents to treat extrapyramidal effects.[85*] Two small open prospective studies supported the use of risperidone for the treatment of symptoms of delirium with minimal risk of sedation or extrapyramidal side effects.[86*,87*] In a third larger open label study of 64 patients, patients with a risperidone intervention achieved a significant reduction in DRS scores during a 7-day observation period with minimal sedation or extrapyramidal effects.[88*] In a recent double blind, comparative delirium intervention study assessing the efficacy of haloperidol versus risperidone, Han and Kim demonstrated in a small sample of 24 oncology patients that

there was no significant difference in clinical efficacy or response rate.[89*]

Breitbart and colleagues recently published the results of a large (N = 82) open trial of olanzapine for the treatment of delirium in hospitalized patients with advanced cancer.[83*] Olanzapine was highly effective in the treatment of delirium, resolving delirium in 76 percent of patients with no incidence of extrapyramidal side effects. Several factors were found to be significantly associated with poorer response to olanzapine treatment for delirium, including age over 70, history of dementia, and hypoactive delirium. The average starting dose was in the 2.5–5 mg range and patients were given up to 20 mg per day of olanzapine. Sedation was the most common side effect. A small comparative study of haloperidol versus olanzapine for the treatment of delirium in 11 patients suggested equivalent efficacy and a favorable side effect profile for olanzapine.[81*] In another open label study, olanzapine significantly reduced DRS scores in 20 patients with lymphoma who experienced delirium, however, side effects were not systematically assessed.[90*] Most recently, a study compared olanzapine to haloperidol in a critical care setting over a 5-day observation period. The authors demonstrated significant improvement in both groups.[91*] Thirteen percent of the patients receiving haloperidol experienced mild parkinsonian side effects while none of the patients receiving olanzapine experienced extrapyramidal side effects.[91]

As a result of increasing clinical experience, more palliative care clinicians are using risperidone in low doses (e.g. 0.5–1.0 mg twice a day, orally) as well as olanzapine (2.5–20 mg/day in divided doses) in the management of delirium in terminally ill patients, particularly in those who have a demonstrated intolerance to the extrapyramidal side effects of the classic neuroleptics.[92] Currently, a limitation on the use of these new agents is the lack of availability of these agents in parenteral formulations. Figure 72.2 illustrates an algorithm that has been developed for use by the Memorial Sloan–Kettering Cancer Center Psychiatry Service for the management of delirium in hospitalized cancer patients.

Clinicians are beginning to examine the efficacy and tolerability of even newer atypical antipsychotics, quetiapine and ziprasidone. A few authors have published their experience with quetiapine for the treatment of delirium. Schwartz and Massand's retrospective review of 11 patients treated with quetiapine compared with patients who received haloperidol demonstrated a significant decline in DRS scores in 10/11 patients with only two patients experiencing sedation with an average dose of quetiapine 200 mg daily.[93*] None of the patients in the quetiapine group demonstrated evidence of extrapyramidal effects in contrast with two patients in the haloperidol group experiencing extrapyramidal side effects.[93] Kim et al. reported on a case series of 12 elderly patients with delirium who received quetiapine for delirium.[94*] There was a significant decline in the DRS scores, however, the authors were unable to determine if

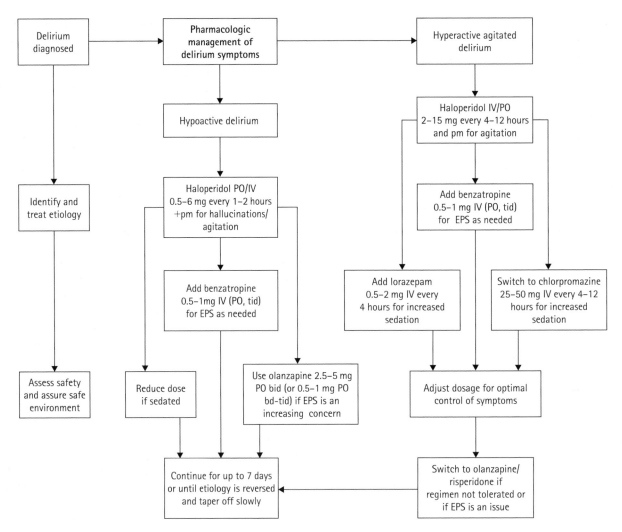

Figure 72.2 *The delirium algorithm. pm, evening; IV, intravenous; PO, per oral; tid, three times daily; EPS, extrapyramidal side effects; bd, twice daily.*

quetiapine treatment or effective resolution of the underlying etiology accounted for a reduction in symptoms.[94] Sasaki *et al.* published a prospective open label trial of 12 patients with postoperative delirium of diverse etiologies who had already received other antipsychotics and/or benzodiazepines without efficacy prior to the introduction of quetiapine.[95*] Although DRS scores significantly improved, the efficacy of quetiapine was difficult to determine as patients continued to receive haloperidol and benzodiazepines for severe agitation.[95] Pae *et al.*'s open label trial in 22 Korean patients with delirium demonstrated significant DRS score reduction in 85 percent of patients.[96*] Three patients experienced sedation and two patients were unable to complete the study (one due to lack of efficacy and one due to oversedation). No patient experienced extrapyramidal side effects.[96] Leso and Schwartz published the first case report of ziprasidone in the treatment of delirium.[97*] A young, human immunodeficiency virus (HIV)+ patient with delirium due to cryptococcal meningitis responded with a reduction in DRS score from 26 to 14

with a total daily dose of ziprasidone 100 mg.[97*] Ziprasidone treatment was discontinued due to hypokalemia and hypomagnesemia and ECG premature ventricular contractions and a calculated 8.4 percent prolongation in QTc interval.[97] Young and Lujan published the first case report of intravenous ziprasidone in the treatment of delirium in a postoperative patient in the intensive care unit who failed to respond to standard haloperidol treatment.[98*] The authors described an effective reduction in dangerous agitation but did not report which measurement scale was used to rate delirium symptoms.[98]

While neuroleptics are most effective in diminishing agitation, clearing the sensorium and improving cognition is not always possible in delirium which complicates the last days of life. Processes causing delirium may be ongoing and irreversible during the active dying phase. Ventafridda and colleagues[99] and Fainsinger and colleagues[26] have reported that 10–20 percent of terminally ill patients experience delirium that can only be controlled by sedation resulting in a significantly decreased level of consciousness.

Lawlor and colleagues report that at least 50 percent of terminal delirium is reversible.[32] The goal of treatment with agents such as midazolam, propofol, and methotrimeprazine is quiet sedation. Midazolam, given by SC or IV infusion in doses ranging from 30 mg to 100 mg per 24 hours, can be used to control agitation related to delirium in the terminal stages.[100*] Propofol, a short-acting anesthetic agent, has also begun to be used primarily as a sedating agent for the control of agitated patients with 'terminal' delirium. In several case reports of propofol used in terminal care, an IV loading dose of 20 mg of propofol was followed by a continuous infusion of propofol with initial doses ranging from 10 mg/h to 70 mg/h with titration of doses up to as high as 400 mg/h over a period of hours to days in severely agitated patients.[101*,102*] Propofol has an advantage over midazolam in that the level of sedation is more easily controlled and recovery is rapid upon decreasing the rate of infusion.[101]

Controversies in the management of terminal delirium

Several aspects of the use of neuroleptics and other pharmacological agents in the management of delirium in the dying patient remain controversial in some circles. Some have argued that pharmacological interventions with neuroleptics or benzodiazepines are inappropriate in the dying patient. Delirium is viewed by some as a natural part of the dying process that should not be altered. In particular, there are clinicians who care for the dying who view hallucinations and delusions which involve dead relatives communicating with, or in fact welcoming dying patients to heaven, as an important element in the transition from life to death. Clearly, there are many patients who experience hallucinations and delusions during delirium that are pleasant and in fact comforting, and many clinicians question the appropriateness of intervening pharmacologically in such instances. Another concern that is often raised is that these patients are so close to death that aggressive treatment is unnecessary. Parenteral neuroleptics or sedatives may be mistakenly avoided because of exaggerated fears that they might hasten death through hypotension or respiratory depression. Many are unnecessarily pessimistic about the possible results of neuroleptic treatment for delirium. They argue that since the underlying pathophysiological process often continues unabated (such as hepatic or renal failure), no improvement can be expected in the patient's mental status. There is concern that neuroleptics or sedatives may worsen a delirium by making the patient more confused or sedated.

Clinical experience in managing delirium in dying patients suggests that the use of neuroleptics in the management of agitation, paranoia, hallucinations and altered sensorium is safe, effective and often quite appropriate.[76] Management of delirium on a case by case basis seems wisest. The agitated, delirious dying patient should probably be given neuroleptics to help restore calm. A 'wait and see' approach, prior to using neuroleptics, may be appropriate with some patients who have a lethargic, or somnolent presentation of delirium, or those who are having frankly pleasant or comforting hallucinations. Such a 'wait and see' approach must, however, be tempered by the knowledge that a lethargic or 'hypoactive', delirium may very quickly and unexpectedly become an agitated or 'hyperactive' delirium that can threaten the serenity and safety of the patient, family and staff. An additional rationale for intervening pharmacologically with patients who have a lethargic or 'hypoactive' delirium is recent evidence that neuroleptics (i.e. haloperidol, chlorpromazine) are effective in controlling the symptoms of delirium in both 'hyperactive' as well as 'hypoactive' subtypes of delirium.[4] In fact neuroleptics improved both the arousal disturbance, as well as cognitive functioning in patients with 'hypoactive' delirium. Also, some clinicians suggest that 'hypoactive' delirium may respond to psychostimulants or combinations of neuroleptics and stimulants.[54] Similarly, hallucinations and delusions during a delirium that are pleasant and comforting can quickly become menacing and terrifying. It is important to remember that by their nature, the symptoms of delirium are unstable and fluctuate over time.

Finally, perhaps the most challenging of clinical problems is management of the dying patient with a 'terminal' delirium that is unresponsive to standard neuroleptic interventions, whose symptoms can only be controlled by sedation to the point of a significantly decreased level of consciousness. Before undertaking interventions, such as midazolam or propofol infusions, where the best achievable goal is a calm and comfortable but sedated and unresponsive patient, the clinician must first take several steps. The clinician must have a discussion with the family (and the patient if there are lucid moments when the patient appears to have capacity) eliciting their concerns and wishes for the type of care that can best honor their desire to provide comfort and symptom control during the dying process. The clinician should describe the optimal achievable goals of therapy as they currently exist. Family members should be informed that the goal of sedation is to provide comfort and symptom control, not to hasten death. They should also be told to anticipate that sedation may result in a premature sense of loss and that they may feel their loved one is in some sort of limbo state, not yet dead, but yet no longer alive in the vital sense. The distress and confusion that family members can experience during such a period can be ameliorated by including the family in the decision making and emphasizing the shared goals of care. Sedation in such patients is not always complete or irreversible; some patients have periods of wakefulness despite sedation, and many clinicians will periodically lighten sedation to reassess the patient's condition. Ultimately, the clinician must always keep in mind the goals of care and communicate these goals to the staff, patients and family members. The clinician must weigh each of the issues outlined above in making decisions on how to best manage the dying patient who presents with delirium that preserves and respects the dignity and values of that individual and family.

Key learning points

- Delirium occurs in up to 85 percent of patients prior to death.

- Delirium is categorized into subtypes based on arousal or motoric disturbance. Hypoactive delirium is as common and as distressing as hyperactive delirium.

- There are typically three or more etiologies for delirium in the palliative care setting.

- In the terminally ill, delirium is reversible in only 50 percent of cases compared with 95 percent of cases in patients with earlier stage disease.

- The management of delirium involves the concurrent search for and treatment of the underlying etiology while actively controlling the symptoms of delirium.

- Delirium often is a harbinger of impending death. Issues of end-of-life care treatment preferences are ideally dealt with prior to the onset of delirium.

- Delirium is associated with high levels of distress in patients, family members, and nurses. Education of family members and nurses in the palliative care setting is important.

- Neuroleptics are effective in controlling the symptoms of delirium.

- Atypical neuroleptics are demonstrating efficacy in controlling the symptoms of delirium with less extrapyramidal side effects.

- Sedation may be necessary in up to 30 percent of patients with delirium unresponsive to neuroleptics.

REFERENCES

1   American Psychiatric Association. *Diagnostic and Statistical Manual of Mental Disorders*. Washington DC: APA, 1994.

● 2   Lipowski Z. *Delirium: Acute Brain Failure in Man*. Springfield, IL: Charles C Thomas, 1980.

◆ 3   Ross C. CNS arousal systems: possible role in delirium. *Int Psychogeriatr* 1991; **3**: 353–71.

● 4   Breitbart W, Marotta R, Platt M. A double-blind comparison trial of haloperidol, chlorpromazine, and lorazepam in the treatment of delirium in hospitalized AIDS patients. *Am J Psychiatry* 1996; **153**: 231–7.

● 5   Massie M, Holland J, Glass E. Delirium in terminally ill cancer patients. *Am J Psychiatry* 1983; **140**: 1048–50.

6   Bruera E, Miller L, McCallion J. Cognitive failure in patients with terminal cancer: a prospective study. *J Pain Symptom Manage* 1992; **7**: 192–5.

7   Fainsinger R, Young C. Cognitive failure in a terminally ill patient. *J Pain Symptom Manage* 1991; 492–4.

8   Leipzig R, Goodman H, Gray G. Reversible narcotic associated mental status impairment in patients with metastatic cancer. *Pharmacology* 1987; **35**: 47–54.

9   Levine P, Silberfarb P, Lipowski Z. Mental disorders in cancer patients: a study of 100 psychiatric referrals. *Cancer* 1978; **42**: 1385–91.

10 Murray G. Confusion, delirium, and dementia. In: Hackett T, Cassem N, eds. *Massachusetts General Hospital Handbook of General Hospital Psychiatry*, 2nd ed. Littleton, MA: PSG Publishing, 1987; 84–115.

11 Posner J. Delirium and exogenous metabolic brain disease. In: Beeson P, McDermott W, Wyngaarden J, eds. *Cecil Textbook of Medicine*. Philadelphia: WB Saunders, 1979; 644–51.

12 Knight E, Folstein M. Unsuspected emotional and cognitive disturbance in medical patients. *Ann Intern Med* 1977; **87**: 723–4.

● 13 Pereira J, Hanson J, Bruera E. The frequency and clinical course of cognitive impairment in patients with terminal cancer. *Cancer* 1997; 835–41.

● 14 Lipowski Z. *Delirium: Acute Confusional States*. New York: Oxford University Press, 1990.

15 Tune L. Post-operative delirium. *Int Psychogeriatr* 1991; **3**: 325–32.

16 Gillick M, Serrel N, Gillick L. Adverse consequences of hospitalization in the elderly. *Soc Sci Med* 1982; **16**: 1033–8.

17 Berman K, Eastham E. Psychogeriatric ascertainment and assessment for treatment in an acute medical ward setting. *Aging* 1974; **3**: 174–88.

18 Warsaw G, Moore J, Friedman S. Functional disability in the hospitalized elderly. *JAMA* 1982; **248**: 847–50.

19 Seymour D, Henschke P, Cape R. Acute confusional states and dementia in the elderly: the role of dehydration/volume depletion, physical illness, and age. *Aging* 1980; **9**: 137–46.

20 Hodkinson H. Mental impairment in the elderly. *J R Coll Phys Lond* 1973; **7**: 305–17.

21 Varsamis J, Zuchowski T, Maini K. Survival rates and causes of death in geriatric psychiatric patients: a six year follow-up study. *Can Psychiatr Assoc J* 1972; **17**: 17–22.

● 22 Breitbart W, Gibson C, Tremblay A. The delirium experience: delirium recall and delirium related distress in hospitalized patients with cancer, their spouses/caregivers, and their nurses. *Psychosomatics* 2002; **43**: 183–94.

23 Bruera E, Fainsinger R, Miller M, Kuehn N. The assessment of pain intensity in patients with cognitive failure: a preliminary report. *J Pain Symptom Manage* 1992; **7**: 267–70.

◆ 24 Trzepacz P, Teague G, Lipowski Z. Delirium and other organic mental disorders in a general hospital. *Gen Hosp Psychiatry* 1985; **7**: 101–6.

25 Coyle N, Breitbart W, Weaver S, Portenoy R. Delirium as a contributing factor to 'Crescendo' pain: three case reports. *J Pain Symptom Manage* 1994; **9**: 44–7.

26 Fainsinger R, MacEachern T, Hanson J. Symptom control during the last week of life in a palliative care unit. *J Palliat Care* 1991; **7**: 5–11.

● 27 Morita T, Tei Y, Inouye S. Impaired communication capacity and agitated delirium in the final week of terminally ill cancer patients: prevalence and identification of research focus. *J Pain Symptom Manage* 2003; **26**: 827–34.

◆ 28 Stiefel F, Breitbart W, Holland J. Corticosteroids in cancer: neuropsychiatric complications. *Cancer Invest* 1989; **7**: 479–91.

29 Bruera E, MacMillin K, Hanson J. The cognitive effects of the administration of narcotic analgesics in patients with cancer pain. *Pain* 1989; **39**: 13–16.

30 Silberfarb P. Chemotherapy and cognitive deficits in patients with cancer. *Annu Rev Med* 1983; **34**: 35–46.

31 Stiefel F, Fainsinger R, Bruera E. Acute confusional states in patients with advanced cancer. *J Pain Symptom Manage* 1992; **7**: 94–8.

● 32 Lawlor P, Gagnon B, Mancini I, *et al*. The occurrence, causes and outcomes of delirium in advanced cancer patients: a prospective study. *Arch Intern Med* 2002; **160**: 786–94.

33 Wise M, Brandt G. Delirium. In: Yudofsky S, Hales R, eds. *Textbook of Neuropsychiatry*, 2nd ed. Washington, DC: American Psychiatric Association, 1992.

◆ 34 Breitbart W, Bruera E, Chochinov H. Neuropsychiatric syndromes and psychological symptoms in patients with advanced cancer. *J Pain Symptom Manage* 1995; **10**: 131–41.

35 Beaver W, Wallenstein S, Houde R. A comparison of the analgesic effect of methotrimeprazine and morphine in patients with cancer. *Clin Pharmacol Ther* 1966; **7**: 436–46.

36 Walsh T. Adjuvant analgesic therapy in cancer pain. In: Foley K, Bonica J, Ventafridda V, eds. *Advances in Pain Research and Therapy*, Vol. 16. New York: Raven Press; 1990: 155–66.

◆ 37 Ross C, Peyser C, Shapiro I, Folstein M. Delirium: Phenomenologic and etiologic subtypes. *Int Psychogeriatr* 1991; **3**: 135–47.

● 38 Breitbart W, Rosenfeld B, Roth A. The Memorial Delirium Assessment Scale. *J Pain Symptom Manage* 1997; **13**: 128–37.

39 Albert M, Levkoff S, Reilley C. The delirium symptom interview: an interview for the detection of delirium symptoms in hospitalized patients. *J Geriatr Psychiatry Neurol* 1991; **5**: 14–21.

40 Folstein M, Folstein S, McHugh P. 'Mini-Mental Status': a practical method for grading the cognitive state of patients for clinicians. *J Psychiatr Res* 1975; **12**: 189–98.

41 Jacobs J, Bernhard M, A D, Strain J. Screening for organic mental syndromes in the medically ill. *Ann Intern Med* 1977; **86**: 40–6.

42 Katzman R, Brown T, Fuld P. Validation of a short orientation-memory-concentration test of cognitive impairment. *Am J Psychiatry* 1983; **140**: 734–9.

◆ 43 Levkoff S, Liptzin B, Cleary P. Review of research instruments and techniques to detect delirium. *Int Psychogeriatr* 1992; **3**: 253–72.

● 44 Trzepacz P, Baker R, Greenhouse J. A symptom rating scale of delirium. *Psychiatry Res* 1988; **23**: 89–97.

45 Williams M. Delirium/acute confusional states: evaluation devices in nursing. *Int Psychogeriatr* 1991; **3**: 301–8.

46 Wolber G, Romaniuk M, Eastman E, Robinson C. Validity of the Short Portable Mental Status Questionaire with elderly psychiatric patients. *J Consult Clin Psychol* 1984; **52**: 712–13.

◆ 47 Smith M, Breitbart W, Platt M. A critique of instruments and methods to detect, diagnose and rate delirium. *J Pain Symptom Manage* 1995; **10**: 35–77.

● 48 Trzepacz P, Mittal D, Torres R, *et al*. Validity of the Delirium Rating Scale-Revised-98 (DRS-98). Paper presented at: 46th Annual Meeting of the Academy of Psychosomatic Medicine; November 18–21, 1999, New Orleans, LA.

● 49 Inouye B, Vandyck C, Alessi C. Clarifying confusion: the confusion assessment method, a new method for the detection of delirium. *Ann Intern Med* 1990; **113**: 941–8.

50 Hart R, Best A, Sessler C, Levenson J. Abbreviated cognitive test for delirium. *J Psychosom Research* 1997; **43**: 417–23.

● 51 Lawlor P, Nekolaichuck C, Gagnon B, *et al*. Clinical utility, factor analysis and further validation of the Memorial Delirium Assessment Scale (MDAS). *Cancer* 2000; **88**: 2859–67.

52 Lichter I, Hunt E. The last 24 hours of life. *J Palliat Care* 1990; **6**: 7–15.

✳ 53 American Psychiatric Association, Practice Guidelines for the Treatment of Patients with Delirium. *Am J Psychiatry* 1999; **156**: S1–S20.

54 Fainsinger R, Bruera E. Treatment of delirium in a terminally ill patient. *J Pain Symptom Manage* 1992; **7**: 54–6.

55 Young D. Neurological complications of cancer chemotherapy. In: Silverstein A, ed. *Neurological Complications of Therapy: Selected Topics*. New York: Futura; 1982: 57–113.

56 Holland J, Fasanello S, Ohnuma T. Psychiatric symptoms associated with L-asparaginase administration. *J Psychiatr Res* 1974; **10**: 105–13.

57 Adams F, Quesada J, Gutterman J. Neuropsychiatric manifestations of human leukocyte interferon therapy in patients with cancer. *JAMA* 1984; **252**: 939–41.

58 Denicoff K, Rubinow D, Papa M. The neuropsychiatric effects of treatment with interleukin-2 and lymphokine-activated killer cells. *Ann Intern Med* 1987; **107**: 293–300.

59 Weddington W. Delirium and depression associated with amphotericin B. *Psychosomatics* 1982; **23**: 1076–8.

60 DeAngelis L, Delattre J, Posner J. Radiation-induced dementia in patients cured of brain metastases. *Neurology* 1989; **39**: 789–96.

● 61 Inouye B, Bogardus Jr S, Charpentier P, *et al*. A multicomponent intervention to prevent delirium in hospitalized older patients. *N Engl J Med* 1999; 669–76.

62 Derogatis L, Feldstein M, Morrow G. A survey of psychotropic drug prescriptions in an oncology population. *Cancer* 1979; **44**: 1919–29.

63 Stiefel F, Kornblith A, Holland J. Changes in the prescription patterns of psychotropic drugs for cancer patients during a 10 year period. *Cancer* 1990; **65**: 1048–53.

64 Goldberg G, Mor V. A survey of psychotropic use in terminal cancer patients. *Psychosomatics* 1985; **26**: 745–51.

65 Jaeger H, Morrow G, Brescia F. A survey of psychotropic drug utilization by patients with advanced neoplastic disease. *Gen Hosp Psychiatry* 1985; **7**: 353–60.

66 Chochinov H, Breitbart W, eds. *Handbook of Psychiatry in Palliative Medicine*. New York: Oxford University Press, 2000.

67 Akechi T, Uchitomi Y, Okamura H. Usage of haloperidol for delirium in cancer patients. *Support Cancer Care* 1996; **4**: 390–2.

68 Fernandez F, Levy J, Mansell P. Management of delirium in terminally ill AIDS patients. *Int J Psychiat Med* 1989; **19**: 165–72.

● 69 Rosen J. Double-blind comparison of haloperidol and thioridazine in geriatric outpatients. *J Clin Psychiatry* 1979; **40**: 17–20.

● 70 Smith G, Taylor C, Linkons P. Haloperidol versus thioridazine for the treatment of psychogeriatric patients: a double-blind clinical trial. *Psychosomatics* 1974; **15**: 134–8.

71 Thomas H, Schwartz E, Petrilli R. Droperidol versus haloperidol for chemical restraint of agitated and combative patients. *Ann Emerg Med* 1992; **21**: 407–13.

72 Tsuang M, Lu L, Stotsky B, Cole J. Haloperidol versus thioridazine for hospitalized psychogeriatric patients: double-blind study. *J Am Geriatr Soc* 1971; **19**: 593–600.

73 Fernandez F, Holmes V, Adams F, Kavanaugh J. Treatment of severe refractory agitation with a Haldol drip. *J Clin Psychiatry* 1988; **49**: 239–41.

74 Breitbart W. Psychiatric management of cancer pain. *Cancer* 1989; **63**: 2336–42.

75 Twycross R, Lack S. *Symptom Control in Far Advanced Cancer: Pain Relief.* London: Pitman, 1983.

◆ 76 Breitbart W. Diagnosis and management of delirium in the terminally ill. In: Portenoy R, Bruera E, eds. *Topics in Palliative Care*, Vol **5**. New York: Oxford University Press, 2001: 303–21.

77 Menza M, Murray G, Holmes V. Controlled study of extrapyramidal reactions in the management of delirious medically ill patients: Intravenous haloperidol versus haloperidol plus benzodiazepines. *Heart Lung* 1988; **17**: 238–41.

78 Oliver D. The use of methotrimeprazine in terminal care. *Br J Clin Pract* 1985; **39**: 339–40.

79 Baldessarini R, Frankenburg F. Clozapine: a novel antipsychotic agent. *N Engl J Med* 1991; **324**: 746–52.

80 Passik S, Cooper M. Complicated delirium in a cancer patient successfully treated with olanzapine. *J Pain Symptom Manage* 1999; **17**: 219–23.

81 Sipahimalani A, Massand P. Olanzapine in the treatment of delirium. *Psychosomatics* 1998; **39**: 422–30.

82 Sipahimalani A, Sime R, Massand P. Treatment of delirium with risperidone. *Int J Geriatr Psychopharmacol* 1997; **1**: 24–6.

● 83 Breitbart W, Tremblay A, Gibson C. An open trial of olanzapine for the treatment of delirium in hospitalized cancer patients. *Psychosomatics* 2002; **43**: 175–6.

84 Schwartz T, Massand P. The role of atypical antipsychotics in the treatment of delirium. *Psychosomatics* 2002; **43**: 171–4.

85 Liu C, Juang Y, Liang H. Efficacy of risperidone in treating the hyperactive symptoms of delirium. *Int Clin Psychopharmacol* 2004; **19**: 165–8.

86 Horikawa N, Yamazaki T, Miyamoto K. Treatment for delirium with risperidone: results of a prospective open trial with 10 patients. *Gen Hosp Psychiatry* 2003; **25**: 289–92.

87 Mittal D, Jimerson N, Neely E. Risperidone in the treatment of delirium: results from a prospective open-label trial. *J Clin Psychiatry* 2004; **65**: 662–7.

88 Parellada E, Baeza I, de Pablo J. Risperidone in the treatment of patients with delirium. *J Clin Psychiatry* 2004; **65**: 348–53.

● 89 Han C, Kim Y. A double-blind trial of risperidone and haloperidol for the treatment of delirium. *Psychosomatics* 2004; **45**: 297–301.

90 Kim K, Pae C, JH C. An open pilot trial of olanzapine for delirium in the Korean population. *Psychiatry Clin Neurosci* 2001; **55**: 515–19.

91 Skrobik Y, Bergeron N, Dumont M. Olanzapine vs haloperidol: treating delirium in a critical care setting. *Intensive Care Med* 2004; **30**: 444–9.

◆ 92 Breitbart W, Chochinov H, Passik S. Psychiatric aspects of palliative care. In: Doyle D, Hanks G, MacDonald N, eds. *Oxford Textbook of Palliative Medicine*, 2nd ed. New York: Oxford University Press, 1998: 933–54.

93 Schwartz T, Massand P. Treatment of delirium with quetiapine. *Prim Care Companion J Clin Psychiatry* 2000; **2**: 10–12.

94 Kim K, Bader G, Kotlyar V. Treatment of delirium in older adults with quetiapine. *J Geriatr Psychiatry Neurol* 2003; **16**: 29–31.

95 Sasaki Y, Matsuyama T, Inouye S. A prospective, open-label, flexible dose study of quetiapine in the treatment of delirium. *J Clin Psychiatry* 2003; **64**: 1316–1321.

96 Pae C, Lee S, Lee C. A pilot trial of quetiapine for the treatment of patients with delirium. *Hum Psychopharmacol* 2004; **19**: 125–7.

97 Leso L, Schwartz T. Ziprasidone treatment of delirium. *Psychosomatics* 2002; **43**: 61–2.

98 Young C, Lujan E. Intravenous ziprasidone for the treatment of delirium in the intensive care unit. *Anesthesiology* 2004; **101**: 794–5.

● 99 Ventafridda V, Ripamonti C, DeConno F. Symptom prevalence and control during cancer patients' last days of life. *J Palliat Care* 1990; **6**: 7–11.

100 Bottomley D, Hanks G. Subcutaneous midazolam infusion in palliative care. *J Pain Symptom Manage* 1990; **5**: 259–61.

101 Mercadante S, DeConno F, Ripamonti C. Propofol in terminal care. *J Pain Symptom Manage* 1995; **10**: 639–42.

102 Moyle J. The use of propofol in palliative medicine. *J Pain Symptom Manage* 1995; **10**: 643–6.

73

Sleeping disorders

FRITZ STIEFEL, DANIELE STAGNO

INTRODUCTION

Sleeping disorders are common in palliative care patients.[1***] The prevalence of insomnia – the most common sleep disorder in palliative care – is reported to range from 23 percent[2] to 70 percent;[3*] the latter percentage has been observed in a recent study, which actively searched for insomnia. Poor sleep affects quality of life and increases perception of symptoms, such as pain, and is therefore an important target of palliative care treatments.[4,5] Both patients and clinicians often consider poor sleep as inevitable in the context of a terminal illness[6*] and there is a trend to prescribe hypnotic drugs with unclear benefits. On the other hand, little attention is paid to the underlying causes of sleep disturbances.[7*]

Sleep disorders can be classified using two diagnostic systems: the International Classification of Sleep Disorders[8] and the Diagnostic and Statistical Manual of Mental Disorders (DSM-IV-TR)[9] (see Box 73.1).

Box 73.1 Classification of sleep disorders according to DSM-IV

Primary sleep disorders

Dyssomnias

- Primary insomnia
- Primary hypersomnia
- Narcolepsy
- Breathing-related sleep disorders
- Circadian rhythm sleep disorders
- Dyssomnias NOS (not otherwise specified)

Parasomnias

- Nightmare disorders
- Sleep terror disorders
- Sleepwalking disorders
- Parasomnias NOS (not otherwise specified)

Sleep disorder related to another mental disorder

Other sleep disorders

- Sleep disorders due to a general medical condition
- Substance-induced sleep disorders

These classification systems may be helpful for the clinician in diagnosing specific sleep disorders and during adjusting management. In palliative care, insomnia due to multiple etiologies – due to the general medical condition, substance-induced and related to another mental disorder – is the most frequently encountered sleep disorder.[1–3] Other forms of primary sleep disorders are relatively rare; this chapter therefore focuses on insomnia.

MEDIATING VARIABLES OF INSOMNIA IN PALLIATIVE CARE

The most important mediating variables of insomnia in palliative care are pain and depression.[10***] Sleep disorders and pain are closely related phenomena. Most epidemiological studies of the impact of pain on sleep are based on self-report; since the definition of normal sleep is not well established, the prevalence of insomnia varies widely. Nevertheless, sleep disorders occur in up to 27 percent of primary care populations[11] and more frequently in the elderly and in patients with advanced medical illness.[12] Pain certainly promotes insomnia, but it is also the individual's emotional, cognitive, and behavioral response that lead to its chronic development.[13] From a clinical point of view, the relation between insomnia and pain appears to be straightforward: pain causes arousal and arousal interferes with the ability to initiate and maintain sleep.[14] However, the few studies investigating this relationship showed a significant, but only moderate positive relationship between pain severity and sleep complaints. Smith *et al.* therefore suggested that the relation may be more complex and not unidirectional; their hypothesis is that pain-related arousal is different from the somatic and/or cognitive arousal of insomnia, even if mediating variables are likely to exist.[15]

One of the best-studied mediating variables in insomnia is depression, but this literature also remains controversial. For example up to 87 percent of chronic pain patients show depressive disorders;[16***] moreover sleep complaints correlate stronger with severity of depression than pain severity.[17–19] On the other hand, Morin *et al.* showed that rating of depression and anxiety did not distinguish patients with chronic pain with or without sleep disturbances.[20*] They suggested that sleep disturbance in patients with chronic pain does not necessarily reflect an underlying emotional disorder. Thus psychiatric morbidity associated with chronic pain seems to be more often a consequence than a cause of pain.[20*,21*]

Many other somatic symptoms (e.g. nausea, dyspnea, or urinary disturbances) and psychiatric disorders (e.g. anxiety, delirium, or substance abuse and withdrawal) may be mediating variables of insomnia. Since the relationships between somatic and psychiatric disturbances and insomnia often remain unsolvable in the individual patient, palliative care physicians have to ensure that both physical and psychiatric disturbances are evaluated and treated.

In recent years there has been increasing emphasis on the relationship between sleep disorders and alterations of immunity.[1] Interferon α (endogenous or exogenous) has now long been incriminated as a causative factor for depression, psychotic disorders, and sleep disorders. Those symptoms are probably mediated by the release of proinflammatory cytokines and an activation of the hypothalamic–pituitary–adrenal (HPA) axis.[22] Insomnia is also negatively correlated with the activity of natural killer cells.[23] Activity of proinflammatory cytokines is increased in people with chronic sleep disturbances[24] and cancer patients especially those with pancreatic cancer.[25,26] Patients receiving antineoplastic drugs as well as radiotherapy show increased sleep disturbances.[1] The mechanisms are unknown, although not surprisingly the immune system may be concerned.

ASSESSMENT

Insomnia is best defined as a complaint by the patient – similar to the definition of pain – of poor or unsatisfactory sleep; this complaint may include different aspects, such as the difficulty to initiate sleep, repeated or lengthy awakenings, early awakening, inadequate total sleep time, poor quality of sleep, or daytime dysfunction such as change of alertness, loss of energy or cognitive, behavioral and emotional changes.[27] A systematic evaluation of insomnia is the key to its adequate management (see Box 73.2).[11]

Box 73.2 Recommendations for the assessment of insomnia in the palliative setting

- Avoid a nihilistic attitude leading to an inadequate prescription of hypnotics

- Try to evaluate the complaints as accurately as possible and identify mediating factors and maladaptive responses to insomnia

- Establish a diagnosis of insomnia if residual daytime effects are present

- Identify possible links between insomnia and somatic and psychological state

- Evaluate if mediating factors of insomnia can be influenced

- Introduce sleep hygiene measures and give the patient written instructions

- Teach nonpharmacological interventions with which you are familiar

- Consider pharmacological treatment if the above mentioned interventions are not successful

- Think about alternatives to benzodiazepines, especially in patients with psychiatric comorbidity and older patients

- Use benzodiazepines, following the recommendations for their use in patients with somatic diseases

- Monitor treatment and continue to offer a therapeutic relationship

---

The first step is an accurate evaluation of the reported symptoms. Although this may be considered as common sense, it has to be remembered that 53 percent of physicians evaluating older patients neglect eliciting any sleep history.[28***] An adequate sleep history – sleep and wakefulness patterns, history of the bed partner, family history of sleep disorders and previous treatments – should be obtained first. Complaints of inadequate sleep in the absence of any residual daytime effects or distress do not indicate significant insomnia.[27] Insomnia causes psychosocial, physical and occupational disturbances, commonly reported as fatigue/lethargy, mood disturbances, cognitive inefficiency, motor impairments, social discomfort, and nonspecific physical symptoms.[29]

Tools have been developed to promote a structured evaluation of insomnia by clinicians; among these is the interview for sleep disorders according to the DSM-III-R,[30] which shows a good interrater reliability and concordance with the electroencephalogram (EEG) (the gold standard to assess sleep disturbances). Another instrument is the Pittsburgh Sleep Quality Index (PSQI),[31,32] a 19-item self-report questionnaire measuring sleep quality. A more specific tool is the Audit of Insomnia In Palliative Care.[3] This 15-item questionnaire is based on key features related to insomnia in the palliative care setting. Questions refer to the presence of sleep disturbance, its physical or psychological causes, sleep pattern, medication, previous and current use of hypnotics, and patients' own suggestions as to what measures may improve their insomnia.

Once the diagnosis of insomnia has been established, mediating somatic and psychiatric disturbances should be identified, since treatment will first attempt to target these factors. Finally, the individual's maladaptive cognitive, behavioral and emotional responses, which may be responsible for a chronic development of insomnia, have to be assessed. Maladaptive responses consist for example of anticipation of insomnia towards bedtime (cognition), excessive time spent in bed without sleeping (behavioral) or irritation upon nighttime wake ups (emotional). Identification of these responses is important to explain sleep hygiene measures and to motivate the patient for nonpharmacological interventions.

MANAGEMENT

Whenever possible, a treatment should target mediating somatic and psychiatric factors. If identification of such factors is not possible or if they are not present (anymore), symptomatic treatment of insomnia will be necessary. Before prescribing hypnotics, sleep hygiene measures and basic behavioral interventions should be considered.

Nonpharmacological management

Recognition of maladaptive psychological and behavioral responses to insomnia has led to the development of non-pharmacological interventions,[33,34] which can also be used in the palliative care setting. Although these interventions are easy to implement, they remain unknown and underused. Among them, sleep hygiene measures are most important and should always be part of the management of insomnia. After verbal discussion, instructions should be given in a written form to the patient and checked during follow-up visits. Sleep hygiene measures have considerable face validity but have not been tested for efficacy in alleviating insomnia.[35***]

SLEEP HYGIENE MEASURES

- Wind down during the second half of the evening; rest for 60–90 minutes before bedtime; avoid intense thinking, discussions, and actions.
- Introduce a pre-sleeping routine.
- Practice relaxation techniques during the day and before bedtime.
- Create an adequate sleeping environment (bed, mattress, external sounds, temperature).
- Keep regular sleep hours, use bed for sleep (and sexual activity) only, avoid excessive time in bed and have a regular getting up time (regardless of the quality of the sleep).

BEHAVIORAL INTERVENTIONS

The American Academy of Sleep Medicine has provided interesting recommendations with different levels of evidence for the nonpharmacological treatment of chronic insomnia.[27] We describe those interventions which can easily be implemented in the palliative care setting; for other, more sophisticated interventions, such as biofeedback, paradoxical intention and cognitive therapy, the reader is referred to the literature.

- **Stimulus control** consists of providing a set of instructions that curtail behaviors incompatible with sleep and ensures that the patient does not spend time in bed awake.[35***] Since the patient may have developed a conditioned response associating the bedroom with poor sleep, the objective is to reassociate the bed and the bedroom with rapid sleep onset. The core instructions are similar to the sleep hygiene measures:
  - Lie down to sleep only when sleepy.
  - Use the bed only for sleep and sex.
  - If unable to fall asleep, get up and go to another room. Stay as long as needed, but when sleepy return to the bedroom to sleep.
  - When in bed and awake for longer than 10 minutes repeat previous step.
- **Imagery training** involves visualization, focusing on pleasant and neutral images. Patients with poor fantasy can remember joyful or peaceful moments of the past.[36]
- **Progressive muscle relaxation** consists of tensing and relaxing different muscle groups throughout the body. These techniques are easy to teach and to learn and are especially helpful for patients with chronic pain who display high levels of arousal.[37]

PHARMACOLOGICAL MANAGEMENT

More than 45 percent of clinicians investigating sleep disorders prescribe a medication after asking a mean of only 2.5 questions.[38] Hypnotic agents are routinely prescribed, but the rational for this practice has not been established.

The current opinion on the use and safety of hypnotics in the treatment of insomnia underlines the lack of strong evidence of major benefits and the existing evidence for potential harm.[38] Hypnotics should be considered only after sleep hygiene measures and nonpharmacological interventions have not been successful. Two consensus conferences[39***],[40***] have concluded that their short-term usage may be useful for acute and situational insomnia, but long-term use remains controversial. For example behavioral therapy and pharmacotherapy produce similar short-term outcomes as recently shown in a comparative meta-analysis of the treatment of persistent insomnia.[41***]

Hypnotics

Nearly half of chronic insomniac individuals who take sleeping pills derive little or no subjective benefits from the medication, although they continue to take the medication for years.[42*]

Benzodiazepines effectively suppress insomnia,[41***] but their use for this indication is a controversial issue. A careful evaluation of the patient, treatment of mediating factors, if possible, and nonpharmacological alternatives to the use of benzodiazepines is therefore mandatory.[43,44] If benzodiazepines are indicated, the following recommendations should be considered: use benzodiazepines only with lowest dosage and short periods (maximum 4 weeks); monitor side effects and do not interrupt their use abruptly.[28,38,43] The most relevant general aspects of the pharmacokinetics of benzodiazepine are summarized in Box 73.3.[43] The box indicates a high interindividual variation and shows that onset, distribution, and excretion are influenced by liver disease or decreased absorption in the gastrointestinal tract. Long-acting substances such as diazepam, nitrazepam or flurazepam can cause hangover, daytime drowsiness, dizziness

---

Box 73.3 Relevant pharmacokinetics of benzodiazepines with regard to their use in patients with an underlying medical condition

- Up to 10-fold interindividual variation

- Age, smoking, liver disease, physical illness, gender, and concomitant drugs influence distribution and elimination

- Long-acting substances associated with daytime side effects, short-acting substances with time-limited effects, amnesia, rebound and withdrawal difficulties

- Most substances metabolized by oxidation (more impaired by physical illness, liver disease, age, and other drugs), few by conjugation

- Most substances with active metabolites

---

and prolonged sedation, especially in terminally ill patients; these side effects are less important with intermediate-acting substances, which are conjugated and without active metabolites (e.g. lorazepam, oxazepam). Short-acting benzodiazepines can lead to early morning insomnia, daytime anxiety, tension or panic, amnesia, rebound and withdrawal difficulties.[45–47] With regard to drug interactions in patients experiencing pain, benzodiazepines have additive effects with morphine and other opioids (e.g. sedation, confusion).

Zolpidem for sleep induction and zopiclone for night awakening, although not belonging to the chemical class of benzodiazepines, share many pharmacological features with this group of drugs. These agents can be prescribed as an alternative to classical benzodiazepines, with similar indications and safety warnings.[48***] Nevertheless, with regard to prescription of zolpidem, zopiclone, and zaleplon no reliable data are available.[49***]

Barbiturates are used rarely; these drugs have a greater tendency to depress respiration and are generally less effective than benzodiazepines. Barbiturates have a high abuse potential and a narrow therapeutic margin, and therefore have been withdrawn from the market in several countries.

A careful evaluation of the risk–benefit ratio should precede a treatment with benzodiazepines. The problem with prescribing benzodiazepines is not the potential abuse, withdrawal symptoms, and drug interactions, but rather the mishandling by clinicians who prescribe them without clear-cut indication or those who use them to get rid of an embarrassing problem.[48]

Antidepressants, neuroleptics, and other psychotropics

Sedative antidepressants such as amitriptyline, trimipramine, doxepin, mianserin, mirtazapine, nefazodone or trazodone are first choice in depressed patients with insomnia.[50–53] Antidepressants are also adjuvant analgesics, drugs with a primary indication other than pain. Although antidepressants have been found to have an analgesic effect independent of the effect on concomitant depression,[54] depression and other symptoms such as insomnia often coexist with pain and have a negative influence on pain perception.[51***] Sedative antidepressants have anticholinergic and other side effects and should therefore be used with caution in patients with somatic diseases; they may also induce or trigger confusional states.

Sedative neuroleptics (such as chlorprothixene, levopromazine, promazine, or thioridazine) are potentially harmful because of adverse effects such as hypotension. For example, levopromazine produces cardiovascular side effects even in young patients.[52,55] In demented patients, pipamperone, clomethiazole or chloral hydrate may be helpful.[52]

Clomethiazole, primarily introduced for the treatment of alcohol withdrawal syndrome[56] can be considered as effective in patients with insomnia due to nocturnal agitation associated with cognitive impairment.[57–60] Clinical experience suggests that sedating antihistamines, such as diphenhy-dramine, hydroxyzine, doxylamine, and promethazine may be of help in some patients, but their efficacy for the treatment of insomnia is not well established and their potential to cause delirium or hypotension make these agents of questionable value. Melatonin, not registered in most European countries, may have some beneficial sleep-regulating activity[61,62] and analgesic adjuvant effects.[63] Compared to the previously mentioned compounds, the sleep-inducing activity of melatonin is relatively scant; however, its excellent tolerability can make it acceptable to patients reluctant to take potent psychotropic drugs.[48] There is a growing literature reporting some benefit of cannabinoids[64] in sleep disorders, but to our knowledge no methodologically sound study has been conducted in palliative care. The same holds for molecules whose purpose is to diminish the expression or the effects of proinflammatory cytokines (tumor necrosis factor, interleukin [IL]-1α/β, IL-6); non-steroidal anti-inflammatory drugs (NSAIDs)[22] and thalidomide[65,66] are under observation.

CONCLUSIONS

Management of insomnia in palliative care is a considerable challenge for the clinician. It requires a careful evaluation, diagnostic skills, familiarity with nonpharmacological interventions and a sound knowledge of pharmacotherapy. In front of patients who are angered and/or saddened by their condition, clinicians are tempted to prescribe psychotropics to offer quick relief. While this may reduce the pressure felt by both the patient and the clinician, it may become a problem, because of the side effects. We therefore would like to invite readers to follow the above mentioned diagnostic and therapeutic strategies.

Key learning points

- Assessment of insomnia and its mediating factors
- Classification systems and specific assessment tools
- Recommendations for clinical evaluation
- Sleep hygiene measures and behavioral interventions
- Pharmacological management of insomnia
- Hypnotics in the palliative care setting

REFERENCES

◆ 1 Savard J, Morin CM. Insomnia in the context of cancer: a review of a neglected problem. *J Clin Oncol* 2001; **19**: 895–908.

2 Ng K, von Gunten CF. Symptoms and attitudes of 100 consecutive patients admitted to an acute hospice/palliative care unit. *J Pain Symptom Manage* 1998; **16**: 307–16.

3 Hugel H, Ellershaw JE, Cook L, *et al.* The prevalence, key causes and management of insomnia in palliative care patients. *J Pain Symptom Manage* 2004; **27**: 316–21.

4 Kupfer DJ. Pathophysiology and management of insomnia during depression. *Ann Clin Psychiatry* 1999; **11**: 267–76.

5 Tamburini M, Selmi S, De Conno F, Ventafridda V. Semantic descriptors of pain. *Pain* 1987; **29**: 187–93.

6 Engstrom CA, Strohl RA, Rose L, *et al.* Sleep alterations in cancer patients. *Cancer Nurs* 1999; **22**: 143–8.

7 Bruera E, Fainsinger RL, Schoeller T, Ripamonti C. Rapid discontinuation of hypnotics in terminal cancer patients: a prospective study. *Ann Oncol* 1996; **7**: 855–6.

8 American Sleep Disorders Association. International Classification of Sleep Disorders, Revised. In: *The International Classification of Sleep Disorders: Diagnostic & Coding Manual.* Rochester, MN: American Sleep Disorders Association, 1997.

9 American Psychiatric Association. *Diagnostic and Statistical Manual of Mental Disorders, 10 edition, Text Revision.* Washington, DC: American Psychiatric Association, 2000.

10 Stiefel F, Stagno D. Management of insomnia in patients with chronic pain conditions. *CNS Drugs* 2004; **18**: 285–96.

11 Lamberg L. Chronic pain linked with poor sleep; exploration of causes and treatment. *JAMA* 1999; **281**: 691–2.

12 Ancoli-Israel S. Epidemiology of sleep disorders. *Clin Geriatr Med* 1989; **5**: 347–62.

13 Edinger JD, Stout AL, Hoelscher TJ. Cluster analysis of insomniacs' MMPI profiles: relation of subtypes to sleep history and treatment outcome. *Psychosom Med* 1988; **50**: 77–87.

14 Lawrence CC, Gilbert CJ, Peters WP. Evaluation of symptom distress in a bone marrow transplant outpatient environment. *Ann Pharmacother* 1996; **30**: 941–5.

15 Smith MT, Perlis ML, Carmody TP, *et al.* Presleep cognitions in patients with insomnia secondary to chronic pain. *J Behav Med* 2001; **24**: 93–114.

16 Smith GR. The epidemiology and treatment of depression when it coexists with somatoform disorders, somatization, or pain. *Gen Hosp Psychiatry* 1992; **14**: 265–72.

17 Pilowsky I, Townley M. Sleep disturbance in pain clinic patients. *Pain* 1985: 27–33.

18 Atkinson JH, Slater MA, Grant I, *et al.* Depressed mood in chronic low back pain: relationship with stressful life events. *Pain* 1988; **35**: 47–55.

19 Haythornthwaite JA, Sieber WJ, Kerns RD. Depression and the chronic pain experience. *Pain* 1991; **46**: 177–84.

20 Morin CM, Gibson D, Wade J. Self-reported sleep and mood disturbance in chronic pain patients. *Clin J Pain* 1998; **14**: 311–14.

21 Wilson KG, Watson ST, Currie SR. Daily diary and ambulatory activity monitoring of sleep in patients with insomnia associated with chronic musculoskeletal pain. *Pain* 1998; **75**: 75–84.

22 Asnis GM, De la Garza R, 2nd, Kohn SR, Reinus JF, Henderson M, Shah J. IFN-induced depression: a role for NSAIDs. *Psychopharmacol Bull* 2003; **37**: 29–50.

23 Irwin M. Effects of sleep and sleep loss on immunity and cytokines. *Brain Behav Immun* 2002; **16**: 503–12.

24 Irwin M, Rinetti G, Redwine L, *et al.* Nocturnal proinflammatory cytokine-associated sleep disturbances in abstinent African American alcoholics. *Brain Behav Immun* 2004; **18**: 349–60.

25 Anforth HR, Bluthe RM, Bristow A, Hopkins S, Lenczowski MJ, Luheshi G, *et al.* Biological activity and brain actions of recombinant rat interleukin-1alpha and interleukin-1beta. *Eur Cytokine Netw* 1998; **9**: 279–88.

26 Ebrahimi B, Tucker SL, Li D, *et al*. Cytokines in pancreatic carcinoma: correlation with phenotypic characteristics and prognosis. *Cancer* 2004; 101: 2727–36.

27 Sateia MJ, Doghramji K, Hauri PJ, Morin CM. Evaluation of chronic insomnia. An American Academy of Sleep Medicine review. *Sleep* 2000; 23: 243–308.

28 Holbrook AM, Crowther R, Lotter A, *et al*. Meta-analysis of benzodiazepine use in the treatment of insomnia. *CMAJ* 2000; 162: 225–38.

29 Zammit GK, Weiner G, Damato N, *et al*. Quality of life in people with insomnia. *Sleep* 1999; 22(Suppl 2): s379–s385.

30 Schramm E, Hohagen F, Grasshoff U, *et al*. Test-retest reliability and validity of the Structured Interview for Sleep Disorders According to DSM-III-R. *Am J Psychiatry* 1993; 150: 867–72.

31 Buysse DJ, Reynolds CF, 3rd, Houck PR, Stack J, Kupfer DJ. Age of illness onset and sleep EEG variables in elderly depressives. *Biol Psychiatry* 1988; 24: 355–9.

32 Buysse DJ, Reynolds CF 3rd, Monk TH, *et al*. Quantification of subjective sleep quality in healthy elderly men and women using the Pittsburgh Sleep Quality Index (PSQI). *Sleep* 1991; 14: 331–8.

33 Chesson AL Jr, Murphy PW, Arnold CL, Davis TC. Presentation and reading level of sleep brochures: are they appropriate for sleep disorders patients? *Sleep* 1998; 21: 406–12.

34 Morin CM, Kowatch RA, Wade JB. Behavioral management of sleep disturbances secondary to chronic pain. *J Behav Ther Exp Psychiatry* 1989; 20: 295–302.

35 Perlis ML, Sharpe M, Smith MS, *et al*. Behavioral treatment of insomnia: treatment outcome and the relevance of medical and psychiatric morbidity. *J Behav Med* 2001; 24: 281–96.

36 Chesson AL Jr, Anderson WM, Littner M, *et al*. Practice parameters for the nonpharmacologic treatment of chronic insomnia. An American Academy of Sleep Medicine report. Standards of Practice Committee of the American Academy of Sleep Medicine. *Sleep* 1999; 22: 1128–33.

37 Morin CM, Hauri PJ, Espie CA, *et al*. Nonpharmacologic treatment of chronic insomnia. An American Academy of Sleep Medicine review. *Sleep* 1999; 22: 1134–56.

38 Holbrook AM, Crowther R, Lotter A, *et al*. The diagnosis and management of insomnia in clinical practice: a practical evidence-based approach. *CMAJ* 2000; 162: 216–20.

39 National Commission on Sleep Disorder Research. *Wake up America: A National Sleep Alert*. Palo Alto: Services DoHaH, 1993.

40 Sackett DL. Rules of evidence and clinical recommendations for the management of patients. *Can J Cardiol* 1993; 9: 487–9.

41 Smith MT, Perlis ML, Park A, *et al*. Comparative meta-analysis of pharmacotherapy and behavior therapy for persistent insomnia. *Am J Psychiatry* 2002: 5–11.

42 Hohagen F, Rink K, Kappler C, *et al*. Prevalence and treatment of insomnia in general practice. A longitudinal study. *Eur Arch Psychiatry Clin Neurosci* 1993; 242: 329–36.

43 Stiefel F, Berney A, Mazzocato C. Psychopharmacology in supportive care in cancer: a review for the clinician. I. Benzodiazepines. *Support Care Cancer* 1999; 7: 379–85.

44 Greenblatt DJ, Shader RI. Dependence, tolerance, and addiction to benzodiazepines: clinical and pharmakinetic considerations. *Drug Metabol Rev* 1978: 13–28.

45 Wysowski DK, Schober SE, Wise RP, Kopstein A. Mortality attributed to misuse of psychoactive drugs, 1979–88. *Public Health Rep* 1993; 108: 565–70.

46 Wysowski DK, Barash D. Adverse behavioral reactions attributed to triazolam in the Food and Drug Administration's Spontaneous Reporting System. *Arch Intern Med* 1991; 151: 2003–8.

47 Wysowski DK, Baum C. Outpatient use of prescription sedative-hypnotic drugs in the United States, 1970 through 1989. *Arch Intern Med* 1991; 151: 1779–83.

48 Buclin T, Mazzocato C, Berney A, Stiefel F. Psychopharmacology in supportive care of cancer: a review for the clinician. IV. Other psychotropic agents. *Support Care Cancer* 2001; 9: 213–22.

49 Hirst A, Sloan R. Benzodiazepines and related drugs for insomnia in palliative care. *Cochrane Database Syst Rev* 2002:CD003346.

50 *The American Psychiatric Publishing Textbook of Consultation-Liaison Psychiatry*, 2nd ed. Washington DC: American Psychiatric Publishing, 2002.

51 Berney A, Stiefel F, Mazzocato C, Buclin T. Psychopharmacology in supportive care of cancer: a review for the clinician. III. Antidepressants. *Support Care Cancer* 2000; 8: 278–86.

52 Hättenschwiler J, Hatzinger M. Diagnostic des troubles du sommeil. *Forum Med Suisse* 2001: 265–76.

53 Mendelson WB, Roth T, Cassella J, *et al*. The treatment of chronic insomnia: drug indications, chronic use and abuse liability. Summary of a 2001 New Clinical Drug Evaluation Unit meeting symposium. *Sleep Med Rev* 2004; 8: 7–17.

54 Portenoy R. Adjuvant analgesics in pain management. In: MacDonald L, ed. *Oxford Textbook of Palliative Medicine*, 2nd ed. Oxford: Oxford University Press; 1998: 361–90.

55 Mazzocato C, Stiefel F, Buclin T, Berney A. Psychopharmacology in supportive care of cancer: a review for the clinician. II. Neuroleptics. *Support Care Cancer* 2000; 8: 89–97.

56 Morgan MY. The management of alcohol withdrawal using chlormethiazole. *Alcohol Alcohol* 1995; 30: 771–4.

57 Ather SA, Shaw SH, Stoker MJ. A comparison of chlormethiazole and thioridazine in agitated confusional states of the elderly. *Acta Psychiatr Scand Suppl* 1986; 329: 81–91.

58 Dehlin O. Hypnotic effect of chlormethiazole in geriatric patients during long-term treatment. *Acta Psychiatr Scand Suppl* 1986; 329: 112–5.

59 Gray PA, Park GR. Chlormethiazole sedation for critically ill patients in renal failure. *Anaesthesia* 1989; 44: 913–5.

60 Overstall PW, Oldman PN. A comparative study of lormetazepam and chlormethiazole in elderly in-patients. *Age Ageing* 1987; 16: 45–51.

61 Zhdanova IV, Lynch HJ, Wurtman RJ. Melatonin: a sleep-promoting hormone. *Sleep* 1997; 20: 899–907.

62 Zhdanova IV, Wurtman RJ, Lynch HJ, *et al*. Sleep-inducing effects of low doses of melatonin ingested in the evening. *Clin Pharmacol Ther* 1995; 57: 552–8.

63 Lissoni P, Paolorossi F, Tancini G, *et al*. Is there a role for melatonin in the treatment of neoplastic cachexia? *Eur J Cancer* 1996; 32A: 1340–3.

64 Walsh D, Nelson KA, Mahmoud FA. Established and potential therapeutic applications of cannabinoids in oncology. *Support Care Cancer* 2003; 11: 137–43.

65 Davis MP, Dickerson ED. Thalidomide: dual benefits in palliative medicine and oncology. *Am J Hosp Palliat Care* 2001; 18: 347–51.

66 Peuckmann V, Fisch M, Bruera E. Potential novel uses of thalidomide: focus on palliative care. *Drugs* 2000; 60: 273–92.

74

Counseling in palliative care

KIMBERLEY MILLER, DAVID W KISSANE

INTRODUCTION

Psychotherapeutic interventions and support may be offered to the individual patient living with advanced cancer, but palliative care also recognizes the needs of the 'second order'[1] or 'hidden'[2] patients among families and caregivers. Although the incidence of distress found in studies varies, approximately 15–40 percent of cancer patients will develop significant anxiety and/or depression,[3–5] rates being less for true major depression.[6] Among caregivers of terminally ill patients, one study using structured psychiatric interviews found that 33 percent had psychiatric morbidity,[7] most commonly major depression, anxiety, or adjustment disorders. When self-report questionnaires are used, these frequencies become higher.[8–10] A systematic review has shown that those experiencing or at risk of psychological distress show a greater effect size in responding to psychological treatments compared with those with minimal or no distress.[11]*** Therefore, identifying and intervening with patients and families at high risk is an important therapeutic and cost minimizing principle.

The approach to counseling will vary according to needs and clinical indications.[12] Services may be delivered individually, some will be more effective when targeting a couple, and meeting with the immediate or extended caregiving family is both helpful and cost-effective. Self-help or professionally led groups are beneficial in promoting support, while focused family therapy and multifamily groups present other options.

In this chapter, the indications for counseling, varied models of intervention, issues for therapists and process challenges in the delivery of the counseling will be reviewed alongside the evidence for effectiveness of outcome.

WHAT ISSUES PRESENT FOR COUNSELING?

Patients present often with a concern or worry, sometimes with a symptom and rarely with a labeled disorder. The concern may be phrased as a question, buried in a bewildered maze of thoughts and feelings or projected as a problem onto another family member. Whatever the presentation – whether emotional, attitudinal, behavioral or conative – each request for help challenges the clinician to recognize what is relevant and organize this meaningfully. Understanding the person with their gamut of life's experiences and influences, successes and failures, accomplishments and omissions, shame and secrets, health or illness is at the heart of being able to respond to the whole person as an unique individual within their culture, family, and social world.[13]

Clinicians respond to such complexity with organizational schemata that structure the phenomena into recognizable patterns and hierarchies. Training, skill, and experience are crucial here if order is to emerge from potential chaos and be channeled constructively towards improved coping and beneficial outcome. Nevertheless, health professionals need to suspend any preconceptions and listen intently, lest the real needs of the patient are ignored with an inherent inability to heal, even if the disease is being treated. During the final weeks and days of life, matters existential, relational and spiritual come to the fore and may be more important ultimately than physical symptom management.[14]

How do clinicians organize patients' concerns to aid comprehension and plan consequent intervention? While listening to the narrative of illness, themes are identified and clustered into groups. Common themes include (i) loss, (ii) emotional response, (iii) meaning, and (iv) coping. Loss is myriad in its presentations during the course of illness,

Table 74.1   *A biopsychosocial and spiritual orientation to common issues that may arise in counseling during palliative care*

Biologic	Psychological	Social	Spiritual
Specific somatic symptoms, e.g. pain, fatigue, insomnia	Emotional responses, e.g. sadness, anger, fear	Instrumental care, e.g. nursing, pharmacy	Meaning of illness, e.g. aging, dying, punishment
Reduced physical function, e.g. frailty, impairment, disability	Adaptation, e.g. courage, acceptance, rejection	Occupational and physical therapies, e.g. respite, aides	Dignity of person, e.g. respect, valuing accomplishments
Altered bodily appearance, e.g. disfigurement	Sense of self, e.g. self-esteem, shame, stigma	Relational, e.g. marital, family, sexual, intimacy	Freedom and control, e.g. choice, mastery
Treatment processes, e.g. radiation, chemotherapy	Decision making, e.g. quality of life and treatment adherence	Financial and supportive e.g. burden, withdrawal	Rituals, e.g. prayer, connection with the sacred

and unless normalized as universal yet forever challenging, grief may not be well supported. When loss corresponds with expectations consonant with the life cycle, acceptance results readily; when illness is out of step with this natural order, distress, resentment, and profound grief develop easily. Identifying relevant emotions and any meaning attributed to illness is pertinent. Concepts of the inevitability of change or transitions associated with aging prove helpful, whereas adaptation as a response invokes some form of coping to optimize outcome and sustain quality of life.

The biopsychosocial and existential/spiritual model is one framework for organizing common issues that present for counseling during palliative care. Its value lies in its integration of the somatic with psychologic, social, and spiritual concerns. Table 74.1 illustrates typical issues without seeking to be exhaustive in its coverage of potential themes.

WHAT DIAGNOSES POTENTIALLY UNDERPIN THESE CONCERNS?

Sometimes therapists offer counseling about specific issues or focused requests like 'What do I say to my children?'. In these circumstances, direct exploration of options and role play will assist readily. Generally, however, the process of making a clinical diagnosis is pivotal to considering all of the therapeutic options available to ease distress and promote healing. The beauty of diagnosis is that it should trigger a comprehensive treatment plan, one based on experience, clinical wisdom, indeed, evidence of effectiveness. In this sense, no counseling should occur in palliative care without a competent, thorough clinical assessment leading to a thoughtful management plan. The clinician is thus always the professional.

Moreover, just as each physical symptom should lead to an assessment, examination, differential diagnosis and continued reevaluation of response to treatment, so too should each emotional theme generate its differential and continued exploration. Thus:

- Is the sadness an expression of grief or depression?
- Is the fear grounded in reality or excessive because of coping style?

- Does a pattern of low self esteem increase embarrassment or sense of stigma?
- Does the loss of meaning constitute demoralization or depression?
- Is concern about being a burden driven by altruism, independence or shame at loss of control?

Before considering what the applicable model of intervention is, these golden rules are vital: always take a careful history, examine the mental state, understand what has predisposed to, precipitated or perpetuated such distress, and formulate why this person is ill in this manner and at this time.

Box 74.1 overviews the common clinical diagnoses that are suitable for counseling. In terms of psychiatric nosological systems, these fall into grief reactions, situational or adjustment disorders, anxiety and depression, existential concerns, relational and V-code categories. Other common diagnoses such as delirium, dementia, psychoses, and a range

---

Box 74.1 Common psychiatric diagnoses that lead to counseling therapies

- Adjustment disorder, e.g. coping with intense grief, social withdrawal

- Anxiety disorder, e.g. panic attacks, nightmares, insomnia

- Depressive disorder, e.g. anhedonia, suicidality

- Demoralization disorder, e.g. loss of meaning, loss of hope

- Relational disorder, e.g. marital and family dysfunction, personality disorders, sexual dysfunction

- Existential disorder, e.g. spiritual despair, concern about being a burden, need to be in control, profound aloneness

- Organic psychiatric disorder, e.g. delirium, medication side effects, alcohol and substance abuse

of other organic states are not suitable for psychotherapy primarily, pharmacotherapy being the mainstay of treatment. For a number of conditions including anxiety and depressive disorders, combinations of psychotropic and psychotherapeutic treatment are indicated.[15]

INDICATIONS FOR COUNSELING

Distress, formal psychiatric disorder, concern about coping, and lack of sufficient social supports are the common indications for counseling.[16] Sometimes it can be as simple as unmet information needs but, in general, we try to distinguish those who can be supported by all members of the multidisciplinary care team from those who warrant referral for specialist counseling. The latter involves particularly clinicians trained in social work, psychology, or psychiatry. Risk factors for poorer coping include:

- *Factors in the person*: past history of depression or psychiatric disorder; cumulative life events; high levels of perceived stress or poor coping.
- *Factors in the illness*: onset at a young age; delay in diagnosis; recent diagnosis with rapid disease progression; long, intensive treatments or complications of treatment; specific cancers – pancreatic, neuroendocrine, lymphomas.
- *Factors in the environment*: poor social supports; family dysfunction; socio-economic deprivation; potential to leave young children behind.

Whenever one or more of these factors are present, consideration of the benefits of supportive counseling proves worthwhile.[17] Once an established psychiatric disorder exists, referral should be axiomatic.

Because of the large research literature showing that psychiatric disorders are often missed (for instance see references 18*, 19*, and 20*), usually through normalization of distress as what is expected, many services utilize a model of screening to assist recognition of those in greater need of psychosocial care.[21,22*] A randomized controlled trial of computer-assisted screening and referral for intervention has demonstrated an ability to reduce depressive disorders in oncology patients.[23**] Many services today use a triage mechanism to refer patients with milder levels of distress to social workers, and those with more severe distress to psychologists or psychiatrists.

MODELS OF COUNSELING

A number of schools of psychotherapy exist, many developed originally for specific clinical circumstances, but generally these are applied eclectically by counselors so that aspects of these different models are combined to suit the clinical predicament of the patient or family. Table 74.2

Table 74.2   *Models of psychotherapy*

Targets of therapy	Categories of therapy
Individual	Psychoeducational
	Supportive-expressive
	Grief therapy
Couple	Existential psychotherapy
	Cognitive–behavioral therapy
Group	Interpersonal psychotherapy
	Psychodynamic therapies
Family	Narrative and dignity therapies
	Spiritual and meaning-centered
	therapies
Community	Systemic therapies

summarizes the common models of psychotherapy. The following case example will illustrate how each psychotherapeutic model can be used.

> Soon after moving back to his hometown with Sue, his girlfriend of 9 years, George, a 29-year-old man was diagnosed with stage IV renal cell carcinoma, involving extensive retroperitoneal and paraaortic lymphadenopathy. They had both just completed their education, and hoped to marry and start a family, while beginning their careers and living closer to their families. Sadly, George's cancer was found to have metastasized quickly to his lungs, bones, and liver. As the cancer progressed, George required regular subcutaneous injections of hydromorphone (Dilaudid) for pain control. He began to feel more helpless and worried that he was placing too large a burden on Sue, who was giving him the injections around the clock, with help from a visiting nurse service. George's underlying fear was that Sue would grow weary of this, her view of him would shift from partner to patient, and that they would drift apart as his health deteriorated.

Psychoeducational interventions

Whether delivered individually, to groups or families, the provision of information about the illness and its treatment is foundational, and a counseling component of all clinical encounters. In their meta-analysis of 116 studies, Devine and Westlake[24***] proved that psychoeducational models have a large effect size, which should not surprising, as the outcome measure in such studies is simply the acquisition of new knowledge. Studies of unmet needs have nevertheless identified information provision as a major concern of patients with cancer,[25*] highlighting its importance at all stages of illness.

In George's case, nursing education covered pain and other symptom management, the nature of his cancer and its treatment, the anticipated process of dying, and how Sue could optimize her role and coordinate care with other members of George's family.

Supportive psychotherapy

Supporting a patient and family through cancer is best done by listening to the story of illness and its treatment, exploring the meaning of the diagnosis and prognosis, allowing the therapist to convey a level of understanding, and thereby developing a trusting relationship with them.[26] The counselor employs typically a range of therapeutic techniques including questions that seek clarification and invite sharing of emotions, comments that affirm, reassure, encourage or explain and suggestions that guide, promote acceptance and optimize support. This approach is the most generic form of counseling and its techniques are found in all other models of psychotherapy. Although cited in group work, the following goals are also pursued in individual supportive therapy: building bonds, expressing emotions about the illness and its impact on relationships, detoxifying death and dying, redefining life priorities, mobilizing supports, and improving coping and communication.[27**,28**,29**] Evidence for its effectiveness in advanced cancer is strongest for supportive-expressive group therapy (SEGT)[30] where randomized controlled trials have demonstrated its ability to reduce emotional distress, anxiety, and depression.[31**]

The unfairness of George's illness occurring out of step with his expected life cycle was acknowledged, their grief at the many losses normalized, their courage affirmed, and their commitment to each other understood. Helping George and Sue to share their feelings and consider how best to support one another led to affirmation of their greater sense of closeness that this tragedy brought. Accompaniment and commitment were key principles in sustaining continuity of care for them.

Grief therapy

Loss is found universally in illness and is experienced through disease, disfigurement, disability, dependency, depression, and death.[32] Although a variant on supportive psychotherapy, the model of counseling developed for the bereaved[33,34] serves well also as a response to the cumulative experience of loss during any journey with advanced disease. Grief is the interest owed on the debt of investment.[35] The tasks involved include promoting the sharing of emotion, normalizing the sadness, educating about the pattern of distress (waves of emotionality) and time course of mourning, interpreting any displacement of anger and encouraging adaptive coping responses. Such counseling techniques should be applied by all clinicians working in palliative medicine.

Counseling the bereaved becomes an important dimension of comprehensive palliative care, those at high risk being identified through recognition of (i) personal vulnerability, such as past history of psychiatric disorder, (ii) relational problems like dependence or ambivalence, (iii) a death experienced as in some way shocking, unexpected or traumatic, and (iv) the presence of family dysfunction or perception of being unsupported or disenfranchised. Group work is especially helpful for the isolated.[36]

Existential psychotherapy

Bred from existentialism, 'the study of the experience of living life to its fullest',[37] concepts of self awareness, freedom and responsibility in making choices in one's life, ultimate aloneness and our human need for relatedness, the meaning of life and the inevitable reality of death[38] are explored and confronted in the dying population. The common sources of existential distress are summarized in Table 74.3 with suitable models of counseling for specific challenges.[39] The counselor helps to define the particular existential challenge that each patient perceives and invites consideration of realistic ways of responding. Built upon processes of confrontation, reaction formation, and inviting choice about those aspects of life that should be most valued, patients are helped to live authentic and purposeful lives with a particular focus on living in the present moment. Many recent end-of-life models of therapy have developed from existential psychotherapy.[40]

In George's case, questions were asked about the meaning of their relationship, what they valued in life and each other, what priorities they had in living life out fully and what benefits Sue found in caring for George. Open acknowledgement of the potential for death helped identify the preciousness of each moment. Grief was checked to the extent that it risked spoiling continued living; the random nature of George's illness was contrasted with their spiritual wonder about life's mysteries.

Cognitive–behavioral therapy

Cognitive–behavioral therapy (CBT) involves teaching the patient to make connections between emotional events or triggers, associated automatic thoughts or beliefs, and resultant feelings or behaviors. This model, well known in

Table 74.3 *Adaptive and maladaptive responses to existential challenges and relevant counseling*

Nature of existential challenge	Features of successful adaptation	Form of existential distress when problematic	Common symptoms experienced	Related psychiatric disorders	Suitable model of therapy
Death	Courageous awareness of and acceptance of dying; saying goodbye	Death anxiety	Fear of the process of dying or the state of being dead; panic at somatic symptoms; distress at uncertainty	Anxiety disorders, panic disorder, agoraphobia, generalized anxiety disorder, acute stress disorder, adjustment disorder with anxious mood	Psychoeducational, cognitive–behavioral therapy, existential psychotherapy, psychodynamic therapy
Loss	Sad at reality of loss yet resigned to the occurrence of illness	Complicated grief	Intense tearfulness, grief and waves of emotionality, progressing into symptoms of depression	Depressive disorders	Supportive psychotherapy, grief therapy, interpersonal psychotherapy
Aloneness	Accompanied and supported by family and friends	Profound loneliness	Isolated, alienated and sense of complete aloneness in life	Dysfunctional family, absence of social support, relationship problems	Interpersonal psychotherapy, family focused therapy, supportive group therapy
Freedom	Acceptance of frailty and reduced independence	Loss of control	Angst at loss of control; obsessional mastery; indecisive, nonadherence to treatments; fear of dependency	Phobic disorders, obsessive-compulsive disorders, substance abuse disorders	Supportive psychotherapy, interpersonal psychotherapy, psychodynamic therapy
Meaning	Sense of fulfillment	Demoralization	Pointlessness, hopelessness, futility, loss of role, desire to die	Demoralization syndrome, depressive disorders	Interpersonal psychotherapy, narrative and dignity-conserving therapies, meaning-centered therapies, existential therapy
Dignity	Sense of worth despite disfigurement or handicap	Worthlessness	Shame, horror, body image concerns, fear of being a burden	Adjustment disorders	Narrative and dignity conserving therapies, supportive psychotherapy, grief therapy
Mystery	Reverence for the unknowable and sacred	Spiritual doubt and despair	Guilt, loss of faith, loss of connection with the transcendent	Adjustment, anxiety and depressive disorders	Meaning-centered therapy, life narrative therapies

the general psychiatry literature for successfully treating anxiety and depressive disorders,[41***,42***,43***] has been further developed specifically for cancer patients.[44,45,46**,47**] Homework is assigned between sessions, allowing the patient to practice identifying thought patterns that accompany distressing experiences associated with their illness. This is reviewed in the session, where cognitive reframing and disputing of negative automatic thoughts is taught, placing a more realistic framework in place. In working with advanced cancer patients, their concerns should not be simply dismissed, shifting to an unrealistic positive stance. Rather, validating their experience remains paramount, while helping them to understand that their pattern, for example that of catastrophizing or overgeneralizing, likely contributes to further psychological distress. In the palliative population, existential themes may be understood through cognitive therapy.[48] Such themes as guilt about prior lifestyle choices, feelings of burden, anxiety about disfigurement, perceived rejection by friends and fear of the dying process are explored and examined.

A focus on problem solving, active coping, including assertiveness training and anger management may also be employed. Additional behavioral interventions include relaxation training through progressive muscular relaxation, guided imagery,[49**,50**] massage,[51**] hypnosis or meditation,[52*] together with activity scheduling, exposure and systematic desensitization as commonly used in the general psychiatry to treat depression and anxiety.

Mind reading and negative predictions were identified as the cognitive distortions being used and alternative explanations were suggested to George. As well, he was urged to clarify this with Sue, who was devastated to learn that he was feeling this way. She explained that providing him with pain relief was a privilege, and that it made her feel helpful. Sue acknowledged that she was tired, but suggested that she was no more tired than he was, and that they were in this together for the long haul. She felt, more than ever before in their relationship, that they were very much partners in this, and reassured him that this was only going to continue to bring them closer together.

Interpersonal psychotherapy

Interpersonal psychotherapy (IPT) focuses pragmatically on one or two of four key domains common to most counseling: grief, role transitions, interpersonal disputes, and interpersonal sensitivity or deficits.[53,54] Therapists help facilitate the mourning process relating to the various losses experienced by patients and families during the cancer illness. This may also occur in the context of role transitions as individuals are aided in coming to terms with the loss of their old roles, while learning to accept the new, generally a movement from health to sickness. Negative attitudes about the new role are disputed and reframed, while self-esteem and mastery over the transition are emphasized.

In examining disputes, expectations in relationships as well as patterns of communication are explored, while parallels to other relationships are made, where appropriate. Often conjoint sessions are needed. Prior to this, role playing or modeling may occur. Interpersonal sensitivity and deficits are generally more entrenched in the personality of the individual, and therefore may not be as workable as other areas in the advanced cancer population. In the general psychiatry population, exploration into social development, specifically issues of trust, occurs and treatment efforts focus on building a therapeutic alliance and minimizing isolation.

George had always been an athlete, playing competitive racket sports, including badminton and tennis, as well as soccer. Determined to continue his active lifestyle for as long as possible into the illness, he did just that. He also began coaching at a local middle school. However, both the pain and fatigue began to interfere with his ability to be active, and he had to stop. A large part of his identity was being an athlete. Now unable to continue an active lifestyle, George felt frustrated and described losing a large part of himself. He felt 'weak', lacked purpose, and became agitated by the lack of distraction these activities provided. The therapist helped clarify the positive and negative aspects of both the old and the new roles, while validating his feelings about the transition. George was able to attend training as an assistant coach, giving more verbal direction than physical. His contribution was affirmed and he was urged to also develop new interests and hobbies, ones that involved less physical activity. George chose to continue coaching from the sidelines, and received great support from others in continuing in the face of advanced disease. The players asked him one day why George was not playing with them anymore, which led to a meaningful discussion about cancer and its limitations, while modeling great courage. He came to enjoy his free time, no longer feeling agitated by it, but blessed that it gave him more time with friends and family. Although he would gladly have turned in his diagnosis for a return to health, George grew to accept that he had purpose in this new role, resulting in feelings of peace and acceptance.

Psychodynamic psychotherapy

Principles from psychodynamic and psychoanalytic psychotherapy are commonly used indirectly in working with advanced cancer patients.[55] Patterns of prior coping and relationship difficulties may play out in the threat of loss, and recognition of such patterns in earlier life may increase understanding and aid resolution of conflicts. Straker recommends identifying and exploring defenses, examining core conflicts, and working with transference and countertransference issues in the cancer population.[56] Defenses such as denial and regression may, in fact, be adaptive and promote functioning. They may serve to alleviate distress such as depression, anxiety or helplessness, assuming they do not result in disruption of appropriate medical treatment or fulfillment of goals, including the organization of one's final affairs. Projected feelings of helplessness may develop in therapists treating patients facing the terminal phase of illness. Making sense of these as a countertransference response increases understanding of what the patient is experiencing, guiding what the focus of therapeutic work might therefore be.

> In reminiscing about his childhood, George recalled how often his mother complained about the extra washing his sporting clothes caused, and how when the washing was not done, he had to miss his beloved events. He felt abandoned by his mother at such times, but retreated from any argument as her verbal lashings were fierce. When George asked the therapist if the sessions were too upsetting for her, she drew a comparison between his fears of being a burden to the therapist and to Sue, akin to how he felt a burden to his mother in childhood. It dawned on George that his fear of Sue retreating from his care was based on his old pattern of relating and not something coming from Sue.

Life narrative and dignity-conserving therapies

The narrative account of the person's life aims to generate an understanding of the patient's reaction to and meaning attributed to their illness from the perspective of their overall philosophy and approach to life.[57–59] Links are made between prior coping during early life experiences and current responses to their cancer experience. The therapist summarizes his or her understanding of the coherent developmental story to promote a sense of accomplishment, fostering celebration and sense of fulfillment while highlighting roles, relationships and any apparent purpose of the patients' life. A shared consensus is sought about all that has been accomplished.[60]

Chochinov has developed a model of dignity-conserving care for patients approaching death (see also Chapter 13 in this book).[61,62] Efforts to improve their self-worth and promote respect are at its core. Each person's illness-related concerns, independence, spiritual, and psychological concerns and how these impact on their sense of dignity are explored. A key goal is to promote hope, autonomy and sense of control, while also addressing spiritual concerns. Dignity-conserving psychotherapy invites the patient to give a narrative account on tape of important aspects of their life that they would most want remembered. This is transcribed, edited and given to the patient, as well as being a legacy for their family. Topics that prompt this life review in the dignity-conserving model include: the individual's life story; how they want their families to remember them; vital roles they have played within their family, job and community; accomplishments they are most proud of; hopes and dreams for relatives and friends; words of advice to pass along to others; things they want to say to family that have not been said before, or that they want to say again; words that might provide comfort to their family and friends.

Meaning-centered psychotherapy

Spiritual suffering arises from doubt about earlier beliefs and religious practices and whether there is any greater meaning to life and death. For the religious, loss of connectedness with the transcendent is problematic; for the atheist, the absence of meaning in the chaos of 'life-considered-random' can render existence pointless. Breitbart and colleagues have developed meaning-centered psychotherapy as a model that promotes a sense of meaning and purpose,[63–65] (and also Gibson CA, Breitbart W. Individual meaning-centered psychotherapy treatment manual. Unpublished document. New York: Memorial Sloan-Kettering Cancer Center, 2004), adopting many principles from Viktor Frankl's 'logotherapy'.[66] Patients are active members in their own treatment, sharing experiences that have helped promote a sense of meaning, peace, and purpose. Exercises are assigned as homework and reviewed at subsequent meetings. The model is being tested in individual and group formats. Sense of personal responsibility, attitudes, creative and experiential values, and the meaning they bring to life are explored.[67]

> George identified the joy that Sue had brought into his life as giving him a special sense of purpose through their relationship together. He lamented nonetheless that they wouldn't reproduce now and that he would not leave a child behind. He told Sue that he wanted her to find someone else after his death and that she should have children early on in this next relationship. Sue told George that she would take some of his gentleness into any future parenting she did, so that he would live on through his influence on her.

Systemic therapies

Whether focused on the marital, parental, or sibling systems, the family-of-origin or current nuclear family, the mutual and reciprocal influence of one party upon another can be an important consideration therapeutically. Furthermore, insight into recurring patterns across generations helps families to vary these 'scripts' and choose a new direction in their relationships. While family therapy is the classical example of a systemic therapy, the concept can also be applied in individual counseling. Family Focused Grief Therapy (FFGT) is one preventive model that targets at risk families during palliative care and continues with the bereaved post death, aiming to optimize family functioning so that complicated grief is reduced.[68] Families with poor communication, reduced cohesion and a muted style of dealing with anger, the so-called sullen families, respond best to FFGT.[69*,70**] Care needs to be exercised with the most dysfunctional or hostile families to respect any salutary solution to family conflict through separations and distance, so that conflict is not rekindled by family meetings. Thus modest goals are set with these very dysfunctional families; FFGT has much to offer families at risk in palliative care, its brief and focused approach delivering cost effectiveness alongside continuity of care into bereavement.

> George and Sue were brought together with their parents and siblings, the broader family rallying to support the young couple. Open communication about the cancer and its treatment ensured their grief was shared, hope fostered, and respite was organized to protect Sue from exhaustion. As teamwork grew, each family's sense of celebration of George's life became apparent, and support was sustained for Sue throughout the subsequent period of bereavement.

THERAPIST AND PROCESS ISSUES

Professionals working with palliative care patients and their families generally include medical practitioners, nurses or nurse practitioners, social workers, psychologists, psychiatrists, pastoral care workers and other integrative medicine or allied health clinicians. Trained volunteers and healthcare aides also play a supportive role. All disciplines should have broad knowledge about palliative medicine, specifically in the understanding of the diagnosis, treatments, and prognosis, as well as a general ability to support dying patients and their families compassionately. The whole of the multidisciplinary treatment team makes a contribution to psychosocial care.

When it comes to developing skill and expertise in the specific models of counseling described in this chapter, formal training is needed. Research confirms that patients respond better to brief interventions provided by well-trained and skilled therapists compared to longer courses of treatment given by less psychologically trained staff.[11***]

The core elements of any counseling comprise the relationship that is established, the explanatory model of intervention used, the procedure for promoting change and the healing that in turn induces further benefit. A number of therapeutic factors are common to all models of intervention. For instance, developing a strong working relationship, often termed a therapeutic alliance, with the patient and their caregivers is foundational. Other key factors include engaging in active listening, allowing patients to ventilate their feelings about their experience, validating their concerns, providing support, and building trust and respect.[71] Exploration of prior losses, especially deaths in the family, and how members coped with their related grief is illuminating.

Irrespective of the model of intervention, some degree of emotional and cognitive learning occurs as each patient is invited to take responsibility for change and well-being. Jerome Frank[72,73] emphasized the restoration of hope and sense of mastery over whatever one can accomplish as being at the heart of all therapeutic improvement. As gains are achieved, consolidation grows from renewed confidence, while response prevention strategies are generally worthwhile. For much of this work, a delicate balance is needed between promoting hope and supporting grief, these two themes often evolving in parallel. Availability, particularly at a time when patients are being told that life-prolonging treatment is no longer an option, can decrease any sense of abandonment. As well, psychological intervention may help patients to adhere to supportive care measures in a way that will improve the quality of life remaining.

Winnicott's model of a facilitating environment is helpful, in which the counselor provides a secure relationship, whose structure creates an experience in which 'holding' and 'containment' of distress are achieved.[74,75] In palliative care, the boundaries under which this structure would be established ordinarily are modified, so that appropriate and compassionate touch is permitted, access and responsiveness are the norm, and the therapist's warmth, empathy and unconditional regard help create the holding frame. Nevertheless, an emphasis still exists on appropriate restriction of therapist self disclosure, here and now feelings being sensitively shared while greater caution is exercised over one's personal life. Disclosure of a gay orientation may be helpful to homosexual patients, but disclosure of personal cancer or illness experiences is generally unwise, the focus of the therapy being truly directed toward the patient.

In the setting of medical illness, most counseling needs to be brief and focused for pragmatic reasons. Given this, the skill and experience of the therapist is especially pertinent, with clinical judgments determining what is worthy of constructive focus and what is wisely left as a long-term or irremediable pattern of behavior. Personality disorders would not be addressed at the individual therapy level and entrenched family conflict might be respected as ultimately a difference of opinion best resolved by accepting distance between relatives. Selection of a model of therapy is usually eclectic and based on clinical experience, combining elements from several models in response to the prevailing symptoms or predicaments that the patient presents.

Flexibility in number, frequency and duration of sessions, location of appointments, and modality of treatment used is a necessary part of working with the palliative care population. Telephone support may substitute for direct patient care. Physical symptoms, side effects of treatments and stage of illness all significantly impact on delivery of services and a change in medical status may necessitate a shift in therapeutic focus. An open flexible approach is best maintained throughout the course of treatment. The potential for psychopharmacological treatment is always considered alongside any counseling and its need monitored.

EFFECTIVENESS OF COUNSELING AND LIMITATIONS

Strong evidence exists from meta-analyses about the effectiveness of psychological interventions for the treatment of anxiety and depression in the medically ill such as those with cancer.[11***,24***,76***] When selectivity is exercised over studies with greater methodological rigor, effect size for anxiety reduction was 0.42 standard deviations (95 percent confidence interval [CI]) 0.08 to 0.74, total sample size 1023 patients) and for depression was 0.36 (95 percent CI 0.06 to 0.66, sample size 1101 patients).[24***] These findings are more robust for anxiety than depression, where treatment with antidepressants is also indicated.

Group therapy is at least as effective as individual counseling. Length of treatment is important, with more than 8 hours of counseling generating an effect size of 1.01 for anxiety compared with 0.41 when only 4–7 hours is given ($P = 0.002$).[24***] Similarly, length of therapy improves outcome in treating depression. More experienced therapists increase the effect size for both anxiety ($d = 0.57$ versus 0.10, $P = 0.054$) and depression ($d = 0.43$ versus -0.18, $P = 0.038$) compared with less experienced counselors.[24***] These findings challenge palliative care services to hire appropriately skilled counselors.

The latter concept may have relevance when one seeks to understand the findings from systematic analyses that palliative care service interventions do not significantly improve the outcome for caregivers of the dying patient.[77***,78***] Community programs the world over have saved costs through engaging unskilled counselors. Another explanation for the apparent absence of proved impact on carers is the absence of targeting 'at risk' carers with preventive interventions. Unless services employ screening to identify high risk individuals and families, many delightful folk, who will otherwise cope admirably, receive expensive therapies and hide the benefit in studies available to those with more limited coping.

Finally, a caveat is needed about the risks of counseling. Just as pharmacotherapy can induce side effects, sometimes with deleterious consequences, so also can counseling cause harm. Research suggests that about 10 percent of counseling interventions generate untoward effects, such as worsening anxiety, depression, or marital and family conflict. This limitation calls for skill and experience being derived from formal training in the models of intervention and in one of the basic psychosocial disciplines, so that therapists can identify any deterioration and introduce corrective strategies. When counseling is delivered by trained and experienced professionals, it has much to offer in ameliorating distress and suffering.

Key learning points

- High rates of distress exist among patients, caregivers and family members during palliative care.

- Counseling interventions have proved efficacy in relieving distress, anxiety, and depression.

- The training and experience of the therapist strongly influences the effectiveness of interventions.

- Outcome is progressively improved by longer interventions.

- Group interventions are at least as efficacious as individual therapies; family group counseling may be more cost effective when applicable.

- Whereas psychoeducational, supportive and grief therapies are the mainstay of psychotherapeutic approaches, interpersonal, narrative and meaning-centered models offer promise in ameliorating existential distress.

REFERENCES

1 Rait D, Lederberg M. The family of the cancer patient. In: Holland JC, Rowland JH, eds. *Handbook of Psychooncology: Psychological Care of the Patient with Cancer*. New York: Oxford University Press, 1989: 585–97.

2 Wiley S. Who cares for family and friends? Providing palliative care at home. Nursing monograph. Darlinghurst (Australia): St Vincent's Healthcare, 1998, 4–7 Available at www.clininfo.health. nsw.gov.au/hospolic/stvincents/stvin98/a2.html (accessed 26 September, 2005).

● 3 Derogatis LR, Morrow GR, Felting D, *et al.* The prevalence of psychiatric disorders among cancer patients. *JAMA* 1983; **249**: 751–7.

4 Massie M, Holland J. Overview of normal reactions and prevalence of psychiatric disorders. In: Holland JC, Rowland JH, eds. *Handbook of Psychooncology: Psychological Care of the Patient with Cancer*. New York: Oxford University Press, 1989: 273–82.

5 Parle M, Jones B, Maguire P. Maladaptive coping and affective disorders among cancer patients. *Psychol Med* 1996; **26**: 735–44.

6 Wilson KG, Chochinov HM, deFaye BJ, Breitbart W. Diagnosis and management of depression in palliative care. In: Chochinov HM, Breitbart W, eds. *Handbook of Psychiatry in Palliative Medicine*. New York: Oxford University Press, 2000: 25–49.

7 Maguire P, Walsh S, Keeling F, *et al.* Physical and psychological needs of patients dying from colo-rectal cancer. *Palliat Med* 1999; **13**: 45–50.

8 Siegel K, Karus DG, Raveis VH, *et al.* Depressive distress among the spouses of terminally ill cancer patients. *Cancer Pract* 1996; **4**: 25–30.

9 Kissane D, Bloch S, Burns WI, *et al.* Psychological morbidity in the families of patients with cancer. *Psychooncology* 1994; **3**: 47–56.

10 Williamson G, Schulz R. Caring for a family member with cancer: past communal behavior and affective reactions. *J Appl Soc Psychol* 1995; **25**: 93–116.

◆ 11 Sheard T, Maguire P. The effect of psychological interventions on anxiety and depression in cancer patients: results of two meta-analyses. *Br J Cancer* 1999; **80**: 1770–80.

✱ 12 National Breast Cancer Centre and National Cancer Control Initiative. *Clinical Practice Guidelines for the Psychosocial Care of Adults with Cancer*. Camperdown: National Breast Cancer Centre, 2003.

13 Cassell EJ. *The Nature of Suffering and the Goals of Medicine*. New York: Oxford University Press, 1991.

14 Sheldon F. *Psychosocial Palliative Care*. Cheltenham: Thornes, 1997.

15 Kissane DW, Smith GC. Consultation-liaison psychiatry in an Australian oncology unit. *Aust N Z J Psychiatry* 1996; **30**: 397–404.

16 Burton M, Watson M. *Counselling People with Cancer*. Chichester: Wiley, 1998.

17 Burton MV. Counselling in routine care: a client-centred approach. In: Watson M, ed. *Cancer Patient Care: Psychosocial Treatment Methods*. Cambridge: British Psychological Society and Cambridge University Press; **1991**: 74–93.

18 Hardman A, Maguire P, Crowther D. The recognition of psychiatric morbidity on a medical ward. *J Psychosom Res* 1989; **33**: 235–9.

19 Clarke DM, Minas IH, Stuart GW. The prevalence of psychiatric morbidity in general hospital patients. *Aust N Z J Psychiatry* 1991; **25**: 322–3.

20 Goldberg DP, Jenkins L, Millar T. The ability of general practitioners to identify psychological distress among patients. *Psychol Med* 1993; **23**: 185–93.

21 Zabora J, Loscalzo MJ. Comprehensive psychosocial programs: a prospective model of care. *Oncol Issues* 1996; **11**: 14–18.

● 22 Zabora J, Brintzenhofezock S, Curbow B, *et al.* The prevalence of psychological distress by cancer site. *Psychooncology* 2001; **10**: 19–28.

● 23 McLachlan SA, Allenby A, Matthews J, *et al.* Randomized trial of coordinated psychosocial interventions based on patient self-assessments versus standard care to improve the psychosocial functioning of patients with cancer. *J Clin Oncol* 2001; **19**: 4117–25.

◆ 24 Devine EC, Westlake SK. The effects of psychoeducational care provided to adults with cancer: Meta-analysis of 166 studies. *Oncol Nurs Forum* 1995; **22**: 1369–81.

25 Newell S, Sanson-Fisher RW, Grigis A, Ackland S. The physical and psychosocial experiences of patients attending an outpatient medical oncology department: a cross-sectional study. *Eur J Cancer Care* 1999; **8**: 73–82.

26 Bloch S. *An Introduction to the Psychotherapies*, 3rd ed. Melbourne: Oxford Medical Publications; 1996.

27 Goodwin P, Leszcz M, Ennis M, *et al.* The effect of group psychosocial support on survival in metastatic breast cancer. *N Engl J Med* 2001; **345**: 1719–26.

28 Koopman C, Hermanson K, Diamond S, *et al.* Social support, life stress, pain and emotional adjustment to advanced breast cancer. *Psychooncology* 1998; **7**: 101–11.

● 29 Spiegel D, Bloom J, Kraemer H, Gottheil E. Effect of psychosocial treatment on survival of patients with metastatic breast cancer. *Lancet* 1989; **2**: 888–91.

30 Spiegel D, Classen C. *Group Therapy for Cancer Patients*. New York: Basic Books, 2000.

31 Cunningham AJ, Edmunds CV, Jenkins, GP, *et al.* A randomized controlled trial of the effects of group psychological therapy on survival in women with metastatic breast cancer. *Psychooncology* 1998; **7**: 508–17.

32 Holland JC, Lewis S. *The Human Side of Cancer*. New York: Harper, 2000.

● 33 Worden JW. *Grief Counseling and Grief Therapy*, 2nd ed. New York: Springer, 1991.

● 34 Christ GH. *Healing Children's Grief*. New York: Oxford University Press, 2000.

35 Yalom ID. *The Gift of Therapy. Reflections on Being a Therapist*. London: Piatkus, 2001.

36 Yalom ID, Vinogradov S. Bereavement groups: techniques and themes. *Int J Group Psychother* 1988; **38**: 419–46.

37 Spira JL. Existential psychotherapy. In: Chochinov HM, Breitbart W, eds. *Handbook of Psychiatry in Palliative Medicine*. New York: Oxford University Press, 2000: 197–214.

38 Fischer C. Existential therapy. In: Covey G, ed. *Theory and Practice of counseling and Psychotherapy*, 2nd ed. San Francisco: Brooks/Cole Publishing, 1982: 67–75.

39 Kissane DW, Yates P. Psychological and existential distress. In: O'Connor M, Aranda S, eds. *Palliative Care Nursing: A Guide to Practice*, 2nd ed. Melbourne: Ausmed, 2003.

● 40 Yalom ID. *Existential Psychotherapy*. New York: Basic Books, 1980.

◆ 41 Clum GA, Clum GA, Surls R. A meta-analysis of treatments for panic disorder. *J Consult Clin Psychol* 1993; **61**: 317–26.

◆ 42 van Balkom AJLM, van Oppen P, Vermeulen AWA, *et al.* A meta-analysis on the treatment of obsessive compulsive disorder: a comparison of antidepressants, behavior and cognitive therapy. *Clin Psychol Rev* 1994; **14**: 359–81.

◆ 43 Gloaquenu K, Cotraux J, Cucherat M, Blackburn IM. A meta-analysis of the effects of cognitive therapy with depressed patients. *J Affect Disord* 1998; **49**: 59–72.

44 Moorey S, Greer S. *Psychological Therapy for Patients with Cancer: A New Approach*. Oxford: Heinemann Medical Books, 1989.

● 45 Moorey S, Greer S. *Cognitive Behaviour Therapy for People with Cancer*, 2nd ed. Oxford: Oxford University Press, 2002.

46 Edelman S, Lemon J, Bell DR, Kidman AD. Effects of group CBT on the survival time of patients with metastatic breast cancer. *Psychooncology* 1999; **8**: 474–81.

47 Kissane DW, Bloch S, Smith GC, *et al.* Cognitive-existential group psychotherapy for women with primary breast cancer: a randomized controlled trial. *Psychooncology* 2003; **12**: 532–46.

48 Kissane DW, Bloch S, Miach P, *et al.* Cognitive-Existential group therapy for patients with primary breast cancer – techniques and themes. *Psychooncology* 1997; **6**: 25–33.

49 Baider LB, Peretz T, Hadani PE, Koch U. Psychological intervention in cancer patients: a randomized study. *Gen Hosp Psychiatry* 2001; **23**: 272–7.

50 Walker LG, Walker MB, Ogston K, *et al.* Psychological, clinical and pathological effects of relaxation training and guided imagery during primary chemotherapy. *Br J Cancer* 1999; **80**: 262–8.

51 Soden K, Vincent K, Craske S, *et al.* A randomized controlled trial of aromatherapy massage in a hospice setting. *Palliat Med* 2004; **18**: 87–92.

52 Carlson L, Ursuliak Z, Goodey E, *et al.* The effects of a mindfulness meditation-based stress reduction program on mood and symptoms of stress in cancer outpatients: 6-month follow-up. *Support Care Cancer* 2001; **9**: 112–23.

● 53 Weissman MM, Markowitz JC, Klerman GL. *Comprehensive Guide to Interpersonal Psychotherapy.* New York: Basic Books, 2000.

54 Klerman GL, Weissman MM, Rounsaville BJ, Chevron ES. *Interpersonal Psychotherapy of Depression.* New York: Basic Books, 1984.

● 55 McDougall J. T*heatres of the Body. A Psychoanalytic Approach to Psychosomatic Medicine.* London: Free Association, 1989.

56 Straker N. Psychodynamic psychotherapy for cancer patients. *J Psychother Pract Res* 1989; **7**: 1–9.

● 57 White M, Epstein D. *Narrative Means to Therapeutic Ends.* New York: Norton, 1990.

● 58 Viederman M. Psychodynamic life narrative in a psychotherapeutic intervention useful in crisis situations. *Psychiatry* 1983; **46**: 236–46.

59 Viederman M, Perry S. Use of the psychodynamic life narrative in the treatment of depression in the physically ill. *Gen Hosp Psychiatry* 1980; **2**: 177–85.

60 White M. *Narratives of Therapists' Lives.* Adelaide: Dulwich, 1997.

61 Chochinov HM. Dignity-conserving care – a new model for palliative care. *JAMA* 2002; **287**: 2253–60.

62 Chochinov HM, Hack T, McClement S, *et al.* Dignity in the terminally ill: a developing empirical model. *Soc Sci Med* 2002; **54**: 433–43.

63 Breitbart W, Heller KS. Reframing hope: meaning-centered care for patients near the end of life. *J Palliat Med* 2003; **6**: 979–88.

64 Breitbart W. Spirituality and meaning in supportive care: spirituality-and meaning-centered psychotherapeutic interventions in advanced cancer. *Support Care Cancer* 2002; **10**: 272–80.

65 Greenstein M, Breitbart W. Cancer and the experience of meaning: a group psychotherapy program for people with cancer. *Am J Psychother* 2000; **54**: 486–500.

● 66 Frankl VF. *Man's Search for Meaning,* 4th ed. Boston: Beacon Press, 1992.

67 Breitbart W, Gibson C, Poppito S, Berg A. Psychotherapeutic interventions at the end of life: a focus on meaning and spirituality. *Can J Psychiatry* 2004; **49**: 366–72.

● 68 Kissane DW, Bloch S. *Family Focused Grief Therapy. A Model of Family-Centered Care during Palliative Care and Bereavement.* Buckingham; Open University Press, 2002.

69 Chan EK, O'Neill I, McKenzie M *et al.* What works for therapists conducting family meetings: treatment integrity in Family Focused Grief Therapy during palliative care and bereavement. *J Pain Symptom Manage* 2004; **27**: 502–12.

70 Kissane DW, McKenzie M, Bloch S, *et al.* Family Focused Grief Therapy: a randomized controlled trial in palliative care and bereavement. *Am J Psychiatry* 2005 (in press).

71 Massie MJ, Popkin MK. Depression. In: Holland JC, Rowland JH, eds. *Handbook of Psychooncology: Psychological Care of the Patient with Cancer.* New York: Oxford University Press, 1989: 518–41.

72 Frank J. The role of hope in psychotherapy. *Int J Psychiatry* 1968; **5**: 383–95.

73 Frank J. The restoration of morale. *Am J Psychiatry* 1974; **131**: 271–4.

74 Davis M, Wallbridge D. *Boundary and Space. An Introduction to the Work of DW. Winnicott.* New York: Brunner/Mazel, 1981.

75 Winnicott DW. *The Maturational Processes and the Facilitating Environment.* London: Karnac Books and The Institute of Psycho-analysis, 1990.

◆ 76 Meyer TJ, Mark MM. Effects of psychosocial interventions with adult cancer patients: a meta-analysis of randomized experiments. *Health Psychol* 1995; **14**: 101–8.

◆ 77 Higginson IJ, Finlay IG, Goodwin DM, *et al.* Is there evidence that palliative care teams alter end-of-life experiences of patienst and their caregivers? *J Pain Symptom Manage* 2003; **25**: 150–68.

◆ 78 Harding R, Higginson IJ. What is the best way to help caregivers in cancer and palliative care? A systematic literature review of interventions and their effectiveness. *Palliat Med* 2003; **17**: 63–74.

Hope in end-of-life care

CHERYL L NEKOLAICHUK

October 29, 2004

the biggest pain to go through in the end . . .
is the gradual drop-away of visitors.
I hope my friends keep their promises.
Promises about sitting with me
and being with me when that time comes . . .

(A patient receiving palliative care. From Nekolaichuk CL.
Understanding the experience of hope in palliative care.
Manuscript in preparation)

INTRODUCTION

The progressive nature of a terminal illness challenges patients to search for the elusive experience of hope. The unpredictable nature of the illness course, marked by debilitating symptoms, body image distortions and multiple losses, propels the terminally ill and their families onto a pathway of uncertainty, fear and, for some, despair. Traditional roles may be reversed or erased, as patients struggle to maintain connections from marginalized positions in society. External messages of 'There is no cure' become internal messages of 'There is no hope', as patients wrestle with their own mortality. In a recent study involving advanced cancer patients, 47.8 percent of participants reported at least some sense of hopelessness,[1] which is not surprising given the adversities many patients face.

Despite these enormous challenges, people who are terminally ill strive to include hope within their caring circles. In interviews with 120 terminally ill cancer patients, 99 percent of respondents rated *having a sense of hope* as a very important existential concern.[2] Based on a review of research studies, Lin and Bauer-Wu[3] identified *living with meaning and hope* as one of six essential themes of psychosocial spiritual

wellbeing in patients with advanced cancer. In a recent qualitative study focusing on information needs, patients with advanced cancer identified the *provision of hope and need for hopeful messages* as one of two most important concerns regarding information content.[4]

Healthcare professionals have equally emphasized the importance of hope in the delivery of palliative care. Numerous position papers and literature reviews highlight the need for intentionally incorporating hope within end-of-life care.[5–12] Janssens and colleagues[13] have further embedded the concept within a philosophy of care framework for palliative care. This framework consists of three realms – medical, psychosocial, and spiritual – with hope as a central existential phenomenon within the spiritual realm.

Although these endorsements are substantive, an intentional integration of hope within end-of-life care remains relatively underdeveloped. To begin to address this issue, we need to consider the following questions:

- What is the nature of hope in palliative care?
- How can we enhance our approaches for assessing hope in people who are terminally ill?
- What types of hope-enhancing strategies and interventions would be most appropriate for this unique population?

Beginning with an overview of the therapeutic value of hope, this chapter will address these three key questions for end-of-life care.

THERAPEUTIC VALUE OF HOPE IN ILLNESS

The therapeutic value of hope in dealing with chronic and life-threatening illnesses is well documented. Hope has been positively linked to effective coping,[14,15] enhanced quality of life,[16,17] spiritual wellbeing,[18] and healing.[19-21] In contrast, hopelessness may be associated with low levels of perceived emotional support,[22,23] depression,[23,24] suicidal intent,[25] desire for hastened death,[26] and pain.[27] Similar to studies in psychiatric populations,[26] recent studies in terminally ill patients identified hopelessness as a strong predictor of suicidal intent.[28,29]

Although these findings are significant, some caution is warranted in making cross-study comparisons. Study samples were quite diverse, including patients with human immunodeficiency virus (HIV)/acquired immune deficiency syndrome (AIDS)[18,22,23,27] and cancer,[14,16,28,29] depressed patients,[20,21,24,25] patients with long-term disabilites,[15,19] and older patients,[17] and were not entirely limited to the terminal illness phase. The use of different measures to assess hope or hopelessness across studies further limits meaningful comparisons. Future research studies, focusing on relationships between hope, symptom expression, and positive health indicators, such as quality of life, wellbeing and coping, need to specifically target the terminally ill, using consistent measurement approaches appropriate for this population.

Nature of hope in palliative care

What does hope mean to you as a healthcare provider?
What does hope mean to the patients for whom you provide care?

Traditionally, within healthcare communities, the concept of hope has been closely linked with treatments and cures.[30,31] When hope for a cure is no longer viable, healthcare professionals and patients may give up hope. Although the situation may be hopeless, there is always hope for the individual.[32] A key challenge is to understand the nature of hope in palliative care. To do so, it is important to begin by understanding the concept of hope in general.

A diversity of definitions and conceptual frameworks for hope exist in the literature. Currently, there is no universal definition for hope. In a recent critique of the hope literature, Nekolaichuk[33] identified seven themes associated with differing perspectives about hope (see Fig. 75.1). Based on these seven themes, the following assumptions about hope were generated:

- *Universality*: Hope is both a universal and an intensely personal experience.
- *Dimensionality*: Hope is a complex concept, ranging from unidimensional to multidimensional aspects of a person's experience.
- *Intangibility*: Hope has both tangible and intangible components, some of which may never be elucidated.
- *Temporality*: Hope appears to imply some sense of temporality, although this may not necessarily be limited to a future orientation. It is also possible that some components of hope may not be bound by time.

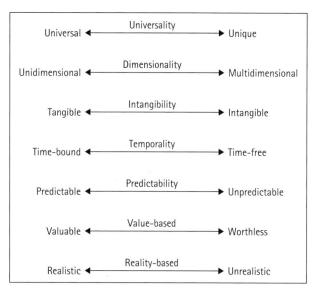

Figure 75.1 *Thematic analysis of the concept of hope.*

- *Predictability*: Hope may have both predictable and unpredictable components to the experience.
- *Value-based*: The value of hope appears to be embedded in personal experience.
- *Reality-based*: Hope appears to be connected with some sense of realism, although the viewpoints of reality remain unclear.

These seven themes provide a helpful framework for understanding the nature of hope in palliative care.

Universality

Although hope is a universal human experience, it is also intensely unique. Thus, it is important to understand the experience from the patient's perspective. A number of qualitative studies, focusing on the terminally ill patient's experience of hope, have been conducted in diverse settings, such as palliative home care,[34,35] inpatients,[36,37] outpatient clinics other than home care,[36,38,39] and nonmedical settings.[32,40-43] The types of sample varied, including people with cancer,[34-37] HIV/AIDS,[32,40-43] and end-stage renal disease.[38] Although most of these studies involved patients directly, one study attempted to understand the experience by interviewing nurses about their perceptions of hope in palliative care patients with cancer.[39]

Dimensionality

A diversity of conceptual frameworks for hope has emerged, ranging from unidimensional to multidimensional models. Of the many diverse frameworks, Dufault and Martocchio's model,[44] qualitatively derived from a sample of older cancer and terminally ill patients, continues to provide a useful initial framework for understanding hope in the terminally ill.

Dufault and Martocchio proposed a multidimensional framework for hope, consisting of six dimensions: cognitive, affective, behavioral, affiliative, contextual, and temporal. Each of these dimensions may be impacted in different ways when a person is facing a terminal illness.

Intangibility

The experience of hope may have both tangible and intangible components. Dufault and Martocchio[44] described these two types of hope as particularized and generalized hopes. Particularized hopes are hopes that are directed towards specific goals. For the terminally ill, particularized hopes may vary as the disease progresses. Patients often describe how their hopes may change over time,[5,45] for example, from a hope for a cure, to a hope for symptom relief, to a hope for special time with family, to a hope for a peaceful death. In contrast, generalized hopes represent an intangible inner experience of hope that is not connected to any specific goal or object. This invisible part of hope, which may be difficult to articulate, is often experienced at a deep, spiritual level.

Temporality

Although most definitions for hope include a future orientation, this may not always be appropriate for the terminally ill.[7] For some people, with strong faith beliefs, hope may be tied to a future beyond this life. For others, however, the experience of hope may be interwoven with past, present and future experiences;[7,44,46,47] may be lived in the present;[16] or may transcend time.[44,48] It is important to have some understanding of how patients view hope in terms of time, potentially deemphasizing the future component.

Predictability

The uncertainty of advancing disease raises fears in most patients who are terminally ill. Although frameworks do differ, some models have included uncertainty as an inherent part of the hope experience.[46,49] Exploring a person's fears, as well as focusing on predictable aspects of a person's life, helps buffer the uncertainties of progressive illness.

Value-based

Few could argue with the potential therapeutic benefits that hope offers to the dying. It is important to acknowledge, however, that not everyone may place a positive value on the experience, particularly if people have been disappointed by hope in the past. For example, this may become an issue when patients place all of their hopes into finding a cure, only to be devastated when they are given the bad news that their condition is incurable. The challenge is to be able to help patients develop a broad hoping repertoire, including hopes beyond a cure.[7]

Reality-based

Often, people may concurrently hold two opposing hopes, such as a hope for a cure and a hope for a peaceful death.[34] This may be troubling for some caregivers and family members, who might view this as unrealistic or unhealthy denial. In contrast, Jevne and Nekolaichuk[50] describe this phenomenon as a normal way for patients to prioritize their hopes:

> It is important to listen to the descriptive words that they [patients] attach to their hopes, acknowledging the range (and depth) of their hopes. One elderly patient who was forced to stop traveling due to a progression of his disease described his hope to travel as a 'forlorn' hope. Another palliative patient who expressed a hope for peace in the world described that particular hope as a 'big' hope. Yet another patient who hung onto a hope for a cure, despite being told that her cancer was incurable, suggested that it 'may not be a very realistic' hope, but that 'miracles do happen.' For a patient who believed in life after death, her hope to be united with God was her 'ultimate' hope. (p. 195)

ASSESSMENT OF HOPE

> How can you tell how hopeful a person is?
> What do you need to know to understand a person's experience of hope?

Although a variety of approaches have been developed for assessing hope in clinical practice (see Farran et al.[49] for an excellent review), few of these approaches have been developed specifically for palliative care.[7,12] Given the frailty of the terminally ill population, assessments need to be relatively brief, psychometrically sound in terms of quantitative measures, and include combined quantitative and qualitative approaches. They also need to be continuous and closely linked with the development of hope-enhancing strategies and interventions. In some cases, the assessment itself may be a type of intervention.

In terms of quantitative assessments, there are two hope measures that show promise. The Herth Hope Index[51] is a well-validated measure that has been used in the terminally ill, most recently being validated in a Swedish sample of palliative patients.[52] Although psychometric findings were favorable, the authors cautioned against its use in Swedish clinical palliative settings, however, due to linguistic, conceptual, and cultural translation difficulties. The Hope Differential-Short, a relatively new measure for capturing the personal experience of hope, was recently validated in a sample of advanced cancer patients.[53] Although further

Table 75.1 *A hope assessment framework for terminally ill patients*

Theme	Questions for the healthcare professional	Questions for the patient
Personal spirit	What is meaningful in this person's life?	What is meaningful in your life? What would give you meaning in your life?
	What is this person's relationship with time?	How has your hope changed over time?
	How might past, present, and future experiences influence this person's experience of hope?	Tell me about a time in your past that has informed you about your hope in some way.
Risk	What is this person's tolerance for uncertainty?	How have you handled times of uncertainty in the past? What are you most afraid of?
	How can I enhance this person's hope, beyond a hope for a cure?	Without taking away your hope for a cure, what else might keep you going in the event that a cure is not possible?
Authentic caring	Who authentically cares about this person?	Who in your world cares about you?
	How can I provide truthful information to this person without destroying all hope?	Who do you care about?

Adapted from Nekolaichuk and Bruera.[7]

validation studies are warranted, this measure provides an innovative approach for individual patient assessments.

Given the complexity of the hope experience, quantitative measures need to be combined with qualitative assessments. One example of a qualitative assessment is Nekolaichuk and Bruera's hope framework for palliative care.[7] This framework is based on an empirically derived model of hope, consisting of three dimensions: personal spirit, risk, and authentic caring.[54] Personal spirit is a predominant personal dimension, represented by a core theme of meaning. Risk, a situational dimension, is primarily represented by an underlying theme of uncertainty. Authentic caring, a relational dimension, is characterized by the complementary themes of credibility and caring. Thus, a person's experience of hope may be associated with finding meaning in life, taking risks in spite of uncertainty and developing caring, credible relationships. An example of how this framework could be used for hope assessment appears in Table 75.1.

HOPE-ENHANCING STRATEGIES AND INTERVENTIONS

How do you enhance hope for someone who appears to have given up?

How do you help repair a patient's hope that others may have inadvertently damaged?

Many people have offered suggestions for hope enhancing strategies and interventions for the terminally ill, based on literature reviews,[55] research studies,[10,45,56–59] theoretical perspectives[60] and clinical experience.[61–63] In a systematic review of nursing literature, Holt[64***] identified 14 hope intervention themes, the six most common being positive relationships, patient self-worth, patient control, goal setting, use of distraction and family support. Many of these

interventions have not been empirically tested, however, particularly in terminally ill patients.

To date, very few intervention studies have focused on hope. Based on a quasi-experimental design, Tollett and Thomas[65*] studied the effect of rational thought on levels of hope in a sample of homeless veterans. Similarly, Rustoen *et al.*[66*] conducted a quasi-experimental study to evaluate the effect of a nursing-based intervention on hope and quality of life in patients with newly diagnosed cancer. Using a quasi-experimental design, Herth[67*] evaluated the effect of a 7-session hope-enhancing nursing intervention program on levels of hope and quality of life in a convenience sample of people with first recurrence of cancer. A follow-up evaluation of this intervention program was also conducted with the treatment group.[68*] Breitbart and Heller[69**] reported on preliminary findings of a meaning-centered psychotherapeutic intervention, suggesting that people in the meaning-centered group had less hopelessness and desire for death, and greater spiritual wellbeing and a sense of meaning, than those in the control group.

Specific hope-enhancing interventions for the terminally ill need to be developed and evaluated. As an example, Jevne and Nekolaichuk[50] developed a hope intervention framework for cancer patients, based on clinical experience, patient interviews and a thematic analysis of the literature. This framework consists of seven hope-enhancing themes: caring, communication, commitment, coping, creating, community, and celebrating. Within each theme, specific strategies for enhancing hope are proposed. An outline of this framework appears in Table 75.2, with sample questions that could be asked of patients (see Jevne and Nekolaichuk[50] for detailed descriptions of additional strategies). Although this framework was developed for cancer patients, many of these strategies could potentially be applied to the terminally ill. Further research is needed to extend its use in this population.

Table 75.2 *The seven Cs: a hope intervention framework*

Theme	Questions for the patient
Caring	Tell me about a time in your life when you experienced a moment of caring.
Communication	Tell me about what it is like to be ill. How has your hope changed since you have become ill?
Commitment	What would be one small thing that you might do on a regular basis to help strengthen your hope?
Coping	What has helped you through difficult times in the past?
Creating	If you were to create a 'hope kit', then what things would you put in it?
Community	How is hope experienced in your community (culture)?
Celebrating	If you were to plan a celebration of hope, then what might you do?

Adapted from Jevne and Nekolaichuk.[50]

SUMMARY

How might we create a space for hope in end-of-life care?

This chapter highlighted three specific challenges for intentionally integrating hope within clinical practice:

- the need to understand the nature of hope in the terminally ill
- the need to develop brief, psychometrically sound and appropriate assessment approaches for a palliative population
- the need to develop and evaluate specific hope-enhancing interventions for the terminally ill.

The lack of well-developed assessment approaches and effective hope-enhancing interventions, targeted specifically for the terminally ill, have impeded progress in this area. Through collaborative efforts involving patients, clinicians, and researchers, appropriate hope assessment frameworks and hope-focused interventions need to be developed and eventually become part of routine end-of-life care.

Key learning points

- Patients, healthcare providers and health researchers have all acknowledged the important role of hope in terminal illness.

- Hope is an inherent part of being human. Although it is a universal human experience, it is also an intensely personal one. It is important to understand what hope means to each person with a terminal illness.

- Hope assessments and interventions are closely intertwined. Assessment is a continuous process and may be a type of intervention. Interventions are closely linked to the types of assessments that are conducted.

- Although many assessment and intervention approaches for hope have been proposed, few have been developed for and validated in the terminally ill.

- Systematic approaches for hope assessment and intervention need to be developed and integrated into routine clinical practice in end-of-life care.

REFERENCES

1 Wilson KG, Graham IG, Viola RA, *et al.* Structured interview assessment of symptoms and concerns in palliative care. *Can J Psychiatry* 2004; **49**: 350–7.

2 Greisinger AJ, Lorimor RJ, Aday LA, *et al.* Terminally ill cancer patients: their most important concerns. *Cancer Pract* 1997; **5**: 147–54.

3 Lin H, Bauer-Wu SM. Psycho-spiritual well-being in patients with advanced cancer: an integrative review of the literature. *J Adv Nurs* 2003; **44**: 69–80.

4 Kirk P, Kirk I, Kristjanson LJ. What do patients receiving palliative care for cancer and their families want to be told? A Canadian and Australian qualitative study. *BMJ* 2004; **328**: 1343.

5 Scanlon C. Creating a vision of hope: the challenge of palliative care. *Oncol Nurs Forum* 1989; **16**: 491–6.

6 Hockley J. The concept of hope and the will to live. *Palliat Med* 1993; **7**: 181–6.

◆ 7 Nekolaichuk CL, Bruera E. On the nature of hope in palliative care. *J Palliat Care* 1998; **14**: 36–42.

8 Bustamante JJ. Understanding hope. Persons in the process of dying. *Int Forum Psychoanal* 2001; **10**: 49–55.

9 Duggleby W. Hope at the end of life. *J Hosp Palliat Nurs* 2001; **3**: 51–7, 64.

◆ 10 Herth KA, Cutcliffe JR. The concept of hope in nursing 3: hope and palliative care nursing. *Br J Nurs* 2002; **11**: 977–83.

◆ 11 Sullivan MD. Hope and hopelessness at the end of life. *Am J Geriatr Psychiatry* 2003; **11**: 393–405.

12 Parker-Oliver D. Redefining hope for the terminally ill. *Am J Hosp Palliat Care* 2002; **19**: 115–20.

13 Janssens RMJ, Zylicz Z, Ten Have HAM. Articulating the concept of palliative care: philosophical and theological perspectives. *J Palliat Care* 1999; **15**: 38–44.

● 14 Herth KA. The relationship between level of hope and level of coping response and other variables in patients with cancer. *Oncol Nurs Forum* 1989; **16**: 67–72.

15 Elliott TR, Witty TE, Herrick S, Hoffman JT. Negotiating reality after physical loss: Hope, depression, and disability. *J Pers Soc Psychol* 1991; **61**: 608–13.

16 Post-White J, Ceronsky C, Kreitzer MJ, *et al.* Hope, spirituality, sense of coherence, and quality of life in patients with cancer. *Oncol Nurs Forum* 1996; **23**: 1571–9.

17 Staats S. Quality of life and affect in older persons: Hope, time frames, and training effects. *Curr Psychol Res Rev* 1991; **10**: 21–30.

18 Carson V, Soeken KL, Shanty J, Terry L. Hope and spiritual well-being: essentials for living with AIDS. *Perspect Psychiatr Care* 1990; **26**: 28–34.

19 Udelman HD, Udelman DL. Hope as a factor in remission of illness. *Stress Med* 1985; **1**: 291–4.

20 Udelman DL, Udelman HD. A preliminary report on anti-depressant therapy and its effects on hope and immunity. *Soc Sci Med* 1985; **20**: 1069–72.

21 Udelman DL, Udelman HD. Affects, neurotransmitters, and immunocompetence. *Stress Med* 1991; **7**: 159–62.

22 Zich J, Temoshok L. Perceptions of social support in men with AIDS and ARC: relationships with distress and hardiness. *J Appl Soc Psychol* 1987; **17**: 193–215.

23 Rabkin JG, Williams JBW, Neugebauer R, *et al.* Maintenance of hope in HIV-spectrum homosexual men. *Am J Psychiatry* 1990; **147**: 1322–6.

● 24 Beck AT, Weissman A, Lester D, Trexler L. The measurement of pessimism: The hopelessness scale. *J Consult Clin Psychol* 1974; **42**: 861–5.

● 25 Beck AT, Steer RA, Kovacs M, Garrison B. Hopelessness and eventual suicide: A 10-year prospective study of patients hospitalized with suicidal ideation. *Am J Psychiatry* 1985; **142**: 559–63.

26 Arnold EM. Factors that influence consideration of hastening death among people with life-threatening illnesses. *Health Soc Work* 2004; **29**: 17–26.

27 Rosenfeld B, Breitbart W, McDonald MV, *et al.* Pain in ambulatory AIDS patients: II. Impact of pain on psychological functioning and quality of life. *Pain* 1996; **68**: 323–8.

28 Breitbart W, Rosenfeld B, Pessin H, *et al.* Depression, hopelessness, and desire for hastened death in terminally ill patients with cancer. *JAMA* 2000; **284**: 2907–11.

● 29 Chochinov HM, Wilson KG, Enns M, Lander S. Depression, hopelessness, and suicidal ideation in the terminally ill. *Psychosomatics* 1998; **39**: 366–70.

● 30 Perakyla A. Hope work in the care of seriously ill patients. *Qual Health Res* 1991; **1**: 407–33.

31 Nuland SB. *How we Die: Reflections on Life's Final Chapter.* New York: Alfred A Knopf, 1994.

● 32 Hall BA. The struggle of the diagnosed terminally ill person to maintain hope. *Nurs Sci Quart* 1990; **3**: 177–84.

◆ 33 Nekolaichuk CL. Diversity or divisiveness? A critical analysis on hope. In: Cutcliffe JRM, McKenna H, eds. *Essential Concepts in Nursing.* Oxford: Elsevier 2005: 179–212.

34 Benzein E, Norberg A, Saveman BI. The meaning of the lived experience of hope in patients with cancer in palliative home care. *Palliat Med* 2001; **15**: 117–26.

35 Appelin G, Bertero C. Patients' experiences of palliative care in the home: a phenomenological study of a Swedish sample. *Cancer Nurs* 2004; **27**: 65–70.

36 Flemming K. The meaning of hope to palliative care cancer patients. *Int J Palliat Nurs* 1997; **3**: 14–18.

37 Salander P, Bergenheim T, Henriksson R. The creation of protection and hope in patients with malignant brain tumors. *Soc Sci Med* 1996; **42**: 985–96.

38 Weil CM. Exploring hope in patients with end stage renal disease on chronic hemodialysis. *Nephrol Nurs J* 2000; **27**: 219–24.

39 Benzein E, Saveman BI. Nurses' perception of hope in patients with cancer: a palliative care perspective. *Cancer Nurs* 1998; **21**: 10–16.

40 Hall BA. Ways of maintaining hope in HIV disease. *Res Nurs Health* 1994; **17**: 283–93.

41 Kylma J, Vehvilainen-Julkunen K, Lahdevirta J. Hope, despair and hopelessness in living with HIV/AIDS: a grounded theory study. *J Adv Nurs* 2001; **33**: 764–75.

42 Ezzy D. Illness narratives: Time, hope and HIV. *Soc Sci Med* 2000; **50**: 605–17.

43 Wong-Wylie G, Jevne RF. Patient Hope: Exploring the interactions between physicians and HIV seropositive individuals. *Qual Health Res* 1997; **7**: 32–56.

● 44 Dufault K, Martocchio BC. Hope: Its spheres and dimensions. *Nurs Clin North Am* 1985; **20**: 379–91.

45 Herth K. Fostering hope in terminally-ill people. *J Adv Nurs* 1990; **15**: 1250–9.

46 Stephenson C. The concept of hope revisited for nursing. *J Adv Nurs* 1991; **16**: 1456–61.

47 Jevne RF, Nekolaichuk CL, Boman J. *Experiments in Hope: Blending Art and Science with Service.* Edmonton: Hope Foundation of Alberta, 1999.

◆ 48 Yates P. Towards a reconceptualization of hope for patients with a diagnosis of cancer. *J Adv Nurs* 1993; **18**: 701–6.

◆ 49 Farran CJ, Herth KA, Popovich JM. *Hope and Hopelessness: Critical Clinical Constructs.* Thousand Oaks, CA: Sage, 1995.

◆ 50 Jevne RF, Nekolaichuk CL. Threat and hope in coping with cancer for health care professionals. In: Jacoby R, Keinan G, eds. *Between stress and hope: From a Disease-Centered to a Health-Centered Perspective.* Westport CT: Praeger Publishers, 2003: 187–212.

● 51 Herth K. Abbreviated instrument to measure hope: Development and psychometric evaluation. *J Adv Nurs* 1992; **17**: 1251–9.

52 Benzein E, Berg A. The Swedish version of Herth Hope Index – an instrument for palliative care. *Scand J Caring Sci* 2003; **17**: 409–15.

53 Nekolaichuk CL, Bruera E. Assessing hope at end-of-life: Validation of an experience of hope scale in advanced cancer patients. *Palliat Support Care* 2004; **2**: 243–53.

● 54 Nekolaichuk CL, Jevne RF, Maguire TO. Structuring the meaning of hope in health and illness. *Soc Sci Med* 1999; **48**: 591–605.

◆ 55 MacLeod R, Carter H. Health professionals' perception of hope: understanding its significance in the care of people who are dying. *Mortality* 1999; **4**: 309–17.

✱ 56 Cutcliffe JR. How do nurses inspire and instil hope in terminally ill HIV patients? *J Adv Nurs* 1995; **22**: 888–95.

57 Herth K. Contributions of humor as perceived by the terminally ill. *Am J Hosp Care* 1990; **7**: 36–40.

✱ 58 Herth K. Engendering hope in the chronically and terminally ill: Nursing interventions. *Am J Hosp Palliat Care* 1995; **12**: 31–9.

59 Kennett CE. Participation in a creative arts project can foster hope in a hospice day centre. *Palliat Med* 2000; **14**: 419–25.

60 Gum A, Snyder CR. Coping with terminal illness: the role of hopeful thinking. *J Palliat Med* 2002; **5**: 883–94.

61 Centers LC. Beyond denial and despair: ALS and our heroic potential for hope. *J Palliat Care* 2001; **17**: 259–64.

62 Aldridge D. Spirituality, hope, and music therapy in palliative care. *Arts Psychother* 1995; **22**: 103–9.

63 Jevne RF. *It all begins with hope*: *Patients, Caregivers and the Bereaved Speak Out*. San Diego, CA: LuraMedia, 1991.

♦ 64 Holt J. A systematic review of the congruence between people's needs and nurses' interventions for supporting hope. *Online J Knowledge Synthesis Nurs* 2001; 8: 10.

65 Tollett JH, Thomas SP. A theory-based nursing intervention to instill hope in homeless veterans. *Adv Nurs Sci* 1995; 18: 76–90.

66 Rustoen T, Wiklund I, Hanestad BR, Moum T. Nursing intervention to increase hope and quality of life in newly diagnosed cancer patients. *Cancer Nurs* 1998; 21: 235–45.

✱ 67 Herth K. Enhancing hope in people with a first recurrence of cancer. *J Adv Nurs* 2000; 32: 1431–41.

✱ 68 Herth K. Development and implementation of a hope intervention program. *Oncol Nurs Forum* 2001; 28: 1009–17.

69 Breitbart W, Heller KS. Reframing hope: meaning-centered care for patients near the end of life. *J Palliat Med* 2003; 6: 979–88.

PART 13

Assessment and management of other problems

76

Dehydration and rehydration

ROBIN L FAINSINGER

INTRODUCTION

There are many facets to the often complicated and controversial topic of dehydration and rehydration of palliative care populations. The ongoing divergent opinion is well illustrated by the following recent statements:

> Research is limited but suggests that artificial hydration in imminently dying patients influences neither survival nor symptom control.[1]
>
> The best available evidence suggests that hydration of advanced cancer patients plays an important role in maintaining cognitive function and is therefore an important factor in the prevention and reversal of delirium in this population.[2]

Superimposed on these conflicting medical comments are other complex issues:

> terminal dehydration is a controversial topic, weighted heavily with historic symbolism, and strong religious, societal, and cultural conflicts.[3]

Some of these issues can be illustrated with the following examples.

SCENARIO 1

A 70-year-old woman living in an isolated rural community in southern Africa develops increasing abdominal discomfort. She has been active and in good health, although she has lost approximately 3 kg of weight over the last 2 months. She develops severe nausea and vomiting and inability to maintain an adequate oral intake. The family's access to transportation that would enable them to travel to the nearest hospital 10 km away is limited. Her extended family nurses her at home and after a few days she is able to resume a reasonable oral intake, her strength improves and she resumes her role with household maintenance and care of her grandchildren.

SCENARIO 2

A 70-year-old woman living in a wealthy country with universal healthcare develops increasing abdominal discomfort. She has been active and in good health, although she notes that she has lost approximately 3 kg of weight over the last few months. Extensive diagnostic imaging and subsequent liver biopsy confirm pancreatic cancer with liver metastases. She develops severe nausea and vomiting and presents to the emergency department of her local hospital with clinical evidence of dehydration. She is rehydrated with intravenous fluids and admitted for investigation. No evidence of bowel obstruction is found on diagnostic imaging. The patient improves, resumes a reasonable oral intake and is discharged home.

SCENARIO 1

Over the course of the next few weeks the woman develops increasing abdominal pain, poor appetite and loss of weight, and intermittent nausea and vomiting. She is fortunate that a mobile health clinic has now started to visit her isolated community on a monthly basis. The nurse practitioner doing the examination notes that the patient looks cachectic and has a very enlarged, tender liver. She suspects that the patient is dying from an unknown gastrointestinal primary with extensive intraabdominal metastatic disease. The family and patient are provided with an explanation of the suspected diagnosis and prognosis. The clinic is able to provide a free prescription of morphine liquid, and an explanation of dietary supplements they could use to prevent constipation.

The nurse practitioner is aware of the options for hydration supplementation including intravenous, hypodermoclysis, and rectal hydration. However for a variety of reasons, including economic and the increased burden this would place on the family caregivers, all of these options are rejected. Instead the family is given suggestions to assist the patient to continue to drink as long as this is comfortable for her, as well as some suggestions to provide mouth care. The nurse practitioner wishes the patient and family well and indicates that they should return for a follow-up visit when the mobile clinic is back in their community. The nonverbal communication in the room indicates that all of them understand that the nurse practitioner does not really expect to see them for a follow-up visit.

SCENARIO 2

Over the next few weeks increasing abdominal pain requires escalating morphine doses to achieve good control. The patient expresses a preference to remain at home as she deteriorates. However the patient and her husband indicate to the family physician that their religious beliefs are that everything possible should be done to maintain life for as long as possible. Intermittent nausea and vomiting results in the oral morphine being changed to the subcutaneous route, and increasing abdominal pain requires increasing the morphine to 100 mg subcutaneously per day. The family physician discusses the option of parenteral hydration. Hypodermoclysis at 1 L overnight is instituted. A daughter and son now arrive to assist and support their father in caring for their mother. The son has worked as a hospice nurse and questions the value of ongoing hydration at this point. The daughter is a nephrologist who believes that hydration is necessary to maintain normal renal function, and avoid the accumulation of morphine metabolites that may cause side effects. The patient and her husband have had extensive discussions over the years with their family physician who has a good understanding of how their spirituality affects their decision making. Although respecting their children's opinions, the couple rely heavily on their family physician to provide information and direction on appropriate management.

These scenarios highlight some of the complexity that surrounds this widely debated and controversial topic. At the center of the discussion, irrespective of the setting and circumstances, is the desire to keep patients as comfortable as possible while avoiding unnecessary management or procedures. However there is no doubt that the definition of 'unnecessary' will have great international variation. Clinicians with the responsibility to make these decisions will need to sort through expressions of opinion, information on pathophysiology and biochemical changes, research looking at a variety of outcomes, differing family and cultural expectations, and consensus statements. This diverse information then has to be individually applied to the specific trajectory and circumstances of patients and their families.

WHAT IS DEHYDRATION?

As has been pointed out in recent reviews, use of the term dehydration in considering this issue, is often inaccurate.[2,4] Fluid deficit is the state of water loss with or without electrolytes, that includes the subtypes of volume depletion and dehydration. Dehydration should be understood as total body water deficit that is predominantly intracellular and associated with hypernatremia. Volume depletion implies a deficit in the intravascular fluid volume and can be isotonic, hyponatremic, or hypernatremic (Fig. 76.1).

A variety of factors can be associated with fluid deficits (Table 76.1). Any of these etiologies for fluid deficit can occur at any stage of a palliative care illness and multiple possible mechanisms can occur simultaneously.

The assessment of risk or presence of fluid deficits is based on a variety of factors that can be determined by history, physical examination, and laboratory findings. The history is of obvious value in determining the possible risk factors listed in Table 76.1. There are sometimes practical difficulties in estimating the accuracy of fluid intake estimates and potential fluid loss through urine and fecal incontinence. Symptoms of fluid deficit can include behavior and cognitive changes, fatigue, thirst, nausea, and a dry mouth. The classic signs of fluid deficit include dry mouth, reduced skin turgor, postural hypotension, tachycardia, reduced jugular venous pressure, sunken eyes, and reduced sweating. However all of these problems need to be interpreted with caution as they can be associated with other causes present in aging, cachexia, advanced cancer, and side effects due to commonly used medications.

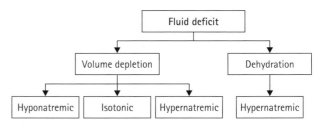

Figure 76.1 *Types of fluid deficit.*

Table 76.1 *Factors associated with fluid deficits*

Decreased intake	Increased fluid loss
Asthenia	Bowel resection
Anorexia	Diarrhea
Coma	Diuretics
Delirium	Diabetes mellitus/insipidus
Dementia	Fistulas
Depression	Fever/sweating
Dysphagia	Hypercalcemia
Nausea	Vomiting

Laboratory evaluation can provide some helpful information in evaluating fluid deficits, but will obviously depend on the setting of care and whether such investigations are acceptable to the patient, family and healthcare team. The common findings present in volume-depleted patients include elevated levels of urea, creatinine, plasma proteins, hematocrit, and sodium. It is worth noting that a systematic review attempted to clarify the physical diagnosis of hypovolemia in adults.[5***] The authors concluded that in patients with vomiting, diarrhea, or deceased oral intake, few findings, with the exception of serum electrolytes, urea, and creatinine values, have proven value.

THE HYDRATION CONTROVERSY

There is no controversy that palliative care populations should be encouraged to maintain an adequate oral intake to prevent fluid deficit. However there are many literature reports illustrating opposing viewpoints on the use of supplemental parenteral hydration. These have been considered from both clinical and ethical viewpoints.[6–16] Historical reviews on this topic have referenced a similar collection of clinical anecdotes and opinions. The arguments for and against hydrating palliative care populations are summarized in Box 76.1.[11,12]

It would appear that the arguments for initiating or maintaining parenteral hydration in palliative care populations originate from the standard medical approach to fluid deficits. Thus it would be reasonable to expect that most patients dying in hospitals will have an intravenous line unless they have undergone rapid deterioration or unanticipated demise. This was originally demonstrated by a Canadian report[17] where 73 of 106 cancer patients dying in a tertiary care hospital were noted to have intravenous fluids administered. A more recent retrospective study on the use of artificial hydration in an acute care hospital in England[1] noted that of 111 patients, 65 percent were hydrated during the last week of life and 46 percent were being hydrated at the time of death. The mean rate of parenteral hydration was 2000 mL/day. The results suggest that artificial hydration is no longer necessarily considered routine hospital practice for dying patients in this setting.

In order to clarify routine practice of physicians involved in end-of-life care in Edmonton, Canada, the routine management of parenteral hydration for patients dying in a palliative care unit, and acute care hospital while receiving or not receiving consult advice from the palliative care program was reported.[18] A retrospective chart review of 50 consecutive patients dying at each of the three sites was included. The majority of patients at all sites received hydration ranging from 66 percent to 98 percent of patients during the last week of life. However the volume of hydration was noted to be significantly lower in the palliative care unit site.

Box 76.1 Hydration in palliative care

Against parenteral hydration

- Symptom distress is not experienced by comatose patients
- Dying is prolonged by parenteral fluids
- There is less urine and thus less problem with incontinence and catheter use
- Decreased gastrointestinal fluid associated with dehydration results in less nausea and vomiting
- Decreased respiratory secretions will result in less cough and pulmonary edema
- The severity of edema and ascites is decreased
- Dehydration can act as a natural anesthetic for the central nervous system
- Parenteral hydration is uncomfortable and limits patient mobility

For parenteral hydration

- Parenteral hydration assists in making dying patients more comfortable
- There is no evidence that parenteral hydration prolongs life
- Fluid deficits can cause restlessness, confusion, and neuromuscular irritability
- Oral hydration is provided to dying patients complaining of thirst, and therefore parenteral hydration should be an option
- Emphasis on the poor quality of life of palliative care populations detracts from efforts to improve comfort and life quality
- Parenteral hydration is considered a minimum standard of care
- Withholding parenteral fluid from palliative care populations may result in withholding therapies to other compromised patient groups

A survey questionnaire of Japanese physicians attempted to clarify attitudes towards terminal dehydration. Results revealed that physicians with more positive attitudes toward intravenous hydration were less involved in end-of-life care and more likely to regard fluid as a necessary physiological requirement, consider it a minimum standard of care, and believe that this was beneficial for palliating symptoms.[19] A Canadian study distributed a questionnaire to 18 palliative care physicians in major Canadian centers in an attempt to clarify the routine practice of physicians involved in end-of-life care.[20] Results demonstrated a wide range of practice. Physicians estimated that they ordered parenteral hydration in a median of 6–10 percent of patients (range 0–100 percent). The route of parenteral hydration was: intravenous hydration, a median of 30 percent (range 0–100 percent), and hypodermoclysis, a median of 70 percent (range 0–100 percent). The estimated average volume range per 24 hours was between 200 mL and 2400 mL.

It is easy to imagine the problems inflicted on advanced palliative care populations by a policy of maintaining intravenous hydration with volumes in excess of 3 L/day. Under this circumstance complications such as increased respiratory and gastrointestinal symptom distress can be anticipated. The literature reports against parenteral hydration would suggest that healthcare professionals looking after palliative care populations have reacted to overuse of intravenous fluids and concluded that no parenteral hydration is the preferred approach. This has been reinforced by anecdotal literature reports noting that many palliative care patients appear to die comfortably without parenteral hydration. Nevertheless a review of the literature indicates that these reports are mostly based on unsubstantiated data.[12] There are other issues worth considering:[11,12,21–24]

- Fluid deficit as a cause of confusion and restlessness in nonterminally ill patients is well recognized. The problems of delirium and agitation have been well reported in palliative care populations.[2]
- Reduced intravascular volume and glomerular filtration rate caused by fluid deficits are well accepted as a cause of prerenal failure.[2,4] Opioid metabolite accumulation in the presence of renal failure, resulting in confusion, myoclonus and seizures, has been well documented.

Reports with regard to agitated delirium and terminal restlessness have frequently appeared in the palliative care literature. Discussion of these problems has generally centered on the need for pharmacological management which often includes sedation.[25–27] Ventafridda et al.[28] reported 9 percent of patients requiring sedation for agitated delirium in a study of unendurable symptoms experienced by patients with cancer during their last days of life. This prompted a report by our group[29] that agitated delirium was the most frequent problem requiring sedation in the last week of life in 10 percent of our patients. A later report noted that the severity of agitated delirium requiring sedation had decreased to 3 percent in our palliative care unit.[30] We speculated that this resulted from a change in our practice to include more frequent use of hypodermoclysis for hydration, switching opioids earlier when toxicity developed, and the use of less sedating treatments such as haloperidol for delirium, decreasing the prevalence and difficulty of managing agitated delirium in this setting.[31]

Reports in the palliative care literature have continued to note innovative approaches to the pharmacological management of symptoms associated with agitated delirium, including the use of intravenous propofol.[32–34] A retrospective chart review of 76 consecutive patients dying at St Luke's Hospice in Cape Town, South Africa, found that 29 percent of patients required sedation for agitated delirium. Although none of these patients were treated with parenteral hydration, patients requiring sedation were noted to require significantly higher doses of opioids during a longer admission.[35]

Further reports on the use of sedation have suggested that agitated delirium appears to be less problematic in a number of different settings in Edmonton,[36] where parenteral hydration is more common practice,[18] compared with requirements for sedation in a number of other international settings.[37] As a result it has been suggested that dehydration could be a reversible component of agitated delirium, that may be ignored by an approach that focuses on a sedative pharmacological solution to this apparently common and certainly distressing situation.[38*] Thus it may be illogical for a patient to receive medications for agitated delirium, myoclonus, and seizures, if in some circumstances these problems could be prevented or corrected by the use of parenteral hydration.

HYDRATION RESEARCH

Research into the use of hydration in palliative care settings has focused on three dimensions:[39]

- The association between biochemical findings and hydration status
- The association between biochemical findings and clinical symptoms
- The association between hydration status and clinical symptoms.

Biochemical findings and hydration status

There is no controversy that dehydration is a cause of renal failure.[40–42,] However while parenteral hydration is accepted standard management in many settings, the impact of fluid deficit and rehydration on the renal function and electrolyte balance of palliative care populations is still questioned.[10,43–46]

Ellershaw et al.[47] undertook biochemical investigation in 82 patients with advanced cancer. The patients were taking oral sips of fluid and no longer able to tolerate oral medication. Our group[48] reported biochemical investigation of 100 consecutive patients, 69 of whom received hypodermoclysis at an average volume of 1203 ± 505 mL/day. A comparison of these two reports[49] has been published (Table 76.2). Morita et al.[50] published further results on the biochemistry of terminally ill cancer patients, and concluded that relatively small amounts of parenteral hydration may result in less abnormal biochemistry, particularly with regard to renal function.

Table 76.2 *Comparison of biochemical findings in patients taking oral fluids (sips)[47] and those receiving hypodermoclysis[48]*

	Fainsinger et al.[48]		Ellershaw et al.[47]	
	Mean	Normal range	Mean	Normal range
Urea (mmol/L)	8.8	3.2–8.2	15.5	2.5–6.5
Creatinine (μmol/L)	101	62–133	177	60–120

Biochemical findings/hydration status and clinical symptoms

Much of the early literature on this issue was based on anecdotal opposing viewpoints and case reports.[51,52] However many reports have now attempted to study this issue more carefully. Burge[45] reported a cross-sectional survey studying the quantitative assessment of the dehydration experience in patients with advanced cancer. The study concluded that parenteral hydration on the basis of fluid intake and laboratory measures were not helpful if the aim was to reduce thirst. McCann et al.[53] studied 48 consecutive patients with regard to symptom prevalence and management of hunger and thirst in terminally ill patients not receiving parenteral hydration. Symptoms of hunger, thirst, and dry mouth were apparently well managed with oral sips and mouth care.

Ellershaw et al.[47] investigated the relationship between symptoms and dehydration in 82 patients not provided parenteral hydration. No significant association was demonstrated between the level of hydration and respiratory tract secretions, thirst, and dry mouth. However they did acknowledge that the effect of renal failure and possible consequences of agitation and confusion were not assessed. Musgrave et al.[54] studied the effect of intravenous fluids on a group of patients with advanced cancer dying in a hospital oncology unit. No relationship was demonstrated between level of thirst, intravenous fluids, and biochemical parameters. A subsequent study[55] also failed to demonstrate any relation between intravenous fluids, fluid balance, and the prevalence of crepitations, ascites, and leg edema. A retrospective chart review of 117 and 162 patients admitted to a palliative care unit in 1988–89 and 1991–92 assessed the impact of a change in practice with regard to management of dehydration and cognitive impairment.[56*] The authors concluded that the data suggested that routine cognitive assessment, opioid rotation and hydration may reduce the frequency of agitated confusion in terminally ill cancer patients. Although hydration may have had a role, it was not possible to determine the relative contribution. A partial replication of this study considered the role of hydration and an incomplete opioid substitution on the prevalence of agitated delirium.[57] However no significant decrease in the occurrence of agitated delirium was noted.

Ashby et al.[58] measured plasma concentrations of morphine and metabolites in 36 hospice patients. They concluded that morphine metabolites may be a causal aggravating factor in nausea and vomiting and cognitive impairment in palliative care patients with significant renal impairment. Lawlor et al.[59*] completed prospective serial assessments of 113 patients with advanced cancer in a delirium study. Univariate analysis demonstrated reversibility associated with psychoactive medications and dehydration. They concluded that although delirium is multifactorial, hydration using hypodermoclysis may be one of the potential useful measures to consider.

A review by Burge[60***] concluded that there is little clinical evidence to guide patients, families, and clinicians in treatment decisions regarding fluid intake during the terminal phase of life. A subsequent systematic review by Viola et al.[61***] summarized existing evidence regarding fluid status effects and fluid therapy. Six studies where selected for inclusion and the authors concluded that given the study limitations it was impossible to draw firm conclusions regarding clinical care.

SOCIAL AND CULTURAL CONSIDERATIONS

There are other important issues to consider in regard to the use of parenteral hydration.[62] Patient and family attitudes, level of comfort with the situation, and education, and healthcare workers' attitudes, level of education and biases in presentation all influence the decision-making process.

Morita et al.[63] studied patients' and family members' perceptions about rehydration to identify factors contributing to decision making. The survey included 121 Japanese hospice patients with insufficient oral intake. Patient performance status, fluid retention symptoms, denial, physician recommendations, patients and family members' beliefs with regard to hydration effect on patient distress, and family anxiety about withholding rehydration were significantly associated with decision making. The main determinants for rehydration were the patient performance status, fluid retention symptoms, denial, and care receiver's beliefs about the effects of rehydration on patient distress.

A Canadian study[64] identified issues of importance to family caregivers with regard to administering parenteral hydration to patients with advanced cancer. Factors influencing caregivers including symptom distress issues, ethical and emotional considerations, information exchanged between health professionals and families, and culture. Perceived benefits of artificial hydration were central to the ethical, emotional, and cultural considerations involved in caregivers' decision making. An article presenting the values of the Jewish faith with regard to terminal dehydration[65] illustrates the difficulty of applying cultural and ethnic research and opinion. Letters in response varied from describing this as an 'excellent article'[66] to 'extremely offensive in its references to Jewish people'.[67]

It has been proposed that terminal dehydration or voluntary cessation of drinking may provide an alternative to physician-assisted suicide. Miller and Meier[68] suggested that terminal dehydration accompanied by standard palliative care management, offers patients a way to escape agonizing, incurable conditions that they consider to be worse than death, without requiring transformation of the law and medical ethics'. Quill et al.[69] suggested that voluntary cessation of 'eating and drinking are clinical options that may be acceptable to a patient and physician and do not require fundamental changes in the law'.

ALTERNATIVE HYDRATION TECHNIQUES

There is universal agreement that the best and most convenient route to correct fluid deficits are increasing or improving oral intake. However where this is impossible or inadequate, there are some circumstances where parenteral hydration may be of benefit. It is often misunderstood that we are not necessarily all seeing patients in the same trajectory of illness. Clinical circumstances evolve,[70] and a physically independent and cognitively intact patient at an early stage of a palliative illness is likely to be viewed very differently to the same patient a number of months later who is now cognitively impaired and physically dependent. However, if a decision is made to use parenteral hydration, there are considerations with regard to the type of fluid, volume and route of administration. There is no doubt that intravenous hydration is the route of choice in acute care institutions. There are obvious disadvantages such as difficulty finding venous access, pain, infection, limitations to mobility, and displaced lines, particularly with confused patients. Nevertheless it should be noted that a report from an Italian palliative care program stated that 82 percent of palliative care patients will have an intravenous line and receive a range of 1–1.5 L of fluid per day.[71] In addition they stated that although hypodermoclysis has been suggested as an alternative, experience suggests that it is not less stressful for palliative care patients and that the intravenous route is preferred.

Nasogastric tubes and gastrostomy

Nasogastric tubes are generally uncomfortable for patients and prolonged used, particularly in palliative care populations should be avoided where possible.[72,73] Percutaneous gastrostomies are commonly used with head and neck or esophageal cancer patients with increasing dysphagia who may benefit from nutrition as well as hydration.[74] As patients deteriorate there is a need to review the goals of care with regard to enteral nutrition. However difficulty with discontinuing management and ease of access can result in ongoing enteral nutrition and hydration in circumstances where this might not otherwise have been instituted.

Hypodermoclysis

The safety of hypodermoclysis has been well documented and reported in noncancer patients.[75*,76*] There have also been studies in palliative care patients demonstrating the ease of administration and minimal toxicity.[48*,77*,78*]

The procedure is simple and associated with minimal pain. A butterfly needle is inserted subcutaneously and attached to a fluid line which can run via gravity or an infusion pump. It requires minimal training for insertion and surveillance, and family caregivers can be trained to supervise this management in the home. Our recent study has suggested increasing acceptance of hypodermoclysis in the acute care setting.[18] It is generally recommended that solutions with some electrolytes are used, as nonelectrolytes solutions have been reported to draw fluid into the interstitial space.[11*,12*,79*] Initial recommendation suggested rates of infusion limited to a maximum of 100–120 mL/h, however, patients can tolerate boluses up to 500 mL/h.[80*]

Traditionally the use of hypodermoclysis was assisted by adding hyaluronidase to promote absorption in a dose ranging from 150 units/L to 750 units/L. Initially smaller volumes of hyaluronidase were demonstrated to be just as effective.[80] However a shortage of hyaluronidase led to clinical experience and anecdotal reports suggesting good absorption of hypodermoclysis without hyaluronidase. This resulted in a report of 24 consecutive patients receiving hypodermoclysis without hyaluronidase.[81*] Hydration was maintained for a mean 12 ± 9 days, with an infusion varying in range between 20 mL/h and 300 mL/h. Three patients were demonstrated to tolerate twice daily boluses of 500 mL over 1 hour. The average infusion site duration was 3.3 ± 3.6 days. These results and the increasing difficulty obtaining hyaluronidase has resulted in the ongoing clinical observation that most patients tolerate hypodermoclysis without requiring the addition of hyaluronidase.

Proctoclysis

As noted intravenous hydration can be uncomfortable, expensive and difficult to maintain in the home, while even hypodermoclysis can be expensive and too complicated in some settings. The potential advantage of the rectal administration of fluid, particularly in resource limited developing countries prompted a trial of rectal hydration in terminally ill cancer patients.[82*] Proctoclysis was offered to 17 adult patients with a fluid deficit where resources were inadequate for the use of hypodermoclysis. Tap water was used and the rectal infusion was increased from 100 mL to a maximum of 400 mL/h, unless fluid leakage occurred before the maximum volume was achieved. The mean daily volume, hourly rate, and duration was reported as 1035 ± 150 mL/day, 224 ± 58 mL/h, and 14 ± 8 days, respectively. Rectal hydration was noted to be well tolerated with minimal side effects in the majority of patients. A follow-up report[83*] included

78 advanced cancer patients receiving rectal hydration. Volumes infused, patient tolerance and side effects were similar to the earlier report, confirming that this is a safe, effective and low cost technique for rehydration in terminally ill palliative care populations.

CONCLUSION

Reconsider the varying circumstances and sociocultural circumstances of the two patients described in the introduction to this chapter. Discussion of management of these two patients, the manner in which information should be presented to them, literature interpretation as reviewed above, and the biases of healthcare providers and the circumstances in which we work will have significant implications on how we consider the issue of fluid deficit and rehydration. We can perhaps achieve consensus that dehydration is a cause of renal failure, and that hypodermoclysis is a safe and effective way of providing rehydration. There may be some agreement that rehydration of palliative care populations may result in better biochemical parameters at the end of life. There is certainly much evidence to recommend that if terminally ill patients are not rehydrated, medications such as opioids should be gradually decreased to avoid accumulation and unnecessary side effects. There is likely to be consensus that the major clinical issue is to consider whether rehydration will cause benefit or harm to palliative care patients unable to sustain adequate oral intake.

The need to consider individual circumstances and predictions of life expectancy in evaluating the potential benefits of rehydration is a recurring theme.[2,11] Although starting from different perspectives, there is some consensus[10,38,61] that:

- Available data are inadequate for final conclusions on this issue.
- Careful individual assessment of the relevance of fluid deficit to each clinical situation is essential.
- Further carefully designed research trials are required.

Key learning points

- Hydration in palliative care is a controversial topic with divergent opinions.
- Fluid deficits can cause confusion and renal failure.
- Hydration research is inconclusive in guiding clinical care.
- Hypodermoclysis is an excellent alternative for rehydration in palliative care populations.
- Diverse clinical and sociocultural circumstances need to be considered.

- Evidence recommends that if terminally ill patients are not rehydrated, medications should be decreased to avoid accumulation and side effects.
- Rehydration may be helpful in some individual situations.

REFERENCES

1 Soden K, Hoy A, Hoy W, et al. Artificial hydration during the last week of life in patients dying in district general hospital. Palliat Med 2002; 16: 542–3.
2 Lawlor P. Delirium and dehydration: Some fluid for thought? Support Care Cancer 2002; 10: 445–54.
3 Huffman JL, Dunn GP. The paradox of hydration in advanced terminal illness. J Am Coll Surg 2002; 194: 835–9.
4 Sarhill N, Walsh D, Nelson K, Davis M. Evaluation and treatment of cancer related fluid deficits: Volume depletion and dehydration. Support Care Cancer 2001; 9: 408–19.
5 McGee S, Abernethy WB, Simel DI. Is this patient hypovolemic? JAMA 1999; 281: 1022–9.
6 Craig GM. On withholding nutrition and hydration in the terminally ill: Has palliative medicine gone too far? J Med Ethics 1994; 20: 139–43.
7 Ashby M, Stoffell B. Artificial hydration and alimentation at the end of life: A reply to Craig. J Med Ethics 1995; 21: 135–40.
8 Dicks B. Rehydration or dehydration? Support Care Cancer 1994; 2: 88–90.
9 Dunlop RJ, Ellershaw JE, Baines MJ, et al. On withholding nutrition and hydration in the terminally ill: Has palliative medicine gone too far? A reply. J Med Ethics 1995; 21: 141–3.
10 Dunphy K, Finlay I, Rathbone G, et al. Rehydration in palliative and terminal care: if not – why not? Palliat Med 1995; 9: 221–8.
11 Fainsinger RL, Bruera E. The management of dehydration in terminally ill patients. J Palliat Care 1994; 10: 55–9.
12 Fainsinger RL, Bruera E. Hypodermoclysis for symptom control vs the Edmonton Injector. J Palliat Care 1991; 7: 5–8.
13 Meares CJ. Terminal dehydration. A review. Am J Hosp Palliat Care 1994; 11: 10–14.
14 Slomka J. What do apple pie and motherhood have to do with feeding tubes and caring for the patient? Arch Intern Med 1995; 155: 1258–63.
15 Smith SA. Patient induced dehydration – can it ever be therapeutic? Oncol Nurs Forum 1995; 22: 1487–91.
16 Wilkes E. On withholding nutrition and hydration in the terminally ill: Has palliative medicine gone too far? A commentary. J Med Ethics 1994; 20: 144–5.
17 Burge FI, King DB, Wilson D. Intravenous fluids and the hospitalized dying: a medical last rite? Can Fam Physician 1990; 86: 883–6.
18 Lanuke K, Fainsinger RL, deMoissac D. Hydration management at the end of life. J Palliat Med 2004; 7: 257–63.
19 Morita T, Shima Y, Adachi I. Attitudes of Japanese physicians towards terminal dehydration: A nation wide study. J Clin Oncol 2002; 20: 4699–704.

20 Lanuke K, Fainsinger RL. Hydration management in palliative care settings – a survey of experts. *J Palliat Care* 2004; **19**: 278–9.

21 Fainsinger RL, Bruera E, Watanabe S. Rehydration in palliative care. *Palliat Med* 1996; **10**: 165–6.

22 Fainsinger RL. Deshydratation et soins palliatifs. In: Roy DJ, Rapin C, eds. *Les annales de soins palliatifs. Vol 3*. Montreal: Centre de Bioethique. Institut de Recherches Cliniques de Montreal, 1995; 171–80.

23 Fainsinger RL. Nutrition and hydration for the terminally ill. *JAMA* 1995; **273**: 1736.

24 MacDonald SM, Fainsinger RL. Symptom control: the problem areas. *Palliat Med* 1994; **8**: 167–8.

25 Burke AL, Diamond PL, Hulbert J. Terminal restlessness – its management and the role of midazolam. *Med J Aust* 1999; **155**: 485–7.

26 Back IN. Terminal restlessness in patients with advanced malignant disease. *Palliat Med* 1992; **6**: 293–8.

27 Lichter I, Hunt E. The last 48 hours of life. *J Palliat Care* 1990; **6**: 7–15.

● 28 Ventafridda V, Ripamonti C, DeConno F, *et al.* Symptom prevalence and control during cancer patients last days of life. *J Palliat Care* 1990; **6**: 7–11.

● 29 Fainsinger RL, Bruera E, Miller MJ, *et al.* Symptom control during the last week of life on a palliative care unit. *J Palliat Care* 1991; **7**: 5–11.

30 Fainsinger RL, MacEacheron T, Miller MJ, *et al.* The use of hypodermoclysis for rehydration in terminally ill cancer patients. *J Palliat Care* 1992; **8**: 70.

31 Fainsinger RL, Tapper M, Bruera E. A perspective on the management of delirium in the terminally ill. *J Palliat Care* 1993; **9**: 4–8.

32 Mercadante S, De Conno F, Ripamonti C. Propofol in terminal care. *J Pain Symptom Manage* 1995; **10**: 639–42.

33 Moyle J. Use of propofol in palliative medicine. *J Pain Symptom Manage* 1995; **10**: 643–6.

34 Morita T, Inoue S, Chihara S. Sedation for symptom control in Japan: the importance of intermittent use and communication with family members. *J Pain Symptom Manage* 1996; **12**: 32–8.

35 Fainsinger RL, Landman W, Hoskings M, Bruera E. Sedation for uncontrolled symptoms in a South African hospice. *J Pain Symptom Manage* 1998; **16**: 145–52.

36 Fainsinger RL, deMoissac D, Mancini I, Oneschuk D. Sedation for delirium and other symptoms in terminally ill patients in Edmonton. *J Palliat Care* 2000; **16**: 5–10.

37 Fainsinger RL, Waller A, Bercovici M, *et al.* A multi-centre international study of sedation for uncontrolled symptoms in terminally ill patients. *Palliat Med* 2000; **14**: 257–65.

● 38 Fainsinger RL, Bruera E. When to treat dehydration in a terminally ill patient? *Support Care Cancer* 1997; **5**: 205–11.

● 39 Morita T, Ichiki T, Tsunoda J, *et al.* Three dimensions of the rehydration – dehydration problem in a palliative care setting. *J Palliat Care* 1999; **15**: 60–1.

40 Badr K, Ichikawa I. Prerenal failure: A deleterious shift from renal compensation to decompensation. *N Engl J Med* 1988; **319**: 623–9.

41 Brady HR, Singer GG. Acute renal failure. *Lancet* 1995; **346**: 1533–40.

42 Weinberg A, Minakar KL. Dehydration. Evaluation and management in older adults. *JAMA* 1995; **274**: 1552–6.

43 Waller A. Letter to the Editor. *Am J Hosp Palliat Care* 1995; **7**: 5–6.

44 Oliver D. Terminal dehydration [letter]. *Lancet* 1994; **ii**: 631.

45 Burge FI. Dehydration symptoms of palliative care cancer patients. *J Pain Symptom Manage* 1993; **8**: 454–64.

46 Waller A, Hershkowitz M, Adunsky A. The effect of intravenous fluid infusion on blood and urine parameters of hydration and on the state of consciousness in terminal cancer patients. *Am J Hosp Palliat Care* 1994; **11**: 22–7.

47 Ellershaw JE, Sutcliffe JM, Saunders CM. Dehydration and the dying patient. *J Pain Symptom Manage* 1995; **10**: 192–7.

48 Fainsinger RL, MacEacheron T, Miller MJ, *et al.* The use of hypodermoclysis for rehydration in terminally ill cancer patients. *J Pain Symptom Manage* 1994; **9**: 298–302.

49 Fainsinger RL. Biochemical dehydration in terminally ill cancer patients. *J Palliat Care* 1999; **15**: 59–61.

50 Morita T, Ichika T, Tsunoda J, *et al.* Biochemical dehydration and fluid retention symptoms in terminally ill cancer patients whose death is impending. *J Palliat Care* 1998; **14**: 60–2.

51 Andrews M, Bell ER, Smith SA, *et al.* Dehydration in terminally ill patients. Is it appropriate palliative care? *Postgrad Med* 1993; **93**: 201–8.

52 Yan E, Bruera E. Parenteral hydration of terminally ill cancer patients. *J Palliat Care* 1991; **7**: 40–3.

53 McCann RM, Hall WJ, Groth-Juncker A. Comfort care for the terminally ill patients. The appropriate use nutrition and hydration. *JAMA* 1994; **272**: 1263–6.

54 Musgrave CF, Bartle N, Opstad J. The sensation of thirst in dying patients receiving IV hydration. *J Palliat Care* 1995; **11**: 17–21.

55 Musgrave CF. Fluid retention and intravenous hydration in the dying. *Palliat Med* 1996; **10**: 53.

● 56 Bruera E, Franco JJ, Maltoni M, *et al.* Changing pattern of agitated impaired mental status in patients with advanced cancer: Association with cognitive monitoring, hydration, and opioid rotation. *J Pain Symptom Manage* 1995; **10**: 287–91.

57 Morita T, Tei U, Ionoue S. Agitated terminal delirium and association with partial opioid substitution and hydration. *J Palliat Med* 2003; **6**: 557–63.

58 Ashby M, Fleming B, Wood M, *et al.* Plasma morphine and glucuronide (M3G & M6G), concentrations in hospice in-patients. *J Pain Symptom Manage* 1997; **14**: 157–67.

● 59 Lawlor PG, Gagnon B, Mancini IL, *et al.* Occurrence, causes, and outcome of delirium in patients with advanced cancer. *Arch Intern Med* 2000; **160**: 786–94.

◆ 60 Burge FI. Dehydration and provision of fluids in palliative care. What is the evidence? *Can Fam Physician* 1996; **42**: 2383–8.

◆ 61 Viola RA, Wells GA, Peterson J. The effects of fluid status and fluid therapy on the dying: a systematic review. *J Palliat Care* 1997; **13**: 41–52.

62 Baumrucker S. Science, hospice, and terminal dehydration. *Am J Hosp Palliat Care* 1999; **16**: 502–3.

63 Morita T, Tsunoda J, Inoue S, *et al.* Perceptions and decision-making on rehydration of terminally ill cancer patients and family members. *Am J Hosp Palliat Care* 1999; **16**: 509–16.

64 Parkash R, Burge F. The family's perspective on issues of hydration in terminal care. *J Palliat Care* 1997; **13**: 23–7.

65 Bodell J, Weng MA. The Jewish patient in terminal dehydration: A hospice ethical dilemma. *Am J Hosp Palliat Care* 2000; **17**: 185–8.

66 Schur TG. Life and afterlife in Jewish tradition. *Am J Hosp Palliat Care* 2000; **17**: 296–7.

67 Rothstein JM. Out of context? *Am J Hosp Palliat Care* 2000; **17**: 297.

68 Miller FG, Meier DE. Voluntary death: A comparison of terminal dehydration and physician-assisted suicide. *Ann Intern Med* 1998; **128**: 559–62.

69 Quill TE, Meier DE, Block SD, *et al.* The debate over physician-assisted suicide: empirical data and conversant views. *Ann Intern Med* 1998; **128**: 552–8.

70 Fainsinger R. Dehydration. In: MacDonald N. ed. *Palliative Medicine. A Case-Based Manual.* New York: Oxford University Press, 1998; 91–9.

71 Mercadante S, Villari P, Ferrera P. A model of acute symptom control unit: Pain relief and palliative unit of LaMaddalena Cancer Centre. *Support Care Cancer* 2003; **11**: 114–19.

72 Fainsinger RL, Spachynski K, Hanson J, *et al.* Symptom control in terminally ill patients with malignant bowel obstruction. *J Pain Symptom Manage* 1994; **9**: 12–18.

73 Ripamonti C, Mercadante S, Groff L, *et al.* Role of octreotide, scopolamine butylbromide and hydration in symptom control of patients with inoperable bowel obstruction and nasogastric tubes: A prospective randomized trial. *J Pain Symptom Manage* 2000; **19**: 23–4.

● 74 Steiner N, Bruera E. Methods of hydration in palliative care patients. *J Palliat Care* 1998; **14**: 6–13.

75 Constans T, Dutertre J, Froge E. Hypodermoclysis in dehydrated elderly patients: local effects with and without hyaluronidase. *J Palliat Care* 1991; **7**: 10–12.

76 Molloy DJ, Cunje A. Hypodermoclysis and the care of old adults. An old solution for new problems? *Can Fam Physician* 1992; **38**: 2038–43.

77 Hays H. Hypodermoclysis for symptom control in terminal cancer. *Can Fam Physician* 1985; **31**: 1253–6.

78 Bruera E, Legris M, Keuhn N, Miller MJ. Hypodermoclysis for the administration of fluids and narcotic analgesics in patients with advanced cancer. *J Pain Symptom Manage* 1990; **5**: 218–20.

79 Turner T, Cassano A. Subcutaneous dextrose for rehydration of elderly patients – An evidence based review. *BMC Geriatrics* 2004; **4**: 2.

80 Bruera E, de Stoutz ND, Fainsinger RL, *et al.* Comparison of two different concentrations of hyaluronidase in patients receiving one hour infusions of hypodermoclysis. *J Pain Symptom Manage* 1995; **10**: 505–9.

81 Centeno C, Bruera E. Subcutaneous hydration with no hyaluronidase in patients with advanced cancer. *J Pain Symptom Manage* 1999; **17**: 305–6.

82 Bruera E, Schoeller T, Pruvost M. Proctoclysis for hydration of terminal cancer patients. *Lancet* 1994; **344**: 1699.

83 Bruera E, Pruvost M, Schoeller T. Proctoclysis for hydration of terminally ill cancer patients. *J Pain Symptom Manage* 1998; **15**: 216–19.

77

Fever, sweats, and hot flashes

SHALINI DALAL, DONNA S ZHUKOVSKY

INTRODUCTION

Fever, sweats, and hot flashes are commonly encountered in the terminally ill and in patients with cancer, and sometimes may be associated with considerable morbidity and mortality. Although infection remains the most common etiology of fever in patients, irrespective of whether they are receiving chemotherapy or not, fever is commonly seen in patients in the absence of infection as well. Fever is also one of the most common symptoms experienced by elderly people at the end of life.[1,2] Similarly, hot flashes are reported by the majority of menopausal women, and in some women can be a major source of distress.[3,4] Less well recognized is the impact of hot flashes on individuals with cancer, particularly women with a history of breast cancer and men with prostate cancer. In women with a history of breast cancer, approximately two-thirds experience hot flashes.[5,6] Optimal management of fevers, chills, sweats, and hot flashes is therefore of vital consideration in symptom management. As detailed in this chapter, it is contingent on meticulous patient assessment, on ascertaining the likely etiology, if possible, and on implementation of appropriate treatment interventions befitting patient-determined goals of care.

FEVERS

Fever, as defined in *Stedman's Medical Dictionary* is a 'complex physiologic response to disease mediated by pyrogenic cytokines and characterized by a rise in core temperature, generation of acute phase reactants, and activation of immune systems'.[7] More commonly, fever is defined as the elevation of core body temperature above normal. Normal average adult core body temperature is 37 °C (98.6 °F) and displays a circadian rhythm with body temperatures being the lowest in the predawn hours, at 36.1 °C (97 °F) or lower, and rising to 37.4 °C (99.3 °F) or higher in the afternoon. In oncology practice, a single reading of temperature of more than 38.3 °C (101 °F) or three readings (each taken at least an hour apart) of temperatures more than 38 °C (100.4 °F) is considered significant.

Pathophysiology of fever

Much like other fundamental aspects of human biology, core body temperature is closely regulated by intricate control mechanisms, involving a complex interplay of autonomic, endocrine, and behavioral responses. Integral to this process is the hypothalamus which functions much like a thermostat, balancing heat production with heat loss. Fever is considered a hallmark of immune system activation, resulting in a regulated rise in body temperature. The regulation of this phenomenon is accomplished by the actions of two types of endogenous immunoregulatory proteins called cytokines, some functioning as pyrogens and others as antipyretics. This is described below and illustrated in Figure 77.1.

A number of exogenous substances, often referred to as exogenous pyrogens, have been found to be capable of evoking fever in animal models.[8] Of these, lipopolysaccharide (LPS), a cell wall product derived from Gram-negative bacteria, has been the most extensively studied. Exogenous pyrogens induce the production of proinflammatory cytokines, such as interleukin (IL)-1β and IL-6, interferon α (INFα) and tumor necrosis factor (TNF), which act as humoral mediators influencing brain structures involved in resetting the hypothalamic set point.[9] Cytokines are thought to exert their effect on the brain via direct and indirect mechanisms.[10–12]

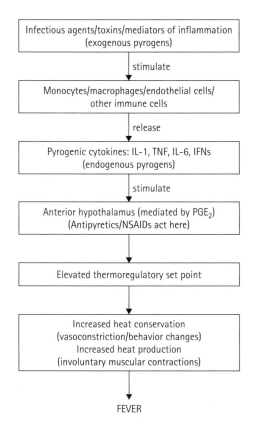

Figure 77.1 *Pathophysiology of fever. IL, interleukin; TNF, tumor necrosis factor; IFN, interferon; PGE, prostaglandin E; NSAID, nonsteroidal anti-inflammatory drug.*

Peripherally produced cytokines reach the central nervous system (CNS) directly by crossing at leaky areas in the blood–brain barrier via circumventricular vascular organs, which are networks of enlarged capillaries surrounding the hypothalamic regulatory centers.[13,14] In disease states such as bacterial infections, the blood–brain barrier can be compromised further, leading to an influx of cytokines from the periphery and which account for several of the neurological manifestations associated with sickness behavior, including fever.[15,16] Cytokines are also produced locally within the CNS,[11] and may account for the hyperpyrexia of CNS hemorrhage. Among the cytokines measurable in the blood plasma during LPS-induced fever, circulating levels of IL-6 have shown the best correlation with fever.[17,18]

Although not fully understood, it is proposed that cytokines stimulate the central production of the inducible enzyme cyclooxygenase (COX)-2, and subsequently stimulate the production of prostaglandins of the E series.[19,20] These prostaglandins activate thermoregulatory neurons of the anterior hypothalamic area to elevate body temperature.[21] Peripherally produced cytokines can also communicate with the brain indirectly in several ways, including the stimulation of terminal fibers of the autonomic nervous system.[22,23] Norepinephrine is the principal neurotransmitter, although several others such as acetylcholine, endorphins, enkephalins, substance P, somatostatin and vasoactive intestinal polypeptide (VIP) have also been implicated.[24]

Etiology of fever (Box 77.1)

INFECTIONS

Nearly two-thirds of fever in patients with prolonged neutropenia may be attributed to infection,[25] a major cause of morbidity in patients with cancer. Fever in a cancer patient should be considered indicative of infection until proved otherwise, with appropriate assessments being instituted in a timely fashion. Febrile neutropenic patients (granulocyte count <500) represent an absolute emergency. In patients with advanced Alzheimer disease, physical consequences of the progression of dementia predispose them to infection and fever, especially to aspiration pneumonia and urinary tract infections.[26–29]

PARANEOPLASTIC FEVERS

Fever may be a common presentation for some malignancies and their progression may parallel the occurrence of fevers. Although Hodgkin disease has classically been associated with Pel–Epstein fevers (recurring periods of fever lasting for 3–10 days at a time), several other malignancies are also associated with paraneoplastic fevers and include acute leukemias, lymphomas, renal cell carcinoma, bone sarcomas, adrenal carcinomas, and pheochromocytomas. Solid tumors such as breast, lung, and colon cancer are less often associated with paraneoplastic fevers. However, the presence of liver metastasis from these tumors may result in fever. In addition, any solid tumor causing obstruction can result in fever.

Malignancy is often found during the work-up of patients presenting with fever of unknown origin. While earlier reports found an incidence of 20 percent, a more recent study reported malignancy as the cause of fever in 15 percent of patients.[30] In patients with cancer presenting with fever of unknown origin, paraneoplastic was found to be the most common etiology.[31] Although the exact mechanism of

---

Box 77.1 Etiology of fever in cancer patients

- Infections
- Tumor (paraneoplastic fever)
- Drug-associated (e.g. cytotoxic agents, antibiotics, IFN)
- Blood transfusion reaction
- Thrombosis
- CNS metastasis
- Radiation-induced (e.g. radiation pneumonitis)

tumor-associated fever is unclear, it is thought to involve inflammatory cytokines such as TNFα, IL-1, and IL-6, which are produced either by host macrophages in response to the tumor or by the tumor itself.[32,33]

TRANSFUSION–ASSOCIATED FEVER

Febrile and allergic nonhemolytic transfusion reactions (NHTRs) are the most common adverse effects of blood transfusion.[34,35] These reactions are generally not life threatening, but they are expensive in their management, evaluation, and associated blood product wastage. The true incidence of febrile NHTRs (FNHTRs) is not well established in patients with cancer. In a large retrospective study, the incidence of side effects following transfusion of 100 000 units of packed red blood cells to more than 25 000 cancer patients over a 4-year period was found to be at 0.3 percent (of these, 51.3 percent were FNHTRs, 36.7 percent were allergic urticarial reactions, and 17 percent were hemolytic reactions).[36] This is comparable to other studies where the incidence has ranged from 0.2 percent to 0.7 percent.[37,38]

The occurrence of fever is usually caused by the presence of antibodies to antigens on the donor's white blood cells and its prevention by using leukodepleted blood components was demonstrated more than two decades ago.[39–41] Some studies have shown a correlation with storage time of platelets and the release of cytokines, as another reason for the occurrence of FNHTRs.[42–44]

Infection may also be a source of fever in patients receiving blood transfusions.[45–47] The prevalence of bacteria is estimated to be about 0.04–2 percent, depending on the type of components, the number and age of the evaluated components, and the detection methods used.[48–51] The last of these studies estimated that 1 in each 1000/2000 units of platelet concentrates (obtained from whole blood or apheresis) is bacterially contaminated. The incidence of bacterial contamination in red cell concentrates is much lower and almost zero for fresh frozen plasma and cryoprecipitate.

DRUG FEVER

Drug-associated fever is usually a diagnosis of exclusion, except for some drugs such as biological response modifiers, amphotericin B, and bleomycin, where the occurrence of fever may be predictable. Other drugs commonly implicated as a cause of fever include antibiotics, cardiovascular drugs, anticonvulsants, cytotoxics, and growth factors. In one retrospective study of 148 episodes of drug fever, antimicrobials were found to be the most common offending agent (31 percent).[52] Cytotoxic agents accounted for 11 episodes (7.4 percent).

In a retrospective chart review of 50 patients who had received at least 100 mg of amphotericin B for at least 3 days, the incidence of fever was 34 percent and chills was 56 percent, with rates of 2.6 and 3.5 mean episodes per patient per treatment course, respectively.[53] Interferon therapy is associated with acute 'flulike syndrome consisting of fever, chills, fatigue, myalgias, arthralgia, and headache, with some variation according to type of IFN, route of administration, schedule, dose, and age of patient.[54] The administration of growth factors is also associated with fever, being more common following granulocyte macrophage colony-stimulating factor (GM-CSF) administration than granulocyte colony-stimulating factor (G-CSF) administration. Bleomycin-associated fever occurs in 20–50 percent of patients and is more common when it is administered intravenously. Fever is also associated with other cytotoxic agents such as cisplatin, streptozocin, 5-fluorouracil, and therapy with monoclonal antibodies.[55–58]

Evaluation of fever

Assessment of fever requires careful history taking, medication review, and a thorough physical examination to include all major body systems. Patients should undergo meticulous evaluation of the skin, and all body orifices including mouth, ears, nose, throat, urethra, vagina and rectum, venipuncture sites, biopsy site, and skin folds (i.e. breast, axilla, abdomen, groin). In nearly two-thirds of neutropenic patients the initial evaluation may not identify a focus of infection.[32] This may relate in part to the high frequency of empirical treatment with broad-spectrum antibiotics, which may make it harder to determine the site of infection. Careful physical examinations should be repeated at least daily in patients with neutropenia, even after the initiation of empirical antibiotics. It must be remembered that immunocompromised patients may be vulnerable to more than one infection and that different organisms may emerge during a single febrile episode.

Interventions for fever

GOALS OF CARE

The presence of fever may be associated with potential metabolic consequences including dehydration and increased oxygen consumption and metabolic rate,[59,60] which may be especially pronounced in debilitated terminally ill patients. If prolonged, fevers may be associated with increased nutritional demands and debilitating fatigue. Although fever may be beneficial for enhancing host defense,[61,62] other factors such as the patient's comfort and physiological responses also deserve consideration. Suppression of fever may help alleviate uncomfortable, constitutional symptoms of fatigue, myalgias, diaphoresis, and chills. In addition to constitutional symptoms, focal findings related to the etiology of fever may also contribute to symptom burden. For example, abscess formation is often associated with pain, while uncomfortable dyspnea and cough can be related to pneumonia. The specific interventions used for fever management are determined by the underlying etiology, together with patient-determined goals of care. Patients with advanced cancer may opt not to treat the underlying etiology of fever and seek only nonspecific palliative measures. For example, individuals seeking comfort-oriented care exclusively may decline parenteral antibiotic treatment of pneumonia to avoid hospitalization and remain at home. For others, treating the underlying etiology of fever with more aggressive interventions, such as surgical drainage of a painful abscess, will offer symptom palliation and potentially contribute to life prolongation. Aggressive treatment of infection does not improve survival rates among persons with severe dementia and has been associated with accelerated progression of the severity of dementia.[63] Antibiotics and other aggressive measures are often associated with numerous deleterious outcomes, including renal failure and ototoxicity, allergic or drug reactions, rash, diarrhea, blood dyscrasias, antibiotic resistance, use of intravenous lines and mechanical restraints, prolonged time to death, and increased costs.[64,65]

NONSPECIFIC INTERVENTIONS

During febrile episodes, increasing fluid intake, removing excess clothing and linens, tepid water bathing or sponging, and use of antipyretics may offer relief. In the very sick, administration of fluids intravenously or subcutaneously may be warranted. Other comfort measures include application of lubricant to dried lips and keeping mucous membranes moist with ice chips. Convective cooling via increasing air circulation by fans or using an airflow blanket may be effective to reduce temperatures and improve patient comfort.[66*] Additionally, ensuring clothes and bed linens are dry should be done and changed as needed.

Antipyretic agents such as acetaminophen (paracetamol), aspirin or nonsteroidal anti-inflammatory drugs (NSAIDS) act by lowering the elevated thermal set point by inhibition of enzyme cyclooxygenase. Although these agents are commonly administered to hospitalized patients to enhance patient comfort,[67] no studies have been done in the cancer population with fever, and carefully controlled efficacy studies have not quantified the degree to which the antipyretics therapy enhances the comfort of febrile patients in other populations. Although theoretically patients with pulmonary and cardiovascular disorders may benefit from antipyretic therapy to minimize the impact of increased metabolic demands, the risk versus benefit of this approach has not been determined. Similarly, antipyretic therapy has not been demonstrated to prevent febrile seizures in children.[68] Several studies have confirmed that increasing the dose of acetaminophen from moderate dosage (10 mg/kg every 4 hours, maximum five doses per day) to relatively higher dosage (15–20 mg/kg every 4 hours, maximum five doses per day) in children failed to reduce the rate of recurrence of febrile seizures.[69]

Fever control may be enhanced by combining physical methods with antipyretics. In children, a randomized placebo-controlled trial of sponging with ice water, isopropyl alcohol or tepid water (with or without acetaminophen) demonstrated that all combinations enhanced fever control, but comfort was greatest in children receiving placebo or sponging, followed by those who received acetaminophen combined with tepid water sponging.[70] Discomfort was found to be greatest when sponging with ice water or isopropyl alcohol with or without concomitant administration. Like acetaminophen, aspirin may be effective in reducing fever, but should be used with caution in patients with or at risk of thrombocytopenia due to its antiplatelet effects. In children, aspirin use is contraindicated due to the risk of Reye syndrome with fever related to certain viral etiologies, including varicella and influenza.[71] Nonsteroidal anti-inflammatory drugs should also be used cautiously in the cancer population, as they inhibit platelet function and may also cause gastrointestinal hemorrhage.

PRIMARY INTERVENTIONS DIRECTED AT THE ETIOLOGY OF FEVER

Infections

Patients should be instructed to seek medical help if a fever develops when the neutrophil count is low or declining. In febrile neutropenic patients broad-spectrum antibiotics should be initiated immediately even before culture results are available,[72] as mortality rate is 70 percent for patients not receiving antibiotics within 48 hours.[73] Initial antibiotic use is guided by knowledge of the treating institution's antimicrobial spectrum and antibiotic resistance pattern, as well as the suspected cause. Although there is general consensus that empirical therapy is appropriate, there is no consensus as to which antibiotics or combinations of antibiotics should be used. The Infectious Diseases Society of America (IDSA) Fever and Neutropenia Guidelines Panel recommends empirical antibiotics based on the patient's clinical condition and risk for complications, and determination of the need of vancomycin in the initial regimen.[74] These four protocols are depicted in Table 77.1.

Treatment regimens are further modified by the duration of fever and individual patient risk factors such as the presence of central lines or other artificial devices, history of steroid use, and history of injection drug use. After a specific pathogen is isolated, antibiotic therapy is then changed to provide optimal therapeutic response. The single most important determinant of successful discontinuation of antibiotics is the neutrophil count. If infection is not identified after 3 days of treatment, if the neutrophil count is $\geq$500 cells/mm^3 for 2 consecutive days, and if the patient is afebrile for $\geq$48 hours, antibiotic therapy may be discontinued. For neutropenic hosts with persistent or recurrent fevers after 1 week of broad-spectrum antibiotic therapy, the addition of an antifungal agent is recommended, as continued granulocytopenia is usually associated with the development of nonbacterial opportunistic infections, particularly candidiasis and aspergillosis.

Table 77.1   *Empiric antibiotic regimens for unexplained neutropenic fever in the cancer population*[35]

Regimen	Route		Antibiotic selection	Comments
1	Oral		Ciprofloxacin *plus* amoxicillin-clavulanate	For use in select *adult* patients: In remission At low risk for serious life-threatening complications Not recommended for patients with comorbidities May be used on an outpatient basis if ready access to care, no signs of focal infection, and no signs or symptoms suggestive of systemic infection other than fever
2	Intravenous	Mono-drug (without vancomycin)	Choose one: cefepime, ceftazidime, imipenem or meropenem	Mono-drug as effective as multiple drug combinations for uncomplicated neutropenic patients Monitor closely for nonresponse, emergence of secondary infection and drug resistance
3	Intravenous	Two-drug regimen (without vancomycin)	Aminoglycoside *plus* antipseudomonal penicillin or ceftazidime or carbapenem	Advantages: Potential synergistic effects against some Gram-negative bacilli Minimal emergence of drug-resistant strains during treatment
4	Intravenous	One or two drug regimen *with* vancomycin	Vancomycin *plus* antibiotics from regimens 2 or 3 above	Restrict to: Institutions with high prevalence of infections with penicillin-resistant Gram-positive bacteria Suspected catheter-related cellulitis or bacteremia Gram-positive bacteremia Evidence of septic shock

Aciclovir is the drug of choice in the treatment of herpes simplex or varicella zoster viral infection. Ganciclovir has activity against cytomegalovirus. Both agents can be used prophylactically in the management of patients at high risk for these infections. Foscarnet is useful in the treatment of cytomegalovirus and aciclovir-resistant herpes simplex virus.

Various investigators have developed models predicting risk groups of febrile neutropenia, with implications for management strategies. Therapeutic options under evaluation include early hospital discharge, home intravenous antibiotic therapy and oral antibiotic regimens. Due to rapid changes in the field, the reader is directed to specialized sources for specific management recommendations of febrile neutropenia.

Paraneoplastic fever

The best management for paraneoplastic fevers remains in the treatment of the underlying neoplasm with definitive antineoplastic therapy. If not possible, NSAIDs have been considered as the mainstay of treatment, with naproxen being the most extensively studied. However, indometacin and diclofenac have also been found to be effective.[75**] Several studies suggesting that neoplastic fevers are more responsive to NSAIDs than are infectious fevers, has led to advocacy of the 'naproxen test' to differentiate between neoplastic and non-neoplastic fevers.[76,77] However, this approach has not been validated.[78] Thalidomide, an immunomodulatory agent, has been shown to have modulatory and/or suppressive effects on several cytokines such as TNFα, IL-1, and IL-6,[79,80] all involved in paraneoplastic fever and which, theoretically, may have a role in treatment of cancer patients with fever and sweats.[81] Despite reports of its antipyretic and antidiaphoretic activity,[82,83] this agent has not been formally tested in clinical studies with cancer patients for fever or sweat control.

Transfusion-associated fever

Many institutions have moved toward leukoreduced transfusions in an effort to decrease incidence of FNHTRs and several countries have even restricted the manufacture and transfusion of blood products to prestorage leukodepleted blood components only. A retrospective analysis conducted at Johns Hopkins Hospital examined the frequency of transfusion reactions associated with transfusion of red blood cells (RBCs), between July 1994 and December 2001.[84] The study directly compared two time periods before and after the initiative towards leukoreduction. In the initial period (July to December 1994) before the initiative to move toward leukoreduction, 96 percent of RBC inventory was non-leukoreduced. In the study period after leukoreduction (July to December 2001) 99.5 percent of RBC inventory was leukoreduced. When comparing these two time periods, the incidence of FNHTRs decreased from 0.37 percent to 0.19 percent ($P = 0.0008$). The trend over the entire 7.5-year study period confirmed the decrease in FNHTRs as the percentage of leukoreduced RBCs increased. The incidence of allergic NHTRs remained unchanged. The decreased incidence of FNHTRs with leukoreduction have been found in other studies as well.[85–88] Common clinical practice prior to blood product transfusions include premedication with acetaminophen, diphenhydramine with or without steroids. The use of erythropoietin for cancer-related anemia may decrease the need of blood transfusions and may be used for cancer-related anemia. The risks versus benefits, and costs, of such prophylactic treatments to avoid or delay transfusion need further investigation.

Drug fever

Drug-associated fever responds to cessation of the offending agent, when possible. Fever and related symptoms with biological response modifier administration is type, route, dose, and schedule dependent. These factors may sometimes be altered for fever control without sacrificing efficacy. Liposomal amphotericin B is as effective as conventional amphotericin B for empirical antifungal therapy in patients with fever and neutropenia, but is associated with decreased toxicity, including occurrence of fever and chills.[89] Fever may also be attenuated by the use of acetaminophen, NSAIDs, and steroid premedication. The same may be true for fever associated with some cytotoxic agents and antimicrobials (i.e. amphotericin). It is common clinical practice to administer meperidine to attenuate severe chills associated with a febrile reaction, although empirical data confirming its efficacy are not available.

Fever versus hyperthermia

Although in the vast majority of patients an elevated body temperature usually represents a fever, there are instances where elevated temperatures could be secondary to hyperthermia. These include heat stroke syndromes, certain metabolic diseases (hyperthyroidism), and drugs that interfere with thermoregulation. With fever, thermoregulatory mechanisms remain intact, but the hypothalamic thermal set point is raised by exposure to endogenous pyrogens,[90] leading to behavioral and physiological responses to elevate body temperature. In contradistinction to fever, during hyperthermia, the setting of the thermoregulatory center remains unchanged at normothermic levels, while body temperature increases in an uncontrolled fashion and overrides the ability to lose heat. Hyperthermia thus results from overwhelming of the peripheral heat-dissipating mechanisms by disease, drugs or from excessive heat, be it external or internal.[91]

Atropine may increase endogenous heat production by interfering with thermoregulation, in that it blocks sweating and vasodilation, thereby raising core temperature. Hyperthermia also occurs with neuroleptic malignant syndrome (NMS), an idiosyncratic reaction to drugs that block the dopamine receptor. Haloperidol, an antipsychotic agent, is the most common offender.[92,93] Atypical antipsychotic medications, including clozapine, risperidone, olanzapine, and quetiapine have also been associated with NMS.[94,95] There are also case reports of other medications causing NMS, including venlafaxine, promethazine and metoclopramide.[96,97] Neuroleptic malignant syndrome typically occurs within several days of the initiation of treatment and dosages and serum concentration of these medications are usually within the therapeutic range. The probability of developing NMS is directly related to the antidopaminergic potency of the neuroleptic agent. In addition, specific polymorphisms of the dopamine D_2 receptor may predispose some patients to NMS.[98]

It is important to make the distinction between fever and hyperthermia since management approaches to these distinct syndromes differ. There is no rapid way to differentiate elevated core temperature due to fever from hyperthermia and a diagnosis of hyperthermia is often made because of a preceding history of heat exposure or use of certain drugs that interfere with normal thermoregulation. On physical examination, the skin is hot but dry in heat stroke syndromes and in patients taking drugs that block sweating.

Antipyretic agents act by lowering the elevated thermal set point and are used in the treatment of fever, but are ineffective in hyperthermia, where the thermal set point is normal. In hyperthermia, drugs that interfere with vasoconstriction such as phenothiazines and those that block muscle contractions or shivering are useful. However, these are not true antipyretics as they can reduce body temperature independently of hypothalamic control. Shivering may be suppressed with intravenous benzodiazepines such as diazepam or lorazepam. Chlorpromazine intravenously (25–50 mg) may also be used for this purpose if NMS is not suspected.

In patients diagnosed with hyperthermia, physical cooling should be started immediately with techniques such as removing bedclothes, sponging the patient with tepid water and use of bed fans. More rapid reductions in body temperature can be achieved by sponging the patient with alcohol or by using hypothermic mattresses or ice packs.

Immersion in ice water is the most effective means of physical cooling, but it should be reserved for true hyperthermic emergencies, such as heat stroke. In true emergencies, treatment may also include the intravenous or intraperitoneal administration of cool fluid, gastric lavage or enemas with ice water, and even extracorporeal circulation. No matter what technique is used, the body temperature must always be monitored closely to avoid hypothermia.

SWEATS

In patients with advanced disease or those receiving palliative care, the prevalence of sweating ranges from 14 percent to 28 percent, is frequently nocturnal and is moderate to severe in intensity.[99–101] Although night sweats have been defined as drenching sweats that require the patient to change bedclothes, this definition may not describe the majority of patients who complain of the symptom. Clinically, hot flashes are often seen in association with sweats and by far this is the most common cause of sweats encountered in clinical medicine, experienced by the majority of perimenopausal and menopausal women and hence this topic will be covered in detail. In the literature, night sweats has also been associated with a variety of medical problems including malignancies (e.g. lymphomas), some infections, tuberculosis, autoimmune diseases, and drugs. Common malignancies associated with night sweats include lymphomas, leukemia, renal cell carcinoma, and Castleman disease. The classic presentation of tuberculosis includes fever, weight loss and night sweats. AIDs-related infections might also cause night sweats, including *Mycobacterium avium* complex (MAC) infection and cytomegalovirus (CMV) syndromes. The differential diagnosis for night sweats is broad and Box 77.2 lists some of these conditions.

Box 77.2 Etiology of night sweats

Malignancy

- Lymphoma
- Leukemia
- Renal cell carcinoma
- Castleman disease
- Other neoplasms

Infections

- Human immunodeficiency virus
- Tuberculosis

- *Mycobacterium avium* complex
- Infectious mononucleosis
- Fungal infections
- Lung abscess
- Endocarditis

Others

- Obstructive sleep apnea
- Gastroesophageal reflux disease
- Chronic fatigue syndrome
- Granulomatous disease
- Diabetes insipidus
- Anxiety
- Rheumatological diseases

Endocrine

- Perimenopausal and postmenopausal women
- Hyperthyroidism
- Diabetes mellitus (nocturnal hypoglycemia)
- Endocrine tumors (pheochromocytoma, carcinoid tumor)
- Orchiectomy

Drugs

- Antipyretics (salicylates, acetaminophen)
- Selective estrogen receptor modulator drugs: tamoxifen and raloxifene
- Leuprolide
- Niacin
- Selective serotonin receptor inhibitors
- Antihypertensives
- Phenothiazines
- Drugs of abuse: alcohol, heroin

Patients presenting with night sweats warrant a detailed evaluation including history and physical examination aimed at revealing associated symptoms to help narrow the broad differential diagnosis and guide further work-up. The prevalence of sweats and their impact on quality of life in the cancer population is not well established and requires further definition.

HOT FLASHES

Hot flashes, experienced by three-quarters of menopausal women, are described as a sudden onset of an uncomfortable sensation of intense heat, accompanied by skin flushing, warmth and sweating, usually of the chest and face.[4] Hot flashes typically last for 2–4 minutes and are often accompanied by palpitations and anxiety, may be triggered by emotional stress, anxiety, alcohol, and certain foods.[102] Factors associated with a greater risk of hot flashes are listed in Box 77.3.[103–106] Approximately two-thirds of women with history of breast cancer experience hot flashes.[5] In postmenopausal women with a history of breast cancer, predictors of hot flash severity include higher body mass index, a high school education or less, younger age at diagnosis, and tamoxifen use.[107,108] For patients starting tamoxifen, hot flashes typically increase in the first 2–3 months, followed by a plateau and then gradual dissipation.[109]

In men treated with androgen ablation for locally advanced or metastatic prostate cancer, 50–88 percent experience hot flashes.[110,111] Patients with other cancers are also affected with hot flashes, however data on this are limited.

Box 77.3 Factors associated with hot flashes

Abrupt menopause

- Chemotherapy
- Drugs
- Radiation
- Surgery

Cancer type

- Breast
- Prostate

Early menopause

Ethnicity

- African women
- Western women

Lack of exercise

High body mass index

Low education

Low estrogen levels

Low socioeconomic status

Smokers

The rapid menopause associated with cancer treatments does not allow for a gradual adjustment of falling estrogen levels and this may explain why hot flushes resulting from cancer treatment tend to be more profound.

Pathophysiology

The prevailing hypothesis relates the development of hot flashes to lowering of estrogen levels leading to complex neuroendocrine mechanisms, including alterations in the level of hypothalamic neurotransmitters, which resets the thermostat to a lower level with a narrower range, as compared with those who do not experience hot flashes.[112,113] A small rise in core body temperature has been found to occur 15 minutes prior to hot flashes in 60 percent of hot flash episodes.[114] This subtle elevation in core body temperature stimulates mechanisms of heat dissipation, resulting in cutaneous vasodilation and sweating, the two central components of the hot flash syndrome.

Two most recognized neurotransmitters involved in hypothalamic thermoregulatory processes are norepinephrine and serotonin. Catecholestrogens (estrogenic metabolites) abundant in the hypothalamus stimulate the production of β-endorphins. Both catecholestrogens and endorphins inhibit the production of hypothalamic norepinephrine. Loss of this negative feedback in low estrogenic states results in rise of norepinephrine levels and an upregulation of certain hypothalamic serotonin receptors responsible for resetting of the thermostat.[115] Norepinephrine is believed to be responsible for the rise in core temperature prior to onset of hot flashes.[114] In men, it is uncertain if low testosterone levels or decline in estrogen levels or both, are responsible for development of the hot flash syndrome.

Assessment and treatment of hot flashes

Hot flashes should be routinely assessed as a component of systematic symptom surveys and if present, a careful assessment of hot flash frequency, intensity, duration, potential triggers, and impact on quality of life is advised in order to construct an individualized treatment plan. Patient self-report diaries with hot flash frequency, intensity, and associated distress can be helpful to clinicians to formulate treatment recommendations.[116] Hot flash score is determined by multiplying the daily frequency of hot flashes by their average severity. Box 77.4 lists the possible options for management of hot flashes.

HORMONE REPLACEMENT THERAPY

Estrogen

Estrogen replacement is effective for treatment of hot flashes in 80–90 percent of patients, regardless of underlying

Box 77.4 Treatment interventions for hot flashes in patients with cancer

Hormonal agents

- Androgens
- Estrogens
- Progestational agents

Nonhormonal agents

- α Adrenergic agents
- Antidepressants
- β Blockers
- Gabapentin
- Veralipride
- Vitamin E

Complementary and alternative medicine (CAM) approaches

- Herbal medications
- Acupuncture
- Behavioral interventions

etiology.[117**,118,119*,120**] However, some women have absolute or relative contraindications to hormone replacement therapy (HRT), and others are reluctant to take hormones due to perceived risks and side effects. The Women's Health Initiative Study evaluated the risks and benefits of estrogen plus progestin therapy in healthy postmenopausal women.[121**] The estrogen plus progestin arm was stopped prematurely in women with an intact uterus at a mean follow-up of 5.2 years (±1.3) due to detection of a 1.26 times increased breast cancer risk (95 percent CI 1.00 to 1.59). Observed benefits of HRT on hip fractures and colon cancer risk were far outweighed by increased risks of venous thromboembolic disease, breast cancer, stroke, and coronary artery disease. Supporting an increased risk of breast cancer with combined HRT is another recent population-based, case–control study of 975 postmenopausal women diagnosed with breast cancer.[122] In this cohort, HRT use was associated with an increased risk of breast cancer, including lobular, ductal and estrogen and progesterone receptor positive tumors.

Progestational agents

Progestational agents have comparable efficacy to estrogens for hot flash reduction. Agents studied include megestrol acetate and transdermal progesterone, and the long-acting intramuscular preparation, depo-medroxyprogesterone acetate (DMPA).[123**,124**,125*]

Despite benefit of amelioration of hot flashes, there is ongoing debate about safety of progesterone in patients with breast, uterine, or prostate cancer. In men with prostate cancer, several investigators have reported a decline in prostate-specific antigen levels after withdrawal of megestrol acetate, raising concerns that its use may be harmful in this population.[126–128] Risk associated with progestin use in women with a history of breast cancer is unknown at this time, as is its effect on outcome of tamoxifen treatment. Some data have suggested that progestational agents may increase epithelial cell proliferation, an undesirable effect in breast cancer.[129,130] There is also some evidence of antitumor activity in breast cancer.[131]

Tibolone

Tibolone, a synthetic steroid compound with combined estrogenic, progestogenic, and androgenic properties, has been reported to reduce hot flashes.[132*,133] A recent study of postmenopausal women receiving tamoxifen after surgery for breast cancer found a significant reduction in the severity of hot flashes with tibolone compared with placebo (0.4 vs. 0.2, respectively, $P = 0.031$) but no change in the daily number of hot flashes with either tibolone or placebo ($P = 0.219$).[134**] Tibolone is not available in the USA.

NONHORMONAL AGENTS

Nonhormonal agents are gaining popularity as therapy for hot flash reduction due to the heightened concerns about the risks of using HRT. These include pharmacotherapies, and complementary and alternative medicine approaches.

Antidepressants

Several large placebo-controlled, randomized trials have shown the beneficial effects of antidepressants from the selective serotonin reuptake inhibitors (SSRIs) and selective serotonin and norepinephrine reuptake inhibitors (SNRIs) class in hot flash management. In the Mayo Clinic study, breast cancer survivors and menopausal women experiencing hot flashes were assigned to receive one of three different dose levels of venlafaxine (37.5 mg, 75 mg, and 150 mg daily), or placebo for 4 weeks.[135**] A dose-related diminution in average hot flashes scores from baseline was noted (27 percent in the placebo subjects vs. 37 percent, 61 percent, and 61 percent for the three venlafaxine groups, respectively). Similar beneficial results have been found in studies with paroxetine and fluoxetine.[136**,137**] Preliminary studies with other newer antidepressants, including citalopram and mirtazapine have also shown good results in standard starting doses.[138*,139*]

Of note, many of the SSRIs can inhibit the cytochrome P450 enzyme system involved in the hepatic metabolism of tamoxifen, a drug commonly used in the treatment of breast cancer. In a prospective study, co-administration of paroxetine with tamoxifen was shown to result in decreased concentrations of 4-hydroxy-N-desmethyl-tamoxifen, an active tamoxifen metabolite (also known as endoxifen).[140] Women with the wild-type CYP2D6 genotype demonstrated greater decreases in endoxifen levels than those with a variant genotype ($P = 0.03$). Given the widespread use of SSRIs for the treatment of mood disorders and hot flashes, the interactions of SSRIs with tamoxifen merit further study.

OTHER NONHORMONAL AGENTS

Several other agents have been found to be useful in hot flash management. In a placebo-controlled, randomized study of 59 postmenopausal women, gabapentin was more effective than placebo in reducing hot flash frequency (45 percent vs. 29 percent, respectively) and hot flash composite score (54 percent vs. 31 percent, respectively).[141**] Clonidine, a central acting α_2-adrenergic receptor agonist has been shown to have modest benefits in hot flash reduction in several studies in healthy postmenopausal women, breast cancer survivors on tamoxifen, and men with prostate cancer, but with significant dose-related side effects.[142**,143**] The North Central Cancer Treatment Group (NCCTG), in a randomized, placebo-controlled crossover trial of vitamin E in women with a history of breast cancer, found a minor decrease with treatment, with a mean reduction of 1 flash/day, without adverse effects.[144**] This reduction is unlikely to be of meaningful clinical benefit. Bellergal, a combination of belladonna and phenobarbital was widely used in the past for hot flash management. Although several reports favor its use over placebo,[145] this therapy cannot be recommended in view of the risk of phenobarbital dependence and dose dependent anticholinergic side effects of belladonna, including dry mouth, constipation, blurry vision, and dizziness.

COMPLEMENTARY AND ALTERNATIVE MEDICINE APPROACHES

Eighty percent of women in the 45–60 age group have reported the use of nonprescription therapies for management of menopausal symptoms.[146] Often perceived to be safer than hormone replacement therapy, CAM may provide users with a sense of personal control over their healthcare.

Soy phytoestrogens are weak estrogens found in plant foods and while dietary supplementation with natural soy products appears to be a benign intervention, long-term effects are not known. Two randomized, placebo-controlled studies show no clinical benefit of soy over placebo for hot flash management.[147**,148**] Breast cancer risk in the general population and risk of recurrence in breast cancer survivors has not yet been clarified, nor has its effect on hormonally mediated antitumor therapies, such as tamoxifen and the aromatase inhibitors. Black cohosh (*Cimicifuga racemosa*) is approved in Germany for the treatment of hot flashes. The anecdotal clinical and observational experience suggests black cohosh may produce 25–30 percent more efficacy than placebo for menopausal symptoms, including hot flashes.[149] In a randomized, double-blind, placebo-controlled study on breast cancer survivors in the USA, however, efficacy of black cohosh was not significantly different from placebo.[150**] The high prevalence of tamoxifen use in study participants may have confounded study results. Red clover, which contains isoflavones (phytoestrogens), and dong quai have not been found to be beneficial in the management of hot flashes.

Acupuncture has been suggested as a remedy for hot flashes. In a randomized controlled study Wyon et al. compared the efficacy of electro-acupuncture with oral estradiol treatment and superficial needle insertion on hot flash reduction in 45 postmenopausal women.[151**] They found that electro-acupuncture decreased the number of hot flashes significantly over time, but not to the same extent as the estrogen treatment. No significant difference in effect was found between electro-acupuncture and the superficial needle insertion. In a small pilot study of prostate cancer patients who underwent castration therapy, a substantial decrease (70 percent reduction) in hot flash symptoms was noted at 10 weeks, with a sustained reduction of 50 percent at 3 months.[152*] Further studies are warranted to determine efficacy and potential mechanisms of action of acupuncture as a modality of therapy for treatment of hot flashes.

Behavioral methods may play a role in hot flash management. Studied methods include relaxation response training[153**] and paced respirations.[154**] These may be used as primary alternatives for patients who do not want to take medications, or as an adjunct for individuals who achieve suboptimal relief with other interventions. The beneficial effects may be related to the decreased adrenergic tone mediated by relaxation techniques. Exercise would similarly be beneficial.

Key learning points

- Fever, chills, and hot flashes are frequently encountered in palliative care patients.
- Fever in patients with cancer should be considered indicative of infection unless proved otherwise. Neutropenic fever is a medical emergency.
- Fever may be associated with potential metabolic consequences including dehydration and fatigue, which may be especially pronounced in debilitated terminally ill patients.
- Paraneoplastic and drug fevers should be considered in the differential diagnosis of fever.
- Cytokines are implicated in the etiology of fever secondary to infections and paraneoplastic fevers.
- Both fever and hyperthermia result in elevation of core body temperatures but differ physiologically and in their management. Many palliative care patients are on drugs which have the potential to cause hyperthermia.
- Patients should be assessed for night sweats and hot flashes. The latter is widely prevalent in some cancers (breast, prostate) and postmenopausal women and may be associated with significant distress.
- Many nonhormonal therapies are available for consideration for hot flash management.

REFERENCES

1   Seah STA, Low JA, Chan YH. Symptoms and care of dying elderly patients in an acute care hospital. *Singapore Med J* 2005; **46**: 210–14.

2   Hall P, Schroder C, Weaver L. The last 48 hours of life in long-term care: a focused chart audit. *J Am Geriatr Soc* 2002; **50**: 501–6.

3   Mckinlay SM, Jeffreys M. The menopausal syndrome. *Br J Prev Soc Med* 1974; **28**: 108–15.

4   Feldman BM, Voda A, Gronseth E. The prevalence of hot flash and associated variables among perimenopausal women. *Res Nurs Health* 1985; **8**: 261–8.

5   Couzi RJ, Helzlsouer KJ, Fetting JH. Prevalence of menopausal symptoms among women with history of breast cancer and attitudes toward estrogen replacement therapy. *J Clin Oncol* 1995; **13**: 2737–44.

6   Carpenter JS, Andrykowski MA, Freedman RR, *et al.* Hot flashes in postmenopausal women treated for breast carcinoma: prevalence, severity, correlates, management, and relation to quality of life. *Cancer* 1998; **82**: 1682–91.

7   *Stedman's Medical Dictionary*, 27th ed. Philadelphia: Lippincott, Williams & Wilkins, 2000: 659.

8   Kluger MJ. Fever: role of pyrogens and cryogens. *Physiol Rev* 1991; **71**: 93–127.

◆ 9   Saper CB. Neurobiological basis of fever. *Ann N Y Acad Sci* 1998; **856**: 90–4.

10   Besedovsky HO, del Rey A, Klusman I, *et al.* Cytokines as modulators of the hypothalamus-pituitary-adrenal axis. *J Steroid Biochem Mol Biol* 1991; **40**: 613–18.

11   Breder CD, Dinarello CA, Saper CD. Interleukin-1 immunoreactive innervation of the human hypothalamus. *Science* 1988; **240**: 321–4.

12   Sternberg EM. Neural-immune interactions in health and disease. *J Clin Invest* 1997; **100**: 2641–7.

13   Stitt, JT. Evidence for the involvement of the organum vasculosum laminae terminalis in the febrile response of rabbits and rats. *J Physiol (Lond)* 1985; **368**: 501.

14   Banks WA, Ortiz L, Plotkin L, *et al.* Human interleukin (IL) 1 alpha, murine IL-1 alpha and murine IL-1 beta are transported from blood to brain in the mouse by a shared saturable mechanism. *J Pharmacol Exp Ther* 1991; **259**: 988–96.

15   Elmquist JK, Scammell TE, Saper CB. Mechanisms of CNS response to systemic immune challenge: the febrile response. *Trends Neurosci* 1997; **20**: 565–70.

16   Plata-Salamán CR. Immunoregulators in the nervous system. *Neurosci Biobehav Rev* 1991; **15**: 185–215.

17   Roth J, Conn CA, Kluger MJ, *et al.* Kinetics of systemic and intrahypothalamic IL-6 and tumor necrosis factor during endotoxin fever in the guinea pig. *Am J Physiol* 1993; **265**: 653–8.

18   LeMay LG, Vander AJ, Kluger MJ. Role of interleukin-6 in fever in the rat. *Am J Physiol* 1990; **258**: 798–803.

19   Elmquist JK, Breder CD, Sherin JE, *et al.* Intravenous lipopoly-sacharide induces cyclooxygenase 2-like immunoreactivity in the rat brain perivascular microglia and meningeal macrophages. *J Comp Neurol* 1997; **381**: 119–29.

20   Li S, Ballou LR, Morham SG, *et al.* Cyclooxygenase-2 mediates the febrile response of mice to interleukin-1 beta. *Brain Res* 2001; **910**: 163–73.

21   Rivest S, Lacroix S, Vallieres L, *et al.* How the blood talks to the brain parenchyma and the paraventricular nucleus of the hypothalamus during systemic inflammatory and infectious stimuli. *Proc Soc Exp Biol Med* 2000; **223**: 22–38.

◆ 22   Blatteis CM, Sehic E. Fever: how may circulating cytokines signal the brain? *Physiol Rev* 1991; **71**: 93–127.

23   Li S, Sehic E, Wang Y. Relationship between complement and the febrile response of guinea pigs to systemic endotoxin. *Am J Physiol* 1999; **277**: 1635–45.

24   Vizi ES. Receptor-mediated local fine-tuning by noradrenergic innervation of neuroendocrine and immune systems. *Ann N Y Acad Sci* 1998; **851**: 388–96.

25   Pizzo PA, Robichaud KJ, Wesley R, *et al.* Fever in the pediatric and young adult patient with cancer: a prospective study of 1001 episodes. *Medicine* 1982; **61**: 153–65.

26   Fabiszewski KJ, Volicer BJ, Volicer L, Effect of antibiotic treatment on outcome of fevers in institutionalized Alzheimer patients. *JAMA* 1990; **263**: 3168–72.

27   Volicer L, Seltzer B, Rheaume Y, *et al.* Eating difficulties in patients with probable dementia of the Alzheimer type. *J Geriatr Psychiatry Neurol* 1989; **2**: 169–76.

28   Parulkar BJ, Barrett DM. Urinary incontinence in adults. *Surg Clin North Am* 1988; **68**: 945–63.

29   Lipsky BA. Urinary tract infections in men: epidemiology, pathophysiology, diagnosis, and treatment. *Ann Intern Med* 1989; **110**: 138–50.

30   Vanderschueren S, Knockaert D, Adriaenssens T, *et al.* From prolonged febrile illness to fever of unknown origin: the challenge continues. *Arch Intern Med* 2003; **163**: 1033–41.

31   Chang JC. How to differentiate neoplastic fever from infectious fever in patients with cancer: usefulness of the naproxen test. *Heart Lung* 1987; **16**: 122–7.

32   Young LS. Fever and septicemia. In: Rubin RH, Young LS, eds. *Clinical Approach to Infection in the Compromised Host*, 2nd ed. New York: Plenum Medical Book Co. 1995; **11**: 75–114.

33   Dinarello CA, Wolff SM. Molecular basis of fever in humans. *Am J Med* 1982; **72**: 799–819.

34   Kasprisin DO, Yogore MG, Salmassi S, *et al.* Blood components and transfusion reactions. *Plasma Ther* 1981; **2**: 25–9.

35   Milner LV, Butcher K. Transfusion reactions reported after transfusions of red blood cells and whole blood. *Transfusion* 1978; **18**: 493–5.

36   Huh YO, Lichtiger B. Transfusion reactions in patients with cancer. *Am J Clin Pathol* 1987; **87**: 253–7.

37   Climent-Peris C, Velez-Rosario R. Immediate transfusion reactions. *P R Health Sci J* 2001; **20**: 229–35.

38   Decary F, Ferner P, Giavedoni L, *et al.* An investigation of nonhemolytic transfusion reactions. *Vox Sang* 1984; **46**: 277–85.

39   Goldfinger D, Lowe C. Prevention of adverse reactions to blood transfusion by the administration of saline-washed red blood cells. *Transfusion* 1981; **21**: 277–80.

40   Schned AR, Silver H. The use of microaggregate filtration in the prevention of febrile transfusion reactions. *Transfusion* 1981; **21**: 675–81.

41   Wenz B. Microaggregate blood filtration and the febrile transfusion reaction. A comparative study. *Transfusion* 1983; **23**: 95–8.

42   Högman C. Adverse effects: bacterial contamination including shelf life. A brief review of bacterial contamination of blood components. *Vox Sang* 1996; **70**: 78–82.

43 Morel P, Deschaseaux M, Bertrand X, *et al.* Transfusion et bactéries: risque résiduel et perspectives de prévention. *Transfus Clin Biol* 2003; **10**: 192–200.

44 Blajchman MA, Goldman M. Bacterial contamination of platelet concentrates: incidence, significance, and prevention. *Semin Hematol* 2001; **38**: 20–6.

45 Andreu G, Morel P, Forestier F, *et al.* Hemovigilance network in France: organization and analysis of immediate transfusion incident reports from 1994 to 1998. *Transfusion* 2002; **42**: 1356–64.

46 Asher D, Atterbury CLJ, Chapman C, *et al. Serious Hazards of Transfusion Annual Report 2000–2001.* Manchester: SHOT Office, 2002.

47 Ness PM, Braine HG, King K, *et al.* Single donor platelets reduces the risk of septic transfusion reactions. *Transfusion* 2001; **1**: 857–61.

48 Blajchman MA, Ali AM. Bacteria in the blood supply: an overlooked issue in transfusion medicine In: Nance SJ, ed. *Blood Safety: Current Challenges.* Bethesda, MD: American Association of Blood Banks, 1992: 213–28.

49 Yomtovian R, Lazarus HM, Goodnough LT, *et al.* A prospective microbiologic surveillance program to detect and prevent the transfusion of bacterially contaminated platelets. *Transfusion* 1993; **33**: 909–19.

50 Soeterboek AM, Welle FM, Marcellis JH, *et al.* Sterility testing of blood products in 1994/1995 by three cooperating blood banks in the Netherlands. *Vox Sang* 1997; **72**: 61–2.

51 Leiby DA, Kerry KL, Campos JM, *et al.* A retrospective analysis of microbial contaminants in outdated random-donor platelets from multiple sites. *Transfusion* 1997; **37**: 259–63.

52 Mackowiak PA, LeMaistre CF. Drug fever: a critical appraisal of conventional concepts. An analysis of 51 episodes diagnosed in two Dallas hospitals and 97% episodes reported in the English literature. *Ann Intern Med* 1987; **106**: 728–33.

53 Clements JS, Peacock. Amphotericin B revisited: reassessment of toxicity. *Am J Med* 1990; **88**: 22–7.

54 Quesada JR, Talpaz M, Rios A, *et al.* Clinical toxicity of interferons in cancer patients: a review. *J Clin Oncol* 1986; **4**: 234–43.

55 Ashford RF, McLachlan A, Nelson I, *et al.* Pyrexia after cisplatin. *Lancet* 1980; **2**: 691–2.

56 Shah KA, Greenwald E, Levin J, *et al.* Streptozocin-induced eosinophilia and fever: a case report. *Cancer Treat Rep* 1982; **66**: 1449–51.

57 Boye J, Elter T, Engert A. An overview of the current clinical use of the anti-CD20 monoclonal antibody rituximab. *Ann Oncol* 2003; **14**: 520–35.

58 Ishii E, Hara T, Mizuno Y, *et al.* Vincristine-induced fever in children with leukemia and lymphoma. *Cancer* 1988; **61**: 660–2.

59 Styrt B, Sugarman B. Antipyresis and fever. *Arch Intern Med* 1990; **150**: 1589–97.

60 Horvath SM, Spurr GB, Hutt BK, *et al.* Metabolic cost of shivering. *J Appl Physiol* 1956; **8**: 595–602.

◆ 61 Kluger MJ. Is fever beneficial? *Yale J Biol Med* 1986; **59**: 89–95.

62 Mackowiak PA. Fever: blessing or curse? A unifying hypothesis. *Ann Intern Med* 1994; **120**: 1037–40.

63 Hurley AC, Volicer BJ, Volicer L. Effect of fever-management strategy on the progression of dementia of the Alzheimer type. *Alzheimer Dis Assoc Disord* 1996; **10**: 5–10.

64 Ahronheim JC, Morrison RS, Baskin SA, *et al.* Treatment of the dying in the acute care hospital. *Arch Intern Med* 1996; **156**: 2094–100.

65 Hurley AC, Mahoney MA, Volicer L. Comfort care in end-stage dementia: what to do after deciding to do no more. In: Olson E, Chichin ER, Libow L, eds. *Controversies in Ethics in Long-Term Care.* New York: Springer, 1995.

66 Creechan T, Vollman K, Kravutske ME. Cooling by convection vs cooling by conduction for treatment of fever in critically ill adults. *Am J Crit Care* 2001; **10**: 52–9.

67 Isaacs SN, Axelrod PI, Lorber B. Antipyretic orders in a university hospital. *Am J Med* 1990; **88**: 31–5.

68 Rosman NP. Febrile convulsions. In: Mackowiak PA, ed. *Fever: Basic Mechanisms and Management*, 2nd ed. Philadelphia: Lippincott-Raven, 1997: 267–77.

69 Schnaiderman D, Lahat E, Sheefer T, Aladjem M. Antipyretic effectiveness of acetaminophen in febrile seizures: ongoing prophylaxis versus sporadic usage. *Eur J Pediatr* 1993; **152**: 747–9.

70 Steele RW, Tanaka PT, Lara RP, *et al.* Evaluation of sponging and of oral antipyretic therapy to reduce fever. *J Pediatr* 1970; **77**: 824–9.

71 Forsyth BW, Horwitz RI, Acampora D, *et al.* New epidemiologic evidence confirming that bias does not explain the aspirin/Reye's syndrome association. *JAMA* 1989; **261**: 2517–24.

◆ 72 Pizzo PA. Management of fever in patients with cancer and treatment-induced neutropenia. *N Engl J Med* 1993; **328**: 1323–32.

73 Pizzo PA. Evaluation of fever in the patient with cancer. *Eur J Cancer Clin Oncol* 1989; **25**: 9–16.

74 Hughes WT, Armstrong D, Bodey GP, *et al.* 2002 guidelines for the use of antimicrobial agents in neutropenic patients with cancer. *Clin Infect Dis* 2002; **34**: 730–51.

75 Tsavaris N, Zinelis A, Krabelis A, *et al.* A randomized trial of the effect of three non-steroidal anti-inflammatory agents in ameliorating cancer induced fever. *J Intern Med* 1990; **228**: 451–5.

76 Chang JC. Utility of Naprosyn in the differential diagnosis of fever of undetermined origin in patients with cancer. *Am J Med* 1984; **76**: 597–603.

77 Chang JC. NSAID test to distinguish between infectious and neoplastic fever in cancer patients. *Postgrad Med* 1988; **84**: 71–2.

78 Vanderschueren S, Knockaert DC, Peetermans WE, *et al.* Diagnostic value of the Naprosyn test in prolonged febrile illness. *Am J Med* 2003; **115**: 572–5.

79 Sampaio EP, Sarno EN, Galilly R, *et al.* Thalidomide selectively inhibits tumor necrosis factor alpha production by stimulated human monocytes. *J Exp Med* 1991; **173**: 699–703.

80 Sampaio EP, Kaplan G, Miranda A, *et al.* The influence of thalidomide on the clinical and immunological manifestation of erythema nodosum leprosum. *J Infect Dis* 1997; **78**: 47–55.

81 Peuckmann V, Fisch M, Bruera E. Potential novel uses of thalidomide. *Drugs* 2000; **60**: 273–92.

82 Calder K, Bruera E. Thalidomide for night sweats in patients with advanced cancer [letter]. *Palliat Med* 2000; **14**: 77–8.

83 Iyer CG, Languillon J, Ramanujam K, *et al.* WHO co-ordinated short-term double blind trial with thalidomide in the treatment of acute lepra reactions in male lepromatous patients. *Bull World Health Organ* 1971; **45**: 719–32.

84   King KE, Shirey RS, Thoman SK, et al. Universal leuko-reduction decreases the incidence of febrile nonhemolytic transfusion reactions to RBCs. Transfusion 2004; **44**: 25–9.

85   Pruss A, Kalus U, Radtke H, et al. Universal leukodepletion of blood components results in a significant reduction of febrile non-hemolytic but not allergic transfusion reactions. Transfus Apheresis Sci 2004; **30**: 41–6.

86   Heddle NM, Klama LN, Griffith L, et al. A prospective study to identify the risk factors associated with acute reactions to platelet and red cell transfusions. Transfusion 1993; **33**: 794–7.

87   Dzik S. Prestorage leukocyte reduction of cellular blood components. Transfus Sci 1994; **15**: 131–9.

88   Heddle NM. Febrile nonhemolytic transfusion reactions to platelets. Curr Opin Hematol 1995; **2**: 478–83.

89   Walsh TJ, Finberg RW, Arndt C, et al. Liposomal amphotericin B for empirical therapy in patients with persistent fever and neutropenia. N Engl J Med 1999; **340**: 764–71.

90   Dinarello CA, Cannon JG, Wolff SM. New concepts on the pathogenesis of fever. Rev Infect Dis 1988; **10**: 168–89.

91   Goodman EL, Knochel JP. Heat stroke and other forms of hyperthermia. In: Mackowiak PA, ed. Fever: Basic Mechanisms and Management. New York: Raven Press, 1991: 267–87.

92   Bhanushali MJ, Tuite PJ. The evaluation and management of patients with neuroleptic malignant syndrome. Neurol Clin 2004; **22**: 389.

93   Hadad E, Weinbroum AA, Ben-Abraham R. Drug-induced hyperthermia and muscle rigidity: a practical approach. Eur J Emerg Med 2003; **10**: 149.

94   Farver DK. Neuroleptic malignant syndrome induced by atypical antipsychotics. Expert Opin Drug Saf 2003; **2**: 21.

95   Kogoj, A, Velikonja I. Olanzapine induced neuroleptic malignant syndrome – a case review. Hum Psychopharmacol 2003; **18**: 301.

96   Nimmagadda SR, Ryan DH, Atkin SL. Neuroleptic malignant syndrome after venlafaxine. Lancet 2000; **355**: 289.

97   Chan-Tack KM. Neuroleptic malignant syndrome due to promethazine. South Med J 1999; **92**: 1017.

98   Mihara K, Kondo T, Suzuki A, et al. Relationship between functional dopamine D2 and D3 receptors gene polymorphisms and neuroleptic malignant syndrome. Am J Med Genet 2003; **117**: 57.

99   Lichter I, Hunt E. The last 48 hours of life. J Palliat Care 1990; **6**: 7–15.

100 Quigley CS, Baines M. Descriptive epidemiology of sweating in a hospice population. J Palliat Care 1997; **13**: 22–6.

101 Ventafridda V, De Conno F, Ripamonti C, et al. Quality of life assessment during palliative care programme. Ann Oncol 1990;1414–20.

102 Kronenberg F. Hot flashes: phenomenology, quality of life, and search for treatment options. Exp Gerontol 1994; **29**: 319–36.

103 Erlik Y. Meldrum DR, Judd HL. Estrogen levels in postmenopausal women with hot flashes. Obstet Gynecol 1982; **59**: 403–7.

104 Chiechi LM, Ferreri R, Granieri M, et al. Climactric syndrome and body weight. Clin Exp Obstet Gynecol 1997; **24**: 163–6.

105 Gold EB, Sternfeld B, Kelsey JL, et al. Relationship of demographic and lifestyle factors to symptoms in a

multi-racial/ethnic population of women 40–55 years of age. Am J Epidemiol 2000; **152**: 463–7.

106 Fuh JL, Wang SJ, Lu SR, et al, The Kinmen Women-Health Investigation(KIWI): a menopausal study of a population aged 40–54. Maturitas 2001; **39**: 117–24.

107 Kronenberg F. Hot flashes: epidemiology and physiology. Ann N Y Acad Sci 1990; **592**: 52–86.

108 Hoskin PJ, Ashley S, Yarnold JR. Weight gain after primary surgery for breast cancer-effect of tamoxifen. Breast Cancer Res Treat 1992; **22**: 129–32.

◆ 109 Loprinzi CL, Zahasky KM, Sloan JA, et al. Tamoxifen induced hot flashes. Clin Breast Cancer 2000; **1**: 52–6.

110 Bucholz NP, Mattarell G, Bucholz MM. Post-orchiectomy hot flushes. Eur Urol 1994; **26**: 120–2.

111 Schow DA, Renfer LG, Rozanski TA, et al. Prevalence of hot flushes during and after neoadjuvant hormonal therapy for localized prostate cancer. South Med J 1998; **91**: 855–7.

112 Freedman RR, Krell W. Reduced thermoregulatory null zone in postmenopausal women with hot flashes. Am J Obstet Gynecol 1999; **181**: 66–70.

113 Rosenberg J, Larsen SH. Hypothesis: pathogenesis of postmenopausal hot flush. Med Hypotheses 1991; **35**: 349–50.

114 Freedman RR, Norton D, Woodward S, et al. Core body temperature and circadian rhythm of hot flashes in menopausal women. J Clin Endocrinol Metab 1995; **80**: 2354–8.

115 Berendson HH. The role of serotonin in hot flushes. Maturitas 2000; **36**: 155–64.

116 Carpenter JS. The Hot Flash Related Daily Interference Scale: a tool for assessing the impact of hot flashes quality of life following breast cancer. J Pain Symptom Manage 2001; **22**: 979–89.

117 Notelovitz M, Lenihan JP, McDermott M, et al. Initial 17 beta-estradiol dose for treating vasomotor symptoms. Obstet Gynecol 2000; **95**: 726–31.

118 Miller JI, Ahmann FR. Treatment of castration-induced menopausal symptoms with low dose diethylstilbestrol in men with advanced prostate cancer. Urology 1992; **40**: 499–502.

119 Smith A. A prospective comparison of treatments for symptomatic hot flushes following endocrine treatment for carcinoma of the prostate. J Urol 1994; **152**: 132–4.

120 Gerber GS, Zayaja CP, Ray P, et al. Transdermal estrogen in the treatment of hot flushes in men with prostate cancer. Urology 2000; **55**: 97–101.

● 121 Women's Health Initiative Investigators. Risks and benefits of estrogen plus progestin in healthy postmenopausal women: Principal results from the Women's Health Initiative randomized controlled trial. JAMA 2002; **288**: 321–33.

122 Li CI, Malone KE, Porter PL, et al. Relationship between long durations and different regimens of hormone therapy and risk of breast cancer. JAMA 2003; **289**: 3254–63.

123 Loprinzi CL, Michalak JC, Quella SK, et al. Megestrol acetate for the prevention of hot flushes. N Engl J Med 1994; **331**: 347–52.

124 Leonetti HB, Longo S, Anasti JN, et al. transdermal progesterone cream for vasomotor symptoms and postmenopausal bone loss. Obstet Gynecol 1999; **94**: 225–8.

125 Lobo RA, McCormick W, Singer F, et al. Depo-medroxyprogesterone acetate compared with conjugated

estrogens for the treatment of postmenopausal women. *Obstet Gynecol* 1984; **63**: 1–5.

126 Dawson NA, McLeod DG. Dramatic prostate specific antigen decrease in response to discontinuation of megestrol acetate in advanced prostate cancer: expansion of the antiandrogen withdrawal syndrome. *J Urol* 1995; **153**: 1946–7.

127 Wehbe TW, Stein BS, Akerley WL. Prostate-specific antigen response to withdrawal of megestrol acetate in a patient with hormone-refractory prostate cancer. *Mayo Clin Proc* 1997; **72**: 932–4.

128 Burch PA, Loprinzi CL. Prostate-specific antigen decline after withdrawal of low-dose megestrol acetate. *J Clin Oncol* 1999; **17**: 1087–8.

129 Hofseth LJ, Raafat AM, Osuch JR, *et al.* Hormone replacement therapy with oestrogen or estrogen plus medroxyprogesterone acetate is associated with increased epithelial proliferation in the normal postmenopausal breast. *J Clin Endocrinol Metab* 1999; **84**: 4459–65.

130 Isaksson E, Sahlin L, Soderqvist G, *et al.* Expression of sex steroid receptors and IGF-1 mRNA in breast tissue: effects of hormonal treatment. *J Steroid Biochem Mol Biol* 1999; **70**: 257–62.

131 Dixon AR, Jackson L. A randomized trial of second-line hormone vs single agent chemotherapy in tamoxifen resistant advanced breast cancer. *Br J Cancer* 1992; **66**: 402–4.

132 Egarter C, Huber J, Leikermoser R, *et al.* Tibolone vs conjugated estrogens and sequential progestogen in the treatment of climacteric complaints. *Maturitas* 1996; **23**: 55–62.

133 Ginsburg J, Prelevic G, Butler D, *et al.* Clinical experience with tibolone (Livial) over 8 years. *Maturitas* 1995; **21**: 71–6.

134 Kroiss R, Fentiman IS, Helmond FA. The effect of tibolone in postmenopausal women receiving tamoxifen after surgery for breast cancer: a randomised, double-blind, placebo-controlled trial. *Br J Obstet Gynaecol* 2005; **112**: 228–33.

135 Loprinzi,CL, Kugler JW, Sloan JA. Venlafaxine in management of hot flashes in survivors of breast cancer: a randomised controlled trial. *Lancet* 2000; **356**: 2059–63.

136 Stearns V, Beebe K. Paroxetine controlled release in the treatment of menopausal hot flashes: A randomized controlled trial. *JAMA* 2003; **289**: 2827–34.

137 Loprinzi CL, Sloan JA, Perez EA, *et al.* Phase III evaluation of fluoxetine for treatment of hot flashes. *J Clin Oncol* 2002; **6**: 578–83.

138 Barton D, Loprinzi CL, Novotny P, *et al.* Pilot evaluation of citalopram for the relief of hot flashes. *J Support Oncol* 2003; **1**: 47–51.

139 Perez DG, Loprinzi CL, Barton DL, *et al.* Pilot evaluation of mirtazapine for the treatment of hot flashes. *J Support Oncol* 2004; **2**: 50–6.

140 Stearns V, Beebe KL, Iyengar M, *et al.* Active tamoxifen metabolite plasma concentrations after coadministration of tamoxifen and the selective serotonin reuptake inhibitor paroxetine. *J Natl Cancer Inst* 2003; **95**: 1758–64.

141 Guttuso T, Kurlan R, McDermott M, *et al.* Gabapentin's effects on hot flashes in postmenopausal women: a randomized controlled trial. *Obstet Gynecol* 2003; **101**: 337–45.

142 Loprinzi CL, Goldberg RM, O'Fallon JR, *et al.* Transdermal clonidine for ameliorating post-orchiectomy hot flashes. *J Urol* 1994; **151**: 634–6.

143 Pandya KJ, Raubertas RF, Flynn PJ, *et al.* Oral clonidine in post-menopausal patients with breast cancer experiencing tamoxifen-induced hot flashes: a University of Rochester Cancer Center Community Clinical Oncology Program study. *Ann Intern Med* 2000; **132**: 788–93.

144 Barton DL, Loprinzi CL, Quella SK, *et al.* Prospective evaluation of vitamin E for hot flashes in breast cancer survivors. *J Clin Oncol* 1998; **16**: 495–500.

145 Bergmans MG, Merkus JM, Corbey R, *et al.* Effect of Bellergal retard on climacteric complaints: a double-blind, placebo-controlled study. *Maturitas* 1987; **9**: 227–34.

146 Eisenberg DM, Davis RB, Ettner SL, *et al.* Trends in alternative medicine in the US; results of a follow up national survey. *JAMA* 1998; **16**: 2377–81.

147 Quella SK, Loprinzi CL, Barton DL, *et al.* Evaluation of soy phytoestrogens for the treatment of hot flashes in breast cancer survivors: A North Central Cancer Treatment Group Trial. *J Clin Oncol* 2000; **18**: 1068–74.

148 Van Patten CL, Olivotto IA, Chambers GK, *et al.* Effect of soy phytoestrogens on hot flashes in postmenopausal women with breast cancer: a randomized, controlled clinical trial. *J Clin Oncol* 2002; **20**: 1149–55.

149 Taylor M. Botanicals: medicines and menopause. *Clin Obstet Gynecol* 2001; **44**: 853–63.

150 Jacobson JS, Troxel AB, Evans J, *et al.* Randomized trial of black cohosh for the treatment of hot flashes among women with a history of breast cancer. *J Clin Oncol.* 2001; **19**: 2739–45.

151 Wyon Y, Wijma K, Nedstrand E, *et al.* A comparison of acupuncture and oral estradiol treatment of vasomotor symptoms in postmenopausal women. *Climacteric* 2004; **7**: 153–64.

152 Hammar M, Frisk J, Grimas O, *et al.* Acupuncture treatment of vasomotor symptoms in men with prostatic carcinoma: a pilot study. *J Urol* 1999; **161**: 853–6.

153 Irvin JH, Domar, AD, Clark C, *et al.* The effects of relaxation response training on menopausal symptoms. *J Psychosom Obstet Gynaecol* 1996; **17**: 202–7.

154 Freedman RR, Woodward S. Behavioral treatment of menopausal hot flushes: evaluation by ambulatory monitoring. *Am J Obstet Gynecol* 1992; **167**: 436–9.

78

Pruritus

VICTORIA LIDSTONE, ANDREW THORNS

INTRODUCTION

Pruritus is defined as 'an unpleasant sensation that provokes the desire to scratch'. It has a prevalence of 27 percent in common tumor sites,[1] and in cholestasis up to 80 percent of patients may complain of itch.[2] In severe cases it can cause undue distress and can be difficult to treat. This chapter will summarize the pathogenesis of pruritus as far as it is known and the causes and effects of pruritus, and will discuss possible treatment options.

PATHOGENESIS OF PRURITUS

The pathogenesis of itch is complex and has not been fully elucidated. Both central and peripheral mechanisms are involved and a number of mediators are being studied to generate future treatment options. Twycross has suggested a clinical classification based on the understandings of the origins of itch[3] (Box 78.1).

Box 78.1 Classification of pruritus based on origin

- Pruritoceptive itch – originating from the skin and transmitted by C fibers, e.g. scabies, urticaria

- Neuropathic itch – originating from disease located along the afferent pathway, e.g. herpes zoster, multiple sclerosis and brain tumors

- Neurogenic itch – originating centrally without any evidence of neural pathology, e.g. itch caused by cholestasis which is due to the action of opioid neuropeptides on μ-opioid receptors

- Psychogenic itch – as in the delusional state of parasitophobia

---

NEURAL PATHWAYS

The neurons responsible for the sensation of itch are a subset of the large population of polymodal C-nociceptors. They are situated close to the dermal–epidermal junction and comprise about 20 percent of the C fiber population in the skin.

The sensation of itch is closely linked to that of pain and for many years it was thought that both were transmitted identically. Both are unpleasant sensory experiences, however, pain sensation results in a reflex withdrawal whereas itch results in a scratch reflex. It is also now known that although the C fibers that are associated with itch are anatomically identical to those that mediate pain, there are some important functional differences. The C fibers responsible for itch are insensitive to mechanical stimuli and are more sensitive to histamine than those responsible for the sensation of pain.[4] Conduction along itch fibers is 50 percent slower than for those fibers transmitting pain and the receptor field is three times larger and more superficial than that associated with pain.[5]

The neural impulse passes via the C fibers to the ipsilateral dorsal root ganglia, and from here to the opposite anterolateral spinothalamic tract, on to the posterolateral ventral thalamic nucleus and through the internal capsule to the somatosensory cortex of the post central gyrus. There is substantial coactivation of the motor areas of the brain which supports the clinical observation that itch is linked to scratching. There does not appear to be a distinct 'itch center'.[6]

The sensation of itch can originate at several points on the neural pathway. Activation of the C fibers in the skin/mucous membranes will trigger itch, and this type of pruritus is mediated by histamine and therefore generally responsive to treatment with H_1 antihistamines, although in the chronic setting this response diminishes, presumably secondary to desensitization at a central level. In addition to pruritogenic stimuli to the skin, itch can originate at any point along the afferent pathway. This may occur with neural damage locally (e.g. postherpetic neuralgia) or centrally (e.g. a space-occupying lesion).[7,8] This neuropathic itch is not usually H_1 antihistamine responsive. In addition pruritus may also be caused by accumulation of toxins (endogenous or exogenous) in the spinal cord or brain; again this type of pruritus is histamine independent. The sensation of itch can be magnified by psychological factors such as stress or anxiety, and conversely, reduced by training and distraction. It appears that the central inhibitory circuits can be altered so affecting the threshold for detecting pruritogenic stimuli.

Central and peripheral mediators

There are many substances known to be involved in the mediation of itch. Histamine is perhaps the best known of these; it is released from mast cells in response to pruritogenic stimuli and acts on the H_1 receptors of the C fibers in the skin causing the characteristic wheal and flare reaction specific to histamine-mediated pruritus. Prostaglandins E_2 and H_2 potentiate pruritus via other mediators including histamine,[9] and, in the case of prostaglandin E_2, also directly.[10] Substance P is synthesized in the cell bodies of C fibers and can directly induce itch as well as modulate the sensation. The release of substance P can be stimulated by tryptase from activated mast cells and neutrophils and this may increase itch. Other neuropeptides, vasoactive intestinal polypeptide (VIP) and calcitonin gene-related protein (CGRP) are found in the free nerve endings and have been implicated in the mediation of itch. An intradermal injection of acetylcholine causes itch in atopic subjects, but pain in nonatopic subjects,[11] which may explain why some atopic subjects experience itch when sweating.

Opioids are thought to mediate itch at several points in the pathway. Peripherally, opioids cause mast cell degranulation and histamine release, but it is at a spinal level that role of opioids appear most interesting. They modulate secondary transmission of the itch sensation by stimulating inhibitory signals to afferent neurons. Centrally opioids have been shown to trigger itch in the laboratory setting by direct action on the floor of the fourth ventricle.

Serotonin induces itch by two mechanisms: indirectly by release of histamine from dermal mast cells, and centrally via a mechanism which may involve opioid neurotransmitters. Both opioid and serotonin receptors appear to alter the central inhibitory circuits and so adjust the itch threshold.

SCRATCH

Scratch is the natural response to itch. In evolutional terms it is likely to have originated when most pruritogens were parasites or insects and served to remove the superficial layers of skin which harbor these.[12] Itch is linked to the motor response of scratching via a spinal reflex and can be inhibited by cortical centers. Scratching stimulates A fibers adjacent to those conducting itch and the A fibers in turn synapse with inhibitory interneurons subsequently causing inhibition of C fibers and a reduced sensation of itch. Scratching provides relief for several minutes; it has been postulated that this occurs due to temporary disruption of the circuits in the relay synapses of the spinal cord which otherwise reinforce the itch sensation.

COMPLICATIONS OF PRURITUS

The commonest complication is excoriation, which can result in secondary infection. The effects of lack of sleep, social unacceptability, and interference with daily functioning should not be overlooked. One study found depressive symptoms in one third of patients with generalized pruritus.[13] The power of suggestion can result in itch and learned behavior can quickly develop. The resultant itch–scratch cycle can be hard to break.

ASSESSMENT OF THE PRURITIC PATIENT

Routine assessment involves careful history and examination, particularly noting whether the itch is generalized or localized, and with careful attention to drug history, exacerbating factors, and previous medical history. Examination should involve detailed description of the site and nature of any skin lesions and ideally photographic records. General first-line investigations may include full blood picture, erythrocyte sedimentation rate (ESR), and renal and liver profiles if clinically indicated. Biopsy of any suspicious lesions should be discussed with a dermatologist or dermooncologist prior to proceeding.

MEASURING ITCH

The subjective nature of this symptom makes it notoriously difficult to quantify, although a number of researchers have designed tools for this purpose but none have been very successful.[14] More recently two validated questionnaires have been developed that attempt to assess the qualitative, temporal, and spatial characteristics of itch, based on the long and short forms of the McGill Pain Questionnaire which show more promise.[6] Also monitoring systems have been developed that provide quantitative data independent of hand/arm movement and these provide the most reliable assessment method to date.[15]

CAUSES OF PRURITUS IN ADVANCED DISEASE

Table 78.1 summarizes the causes of pruritus that may be relevant in patients with advanced disease. These can be divided into general causes of pruritus and those specifically related to disease (e.g. malignancy, human immunodeficiency virus [HIV]) and in either case pruritus may be localized or generalized.

Senile itch is experienced by 50–70 percent of those over the age of 70 years. The majority have xerosis and skin atrophy, in others the cause is unknown. It is best treated with general measures (see below) and the application of emollient cream. Pruritus can be iatrogenic and the following drugs are commonly culprits: opioids, aspirin, etretinate, amfetamines, and drugs that can cause cholestasis such as erythromycin, hormonal treatment, and phenothiazines.

Iron deficiency with or without anemia can cause pruritus[16] and responds to iron replacement. Pruritus occurs in up to 11 percent of patients with thyrotoxicosis, particularly long-term untreated Graves disease, and less commonly in hypothyroidism. The link between diabetes mellitus and pruritus is controversial.

Other common causes of pruritus are discussed in the management section.

MANAGEMENT OF PRURITUS

Removal of causative agents (e.g. drugs) and appropriate investigation and treatment of underlying disease are essential first-line measures in the treatment of pruritus. Management can be divided into general and pharmaceutical measures suitable for all causes, and pharmacological measures which are more cause specific. When considering any interventions for pruritus a strong placebo response is common.

Evidence for the use of different systemic agents in the treatment of pruritus is limited, and largely pertains to the treatment of opioid-induced pruritus, particularly following neuro-axial administration. This topic is outside the scope of this chapter but is covered well in a recently published systematic review.[17] In the context of treating pruritic patients with advanced disease there are few useful trials and the use of many agents remains historical or originates from case reports. This is not to say these agents are not helpful, just that the evidence either confirming or refuting their use is, thus far, unavailable.

Some of the main groups of drugs used to systemically treat pruritus and the evidence for their efficacy are summarized in Table 78.2, and discussed in more detail below.

Table 78.1 *Causes of pruritus*

Localized	Generalized
Dry skin (xerosis)	Primary skin diseases
Infestation, e.g. scabies	Metabolic disorders: hypothyroidism and hyperthyroidism, carcinoid
Insect bites	syndrome, diabetes mellitus and insipidus
Candida	Renal disorders: renal failure with uremia
Eczema	Liver disorders: cholestasis
Contact dermatitis	Infection: HIV, syphilis
Bullous pemphigoid	Hematological disorders: polycythemia vera, iron deficiency anemia
Dermatitis herpetiformis	Neurological disorders: cerebrovascular accident multiple sclerosis,
Urticaria	brain abscess/tumors
	Drug-induced (see text)
	Senile pruritus
	Aquagenic
	Psychogenic
Cancer-specific pruritus	
Melanomatosis	Chronic lymphocytic leukemia
Mycosis fungoides	Hodgkin and non-Hodgkin lymphoma
Carcinoma *in situ*: vulval, anal	Mycosis fungoides
Paraneoplastic syndrome: prostatic, rectal/	Cutaneous T cell lymphoma
colonic, cervical carcinomas; glioblastoma	Multiple myeloma
Metastatic infiltration of skin	Paraneoplastic syndrome: breast, colonic, lung, stomach carcinomas and others

Table 78.2 *Evidence for the systemic treatment of pruritus*

Cause	Treatment											
	H$_1$ receptor antagonists	H$_2$ receptor antagonists	5-HT$_3$ receptor antagonists	Opioid receptor antagonists	NSAIDs	SSRIs	17-α alkyl androgen	Cholestyramine	Thalidomide	UVB	Psoralen + UVA	Capsaicin cream (localized)
Solid tumor		+			+							
Hematologic malignancy		+			+ CT			+				
Skin malignancy		+			+							
Paraneoplastic			+			+ RCT			+			
Opioid-induced			+ RCT	+								
Uremia	–	–	+ RCT – RCT	+ RXT – RCT				+	+ RXDB	+ RCT		+ [18]
Cholestasis			+ RPCDBX	+ DBPC 4 × CT			+	+		+		
Atopy	+											
Notalgia paresthetica											+	
HIV										+	+	
Polycythemia											+	
Central lesions/multiple sclerosis					+							

+, evidence supporting use; –, evidence against use.

More robust evidence is detailed as: CT, controlled trial; RCT, randomized controlled trial; RXT, randomized crossover trial; DBPC, double blind, placebo controlled trial; RPCDBX, randomized, placebo controlled, double blind, crossover trial; RXDB, randomized crossover, double blind trial.

SSRIs, selective serotonin reuptake inhibitors; NSAIDs, non-steroidal anti-inflammatory drugs.

General management techniques

These measures are widely accepted as essential although the evidence for their efficacy is largely anecdotal. Exacerbating factors such as heat, dehydration, anxiety and boredom should be avoided. Particular attention should be paid to measures that keep the skin well hydrated and avoid sweating. Patients should wear light clothes, use fans to maintain a passage of air, take tepid baths or shower avoiding hot water, and use emulsifying ointment or aqueous cream instead of soap. Skin hydration should be maintained with regular use of emollients. Alcohol and spicy foods may worsen itch.

Patients should be advised to gently rub the skin rather than scratching it, and to keep nails short and wear cotton gloves at night to limit the damage to the skin. Sweating may exacerbate itch; the general measures described above may help reduce sweating, otherwise an antimuscarinic agent may be required.

Exposure to ultraviolet (UV) B light may help in both cholestatic, uremic and acquired immune deficiency syndrome (AIDS)-related pruritus. Although the nontoxic nature of this treatment makes it an attractive alternative, it may not be a suitable treatment for a very sick patient. The antipruritic effect is thought to be due to a reduction in the vitamin A content of the skin, inhibition of the release of histamine, and inhibition of dermal mast cell proliferation.[19,20]

Sedatives such as benzodiazepines do not relieve itch but may help improve associated anxiety and insomnia.[21] Behavioral treatments and hypnotherapy may help ease associated psychological issues and break the cycle of itching and scratching.[22] Transcutaneous electronic nerve stimulation (TENS) and acupuncture have been successful in case reports.[23,24]

Topical agents

Topical agents generally provide some relief but may be inconvenient to apply in generalized pruritus, and are probably best reserved for localized symptoms. A number of topical agents have been suggested such as: zinc oxide, calamine, glycerin, and salicylates but their mechanisms are not understood and their effectiveness is unproved. One double blind, controlled trial of crotamiton (Eurax®) showed it to be ineffective.[25] Polidocanol bath oil has been shown to reduce itch in uremia,[26] and 3 percent polidocanol/5 percent urea cream has been shown to reduce itch in psoriasis.[27]

Corticosteroid creams may help localized areas of inflamed skin. Local anesthetic creams can be helpful but may cause skin sensitization. Lidocaine is the least likely to have this effect but systemic absorption prevents its use over large areas or for prolonged periods. Topical counterirritants such as menthol 0.25–2 percent or camphor 1–3 percent may be useful.

Capsaicin 0.025 percent may be useful; it acts by depleting substance P in C fibers on repeated application, reducing pain and itch. It needs to be applied four times a day and has been shown to be helpful in uremic pruritus.[28] Application can cause an initial burning sensation which prohibits widespread application and decreases compliance; for these reasons it is best reserved for localized pruritus.

Strontium nitrate cream is an effective antipruritic, which may act by selectively blocking C-fiber transmission.[29] Doxepin, a tricyclic antidepressant with potent antihistaminic action now produced in a topical form, has been shown to be effective in atopic dermatitis and chronic urticaria. The topical form has been shown to be less effective than the systemic form;[30] its place in other causes of pruritus has not been established.

Systemic agents

Antihistamines are active at either the H_1 or H_2 receptor. H_1 receptor antagonists are often used as the first choice for any form of generalized pruritus, however there is little evidence for their use other than in urticaria or allergy. The more sedative agents such as chlorphenamine are believed to be more effective either because of a more potent central action or because the sedation itself helps to improve the insomnia caused by the itch. H_2 antihistamines such as cimetidine have been shown to be beneficial in the pruritus associated with lymphoproliferative disorders (see below). Doxepin, which acts at H_1 and H_2 receptors is effective in atopic dermatitis as discussed above.

The 5-hydroxytryptamine 3 (5-HT_3) receptor antagonists have shown promising results in the treatment of opioid-induced pruritus, particularly when the opioids are delivered by the neuro-axial route; early results in cholestatic and uremic pruritus showed some benefit too[31,32] but more recent randomized trials have shown minimal or no benefit.[33**,34**,35**]

The serotonin selective reuptake inhibitor (SSRI) paroxetine is helpful in paraneoplastic pruritus but the effect may only be temporary, lasting about 6 weeks,[36] and may also be associated with initial nausea and vomiting. Mirtazapine is a norepinephrine and specific serotonin antidepressant and its actions include blocking H_1, 5-HT_2 and 5-HT_3 receptors. It has been shown to be a helpful antipruritic agent in cholestasis, uremia, and lymphoma.[37]

Specific management strategies

CANCER-SPECIFIC PRURITUS

Pruritus is associated with hematological malignancies such as Hodgkin lymphoma and polycythemia rubra vera. Pruritus occurs in about 50 percent of patients with polycythemia and is commonly aquagenic pruritus; in almost 100 percent of patients with cutaneous T cell lymphoma; and in 30 percent of patients with Hodgkin disease and is more common in the nodular sclerosing subtype with mediastinal mass.[38] Its presence may precede overt disease by up to 5 years.[39] In pruritus secondary to polycythemia vera the use of disease-modifying therapy often reduces pruritus and should be considered first,[40] aspirin, paroxetine, and cimetidine have been shown to be helpful.[41**,42,43]

In Hodgkin disease cimetidine[44] and topical 5 percent sodium cromoglycate[45] have been reported as helpful. Corticosteroids have been used historically and are felt to be effective but evidence is lacking. Although cimetidine is an H_2 receptor antagonist, its action is not thought to be a direct antihistaminic effect as it has little effect on itching caused by histamine, but is thought to be related to its inhibitory action on CYP2D6 liver enzymes which are involved in the synthesis of endogenous opioids and possibly other pruritogens.[46] See Figure 78.1 for a suggested approach to treatment.

Mycosis fungoides often presents in the early stages with pruritic dermatitis that may precede cutaneous lesions by up to 10 years.[48] Tumor-modifying treatments are effective in reducing pruritus and mycosis fungoides cells are very radiosensitive. Ciclosporin is also effective but long-term effects of treatment are currently unevaluated.[49]

Tumors of the anus and vulva can present with local itch. Pruritus can also present as part of a paraneoplastic syndrome in association with some solid tumors including lung, colon, breast, stomach, and prostate. In these cases it is usually generalized rather than localized with a few notable exceptions:

gliomas and carcinomas of the cervix, rectum, sigmoid colon, and prostate, which may manifest with pruritus of the face, nostrils, vulvae, anus, and scrotum, respectively. It may be the presenting symptom in these diseases, and, as for Hodgkin disease may appear some years before the tumor is identifiable. However research has shown that patients with generalized pruritus followed-up for 6 years did not have a higher overall incidence of malignancy and that follow-up screening was therefore not warranted in this group of patients.[50]

Paroxetine, an SSRI antidepressant has been shown to relieve itch in a case series of advanced cancer patients with paraneoplastic itch and in a randomized controlled trial for severe nondermatological pruritus, probably due to down regulation of 5-HT_3 receptors, but side effects (nausea, vomiting and sedation) may limit its use.[36**,51**] See Figure 78.2 for a suggested approach to management.

OPIOID-INDUCED PRURITUS

Opioids provide good pain control for the majority of patients, and are used frequently in advanced disease in accordance with the World Health Organization (WHO) analgesic ladder guidelines. Itch is a well-recognized side effect of opioids although the exact etiology is currently unknown. Pruritus occurs in about 1 percent of patients on opioids delivered subcutaneously, orally or intravenously, and up to 90 percent of

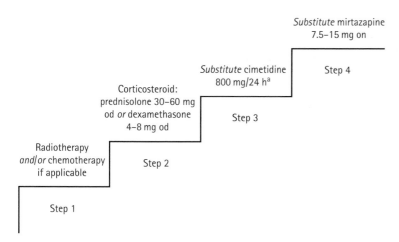

Figure 78.1 Treatment of pruritus in Hodgkin lymphoma. [a]Alternative H_2 receptor antagonists probably equally effective. od, once daily; on, every night. Redrawn with permission from Twycross and Zylicz. Prog Palliat Care 2002; 10: 285–9[47] with permission.

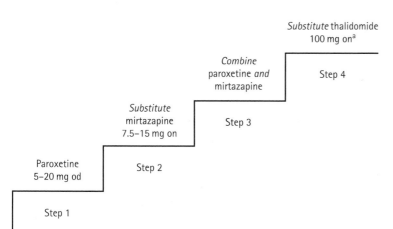

Figure 78.2 Treatment of paraneoplastic pruritus. [a]Undesirable effects include peripheral neuropathy and congenital malformations (shortened or absent limbs). Redrawn with permission from Twycross and Zylicz. Prog Palliat Care 2002; 10: 285–9[47] with permission.

patients receiving neuro-axial opioids. Experience suggests that pruritus tends to be generalized in patients on nonspinal opioids, although in children it is more common in the facial area, particularly the nose. In neuro-axial delivery, the pruritus spreads upwards from the level of injection, is commonly maximal in the face, and may be limited to the nose.[52] Postulated mechanisms include a direct central effect,[53] and related histamine release[54] and more recently serotonin release.[55] There is some evidence that itch is more common with the naturally occurring opioids and is also related to the route of administration, being commoner with neuro-axial opioids than oral opioids. Previous researchers have reported itch with epidural morphine,[56] intravenous and oral morphine,[57] and epidural fentanyl,[58] and oral oxycodone.[59]

In the treatment of opioid-induced pruritus opioid antagonists are useful in reducing pruritus but may reverse the analgesic effects,[60] making them an unhelpful choice of treatment for most patients with advanced disease. One study suggests that using an agonist-antagonist drug such as nalbuphine can reduce pruritus without compromising its analgesic effect.[61] One disadvantage of opioid antagonists is that they are generally expensive. Opioid rotation, in particular changing to hydromorphone, may be a more practical solution and may be effective.[57]

Ondansetron has been shown to be useful in opioid-induced itch[62] at traditional antiemetic doses, although most studies pertain to its success in treating the pruritus associated with neuro-axial opioids.

CHOLESTASIS

Cholestasis may occur in the general population as a result of gallstones, drugs or intrahepatic disease, as well as obstruction from primary or secondary tumors involving the biliary tree. Pruritus is a common sequela of cholestasis, starting on the palmar and planter surfaces and becoming more generalized. Accumulation of bile salts have long been suspected as an etiological factor and although they may have a role to play the evidence for a central mechanism related to increased opioidergic tone and activation of itch centers

in the brain is gathering pace.[3] Treatment of cholestatic pruritus with the opioid antagonists naltrexone, naloxone, and nalmefene follow this body of evidence and are successful.[63**,64*,65*] It is interesting to note that opioid withdrawal effects were noted even in opioid-naïve patients with cholestatic pruritus; this may be an effect of high levels of endogenous opioids. Pain may also be a complication of using opioid antagonists for symptom control.[66] It has been suggested that these side effects may be avoided by titrating an infusion of naloxone to establish an effective dose before switching to an oral form.[67]

Treatment of cholestatic pruritus with 5-HT$_3$ antagonists was supported by early evidence but recent robust trials have found little or no benefit.[31,33**,34**] These drugs are used at traditional antiemetic doses and are relatively expensive, and constipation can be a troublesome side effect.

The most effective method of relieving pruritus secondary to cholestasis is to relieve the obstruction. This may be possible by treating the underlying disease with surgery or chemotherapy or high-dose dexamethasone but where this is not possible the treatment of choice is a biliary stent (Fig. 78.3), even in the terminally ill. Cholestyramine binds bile salts in the gut and has traditionally been used for the treatment of cholestatic pruritus, although evidence for benefit is limited to one small, open label study completed nearly 40 years ago.[68] As a result of this mechanism of action it is ineffective in complete biliary obstruction. Its use is limited because it is unpalatable and relatively large quantities must be consumed for effect, although helped by mixing with fruit juice. Charcoal has been used along the same therapeutic line, with similar success and similar consumer acceptability problems. Rifampicin is a hepatic enzyme inducer and also inhibits reuptake of bile acids by hepatocytes. It is thought to interrupt the enterohepatic circulation of bile acids and therefore reduce the impact of bile acids on the metabolic processes of the liver, and has been shown to reduce pruritus in cholestasis.[69**] However the presence of severe idiosyncratic side effects in one study may limit its use.[70]

The 17-α alkyl androgens have also been used historically with some effect.[71] The action is not fully understood, but the

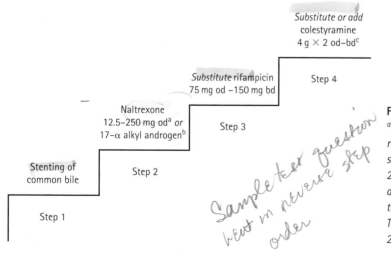

Substitute or add
colestyramine
4 g × 2 od–bd[c]

Substitute rifampicin
75 mg od –150 mg bd

Step 4

Naltrexone
12.5–250 mg od[a] or
17–α alkyl androgen[b]

Step 3

Stenting of
common bile

Step 2

Step 1

Figure 78.3   *Treatment of cholestatic pruritus.* [a]*Contraindicated in patients needing opioids for pain relief.* [b]*For example, methyltestosterone 25 mg sublingually od (not available in UK), danazol 200 mg mg od–tds.* [c]*Not of benefit in complete large duct biliary obstruction. od, once daily; bd, twice daily; tds, three times daily. Redrawn with permission from Twycross and Zylicz.* Prog Palliat Care *2002;* **10:** *285–9[47] with permission.*

17-α alkyl androgens are directly toxic to hepatocytes and may limit the capacity of the liver's enkephalin production.[72] Care should be taken when considering long-term use of 17-α alkyl androgens in patients with years to live as they have the potential to cause masculinization in women and also, occasionally serious liver impairment. Other experimental options have been explored including: propofol, S-adenosylmethionine (SAMe), anti-oxidants, tetrahydrocannabinol, macrolide antibiotics, plasmapheresis and albumin dialysis.[73]

CHRONIC RENAL FAILURE

Renal failure may occur as a primary disorder or secondary to a cancer either as a result of direct tumor infiltration of the kidney or ureteric obstruction caused by tumor mass, metastases, or lymph nodes. It is chronic renal failure that is likely to be associated with pruritus. Pruritus may be generalized or be limited to the back and the forearm at the site of the arteriovenous shunt.[74] The pathogenesis of pruritus in this setting has not been fully defined but is thought to be multifactorial. The skin of these patients is atrophic and dry,[75] cytokine production in the skin may contribute, and interleukin-1 may cause release of pruritogens. Mast cells are more numerous in patients with pruritic uremia[76] and although plasma histamine levels have been shown to be much increased in this group of patients, antihistamines *per se* are ineffectual in improving the pruritus.[77]

Pruritus is more common in uremic patients receiving dialysis than those who are not, and a recent study supports the idea that the itch is caused by accumulation of pruritogenic metabolites rather than hypersensitivity to dialysis equipment.[78] Pruritus is reduced by the use of more permeable membranes in hemodialysis, suggesting that this facilitates clearing of pruritogens.

Pruritus is local in 70 percent of patients and for these patients capsaicin cream can be effective and practical.[28] The efficacy of opioid antagonists is under dispute: opioid antagonists have been found to be effective by some researchers,[79**] and not by others.[32**] Ondansetron has been used to treat uremic pruritus but the evidence for success is conflicting.[35**,80] There is some good evidence of thalidomide having an antipruritic effect in uremia.[81**] Postulated mechanisms for its antipruritic effect include: reduction of tumor necrosis factor synthesis by monocytes; anti-inflammatory action; and interference with cytokine production. It has also been shown to be effective in the pruritus of various primary skin conditions, senile pruritus, and primary biliary cirrhosis.[82] UVB phototherapy may also be effective.[20]

Homeopathic treatments have also been shown to be effective: in one controlled trial patients reported a 49 percent reduction in pruritus score.[83] An approach to management is suggested in Figure 78.4.

HIV/AIDS

There are many causes of pruritus in HIV-positive patients,[84] and itch can be the first symptom of disease even in the absence of apparent skin lesions. Pruritus in HIV may be related to cytokine-induced prostaglandin 2 synthesis, and increased plasma cytokine levels are not uncommon in patients with HIV.[85,86] Localized pruritus may occur with peripheral neuropathy.[6] Exposure to UVB light has been shown to be effective.[87] Treatment should relate to the specific cause, but in the absence of an obvious cause indometacin 25 mg three times daily may be helpful.[58]

CENTRAL LESIONS AND MULTIPLE SCLEROSIS

Historically pruritus in this group of patients has been treated effectively with anti-epileptic drugs such as carbamazepine. Gabapentin may be a better tolerated choice and does not interfere with other medication by inducing liver enzymes.[88] NSAIDS such as ibuprofen may also be helpful.[89]

SUMMARY

Pruritus can be a troublesome symptom in patients with advanced disease and may have a substantial effect on

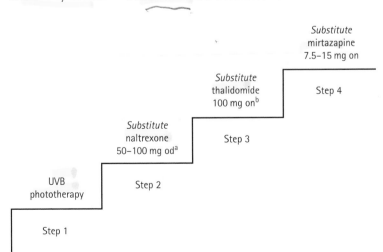

? gabapentin - possible referred to in sample text

Figure 78.4 *Treatment of uremic pruritus. [a]Benefit disputed; contraindicated in patients needing opioids for pain relief. [b]Undesirable effects include peripheral neuropathy and congenital malformations (shortened or absent limbs). od, once daily; on, every night. Redrawn with permission from Twycross and Zylicz. Prog Palliat Care 2002;**10**: 285–9[47] with permission.*

Substitute
mirtazapine
7.5–15 mg on
Step 4

Substitute
thalidomide
100 mg on[b]

Substitute
naltrexone
50–100 mg od[a]
Step 3

UVB
phototherapy
Step 2

Step 1

quality of life despite the apparent trivial nature of the symptom relative to a life-limiting diagnosis. Careful history and examination may reveal an easily reversible cause; where this is not the case intervention may be helpful. First and foremost, management should include patient education and life-style changes to recognize and avoid triggering factors, and to include important general measures for maximal skin hydration in daily routine. Alongside these measures investigation and treatment of the underlying cause, where possible, is helpful. Topical or systemic medication should be used appropriate to the cause when required. The relatively limited etiological understanding of pruritus has hindered logical management but there is now a more compre- hensive body of evidence slowly but surely being created. Development of further useful interventions depends on continued investigation of the complex mechanisms by which pruritus is created, and more detailed evaluation of currently available interventions.

Key learning points

- Pruritus may be directly related to advanced disease (e.g. cancer, multiple sclerosis), indirectly related (e.g. cholestasis, uremia), or associated with the treatment of advanced disease.

- Pruritus may significantly impact on sleep, social acceptance, and daily functioning; and has been shown to be associated with depression.

- Initial management should include patient education and lifestyle changes to encourage identification and avoidance of triggering factors.

- The use of emollients to keep the skin continually hydrated cannot be overemphasized and must continue on a long-term basis. In addition large numbers of other topical agents are available and there is a reasonable evidence base supporting their use.

- Diagnosis of the underlying cause of pruritus is important and treatment of underlying disease will in many cases resolve the pruritus.

- If topical measures and lifestyle changes are not adequate, systemic treatment may be necessary and this chapter provides some evidence-based suggestions for first, second, and third line treatments based on etiology.

- The historical use of histamine antagonists in the treatment of all pruritus has now been modified by the growing evidence base in this area, and these drugs are now only recommended for use in the treatment of urticaria, allergy, and lymphoproliferative pruritus.

REFERENCES

1   Portenoy RK, Thaler HT, Kornblith AB, et al. Symptom prevalence, characteristics and distress in a cancer population. Qual Life Res 1994; **3**: 183–9.

◆ 2   Connolly CS, Kantor GR, Menduke H. Hepatobiliary pruritus: What are effective treatments? J Am Acad Dermatol 1995; **33**: 801–5.

✱ ◆ 3   Twycross R, Greaves MW, Handwerker H, et al. Itch: scratching more than the surface. Q J Med 2003; **96**: 7–26.

4   Schelmz M, Michael K, Weidner C, et al. Which nerve fibres mediate the axon reflex flare in human skin? Neuroreport 2000; **11**: 645–8.

5   Schmelz M, Schmidt R, Bickel A, et al. Specific C-receptors for itch in human skin. J. Neurosci 1997; **17**: 8003–8.

6   Yosipovitch G, Greaves M, Schmelz M. Itch. Lancet 2003; **361**: 690–4.

7   Oaklander AL, Cohen SP, Raju SV. Intractable postherpetic itch and cutaneous deafferentation after facial shingles Pain 2002; **96**: 9–12.

8   King CA, Huff FJ, Jorizzo JL. Unilateral neurogenic pruritus: paroxysmal itching associated with central nervous system lesions. Ann Intern Med 1982; **97**: 222–3.

9   Greaves MW, McDonald-Gibson W. Itch: the role of prostaglandins. Br Med J 1973; **22**: 608–9.

10   Woodward DF, Nieves AL, Hawley SB. et al. The pruritogenic and inflammatory effects of prostanoids in the conjunctiva. J Ocul Pharmacol Ther 1995; **11**: 339–47.

11   Vogelsang M, Heyer G, Hornstein OP. Acetylcholine induces different cutaneous sensations in atopic and non-atopic subjects. Acta Derm Venereol 1995; **75**: 434–6.

◆ 12   Krajnik M, Zylicz Z. Understanding pruritus in systemic disease. J Pain Symptom Manage 2001; **21**: 151–68.

13   Sheehan-Dare RA, Henderson MJ, Cotterill JA. Anxiety and depression in patients with chronic urticaria and generalised pruritus. Br J Dermatol 1990; **123**: 769–74.

14   Wahlgren CF. Measurement of itch. Semin Dermatol 1995; **14**: 277–84.

15   Molenaar HAJ, Oosting J, Jones EA. Improved device for measuring scratching activity in patients with pruritus. Med Biol Eng Comput 1998; **36**: 220–4.

16   Vickers CF. Iron deficiency pruritus. JAMA 1977; **238**: 129.

17   Kjellberg F, Tramer MR. Pharmacological control of opioid-induced pruritus: a quantitive systematic review of randomised trials. Eur J Anaesthesiol 2001; **18**: 346–57.

18   Wallengren J. Treatment of notalgia paraesthetica with topical capsaicin. J Am Acad Dermatol 1991; **24**: 286–8.

19   Szeptietowski JC, Morita A, Tsuji T. Ultraviolet B induces mast cell apoptosis: a hypothetical mechanism of ultraviolet B treatment for uraemic pruritus. Med Hypotheses 2002; **58**: 167–70.

20   Gilchrest BA, Rowe JW, Brown RS, et al. Relief of uraemic pruritus with ultraviolet phototherapy. N Engl Med J 1977; **297**: 136–8.

21   Ebata T, Izumi H, Aizawa H, et al. Effects of nitrazepam on nocturnal scratching in adults with atopic dermatitis: a double blind placebo-controlled crossover study. Br J Dermatol 1998; **138**: 631–4.

22   Pittelkow MR, Loprinzi CL. Pruritus and sweating. In: Doyle D, Hanks GWC, MacDonald N, eds. Oxford Textbook of Palliative Medicine, 2nd ed. New York: Oxford University Press, 1998: 633.

23 Monk BE. Transcutaneous electronic nerve stimulation in the treatment of generalised pruritus. *Clin Exp Dermatol* 1993; **18**: 67–8.

24 Bjorna H, Kaada B. Successful treatment of itching and atopic eczema by transcutaneous nerve stimulation. *Acupunct Electro-ther Res* 1987; **12**: 101–12.

25 Smith EB, King CA, Baker MD. Crotamiton and pruritus. *Int J Dermatol* 1984; **23**: 684–85.

26 Wasik F, Szeptietowski JC, Szeptietowski T, Weyde W. Relief of uraemic pruritus after balneological therapy with a bath oil containing polidocanol. An open clinical study. *J Dermatol Treat* 1996; **7**: 231–3.

27 Freitag G, Hoppner T. Results of a postmarketing drug monitoring survey with a polidocanol-urea preparation for dry itching skin. *Curr Med Res Opin* 1997; **13**: 529–37.

28 Breneman DL, Cardone JS, Blumsack RF *et al.* Topical capsaicin for treatment of haemodialysis related pruritus. *J Am Acad Dermatol* 1992; **26**: 91–4.

29 Zhai H, Hannon W, Hahn, GS, Harper RA *et al.* Strontium nitrate decreased histamine induced itch magnitude and duration in man. *Dermatology* 2000; **200**: 244–6.

30 Smith PF, Corelli RL. Doxepin in the management of pruritus associated with allergic cutaneous reactions. *Ann Pharmacother* 1997; **31**: 633–5.

◆ 31 Jones EA, Bergasa NV. Evolving concepts of the pathogenesis and treatment of the pruritus of cholestasis. *Can J Gastroenterol* 2000; **14**: 33–40.

32 Kirschner D, Nagel W, Gugeler N, *et al.* Naltrexone does not relieve uremic pruritus: results of a randomised, double blind, placebo-controlled study. *J Am Soc Nephrol* 2000; **11**: 514–19.

33 Muller C, Pongratz S, Pidlich J, *et al.* Treatment of pruritus in chronic liver disease with the 5HT3 antagonist ondansetron: a randomised, placebo-controlled double-blind cross over trial. *Eur J Gasterenterol Hepatol* 1998; **10**: 865–70.

34 O'Donohue JW, Haigh C, Williams R. Ondansetron in the treatment of pruritus of cholestasis: a randomised controlled trial. *Gastroenterology* 1997; **112**: A1349.

35 Murphy M, Reaich D, Pai P, *et al.* A randomised, placebo-controlled, double blind trial of ondansetron in renal itch. *Br J Dermatol* 2001; **145**(Suppl 59): 20–1.

36 Zylicz Z, Smits C, Krajnik M. Paroxetine for pruritus in advanced cancer. *J Pain Symptom Manage* 1998; **16**: 121–4.

37 Davis MP, Frandsen J L, Walsh D, *et al.* Mirtazapine for pruritus *J Pain Symptom Manage* 2003; **25**: 288–91.

38 Lober CW. Should the patient with generalized malignancy be evaluated for malignancy? *J Am Acad Dermatol* 1988; **19**: 350–2.

39 Goldman BD, Koh HK. Pruritus and malignancy. In: Bernhard JD, ed. *Itch. Mechanisms and Management of Pruritus.* New York: McGraw-Hill, 1994: 299–319.

◆ 40 Terrifi A. Polycythaemia vera: a comprehensive review and clinical recommendations. *Mayo Clin Proc* 2003; 78;174–94.

41 Jackson N, Burt D, Crocker J, Boughton B. Skin mast cells in polycythameia vera: relationship to pathogenesis and treament of pruritus. *Br J Dermatol* 1987; **116**: 21–9.

42 Terrifi A, Fonseca R. Selective serotonin reuptake inhibitors are effective in the treatment of polycythaemia vera associated pruritus. *Blood* 2002; **99**: 26–7.

43 Weick JK, Dinovan PB, Najean Y, *et al.* The use of cimetidine for the treatment of pruritus in polycythaemia rubra vera. *Arch Intern Med* 1982; **142**: 241–2.

44 Aymard JP, Lederlin P, Witz F, *et al.* Cimetidine for pruritus in Hodgkin's Disease. *Br J Med* 1980; **280**: 151–2.

45 Leven A, Naysmith A, Pickens S, *et al.* Sodium cromoglycate and Hodgkin's disease. *Br J Med* 1977; **2**: 896.

46 Martinez C, Albet C, Agundez JA, *et al.* Comparative in vitro and in vivo inhibition of cytochrome p450, CYP1A2, CYP2D6 and CYP3A by H2 receptor antagonists. *Clin Pharmacol Ther* 1999; **65**: 369–76.

47 Twycross R, Zylicz Z. OICPC Therapeutic Highlights. Itch: Scratching more than the surface. *Prog Palliat Care* 2002; **10**: 285–9.

48 Pujol RN, Gallardo F, Llistosella E, *et al.* Invisible mycosis fungiodes: a diagnostic challenge. *J Am Acad Dermatol* 2002; **47**(2 Suppl): S168–S71.

49 Totterman TH, Scheynius A, Killander A, *et al.* Treatment of therapy resistant Sezary syndrome with cyclosporin A: suppression of pruritus, leukaemic T cell activation markers and tumour mass. *Scand J Haematol* 1985; **34**: 196–203.

50 Paul R, Jansen C. Itch and malignancy prognosis in generalised pruritus: A 6 year follow-up of 125 patients. *J Am Acad Dermatol* 1987; **16**: 1179–82.

51 Zylicz Z, Krajnik M, van Sorge A, Constantini M. Paroxetine in the treatment of severe non-dermatological pruritus: A randomised controlled trial. *J Pain Symptom Manage* 2003; **26**: 1105–12.

52 Ballantyne JC, Loach AB, Carr DB. Itching after epidural and spinal opiates. *Pain* 1988; **33**: 149–60.

53 Stoelting RK. Pharmacology and physiology. In: Capan LM, Miller SM, Turndorf H, eds. *Anaesthetics Practice*, 2nd ed. Philadelphia: Lippincott, 1991.

54 Etches RC. Complications of acute pain management. *Anaesth Clin North Am* 1992; **10**: 417–33.

55 Larijani G, Goldberg ME, Rogers KH. Treatment of opioid induced pruritus with ondansetron – report of four patients. *Pharmacotherapy* 1996; **16**: 958–60.

56 Chaplan S, Duncan SR, Brodsky JB, Brose WG. Morphine and Hydromorphone epidural analgesia. *Anaesthesiology* 1992; **77**: 1090–4.

57 Katcher J, Walsh D. Opioid induced itching: morphine sulfate and hydromorphone hydrochloride. *J Pain Symptom Manage* 1999; **17**: 70–2.

58 Davies GG, From R. A blinded study using nalbuphine for prevention of pruritus induced by epidural fentanyl. *Anaesthesiology* 1988; **69**: 763–5.

59 Glare P, Walsh TD. Dose ranging study of oxycodone for chronic pain in advanced cancer. *J Clin Oncol* 1993; **11**: 973–8.

60 Wang JJ, Ho ST, Tzeng JI. Comparison of intravenous nalbuphine infusion versus naloxone in the prevention of epidural morphine related side effects. *Reg Anesth Pain Med* 1998; **23**: 479–84.

61 Cohen SE, Ratner EF, Kreitzman TR, *et al.* Nalbuphine is better than naloxone for treatment of side effects after epidural morphine. *Anesth Analg* 1992; **75**: 747–52.

62 Borgeat A, Stirnemann HR. Ondansetron is effective to treat spinal or epidural morphine-induced pruritus. *Anaesthesiology* 1999; **90**: 432–6.

63 Wolfhagen FH, Sternieri E, Hop WC, *et al.* Oral naltrexone treatment for cholestatic pruritus: a double blind placebo controlled study. *Gastroenterology* 1997; **113**: 1264–9.

64 Bergasa NV, Talbot TL, Alling DW, *et al.* A controlled trial of naloxone infusions for the pruritus of chronic cholestasis. *Gastroenterology* 1992; **102**: 544–9.

65 Bergasa NV, Talbot TL, Alling DW, *et al.* Oral nalmefene therapy reduces scratching activity due to pruritus of cholestasis: a controlled study. *J Am Acad Dermatol* 1999; **41**: 431–4.

66 McRae CA, Prince MI, Hudson M, *et al.* Pain as a complication of opiate antagonists for symptom control in cholestasis. *Gastroenterology* 2003; **125**: 591–6.

67 Jones EA, Neuberger J, Bergasa NV. Opiate antagonist therapy for the pruritus of cholestasis: the avoidance of opioid withdrawal-like reactions. *Quart J Med* 2002; **95**: 547–52.

68 Datta DV, Sherlock S. Cholestyramine for long-term relief of the pruritus complicating intrahepatic cholestasis. *Gastroenterology* 1966; **50**: 323–32.

69 Ghent C, Curruthers S. Treatment of pruritus in primary biliary cirrhosis with rifampicin. Results of a double-blind randomised cross-over trial. *Gasterenterology* 1988; **94**: 488–93.

70 Prince MI, Burt AD, Jones DE. Hepatitis and liver dysfunction with rifampicin therapy for pruritus in primary biliary cirrhosis. *Gut* 2002; **50**: 436–9.

71 Twycross RG, Lack SA. *Therapeutics in Terminal Cancer*, 2nd ed. Pitman, 1990: 151.

72 Bergasa NV, Sabol SL, Yound WS, *et al.* Cholestasis is associated with preproenkephalin mRNA expression in the adult rat liver. *Am J Physiol* 1995; **268**: G346–G354.

73 Mela M, Mancuso A, Burroughs K. Review article: pruritus in cholestatic and other liver diseases. *Aliment Pharmacol Ther* 2003; **17**: 857–70.

74 Szepietowski JC. Selected elements of the pathogenesis of pruritus in haemodialysis patients: my own study. *Med Sci Monitor* 1996; **2**: 343–7.

75 Young Aw, Sweeney EW, David DS, *et al.* Dermatologic evaluation of pruritus in patients on hemodialysis. *N Y State J Med* 1973; **73**: 2670–4.

76 Matsumoto M, Ichimaru K, Horie A. Pruritus and mast cell proliferation of the skin in end stage renal failure. *Clin Nephrol* 1985; **23**: 285–8.

77 Szepietowski JC, Schwartz RA. Uremic pruritus. In: Demis J, ed. *Clinical Dermatology*, 26th ed. New York: Lippincott, Williams & Wilkins, 1999: Unit 29–2B.

78 Hagermark O, Wahlgren CF. Some methods for evaluating clinical itch and their application for studying pathophysiological mechanisms. *J Dermatol Sci* 1992; **4**: 55–62.

79 Peer G, Kivity S, Agami O, *et al.* Randomised crossover trial of naltrexone in uraemic pruritus. *Lancet* 1996; **348**: 1552–4.

80 Balaskas EV, Bamihas HI, Karamouzis M, *et al.* Histamine and serotonin in uremic pruritus: effect of ondansetron in CAPD-pruritic patients. *Nephron* 1998; **78**: 395–402.

81 Silva SR, Viana PC, Lugon NV, *et al.* Thalidomide for the treatment of uraemic pruritus: a crossover randomised double-blind trial. *Nephron* 1994; **67**: 270–3.

82 Daly BM, Shuster S. Antipruritic action of thalidomide. *Acta Dermatol Venereol* 2000; **80**: 24–5.

83 Cavalcanti AM, Rocha LM, Carillo R, *et al.* Effects of homeopathic treatment on pruritus of haemodialysis patients: a randomised placebo-controlled double-blind trial. *Homeopathy* 2003; **92**: 177–81.

84 Cockerall CJ. The itches of HIV infection and AIDS. In: Bernhard J, ed. *Itch: Mechanisms and Management of Pruritus.* New York: McGraw-Hill, 1994: 347–65.

85 Smith CJ, Skelton HG, Yeager J, *et al.* Pruritus in HIV-1 disease: therapy with drugs which may modulate the pattern of immune dysregulation. *Dermatology* 1997; **195**: 353–8.

86 Breur-McHam JN, Marshall GD, Lewis DE, Duvic M. Distinct Serum Cytokines in AIDS related skin diseases. *Viral Immunol* 1998; **11**: 215–20.

87 Lim HW, Vallurupalli S, Meola T, Soter NA. UVB phototherapy is an effective treatment for pruitus in patients infected with HIV. *J Am Acad Dermatol* 1997; **37**: 414–17.

88 Zylicz Z. Neuropathic pruritus. In: Zylicz Z, Twycross R, Jones EA, ed. *Pruritus in Advanced Disease.* Oxford: Oxford University Press, 2004: 117–31.

89 Khan OA. Treatment of paroxysmal symptoms in multiple sclerosis with ibuprofen. *Neurology* 1994; **44**: 571–2.

79

Infections

PAULA S PROVINCE, RUDOLPH M NAVARI

INTRODUCTION

Patients receiving palliative care are at high risk for infections as a result of their underlying disease, poor nutritional state, and/or a direct suppression of the hematological system due to chemotherapy or radiation treatments, viral infection, or corticosteroids.[1*] An infectious complication may occur due to an alteration in the phagocytic, cellular, or humoral immunity, an alteration or breach of skin or mucosal defense barriers, indwelling catheters, or a splenectomy. A high index of suspicion, an awareness of the possibility of unusual infectious agents, consideration of the empirical institution of antimicrobials, and constant surveillance of the hematological status of the patients are necessary to provide optimal management of infections in this patient population.

In addition to the high risk of infections, patients in palliative care also experience a high incidence and a wide variety of infections.[1*,2***] Several retrospective studies have shown that a large number of patients receiving hospice or palliative care are treated with antibiotics for suspected or documented infections.[3*,4*,5*,6*] The benefits and burdens of the use of antimicrobials in this patient population are topics of much discussion.[3*,4*,6*,7***] Two prospective studies have suggested that symptom control may be the main objective in the decision to use antimicrobials to treat clinically suspected or documented infections in patients receiving palliative or hospice care.[9*,10*] The use of symptom control as the main determinant of whether to use antimicrobials in any given clinical situation is markedly affected, however, by the uncertainty of predicting which patients will achieve symptom relief and which patients will experience only the additional burdens of treatment. Determining whether fever is due to infection, tumor, or other causes, and deciding which symptoms from suspected infections

might respond to various antimicrobial interventions can be difficult clinical judgments, particularly in a patient population which has multiple active medical problems and where the goal of treatment is symptom control. These are crucial issues in patients receiving palliative care in that studies have shown that incurably ill patients often receive nonpalliative interventions at the end of life.[8*]

This chapter will discuss the incidence and the type of infections seen in various palliative care clinical settings (Table 79.1) and the judicious use of antimicrobials, and will also suggest the use of symptom control as a major criterion for treatment. The chapter concludes by suggesting guidelines for the approach to infections in palliative care.

INCIDENCE AND TYPE OF INFECTIONS

Patients who are receiving palliative care or hospice care have a high frequency of infections due to the underlying disease, the use of indwelling urinary catheters and vascular access devices, as well as the generally poor functional status of the patients, characterized by impaired cognition and immobility. There have been a number of reports on the use of antimicrobials in patients receiving hospice and palliative care.[1*,3*,4*,6*,9*,10*]

Vitetta et al.[3*] performed a retrospective chart review on the prevalence of infections in 102 patients (92 percent with terminal malignant illness) who died after admission to a tertiary care inpatient palliative care unit. Thirty-seven patients were diagnosed with 42 infections. The urinary tract, respiratory tract, blood, skin and subcutaneous tissues, and eyes were the most common sites of infection. Escherichia coli was the most common organism. Of the 37 patients, 35 were treated with antibiotics and symptom improvement was noted in half

Table 79.1 *Summary of studies of infections in patients receiving palliative care*

Study (type)	Location of care (No. of patients)	Percentage of patients with infection (n/N)	Measurement of symptom control	Conclusions
Ahronheim et al.[8] (retrospective)	Teaching hospital (84)	83 (70/84) received antibiotics	Not done	Nonpalliative interventions are frequently used at the end of life. Cancer patients receive more diagnostic tests and dementia patients receive more enteral tube feeding. Many patients received systemic antibiotics (88%)
Chen et al.[5] (retrospective)	Hospice and palliative care unit (535)	68.8 (93/135) febrile 84.9 (79/93) treated with antibiotics	Significantly greater proportion of clinical improvement when patients were treated with antibiotics 3 days post-initial fever (54.4%)	Based on mean survival rate, appropriate antibiotic use may diminish fever, ultimately decreasing fever related discomfort. Reasons to withhold antibiotics include poor Karnofsky Performance Status, or poor prognosis at time of fever. From study, it is known that antibiotics may reduce fever but it is not known if antibiotics increase the quality of life
Clayton et al.[10] (prospective)	Palliative care unit (913)	4.49 (41/913) received antibiotics	43 courses of parenteral antibiotics given. In 62% (27/43), parenteral antibiotics were considered helpful. Of 'helpful' outcomes, 22 patients had documented symptomatic benefit and 5 had no documented response, but clinical signs showed improvement	In specific circumstances, particularly in urinary tract infections, there appeared to be a beneficial role for the use of parenteral antibiotics, even in the terminal phase
Fabiszewski et al.[11] (prospective)	Hospital intermediate care unit (104)	72.1 (75/104) developed fever; 172 fever episodes in 75 patients	In the antibiotic group, 64 episodes of fever were treated with antibiotics and 28 without use of antibiotics. The palliative group had 1 instance of antibiotics use	Use of antibiotics to treat fevers in Alzheimer patients is complicated by several factors (increased susceptibility to infection, poor communication, and normal fever accompaniment to disease). The use of antibiotics did not influence the outcome of patients with advanced dementia, but treatment of patients in less advanced stages may be beneficial
Homsi et al.[1] (retrospective)	Acute care palliative medicine unit (393)	29.3 (115/393)	Not done	Infections are an underrecognized but common complication in non-neutropenic palliative care patients with advanced solid tumors. Infections are associated with significant mortality, increased morbidity, and are frequently responsible for hospital admission.

Study	Setting (n)	Overall rate of infection		Conclusion
Nagy-Agren and Haley[7] (evaluation of mainly retrospective studies)	Palliative care units, hospice, teaching hospitals, hem/onc units, home; 8 reports and 957 patients	Overall, rate of infection among studies was 41.6%	Considered by one study	Decision on whether or not to use antibiotics in the palliative care setting is very individualized and can be influenced by factors such as potential adverse side-effects, the need for laboratory monitoring, and the comfort and convenience of the patient. Studies show that increased education of the public and health professionals is necessary to develop more universal guidelines concerning this issue
Oneschuk et al.[6] (retrospective)	Acute care hospital, Tertiary palliative care unit, and hospice settings (150)	44 (66/150) of patients given antibiotics	Not done	There was a great deal of variability in the numbers and types of antibiotics prescribed in the different locations of care. Results also indicate the need for further investigation into this area because of the high number of patients receiving antibiotics at the time of death
Pereira et al.[4] (retrospective)	Acute palliative care unit (100)	55 (55/100); 74 total infections	Not done	The study found a high frequency of symptomatic infections in patients with advanced cancer, most often caused by respiratory and urinary tract infections. The goal of antibiotic therapy in a palliative setting should be one of symptom control rather than decreasing mortality/morbidity. Patient discomfort level should be avoided or at least minimized
Vitetta et al.[3] (retrospective)	Hospice (102)	36.3 (37/102); overall rate of infection was 41.6%	36 patients were evaluated for symptom control. Appropriate infection man-agement resulted in enhanced palliative symptom control in 8/17 patients with urinary tract infections, 3/9 patients with respiratory tract infections, 1/5 patients with skin infections, and 1/5 patients with bacteremia	Multiple factors contribute to terminally ill patients' heightened risk of infections, especially urinary tract and respiratory infections. Results are suggestive, however, that appropriate management of such infections via antibiotic treatment will enhance palliative symptom control
White et al.[9] (prospective)	Outpatient hospice and palliative care program (255)	45.9 (117/255)	A positive symptom response was seen in 25/30 patients with urinary tract infections, 10/26 of patients with lower respiratory infections, 4/9 patients with skin infections, 4/9 patients with oral infections, and 0/3 patients with bacteremia	This study showed that symptom control may be the main indication for the use of antimicrobials in patients receiving hospice or palliative care. Antimicrobials were most effective in treating urinary tract infections. Patient survival was not affected by the use of antimicrobials

of the patients treated; 2 of 37 patients were not treated with antibiotics due to survival limited to the day of admission. Pereira et al.[4*] reported a retrospective chart review of the prevalence of infections in 100 consecutive admissions to a tertiary care palliative care unit. There were 74 infections in 55 patients. The urinary tract, respiratory tract, skin and subcutaneous tissue, blood, and mouth were the most common infection sites. E. coli, Staphylococcus aureus, and Enterococcus were the most common organisms. Twenty-one of the 74 infections were not treated, and the reasons for not using antimicrobials were documented in 10 patients: very poor general condition (n = 5), not able to take oral antimicrobials and refusal of parenteral antimicrobials (n = 3), and family refusal in (n = 2). The retrospective nature of the study did not allow for an adequate analysis of the symptom response to antibiotic therapy. Homsi et al.[1*] reported a retrospective analysis of 393 patients with advanced cancer who were admitted to an acute care palliative medicine unit over an 8-month period. A total of 115 patients had at least one positive bacteriological culture and 100 patients were evaluable. Of these, 66 patients had a urinary tract infection, 31 patients had bacteremia, and 21 patients had pneumonia. E. coli, Staphylococcus spp., Enterococcus, and Klebsiella pneumoniae were cited as the most common organisms. Symptom response was not reported in this study.

Oneschuk et al.[6*] retrospectively examined the frequency and types of antibiotics prescribed in the last week of life in three palliative care settings: acute care hospital, tertiary palliative care unit, and hospice inpatient unit. Of 50 patients in each setting, 29 (58 percent) in the acute care hospital, 26 (52 percent) in the palliative care unit, and 11 (22 percent) in the inpatient hospice unit received antibiotics in the last week of life. The types of infection, the specific organisms, and symptom response were not reported. Clayton et al.[10*] prospectively studied all patients receiving parenteral antibiotics in a palliative care unit. Of 913 consecutive admissions over a 13-month period, 41 patients received 43 courses of parenteral antibiotics. The most common sites of infection were urinary tract infections (37 percent), lower respiratory tract infection (26 percent), soft tissue/skin infections (16 percent). The predominant organisms were not reported, and the use of antibiotics was considered 'helpful' in 27 of the 43 antibiotics courses (62 percent).

White et al.[9*] studied 255 patients with advanced cancer at the time they entered a community-based outpatient hospice and palliative care program and prospectively documented the use and effectiveness of the antimicrobials employed during the palliative care period. The 117 patients had a total of 129 infections with the most common sites being urinary tract, respiratory tract, mouth/pharynx, and skin/subcutaneous tissues. The most common organisms in this patient population were E. coli, S. aureus, Enterococcus spp., and K. pneumoniae. The use of antimicrobials controlled symptoms in the majority of the urinary tract infections, but were less effective in controlling symptoms of the other sites of infection. Survival was not affected by the patients' choice of whether to use antimicrobials, the prevalence of infections, or the actual use of antimicrobials.

These studies, carried out in a wide variety of palliative care settings, have suggested that 30–55 percent of patients receiving palliative care have at least one or more infections which are considered for antimicrobial treatment. The most common clinical conditions are urinary tract infections, upper and lower respiratory tract infections, skin and subcutaneous tissues infections, and a fewer number of patients with bacteremia. The most common organisms are E. coli, Staphylococcus spp., Enterococcus, and K. pneumoniae. Most patients are treated with antimicrobials when an infection is suspected, with varying responses.

EVALUATION OF FEVER

In patients with advanced cancer, fever is common and it may or may not have an infectious etiology. It must be noted that fever may be the only manifestation of an infection in an immunocompromised patient, and there is no pattern of fever that can be used to definitively rule out an infectious etiology. Fever may also be modified by the use of specific medications such as corticosteroids or nonsteroidal anti-inflammatory agents.

Fever in patients with advanced or terminal cancer must be evaluated in terms of the underlying disease, the specific risk for a local or systemic infection, the urgency for empirical antimicrobial therapy, the presence or absence of neutropenia, and any signs or symptoms which may suggest a site of infection. Attention should be directed to the most common sites of infection such as the oral cavity, lungs, perirectal area, urinary tract, skin, and soft tissues. In most patients with fever and neutropenia the initial evaluation does not identify a site of infection.

Depending on the status of the patient at the time of the fever, an initial evaluation may include, in addition to the history and physical examination, a hematological profile, cultures of nose and throat, urine, blood, stool, and cerebrospinal fluid, and radiological evaluation of the chest and sinuses. Whether or not antimicrobials are begun at the time of the initial fever, patients should be carefully reevaluated at least every 24 hours. It must be remembered that in patients with profound and prolonged neutropenia, multiple sites of infection and multiple organisms may be present.

The approach to fever in patients receiving palliative care should be similar to that outlined above, with symptom control, accomplished through a minimum of interventions, as the primary goal. Chen et al.[5*] retrospectively studied 535 admissions to a hospice and palliative care unit and identified 93 fever episodes, of which 79 episodes were treated with antibiotics. Although the use of antibiotics appeared to decrease fever-related discomfort, it was not clear that quality of life was improved.

TREATMENT WITH ANTIMICROBIALS

Studies suggest that antimicrobials are initiated in the overwhelming majority (70–90 percent) of patients receiving palliative care when they have fever or a suspected or documented infection.[1*,5*] The response rate to antibiotics appears to be varied with symptom improvement in the majority of urinary tract infections, but symptom improvement in less than half of the patients with infections of other organ systems.[9*]

The decision making process in the use of antimicrobials in patients receiving palliative care is highly complex. In most situations, the approach should be individualized for each patient based on the desires of the patient, the control of symptoms, and quality of life issues. Issues to be considered include the potential benefit of the use of antimicrobials compared to the potential toxicities that may result from the extent of the investigation of a suspected infection, the number of diagnostic tests to be employed, and the means to be employed to treat a suspected or documented infection. It may be appropriate to treat a fever with an antipyretic alone in a patient whose death is imminent rather than proceed with an extensive laboratory workup and the initiation of antimicrobials. Alternatively, the pain resulting from a symptomatic, localized skin or soft tissue infection may be treated more successfully with both antibiotics and pain medications. For patients receiving hospice care at home or in an institution such as a hospital palliative care unit or a chronic care facility, consideration should be given to initiating oral or parenteral antibiotics based on only clinical indications without the use of laboratory or imaging criteria. Mobilization of the patients for diagnostic interventions may be associated with significant discomfort.

Table 79.2 suggests an approach to the management of common infections in patients receiving palliative care.

Patients with uncomplicated cystitis can be effectively and inexpensively treated with a 3-day course of oral trimethoprim-sulfamethoxazole or a fluoroquinolone. Acute uncomplicated pyelonephritis can often be managed with a 7-day course of an oral fluoroquinolone.[12] For community-acquired bacterial pneumonia, an oral macrolide (erythromycin, azithromycin, or clarithromycin), doxycycline, or a fluoroquinolone with good anti-pneumococcal activity (levofloxacin, gatifloxacin, or moxifloxacin) is recommended.[12,13] For patients who require parenteral antibiotics, cefotaxime or ceftriaxone may be reasonable first choices. An antipneumococcal fluoroquinolone may be added to cover *Legionella*, *Mycoplasma*, and *Chlamydia*. These agents would not require monitoring of blood levels.[12,13]

Issues that patients, families, and physicians consider when making decisions concerning the use of a respirator, cardiac resuscitation, dialysis, etc. should, in general, also apply to the use of antimicrobials. Antimicrobial use in patients receiving palliative care may be a part of symptomatic care, may or may not result in prolongation of life, and/or may be associated with symptom producing interventions such as laboratory testing, venous access, and direct antimicrobial toxicities. The goal of antimicrobial therapy in palliative care is symptom control, in contrast to the goal of decreased morbidity and mortality in acute medical or surgical situations.

SYMPTOM CONTROL

There has been much discussion in the literature about the use of symptom control as criterion for use of antimicrobials in patients receiving palliative care. However, there have been only a few studies which have evaluated the effects of antimicrobials on the symptoms associated with infections

Table 79.2 *Management of common infections in patients receiving palliative care*

Infection	Signs/symptoms	Antimicrobial(s)	Diagnostic[a]
Urinary tract	Dysuria, fever, frequency, pain	Oral trimethoprim-sulfamethoxazole or fluoroquinolone	Urine analysis, culture and sensitivity
Oral/upper respiratory	Fever, mucositis, odynophagia, pain	Fluconazole, nystatin	Mouth swab for culture and sensitivity, endoscopy
Lower respiratory	Cough, dyspnea, fever, sputum production	Oral macrolides (erythromycin, azithromycin, clarithromycin), doxycycline, fluorquinolone (levofloxacin, gatifloxacin, moxifloxacin), or parenterals (cefotaxime, ceftriaxone)	Sputum culture and sensitivity, chest X-ray, bronchoscopy
Skin/subcutaneous	Fever, pain, skin rash/discoloration	Cephalexin	Skin culture and sensitivity, blood cultures
Bacteremia	Fever, disorientation, dyspnea, hypotension, tachycardia	Cefotaxime or ceftriaxone	Blood cultures

[a] The decision to use any diagnostic intervention should be evaluated in terms of potential benefit to the patient in symptom control versus the potential toxicities of the diagnostic interventions.

in patients with advanced cancer. Bruera[14] reported a marked improvement in pain with the use of antimicrobials for seven patients with infected, ulcerated head and neck neoplasms. Green et al.[15] described improved symptom control with the use of antibiotics in two patients with advanced cancer. One patient had severe respiratory distress from pneumonia and one patient had sepsis-induced delirium.

In a retrospective study of 102 patients admitted to a tertiary care palliative care unit, Vitetta et al.[3*] reported on antibiotic-induced symptom control in 36 patients. Antibiotic-associated positive symptom response was seen in 8 of 17 patients with urinary tract infections, 3 of 9 patients with respiratory tract infections, 1 of 5 patients with subcutaneous skin infections, and 1 of 5 patients with bacteremia. Clayton et al.[10*] reported that the use of parenteral antibiotics was 'helpful' (overall condition improved or symptoms and/or signs of infection improved) in 27 of 43 infections in 41 patients in an inpatient palliative care unit. Antibiotic response was seen in 14 of 16 patients with urinary tract infections, 6 of 11 patients with lower respiratory tract infections, 2 of 2 patients with purulent terminal respiratory secretions, 5 of 7 patients with soft tissue/wound infections, and none of 7 patients with other suspected infections. The types of infections and the response rates followed a similar pattern to that found in Vitetta et al.'s[3*] study, with a somewhat higher response rate possibly due to the use of parenteral rather than oral antibiotics. In a prospective study by White et al.[9*] of antibiotic choices by patients with advanced cancer receiving outpatient hospice care, antibiotic associated positive symptom response was seen in 25 of 30 patients with urinary tract infections, 10 of 26 patients with respiratory tract infections, 4 of 9 patients with mouth/pharyngeal infections, 4 of 9 patients with subcutaneous skin infections, and none of 3 patients with bacteremia.

The types of infections and the responses recorded appear similar in the above studies, despite major differences in the types of palliative care settings. In these studies, it appeared that the majority of the organisms cultured were sensitive to the antimicrobials used, suggesting that the lack of symptom response in some patients may have been due to comorbid condition such as an immunocompromised state, malnutrition, the failure of host barriers, decreased level of consciousness or immobility, or the presence of a neoplasm in the symptomatic organ. Regardless of the reason for the lack of symptom response, it is essential that treating clinicians be aware of the limitations of the use of antimicrobials in palliative care.

PATIENT SURVIVAL

Although symptomatic care, and not survival, is the main issue in palliative and hospice care, survival may be an issue for some patients, families, and healthcare professionals. Survival was not affected by the patients' choice of whether to use antimicrobials, the prevalence of infections, or the actual use of antimicrobials in the recent study by White et al.[9*] Also, antimicrobial use did not affect survival in patients severely affected with Alzheimer disease who were treated for fever.[11*] Vitetta et al.[3*] and Chen et al.,[5*] however, showed that terminally ill hospice patients with documented infections treated with antibiotics had a longer median survival. The proposed explanation for the increased survival was that the probability of infection increases with the duration of survival rather than an increased survival due to the use of antimicrobials.

The effect of the use of antimicrobials on survival is important information for patients entering hospice care. This information might strongly influence their choice of whether to receive antimicrobials.

GUIDELINES FOR ANTIBIOTIC USE

Based on the data generated in the current and previous studies, we suggest the following guidelines in patients with advanced cancer receiving hospice care:

- On entry into hospice care, discussions should be held with the patient and family on their wishes in the treatment of infections, just as is done with cardiopulmonary resuscitation, use of a respirator, blood transfusions, etc.
- Strong consideration should be given to symptom control as the major indication for the use of antimicrobials for the treatment of infections. In a previous study,[9*] the majority of patients chose either no antimicrobials or symptomatic use only.
- One recent prospective study[9*] and two other studies in the literature[10*,3*] suggest that antimicrobial treatment of urinary tract infections improve symptoms in a large majority of patients, but antimicrobial treatment of respiratory tract infections, mucositis, and skin infections is much less successful in symptom control. Sepsis/bacteremia is very poorly controlled by antimicrobials in this patient population
- Overall survival appears to be unaffected by antimicrobial use.
- Patients and families should be informed of the effects of antimicrobials on symptom control of various infections and on survival.
- Each patient's specific situation and condition must be evaluated in the decision to employ antimicrobials for a suspected or documented infection.

Key learning points

- Patients in palliative care settings experience a high incidence of infections.
- The most common sites of infection in patients receiving palliative care are the urinary tract, respiratory tract, skin

and subcutaneous tissues, mouth and blood. The most common pathogens are *E. coli*, *Staphylococcus* spp., *Enterococcus*, and *K. pneumoniae*.

- Although the use of antimicrobials improves symptoms in the majority of patients with urinary tract infections, symptom control is less successful with antimicrobial use in infections of the respiratory tract, mouth/pharynx, skin/subcutaneous tissue, or blood.

- Physicians should be aware of the limitations of the use of antimicrobials in patients receiving palliative care

- Strong consideration should be given to the use of symptom control as the major indication for the use of antimicrobials for the treatment of infections.

- Antimicrobial use has not been shown to affect patients' survival and this information is very valuable to physicians, patients, and caregivers when making decisions about the use of antimicrobials.

- Each patient's specific situation and condition in the palliative care setting must be evaluated in the decision to employ antimicrobials for a suspected or documented infection.

REFERENCES

- 1   Homsi J, Walsh D, Panta R, *et al.* Infectious complications of advanced cancer. *Support Care Cancer* 2000; **8**: 487–92.
- 2   Viscoli C. Management of infection in cancer patients: studies of the EORTC International Antimicrobial Therapy Group (IATG). *Eur J Cancer* 2002; **38**: S82–S87.
- 3   Vitetta L, Kenner D, Sali A. Bacterial infections in terminally ill hospice patients. *J Pain Symptom Manage* 2000; **20**: 326–34.
- 4   Pereira J, Watanabe S, Wolch G. A retrospective study of the frequency of infections and patterns of antibiotic utilization on a palliative care unit. *J Pain Symptom Manage* 1998; **16**: 374–81.
- 5   Chen L, Chou Y, Hsu P, *et al.* Antibiotic prescription for fever episodes in hospice patients. *Support Care Cancer* 2002; **10**: 538–41.
- 6   Oneschuk D, Fainsinger R, Demoissac D. Antibiotic use in the last week of life in three different palliative care settings. *J Palliat Care* 2002; **18**: 25–8.
- 7   Nagy-Agren S, Haley HB. Management of infections in palliative care patients with advanced cancer. *J Pain Symptom Manage* 2002; **24**: 64–70.
- 8   Ahronheim JC, Morrison S, Baskin SA, *et al.* Treatment of the dying in the acute care hospital. *Arch Intern Med* 1996; **156**: 2094–100.
- 9   White PH, Kuhlenschmidt HL, Vancura BG, Navari RM. Antimicrobial use in patients with advanced cancer receiving hospice care. *J Pain Symptom Manage* 2003; **25**: 438–43.
- 10 Clayton J, Fardell B, Hutton-Potts J, *et al.* Parenteral antibiotics in a palliative care unit: prospective analysis of current practice. *Palliat Med* 2003; **17**: 44–8.
- 11 Fabiszewski KJ, Volicer B, Volicer L. Effect of antibiotic treatment on outcome of fevers in institutionalized Alzheimer patients. *JAMA* 1990; **263**: 3168–172.
- 12 The choice of antibacterial drugs. *Med Letts Drugs Ther* 2001; **43**: 69–78.
- 13 Gemifloxacin clinical studies. *Med Letts* 2004; **46**: 78–9.
- 14 Bruera E. Intractable pain in patients with advanced head and neck tumors: a possible role of local infection. *Cancer Treat Rep* 1986; **70**: 691–2.
- 15 Green K, Webster H, Watanabe S, Fainsinger R. Case Report: management of nosocomial respiratory tract infections in terminally ill cancer patients. *J Palliat Care* 1994; **10**: 31–4.

80

Pressure ulcers/wounds

KATHRYN G FROILAND

INTRODUCTION

Skin is an essential organ for physical protection from environmental trauma and for emotional wellbeing. It functions as a protective barrier providing immunity, thermoregulation, sensation, and synthesis of vitamin D. It performs individual identification and communication roles. Impairment of any of these functions can result in loss of integrity of the skin, which can lead to life-threatening consequences. Age, nutritional status, hydration status, prior sun exposure, current medications, and even the soap used for bathing, can affect normal skin function and its ability to heal as breakdown occurs.

Skin breakdown in a patient with cancer can be especially difficult to prevent and treat effectively. Prevention of skin breakdown is essential at all phases of cancer management. The challenges include: immunosuppression, infection, edema, prior irradiation of tissue, malnutrition, dehydration, neuropathy, incontinence, and several comorbid conditions (e.g. diabetes mellitus, peripheral vascular disease, autoimmune disorders). These challenges can compromise the ability to heal and may actually prevent healing from occurring. Management of all of these factors must be optimized to progressively heal areas of skin breakdown. Healing often reflects progress in gaining control of the primary cancer disease process. As the cancer becomes resistant to treatment, the potential for skin breakdown increases, and wounds become more difficult to heal.

PATHOPHYSIOLOGY

Pressure ulcers are localized areas of tissue necrosis that develop when soft tissue is compressed between a bony prominence and an external surface for a prolonged period of time.[1***] The coccyx, sacrum, and heel are most vulnerable, as less soft tissue is present between the bone and skin in these areas than in other areas of the body. Sixty percent of these ulcers develop in the area of the pelvis.[2*] However, they may develop in conjunction with any improperly filling assistive device. The risk of pressure ulcer formation increases for those who experience atrophy of subcutaneous and muscle tissue layers. Pressure ulcers can be classified in stages that identify tissue layers.

Stage 1: An observable, pressure-related alteration of intact skin whose indicators, compared with the adjacent or opposite area on the body, may include changes in one or more of the following: skin temperature (warmth or coolness), tissue consistency (firm or boggy feeling), and sensation (pain, itching). The ulcer appears as a defined area of persistent redness in lightly pigmented skin, whereas in darker skin tones the ulcer may appear with persistent red, blue, or purple hues. It appears as nonblanchable erythema of intact skin.

Stage 2: Partial-thickness skin loss involving epidermis, dermis, or both. The ulcer is superficial and presents clinically as an abrasion, blister, or shallow crater.

Stage 3: Full-thickness skin loss involving damage or necrosis of subcutaneous tissue, which may extend down to, but not through, underlying fascia. The ulcer presents clinically as a deep crater with or without undermining of adjacent tissue.

Stage 4: Full-thickness skin loss with extensive destruction, tissue necrosis, or damage to muscle, bone, or supporting structures (e.g. tendon, joint capsule). These lesions appear as deep craters; undermining and sinus tracts are common. NB: If the wound involves necrotic tissue, staging cannot be confirmed until the wound base is visible.[1***]

Patients with cancer are at greater risk of pressure ulcer development because they often are older than the population average and have concurrent chronic illnesses. Poorly controlled pain and fatigue may contribute to self-limited mobility during the course of the disease and its treatment. Poor nutritional status is a common finding for patients with cancer, which further impairs their ability to maintain skin integrity and their wounds to heal. The situation may be further complicated if the wound is infected or the patient is incontinent.

Friction and shear are extrinsic forces that may exacerbate the effects of pressure on the skin. Friction causes damage to the epidermal and upper dermal layers of the skin caused when two surfaces rub against each other. This may occur when a patient is dragged rather than lifted. Moisture from perspiration or incontinence adds to the force of friction. Shearing force results when friction acts synergistically with gravity. Separation of the skin from underlying structures results when gravity pulls the body downward while resistance from the surface holds the skin in place. Deeper fascia level tissue and blood vessels are primarily affected by shear.[3**]

Although a pressure ulcer can occur at any time during the cancer care continuum, a Kennedy terminal ulcer may develop as a person is dying. These ulcers begin as stage 2 blisters, and progress rapidly to stages 3–4 pressure ulcers. They usually occur on the sacral area, are large, superficial, and then change in color from red, to yellow, and finally become black. They have been observed most often in older patients rather than in children. The ulcer tends to progress quickly and appears to be a hallmark sign of impending death within 8–24 hours, although some patients have lived up to 2 weeks following the development of the ulceration. Causation may be due to a decline in peripheral perfusion during the dying process. The skin is the largest organ of the body. As the only organ visible to the outside observer, it may reflect the gradual shutdown of function of the internal organs. The ultimate result is multisystem organ failure. Skin organ failure in the form of pressure ulceration over bony prominences occurs over a relatively short period of time and coincides with the patient's death.[4*]

ASSESSMENT AND DIAGNOSIS

Wounds do not exist in isolation. The healthcare professional must assess the patient as a whole being to determine the events leading up to the development of a pressure ulcer. This holds true in assessing patients with any type of wound including vascular wounds, diabetic foot ulcers, malignant cutaneous wounds, surgical wounds, burns, or wounds due to trauma. Information on the current status of the underlying cancer disease and its treatment to this point in time is essential. The history of the wound and its management is also necessary for classification and identification of previous unsuccessful treatment strategies. Reasons for delayed healing or progressive deterioration of

the wound may be explained by thorough evaluation of the patient's past history and physical status. Remember to position the patient comfortably and medicate if necessary prior to wound assessment and care. Wound assessment and documentation should include the following aspects:

- degree of tissue layer destruction and color
- anatomical location
- length, width, depth, and tunneling using consistent units of measure
- appearance of the wound bed and surrounding skin
- drainage and bleeding – specifying amount, color, odor
- pain or tenderness of wound and surrounding skin
- temperature of tissue.[5***]

Wound dimensions can be measured by using a sterile cotton-tipped applicator and a wound measuring guide or ruler. The thumb and forefinger are placed at the point on the applicator that corresponds to the wound's length, width, or depth. Measurements are commonly recorded in centimeters. The depth of tunneling can be measured in the same fashion. The direction of tunneling also can be described. The cotton-tipped applicator is again used to assess the wound for tunneling. The wound is compared to the face of a clock, with 12 o'clock pointing toward the head. Beginning at the 12 o'clock position progress in a clockwise direction assessing the wound. Document the direction of the existing tunnel(s) according to their corresponding positions on a clock face.[5***] Accurate measurement of the wound serves to describe and then classify the wound.

Potential for further breakdown of the surrounding skin should be assessed so as to plan preventive measures. Excessive dryness, moisture, or nonviable tissue may result in pruritus, pain, and loss of skin integrity. Assessment of the wound for the presence of foreign objects is advised, as these objects may cause infection or delayed healing.

MANAGEMENT

Prevention

A comprehensive program for prevention of the development of pressure ulcers is advised. Monetary savings in the limited use of wound dressings and treatments, specialized beds, as well as the cost of excess caregiver time, enforces the need for prevention. Any value placed on patient suffering argues for the need for a plan that is comprehensive, but easily implemented.

Risk assessment tools such as the Braden scale or Norton scale for adults, and the Braden Q scale for children, are easy to use and provide basic information useful in developing an individualized plan of care. These scales assess general physical condition, mental status, activity, mobility, incontinence, and nutritional status.[5***]

Following assessment of risk, preventative measure can be implemented. Basic, but essential measures include:

- Inspecting skin at least daily.
- Keeping skin clean and dry:
  - cleanse skin with cleansers or soaps with neutral pH to maintain skin's acid mantle
  - apply barrier ointment to protect skin from stool or urine
  - consider use of absorbent pads or containment devices for the incontinent patient.
- Preventing friction and shear injuries:
  - use lifting pads and turning sheets when transferring patients
  - apply lubricants, thin film dressings, or protectors to heels and elbows.
- Mobilizing patients if tolerable, or performing range-of-motion exercises for bed-bound patients.
- Reducing pressure on tissues:
  - turn and reposition at least every 2 hours
  - shift weight if chair-bound every 15 minutes
  - avoid positioning on trochanters
  - use supports (foam wedges, pillows, heel supports)
  - consider use of special mattresses
  - avoid massaging skin over bony prominences[6***]
  - avoid using foam or rubber rings (i.e. donuts), as they concentrate the intensity of pressure to surrounding tissues
  - avoid using sheepskin as it does not relieve pressure.[3**]
- Monitoring nutritional status:
  - assess current and usual weight
  - assess history of involuntary weight loss or gain
  - assess nutritional intake versus protein, calorie, and fluid needs
  - assess appetite
  - assess dental health
  - assess oral and gastrointestinal history; chewing or swallowing difficulty, and ability to feed him/herself
  - assess drug/nutrient interactions
  - assess for prior medical/surgical interventions affecting intake or absorption of nutrients
  - assess psychosocial factors affecting food intake.[7**]
- Assessing laboratory parameters for nutritional status. Standard measurements of protein status: albumin, transferrin, prealbumin, total lymphocyte count.

By using an assessment tool for screening, at-risk individuals can be identified early. Incorporating these measures will improve outcomes by reducing the incidence of pressure ulcers and the stress that they incur on the individual and their caregivers.

Treatment

Healing wounds caused by pressure or any other source is the ultimate goal of any treatment plan. However, healing may be unattainable if the patient's cancer disease, effects of treatment, or other medical condition cannot be controlled. Healing may be delayed while the patient is immunosuppressed, malnourished, or infected. Maintaining the wound as is and preventing further deterioration are realistic goals for a patient with aggressive end-stage disease. Palliation of the symptoms of pain, odor, itching, and managing exudate and bleeding are appropriate goals in this situation.

Prevention strategies of reducing the effects of friction, shear, and pressure must be evaluated and used to prevent further skin breakdown. The patient may become incontinent of urine and/or stool. Establishing a bowel and bladder program may be feasible if the cause can be manipulated. Gentle pH balanced skin cleansers should be used at each soiling episode. Skin barriers (e.g. creams, ointments, films), may protect and maintain intact skin. Absorbent underpads and diapers should wick moisture away from the skin rather than trapping it against the skin causing maceration. Urinary collection pouches are available for the bed-bound female. Condom catheters can be safely used for males. If urinary or fecal incontinence causes contamination or infection of the pressure ulcer, use of an indwelling device is indicated. Indwelling urinary catheters are accessible and easy to care for. Although various types of rectal catheters have been used with considerable morbidity and difficulty, a promising device has recently become available. This catheter keeps the wound clean while minimizing pressure to vulnerable bowel mucosa. It is easily inserted and can be maintained in the rectum up to 29 days. It has been tested in several acute care settings in patients with various types of wounds. Nosocomial infections have been reduced in these high-risk patients.[8*]

A critical area of need and intervention in a patient with a pressure ulcer is to correct nutritional deficiencies. Protein and calorie malnutrition results in decreased fibroblast proliferation and angiogenesis which impairs collagen synthesis and inhibits wound repair.[7***] General recommendations for calorie and protein requirements for patients with pressure ulcers are 35–49 kcal/kg of body weight per day, and 1.0–1.5 g protein/kg of body weight perday.[1***] Various dietary supplements (e.g. amino acid supplements) have been used, however, none of the available data support their use.[9*] Facilitation of weight gain with oxandrolone, an anabolic steroid, and glutamine has been studied in a small series of patients with weight loss and pressure ulcers.[10*,11*] Involving a dietician, nutritionist, and/or nutritional pharmacist in treatment planning is advisable.

Wound care management should be simplified to be comfortable for the patient and achievable for the caregiver. Management techniques must address the following aspects of care:

- manipulation of the cellular environment
- prevention or treatment of infection
- debridement of nonviable tissue

- promotion of closure of a clean wound
- protection of wound edges from the effects of excess moisture.

Topical wound care is designed to keep the wound moist, clean, warm, and protected from trauma and infection. The choice of an appropriate product(s) depends on:

- amount and character of exudate
- debridement needs
- odor control needs
- compression needs
- frequency of assessment
- ease of use by caregiver
- cost and accessibility.

Warmed saline is the preferred cleansing solution for chronic wound care. It cleans the wound gently without harming viable tissue. It can be applied via soaked gauze or by irrigating by pouring solution, using a spray bottle or piston syringe. Pressures of 34.5–55.2 kPa (5–8 psi) are adequate for cleansing, although 34.5–103.4 kPa (5–15 psi) may be necessary to remove thick exudate. Devices delivering higher pressures should be avoided as they may cause tissue damage and bleeding. Use of commercial wound cleaning products and antiseptic agents is controversial. They require significant dilution to maintain phagocytic function and white blood cell viability. Guidelines can be found online through the National Guidelines Clearinghouse (www.guidelines.gov). Saline remains acceptable as readily available, comforting, inexpensive, and harmless to the wound bed.

Odor is one of the most distressing symptoms for the patient to cope with. This concern should be addressed even when others cannot detect it. Necrotic tissue, infected tissue, or saturated dressings are sources of odor. There exist several methods of debridement to remove necrotic, devitalized tissue. Surgical or sharp debridement is the fastest method. It is invasive, may require anesthesia, and should not be done if vasculature of the cutaneous tumor places the patient at risk for excessive bleeding. Licensure regulations and institutional policies require that a trained wound care professional perform this type of debridement. Mechanical debridement involves physical force to remove debris and necrotic tissue. It cannot discriminate between viable and nonviable tissue. Although commonly used in the past, wet-to-dry dressings are not recommended as they cause pain, bleeding, and tissue damage upon removal. Enzymatic debridement uses enzymes to dissolve necrotic tissue from the wound. Topical gels and solutions are directly applied to the eschar or applied following scoring of the eschar to allow penetration into the tissue. Enzymes are categorized as collagenases, fibrinolytics, and proteolytics. Autolytic debridement is a process that creates a moist environment allowing the wound bed to rid itself of dead tissue by endogenous proteolytic enzymes and phagocytic cells present in the wound and its drainage. Creation of this environment is achieved by application of an occlusive, semiocclusive, or moisture interactive dressing and/or an autolytic debriding gel directly applied to the wound surface. This process is potentially more time consuming; however, it can be effective and less traumatic than surgical, sharp, or mechanical methods. Biological debridement (larvae therapy) has resurfaced as a method useful in digesting necrotic tissue and pathogens. Consideration of this method may be appropriate when surgical debridement is not an option.[12***] It is recommended that dry, stable, black eschar on heels should not be debrided if the heel is nontender, nonfluctuant, nonerythematous, and nonsuppurative.[1***]

Chronic wounds are contaminated with surface aerobic pathogens. Wounds may become infected (greater than 10^5 colony-forming units of bacteria) by bacteria that may/may not be normal flora. Odor is associated with anaerobic infection. If infection is suspected, a quantitative culture can be obtained by tissue biopsy or swab culture technique. Use of topical antibiotics is controversial and not supported by clinical research.[7**] Systemic antibiotics are warranted if the patient has bacteremia, sepsis, advancing cellulitis, or osteomyelitis.[1***]

Adjunctive therapies in wound management have become available in recent years. Several of these therapies are listed below:

- Growth factors
- Electrical stimulation
- Ultrasound
- Electromagnetic therapy
- Noncontact normothermic wound therapy or radiant heat dressing
- Vacuum-assisted wound closure therapy
- Hyperbaric oxygen therapy[7***]

Surgical closure of stage 3 and stage 4 pressure ulcers may be appropriate if the wound does not respond to conservative therapy.

The shape of the wound and volume of exudate must be matched to the dressing chosen for containment. Changing dressings more than twice a day can be burdensome for the caregiver. Alginate, hydrofiber, or foam dressings absorb higher volumes of drainage than hydrocolloids or gauze. Collection of very heavily exudative wound drainage may be accomplished by using a drainable ostomy or wound collection device. These plastic odor-controlling pouches are available in many sizes, have a protective barrier applied to intact surrounding skin, and require changing as infrequently as once a week. Pouches are drained as needed and are less bulky than dressings. Mobility may be facilitated with the use of these products. Charcoal-containing dressings can be used to filter odorous exudate. Silver ion-containing dressings and powders may also be useful in managing odorous and potentially infected wounds. Thousands of wound care products are commercially available. Consultation with a certified wound care specialist is advised for continuity and cost-effective wound care management.

The feasibility of any wound treatment plan must be evaluated. Consideration of the wound's healing potential, accessibility of therapy, cost, and the patient's wishes must be realistically addressed. Management of pain caused by the wound, the removal and application of dressings, and distress caused by seeing the wound must also be acknowledged and resolved. Educating patients and their caregivers in the cause of the wound, its treatment, and in ways to minimize progression must be included in any wound management plan.

Care of a patient with any wound takes time for thorough assessment and ongoing management. Periodic assessment of the wound is necessary, as its characteristics may evolve or the condition and desires of the patient may change. Management goals and treatment plans require review and alteration over time. Patients may present with more than one wound, or more than one type of wound, adding to the complexity of management. Emotional and social issues, pain control, and management of other symptoms of the disease process are challenges that the interdisciplinary palliative care team must address. Of utmost importance, the patients and their families or caregivers need our encouragement, praise, and guidance throughout the course of caring for the wound.

Key learning points

Managing patients with pressure ulcers in the palliative care setting involves:

- Recognizing the multiple functions of the skin.

- Identifying impediments to healing in the patient with cancer.

- Identifying patients at risk for developing pressure ulcers.

- Implementing preventative measures for patients at risk.

- Assessing the wound is just as important as assessing patients and their cancer disease.

- Setting realistic treatment goals based on wound characteristics and the patient's healing potential.

REFERENCES

✱ 1 Agency for Healthcare Research and Quality, Panel for the prediction and prevention of pressure ulcers in adults. *Pressure Ulcers in Adults: Prediction and Prevention. Clinical Practice Guideline*. Rockville, MD: Agency for Healthcare Research and Quality, 1994. Publication no. 92–0047.

◆ 2 Barczak CA, Barnett RI, Childs EJ, Bosley LM. Fourth national pressure ulcer prevalence survey. *Adv Wound Care* 1997; **10**: 18–26.

● 3 Pieper B. Mechanical forces: pressure, shear, and friction. In: Bryant RA, ed. *Acute and Chronic Wounds: Nursing Management*, 2nd ed. St. Louis: Mosby, Inc, 2000: 221–64.

● 4 Kennedy KL. The Kennedy terminal ulcer. In: Milne CT, Corbett LQ, Dubec DL, eds. *Wound, Ostomy, and Continence Nursing Secrets*. Philadelphia: Hanley & Belfus, Inc., 2003: 198–99.

◆ 5 Hess CT. *Clinical Guide: Wound Care*, 4th ed. Springhouse, PA: Springhouse Corporation, 2002.

◆ 6 Heidrich DE. Skin lesions. In: Kuebler KK, Esper P, eds. *Palliative Practices from A to Z for the Bedside Clinician*. Pittsburgh, PA: Oncology Nursing Society, 2002: 221–6.

✱ 7 Wound, Ostomy, Continence Nurses Society. *Guideline for Prevention and Management of Pressure Ulcers*. Glenview, IL: WOCN, 2003, www.wocn.org (accessed September 21, 2004).

✱ 8 Zassi Medical Evolutions. *Bowel Management System*. Fernandina Beach, FL: Zassi, 2004, www.zassimedical.com (accessed September 24, 2005).

◆ 9 Langkamp-Henken B, Herrlinger-Garcia K, Stechmiller J, *et al.* Arginine supplementation is well tolerated but does not enhance nitrogen-induced lymphocyte proliferation in elderly nursing home residents with pressure ulcers. *J Parent Enteral Nutr* 2000; **24**: 280–7.

◆ 10 Demling D, DeSanti L. Closure of the 'non-healing wound' corresponds with correction of weight loss using the anabolic agent oxandrolone. *Ostomy Wound Manage* 1998; **44**: 58–60, 62, 64.

◆ 11 Spungen AM, Koehler KM, Modeste-Duncan R, *et al.* 9 clinical cases of non-healing pressure ulcers in patients with spinal cord injury treated with an anabolic agent: a therapeutic trial. *Adv Skin Wound Manage* 2001; **14**:139–44.

◆ 12 Hayden BK. Skin ulcerations. *CancerSourceMD.com* 2004; www.cancersourcemd.com/tools/print/print.cfm?contentID=28316 (accessed September 24, 2005).

Mouth care

FLAVIO FUSCO

INTRODUCTION

In the palliative care patient, the oral cavity represents the true 'target organ'. The mouth plays a fundamental role in a many aspects of life: nutrition, hydration, phonation, speech articulation processes, relational and communication activities, and emotional, affective and sexual relations.[1] Several studies have shown that oral complications and abnormalities of the oral microflora can be found in significant numbers of terminally ill cancer patients, affecting their quality of life. Sixteen of 99 consecutive patients with advanced cancer, followed in a palliative care program, reported experiencing mouth pain at a mean (SD) intensity of 5.5 ± 2.21 on a 0 (no pain) to 10 (worst possible pain) numerical scale, and 88 patients reported dry mouth at a mean intensity of 6.2 ± 2.21.[2*]

Sweeney and Bagg[3*] studied the prevalence of oral signs and symptoms among a group of 70 terminally ill cancer patients: 68 patients (97 percent) complained of oral dryness during the day and 59 patients (84 percent) complained of oral dryness at night. Oral soreness was reported by 22 patients (31 percent). Forty-six patients (66 percent) had difficulty talking and 36 (51 percent) reported difficulty eating. Oral mucosal abnormalities were detected in 45 patients (65 percent), most commonly erythema (20 percent), coated tongue (20 percent), atrophic glossitis (17 percent), angular cheilitis (11 percent) and pseudomembranous candidiasis (9 percent).

This chapter describes the major and more frequent oral problems experienced by patients with advanced cancer followed in palliative care programs. Aspects of their management will also be discussed.

INFECTIONS

Fungal and viral infections frequently develop in patients with advanced cancer.

Fungal infections

The most common oral infection is oral candidiasis: high levels of *Candida* have been reported among terminally ill patients, with correspondingly high levels of mucosal disease.[4] Debilitated patients, such as those receiving antibiotics, steroids, cytotoxic therapies, are particularly susceptible to oral candidiasis. Other general factors, such as diabetes mellitus, or predisposing local factors (e.g. poor denture hygiene, presence of xerostomia) are also important in the pathogenesis of oral candidiasis.

There are more than 150 species of *Candida* but only 10–15 of them are regarded as important pathogens for humans. *Candida albicans* is one of these candidal species, which is found in the oral cavity and responsible for most oral candidal infections.

The *pseudomembranous form* (thrush) is a classic clinical feature, characterized by creamy white, curdlike patches on the tongue and other oral mucosal surfaces. The patches can be removed by scraping and leave a raw, bleeding, and painful surface. Besides the classic lesion, other manifestations include:

- *Acute atrophic candidiasis* or 'antibiotic-related stomatitis'. This is a nonspecific atrophy of the tongue, associated with burning sensation, dysphagia, and mouth pain.

- *Chronic atrophic candidiasis* (erythematous candidiasis) or 'denture sore mouth'. This is a chronic inflammatory reaction with epithelial thinning under the dental plates.
- *Angular cheilitis*. This is an inflammatory reaction at the corners of the mouth (not due exclusively to *Candida* but to mixed infection with *Staphylococcus aureus* or, less frequently, β-hemolytic streptococci.
- *Candida leukoplakia* (hyperplasic candidiasis). In this the lesions are firm, adherent plaques involving the cheek, lips, and tongue.

The diagnosis can be made by the clinical appearance of the lesion, by scraping (using either a potassium hydroxide smear or a Gram stain to show masses of hyphae, pseudo-hyphae, and yeast forms). Other simple methods are swabs, imprint cultures, or culture of oral rinses.

TREATMENT OF ORAL FUNGAL INFECTIONS

Specific antifungal treatment may be provided either topically and systemically. Nystatin in the form of suspension (100 000 units/mL, 1–5 L), pastilles, or tablets (100 000 units) is a traditional local treatment. Duration of treatment is usually 10–14 days but some patients need to continue the treatment for at least 2 weeks after clinical resolution. Miconazole gel is useful for the management of angular cheilitis; it has weak activity against Gram-positive cocci as well as yeasts.[5] In a randomized, double-blind trial, a 50 g clotrimazole troche was found to be effective and safe in the treatment of oropharyngeal candidiasis.[6**] Ketoconazole is available in a number of oral and topical forms. The slow therapeutic response, variable absorption, and frequent adverse effects (anorexia, nausea, vomiting, liver toxicity) make it a poor choice in patients with advanced cancer. Fluconazole is a triazole with established therapeutic efficacy in candidal infections. It is both an oral and a parenteral fungistatic agent that inhibits ergosterol synthesis in yeasts. Fluconazole 50–100 mg once daily is one of the most effective treatments for oropharyngeal candidiasis; daily doses of 100–200 mg are recommended for esophageal candidiasis. Extensive clinical studies have demonstrated fluconazole's remarkable efficacy, favorable pharmacokinetics, and reassuring safety profile, all of which have contributed to its widespread use.[7,8**] Itraconazole, structurally similar to ketoconazole, has a broader spectrum of action and it is available in parenteral and oral formulations. To achieve the highest plasma concentration, the tablet is given with food and acidic drinks, whereas the solution is taken in the fasted state.

The most common triazole-related adverse effects are dose-related nausea, abdominal discomfort and diarrhea, but these symptoms rarely necessitate stopping therapy.[9] Ketoconazole and itraconazole may seriously interact with some of the substrates of CYP3A4. In a double-blind, randomized, three-phase crossover study, Varhe *et al.*[10**] reported that ketoconazole and itraconazole seriously affect the pharmacokinetics of triazolam and increase the intensity and duration of its effects, with potentially hazardous consequences. Azoles have also been implicated in fatal interactions with antihistamines (polymorphic ventricular tachycardia). Caution should be used when fluconazole and methadone are administrated concurrently.[11**,12]

Several recent studies have showed an emerging high prevalence of non-*C. albicans* yeasts and azole resistance in the oral flora of patients with advanced cancer. Bagg *et al.*[13*] examined the oral mycological flora of 207 patients receiving palliative care. A total of 194 yeasts were isolated, of which 95 (49 percent) were *C. albicans*. There was a high prevalence of *C. glabrata* (47 isolates) of which 34 (72 percent) were resistant to both fluconazole and itraconazole. Other non-*C. albicans* species, such as *C. parapsilosis*, *C. krusei*, and, more recently, *C. dubliniensis* are less susceptible than *C. albicans* to fluconazole.[14]

Viral infections

Herpes simplex virus 1 (HSV-1) is the commonest cause of viral infection of the oral mucosa. Herpes viruses are characterized by their ability to establish and maintain latent infections, which can get reactivated. Several stimuli, such as radiotherapy or chemotherapy, can trigger the reactivation of herpes viruses.

Small vesicles usually appear on the pharyngeal and oral mucosa; these rapidly ulcerate and increase in number, often involving the soft palate, buccal mucosa, tongue, and floor of the mouth. Anorexia, fever, mouth pain, and dysphagia may be present. The disease generally runs its course over 10–14 days.

TREATMENT OF ORAL VIRAL INFECTIONS

Aciclovir triphosphate is available as a topical 5 percent ointment, and as intravenous and oral formulations. In the immunocompromised patient, aciclovir is useful for both treatment and suppression of recurrent mucocutaneous HSV lesions.[15**] Penciclovir, a novel acyclic nucleoside analog, has shown efficacy against HSV types 1 and 2 and seems to have a pharmacological advantage due to a prolonged half-life of its active form in HSV-infected cells.[16,17**]

Al-Waili[18*] carried out an interesting, small, prospective, randomized trial that compared topical application of honey with aciclovir cream in patients with recurrent episodes of labial and genital herpes simplex lesions. For labial herpes, the mean duration of attacks, occurrence of crust, healing time, and pain duration were significantly lower when treated with honey when compared with aciclovir treatment ($P < 0.05$).

XEROSTOMIA

Xerostomia, defined as the subjective feeling of oral dryness, is one of the five most common symptoms affecting patients with advanced cancer, with a reported prevalence between 30 percent and 97 percent.[1,19,20] Indeed, despite the high prevalence of this distressing symptom – which may contribute to mouth pain and oral infections – there has been relatively little research into this 'orphan topic in supportive care'.[21]

There are many general causes of xerostomia (Box 81.1), but drug therapies are probably the most important, via a number of different mechanisms: the direct effects include interference with the nerve supply to the salivary glands (e.g. antidepressants), or with the productive capacity of salivary glands (e.g. diuretics, opioids). The indirect effects include imbalance with the normal stimuli to the secretion of saliva.[22*]

The effects of xerostomia on patient's symptoms are numerous: the absence of protective effect of saliva on the oral mucosa facilitates exogenous bacterial colonization and infections, and the loss of lubrication makes swallowing and chewing difficult and painful. Another feature of xerostomia is taste alteration with a subsequent loss of appetite. The sensations of burning, soreness, and dryness may have a considerable effect on speech, with subsequent fall in mood state and relational abilities. Saliva also plays an important role in preventing loss of tooth substance by its antimicrobial, buffering, and cleansing activities; thus, dental caries and dental erosions are often seen in terminally ill patients.[3,20]

MANAGEMENT OF XEROSTOMIA

The primary management of xerostomia involves treatment of the underlying cause. Take a detailed treatment history. Discontinuation or substitution of regimens of xerostomic drugs may sometimes be possible. Patients with ill-fitting dentures can be advised to see their dentist: relining of dentures can improve their fit and function and help to lessen oral pain and dryness caused by the lack of support for dentures. Dentate patients should receive preventive or dietary advice, as well as treatment for any caries present.

The secondary management of xerostomia involves the use of salivary substitutes and stimulants. Pilocarpine is a muscarinic agonist, although it does have some effect on the β-adrenergic receptors in the salivary and sweat glands. There have been a number of double-blind, randomized controlled studies that have shown that pilocarpine is an effective treatment for radiation and drug-induced xerostomia. Davies et al.,[23**] in a multicenter, crossover study, compared a mucin-based artificial saliva with oral formulation of pilocarpine hydrochloride in 70 patients with advanced disease and xerostomia. The pilocarpine formulation was found to be more effective than artificial saliva but it was found to be associated with more side effects such as sweating, lacrimation, and dizziness. Extreme caution in the use of pilocarpine is important due to reported side effects of glaucoma, cardiac disturbances, and sweating. For this reason, other studies have explored the possibility of using other saliva stimulants. Davies[24**] carried out a prospective, open, crossover, randomized study comparing a mucin-based artificial saliva with a low-tack, sugar-free chewing gum in the management of xerostomia in 43 patients with advanced cancer. Chewing gum is a saliva stimulant. It produces an increase in salivary flow due to a combination of stimulation of chemo- and mechanoreceptors. In this study, both artificial saliva and chewing gum were effective in the management of xerostomia, but 61 percent of the patients preferred the chewing gum to the artificial saliva. The use of chewing gum may be limited by the presence of jaw and oral discomfort, headaches, and swallowing difficulties.

A variety of saliva substitutes is now commercially available. The substitutes contain different synthetic polymers as thickening agents, e.g. carboxymethylcellulose, polyacrylic acid, and xanthan gum, but conflicting results have been

---

> ## Box 81.1 Main causes of xerostomia in patients with advanced cancer
>
> **Related to cancer itself**
>
> - Head and neck cancer
> - Obstruction/compression/destruction of the salivary glands
>
> **Related to dehydration**
>
> - Anorexia, poor fluid intake
> - Diarrhea, vomiting
> - Hemorrhage
> - Fever
> - Oxygen supply
>
> **Related to treatment**
>
> - Radiotherapy
> - Oral and jaw surgery
> - Drug therapy: anticholinergics; antihistamines; antihypertensive/diuretics; opioid analgesics; non-steroidal anti-inflammatory drugs (NSAIDs); corticosteroids; proton pump inhibitors
>
> **Related to concurrent disorders**
>
> - Sjögren syndrome
> - Diabetes (mellitus and insipidus)
> - Sarcoidosis
> - Thyroid dysfunctions
> - Anxiety/depression states

reported.[1,3,20,25] Recent developments – still in the experimental stage – include bioactive salivary substitutes and mouthwashes containing antimicrobial peptides to protect the oral tissues against microbial colonization and to suppress and cure mucosal and gingival inflammation.[25]

A randomized controlled trial of standard fractionated radiation with or without amifostine ($200 \, mg/m^2$) before each fraction of radiation, was conducted in 315 patients with head and neck cancer. Amifostine administration was associated with a reduced incidence of grade ≥ 2 xerostomia over 2 years of follow-up ($P = 0.002$), an increase in the proportion of patients with meaningful ($>0.1 \, g$) unstimulated saliva production at 24 months ($P = 0.011$), and reduced mouth dryness scores on a patient benefit questionnaire at 24 months ($P < 0.001$).[26**]

CHEMOTHERAPY/RADIATION–INDUCED STOMATITIS

The oral mucosa is frequently damaged during chemotherapy/radiotherapy in patients with cancer, leading to a high incidence of oral and esophageal mucositis. Patients with mucositis often experience considerable pain and discomfort. The incidence of oral mucositis ranges from 15 percent to 40 percent in patients receiving stomatotoxic chemotherapy or radiotherapy and from 70 percent to 90 percent in bone marrow recipients.

Raber-Durlacher et al.[27*] reported a retrospective analysis of the incidence and the severity of chemotherapy-associated oral mucositis in 150 patients with various solid tumors. Eighty-seven episodes of mucositis occurred in 47 (31 percent) patients. Twenty-six patients each experienced only one episode, whereas 21 patients had up to eight episodes of mucositis. Multivariate analysis identified the administration of paclitaxel, doxorubicin, or etoposide as independent risk factor (adjusted rate ratios 8.06, 7.35, and 6.70, respectively), whereas low body mass was associated with a slightly increased risk (adjusted rate ratio 0.92). Other anticancer drugs, such as alkylating agents, vinca alkaloids, antimetabolites and antitumor antibiotics are especially liable to cause stomatitis, and it is important to carefully consider their use in patients with advanced cancer.[28]

Both chemotherapy and radiotherapy interfere with cellular mitosis and reduce the regenerative properties of the oral mucosa. A poor nutritional status further interferes with mucosal regeneration; oral infections can exacerbate the mucositis and may lead to systemic infections. If the patient develops both severe mucositis and thrombocytopenia, oral bleeding may occur, and this may be difficult to treat. Direct stomatotoxicity is usually seen 5–7 days after the start of chemotherapy or radiotherapy; in non-immunocompromised patients, oral lesions heal within 2–3 weeks. The most common sites include the buccal, labial and soft palate mucosa, as well as the floor of the mouth and the ventral surface of the tongue.[28]

MANAGEMENT OF CHEMOTHERAPY/ RADIATION–INDUCED STOMATITIS

Chlorhexidine, amifostine, hematological growth factors, pentoxifylline, sucralfate, glutamine, and several other agents have been investigated for prevention of oral mucositis. Results have been conflicting, inconclusive, or of limited benefit. Topical anesthetics, mixtures (also called cocktails), and mucosal-coating agents have been used despite the lack of experimental evidence supporting their efficacy. Of the current available topical products, the supporting evidence is strongest for ice chips and benzydamine in the prophylaxis of mucositis.[29*,30***] Promising investigational approaches have recently emerged: the candidate that is most advanced in terms of drug development is recombinant human keratinocyte growth factor (rHuKGF; palifermin), which in phase III clinical trials has been shown to reduce the severity and duration of oral mucositis and improve clinical outcome.[29*]

Biswal et al.[31**] carried out the first prospective, randomized trial to evaluate the effect of pure natural honey in radiation-induced mucositis. Forty patients received topical application of honey along with radiotherapy to the head and neck region or radiotherapy alone. A significant reduction in symptomatic grade 3–4 mucositis (Radiation Therapy Oncology Group [RTOG] grading system) was found in the honey group compared with the control group ($P = 0.0005$). Fifty-five percent of patients treated with topical honey showed no change or a positive gain in body weight compared with 25 percent in the control arm, the majority of whom lost weight. Recent articles have reported successful use of topical opioids, prepared with taste supplements, in treating persistent mucosal pain in palliative care patients.[32,33*]

ALTERED TASTE SENSATIONS

A reduction (hypogeusia), distortion (dysgeusia), or absence (ageusia) of normal taste sensation is common in patients with cancer, and can be the result of the disease itself and/or its treatment (drug therapy, chemotherapy, radiotherapy). Between 25 percent and 50 percent of patients with cancer are reported to experience taste changes. Typically, patients appeared to have difficulty in differentiating sour and bitter tastes, which are affected more than salty and sweet tastes. Women appeared to report greater changes in taste than men.[1,34,35] Zinc deficiency has been linked with abnormalities in taste sensation.

MANAGEMENT OF ALTERED TASTE SENSATIONS

Ripamonti et al.[36**] in a randomized, double-blind, placebo-controlled trial, described the beneficial effects of oral zinc sulfate tablets (45 mg three times a day) in 18 patients with cancer receiving external radiotherapy to the head and neck region (ERT). One month after ERT was terminated, the patients receiving zinc sulfate had a quicker recovery of taste acuity than those receiving placebo.

Nonpharmacological treatment includes mouth care, dental hygiene improvement, and dietary advice. The urea content in the diet can be reduced by eating white meats and eggs. This masks the bitter taste of food. Food should be eaten cold or at room temperature.

ORAL LESIONS IN PATIENTS WITH HIV/AIDS

Oral candidiasis, hairy leukoplakia, Kaposi sarcoma, necrotizing ulcerative gingivitis, linear gingival erythema, necrotizing ulcerative periodontitis, and oral non-Hodgkin lymphoma are strongly associated with human immunodeficiency virus (HIV) infection and may be present in up to 80 percent of people with acquired immune deficiency syndrome (AIDS).[37] These lesions parallel the decline in number of CD4 cells and an increase in viral load. Cross-sectional studies have shown an association between low CD4 lymphocyte count with the presence of oral Kaposi sarcoma, non-Hodgkin lymphoma, and necrotizing ulcerative peridontitis.[38*]

Highly active antiretroviral therapy (HAART) with protease inhibitors (PIs) has reduced the frequency of occurrence and the severity of many oral lesions such as oral candidiasis and hairy leukoplakia. Interestingly, the prevalence of Kaposi sarcoma has not changed, and HAART may predispose to human papilloma virus infection and potentially increase the risk of later oral squamous cell carcinoma.[39*,40] Regimens based on PIs may also have adverse effects including oral problems such as paresthesia, taste disturbance, and xerostomia, and may interact with a number of drugs used in oral healthcare.[41]

MANAGEMENT OF ORAL LESIONS IN PATIENTS WITH HIV/AIDS

At the end of 2005, the great majority of HIV/AIDS-affected people are in the developing world and do not have affordable access to HAART and/or conventional antifungal therapy (clotrimazole, fluconazole, itraconazole). For this reason some less expensive and more readily available alternatives are been tested. In Malawi, gentian violet was found to be as effective as nystatin for the management of oral candidiasis; topical chlorhexidine, in a pilot study, has also shown promise in the prevention of oral candidiasis in HIV-infected children; the essential oral oil solution of *Melaleuca alternifolia* (tea tree oil) has been successfully used to treat fluconazole-refractory oropharyngeal candidiasis in AIDS patients.[37,42,43] In poor resource-limited settings, thalidomide may be a cheap palliative therapy for mucocutaneous Kaposi sarcoma in children.[37]

OSTEONECROSIS OF THE JAW: AN EMERGING PROBLEM

Osteonecrosis of the jaw has been recently shown to be associated with the use of pamidronate and zoledronic acid, two bisphosphonates that inhibit bone resorption and thus bone renewal by suppressing the recruitment and activity osteoclasts. People at risk include those with multiple myeloma and cancer metastatic to bone who are receiving intravenous bisphosphonates. The risk of developing complication appears to increase with time of use of the medication.[44***,45*]

Bamias et al.[46*] studied the incidence, characteristics, and risk factors for the development of osteonecrosis of the jaw among 252 patients with advanced cancer. The incidence increased with time to exposure from 1.5 percent among patients treated for 4–12 months to 7.7 percent in those treated for 37–48 months. The cumulative hazard was significantly higher with zoledronic acid compared with pamidronate alone or pamidronate and zoledronic acid sequentially ($P < 0.001$). In addition, some authors have reported a few cases of osteonecrosis of the jaw in patients taking oral doses of alendronate for the treatment of osteoporosis or osteopenia.[47*,48]

Comorbid factors may play a role, such as the presence of diabetes mellitus, the degree of immunosuppression, the use of other medications (chemotherapeutic agents, corticosteroids). Other drug-related risk factors include the use of antiangiogenic agents such as thalidomide and bortezomib in patients with multiple myeloma.[49] Local comorbid factors include oral health status, presence of infection, and history of radiation therapy.

A recent internet-based survey evaluated the incidence of bisphosphonate-associated osteonecrosis in 1203 patients receiving intravenous bisphosphonate therapy for the treatment of myeloma or breast cancer. This study showed that 81 percent of the patients with myeloma and 69 percent of the patients with breast cancer who developed osteonecrosis had underlying dental disease, such as infection, or had had a dental extraction, compared with 33 percent of the patients who did not develop osteonecrosis.[45*]

The most common initial complaint is the sudden presence of intraoral discomfort and roughness that may traumatize the oral soft tissues surrounding the area of necrotic bone. The classic clinical features are a growing, painful and unilateral swelling with jaw pain, and difficulty chewing and brushing teeth.[50] The mandible and maxilla, with or without oroantral fistulas, are the main areas affected by osteonecrosis.

MANAGEMENT OF OSTEONECROSIS OF THE JAWS

The treatment in patients receiving oral or intravenous bisphosphonate therapy is principally preventive in nature.[44***] Ruggiero et al.[47*] in a case series of 63 patients, reported that despite several treatment modalities, such as minor debridement, major surgical sequestrectomies, partial or complete maxillectomies and hyperbaric oxygen therapies, no healing occurred in any of the patients treated. For this reason, preventive measures prior to the initiation of intravenous bisphosphonate therapy are of paramount importance, with the dentist and oncologist working collaboratively. Box 81.2 summarizes the potential preventive measures in osteonecrosis of the jaw. There is no scientific evidence to support discontinuation of bisphosphonate therapy to promote healing of necrotic osseous tissues in the oral cavity.[44***]

Box 81.2 Bisphosphonate–associated osteonecrosis of the jaw: preventive measures

- Clinical dental examination: comprehensive extraoral and intraoral examination; full-mouth radiographic series plus panoramic radiograph; evaluation of third molars

- Removal of abscessed and nonrestorable teeth

- Restoration of periodontal health status (pocket elimination, plaque reduction)

- Caries control, elimination of defective restorations

- Oral hygiene and self-care education

- Functional rehabilitation of salvageable dentition (endodontic therapy)

- Properly fitting dentures

- Scheduled periodic follow-up visits

Systemic antibiotic therapy to control secondary infection and pain may be beneficial and should be administered whenever active infection is present. Antibiotics that have been found useful for osteonecrosis include penicillin or amoxicillin, and in presence of penicillin-related allergy, clindamycin or erythromycin ethylsuccinate. A 0.12 percent chlorhexidine antiseptic mouthwash, or minocycline hydrochloride, can be useful for periodontal pockets.[51*,52*]

Key learning points

- Oral lesions are frequently experienced by patients with advanced cancer.

- The most common problems are xerostomia, fungal infections, treatment-related mucositis, and taste disturbances.

- Azole resistance may become a clinical problem in the treatment of oral fungal infections.

- Improving dental and oral hygiene, good fluid intake, ice chips and dietary advice are the mainstay of nonpharmacological prophylaxis and treatment of xerostomia, mucositis, and taste alterations in palliative care patients.

- Honey may be a cheaper and worldwide-available choice for treating herpes simplex lesions and radiation-induced mucositis.

- In poor resourced-limited settings, mouth care for people with AIDS is a basic clinical strategy.

- Bisphosphonate-related osteonecrosis of the jaw is an emerging and challenging problem in palliative care: prevention of the osteonecrosis is the best approach to management of this complication.

REFERENCES

- 1 De Conno F, Sbanotto A, Ripamonti C, Ventafridda V. Mouth care. In: Doyle D, Hanks G, Cherny N, Calman K, eds. *Oxford Textbook of Palliative Medicine*, 3rd ed. Oxford: Oxford University Press, 2004.

- 2 Oneschuk D, Hanson J, Bruera E. A survey of mouth pain and dryness in patients with advanced cancer. *Support Care Cancer* 2000; **8**: 372–6.

- 3 Sweeney MP, Bagg J. The mouth and palliative care. *Am J Hosp Palliat Care* 2000; **17**: 118–24.

4 Finlay IG. Oral symptoms and candida in the terminally ill. *Br Med J* 1986; **292**: 592–93.

5 Roed-Petersen B. Miconazole in the treatment of oral candidosis. *Int J Oral Surg* 1978; **7**: 558–63.

6 Yap BS, Bodey GP. Oropharyngeal candidiasis treated with a troche form of clotrimazole. *Arch Intern Med* 1979; **139**: 656–7.

7 Meunier F. Fluconazole treatment of fungal infections in the immunocompromised host. *Semin Oncol* 1990; **17**(Suppl 6): 19–23.

- 8 Goodman JL, Winston DJ, Greenfield RA, *et al.* A controlled trial of fluconazole to prevent fungal infections in patients undergoing bone marrow transplantation. *N Engl J Med* 1992; **326**: 845–51.

- 9 Perfect JR, Lindsay MH, Drew RH. Adverse drug reactions to systemic antifungals. *Drug Saf* 1992; **7**: 323–63.

- 10 Varhe A, Olkkola KT, Neuvonen PJ. Oral triazolam is potentially hazardous to patients receiving systemic antimycotics ketoconazole or itraconazole. *Clin Pharmacol Ther* 1994; **56**: 601–7.

- 11 Cobb MN, Desai J, Brown LS Jr, *et al.* The effect of fluconazole on the clinical pharmacokinetics of methadone. *Clin Pharmacol Ther* 1998; **63**: 655–62.

12 Y, Pereira J, Watanabe S. Methadone and fluconazole: respiratory depression by drug interaction. *J Pain Symptom Manage* 2002; **23**: 148–53.

- 13 Bagg J, Sweenwy MP, Lewis MAO, *et al.* High prevalence of non-albicans yeasts and detection of anti-fungal resistance in the oral flora of patients with advanced cancer. *Palliat Med* 2003; **17**: 477–81.

14 Davies A, Brailsford S, Broadley K, Beighton D. Resistance amongst yeasts isolated from the oral cavities of patients with advanced cancer. *Palliat Med* 2002; **16**: 527–31.

15 Rooney JF, Straus SE, Manix ML, *et al.* Oral acyclovir to suppress frequently recurrent herpes labialis. A double-blind, placebo controlled trial. *Ann Intern Med* 1993; **118**: 268–72.

16 Schmid-Wendtner MH, Korting HC. Penciclovir cream improved topical treatment for herpes simplex infection. *Skin Pharmacol Physiol* 2004; **17**: 214–18.

17 Raborn GW, Martel AY, Lassonde M, *et al.* Effective treatment of herpes simplex labialis with penciclovir cream: combined results from two trials. *J Am Dent Assoc* 2002; **133**: 303–9.

18 Al-Waili NS. Topical honey application vs. acyclovir for the treatment of recurrent herpes simplex lesions. *Med Sci Monit* 2004; **10**: MT94–98.

19 Ventafridda V, De Conno F, Ripamonti C, *et al.* Quality-of-life assessment during a palliative care program. *Ann Oncol* 1990; **1**: 415–20.

20 Sweeney MP, Bagg J, Baxter WP, Aitchinson TC. Oral disease in terminally ill cancer patients with xerostomia. *Oral Oncol* 1998; **34**: 123–6.

21 Senn HJ. Orphan topics in supportive care: how about xerostomia? *Support Care Cancer* 1997; **5**: 261–2.

● 22 Davies AN, Broadley K, Beighton D. Xerostomia in patients with advanced cancer. *J Pain Symptom Manage* 2001; **22**: 820–5.

● 23 Davies AN, Daniels C, Pugh R, Sharma K. A comparison of artificial saliva and pilocarpine in the management of xerostomia in patients with advanced cancer. *Palliat Med* 1998; **12**: 105–11.

● 24 Davies AN. A comparison of artificial saliva and chewing gum in the management of xerostomia in patients with advanced cancer. *Palliat Med* 2000; **14**: 197–203.

● 25 Nieuw Amerongen NV, Veerman EC. Current therapies for xerostomia and salivary gland hypofunction associated with cancer therapies. *Support Care Cancer* 2003; **11**: 226–31.

26 Wasserman TH, Brizel DM, Henke M, *et al.* Influence of intravenous amifostine on xerostomia, tumour control, and survival after radiotherapy for head-and-neck cancer: 2-year follow-up of a prospective, randomised, phase III trial. *Int J Radiat Oncol Biol Phys* 2005; **63**: 985–90.

27 Raber-Durlacher JE, Weijl NI, Abu Saris M, *et al.* Oral mucositis in patients treated with chemotherapy for solid tumours: a retrospective analysis of 150 cases. *Support Care Cancer* 2000; **8**: 366–71.

28 Pico JL, Avila-Garavito A, Naccache P. Mucositis: its occurrence, consequences, and treatment in the oncology setting. *Oncologist* 1998; **3**: 446–51.

● 29 Peterson DE, Cariello A. Mucosal damage: a major risk factor for severe complications after cytotoxic therapy. *Semin Oncol* 2004; **31**: 35–44.

◆ 30 Scully C, Epstein J, Sonis S. Oral mucositis: a challenging complication of radiotherapy, chemotherapy and radiochemotherapy. Part 2: diagnosis and management of mucositis. *Head Neck* 2004; **26**: 77–84.

● 31 Biswal BM, Zakaria A, Ahmad NM. Topical application of honey in the management of radiation mucositis. A preliminary study. *Support Care Cancer* 2003; **11**: 242–8.

32 Krajnik M, Zylicz Z, Finlay I, *et al.* Potential uses of topical opioids in palliative care report of 6 cases. *Pain* 1999; **80**: 121–5.

33 Cerchietti LC, Navigante AH, Korte MW, *et al.* Potential utility of peripheral analgesic properties of morphine in stomatitis-related pain: a pilot study. *Pain* 2003; **105**: 265–73.

● 34 Twycross RG, Lack SA, eds. *Control of Alimentary Symptoms in Far Advanced Cancer.* Edinburgh: Churchill Livingstone, 1986: 57–65.

● 35 Ripamonti C, Fulfaro F. Taste disturbance. In: Davies A, Finlay I, eds. *Oral Care in Advanced Disease.* Oxford: Oxford University Press, 2004: 115–24.

36 Ripamonti C, Zecca E, Brunelli C, *et al.* A randomised, controlled clinical trial to evaluate the effects of zinc sulfate on cancer patients with taste alterations caused by head and neck irradiation. *Cancer* 1998; **82**: 1938–45.

◆ 37 Coogan MM, Greensoan J, Challacombe SJ. Oral lesions in infection with human immunodeficiency virus. *Bull World Health Organ* 2005; **83**: 700–6.

38 Glick M, Muzyka BC, Lurie D, Salkin M. Oral manifestation associated with HIV-related disease as markers for immune suppression and AIDS. *Oral Surg Oral Med Oral Pathol* 1994; **77**: 344–9.

39 Ramirez-Amador V, Esquivel-Pedraza L, Sierra-Madero J, *et al.* The changing clinical spectrum of human immunodeficiency virus (HIV)-related oral lesions in 1,000 consecutive patients. A twelve-year study in referral center in Mexico. *Medicine* 2003; **82**: 39–50.

40 Frezzini C, Leao JC, Porter S. Current trends of HIV disease of the mouth. *J Oral Pathol Med* 2005; **34**: 513–31.

● 41 Porter SR, Scully C. HIV topic update: protease inhibitor therapy and oral health care. *Oral Dis* 1998; **4**: 159–63.

42 Barasch A, Safford MM, Dapkute-Marcus I, Fine DH. Efficacy of chlorhexidine gluconate rinse for treatment and prevention of oral candidiasis in HIV-infected children: a pilot study. *Oral Surg Oral Med Oral Pathol Oral Radiol Endodont* 2004; **97**: 204–7.

43 Vazquez JA, Zawawi AA. Efficacy of alcohol-based and alcohol-free melaleuca oral solution for the treatment of fluconazole-refractory oropharyngeal candidiasis in patients with AIDS. *HIV Clin Trials* 2002; **3**: 379–85.

✱ 44 Migliorati CA, Casiglia J, Epstein J, *et al.* Managing the care of patients with bisphosphonates-associated osteonecrosis. An American Academy of Oral Medicine position paper. *J Am Dent Assoc* 2005; **136**: 1658–68.

45 Durie BGM, Katz M, Crowley J. Osteonecrosis of the jaw and bisphosphonates. *N Engl J Med* 2005; **353**: 99–100.

46 Bamias A, Kastritis E, Bamia C, *et al.* Osteonecrosis of the jaw in cancer after treatment with bisphosphonates: incidence and risk factors. *J Clin Oncol* 2005; **23**: 8580–7.

47 Ruggiero SL, Mehrotra B, Rosenberg TJ, Engroff SL. Osteonecrosis of the jaw associated with the use of bisphosphonates: a review of 63 cases. *J Oral Maxillofac Surg* 2004; **62**: 527–34.

48 Purcell PM, Boyd IW. Bisphosphonates and osteonecrosis of the jaw. *Med J Aust* 2005; **182**: 417–18.

49 Clerc D, Fernand JP, Mariette X. Treatment of multiple myeloma. *Joint Bone Spine* 2003; **70**: 173–86.

50 Sanna G, Zampino MG, Pelosi G, *et al.* Jaw vascular bone necrosis associated with long-term use of bisphosphonates. *Ann Oncol* 2005; **16**: 1207–13.

51 Migliorati CA, Schubert MM, Peterson DE, Seneda LM. Bisphosphonate-associated osteonecrosis of mandibular and maxillary bone. An emerging oral complication of supportive cancer therapy. *Cancer* 2005; **104**: 83–93.

52 Marx RE, Sawatari Y, Fortin M, Broumand V. Bisphosphonate-induced exposed bone (osteonecrosis/osteopetrosis) of the jaws: risk factors, recognition, prevention, and treatment. *J Oral Maxillofac Surg* 2005; **63**: 1567–75.

82

Fistulas

FABIO FULFARO, CARLA RIPAMONTI

INTRODUCTION

A fistula is an abnormal communication between two digestive organs (internal fistula) or between the skin and a hollow organ (external fistula).[1] Fistulas may be classified according to the amount of the output: low output (<200 mL/24-h period), moderate output (200–500 mL/day), and high output (>500 mL/day).[2] Fistulas may be single or multiple.[3] The most frequent causes of fistulas in oncological patients are given in Box 82.1.[4–16]

Box 82.1 Causes of fistulas in patients with cancer

Causes related to treatments

- Surgery
- Radiotherapy
- Chemotherapy
- Photodynamics
- Endoscopy
- Invasive diagnostic procedures

Causes related to cancer

- Tumoral local progression
- Locoregional relapse of the disease

Mixed causes (related to treatments and to cancer)

The development of a fistula produces various complications (Box 82.2). Sepsis is the most frequent cause of death in patients with fistulas.[17] Nutritional status as well as a condition of impaired tissue vascularity may be predisposing factors.[18,19]

Box 82.2 Frequent complications of fistulas

- Infection → sepsis
- Hydro-electrolytic losses: electrolyte imbalance, dehydration
- Malnutrition
- Skin lesions
- Hemorrhages
- Delay in oncological treatments
- Psychosocial problems

GENERAL PRINCIPLES OF TREATMENT

Prior to planning a treatment, it is important to define the objectives to be achieved. In patients with advanced cancer, treatment will be conservative, whereas for a patient with a longer survival expectancy, more invasive treatment may be performed. Box 82.3 shows the possible conservative[20–22] and nonconservative treatments.[19,23,24]

Box 82.3 General management of fistulas

Conservative treatment

- Skin care and local disinfection

- Pouching of secretions (particularly gastric and pancreatic)

- Control of odor, delicate fistula areas, use of antibiotics against anaerobic bacteria (metronidazole)

- Control of local itching and pain

- Control of infections (specific antibiotic treatment, care in the use of corticosteroids, radiotherapy, and chemotherapy)

- Control of nutrition and electrolytes (particularly in high-output fistulas) and eventual total parenteral nutrition (TPN) and antisecretory treatments (scopolamine, octreotide)

- Treatment of site-related symptoms (antiemetic, antispastic, antihemorrhagic, antisecretory, use of vasopressin for urinary incontinence, use of urinary catheters)

- Control of psychological conditions (distortion of body image, isolation, social discomfort).

Nonconservative treatment

- Surgical resection of fistula

- Surgical repair with corrective procedures or with myocutaneous flaps

- Colonic and/or urinary diversion

- Endoscopic treatments with metallic stents

GASTROINTESTINAL FISTULAS

Gastrointestinal fistulas may be classified as external (enterocutaneous fistulas) and internal (communication between hollow organs), or according to the anatomical site of onset: esophageal, gastric and duodenal, pancreatic, enteric and colonic.[18]

Esophageal fistulas

Esophageal fistulas may be classified as esophagorespiratory (particularly esophagotracheal) and esophagocardiovascular. As far as the former are concerned, most of them are due to esophageal carcinoma (75 percent) and lung cancer (16 percent).[25,26] Some rare cases due to Hodgkin disease are cited in the literature.[27] Symptoms may be dysphagia,

coughing, aspiration, suffocation, and fever. When the patient's clinical condition allows it, surgery may be performed[28] with an eventual gastrostomy and/or jejunostomy, the use of metallic stents[29,31] and/or palliative radiotherapy. Chemotherapy is indicated particularly in the presence of lymphomas. From a prognostic point of view, patients with esophagorespiratory fistulas are at high risk of developing lung abscesses, empyema, and pneumonia ab ingestis.[28]

Esophagocardiovascular fistulas are rare in patients with cancer and also include the aortoesophageal fistula, which is mainly caused by the rupture of a thoracic aneurysm into the esophagus, and the esophagocardiac fistula.[4,28]

Gastric and duodenal fistulas

More than 90 percent of gastric and duodenal fistulas are a consequence of surgery in those areas.[32] Postoperative fistulas are frequently due to an 'anastomotic leak' and abscess formation. Cancers of the transverse colon, stomach, and duodenum are more prone to fistulization. Other rare causes are lymphomas and the placing of pumps for chemotherapy infusion in the gastroduodenal artery.[10] Whereas external fistulas are easily diagnosed, internal fistulas that can cause diarrhea and nutritional deficit are less detectable.

Most postoperative gastrointestinal fistulas heal spontaneously within 4–5 weeks. Factors associated with poor healing or delayed healing include multiple fistulous tracts, malnutrition, acute infection or sepsis, decreased level of serum transferrin (unfavorable $<200\,mg/dL$),[33,34] cancer progression, and previous radiotherapy in the involved areas.[17] Treatment of gastric and duodenal fistulas may be medical, endoscopic, and/or surgical. Nutritional support[35*] and treatment of infection[36*] are essential in the management of postoperative fistulas.

With regard to endoscopic treatment, some authorities have reported obliteration of the fistula tract with adhesive fibrin tissue.[37*] For patients with persistent fistulas and a good performance status, three different surgical approaches have been described: exclusion, resection, and 'closure of the leak'.[32] Exclusion of a fistula is not the treatment of choice and is reserved for very ill patients. The procedure involves resection of the diseased segment and exteriorization of the proximal and distal segments. In this way an uncontrolled anastomotic leak is converted into a controlled external fistula. The procedure of choice is the resection of the anastomotic leak with the formation of a new anastomosis. Major contraindications to this procedure are ischemia or tension on the anastomosis. If the anastomotic leak cannot be resected then closure of the leak with a serosal patch or Roux-en-Y anastomosis is the preferred surgical alternative.[32]

Pancreatic fistulas

Pancreatic fistulas are more frequently external and are usually complications of upper abdominal invasive procedures on the pancreas or surrounding area[38] and occur in 6 percent to 25 percent of pancreaticoduodenectomies.[39] Fistulas are more frequent during the first postoperative week and associated with high levels of serum amylase. Internal fistulas, which most commonly involve the peritoneum, are rare. They are usually diagnosed by radiological examination (fistulography, computed tomography [CT] scan), ultrasonography and/or by endoscopic retrograde cholangiopancreatography (ERCP).[40]

Postoperative external fistulas heal spontaneously in 80 percent of cases with conservative treatment incorporating skin care, drainage and collection of pancreatic secretion, control of infection and parenteral nutrition (to reduce pancreatic secretion).[40] Octreotide, in doses of 50–200 µg three times daily, have been used in conservative treatment to reduce gastrointestinal secretion.[41,42] Many authors have suggested the use of subcutaneous injection of octreotide at doses of 50–200 µg three times daily according to output.[43] Recently, Barnett et al.[44] have expressed some concern about the use of octreotide in the treatment of pancreatic fistula.

Surgical approaches are reserved for situations of failure of conservative management in patients with good performance status and favorable tumor anatomy.[40] Placement of an endoscopic stent has proved effective in certain studies but a longer follow-up is necessary to evaluate possible long-term complications.[40*] Another surgical approach involves creating a subcutaneous fistulojejunostomy.[45*]

Small bowel and colonic fistulas

Intestinal fistulas are classified as internal, external, or mixed; the most common are external (enterocutaneous).[46] Most of them are a consequence of postoperative complications following surgery on gastrointestinal cancers with diastasis of the anastomotic wound and damage to the bowel and its vascularization.

The severity of the consequences of an enterocutaneous fistula depends on the site and the amount of secretion, for example, large volumes of secretion and small bowel fistulas may be associated with severe fluid and electrolyte abnormalities and malabsorption. In a series of 25 cancer patients with enterocutaneous fistulas, the most frequent site was the jejunum-ileum, and mortality was correlated to previous radiotherapy, the site, fistula output, and the presence of hypoalbuminemia. In 63 percent of patients, the presence of a fistula resulted in suspension of any ongoing anticancer treatment.[46] A rare presentation of an enterocutaneous fistula may be subcutaneous emphysema.[47]

Enterocutaneous fistulas may heal spontaneously with adequate supportive therapy including TPN, prevention, and treatment of infective complications (in 70 percent of these cases). Limited data support the use of octreotide to reduce secretion volume.[48,49**] The use of TPN allows an adequate fluid intake, normalization of electrolytes as well as catabolic blockage. Factors which negatively influence spontaneous

closure of the fistula include the presence of cancer together with sepsis, malnutrition, distal obstruction to the fistula, and the epithelialization of the fistulous tract.[50] Surgery is indicated whenever conservative treatment has not been effective and when the patient's condition allows it.[50*] Recently, a case of enterobiliary fistula following radiofrequency on the liver was reported.[51]

Colonic fistulas, although considered uncommon, can also be classified as external, internal (colocutaneous), and mixed.[52] Among the internal fistulas, the most common are colovesical, followed by colovaginal and coloenteric. The most evident sign of colocutaneous fistulas is the passage of air and feces through an incision in the abdominal wall following surgery. Other signs and symptoms are sepsis, fever, tachycardia, leukocytosis, and pain due to abscess with local peritonitis. Patients with an internal fistula complain of a variety of symptoms depending on the viscera involved. Patients with colovesical fistulas frequently have cystitis, high fever, shivering and sweating and, if the fistulous tract is wide, pneumaturia and fecaluria. Patients with colovaginal fistulas suffer from increased vaginal secretion, sometimes associated with the passage of feces. Patients with coloenteric fistulas suffer from abdominal pain and severe diarrhea.[53]

An internal colovesical fistula is diagnosed by means of cystoscopy, a colovaginal fistula is diagnosed by means of a fistulogram and/or a vaginogram, and a coloenteric fistula is diagnosed by means of an abdominal CT scan with contrast. Colocutaneous fistulas may be conservatively treated even if the rate of healing is lower than of enteric fistulas, particularly in the presence of a malignancy or a distal occlusion. Some patients may require a surgical bowel diversion. In the presence of a malignancy, a partial cystectomy together with the removal of the sigmoid colon is indicated for colovesical fistulas. Radiotherapy-induced fistulas may be complex and often involve more than one organ, for example, either the colon or the rectum with the bladder, the vagina, the small bowel and the skin. These fistulas are more difficult to treat because of the low rate of spontaneous healing and the high rate of relapse.[54*] It is possible to treat coloenteric fistulas with stents.[53*]

HEAD AND NECK FISTULAS

As regards patients with head and neck cancer, the most frequent fistulas are pharyngocutaneous; these are the most common complications resulting from total laryngectomy. It has been observed that 12–16 percent of the patients undergoing laryngectomy develop fistulas 11–14 days after surgery.[55–57] Although spontaneous closure of the fistula occurs in two-thirds of the cases, about 20 percent of patients have to undergo surgery with direct suture of pharyngeal mucosa or reparative surgery by means of a deltopectoral flap or a pectoralis major myocutaneous flap.[58,59]

Negative prognostic factors that give rise to fistulas are: hemoglobin levels lower than 12.5 g/dL, concomitant heart pathology, extension of surgery, the surgeon's experience, tumor size, and the use of catgut.[55,60,61] Previous radiotherapy to the head and neck increases the risk of developing fistulas by 10–12 percent and the healing rate is lower.[62,63] In some groups of patients treated with radiotherapy, the percentage of fistulization increases up to 30 percent after total laryngectomy with prolonged hospitalization.[64]

Some authors have suggested using growth factors with the aim of preventing infection and sepsis.[65*] The concomitant use of oxygen therapy and radiotherapy favors neovascularization and prevents fistulas from occurring.

Another relatively frequent group of fistulas are the esophagotracheal fistulas (see Esophageal fistulas above). Rarer fistulas are the tracheocutaneous, which are often related to long-term tracheostomy, salivary fistulas,[66] oroantral fistulas,[67] and chylous fistulas.[68]

BRONCHOPLEURAL FISTULAS

Bronchopleural fistulas are often related to pneumonectomy for the treatment of lung cancer.[69,70] The incidence is about 8–10 percent.[71] Significant risk factors involved in the development of fistulas are: preoperative infection, diagnostic pneumonectomy and the presence of subcarinal metastatic lymph nodes, preoperative radiotherapy, and diabetes.

From a pathophysiological view, it is difficult to preserve bronchial arteries in the dissection of the metastatic subcarinal lymph nodes which adhere to the bronchial tree. Ligation of the bronchial arteries or the protrusion of the bronchial stump into the pleura reduces the blood flow to very low levels, thus favoring fistula development.[71] The most common signs and symptoms are: air in the pleural cavity, dyspnea, anterior chest pain.[72] The diagnosis is usually made by a bronchoscopy, even though scintigraphic techniques using xenon-133 and technetium-99m have given good results.[73] Surgery is the first choice of treatment whenever possible.[74*] In the case of fistulas smaller than 3 mm, however, successful results with reparative endoscopy have been reported.[74,75] A thorough follow-up in the first 3 months after pneumonectomy is indicated as a preventive measure.[74]

GENITOURINARY FISTULAS

The incidence of fistulas in the genitourinary tract is about 2 percent in patients with cancer. The most frequent causes are: surgery (hysterectomy, prostatectomy, rectal resections, pelvic evisceration,[76,77]), radiotherapy on the pelvic organs[78] and locoregional relapses. Signs and symptoms are characteristically urinary incontinence, pain and itching at the fistula site, pneumaturia, sometimes fecaluria, GI disorders, hemorrhage, and are often present with psychological distress.[79] For diagnostic reasons, the following are often used: CT, nuclear magnetic resonance (NMR), cystoscopy, charcoaluria, and barium enema.[80–82]

As far as the anatomical site is concerned, the most frequent fistulas in this group of patients are: rectovaginal, enterovesical, vesicovaginal, ureterovaginal, urethrocutaneous, rectoureteral. The rarer ones are the vesicocutaneous and the vescicouterine.[83,84] The rectovaginal and enterovesical fistulas are often the consequence of radiotherapy on the pelvis, with necrosis of the vaginal and rectal walls or hysterectomies.[82,85,86]

Carcinomas of the rectum, uterine cervix, and vagina are those most at risk of fistulization due to the site of disease.[87] When the fistula is in the lower part of the rectum, fecal incontinence due to involvement of anal sphincter may be present. Surgical treatment consists of a colon or urinary ostomy.[88*] Profuse hemorrhages can be controlled by embolization.[89]

Vescicovaginal fistulas are often the outcome of hysterectomies[90] and the two orifices are 1 cm above the trigone for the bladder and in the anterior wall for the vagina. These fistulas heal with the use of a catheter from 12 to 20 days with closed drainage to prevent infection.[91]

Ureterovaginal fistulas are often the result of radical hysterectomy via laparotomy. The risk of renal damage should always be taken into consideration and the areas most at risk of fistulization are the common iliac artery, uterine artery, and sacrouterine ligament. The treatment of the fistulas in these areas involves the use of the ureteral catheter of Finney, when possible, or eventually an ureteroneocystostomy may be indicated.[92]

Urethrocutaneous fistulas more frequently involve the prostatic urethra than the bulbar urethra. These fistulas are the result of a perineal prostatectomy and there is often a concomitant prostatic abscess. The cutaneous orifice is usually central and in a pre-anal area. The urethral orifice is located above the urogenital diaphragm and may reach the bladder.[93] Urethrorectal fistulas are often associated with carcinoma of the rectum, prostate and bladder with concomitant abscess. The rectal orifice is suprasphinteric, concealed behind a mucosal fold or in the Morgagni cyst. The urethral orifice is situated in the prostatic urethra.[93]

Vescicocutaneous fistulas are rarer and are usually related to lesions of the bladder fundus on the laparotomy wound. The cutaneous orifice is suprapubic. Treatment aimed at achieving continence is important in these fistulas.[94,95*]

CONCLUSIONS

In patients with cancer fistulas are complications that need consideration due to delays that can be caused in the treatment of cancer as well as in the worsening of patients' clinical and psychological status. Prior to planning conservative treatment rather than an invasive one, it is mandatory to assess patients' chances of survival as well as their quality of life. Considerable effort should be made by caregivers to manage all the different symptoms related to this complication in patients with cancer.

Key learning points

- A fistula is an abnormal communication between two digestive organs (internal fistula) or between the skin and a hollow organ (external fistula).

- In oncological patients, the most frequent causes of fistulas are related to cancer and/or treatments.

- The development of a fistula produces various complications: infections, electrolyte imbalance, dehydration, malnutrition, cutaneous lesions, bleeding, delay in oncological treatments, and psychosocial problems.

- In patients with advanced cancer, treatment will be conservative, whereas for a patient with a longer survival expectancy a more invasive treatment may be undertaken.

- Conservative treatment includes: skin care and local disinfection, control of local itching and pain, control of nutrition and electrolytes, control of infections, pouching of secretions, control of psychosocial distress. Nonconservative treatments are: surgical resection of fistula, surgical repair with corrective procedures or with myocutaneous flaps, colonic and/or urinary diversion, and endoscopic treatments with metallic stents.

REFERENCES

● 1 Doughty D. Principles of fistula and stoma management. In: Berger A, Portenoy RK, Weissman, DE, eds. *Principles and Practice of Supportive Oncology*. Philadelphia: Lippincott Raven, 1998: 285–94.

● 2 Benson DW, Fisher JE: Fistulas. In: Fischer JE, ed. *Total Parenteral Nutrition*, 2nd ed. Boston: Little, Brown & Co, 1991: 253–62.

✱ 3 Oneschuk D, Bruera E. Successful management of multiple enterocutaneous fistulas in a patient with metastatic colon cancer. *J Pain Symptom Manage* 1997; **14**: 121–4.

4 Allgaier HP, Schwacha H, Technau K, Blum HE. Fatal esophagoaortic fistula after placement of a self-expanding metal stent in a patient with esophageal carcinoma. *N Engl J Med* 1997; **337**: 1778.

5 Bonomi P, Faber LP, Warren W, *et al.* Postoperative bronchopulmonary complications in stage III lung cancer patients treated with preoperative paclitaxel-containing chemotherapy and concurrent radiation. *Semin Oncol* 1997; **24**(4 Suppl 12): S123–S129.

6 Bubenik O, Lopez MJ, Greco AO, *et al.* Gastrosplenic fistula following successful chemotherapy for disseminated histiocytic lymphoma. *Cancer* 1983; **52**: 994–6.

7 De Villa VH, Calvo FA, Bilbao JI, *et al.* Arteriodigestive fistula: a complication associated with intraoperative and external beam radiotherapy following surgery for gastric cancer. *J Surg Oncol* 1992; **49**: 52–7.

8 Gabrail NY, Harrison BR, Sunwoo YC. Chemo-irradiation induced aortoesophageal fistula. *J Surg Oncol* 1991; **48**: 213–15.

9 Hiltunen KM, Airo I, Mattila J, Helve O. Massively bleeding gastrosplenic fistula following cytostatic chemotherapy of a malignant lymphoma. *J Clin Gastroenterol* 1991; **13**: 478–81.

10 Kernstine KH, Kryjeski SR, Hall LJ, *et al.* Gastroduodenal artery-duodenal fistula: a complication of continuous floxuridine (FUDR) infusion into the gastroduodenal artery. *J Surg Oncol* 1990; **45**: 59–62.

11 Luketich JD, Westkaemper J, Sommers KE, *et al.* Bronchoesophagopleural fistula after photodynamic therapy for malignant mesothelioma. *Ann Thorac Surg* 1996; **62**: 283–4.

12 Noda M, Kusunoki M, Yanagai H, *et al.* Hepatic artery-biliary fistula during infusion chemotherapy. *Hepatogastroenterology* 1996; **43**: 1387–9.

13 Schowengerdt CG. Tracheoesophageal fistula caused by a self-expanding esophageal stent. *Ann Thorac Surg* 1999, **67**: 830–1.

14 Stein ME, Bernstein Z, Drumea K, *et al.* Intra-abdominal abscess and tumor-enteric fistula formation: an unusual complication of chemotherapy for advanced testicular choriocarcinoma. *Ann Oncol* 1996; **7**: 536–7.

15 Wakefield T, Eckhauser F, Strodel W, Knol J. Colocutaneous fistula complicating Tenckhoff catheter placement for intraperitoneal chemotherapy. *J Surg Oncol* 1984; **27**: 205–7.

16 Yamazaki T, Sakai Y, Hatakeyama K, Hoshiyama Y. Colocutaneous fistula after percutaneous endoscopic gastrostomy in a remnant stomach. *Surg Endosc* 1999; **13**: 280–2.

◆ 17 Campos AC, Meguid MM, Coelho JC. Factors influencing outcome in patients with gastrointestinal fistula. *Surg Clin N Am* 1996; **76**: 1191–98.

◆ 18 Berry SM and Fischer JE. Classification and pathophysiology of enterocutaneous fistulas. *Surg Clin North Am* 1996; **76**: 1009–18.

19 Amodeo C, Caglia P, Gandolfo L, *et al.* Role of nutritional support in the treatment of enteric fistulas. *Chir Ital* 2002; **54**: 379–83.

◆ 20 Dudrick SJ, Maharaj AR, McKelvey AA. Artificial nutritional support in patients with gastrointestinal fistulas. *World J Surg* 1999; **23**: 570–6.

✱ 21 Mercadante S. Treatment of diarrhoea due to enterocolic fistula with octreotide in a terminal cancer patient. *Palliat Med* 1992; **6**: 257–9.

22 Spiliotis J, Briand D, Gouttebel MC, *et al.* Treatment of fistulas of the gastrointestinal tract with total parenteral nutrition and octreotide in patients with carcinoma. *Surg Gynecol Obstet* 1993; **176**: 575–80.

23 Ahmed HF, Hussain MA, Grant CE, Wadleigh RG. Closure of tracheoesophageal fistulas with chemotherapy and radiotherapy. *Am J Clin Oncol* 1998; **21**: 177–9.

24 Russo P, Saldana EF, Yu S, *et al.* Myocutaneous flaps in genitourinary oncology. *J Urol* 1994; **151**: 920–4.

◆ 25 Reed MF, Mathisen DJ. Tracheoesophageal fistula. *Chest Surg Clin North Am* 2003; **13**: 271–89.

◆ 26   Chauhan SS, Long JD. Management of tracheoesophageal fistulas in adults. *Curr Treat Options Gastroenterol* 2004; **7**: 31–40.

27   Tse DG, Summers A, Sanger JR, Haasler GB. Surgical treatment of tracheomediastinal fistula from recurrent Hodgkin's lymphoma. *Ann Thorac Surg* 1999; **67**: 832–4.

◆ 28   Fernando HC, Benfield JR. Surgical management and treatment of esophageal fistula. *Surg Clin North Am* 1996; **76**: 1123–35.

29   Raijman I, Siddique I, Ajani J, Lynch P. Palliation of malignant dysphagia and fistulae with coated expandable metal stents: experience with 101 patients. *Gastrointest Endosc* 1998; **48**: 172–9.

30   Saxon RR, Morrison KE, Lakin PC, et al. Malignant esophageal obstruction and esophagorespiratory fistula: palliation with a polyethylene-covered Z-stent. *Radiology* 1997; **202**: 394–404.

31   Miwa K, Mitsuoka M, Tayama K, et al. Successful airway stenting using silicone prosthesis for esophagobronchial fistula. *Chest* 2002; **122**:1485–7.

● 32   Chung MA, Wanebo HJ. Surgical management and treatment of gastric and duodenal fistulas. *Surg Clin North Am* 1996; **76**: 1137–45.

✱ 33   Kuvshinoff BW, Brodish RJ, McFadden DW, Fischer JE. Serum transferrin as a prognostic indicator of spontaneous closure and mortality in gastrointestinal cutaneous fistulas. *Ann Surg* 1993; **217**: 615–22.

◆ 34   Falconi M, Pederzoli P. The relevance of gastrointestinal fistulae in clinical practice: a review. *Gut* 2001; **49**(Suppl 4): 2–10.

● 35   Meguid MM, Campos AC. Nutritional management of patients with gastrointestinal fistulas. *Surg Clin North Am* 1996; **76**: 1035–80.

◆ 36   Rolandelli R, Roslyn JJ. Surgical management and treatment of sepsis associated with gastrointestinal fistulas. *Surg Clin North Am* 1996; **76**: 1111–22.

✱ 37   Shand A, Reading S, Ewing J, et al. Palliation of malignant gastrocolic fistula by endoscopic human fibrin sealant injection. *Eur J Gastroenterol Hepatol* 1997; **9**: 1009–111.

38   Siewert JR, Bottcher K, Stein HJ, et al. Problem of proximal third gastric carcinoma. *World J Surg* 1995; **19**: 523–31.

● 39   Kozarek RA, Traverso LW. Pancreatic fistulas: etiology, consequences, and treatment. *Gastroenterologist* 1996; **4**: 238–44.

◆ 40   Ridgeway MG, Stabile BE. Surgical management and treatment of pancreatic fistulas. *Surg Clin North Am* 1996; **76**: 1159–73.

41   Martineau P, Shwed JA, Denis R. Is octreotide a new hope for enterocutaneous and external pancreatic fistulas closure? *Am J Surg* 1996; **172**: 386–95.

42   Niv Y, Charash B, Sperber AD, Oren M. Effect of octreotide on gastrostomy, duodenostomy, and cholecystostomy effluents: a physiologic study of fluid and electrolyte balance. *Am J Gastroenterol* 1997; **92**: 2107–11.

43   Berberat PO, Friess H, Uhl W, Buchler MW. The role of octreotide in the prevention of complications following pancreatic resection. *Digestion* 1999; **60**(Suppl 2): 15–22.

44   Barnett SP, Hodul PJ, Creech S, et al. Octreotide does not prevent postoperative pancreatic fistula or mortality following pancreaticoduodenectomy. *Am Surg* 2004; **70**: 222–6.

45   Shibuya T, Shioya T, Kokuma M, et al. Cure of intractable pancreatic fistula by subcutaneous fistulojejunostomy. *J Gastroenterol* 2004; **39**: 162–7.

◆ 46   Chamberlain RS, Kaufman HL, Danforth DN. Enterocutaneous fistula in cancer patients: etiology, management, outcome, and impact on further treatment. *Am Surg* 1998; **64**: 1204–11.

47   Correoso LJ, Mehta R. Subcutaneous emphysema: an uncommon presentation of enterocutaneous fistula. *Am J Hosp Palliat Care* 2003; **20**: 462–4.

◆ 48   Dorta G. Role of octreotide and somatostatin in the treatment of intestinal fistulae. *Digestion* 1999; **60**(Suppl 2): 53–6.

✱ 49   Sancho JJ, Di Costanzo J, Nubiola P, et al. Randomized double-blind placebo-controlled trial of early octreotide in patients with postoperative enterocutaneous fistula. *Br J Surg* 1995; **82**: 638–41.

50   D'Harcour JB, Boverie JH, Dondelinger RF. Percutaneous management of enterocutaneous fistulas. *AJR Am J Roentgen* 1996; **167**: 33–8.

51   Bessoud B, Doenz F, Qanadli SD, et al. Enterobiliary fistula after radiofrequency ablation of liver metastases. *J Vasc Interv Radiol* 2003; **14**: 1581–4.

◆ 52   Lavery IC. Colonic fistulas. *Surg Clin North Am* 1996; **76**: 1183–90.

53   Grunshaw ND, Ball CS. Palliative treatment of an enterorectal fistula with a covered metallic stent. *Cardiovasc Intervent Radiol* 2001; **24**: 438–40.

54   Levenback C, Gershenson DM, McGehee R, et al. Enterovesical fistula following radiotherapy for gynecologic cancer. *Gynecol Oncol* 1994; **52**: 296–300.

◆ 55   Redaelli de Zinis LO, Ferrari L, Tomenzoli D, et al. Postlaringectomy pharyngocutaneous fistula: Incidence, predisposing factors, and therapy. *Head Neck* 1999; **21**: 131–8.

● 56   Makitie AA, Irish J, Gullane PJ. Pharyngocutaneous fistula. *Curr Opin Otolaryngol Head Neck* Surg. 2003; **11**: 78–84.

57   Smith TJ, Burrage KJ, Ganguly P, et al. Prevention of postlaryngectomy pharyngocutaneous fistula: the Memorial University experience. *J Otolaryngol* 2003; **32**: 222–5.

58   Chambers PA, Worrall SF. Closure of large orocutaneous fistulas in end-stage malignant disease. *Br J Oral Maxillofac Surg* 1994; **32**: 314–15.

◆ 59   Drezner DA, Cantrell H. Surgical management of tracheocutaneous fistula. *Ear Nose Throat J* 1998; **77**: 534–7.

◆ 60   Soylu L, Kiroglu M, Aydogan B. Pharyngocutaneous fistula following laryngectomy. *Head Neck* 1998; **20**: 22–5.

61   Weingrad DN, Spiro RH. Complications after laryngectomy. *Am J Surg* 1983; **146**: 517–20.

62   Viani L, Stell PM, Dalby JE. Recurrence after radiotherapy for glottic carcinoma. *Cancer* 1991; **67**: 577–84.

63   Grau C, Johansen LV, Hansen HS, et al. Salvage laryngectomy and pharyngocutaneous fistulae after primary radiotherapy for head and neck cancer: *Head Neck* 2003; **25**: 711–16.

64   McCombe AW, Jones AS. Radiotherapy and complications of laryngectomy. *J Laryngol Otol* 1993; **107**: 130–2.

65   Cody DT, Funk GF, Wagner D, et al. The use of granulocyte colony stimulating factor to promote wound healing in a neutropenic patient after head and neck surgery. *Head Neck* 1999; **21**: 172–5.

66   Cavanaugh K, Park A. Postparotidectomy fistula: a different treatment for an old problem. *Intern J Ped Otorhinolaryngol* 1999; **47**: 265–8.

67   Aksungur EH, Apaydin D, Gonlusen G, et al. A case of oroantral fistula secondary to malignant fibrous histiocytoma. *Eur J Radiol* 1994; **18**: 212–13.

68 De Gier HH, Balm AJ, Bruning PF, *et al*. Systematic approach to the treatment of chylous leakage after neck dissection. *Head Neck* 1996; **18**: 347–51.

69 Hollaus PH, Lax F, el-Nashef BB, *et al*. Natural history of bronchopleural fistula after pneumonectomy: a review of 96 cases. *Ann Thorac Surg* 1997; **63**: 1391–6.

● 70 Yano T, Yokoyama H, Fukuyama Y, *et al*. The current status of postoperative complications and risk factors after a pulmonary resection for primary lung cancer. A multivariate analysis. *Eur J Cardiothorac Surg* 1997; **11**: 445–9.

71 Haraguchi S, Koizumi K, Gomibuchi M, *et al*. Analysis of risk factors for development of bronchopleural fistula after pneumonectomy for lung cancer. *Nippon Kyobu Geka Gakkai Zasshi* 1996; **44**: 1835–9.

72 Butt A, Pankey GA, Figueroa JE. A draining chest wall abscess. *Infect Med* 1997; **14**: 935–8.

73 Raja S, Rice TW, Neumann DR, *et al*. Scintigraphic detection of post-pneumonectomy bronchopleural fistulae. *Eur J Nucl Med* 1999; **26**: 215–19.

74 Hollaus PH, Lax F, Janakiev D, *et al*. Endoscopic treatment of postoperative bronchopleural fistula: experience with 45 cases. *Ann Thorac Surg* 1998; **66**: 923–7.

◆ 75 Varoli F, Roviaro G, Grignani F, *et al*. Endoscopic treatment of bronchopleural fistulas. *Ann Thorac Surg* 1998; **65**: 807–9.

◆ 76 Bladou F, Houvenaeghel G, Delpero JR, Guerinel G. Incidence and management of major urinary complications after pelvic exenteration for gynecological malignancies. *J Surg Oncol* 1995; **58**: 91–6.

77 Magrina JF. Complications of irradiation and radical surgery for gynecologic malignancies. *Obstet Gynecol Surg* 1993; **48**: 571–5.

78 Tabakov ID, Slavchev BN. Large post-hysterectomy and post-radiation vesicovaginal fistulas: repair by ileocystoplasty. *J Urol* 2004; **171**: 272–4.

● 79 Bahadursingh AM, Longo WE. Colovaginal fistulas. Etiology and management. *J Reprod Med* 2003; **48**: 489–95.

80 Blomlie V, Rofstad EK, Trope C, Lien HH. Critical soft tissues of the female pelvis: serial MR imaging before, during and after radiation therapy. *Radiology* 1997; **203**: 391–7.

● 81 Larsen A, Bjerklund Johansen TE, Solheim BM, Urnes T. Diagnosis and treatment of enterovesical fistula. *Eur Urol* 1996; **29**: 318–21.

82 Lee BH, Choe DH, Lee HJ, *et al*. Device for occlusion of rectovaginal fistula: clinical trials. *Radiology* 1997; **203**: 65–9.

83 Memon MA, Zieg DA, Neal PM. Vesicouterine fistula twenty years following brachytherapy for cervical cancer. *Scand J Urol Nephrol* 1998; **32**: 293–5.

◆ 84 Saclarides TJ. Rectovaginal fistula. *Surg Clin North Am* 2002; **82**: 1261–72.

◆ 85 Munoz M, Nelson H, Harrington J, *et al*. Management of acquired rectourinary fistulas: outcome according to cause. *Dis Colon Rectum* 1998; **41**: 1230–8.

86 Pesce F, Righetti R, Rubilotta E, Artibani W. Vesico-crural and vesicorectal fistulas 13 years after radiotherapy for prostate cancer. *J Urol* 2002; **168**: 2118–19.

◆ 87 Rinnovati A, Milli I, Francalanci R. Entero-vesical fistulae in surgical practice. *Minerva Urol Nefrol* 2002; **54**: 45–9.

88 Fengler SA, Abcarian H. The York Mason approach to repair of iatrogenic rectourinary fistulae. *Am J Surg* 1997; **173**: 213–17.

89 Dushnitsky T, Ziv Y, Peer A, Halevy A. Embolization – an optional treatment for intractable hemorrhage from a malignant rectovaginal fistula: report of a case. *Dis Colon Rectum* 1999; **42**: 271–3.

90 Langkilde NC, Pless TK, Lundbeck F, Nerstrom B. Surgical repair of vesicovaginal fistulae – a ten-year retrospective study. *Scand J Urol Nephrol* 1999; **33**: 100–3.

91 Nesrallah LJ, Srougi M, Gittes RF. The O'Conor technique: the gold standard for supratrigonal vesicovaginal fistula repair. *J Urol* 1999; **161**: 566–8.

◆ 92 Emmert C, Kohler U. Management of genital fistulas in patients with cervical cancer. *Arch Gynecol Obstet* 1996; **259**: 19–24.

93 Harpster LE, Rommel FM, Sieber PR, *et al*. The incidence and management of rectal injury associated with radical prostatectomy in a community based urology practice. *J Urol* 1995; **154**: 1435–8.

● 94 Turner-Warwick R. Urinary fistulae in the female. In: Walsh PC, Gittes RF, Perlmutter AD, Stanley TA, eds. *Campbell's Urology*, 5th ed. Philadelphia: WB Saunders, 1986: 2718–38.

◆ 95 Davies Q, Luesley DM. Urological problems and the treatment of gynecological cancer. *Curr Opin Obstet Gynecol* 1998; **10**: 401–3.

83

Lymphedema

YING GUO, BENEDICT KONZEN

INCIDENCE AND CLASSIFICATION OF LYMPHEDEMA

Lymphedema is a chronic, progressive, incurable condition, affecting at least 3 million Americans, and 140–250 million patients worldwide. Filariasis, a parasitic infestation is the most common cause. Lymphedema is an accumulation of lymphatic fluid in the interstitial tissue that causes swelling, most often in the upper or lower extremity(ies), and occasionally in face, neck, trunk, and external genitalia. Lymphedema negatively affects the activities of daily living, vocational, domestic, psychosocial, sexual lives, and quality of life of patients.[1*,2,3*,4*,5*] In addition, it puts patients at increased risk for life-threatening infections and malignancies.[6] Lymphedema is classified as primary and secondary lymphedema.

Primary lymphedema

Primary lymphedema is caused by a congenital abnormality or dysfunction in the lymphatic system and can be further classified according to age of onset. Primary lymphedema is rare, affecting 1.15 per 100 000 younger than 20 years of age.[7] The congenital form is detected at birth or in the first year of life and may either be sporadic or familial. The onset of lymphedema praecox is between the ages of 1 and 35 years. The onset of lymphedema tarda occurs after 35 years of age.

Alternatively, primary lymphedema can be classified according to the abnormality found in the lymphatics. Thus, it may be aplastic, hypoplastic, or hyperplastic. These terms suggest an abnormality in the development of the lymphatic system. Whereas this is true for congenital lymphedema, cases of later-onset primary lymphedema might be due to an acquired abnormality.

Secondary lymphedema

Secondary lymphedema is edema that occurs due to a reduction in lymph flow by an acquired cause. The causes of secondary lymphedema include trauma, recurrent infection, and malignancy and its treatment (surgery, radiation). In the developed world, the most common cause of secondary lymphedema is malignancy (including that resulting from cancer treatment). Lymphedema is common in the developing world secondary to infection with the parasitic nematode *Wucheria bancrofti* (otherwise known as filariasis), making this the most common cause of lymphedema worldwide.[8] Cancer-related lymphedema usually occurs at proximal limb segments (i.e. lymph nodes) due to infection, ligation, malignancy, scar tissue, and radiation therapy.[9] The pelvic and inguinal nodes in the lower extremities and the axillary nodes of the upper extremities are the primary sites of obstruction.

This chapter will be emphasizing on secondary lymphedema related to cancer and its treatment, which is frequently overlooked. The reported incidence of lymphedema secondary to postmastectomy radiotherapy ranges from 2.4 percent to 54 percent.[10*,11*,12–17] The incidence of lower limb lymphedema secondary to gynecological cancer has been reported to be 18 percent.[18*] Lymphedema is uncommon from cancer of the abdominal and pelvic urological organs and its treatment, because of the rich anastomotic networks and bilateral lymphatic drainage from the midline organs. In patients with penile carcinomas, lymph node metastasis is reported in up to 35 percent[19] and following treatment by groin node dissection, lymphedema developed in 50–100 percent of patients.[19,20] The incidence and prevalence of lymphedema in other urological cancers remains largely unknown.[21]

In the pre–prostatic-specific antigen era, chronic lymphedema was reported as a complication of bilateral pelvic lymphadenectomy for prostate cancer in 15 of 82 patients (18 percent), 10 of whom had additional radiotherapy.[22] Greskovich *et al.* reported transient lymphedema in 2 of 65 patients who underwent staging lymphadenectomy prior to radiotherapy.[23]

PATHOPHYSIOLOGY

Lymphedema occurs when lymphatic fluid load exceeds the lymphatic transport capacity and an abnormal amount of protein-rich fluid collects in the tissues of the affected area. In most cases, the transport capacity is impaired, but in patients with venous insufficiency, the lymphatic load is increased. The lymphatic drainage system is separate from the general circulatory system and is the conduit for returning tissue fluids to the circulation.[24] The superficial lymphatic system begins with initial lymphatics, which are formed from one-layer endothelial cells, overlapping each other but not forming a continuous connection. Each of the cells is attached to the surrounding tissue by anchoring filaments. When there is a change in tissue pressure, caused by arterial pulsation, muscle contraction, or respiration, or when the skin is lightly stretched, the anchoring filaments pull on the cells of the initial lymphatics. Because of this, the gap between the cells opens, and fluid drains into the vessels.[25] Initial lymphatics combine to form larger vessels called precollectors and collectors, which in turn lead to the lymph nodes in the axillary and inguinal regions. The collector vessels of the lymphatic system contain smooth muscle and valves to regulate flow.[25] The regional lymph nodes drain fluid from the ipsilateral limb and torso quadrant. Deep lymph nodes for visceral drainage are located along major arteries. Major somatic drainage areas are connected via subcutaneous collateral channels, both anteriorly and posteriorly. Lymph drains from the lower limbs into the lumbar lymphatic trunk, which joins the intestinal lymphatic trunk and cisterna chyli to form the thoracic duct. Lymph returns to the blood circulation at the venous angles, which are formed by the junctures of the internal jugular and subclavian veins. Most of the lymph in the body drains via the thoracic duct, which enters the circulation at the left venous angle. Only the right upper torso, arm, face, and neck drain into circulation on the right side via the right lymphatic duct, which empties into the right subclavian vein.[24] An important function of the lymphatic system is the prevention of infection. The lymphatic system is responsible for picking up excess interstitial water and protein as well as other cells, including bacteria, which can enter the tissue through small cuts or breaks in the skin. Bacteria and other antigens are transported by the lymphatic system from the interstitium to lymphocytes in the lymph nodes, where an immune response may be initiated. Physiologically, most of the interstitial fluid generated daily (18 L) arises from the blood capillaries; 14–16 L subsequently returns directly to the venous circulation. The remaining 10–20 percent, approximately 2 L/day, passes through the lymphatic transport.

Histologically, the reparative process in the traumatized lymphatic vessels after mastectomy demonstrates fibrosis and an accompanying reduction in vessel diameter. With the subsequent ligation or interruption in lymph channels and lymphadenectomy, the body attempts a regenerative process with the formation of collateral circulation. Radiation treatment may lead to fibrosis. Non-irradiated lymph nodes develop compensatory dilated sinuses to handle lymph volume. This may be associated anatomically with lymph node hyperplasia. If the lymphatic system fails locally, protein subsequently accumulates in the interstitium. If no intervention occurs at this point, fibrosclerosis will follow along with inflammation, scarring, and loss of regional lymphatic integrity.[26]

The frequency with which lymphedema occurs after cancer therapy depends on multiple factors (Box 83.1).

Box 83.1 Factors affecting development of cancer-related lymphedema

Extent of lymphatic system damage

- Recurrence of tumor
- Lymph node dissection
- Radiation

Inherent compensatory ability of the lymphatic system

- Age
- Obesity
- Infection
- Heart failure
- Venous insufficiency
- Other factors that affect lymph load

Extent of lymphatic system damage

In a study by Kiel and Rademacher in 1996, in the absence of lymph node dissection, the incidence of edema after breast cancer treatment was 21 percent; with 11–15 nodes removed, edema was present in 27 percent; with more than 15 lymph nodes removed it was 44 percent.[27] Lymphatics have excellent regenerative capabilities. Even after radical lymph node excision for malignancy, lymphedema does not always happen. When it does occur, it is often a late complication. The reasons for this late development are uncertain, but gradual failure of distal lymphatics, which have to 'pump' lymph at a greater pressure through damaged proximal ducts, has been postulated.

The transected lymphatics will regenerate after node clearance procedures. If combined with radiotherapy, however, the risk of lymphedema is higher, as fibrous scarring reduces regrowth of ducts. In approximately 10 percent of patients with cancer, the onset of lymphedema heralds local recurrence of tumor or is the result of metastases.[26]

Inherent compensatory ability of the lymphatic system

A patient's weight and age may affect the development of lymphedema. When compared with their younger counterparts, breast cancer patients older than 55 were shown to have an increased lymphedema risk (14 percent vs. 22 percent, respectively).[27,28] Comorbidities, such as heart failure, renal insufficiency, and venous insufficiency may contribute to the onset and progression of lymphedema. Recurrent cellulitis can further compromise the fluid return. Any situation that causes an increase in lymphatic load can predispose patients to development or worsening of lymphedema. The onset of lymphedema may be provoked in a variety of common situations that occur on a daily basis: muscle fatigue resulting from overuse; vasodilatation following exposure heat; local trauma; vigorous massage; constriction or a 'tourniquet effect', which causes swelling distal to that point; or sustained dependency of the limb. Other situations that may increase lymphatic load include airplane flights and higher altitudes; these situations involve decreased atmospheric pressure and may result in increased filtration into the tissue from the blood capillaries.

COMMON COMPLICATIONS

Lymph fluid reflux

Overdistended lymph vessels cause valvular insufficiency and retrograde flow, and patients present with blister like formation on the surface of the skin, called lymphatic cysts. Lymphatic cysts are usually found in axillary, cubital, genital, and popliteal areas, and easily break open and lead to infection or fistulas. Treatment should include prevention of infection.

Musculoskeletal complications

Lymphedema can lead to musculoskeletal pain, nerve compression, and decreased range of motion. Swelling and pain can interfere with mobility and influence the affected patient's perception of themselves.[1*]

Infection

Bacterial and fungal infections are common in stage 2 and 3 (see below) lymphedema. Clinical signs and symptoms of cellulitis (erysipelas) are fever, erythema, warmth, and tenderness. Patients should be treated with either oral or intravenous antibiotics. In general, an antibiotic needs to cover the normal skin flora (i.e. Gram-positive cocci) and have good skin penetration. Intravenous antibiotics are considered when there is more significant local or systemic infection. Some patients develop chronic infections that may necessitate ongoing antibiotic therapy. Fungal infections cause skin itching, crusting, maceration between the toes, and typical fungal nail changes. Systemic or local antifungal treatment can be used. Recurrence of infection/inflammation indicates reduced local immunity.[29] It is reasonable to emphasize the importance of lymphedema limb care.[30] Decongestive lymphatic therapy is contraindicated until the infection subsides.

Hyperkeratosis

Hyperkeratosis presents as thickening of skin and wartlike papillomas. Care must be taken to avoid skin breakdown and infection.

Malignancies

Lymphangiosarcoma is a rare late complication of lymphedema,[31] also described as Stewart–Treves syndrome[32] and Milroy disease.[33] In patients with longstanding lymphedema and cellulitis that does not respond to systemic antibiotics, physicians should consider a skin biopsy. Treatment is primarily radiotherapy, with surgery reserved for patients with discrete, nonmetastatic disease.

DIAGNOSIS

History and physical examination (Box 83.2)

The history should include full medical history, all anticancer therapies, past surgeries, postoperative complications, radiation treatment, the time interval from radiation or surgery to the onset of symptoms, and intervening variables in the presence or severity of symptoms. History of trauma or infection should be determined, and information concerning current medications elicited, which may be important. Quality and behavior of edema (fluctuation with position, progression over time) and associated symptoms should be assessed. Edema is not detectable clinically until the interstitial volume exceeds 30 percent above normal. Post-mastectomy and radiation lymphedema initially presents as mild edema in the hand or forearm, often in the dorsal epicondylar region (Fig. 83.1). Other complaints related to lymphedema are heaviness or fullness related to the weight of the limb, skin feeling tight, decreased flexibility in the hand, wrist or ankle, difficulty fitting into clothing in one specific area, or ring/wristwatch/bracelet tightness.

Box 83.2 Clinical features of lymphedema

History

- Medical history (anticancer therapies, past operations, postoperative complications, radiation treatment)

- Edema (onset, fluctuation, progression)

- Associated symptoms

- Infection and trauma

- Function

- Social history

- Psychological impact

Physical examination

- Edema: skin texture, color, infection, scar; volume

- Neurological examination

- Range of motion

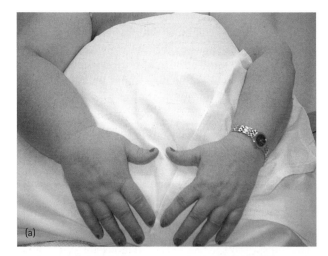

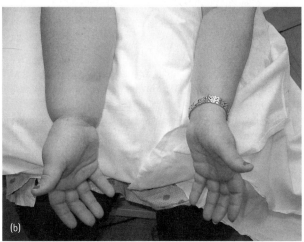

Figure 83.1 *(a,b) Right upper extremity lymphedema.*

Associated clinical features of lower limb lymphedema include tightness of or inability to wear shoes, itching of the legs or toes, burning sensation in the legs, sleep disturbances and loss of hair. Ambulation is affected because of the limb size and weight, causing an inability to wear clothing. Impact on activities of daily living, hobbies, work, and psychological status of the patient needs to be assessed as well.

On examination, the affected limb will be swollen with enhanced skin creases, hyperkeratosis, and papillomatosis. Lymphedema is traditionally described as non-pitting, but in early cases pitting may be present. The Stemmer sign – inability to pinch the skin at the base of the second toe due to the thickened skin folds – is a useful clinical sign.[34] Cutaneous fungal or bacterial infections are not unusual in patients with lymphatic obstruction. Skin folds should be frequently inspected for ulcers and infections. A neurological examination should be conducted for possible nerve entrapment and plexus involvement, and range of motion of different joints also needs to be assessed. In established cases of lymphedema, the clinical features are diagnostic and diagnostic investigations are not required.

Skin condition and measurement of volume

The initial assessment of lymphedema and follow-up of the response to treatment should include the measurement of volume and assessment of skin condition.[35] The most commonly used assessment tool involves measuring the contralateral limb circumference at several points along the limb. However, when the disease affects both sides, this type of comparison may not be accurate.[36*] Multiple transverse tapes, placed at 4 cm intervals in a device, can be used to measure the circumference accurately; this is a simple and convenient method.[37] Volume can be calculated from surface measurements.[38] Truncal swelling can be measured with skinfold calipers.

Water displacement volumetry, although no longer commonly used, measures limb volume[35] and is more accurate than the calculation of leg volume from circumferential measurements with a tape measure.[35] The optoelectronic Perometer, a device designed for the measurement of limb volume, has been validated as a reliable and convenient tool for the measurement of limb volume[39] (Fig. 83.2). Bioelectrical impedance has been used successfully for the evaluation of swelling in patients with postmastectomy lymphedema[40] and lower extremity lymphedema.[41*]

Skin condition can be measured by recording deformation of tissue by a mass (tonometry) and the step compression method. In lymphedema, the tissue tonicity (degree of tissue resistance to mechanical compression) is either higher or lower compared with the nonedematous leg.[35]

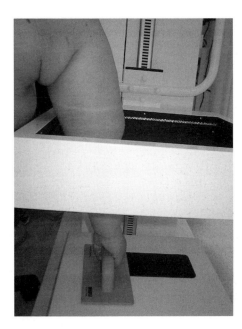

Figure 83.2 *Measurement of limb volume with the Perometer.*

Measurement of tissue tonometry is more useful in assessing the response to treatment than in the initial assessment of disease.

Imaging studies

Lymphangioscintigraphy (LAS) permits high-resolution imaging of peripheral lymphatic vessels and provides insight into lymph flow dynamics. It is indispensable for patients with known or suspected lymphatic circulatory disorders in confirming the diagnosis and delineating the pathogenesis and evolution of lymphedema. In addition, LAS helps evaluate lymphatic truncal anatomy and radiotracer transport. It is also useful in preoperative evaluation, especially for microvascular anastomoses. The procedure involves intradermal injection of a radioactive tracer and does not adversely affect the lymphatic vascular endothelium. Using a combination of mobile scanners integrated with computer imaging, lymphatic vessels and nodes are visualized, and the speed of lymph node uptake and the rate of lymph transport can be measured.[42] Patients with a provisional diagnosis of peripheral lymphatic dysfunction or idiopathic edema should undergo diagnostic LAS to verify diagnostic accuracy, pinpoint the specific abnormality, and help guide subsequent therapy.[43] Conventional oil-contrast lymphography is no longer commonly used, because it is associated with complications such as allergic and inflammatory reactions, pulmonary embolism and damage to the endothelial lining of the lymphatic vessel.

Magnetic resonance imaging and computed tomography complements LAS in monitoring the progression of cancer. Ultrasonography has proved useful in the setting of filariasis and differential diagnosis of venous obstruction.

Dual X-ray absorptiometry or bi-photonic absorptiometry is useful in assessing the chemical component of limb swelling (percentage of fat, water, and lean mass).[44]

DIFFERENTIAL DIAGNOSIS

Lipedema

The clinical features of lipedema (also known as lipomatosis of the leg) include early age of onset, female exclusivity, and positive family history in some patients.[45,46] The clinical signs include elastic symmetrical enlargement of both legs with sparing of the feet.

Deep vein thrombosis and chronic venous disease

Deep vein thrombosis (DVT) results in obstruction to venous flow. The clinical picture is thus one of a swollen, warm, and tender extremity. The resulting edema is pitting in nature and is usually much softer than in established lymphedema. Often, there are underlying risk factors, such as recent surgery or immobility, malignancy, a preceding long flight, or thrombophilia. The diagnosis is confirmed with duplex scanning or venography, and treatment is with anticoagulation. Chronic venous stasis results in hyperpigmentation, and varicose veins, and in severe cases, venous ulceration may be more difficult to differentiate from lymphedema. Untreated venous insufficiency can progress to a combined venous/lymphatic disorder which is treated in the same way as lymphedema.

Heart failure or renal failure

These conditions need appropriate medical management.[47]

STAGING OF LYMPHEDEMA

Generally, lymphedema is staged using a three-stage scale. However, an increasing number of workers are recognizing stage 0. In this stage, swelling is not evident, despite alteration in lymph transport. In stage 1, there is early accumulation of a high-protein–laden fluid (vs. venous edema) that subsides with limb elevation. Pitting of the extremity may be present. In stage 2, limb elevation alone rarely reduces tissue swelling and pitting is present. In late stage 2, fibrosis is present and there may or may not be pitting of the extremity. Stage 3 is characterized by lymphostatic elephantiasis. Pitting is absent and the trophic skin is characteristically acanthotic with warty overgrowth (Table 83.1).[34] The severity of unilateral lymphedema in each stage can be further assessed by the grading system given in Table 83.2.

Table 83.1 *Staging of lymphedema*

Stage	Edema	Elevation helps	Pitting	Fibrosis	Acanthosis
0	−	+	−	−	−
1	+	+	±	−	−
2 (early)	+	±	+	−	−
2 (late)	+	−	±	+	−
3	+	−	−	+	+

+, present; −, absent.

Table 83.2 *Grading of lymphedema based on severity*

Severity of lymphedema	Volume increase (%)
Minimal	<20
Moderate	20–40
Severe	>40

TREATMENT

As with most chronic problems, the responsibility for managing lymphedema lies with the patient. Education about the etiology of lymphedema and principles of management is the first and most important part of patient care. Management of this condition by decongesting the reduced lymphatic pathways to reduce the size of the limb and preventing infection, encouraging the development of collateral drainage routes, and stimulating the function of remaining patent routes, will result in longlasting lymphedema control. In 1995, the International Society of Lymphology Executive Committee developed a consensus document that offered an integrated view of the management of lymphedema.[48] However, controversy still exists about the efficacy and application of treatment approaches in different situations.

The most commonly used method is called decongestive lymphatic therapy (DLT) (or combined physical therapy [CPT], or complete/complex decongestive therapy [CDT], or complex decongestive physiotherapy [CDP]) and involves a two-phase treatment program.[49] In the first phase, intensive every other day physical therapy visits are recommended for a course of 4–6 weeks, although daily treatment is more effective; these treatments usually include:

- manual lymph drainage (MLD) and teaching the patient about MLD
- multilayer bandaging
- care of the skin
- exercises to promote lymph drainage.

The goals of this phase are to reduce the size of the limb, and improve the texture and the health of the skin. Ko *et al.* used CDP in 299 patients with both upper and lower extremity lymphedema for 15.9 days.[50*] Lymphedema reduction averaged 59.1 percent after upper extremity CDP and 67.7 percent after lower extremity treatment. When followed up at 9 months, improvement was maintained in 86 percent of patients. At least 90 percent of the initial reduction was maintained. Incidence of infection also decreased by approximately 50 percent.[50*] Outcomes of different studies vary because of the skills of the treating therapists, patient compliance, exercise protocols, duration of DLT, number of treatments per week, etc.

In lymphedema that is the result of tumor-obstructing lymphatics DLT may be used palliatively. This treatment is usually conducted in conjunction with chemoradiation. In the past, controversy existed as to whether massage and mechanical compression would promote metastasis. In practice, disease is already present and the goal simply is palliation of morbid swelling.[42,50*,51,52]

In the second phase of treatment the patients are usually recommended to:

- wear strong compression hosiery to maintain the reduction in swelling
- carry out regular daily exercise
- perform regular MLD, where possible.

The goal of the second phase is to preserve and optimize the improvements made in the first phase. The role of weight control and regular exercises in the management of lymphedema is thought to be important.

Relative contraindications to DLT include significant congestive heart failure, acute deep vein thrombosis, acute or untreated infection or inflammation of the affected limb, and active malignancy.

Skin care

Skin care should include routine skin inspection (for ingrown toenails, cuticle integrity, abrasions, bruising, ulcerations, impaired circulation); use of skin emollients; avoidance of extremes in heat and cold including sun exposure. In the clinician's office or hospital setting, blood pressure measurements, venipuncture or injections should not be undertaken on the affected side. The patient is counseled on limiting excessive exercise and avoiding trauma to the affected region from clothing (brassiere, purse straps).

In the early pitting stage, many patients benefit from elevating the limb during the night, at or above relative to the heart level.

Manual lymphatic drainage

This is a therapeutic technique used to increase lymph flow. It consists of movement of the therapist's hands over the patient's skin and subcutaneous tissue. The pressure applied is very gentle, and the movements are slow to correspond with the slow lymphatic pulsations. The massage sequence begins at the center of the body and moves to the periphery, and from unaffected side to affected side. The rationale for this is that the lymph nodes must be emptied before they can receive more lymph from the periphery. Each maneuver is performed in a distal to proximal direction. Patients and also family members or friends can be trained in this gentle form of self-massage. Andersen *et al.* conclude from their study that MLD provided no extra benefit.[53**]

The use of massage (classic massage or effleurage) is not recommended, since it may be excessively vigorous and cause damage to the lymphatic vessels.

Exercise

When combining with nonelastic compression bandage, it has been hypothesized that the contraction of muscle against the elastic bandage provides increased subcutaneous tissue pressure and thus encourages movement of interstitial fluid into the lymphatic system.[54]

Compression bandages and garments

Wrapping the limb with low-stretch bandages in conjunction with padding and foam provides the ideal type of compression in patients with lymphedema. It allows a low resting pressure and a high working pressure during muscle contraction to facilitate lymphatic flow. The bandage accommodates the change of volume over time and provides 'custom-made' compression. The disadvantages of this technique are:

- it is difficult to apply
- it requires training
- it is cumbersome.

One study showed that compression bandaging prior to use of compression garments is more effective than compression garments alone.[55**] Once the extremity reaches its smallest achievable size, a customized low-stretch elastic compression garment can be fitted and used during normal activities. Compression garments provide gradient pressure ranging from 20 mm Hg to 60 mm Hg. Replacements are needed every 6 months. Proper fitting is necessary to avoid a tourniquet effect.[56,57*] Hornsby investigated the use of

hosiery on its own compared with control. Although this was a small study the results suggest that wearing a compression sleeve is beneficial and that the high dropout rate in the control group may have reflected the subjects' lack of progress.[58]

Contraindications include concurrent presence of arterial disease, allergy, ulceration or a painful post-phlebitic syndrome.

Pneumatic compression

Controversy exists regarding the use of pneumatic compression pumps. Some schools of thought that support the utilization of pumps generally suggest using relatively low pressures (40 mm Hg maximum distal pressure) as part of a comprehensive program.[59,60] Pressures greater than 50–60 mm Hg may cause injury to lymphatic vessels.[61] The extremity is placed into a long inflatable sleeve that is connected to a pump that inflates the sleeve to a predetermined pressure. External compression therapy is applied with a sequential gradient 'pump'. In between pump use, the extremity should be wrapped with elastic compression bandage or have temporary compression garments applied to reduce recurrence of lymph in the extremity. It may take months to obtain a demonstrable reduction in the size of the extremity.[62*]

Surgery

Controversy exists regarding surgical intervention in the treatment of lymphedema. Patients with severe lymphedema and minimal improvement with compression therapy may benefit from a lymph-reducing surgical procedure. The patient needs to be informed fully about the intended procedure: the risks; the possible impairment; and disability. Complications such as shunt failure, hypertrophic scarring, sensory loss, aggravation of edema distal to the resection, and gross deformity of the limb, have been reported in surgically treated patients.[63*]

Two types of procedure are available: excisional procedures (or debulking procedures) with or without skin grafting and drainage procedures (or microsurgical procedures). Excisional therapy involves removing a large section of skin and subcutaneous tissue down to the muscle fascia and reapproximating the wound edges. Problems associated with this procedure are in relation to wound healing. In addition, this method does not treat the underlying problem of lymphatic outflow obstruction. Excisional therapy with skin grafting involves completely degloving the overlying tissue on the affected extremity and split-thickness grafting directly onto the muscular bed. By removing all overlying lymphatic tissue within the dermal and subcutaneous space down to the muscle bed, lymphedema in the area of grafting is no longer a concern. The result is one of marked reduction in the size of the extremity, but any tissue distal to this is left with more exaggerated lymphedema than in the preoperative state. Skin grafting has a 5–10 percent incidence of failure. Frequent complications are protracted lymph leakage and poor healing.

A drainage procedure for lymphatic obstruction may be considered in patients with lymphatic obstruction at the level of the upper leg or more proximal extremity and for those who have short-segment obliteration of lymphatic channels.[64*] The procedure is contraindicated in patients with distal or obliterative disease and those with combined proximal and distal obliterative disease. The drainage procedure currently favored for the treatment of limited lymphatic obstruction is a surgical lymphovenous microvascular anastamosis.[65] Patients still need to wear compression garments for life. Liposuction combined with constant use of compression garment has been reported.[66*]

Drug therapy

Coumarin (5,6-benzo-α-pyrone, or 1,2-benzopyrone) and related drugs have been reported to reduce lymphedema, possibly through stimulation of proteolysis by tissue macrophages. In addition to findings that it decreases the pain and discomfort caused by lymphedema, coumarin has been reported to reduce the incidence of cellulitis or lymphangitis and to soften slowly the brawny edema that is often found in conjunction with lymphedema. In 1993, Casley-Smith et al. reported the results of a double-blind, crossover trial of coumarin in 31 women with postmastectomy lymphedema and 21 men and women with lymphedema of the leg of various causes.[67**] Coumarin was reported to be more effective than placebo in reducing the volume of edema fluid in the arm, in reducing skin temperature, and in increasing the softness of the limb tissue. In 1999, Loprinzi et al. studied 140 women with chronic lymphedema of the ipsilateral arm after treatment for breast cancer. The volumes of the arms at 6 and 12 months were virtually identical, regardless of whether coumarin or placebo was given first, and no significant differences in symptoms were found between the two treatment groups. Coumarin was well tolerated, except that it resulted in serological evidence of liver toxicity in 6 percent of the women.[68**] It appears that at present there is no drug that will reduce chronic lymphedema and allow the reduction to be maintained.[68**,69***]

Psychosocial support

For a patient with lymphedema, physical and emotional challenges are profound. In a study by Tobin et al., patients with arm edema experienced greater functional impairment, and increased difficulty adjusting to their illness, home life, and personal/familial relationships.[1*] The openly exposed lymphedematous limb is a constant reminder to the patient and the community at large of the occurrence of a cancer and that the patient is physically different from the norm. As a result, the patient may lose interest in dressing up or general appearance. This loss of self-esteem may also contribute to difficulties with interpersonal relationships, social activities, and intimacy.[70] Efforts may be made to strengthen patients' coping skills, eventually in a multidisciplinary approach by palliative and rehabilitation professionals.

Key learning points

Lymphedema occurs when lymphatic fluid exceeds the lymphatic transport capacity.
    Lymphedema is classified as:

- primary

- secondary: filariasis, cancer and its treatment, other causes.

Stages of lymphedema are: 0, 1, 2, and 3.
It is graded as: mild, moderate, severe.
Diagnosis of lymphedema is based on:

- History: medical and surgical history, edema and associated symptoms, function, psychosocial effect.

- Physical examination:

    - Volume measurement (circumference, water displacement volumetry, optoelectronic Perometer, bioelectrical impedance, skinfold calipers)

    - Assessment of skin condition (texture, color, tonometry)

- Imaging studies: LAS, magnetic resonance imaging and computed tomography, ultrasonography (differential diagnosis of deep venous thrombosis), dual X-ray absorptiometry or bi-photonic absorptiometry

Treatment:

- Goal: development of collateral drainage routes, stimulating the function of remaining patent routes, decrease volume and improve skin condition, prevent complications.

- Methods: skin care, MLD, exercise, compression bandaging/compression garment, pneumatic compression, surgery and drug therapy, psychosocial support.

REFERENCES

1   Tobin MB, Lacey HJ, Meyer L, Mortimer PS. The psychological morbidity of breast cancer-related arm swelling. Psychological morbidity of lymphoedema. Cancer 1993; **72**: 3248–52.

2   Cohen SR, Payne DK, Tunkel RS. Lymphedema: strategies for management. Cancer 2001; **92**(4 Suppl): 980–7.

3 Velanovich V, Szymanski W. Quality of life of breast cancer patients with lymphedema. *Am J Surg* 1999; **177**: 184–7.

4 Passik SD, McDonald MV. Psychosocial aspects of upper extremity lymphedema in women treated for breast carcinoma. *Cancer* 1998; **83**: 2817–20.

5 Kwan W, Jackson J, Weir LM, *et al*. Chronic arm morbidity after curative breast cancer treatment: prevalence and impact on quality of life. *J Clin Oncol* 2002; **20**: 4242–8.

6 Mortimer PS. The pathophysiology of lymphedema. *Cancer* 1998; **83**: 2798–802.

7 Smeltzer DM, Stickler GB, Schirger A. Primary lymphedema in children and adolescents: a follow-up study and review. *Pediatrics* 1985; **76**: 206–17.

8 Board J, Harlow W. Lymphoedema 2: classification, signs, symptoms and diagnosis. *Br J Nurs* 2002; **11**: 389–95.

9 Brennan MJ. Lymphedema following the surgical treatment of breast cancer: a review of pathophysiology and treatment. *J Pain Symptom Manage* 1992; **7**: 110–16.

10 Cambria RA, Gloviczki P, Naessens JM, Wahner HW. Noninvasive evaluation of the lymphatic system with lymphoscintigraphy: a prospective, semiquantitative analysis in 386 extremities. *J Vasc Surg* 1993; **18**: 773–82.

11 Ryttov N, Holm NV, Qvist N, Blichert-Toft M. Influence of adjuvant irradiation on the development of late arm lymphedema and impaired shoulder mobility after mastectomy for carcinoma of the breast. *Acta Oncol* 1988; **27**: 667–70.

12 Ragaz J, Jackson SM, Le N, *et al*. Adjuvant radiotherapy and chemotherapy in node-positive premenopausal women with breast cancer. *N Engl J Med* 1997; **337**: 956–62.

13 Johansson S, Svensson H, Denekamp J. Dose response and latency for radiation-induced fibrosis, edema, and neuropathy in breast cancer patients. *Int J Radiat Oncol Biol Phys* 2002; **52**: 1207–19.

14 Schunemann H, Willich N. Lymphoedema of the arm after primary treatment of breast cancer. *Anticancer Res* 1998; **18**: 2235–6.

15 Hinrichs CS, Watroba NL, Rezaishiraz H, *et al*. Lymphedema secondary to postmastectomy radiation: incidence and risk factors. *Ann Surg Oncol* 2004; **11**: 573–80.

16 Hojris I, Andersen J, Overgaard M, Overgaard J. Late treatment-related morbidity in breast cancer patients randomized to postmastectomy radiotherapy and systemic treatment versus systemic treatment alone. *Acta Oncol* 2000; **39**: 355–72.

17 Erickson VS, Pearson ML, Ganz PA, *et al*. Arm edema in breast cancer patients. *J Natl Cancer Inst* 2001; **93**: 96–111.

18 Ryan M, Stainton MC, Slaytor EK, *et al*. Aetiology and prevalence of lower limb lymphoedema following treatment for gynaecological cancer. *Aust N Z J Obstet Gynaecol* 2003; **43**: 148–51.

19 Cabanas RM. An approach for the treatment of penile carcinoma. *Cancer* 1977; **39**: 456–66.

20 Catalona W. Modified inguinal lymphadenectomy for carcinoma of the penis with preservation of saphenous veins: technique and preliminary results. *J Urol* 1988; **140**: 306–10.

21 Okeke AA, Bates DO, Gillatt DA. Lymphoedema in urological cancer. *Eur Urol* 2004; **45**: 18–25.

22 Lieskovsky G, Skinner DG, Weisenburger T. Pelvic lymphadenectomy in the management of carcinoma of the prostate. *J Urol* 1980; **124**: 635–8.

23 Greskovich FJ, Zagars GK, Sherman NE, Johnson DE. Complications following external beam radiation therapy for prostate cancer: an analysis of patients treated with and without staging pelvic lymphadenectomy. *J Urol* 1991; **146**: 798–802.

◆ 24 Brennan MJ, DePompolo RW, Garden FH. Focused review: postmastectomy lymphedema. *Arch Phys Med Rehabil* 1996; **77**: S74–S80.

25 Szuba A, Rockson SG. Lymphedema: anatomy, physiology, and pathogenesis. *Vasc Med* 1997; **2**: 321–6.

✱ 26 Weissleder H, Schuchhardt C. Lymphedema in tumor management. In: Weissleder H, Schuchhardt C, eds. *Lymphedema: Diagnosis and Therapy.* Cologne: Viavital Verlag, 2001: 187–213.

27 Kiel KD, Rademacher AW. Early-Stage breast cancer: arm edema after wide-excision and breast irradiation. *Radiology* 1996; **198**: 279–83.

28 Garcia Hidalgo L. Dermatological complications of obesity. *Am J Clin Dermatol* 2002; **3**: 497–506.

29 Mallon E, Powell S, Mortimer P, Ryan TJ. Evidence for altered cell-mediated immunity in postmastectomy lymphoedema. *Br J Dermatol* 1997; **137**: 928–33.

◆ 30 Badger C, Seers K, Preston N, Mortimer P. Antibiotics/anti-inflammatories for reducing acute inflammatory episodes in lymphoedema of the limbs. *Cochrane Database Syst Rev* 2004; **2**: CD003143.

31 Lewis JM, Wald ER. Lymphedema praecox. *J Pediatr* 1984; **104**: 641–8.

32 Stewart FW, Treves N. Lymphangiosarcoma in postmastectomy lymphedema: a report of six cases in elephantiasis chirurgica. *Cancer* 1948; **1**: 64–81.

33 Brostrom LA, Nilsonne U, Kronberg M, Soderberg G. Lymphangiosarcoma in chronic hereditary oedema (Milroy's disease). *Ann Chir Gynaecol* 1989; **78**: 320–3.

34 Mortimer PS. Investigation and management of lymphoedema. *Vasc Med Rev* 1990; **1**: 1–20.

35 Stanton AW, Badger C, Sitzia J. Non-invasive assessment of the lymphedematous limb. *Lymphology* 2000; **33**: 122–35.

36 Berard A, Zuccarelli F. Test-retest reliability study of a new improved Leg-O-meter, the Leg-O meter II, in patients suffering from venous insufficiency of the lower limbs. *Angiology* 2000; **51**: 711–7.

37 Imran D, Mandal A. Measurement of lymphedema using a simple device. *Plast Reconstr Surg* 2004; **113**: 456–7.

38 Sitzia J. Volume measurement in lymphoedema treatment: examination of formulae. *Eur J Cancer Care (Engl)* 1995; **4**: 11–16.

39 Stanton AW, Northfield JW, Holroyd B, *et al*. Validation of an optoelectronic limb volumeter (Perometer). *Lymphology* 1997; **30**: 77–97.

40 Ward LC. Regarding edema and leg volume: methods of assessment. *Angiology* 2000; **51**: 615–16.

41 Moseley A, Piller N, Carati C. Combined opto-electronic perometry and bioimpedance to measure objectively the effectiveness of a new treatment intervention for chronic secondary leg lymphedema. *Lymphology* 2002; **35**: 136–43.

42 Zuther JE. Lymphedema management. In: Von Rohr M, Berger J, eds. *The Comprehensive Guide for Practitioners.* New York: Thieme, 2005: 68–9.

43 Witte CL, Witte MH, Unger EC, *et al*. Advances in imaging of lymph flow disorders. *Radiographics* 2000; **20**: 1697–719.

* 44 Consensus Document of the International Society of Lymphology, 2004: 1–7. www.u.arizona.edu/˜witte/2003 consensus.htm (accessed October 21, 2005).

45 Rudkin GH, Miller TA. Lipedema: a clinical entity distinct from lymphedema. *Plast Reconstr Surg* 1994; **94**: 841–7.

46 Harwood CA, Bull RH, Evans J, Mortimer PS. Lymphatic and venous function in lipoedema. *Br J Dermatol* 1996; **134**: 1–6.

47 Gniadecka M. Localization of dermal edema in lipodermatosclerosis, lymphedema, and cardiac insufficiency. High-frequency ultrasound examination of intradermal echogenicity. *J Am Acad Dermat* 1996; **35**: 37–41.

* 48 International Society of Lymphology Executive Committee. The diagnosis and treatment of peripheral lymphedema. *Lymphology* 1995; **28**: 113–17.

49 Casley-Smith JR, Boris M, Weindorf S, *et al.* Treatment for lymphedema of the arm: the Casley-Smith method. *Cancer* 1998; **83**: 2843–60.

50 Ko DS, Lerner R, Klose G, Cosimi AB. Effective treatment of lymphedema of the extremities. *Arch Surg* 1998; **133**: 452–7.

51 Mortimer PS. Managing lymphoedema. *Clin Exp Dermatol* 1995; **20**: 98–110.

52 Foldi E, Foldi M, Weissleder H. Conservative treatment of lymphoedema of the limbs. *Angiology* 1985; **36**: 171–80.

53 Andersen L, Hojris I, Erlandsen M, Andersen J. Treatment of breast-cancer-related lymphedema with or without manual lymphatic drainage – a randomized study. *Acta Oncologica* 2000; **39**: 399–405.

54 LeDuc O, Peeters A, Bourgeois P. Bandages: scintigraphic demonstration of its efficacy on colloidal protein reabsorption during muscle activity. In: Nishi M, Uchino S, Yabuki S, eds. *Progress in Lymphology.* New York: Elsevier Science, 1990: 421–3.

55 Badger CMA, Peacock JL, Mortimer PS. A randomized, controlled, parallel-group clinical trial comparing multilayer bandaging followed by hosiery versus hosiery alone in the treatment of patients with lymphedema of the limb. *Cancer* 2000; **88**: 2832–7.

56 Bertelli G, Venturini M, Forno G, *et al.* An analysis of prognostic factors in response to conservative treatment of postmastectomy lymphedema. *Surg Gynecol Obstet* 1992; **175**: 455–60.

57 Yasuhara H, Shigematsu H, Muto T. A study of the advantages of elastic stockings for leg lymphedema. *Int Angiol* 1996; **15**: 272–7.

58 Hornsby R. The use of compression to treat lymphoedema. *Prof Nurse* 1995; **11**: 127–8.

◆ 59 Brennan MJ, Miller LT. Overview of treatment options and review of the current role and use of compression garments, intermittent pumps, and exercise in the management of lymphedema. *Cancer* 1998; **83**: 2821–7.

◆ 60 Leduc O, Leduc A, Bourgeois P, *et al.* The physical treatment of upper limb edema. *Cancer* 1998; **83**: 2835–9.

61 Eliska O, Eliskova M. Lymphedema: morphology of the lymphatics after manual massage. In: Witte MH, Witte CL, eds. *Progress in Lymphology.* Zurich: International Society of Lymphology 1994: 132–5.

62 Pappas CJ, O'Donnell TF Jr. Long-term results of compression treatment for lymphedema. *J Vasc Surg* 1992; **16**: 555–63.

63 Savage RC. The surgical management of lymphedema. *Surg Gynecol Obstet* 1984; **159**: 501–8.

64 Brorson H, Svensson H. Liposuction combined with controlled compression therapy reduces arm lymphedema more effectively than controlled compression alone. *Plast Reconstr Surg* 1998; **102**: 1058–67.

65 Campisi C. Boccardo F. Lymphedema and microsurgery. *Microsurgery* 2002; **22**: 74–80.

66 Brorson H. Liposuction in arm lymphedema treatment. *Scand J Surg* 2003; **92**: 287–95.

67 Casley-Smith JR, Morgan RG, Piller NB. Treatment of lymphedema of the arms and legs with 5,6-benzo-(alpha)-pyrone. *N Engl J Med* 1993; **329**: 1158–63.

68 Loprinzi CL, Kugler JW, Sloan JA, *et al.* Lack of effect of coumarin in women with lymphedema after treatment for breast cancer. *N Engl J Med* 1999; **340**: 346–50.

◆ 69 Badger C, Preston N, Seers K, Mortimer P. Benzo-pyrones for reducing and controlling lymphoedema of the limbs. *Cochrane Database Syst Rev* 2004; **2**: CD003140.

70 Carter BJ. Women's experiences of lymphedema. *Oncol Nurs Forum* 1997; **24**: 875–82.

PART 14

Emergencies in palliative medicine

84

Hypercalcemia

D SCOTT ERNST, GARY WOLCH

INTRODUCTION

Hypercalcemia is a common metabolic complication of malignant disease and is most frequently associated with the prevalent cancers of the breast and lung.[1] Because of the ensuing complications, it is responsible for a significant number of hospitalizations.[2*] Signs and symptoms of hypercalcemia may be subtle and can easily be missed unless the index of suspicion is sufficiently raised.[3] Control of distressing symptoms in patients with advanced cancer is often made more difficult by hypercalcemia symptomatology, which often exacerbates existing palliative issues. Furthermore, hypercalcemia is a readily treatable condition and the management can significantly improve patients' overall palliation.[4,5] Recent developments in the therapeutic armamentarium have simplified management, often allowing for outpatient treatment.[6*]

EPIDEMIOLOGY

Hypercalcemia of malignancy (HCM) was first recognized over 80 years ago by Zondec and has become increasingly recognized with the advent of routine serum calcium measurement.[7*] Still the most common cause of hypercalcemia remains hyperparathyroidism. Primary hyperparathyroidism (PHPTH) is found in approximately 250 new cases per million persons per year compared with 150 new cases per million per year of HCM.[8*,9] The incidence of HCM varies between 0.6 percent and 5 percent of all patients with cancer.[10] It occurs preferentially in certain types of malignancy, with over 50 percent of cases associated with carcinoma of either the lung or breast.[1,11*] The incidence of HCM varies widely and depends on the primary site, histological subtype, and the presence or absence of bone metastases. For instance, HCM occurs in approximately 7 percent of squamous carcinomas of the lung and is rare in primary small cell carcinoma of the lung.[12] It occurs in 15–20 percent of patients with untreated multiple myeloma, whereas more common cancers, such as carcinoma of the colon, uterus and cervix, are rarely associated with hypercalcemia.[3] Patients who have advanced carcinoma of the prostate and who often have widespread metastatic bone disease, rarely develop HCM. Other tumor types which are well known to be associated with HCM include renal cell carcinoma, carcinomas of the head and neck, ovarian cancer and non-Hodgkin lymphomas.[13]

PATHOGENESIS

Hypercalcemia of any etiology can theoretically result from one of or a combination of three different mechanisms:

- enhanced calcium absorption from the gastrointestinal tract
- impaired calcium excretion from the kidney
- accelerated calcium resorption from bone.[14]

In HCM, calcium absorption is generally impaired and dietary factors have little influence on serum levels.[15*]

Two broad categories of HCM have been recognized.[16] In patients with extensive lytic bone metastases, tumor cells have been found to release a variety of cytokines which act locally to induce osteolysis and release calcium into the systemic circulation. Hypercalcemia may also develop in the absence of bone metastasis and results from the secretion of a hormone produced by the tumor which acts to promote calcium reabsorption in the kidney and to enhance bone resorption, so called humoral hypercalcemia of malignancy. The predominant humoral factor is now thought to be parathyroid hormone-related protein (PTHrP). There may be considerable overlap between these two mechanisms which may explain variable responses to therapy.[17]

Osteolysis

In those patients with bone metastasis, the interaction between the tumor and the resident cells within bone can result in the development of hypercalcemia. Osteoclasts have become recognized as the predominate mediators of osteolysis.[18,19] Tumor cells also release a variety of factors, such as interleukin (IL)-1, IL-6, tumor necrosis factor α and macrophage inflammatory protein-1α, which stimulate the osteoclast to resorb bone.[20] The bone matrix itself is a rich source of growth factors such as transforming growth factor β (TGFβ), insulinlike growth factors (IGFs), and platelet-derived growth factors (PDGFs).[21] These cytokines can in turn stimulate local tumor growth and the release of additional factors from the tumor cells to further incite osteoclast activation.[18,22] In multiple myeloma, extensive osteoclast-mediated bone resorption typically occurs. A wide spectrum of cytokines, osteoclast-activating factors (OAFs), have been implicated in the pathogenesis of the lytic bone disease and of hypercalcemia.[18,23,24,25]

PTH–related protein

In many cases of HCM, the biochemical changes are suggestive of overstimulation by parathyroid hormone (PTH).[26,27*] Not only is calcium resorption from bone increased, but renal tubular reabsorption of calcium is also enhanced. Phosphaturia with consequent hypophosphatemia develops and nephrogenous cyclic AMP levels are increased. PTHrP is a 16 kDa peptide with 61 percent sequence homology with PTH,[28*,29*] and it has four times the bioactivity of PTH and competitively binds with the PTH receptor.[30] PTHrP gene expression is present in several normal tissues including skin, breast, liver and brain.[31] The physiological role of PTHrP is not well established, but it likely acts as a paracrine factor which regulates extracellular calcium homeostasis.[16]

PTHrP appears to be the central mediator of HCM.[32*] PTHrP levels are frequently elevated in patients with humoral hypercalcemia of malignancy and in approximately two-thirds of patients with bone metastasis.[29] It is most often associated with squamous cell carcinomas and rarely found in patients with hematological malignancies such as multiple myeloma and lymphomas.[33] It was found to be elevated in 30–50 percent of breast cancer patients with HCM irrespective of known bone involvement. Furthermore, circulating PTHrP may be generated at specific sites

of bone metastases.[34] Of clinical relevance, patients with HCM mediated by PTHrP tend to be more resistant to therapy.

Renal mechanisms

The kidneys play a central role in regulation of calcium homeostasis.[35] The parathyroid glands are also very sensitive to any fluctuation in calcium levels, and by reducing PTH secretion can retard bone resorption and intestinal absorption of calcium, and can promote renal calciuresis. In HCM, the influx of calcium from osteolysis and/or PTHrP secretion often leads to impairment of the kidney's ability to effectively eliminate the excess calcium. Furthermore, the hypercalcemia-induced nausea and anorexia can reduce fluid intake and diminish intravascular volume. With volume depletion, sodium resorption in the proximal tubule is enhanced and calcium resorption is augmented because of the tight linkage between sodium and calcium transport within the nephron. Consequently, the combined factors of hypercalcemia, volume depletion, and impaired renal excretion of calcium lead to a perpetuating vicious circle which persists until effective therapy is introduced.

DIFFERENTIAL DIAGNOSIS

Although the differential diagnosis of hypercalcemia is extensive, most cases can be accounted for by PHPTH or by HCM.[36] Box 84.1 lists the broad differential diagnosis for hypercalcemia. PHPTH is a common, benign disorder and accounts for the majority of cases among the general population. If symptomatic, treatment with surgery alone is curative.[37***,38*] Although PHPTH is the most common outpatient cause of hypercalcemia, malignancy is the most common inpatient cause. Indeed, benign causes of hypercalcemia are not uncommon in patients.[36] Hutchesson et al. reported a 15 percent rate of concurrent PHPTH and malignancy-related hypercalcemia.[39*] HCM is usually associated with clinical signs suggestive of an underlying malignancy and the biochemical abnormalities usually progress over a short period of time. When a level of clinical uncertainty exists, the two conditions can usually be distinguished by obtaining an immunoradiometric assay for PTH.[40]

CLINICAL PRESENTATION

Symptoms are often not well correlated with serum calcium or bone destruction and are more likely to depend on the rate of onset rather than the absolute serum calcium levels[41] (Table 84.1). The initial symptoms may be very mild and

Box 84.1 Differential diagnosis of hypercalcemia

Primary hyperparathyroidism

- Sporadic
- Familial

Malignancy

- Local osteolysis (e.g. multiple myeloma, breast carcinoma)
- Humoral HCM (e.g. squamous cell carcinomas of the lung, renal cell carcinoma)
- Vitamin D-related (e.g. Hodgkin lymphoma)

Other endocrinopathies

- Thyrotoxicosis
- Adrenal insufficiency
- Pheochromocytoma
- Acromegaly

Medications

- Thiazide diuretics
- Lithium
- Milk-alkali syndrome
- Vitamin D

Other

- Sarcoidosis and granulomatous diseases
- Acute renal failure
- Immobilization

can be difficult to distinguish from those of the underlying disease or from the side effects of cancer therapy. Early recognition is important because, if left untreated, the symptoms can rapidly progress and become severe.[14] The most common symptom is fatigue (75 percent).[42] Other frequent manifestations include: anorexia (64 percent), weight loss (64 percent), bone pain (58 percent) and constipation (58 percent). The mnemonic, 'stones, bones, abdominal moans, and psychic groans' is a simple means of remembering the signs and symptoms of hypercalcemia irrespective of the underlying cause.[36]

The clinical manifestations of the altered renal function include polydipsia and polyuria. Nausea and vomiting may also be present.[35] Nephrolithiasis may develop, particularly if the hypercalcemia occurs over a protracted period of time. Signs of volume contraction, such as postural hypotension, tachycardia, mucosal dryness, and altered skin turgor are commonly seen and should be specifically addressed in the clinical evaluation.

Neurological and cognitive symptoms may be particularly subtle and readily overlooked.[38*] Patients may experience changes in concentration, memory, or mood.[43*] Drowsiness, confusion, and acute delirium may develop and may progress rapidly to coma and death. Slight changes in serum calcium can produce symptoms, particularly in older and debilitated patients.

The laboratory evaluation of HCM should include serum electrolytes, phosphorus, creatinine, albumin, and total serum calcium or serum ionized calcium (where available). Direct measurement of serum ionized calcium is considered the gold standard in the diagnosis of HCM.[44] Total serum calcium results must be interpreted in view of the existence in three forms of calcium in plasma: bound to albumin and other proteins (approximately 40 percent), chelated to serum anions (13 percent), and as free ionized calcium (47 percent).[45,46] Serum (free) ionized calcium is the biologically active component of total calcium, and is responsible for the deleterious effects of HCM. In patients with hypoalbuminemia for various reasons, including malnutrition and chronic illness, measured serum calcium will underestimate actual total calcium.[35] Serum calcium should

Table 84.1 *Classification and symptoms of hypercalcemia*

Severity	Serum calcium level mmol/L (mg/dL)	Associated symptoms
Mild	<3.0 (<12)	Anorexia, mild nausea, constipation, fatigue, subtle mental status alteration, bone pain
Moderate	3.0–3.5 (12–14)	Similar to mild HCM + abdominal pain, nephrolithiasis, nephrocalcinosis, progressive renal dysfunction
Severe	>3.5 (>14)	Similar to moderate HCM + dehydration, severe nausea/vomiting, pancreatitis, marked changes in mental status, coma, cardiac dysrhythmias

HCM, hypercalcemia of malignancy.

be adjusted in accordance with serum albumin using the following formulae:

- In Imperial Units: corrected calcium (mg/dL) = serum calcium + 0.8 mg/dL (4 g/dL − serum albumin)
- In SI Units: corrected calcium (mmol/L) = serum calcium + 0.2 mmol/L (40 g/L − serum albumin)

(Note: serum calcium measurements given in mmol/L can be multiplied by 4 to convert to mg/dL).

TREATMENT OF HYPERCALCEMIA OF MALIGNANCY

The classification of HCM as an 'oncological emergency' arises from the potential complications which may ensue if this condition remains unrecognized or undertreated. In the absence of effective treatment, progressive dehydration and deteriorating renal function may lead to progressive hypercalcemia and possibly coma and/or death.[35] Dysrhythmias and cardiac arrest may occur with rapid escalations of serum calcium.

Treatment of HCM must be recognized as only a temporizing measure, with treatment of the underlying cancer remaining the most definitive method of preventing recurrence. Indeed, since hypercalcemia is often an end-stage manifestation of malignancy, it may be appropriate to withhold treatment depending on patient and family goals.[35]

Hydration and diuretics

Hydration is the cornerstone of the HCM therapy. Fluid therapy is essential to reverse the impending cycle of decreased glomerular filtration, impaired renal calcium excretion, and nephrocalcinosis. Rehydration should begin with isotonic saline solution, and should be pursued aggressively often requiring up to 6 L daily. Mild hypercalcemia in asymptomatic patients may allow for outpatient oral rehydration, although many patients require hospitalization for intravenous hydration along with calcium-lowering agents. Adequate rehydration can be assessed by monitoring urine output along with urine/serum osmolality. Attempts should be made to restore urine output to approximately 2 L/day. Frequent clinical assessments help to avoid the complication of congestive heart failure, as a result of excessive hydration. Electrolytes should be monitored, as patients with HCM may have concurrent hypokalemia and hypomagnesemia, both of which may be exacerbated by volume expansion.[47]

Loop (sulfonylurea) diuretics, such as furosemide and ethacrynic acid, inhibit the Na/K/Cl transporter in the loop of Henle and increase delivery of sodium to the distal nephron, which in turn promotes calcium excretion.[48] Despite their ability to promote calciuresis, loop diuretics should be administered with caution because of the risk of hypokalemia, alkalosis, hypomagnasemia, and recurrent hypovolemia. The effectiveness and favorable side effect profile of newer agents has minimized the role of loop diuretics in the treatment of HCM.

Bisphosphonates

Bisphosphonates are synthetic pyrophosphate analogs characterized by a phosphorus-carbon-phosphorus bond which renders them resistant to enzymatic hydrolysis[49***] (Table 84.2). Bisphosphonates are potent inhibitors of normal and pathological bone resorption. Although their mechanism of action is complex and not fully understood, bisphosphonates exert their hypocalcemic effect principally through inhibition of osteoclast activity.[50***] The agents are avidly taken up within the bone matrix from the circulation and over subsequent months are slowly released into the

Table 84.2 Bisphosphonates

Bisphosphonate	Bisphosphonate-R2 side chain	Relative potency	Recommended dose
Non-nitrogen-containing			
Etidronate	$-CH_3$	1	7.5 mg/kg per day by intravenous infusion over 2–4 hours (500 mL diluent) on 3 consecutive days
Clodronate	$-Cl$	10	1500 mg by intravenous or subcutaneous infusion over 4 hours (500 mL diluent)[a]
Nitrogen-containing			
Pamidronate	$-CH_2CH_2NH_2$	100	60–90 mg by intravenous infusion over 2–4 hours (250–500 mL diluent)[a]
Alendronate	$-(CH_2)_3NH_2$	500	5–15 mg by intravenous infusion over 2 hours (250 mL diluent)
Ibandronate	$-CH_2CH_2N(CH_3)-(pentyl)$	5 000	2–6 mg by intravenous infusion over 2 hours (500 mL diluent)[a]
Zoledronic acid	$-CH_2-imidazole$	10 000	4 mg by intravenous infusion over at least 15 min (100 mL diluent)

[a]Smaller volumes and shorter infusion times have been used without significant renal toxicity.

resorptive lacunae.[51***] Once taken up into the osteoclast, the bisphosphonates appear to inhibit protein synthesis and proton production diminishing further bone resorption.[52] Osteoclast apoptosis can be induced *in vivo* and *in vitro* by the bisphosphonates, further retarding bone resorption.[53] The osteoblast may be the initial target of some bisphosphonates. By modulating osteoblastic stimulatory factors, osteoclast function and recruitment are impaired.[50***,54,55] The nature of the side chains stemming from the central carbon determine the potency of the bisphosphonate.[56***] Nitrogen-containing bisphosphonates are more potent inhibitors of bone resorption due to their ability to inhibit the mevalonate biosynthetic pathway within the ostoclarks. The inhibition of this pathway potently decreases osteoclast function and survival.[55]

Intravenous bisphosphonates have become the standard of care for the treatment of HCM unresponsive to hydration alone and can be utilized irrespective of the predominant underlying pathogenic mechanism.[50***,57] Due to their limited enteral absorption (1–2 percent) and gastrointestinal side effects, oral bisphosphonates are rarely indicated for the management of HCM, although they may be used for maintenance of normocalcemia. The ability of bisphosphonates to reverse HCM has minimized the role of other therapeutic agents such as gallium nitrate, calcitonin, and plicamycin.[50***] The combination of a parenterally administered bisphosphonate and adequate hydration will normalize serum calcium in the majority of patients.[55] Normalization of calcium levels often takes 3–5 days following infusion.

TOXICITY

Although the side effects from bisphosphonates may be similar to those produced by the hypercalcemia, a consistent toxicity profile for bisphosphonate therapy has emerged. The majority of these adverse events occur infrequently and are self-limiting (Box 84.2).[58***]

Box 84.2   Side effects of bisphosphonates

More common

- Fever

Occasional

- Renal toxicity
- Nausea and vomiting

Rare

- Symptomatic hypocalcemia
- Symptomatic hypophosphatemia
- Infusion site reaction

Fever is the most commonly reported adverse event.[56,58***,59**] Fever appears to be more common, with the nitrogen-containing bisphosphonates, occurring in up to 44 percent of patients. Patients may benefit from prophylactic acetaminophen prior to aminobisphosphonate infusion. High systemic bisphosphonate concentrations following rapid intravenous administration may result in the formation of insoluble bisphosphonate– calcium complexes in the kidney and may lead to renal tubule damage, further aggravating renal dysfunction. Although renal complications are rare, cases of acute renal failure have been reported with bisphophonate use.[59**] This risk can be minimized by giving lower doses over a prolonged infusion period. The potential for symptomatic hypocalcemia with bisphosphonate use is small given the intrinsic stimulation of PTH secretion that occurs.[60**] Occasional vision-threatening ocular side effects (uveitis/scleritis) have been reported.[61*]

NON–NITROGEN-CONTAINING BISPHOSPHONATES

Etidronate

Etidronate was one of the earliest bisphosphonate products to be used clinically.[49***] Etidronate (see Table 84.2) administered intravenously over 3 days is the recommended treatment regimen, although a multicenter study has demonstrated the safety and effectiveness of a single 24-hour infusion.[36,62*] The oral formulation of etidronate maintains an indication for the short-term (30–90 days) maintenance of normocalcemia following intravenous infusion. Because of its relative low potency and the observation that it may inhibit normal bone mineralization, etidronate's role in HCM therapy is primarily historical.[63]

Clodronate

The effectiveness of clodronate for the treatment of HCM was first reported in 1980.[56] A double blind, randomized controlled trial published in 1995 demonstrated the superiority of hydration plus clodronate over hydration alone in the treatment of HCM.[64***] In this study, 44 female breast cancer patients with serum ionized calcium >1.6 (normal range 1.09–1.3) were randomized to receive either clodronate (300 mg intravenously in 500 mL normal saline) daily for up to 7 days, or placebo. A significantly larger number of patients achieved normocalcemia in the clodronate group than in the placebo group (17/21 vs. 4/19). The median 'time to normocalcemia' in the clodronate group was 5 days (range 3–7).

To reduce the number of infusion days, O'Rourke *et al.* reported on a cohort of 30 HCM patients with different tumor types, in whom hypercalcemia (>2.63 mmol/L) persisted following 3 days of intravenous hydration.[65*] All were given 1500 mg of clodronate (intravenously in 500 mL of normal saline over 4 hours). Serum calcium normalized in 54 percent of patients by day 3, and 80 percent by day 10. A single 1500 mg infusion of clodronate is as efficient as the 5-day regimen.[50***]

Bisphosphonate use for HCM may be required in settings where symptom palliation is the primary goal. For these terminally ill patients, securing intravenous access may be an obstacle to bisphosphonate therapy. Subcutaneous clodronate infusion has recently been shown to be a safe and reliable alternative for the management of HCM in this population (see Table 84.2 for recommended administration).[66*] Continued experience with this technique has allowed for smaller volumes and shorter durations of infusion without added toxicity.[67*]

NITROGEN-CONTAINING BISPHOSPHONATES

Pamidronate

Pamidronate was the first of the nitrogen-containing bisphosphonates to be available for clinical use. Early studies of pamidronate utilized doses (30–45 mg) at the lower end of the therapeutic range.[68**] Subsequently, a dose–response study found that the majority of patients who failed to achieve normocalcemia with pamidronate had high initial calcium levels (>3.5) and received low-dose pamidronate (30 mg or 45 mg). Higher doses of pamidronate (60–90 mg) were almost universally effective.[69*] Dose adjustments for pamidronate based on initial calcium levels are unnecessary. Pamidronate 90 mg will achieve normocalcemia in over 90 percent of patients and prevent an inadequate response in those with enhanced renal calcium re-absorption.[70***,71]

Pamidronate and clodronate at recommended dosages (see Table 84.2) are equally efficacious, although pamidronate has a longer duration of effect.[58***,64***]

Alendronate

Alendronate has superior antiresorptive potency compared with etidronate and clodronate. In a small randomized controlled trial, intravenous alendronate (10 mg) reversed HCM in a majority of patients.[72*] Intravenous alendronate (7.5 mg) and intravenous clodronate (600 mg) have comparable efficacy in the treatment of HCM. Comparison studies with other nitrogen-containing bisphosphonates are unavailable.

The recommended intravenous alendronate dosage range is 5–15 mg, with a trend toward superior efficacy at the higher doses.[73**] Alendronate may be infused safely over 2 hours.[74**] The availability of intravenous alendronate is limited in many countries, and some national regulatory bodies have not approved its use for HCM.

Ibandronate

In the early 1990s investigators began screening hundreds of new bisphosphonates for their effect on bone resorption in animal models.[75***] Ibandronate emerged as a bisphosphonate with a bone resorption potency 50 and 500 times that of pamidronate and clodronate, respectively.[76*]

As pamidronate had already been widely used for HCM when ibandronate (intravenous) was introduced, a comparison trial in 66 cancer patients (most commonly breast, lung, and head/neck) with hypercalcemia was undertaken.[60**]

A range of ibandronate and pamidronate doses were administered commensurate with the initial calcium level. Normocalcemic response rates for ibandronate and pamidronate were 76.5 percent and 75.8 percent, respectively. The median time to relapse was significantly longer for ibandronate than pamidronate (14 vs. 4 days, respectively). Ibandronate appeared to be as effective as pamidronate, and potentially achieved a longer duration of response.

The optimal dose of ibandronate has not been established. In a dose–response study by Ralston, ibandronate 2 mg was significantly less effective than a 4 mg or 6 mg dose.[76*] The duration of ibandronate infusions in the published HCM literature range from 1 to 4 hours. Shorter infusion times and rapid bolus injection have been shown to be safe in other patient populations.[77*] Ibandronate (intravenous form) has been approved for the treatment of HCM by the European Union since 1997.[60**]

Zoledronic acid

Phase I clinical trials were first reported for the bisphosphonate zoledronate in 1996.[78*] Animal model studies found the antiresorptive potency of zoledronate to be at least 100 times that of pamidronate.[57*] The recommended dosage and administration of zoledronic acid is 4 mg (with 100 mL of normal saline) given intravenously over a minimum of 15 minutes. Higher doses and shorter infusion times have been associated with renal dysfunction.[79***]

Zoledronic acid has gained worldwide regulatory approval for the treatment of HCM based upon the pooled results of two identical, randomized, double blind, comparison trials of zoledronic acid and pamidronate.[59**] A total of 275 cancer patients with HCM were randomized to zoledronic acid 4 mg or 8 mg, or pamidronate 90 mg. Normocalcemia by day 10 was achieved in 88.4 percent, 86.7 percent, and 69.7 percent of patients in the zoledronic acid 4 mg and 8 mg, and pamidronate 90 mg arms, respectively. The median duration of response was 32, 43, and 18 days in the zoledronic acid 4 mg and 8 mg, and pamidronate 90 mg arms, respectively. Although the study was designed to show equivalence between the three arms, the response rate to pamidronate was significantly lower than expected and an advantage to using zoledronic acid is inferred.

Gallium nitrate

The hydrated nitrate salt of gallium was historically utilized in the treatment of lymphoma, where it was found to cause hypocalcemia in cancer patients.[56] Gallium nitrate impairs the ability of osteoclasts to resorb bone by interfering with a membrane proton pump and binds to the surface of hydroxyapatite decreasing its solubility.[80*,81***]

A randomized, double blind comparison of pamidronate versus gallium nitrate for HCM was presented at the European Organization for Research and Treatment of Cancer (EORTC) symposium in March 1996.[82**] In this study patients were randomized to receive either gallium nitrate (200 mg/m², 5-day continuous intravenous infusion) or pamidronate (60–90 mg, 24-hour intravenous infusion) along with an intravenous placebo infusion for 4 days. Normocalcemia was achieved in 72 percent and 59 percent of patients in the gallium nitrate and pamidronate groups, respectively. Gallium nitrate has been shown to have a superior rate and duration of response to that of etidronate and calcitonin in treating HCM. Nephrotoxicity is a concern with gallium nitrate use, although the incidence of renal dysfunction with gallium nitrate is similar to that of comparator agents.[80*]

Calcitonin

Calcitonin plays a physiological role in maintaining the skeletal integrity by inhibiting osteoclast function. Although calcitonin is found in many tissues, calcitonin is primarily released into the circulation from the C cells (parafollicular cells) within the thyroid in response to elevations in serum calcium.[83] Synthetic salmon calcitonin is preferred over the human variety due to its greater hypocalcemic potency, along with a slower rate of degradation and clearance.[84***]

Calcitonin remains useful in the first few days of severe and life-threatening HCM. Unlike bisphosphonates which exert their effect mainly on bone, calcitonin inhibits both osteoclast activity and renal tubular calcium reabsorption.[49***] A dosage of 1–8 units/kg subcutaneously every 6–12 hours is recommended and can be administered parenterally or intranasally. Calcitonin's effect is rapid in onset (within 48 hours of administration); however, the net effect in reducing serum calcium tends to be modest in magnitude (0.5–1 mmol/L) and exhibits tachyphylaxis due to downregulation of osteoclastic calcitonin receptors.[56***] Side effects include nausea, flushing, abdominal pain, and local irritation at the injection site. Calcitonin is indicated in the first 48 hours of severe and life-threatening hypercalcemia, and it is used in conjunction with hydration and bisphosphonates.

Other agents

Corticosteroids have a negligible role in the treatment of HCM associated with solid tumors. In patients with multiple myeloma or lymphoma, in whom the underlying malignancy is considered to be steroid responsive, a trial of corticosteroids may be indicated.[67*] Although plicamycin (mithramycin) remains indicated in the treatment of HCM, its poor rate of inducing normocalcemia (range 30–50 percent), limited duration of response, and significant adverse effects, make it an undesirable agent for HCM.[56***,67***] Oral and intravenous phosphate use in the treatment of HCM has become obsolete due to the advent of safer and more potent therapies.[35]

REFERENCES

◆ 1   Heath DA. Hypercalcemia of malignancy. *BMJ* 1989; **298**: 1468–9.

2   Vassilopoulou-Sellin R, Newman B, Taylor S, Guinee V. Incidence of hypercalcemia in patients with malignancy referrred to a comprehensive cancer center. *Cancer* 1993; **71**: 1309–12.

3   Lamy O, Jenzer-Closuit A, Burckhardt P. Hypercalcemia of malignancy: an underdiagnosed and undertreated disease. *J Intern Med* 2001; **250**: 73–9.

4   Morita T, Tei Y, Shishido H, Inoue S. Treatable complications of cancer patients referred to an in-patient hospice. *Am J Hosp Palliat Care* 2003; **20**: 389–91.

5   Falk S, Fallon M. ABC of palliative care: emergencies. *BMJ* 1997; **315**: 1525–8.

6   Roemer-Becuwe C, Vigano A, Romano F, *et al.* Safety of subcutaneous clodronate and efficacy in hypercalcemia of malignancy: a novel route of administration. *J Pain Symptom Manage* 2003; **26**: 843–8.

● 7   Zondek H, Petow H, Siebert W. Die Bedeutung der calcium-bestimmung im blute fur die diagnose der niereninsuffizienz. *Z Klin Med* 1924; **99**: 138.

8   Heath H, Hodgson S, Kennedy M. Primary hyperparathyroidism: incidence, morbidity and potential economic impact in a community. *N Engl J Med* 1980; **302**: 189–93.

9   Mundy GR. Malignancy and the skeleton. *Horm Metab Res* 1997; **29**: 120–7.

10   Fiskin R, Heath D, Somers S, Bold A. Hypercalcemia in hospital patients. *Lancet* 1981; **i**: 202–7.

11   Frolich A. Prevalence of hypercalcaemia in normal and in hospital populations. *Dan Med Bull* 1998; **45**: 436–9.

12   Burt M, Brennan M. Incidence of hypercalcemia and malignant neoplasm. *Arch Surg* 1980; **115**: 704–7.

13 Singer FR. Pathogenesis of hypercalcemia of malignancy. *Semin Oncol* 1991; **18**: 4–10.

◆ 14 Warrell R. Etiology and current management of cancer related hypercalcemia. *Oncology* 1992: 37–43.

15 Adams J, Fernandez M, Gacad M, *et al.* Vitamin D metabolite mediated hypercalcemia and hypercalcuria in patients with AIDS and non-AIDS-associated lymphoma. *Blood* 1990; **73**: 235–9.

◆ 16 Bayne MC, Illidge TM. Hypercalcaemia, parathyroid hormone-related protein and malignancy. *Clin Oncol* 2001; **13**: 372–7.

17 Ralston S, Fogelman I, Gardner M, *et al.* Relative contribution of humoral and metastatic factors to the pathogenesis of hypercalcemia of malignancy. *BMJ* 1984; **288**: 1405–8.

18 Roodman G. Biology of osteoclast activation in cancer. *J Clin Oncol* 2001; **19**: 3562–71.

● 19 Fallon M. Alteration in the pH of osteoclast resorbing fluid reflects changes in bone degradation activity. *Calcif Tissue Int* 1984; **36**: 458–61.

20 Dodwell D. Malignant bone resorption; cellular and biochemical mechanisms. *Ann Oncol* 1992; **3**: 257–67.

21 Pfeilschifter J, Mundy G. Modulation of transforming growth factor beta activity in bone cultures by osteotropic hormones. *Proc Natl Acad Sci U S A* 1987; **84**: 2024–8.

22 Felix R, Fleisch H, Elford P. Bone resorbing cytokines enhance release of macrophage colony stimulating activity by the osteoblastic cell. *Calcif Tissue Int* 1989; **44**: 356–60.

23 Garrett I, Durie B, Nedwin G, *et al.* Production of the bone resorbing cytokine lymphotoxin by cultured human myeloma cells. *N Engl J Med* 1987; **317**: 526–32.

24 Black K, Garret IR, Mundy G. Chinese hamster ovarian cells transfected with the murine interleukin-6 gene cause hypercalcemia as well as cachexia, leukocytosis and thrombocytosis in tumour-bearing nude mice. *Endocrinology* 1991; **128**: 2657–9.

25 Cozzolino F, Torcia M, Aldinucci D. Production of interleukin-1 by bone marrow myeloma cells. *Blood* 1989; **74**: 380–7.

◆ 26 Rabbani SA. Molecular mechanism of action of parathyroid hormone related peptide in hypercalcemia of malignancy: therapeutic strategies [review]. *Int J Oncol* 2000; **16**: 197–206.

27 Stewart AF, Horst R, Deftos LJ, *et al.* Biochemical evaluation of patients with cancer-associated hypercalcemia: evidence for humoral and non-humoral groups. *N Engl J Med* 1980; **303**: 1377–83.

● 28 Suva L, Winslow GA, Wettenhall REH, *et al.* A parathyroid hormone-related protein implicated in malignant hypercalcemia; cloning and expression. *Science* 1987; **237**: 893–6.

29 Grill V, Body J, Johanson N, *et al.* Parathyroid hormone-related protein: elevated levels in both humoral hypercalcemia of malignancy and hypercalcemia compli-cating metstatic breast cancer. *J Clin Endocrinol Metab* 1991; **73**: 1309–15.

◆ 30 Karaplis AC, Goltzman D. PTH and PTHrP effects on the skeleton. *Rev Endocr Metab Disord* 2000; **1**: 331–41.

● 31 Ikeda K, Weir E, Mangin M, *et al.* Tissue-specific and developmental expression of mRNAs encoding a PTH-like peptide [abstract]. *J Bone Mineral Res* 1988; **3**: 578.

32 Burtis W, Brady TG, Orloff JJ, *et al.* Immunochemical characterization of circulating parathyroid hormone-related protein in patients with humoral hypercalcemia of cancer. *N Engl J Med* 1990; **322**: 1106–12.

◆ 33 Budayr AA, Nissenson RA, Klein RF, *et al.* Increased serum levels of a parathyroid hormone-like protein in malignancy-associated hypercalcemia. *Ann Intern Med* 1989; **111**: 807–12.

34 Powel G, Southby J, Danks J, *et al.* Localization of parathyroid hormone-related protein in breast cancer metastases; increased incidence in bone compared to other sites. *Cancer Res* 1991; **51**: 3059–61.

35 Davis K, Attie M. Management of severe hypercalcemia. *Crit Care Clin* 1991; **7**: 175–90.

36 Carrol M, Schade D. A practical approach to hypercalcemia. *Am Fam Physician* 2003; **67**: 1959–66.

✱ 37 NIH conference: diagnosis and management of asymptomatic primary hyperparathyroidism: concensus development conference statement. *Ann Intern Med* 1991; **114**: 593–7.

38 Ralston S, Gallacher SJ, Patel U, *et al.* Cancer-associated hypercalcemia: morbidity and mortality. Clinical experience in 126 treated patients. *Ann Intern Med* 1990; **112**: 499–504.

39 Hutchesson A, Bundred N, Ratcliffe W. Survival in hypercalcemic patients with cancer and co-existing primary hyperparathyroidism. *Postgrad Med J* 1995; **71**: 28–31.

40 Logue F, Perry B, Chapman R, *et al.* A two site immunoradiometric assay for PTH using N and C terminal specific monoclonal antibodies. *Ann Clin Biochem* 1991; **28**: 160–6.

41 Bajorunas DR. Clinical manifestations of cancer-related hypercalcemia. *Semin Oncol* 1990; **17**: 16–25.

42 Nelson K, Walsh D, Abdullah O, *et al.* Common complications of advanced cancer. *Semin Oncol* 2000; **27**: 34–44.

43 Solomon B, Schaaf M, Smallridge R. Psychologic symptoms before and after parathyroid surgery. *Am J Med* 1994; **96**: 101–6.

44 Ratcliffe W, Hutchesson A, Bundred N, Ratcliffe J. Role of assays for parathyroid-hormone-related protein in the investigation of hypercalcemia. *Lancet* 1992; **339**: 164–7.

45 Clase C, Norman G, Beecroft M, Churchill D. Albumin-corrected calcium and ionized calcium in stable hemodialysis patients. *Nephrol Dial Transplant* 2000; **15**: 1841–6.

46 Riancho J, Arjona R, Sanz J, *et al.* Is the routine measurement of ionized calcium worthwhile in patients with cancer? *Postgrad Med J* 1991; **67**: 350–3.

◆ 47 Mundy GR. Hypercalcemia of cancer. *N Engl J Med* 1984; **310**: 1718–27.

◆ 48 Inzucchi S. Management of hypercalcemia diagnostic workup, therapeutic options for hyperparathyroidism and other common causes. *Postgrad Med* 2004; **115**: 5–27.

◆ 49 Patel S, Lyons A, Hosking D. Drugs used in the treatment of metabolic bone disease. Clinical pharmacology and therapeutic use. *Drugs* 1993; **46**: 594–617.

◆ 50 Body JJ, Bartl R, Burckhardt P, *et al.* Current use of bisphosphonates in oncology. *J Clin Oncol* 1998; **16**: 3890–9.

51 Plosker G, Goa K. Clodronate: a review of its pharmacological properties and therapeutic efficacy in resorptive bone disease. *Drugs* 1994; **47**: 945–82.

52 Carano A, Teitelbaum S, Konsek J, *et al.* Bisphosphonates directly inhibit the bone resorption activity of isolated osteoclasts in vitro. *J Clin Invest* 1990; **85**: 456–61.

53 Hughes D, Wright K, Uy Hea. Bisphosphonates promote apoptosis in murine osteoclasts in vitro and in vivo. *J Bone Miner Res* 1995; **10**: 1478–87.

54 Sahni M, Guenther H, Fleisch H, *et al*. Bisphosphonates act on rat bone resorption through the mediation of osteoblasts. *J Clin Invest* 1993; **91**: 2004–11.

◆ 55 Major P. Use of zoledronic acid, a novel, highly potent bisphosphonate, for the treatment of hypercalcemia of malignancy. *Oncologist* 2002; **7**: 481–91.

◆ 56 Watters J, Gerrard G, Dodwell D. The management of malignant hypercalcemia. *Drugs* 1996; **52**: 837–48.

57 Berenson J, Hirschberg R. Safety and convenience of a 15-minute infusion of zoledronic acid. *Oncologist* 2004; **9**: 319–29.

◆ 58 Saunders Y, Ross J, Broadley K, Patel S. Systematic review of bisphosphonates for hypercalcemia of malignancy. *Palliat Med* 2004; **18**: 418–31.

59 Major P, Lortholary A, Hone J, *et al*. Zoledronic acid is superior to pamidronate in the treatment of hypercalcemia of malignancy: a pooled analysis of 2 randomized, controlled clinical trials. *J Clin Oncol* 2001; **19**: 558–67.

60 Pechersorfer M, Steinhauer E, Rizzoli R, *et al*. Efficacy and safety of ibandronate in the treatment of hypercalcemia of malignancy: a randomized multicentric comparison to pamidronate. *Support Care Cancer* 2003; **11**: 539–47.

61 Fraunfelder F, Fraunfelder F, Jensvold B. Scleritis and other ocular side effects associated with pamidronate disodium. *Am J Ophthalmol* 2003; **135**: 219–22.

62 Flores J, Rude R, Chapman R, *et al*. Evaluation of a 24-hour infusion of etidronate disodium for the treatment of hypercalcemia of malignancy. *Cancer* 1994; **73**: 2527–34.

63 Flora A, Hassing GS, Parfitt A, Villanueva A. Comparative skeletal effects of 2 diphosphonates in dogs. *Metab Bone Dis Rel Res* 1980; **2**: 389–407.

64 Purohit O, Radstone C, Anthony C, *et al*. A randomised double-blind comparison of intravenous pamidronate and clodronate in the hypercalcemia of malignancy. *Br J Cancer* 1995; **72**: 1289–93.

65 O'Rourke N, McCloskey E, Vasikaran S, *et al*. Effective treatment of malignant hypercalcemia with a single intravenous infusion of clodronate. *Br J Cancer* 1993; **67**: 560–3.

66 Walker P, Watanabe S, Lawlor P, *et al*. Subcutaneous clodronate: a study evaluating efficacy in hypercalcemia of malignancy and local toxicity. *Ann Oncol* 1997; **8**: 915–16.

67 Kovacs C, MacDonald S, Chik C, Bruera E. Hypercalcemia of malignancy in the palliative care patient: a treatment strategy. *J Pain Symptom Manage* 1995; **10**: 224–32.

68 Ralson S, Gallagher S, Patel U, *et al*. Comparison of three intravenous bisphosphonates in cancer associated hypercalcemia. *Lancet* 1989; **2**: 1180–2.

69 Thiebaud D, Jaeger P, Jacquet A, Burckhardt P. Dose-response in the treatment of hypercalcemia of malignancy by a single infusion of the bisphosphonate AHPrBP. *J Clin Oncol* 1988; **6**: 762–8.

◆ 70 Body JJ. Current and future directions in medical therapy: hypercalcemia. *Cancer* 2000; **88**: 3054–8.

71 Gucalp R, Ritch P, Wiernik P, *et al*. Comparative study of pamidronate sodium and etidronate in the treatment of cancer-related hypercalcemia. *J Clin Oncol* 1992; **10**: 134–42.

72 Rizzoli R, Buchs B, Bonjour J. Effect of a single infusion of alendronate in malignant hypercalcemia: dose dependency and comparison with clodronate. *Int J Cancer* 1992; **50**: 706–12.

73 Nussbaum SR, Warrell RP, Rude R, *et al*. Dose-response study of alendronate sodium for the treatment of cancer-associated hypercalcemia. *J Clin Oncol* 1993; **11**: 1618–23.

74 Zysset Eea, Ammann P, Jenzer A, *et al*. Comparison of rapid versus slow infusion of alendronate in the treatment of hypercalcemia of malignancy. *Bone Miner* 1992; **18**: 237–49.

● 75 Muhlbauer R, Bauss F, Schenk R, *et al*. BM 21.0955, a potent new bisphosphonate to inhibit bone resorption. *J Bone Miner Res* 1991; **6**: 1003–11.

76 Ralston H. Dose-response study of ibandronate in the treatment of cancer-associated hypercalcemia. *Br J Cancer* 1997; **75**: 295–300.

77 Pecherstorfer M, Diel I. Rapid administration of ibandronate does not affect renal functioning: evidence from clinical studies in metastatic bone disease and hypercalcemia of malignancy. *Support Care Cancer* 2004; **12**: 877–81.

● 78 Berenson J, Lipton A, Rosen L, *et al*. Phase 1 clinical study of a new bisphosphonate, zoledronate, in patients with osteolytic bone metastases. *Blood* 1996; **88**: 586a.

◆ 79 Perry CM, Figgitt DP. Zoledronic acid: a review of its use in patients with advanced cancer. *Drugs* 2004; **64**: 1197–211.

◆ 80 Leyland-Jones B. Treatment of cancer-related hypercalcemia: the role of gallium nitrate. *Semin Oncol* 2003; **20**: 13–19.

◆ 81 Todd PA, Fitton A. Gallium nitrate. A review of its pharmacological properties and therapeutic potential in cancer related hypercalcaemia. *Drugs* 1991; **42**: 261–73.

82 Warrell RP. Gallium nitrate for the treatment of bone metastases. *Cancer* 1997; **80**: 1680–5.

83 Becker KL, Snider R, Moore C, *et al*. Calcitonin in extrathyroidal tissues of man. *Acta Endocrinol* 1979; **92**: 746–50.

◆ 84 Clissold S, Fitton A, Chrisp P. Intranasal salmon calcitonin: a review of its pharmacological properties and potential utility in metabolic bone disorders associated with aging. *Drugs* 1991; **1**: 405–23.

85

Hemorrhage

SRIRAM YENNURAJALINGAM, EDUARDO BRUERA

INTRODUCTION

Patients in palliative care who have advanced cancer experience a wide variety of bleeding problems. Bleeding occurs in approximately 10 percent of patients with advanced cancer[1,2] and is manifested as hemoptysis, hematuria, vaginal bleeding, rectal bleeding, hematemesis, melena, or bleeding from tumors fungating through the skin. It is the immediate cause of death in 6 percent of cancer patients and its management may pose a challenge to the healthcare provider. Bleeding is very distressing to the patient and his or her family.[3] Many of these patients require admission to the palliative care unit for various reasons such as transfusions, administration of medications like midazolam, or psychological reasons. In addition, it is difficult to predict which patients will suffer a catastrophic event; hence, a clear plan of action must be established in advance to prepare for a possible distressing circumstance.

This chapter will focus on the causes and management of bleeding in patients with advanced cancer.

CLINICAL PRESENTATION AND UNDERLYING PATHOPHYSIOLOGY OF BLEEDING IN PATIENTS WITH ADVANCED CANCER

Hemoptysis

Hemoptysis, a common symptom of bronchial carcinoma, is present in approximately 50 percent of patients at presentation[4] and may also accompany pulmonary metastasis.

Although rarely of hemodynamic significance, hemoptysis is distressing for the patient and an indication for local radiotherapy.[5**] There is no proved advantage, in terms of survival, for treating asymptomatic patients with inoperable lung cancer, but some evidence suggests that tumors greater than 10 cm in diameter, whether primary or metastasized, carry a significant risk of hemorrhage. It has been suggested that patients with such lesions should receive prophylactic treatment.[6]

Vaginal bleeding

Ninety percent of patients with endometrial cancer report vaginal bleeding at the time of their diagnosis. Vaginal bleeding is rarely excessive and can be managed conservatively. Occasionally, a patient with uterine tumor may present in the form of a major hemorrhage requiring urgent resuscitation and vaginal packing before urgent treatment to stop the hemorrhage is investigated. Hemorrhage in patients with advanced or metastatic cancer may be due to recurrent or locally advanced tumors of the cervix or uterus. Local infiltrations of advanced cancers of the bladder and rectum or mucosal deposits along the vaginal wall are the typical pattern of spread from endometrial cancer. Radiotherapy using either external beam irradiation or intracavitary treatment is of value in obtaining definitive control of bleeding.

Gastrointestinal hemorrhage

Symptomatic gastrointestinal hemorrhage may arise from either the upper or lower gastrointestinal tract and result in hematemesis and melena, or rectal bleeding. Rectal bleeding is reported by 10 to 20 percent of patients with colorectal cancer. The underlying tumor may be a primary neoplasm arising within the gastrointestinal tract, most commonly from the stomach, large bowel, or rectum, or as a result of direct invasion of a locally advanced tumor from adjacent structures such as the uterus, bladder, or the prostate that has invaded the rectum. Modest doses of radiation at the bleeding sites will often control the bleeding effectively and durably.

Hematuria

Hematuria is a frequent symptom and sign of underlying urological disease. In patients with advanced cancer, hematuria may be secondary to an underlying malignancy, a possible major coagulation disorder, or as a result of interventions such as pelvic irradiation and cyclophosphamide treatment. Hematuria usually manifests as the passage of brown or red urine or could involve the passage of large clots, clot retention, or colic.

Patients who retain clots require immediate intervention before specific studies are initiated. On clinical confirmation of a palpable bladder as a result of a clot, complete evacuation can be achieved by inserting a multi-eyed Robinson catheter (24 F or 26 F) into the urethra. Once the catheter has passed into the bladder, vigorous irrigation with water or saline using a Toomey syringe will permit removal of all clots. Irrigation of the bladder can be uncomfortable, however, and may require analgesia. Unsuccessful initial placement of the catheter or continued bleeding and recurrent obstruction of the irrigating catheter are the specific indications for endoscopic evaluation. If the bleeding is refractory to conservative measures, instillation of silver nitrate, alum, or aminocaproic acid into the bladder, with formalin under general anesthesia (with help from a urologist) may be tried. Bleeding as a result of radiation cystitis may be stopped by hyperbaric oxygen, and in chronic cases, oral pentosan polyphosphate may be used. For palliation, local irradiation and oral tranexamic acid may be helpful.

Causes of bleeding due to cancer may be anatomical, generalized, or combined (Box 85.1). Bleeding may involve damage to local vessels, invasion of vessels, mucositis, a systemic process such as disseminated intravascular coagulation (DIC), or abnormalities in platelet number and function. The underlying causes of these abnormalities are varied and include liver failure, medications such as anticoagulants, chemotherapy, radiotherapy, surgery, and the cancer itself.

Disseminated intravascular coagulation

Disseminated intravascular coagulation, also called consumption coagulopathy and defibrination syndrome, is a systemic process producing both thrombosis and hemorrhage.

Box 85.1 Etiology of bleeding in patients with cancer

Anatomical

- Local tumor invasion (tumor erosion to a major vessel)
- Tumor surface bleeding
- Mucositis (infection, drug-related, chemotherapy-induced, radiation-therapy–induced, peptic-acid–related, and stress)

Generalized

- Platelet disorders
  (i) Thrombocytopenia – due to bone marrow involvement by the tumor (hematological malignancies), drug-induced, radiation-therapy–induced, viral, vitamin deficiency, autoimmune
  (ii) Platelet function defect – drug-induced, uremic, paraprotein effect
- Bone marrow involvement by the tumor (hematological malignancies)
- Bone marrow suppression (chemotherapy or radiotherapy)
- Disseminated intravascular coagulation (sepsis, prostate cancer, etc.)
- Liver failure
- Medications (anticoagulants, acetylsalicylic acid, nonsteroidal anti-inflammatory drugs, etc.)
- Concomitant disease (liver cirrhosis, von Willebrand disease, etc.)

Combined

- Local and systemic factors

It is initiated by a number of defined disorders and consists of the following components:

1 exposure of blood to procoagulants such as tissue factor and procoagulant
2 formation of fibrin in the circulation
3 fibrinolysis
4 depletion of clotting factors
5 end-organ damage.

Common manifestations of acute DIC, in addition to bleeding, include thromboembolism and dysfunction of the kidney, liver, lungs, and central nervous system (CNS). In one series of 118 patients with DIC, the main clinical manifestations were bleeding (64 percent), renal dysfunction

(25 percent), hepatic dysfunction (19 percent), respiratory dysfunction (16 percent), shock (14 percent), thromboembolism (7 percent), and CNS involvement (2 percent).[7]

Petechiae and ecchymoses are common in conjunction with blood oozing from wound sites, intravenous lines, catheters, and, in some cases, mucosal surfaces. Such bleeding can be life threatening if it involves the gastrointestinal tract, lungs, or CNS. In patients who develop DIC after surgical procedures, hemorrhage may develop around indwelling lines, catheters, drains, and tracheotomies, and blood may accumulate in serous cavities.

Although malignancy often causes chronic DIC, it can also produce acute DIC, particularly in patients with acute promyelocytic leukemia. Disseminated intravascular coagulation is often present at the time of diagnosis or soon after the initiation of cytotoxic chemotherapy in patients with this disorder. It can cause pulmonary or cerebrovascular hemorrhage in up to 40 percent of patients, and some studies have shown early hemorrhagic death in 10–20 percent of these patients.[8] The induction of tumor cell differentiation with all-*trans*-retinoic acid can rapidly alleviate the coagulopathy.[8]

CHRONIC DISSEMINATED INTRAVASCULAR COAGULATION

Compensated or chronic DIC develops when blood is continuously or intermittently exposed to small amounts of tissue factor, and compensatory mechanisms in the liver and bone marrow are largely unable to replenish the depleted coagulation proteins and platelets, respectively. Under these conditions, the patient is either asymptomatic with increased levels of fibrin degradation products or has manifesations of venous or arterial thrombosis, or both. Patients with chronic DIC may also have minor bleeding from the skin and mucosal membranes.

Malignancies, particularly solid tumors, are the most common cause of chronic DIC. Venous thromboses commonly present as deep venous thrombosis in the extremities or superficial migratory thrombophlebitis (Trousseau syndrome), where arterial thromboses can produce digital ischemia, renal infarction, or stroke. Arterial ischemia can also be due to embolization from nonbacterial thrombotic (marantic) endocarditis.

The diagnosis of acute DIC is suggested by the history (e.g., sepsis, trauma, malignancy), clinical presentation, moderate to severe thrombocytopenia (less than 100 000 platelets/μL), and the presence of microangiopathic changes on the peripheral blood smear. The diagnosis is confirmed by the findings of increased thrombin generation (e.g. decreased fibrinogen) and increased fibrinolysis (e.g. elevated fibrin degradation products and D-dimer). The extent of these abnormalities may correlate with the extensiveness of organ involvement. The laboratory values in the abovementioned studies are variable in chronic DIC because a slower rate of the consumption of coagulation factors may be offset by enhanced synthesis of these proteins. In such patients, the diagnosis may be largely based upon the finding of microangiopathy in the peripheral blood smear and increased levels of fibrin degradation products and, in particular, D-dimer.

TREATMENT

Treatment of the underlying disease (e.g. sepsis) is of central importance in controlling acute or chronic DIC. Hemodynamic support is essential, but many patients do not require specific therapy for the coagulopathy, because it is either short lived or not severe enough to pose a major risk for bleeding or thrombosis. In select instances, blood component replacement therapy or heparin may be of value, although there are no controlled studies showing the definitive benefit of either. In contrast, the administration of antifibrinolytic agents, such as ε-aminocaproic acid (EACA) or aprotinin, are generally contraindicated, because blockage of the fibrinolytic system may increase the risk of thrombotic complications.[9*] Disseminated intravascular coagulation associated with acute promyelocytic leukemia responds to treatment with all-*trans*-retinoic acid.

Platelet transfusion and fresh frozen plasma

Patients with DIC bleed because of thrombocytopenia and coagulation factor deficiency. There is no evidence to support the administration of platelets and coagulation factors in patients who are not bleeding or at high risk of bleeding. However, treatment is justified in patients who have serious bleeding, are at high risk for bleeding (e.g. after surgery), or require invasive procedures.

Patients with marked thrombocytopenia (less than 20 000 platelets/μL) or those with moderate thrombocytopenia (less than 50 000 platelets/μL) and serious bleeding should be given platelet transfusions (1–2 units/10 kg per day). Such patients typically show a less-than-expected rise in platelet count, due to the ongoing consumption. With respect to replacement therapy, patients who are actively bleeding with a significantly elevated prothrombin time, international normalized ratio (INR), or a fibrinogen concentration <50 mg/dL, or both should receive fresh frozen plasma or cryoprecipitate, the latter for fibrinogen replacement. It is preferable to keep the fibrinogen level above 100 mg/dL.

Heparin

The administration of heparin or other anticoagulants to interrupt the underlying coagulopathy in DIC would appear to be a logical therapeutic approach. However, there are no controlled trials indicating a benefit to these, and there is little evidence that the use of heparin improves organ function.[10,11]

THROMBOCYTOPENIA AND HEMORRHAGIC RISK IN PATIENTS WITH CANCER

The direct relationship between the platelet count and bleeding episodes in patients with malignant diseases was first documented in 1962 by Gaydos *et al.*,[12] in patients with acute leukemia. Since then it has become well known that a spontaneous hemorrhage rarely occurs when the patient's platelet count exceeds 50 000/μL, but the risk of bleeding increases considerably as the count falls below 20 000/μL. The most feared complication of thrombocytopenia is intracranial hemorrhage. In this study major bleeding rarely occurred when the platelet count exceeded 20 000/μL but gradually the incidence increased as the platelet count ranged between 20 000/μL and 5000/μL, and became more dramatic when the platelet count fell below 5000/μL. In particular, Gaydos *et al.* observed that bleeding episodes associated with thrombocytopenia frequently follow a decline in platelet count, especially in cases in which the bleeding occurred when platelet counts exceeded 5000/μL. Moreover, no intracranial bleeding was observed at a platelet count exceeding 10 000/μL. Despite these data, Gaydos *et al.*'s study has been widely misinterpreted and overinterpreted, and for years it became the practice to administer platelets prophylactically to maintain the platelet count above a level of 20 000/μL.[13] Aspirin, nonsteroidal antiinflammatory drugs (NSAIDs) and some antibiotics, such as high-dose penicillin, taken by patients with malignant disease may impair platelet function. In 1978, Slichter and Harker[14] published that the threshold for spontaneous bleeding, as measured by fecal blood loss, was at approximately 5000 platelets/μL in patients with aplastic anemia. This finding was confirmed by the randomized study of Solomon *et al.*[15] showing that patients routinely transfused with platelets at 20 000/μL fared no better than those who were transfused only if they were bleeding or if their platelet count was decreasing rapidly.

The incidence of hemorrhagic complications in patients with solid tumors was first studied by Belt *et al.*[16] in a cohort of 718 patients receiving myelosuppressive chemotherapeutic agents. (Seventy-five patients [10.4 percent] experienced one or more episodes of hemorrhage. Bleeding was due to tumor invasion in 25/75 patients [33.3 percent] and DIC in 7 patients [9.3 percent] and was unrelated to malignant neoplasms or drug treatment in 6 patients [8 percent]. Thirty-seven patients [49.3 percent] had hemorrhages associated with drug-induced thrombocytopenia.) These results confirmed that there was a quantitative relation between the incidence of hemorrhage and the platelet count for both the group with thrombocytopenia and the group with hemorrhage resulting from all causes. However, the incidence of hemorrhage was low until the platelet count decreased below 10 000/μL, and fatal bleeding was unlikely to occur at platelet counts above 5000/μL.[16]

In 1984, Dutcher *et al.*[17] reviewed the records of 1274 patients treated between 1972 and 1980 on protocols known to produce significant myelosuppression to evaluate the incidence of thrombocytopenia and bleeding among patients with solid tumors, who had been treated intensively with chemotherapy. Of these, 301 patients experienced 5063 days of thrombocytopenia <50 000 platelets/μL and 670 days of severe thrombocytopenia <20 000 platelets/μL. The median number of days with thrombocytopenia was 6 (range 1–250). There were only 44 episodes of clinically detectable serious bleeding, primarily gastrointestinal (26/44), during thrombocytopenia and all but 7 episodes first occurred at platelet counts between 20 000/μL and 50 000/μL. Fifteen of the 44 bleeding episodes were associated with coagulation abnormalities, 24 occurred during serious infection, and 12 occurred at the sites of tumors. Of the 301 patients, 147 (49 percent) received platelet transfusions. In 86 patients with thrombocytopenia who had CNS tumors, there was no evidence of CNS bleeding during thrombocytopenia. Hemorrhagic deaths were uncommon; of the 12 patients who died of bleeding, seven had normal platelet counts.[17]

Ten years later, Goldberg *et al.*[18] retrospectively studied the clinical impact of thrombocytopenia in patients with gynecological cancer who received chemotherapy. Thrombocytopenia, which was defined as having a platelet count below 100 000/μL, occurred in 182/501 (36.3 percent) patients. No intracranial or life-threatening bleeding occurred in any patient. Of these 182 patients, 139 (76.4 percent) had no clinical bleeding. Minor bleeding occurred in 34 patients (18.7 percent) and 44 cycles of chemotherapy (5.4 percent). Major bleeding occurred in nine patients (4.9 percent) and 10 cycles (1.3 percent). Of the major bleeding events, five occurred in 49 patients with platelet counts between 0 μL and 10 000/μL. Forty-three of these patients received platelet transfusions, and 38 of these 43 patients (88.3 percent) had no bleeding. Of the remaining five patients, two received prophylactic transfusions with no effect. Three major bleeding events occurred in patients with platelet counts that ranged from 11 000/μL to 20 000/μL, but these were due to chronic instrumentation or trauma. In patients with platelet counts exceeding 20 000/μL, major bleeding occurred only from necrotic metastatic lesions. Therefore, in this study, platelet counts of 10 000/μL were not associated with spontaneous major bleeding.[18]

To evaluate the conservative management of chemotherapy-induced thrombocytopenia, prophylactic transfusions were administered only to patients with platelet counts <5000/μL. Fanning *et al.*[19] evaluated 179 episodes of thrombocytopenia in 46 women with gynecological cancers who were enrolled in four dose-intense chemotherapy trials. Of the 179 episodes of thrombocytopenia evaluated, 100 were severe (<20 000/μL). None of the 179 episodes of thrombocytopenia resulted in major bleeding, including 70 that occurred in patients with platelet counts below <20 000/μL who were not receiving prophylactic platelet transfusions and 14/70 in patients who had platelet counts between 5000/μL and 10 000/μL.[19]

From these studies, it is evident that the risk of bleeding depends not only on the platelet count, but also on the underlying disease, the use of drugs interfering with platelet function, and complications such as fever and infection or the presence of coagulation defects. As a consequence, it is not just the absolute platelet count, but rather the number of functional platelets that is important for the prevention of bleeding. Despite this, there are no studies showing that the bleeding time may aid in defining the risk of bleeding.

CLINICAL APPROACH (BOX 85.2)

A broad, open, and inquisitive frame of mind is a must when approaching the bleeding patient. The history and physical examination should provide important baseline information. Key laboratory tests must be quickly ordered and interpreted. Using this database, one can quickly determine whether the hemorrhagic disorder is congenital or acquired, severe or mild, and progressive or stable. Hemostasis may fail because of the deficiencies of platelets, the plasma coagulation protein system, or endothelial disturbances.

Box 85.2 Management of hemorrhage

- Identify patients at risk, if possible (such as patients who have already had a previous episode of bleeding)

- Identify the cause (detailed history and laboratory tests including cancer history, surgical history, medications, platelet disorder, coagulation disorders to determine whether it is anatomical, generalized, or both)

- Formulate a management plan and communicate it to the patient, family, and the medical team. Emphasize a caring approach and empathic listening to the fears of the patient and family that may help to resolve any conflicts arising from the situation

- Provide dark towels and a dark basin at the patient's bedside

- Prepare an emergency pack of a sedating drug (e.g. midazolam 5 mg in a prefilled syringe) to be given subcutaneously or intravenously

- Treat the bleeding, if appropriate, with several local modalities (such as topical hemostatic agents, radiotherapy, or interventional radiology) or systemic treatments (such as tranexamic acid)

- Consider transfusions or erythropoietin for the management of hypovolemia and anemia

---

In the palliative setting, many factors must be considered with regard to the management of bleeding. The clinician has to not only consider the underlying cause and the clinical presentation, including the severity and nature of each event, but also take into account other salient factors such as the setting of care, availability of various resources, overall disease burden, predicted life expectancy, the patient's overall quality of life, and wishes of the patient and family.

The choice of treatment modality must balance the risk of aggressive management with increased treatment-related toxicity, i.e. against the failure to use treatments that have potential symptomatic benefit. Although the staff providing palliative care can initiate many simple treatments, a definitive approach to management requires an interdisciplinary approach and sometimes expertise of various specialists.

As an example of the need to set priorities, it is evident that interventional radiology or surgical ligation of the pelvic vessel would be less likely to be considered in a homebound, cachectic patient who has expressed the desire to remain at home, particularly if the patient has an estimated life expectancy ranging from a few days to a few weeks. On the other hand, if the same patient presented soon after significant hemorrhaging began, it would be reasonable to at least consider the aforementioned treatments, particularly if specialists with the required skills and equipment are available. The patients and families facing the prospect or reality of massive bleeding require extensive psychological support.

Management of bleeding

General management of bleeding needs to be individualized and depends on the underlying cause, the likelihood of reversing or controlling the underlying cause, and the burden-to-benefit ratio of the treatment. If the patient's disease burden and life expectancy warrant it, then the management of a bleeding episode consists of general resuscitative measures, such as volume and fluid replacement, and specific measures to stop the bleeding. On the other hand, palliative measures may be most appropriate in end-stage patients. Appropriate management involves a detailed assessment via a history that includes a review of prior bleeding episodes, past illness, psychosocial stressors (including level of family support), and medications such as NSAIDs and anticoagulants. Physical examination should focus on whether the bleeding is focal or occurring at multiple sites. Investigations such as a hemogram and clotting profile may reveal a systemic disease, whereas endoscopic studies or angiography may reveal the site of the bleeding.

LOCAL INTERVENTIONS (BOX 85.3)

Packing can be used with or without pressure to achieve hemostasis when bleeding originates in the nose, vagina, or rectum. Surgical swabs of various sizes may be used for this purpose. Nonadherent dressings should be used. A variety of hemostatic agents and dressings, mostly designed for surgical procedures, are beneficial for exterior topical use in patients with advanced cancer.[21] Thromboplastin, a

Box 85.3 Local measures

- Epinephrine – may be used topically, but its liberal use is discouraged

- Prostaglandins E_2 and F_2 – used in intractable hemorrhagic cystitis

- Silver nitrate – induces chemical cauterization and has been used to control hemorrhages in the bladder and epistaxis

- 2–4 percent formalin – acts as a chemical cautery and has been used to control intractable rectal and bladder hemorrhaging

- Aluminum astringents – an example is 1 percent alum, which can be delivered by continuous irrigation of the bladder

- Sucralfate – controls cancer-related gastrointestinal bleeding and cutaneous oozing

- Tranexamic acid – controls bleeding when used locally[20*]

natural blood-clotting agent obtained from bovine plasma, is available as a powder for topical preparation.[22*]

Absorbable gelatin is available as a sterile spongelike dressing or sterile powder that can be applied dry or saturated with sterile sodium solution and is absorbed within 4–6 weeks. When the gelatin is applied, fibrin is deposited in the interstices of the foam, resulting in the swelling of the sponge, thereby forming a large synthetic clot. When the gelatin is applied to nasal, rectal, or vaginal mucosa, it liquefies within 2–5 days. Other bioabsorbable topical hemostatic agents include fibrin sealants and oxidized cellulose.[23**,24*] Fibrin sealants are derived from human plasma and reproduce the final steps in the coagulation pathway to form a clot. The inherent hemostatic activity of absorbable collagen agents provokes a clotting cascade when the bovine-derived mesh comes into contact with blood, and forms a clot. Other available hemostatic agents are oxidized cellulose compounds and highly absorbent alginate dressings derived from seaweed. Vasoconstricting or cauterizing agents are used to manage localized capillary-based bleeding.

RADIOTHERAPY

External beam radiotherapy is used to decrease the hemoptysis caused by lung cancer and is effective in 80 percent of patients.[5**,6**,25***] It also controls bleeding in 85 percent of patients with rectal bleeding and 60 percent of those with hematuria from bladder cancer.[6**,26**] Radiotherapy should

also be considered for treating bleeding from cancerous lesions in the vagina, skin, rectum, and bladder. Although radiotherapy can be useful in controlling the bleeding in patients with head and neck cancers, many patients have already received the maximal allowable doses of radiotherapy by the time bleeding occurs and cannot receive further radiation. Single or reduced fraction regimens appear to be as effective as multiple fractions in controlling bleeding. Upper gastrointestinal hemorrhaging from a malignant process is less amenable to radiotherapy.

ENDOSCOPY (TABLE 85.1)

Endoscopy-based treatments have, for a long time, been used to manage the bleeding from upper gastrointestinal varices, particularly after systemic therapies with agents such as vasopressin or somatostatin analogs have failed.[27, 28*]

INTERVENTIONAL RADIOLOGY

Embolization may be useful in well-selected patients whose blood vessels are accessible by catheter, and have not resulted in ischemia. The benefits of embolization have been reported in patients with cancers involving head and neck, pelvis, lung, liver, and gastrointestinal tract.[29–42*]

Transcutaneous arterial embolization is the technique used in some of these patients to control bleeding in select cases of intractable hemorrhage resulting from advanced pelvic urological malignancies, carotid artery rupture due to cancer, and spontaneous rupture of hepatocellular carcinoma.

Table 85.1 *Endoscopic interventions*

Procedure	What it does
Upper gastrointestinal endoscopy	Argon beam plasma coagulation has been shown to control bleeding in esophagogastric cancer
Cystoscopy	Cystoscopic-assisted cautery by either heat or laser probes has been used in the treatment of hematuria patients with bladder cancer
Bronchoscopy	In case of hemoptysis, bronchoscopy allows for ice-cold saline lavages and/or the use of balloon tamponade, laser photocoagulation, or topical application of thrombin or fibrinogen at the site of the bleeding
Colonoscopy	Techniques such as bipolar electrocoagulation, heater probe, argon, and Nd:YAG lasers are used to control bleeding in the lower gastrointestinal tract

SURGERY

Surgery may be appropriate for select patients for whom conservative measures have failed, and for those who are deemed fit for surgery. Bleeding has been controlled with surgery in patients with head and neck cancers who presented with acute or imminent carotid artery rupture and in radiation proctitis in whom the bleeding was not controlled by topically applied formalin.[43,44*]

SYSTEMIC INTERVENTIONS

Vitamin K

Vitamin K (phytonadione, menadiol) may be useful in the treating a derangement in vitamin K-dependent coagulation factors, such as factors II, VII, IX, and X, or for treating bleeding in patients with advanced cancer caused by excessive therapy with warfarin. The preferable route of administration would be oral or subcutaneous, but the intravenous route should be considered when rapid correction is required. The recommended doses vary from 2.5 mg to 10 mg depending on the severity.[45**]

Vasopressin/desmopressin

Vasopressin/desmopressin is a hormone in the posterior pituitary gland that causes splanchnic arteriolar constriction and reduction in portal pressure when it is injected intravenously or intraarterially. It has been used in a controlled trial to manage bleeding in selected patients with upper gastrointestinal bleeding related to a malignancy.[46*]

Somatostatin analogs

Octreotide, an analog of somatostatin, has been used in palliative care for reducing secretions in patients with a gastrointestinal obstruction. It also reduces the splanchnic flow and pressure by causing venous dilatation, thereby reducing portal pressure and portal venous flow and may reduce bleeding.[47***] Its use for controlling bleeding in cancer patients has not been reported.

Antifibrinolytic agents

Tranexamic acid and EACA are synthetic antifibrinolytic agents that block the binding sites of plasminogen, thereby inhibiting the conversion of plasminogen into plasmin by tissue plasminogen activator. The end result is the decreased lysis of fibrin clots.[48,49] Tranexamic acid and EACA have been administered orally and intravenously. Tranexamic acid is 10 times more potent than EACA in vitro. The suggested intravenous dose of tranexamic acid is 10 mg/kg three to four times a day, infused over about 1 hour. The suggested intravenous dose of EACA is 4–5 g in 250 mL over the first hour and then 1 g/hour in 50 mL administered continuously for 8 hours, or until the bleeding is controlled.[50*] The most common adverse effects of tranexamic acid and EACA are gastrointestinal in nature (nausea, vomiting, and diarrhea) and occur in 25 percent of cases. The adverse effects appear to be dose dependent. Thromboembolism is uncommon.[51,52]

BLOOD PRODUCTS

Transfusions of blood products should be undertaken on a selective basis. There is no scientific basis for the 20 000/μL cut to transfuse platelets. Lassauniere and colleagues proposed criteria for platelet transfusions in patients with advanced hematological malignancies.[53***] These criteria include continuous bleeding of the mouth or gums, epistaxis, extensive and painful hematomas, severe headaches, or disturbed vision of recent onset, as well as continuous bleeding through the gastrointestinal, gynecological, or urinary systems. The continuation of platelet transfusion in patients with end-stage thrombocytopenia poses an ethical dilemma. Even through the ongoing transfusions may be futile, the patients and their families may perceive the cessation of transfusions as the withdrawal of life-sustaining therapy. Sensitive and empathic discussions between patients, their families, the attending physician and the health team are essential in order to explore their expectations, fears, and concerns and to engage in advanced end-of-life planning while ensuring ongoing support and providing optimal comfort care.

Transfusions of fresh frozen plasma are indicated in patients:

- who are bleeding and have specific deficiencies in certain coagulation factors
- in whom the effects of warfarin urgently need to be reversed
- who require urgent invasive interventions such as thoracenteses or surgery
- with DIC, when appropriate.

Transfusions of packed red cells are indicated when anemia resulting from blood loss causes or aggravates symptoms such as fatigue and dyspnea.

CONCLUSIONS

Massive bleeding, which occurs in 6–10 percent of patients in palliative care settings, can be extremely distressing for both the patients and caregivers. These episodes require an individualized approach based on the specific needs of the patient and family, which include the level of distress, the stage of disease, and the expertise available. A multidisciplinary approach that makes use of various modalities may be required. Treatments range from simple hemostatic techniques to more invasive and sophisticated modalities. Minimal management requires the identification of patients at risk and preparatory measures to empower caregivers to deal appropriately with massive bleeding if it occurs.

Key learning points

- Bleeding occurs in approximately 10 percent of patients with advanced cancer.

- It is the immediate cause of death in 6 percent of patients with cancer.

- Bleeding is very distressing to the patient and his or her family.

- Thorough clinical assessment is essential to identify the risk of bleeding and the cause when it occurs.

- Formulate a management plan and communicate it to the patient, family, and the medical team.

- Emphasize a caring approach and empathic listening to the fears of the patient and family that may help to resolve any conflicts arising from the situation.

REFERENCES

◆ 1   Smith AM. Emergencies in palliative care. *Ann Acad Med Singapore* 1994; **23**: 186–90.

◆ 2   Hoskin P, Makin W, eds. *Oncology for Palliative Medicine.* Oxford: Oxford University Press, 1998: 229–34.

◆ 3   Gagnon B, Mancini I, Pereira J, Bruera E. Palliative management of bleeding events in advanced cancer patients. *J Palliat Care* 1998; **14**: 50–4.

◆ 4   Devita VT, Hellman S, Rosenberg SA, eds. *Cancer. Principles and Practice of Oncology,* 4th ed. Philadelphia: JB Lippincott Co., 1993.

● 5   MRC Lung Cancer Working Party. Inoperable non-small cell lung cancer (NSCLC): a Medical Research Council randomized trial of palliative radiotherapy with two fractions. *Cancer* 1991; **63**: 265–70.

◆ 6   Hoskin P. Radiotherapy in symptom management. In: Doyle D, Hanks G, Cherney M, Calman K, eds. *Oxford Textbook of Palliative Medicine,* 3rd ed. Oxford University Press, 2003: 239–55.

● 7   Siegal T, Seligsohn U, Aghai E, Modan M. Clinical and laboratory aspects of disseminated intravascular coagulation (DIC): A study of 118 cases. *Thromb Haemost* 1978; **39**: 122–34.

● 8   Barbui T, Finazzi G, Falenga A. The impact of all-trans-retinoic acid on the coagulopathy of acute promyelocytic leukemia. *Blood* 1998; **91**: 3093–102.

● 9   Garcia-Avello A, Lorente JA, Cesar-Perez J, *et al.* Degree of hypercoagulability and hyperfibrinolysis is related to organ failure and prognosis after burn trauma. *Thromb Res* 1998; **89**: 59–64.

◆ 10 Feinstein DI. Diagnosis and management of disseminated intravascular coagulation: The role of heparin therapy. *Blood* 1982; **60**: 284–7.

● 11 Corrigan JJ Jr, Jordan CM. Heparin therapy in septicemia with disseminated intravascular coagulation. Effect on mortality and on correction of hemostatic defects. *N Engl J Med* 1970; **283**: 778–9.

● 12 Gaydos LA, Freireich EJ, Mantel N. The quantitative relation between platelet count and hemorrhage in patients with acute leukemia. *N Engl J Med* 1962; **266**: 905–9.

◆ 13 Ford JM. Should prophylactic platelets be given to patients with acute leukemia? In: Lister TA, Malpas JS, eds. *Platelet Transfusion.* Baltimore, CO: University Park, 1980: 45–9.

◆ 14 Slichter SJ, Harker LA. Thrombocytopenia: mechanisms and management of defects in platelet production. *Clin Haematol* 1978; **7**: 523–9.

◆ 15 Solomon J, Bofenkamp T, Fahey JL, *et al.* Platelet prophylaxis in acute non-lymphoblastic leukemia. *Lancet* 1978; **i**: 267.

● 16 Belt RJ, Leite C, Haas CD, Stephens RL. Incidence of hemorrhagic complications in patients with cancer. *J Am Med Assoc* 1978; **239**: 2571–4.

● 17 Dutcher JP, Schiffer CA, Aisner J, *et al.* Incidence of thrombocytopenia and serious hemorrhage among patients with solid tumors. *Cancer* 1984; **53**: 557–62.

● 18 Goldberg GL, Gibbon DG, Smith HO, *et al.* Clinical impact of chemotherapy-induced thrombocytopenia in patients with gynecologic cancer. *J Clin Oncol* 1994; **12**: 2317–20.

◆ 19 Fanning J, Hilgers RD, Murray KP, *et al.* Conservative management of chemotherapeutic-induced thrombocytopenia in women with gynecologic cancers. *Gynecol Oncol* 1995; **59**: 191–3.

  20 Waly NG. Local antifibrinolytic treatment with tranexamic acid in hemophilic children undergoing dental extractions. *Egypt Dent J* 1995; 41: 961–8.

◆ 21 Woodruff R. Haematological problems. In: Woodruff R, ed. *Palliative Medicine: Symptomatic and Supportive Care for Patients with Advanced Cancer and AIDS.* Melbourne: Aperula Pty Ltd., 1993: 228–52.

◆ 22 Thrombostat. Compendium of Pharmaceuticals and Specialities. Ottawa, Canada: Canadian Pharmacists Association, 1997; **32**: 1587.

● 23 Shinkwin CA, Beasley N, Simo R, *et al.* Evaluation of surgical Nu-knit, Merocel and Vaseline gauze nasal packs: a randomized trial. *Rhinology* 1996; **34**: 41–3.

◆ 24 Mankad PS, Codispoti M. Role of fibrin sealants in hemostasis. *Am J Surg* 2001; **182**(suppl 2): 21S–28S.

◆ 25 Brundage MD, Bezjak A, Dixon P, *et al.* The role of palliative thoracic radiotherapy in non-small cell lung cancer. *Can J Oncol* 1996; **6**(suppl 1): 25–32.

● 26 Langendijk JA, ten Velde GP, Aaronson NK, *et al.* Quality of life after palliative radiotherapy in non-small cell lung cancer: a prospective study. *Int J Radiat Oncol Biol Phys* 2000; **47**: 149–55.

● 27 Srinivasan V, Brown CH, Turner AG. A comparison of two radiotherapy regimens for the treatment of symptoms from advanced bladder cancer. *Clin Oncol (R Coll Radiol)* 1994; **6**: 11–13.

◆ 28 Akhtar K, Byrne JP, Bancewicz J, Attwood SE. Argon beam plasma coagulation in the management of cancers of the esophagus and stomach. *Surg Endosc* 2000; **14**: 1127–30.

◆ 29 Loftus EV, Alexander GL, Ahlquist DA, Balm RK. Endoscopic treatment of major bleeding from advanced gastroduodenal malignant lesions. *Mayo Clin Proc* 1994; **69**: 736–40.

◆ 30 Kvale PA, Simoff M, Prakash UB. Lung cancer. Palliative care. *Chest* 2003; **123**(Suppl 1): 284S–311S.

◆ 31 Patel U, Pattison CW, Raphael M. Management of massive haemoptysis. *Br J Hosp Med* 1994; **52**: 74, 76–8.

◆ 32 Bates MC, Shamsham FM. Endovascular management of impending carotid rupture in a patient with advanced head and neck cancer. *J Endovasc Ther* 2003; **10**: 54–7.

● 33 Sakakibara Y, Kuramoto K, Jikuya T, *et al.* An approach for acute disruption of large arteries in patients with advanced cervical cancer: endoluminal balloon occlusion technique. *Ann Surg* 1998; **227**: 134–7.

◆ 34 Morrissey DD, Andersen PE, Nesbit GM, *et al.* Endovascular management of hemorrhage in patients with head and neck cancer. *Arch Otolaryngol Head Neck Surg* 1997; **123**: 15–19.

● 35 Nabi G, Sheikh N, Greene D, Marsh R. Therapeutic transcatheter arterial embolization in the management of intractable haemorrhage from pelvic urological malignancies: preliminary experience and long-term follow-up. *BJU Int* 2003; **92**: 245–7.

◆ 36 Wells I. Internal iliac artery embolization in the management of pelvic bleeding. *Clin Radiol* 1996; **51**: 825–7.

● 37 Yamashita Y, Harada M, Yamamoto H, *et al.* Transcatheter arterial embolization of obstetric and gynecological bleeding: efficacy and clinical outcome. *Br J Radiol* 1994; **67**: 530–4.

◆ 38 Hayes MC, Wilson NM, Page A, Harrison GS. Selective embolization of bladder tumors. *Br J Urol* 1996; **78**: 311–12.

● 39 Jenkins CN, McIvor J. Survival after embolization of the internal iliac arteries in ten patients with severe haematuria due to recurrent pelvic carcinoma. *Clin Radiol* 1996; **51**: 865–8.

● 40 Kawaguchi T, Tanaka M, Itano S, *et al.* Successful treatment of bronchial bleeding from invasive pulmonary metastasis of hepatocellular carcinoma: a case report. *Hepatogastroenterology* 2001; **48**: 851–3.

● 41 Recordare A, Bonariol L, Caratozzolo E, *et al.* Management of spontaneous bleeding due to hepatocellular carcinoma. *Minerva Chir* 2002; **57**: 347–56.

● 42 Srivastava DN, Gandhi D, Julka PK, Tandon RK. Gastrointestinal hemorrhage in hepatocellular carcinoma: management with transhepatic arterioembolization. *Abdom Imaging* 2000; **25**: 380–4.

● 43 Yegappan M, Ho YH, Nyam D, *et al.* The surgical management of colorectal complications from irradiation for carcinoma of the cervix. *Ann Acad Med Singapore* 1998; **27**: 627–30.

● 44 Witz M, Korzets Z, Shnaker A, *et al.* Delayed carotid artery rupture in advanced cervical cancer: a dilemma in emergency management. *Eur Arch Otorhinolaryngol* 2002; **259**: 37–9.

● 45 Nee R, Doppenschmidt D, Donovan DJ, Andrews TC. Intravenous versus subcutaneous vitamin K1 in reversing excessive oral anticoagulation. *Am J Cardiol* 1999; **83**: 286–8, A6–A7.

◆ 46 Allum WH, Brearley S, Wheatley KE, *et al.* Acute haemorrhage from gastric malignancy. *Br J Surg* 1990; **77**: 19–20.

◆ 47 Gotzsche PC, Hrobjartsson A. Somatostatin analogues for acute bleeding oesophageal varices. *Cochrane Database Syst Rev* 2005; CD000193.

◆ 48 Garewal HS, Durie BG. Anti-fibrinolytic therapy with aminocaproic acid for the control of bleeding in thrombocytopenic patients. *Scand J Haematol* 1985; **35**: 497–500.

◆ 49 Fricke W, Alling D, Kimball J, *et al.* Lack of efficacy of tranexamic acid in thrombocytopenic bleeding. *Transfusion* 1991; **31**: 345–8.

◆ 50 Herfindal ET, Gourley DR, eds. *Textbook of Therapeutics: Drug and Disease Management,* 6th ed. Baltimore: Williams and Wilkins, 1996.

● 51 Hashimoto S, Koike T, Tatewaki W, *et al.* Fatal thromboembolism in acute promyelocytic leukemia during all-trans retinoic acid therapy combined with antifibrinolytic therapy for prophylaxis of hemorrhage. *Leukemia* 1994; **8**: 1113–15.

● 52 Woo KS, Tse LK, Woo JL, Vallance-Owen J. Massive pulmonary thromboembolism after tranexamic acid antifibrinolytic therapy. *Br J Clin Pract* 1989; **43**: 465–6.

✱ 53 Lassauniere JM, Bertolino M, Hunault M, *et al.* Platelet transfusions in advanced hematological malignancies: a position paper. *J Palliat Care* 1996; **12**: 38–41.

86

Spinal cord compression

NORA A JANJAN, ANITA MAHAJAN, ERIC L CHANG

INTRODUCTION

In the past decade, 11 million cases of cancer were diagnosed and 5 million people have died from cancer in the US. Approximately half the patients diagnosed with cancer will develop metastatic disease. Over 70 percent of all cancer patients develop symptoms from either their primary or metastatic disease.[1–5] Prognosis is influenced by the overall metastatic burden, and the number and location of the sites involved by disease. When metastases are found also in the lung, liver and/or central nervous system, the prognosis is especially poor.[6–15]

Spinal cord compression generally results from bone metastases rather than as a result of leptomeningeal or intramedullary metastases. Prognosis after the development of metastatic disease is important to the type of radiation therapy administered. After bone metastases are diagnosed, the median survivals are 12 months for breast cancer, 6 months with prostate cancer, and 3 months with lung cancer.[7–9] The site of the primary disease and the presence of a solitary metastatic site are predictive of a more prolonged survival.[16–19] The distribution of bone metastases in prostate cancer has prognostic significance. The rate of survival is significantly longer when the metastases are restricted to the pelvis and lumbar spine, and among patients who respond to salvage hormone therapy.[10–12] Any metastatic involvement outside the pelvis and lumbar spine results in lower rates of survival irrespective of response to salvage hormone therapy.

A bone scan index (BSI) has been formulated based on the weighted proportion of tumor involvement in individual bones. The BSI was then related to known prognostic factors and survival in patients with androgen-independent prostate cancer.[13] In multivariable proportional hazards analyses, only the BSI, age, hemoglobin level, and lactate dehydrogenase level were associated with survival. Survival rates were 18.3 months for a BSI of <1.4 percent, 15.5 months for a BSI of 1.4–5.1 percent, and 8.1 months for a BSI > 5.1 percent. Elevations in the bone resorption marker N-telopeptide (NTx) have been associated with a 20 times higher risk for the development of a skeletal complications within 3 months, and shorter times to first disease progression and death.[20,21] These identified prognostic factors should be considered, as a surrogate to a staging system for metastatic disease, so that palliative treatment is appropriate to prognosis based on the extent of disease.

Bone metastases are the most common cause of cancer-related pain, and over 70 percent of patients with bone metastases have symptoms. Among hospitalized patients, over 50 percent of patients experience severe pain due to bone metastases.[4] One of the most important goals in the treatment of bone metastases is to relieve suffering and return the patient to independent function.[22,23] The location of the metastasis influences the types of palliative intervention necessary, especially in weight-bearing bones and bones responsible for ambulation and activities of daily living. Complete pain relief after radiation is achieved in 88 percent of limb lesions, 73 percent of spine metastases, and 67 percent of pelvic metastases.[24]

Bone scans are the most sensitive and specific method of detecting bone metastases, but magnetic resonance imaging (MRI) is the best available technique for evaluating the bone marrow, neoplastic invasion of the vertebrae, the central nervous system and peripheral nerves.[25–27] In a study of melanoma patients, positron emission tomography (^{18}F-fluorodeoxyglucose PET) also found unsuspected spinal cord compression, later confirmed on MRI.[28] Bone or other metastases rarely fail to be detected when radiographic diagnosis is pursued. When radiographic confirmation of malignancy is equivocal, bone biopsy should be considered.[29]

Pain, risk for pathological fracture, and spinal cord compression are the most common indications to treat bone metastases with localized therapy including radiation and surgery. Because external beam radiation provides treatment only to a localized symptomatic site of disease, it is frequently used in coordination with systemic therapies such as chemotherapy, hormonal therapy, and bisphosphonates.

PRINCIPLES OF RADIATION THERAPY

Radiotherapy techniques vary considerably based upon the involved and adjacent normal structures. Basic to an understanding of applied techniques and potential morbidity during a course of radiation are the following principles:[30] radiation therapy is delivered in units designated as the Gray. Relating this to the previously used term rad, equivalent doses can be expressed as 1 Gray (Gy), 100 centigray (cGy) and 100 rad; 1 rad equals 1 cGy.

Radiation for spinal cord compression is delivered by external beam therapy (linear accelerators, cobalt-60 units) that is administered with a prescribed number of daily fractions over several weeks. A variety of radiation energies and biological characteristics are now available to help localize treatment to the areas at risk and exclude uninvolved normal tissues.

External beam irradiation

Included within the classification of external beam radiation are *photons* that are penetrating forms of radiation, and *electrons*, delivering treatment to superficial areas. Other specialized types of external radiation beams are available at only a few centers and they include *proton beam* therapy (administering radiation with high precision to well-defined small areas of tumor involvement, e.g. pituitary or midbrain lesions) and *neutrons* (used by a few centers to treat bulky unresectable or recurrent tumors). Generally photons are used to treat spinal cord compression. Occasionally, electron beam therapy is used in children, and proton beam radiation is now becoming available for the treatment of spinal cord tumors at many centers in the USA.

The concept of integral dose relates the amount of radiation deposited to uninvolved normal tissues located between the skin surface and tumor; the goal in any radiation plan is to minimize integral dose by selecting the appropriate beam energy (Table 86.1). The D_{max} radiation dose is the depth at which 100 percent of the prescribed radiation is deposited. Higher-energy photon radiation, e.g. 18 MeV photons, reduces integral dose because it deposits more radiation to deeper structures while delivering relatively little radiation to superficial tissues.

Multiple radiation portals, each of which is treated daily, are also routinely used in radiotherapy to reduce integral dose. Table 86.2 gives an example of the impact on integral

radiation dose when 200 cGy are prescribed at 10 cm depth from a 6 MeV linear accelerator. When only the posterior radiation portal is used to deliver radiation in the example, the integral dose is high because more superficial tissues receive nearly 50 percent more than the prescribed radiation dose at the site of the tumor located 10 cm below the skin surface; at 1.5 cm from the skin surface the daily radiation dose is 294 cGy per fraction and the total dose is 5880 cGy as compared to the 200 cGy per fraction and total radiation dose of 4000 cGy at the tumor. Radiation tolerance is primarily based on the daily radiation dose; as the

Table 86.1 *The concept of integral dose is demonstrated by the following radiation dose distributions for three different energies including cobalt-60, 6 and 18 MeV photons. D_{max}, the maximum dose, refers to the depth at which 100 percent of the prescribed dose is located below the skin surface. The greater the D_{max}, the greater the skin sparing associated with less of an integral dose*

Skin surface (cm)	Cobalt-60 (%)	6 MeV (%)	18 MeV (%)
0.5	100	30	25
1.0	98	90	50
1.5	95	100	90
2.0	93	98	96
2.5	90	97	98
3.0	88	95	98
3.5	85	92	100
5.0	80	88	96
10.0	55	68	80

Table 86.2 *The impact on integral radiation dose when 200 cGy are prescribed at midline (10 cm depth; patient diameter is 20 cm) from an 6 MeV linear accelerator*

Distance from skin surface (cm)	6 MeV photons (%)
0.5	30
1.0	90
1.5	100
2.0	98
2.5	97
3.0	95
3.5	92
5.0	88
10.0	68
15.0	51
16.5	48
17.5	44
18.5	42
19.5	40

Radiation dose = 200 cGy at 10 cm depth; percentage depth dose = 68%.
Radiation dose at 1.5 cm (D_{max} or 100%) is the radiation dose prescribed/0.68.
Radiation dose at other depths is the D_{max} dose $\times$ % isodose (see Table 86.1).

daily radiation dose increases, the total radiation dose that can be given to normal tissues decreases. Because of this, treatment with a posterior field alone would result in significant side effects due to the high integral dose manifested by skin fibrosis that outlines the radiation field. It is important to realize that giving the first half of the radiation course from the anterior (AP) field alone, and the second half of the radiation course from the posterior (PA) field alone would not reduce radiation side effects. Although the total

radiation dose would be more even using an AP field during the first half and a PA field during the last half of a radiation dose, side effects still may be severe because of the high daily (integral) dose of radiation.

When the radiation is delivered each day from an AP and PA radiation portal, the radiation dose given in the portal is the sum of the radiation dose from each field (Fig. 86.1). The integral dose in the case presented decreases significantly with AP and PA treatment fields because the daily radiation dose throughout the treatment field is within 6 percent (with a daily dose of 211 cGy per fraction at 16.5 cm below the anterior skin surface) of the prescribed dose of 200 cGy per fraction (Fig. 86.2). Likewise, the maximum total radiation dose in the field is 4220 cGy, just 220 cGy more than the prescribed radiation dose at the tumor (Fig. 86.3). Newer treatment approaches, like conformal radiation therapy, exploit this relation by treating up to eight different radiation fields each day. Reducing integral dose is a principal concept of radiation treatment planning because it allows higher radiation doses to the tumor and less radiation to the surrounding normal tissues.

A wide variety of photon energies are available. This allows selective administration of treatment to the tumor and minimizes radiation to uninvolved tissues. As a standard, available photon beam energies range from cobalt-60 to 22 MeV photons. Cobalt-60 delivers 100 percent of the prescribed radiation dose, indicated as the maximum radiation dose (D_{max}), 0.5 cm below the skin surface; 6 MeV X-rays from a linear accelerator have a D_{max} of 1.5 cm, and 18 MeV photons have a D_{max} of 3.5 cm below the skin. Tissues 0.5 cm below the skin surface treated with 18 MeV photons receive only 30 percent of the prescribed radiation dose (Fig. 86.4). This demonstrates the relation in radiation physics that there is more sparing of superficial structures (skin and subcutaneous tissues) from radiation with higher photon energies even though the beam deeply penetrates into the tissue. In contrast to the 18 MeV linear accelerators currently available, the low radiation energy of orthovoltage radiation ranges between 125 keV and 250 keV.

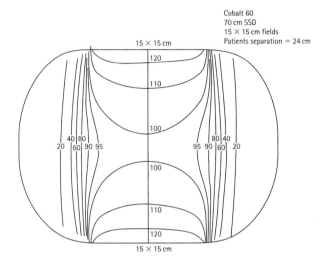

Figure 86.1 *The radiation isodose distribution for a 15 cm × 15 cm radiation field using anterior and posterior (AP and PA) parallel opposed portals with cobalt-60. In this case the patient has a 24 cm diameter. Each number represents a percentage of the prescribed radiation dose. If 200 cGy was prescribed to the 100 percent isodose line, then 240 cGy would be delivered to the 120 percent isodose line near the skin surface and only 180 cGy would be given at the edge of the radiation field at the 90 percent isodose line. The edges of the field receive less radiation dose because there is less opportunity for radiation dose contributed by interactions with adjacent radiated tissue at the blocked edge than in the middle of the field.*

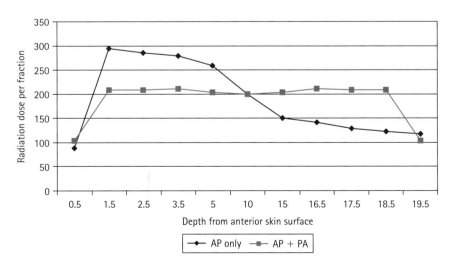

Figure 86.2 *Graphic comparison of the integral radiation dose, defined as the radiation dose deposited between the skin surface and the tumor. In this case, the tumor is 10 cm below the skin surface. If radiation were only given from the anterior treatment portal the radiation dose to the skin would result in complications because of the high radiation dose per fraction as well as the high total dose of radiation.*

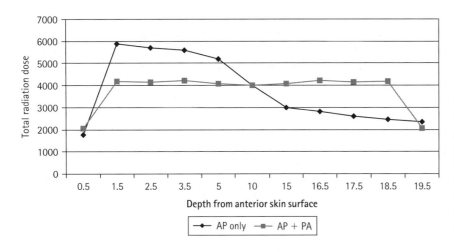

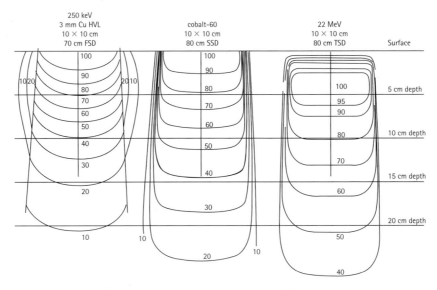

Figure 86.3   *Graphic comparison of the total radiation dose given when a single anterior radiation field is used instead of parallel opposed radiation fields (AP and PA fields) treated every day. With the AP field alone, the skin would receive 30 percent more radiation than the parallel opposed treatment approach to achieve the same radiation dose at the tumor.*

Figure 86.4   *The different radiation isodose distributions for 10 cm × 10 cm radiation fields. The three beams compared include orthovoltage radiation with a 250 keV radiation beam (left), a cobalt-60 unit (middle), and a 22 MeV linear accelerator (right). The 250 keV unit has no skin sparing and little depth of penetration of the radiation beam. The cobalt-60 unit is ideal for treating head and neck cancers in that adequate radiation is given to superficial lymph nodes and scars in the postoperative setting. Because the diameter of the head and neck region is limited, a highly penetrating photon beam is not advisable. Photons of 22 MeV are ideal for deep-seated tumors such as in the pelvis and abdomen because of skin sparing and deep penetration of the photon beams.*

Using conventional radiation techniques, radiation for vertebral metastases commonly were prescribed to 5 cm below the skin surface using cobalt-60 or 6 MeV photons. However, mean depths from MRI scans of 20 patients equaled 5.5 cm for the posterior spinal canal, 6.9 cm for the anterior spinal canal, and 9.6 cm for the anterior vertebral body. Based on the radiation dose distributions, a metastatic lesion in the anterior vertebral body could receive a radiation dose that is significantly lower than that prescribed.[31]

External beam irradiation is administered from specialized machines which emit gamma rays from a housed isotope (cobalt-60) or X-rays (linear accelerators), which are more than 1000 times as powerful as those used in diagnostic radiology, and are generated by electricity. The availability of higher-energy radiation beams, and the development of

a variety of different radiation energies was critical to the advancement of radiation therapy. These advancements allowed more precise deposition of the radiation in the area of the tumor while sparing surrounding uninvolved normal tissues.

Radiation beams diverge as they penetrate through the beam such that the field that exits the body is larger than the field that enters the body. If spinal metastases occur near a previously radiated area of the spinal cord, the new radiation field must be matched to the prior radiation field, accounting for the divergence of the radiation beam. Extreme precision is required when administering radiation, especially when the radiation treatment must match a previously radiated segment of the spinal cord.[32,33] A computed tomography (CT) scanner on rails with a linear accelerator has been

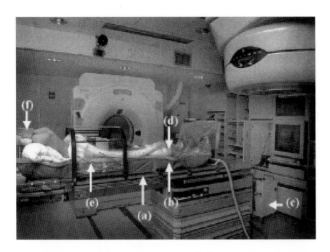

Figure 86.5 *A computed tomography (CT) scanner on rails with a linear accelerator has been used to verify the position of the patient immediately before the administration of the radiation treatment. (a) A carbon fiber base plate; (b) a whole-body vacuum cushion; (c) a vacuum system; (d) a plastic fixation sheet; (e) a stereotactic localizer; and (f) an arm-support system.*
Reprinted from Shiu *et al.* Near simultaneous computed tomography image-guided stereotactic spinal radiotherapy. *Int J Radiat Oncol Biol Phys* 2003; **57**: 605–13[32] with permission from Elsevier.

used to verify the position of the patient immediately before the administration of the radiation treatment; once the patient position is verified on the treatment table by a CT scan, the treatment table is rotated to administer the intensity modulated radiation therapy (IMRT) treatment (Fig. 86.5). Treatment accuracy is within 1 mm of the planned treatment center and the dose variation in the high-dose region is 2 percent or less. Five IMRT treatments delivered 30 Gy to the tumor, limiting the spinal cord radiation dose to 10 Gy or less (Fig. 86.6).

Stereotactic radiosurgery provides a high dose of photon radiation to a small, well-defined area. Using radiosurgery, the vertebral body can receive 20 Gy while less than 0.5 cm^3 of the spinal cord is exposed to 8 Gy of radiation.[34,35] Combined with kyphoplasty, radiosurgery is able to relieve pain in 92 percent of patients during a 7–20-month follow-up period.

Proton beam therapy and 'radiosurgery' are more limited in application and availability, however, the concept is to precisely deposit a large amount of radiation to a well defined volume of tumor while sparing intervening tissues. Precision of proton beam therapy is to the level of the millimeter, requiring exact mapping of the tumor volume and potential microscopic areas of involvement. An additional advantage of proton irradiation is the improvement of relative biological effectiveness of this type of radiation because of the characteristic Bragg–Peak distribution of radiation within a narrow volume of tissue (Fig. 86.7). Chordomas and localized intracranial tumors, especially

around the optic chiasma, have been treated with proton irradiation. Because of its precision, research is ongoing to define further applications of proton therapy, especially in pediatric tumors and previously irradiated recurrent tumors.

The clinical status of the patient is accounted for in the treatment set-up and in the number of radiation treatments that are prescribed. The radiation dose-fractionation schedule and technique also considers the site and volume irradiated, and the integration of other therapies. Conformal, IMRT and proton therapy are all techniques that can better localize radiation dose and reduce side effects, especially in a previously irradiated area.

Reirradiation

Issues regarding reirradiation are especially important in palliative therapy. Experimental data suggest that acute responding tissues recover from radiation injury in a few months and can tolerate additional radiation therapy. However, there is considerable variability in recovery from radiation among late-reacting tissues such as the spinal cord.[36,37] This recovery depends on the technique used, the organ irradiated, the volume irradiated, the initial total dose of radiation, the radiation dose given with each fraction, and the time interval between the initial and second courses of radiation.[38]

Correlating with existing clinical experience, limited toxicities occur with reirradiation when there is careful attention to treatment techniques and radiobiological factors. Radiotherapeutic techniques that localize the radiation dose to the recurrent tumor and limit the dose to the surrounding normal tissues allow the reirradiation of recurrent tumors. Other techniques include conformal external beam radiation, IMRT, and proton therapy.[39,40]

Conformal radiation therapy/IMRT

Conformal radiation techniques precisely localize the radiation dose using external beam radiation from a linear accelerator. Because very low doses of radiation are given through a number of beams, no one area of normal tissues receives a significant dose of radiation. The tumor, though, is given the sum of the radiation from the beams and receives a high dose of radiation. This technique has allowed high doses of radiation to be given, and has allowed for reirradiation of normal tissues without significant side effects.

Intensity modulated radiation therapy is a form of conformal external beam radiation that even more precisely administers radiation. It is possible to deliver different doses of radiation to specific areas in a single radiation fraction. For example, with IMRT the center of the tumor may receive 2.20 Gy with each radiation treatment to a total dose of 66 Gy over 30 fractions in 6 weeks, while the periphery of the tumor may receive 2.0 Gy with each radiation treatment

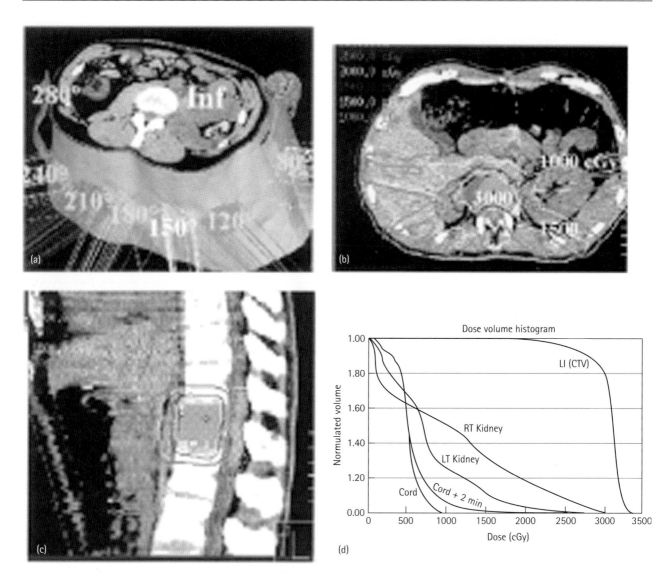

Figure 86.6 *(a–d) Five intensity modulated radiation therapy (IMRT) treatments delivered 30 Gy to the tumor in the patient in* **Figure 86.5**, *limiting the spinal cord radiation dose to 10 Gy or less.*

to a total dose of 60 Gy. At the same time, the normal tissues within 2 cm of the tumor (clinical tumor volume to account for possible microscopic tumor extension) may receive 1.8 Gy with each radiation treatment to a total dose of 54 Gy. Thus, IMRT provides the radiobiological advantage of giving a high daily dose of radiation localized within a tumor while giving a well-tolerated lower daily dose of radiation to the surrounding tissues at the same time. By localizing high daily and total doses of radiation in the tumor, IMRT is able to kill more cancer cells with higher radiation doses without harming the surrounding tissues. Any shape or configuration of radiation dose, like an hourglass, can be designed with IMRT. Because of these factors, this radiotherapeutic tool is extremely helpful in delivering high radiation doses to inoperable tumors over a shorter period of time, and in treating tumors that recur in a previously irradiated field.

Normal tissue tolerance with radiation

A balance is required between the dose required to kill the tumor and the radiation dose tolerated by the normal tissues. The concept of fractionated radiation allows treatment of the cancer while not exceeding the tolerance of the surrounding normal tissues. The four 'Rs' of radiation biology are repair of sublethal damage, reoxygenation, repopulation, and reassortment of cells within the cell cycle.[36] These four factors are key to deciding the radiation schedule to optimize tumor regression while minimizing effects to normal tissues.

With fractionated radiation normal tissues are able to *repair* sublethal radiation effects between treatments. With large daily doses of radiation, a large number of tumor cells are killed, but repair of normal tissues is lower (Fig. 86.8). Because the normal tissues are unable to repair the radiation

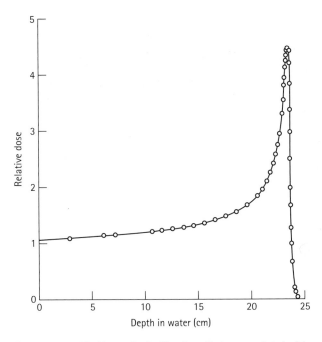

Figure 86.7 *The Bragg–Peak effect in radiation associated with proton radiation. Only the designated tumor area receives radiation and the surrounding normal tissues are spared radiation. Although currently used to treat intracranial tumors and children, proton radiation may have application in palliative care for the re-treatment of tumors.*

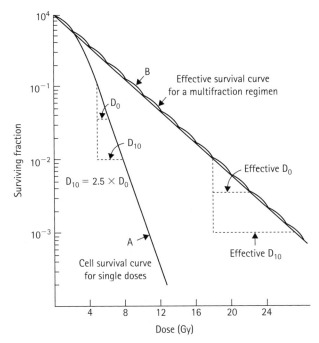

Figure 86.8 *Cell survival curve for single and multiple fraction radiation schedules. A large single dose of radiation, like a single 8 Gy radiation fraction, proportionally kills more tumor cells than equivalent total doses of radiation spread out over multiple fractions, like four 2 Gy fractions, because of repopulation of tumor cells and repair of sublethal damage.*

damage of large daily doses of radiation, the total radiation dose that can be given is also much lower.[36]

Equivalent normal tissue effects can be achieved with a variety of radiation treatment schedules. The following clinical radiation schedules are used to treat spine metastases: 2000 cGy is delivered in five fractions, 3000 cGy is administered in 10 fractions, 3500 cGy in 14 fractions or 4000 cGy in 20 fractions. The late radiation effects on the spinal cord would be equal to giving 2800 cGy, 3600 cGy, and 3900 cGy, respectively, at 200 cGy per fraction. This shows that as the radiation dose per fraction increases, the late radiation toxicities biologically exceed the total radiation dose administered. This effect is more exaggerated as the radiation dose per fraction increases from the standard 200 cGy per fraction.[41] Relating back to the example on integral dose in Table 86.2, administration of 5880 cGy at 294 cGy per fraction would result in severe long-term radiation effects because this would be biologically equal to a total radiation dose of 7200 cGy at 200 cGy per fraction to a large area of small bowel.[42]

The total dose of radiation necessary to eradicate a tumor is a function of the volume of disease and the number of tumor cells killed with each radiation fraction. The tumor volume is the sum of viable and nonviable cells. In most tumors, the potential number of tumor cells is directly proportional to the tumor volume. In some tumors, e.g. soft tissue sarcomas, there is a large necrotic fraction and the rate of cell loss and removal of dead tumor cells from the tumor volume is low. The viable cells may be less responsive to radiation because of the low oxygen tension in the nearby necrotic region. The radiosensitivity of cells also varies during the cell cycle. Cells are most resistant to radiation when they are in the late S-phase, and in the late G1/G0 phase. Radiation resistance results from either rapidly proliferating tumors that spend most of their time in S-phase or a slowly proliferating tumor where many cells are in G1/G0.

Less total radiation dose is required to control microscopic residual disease than bulk disease. For example, the 2-year rate of local control following radiation alone in the treatment of cervical node metastases in head and neck cancer is directly related to the node diameter and total dose. Using 200 cGy per daily fraction of radiation, over 95 percent of patients with only microscopic residual cancer achieve tumor control, and over 85 percent of patients with lymph node diameters of less than 2 cm in size are controlled with a median dose of 6600 cGy. But only 69 percent of nodes measuring between 2.5 cm and 3.0 cm are controlled after 6900 cGy and 59 percent of nodes larger than 3.5 cm are controlled after 7000 cGy. Large tumors have a large hypoxic fraction of cells.[36] Hypoxic cells are relatively resistant to radiation effects; it takes three times the dose of radiation to control hypoxic tumors as it does well-oxygenated tumors (Fig. 86.9). With fractionated radiation, hypoxic areas are able to reoxygenate to some degree during the course of treatment.

Additionally, tumor cells and normal tissues vary widely in their tolerance to radiation because of cellular repopulation.

Radiation doses need to be high enough to kill tumor cells but low enough to allow normal tissues to repair and repopulate. Very low doses of radiation have limited acute effects on normal tissues. No inflammation of the skin or mucosa occurs when the radiation dose is less than 2000 cGy when given in 200 cGy fractions over 2 weeks. But this total dose of radiation is not sufficient to permanently kill tumor cells due to repopulation of the tumor cells. In the past, a course of radiation was interrupted after 2 weeks of treatment to minimize the side effects of treatment. These so-called 'split-courses of radiation' that allowed repair and repopulation of normal tissues and improved tolerance to radiation have been abandoned because tumor control rates were compromised by tumor repopulation during the interruption in the treatment.[43,33] In fact, tumor repopulation was found during radiobiological evaluations to be accelerated after 2 weeks of radiation because of tumor reoxygenation.

Tolerance to radiation also depends on the type of tissue treated. There are two types of normal tissue:

- *Acute reacting tissues.* These are rapidly proliferating tissues, e.g. mucosal surfaces, and usually develop an inflammatory radiation reaction during the course of treatment.

- *Late reacting tissues.* These do not proliferate, e.g. brain and spinal cord, liver, and muscle, and generally do not develop a significant inflammatory reaction during the radiation course.

Acute radiation reactions do not predict the extent of late radiation effects. Scar tissue is the most common form of late radiation effect. These effects are similar to those seen in wound healing. The alpha-beta ratio is a calculation that relates to the ability of normal tissues to repair the damage caused by radiation.[36] With low daily doses of radiation over several weeks, more acute radiation effects are seen during the course of radiation. When high daily doses of radiation are given over a short period of time, the most significant radiation side effects occur months to years later after the radiation is completed.

Relating normal tissue tolerance to a 5 percent risk of a treatment-related complication at 5 years, the tolerance doses (TD 5/5) of each organ have been reported by a National Cancer Institute task force. The TD 5/5 ranges from 1000 cGy for the eye, to 1750 cGy for the lung, 4500 cGy for the brain, and 7000 cGy for the larynx when the entire organ is treated. Radiation tolerance is a function both of the type and the volume of tissue irradiated. When only a third of the organ is irradiated, these values equal 4500 cGy for the lung, 6000 cGy for the brain and 7900 cGy for the larynx. The normal tissue tolerance for spinal cord is more limited.

RADIATION TOLERANCE OF THE SPINAL CORD

The potential for the development of radiation myelitis with total radiation doses which exceed 40 Gy at 2 Gy per fraction represents the limiting factor in the treatment of large tumor burdens near or involving the spinal canal. Furthermore, the length of spinal cord that needs to be irradiated significantly affects the radiation tolerance of the spinal cord.[45–49] Changes seen in the bone marrow on MRI after palliative radiotherapy initially includes decreased cellularity, edema, and hemorrhage followed by fatty replacement and fibrosis. These well-defined changes on MRI after radiotherapy can be distinguished from those seen with progressive disease.[50–52]

Clinical and experimental experience has failed to demonstrate any difference in radiosensitivity in different segments of the spinal cord.[45,48] The risk of radiation myelitis in the cervicothoracic spine is less than 5 percent when 6000 cGy is administered at 172 cGy per fraction, or 5000 cGy is given with daily fractions of 200 cGy per fraction. Especially among patients who have received chemotherapy or need to have a significant length of spinal cord irradiated, the total dose to the spinal cord is generally limited to 4000 cGy administered at 200 cGy per fraction to minimize any risk of irreversible radiation injury to the spinal cord. A steep curve based on total radiation dose predicts the risk of developing radiation myelopathy; a small increase in total radiation dose can result in a large increased risk for radiation myelopathy.[45,47,49]

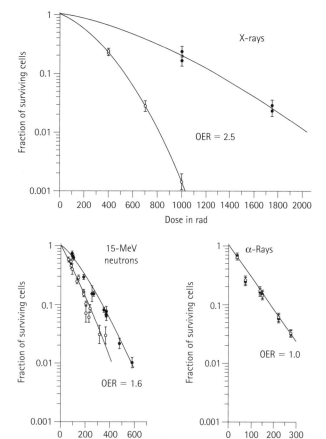

Figure 86.9 *Influence of oxygen on the ability of radiation to kill tumor cells. Open symbols represent hypoxic cells; closed symbols represent oxygenated cells. OER, oxygen enhancement ratio.*

Re-treatment of a previously irradiated segment of spinal cord results in high risk for radiation-induced myelopathy because other neurological pathways cannot compensate for an injury to a specific level of the spinal cord. Experimental data also have shown that the time course and the extent of long-term recovery from radiation are dependent on the specific type and age of tissue.

The radiation tolerance of the spinal cord can be compromised by prior injury. Difficulty arises in separating traumatic, pathological, and radiotherapeutic injury to spinal cord compression. Vasogenic edema of the spinal cord and nerve roots can be caused by compression injury. Metastatic epidural compression results in vasogenic spinal cord edema, venous hemorrhage, loss of myelin, and ischemia. Other consequences of pathological compression include hemorrhage, loss of myelin, and ischemia.[45-49]

PALLIATIVE RADIATION

With palliative radiation, shorter external beam radiation schedules are generally used that administer a higher radiation dose with each radiation fraction. This is known as *hypo*fractionation (Table 86.3). Tumor cell kill is proportional to the radiation dose that is administered. Therefore, symptomatic relief is more quickly achieved because of the large number of tumor cells that are killed in a short period of time with large daily doses of radiation (see Fig. 86.8).

A shorter course of therapy also has a significant impact on quality of life. This short course of treatment not only provides more prompt relief of tumor-related symptoms, but it limits the amount of time needed for the patient to come back and forth for radiation treatments. This is particularly important because the median survival is less than 6 months among patients with poor prognostic factors. However, higher radiation doses, that provide more durable pain relief, are considered warranted for patients with good prognostic factors who require treatment over the spine and other critical sites. It is important to recognize that palliative radiation only results in tumor regression and does not eradicate the tumor. With prolonged survival, the site of metastatic disease may require re-treatment due to regrowth of the tumor.

In contrast to the low daily radiation doses (1.8–2 Gy) given with each treatment during conventional radiation schedules to total radiation doses of 50–60 Gy over 5–6

Table 86.3   *(A) Single anterior radiation field delivering 200 cGy at midline (10 cm)*

Depth from anterior skin surface (cm)	Dose from AP	Total dose × 20 fractions
0.5	88 cGy [294 × 0.30]	1760 cGy [88 × 20]
1.5	294 cGy [200/0.68]	5880 cGy [294 × 20]
2.5	285 cGy [294 × 0.97]	5700 cGy [285 × 20]
3.5	279 cGy [294 × 0.92]	5580 cGy [279 × 20]
5.0	259 cGy [294 × 0.88]	5180 cGy [259 × 20]
10.0	200 cGy [294 × 0.68]	4000 cGy [200 × 20]
15.0	150 cGy [294 × 0.51]	3000 cGy [165 × 20]
16.5	141 cGy [294 × 0.48]	2820 cGy [144 × 20]
17.5	129 cGy [294 × 0.44]	2580 cGy [129 × 0]
18.5	123 cGy [294 × 0.42]	2460 cGy [126 × 20]
19.5	118 cGy [294 × 0.40]	2360 cGy [118 × 20]

(B) Parallel opposed (AP and PA) radiation fields treated each day delivering 200 cGy at midline (10 cm)

Depth from anterior skin surface (cm)	Dose from AP	Dose from PA	Total dose per fraction (AP + PA)	Total dose × 20 fractions (AP + PA)
0.5	44 cGy [147 × 0.30]	59 cGy [147 × 0.40]	103 cGy	2060 cGy
1.5	147 cGy [100/0.68]	62 cGy [147 × 0.42]	209 cGy	4180 cGy
2.5	143 cGy [147 × 0.97]	65 cGy [147 × 0.44]	208 cGy	4160 cGy
3.5	140 cGy [147 × 0.92]	71 cGy [147 × 0.48]	211 cGy	4220 cGy
5.0	129 cGy [147 × 0.88]	75 cGy [147 × 0.51]	204 cGy	4080 cGy
10.0	100 cGy [147 × 0.68]	100 cGy [147 × 0.68]	200 cGy	4000 cGy
15.0	75 cGy [147 × 0.51]	129 cGy [147 × 0.88]	204 cGy	4080 cGy
16.5	71 cGy [147 × 0.48]	140 cGy [147 × 0.92]	211 cGy	4220 cGy
17.5	65 cGy [147 × 0.44]	143 cGy [147 × 0.97]	208 cGy	4160 cGy
18.5	62 cGy [147 × 0.42]	147cGy [100/0.68]	209 cGy	4180 cGy
19.5	59 cGy [147 × 0.40]	44 cGy [147 × 0.30]	103 cGy	2060 cGy

weeks, large daily radiation fractions are given with hypofractionated radiation schedules used for palliative radiation. Because of normal tissue tolerance to radiation, the total radiation dose that can be administered is low when high doses of radiation are given with each daily fraction. Hypofractionated radiation schedules can range from 2.5 Gy per fraction administered over 3 weeks for a total radiation dose of 35 Gy to a single 8 Gy dose of radiation.[53,54] Most frequently, 30 Gy is administered in 10 fractions over 2 weeks. The decision for the radiation schedule depends on the radiation tolerance of the tissues in the field and the prognosis. The radiation schedule used to relieve symptoms must be indexed to the types of tissues treated, the potential for tumor resection, and/or overall prognosis.

Radiopharmaceuticals are another systemic option that treat diffuse symptomatic bone metastases. Radiopharmaceuticals, such as strontium-89 or samarium-153, can also be used to treat bone metastases when symptoms recur in a previously irradiated site but are contraindicated with epidural disease because the radiation is deposited directly at the involved area in the bone.[55–60] Radiopharmaceuticals can also act as an adjuvant to localized external beam irradiation and reduce the development of other symptomatic sites of disease.

Control of cancer-related pain with the use of analgesics is imperative to allow comfort during and while awaiting response to antineoplastic interventions. Pain represents a sensitive measure of disease activity. Patients should be closely followed up to ensure control of cancer and treatment-related pain, and to initiate diagnostic studies to determine the cause of persistent, progressive or recurrent symptoms. The limited radiation tolerance of the normal tissues, like the spinal cord, that are adjacent to a bone metastasis make it impossible to administer a large enough dose of radiation to eradicate a measurable volume of tumor. Palliative radiation should result in sufficient tumor regression off critical structures to relieve symptoms. Symptoms that recur after palliative radiation most commonly result from localized regrowth of tumor in the radiation field.

Localized bone metastases

Radiation of localized bone metastases relieves symptoms and helps prevent spinal cord compression and pathological fractures. There has been much controversy about palliative radiation schedules for localized symptomatic bone metastases. The Radiation Therapy Oncology Group (RTOG) conducted a prospective trial that included a variety of treatment schedules. In order to account for prognosis, patients were stratified on the basis of whether they had a solitary or multiple sites of bony metastases. The initial analysis of the study concluded that low-dose, short-course treatment schedules were as effective as high-dose protracted treatment programs.[61] For solitary bone metastases, there was no difference in the relief of pain when 20 Gy using 4 Gy fractions was compared with 40.5 Gy delivered as 2.7 Gy per fraction. In patients with multiple bone metastases, the following dose

schedules were compared: 30 Gy at 3 Gy per fraction, 15 Gy given as 3 Gy per fraction, 20 Gy using 4 Gy per fraction, and 25 Gy using 5 Gy per fraction. No difference was identified in the rates of pain relief between these treatment schedules (Table 86.4). Partial relief of pain was achieved in 83 percent, and complete relief occurred in 53 percent of the patients studied. Over 50 percent of these patients developed recurrent pain, and 8 percent of patients developed a pathological fracture.

In a reanalysis of the data, a different definition for complete pain relief was used and excluded the continued administration of analgesics. Using this definition, the relief of pain was significantly related to the number of fractions and the total dose of radiation that was administered.[62] Complete relief of pain was achieved in 55 percent of patients with solitary bone metastases who received 40.5 Gy at 2.7 Gy per fraction as compared with 37 percent of patients who received a total dose of 20 Gy given as 4 Gy per fraction. A similar relation was observed in the reanalysis of patients who had multiple bone metastases. Complete relief of pain was achieved in 46 percent of patients who received 30 Gy at 3 Gy per fraction versus 28 percent of patients treated to 25 Gy using 5 Gy fractions.

Three important issues are identified from this RTOG experience. First, the results of the reanalysis demonstrate the importance of defining what represents a response to therapy. Second, this revised definition of response showed that the total radiation dose did influence the degree that pain was relieved. Third, the RTOG experience identified the amount of time that was needed to experience relief of pain after radiation for bone metastases (Tables 86.5 and 86.6). It is important to note that only half of the patients who were going to respond had relief of symptoms at 2 weeks to 4 weeks after radiation.[61,62] This underscores the need for continued analgesic support after completing radiation. Consistently, it took 12 weeks to 20 weeks after radiation to accomplish the maximal level of relief. That period of time may reflect the time needed for reossification.

Radiographic evidence of recalcification is observed in about a fourth of cases, and in 70 percent of the time recalcification is seen within 6 months of completing radiation and other palliative therapies.[63–65] Therefore, it is critical to determine the time and parameters of response. Pretreatment characteristics also can influence the level of response. Neuropathic pain is a significant clinical variable that reduces the response to palliative radiation.[67,68]

The projected length of survival is the critical issue for radiation dose and schedule for palliative radiation. In one study, only 12 of 245 patients were alive at the time of analysis with approximately 50 percent alive at 6 months, 25 percent at 1 year, 8 percent at 2 years, and 3 percent at 3 years after palliative radiation. For breast cancer patients the survival rates at these time points after palliative radiation were 60 percent, 44 percent, 20 percent, and 7 percent, respectively. For prostate cancer, the survival rates were 60 percent at 6 months, 24 percent at 1 year, and there were no patients who survived 2 years.[69] In the RTOG trial

Table 86.4 *(A) Different radiation schedules. Arrows represent a comparison to conventional fractionation*

	Conventional	Hyperfractionation	Accelerated	Hypofractionation
Intent	Curative	Curative	Curative	Palliative
No. of fractions per day	1	2 (↑)	1/day for the first 3 to 4 weeks of XRT (↔) Then 2/day (large field + boost field around the tumor) for the last 1 to 2 weeks of XRT (↑)	1 [↔]
No. of fractions	25–30	60–70 (↑)	30–35 (↑)	1–15 (↓)
Dose per fraction	1.8–2 Gy	1.2 Gy BID (↓)	1.8 to 2 Gy to a large field (↔) 1.5 Gy to a boost field (↓)	8 Gy (1 fraction) to 2.5 Gy (15 fractions) (↑)
No. of weeks	5–6	7–9 (↑)	5–6 (↔)	1–3 (↓)
Total radiation dose	45–60 Gy	70–84 Gy (↑)	52–65 Gy (↑)	8–35 Gy (↓)

(B) Relative relations of radiation dose per fraction, and total dose in a variety of radiation schedules. When a high dose of radiation is given per fraction, the total dose must be low and given in a small number of fractions

	Low		High
Hypofractionation	Conventional fractionation	Hyperfractionation	Accelerated fractionation
20–30 Gy	50–60 Gy	70–80 Gy	55–65 Gy
5–10 fractions	25–30 fractions	60–70 fractions	28–35 fractions
1–2 weeks	5–6 weeks	7–8 weeks	5–6 weeks

Table 86.5 *Dose–response evaluation from the reanalysis of the RTOG Bone Metastases Protocol.[90] Listed are the dose per fraction (dose/fx), total radiation dose, the radiobiological equivalent dose if administered at 2 Gy/fx, the complete response rate (CR) using the definition that excludes the use of analgesics and that accounts for re-treatment*

	Dose/fx (Gy)	Total dose (Gy)	Tumor dose at 2 Gy/fx	CR (%)	P value
Solitary bone metastases					0.0003
	2.7	40.5	42.9	55	
	4.0	20.0	23.3	37	
Multiple bone metastases					0.0003
	3.0	30	32.5	46	
	3.0	15.0	16.2	36	
	4.0	20.0	23.3	40	
	5.0	25.0	31.25	28	

Table 86.6 *Percentage of patients who responded to radiation relative to time, designated in weeks after completion of radiation therapy. This prospective trial, conducted by the RTOG, randomized radiation dose and number of fractions and stratified the randomization on the basis of solitary or multiple bone metastases.[79,80] Also listed is the radiobiological equivalent dose if administered at 2 Gy per fraction*

Total dose (Gy)	Dose per fraction (Gy)	Tumor dose at 2 Gy/fx	Weeks after radiation therapy (%)			
			<2	2–4	4–12	12–20
Solitary metastasis						
40.5	2.7	42.9	7	29	53	77
20.0	4	23.3	16	50	66	82
Multiple metastasis						
30.0	3	32.5	19	48	73	84
15.0	3	16.2	34	70	84	93
20.0	4	23.3	28	53	75	88
25.0	5	31.25	22	41	72	80

the median survival for solitary bone metastases was 36 weeks and was 24 weeks for multiple bone metastases.[61,62] The RTOG study also demonstrated that the level of pain correlated with prognosis among patients with multiple bone metastases. This survival difference may be an important observation because unrelieved pain and the resultant sequelae of immobility may contribute to mortality as well as morbidity.

Spinal cord compression

The time from the original diagnosis to the development of metastatic spinal disease averages 32 months, and the average time is reported to be 27 months from diagnosis of skeletal metastases to spinal cord compression. Median survival among patients with spinal cord compression ranges between 3 and 7 months with a 36 percent probability for a 1-year survival. The vertebral column is involved by metastatic tumor in 40 percent of patients who die of cancer, and approximately 70 percent of vertebral metastases involve the thoracic spine, 20 percent the lumbosacral region, and 10 percent the cervical spine. From a tumor registry of 121 435 patients, the cumulative probability of at least one episode of spinal cord compression occurring in the last 5 years of life was 2.5 percent.[72] The diagnosis of spinal cord compression was associated with a doubling of the time spent in hospital in the last year of life.

The demographics of spinal cord compression were: 37 percent of patients had breast cancer, 28 percent had prostate cancer, 18 percent had lung cancer, and 17 percent had other solid tumors. The time between primary tumor diagnosis and development of spinal cord compression is dependent on tumor type with the shortest time associated with lung cancer and the longest time for breast cancer. Lung cancer patients have the most severe functional deficit with more than 50 percent totally paralyzed. Breast cancer patients are ambulatory 59 percent of the time. More severe disturbances in gait occurred when the time between the interval from the diagnosis of the primary tumor and spinal cord compression was short.[70–75] The mean survival time after the diagnosis of spinal cord compression is 14 months for breast cancer, 12 months in prostate cancer, 6 months in malignant melanoma, and 3 months in lung cancer.[70–72]

In a series of 153 consecutive patients with spinal cord compression, total paralysis was present in 28 percent of patients presenting for radiation, 20 percent were able to move their legs but could not walk, 12 percent were able to walk with assistance, and 40 percent could walk unassisted. Sensory exam of the legs was normal in 34, slight disturbances were present in 84, and total lack of pain perception occurred in 35 patients. After radiation, 26 percent were totally paralyzed, 13 percent were able to move their legs without being able to walk, 11 percent were able to walk with assistance, and 50 percent had unassisted gait.[76] Survival in this series was dependent on time from primary tumor diagnosis,

ambulatory function at diagnosis and after radiation therapy, and median survival was 3.5 months. The type of primary tumor also has a direct influence on the interval between the diagnosis of the primary tumor and the diagnosis of spinal cord compression due to metastatic disease.[77] Factors such as age, discharge destination, primary tumor site, other metastases, comorbidities, and hemoglobin and albumin levels had no significant influence on survival time in a study of 60 consecutive patients with metastatic spinal cord compression.[78]

RADIATION SCHEDULE FOR SPINAL CORD COMPRESSION BASED ON PROGNOSIS

The time under radiation needs to be considered as the opportunity cost of palliative treatment.[79] If the median survival of a patient with spinal cord compression is 6 months (180 days), the patient will spend 0.6 percent of the remaining survival time under radiation treatment when a single fraction of radiation is given. If 10 radiation fractions are given, 8 percent of the remaining survival and if 20 fractions are prescribed 16 percent of the remaining survival will be consumed by radiation therapy. Even if re-treatment with a second single fraction is required, the patient will continue to spend about 1 percent of the survival time under radiation therapy. For lung cancer patients with a 3 month survival rate, 1 percent of the remaining time is spent with a single fraction of radiation as compared to 16 percent if 10 fractions are given, or 30 percent if 20 fractions are prescribed.

A more protracted course of radiation is still used for patients with a more prolonged prognosis who require treatment over the spine and other critical sites. With a more limited prognosis, metastatic spinal cord compression has been treated either with a single 8 Gy fraction or five 4 Gy fractions. The median time to recurrence was 6 months among 62 patients with a range of 2–40 months.[73] Re-treatment consisted of another single 8 Gy fraction, or five more fractions of either 3 Gy or 4 Gy. Motor function improved in 40 percent, and it was stable in an additional 45 percent; 38 percent of the nonambulatory patients regained the ability to walk.[80,81] Use of a single fraction of radiation provided sufficient tumor regression for neurological improvement while minimizing time under radiation.

Arguments against the use of a single fraction of radiation in patients with a more limited prognosis involve gastrointestinal toxicity from the exit dose of radiation. Using a single posterior radiation field, about two-thirds of the radiation dose causes toxicity as it exits through the esophagus, stomach, and bowel (Fig. 86.10). Acute radiation toxicities are a function of the dose per fraction, total dose, and the area and volume of tissue irradiated. If mucosal surfaces like the upper aerodigestive tract, bowel and bladder can be excluded from the radiation portals, acute radiation side effects can be significantly reduced whether a single or multiple fractions are prescribed.[82–90] Gastrointestinal toxicities, like esophagitis, nausea and vomiting, and small bowel

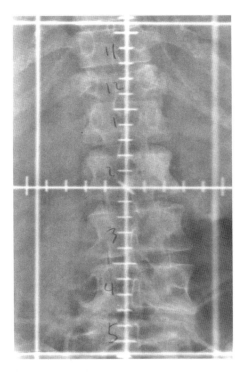

Figure 86.10 *Typical radiation portal to treat disease involvement in the vertebral bodies and epidural region.*

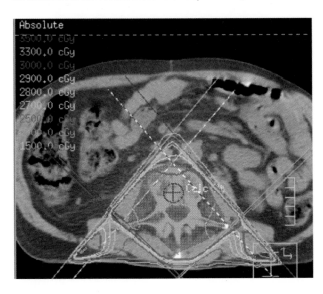

Figure 86.11 *Radiation plan that reduces exit beam and toxicity to adjacent visceral structures.*

toxicity, can be avoided when a high dose of radiation, is administered with the use of more conformal radiation that localizes the radiation to the vertebra and minimizing dose to adjacent normal structures (Fig. 86.11).

RESPONSE TO RADIATION THERAPY

Pain is the initial symptom in approximately 90 percent of patients with spinal cord compression, and the development of spinal cord compression is associated with a poor overall prognosis. Paraparesis or paraplegia occurs in over 60 percent, sensory loss is noted in 70 percent to 80 percent, and 14 percent to 77 percent have bladder and/or bowel disturbances.[73,77,91–100] Among 102 consecutive patients with metastatic spinal cord compression, only 51 percent were fully ambulatory at the time of radiotherapy, and 41 percent had paraparesis. Median survival was 3.5 months, with normal gait returning in 58 percent, 2 weeks after completing radiation, and in 71 percent, 2 months after radiation. No paraplegic patient regained function.[91]

The rate of development of motor symptoms correlates with the possibility of recovering neurological function after radiation therapy. Weakness can signal the rapid progression of symptoms and 30 percent of patients with weakness become paraplegic within 1 week. Rapid development of weakness, defined as occurring in less than 2 months, most commonly occurs in lung cancer whereas breast and prostate cancers can progress more slowly. Neurological deficits can develop within a few hours in up to 20 percent of patients with spinal cord compression.[70–72,76,77,91,93,95–100] Motor function improved among 86 percent of patients who had >14-day time to development of symptoms. Only 29 percent improved when motor deficits developed over 8 to 14 days before the diagnosis of spinal cord compression. Improvements occurred in only 10 percent if motor deficits developed over 1 to 7 days. The severity of weakness at the time that radiation therapy is initiated is the most significant factor for recovery of function. Ninety percent of patients who are ambulatory at presentation will be ambulatory after radiation. Only 13 percent of paraplegic patients will regain function, particularly if paraplegia is present for more than 24 hours before the initiation of radiation.

The degree and rate of pain relief is also dependent on the level of pain at the time radiation is administered.[77,76,77,91,93,95–100] Pain relief is accomplished in 73 percent of patients, and the mean time to pain relief was 35 days in 108 breast cancer patients. Recurrent symptoms at a different spinal level occur in more than three-fourths of patients and within 6 months of radiation.[72]

Without motor impairment, corticosteroids are unnecessary when radiation therapy is administered to relieve pain from vertebral involvement.[101] Elimination of steroids from the standard treatment avoids cortisone side effects above all in those patients with diabetes, hypertension, peptic ulcer, and other steroid-sensitive medical problems. However, corticosteroids should be initiated with clinical and/or radiographic evidence of spinal cord compromise prior to the start of radiotherapy to reduce disease-related edema and pain. Oral dexamethasone (4 mg) generally is administered four times daily, but intravenous dexamethasone should be considered with severe and/or rapid neurological impairment. Experimental studies have shown that high-dose steroids are more effective than lower doses in reversing edema and improving neurological function.

Consistent with this are clinical data including a well-designed randomized trial that administered radiation therapy either with high-dose corticosteroids or placebo. In that trial the group that received corticosteroids were more likely to retain or regain ambulation.[102] Pain relief is also more rapid and complete with high-dose steroids (initial bolus of 100 mg followed by 4 mg dexamethasone four times daily for the duration of radiation therapy) among patients suspected to have spinal cord compression.

The radiation tolerance of the spinal cord can be compromised by prior injury. Difficulty arises in separating the pathological and radiotherapeutic injury to spinal cord compression. Vasogenic edema of the spinal cord and nerve roots can be caused by compression injury. Metastatic epidural compression results in vasogenic spinal cord edema, venous hemorrhage, loss of myelin, and ischemia. Vasogenic edema results in an increased synthesis of prostaglandin E_2 that can be inhibited by steroids or nonsteroidal anti-inflammatory agents. Other consequences of pathological compression include hemorrhage, loss of myelin, and ischemia.[45–47]

A statistically significant improvement in functional outcome occurs with laminectomy and radiotherapy in treatment of epidural spinal cord compression over either modality alone for selected clinical presentations. Laminectomy has been recommended to promptly reduce tumor volume in an attempt to relieve compression and injury of the spinal cord and provide stabilization to the spinal axis. The rate of tumor regression following radiotherapy is too slow in these cases to effect recovery of lost neurologic function, and radiation therapy cannot relieve compression of the spinal column due to vertebral collapse. After radiation alone to treat a partial spinal cord block, 64 percent of patients regain ambulation, 33 percent have normalization of sphincter tone, 72 percent are pain free, and median survival is 9 months.[70,76,86,89,90,103,104] With a complete spinal cord block only 27 percent will have improvement in motor function and 42 percent will continue to have pain after radiation alone. In paraparetic patients who undergo laminectomy and radiation, 82 percent regain the ability to walk, 68 percent have improved sphincter function, and 88 percent have relief of pain.

Laminectomy is indicated with rapid neurological deterioration, tumor progression in a previously irradiated area, stabilization of the spine, paraplegic patients with limited disease and good probability of survival, and to establish a diagnosis. Adjuvant radiotherapy is often given after laminectomy to treat microscopic residual disease after neurosurgical intervention.[70,84–86,88–90,103,104] Surgical restoration of the vertebral alignment may be required due to neurologic compromise and pain caused by progressive vertebral collapse. Vertebral collapse may occur due to cancer or vertebral instability after cancer therapy, e.g. radiation (Fig. 86.12). Appropriate diagnostic studies and intervention should be pursued with persistent pain because the neurological compromise and pain from vertebral instability

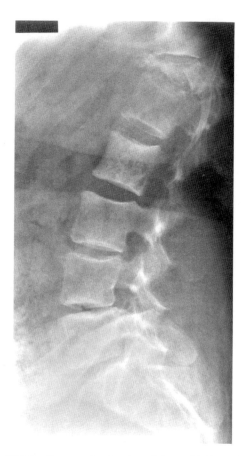

Figure 86.12 *Compression fraction of the twelfth thoracic vertebral body following an initial pain-free interval after palliative radiation. Vertebral weakness with rapid tumor regression resulted in the compression fracture which caused recurrent back pain due to spinal instability.*

can be as devastating as that with epidural spinal cord metastases.[89,104]

Based on clinical and radiographic grounds, leptomeningeal carcinomatosis must also be considered in the diagnostic evaluation. Leptomeningeal carcinomatosis occurs more commonly than expected. For example, only half of breast cancer patients with leptomeningeal carcinomatosis will be diagnosed before death.[70,75,84,90,97] Radiation therapy is indicated in localized regions of nodular leptomeningeal involvement.[97]

THERAPEUTIC RECOMMENDATIONS

The primary goals of palliative treatment are to efficiently relieve disease-related symptoms and maintain function, while minimizing treatment-related symptoms and time under therapy. Spine metastases cause significant pain and can result in irreversible paralysis. Patients with known vertebral metastases require frequent clinical evaluation to identify any change in symptoms and/or radiographic findings suggesting risk for spinal cord compromise. Early detection of vertebral compromise is paramount to preventing an oncological emergency with severe pain and neurological compromise from spinal cord compression. Emergent oncological care involves either surgical decompression and/or radiation therapy.

To prevent disease progression resulting in spinal cord compression, radiation should be considered to treat extensive and/or painful vertebral metastases, and with limited asymptomatic epidural involvement. Radiopharmaceuticals, administered by a single injection, are an important option with multifocal bone metastases, especially if symptoms and disease recurs in a previously irradiated area in the absence of epidural involvement.

Radiation remains an important modality in palliative care. A number of clinical, prognostic and therapeutic factors must be considered to determine the most optimal treatment regimen in palliative radiotherapy in general. Symptoms that persist after palliative radiation should be evaluated to exclude progression of disease in the treated area, and possible extension of disease outside the radiation portal especially if there is an associated paraspinal mass. Pain may also persist due to reduced cortical strength after treatment of spinal metastases that can result in vertebral compression or stress microfractures.

A wide range of radiotherapeutic options are available for the treatment of spinal cord compression. Radiobiological principles, the radiation tolerance of adjacent normal tissues, and the clinical condition influence the selection of radiation technique, dose, and fraction size. As a late-reacting tissue, the radiobiological tolerance of the spinal cord to radiation is finite. Technological advances, however, have increased our ability to treat spinal metastases with greater precision, and have allowed consideration of retreatment with radiation to selected patients.

Prevention or early treatment of symptoms is often the most important care administered. The treatment of vertebral metastases and spinal cord compression to prevent or relieve symptoms of pain and paralysis is one of the most important services rendered to cancer patients.

Key learning points

- Spinal cord compression results in significant morbidity, constitutes an oncological emergency, and is associated with a poor overall prognosis.

- Early diagnosis and treatment prevents lasting neurological dysfunction.

- New therapeutic modalities are now available to prevent and treat spinal cord compression.

REFERENCES

1 Cleeland CS, Gonin R, Hatfield AK, et al. Pain and its treatment in outpatients with metastatic cancer. N Engl J Med 1994; **330**: 592–6.
2 Jacox AK, Carr DB, Payne R, eds. Management of Cancer Pain. Clinical practice guideline no. 9, Rockville, MD: Agency for Health Care Policy and Research (AHCPR publication no. 94-0592); 1994.
3 Jacox A, Carr DB, Payne R. New Clinical Practice Guidelines for the management of pain in patients with cancer. N Engl J Med 1994; **330**: 651–5.
4 Brescia FJ, Portenoy RK, Ryan M, et al. Pain, opioid use, and survival in hospitalized patients with advanced cancer. J Clin Oncol 1992; **10**: 149–55.
5 Dale RG, Jones B. Radiobiologically based assessments of the net costs of fractionated radiotherapy. Int J Radiat Oncol Biol Phys 1996; **36**: 739–46.
6 Vigano A, Bruera E, Jhangri GS, et al. Clinical survival predictors in patients with advanced cancer. Arch Intern Med 2000; **160**: 861–8.
7 Sherry MM, Greco FA, Johnson DH, Hainsworth JD. Breast cancer with skeletal metastases at initial diagnosis-distinctive clinical characteristics and favorable prognosis. Cancer 1986; **58**: 178–82.
8 Sherry MM, Greco FA, Johnson DH, Hainsworth JD. Metastatic breast cancer confined to the skeletal system. Am J Med 1986; **81**: 381–6.
9 Plunkett TA, Smith P, Rubens RD. Risk of complications from bone metastases in breast cancer: implications for management. Eur J Cancer 2000; **36**: 476–2.
10 Lai PP, Perez CA, Lockett MA. Prognostic significance of pelvic recurrence and distant metastases in prostate carcinoma following definitive radiotherapy. Int J Radiat Oncol Biol Phys 1992; **24**: 423–30.
11 Yamashita K, Denno K, Ueda T, et al. Prognostic significance of bone metastases in patients with metastatic prostate cancer. Cancer 1993; **71**: 1297–302.
12 Knudson G, Grinis G, Lopez-Majano V, et al. Bone scan as a stratification variable in advanced prostate cancer. Cancer 1991; **68**: 316–20.
13 Sabbatini P, Larson SM, Kremer A, et al. Prognostic significance of extent of disease in bone in patients with androgen-independent prostate cancer. J Clin Oncol 1999; **17**: 948–57.
14 Greenwald HP, Bonica JJ, Bergner M. The prevalence of pain in four cancers. Cancer 1987; **60**: 2563–9.
15 Borre M, Nerstrom B, Overgaard J. The natural history of prostate carcinoma based on a Danish population treated with no intent to cure. Cancer 1997; **80**: 917–28.
16 Grabowski CM, Unger JA, Potish RA. Factors predictive of completion of treatment and survival after palliative radiation therapy. Radiology 1992; **184**: 329–32.
17 Reuben DB, Mor V, Hiris J. Clinical symptoms and length of survival in patients with terminal cancer. Arch Intern Med 1988; **148**: 1586–91.
18 Fielding LP, Henson DE. Multiple prognostic factors and outcome analysis in patients with cancer-communication from the American Joint Committee on Cancer. Cancer 1993; **71**: 2426–9.
19 Portenoy RK, Miransky J, Thaler HT, et al. Pain in ambulatory patients with lung or colon cancer. Cancer 1992; **70**: 1616–24.

20 Brown JE, Thomson CS, Ellis SP, *et al*. Bone resorption predicts for skeletal complications in metastatic bone disease. *Br J Cancer* 2003; **89**: 2031–7.

21 Brown J, Cook R, Major P, *et al*. Bone turnover markers as predictors of skeletal complications in prostate cancer, lung cancer and other solid tumors. *J Natl Cancer Inst* 2005; **97**: 59.

22 Powers WE, Ratanatharathorn V. Palliation of bone metastases. In: Perez CA, Brady LW, eds. *Principles and Practice of Radiation Oncology*, 3rd ed. Philadelphia: Lippincott Raven, 1998; 2199–219.

23 Bunting RW, Boublik M, Blevins FT, *et al*. Functional outcome of pathologic fracture secondary to malignant disease in a rehabilitation hospital. *Cancer* 1992; **69**: 98–102.

24 Arcangeli G, Micheli A, Arcangeli F, *et al*. The responsiveness of bone metastases to radiotherapy: the effect of site, histology and radiation dose on pain relief. *Radiother Oncol* 1989; **14**: 95–101.

25 Steiner RM, Mitchell DG, Rao VM, Schweitzer ME. Magnetic resonance imaging of diffuse bone marrow disease. *Radiol Clin North Am* 1993; **31**: 383–409.

26 Algra PR, Bloem JL, Tissing H, *et al*. Detection of vertebral metastases: comparison between MR imaging and bone scintigraphy. *Radiographics* 1991; **11**: 219–32.

27 Le Bihan DJ. Differentiation of benign versus pathologic compression fractures with diffusion-weighted MR imaging: a closer step toward the 'holy grail' of tissue characterization? *Radiology* 1998; **207**: 305–307.

28 Francken AB, Hong AM, Fulham MJ, *et al*. Detection of unsuspected spinal cord compression in melanoma patients by 18F-fluorodeoxyglucose-positron emission tomography. *Eur J Surg Oncol* 2005; **31**: 197–204.

29 Nielsen OS, Munro AJ, Tannock IF. Bone metastases: pathophysiology and management policy. *J Clin Oncol* 1991; **9**: 509–24.

30 Khan FM. Dose distribution and scatter analysis. In: *The Physics of Radiation Therapy*. Baltimore: Williams and Wilkins, 1984; 157–78.

31 Barton R, Robinson G, Gutierrez E, *et al*. Palliative radiation for vertebral metastases: the effect of variation in prescription parameters on the dose received at depth. *Int J Radiat Oncol Biol Phys* 2002; **52**: 1083–91.

32 Shiu AS, Chang EL, Ye JS, *et al*. Near simultaneous computed tomography image-guided stereotactic spinal radiotherapy: An emerging paradigm for achieving true stereotaxy. *Int J Radiat Oncol Biol Phys* 2003; **57**: 605–13.

33 Chang EL, Shiu AS, Lii MF, *et al*. Phase I clinical evaluation of near-simultaneous computed tomographic image-guided stereotactic body radiotherapy for spinal metastases. *Int J Radiat Oncol Biol Phys* 2004; **59**: 1288–94.

34 Gerszten PC, Germanwala AN, Burton SA, *et al*. Combination kyphoplasty and spinal radiosurgery; a new treatment paradigm for pathological fractures. *Neurosurg Focus* **18**: E8; 2005.

35 Gerszten PC, Burton SA, Ozhasoglu C, *et al*. Stereotactic radiosurgery for spinal metastases from renal cell carcinoma. *J Neurosurg Spine* 2005; **3**: 288–95.

36 Hall E. Dose response relationships for normal tissues. In: *Radiobiology for the Radiologist*, 4th ed. Philadelphia: JB Lippincott, 1994: 45–75.

37 Nieder C, Milas L, Ang KK. Tissue tolerance to reirradiation. *Semin Radiat Oncol* 2000; **10**: 200–9.

38 Morris DE. Clinical experience with retreatment for palliation. *Semin Radiat Oncol* 2000; **10**: 210–21.

39 Mohiuddin M, Marks GM, Lingareddy V, Marks J. Curative surgical resection following reirradiation for recurrent rectal cancer. *Int J Radiat Oncol Biol Physics* 1997; **39**: 643–9.

40 Mohiuddin M, Regine WF, Stevens J, *et al*. Combined intraoperative radiation and perioperative chemotherapy for unresectable cancers of the pancreas. *J Clin Oncol* 1995; **13**: 2764–8.

41 Barton M. Tables of equivalent dose in 2 Gy fractions: a simple application of the linear quadratic formula. *Int J Radiat Oncol Biol Phys* 1995; **31**: 371–8.

42 Minsky BD, Conti JA, Huang Y, Knopf K. Relationship of acute gastrointestinal toxicity and the volume of irradiated small bowel in patients receiving combined modality therapy for rectal cancer. *J Clin Oncol* 1995; **13**: 1409–16.

43 Cox JD, Pajack TF, Asbell S, *et al*. Interruptions of high-dose radiation therapy decrease long-term survival of favorable patients with unresectable non-small cell carcinoma of the lung: analysis of 1244 cases from 3 Radiation Therapy Oncology Group (RTOG) trials. *Int J Radiat Oncol Biol Phys* 1993; **27**: 493–8.

44 Cox JD, Pajak TF, Marcial VA, et al. Interruptions adversely affect local control and survival with hyperfractionated radiation therapy of carcinomas of the upper respiratory and digestive tracts. New evidence for accelerated proliferation from Radiation Therapy Oncology Group Protocol 8313. *Cancer* 1992; **69**: 2744–8.

45 Jeremic B, Djuric L, Mijatovic L. Incidence of radiation myelitis of the cervical spinal cord at doses of 5500 cGy or greater. *Cancer* 1991; **68**: 2138–41.

46 Wen PY, Blanchard KL, Block CC, *et al*. Development of Lhermitte's sign after bone marrow transplantation. *Cancer* 1992; **69**: 2262–6.

47 Powers BE, Thames HD, Gillette SM, *et al*. Volume effects in the irradiated canine spinal cord: do they exist when the probability of injury is low? *Radiother Oncol* 1998; **46**: 297–306.

48 Maranzano E, Bellavita R, Floridi P, *et al*. Radiation induced myelopathy in long-term surviving metastatic spinal cord compression patients after hypofractionated radiotherapy: a clinical and magnetic resonance imaging analysis. *Radiother Oncol* 2001; **60**: 281–8.

49 Ridet JL, Pencalet P, Belcram M, *et al*. Effects of spinal cord x-irradiation on the recovery of paraplegic rats. *Exp Neurol* 2000; **161**: 1–14.

50 Algra PR, Heimans JJ, Valk J, *et al*. Do metastases in vertebrae begin in the body or the pedicles? Imaging study in 45 patients. *AJR Am J Roentgenol* 1992; **158**: 1275–9.

51 Sugimura H, Kisanuki A, Tamura S, *et al*. Magnetic resonance imaging of bone marrow changes after irradiation. *Investig Radiol* 1994; **29**: 35–41.

52 Yankelevitz DF, Henschke C, Knapp PH, *et al*. Effect of radiation therapy on thoracic and lumbar bone marrow: evaluation with MR imaging. *Am J Roentgenol* 1991; **157**: 87–92.

53 Cox JD. Fractionation: a paradigm for clinical research in radiation oncology. *Int J Radiat Oncol Biol Phys* 1987; **13**: 1271–81.

54 Cox JD. Large-dose fractionation (hypofractionation). *Cancer* 1985; **55** (9 Suppl): 2105–11.

55 Porter AT, McEwan AJB, Powe JE, *et al*. Results of a randomized Phase III trial to evaluate the efficacy of Strontium 89 adjuvant to local field external beam irradiation in the management of endocrine resistant metastatic prostate cancer. *Int J Radiat Oncol Biol Phys* 1993; **25**: 805–13.

56 Robinson RG, Preston DF, Schiefelbein M, Baxter KG. Strontium 89 therapy for the palliation of pain due to osseous metastases. *JAMA* 1995; **274**: 420–4.

57 Serafini AN, Houston SJ, Resche I, *et al*. Palliation of pain associated with metastatic bone cancer using samarium-153 lexidronam: a double-blind placebo-controlled clinical trial. *J Clin Oncol* 1998; **16**: 1574–81.

58 Sciuto R, Maini CL, Tofani A, *et al*. Radiosensitization with low-dose carboplatin enhances pain palliation in radioisotope therapy with strontium-89. *Nucl Med Commun* 1996; **17**: 799–804.

59 Alberts AS, Smit BJ, Louw WKA, *et al*. Dose response relationship and multiple dose efficacy and toxicity of samarium-153-EDTMP in metastatic cancer to bone. *Radiother Oncol* 1997; **43**: 175–9.

60 Anderson PM, Wiseman GA, Dispenzieri A, *et al*. High-dose samarium-153 ethylene diamine tetramethylene phosphonate: low toxicity of skeletal irradiation in patients with osteosarcoma and bone metastases. *J Clin Oncol* 2002; **20**: 189–96.

61 Tong D, Gillick L, Hendrickson FR. The palliation of symptomatic osseous metastases-final results of the study by the Radiation Therapy Oncology Group. *Cancer* 1982; **50**: 893–9.

62 Blitzer PH. Reanalysis of the RTOG study of the palliation of symptomatic osseous metastasis. *Cancer* 1985; **55**: 1468–72.

63 Ford HT, Yarnold JR. Radiation therapy – Pain relief and recalcification. In: Stoll BA, Parbhoo S, eds. *Bone Metastases: Monitoring and Treatment*. New York, NY: Raven Press, 1983: 343–54.

64 Hortobagyi GN, Libshitz HI, Seabold JE. Osseous metastases of breast cancer-clinical, biochemical, radiographic, and scintigraphic evaluation of response to therapy. *Cancer* 1984; **53**: 577–82.

65 Vogel CL, Schoenfelder J, Shemano I, *et al*. Worsening bone scan in the evaluation of antitumor response during hormonal therapy of breast cancer. *J Clin Oncol* 1995; **13**: 1123–8.

66 Rutten EHJM, Crul BJP, van der Toorn PPG, *et al*. Pain characteristics help to predict the analgesic efficacy of radiotherapy for the treatment of cancer pain. *Pain* 1997; **69**: 131–5.

67 Kelly JB, Payne R. Pain syndromes in the cancer patient. *Neurol Clin* 1991; **9**: 937–53.

68 Portenoy RK. Cancer pain management. *Semin Oncol* 1993; **20**: 19–35.

69 Gaze MN, Kelly CG, Kerr GR, *et al*. Pain relief and quality of life following radiotherapy for bone metastases: a randomised trial of two fractionation schedules. *Radiother Oncol* 1997; **45**: 109–16.

70 Boogerd W, van der Sande JJ, Kroger R. Early diagnosis and treatment of spinal metastases in breast cancer: a prospective study. *J Neurol Neurosurg Psychiatry* 1992; **55**: 1188–93.

71 Bach F, Agerlin N, Sorensen JB, *et al*. Metastatic spinal cord compression secondary to lung cancer. *J Clin Oncol* 1992; **10**: 1781–7.

72 Prie L, Lagarde P, Palussiere J, *et al*. Radiation therapy of spinal metastases in breast cancer: retrospective analysis of 108 patients. *Cancer/radiotherapie* 1997; **1**: 234–9.

73 Rades D, Stalpers LJA, Veninga T, Hoskin PJ. Spinal reirradiation after short-course RT for Metastatic Spinal Cord Compression. *Int J Radiat Oncol Biol Phys* 2005; **63**: 872–5.

74 Rades D, Blach M, Bremer M, *et al*. Prognostic significance of the time of developing motor deficits before radiation therapy in metastatic spinal cord compression: one-year results of a prospective trial. *Int J Radiat Oncol Biol Phys* 2000; **48**: 1403–8.

75 Rades D, Heidenreich F, Karstens JH. Final results of a prospective study of the prognostic value of the time to develop motor deficits before irradiation in metastatic spinal cord compression. *Int J Radiat Oncol Biol Phys* 2002; **53**: 975–9.

76 Turner S, Marosszeky B, Timms I, Boyages J. Malignant spinal cord compression: A prospective evaluation. *Int J Radiat Oncol Biol Phys* 1993; **26**: 141–6.

77 Helweg-Larsen S, Soelberg Sorensen P, Kreiner S. Prognostic factors in metastatic spinal cord compression: a prospective study using multivariate analysis of variables influencing survival and gait function in 153 patients. *Int J Radiat Oncol Biol Phys* 2000; **46**: 1163–9.

78 Guo Y, Young B, Palmer JL, *et al*. Prognostic factors for survival in metastatic spinal cord compression: a retrospective study in a rehabilitation setting. *Am J Phys Med Rehab* 2003; **82**: 665–8.

79 Chow E, Coia L, Wu J, *et al*. This house believes that multiple-fraction radiotherapy is a barrier to referral for palliative radiotherapy for bone metastases. *Curr Oncol* 2002; **9**: 60–6.

80 Milker-Zabel S, Zabel A, Thilmann C, *et al*. Clinical results of retreatment of vertebral bone metastases by stereotactic conformal radiotherapy and intensity-modulated radiotherapy. *Int J Radiat Oncol Biol Phys* 2003; **55**: 162–7.

81 Grosu AL, Andratschke N, Nieder C, Molls M. Retreatment of the spinal cord with palliative radiotherapy. *Int J Radiat Oncol Biol Phys* 2002; **52**: 1288–92.

82 Chow E, Lutz S, Beyene J. A single fraction for all, or an argument for fractionation tailored to fit the needs of each individual patient with bone metastases? *Int J Radiat Oncol Biol Phys* 2003; **55**: 565–7.

83 Haddad P, Wong R, Wilson P, *et al*. Factors influencing the use of single versus multiple fractions of palliative radiotherapy for bone metastases: a 5-yr review and comparison to a survey. *Int J Radiat Oncol Biol Phys* 2003; **57** (Suppl): S278.

84 Boogerd W, van der Sande JJ. Diagnosis and treatment of spinal cord compression in malignant disease. *Cancer Treat Rev* 1993; **19**: 129–50.

85 Byrne TN. Spinal cord compression from epidural metastases. *N Engl J Med* 1992; **327**: 614–19.

86 Grant R, Papadopoulos SM, Greenberg HS. Metastatic epidural spinal cord compression. *Neurol Clin* 1991; **9**: 825–41.

87 Maranzano E, Latini P, Checcaglini F, *et al*. Radiation therapy in metastatic spinal cord compression–a prospective analysis of 105 consecutive patients. *Cancer* 1991; **67**: 1311–17.

88 Janjan NA. Radiotherapeutic management of spinal metastases. *J Pain Symptom Manage* 1996; **1**: 47–56.

89 Loblaw DA, Laperriere NJ. Emergency treatment of malignant extradural spinal cord compression: an evidence-based guideline. *J Clin Oncol* 1998; **16**: 1613–24.

90 Boogerd W. Central nervous system metastasis in breast cancer. *Radiother Oncol* 1996; **40**: 5–22.

91 Hoskin PJ, Grover A, Bhana R. Metastatic spinal cord compression; radiotherapy outcome and dose fractionation. *Radiother Oncol* 2003; **68**: 175–80.

92 Bates T, Yarnold JR, Blitzer P, *et al*. Bone metastases consensus statement. *Int J Radiat Oncol Biol Phys* 1992; **23**: 215–16.

93 Bates T. A review of local radiotherapy in the treatment of bone metastases and cord compression. *Int J Radiat Oncol Biol Phys* 1992; **23**: 217–21.

94 Tow B, Seang BT, Chong TT, Chen J. Predictors for survival in metastases to the spine. *Spine* 2005; **5**: 73S.

95 Wada E, Yamamoto T, Furuno M, *et al.* Spinal cord compression secondary to osteoblastic metastasis. *Spine* 1993; **18**: 1380–1.

96 Kim RY, Smith JW, Spencer SA, *et al.* Malignant epidural spinal cord compression associated with a paravertebral mass: its radiotherapeutic outcome on radiosensitivity. *Int J Radiat Oncol Biol Phys* 1993; **27**: 1079–83.

97 Russi EG, Pergolizzi S, Gaeta M, *et al.* Palliative radiotherapy in lumbosacral carcinomatous neuropathy. *Radiother Oncol* 1993; **26**: 172–3.

98 Saarto T, Janes R, Tenhunen M, Kouri M. Palliative radiotherapy in the treatment of skeletal metastases. *Eur J Pain* 2002; **6**: 323–30.

99 Loblaw DA, Laperriere NJ, Mackillop WJ. A population-based study of malignant spinal cord compression in Ontario. *Clin Oncol* 2003; **15**: 211–17.

100 Altehoefer C, Ghanem N, Hogerle S, *et al.* Comparative detectability of bone metastases and impact on therapy of magnetic resonance imaging and bone scintigraphy in patients with breast cancer. *Eur J Radiol* 2001; **40**: 16–23.

101 Maranzano E, Latini P, Beneventi S, *et al.* Radiotherapy without steroids in selected metastatic spinal cord compression patients. A phase II trial. *Am J Clin Oncol* 1996; **19**: 179–83.

102 Quinn JA, De Angelis LM. Neurologic emergencies in the cancer patient. *Semin Oncol* 2000; **27**: 311–21.

103 Hatrick NC, Lucas JD, Timothy AR, Smith MA. The surgical treatment of metastatic disease of the spine. *Radiother Oncol* 2000; **56**: 335–9.

104 Landmann C, Hunig R, Gratzi O. The role of laminectomy in the combined treatment of metastatic spinal cord compression. *Int J Radiat Oncol Biol Phys* 1992; **24**: 627–31.

87

Superior vena cava syndrome

MARÍA LUISA DEL VALLE, CARLOS CENTENO

INTRODUCTION

Superior vena cava syndrome (SVCS) is an array of symptoms resulting from the impairment of blood flow through the superior vena cava to the right atrium. It is present at diagnosis in 10 percent of patients with small cell lung cancer and less than 2 percent of patients with nonsmall cell lung cancer. There are no reliable data on the risk of subsequent development of SVCS in patients with lung cancer or on its prevalence in a terminal setting. However, clinically relevant SVCS can develop in more than 10 percent of patients with right-sided malignant intrathoracic tumors.[1]

ETIOLOGY

The spectrum of underlying conditions associated with SVCS has shifted from tuberculosis and other benign diseases such as mediastinal fibrosis or histoplasmosis to malignant disorders. Almost 95 percent of SVCS cases described in recent studies are due to cancer. The most common cause is small cell lung cancer,[2*] followed by nonsmall cell lung carcinoma – in different proportions for each histological subtype (Table 87.1). Additional causes of

Table 87.1 *Histologic subtypes of lung cancer in superior vena cava syndrome*

Histology	Patients (%)
Small cell	40
Squamous	25
Adenocarcinoma	15
Large cell	10
Unknown	10

SVCS include cancers, such as germ cell tumors, lymphoma, thymoma, esophageal cancer or mediastinal metastases from other tumors, and nonmalignant diseases, such as sarcoidosis.[3] A nonmalignant cause of SVCS in patients with cancer that is becoming more frequent is thrombosis, sometimes due to intracaval catheters.

PHYSIOPATHOLOGY

Superior vena cava syndrome results from the compression of the superior vena cava by:

- tumor arising in the mediastinum or in the right main or upper lobe bronchus
- large-volume mediastinal lymphadenopathy (most commonly from the right paratracheal or precarinal lymph nodes).[4]

The superior vena cava is formed by the junction of the left and right brachiocephalic veins in the mid-third of the mediastinum. It extends caudally for 6–8 cm, coursing anterior to the right mainstem bronchus and terminating in the superior right atrium. It is joined posteriorly by the azygos vein as it loops over the right mainstem bronchus and lies posterior to and to the right of the ascending aorta. The right mediastinal parietal pleura is lateral to the superior vena cava, creating a confined space, and the superior vena cava lies adjacent to the right paratracheal, azygos, right hilar and subcarinal lymph node groups. It is a thin-walled vessel and the blood flows in it under low pressure. Thus, when the nodes or ascending aorta enlarge and the superior vena cava is compressed, partial occlusion may occur leading to slowing of blood flow, and eventually, complete superior vena cava occlusion may develop.

The severity of the syndrome depends on the rapidity of onset of the obstruction and its location. The more rapid the onset, the more severe the symptoms because the collateral veins do not have time to distend to accommodate the increased blood flow. If the obstruction is above the entry of the azygos vein, the syndrome is less pronounced because the azygous system can readily distend to accommodate the shunted blood, allowing a reduction of the venous pressure in the head, arms, and upper thorax. If the obstruction is below the entry of the azygos vein, more florid and severe symptoms and signs are seen because the blood pressure increases in order to return to the heart via the upper abdominal veins and the inferior vena cava.[5] Other patterns of venous collateral return have been described, but their significance is less relevant.[6]

CLINICAL PRESENTATION

The diagnosis of SVCS is usually made clinically in the first instance. The most frequent symptoms that prompt suspicion of this syndrome include swelling of the face, neck, upper trunk and extremities, coughing, and dyspnea. Several other symptoms may be associated, such as chest pain, dysphagia and less frequently, lethargy and headache. More rarely, cyanosis, Horner syndrome, and paralysis of the vocal chords may also be present. Physical signs usually noted on presentation are neck and thoracic vein distension, edema of the face and upper extremities, venous regurgutation, hoarseness, and tachypnea (Table 87.2).

Although SVCS may present with different manifestations depending on the severity of obstruction and the rate of progression of disease, there is no commonly accepted scoring system to assess its risk and provide adequate treatment.

DIAGNOSIS

Once SVCS is recognized, prompt clinical attention is important. In the absence of a histological diagnosis, however, it

Table 87.2 *Most frequent symptoms and physical signs in superior vena cava syndrome*

Symptoms	Percent	Signs	Percent
Dyspnea	65	Venous distension of neck	65
Swelling of the face and neck	50	Venous distension of upper trunk	55
Cough	25	Facial edema	45
Swelling of the extremities	20	Cyanosis	20
Chest pain	15	Venous regurgitation	20
Dysphagia	10	Arm edema	15

is advisable that this should be established prior to initiating therapy. Usually there is time to obtain a histological diagnosis, chiefly because 3–5 percent of the patients diagnosed with SVCS do not have cancer. Even when SVCS is evidently an oncological complication, generally no emergent therapeutic interventions are required. This is because this syndrome usually presents with slow progressive development of clinical manifestations as a chronic or at least, as a subacute disease. In fact, up to 75 percent of patients present symptoms and signs of SVCS for over a week before seeking medical attention.[7] In addition, it must be borne in mind that SVCS is rarely lethal by itself. Cancer patients diagnosed with SVCS (even more, those patients with advanced and refractory tumors) do not die because of this syndrome itself but from the extent of underlying disease. Only in exceptional cases, where tracheal obstruction or cerebral edema is present, could SVCS be considered as an oncological emergency requiring immediate therapy. In the rest, treatment prior to definitive diagnosis does not seem to be justified.[8]

The initial evaluation of the patient should include a chest radiograph to look for mediastinal masses and other possible associated findings, such as pleural effusion, lobar collapse, or cardiomegaly. Computed tomography (CT) or magnetic resonance imaging (MRI) is of a great value in defining the extent of the disease and even in planning the treatment.[9] Both yield the most useful diagnostic information and can define the anatomy of the involved mediastinal nodes. They might assist in radiotherapy planning or act as a baseline for assessment of response to treatment such as chemotherapy. Venous patency and the presence of thrombus are assessed by using contrast and rapid scanning techniques.[10] For example, contrast-enhanced spiral or multislice CT and MRI are now able to identify accurately the level of the obstruction and the presence of associated intravascular thrombus. Depending on local expertise, contrast and nuclear venography and ultrasound may help in further assessment of the nature and location of the obstruction.

After the first clinical and radiographic approach, a histological diagnosis is essential for appropriate treatment planning. This is because in SVCS due to cancer, the treatment depends on tumor histology. When the syndrome appears within the framework of a tumoral disease but without defined histology, the biopsy specimen should be taken from the most accessible site that is clinically involved with disease. The protocol for biopsy is based on the location of the tumor, the performance status of the patient, and the expertise available. It may include bronchoscopy, biopsy of palpable cervical or supraclavicular lymph nodes or needle biopsy of a lung mass or mediastinal nodes using either CT or ultrasound guidance. In a number of patients, more aggressive tools such as mediastinoscopy, mediastinotomy, median sternotomy, video-assisted thoracoscopy, or conventional thoracotomy may be required.

TREATMENT

The treatment of SVCS depends on the cause of the obstruction, the severity of the symptoms, the prognosis of the patient, and the patient's preferences and goals for therapy. In patients with advanced cancer, treatment is generally purely symptomatic. Yet in some patients, the best palliation, measured as both symptom control and quality of life and even prolongation of survival, is achieved not only by 'symptomatic' treatment but also by treatment specifically directed against the tumor.

It is advisable to withhold both radiation therapy and chemotherapy until the etiology of the obstruction is clear. Since treatment of a malignant obstruction may depend on tumor histology, a histological diagnosis, if not made earlier, should be made immediately prior to initiation of treatment.[11] Unless there is airway obstruction or cerebral edema, there appears to be no detriment in outcome when treatment is delayed until these data are obtained.

Response rates to therapy are difficult to evaluate. Radiographic measures of tumor may not directly correlate with the severity of symptoms or the clinical status of patients and criteria for relief are not well defined. As the diagnosis of SVCS is made clinically, the clinical response and subsequent relapse need to be assessed in the same way. Although a number of studies have described the range of symptoms prior to treatment, response assessment was limited to whether SVCS had been relieved or not. In other studies different scoring systems have been proposed,[12,13*] but as of now there is no standard scoring system.

Medical management

A patient with sufficient collateral blood flow and minimal symptoms may not need treatment other than postural advice and appropriate prevention of further complications such as thrombosis. If the occlusion is small enough to allow sufficient collateral circulation, the symptoms and signs may stabilize and the patient may be comfortable enough without further therapy.

As mentioned above, in 10 percent of patients with small cell lung cancer and less than 2 percent with nonsmall cell lung cancer SVCS is present at diagnosis. In these patients the specific treatment directed toward relieving SVCS is commenced at the same time as treatment for the disease. This is preferred even when medical management may be adequate at least until the time the antitumor therapy works. However, a proportion of patients have SVCS relapse after the initial antitumor treatment, usually chemotherapy. In such patients only second-line therapy may be suitable, but it is hardly successful. Thus in most patients, palliative therapy is preferred as the tumor becomes resistant to treatment. In symptomatic advanced cancer patients with poor performance status or in patients who do not want aggressive treatment, palliation may be achieved by medical interventions such as postural advice, since a raised head may help blood to flow better through the superior vena cava to the heart, and drugs.[14]

Traditionally, treatment has included systemic steroids (prednisolone or dexamethasone) to alleviate respiratory compromise. These are also recommended to prevent radiation-induced edema when radiotherapy is used but there is no strong evidence of such an inflammatory reaction or edema after radiotherapy for SVCS. There are no definitive studies that prove the effectiveness of steroids,[15*] although they are potentially useful to treat respiratory compromise. If steroids are to be prescribed, high doses should be used for a limited duration. Diuretics have been used in the treatment of SVCS with anecdotal reports of benefit. There may be symptomatic relief of edema but ultimately these can lead to systemic complications, such as dehydration.

Other usual measures such as oxygen or antithrombotic therapy are not established enough but may help to alleviate some problems. For instance, oxygen may palliate dyspnea in some cancer patients.[16] Low-molecular weight heparin may prevent further thrombosis in a cancer patient with slow flow in the vena cava.

Chemotherapy

Chemotherapy is the anticancer treatment of choice for sensitive tumors such as small cell lung cancer, lymphoma, and germ-cell tumors. In these cases, SCVS does not appear to be an independent prognostic factor, and its presence should not be used to change the treatment approach. The response rates to chemotherapy in sensitive tumors such as small cell lung cancer approaches 80 percent,[17,18] but in more than 15 percent of those there was a recurrence of SVCS.

In tumors which are less chemosensitive, such as nonsmall cell lung cancer, chemotherapy can relieve SVCS in 60 percent of the patients.[19,20**] The proportion of recurrences of SVCS after response to chemotherapy is about 20 percent.

Radiation therapy

If the obstruction of the superior vena cava is caused by a tumor that is or has become refractory to chemotherapy, radiation therapy remains highly effective as symptomatic treatment.[21] Historically, treatment started with larger fractions of 4 Gy for the first few days, because it was thought that this led to a more rapid response, and then continued with smaller fractions until the desired total dose was reached.[22**,23] However, there is no obvious need for large radiation fraction sizes in the first few days.[24] Many fractionation schemes have been used,[25,26] with doses ranging from 20 Gy in five fractions to 50 Gy in 25 fractions. Single dose (6–8 Gy) has been recommended for rapid relief in patients with poor performance status or short life expectancy. Overall, in 60 percent of nonsmall cell lung cancer and 80 percent of small cell lung cancer, SVCS responds to radiotherapy.[27]

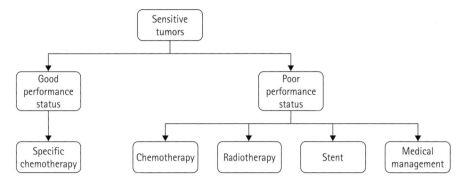

Figure 87.1 *Algorithm of treatment of malignant superior vena cava syndrome in patients with potentially sensitive tumors.*

There are no definitive data regarding a fractionation scheme of choice. The fractionation scheme will depend on histology, previous therapy, disease extent, prognosis, and performance status. In previously treated patients with short life expectancy who have now become resistant, and in disseminated disease and poor performance status, a short-term schedule would be preferable with a total dose of 20–30 Gy, or a single-fraction treatment. However, patients in whom the disease is limited to the thorax or in those with good performance status might benefit by conventional fractionation treatment and higher total doses (50–60 Gy).

In lung cancer, there appears to be no distinction between radiotherapy and chemotherapy with regard to speed of palliation. Median time to response ranges from 10 to 15 days, with 75 percent of responses occurring within 3 weeks of starting treatment.[24]

Stent placement

There has been rapid increase in experience with intravascular expandable stent to reopen the occluded superior vena cava. However, no prospectively designed comparative studies have been published. The procedure allows rapid restoration of the normal flow pattern with rapid resolution of symptoms. Response rates are very high, at around 95 percent, with phlebographic resolution in the majority of patients,[28,29] independent of the type of stent used (Wallstent, Gianturco, or Palmaz). Following stent insertion, relief of headache can be immediate,[30] and facial edema may be resolved within 24 hours.[31] The proportion that relapse following stent placement approaches 10 percent, frequently due to thrombus within the stent.

There is no agreement about the optimal timing of this procedure: at diagnosis, as the first choice treatment, or after failure of other treatment modalities. Nevertheless, we should not forget that there is associated morbidity (hematoma, bleeding or stent migration), and that stenting is time consuming and costly. Thrombolytic agents such as streptokinase or urokinase can be administered prior to stent insertion to help with this procedure.[32] Morbidity following stent insertion is greater if thrombolytics are administered. In any case the relapse rate with thrombolytics administered prior to stent insertion does not seem to increase when those drugs are not used.[33***] In the same way,

there is no agreement on the need for the indication or the duration of anticoagulant or antiaggregant therapy after stent placement. However, this policy seems to be related to a lower rate of reocclusion[34] but there is not enough evidence to reach solid conclusions.

In summary, stenting of superior vena cava syndrome is an effective procedure resulting in rapid alleviation of symptoms in almost all patients and allowing for full dose anticancer treatment after stent insertion.

Surgery

There are just a few reports on palliative surgery for malignant SVCS. Surgical bypass is more appropriate for patients with a benign obstruction, although surgical bypass has also been used for some selected patients with malignant obstructions.[35] The indications are limited by the prognosis of patients and the severe complications of the procedure.

Clinical management

In patients with good performance status, several variables have to be considered before the choice of treatment can be made. Tumor histology, extent of disease, prognosis, and type of the vena cava obstruction influence the choice. In very sensitive tumors where systemic therapy modifies survival and may even result in cure, such as lymphoma, germ-cell tumor and even limited disease small cell lung cancer, aggressive therapy aimed at achieving a quick response and improving survival is warranted. In these cancers, radiotherapy can be included as part of the protocol to improve local control. In extensive small cell lung cancer, chemotherapy is the treatment of choice even when cure is not possible (Fig. 87.1).

In other tumors where the benefit of chemotherapy is not so impressive, such as locally advanced or metastatic cancer, radiotherapy is the anticancer treatment of choice for SVCS. Systemic therapy may produce relevant palliation of symptoms in some cases. In patients with potentially sensitive disease but with poor performance status chemotherapy remains a choice.[36] Stent insertion appears to provide relief in a higher proportion and more rapidly (Fig. 87.2). Even when the response is more frequent and faster, stenting is a more aggressive approach than just single-fraction palliative

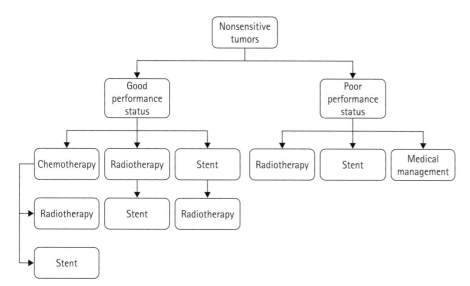

Figure 87.2 *Algorithm of treatment of malignant superior vena cava syndrome in patients with non-sensitive tumors.*

radiotherapy for patients with very poor survival expectancy. There are no data supporting a particular schedule or timing for the combination of different treatments, in particular, local approaches such as radiotherapy and stents.

However, a majority of such patients will require only palliative treatment that is not directed at the tumor. These people can achieve significant relief with medical treatment and a short-term radiotherapy schedule.

Key learning points

- In the absence of histological diagnosis, it is advisable that this should be established prior to initiating therapy because between 3 percent and 5 percent of the patients diagnosed with SVCS do not have cancer.

- Almost 95 percent of SVCS cases described in recent studies are due to cancer.

- No emergent therapeutic interventions are required, and SVCS is rarely lethal by itself. Only in exceptional cases where tracheal obstruction or cerebral oedema is present, could it be considered as an oncological emergency.

- There is no standard scoring system as yet: diagnosis, response and subsequent relapse of SVCS are usually clinically assessed.

- Anticancer therapy, chemotherapy and/or radiotherapy form the basis of treatment (scheme depends on histology and clinical situation).

- Patients with poor performance status or short life expectancy may be managed by medical treatment and a short-term radiotherapy schedule.

- Stent insertion appears to provide relief in a higher proportion and more rapidly. There is no agreement about the timing of stenting.

REFERENCES

✱ 1 Kvale PA, Simoff M, Prakash UBS. Palliative care. *Chest* 2003; **123**: 284S–311S.

◆ 2 Yellin A, Rosen A, Reichert N, *et al.* Superior vena cava syndrome. The myth – the facts. *Am Rev Respir Dis* 1990; **141**: 1114–18.

● 3 Goodwin RA, Nickell JA, Des Prez RM. Mediastinal fibrosis complicating healed primary histoplasmosis and tuberculosis. *Medicine (Baltimore)* 1972; **51**: 227–46.

◆ 4 Yahalom J. Oncologic emergencies: superior vena cava syndrome. In: DeVita VT, Hellman S, Rosemberg SA, eds. *Cancer: Principles and Practice of Oncology*, 6th ed. Philadelphia: JB Lippincot, 2001: 2111–18.

● 5 Netter FH. *The CIBA Collection of Medical Illustrations. Respiratory System.* Newark, NJ: CIBA Pharmaceutical Company, 1980.

● 6 Standford W, Jolles H, Ell S, Chiu LC. Superior vena cava obstruction: a venographic classification. *Am J Roentgenol* 1987; **148**: 259–62.

◆ 7 Schraufnagel DE, Hill R, Leech JA, *et al.* Superior vena caval obstruction. Is it a medical emergency? *Am J Med* 1981; **70**: 1169–74.

◆ 8 Gauden SJ. Superior vena cava syndrome induced by bronchogenic carcinoma: is this an oncologic emergency? *Austral Radiol* 1993; **37**: 363–6.

● 9 Betchtold RE, Wolfman NT, Karstaedt N, Choplin RH. Superior vena caval obstruction: detection using CT. *Radiology* 1985; **157**: 485–487.

✱ 10 Abner A. Approach to the patient who presents with superior vena cava obstruction. *Chest* 1993; **103**: 394S–397S.

◆ 11 Chen JC, Bongard F, Klein SR: A contemporary perspective on superior vena cava syndrome. *Am J Surg* 1990, **160**: 207–11.

◆ 12 Kishi K, Sonomura T, Mitsuzane K, *et al.* Self expandable metallic stent therapy for superior vena cava syndrome: clinical observations. *Radiology* 1993; **189**: 531–5.

◆ 13 Nicholson AA, Teles DF, Arnold A, *et al.* Treatment of malignant superior vena cava obstruction: metal stents or radiation therapy. *J Vasc Intervent Radiol* 1997; **8**: 781–8.

◆ 14 Baker GL, Barnes HJ: Superior vena cava syndrome: etiology, diagnosis, and treatment. *Am J Crit Care* 1992, **1**: 54–64.

◆ 15 Ostler PJ, Clarke DP, Watkinson AF, Gaze MN. Superior vena cava obstruction: a modern management strategy. *Clin Oncol* 1997; **9**: 83–9.

✽ 16 Thomas JR, von Gunten CF. Clinical management of dyspnoea. *Lancet Oncol* 2002; **3**: 223–8.

◆ 17 Urban T, Lebeau B, Chastang C, *et al.* Superior vena cava syndrome in small cell lung cancer. *Arch Intern Med* 1993; **153**: 384–7.

● 18 Würschmidt F, Bünemann H, Heilman HP. Small cell lung cancer with and without superior vena cava syndrome: a multivariate analysis of prognostic factors in 408 cases. *Int J Radiat Oncol Biol Phys* 1995; **33**: 77–82.

● 19 Tanigawa N, Sawada S, Mishima K, *et al.* Clinical outcome of stenting in superior vena cava syndrome associated with malignant tumors. Comparison with conventional treatment. *Acta Radiol* 1998; **39**: 669–74.

● 20 Pereira JR, Martins SJ, Ikari FK, *et al.* Neoadjuvant chemotherapy versus radiotherapy alone for superior vena cava syndrome (SCVS) due to non small cell lung cancer (NSCLC): preliminary results of randomized phase II trial. *Eur J Cancer* 1999; **35** (suppl 4): 260.

◆ 21 Davenport D, Ferree C, Blake D, Raven M. Response of superior vena cava syndrome to radiation therapy. *Cancer* 1976; **38**: 1577–1580.

● 22 Levitt SH, Jones TK, Bogardus CR. Treatment of malignant superior vena caval obstruction. A randomized study. *Cancer* 1969; **24**: 447–51.

● 23 Fisherman WH, Bradfield JS. Superior vena caval syndrome: response with initial high daily dose irradiation. *South Med J* 1973; **66**: 677–80.

◆ 24 Chan RH, Dar AR, Yu E, *et al.* Superior vena cava obstruction in small-cell lung cancer. *Int J Radiat Oncol Biol Phys* 1997; **38**: 384–7.

● 25 Sorensen JB, Stenbygaard LE, Dahlberg J, Engelholm SA. Short fractionation radiotherapy for superior vena cava syndrome (SVCS) in 148 lung cancer patients. *Lung Cancer* 1997; **18** (Suppl 1): 125.

◆ 26 Amstrong BA, Perez CA, Simpson JR, Hederman MA. Role of irradiation in the management of superior vena cava syndrome. *Int J Radiat Oncol Biol Phys* 1987; **13**: 531–9.

◆ 27 Rodríguez CI, Njo KH, Karim AB. Hypofractionated radiation therapy in the treatment of superior vena cava syndrome. *Lung Cancer* 1993; **10**: 221–8.

◆ 28 Wilson E, Lynn A, Khan S. Radiological stenting provides effective palliation in malignant central venous obstruction. *Clin Oncol* 2000; **12**: 331.

● 29 Urruticoechea A, Mesia R, Domínguez J, *et al.* Treatment of malignant superior vena cava syndrome by endovascular stent insertion. Experience on 52 patients with lung cancer. *Lung Cancer* 2004; **43**: 209–14.

● 30 Irving JD, Dondelinger RF, Reidy JF, *et al.* Gianturco self expanding stents: clinical experience in the vena cava and large veins. *Cardiovasc Intervent Radiol* 1992; **15**: 328–33.

● 31 Hennequin LM, Fade O, Fays JG, *et al.* Superior vena cava stent placement: results with the Wallstent endoprosthesis. *Radiology* 1995; **196**: 353–61.

● 32 Kee ST, Kinoshita L, Razavi MK, *et al.* Superior vena cava syndrome: treatment with catheter directed thrombolysis and endovascular stent placement. *Radiology* 1998; **206**: 187–93.

◆ 33 Rowell NP, Gleeson FV. Steroids, radiotherapy, chemotherapy and stents for superior vena caval obstruction in carcinoma of the bronchus (Cochrane Review). In: *Cochrane Library*, Issue **1**, 2004.

◆ 34 Dyet JF, Nicholson AA, Cook AM. The use of Wallstent endovascular prosthesis in the treatment of malignant obstruction of the superior vena cava. *Clin Radiol* 1993; **48**: 381–5.

● 35 Doty DB. Bypass of superior vena cava: Six years' experience with spiral vein graft for obstruction of superior vena cava due to benign and malignant disease. *J Thorac Cardiovasc Surg* 1982; **83**: 326–38.

◆ 36 Bowcock SJ, Shee CD, Rassam SMB, Harper PG. Chemotherapy for cancer patients who present late. *BMJ* 2004; **328**: 1430–32.

88

Seizures

FABIO SIMONETTI, AUGUSTO T CARACENI

INTRODUCTION

Seizures are not infrequently encountered in palliative medicine. They may be caused by metastatic cerebral lesions in advanced cancer, by acquired immune deficiency syndrome (AIDS), or as a consequence of metabolic derangement or drug toxicity. Nonstructural causes of seizures are quite common,[1] and they can occur in patients with brain metastases (Table 88.1).

DEFINITIONS AND CLASSIFICATION OF SEIZURES[2]

Epileptic seizures are classified according to their electroencephalographic features into partial seizures (when an initiating focus can be identified in a specific brain area) and generalized seizures (when the seizure seems to have bilateral onset). Partial seizures can evolve into generalized tonic-clonic seizures, and in this case the term secondarily generalized seizures is used.

Depending on the level of consciousness during attacks, seizures can be classified as follows:

- *Simple partial seizures.* These are associated with a normal level of consciousness. Only a selective area of the cortex participates in the seizure activity causing symptoms that are therefore typical of the function of the cortical area involved: partial motor, sensory, autonomic, and affective may occur. At times when symptoms of this kind precede the onset of a generalized seizure they are called an 'aura'.

- *Complex seizures.* These are associated with impaired consciousness and may be:
  - *Absence (petit mal) seizures.* These are typical of infancy and can last for 5–10 seconds and occur ten to hundreds of times a day. The patient stops whatever they are doing, with fixed unresponsive eyes. If the seizure lasts for more than 10 seconds he or she may blink or smack the lips repetitively. Atypical absences can be of longer duration and can be associated with flaccidity or muscle rigidity and usually have onset after age of five.
  - *Partial complex seizures.* These combine focal symptoms with an altered state of consciousness. These are the most common type of seizures seen in adults and probably also the most common in the palliative care setting. The patient seems to be awake but has no contact with the environment. He or she does not answer questions appropriately, the eyes can be fixed or rolling purposelessly around, the patient is immobile or engaged in repetitive behaviors (motor automatisms), repeats words or sentences and may be grimacing, snapping fingers, chewing, running or undressing. If physically restrained, the patient can become hostile or aggressive. These attacks can be preceded by auras that are similar to simple partial seizures. The seizure lasts on average 3 minutes and is followed by a post-ictal phase with symptoms as somnolence, delirium, or headache, which can last for several hours. After complete recovery the patient has no recollection of the event, but sometimes may remember the aura.
  - *Generalized tonic-clonic (grand mal) seizures.* These start with a sudden loss of consciousness, at times

Table 88.1 *Causes of seizures in palliative care*

Cause	Comment
Brain metastases	More frequent when involving gray matter
	Due to bleeding
	Particularly frequent with melanoma
Meningeal metastases	Due to cerebral cortex infiltration
AIDS	Frequent in AIDS dementia complex (50%)
	Due to CNS infection
	Due to primary brain lymphoma
	Metabolic
	In 20% of cases cause remains unknown
Drug toxicity	Chemotherapy with vincristine, ifosfamide,[a] thiothepa, methotrexate, busulfan
	Antiviral therapy
	Opioids (very high doses)
	Quinolonic antibiotics
	Penicillin and derivatives
	Imipenem
	Neuroleptics and tricyclic antidepressants can lower seizure threshold
	Theophylline, aminophylline, terbutaline
	Antiarrhythmics
	Immunosuppressants
Drug withdrawal	Alcohol
	Opioids
	Benzodiazepine
Brain radiation (both whole brain and stereotactic)	Acute worsening of brain edema
	Necrosis or local bleeding
CNS infection	Encephalitis
	Brain abscess
	Meningitïs
	Frequent in immunocompromised patients post bone marrow transplant
Metabolic	Electrolyte derangement (severe and sudden hyponatremia, hypocalcemia, hypophosphatemia)
	Renal failure with very high uremia
	Liver failure
	Thyroid disturbances
	Hypoglycemia
Neurologic disease	Primary brain tumor
	Multiple sclerosis
	Tuberous sclerosis
	Cerebrovascular accident
	Leukodystrophies
	Alzheimer disease

[a] Ifosfamide high dose infusion typically causes nonconvulsive status epilepticus.

accompanied by shouting (due to forced air expiration by sudden contraction of the diaphragm). Diffuse muscle rigidity and cyanosis follow, and after a minute myoclonus and muscle fasciculations occur for 1–2 minutes. In this phase the patient can bite his or her tongue. At the end, the post-ictal phase, the patient is in deep sleep, and breathing slowly and deeply when they gradually awaken, and often complain of headache.

Absence and tonic-clonic seizures are the most typical clinical manifestations of generalized seizures which also include *clonic seizures* (rhythmic contractions of upper limb, neck and face muscles), *myoclonic seizures* (brief segmental contractions of the limbs, occurring alone or in clusters without loss of consciousness), *tonic seizures* (sudden generalized muscle rigidity associated with loss of consciousness and falls), and *atonic seizures* (sudden muscle tone resolution).

TREATMENT OF SEIZURES[3,4]

Prophylactic anticonvulsant treatment in patients with brain tumors or metastases is controversial and in fact few studies have addressed the efficacy of prophylactic anticonvulsant therapy in these patients. In noncontrolled clinical series prophylactic treatment has not been shown to give any advantage. One randomized clinical trial confirmed that in patients with brain metastases who had never had seizures prophylactic treatment did not prevent seizure development.[3,4**] In patients with primary brain tumors without seizures it is suggested that anticonvulsant therapy be withdrawn 1 week after surgery.[4] Metastases from melanoma, choriocarcinoma, and cancer of the testis are more often associated with seizures, possibly because these lesions are often hemorrhagic and, in the case of melanoma, tend to invade the cortical gray matter. Many anticonvulsants have potentially serious side effects and may interact with chemotherapeutic drugs and steroids. They can be sedative and can produce cognitive impairment. Prophylaxis is therefore only recommended in patients who have already had seizures. Seizures worsen brain edema and vice versa, therefore, in patients who develop new seizures in spite of anticonvulsant therapy it is advisable to optimize antiedema therapies before modifying the anticonvulsant regimen.

It is worth emphasizing that in every other case of seizures secondary to medical or metabolic causes in palliative care patients without brain tumor lesions there is no indication to start long-term anticonvulsant therapy.

Pharmacological therapy[5–8]

This section summarizes the general characteristics of anticonvulsants. One must bear in mind that blood levels, when available, should be monitored because of the unpredictability of metabolic changes and drug interactions, although it should also be remembered that clinical response and not blood levels will guide dosage.

PHENYTOIN

Phenytoin is a first-line drug in simple and complex partial seizures and in generalized tonic-clonic seizures. It is metabolized by a saturable hepatic enzyme so it has non-linear kinetics making dosage adjustments difficult. It is available in two different intravenous formulations (phenytoin and fosphenytoin) suitable for emergencies or when administration by the oral route is not possible. The dose varies from 4 mg/kg per day to 8 mg/kg per day. Its long half-life allows the dose to be given once daily, but it may be divided into two to three doses daily to avoid gastric discomfort.

Phenytoin has some drawbacks. Blood levels of phenytoin are quite variable as a consequence of the administration of many other drugs interfering with liver metabolism, absorption, or protein binding. Interference has been demonstrated with ciclosporin, cisplatinum, and paclitaxel. Significant pharmacokinetic interactions can occur with concurrent dexamethasone which can reduce phenytoin plasma levels by 50 percent. Advantages of phenytoin include the lack of sedative effects and good tolerability even at higher than recommended doses.

Side effects due to long-term use include ataxia, gastrointestinal disturbances, gingival hypertrophy, hirsutism, osteoporosis, and megaloblastic anemia. Severe allergic reactions involving rash, hypersensitivity reactions, liver toxicity and myelo-suppression have been reported but are rare.

PHENOBARBITAL

Phenobarbital is effective in both partial and generalized tonic-clonic seizures. It is metabolized by liver cytochrome P450, and has very slow plasma clearance (4–5 days), that can be affected by liver disease. It is a safe drug with a wide therapeutic index but it can cause drowsiness, ataxia, and severe rash (Stevens–Johnson syndrome and Lyell syndrome). It interferes with the metabolism of several chemotherapeutic agents and long-term use is associated with pseudorheumatism which can worsen the symptoms of a concurrent steroid-induced osteoporosis.

It is available in oral and parenteral formulations; the dose varies from 1 mg/kg per day to 5 mg/kg per day, given once daily. It can be used in subcutaneous infusions.

SODIUM VALPROATE

Sodium valproate is active in most types of generalized seizure (tonic, myoclonic, absence, tonic-clonic) including secondarily generalized partial seizures. It is also effective in treating neuropsychiatric disturbances commonly seen in palliative care situations. Doses start at 250–500 mg/day and are increased by 250 mg per week up to 1000–3000 mg/day. In children the initial dose is 10–15 mg/kg per day, increased by the same incremental doses. It has the potential for drug–drug interactions.

Common side effects of sodium valproate include tremors, weight gain, sedation, ataxia, gastrointestinal symptoms and thrombocytopenia. Liver enzymes and blood ammonia can be increased. Severe liver toxicity can occur (usually in the first 6 months of therapy); most cases occur in children and in association with other anticonvulsants.

CARBAMAZEPINE

Carbamazepine is effective in the treatment of simple and complex partial seizures, and in tonic-clonic generalized seizures. It is available only in oral formulations and the dose should start at 200 mg/day, increasing by 200 mg per week.

Acute intoxication can cause stupor and coma, convulsions, and respiratory depression. After chronic administration sedation, vertigo, ataxia, double vision, and myelo-suppression can occur. Severe myelotoxicity has been found (1 case of aplastic anemia/200 000 patients).

CLONAZEPAM

Clonazepam is approved by the US Food and Drug Administration (FDA) for the prophylaxis of absence, atypical absence, and myoclonic epilepsy. It can also be used as a temporary treatment to control and prevent seizures not controlled by ongoing therapy. In children initial doses start at 0.01–0.03 mg/kg per day and are increased by 0.25–0.5 mg every 3 days. The most relevant side effect is sedation. Paradoxical excitation is rare.

NEWER ANTIEPILEPTIC DRUGS[9,10]

Oxcarbazepine

Oxcarbazepine can be used as monotherapy in patients with refractory partial epilepsy. It is chemically related to carbamazepine, but it has less pharmacological interaction liability because it is a poor inducer of liver enzymes, although a decrease in serum ethinyl estradiol has been seen. Its mechanism of action also seems to be linked to sodium channel modulation. It is approved for partial seizures in adults both as monotherapy and add-on therapy. Side effects are similar to carbamazepine but it is usually better tolerated. Initial doses range from 300 mg to 600 mg in two to three daily doses and is usually titrated up to 600–1800 mg per day. Patients taking this drug can have clinically significant hyponatremia (more common in older people) and rash.

Gabapentin

Gabapentin is approved for adjunctive therapy of partial seizures with or without secondary generalization. Its use is facilitated by the lack of binding to plasma protein and pharmacological metabolic interferences. Because of its short half-life multiple doses are required per day. Elimination is renal and influenced only by renal function. Daily doses are 900–1880 mg/day in three divided doses but doses as high as 3600–6000 mg/day in adults have been used without severe side effects. Gabapentin is also considered effective as monotherapy in epilepsy but its use in neurooncology has never been studied. There are no serious adverse events, minor events include sedation, ataxia, weight gain, peripheral edema, dizziness, and behavioral changes.

Topiramate

Topiramate is indicated in partial and generalized seizures in children and adults. Initial dose should be low (25 mg) and increased by 25–50 mg per week. Minimal daily doses range from 200 mg to 400 mg. In children the initial dose is 0.5–1 mg/kg per day, and it is increased weekly by the same amount up to 5–9 mg/kg. Side effects are of the central type, sedation, unsteadiness, memory and concentration problems; serious adverse events include nephrolithiasis, open angle glaucoma, and hypohidrosis. Topiramate 6 mg/kg per day is effective in reducing drop attacks (tonic and atonic seizures) in patients with the Lennox–Gastaut syndrome.

Topiramate can also be used as monotherapy in patients with refractory partial epilepsy and at 6 mg/kg per day is effective for the treatment of refractory generalized tonic-clonic convulsions and in other seizure types in adults and children. Topiramate causes a decrease in the serum concentration of ethinyl estradiol.

Lamotrigine

Lamotrigine has been approved for partial seizures in adults in association with other drugs. It is effective also as monotherapy in patients with refractory partial epilepsy and also for the treatment of absence seizures in children. It is metabolized by the liver and has significant interactions with all the classic anticonvulsants (phenobarbital, phenytoin, carbamazepine). Serious adverse events are rashes including Stevens–Johnson syndrome and toxic epidermolysis, more so in children and with concomitant valproate use. They are related to a rapid titration of the drug dose. With slow initiation of therapy the risk of skin rash is comparable with that seen with phenytoin. It is therefore important to titrate the dose slowly with weekly increments of 25 mg or 50 mg up to 300–500 mg/day. In patients who are already taking liver enzyme-inducing antiepileptic drugs (with the exception of valproic acid) the starting dose should be 50 mg/day for 2 weeks, then increased by 100 mg/day (in two divided doses) to a maintenance dose of 300–500 mg/day. If added to a regimen consisting of valproic acid, lamotrigine should be started at 25 mg every other day for 2 weeks and titrated even more carefully. Nonserious adverse events include tics, predominantly in children and insomnia. It is available only in oral formulation. A decrease in lamotrigine serum concentrations has been observed with oral contraceptives.

Summary and practical guidelines for management in palliative care

The ideal antiepileptic drug for palliative care is not easy to establish as the classic anticonvulsants cause a variety of metabolic interactions and significant side effects. Among the newer drugs there is little experience in this indication. On the basis of our experience we suggest some practical management guidelines:

- The need for slow titration schedules limits the usefulness of topiramate and lamotrigine, which is also a strong inducer of liver enzymes.[7,8] In our experience oxcarbazepine and valproate seem to have a more favorable profile compared with other available drugs.
- Prophylactic treatment should be started only in patients with structural brain disease who have had a seizure before. In cases of metabolic or toxic causes that have been successfully managed there is no need for prophylaxis.
- In case of brain lesions we do not counsel the family or patients about the risk of seizures unless risk is very high, such as in case of brain metastases from melanoma, for which we also recommend prophylaxis.
- If the patient had a seizure due to structural brain lesion, the family should be informed about how to react in case of another seizure. They should position the patient on one side to protect from injury and aspiration and they should not try to force open the mouth in case of 'morsus'.
- The seizure is usually a self-limiting event, and the family should wait for spontaneous resolution unless the seizures are prolonged (more than a few minutes) or repetitive. Although recovery from a seizure or recognition of recurrence may be difficult for family members, in these circumstances they can be instructed to use rectal diazepam preparations while waiting for medical assistance. If in the same situation medical or nursing care is available lorazepam 2–4 mg intravenously should be given if intravenous access is available.
- In patients with poor oral intake phenobarbital subcutaneous infusion is the best alternative for home and hospice care. Midazolam can be added in case of difficult-to-control seizures.
- Blood levels should be checked only if under- or overdosing are suspected, which lead to poor seizure control or toxicity, respectively. Toxicity from antiepileptic agents can be difficult to distinguish from worsening of the underlying brain disease. If feasible, it is also advisable to check blood levels at least once after initial titration of phenobarbital, carbamazepine, phenytoin, oxcarbazepine, or sodium valproate.

STATUS EPILEPTICUS

The most commonly accepted definition of status epilepticus (SE)[2] is continuous seizure activity persisting for more than 30 minutes or two or more seizures without full recovery of neurological function in between. Another definition of SE is continuous generalized seizures lasting longer than 5 minutes or, of course, two or more seizures during which the patient does not return to baseline consciousness; this is more practical in palliative care setting because patients are usually more ill; moreover if a seizure lasts more than 5 minutes the likelihood of spontaneous termination decreases. A patient who has not responded to first-line therapy in an hour is said to be in *refractory status epilepticus*.

Clinical characteristics

Status epilepticus may be characterized by motor convulsions (convulsive SE) or by absence of motor phenomena (nonconvulsive SE); and may affect the whole brain (generalized SE) or only part of the brain (partial SE). Depending on the type of seizures SE can be also defined as:

- Tonic-clonic SE
- Tonic SE
- Clonic SE (only in children)
- Myoclonic SE
- Simple partial SE or SE epilepsia partialis continua (without impairment of consciousness)
- Nonconvulsive status epilepticus (NCSE).

NONCONVULSIVE STATUS EPILEPTICUS

This particular condition is characterized by electro-encephalogram (EEG) seizure activity without convulsive activity. It is a significant cause of impaired consciousness in patients with complex toxic-metabolic encephalopathies, occurring in 8 percent[11*] of comatose patients according to recent data. According to some authors most patients with altered state of consciousness and mild motor signs have EEG findings compatible with SE. Manifestations of NCSE include absence type NCSE and partial complex NCSE. Although no data are available we consider this condition not to be totally rare in palliative care and its differential diagnosis may apply more often than usually thought.

Partial complex NCSE is a particularly challenging situation. Seizure activity fluctuates and recurs, often originating from temporal cortical areas and causes a confusional state with variable clinical findings. This condition can be continuous, with longlasting delirium, with or without psychotic behaviors and automatisms, and, in this case, is sustained by continuous focal seizures, or discontinuous with recurrent partial complex seizures, but with recovery of consciousness between the single seizure episodes. Clinical aspects may be baffling with minimal abnormalities in answering questions but affective manifestations of fear or paranoid ideation.

Duration can vary from 30 minutes to 2 weeks. In 40 percent of cases the episode is shorter than 24 hours; in another 40 percent the episode lasts from 1 to 10 days. In one case report a partial complex status lasted for 7.5 months.[12*]

Treatment

Convulsive SE is a neurological emergency associated with significant mortality and morbidity and thus requires rapid and aggressive treatment.[13] In terminally ill patients the treatment must be weighted. The first priority is that the cardiocirculatory and respiratory functions are supported. Intravenous infusion of benzodiazepines and phenytoin are the first-line pharmacological approaches (Fig. 88.1). Treatment has a high rate of success (80 percent) if initiated within 30 minutes. If delayed for more than 2 hours these drugs fail in 60 percent of cases.

CHARACTERISTICS OF DRUGS USED IN SE

The drugs used for the acute control of epileptic seizures also have other indications in palliative care when they are used primarily for their sedative effects.

Lorazepam

Lorazepam is considered the drug of choice.[15**] The mean time to clinical effect is 3 minutes, the half-life is 10–15 hours but effective brain levels are maintained for 8–24 hours. It has no active metabolites. It should be infused intravenously not faster than 2 mg/minute. It is rapidly absorbed after rectal administration. Intramuscular administration is not recommended. In acute administration the main risk is respiratory depression. Refrigeration is usually necessary, but some authors have observed that lorazepam retained 90 percent of its original concentration when stored without refrigeration in ambulances for 5 months.

Diazepam

Diazepam enters the brain in a few seconds but because of its high lipid solubility, redistribution to all body tissues is rapid with a consequent fall of brain concentrations. Its anticonvulsant effect is therefore very brief and a second dose may be necessary after only 20–30 minutes. Rectal formulations are available. Recommended doses are 10 mg in adults and 5 mg (0.5 mg/kg) in children. Rectal administration at these doses does not cause respiratory depression. After intramuscular administration absorption is variable and unpredictable and this route should generally be avoided.

Phenytoin

The onset of action of phenytoin is short (10–20 minutes), it has no sedative effects, does not cause respiratory depression, and has a long duration of action.

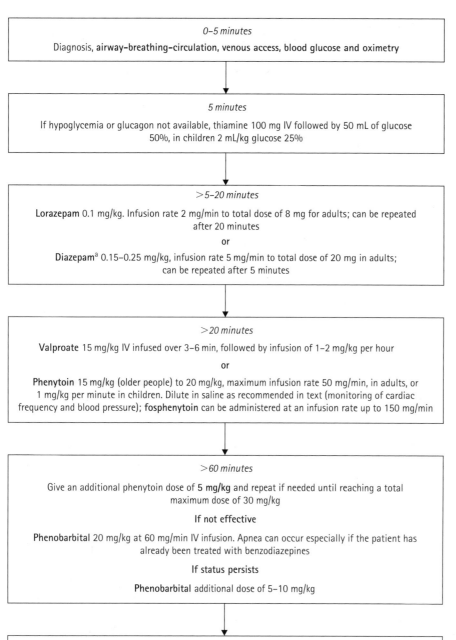

Figure 88.1 *Algorithm for the management of status epilepticus. ᵃDiazepam is now considered an undesirable second choice. ᵇSolution should be freshly prepared every 6 hours. IV, intravenous. Modified from Working Group on Status Epilepticus recommendations.[14]*

It should be used in benzodiazepine-refractory SE by intravenous infusion, at 20 mg/kg, not more than 50 mg/minute. In older patients the dose should be reduced to 15 mg/kg. After a loading dose has been infused the duration of the therapeutic effect is about 24 hours. Blood levels can be checked 120 minutes after the end of the infusion. A loading dose of 15–20 mg/kg can be also administered orally but poor gastric tolerability limits the use of this route in some patients.

After diluting phenytoin in saline, the solution should be infused within 1 hour. A concentration of 6.7 mg/mL (1000 mg/130 mL) is suggested although the drug is stable in solutions of up to 10 mg/mL. Side effects may be related to excessively fast infusion rates, as may be required in emergency situations and include cardiac arrhythmias, arterial hypotension and central nervous system depression. The 'purple glove syndrome' is due to the high pH of the drug (−13) causing local toxicity at the site of infusion which manifests with blue discoloration, and distal edema, 2 hours after administration.[16]

Sodium valproate

The availability of a parenteral formulation of valproate provides an alternative to phenytoin. Many reports confirm the efficacy and safety of valproate infusion (up to 6 mg/kg per minute and dose of up to 30 mg/kg followed by a maintenance dose of 1–2 mg/kg per hour) in emergency situations.[17*]

Midazolam

Midazolam is water soluble, has a very short half-life, and has no active metabolites. Its onset of action is 3 minutes, 5 minutes, and 15 minutes after intravenous, intramuscular, and oral administration, respectively. The good intramuscular and subcutaneous absorption is an important advantage in cases of difficult venous access and therefore can be indicated is some palliative care settings. In refractory SE the initial dose is 0.2 mg/kg, followed by 0.05–0.5 mg/kg per hour intravenous infusion.[18*,19*]

Propofol

Propofol has an effect on γ-aminobutyric acid (GABA) receptors similar to that of benzodiazepines and barbiturates. Its use requires intensive care support and is reserved for SE which is refractory to standard treatment. Hypotensive effects should be carefully managed. A loading dose of 3–5 mg/kg IV followed by a continuous infusion at a rate which can cause a burst suppression pattern on the EEG, usually 30–100 μg/kg per minute (maximum dose = 108 g in 9 days in one patient who had one single asymptomatic episode of hypertriglycidemia without rhabdomyolysis).[20*]

Phenobarbital

This is an option if benzodiazepines and phenytoin fail. The peak clinical effect is delayed for 20–60 minutes after administration.

Thiopental

Thiopental is highly lipid soluble and for this reason undergoes rapid redistribution, resulting in a state of coma that is less prolonged than with phenobarbital. It is partially metabolized to pentobarbital. Thiopental lowers the intracranial pressure but is associated with severe hypotension, edema, ileus, sepsis, immune depression and an increase in P_{CO_2}.

Awakening is complicated by longlasting side effects and function recovery has a long and variable profile: recovery of motor function occurs within 1–72 hours after the end of treatment, eye-opening after 1–3 days, and cognitive function after 2–18 days.

Differential diagnosis

It is important to keep in mind that acute conditions with an altered state of consciousness at times associated with motor or behavioral abnormalities are often erroneously considered seizures. The most frequently occurring of these conditions are listed in Box 88.1.[21]

Box 88.1 Differential diagnosis of seizures

- Psychiatric disturbances: somatoform reactions, anxiety panic attacks, psychotic dissociative episodes, Munchausen syndrome

- Cardiovascular disorders: syncope, arrhythmia, transient ischemic attacks

- Headache: hemicrania comitata, basilar migraine

- Movement disorders: tremor, dyskinesia, tic, myoclonus

- Parasomnias and sleep disturbances: nightmares, somnambulism, narcolepsy, cataplexy, nocturnal paroxysmal dystonia

- Gastrointestinal symptoms: nausea or colic

- Delirium

- Progressive worsening of intracranial hypertension or herniation with opisthotonus or other acute neurological findings

---

Key learning points

- Secondary epilepsy is common in palliative care and has complex multifactorial etiologies.

- Prophylactic anticonvulsants in patients with primary or metastatic brain tumor who have never had seizures is not recommended.

- All anticonvulsants offer effective protection against seizures in patients with brain tumor and a seizure disorder but have varying profiles of toxicity and metabolic interactions. Sodium valproate, oxcarbazepine and topiramate offer a favorable therapeutic index in these patients.

- Generalized SE is a medical emergency while nonconvulsive SE is an important differential diagnosis in patients with changes in behavior and mental status.

- Lorazepam and sodium valproate are first-line therapies of generalized SE with low risk of administration. Midazolam is an important alternative if venous access is not available.

REFERENCES

◆ 1 Delanty N, Vaughan CJ, French JA. Medical cause of seizure. *Lancet* 1998; **352**: 383–90.

2　Victor M, Ropper AH. *Adams and Victor's Principles of Neurology, 7th ed.* New York: McGraw-Hill, 2001.

● 3　Forsyth PA, Weaver S, Fulton D, *et al.* Prophylactic anticonvulsants in patients with brain tumour. *Can J Neurol Sci* 2003; **30**: 106–12.

✱ 4　Glantz MJ, Cole BF, Forsyth PA, *et al.* Practice parameter: anticonvulsivant prophylaxis in patients with newly diagnosed brain tumors. Report of the Quality Standards Subcommittee of the American Academy of Neurology. *Neurology* 2000; **54**: 1886–93.

◆ 5　Bergin AM, Connolly M. New antiepileptic drug therapies. *Neurol Clin North Am* 2002; **20**: 1163–82.

◆ 6　Bazil CW, Pedley TA. Clinical pharmacology of antiepileptic drugs. *Clin Neuropharmacol* 2003; **1**: 38–52.

◆ 7　Vecht CJ, Wagner L, Wilms EB. Interactions between antiepileptic and chemotherapeutic drugs. *Lancet Neurol* 2003; **2**: 404–9.

◆ 8　Patsalos PN, Perucca E. Clinically important drug interactions in epilepsy: general features and interactions between antiepileptic drugs. *Lancet Neurol* 2003; **2**: 473–81.

✱ 9　French JA, Kanner AM, Bautista J. Efficacy and tolerability of the new antiepileptic drugs I: Treatment of new onset epilepsy. Report of the Therapeutics and Technology Assessment Subcommittee and Quality Standards Subcommittee of the American Academy of Neurology and the American Epilepsy Society. *Neurology* 2004; **62**: 1252–60.

✱ 10　French JA, Kanner AM, Bautista J. Efficacy and tolerability of the new antiepileptic drugs II: Treatment of refractory epilepsy. Report of the Therapeutics and Technology Assessment Subcommittee and Quality Standards Subcommittee of the American Academy of Neurology and the American Epilepsy Society. *Neurology* 2004; **62**: 1261–73.

● 11　Towne AR, Waterhouse EJ, Boggs JG, *et al.* Prevalence of nonconvulsive status epilepticus in comatose patients. *Neurology* 2000; **54**: 340–5.

● 12　Roberts MA, Humphrey PRD. Prolonged complex partial status epilepticus: a case report. *J Neurol Neurosurg Psychiatry* 1988; **51**: 586–92.

◆ 13　Shorvon S. The management of status epilepticus. *J Neurol Neurosurg Psychiatry* 2001; **70** (Suppl II): ii22–ii27.

✱ 14　Working Group on Status Epilepticus. Treatment of convulsive status epilepticus. Recommendations of the Epilepsy Foundation of America's Working Group on Status Epilepticus. *JAMA* 1993; **270**: 854–9.

● 15　Alldredge BK, Gelb AM, Isaacs SM, *et al.* A comparison of lorazepam, diazepam, and placebo for the treatment of out-of-hospital status epilepticus. *N Engl J Med* 2001; **345**: 631–7.

◆ 16　Wheless J. Pediatric use of intravenous and intramuscular phenytoin: lesson learned. *J Child Neurol* 1998; **13** (Suppl 1): S11–S14.

● 17　Wheless JW, Vazquez BR, Kanner AM, *et al.* Rapid infusion with valproate sodium is well tolerated in patients with epilepsy. *Neurology* 2004; **63**: 1507–8.

● 18　Yoshikawa H, Yamazaki S, Abe T, Oda Y. Midazolam as a first-line agent for status epilepticus in children. *Brain Dev* 2000; **22**: 239–42.

● 19　Prasad A, Worrall BB, Bertram EH, Bleck TP. Propofol and midazolam in the treatment of refractory status epilepticus. *Epilepsia* 2001; **42**: 380–6.

● 20　Rossetti A, Reichhart MD, Schaller M-D, *et al.* Propofol treatment of refractory status epilepticus: a study of 31 episodes. *Epilepsia* 2004; **45**: 757–63.

◆ 21　Krumholz A. Nonepileptic seizures: diagnosis and management. *Neurology* 1999; **53** (Suppl 2): S76–S83.

89

Acute pain syndromes*

MELLAR P DAVIS

WHAT IS ACUTE PAIN?

There is an implicit understanding of what acute pain is (or at least an assumed understanding), yet few reviews define acute cancer pain and most treatment strategies intermingle chronic and acute cancer pain management without a clear separation. Almost all published reviews are about postoperative or procedural-related pain management. If we can borrow from the cardiology nomenclature of unstable angina, then acute cancer pain (unrelated to procedures) is a new onset or a change in the pattern of chronic pain which evolves over hours to days. Acute pain in cancer usually signifies new metastases, a complication from existing metastases, an indirect complication from treatment such as herpes zoster or mucositis, an evolving chronic comorbidity or developing comorbidity. Patients are more likely to seek medical attention in the emergency rooms with acute cancer pain than with chronic cancer pain (unless chronic cancer pain is grossly under-treated). The change in pain may be related to the frequency of breakthrough pain or a sharp increase in the intensity of the underlying chronic pain, a change in pain referral pattern or new pain upon chronic pain, or associated new symptoms (such as nausea and vomiting) upon a background of chronic (abdominal) pain. The general assumption most physicians have is that acute pain is severe, however some patients will experience acute, mild, or moderate pain or the pattern of pain may change but severity remains the same (e.g. continued moderate back pain but new onset of radicular pain with spinal cord compression).

TEMPORAL CLASSIFICATION OF PAIN

Acute pain has most often been classified as transient pain due to procedures or postoperative pain. But acute pain may also crescendo 'acute on chronic' pain from rapidly evolving tumor cancer complications such as hemorrhage or infection within the tumor, pathological fracture, bowel obstruction, or perforation of the hollow viscous. Acute pain draws attention to the injury typified by a 'fight or flight' response. The 'fight or flight' response results in pupillary dilation, sweating, tachycardia, tachypnea, or shunting of blood from viscera.[1] Responses to chronic pain differ significantly from acute pain. Chronic persistent pain is generally purposeless, poorly related to the degree of tissue injury and has a significant component of neuroplasticity resulting in abnormal pain processing. Patients tend to be somnolent, hypokinetic and anorexic. Libido is reduced (independent of opioids), constipation, anhedonia, and somatic preoccupation and personality changes may supervene.[1] In one sense breakthrough pain is a type of acute pain (usually upon a background of chronic pain) but is not 'acute pain syndrome' and is generally discussed under chronic cancer pain.

The temporal nature and severity of pain dictate the speed with which the cycle of assessment, analgesic choice, application and reassessment occurs.[2] Among the errors cited in treatment strategies, failure to escalate in a timely fashion with adequate doses of opioids is common.[2] This may

---

*A World Health Organization project in palliative medicine.

be due in part to the use of chronic pain dosing strategies in the management of acute pain. Chronic pain is evaluated at intervals of days whereas acute pain requires reassessment within minutes to hours. The strategy of continuous opioid parenteral infusion or every 4-hour oral dosing with provision for breakthrough for chronic pain is simply inadequate for acute pain.[3] Parenteral titrated opioids are preferred in the face of crescendo pain.[4] The importance of providing expedited pain relief in acute pain syndromes goes beyond the ethical principle of limiting suffering. The neurohumoral response to acute pain particularly in the setting of comorbidities and limited cardiopulmonary function leads to quick demise of the patient. Immobility due to acute pain increases the risk for thromboembolism. Acute oropharyngeal pain from mucositis accelerates nutritional deficiency. Acute pain leads to anxiety and fear which worsens pain and may precipitate an existential crisis.[5] Uncontrolled acute pain, if treated ineffectively will lead to abnormal central pain processing through neuroplasticity, which ends up as refractory chronic pain. Uncontrolled acute pain increases medical expenditures and prolongs hospitalization.[5,6] Acute crescendo pain accounts for only 4 percent of cancer pain visits to the emergency room but its overall incidence is relatively underreported.[7]

ASSESSMENT OF ACUTE PAIN SYNDROMES

The management of cancer pain depends on a comprehensive assessment. This needs to characterize the symptoms in terms of phenomenology and pathogenesis, and assess the relationship between pain and disease and clarify the impact of pain and co-morbid conditions on the patient's quality of life.[8]

Acute pain as transient flares of pain due to procedures is unlikely to influence overall quality of life but acute pain as a complication of cancer will significantly affect a patient's quality of life. A pain history should include documentation of the temporal pattern, location, severity, quality, and palliative factors to pain. Procedural-related pain is quite obvious. The focus of assessment in this situation will be pain severity, duration, and response to analgesia. However, acute or chronic or crescendo pain will require a full history as has been outlined for chronic cancer pain.[8]

Cancer pain syndromes are well defined for chronic cancer pain.[8–11] Most cancer pain classification systems are based upon chronic pain where the prevalence and etiology are well defined. This is not true for acute pain syndromes. Acute pain syndromes have been listed by various authors but remain incomplete due to lack of definition.[8,10] Prevalence of acute pain in cancer pain is less well defined. Boxes 89.1 and 89.2 represent the author's attempt to classify acute pain based upon clinical experience and from the literature.[12,13]

Box 89.1 Acute pain syndrome in advanced cancer

Directly related to cancer

- Destruction of joints
- Pathologic fracture of long bone
- Vertebral fracture with mechanical instability and/or cord compression
- Visceral infiltration with obstruction of a hollow organ
- Visceral perforation and secondary peritonitis
- Hepatic capsule infiltration and/or rupture or acute bleed
- Splenic infarct
- Pulmonary artery tumor infiltration and pulmonary infarct
- Bronchopleural fistula with empyema
- Cerebral or brain stem metastases with bleed or infection
- Secondary tumor infection (particularly oropharyngeal carcinoma)
- Tumor-induced pericarditis or cardiac tamponade
- Budd–Chiari syndrome from hepatic venous cancer invasion

Acute pain related to treatment or procedures

- Acute postoperative pain
- Postradiation: mucositis, esophagitis, brachial plexopathy, arachnoiditis (Lhermitte syndrome), enteritis, cystitis, proctitis
- Chemotherapy: extravasation, endophlebitis, neuropathy (oxaliplatin, taxanes, vinca alkaloids), acute jaw pain (vincristine), mucositis (radiation or chemotherapy)
- Steroid withdrawal and arthralgia-myalgia
- Dexamethasone-induced rectal pain
- Luteinizing hormone-releasing hormone agonist or hormone-induced bone pain flare (prostate cancer and breast cancer)
- Chemical pleuritis from pleurodesis
- Hepatic pain from hepatic artery embolization and/or chemotherapy
- Chest pain from pericardiocentesis + sclerosis

- Paracentesis and chemotherapy lavage
- Post lumbar puncture headaches
- Post bone marrow biopsy pain
- Venipuncture
- Stent placement (biliary or ureteral, esophageal)
- Percutaneous endoscopic gastrostomy tube placement
- Nephrostomy tube placement
- Transhepatic biliary drainage tube

Indirect complications of cancer

- Pulmonary embolism
- Venous thrombosis
- Arterial thrombosis
- Marantic endocarditis with multiple infarcts
- Shingles
- Oropharyngeal candidosis
- Clostridium enterocolitis
- Acute myalgias from sepsis
- Ascending cholangitis
- Pyelonephritis
- Graft vs. host disease
- Hepatic venous occlusive disease after bone marrow transplant
- Typhlitis

Box 89.2 Acute neuropathic pain syndromes

- Vinca-induced lancinating pain
- Oxaliplatin-induced cold sensitivity
- Lhermitte syndrome from cord compression
- Funicular pain from cord compression
- Radiculopathy from plexopathy, vertebral collapse or spinal cord compression
- Postherpetic neuralgia

Unidimensional pain scales, either verbal rating scales or visual numerical rating scales (VNRS), visual analog scales (VAS) or category scales (CS) are used to assess acute pain severity and pain response.[8,14] A pain relief scale is frequently combined with unidimensional scales to assess the adequacy of response. The algorithm of assessment, treatment, and reassessment is more rapid than with chronic pain since the acute nature, pain severity and dosing strategy dictates the need for a quick response.[2] Failure to escalate analgesics in a timely manner can be due to failure to reassess at appropriate intervals.[2] A lack of uniform and timely assessment influences comparisons of opioid dosing strategies for acute pain.

RESPONSE CRITERIA

The response criteria in acute pain are defined by several parameters (Box 89.3). Area under the curve (AUC) for time-analgesic response for pain intensity is one parameter. This requires measurements prior to intervention and at multiple occasions thereafter.[15] This is similar to pharmacokinetics during drug trials with subjective pain relief substituted for plasma drug levels. The sum of pain intensity differences is measured by calculating the AUC. Both of these measures reflect a cumulative response to analgesics but do not provide information about the onset to peak pain relief or duration of relief, both of which are clinically relevant to acute pain.[15] 'Half pain relief' (the percentage of patients who obtain at least a 50 percent relief of their pain) over a 4–6-hour interval as an outcome distinguishes effectiveness of analgesics for acute pain. 'Half pain relief' is governed by three factors: analgesic potency, analgesia dose, and frequency of dosing. To adequately detect a difference between two different methods of pain control, either timing frequency, route, dose, or drug should vary as a single variable and an adequate number of patients should be included in each arm (estimated to be 40) of the study.[15] This is a rarity in cancer pain trials.

Box 89.3 Outcome measures for acute pain

- Peak pain relief
- Number of patients who experience 50 percent reduction in pain intensity
- Summed pain intensity differences (numerical or visual analog scale)
- Total pain relief (numerical or visual analog scale)
- The proportion of patients with 50 percent pain relief
- The proportion of patients who rate their relief as good or excellent
- Time to analgesia (or the time to rescue dose after pain intervention)[15]

The clinically significant changes in VAS or VNRS for acute pain are debated in the literature. There is a significant difference in opinion about the degree of change in unidimensional scales which is relevant to pain relief. That is, if patients have severe pain (VNRS > 7 or a VAS > 70) do these scales need to change to a greater degree for the similar degree of pain relief as compared with mild or moderate pain to be able to detect a meaningful change in pain severity? Gallagher et al. found that a significant detectable difference in VAS for acute abdominal pain was 16 mm (VAS).[16] Myles et al. found that the VAS was linear for mild to moderate acute postoperative pain. The change in the VAS scale with pain relief represented a linear magnitude in change of pain intensity by unidimensional scales.[17] Kelly found that the minimal significant difference in VAS appeared not to vary with pain intensity. Mild pain required an 11 mm decrease in VAS, which was 15 mm for moderate pain and 11 mm for severe pain.[18] Farrar and colleagues found that a ≥ 2.0 difference in the VRNS (0–10) was indicative of perceived significant pain relief with oral transmucosal fentanyl citrate for acute breakthrough cancer pain.[19,20] On the other hand, Cepeda et al. found a nonlinear relation between decreases in pain intensity and pain relief. Minimally detectable pain relief required a decrease in the VNRS of 1.8 for severe pain. The VNRS decreased on an average of 2.4 or greater to detect 'much pain relief' when patients had moderate pain and average of 4.0 if patients had severe intense pain. Pain had to decrease by 3.5 (VNRS) for 'very much pain relief' if the initial pain was moderate and by 5.2 if pain was severe.[21] Aubrun and colleagues found that the relation between VNRS and morphine was not linear but sigmoid. Higher pain intensity required greater doses of morphine in order to reduce the VNRS to the same degree.[22] A nonlinear relation was found by Bird and Dickson.[23] This appears to be independent of gender and age. Acute pain perception differs with age; procedural-related pain is perceived by older patients as less painful than younger patients.[24] In general, the VNRS and VAS correlate but there is a tendency for the VNRS to be higher than the VAS for pain intensity. However, wide interindividual differences exist in distribution between VAS and VNRS.[25]

Satisfaction scales are inaccurate in determining pain response. Patients tend to be satisfied with pain treatment even when pain is not relieved.[26] The VAS cannot adequately discriminate between those patients in acute pain who do and do not want analgesics.[27] Patients can present with severe pain and refuse or be reluctant to take analgesics.

BARRIERS TO ACUTE PAIN MANAGEMENT

The reluctance on the part of the patients in acute pain to take opioids may be due to fear of addiction, sedation, or adverse effects. Pain intensity is perceived as the need for prolonged hospitalization which will be 'shortened' if analgesics are minimized or avoided.[28] Pain may signify that the cancer is progressing and this perception can be 'minimized' by avoiding analgesics as a means of denial. Patients hope that pain will spontaneously resolve. Acute pain management involves high technology, and for some, the use of patient-controlled analgesia (PCA) devices. A significant number of patients have fears about the technology of PCA or fear of self-induced overmedication.[28] Half of the patients are concerned about opioid dose titrations and half receive anxiolytics and adjuvants during acute pain management for that reason.[28]

The majority entering an emergency room with acute cancer pain will not receive sufficient opioids for pain relief (77 percent).[3] This is not related to pain intensity and in fact relief is inversely related to the initial intensity of the pain upon entering the emergency room. Patients with mild to moderate pain are more likely to have their pain ignored and undertreated. Usually no analgesics are given prior to procedures or examinations. There is a lack of training for emergency room physicians in acute pain management. Patients refuse analgesics 15 percent of the time for fear of masking important clinical findings and physicians provide minimal analgesics for the same reason despite randomized trials which have demonstrated that effective analgesics do not prevent good assessment.[3,29,30] Finally, the wrong treatment strategy is chosen to manage acute pain, such as continuous infusions of opioids, resulting in a delayed onset to analgesia.

Physicians initially underrate acute pain relative to the patient's rating. The physician's assessment will be more congruent with the patient's perceived pain severity if assessment is repeated.[31–33]

TREATMENT

The traditional method of fixed doses of oral immediate-release morphine every 4 hours or parenteral continuous infusion with rescue dosing is largely inadequate in acute pain management.[3,34] Patient-controlled analgesia developed in the 1970s and 1980s established the fundamental acute dosing strategy of small opioid doses administered at short intervals. In postoperative patients, PCA is both safe and effective. Opioids are titrated against pain intensity, then PCA is used as maintenance. Excessive self-administered doses by PCA are limited by sedation (which occurs before respiratory depression). Two insights are gained with PCA: (i) most patients like to participate in the management of pain and (ii) there is an 8–10-fold difference in opioid requirement between individuals in acute pain such that there is no 'standard' dose.[3,35] Age, not body weight, predicts opioid doses in acute pain management.[3] Women in certain studies required 30 percent (median) more morphine than men.[36,37]

The goals in acute pain management are pain relief balanced by side effects whereas the goals in chronic pain management balance pain relief with function (i.e. activities of daily living and social interactions).

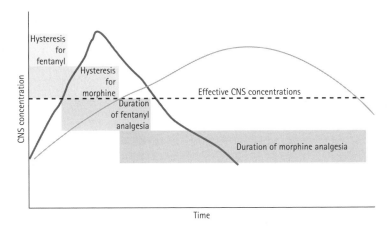

Figure 89.1 *The physicochemical properties of an opioid will determine in part the onset to analgesia (time to effective central nervous system (CNS) concentrations or hysteresis) and duration of effect. Lipophilic opioids initially will have a rapid onset to active and rapid redistribution whereas hydrophilic opioids will have a delayed hysteresis but slower egress from the CNS. The level of P-glycoprotein may also play a role in determining CNS levels for certain opioids.*[38]

Pharmacology and the management of acute pain

Opioid pharmacology is important in the understanding of treatment strategies for acute pain and opioid titration (Box 89.4). The time course to analgesia is not reflected by the change in opioid blood concentrations. Opioid blood concentrations play little role in the management of acute pain, nor do blood levels provide insight into the clinical use of opioids.[3] There is a temporal delay between the drug concentration in plasma and the time to analgesia (frequently called drug hysteresis) related in part to the partition coefficient (lipid solubility) of the opioid (Fig. 89.1 and Box 89.5). The longer the effect delay (hysteresis) the greater the dissimilarity between plasma levels and analgesia. Among phenylpiperdine opioids (alfentanil, fentanyl, and sufentanil) there is a strong association between lipid solubility and minimal effective plasma concentrations, suggesting that the onset to analgesia and potency are related to the ability to cross the blood–brain barrier.[3,38,39] The ability to approach the opioid receptor from multiple directions through the lipid membrane by lipophilic opioids is another factor. Lipophilic opioids give greater access to opioid receptors relative to hydrophilic opioids which are limited to the aqueous phase.

Box 89.4   Factors influencing opioid responses in acute pain

- Differences in tissue damage
- Variability in opioid pharmacokinetics (which range twofold to fourfold between individuals)
- Differences in permeability due to the blood–brain barrier (partition coefficient of each opioid)
- Differences in opioid receptor genetics between individuals
- Variability in perception, meaning of, and attitude toward the pain experience[3]

Box 89.5   Effect delay[3,30,38]

- Morphine – 17–34 minutes
- Fentanyl – 6 minutes
- Alfentanil – 1 minute

P-glycoprotein acts as an efflux pump along the blood–brain barrier that extrudes morphine and morphine 6-glucuronide from the CNS. Morphine 6-glucuronide is several-fold more potent than morphine but its CNS concentrations are significantly less than morphine due to its hydrophilic character and perhaps P-glycoprotein.[38]

The effect delay for morphine has been based on the vocalization responses to electrical stimulation in rats and by the experiences with PCA in humans. However, the published experience of Mercandante and colleagues suggests that by morphine titration 2 mg every 2 minutes the onset to analgesia is less than 10 minutes.[40] Continuous infusions of opioids produce steady state concentrations at 5 half-life intervals resulting in a slow onset to analgesia and an unacceptably long time to reach effective CNS concentrations[3] (Fig. 89.2). Such an approach subjects patients to prolonged, uncontrolled pain.

The onset to analgesia does not correlate with duration of effective analgesia. The CNS dwell time of morphine is much longer than fentanyl, as fentanyl is rapidly redistributed from the CNS. Opioids with short CNS dwell times produce poor pain control with intermittent injections alone.[3] Thus, the need for rescue doses (which reflects CNS levels below effective analgesia) differs between lipophilic opioids and hydrophilic opioids. Traditional methods using 1–2-hour intervals are suitable for opioids with longer CNS dwell times. With PCA, lockout intervals of 6–10 minutes if demand only or continuous infusion plus patient activated rescue doses are more suitable for fentanyl and other lipophilic opioids.[3]

Patient-controlled analgesia has been recommended for unstable acute cancer pain. The cardinal principle of PCA is

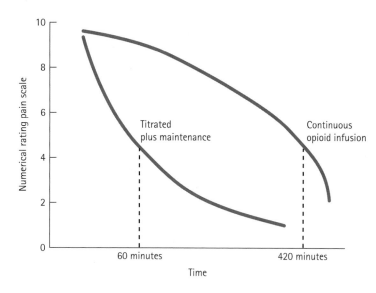

Figure 89.2 *Parenteral titration or bolus infusions of morphine will achieve effective central nervous system concentrations quickly depending upon the dosing strategy. Continuous infusions of morphine require 420 minutes to relative onset of analgesia.[3]*

patient-directed opioid titration to analgesia. Patients vary widely in the dose needed for pain control.[3] However, in reality, patients frequently wait to activate the device until pain resurges to its original intensity, and some will not activate the device at all for fear of causing sedation. This delays analgesia despite the prescribed short lockout intervals. In fact the present evidence suggests that oral titration at 2-hour intervals produces pain relief in the same time as PCA. Physician-controlled titration to relief followed by maintenance increases pain relief in a significantly shorter time compared with PCA alone.[40] In studies using PCA patients were not titrated to pain control prior to using PCA and thus differ from usual guidelines for postoperative pain.[41,42]

MANAGEMENT OF ACUTE PAIN IN CANCER: REVIEW OF THE LITERATURE

Severe, unstable, or crescendo pain requires aggressive opioid titration.[43] Titration schedules can consist of either planned dose escalation of opioids at fixed intervals or loading doses of opioids to pain relief followed by maintenance.[3] The evidence supporting dosing strategies is weak due to the paucity of randomized trials.[44,45] The French National Federation of Cancer Centers working group recommends that 'in the presence of very unstable intense pain, preference should be given to intravenous or subcutaneous patient controlled analgesia' as an expert opinion with little evidence for such recommendations.[46] On the other hand reviews of PCA for acute pain state that PCA is essentially a maintenance therapy and therefore acute pain should be controlled prior to starting PCA.[47,48] Discrepancies between guidelines and expert opinion are due to the lack of strong evidence to support such guidelines.

A systematic review of opioid dosing strategy for acute pain has been published.[3,40–42,45] Since that publication, three additional studies have become available for

review.[7,45,49,50] A total of 12 studies are now available in the English literature, providing clinical evidence with regards to dosing strategies. Eight of the 12 trials were prospective, two retrospective, and only two were randomized. Evidence-based guidelines and meta-analyses are not possible due to population heterogeneity and study methodologies. Patients were opioid naïve or on weak opioids and in some studies patients were on potent opioids.[45] Routes, dosing schedules, and outcome parameters also differed. While there are no strong evidence-based recommendations some wisdom can be gleaned from these 12 studies. All reported methods and strategies were safe. Respiratory depression was not observed. Drop-out due to toxicity from opioid titration was rare but some patients developed nausea and mild sedation. Hallucinations, myoclonus, constipation, and hypotension were not observed during titration.

Traditional intravenous titration for acute or crescendo cancer pain

All six trials that studied intravenous titration for acute or crescendo cancer pain used a numerical rating scale. 'Responses' differed and ranged from 'initial onset of analgesia' to <5 out of 10 on a VNRS to complete pain relief.[40,45,49,51–53] Time to response ranged between 9.7 to 89 minutes and all were within 100 minutes (Tables 89.1 and 89.2).

Traditional titration leads to rapid pain relief within 2 hours and in several studies within minutes of starting titration. Responses occurred in over 80 percent. This is true both for opioid-tolerant and opioid-naïve patients. Assessment is done frequently, usually at several minute intervals. Close monitoring is necessary with traditional opioid titration.

For maintenance, the total titrated dose is the 4-hourly dose. The titrated dose can be converted to the oral morphine dose by using a 1:3 ratio (parenteral:oral). If patients require high doses of morphine the recommended ratio is 1:2.[40]

Table 89.1   *Intravenous titration for acute or crescendo cancer pain*

Study	Method	Pretrial opioid	Dose	Pain measure and response
Hagen et al.[51]	Prospective case series	Morphine	Morphine 10–20 mg/15 minutes Double the dose every 30 minutes if no response	VNRS; response: ≤5
Kumar et al.[53]	Retrospective case series	NSAIDs, 'weak' opioids	Morphine 1.5 mg/10 minutes	VNRS; response: complete relief
Harris et al.[52]	Prospective randomized trial	NSAIDs, 'weak' opioids	Morphine 1.5 mg/10 minutes	VNRS; response: complete relief
Mercadante et al.[40]	Prospective case series	NSAIDs, 'weak' potent opioids	Morphine 2 mg/2 minutes	VNRS; initial onset of significant analgesia
Soares et al.[49]	Prospective case series	Oral morphine	Fentanyl 10% of MEDD 95 minutes × 2 then 5% increase 95 minutes × 2	VNRS <4 on 0–10 scale
Davis et al.[45]	Retrospective case series	Morphine	Morphine 1 mg/min × 10 minute followed by 5-minute respite then repeat × 3	VNRS; response: pain relief

NSAID, nonsteroidal anti-inflammatory drug; VNRS, visual numeric rating scale; MEDD, mean equivalent daily dose.

Table 89.2   *Intravenous titration for acute pain*

Study	No. of patients	Response time
Hagen et al.[51]	9	89 minutes
Kumar et al.[53]	491	<100 minutes
Harris et al.[52]	62	<1 hour
Mercadante et al.[40]	49	9.7 minutes
Soares et al.[49]	18	11 minutes
Davis et al.[45]	3	20 minutes

Maintenance doses will also depend upon chronic opioid doses in opioid-tolerant patients.[54] Our group has used fentanyl 20 μg or hydromorphone 0.2 mg in substitution for morphine 1 mg in those who cannot take morphine.[54,55]

Patient-controlled analgesia in acute cancer pain

Patient-controlled analgesia has been used to improve relief from cancer pain, and in a small number of studies PCA has been used for relief of acute crescendo cancer pain. It has been stated that PCA improves the titration of opioids to pain relief and minimizes individual pharmacokinetic and pharmacodynamic differences. It reduces patient anxiety about delays in dosing and is said to foreshorten the slow onset to pain relief associated with continuous infusions. Overdose is minimized by small bolus doses and mandatory lockout intervals.[56–58]

A syringe driver, disposable plastic cylinder, or a battery operated computer-driven pump and multiple routes, intranasal, subcutaneous, intravenous, and spinal can be used for PCA.[57] However, regardless of technique, if the patient receives an adequate dose in a timely fashion, a good outcome will occur. The proposed success of PCA over conventional (traditional) methods is related to (i) the nurse to patient ratio, and (ii) the dedication of the nursing staff to pain control. The assessed response benefit of PCA may be missed if assessment is not related to the timing of the dose.[47] Assessment at 2–4-hour intervals or once daily (as occurs in most acute cancer pain trials) will miss the temporal benefits to PCA.[47] The risk of respiratory depression is small (ranges between 0.1 and 0.8 percent). Patient satisfaction, rather than pain relief with PCA is misleading as an outcome measure. Patients generally do not like to criticize those caring for them even if pain is suboptimally controlled. Expectations for pain relief by patients may be low and some pain relief may be better than anticipated.[47] Continuous infusion PCA with demand rescue dosing should be avoided in opioid-naïve patients.

Contraindications to PCA include: dementia or delirium, renal failure, dehydration, obesity, and obstructive sleep apnea.[47] A prescription for PCA requires (i) drug, (ii) bolus dose, (iii) background infusion (if applicable), (iv) lockout interval, and (v) maximum hourly or 4-hourly dose.[47] Patients cannot be expected to activate the demand device frequently to make up for inadequately small bolus doses to sustain pain relief.[47] However most importantly, PCA is essentially a maintenance therapy and pain should be under control prior to PCA.[47] PCA is not a 'one-size-fits-all' nor a 'set-and-forget' technology.[47] Patients need close observation and individualization. Appropriate doses based upon titration and short intervals make up for wide individual differences in opioid requirements. However, most PCA prescriptions are generally done without individualization, or differences in opioid physicochemical properties which influence effect delays, opioid clearance, opioid redistribution, and duration of pain relief.[47]

Table 89.3 *Patient-controlled analgesia in acute crescendo cancer pain*

Study	Method	Pretrial opioid	Dose	Pain measure and response
Radbruch et al.[42]	Prospective case series	Weak opioids	Morphine 1 mg/5-minute lockout interval	VNRS; response not defined; characterized by a decrease in VNRS at 24 hours
Zech and Lehmann[67]	Prospective case series	Morphine	Fentanyl 50 μg/5-minute lockout interval	VAS; response not defined but characterized by a decrease in VAS
Kornick et al.[50]	Prospective case series	Transdermal fentanyl	Fentanyl 100% of the transdermal fentanyl dose plus 50–100% of the hourly fentanyl dose lockout interval 15–20 minutes	VNRS; response not defined but characterized by a reduction in the VNRS score

VNRS, visual numerical rating scale; VAS, visual analog scale.

Table 89.4 *Acute pain management by patient-controlled analgesia for acute crescendo pain*

Study	No. of patients	Time to response
Radbruch et al.[42]	28	300 minutes (subset)
Zech and Lehmann[67]	20	24 hours (VAS from 68 to 34)
Kornick et al.[50]	9	Mild pain at rest 1.5 days
		Mild pain with movement 3 days

VAS, visual analog scale.

PCA AND ACUTE TRANSIENT PAIN

Transient procedural pain is frequently treated with PCA patterned after postoperative pain management and is most studied in mucositis associated with bone marrow transplantation. Interpreting PCA trials with mucositis induced by bone marrow transplantation is fraught with some difficulties.[59] Simply by participating in a trial, and assessment and management by the nursing staff, the control group will improve (Hawthorne effect).[60,61] The overall findings demonstrate that PCA has little advantage over conventional continuous opioid infusions in the treatment of painful mucositis.[61**,62**,63*,64**,65***] Morphine consumption is less with PCA than continuous morphine infusion, but is probably not a major measure of success. Patients develop rapid tolerance when alfentanil or sufentanil are used with PCA.[66**]

PCA MANAGEMENT OF CRESCENDO CANCER PAIN

There have been three trials on the management of acute crescendo pain (Tables 89.3 and 89.4).[42*,50,67*] These three studies illustrate the difficulty in evaluating the efficacy of PCA for crescendo pain. In all three studies assessments were done only once daily and unrelated to the dose. A small subset of patients were evaluated more frequently. All three used PCA without previous titration to pain control. Morphine and fentanyl were prescribed with the same demand interval despite differences in physicochemical properties.

Response to PCA appears to be slower than to traditional titration despite similar dosing intervals. This may be related to the need to frequently activate the device and the reluctance of the patient to activate the device until pain recurs. Many patients will lack a fundamental knowledge of PCA and require getting used to activating the device to effectively use PCA.

Oral opioid dose titration for acute crescendo pain

Oral titration studies have used morphine, except for one retrospective study which used oral transmucosal fentanyl citrate (Tables 89.5 and 89.6).[7*,45***,68**,69*] Morphine dosing intervals were at 12-hour intervals for sustained release and 4 or 2 hours for immediate release. Planned dose escalation depended upon pain relief at the time of the next dose or at 24-hour intervals. Oral transmucosal fentanyl citrate was prescribed at 30-minute intervals until pain relief.

The European Association of Palliative Care (EAPC) working group has recommended daily assessments during oral titration due to steady state concentrations of oral morphine (4–5 half-lives with a 4-hour single dose half-life). During titration the 4-hourly dose is used every 1–2 hours based upon consensus recommendation.[70] The only evidence for short oral titration intervals is a 2-hour interval in Lichter's study.[41*] The recommendation by the EAPC is the same dose hourly whereas Lichter used planned dose increments based upon hourly or every 2-hourly assessments.[41*] The 'titration' strategies of the EAPC appear to be based upon breakthrough pain whereas strategies in the Lichter study were based upon acute uncontrolled pain.[44*] This author has given fixed doses of morphine at 15–30-minute intervals until pain control in home hospice patients with severe crescendo with success (and with a hospice nurse in the home). At the present time there is little to guide us on the particular safe and effective oral dosing strategies (whether fixed doses at frequent intervals or dose escalation at fixed intervals).

Table 89.5 *Oral opioid titration for crescendo cancer pain*

Study	Method	Pretrial opioid	Dose	Pain assessment and response
Klepstad et al.[68]	Randomized controlled, double blind trial	Codeine and dextropropoxyphene	IR morphine or SR morphine at 4 or 24-hour intervals starting with 60 mg titrating to 90, 120, 180, 240, 360 mg depending upon response daily	VAS and VRS; response was less than 3 on a VRS (1–7)
Klepstad et al.[69]	Prospective case series	Codeine and dextropropoxyphene	IR morphine 10 mg every 4 hours × 6 increase by 33–50% every 24 hours	VAS and VRS; response was less than 3 on a VRS (1–7)
Lichter[41]	Prospective case series	Weak or potent nonmorphine opioid	IR morphine every 4-hour intervals starting with 5 mg and titrating to 10, 15, 20, 30, 40, 60, 80, 120, 160, 200 mg at 4-hour intervals or 2-hour intervals	Qualitative descriptor
Burton et al.[7]	Retrospective	Morphine	Fentanyl 200–600 μg every 30 minutes	VNRS

VAS, visual analog scale; VRS, verbal rating scale; VNRS, visual numerical rating scale; IR, immediate release; SR, sustained release.

Table 89.6 *Oral opioid titration for acute crescendo cancer pain*

Study	No. of patients	Time to response
Klepstad et al.[68]	120	2.1 days (SR) 1.7 days (IR)
Klepstad et al.[69]	40	2.3 days
Lichter[41]	50	1 day (every 4 hours) 6 hours (every 2 hours)
Burton et al.[7]	39	<30 minutes in 35 patients

IR, immediate release; SR, sustained release.

- Assessment of the underlying cause is not impeded by effective opioid titration.

- Further studies are needed to develop guidelines for the management of acute crescendo cancer pain.

ACKNOWLEDGMENTS

The author would like to acknowledge Becky Phillips for her skills in preparing the manuscript and Deborah Davis for her editorial skills.

Key learning points

- Transient pain in patients with cancer occurs due to investigational procedures, interventions, or complications from treatment and cancer.

- Opioid dosing strategies on an as needed basis or by PCA are reasonable for procedure-related pain.

- Acute unstable and crescendo pain is managed by opioid titration followed by maintenance opioid dosing for quick pain relief.

- Titration consists of either small frequent doses to analgesia or planned dose escalation at fixed intervals.

- Response is assessed at short intervals (minutes to hourly).

- The effective titrated dose at which pain relief occurs provides the basis for maintenance doses.

- The pre-titration opioid dose in the opioid-tolerant patient needs to be added to maintenance doses.

- Rapid opioid titration is safe in those monitored closely.

REFERENCES

1 Twycross R. Cancer pain classification. *Acta Anaesthesiol Scand* 1997; **41**(1 Pt 2): 141–5.

2 Du Pen SL, Du Pen AR, Polissar N, *et al.* Implementing guidelines for cancer pain management: results of a randomized controlled clinical trial. *J Clin Oncol* 1999; **17**: 361–70.

◆ 3 Upton RN, Semple TJ, Macintyre PE. Pharmacokinetic optimisation of opioid treatment in acute pain therapy. *Clin Pharmacokinet* 1997; **33**: 225–44.

4 Ripamonti C, Zecca E, De Conno F. Pharmacological treatment of cancer pain: alternative routes of opioid administration. *Tumori* 1998; **84**: 289–300.

5 Manfredi PL, Chandler S, Pigazzi A, Payne R. Outcome of cancer pain consultations. *Cancer* 2000; **89**: 920–4.

6 Chandler S, Payne R. Economics of unrelieved cancer pain. *Am J Hosp Palliat Care* 1998; **15**: 223–6.

● 7 Burton AW, Driver LC, Mendoza TR, Syed G. Oral transmucosal fentanyl citrate in the outpatient management of severe cancer pain crises: a retrospective case series. *Clin J Pain* 2004; **20**: 195–7.

◆ 8 Portenoy RK, Lesage P. Management of cancer pain. *Lancet* 1999; **353**: 1695–700.

9   Gutgsell T, Walsh D, Zhukovsky DS, *et al.* A prospective study of the pathophysiology and clinical characteristics of pain in a palliative medicine population. *Am J Hosp Palliat Care* 2003; **20**: 140–8.

◆ 10 Portenoy RK. Cancer pain: pathophysiology and syndromes. *Lancet* 1992; **339**: 1026–31.

11 Caraceni A, Portenoy RK. An international survey of cancer pain characteristics and syndromes. IASP Task Force on Cancer Pain. International Association for the Study of Pain. *Pain* 1999; **82**: 263–74.

12 Gordin V, Weaver MA, Hahn MB. Acute and chronic pain management in palliative care. *Best Pract Res Clin Obstet Gynaecol* 2001; **15**: 203–34.

13 Zekry HA, Bruera E. Regional pain syndromes in cancer patients. *Curr Rev Pain* 2000; **4**: 179–86.

14 De Conno F, Caraceni A, Gamba A, Mariani L, Abbattista A, Brunelli C, *et al.* Pain measurement in cancer patients: a comparison of six methods. *Pain* 1994; **57**: 161–6.

15 Moore A, Edwards J, Barden J, McQuay H. *Bandolier's Little Book of Pain.* Oxford: Oxford University Press, 2003.

16 Gallagher EJ, Bijur PE, Latimer C, Silver W. Reliability and validity of a visual analog scale for acute abdominal pain in the ED. *Am J Emerg Med* 2002; **20**: 287–90.

17 Myles PS, Troedel S, Boquest M, Reeves M. The pain visual analog scale: is it linear or nonlinear? *Anesth Analg* 1999; **89**: 1517–20.

18 Kelly AM. The minimum clinically significant difference in visual analogue scale pain score does not differ with severity of pain. *Emerg Med J* 2001; **18**: 205–7.

19 Farrar JT, Berlin JA, Strom BL. Clinically important changes in acute pain outcome measures: a validation study. *J Pain Symptom Manage* 2003; **25**: 406–11.

20 Farrar JT, Portenoy RK, Berlin JA, Kinman JL, Strom BL. Defining the clinically important difference in pain outcome measures. *Pain* 2000; **88**: 287–94.

21 Cepeda MS, Africano JM, Polo R, Alcala R, Carr DB. What decline in pain intensity is meaningful to patients with acute pain? *Pain* 2003; **105**: 151–7.

22 Aubrun F, Langeron O, Quesnel C, *et al.* Relationships between measurement of pain using visual analog score and morphine requirements during postoperative intravenous morphine titration. *Anesthesiology* 2003; **98**: 1415–21.

23 Bird SB, Dickson EW. Clinically significant changes in pain along the visual analog scale. *Ann Emerg Med* 2001; **38**: 639–43.

24 Li SF, Greenwald PW, Gennis P, *et al.* Effect of age on acute pain perception of a standardized stimulus in the emergency department. *Ann Emerg Med* 2001; **38**: 644–7.

25 Holdgate A, Asha S, Craig J, Thompson J. Comparison of a verbal numeric rating scale with the visual analogue scale for the measurement of acute pain. *Emerg Med (Fremantle)* 2003; **15**: 441–6.

26 Mamie C, Morabia A, Bernstein M, Klopfenstein CE, Forster A. Treatment efficacy is not an index of pain intensity. *Can J Anaesth* 2000; **47**: 1166–70.

27 Blumstein HA, Moore D. Visual analog pain scores do not define desire for analgesia in patients with acute pain. *Acad Emerg Med* 2003; **10**: 211–14.

28 Rapp SE, Wild LM, Egan KJ, Ready LB. Acute pain management of the chronic pain patient on opiates: a survey of caregivers at University of Washington Medical Center. *Clin J Pain* 1994; **10**: 133–8.

29 Thomas SH, Silen W. Effect on diagnostic efficiency of analgesia for undifferentiated abdominal pain. *Br J Surg* 2003; **90**: 5–9.

30 American Pain Society. *Principles of Analgesic Use in the Treatment of Acute Pain and Cancer Pain,* 3rd ed. Skokie, IL: American Pain Society, 1992.

31 Thomas SH, Borczuk P, Shackelford J, *et al.* Patient and physician agreement on abdominal pain severity and need for opioid analgesia. *Am J Emerg Med* 1999; **17**: 586–90.

32 Luger TJ, Lederer W, Gassner M, *et al.* Acute pain is underassessed in out-of-hospital emergencies. *Acad Emerg Med* 2003; **10**: 627–32.

33 Klopfenstein CE, Herrmann FR, Mamie C, *et al.* Pain intensity and pain relief after surgery. A comparison between patients' reported assessments and nurses' and physicians' observations. *Acta Anaesthesiol Scand* 2000; **44**: 58–62.

34 Ferrante FM. Principles of opioid pharmacotherapy: practical implications of basic mechanisms. *J Pain Symptom Manage* 1996; **11**: 265–73.

◆ 35 Macintyre PE. Intravenous patient-controlled analgesia: one size does not fit all. *Anesthesiol Clin North Am* 2005; **23**: 109–23.

36 Cepeda MS, Carr DB. Women experience more pain and require more morphine than men to achieve a similar degree of analgesia. *Anesth Analg* 2003; **97**: 1464–8.

37 Green CR, Wheeler JR, LaPorte F. Clinical decision making in pain management: Contributions of physician and patient characteristics to variations in practice. *J Pain* 2003; **4**: 29–39.

◆ 38 Bernards CM. Clinical implications of physiochemical properties of opioids. In: Stein C, ed. *Opioids in Pain Control: Basic and Clinical Aspects.* Cambridge: Cambridge University Press, 1999: 166–87.

39 Birkett DJ. *Pharmacokinetics Made Easy.* North Ryde, NSW: McGraw-Hill Australia, 2002.

● 40 Mercadante S, Villari P, Ferrera P, *et al.* Rapid titration with intravenous morphine for severe cancer pain and immediate oral conversion. *Cancer* 2002; **95**: 203–8.

● 41 Lichter I. Accelerated titration of morphine for rapid relief of cancer pain. *N Z Med J* 1994; **107**: 488–90.

● 42 Radbruch L, Loick G, Schulzeck S, *et al.* Intravenous titration with morphine for severe cancer pain: report of 28 cases. *Clin J Pain* 1999; **15**: 173–8.

43 Benedetti C, Brock C, Cleeland C, *et al.* NCCN Practice Guidelines for Cancer Pain. *Oncology (Huntingt)* 2000; **14**(11A): 135–50.

44 Rostaing-Rigattieri S, Rousselot H, Krakowski I, *et al.* Standards, Options et Recommandations 2002 pour les traitements antalgiques medicamenteux des douleurs cancereuses par exces de nociception chez l'adulte, mise a jour: place des opioides forts (morphine orale exclue) et rotation des opioides. *Bull Cancer* 2003; **90**: 795–806.

◆ 45 Davis MP, Weissman DE, Arnold RM. Opioid dose titration for severe cancer pain: a systematic evidence-based review. *J Palliat Med* 2004; **7**: 462–8.

◆ 46 Krakowski I, Theobald S, Balp L, *et al.* Summary version of the Standards, Options and Recommendations for the use of analgesia for the treatment of nociceptive pain in adults with cancer (update 2002). *Br J Cancer* 2003; **89**(Suppl 1): S67–S72.

◆ 47 Macintyre PE. Safety and efficacy of patient-controlled analgesia. *Br J Anaesth* 2001; **87**: 36–46.

◆ 48 Etches RC. Patient-controlled analgesia. *Surg Clin North Am* 1999; **79**: 297–312.

● 49 Soares LGL, Martins M, Uchoa R. Intravenous fentanyl for cancer pain: a 'fast titration' protocol for the emergency room. *J Pain Symptom Manage* 2003; **26**: 876–81.

● 50 Kornick CA, Santiago-Palma J, Schulman G, *et al.* A safe and effective method for converting patients from transdermal to intravenous fentanyl for the treatment of acute cancer-related pain. *Cancer* 2003; **97**: 3121–4.

● 51 Hagen NA, Elwood T, Ernst S. Cancer pain emergencies: a protocol for management. *J Pain Symptom Manage* 1997; **14**: 45–50.

● 52 Harris JT, Suresh Kumar K, Rajagopal MR. Intravenous morphine for rapid control of severe cancer pain. *Palliat Med* 2003; **17**: 248–56.

53 Kumar KS, Rajagopal MR, Naseema AM. Intravenous morphine for emergency treatment of cancer pain. *Palliat Med* 2000; **14**: 183–8.

● 54 Davis MP. Acute pain in advanced cancer: an opioid dosing strategy and illustration. *Am J Hosp Palliat Care* 2004; **21**: 47–50.

◆ 55 Walsh D. Pharmacological management of cancer pain. *Semin Oncol* 2000; **27**: 45–63.

● 56 White PF. Use of patient-controlled analgesia for management of acute pain. *JAMA* 1988; **259**: 243–7.

57 Kendall JM, Reeves BC, Latter VS. Multicentre randomised controlled trial of nasal diamorphine for analgesia in children and teenagers with clinical fractures. *BMJ* 2001; **322**: 261–5.

58 Semple D, Aldridge LA, Doyle E. Comparison of i.v. and s.c. diamorphine infusions for the treatment of acute pain in children. *Br J Anaesth* 1996; **76**: 310–12.

59 McGuire DB, Altomonte V, Peterson DE, *et al.* Patterns of mucositis and pain in patients receiving preparative chemotherapy and bone marrow transplantation. *Oncol Nurs Forum* 1993; **20**: 1493–502.

60 Chapman CR, Donaldson GW, Jacobson RC, Hautman B. Differences among patients in opioid self-administration during bone marrow transplantation. *Pain* 1997; **71**: 213–23.

● 61 Zucker TP, Flesche CW, Germing U, *et al.* Patient-controlled versus staff-controlled analgesia with pethidine after allogeneic bone marrow transplantation. *Pain* 1998; **75**: 305–12.

● 62 Pillitteri LC, Clark RE. Comparison of a patient-controlled analgesia system with continuous infusion for administration of diamorphine for mucositis. *Bone Marrow Transplant* 1998; **22**: 495–8.

● 63 Mackie AM, Coda BC, Hill HF. Adolescents use patient-controlled analgesia effectively for relief from prolonged oropharyngeal mucositis pain. *Pain* 1991; **46**: 265–9.

● 64 Hill HF, Chapman CR, Kornell JA, *et al.* Self-administration of morphine in bone marrow transplant patients reduces drug requirement. *Pain* 1990; **40**: 121–9.

◆ 65 Worthington HV, Clarkson JE, Eden OB. Interventions for treating oral mucositis for patients with cancer receiving treatment. *Cochrane Database Syst Rev* 2004: CD001973.

66 Hill HF, Coda BA, Mackie AM, Iverson K. Patient-controlled analgesic infusions: alfentanil versus morphine. *Pain* 1992; **49**: 301–10.

67 Zech DF, Lehmann KA. Transdermal fentanyl in combination with initial intravenous dose titration by patient-controlled analgesia. *Anticancer Drugs* 1995; **6**(Suppl 3): 44–9.

● 68 Klepstad P, Kaasa S, Jystad A, *et al.* Immediate- or sustained-release morphine for dose finding during start of morphine to cancer patients: a randomized, double-blind trial. *Pain* 2003; **101**: 193–8.

● 69 Klepstad P, Kaasa S, Skauge M, Borchgrevink PC. Pain intensity and side effects during titration of morphine to cancer patients using a fixed schedule dose escalation. *Acta Anaesthesiol Scand* 2000; **44**: 656–64.

◆ 70 Hanks GW, Conno F, Cherny N, *et al.* Morphine and alternative opioids in cancer pain: the EAPC recommendations. *Br J Cancer* 2001; **84**: 587–93.

90

Suicide

WILLIAM BREITBART, CHRISTOPHER GIBSON, JENNIFER ABBEY, NICOLE IANNARONE, RONI BORENSTEIN

INTRODUCTION

Suicide is a tragic, but often preventable response, to the emotional challenges of terminal physical illness. Whitlock[1***] points out that when we consider the stressors that an individual must face in confronting such illnesses we might expect suicide to be a more common reaction, while in reality it is relatively uncommon. Such a realization may indicate that suicide in the terminally ill is a pathologic, and thus potentially treatable, coping response. The purpose of this chapter is to examine the prevalence of suicide in this population, factors that contribute to it, and potential interventions both to prevent it as well as to deal with the trauma that completed suicides have on family and significant others.

SUICIDAL IDEATION IN THE TERMINALLY ILL

Thoughts of suicide probably occur quite frequently, particularly in the setting of advanced physical disease, and may serve as a 'steam valve' for ideations often expressed by patients as 'no matter how bad things become, I always have a way out'. However, published reports have suggested that suicidal ideation is relatively infrequent in illnesses such as cancer and is limited to those who are significantly depressed. Silberfarb et al.[2**] found that only 3 of 146 patients with breast cancer had suicidal thoughts, while none of the 100 cancer patients interviewed in a Finnish study expressed suicidal thoughts.[3] A study conducted at St Boniface Hospice in Winnipeg, Canada, demonstrated that only 10 of 44 terminally ill cancer patients were suicidal or

desired an early death, and all 10 were suffering from clinical depression.[4]

At Memorial Sloan–Kettering Cancer Center (MSKCC), suicide risk evaluation accounted for 8.6 percent of psychiatric consultations, usually requested by staff in response to a patient verbalizing suicidal wishes.[5] Among 185 cancer patients with pain studied at MSKCC, suicidal ideation was found in 17 percent of the study population.[5] It should be noted that the actual prevalence of suicidal ideation may be considerably higher than these figures suggest, in that patients often disclose these thoughts only after a stable, ongoing physician–patient relationship has been established. It has been our experience that once patients develop such a trusting and safe relationship, they almost universally reveal occasional persistent thoughts of suicide as a means of escaping the threat of being overwhelmed by their illness.

SUICIDE AND TERMINAL ILLNESS

Patients suffering from terminal illnesses, such as cancer and acquired immune deficiency syndrome (AIDS), are at increased risk of suicide relative to the general population, particularly in the terminal stage of illness. Unfortunately, the frequency of suicide attempts in illnesses such as cancer has not been well studied. However, a recent study by Hem and colleagues examining data from the Cancer Registry of Norway is a step forward in this area.[6*] This study revealed standardized mortality ratios (SMRs) of 1.55 for males and 1.35 for females. In addition, risk was found to be greatest in the first months following diagnosis and was significantly increased in male patients with respiratory cancers. While the overall frequency of suicidal thinking in the cancer setting may be in question, its relationship to suicide attempts or completions is clearer. Bolund[7*] reports that fully half of all Swedish cancer suicides had previously conveyed suicidal thoughts or plans to their relatives. In addition, many of the completed cancer suicides had been preceded by an attempted suicide. This is consistent with the statistics of suicide in general, which show that a previous suicide attempt greatly increases the risk of completed suicide.[8*,9,10] A family history of suicide is of increasing relevance in assessing suicide risk.

Factors associated with increased risk of suicide in patients with advanced physical disease[5,11***] are listed in Box 90.1. Patients with advanced illness are at highest risk, perhaps because they are most likely to have such complications as pain, depression, delirium, and deficit symptoms. Psychiatric disorders are frequently present in hospitalized patients who are suicidal. For example, a review of consultation data from the psychiatry service at MSKCC revealed that one-third of suicidal cancer patients had a major depression, about 20 percent suffered from a delirium, and 50 percent were diagnosed as having an adjustment disorder with both anxious and depressed features at the time of evaluation.[5,11***]

Box 90.1   Factors associated with increased risk of suicide in patients with advanced physical disease

- Pain – aspects of suffering
- Advanced illness – poor prognosis
- Depression – hopelessness
- Delirium – disinhibition
- Control – helplessness
- Preexisting psychopathology
- Substance/alcohol abuse
- Suicide history – family history
- Fatigue – exhaustion
- Lack of social support – social isolation

Physically ill patients commit suicide most frequently in the advanced stages of disease.[7*,12*,13*,14] Eighty-six percent of suicides studied by Farberow et al.[15**] occurred in the preterminal or terminal stages of illness, despite greatly reduced physical capacity. Poor prognosis and advanced illness usually go hand in hand. It is thus not surprising that in Sweden, those who were expected to die within a matter of months were the most likely to commit suicide. Of 88 cancer suicides, 14 had an uncertain prognosis, and 45 had a poor prognosis.[16**] With advancing disease, the incidence of significant cancer pain increases. Uncontrolled pain in cancer patients is a dramatically important risk factor for suicide. The vast majority of cancer suicides in several studies showed that these patients had severe pain which was often inadequately controlled and poorly tolerated.[7*,17*]

Depression is a factor in 50 percent of all suicides. Those suffering from depression are at 25 times greater risk of suicide than the general population.[18*,19] The role depression plays in suicides among the seriously medically ill is equally significant. Approximately 25 percent of all patients with cancer experience severe depressive symptoms, with about 6 percent fulfilling the Diagnostic and Statistical Manual (DSM)-III criteria for the diagnosis of major depression.[20,21] Among those with advanced illness and progressively impaired physical function, symptoms of severe depression rise to 77 percent.[22***] Depression also appears to be important in terms of patient preferences for life-sustaining medical therapy. Ganzini and colleagues reported that among older depressed patients, an increase in desire for life-sustaining medical therapies followed treatment of depression in those subjects who had been initially more severely depressed, more hopeless, and more likely to overestimate the risks and to underestimate the benefits of treatment.[23*] They concluded that whereas patients with mild to moderate depression are unlikely to alter their decisions regarding life-sustaining medical treatment in spite of treatment for their depression, severely depressed patients – particularly those who are hopeless – should be encouraged to defer advance treatment directives. In these patients, decisions about life-sustaining therapy should be discouraged until after treatment of their depression.

Hopelessness is the key variable that links depression and suicide in the general population. Further, hopelessness is a significantly better predictor of completed suicide than is depression alone.[24] In a recent study[25] Chochinov and colleagues demonstrated that hopelessness was correlated more highly with suicidal ideation in terminally ill patients than was the level of depression. With the typical cancer suicide being characterized by advanced illness and poor prognosis, hopelessness is commonly experienced. In Scandinavia, the highest incidence of suicide was found in cancer patients who were offered no further treatment, and no further contact with the healthcare system.[7*,14] Being left to face illness alone creates a sense of isolation and abandonment that is critical to the development of hopelessness. The prevalence of organic mental disorders among seriously medically ill patients requiring psychiatric consultation has been found to range from 25 percent to 40 percent[26*,27*] and as high as 85 percent during the terminal stages of illness.[28] Although earlier work suggested that delirium was a protective factor in regard to suicide,[12*] clinical experience has found these confusional states to be a major contributing factor in impulsive suicide attempts, especially in the hospital setting.

Loss of control and a sense of helplessness in the face of one's illness are important factors in suicide vulnerability. Control refers to both the helplessness induced by symptoms or deficits due to the illness or its treatments, as well as the excessive need on the part of some patients to be in control of all aspects of living or dying. Farberow noted that patients who were accepting and adaptable were much less likely to commit suicide than patients who exhibited a need to be in control of even the most minute details of their care.[15**] This need to control may be prominent in some patients and cause distress with little provocation. However, it is not uncommon for illness-related events to induce a great sense of helplessness even in those who are not typically controlling individuals. Impairments or deficits induced by the patient's illness or its treatments often include loss of mobility, paraplegia, loss of bowel and bladder function, amputation, aphonia, sensory loss, and inability to eat or swallow. Most distressing to patients is the sense that they are losing control of their minds, especially when they are confused or sedated by medications. The risk of suicide is increased in patients with such physical impairments, especially when accompanied by psychological distress and disturbed interpersonal relationships due to these deficit factors.[17*]

Fatigue, in the form of emotional, spiritual, financial, familial, communal, and other resource exhaustion increases risk of suicide in the seriously physically ill patient.[5] Due to advancements in treatment, illnesses such as cancer now often follow more of a chronic course. Increased survival is accompanied by increased number of hospitalizations, complications, and expenses. Symptom control thus becomes a prolonged process with frequent advances and setbacks. The dying process also can become extremely long and arduous for all concerned. It is not uncommon for both family members and healthcare providers to withdraw prematurely from the patient under these circumstances. A suicidal patient can thus feel even more isolated and abandoned. The presence of a strong support system for the patient that may act as an external control of suicidal behavior reduces the risk of suicide significantly.

Holland[29***] advises that it is extremely rare for a cancer patient to commit suicide without some degree of premorbid psychopathology that places them at increased risk. Farberow et al.[12*] described a large group of cancer suicides as the 'dependent dissatisfied'. These patients were immature, demanding, complaining, irritable, hostile, and difficult to manage on the ward. Staff often felt manipulated by these patients and became irritable due to what they saw as excessive demands for attention. Suicide attempts or threats were often seen as 'hysterical' or manipulative. Consultation data from MSKCC on suicidal cancer patients showed that half had a diagnosable personality disorder.[30]

ASSESSMENT AND MANAGEMENT OF THE SUICIDAL PATIENT

Assessment of suicide risk and appropriate intervention are critical. Early and comprehensive psychiatric involvement with high-risk individuals can often avert suicide in the cancer setting.[31**] A careful evaluation includes a search for the meaning of suicidal thoughts, as well as an exploration of the seriousness of the risk. The clinician's ability to establish rapport and elicit a patient's thoughts is essential as he or she assesses history, degree of intent, and quality of internal and external controls. The clinician should listen sympathetically, not appearing critical or stating that such thoughts are inappropriate. This is critical, in that allowing the patient to discuss suicidal thoughts often decreases the risk of suicide. The myth that asking about suicidal thoughts 'puts the idea in their head', is one that should be dispelled.[32***] Patients often reconsider and reject the idea of suicide when the physician acknowledges the legitimacy of their option and the need to retain a sense of control over aspects of their death.

The suicide vulnerability factors presented in Box 90.1 should be used as a guide to evaluation and management. Once the setting has been made secure, assessment of the relevant mental status and adequacy of pain control can begin. Analgesics, neuroleptics, or antidepressant drugs should be used when appropriate to treat agitation, psychosis, major depression, or pain. Underlying causes of delirium or pain should be addressed specifically when possible. Initiation of a crisis-intervention–oriented psychotherapeutic approach, mobilizing as much of the patient's support system as possible is important. A close family member or friend should be involved in order to support the patient, provide information, and assist in treatment planning. Psychiatric hospitalization can sometimes be helpful but is usually not desirable in the terminally ill patient. Thus, the medical hospital or home is the setting in which management most often takes place. Whereas it is appropriate to intervene when medical or psychiatric factors are clearly the driving force in a cancer suicide, there are circumstances when usurping control from the patient and family with overly aggressive intervention may be less helpful. This is most evident in those with advanced illness where comfort and symptom control are the primary concerns.

Ultimately the palliative care clinician may not be able to prevent all suicides in all terminally ill patients that he or she cares for. The emphasis of intervention should be to aggressively attempt to prevent suicide that is driven by the desperation of uncontrolled physical and psychological symptoms such as uncontrolled pain, unrecognized delirium, and unrecognized and untreated depression. Prolonged suffering caused by poorly controlled symptoms may lead to such desperation, and it is the appropriate role of the palliative care team to provide effective management of physical and psychological symptoms as an alternative to desire for death, suicides, or requests for assisted suicide by their patients.

REQUESTS FOR ASSISTED SUICIDE

A growing body of literature has emerged on the type of physical and psychological concerns that may give rise to a desire for hastened death and request for assisted suicide. Even if relatively little empirical research has addressed this issue, especially with medically ill patients, some authors found rates of support for legalization of assisted suicide that were roughly comparable to those published in studies on the general population. In Breitbart *et al.*'s survey study 64 percent of AIDS patients supported legalization of assisted suicide.[33*] In another study 55 percent of terminally ill AIDS patients indicated a possible interest in assisted suicide. In a 1996 study of oncology patients, 25 percent reported that they had thought seriously about euthanasia and 12 percent had discussed this option with their physicians.[34*] A number of social variables, such as fear of becoming a burden to family and friends and experience with the death of a friend or family, have been significant predictors of interest in assisted suicide among ambulatory patients with AIDS.[33*] This joins a growing evidence of research demonstrating an important relation between social support and desire for death, when no relation was found with pain, physical symptoms, or stage of disease.[32***]

DESIRE FOR HASTENED DEATH

Desire for hastened death may be thought of as a unifying construct underlying requests for assisted suicide or euthanasia, as well as suicidal thoughts in general. Literature has emerged on the type of physical and psychological concerns that may give rise to a desire for hastened death. Several studies have demonstrated that depression plays a significant role in the terminally ill patient's desire for hastened death. The precise intensity of this association between depression and desire for hastened death is still being investigated. Chochinov *et al.* found that of 200 terminally ill patients in a palliative care facility, 44.5 percent acknowledged at least a fleeting desire to die – these episodes were brief and did not reflect a sustained or committed desire to die.[35**] However, 17 patients (8.5 percent) reported an unequivocal desire for death to come soon and indicated that they held this desire consistently over time. Among this group, 10 (58.8 percent) received a diagnosis of depression, compared to a prevalence of 7.7 percent in patients who did not endorse a genuine, consistent desire for death. Patients with depression were approximately six to seven times more likely to have a desire for hastened death than patients without depression. Patients with a desire for death were also found to have significantly more pain and less social support than those patients without a desire for death. Breitbart *et al.*[36**] recently studied the relationships between depression, hopelessness, and desire for death in a sample of 92 terminally ill cancer patients. Sixteen patients (17 percent) were

classified as having a high desire for death, based on their scores on a validated self-report measure of desire for hastened death called the Schedule of Attitudes Toward Hastened Death,[37**,38**] and 16 percent met criteria for a current major depressive episode. Of the patients who met criteria for major depressive episode, 7 (47 percent) were classified as having a high desire for hastened death while only 12 percent without a desire for death met criteria for depression. Thus, patients with a major depression were four times more likely to have a high desire for hastened death. In addition, Breitbart and colleagues found that both depression and hopelessness, characterized as a pessimistic cognitive style rather than an assessment of one's poor prognosis, appear to be unique and synergistic determinants of desire for hastened death.[39***] No significant association with the presence or the intensity of pain was found. Desire for hastened death also appears to be primarily a function of psychological distress and social factors such as social support, spiritual wellbeing, quality of life, and perception of oneself as a burden to others. Recent data suggest that among dying patients 'will to live', as measured with a visual analog scale, tends to fluctuate rapidly over time and is correlated with anxiety, depression and shortness of breath as death approaches.[40]

INTERVENTIONS FOR DESPAIR AT THE END OF LIFE

The response of a clinician to despair at the end of life as manifest by a patient's expression of desire for death or request for assisted suicide has important and obvious implications on all aspects of care which impact on patients, family, and staff.[41***] These issues must be addressed both rapidly and thoughtfully, offering the patient a nonjudgmental willingness to engage in a discussion of the factors that contribute to the suffering and despondency that leads patients to express such a desire for death. Some investigators speak of this suffering in using such terms as 'spiritual' suffering, 'demoralization', loss of 'dignity', 'loss of meaning',[42***,43,44,45*,46] and have developed interventions based on these concepts/themes.

Palliative care practitioners have begun to deal with the issue of spirituality in the dying and interventions for spiritual suffering. Rousseau[43] outlines an approach for the treatment of spiritual suffering composed of the following steps

1. controlling physical symptoms
2. providing a supportive presence
3. encouraging life review to assist in recognizing purpose, value, and meaning
4. exploring guilt, remorse, forgiveness, reconciliation
5. facilitating religious expression
6. reframing goals
7. encourage meditative practices, focus on healing rather than cure.

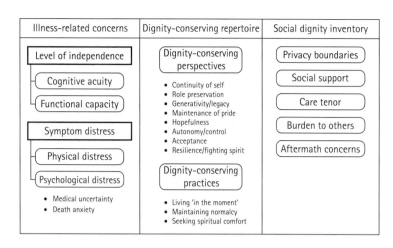

Figure 90.1 *Major dignity categories, themes and sub-themes. Adapted from Chochinov et al.[45]*

Rousseau has presented an approach to spiritual suffering, which is an interesting blend of basic psychotherapeutic principles. Psychotherapeutic techniques that are particularly adaptive to psychotherapy with the dying such as life narrative and life review are also included. There is an emphasis on facilitating religious expression and confession that in fact may be extremely useful to many patients, but is not applicable to all patients and not necessarily an intervention that many clinicians feel comfortable providing. What Rousseau's work suggests is that novel psychotherapeutic interventions aimed at improving spiritual wellbeing, sense of meaning and diminishing hopelessness, demoralization, and distress, are critically necessary to develop at this stage in the development of palliative medicine.

Kissane and colleagues[44] have described a syndrome of 'demoralization' in the terminally ill which they propose is distinct from depression, and consists of a triad of hopelessness, loss of meaning, and existential distress expressed as a desire for death. It is associated with life-threatening medical illness, disability, bodily disfigurement, fear, loss of dignity, social isolation, and feelings of being a burden. Because of the sense of impotence and hopelessness, those with the syndrome predictably progress to a desire to die or commit suicide. Kissane and his group describe a treatment approach for demoralization syndrome.[44] This approach emphasizes a multidisciplinary, multimodal approach consisting of:

- ensuring continuity of care and active symptom management
- ensuring dignity in the dying process
- utilizing various types of psychotherapy to help sustain a sense of meaning, limit cognitive distortions and maintain family relationships (i.e. meaning-based, cognitive–behavioral, interpersonal, and family psychotherapy interventions
- using life review and narrative, and attention to spiritual issues
- using pharmacotherapy for comorbid anxiety, depression, delirium.

Ensuring 'dignity' in the dying process is a critical goal of palliative care. Despite use of the term 'dignity' in arguments for and against a patient's self-governance in matters pertaining to death, there is little empirical research on how this term has been used by patients who are nearing death. Chochinov et al.[45*] examined how dying patients understand and define the term 'dignity', in order to develop a model of dignity in the terminally ill (see Fig. 90.1). A semi-structured interview was designed to explore how patients cope with their advanced cancer and to detail their perceptions of dignity. Three major categories emerged from a detailed qualitative analysis, including illness-related concerns (concerns that derive from or are related to the illness itself, and threaten to or actually do impinge on the patient's sense of dignity); dignity-conserving repertoire (internally held qualities or personal approaches or techniques that patients use to bolster or maintain their sense of dignity); and social dignity inventory (social concerns or relationship dynamics that enhance or detract from a patient's sense of dignity). These broad categories and their carefully defined themes and sub-themes form the foundation for an emerging model of dignity amongst the dying. The concept of dignity and the notion of dignity-conserving care offer a way of understanding how patients face advancing terminal illness, and presents an approach that clinicians can use to explicitly target the maintenance of dignity as a therapeutic objective and principle of bedside care for patients nearing death. Chochinov, in fact, describes his technique of 'dignity-conserving care' in a recent review[47] which interested readers can read for further details (see also Chapter 13).

Interventions for hopelessness and loss of meaning and purpose in the terminally ill are of particular importance when addressing the issues of desire for death and despair at the end of life. Breitbart and colleagues[42***,46] have developed an intervention they term 'meaning-centered' group psychotherapy for advanced cancer patients; an intervention based on the concepts and principles of Viktor Frankl's writings and logotherapy. The intervention is designed to help patients with advanced cancer sustain or enhance a sense of meaning, peace and purpose in their lives even as they approach the end of life. Meaning-centered group psychotherapy is a manualized, 8-week (one and a half hour weekly sessions) intervention which uses a mixture of didactics, discussion, and experiential exercises that focus around particular themes related to meaning and advanced cancer. The session themes include:

Session 1 – Concepts of meaning and sources of meaning
Session 2 – Cancer and meaning
Session 3 – Meaning and historical context of life
Session 4 – Storytelling, life project
Session 5 – Limitations and finiteness of life
Session 6 – Responsibility, creativity, deeds
Session 7 – Experience, nature, art, humor
Session 8 – Termination, goodbyes, hopes for the future

Patients are assigned readings and homework that are specific to each session's theme and which are utilized in each session. While the focus of each session is on issues of meaning/peace and purpose in life in the face of advanced cancer and a limited prognosis, elements of support and expression of emotion are inevitable in the context of each group session (but limited by the focus on experiential exercises, didactics and discussions related to themes focusing on meaning). Currently this intervention is undergoing a randomized controlled trial for efficacy.

Most palliative care clinicians believe that aggressive management of physical and psychological symptoms and syndromes that have been demonstrated to contribute to desire for death will naturally prevent such expressions of distress or requests for assisted suicide. For instance, there is a general consensus that individuals with major depression can be effectively treated in the context of terminal illness. No research has yet addressed if such treatment for depression directly influences desire for hastened death. There are currently two large trials in cancer and AIDS populations examining this specific question.[36**] Because depression and hopelessness are not identical constructs (although highly correlated) clinical interventions, such as those described above, developed to more specifically address hopelessness and related constructs such as dignity, loss of meaning, demoralization, and spiritual suffering or distress will be important to test empirically and utilize in general palliative care practice if they prove effective.

INTERVENTIONS FOR FAMILY MEMBERS FOLLOWING A COMPLETED SUICIDE

When a terminally ill patient chooses to end his or her own life, the treatment team must quickly turn its attention to addressing the needs of the patient's family so as to reduce the chances of complicated bereavement. In order to provide effective support, it is essential that the team is aware of the unique reactions commonly found among suicide survivors. A number of studies have compared the bereavement patterns of suicide survivors and nonsuicide survivors.[48**,49,50*]

Findings from these studies indicate that there are several distinguishing themes that arise in suicide bereavement.

Foremost among them is the desire for the survivor to make meaning of the suicide, or to answer the question 'Why?'.[48**,49,51] Van Dongen[52] calls this process 'agonizing questioning' given the impossibility of ascertaining the answer from the now deceased. Second, survivors often express feelings of guilt, blame, and responsibility for the death.[48**,49] Often they engage in a struggle to retrace the days and months leading up to the suicide in order to pick up clues that they 'missed'. Another documented theme is a heightened feeling of rejection or abandonment, which is often accompanied by anger toward the deceased.[48**,49,53**] Finally, perceived feelings of stigmatization, shame, and embarrassment are well documented.[48**,53**] These feelings may be warranted as there is much evidence in the literature showing that suicide survivors are in fact viewed more negatively by others in their social network in comparison with other mourners.[49] One study by Allen and colleagues[54**] found that individuals bereaved by suicide were viewed as more psychologically disturbed, less likable, more blameworthy, and more in need of professional mental healthcare than those bereaved by other causes. As a result it is not surprising that these individuals struggle with isolation and lack of social support at a time when it is needed most.

Although the aforementioned themes are likely to arise to some extent in all suicide survivors, some may be more or less likely when the suicide is completed by a terminally ill patient. First, on the positive side, family members of a terminally ill suicide completer may not struggle as restlessly with the meaning of the suicide, particularly if their loved one was in a large amount of physical pain or was somehow physically incapacitated. Second, family members may not feel as much responsibility for the suicide as there is a clear external factor, namely the terminal illness, to which one can assign blame. Finally, given that the suicide may not be as unexpected among such a population, the family member may have already started the anticipatory grieving process and may not feel as rejected and abandoned as other survivors. On the other hand, although suicide among the terminally ill may be more socially accepted and thus less stigmatizing for the survivor, this group may receive fewer offers of professional support in comparison with other mourners. Additionally, guilt feelings may be more common among this group of survivors as a consequence of the simultaneous feeling of relief they may experience at the end of a possibly long caregiving period.

Armed with an understanding of the key issues for suicide survivors in general, and for survivors of a terminally ill patient's suicide more specifically, the treatment team can now begin to intervene on behalf of the family. First and foremost, the physician and mental health professional on the team should contact the family immediately after hearing of the suicide. This will communicate that the treatment team does not criticize or blame the family, and that they will not abandon the family just because the patient has passed away.

Similarly, efforts should be made to attend the funeral or memorial services. These acts will serve to diffuse the family's feelings of isolation and stigmatization. Second, attempts should be made to connect the family member to a support group specifically designed for suicide survivors. Jordan[49] (p. 97) argues that groups limited to suicide survivors seem more likely to cohere quickly and to 'avoid a replication of the empathic failure that too often occurs for survivors in their larger social networks'. Such groups should focus on areas such as facilitating integration of the loss by understanding why and how the suicide occurred, exploring the meaning of the loss for the survivor, and providing space for the expression of all types of feelings both positive and negative.[51] Effective support groups for suicide survivors should also include a psychoeducational component, which has been found to reduce survivor anxiety and bolster coping strategies.[51] Psychoeducational resources and materials should also be designed to support and educate those in the survivor's support network so as to reduce their negatively held stereotypes about this group of mourners. A third objective of the treatment team should be to encourage the family to engage in a grieving ritual for the survivor. Some cultures restrict the use of traditional grieving rituals which can leave the survivor with no closure.[51] Developing their own unique ritual can be a liberating experience for the family. Finally, survivors are at risk for increased suicidality of their own, although possibly less so when it is a terminally ill patient that takes his or her own life. Nevertheless, the treatment team should proactively assess the family member's risk, and make an appropriate referral if warranted.

Key learning points

- Suicide is a tragic but often preventable response to terminal physical illness.

- Existing data on the frequency of suicidal ideation in the terminally ill may be misleading, in that patients often disclose these thoughts only after a stable, ongoing physician–patient relationship has been established.

- Patients suffering from terminal illnesses, such as cancer and AIDS, are at increased risk of suicide relative to the general population, particularly in the terminal stage of illness.

- Psychiatric disorders (such as major depression, delirium, and adjustment disorders) are frequently present in hospitalized patients who are suicidal. Depression is a factor in 50 percent of all suicides.

- Physically ill patients commit suicide most frequently in the advanced stages of disease.

- Loss of control and a sense of helplessness in the face of illness are important factors in suicide vulnerability.

- The prevalence of organic mental disorders, such as delirium, among seriously medically ill patients has been found to range from 25 percent to 85 percent during the terminal stages of illness. Clinical experience has found these confusional states to be a major contributing factor in impulsive suicide attempts, especially in the hospital setting.

- Assessment of suicide risk and appropriate intervention is critical. Early and comprehensive psychiatric involvement with high risk individuals can often avert suicide in the medical setting.

- The clinician's ability to establish rapport and elicit a patient's thoughts is essential. Allowing the patient to discuss suicidal thoughts often decreases the risk of suicide. The myth that asking about suicidal thoughts 'puts the idea in their head', is false and should be dispelled.

- Analgesics, neuroleptics, or antidepressant drugs should be used when appropriate to treat any agitation, psychosis, major depression, or pain that are contributing to the patient's suicidal ideation.

- Novel psychotherapeutic interventions aimed at improving spiritual wellbeing, sense of meaning and diminishing hopelessness, demoralization, and distress are being developed which may prove effective in reducing suicidal ideation and attempts. Interventions for hopelessness, loss of meaning and purpose in the terminally ill are of particular importance when addressing the issues of desire for death and despair at the end of life.

- In cases of completed suicide, clinicians need to be sensitive to the needs of the patient's family and loved ones. These individuals may require some form of intervention to assist them in coping. Such individuals may also be at a potentially higher risk for suicide themselves.

REFERENCES

1 Whitlock FA. Suicide and physical illness. In: Roy A, ed. *Suicide*. Baltimore: Williams & Willkins, 1986: 151–70.

2 Silberfarb PM, Maurer LH, Cronthamel CS. Psychosocial aspects of breast cancer patients during different treatment regimens. *Am J Psychiatry* 1980; **137**: 450–5.

3 Achte KA, Vanhkouen ML. Cancer and the psyche. *Omega* 1971; **2**: 46–56.

● 4 Brown JH, Henteleff P, Barakat S, Rowe JR. Is it normal for terminally ill patients to desire death? *Am J Psychiatry* 1986; **143**: 208–11.

◆ 5 Breitbart W. Suicide in cancer patients. *Oncology* 1987; **1**: 49.

6 Hem E, Loge J, Haldorsen T, Ekeberg, O. Suicide risk in cancer patients from 1960 to 1999. *J Clin Oncol* 2004; **22**: 4209–16.

● 7 Bolund C. Suicide and cancer: II. Medical and care factors in suicide by cancer patients in Sweden. 1973–1976. *J Psychosoc Oncol* 1985; **3**: 17–30.

8 Zweig R, Hinrichsen G. Factors associated with suicide attempts by depressed older adults: a prospective study. *Am J Psychiatry* 1993; **150**: 1687–92.

◆ 9 Dubovsky SL. Averting suicide in terminally ill patients. *Psychosomatics* 1978; **19**: 113–15.

10 Murphy GE. Suicide and attempted suicide. *Hosp Pract* 1977; **12**: 78–81.

◆ 11 Breitbart W. Cancer pain and suicide. In: Foley KM, Bonica JJ, Ventafridda V, eds. *Advances in Pain Research and Therapy*, Vol. 16. New York: Raven Press, 1990: 399–412.

● 12 Farberow NL, Shneidman ES, Leonard CV. Suicide among general medical and surgical hospital patients with malignant neoplasms. *Med Bull Vet Adm* 1963; MB-9: 1–11.

● 13 Fox BH, Stanek EJ, Boyd SC, Flannery JT. Suicide rates among cancer patients in Connecticut. *J Chronic Dis* 1982; **35**: 85–100.

● 14 Louhivuori KA, Hakama J. Risk of suicide among cancer patients. *Am J Epidemiol* 1979; **109**: 59–65.

15 Ayd F. Amoxapine: a new tricyclic antidepressant. *Int Drug Ther Newsltr* 1979; **14**: 33–40.

16 Lloyd AH. Practical consideration in the use of maprotiline (Ludiomil) in general practice. *J Int Med Res* 1977; **5**: 122–5.

● 17 Farberow NL, Ganzler S, Cuter F, Reynolds D. An eight year survey of hospital suicides. *Suicide Life Threat Behav* 1971; **1**: 198–201.

● 18 Robins E, Murphy G, Wilkinson RH Jr, *et al.* Some clinical considerations in the prevention of suicide based on 134 successful suicides. *Am J Public Health* 1950; **49**: 888–9.

● 19 Guze S, Robins E. Suicide and primary affective disorders. *Br J Psychiatry* 1970; **117**: 437–8.

● 20 Chochinov HMC, Wilson K, Enns M, Lander S. Prevalence of depression in the terminally ill: effects of diagnostic criteria and symptom threshold judgments. *Am J Psychiatry* 1994; **151**: 4.

◆ 21 Massie MJ, Holland JC, Straker N. Psychotherapeutic interventions. In: Holland JC, Rowland JH, eds. *Handbook of Psychooncology: Psychological Care of the Patient With Cancer*. New York: Oxford University Press 1989: 455–69.

◆ 22 Breitbart W, Jaramillo JR, Chochinov HM. Palliative and terminal care. In Holland JC, *et al.*, eds. *Psycho-Oncology*. New York: Oxford University Press, 1998: 437–49.

● 23 Ganzini L, Lec MA, Heintz RT, *et al.* The effect of depression treatment on elderly patients' preferences for life-sustaining medical therapy. *Am J Psychiatry* 1994; **151**: 1613–16.

◆ 24 Beck AT, Kovacs M, Weissman A. Hopelessness and suicidal behavior: an overview. *JAMA* 1975; **234**: 1146–9.

● 25 Chochinov HM, Wilson KG, Enns M, Lander S. Depression, hopelessness, and suicidal ideation in the terminally ill. *Psychosomatics* 1998; **39**: 366–70.

26 Derogatis LR, Marrow GR, Fetting J, *et al.* The prevalence of psychiatric disorders among cancer patients. *JAMA* 1983; **249**: 751–7.

27 Levine PM, Silberfarb PM, Lipowski ZJ. Mental disorders in cancer patients. *Cancer* 1978; **42**: 1385–90.

28 Massie MJ, Holland JC, Glass E. Delirium in terminally ill cancer patients. *Am J Psychiatry* 1983; **140**: 1048–50.

29 Holland JC. Psychological aspects of cancer. In: Holland JF, Frei E, eds. *Cancer Medicine*, 2nd ed. Philadelphia: Lea and Febiger, 1982.

30 Gillick MR, Serrel NA, Gillick LS. Adverse consequences of hospitalization in the elderly. *Soc Sci Med* 1982; **16**: 1033–1038.

31 Warot D, Corruble E, Payan C, *et al.* Subjective effects of modafinil, a new central adrenergic stimulant in healthy volunteers: a comparison with amphetamine, caffeine, and placebo. *Eur Psychiatry* 1993; **8**: 201–8.

◆ 32 Rosenfeld B, Krivo S, Breitbart W, *et al.* Suicide, assisted suicide, and euthanasia in the terminally ill. In Chochinov HM, Breitbart W, eds. *Handbook of Psychiatry in Palliative Medicine*. New York: Oxford University Press, 2000: 51–62.

● 33 Breitbart W, Rosenfeld B, Passik SD. Interest in physician-assisted suicide among ambulatory HIV-infected patients. *Am J Psychiatry* 1996; **153**: 238–42.

● 34 Emmanuel EJ, Fairclough DL, Daniels ER, Clarridge BR. Euthanasia and physician-assisted suicide: Attitudes and experiences of oncology patients, oncologists and the public. *Lancet* 1996; **347**: 1805–10.

● 35 Chochinov HMC, Wilson KG, Enns M, *et al.* Desire for death in the terminally ill. *Am J Psychiatry* 1995; **152**: 1185–91.

● 36 Breitbart W, Rosenfeld B, Pessin H, *et al.* Depression, hopelessness, and desire for hastened death in terminally ill patients with cancer. *JAMA* 2000; **284**: 2907–11.

● 37 Rosenfeld B, Breitbart W, Stein K, *et al.* Measuring desire for death among patients with HIV/AIDS: the Schedule of Attitudes Toward Hastened Death. *Am J Psychiatry* 1999; **156**: 94–100.

● 38 Rosenfeld B, Breitbart W, Galietta M, *et al.* The Schedule of Attitudes Toward hastened Death: measuring desire for hastened death in terminally ill cancer patients. *Cancer* 2000; **88**: 2868–75.

39 Chochinov HM, Holland JC. Bereavement. In: Holland JC, Rowland JH, eds. *Handbook of Psychooncology: Psychological Care of the Patient With Cancer*. New York: Oxford University Press, 1989: 612–27.

● 40 Chochinov HM, Tataryn D, Clinch JJ, Dudgeon D. Will to live in the terminally ill. *Lancet* 1999; **354**: 816–19.

◆ 41 Breitbart W, Chochinov HM, Passik S. Psychiatric aspects of palliative care. In: Doyle D, Hanks GEC, McDonald N, eds. *Oxford Textbook of Palliative Medicine*, 3rd ed. Oxford: Oxford University Press, 2004: 933–54.

42 Breitbart W. Spirituality and meaning in supportive care: spirituality and meaning-centered group psychotherapy interventions in advanced cancer. *Support Care Cancer* 2002; **10**: 272–80.

43 Rousseau P. Spirituality and the dying patient. *J Clin Oncol* 2000; **18**: 2000–2.

◆ 44 Kissane D, Clarke DM, Street AF. Demoralization syndrome – a relevant psychiatric diagnosis for palliative care. *J Palliat Care* 2001; **17**: 12–21.

45 Chochinov HM, Hack T, McClement S, *et al.* Dignity in the terminally ill: an empirical model. *Soc Sci Med* 2002; **54**: 433–43.

46 Greenstein M, Breitbart W. Cancer and the experience of meaning: A group psychotherapy program for people with cancer. *Am J Psychother* 2000; **54**: 486–500.

◆ 47 Chochinov HM. Dignity-conserving care – a new model for palliative care. *JAMA* 2002; **287**: 2253–60.

48 Bailey SE, Kral MJ, Dunham K. Survivors of suicide do grieve differently: empirical support for a common sense proposition. *Suicide Life Threat Behav* 1999; **29**: 256–72.

49 Jordan JR. Is suicide bereavement different? A reassessment of the literature. *Suicide Life Threat Behav* 2001; **31**: 91–103.

● 50 Barrett TW, Scott TB. Suicide bereavement and recovery patterns compared with non-suicide bereavement patterns. *Suicide Life Threat Behav* 1990; **20**: 1–15.

51 Barlow CA, Morrison H. Survivors of suicide: Emerging counseling strategies. *J Psychosoc Nurs Mental Health Serv* 2002; **40**: 28–39.

52 Van Dongen CJ. Survivors of a family member's suicide: implications for practice. *Nurse Pract* 1991; **16**: 31–6.

● 53 Harwood D, Hawton K, Hope T, Jacoby R. The grief experiences and needs of bereaved relatives and friends of older people dying through suicide: a descriptive and case-control study. *J Affective Disord* 2001; **72**: 185–94.

54 Allen BG, Calhoun LG, Cann A, Tedeschi RG. The effects of cause of death on responses to the bereaved: suicide compared to accidental and natural causes. *Omega* 1993; **28**: 39–48.

PART 15

Specific conditions and situations

91

Cancer: radiotherapy

ELIZABETH A BARNES, EDWARD CHOW

INTRODUCTION

Radiotherapy plays an important role in the multidisciplinary management of patients with cancer. It is a local treatment, and can be used with curative intent for a localized tumor, in the adjuvant setting after surgery, and with palliative intent to relieve symptoms resulting from tumor mass effect. Approximately half of all radiotherapy treatment is given with palliative as opposed to curative intent.[1] The goal of palliative radiotherapy is to use a short treatment schedule to provide effective and durable symptom relief with minimal treatment-related side effects.

Radiotherapy is used to treat cancer with ionizing radiation resulting in damage to cellular DNA (Fig. 91.1). When radiation passes through a living cell, it causes damage by direct and indirect effects. Direct effects include damage to the DNA strand (base deletions, single, and double-strand breaks). Indirect effects result from ionization of water molecules causing free radicals, which in turn damage the DNA. Repair of DNA damage is possible both in normal and malignant cells, but malignant cells often have defective DNA repair and so significant damage can accumulate. Lethally damaged cells do not show morphological evidence of radiation damage until they attempt to divide.

Radiotherapy delivery is broadly classified as external beam radiation or brachytherapy. External beam treatment involves high energy γ rays produced from a linear accelerator, or from a radioactive cobalt source housed within the head of the treatment machine. Brachytherapy involves delivering radiation over a short distance from a radiation source that is placed on or into a body surface, tissue or cavity. Another form of brachytherapy involves using

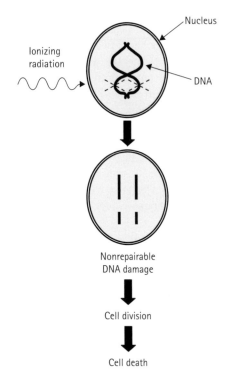

Figure 91.1 *Radiation damaging nuclear DNA resulting in cell death.*

radioactive isotopes that have affinity to specific tissues, e.g. bone or thyroid, and are injected into the blood stream and deposit radiation locally.

When a patient is seen in consultation for palliative radiotherapy, the radiation oncologist takes into consideration tumor factors such as histology and tumor location, and patient factors such as symptom burden and life expectancy to determine whether treatment is appropriate. Repeat radiotherapy to the same site may be possible depending on the previous treatment parameters (dose and fractionation), time since previous radiotherapy, and the radiation tolerance of structures within the radiotherapy field. As radiotherapy is a local treatment, the objective is to treat the tumor while minimizing dose to surrounding normal tissue. Immobilization of the patient is first required; usually this involves having the patient lie still in the supine position. External beam treatment planning (simulation) involves localizing the tumor clinically if a superficial lesion, or using fluoroscopy or computed tomography (CT) if deep seated. After treatment field planning and radiation dose calculation, the patient then receives treatment from a linear accelerator or cobalt unit in a heavily shielded room. It is important to remember that the patient must be able to lie still, unattended, on the simulator and treatment tables (which are hard and narrow) for approximately 15 minutes at a time. This may be difficult for patients who are delirious, orthopneic, or have uncontrolled pain.

Radiotherapy services are closely linked to the level of medical care of a given country. Of the 6805 radiotherapy units worldwide, 4572 (67 percent) are in developed countries, even though they have just 21 percent of the population.[2] Moreover, 56 of the 129 developing countries (43 percent) do not have any radiotherapy facilities, with the problem being worst in Africa. The incidence of cancer is projected to rise worldwide by around 50 percent in the next 20 years, mostly in developing countries. Therefore, the lack of radiotherapy services will worsen unless there is appropriate planning and financial investment. In contrast, there is greater access to radiotherapy in resource-rich countries (such as the USA) that have both state funded and freestanding radiotherapy centers, and so patterns of practice tend to differ.

The unit of radiation dose for many years was the rad (radiation absorbed dose). This has now been replaced by the SI unit gray (Gy), (1 rad = 0.01 Gy = 1 centigray [cGy]). Typically one radiotherapy treatment (fraction) is given per day, 5 days a week (Monday through Friday). Large doses per fraction are poorly tolerated and increase the risk of late tissue toxicity. Small doses per fraction delivered over many days are used to take advantage of the observation that cancers have impaired DNA repair as compared with normal tissue. Therefore during treatment normal tissue can recover through repair and repopulation, while DNA damage in malignant cells accumulates and is fatal when the cell tries to divide. The differential toxicity between cancer and normal tissue is not complete, and normal tissues have a tolerance dose beyond which they are irreversibly damaged. This dose is lower for spinal cord and bowel than muscle and bone. The optimal dose of radiation is one that will produce the maximal probability of tumor control with minimal complications. In curative

treatment regimens a high total dose needs to be delivered (5000–8000 cGy), which is accomplished by using small daily fractions (180–200 cGy). For symptom palliation a high total dose is not required, therefore palliative fractionation schedules can be shorter and use a higher dose per fraction. This serves to minimize patient visits to the cancer center and treatment-related side effects. Commonly used palliative radiotherapy regimens include 800 cGy in a single fraction, 2000 cGy in five fractions (400 cGy per fraction) and 3000 cGy in 10 fractions (300 cGy per fraction). Treatment-related side effects are defined as acute (≤90 days after treatment start) or late (>90 days). As radiotherapy is a local treatment, apart from fatigue, side effects depend on the area treated. Acute toxicity is self-limiting and tends to resolve within 2 weeks of treatment completion. Late toxicity is usually not a problem in the palliative setting, given the low total radiotherapy doses used and the limited life expectancy of patients with advanced cancer. However, the radiation tolerance of normal tissue such as spinal cord needs to be respected, especially when retreating, as patients can live longer than expected.

BONE METASTASES

Bone metastases are common in patients with advanced cancer, and are the most common cause of cancer pain.[3] Palliation of bone metastases comprises a significant workload in a radiotherapy department, accounting for 40 percent of palliative radiotherapy courses.[1] Radiotherapy is used in the management of bone metastases for relief of bone pain, prevention of impending fractures, and promotion of healing pathological fractures. Prophylactic surgical fixation should be considered for good performance status patients with bone lesions at high risk of fracture, as prophylactic surgery is easier to perform than surgery after a pathological fracture, and is associated with better functional outcomes and increased survival.[4,5] High-risk lesions include those with >50 percent cortical destruction of a long bone; femoral lesions >25 mm in the neck, subtrochanteric, intertrochanteric, or supracondylar regions; and diffuse lytic involvement of a weight bearing bone especially if painful.[7*] Postoperative radiotherapy is routinely given and has been shown to improve functional status, decrease pain, and reduce the risk of refracture.[6*] Database analysis from a recent bone metastases trial found the risk of femoral fracture was most dependent on the amount of axial cortical involvement, and recommended prophylactic fixation for lesions >30 mm, or in nonsurgical candidates multiple fraction radiotherapy to decrease fracture occurrence.[8**]

Two recent meta-analyses have shown the overall and complete pain response rates to bone radiotherapy are 59–62 percent and 32–34 percent, respectively.[9***][10***] The median time to pain relief is 3 weeks,[11**] and the median duration of pain relief is 12–24 weeks.[9***] Acute toxicity is mild, seen in 10–17 percent of patients, and late toxicity is rare (4 percent).[12**] Toxicity is site specific, for example acute toxicity from cervical spine radiotherapy can result in dysphagia, thoracic and lumbar spine radiotherapy nausea and vomiting, and pelvic radiotherapy diarrhea. Prophylactic ondansetron can be used to reduce emesis when treating over the epigastrium, lumbothoracic spine, or a large pelvic field.[9***] Re-treatment can be considered for patients who experience initial pain relief followed by a relapse, have incomplete pain relief, or no pain relief. Re-treatment offers effective palliation, with a response rate of 63 percent.[13**] Generally a 4-week interval is given before considering re-treatment, to allow enough time to derive benefit from the first treatment. There is an ongoing international phase III randomized trial of single versus multiple fractions for reirradiation of painful bone metastases to determine the optimal dose fractionation regimen for re-treatment.[14]

Despite the frequent use of palliative bone radiotherapy, and the fact that numerous randomized trials have been conducted on dose fractionation schedules, there is still no uniform consensus on the optimal radiotherapy schedule for uncomplicated bone metastases. The most commonly employed schedules are a single 800 cGy, 2000 cGy in five daily fractions, or 3000 cGy in 10 daily fractions. Two recent meta-analyses show no significant difference in overall or complete response rates or duration of pain relief between single and multiple fractions.[9***,10***] Furthermore, no difference in quality of life, analgesic use, or acute toxicity were observed. However, the observed re-treatment rates were higher with the use of a single fraction at 20–25 percent compared with 7–12 percent following multiple fraction regimens.[9***,10***] Physician training, department policy, resource availability, and reimbursement can influence practice patterns.[15] In the USA, where radiation is reimbursed on a per fraction basis, there is a tendency to use protracted fractionation regimens. In Europe, where radiation is paid for on a global, or per episode basis and where the recent large randomized trials demonstrating equivalence were performed, single fractions are more commonly used. Practice in the USA may change with the results of RTOG 97–14, which was recently published.[12**] This compared a single 8 Gy fraction to 30 Gy in 10 fractions for good performance status breast and prostate cancer patients with painful bone metastases. No difference was found in overall response rate between the two arms, with pain improvement seen in 66 percent of patients at 3 months.

The optimal palliative radiotherapy treatment regimen is one that provides prompt and effective pain relief with minimal toxicity and patient inconvenience. A single fraction has the advantage of requiring only one visit, which is especially beneficial for patients with poor performance status and those who live at a distance from the center. For patients with longer life expectancy, receiving multiple fractions upfront may avoid the need for re-treatment, and

therefore the choice of fractionation schedule should be discussed with the patient.[16,17]

Patients with bone metastases often have diffuse bony disease, for which half-body irradiation (HBI) and systemic radionuclides can be useful treatment modalities to simultaneously target all bony lesions. HBI encompasses either the upper half (base of skull to iliac crest), or lower half (iliac crest to ankles) of the body in a single large radiotherapy field.[18**] Single fraction HBI has been shown to provide pain relief in 70–80 percent of patients.[19*,20*] The onset of pain relief is quicker than with local radiotherapy, occurring within 24–48 hours, suggesting that cells of the inflammatory response pathway may be the initial target tissue, since tumor cell activities are unlikely to be halted so quickly. The dose delivered is typically a single fraction of 6 Gy to the upper body (reduced dose due to potential for lung toxicity), and 8 Gy to the lower body. Addition of a single fraction of HBI to local radiotherapy has been shown to delay the time to disease progression and time to re-treatment.[21**] An international phase III trial looked at different fractionation regimens (15 Gy in five fractions over 5 days, 8 Gy in two fractions over 1 day, and 12 Gy in four fractions over 2 days) to determine the most effective and least burdensome treatment regimen.[18**] Results showed the 2 and 5-day regimens gave similar results (except for prostate primaries where the 2-day arm was inferior), with pain relief seen in 91 percent of patients by day 3. The 1-day regimen provided inferior pain relief and quality of life; and therefore except for prostate primaries, the 2-day regimen can be recommended for patients with widespread bony disease. Half-body irradiation is associated with acute gastrointestinal toxicity (nausea, vomiting, diarrhea), thought to be more pronounced with use of a single fraction.[22] Acute toxicity usually requires intravenous fluids and premedication with antiemetics and corticosteroids, and in some cases an overnight stay in hospital for observation. Reversible myelosuppression occurs, therefore sequential treatment of upper and lower body requires a 4–6-week interval for counts to recover.

Systemic radionuclides are deposited at the site of osteoblastic bony metastases, mirroring the uptake seen on bone scan, and emit radiation with a mean range <3 mm.[23,24] Radionuclides have been mainly studied in patients with hormone refractory prostate cancer, as these bone metastases tend to be osteoblastic rather than osteolytic. Patients with lung or breast primaries typically have mixed osteoblastic and osteolytic bone metastases, and therefore the use of radionuclides is less applicable. Strontium-89 and samarium-153 are the agents most commonly utilized in clinical practice, and can be given in a single intravenous injection on an outpatient basis. Efficacy of the various radionuclides is thought to be similar, although comparative trials have not been conducted. Contraindications for use are fracture, spinal cord compression, lesions with extraosseous component, renal failure, inadequate hemogram, life expectancy <2 months, and chemotherapy within 1 month.[24] A randomized trial comparing strontium to local or wide field radiotherapy in patients with metastatic prostate cancer found similar response rates in all arms (65 percent), and strontium decreased the incidence of new painful sites.[25**] Strontium toxicity consists mainly of reversible myelosuppression, with a decrease in platelet and leukocyte counts of 30–40 percent at nadir, occurring at 4–8 weeks.[25**] Cancer Care Ontario Guidelines (CCOG) for patients with hormone refractory prostate cancer recommend strontium for use in patients with multiple uncontrolled painful sites of bone metastases on both sides of the diaphragm not adequately controlled with analgesics, and where the use of multiple single fields of radiotherapy is not possible.[26***] A randomized trial of strontium versus placebo as an adjunct to local radiotherapy in patients with metastatic prostate cancer found strontium improved quality of life and decreased analgesic requirement at 3 months, as well as reduction in the lifetime need for radiotherapy and rate of new painful sites.[27**] The CCOG guidelines, however, do not recommend the use of strontium in this adjuvant setting as the clinical significance of these findings is uncertain.[26***]

There is limited evidence to compare the efficacy of radionuclides with HBI.[26***] The pain relief achieved with HBI and radionuclides appears to be comparable, however the onset of pain relief is faster with HBI.[18**] Both are associated with transient myelosuppression, but with HBI acute gastrointestinal toxicity is worse, and there are concerns of late toxicity to visceral structures. Systemic radionuclides may be preferred in the setting of diffuse blastic disease, however, its use is limited by cost and resource availability. Half-body irradiation remains an effective treatment option for patients with diffuse lytic disease refractory to other therapies.

BRAIN METASTASES

Brain metastases occur in approximately 25 percent of cancer patients, and are most commonly seen in patients with lung, breast, and gastrointestinal primaries.[28,29] Brain metastases are associated with major neurological morbidity and shortened survival, with a median survival of 1–2 months with corticosteroids alone,[30] and 4–6 months with whole-brain radiotherapy (WBRT).[31] Treatment typically consists of corticosteroids to reduce peritumoral edema, followed by WBRT. The goal of radiotherapy is to provide neurological symptom relief, allow corticosteroid tapering, and possibly improve survival. The acute side effects of treatment include fatigue, alopecia, and erythema of the scalp. Long-term toxicity is limited and rarely a concern for these patients with limited life expectancy. A recent practice guidelines report found no benefit with respect to

survival or symptom control for doses higher than 2000 cGy in five fractions or 3000 cGy in 10 fractions.[32***]

A single brain metastasis is present in 30–40 percent of patients.[33] For these patients with good performance status and minimal or no evidence of extracranial disease, surgical excision followed by WBRT has been shown to improve survival over WBRT alone.[32***,34**,35**] Postoperative WBRT after surgical excision of a single metastasis can improve local control.[32***,36**] The addition of a stereotactic radiosurgery boost to WBRT for patients with good performance status has been recently shown to improve survival for patients with a single brain metastasis, and to improve functional autonomy for patients with two to three metastases.[37**]

A single institution observational study of all patients receiving WBRT for symptomatic brain metastases found at 1 month only 15–39 percent of patients benefited from treatment (depending on the criteria used), and 27 percent died at or soon after 1 month.[38*] This emphasizes the importance of appropriately selecting patients for treatment, as patients with poor performance status and rapidly progressive extracranial disease may not derive a clinical benefit from radiotherapy.[32***]

LUNG CANCER

Lung cancer is one of the most common causes of cancer death worldwide. Nonsmall cell lung cancer (NSCLC) accounts for 80 percent of lung cancers, and small cell lung cancer (SCLC) 20 percent. The latter is typically treated with chemotherapy, given the propensity for widespread dissemination at diagnosis. More than two-thirds of NSCLC patients present with incurable locally advanced or metastatic disease.[39**] The overall prognosis of patients is poor, with a median survival of less than 1 year.

The use of chemotherapy for NSCLC has been increasing over the past two decades, but radiotherapy remains an important treatment modality for patients with predominantly intrathoracic disease, who are unable to receive or decline chemotherapy, or have chemoresistant disease.[40] Thoracic symptoms can be effectively palliated with local radiotherapy, with up to 90 percent of patients obtaining relief from hemoptysis and chest pain, and up to 65 percent obtaining relief from cough and dyspnea.[39**,41**] Symptom palliation with radiotherapy has been found to last for over half of the patient's lifetime.[42**] Reirradiation using techniques to spare spinal cord can provide effective and durable symptom palliation.[43*] In locally advanced NSCLC patients with asymptomatic pulmonary disease, no advantage has been shown with respect to overall survival, quality of life or symptom control to immediate versus delayed thoracic radiotherapy.[44**] For patients with total atelectasis secondary to obstruction of the mainstem bronchus, receiving radiotherapy within 2 weeks of atelectasis results in higher rates of complete reexpansion (71 percent vs. 23 percent after 2 weeks).[45*] Intraluminal brachytherapy with a high dose rate applicator can offer effective palliation of symptoms arising from endobronchial disease in 1–3-fraction outpatient treatments.[46*] This is also a treatment option for patients with endobronchial tumor recurrence who have received maximal doses of external beam radiotherapy.

Several studies have investigated optimal fractionation regimens for palliative thoracic radiotherapy. A systemic review published in 2003 of 12 randomized trials stated a meta-analysis could not be performed due to the large heterogeneity in radiotherapy regimens, outcome measures and patient characteristics.[47***] However, they found no strong evidence that higher doses offered better symptom palliation, but good evidence to suggest that toxicity is greater. There is a suggestion that higher doses of radiotherapy for good performance status patients with locally advanced nonmetastatic lung cancer may lead to a modest (6 percent at 1 year, 3 percent at 2 years) increase in survival.[48***] The fractionation regimens in these trials include common palliative schedules such as a single dose of 10 Gy, a total dose of 17 Gy in 2 fractions 1 week apart, 20 Gy in 5 fractions, 30 Gy in 10 fractions, and more radical doses such as 60 Gy in 30 fractions. Of note, none of these trials examined the role of chemotherapy, which is now playing an increasingly important role in patient management. Good performance status patients with locally advanced nonmetastatic disease can be considered for radical chemoradiotherapy.[49] For patients treated with palliative intent, chemotherapy has been shown to improve survival, symptom relief, and quality of life compared to best supportive care.[49] Whether combining radiotherapy with chemotherapy improves symptom relief or quality of life for selected NSCLC patients is unknown.

PELVIC DISEASE

Locally advanced and recurrent pelvic malignancies (i.e. genitourinary, gastrointestinal, and gynecological primaries) can result in many disabling symptoms. These include hemorrhage; necrotic vaginal discharge; local pelvic and neuropathic pain due to adenopathy, invasion of bone and lumbosacral plexus; lower extremity edema; fistula formation; gastrointestinal tract obstruction; and renal failure due to ureteric obstruction.

Effective symptom palliation has been seen following one to three fractions of 10 Gy given 4 weeks apart to the pelvis.[50*,51*,52*] RTOG 7905 examined combining three fractions with misonidazole (a radiosensitizer) in patients with gynecologic, bowel, and prostate cancers, and found the overall and complete response rate to treatment was 62 percent and 38 percent, respectively.[53*] A dose–response relationship has been reported, with repeat fractions giving more effective symptom palliation.[50*,53*] However, RTOG

7905 found three fractions gave a very high rate (49 percent) of late complications,[53*] while one to two fractions is associated with a late complication rate of 0–10 percent.[50*,53*] Given the high complication rate, RTOG 8502 explored using 370 cGy twice a day for 2 days, with a rest interval of 2–4 weeks, repeated three times to a total dose of 4440 cGy.[54*] This regimen was associated with a much lower risk of late toxicity (6 percent), yet gave similar symptom palliation with approximately 50 percent of patients having complete pain relief, and 90 percent complete resolution of bleeding or obstruction.[55,56*] As the incidence of late toxicity increases with time, patients with a life expectancy greater than 9 months should receive the second RTOG schedule, or other treatment schedules using lower dose per fraction, or one to two fractions of 10 Gy.

Patients with muscle invasive bladder cancer are typically smokers, older (>70 years of age), and often have numerous medical comorbidities. For patients unable to tolerate radical treatment, and for patients with locally advanced incurable disease, palliative radiotherapy with the goal of symptom relief can be given. A large randomized trial was conducted comparing the efficacy and toxicity of two palliative radiotherapy schedules (35 Gy in 10 fractions, and 21 Gy in three fractions on alternate days over 1 week).[57**] There was no difference between the two arms, with 68 percent overall improvement in bladder symptoms at 3 months, median survival of 7.5 months, and late bowel toxicity rate of <1 percent. Improvement at 3 months of individual symptoms was 88 percent for hematuria, 82 percent for frequency, 72 percent for dysuria, 64 percent for nocturia, and this was maintained in many patients for the duration of their survival. Other groups have reported using 5–6-weekly fractions of 6 Gy with effective symptom palliation,[58*,59*] late bowel (2 percent) and bladder (11 percent) toxicity was reported in one trial.[58*] Another trial reported that by using 5.75 Gy vs. 6.5 Gy in 6-weekly fractions the incidence of late bowel toxicity was reduced from 15 percent to 0 percent.[60*] Of interest, the radiotherapy treatment volume in these bladder cancer trials consisted of the bladder with a small margin (usually 100 cm^3), which was smaller than the volumes treated in the RTOG trials (usually 225 cm^3). This may partially explain the higher bowel complication rate seen in the RTOG trials. Using modern CT-based radiation treatment planning to treat the tumor while minimizing bowel and other structures can reduce treatment toxicity and allow for dose escalation.

Paraaortic adenopathy from pelvic primaries can result in lower back pain which can be palliated with local radiotherapy. Recurrent ovarian cancer is typically treated with chemotherapy, however radiotherapy offers very good symptom palliation with response rates >70 percent, even in patients with platinum resistant disease.[61*,62*] Patients with metastatic rectal cancer can suffer from severe pelvic pain and bowel obstruction due to their primary disease, and palliative resection or diverting colostomy is often recommended. Palliative chemoradiotherapy with concurrent 5-fluorouracil (5-FU) has been shown to provide symptom relief in 94 percent of patients, and gives a 1-year colostomy-free survival rate of 87 percent.[63*] The study recommended radiotherapy regimens of 36 Gy/12 fraction/3 weeks, 35 Gy/14 fraction/3 weeks, or 30 Gy/6 fraction/2 weeks. A review addressing the question of the most effective dose fractionation for symptom relief in patients with pelvic recurrence from colorectal or rectal cancer included studies using doses ranging from 1500 cGy to 7000 cGy, but could not provide a definitive answer.[64***]

HEAD AND NECK CANCER

Patients with locally advanced head and neck cancer can have many devastating symptoms due to their disease. These include pain, dysphagia, hoarseness, otalgia, and respiratory distress.[65**] Tracheostomy placement may be required to maintain the airway, and patients commonly have malnutrition and may require a feeding tube. Radiotherapy with concurrent chemotherapy can be offered to patients with advanced inoperable disease with curative intent, but treatment is associated with high rates of acute toxicity, and 3-year survival rates are approximately 40 percent.[66**] Patients with incurable disease or those not able to tolerate radical treatment can be offered palliative radiotherapy. An expert panel in 1996 found there were insufficient data in the medical literature on the role of palliative radiotherapy for head and neck cancer with regards to symptomatic outcomes, toxicity, and palliative radiotherapy treatment regimes.[67***] A recent study from India reported on over 500 patients with nonmetastatic stage IV head and neck cancer treated with a short course of palliative radiotherapy (2000 cGy in five fractions).[65**] At 1 month the partial response rate was 37 percent, and >50 percent symptom relief was seen in 47–76 percent of patients. Median survival was 200 days. Patients with good performance status achieving partial response at 1 month were advised to have further radiotherapy with radical intent, and this treatment resulted in a median survival of 400 days and a disease-free rate of 10 percent.

ESOPHAGEAL CANCER

More than half of patients with esophageal cancer present with inoperable disease and require palliation of dysphagia.[68] External beam radiotherapy, intraluminal brachytherapy, photodynamic therapy, laser ablation, and stent placement are among the treatment options.[69**] Palliative external beam radiotherapy regimens that have been explored include 3000 cGy in 10 fractions with a single course of concurrent 5-FU and mitomycin C, which gave complete relief of dysphagia in 68 percent of patients at a median interval of 5 weeks, with 73 percent remaining dysphagia free until death.[70*] Another study using 4000 cGy in two daily fractions of 200 cGy over 2 weeks again found good relief of dysphagia, with a response rate of 67 percent seen at a median of 4 weeks, and a favorable toxicity profile.[71*] High dose rate brachytherapy given in one to three fractions palliates dysphagia in 50 percent of patients, although care needs to be taken with the dose delivered due to the risk of bleeding, and fistula and stricture formation.[72*] A randomized trial comparing a single fraction of brachytherapy with stent placement found dysphagia relief was faster with stent placement, although the overall response was better with brachytherapy.[73**] Higher complication rates were seen with stent placement, and quality-of-life outcomes favored the brachytherapy group. The need for reintervention was similar in both groups (40 percent), and there was no difference in median survival. Palliation of dysphagia needs to be individualized based on patient factors, local expertise, and resource availability.

SKIN CANCER

Skin cancers are classified into two main groups: melanoma and nonmelanoma (basal cell and squamous cell carcimoma).[74] Basal and squamous cell carcinomas are common in older patients, and are often seen in sun-exposed areas of the face and limbs. Neglect in older people can lead to patients presenting with large destructive lesions invading surrounding soft tissue and bone. This can result in pain, bleeding, ulceration, and secondary infection. A short course of palliative radiotherapy can reduce bleeding and allow ulcerative lesions to dry out, making dressing changes and nursing care easier. Melanoma is an aggressive disease with high rates of distant metastases. While often considered radiation resistant, palliative radiotherapy does provides effective and durable palliation. Fractional doses of ≥400 cGy are thought to be more effective than <400 cGy, with response rates of 82 percent vs. 36 percent, respectively.[75***] Examples of radiotherapy regimens using high dose per fraction are 8 Gy days 0–7–21,[76*] and four to five fractions of 6 Gy delivered twice weekly.[75***]

Key learning points

- Local radiotherapy can provide effective palliation of distressing symptoms.

- A short course of radiotherapy (one to five treatments) can be used to minimize treatment-related side effects and limit patient visits to the cancer center.

- A single 8 Gy treatment is recommended for symptomatic relief of uncomplicated bone metastasis, with an expected overall and complete response rate of 60 percent and 32 percent, respectively.

- Patients with symptomatic multiple brain metastases and reasonable performance status are recommended to receive WBRT – suggested radiotherapy schedules are 2000 cGy in five fractions or 3000 cGy in 10 fractions.

- Radiotherapy can also be used to palliate hemorrhage (hemoptysis, hematuria, vaginal bleeding, infiltrating skin lesions), cough, dyspnea, dysphagia, and pain due to tumor infiltration.

REFERENCES

1 Hoegler D. Radiotherapy for palliation of symptoms in incurable cancer. *Curr Probl Cancer* 1997; **21**: 129–83.

2 Stewart BW, Kleihues P, eds. *World Cancer Report.* Lyon: International Agency for Research on Cancer Press, 2003.

◆ 3 Mercadante S. Malignant bone pain: pathophysiology and treatment. *Pain* 1997; **69**: 1–18.

4 Springfield DS. Pathologic fractures. In: Rockwood and Green, eds. *Fractures in Adults.* Baltimore: Lippincott Williams Wilkins, 2001: 557–83.

5 Hardman PD, Robb JE, Kerr GR, *et al.* The value of internal fixation and radiotherapy in the management of upper and lower limb bone metastases. *Clin Oncol (R Coll Radiol)* 1992; **4**: 244–8.

6 Townsend PW, Smalley SR, Cozad SC, *et al.* Role of postoperative radiation therapy after stabilization of fractures caused by metastatic disease. *Int J Radiat Oncol Biol Phys* 1995; **31**: 43–9.

7 Parrish FF, Murray JA. Surgical treatment for secondary neoplastic fractures. A retrospective study of ninety-six patients. *J Bone Joint Surg (Am)* 1970; **52**: 665–86.

8 van der Linden YM, Kroon HM, Dijkstra SP, *et al.* Simple radiographic parameter predicts fracturing in metastatic femoral bone lesions: results from a randomised trial. *Radiother Oncol* 2003; **69**: 21–31.

∗ 9 Wu JS, Wong R, Johnston M, *et al.* Cancer Care Ontario Practice Guidelines Initiative Supportive Care Group. Meta-analysis of dose-fractionation radiotherapy trials for the palliation of painful bone metastases. *Int J Radiat Oncol Biol Phys* 2003; **55**: 594–605.

◆ 10 Sze WM, Shelley MD, Held I, *et al.* Palliation of metastatic bone pain: single fraction versus multifraction radiotherapy– a systematic review of randomised trials. *Clin Oncol (R Coll Radiol)* 2003; **15**: 345–52.

● 11 Steenland E, Leer JW, van Houwelingen H, *et al.* The effect of a single fraction compared to multiple fractions on painful bone metastases: a global analysis of the Dutch Bone Metastasis Study. *Radiother Oncol* 1999; **52**: 101–9.

● 12 Hartsell WF, Scott C, Bruner DW, *et al.* Randomized trial of short versus long-course radiotherapy for palliation of painful bone metastases. *J Natl Cancer Inst* 2005; **97**: 798–804.

● 13 van der Linden YM, Lok JJ, Steenland E, *et al.* Single fraction radiotherapy is efficacious: a further analysis of the Dutch Bone Metastasis Study controlling for the influence of retreatment. *Int J Radiat Oncol Biol Phys* 2004; **59**: 528–37.

14 Kachnic L, Berk L. Palliative single-fraction radiation therapy: how much more evidence is needed? *J Natl Cancer Inst* 2005; **97**: 786–8.

15 van der Linden YM, Leer JW. Impact of randomized trial-outcome in the treatment of painful bone metastases; patterns of practice among radiation oncologists. A matter of believers vs. non-believers? *Radiother Oncol* 2000; **56**: 279–81.

16 Shakespeare TP, Lu JJ, Back MF, *et al.* Patient preference for radiotherapy fractionation schedule in the palliation of painful bone metastases. *J Clin Oncol* 2003; **21**: 2156–62.

17 Szumacher E, Franssen E, Lewellin Thomas H. Patient's decisional preferences in palliative radiotherapy for bone metastases (preliminary results). 21st Annual ESTRO Meeting Programme book. Praha, September 17–21, 2002.

● 18 Salazar OM, Sandhu T, da Motta NW, *et al.* Fractionated half-body irradiation (HBI) for the rapid palliation of widespread, symptomatic, metastatic bone disease: a randomized Phase III trial of the International Atomic Energy Agency (IAEA). *Int J Radiat Oncol Biol Phys* 2001; **50**: 765–75.

● 19 Salazar OM, Rubin P, Hendrickson FR, *et al.* Single-dose half-body irradiation for palliation of multiple bone metastases from solid tumors – final Radiation Therapy Oncology Group Report. *Cancer* 1986; **58**: 29–36.

20 Hoskin PJ, Ford HT, Harmer CL. Hemibody irradiation (HBI) for metastatic bone pain in two histologically distinct groups of patients. *Clin Oncol (R Coll Radiol)* 1989; **1**: 67–9.

● 21 Poulter CA, Cosmatos D, Rubin P, *et al.* A report of RTOG 8206: A phase III study of whether the addition of single dose hemibody irradiation to standard fractionated local field irradiation is more effective than local field irradiation alone in the treatment of symptomatic osseous metastases. *Int J Radiati Oncol Biol Phys* 1992; **23**: 207–14.

22 Salazar OM, Scarantino CW. Theoretical and practical uses of elective systemic (half-body) irradiation after 20 years of experimental designs. *Int J Radiat Oncol Biol Phys* 1997; **39**: 907–13.

◆ 23 Silberstein EB. Systemic radiopharmaceutical therapy of painful osteoblastic metastases. *Semin Radiat Oncol* 2000; **10**: 240–249.

◆ 24 McEwan AJB. Use of radionuclides for the palliation of bone metastases. *Semin Radiat Oncol* 2000; **10**: 103–14.

● 25 Quilty PM, Kirk D, Bolger JJ, *et al.* A comparison of the palliative effects of strontium-89 and external beam radiotherapy in metastatic prostate cancer. *Radiother Oncol* 1994; **31**: 33–40.

∗ 26 Tsao MN, Lloyd NS, Wong RK, *et al.* Supportive Care Guidelines Group of Cancer Care Ontario's Program in Evidence-based Care. Radiotherapeutic management of brain metastases: a systematic review and meta-analysis. *Cancer Treat Rev* 2005; **31**: 256–73.

● 27 Porter AT, McEwan AJB, Powe JE *et al.* Results of a randomized phase-III trial to evaluate the efficacy of strontium-89 adjuvant to local field external beam irradiation in the management of endocrine resistant metastatic prostate cancer. *Int J Radiat Oncol Biol Phys* 1993; **25**: 805–13.

28 Johnson JD, Young B. Demographics of brain metastasis. *Neurosurg Clin North Am* 1996; **7**: 337–44.

29 Walker AE, Robins M, Weinfeld FD. Epidemiology of brain tumors: the national survey of intracranial neoplasms. *Neurology* 1985; **35**: 219–26.

◆ 30 Weissman DE. Glucocorticoid treatment for brain metastases and epidural spinal cord compression: a review. *J Clin Oncol* 1988; **6**: 543–51.

● 31 Diener-West M, Dobbins TW, Phillips TL, Nelson DF. Identification of an optimal subgroup for treatment evaluation of patients with brain metastases using RTOG study 7916. *Int J Radiat Oncol Biol Phys* 1989; **16**: 669–73.

✱ 32 Brundage MD, Crook JM, Lukka H. Use of strontium-89 in endocrine-refractory prostate cancer metastatic to bone. Provincial Genitourinary Cancer Disease Site Group. *Cancer Prev Control* 1998; **2**: 79–87.

33 Lohr F, Pirzkall A, Hof H, *et al.* Adjuvant treatment of brain metastases. *Semin Surg Oncol* 2001; **20**: 50–6.

● 34 Patchell RA, Tibbs PA, Walsh JW, *et al.* A randomized trial of surgery in the treatment of single metastases to the brain. *N Engl J Med* 1990; **322**: 494–500.

● 35 Noordijk EM, Vecht CJ, Haaxma-Reiche H, *et al.* The choice of treatment of single brain metastasis should be based on extracranial tumor activity and age. *Int J Radiat Oncol Biol Phys* 1994; **29**: 711–17.

● 36 Patchell RA, Tibbs PA, Regine WF, *et al.* Postoperative radiotherapy in the treatment of single metastases to the brain: a randomized trial. *JAMA* 1998; **280**: 1485–9.

● 37 Andrews DW, Scott CB, Sperduto PW, *et al.* Whole brain radiation therapy with or without stereotactic radiosurgery boost for patients with one to three brain metastases: phase III results of the RTOG 9508 randomised trial. *Lancet* 2004; **363**: 1665–72.

● 38 Bezjak A, Adam J, Panzarella T, *et al.* Radiotherapy for brain metastases: defining palliative response. *Radiother Oncol* 2001; **61**: 71–6.

● 39 Sundstrom S, Bremnes R, Aasebo U *et al.* Hypofractionated palliative radiotherapy (17 Gy per two fractions) in advanced non-small cell lung carcinoma is comparable to standard fractionation for symptom control and survival: A national phase III trial. *J Clin Oncol* 2004; **22**: 801–10.

◆ 40 Shepherd FA. Chemotherapy for non-small cell lung cancer: have we reached a new plateau? *Semin Oncol* 1999; **26**: 3–11.

● 41 A Medical Research Council (MRC) randomised trial of palliative radiotherapy with two fractions or a single fraction in patients with inoperable non-small-cell lung cancer (NSCLC) and poor performance status. Medical Research Council Lung Cancer Working Party. *Br J Cancer* 1992; **65**: 934–41.

● 42 Inoperable non-small-cell lung cancer (NSCLC): a Medical Research Council randomised trial of palliative radiotherapy with two fractions or ten fractions. Report to the Medical Research Council by its Lung Cancer Working Party. *Br J Cancer* 1991; **63**: 265–70.

43 Kramer GW, Gans S, Ullmann E, *et al.* Hypofractionated external beam radiotherapy as retreatment for symptomatic non-small-cell lung carcinoma: an effective treatment? *Int J Radiat Oncol Biol Phys* 2004; **58**: 1388–93.

● 44 Falk SJ, Girling DJ, White RJ, *et al.* Medical Research Council Lung Cancer Working Party. Immediate versus delayed palliative thoracic radiotherapy in patients with unresectable locally advanced non-small-cell lung cancer and minimal thoracic symptoms: randomised controlled trial. *BMJ* 2002; **325**: 465.

45 Reddy SP, Marks JE. Total atelectasis of the lung secondary to malignant airway obstruction. Response to radiation therapy. *Am J Clin Oncol* 1990; **13**: 394–400.

46 Kelly JF, Delclos ME, Morice RC, *et al.* High-dose-rate endobronchial brachytherapy effectively palliates symptoms due to airway tumors: the 10-year M. D. Anderson cancer center experience. *Int J Radiat Oncol Biol Phys* 2000; **48**: 697–702.

✱ 47 Macbeth F, Toy E, Coles B, *et al.* Palliative radiotherapy regimens for non-small cell lung cancer. *Cochrane Database Syst Rev* 2001; **3**: CD002143.

✱ 48 Toy E, Macbeth F, Coles B, *et al.* Palliative thoracic radiotherapy for non-small-cell lung cancer: a systematic review. *Am J Clin Oncol* 2003; **26**: 112–20.

◆ 49 Socinski MA. The role of chemotherapy in the treatment of unresectable stage III and IV nonsmall cell lung cancer. *Respir Care Clin North Am* 2003; **9**: 207–36.

50 Onsrud M, Hagen B, Strickert T. 10-Gy single-fraction pelvic irradiation for palliation and life prolongation in patients with cancer of the cervix and corpus uteri. *Gynecol Oncol* 2001; **82**: 167–71.

51 Chafe W, Fowler WC, Currie JL, *et al.* Single-fraction palliative pelvic radiation therapy in gynecologic oncology: 1,000 rads. *Am J Obstet Gynecol* 1984; **148**: 701–5.

52 Halle JS, Rosenman JG, Varia MA, *et al.* 1000 cGy single dose palliation for advanced carcinoma of the cervix or endometrium. *Int J Radiat Oncol Biol Phys* 1986; **12**: 1947–50.

● 53 Spanos WJ Jr, Wasserman T, Meoz R, *et al.* Palliation of advanced pelvic malignant disease with large fraction pelvic radiation and misonidazole: final report of RTOG phase I/II study. *Int J Radiat Oncol Biol Phys* 1987; **13**: 1479–82.

● 54 Spanos W Jr, Guse C, Perez C, *et al.* Phase II study of multiple daily fractionations in the palliation of advanced pelvic malignancies: preliminary report of RTOG 8502. *Int J Radiat Oncol Biol Phys* 1989; **17**: 659–61.

55 Spanos WJ Jr, Pajak TJ, Emami B, *et al.* Radiation palliation of cervical cancer. *J Natl Cancer Inst Monogr* 1996; **21**: 127–30.

● 56 Spanos WJ Jr, Clery M, Perez CA, *et al.* Late effect of multiple daily fraction palliation schedule for advanced pelvic malignancies (RTOG 8502). *Int J Radiat Oncol Biol Phys* 1994; **29**: 961–7.

● 57 Duchesne GM, Bolger JJ, Griffiths GO, *et al.* A randomized trial of hypofractionated schedules of palliative radiotherapy in the management of bladder carcinoma: results of medical research council trial BA09. *Int J Radiat Oncol Biol Phys* 2000; **47**: 379–88.

58 Jose CC, Price A, Norman A, *et al.* Hypofractionated radiotherapy for patients with carcinoma of the bladder. *Clin Oncol (R Coll Radiol)* 1999; **11**: 330–3.

59 McLaren DB, Morrey D, Mason MD. Hypofractionated radiotherapy for muscle invasive bladder cancer in the elderly. *Radiother Oncol* 1997; **43**: 171–4.

60 Rostom AY, Tahir S, Gershuny AR, *et al.* Once weekly irradiation for carcinoma of the bladder. *Int J Radiat Oncol Biol Phys* 1996; **35**: 289–92.

61   Gelblum D, Mychalczak B, Almadrones L, *et al*. Palliative benefit of external-beam radiation in the management of platinum refractory epithelial ovarian carcinoma. *Gynecol Oncol* 1998; **69**: 36–41.

62   Tinger A, Waldron T, Peluso N, *et al*. Effective palliative radiation therapy in advanced and recurrent ovarian carcinoma. *Int J Radiat Oncol Biol Phys* 2001; **51**: 1256–63.

● 63   Crane CH, Janjan NA, Abbruzzese JL, *et al*. Effective pelvic symptom control using initial chemoradiation without colostomy in metastatic rectal cancer. *Int J Radiat Oncol Biol Phys* 2001; **49**: 107–16.

◆ 64   Wong R, Thomas G, Cummings B, *et al*. In search of a dose-response relationship with radiotherapy in the management of recurrent rectal carcinoma in the pelvis: a systematic review. *Int J Radiat Oncol Biol Phys* 1998; **40**: 437–46.

● 65   Mohanti BK, Umapathy H, Bahadur S, *et al*. Short course palliative radiotherapy of 20 Gy in 5 fractions for advanced and incurable head and neck cancer: AIIMS study. *Radiother Oncol* 2004; **71**: 275–80.

● 66   Calais G, Bardet E, Sire C, *et al*. Radiotherapy with concomitant weekly docetaxel for Stages III/IV oropharynx carcinoma. Results of the 98–02 GORTEC Phase II trial. *Int J Radiat Oncol Biol Phys* 2004; **58**: 161–6.

67   Hodson DI, Bruera E, Eapen L, *et al*. The role of palliative radiotherapy in advanced head and neck cancer. *Can J Oncol* 1996; **6**(Suppl 1): 54–60.

68   Sagar PM, Gauperaa T, Sue-Ling H, *et al*. An audit of the treatment of cancer of the oesophagus. *Gut* 1994; **35**: 941–5.

● 69   Polinder S, Homs MY, Siersema PD, Steyerberg EW, Dutch SIREC Study Group. Cost study of metal stent placement vs single-dose brachytherapy in the palliative treatment of oesophageal cancer. *Br J Cancer* 2004; **90**: 2067–72.

70   Hayter CR, Huff-Winters C, Paszat L, *et al*. A prospective trial of short-course radiotherapy plus chemotherapy for palliation of dysphagia from advanced esophageal cancer. *Radiother Oncol* 2000; **56**: 329–33.

71   Wong R, Davey P, DeBoer G, *et al*. Accelerated fractionation radiotherapy for the palliation of dysphagia in esophageal cancer–a university of Toronto study. *Int J Radiat Oncol Biol Phys* 2003; **57**: S219.

72   Sur RK, Donde B, Levin VC, Mannell A. Fractionated high dose rate intraluminal brachytherapy in palliation of advanced esophageal cancer. *Int J Radiat Oncol Biol Phys* 1998; **40**: 447–53.

73   Homs MYV, Essink-Bot M, Borsbom GJJM *et al*. Quality of life after palliative treatment for oesophageal carcinoma – a prospective comparison between stent placement and single dose brachytherapy. *Eur J Cancer* 2004; **40**: 1862–71.

74   Hoskin P, Makin W. Skin tumours. In: Hoskin P, Makin W, eds. *Oncology for Palliative Medicine*. Oxford: Oxford University Press, 2003: 235–43.

✱ 75   Ballo MT, Ang KK. Radiotherapy for cutaneous malignant melanoma: rationale and indications. *Oncology (Huntingt)* 2004; **18**: 99–107.

76   Johanson CR, Harwood AR, Cummings BJ, Quirt I. 0-7-21 radiotherapy in nodular melanoma. *Cancer* 1983; **51**: 226–32.

92

Cancer: chemotherapy

XIPENG WANG, JOHN J KAVANAGH

INTRODUCTION

In modern medicine, chemotherapy is one of the most important approaches for managing malignant disease, regardless of whether the goal of that management is cure or palliation of symptoms. However, nearly all forms of chemotherapy are associated with side effects, some of which can be serious or even life threatening, either in their own direct effects or indirectly if chemotherapy must be discontinued because of intolerable toxicity. The extent of toxicity depends both on the chemotherapeutic protocol and on the condition of the patient; poor nutritional status or cachexia, advanced age, and extent of organ involvement by primary or metastatic tumor can all affect the ability to tolerate chemotherapy.

Control of chemotherapy-related symptoms is a vital aspect of cancer therapy and an important clinical goal. Effective control of symptoms associated with chemotherapy, regardless of whether that therapy is delivered with curative or with palliative intent, can enhance the benefits to patients in terms of effectiveness, as the ability to tolerate chemotherapy increases the chances of completing planned regimens, as well as maintaining quality of life by diminishing adverse effects and protecting organ function. Hence, offering symptom-related palliation during cancer chemotherapy can help to guarantee that the chemotherapy is effective as well as enhancing the psychological and physiological state of the patients. Chemotherapy itself is increasingly being used for palliative care, the goal of which is not to prolong survival but rather to improve tumor-related symptoms, where the palliation/toxicity trade-off from treatment clearly favors symptom relief.[1]

The next section of this chapter will review some of the symptoms commonly associated with use of chemotherapeutic agents, with descriptions of efforts to address those symptoms or their underlying causes. The remainder of the chapter will describe principles for the use of chemotherapy for symptom control in advanced disease and the experience with palliative chemotherapy for lung, breast, prostate, and ovarian cancer.

SYMPTOMS RELATED TO USE OF CHEMOTHERAPY AGENTS

Fatigue

Fatigue is often cited by patients with malignancies as being a major obstacle to normal functioning and good quality of life. Between 70 percent and 80 percent of patients undergoing chemotherapy will experience fatigue.[2–5] Severe fatigue is almost universal with the use of biological response modifiers such as interferons and interleukins.[6,7] In cyclic chemotherapy, fatigue often peaks within a few days of the beginning of each cycle and declines until the next cycle is begun.[8–10] The etiology of chemotherapy-related fatigue, and factors that predispose patients to experience the more severe forms, are not well understood.

Strategies for managing fatigue should be based on educating patients about the nature of the fatigue and the available therapeutic options and anticipated outcomes, and on establishing a collaboration among patients, families, and medical professionals. For every patient receiving chemotherapy who is experiencing fatigue, we first assess the characteristics of the fatigue, such as its severity, patterns of onset, duration, and exacerbating and palliative factors. Next we evaluate possible contributing factors, including the underlying disease, the chemotherapeutic regimen and associated side effects of its component agents, sleep disturbances, and psychological factors such as depression. The third step is to correct any existing pathophysiological disorders such as anemia, electrolyte imbalances, myelosuppression, or organ dysfunction and to provide treatment for sleep disorders or psychological problems. Both pharmacological and nonpharmacological interventions are used as appropriate.[11***,12]

TREATMENT OF UNDERLYING CAUSES: ANEMIA

Some evidence exists that links chemotherapy-induced anemia with both fatigue and interference with quality of life. Two large, prospective, nonrandomized, community oncology trials evaluated the effectiveness of epoetin alfa for treating the anemia associated with cancer chemotherapy.[13,14] In those studies, more than 4000 patients with cancer were given epoetin alfa 10 000 units three times weekly for a maximum of 16 weeks. If the hemoglobin level had not increased by at least 1.0 g/dL at 4 weeks, the dose was increased to 20 000 units three times weekly. Overall, patients experienced significant improvements in energy level, activity level, functional status, and quality of life. These improvements were independent of antitumor response and correlated significantly with hemoglobin levels.

PHARMACOLOGICAL INTERVENTIONS

A few randomized controlled trials have been done to test pharmacological therapies for cancer-related (if not strictly chemotherapy-related) fatigue.[15,16] Three classes of drug have been used for cancer-related fatigue: psychostimulants, antidepressants, and corticosteroids. Psychostimulants (e.g. methylphenidate, pemoline, or dextroamfetamine) or antidepressants (e.g. selective serotonin reuptake inhibitors, tricyclics [nortriptyline, desipramine], or bupropion) can sometimes induce increases in energy that seem disproportionate to changes in mood. Methylphenidate has been the most extensively evaluated of the central nervous system (CNS) stimulants and often is the first drug given for cancer-related fatigue. Regimens usually begin with 5–10 mg taken once or twice daily, with the dose increased as needed to control the fatigue. Most patients seem to require less than 60 mg per day. Adverse effects such as anorexia, insomnia, tremulousness, anxiety, or delirium have been rare. Corticosteroids such as dexamethasone or prednisone have been given in low doses to control fatigue in patients with advanced cancer, but no comparative trials have been done for chemotherapy-related fatigue. Empirical therapy with selective serotonin reuptake inhibitors may be useful for fatigue that does not respond to psychostimulants or corticosteroids, but no randomized trials have been conducted and little information is available regarding use of these drugs for patients who are not depressed.[17]

NONPHARMACOLOGICAL INTERVENTIONS

Nonpharmacological management strategies for chemotherapy-related fatigue can be useful, particularly if they are used in combination with education and counseling to patients and their families. Moderate exercise can be beneficial in relieving fatigue,[18,19] as can counseling on modifying activity and sleep patterns and stress management techniques.

Nausea, vomiting, and retching

The triad of nausea, vomiting, and retching (NVR) is both a common and a greatly feared side effect of antineoplastic chemotherapy that can significantly affect daily functioning, quality of life, and compliance with therapy.[20] The mechanism of chemotherapy-related NVR probably involves stimulation of the chemoreceptor trigger zone (CTZ) in the area postrema of the cerebral cortex, which is sensitive to emetic toxins in the cerebrospinal fluid and blood. Several chemotherapeutic agents in current use are quite emetogenic; carmustine, cisplatin, cyclophosphamide, cytarabine, mechlorethamine, melphalan, and streptozocin, for example, can induce NVR in up to 90 percent of patients.

Management strategies for NVR rely on identifying both the causative agent and the pattern of expression of symptoms. Dopamine, acetylcholine, histamine, serotonin (5-hydroxytryptamine [5-HT]), and, most recently, substance P and other neurokinins have been implicated in NVR, and receptor antagonists, particularly those to 5-HT$_3$ and neurokinin-1, are being tested for their ability to reduce or eliminate chemotherapy-related NVR. Typical patterns of NVR have been classified as acute (occurring within 24 hours of treatment), delayed (occurring more than 24 hours after treatment), or anticipatory (occurring before, during, or after treatment). Anticipatory NVR is a conditioned response that can be linked to visual, gustatory, olfactory, and environmental factors. Attempts to manage chemotherapy-related NVR have included both pharmacological and nonpharmacological interventions.

PHARMACOLOGICAL INTERVENTIONS

5-HT$_3$ receptor antagonists

Use of 5-HT$_3$ receptor antagonists has significantly improved the management of NVR, particularly when such agents are given in combination with dexamethasone.[21] Granisetron, ondansetron, and dolasetron are widely used in the USA for preventing chemotherapy-related NVR; these agents are effective for acute NVR, but most studies have failed to show a benefit for delayed NVR.[22***] The most common dosages are as follows:[23]

- dolasetron – 100 mg per oral (PO) or intravenously (IV), given once
- granisetron – 1–2 mg PO, given once, or 8 mg given IV once
- ondansetron – 16–24 mg PO given once or 8 mg PO every 12 hours for 2 doses.

Clinical experience indicates that the antiemetic efficacy of 5-HT$_3$ antagonists (given as single-agent therapy or in combination with dexamethasone) is not always maintained over multiple chemotherapy cycles. Moreover, failure to control delayed NVR from previous chemotherapy cycles can adversely affect antiemetic effectiveness during the acute phase of current cycles.[24] One randomized study showed that use of 5-HT$_3$ receptor antagonists before chemotherapy could reduce the incidence of post-treatment vomiting but had no effect on the duration of post-treatment vomiting or the incidence of anticipatory nausea or vomiting.[25]

Other antiemetic agents

Neurokinin receptor antagonists are being studied for the prevention of chemotherapy-related NVR owing to the possible involvement of substance P, which is secreted by the gastrointestinal tract and is a ligand for neurokinin receptors, in NVR. Neurokinin receptor antagonists, given in combination with dexamethasone, may be more effective than 5-HT$_3$ receptor antagonists for preventing delayed NVR after chemotherapy;[26] a neurokinin-1 receptor antagonist, aprepitant, was recently approved for use in combination with dexamethasone and 5-HT$_3$ receptor antagonists for this indication and is currently in phase III trials.[27] Metoclopramide, the prototype substituted benzamide (a selective dopamine antagonist), has also shown modest effectiveness in some but not all studies.

NONPHARMACOLOGICAL INTERVENTIONS

Acupuncture and acupressure may have some modest effects on chemotherapy-induced NVR.[28] Some types of behavioral modification skills may also be helpful.[29] Other possible interventions include modifying the patients' diet and environment so as to diminish visual, auditory, and olfactory stimuli that initiate nausea. Other treatments such as music therapy and progressive muscle relaxation may also be helpful in inducing relaxation and reducing anxiety.

Gastrointestinal effects: diarrhea and constipation

Both cancer and chemotherapy can affect bowel function and lead to diarrhea or constipation. Chemotherapeutic agents that often cause bowel hyperreactivity and diarrhea include capecitabine, cytarabine, dactinomycin, 5-azacytidine, fluorouracil, hydroxyurea, irinotecan, methotrexate, mitotane, raltitrexed, and topotecan. Chemotherapy-related diarrhea is managed pharmacologically with loperamide with a 4 mg starting dose, to be followed by 2 mg after each episode, for 12 mg or more per day.[30] Persistent diarrhea requires interventions to minimize the further complications of dehydration, electrolyte imbalance, weakness, decreased caloric intake, and weight loss. Octreotide has been successful in treating chemotherapy-related diarrhea that is refractory to other forms of therapy. Recommendations for supportive care include eating a low-residue diet of high protein

and caloric content; avoiding consumption of irritating or stimulating foods and beverages; consuming foods and liquids that are high in potassium (e.g. asparagus, bananas, Gatorade); drinking at least 3 L of noncarbonated fluid each day; eating small and frequent meals; and resuming consumption of milk products slowly after the symptoms subside.[31]

Constipation, in contrast, is associated mainly with the vinca alkaloids, and the clinical emphasis is on prevention rather than treatment. Dietary changes and use of bulk laxatives are usually insufficient, and a prophylactic bowel program is recommended.[31] Senna compounds, anthraquinone cathartics that stimulate longitudinal peristalsis in the colon, have been consistently shown to prevent or reverse opioid-induced constipation. If use of such compounds does not result in bowel movements, more aggressive therapy is indicated with rectal suppositories or osmotic laxatives with saline, sorbitol, or lactulose.

Stomatitis

Oral mucositis is another common complication of cancer chemotherapy, occurring in approximately 40 percent of patients receiving standard-dose chemotherapy. The severity varies, but severe (grade 3–4) oral or gastrointestinal mucositis increases the risk of bleeding, susceptibility to infection, and the need for hospitalization. The agents most commonly associated with mucositis are dactinomycin, daunorubicin, docetaxel, paclitaxel, doxorubicin, fluorouracil, methotrexate, raltitrexed, and high-dose busulfan, etoposide, melphalan, and thiotepa.

Principles for managing oral mucositis are to maintain the integrity of the oral mucosa, prevent secondary infection, provide pain relief, and allow adequate dietary intake to be maintained. Preventive oral care should begin in tandem with the chemotherapy so as to prevent or minimize oral complications.[32] Patients with evidence of mucositis can benefit from oral oxygen therapy, delivered every 2 hours or every hour if mucositis is severe; oral infections can be treated with topical antifungal or antiviral agents. Serious oral ulcerations can be treated with topical or systemic analgesics and topical protective agents.[33]

Anorexia

Chemotherapeutic agents can directly or indirectly lead to loss of appetite and anorexia through the induction of nausea and vomiting, stomatitis, diarrhea, or constipation.[34] Pharmacological management strategies for anorexia include the use of megestrol acetate and steroids. Megestrol acetate (given in suspension in doses of 480–840 mg/day) has led to significant improvements in appetite.[35] Steroids can also be helpful in treating anorexia. Nonpharmacological treatment strategies are to assess nutritional intake and physiological nutritional status, consider patients' likes and dislikes regarding food and fluids, encourage consumption of small, frequent meals consisting of foods that the patients enjoy, use of nutritional supplements that are high in protein and calories, and control of symptoms, particularly nausea and vomiting.

Cutaneous reactions

Cancer chemotherapy can also lead to skin changes such as dermatitis, nail changes, hyperpigmentation, urticaria, acral erythema, and photosensitivity reactions. Most cutaneous reactions are self-limited, lasting only as long as the chemotherapy. Rashes and erythema can occur with a variety of chemotherapy drugs, including carboplatin, aminoglutethimide, carmustine, cytarabine, daunorubicin, methotrexate, and trimetrexate, among others. Palmar–plantar erythrodysesthesia, characterized by demarcated, tender erythematous plaques on the palms and soles of the feet, can range from mild to extremely painful; this syndrome is associated with use of cyclophosphamide, cytarabine, docetaxel, doxorubicin, liposomal doxorubicin, capecitabine, etoposide, fluorouracil, hydroxyurea, lomustine, mercaptopurine, methotrexate, mitotane, and paclitaxel. Management is focused on prevention and on pain relief with systemic and local therapies as needed. Extravasation of chemotherapeutic agents from vessels into the interstitium and surrounding tissue can produce local skin burning, erythema, pain, edema, induration, ulceration, and necrosis; symptoms can occur immediately or not appear for days or weeks after the chemotherapy. Extravasation of some agents, e.g. dactinomycin, daunorubicin, doxorubicin, epirubicin, idarubicin, and mitomycin, can cause long-term skin injury, whereas others such as carmustine, cisplatin, etoposide, fluorouracil, mechlorethamine, plicamycin, vinblastine, vincristine, and vinorelbine tend to cause short-lasting skin injury. Extravasation of vinca alkaloids (vinblastine, vincristine, vindesine) should be treated with hyaluronidase and local heat; extravasation or skin irritation from any of the other agents should be treated with 15–20-minute applications of ice at least four times a day during the 24–48 hours of chemotherapy.

Cardiopulmonary toxicity

The severity of pulmonary toxicity from chemotherapy varies widely, ranging from mild asymptomatic episodes to life-threatening respiratory insufficiency. The predominant clinical patterns range from interstitial pneumonitis with pulmonary fibrosis to acute hypersensitivity, noncardiogenic pulmonary edema, or acute pulmonary syndromes.[36] Common symptoms include tachypnea, dyspnea, cough, chills, and myalgia. Drugs with pulmonary toxicity include bleomycin, carmustine, mitomycin C, cyclophosphamide and other alkylating agents, vinca alkaloids, doxorubicin, methotrexate, procarbazine, cytarabine, gemcitabine, retinoic acid, and some biological agents (e.g. interleukin-2).

Acute pulmonary toxicity, which often manifests as acute shortness of breath, can result from the combination of mitomycin C and a vinca alkaloid. Onset can occur within 2 hours of receiving a vinca alkaloid with or without concomitant administration of mitomycin C. Symptoms include severe tachypnea and dyspnea, possibly with wheezing, rales, and rhonchi. Chest X-rays may show bilateral infiltrates and pleural effusions. Patients being given this combination of drugs should be monitored for the appearance of pulmonary symptoms during the first 2 hours of treatment. If symptoms appear, the chemotherapeutic agents should be discontinued immediately and supportive measures such as oxygen, bronchodilators, or corticosteroids provided. Chest-X ray, blood gases, and electrocardiogram should be obtained and psychological counseling provided if necessary. Cytarabine, cyclophosphamide, methotrexate, mitomycin are also associated with pulmonary toxicity, although this reaction is less common.[37] Docetaxel can produce fluid retention, which can result in pulmonary edema, or pleural effusion.

Cardiomyopathy is the most common form of chemotherapy-associated cardiac toxicity. Other less common cardiac reactions include myocardial ischemia, pericarditis, arrhythmias, miscellaneous electrocardiographic changes, and angina. Doxorubicin and other anthracyclines are the most likely to cause cardiomyopathy, which is both cumulative and dose related. Other chemotherapeutic agents that can lead to cardiomyopathy include cyclophosphamide, ifosfamide, fluorouracil, paclitaxel, etoposide, amsacrine, vinca alkaloids, and some biological agents (interferon alfa or gamma, interleukin-2). Doxorubicin produces intracellular free radicals that can damage the myocardial membrane. Given its cumulative toxicity, the probability of developing congestive heart failure after doxorubicin increases from about 3 percent at $400\,\mathrm{mg/m^2}$ to 18 percent at $700\,\mathrm{mg/m^2}$.[38] Patients with severely reduced left ventricular ejection fraction (i.e. less than 30 percent) should not be treated with anthracyclines; further, anthracyclines should be discontinued in any patient whose left ventricular ejection fraction declines by 10–15 percent during the course of treatment.[36] Management of anthracycline cardiotoxicity is based on prevention and early detection. Cardiac function should be assessed before treatment is begun and monitored during and after therapy by multigated acquisition (MUGA) scanning or echocardiography. Long-term follow-up monitoring is also recommended. Management of chemotherapy-induced cardiac dysfunction is the same as conventional therapy for heart failure.

Bladder toxicity

Contact with acrolein, the major metabolic byproduct of cyclophosphamide and ifosfamide, can cause mucosal erythema, inflammation, ulceration, necrosis, and diffuse small-vessel hemorrhagic oozing, particularly in the bladder mucosa. Standard doses of cyclophosphamide, especially those given orally, produce bladder toxicity in less than 10 percent of cases. High-dose cyclophosphamide, on the other hand, puts patients at high risk of developing hemorrhagic cystitis,[39] the symptoms of which are hematuria and dysuria. Pharmacological treatment is with mesna, which binds acrolein and reduces its toxic effects on the bladder mucosa, as well as discontinuation of chemotherapy and hydration. Fulguration (cautery) may be necessary to stop the bleeding in some cases.

Neuropathy

Neurotoxicity is most commonly associated with vinca alkaloids, paclitaxel, cisplatin, and high-dose cyclophosphamide.[40] Central nervous system neurotoxicity can manifest as encephalopathy, seizures, cerebellar dysfunctions, ophthalmological or ototoxicity, and mental status changes; peripheral manifestations can include peripheral neuropathies with sensory or motor dysfunctions. The only effective therapy is discontinuation of the causative chemotherapy agent.

PALLIATIVE CHEMOTHERAPY

Despite its own side effects, chemotherapy can be effective in palliative as well as curative treatment, depending on the type and stage of malignancy. Palliative chemotherapy is, by definition, not intended to cure, but increasing evidence suggests that it can reduce morbidity related to the malignancy, particularly that of metastatic disease that involves or impinges on vital organs. Tumor shrinkage induced by palliative chemotherapy has shown some benefit in terms of reducing pain, dyspnea, coughing, metabolic abnormalities, and bleeding in the bowel and genital tract. These and other symptoms can be controlled to some extent by reducing tumor involving the bronchial tract or bowel, by stabilizing hypercalcemia, and by relieving pressure on vital organs. The mechanisms by which chemotherapeutic agents relieve pain are not well understood, but cytotoxic drugs that alter peripheral nerve function and can cross the blood–brain barrier could affect neurotransmitter function in both the central and peripheral and central nervous systems, which could influence pain and other symptoms independent of their effect on the tumor.

Key to the success of palliative chemotherapy for patients with advanced disease is that everyone – the patient, the family, and the physician – understand the purpose of the treatment in terms of the kinds of response that can be expected, particularly with regard to survival. In one study of patients with metastatic colon or lung cancer, those who believed that they had a significant chance of dying within 6 months were less likely to choose a possibly life-extending therapy over comfort care; specifically, if the likelihood of 6-month survival was stated to be 90 percent, 75 percent, 25 percent, or 10 percent, the corresponding proportions

of patients who would choose life-extending therapy were 51 percent, 29 percent, 31 percent, and 21 percent. Finally, patients in that study tended to overestimate their chances of surviving for 6 months relative to the estimates of their physicians.[41]

The possibility of palliative chemotherapy benefit varies among cancer types based on relative sensitivities to systemic chemotherapy. Tumors with low, moderate, and high sensitivity are listed in Table 92.1. For patients in group I, who are even in late stage, the opportunity of palliative chemotherapy should not be missed. Tumors in group II are not curable by chemotherapy once disease has disseminated. Some patients with small cell lung cancer (SCLC) and ovarian cancer might get the benefit of prolongation of comfortable life and increased quality of life. So systemic chemotherapy should be considered in this group of patients, which is dependent on patient preference and physical condition. Patients in group III have disseminated disease and tumor insensitive to chemotherapy. Palliative care is a difficult objective. Careful clinical decision making is necessary. However, in one randomized trial of chemotherapy in patients with advanced nonsmall cell lung cancer (NSCLC), the patients not only had an increased chance of prolonged survival (albeit only for a few months) but also required less hospital care and palliative radiotherapy.[42] Indeed, another similar study showed modest benefit in NSCLC.[43] Patients with group III tumors who have a good performance status should be given the opportunity to participate in clinical trials.

Another key question concerns when to consider starting palliative chemotherapy and how long that therapy should last. When curative therapy is not possible, as is the case for most metastatic malignancies, then multiple factors must be weighed in this decision. If the goal of palliative chemotherapy is to relieve or prevent tumor-induced symptoms, then it should be considered when patients are either experiencing symptoms or expected to develop symptoms shortly. Decisions in the latter case, when patients may have low-volume disease in nonvital organs or areas, can be quite difficult. The possible benefit in terms of tumor response must be weighed carefully against the toxicity of the chemotherapy. In some cases, close monitoring could allow treatment to be withheld until symptomatic progression becomes evident or imminent. For some chemosensitive tumors, chemotherapy could be the sole treatment modality for relieving symptoms, even in oncological emergencies such as superior vena cava syndrome, epidural spinal cord compression, or airway obstruction. On the other hand, chemoresistant tumors may be more appropriately managed by local treatment such as radiotherapy or surgery.[44] Stable disease can be very hard to manage; slow-growing tumors that are resistant to chemotherapy may not demonstrate apparent growth until after many months of treatment. It can be difficult to determine whether tumors are merely slow-growing or whether they are responding to the chemotherapy. If the treatment is not associated with significant side effects, it would be

Table 92.1 *Response of advanced or disseminated cancers to systemic chemotherapy*

Group I	Group II	Group III
Highly sensitive – systemic therapy must be considered	Sensitive – systemic therapy	Low sensitivity – poor response
Germ cell tumors	Prostate cancer	Esophageal cancer
Testicle	Breast cancer	Nonsmall cell lung cancer
Choriocarcinoma	Small cell lung cancer	Melanoma
Acute lymphocytic leukemia	Chronic myelogenous leukemia	Renal cell cancer
Acute myelogenous leukemia	Ovarian cancer	Pancreatic cancer
Pediatric tumors	Bladder cancer	Hepatocellular cancer
Ewing sarcoma	Endometrial cancer	
Wilm tumor	Neuroendocrine cancer	
Rhabdomyosarcoma	Kaposi sarcoma	
Lymphomas	Multiple myeloma	
Hodgkin disease	Neuroblastoma	
Non-Hodgkin lymphoma	Gastric carcinoma	
	Cervical carcinoma	
	Head and neck cancer	
	Colorectal cancer	

reasonable to discuss with the patient the possibility of discontinuing treatment until the tumor shows some progression and then resuming treatment at that time. The experience with use of palliative chemotherapy for various types of advanced disease is described briefly below.

Lung cancer

Nonsmall cell lung cancer is a cruel disease for which few treatments are effective in terms of cure and quality of life becomes quite poor as the disease progresses. Four prospective randomized trials have been conducted that compared single-agent palliative chemotherapy (with vinorelbine, gemcitabine, docetaxel, or paclitaxel) with supportive care for patients with previously treated or untreated NSCLC.[45**,46**,47**,48**] In these studies, vinorelbine or gemcitabine led to substantial improvements in quality of life and reductions in disease-related symptoms relative to supportive care. Treatment with paclitaxel or docetaxel not only led to improved quality of life but also extended overall survival time and time to disease progression. Other drugs may also be effective in palliating symptoms of NSCLC; irinotecan can reduce symptoms and prolong survival, and gefitinib (Iressa®), an epidermal growth factor receptor tyrosine kinase inhibitor, was shown in a phase I study to extend the disease-free interval and survival time as well as improving quality of life in patients with NSCLC.[49*]

Breast cancer

Palliative chemotherapy can lead to remarkable improvement in symptoms for some, but not all, women with metastatic breast cancer. Agents like docetaxel, epirubicin, capecitabine, and trastuzumab (Herceptin®) can be used for metastatic breast cancer as well as for earlier-stage disease. Perhaps not surprisingly, patients with metastatic breast cancer who responded to palliative chemotherapy are more likely to conclude that the treatment was worthwhile regardless of its toxicity. The introduction of taxanes has greatly influenced the treatment approach for breast cancer that recurs or progresses after anthracycline chemotherapy. Docetaxel in particular has been shown to extend the time to progression and overall survival time, and to alleviate malignancy-related symptoms, with improvements in quality of life comparable with those from vinblastine plus mitomycin[50**] or vinorelbine.[51**] Several approaches to palliative chemotherapy are currently being tested. In one study, the response rate and survival time were significantly higher, and pain control, mobility, and anxiety improved more, in a group given high-dose chemotherapy than in a group given lower-dose chemotherapy, despite the greater toxicity of the higher-dose regimen.[52] Other approaches involve comparing the use of single agents in sequence versus in combinations. One study showed that patients given single-agent epirubicin followed by single-agent mitomycin had similar survival time but less treatment-related toxicity and better quality of life than did patients given cyclophosphamide plus epirubicin plus cyclophosphamide followed by mitomycin plus vinblastine sulfate.[53**] Another approach, intermittent therapy, seeks to minimize treatment toxicity by discontinuing treatment after remission is achieved and beginning again when disease reappears; however, some authors have found intermittent therapy to be associated with poor physical wellbeing, mood, appetite, and quality of life.

Table 92.2 *Common paraneoplastic syndromes and associated cancers*

Paraneoplastic syndrome	Cancer type
Hypercalcemia	All types of lung cancer; breast cancer; multiple myeloma
Syndrome of inappropriate antidiuresis	Small cell lung cancer; carcinoid tumors; cancer of esophagus, pancreas, duodenum, colon, adrenal cortex, and prostate; thymomas; lymphomas
Cushing syndrome (adrenocorticotropic hormone, corticotropic hormone)	Primary adrenal tumors, pituitary adenoma, and all types of lung cancer
Hypocalcemia	Osteoblastic metastases of breast, prostate, and lung
Hypophosphatemia	Mesenchymal tumors
Hyperthyroidism	Gestational trophoblastic disease; testicular tumors
Acromegaly	Pancreatic islet cell tumors; bronchial carcinoids
Calcitoninemia	Medullary thyroid carcinoma; small cell lung cancer; carcinoid; breast cancer; colon cancer; gastric cancer
Extrapancreatic hypoglycemia	Fibrosarcomas; mesotheliomas; hepatomas; adrenal cortical carcinoma; gastrointestinal adenocarcinomas

Prostate cancer

Metastatic prostate cancer embodies some of the classic difficulties in clinical decision making regarding when (or whether) to institute palliative treatment and balancing the toxicity of treatments with the potential benefits. Metastatic prostate cancer usually occurs in older men, many of whom have other medical problems or are in otherwise poor physical condition. Some evidence exists to suggest that changes in serum prostate-specific antigen level may reflect the tumor's response to chemotherapy; in some studies, reductions of more than 50 percent correlated with improved survival and control of symptoms, but smaller declines have not been associated with clinically meaningful results. Some well-designed phase III studies have shown that palliative chemotherapy can be beneficial in hormone-refractory prostate cancer. Glucocorticoids can also be effective in some cases; in one study, mitoxantrone given with hydrocortisone or prednisone yielded modest improvements in quality of life compared with glucocorticoids alone.

Ovarian cancer

Ovarian cancer has become the fourth most common cancer in developed countries, and in most cases disease is advanced at diagnosis. During the past 20 years, use of platinum-based and taxane-based chemotherapy regimens have led to improved overall 5-year survival rates and longer disease-free intervals for women with advanced ovarian cancer. Chemotherapy can be useful for reducing the common symptoms of bloating or abdominal fullness, particularly in cases when surgery is contraindicated. In one study, palliative carboplatin was more effective in improving quality of life and relieving tumor-related symptoms than was cisplatin for patients with relapsed ovarian cancer.[54] In

endometrioid ovarian cancer, oral megestrol acetate has shown definite activity in patients with platinum-refractory disease, with only minimal toxicity and fair quality of life during treatment.[55] Deciding when to provide palliative chemotherapy versus a second challenge with platinum compounds, whether to use single agents or combinations of agents, and whether to use concomitant versus sequential therapy is particularly difficult in relapsed ovarian cancer. In one study conducted at an outpatient clinic, patients with ovarian cancer (as opposed to other types of gynecological cancer) for whom therapy was prolonged and who had little education and little social support showed the most significant impairments in quality of life and needed the most additional support and resources.[56]

Paraneoplastic syndromes

Under various conditions, patients with advanced malignancy could present diverse endocrine and metabolic disorders. Primary cancerous and metastatic sites initiate pathological effects through the excess or lack production of hormones, cytokines, and growth factors, the so called 'paraneoplastic syndromes'. Table 92.2 lists the most frequent paraneoplastic syndromes and associated cancer types.

Hypercalcemia is the most frequent metabolic disorder, and it is estimated that as many as 8–10 percent of patients with malignancy will present this disorder during their disease course. Two mechanisms contribute to the development of hypercalcemia in most patients with malignancy: osteolytic hypercalcemia (tumor invasion of bone tissues releases large amounts of calcium from destroyed areas of bone) and humoral hypercalcemia. Parathyroid hormone-related protein (PTHrP), tumor necrosis factor α, interleukin (IL)-1, prostaglandin E, and IL-6, which are produced by tumor tissue, may increase the level of calcium, in particular

PTHrP may mimic the role of parathyroid hormone in calcium metabolism.[57**,58] Renal tubular reabsorption of filtered calcium is increased in addition to the increased generalized osteoclastic activity throughout the skeleton. Although the diagnosis of hypercalcemia is not very difficult, it is often delayed. The symptoms of hypercalcemia are often vague and nonspecific. Furthermore, there is poor correlation between calcium level and degree of symptomatology. The most common symptoms include nausea, anorexia, vomiting, constipation, cramping abdominal pain, and bone pain, which are frequently thought of as symptoms of advanced malignancy and overlooked. Patients with symptomatic hypercalcemia should be managed in an emergent manner. Most patients are severely dehydrated, so immediate fluid resuscitation is indicted. Bisphosphonates are the most frequently used antiresorptive agents. These interfere with osteoclast function and inhibit calcium release from bone. If hypercalcemia does not respond adequately to the above approaches, loop diuretics can be administered for severe hypercalcemia that fails to respond. Calcitonin (6–8 IU/kg every 6–12 hours subcutaneously or intramuscularly) should be added to the regimen (see also Chapter 84). The role of palliative chemotherapy in controlling hypercalcemia is not well understood because no such clinical trials have been performed as yet. Chemotherapy could be directed at removal of the source of the hypercalcemia.

Syndrome of inappropriate antidiuretic hormone secretion (SIADH) is most commonly associated with SCLC. The abnormal production of ADH or ADH-like substances by cancer cells may result in an increase in intravascular volume, enhancing renal perfusion and decreasing proximal tubular resorption of sodium. The treatment of the underlying cancer is the most effective management of ectopic serious SIADH. Administration of systemic chemotherapy is associated with an improvement in this syndrome within 6 weeks of treatment in 80 percent of patients with SCLC.[59] Supportive management also may be undertaken while awaiting a response to the treatment of the underlying cancer.

Cancer associated with Cushing syndrome could be classified into endogenous and ectopic Cushing syndrome. The former includes excessive production of glucocorticoid by a primary adrenal neoplasm and overproduction of adrenocorticotropic hormone (ACTH) by a pituitary adenoma. Ectopic Cushing syndrome implies increased production of ACTH or corticotropic hormone (CRH) is from the tumor. There are subtle clinical differences between the two types of Cushing syndrome. The treatment of the underlying malignancy is the primary management of paraneoplastic Cushing syndrome. Symptom control in hypercortisolism can be accomplished with the use of steroid synthesis inhibitors, such as ketoconazole, mitotane, metyrapone, and aminoglutethimide.

Increasing knowledge of the pathology of cancer and the body's response to disease will improve our understanding of the mechanisms underlying paraneoplastic syndromes. Overall, the principal aim of management is to treat the underlying cancer disease and control the symptoms associated with metabolic disorders.

SUMMARY

Use of chemotherapy, whether for curative or palliative purposes, requires balancing the likelihood of the intended effect with the adverse effects of the treatment. By controlling the symptoms associated with toxicity, one can ensure that patients are able to complete the treatment – whether curative or palliative – as planned. Used effectively, palliative chemotherapy can control tumor-related symptoms and sustain good physiological and psychological functions; its ultimate objective is to maintain patients' quality of life at the highest possible level. Certainly in the past attention was focused solely on curing the disease, with the 'objective' endpoints of clinical (and pathologic) tumor response, the length of the progression-free interval, and overall survival – none of which take into account the importance of the patient's quality of life during and after the treatment process. As one author in 1996 put it, 'Palliative care is a vast wasteland in American medicine, and nowhere is it less well understood or more neglected than in the academic health science center'.[60] Thankfully, things have changed since then. Palliative care is coming to be understood as an important part of the entire range of traditional cancer management – surgery, chemotherapy, radiotherapy, or biotherapy – and palliation of symptoms has a role in therapy intended to be curative as well. Nowadays the term 'palliative chemotherapy' is no longer considered a contradiction in terms. Overall, oncologists should not overlook the possibility of palliative chemotherapy; more clinical trials should be designed with the endpoint of relieving symptoms rather than curing disease. Such trials represent substantial challenges for appropriate design and conduct, but they will ultimately allow clinicians to provide better care for patients with cancer.

Key learning points

- Control of chemotherapy-related symptoms is a vital aspect of cancer treatment.

- Chemotherapy-related toxicity affects almost all the systems in the human body.

- The goal of palliative chemotherapy is to relieve or prevent tumor-induced symptoms.

- The relative sensitivities to systemic chemotherapy determine the possibility of palliative chemotherapy.

- What is the most appropriate chemotherapeutic regimen for different types of cancer is not known.

REFERENCES

◆ 1 Archer VR, Billingham LJ, Cullen MH. Palliative chemotherapy: no longer a contradiction in terms *Oncologist* 1999; **4**: 470–7.

2 Cella D, Peterman A, Passik S, *et al.* Progress toward guidelines for the management of fatigue. *Oncology* 1998; **12**: 1–9.

◆ 3 Portenoy RK, Thaler HT, Kornblith AB, *et al.* Pain in ovarian cancer: prevalence, characteristics, and associated symptoms. *Cancer* 1994; **74**: 907–15.

● 4 Yellen SB, Cella DF, Webster MA, *et al.* Measuring fatigue and other anemia-related symptoms with Functional Assessment of Cancer Therapy (FACT) measurement system. *J Pain Symptom Manage* 1997; **13**: 63–74.

● 5 Yogelzang N, Breibart W, Cella D, *et al.* Patient, caregiver, and oncologist perceptions of cancer-related fatigue: results of a tripart assessment survey. *Semin Hematol* 1997; **34**(Suppl 2): 4–12.

6 Dean GE, Spears L, Ferrell B, *et al.* Fatigue in patients with cancer receiving interferon alpha. *Cancer Pract* 1995; **3**: 164–71.

7 Piper BF, Rieger PT, Brophy L, *et al.* Recent advances in management of biotherapy-related side effects: fatigue. *Oncol Nurs Forum* 1989; **16**(Suppl 6): 27–34.

8 Berger A. Patterns of fatigue and activity and rest during adjuvant breast cancer chemotherapy. *Oncol Nurs Forum* 1998; **25**: 51–62.

9 Broeckel JA, Jacobsen PB, Horton J, *et al.* Characteristics and correlates of fatigue after adjuvant chemotherapy for breast cancer. *J Clin Oncol* 1998; **16**: 1689–96.

● 10 Richardson A, Ream E, Wilson-Barnett J. Fatigue in patients receiving chemotherapy: patterns of change. *Cancer Nurs* 1998; **21**: 17–30.

✱ 11 Portenoy RK, Itri L. Cancer-related fatigue: guidelines for evaluation and management. *Oncologist* 1999; **4**: 1–10.

12 Berger A. Treating fatigue in cancer patients. *Oncologist* 2003; **8**(Suppl): 10–14.

13 Glaspy J, Bukowski R, Steinberg D, *et al.* The impact of therapy with epoetin alfa on clinical outcomes during cancer chemotherapy in community oncology practice. *J Clin Oncol* 1997; **15**: 1218–34.

◆ 14 Demetri GD, Kris M, Wade J, *et al.* Quality-of-life benefit in chemotherapy patients treated with epoetin alfa is independent of disease response or tumor type: results from a prospective community oncology study. *J Clin Oncol* 1998; **16**: 3412–25.

● 15 Bruera E, Driver L, Barnes EA, *et al.* Patient-controlled methylphenidate for the management of fatigue in patients with advanced cancer: a preliminary report. *J Clin Oncol* 2003; **21**: 4439–43.

16 Sarhill N, Walsh D, Nelson KA, *et al.* Methylphenidate for fatigue in advanced cancer: a prospective open-label pilot study. *Am J Hosp Palliat Care* 2001; **18**: 187–92.

17 Caldwell PK. Anxiety medications in palliative care. *Am J Nurs* 2003; **103**: 15; author reply 15.

18 Dimeo F, Rumberger BG, Keul J. Aerobic exercise as therapy for cancer fatigue. *Med Sci Sports Exerc* 1998; **30**: 475–8.

19 Schwartz AL. Patterns of exercise and fatigue in physically active cancer survivors. *Oncol Nurs Forum* 1998; **25**: 485–91.

◆ 20 Osoba D, Zee B, Warr D, *et al.* Effect of postchemotherapy nausea and vomiting on health-related quality of life. The Quality of Life and Symptom Control Committees of the National Cancer Institute of Canada Clinical Trials Group. *Support Care Cancer* 1997; **5**: 307–13.

21 Goodin S, Cunningham R. 5-HT(3)-receptor antagonists for the treatment of nausea and vomiting: a reappraisal of their side-effect profile. *Oncologist* 2002; **7**: 424–36.

22 Hesketh PJ. Comparative review of 5-HT3 receptor antagonists in the treatment of acute chemotherapy-induced nausea and vomiting. *Cancer Invest* 2000; **18**: 163–73.

◆ 23 Rhodes VA, McDaniel RW. Nausea, vomiting, and retching: complex problems in palliative care. *CA Cancer J Clin* 2001; **51**: 232–48; quiz 49–52.

24 de Wit R, van den Berg H, Burghouts J, *et al.* Initial high anti-emetic efficacy of granisetron with dexamethasone is not maintained over repeated cycles. *Br J Cancer* 1998; **77**: 1487–91.

● 25 Morrow GR, Roscoe JA, Hynes HE, *et al.* Progress in reducing anticipatory nausea and vomiting: a study of community practice. *Support Care Cancer* 1998; **6**: 46–50.

26 Van Belle S, Lichinitser MR, Navari RM, *et al.* Prevention of cisplatin-induced acute and delayed emesis by the selective neurokinin-1 antagonists, L-758,298 and MK-869. *Cancer* 2002; **94**: 3032–41.

◆ 27 Hesketh PJ. New treatment options for chemotherapy-induced nausea and vomiting. *Support Care Cancer* 2004; **12**: 550–4.

28 Collins KB, Thomas DJ. Acupuncture and acupressure for the management of chemotherapy-induced nausea and vomiting. *J Am Acad Nurse Pract* 2004; **16**: 76–80.

29 King CR. Nonpharmacologic management of chemotherapy-induced nausea and vomiting. *Oncol Nurs Forum* 1997; **24**: 41–8.

◆ 30 Mercadante S. Diarrhea, malabsorption and constipation. In: Berger A, Portenoy R, Weissman D, eds. *Principles and Practice of Palliative and Supportive Oncology*, 2nd ed. Philadelphia: Lippincott Williams & Wilkins, 2002: 233–49.

31 Fischer DS, Knobf MT, Durivage HJ, *et al. The Cancer Chemotherapy Handbook*, 6th ed. Mosby, 2003: 497–8.

◆ 32 Wilkes JD. Prevention and treatment of oral mucositis following cancer chemotherapy. *Semin Oncol* 1998; **25**: 538–51.

◆ 33 Kostler WJ, Hejna M, Wenzel C, Zielinski CC. Oral mucositis complicating chemotherapy and/or radiotherapy: options for prevention and treatment. *CA Cancer J Clin* 2001; **51**: 290–315.

◆ 34 Stepp L, Pakiz TS. Anorexia and cachexia in advanced cancer. *Nurs Clin North Am* 2001; **36**: 735–44, vii.

35 Tomiska M, Tomiskova M, Salajka F, *et al.* Palliative treatment of cancer anorexia with oral suspension of megestrol acetate. *Neoplasma* 2003; **50**: 227–33.

◆ 36 Davies MJ, Schultz MZ. Cardiopulmonary toxicity of cancer therapy. In: Berger A, Portenoy R, Weissman D, eds. *Principles and Practice of Palliative and Supportive Oncology*, 2nd ed. Philadelphia: Lippincott Williams & Wilkins, 2002: 413–40.

37 Cooper JA Jr, Matthay RA. Drug-induced pulmonary disease. *Dis Mon* 1987; **33**: 61–120.

38 Von Hoff DD, Layard MW, Basa P, *et al.* Risk factors for doxorubicin-induced congestive heart failure. *Ann Intern Med* 1979; **91**: 710–17.

◆ 39 Patterson WP, Reams GP. Renal toxicities of chemotherapy. *Semin Oncol* 1992; **19**: 521–8.

40 Arany I, Safirstein RL. Cisplatin nephrotoxicity. *Semin Nephrol* 2003; **23**: 460–4.

41 Weeks JC, Cook EF, O'Day SJ, *et al.* Relationship between cancer patients' predictions of prognosis and their treatment preferences. *JAMA* 1998; **279**: 1709–14.

42 Jaakkimainen L, Goodwin PJ, Pater J, *et al.* Counting the costs of chemotherapy in a National Cancer Institute of Canada randomized trial in nonsmall-cell lung cancer. *J Clin Oncol* 1990; **8**: 1301–9.

43 Rapp E, Pater JL, Willan A, *et al.* Chemotherapy can prolong survival in patients with advanced non-small-cell lung cancer – report of a Canadian multicenter randomized trial. *J Clin Oncol* 1988; **6**: 633–41.

44 Sinoff CL, Blumsohn A. Spinal cord compression in myelomatosis: response to chemotherapy alone. *Eur J Cancer Clin Oncol* 1989; **25**: 197–200.

45 Effects of vinorelbine on quality of life and survival of elderly patients with advanced non-small-cell lung cancer. The Elderly Lung Cancer Vinorelbine Italian Study Group. *J Natl Cancer Inst* 1999; **91**: 66–72.

46 Anderson H, Hopwood P, Stephens RJ, *et al.* Gemcitabine plus best supportive care (BSC) vs BSC in inoperable non-small cell lung cancer – a randomized trial with quality of life as the primary outcome. UK NSCLC Gemcitabine Group. Non-Small Cell Lung Cancer. *Br J Cancer* 2000; **83**: 447–53.

● 47 Roszkowski K, Pluzanska A, Krzakowski M, *et al.* A multicenter, randomized, phase III study of docetaxel plus best supportive care versus best supportive care in chemotherapy-naive patients with metastatic or non-resectable localized non-small cell lung cancer (NSCLC). *Lung Cancer* 2000; **27**: 145–57.

● 48 Shepherd FA, Dancey J, Ramlau R, *et al.* Prospective randomized trial of docetaxel versus best supportive care in patients with non-small-cell lung cancer previously treated with platinum-based chemotherapy. *J Clin Oncol* 2000; **18**: 2095–103.

49 LoRusso PM, Herbst RS, Rischin D, *et al.* Improvements in quality of life and disease-related symptoms in phase I trials of the selective oral epidermal growth factor receptor tyrosine kinase inhibitor ZD1839 in non-small cell lung cancer and other solid tumors. *Clin Cancer Res* 2003; **9**: 2040–8.

50 Nabholtz JM, Senn HJ, Bezwoda WR, *et al.* Prospective randomized trial of docetaxel versus mitomycin plus vinblastine in patients with metastatic breast cancer progressing despite previous anthracycline-containing chemotherapy. 304 Study Group. *J Clin Oncol* 1999; **17**: 1413–24.

51 Launois R, Reboul-Marty J, Henry B, Bonneterre J. A cost-utility analysis of second-line chemotherapy in metastatic breast cancer. Docetaxel versus paclitaxel versus vinorelbine. *Pharmacoeconomics* 1996; **10**: 504–21.

52 Slater S. Non-curative chemotherapy for cancer – is it worth it? *Clin Med* 2001; **1**: 220–2.

53 Joensuu H, Holli K, Heikkinen M, *et al.* Combination chemotherapy versus single-agent therapy as first- and second-line treatment in metastatic breast cancer: a prospective randomized trial. *J Clin Oncol* 1998; **16**: 3720–30.

54 Lakusta CM, Atkinson MJ, Robinson JW, *et al.* Quality of life in ovarian cancer patients receiving chemotherapy. *Gynecol Oncol* 2001; **81**: 490–5.

55 Wilailak S, Linasmita V, Srisupundit S. Phase II study of high-dose megestrol acetate in platinum-refractory epithelial ovarian cancer. *Anticancer Drugs* 2001; **12**: 719–24.

56 Miller BE, Pittman B, Case D, McQuellon RP. Quality of life after treatment for gynecologic malignancies: a pilot study in an outpatient clinic. *Gynecol Oncol* 2002; **87**: 178–84.

57 Yoneda T, Nakai M, Moriyama K, *et al.* Neutralizing antibodies to human interleukin 6 reverse hypercalcemia associated with a human squamous carcinoma. *Cancer Res* 1993; **53**: 737–40.

58 Stashenko P, Dewhirst FE, Peros WJ, *et al.* Synergistic interactions between interleukin 1, tumor necrosis factor, and lymphotoxin in bone resorption. *J Immunol* 1987; **138**: 1464–8.

◆ 59 Thomas L, Kwok Y, Edelman MJ. Management of paraneoplastic syndromes in lung cancer. *Curr Treat Options Oncol* 2004; **5**: 51–62.

60 Rowe J. Healthy care myths at the end of life. *Bull Am Coll Surg* 1996; **81**: 11–18.

93

Physical medicine and rehabilitation

BENEDICT KONZEN, KI SHIN

INTRODUCTION

Some may mistakenly think that the fields of palliative medicine and rehabilitation medicine have divergent goals. Yet, both fields have a common focus in the relief of suffering and the improvement of quality of life. They differ in their historical roots. Palliative medicine grew out of observations made in the care of dying patients in hospice programs. It later grew to include other serious and life-threatening illnesses of uncertain prognosis. Rehabilitation medicine had its roots in restoration of impaired physical and cognitive functioning – 'fixed deficits' often incurred as a result of trauma. As a field it later grew to include patient with progressive acute on chronic deficits, for example, patients with cancer.

The assertion has been made that rehabilitating patients with cancer or other diseases with terminal prognoses is a poor allocation of scarce medical resources. However, when economic and psychological costs are included in the equation, the argument for such treatment is strengthened. In addition to the economic argument, both moral and spiritual arguments can also be made. Every human being values the ability to make decisions; to participate actively in their home; and to have value in the eyes of their peers, family and community. These needs may become more urgent for the patient with cancer or other serious illness. Rehabilitation medicine and palliative medicine share the goals of permitting a patient the opportunity to reflect on an ongoing life; understand the implication of their disease process as it impacts themselves, their caregiver, family, and friends; and move forward both physically and mentally. Despite illness, the physiatrist's goal is to promote physical functioning; where this is impeded, the physiatrist works with caregiver and family as adjuvant supports. The palliative medicine physician, primarily, and in association the physiatrist, both attempt to reduce the pain, asthenia, fatigue, and symptoms related to ongoing medical treatment, the final goal being living completely and fully – whether that be in a physical, cognitive, or spiritual sense. In this chapter, we will explore the role that rehabilitation medicine plays in the overall care of the palliative medicine patient.

The fields of both physical medicine and palliative care medicine arose out of specific medical care needs. Physical medicine was not formally recognized as a medical specialty until 1950. However, the historical record is long in its documentation of administering physiatric care to patients with mechanical or neurological trauma – often the result of accident or wars. The tenets of physical medicine foster the belief that despite injury, attempts at reestablishing premorbid functioning are not only desirable, but hopefully, obtainable. Palliative medicine seeks to advance all forms of medical care by treating the acute and chronic symptoms of disease. In addition, the field not only focuses on the individual, but advances the notion that care requires the additional interaction of spouse, family, acquaintances, and healthcare professionals. Both fields require a host of healthcare professionals – physicians, physician assistants, advance practice nurses, floor nursing, psychologists, and psychology nurses. Equally important are the roles played by case managers, social workers, and chaplains. The healthcare team does not exist independently. There continues to be a daily interchange between these team members. Indeed, team members must be strongly linked in purpose, but flexible enough to understand an individual's idiosyncrasies. Cultural diversity, religious belief, language, and perceptions of health, values, success, and disappointment are all unique characteristics in the patient being cared for. The field of physical medicine attempts to restore a prior level of functioning. The physiatrist is aware that family interaction is critical. Neurological injury such as a traumatic brain injury, stroke or tumor may leave a previously accomplished, mentally adept individual dependent on others. The prior relationship of husband/wife or significant others may be inextricably altered into patient/caregiver roles.

A united team approach of health professionals establishes a support network for ongoing medical care, teaching, and training. Whether in the outpatient clinic setting or on the acute inpatient unit, both rehabilitation and palliative medicine teach patients and their families anticipated and future care needs. As a supervised team, patients and their families can practice new tasks, and troubleshoot and modify unsafe behaviors. In addition, a close-knit team network can promote diversity of ideas as well as solutions. Both fields have a role to play throughout a person's disease state and life. Activity without symptoms of pain, nausea, fatigue, or discomfort will only enhance function. Activities with family and friends help to dissipate isolation and depression. Despite the timeline of a patient's disease, the palliative medicine physician's role remains interactive. Symptom management has both physical and spiritual components. Not only are nausea, fatigue, depression, anxiety, pain, constipation, asthenia addressed; but attempts are also made to assist the patient in coming to terms with both resolved and unresolved issues – including the fear of dying, abandonment, unfulfilled dreams/expectations, and disputes. In essence, both physical medicine and palliative medicine take an integrative look at the components which define us as human: physical, mental, social, and spiritual. When disease intervenes, these two fields attempt to restore a homeostatic balance, with an eventual goal of finding peace after, hopefully, a prosperous life lived.

CANCER FROM THE REHABILITATIONIST'S PERSPECTIVE

In traditional rehabilitation, causes of disability such as stroke, amputation, brain/spinal cord injury often have a defined deficit. Patients undergo acute treatment. A return to community functioning is often anticipated. In cancer care, initial and ongoing medical treatment is not necessarily curative. The rehabilitationist addresses deficits that may be progressive over time. Traditionally, in rehabilitation medicine, therapies continue until maximal functional improvement has been obtained. However in a chronic, potentially relapsing disease state such as cancer, the therapist deals with a patient who may have had recent surgery, chemotherapy, and radiation. There may be ongoing functional loss. Despite such losses, it has been shown repeatedly that patients with cancer – even during treatment – benefit from rehabilitation.[1]

Cancer rehabilitation initially arose through the work of three physiatrists, Herbert Dietz, Harold Rusk, and AE Gunn.[2] Financial support was provided by the National Cancer Institute (NCI). Modest gains continued through the 1980s until the focus of the NCI shifted from patient rehabilitation to the cure of cancer.[2] DeLisa[3] further comments on three additional factors limiting the role of cancer rehabilitation:

- oncologist not being aware of the potential benefits of rehabilitation
- failure of physiatry residency programs to incorporate cancer rehabilitation into the curriculum
- trend toward moving rehabilitation from an inpatient service to an outpatient arena.

One of the earliest cancer rehabilitationists was Dietz.[4] In 1969, he proposed four goals for the cancer rehabilitationist:

1 Prevent disability whenever possible.
2 Where disability occurs, attempt to restore the individual to the premorbid state of functioning.
3 Institute supports in order to reduce future disability.
4 Palliate to reduce complications, maintain independence and provide comfort.

Dietz felt that the effects of cancer were wide-reaching, affecting the socioeconomic, vocational, and emotional aspects of an individual's life. Therefore a team approach initially involving physiatrist, therapists, nursing, and social work was recommended. This has since broadened in scope to also include chaplaincy, case management, speech pathology, pharmacy, medical oncology, surgery, and radiation therapy.[4]

In his initial study, Dietz interviewed 1019 patients with cancer. He devised a scale ranging from 0 to 4 with which to rate the benefit of physical therapy on patients receiving treatment; 0 represented no clinical benefit and 4 represented individuals who were fully independent with no ongoing disability. Of patients being discharged from inpatient rehabilitation, the largest percentage was rated at a 2, i.e. moderate improvement with an appropriate response to rehabilitative care (Table 93.1).[4] Dietz maintained that rehabilitation care was essential for patients with incurable and terminal disease. Since the overall goal was the maintenance of function and overall range of motion, therapies should be instituted immediately.[4]

A specific study lends further credence to the role of rehabilitation in cancer care. In 1991, O'Toole and Goden investigated functioning in 70 patients with cancer. Of these, 14 percent were ambulatory at the time of admission to inpatient rehabilitation. At discharge, 80 percent could ambulate independently. Urinary continence likewise improved from 38 percent to 87 percent. However, 3 months

Table 93.1 *Response to inpatient rehabilitation and functional improvement (N = 1019)*

Level achieved	No.
0 (no improvement)	211
1 (slight improvement)	110
2 (moderate improvement)	320
3 (marked improvement)	270
4 (fully independent)	108

Source: Dietz (1969).[4]

after discharge, 33 percent had either died or were lost to follow-up. Of the remaining 37 patients, 27 had maintained or improved functioning.[5] Of significance in this investigation, was O'Toole and Goden's correlation between the Karnofsky performance scale – a measure of functional performance used by oncologists (Box 93.1) – and the Functional Independence Measure (FIM) score – a measure of functioning used by rehabilitationists. The conclusion was that patients with scores as low as 30 (severely disabled, inpatient hospital stay indicated, death not imminent) still were candidates for rehabilitation services.[5]

Box 93.1 Karnofsky scale

- 100 – Normal. No complaints; no evidence of disease; able to work

- 90 – Able to carry on normal activity. Minor symptoms; able to work

- 80 – Normal activity with effort. Some symptoms; able to work

- 70 – Cares for self. Unable to carry on normal activity; independent; not able to work

- 60 – Disabled; dependent. Requires occasional assistance; cares for most needs

- 50 – Moderately disabled; dependent. Requires considerable assistance and frequent care.

- 40 – Severely disabled; dependent. Requires special care and assistance

- 30 – Severely disabled. Hospitalized, death not imminent

- 20 – Very sick. Active supportive treatment needed

- 10 – Moribund. Fatal processes are rapidly progressing.

Adapted from Karnofsky et al., 1948, taken from: www.anapsid.org/cnd/files/karnofskyscale.pdf[6]

FUNCTIONAL AREAS ASSESSED

Functional areas assessed by the FIM (Table 93.2) are eating, grooming, bathing, upper and lower body dressing; toileting; bladder and bowel management; transfers; and locomotion. The FIM scores also assess comprehension, expression, social interaction, problem solving and memory.

Marciniak et al. from the Rehabilitation Institute of Chicago reviewed 159 patients over a 2-year period and looked at motor function. They found that metastatic disease did not affect functional outcome. Furthermore, radiation therapy was associated with greater functional improvement than when it was not provided or completed before starting rehabilitation.[8] According to Sliwa and Marciniak[1] the most common cause of functional decline in patients with cancer is deconditioning. Prolonged bed rest along with chemotherapy and/or radiation can lead to significant functional limitations. The degree of impairment is based on the duration and degree of immobilization. In general, healthy individuals on complete bed rest exhibit a 1–1.5 percent loss in strength per day or 10 percent per week.[9] Loss of proximal lower extremity strength is often greater than that seen in the upper extremities. This impedes sitting, standing, and ambulation.[10] Urinary calcium excretion increases. Diaphragmatic and intercostal muscle activity is reduced. Maximal oxygen consumption decreases by as much as 15 percent when healthy individuals resume exercise in an upright position after 10 days of bed rest.[11] Indeed, it may take up to one month to reestablish the normal postural response.[11] Healthy young men lose 300–500 mL of plasma volume within the first week of bed rest.[12] As plasma volume declines, blood viscosity increases leading to the risk of deep venous thrombosis.[1] In addition, there may be a hypotensive response. Both stroke volume and cardiac output decline.[12] From a neurological perspective, balance and coordination decline.[13] There may even be sensory deprivation.[14] Effective bladder evacuation is inhibited by recumbency. Inactivity results in impaired colonic function and possibly constipation with anorexia.[1] Lastly, hospitalized patients are at high risk (7.7 percent) of developing a pressure ulcer as sustained pressure over bony prominences results in ischemic injury.[15]

Table 93.2 *Functional Independence Measure (FIM)*

Score range	Interpretation	Patient's effort	In everyday parlance
1	Total assistance	Less than 25%	Completely dependent
2	Maximal assistance	25–49%	Completely dependent
3	Moderate assistance	50–74%	Needs hands-on help
4	Minimal contact assist	75%+	Needs minimal hands-on
5	Supervision/set-up	75%+	Needs cues; can do task
6	Modified independent	100%	Completes task without cues but needs assistive device, independent
7	Totally independent	100%	No helper needed, task done safely without device

From: www.medfriendly.com/functionalindependencemeasure.html[7]

Neurological impairment in patients with cancer may be an increasing cause of disability. There may be both central and peripheral nerve involvement either by tumor, metastatic disease, side effect of therapy (chemotherapy/radiation) or by concurrent, related issues such as paraneoplastic syndromes, infection or vasculitis.[1] Intracranial metastases are found in approximately 25 percent of patients who die from cancer. The origins of these metastases are frequently from lung, breast, and skin.[16,17] In a study of 363 cancer patients with brain metastases, 59 percent presented with hemiparesis.[18,19] Two recent studies have investigated neurooncological patients who had completed inpatient rehabilitation. Huang et al.[20] noted that there was concordance in functional return and rate of discharge to the community between the brain tumor patients and stroke patients. Indeed, length of stay was shorter for the former. In a second study, O'Dell et al.[21] compared patients with brain tumors and traumatic injuries. With comparable age, gender, and functional admission status, both groups made similar daily functional gains and 82.5 percent of patients with brain tumors were discharged home. On evaluation of functional status after inpatient rehabilitation, Sherer et al.[22] found that with a mean treatment time of 2.6 months, patients maintained these gains at a mean follow-up time of 8 months.

Of great concern to the rehabilitationist is metastatic disease of the spine. Although direct spinal cord involvement by metastatic tumor is rare, most spinal cord damage is the result of epidural compression by the tumor itself or vertebral body metastases resulting in bony compression. In only a small percentage of vertebral metastatic lesions will symptoms of compression be noted.[1] Many individuals are either asymptomatic or simply present with pain. However, in a study of 211 cancer patients,[23] 74 percent of individuals with metastatic cord compression were noted to have significant weakness at presentation. Close monitoring of functional status is essential. Involvement of the cervical spine may lead to plegia. Thoracolumbar involvement may lead to paraplegia and a neurogenic bowel/bladder. Typically, in the non-cancer patient this level of injury would still allow an individual to functional independently at the wheelchair level. In the case of the oncology patient, however, the activity of the tumor, interrelated surgery/chemotherapy or radiation – and ensuing comorbidities – may alter the ultimate functional outcome of the cancer patient.[24]

REHABILITATIVE INTERVENTIONS

One of the most important tasks for the rehabilitationist and patient with cancer is the establishment of appropriate goals. Patients vary in their understanding of disease and its implications. Functionally, they will have a unique response to surgical, chemotherapeutic, or radiation treatment. Initial and final expectations of treatment may be diametrically opposed. The rehabilitationist needs to modify general principles of rehabilitation to accommodate for persistent disease and the possibility of imminent or future decline. Challenges unique to patients with cancer would include chemotherapy-induced neuropathies, progressive lymphedema, pathological fractures requiring surgical stabilization, and metastatic disease compromising neurological functioning.[24]

Compensatory strategies in the care of patients with cancer make use of assistive devices. Reachers allow paraparetic, hemiparetic/hemiplegic patients to retrieve objects. Dressing and bathing aids compensate for diminished force and coordination. Orthotics can enhance stability and safety in the patient with motor deficits by protecting and stabilizing joints which are controlled by paretic muscles (e.g. ankle foot orthoses in the treatment of a 'drop foot'). In terms of home and community accessing, mobility can be restored with the use of wheelchairs and scooters.[24]

Sensory deficits are often seen in spinal cord compression and leptomeningeal disease (53 and 50 percent, respectively).[24] Anatomically, they are associated with brachial and lumbosacral plexopathies secondary to tumor encroachment or radiation effect. Chemotherapeutic agents such as cisplatin, vincristine and taxanes have also been associated with sensory neuropathies. In addition to instruction in compensatory strategies, assistive devices, and the use of orthotic devices, therapists work on enhancing stability by broadening a patient's base of support, enhancing tactile input, and instituting safety awareness of the insensate extremity while further educating patients on the use of alternative senses such as vision.[24]

In a large series of patients with brain metastases, cognitive dysfunction was found in 58 percent.[18,19] Such deficits can increase caretaker burden, render patients unsafe and limit effective communication. Deficits arising from neurological tumors include apraxia, alexia, aphasia, and agnosia. Patients may experience inattention, difficulties with concentration and disturbance in short-term memory. Strategies are limited, but may include memory notebooks or computerized prosthetics.[24] In cases of cerebellar dysfunction where ataxia and truncal instability destabilize the patient, therapists use devices with a broad support base such as wide-based quadruped canes, standard walkers, and hemiwalkers.[24]

Discussion continues about what is the most distressing experience among cancer patients, whether it is uncontrolled pain or fatigue. Santiago-Palma and Payne[25] noted that in approximately 70 percent of patients, fatigue was chronic or was acute during chemoradiation therapy. Specifically, fatigue may be the result of cachexia, infection, anemia or other metabolic/endocrine disorders.[25] Metastatic disease to the lungs and pleural effusions may result in significant dyspnea with concurrent decline in endurance.[25] In 2001, Winningham[26] identified 'cancer-related fatigue syndrome' (CRFS) as the most distressing experience among cancer patients. Winningham looked at fatigue from a metabolic/cellular level. She proposes that fatigue is amenable to rehabilitative efforts. Indeed, treatment for cancer-related fatigue may lie in endurance exercise training. When oxidative metabolism is maximized – as during exercise – there is improvement in muscle mass, plasma volume, pulmonary ventilation/perfusion, cardiac reserve, and a subsequent increased concentration of oxidative muscle enzymes. Interleukin-1 and other myotoxic cytokines are downregulated.[27] Finally, resistance exercise reduces steroid-induced loss of muscle mass.[26] Optimization of oxidative capacity, however, requires sound nutritional support. Even with nutritional intervention in the form of supplements, oral intake may be insufficient. The patient may have alteration to nutrient processing secondary to mechanical (surgical) intervention or cachexia.[28,29]

Pain is a prevalent finding in patients with cancer. In 70–90 percent of patients with advanced disease, significant pain is present.[25] From a symptom-control perspective, pain was controlled without excessive sedation in 85–90 percent of patients with cancer when the right combination of nonpharmacological techniques, pharmacological therapy, and radiopharmaceuticals were used.[30] Current recommendations suggest use of nonopioid agents initially for mild pain with addition of opioids for moderate or severe pain.[30] From the rehabilitationist's perspective, additional useful adjuvant therapy might include massage, and heat and cold modalities with certain restrictions. Physical therapy should educate a patient regarding proper seating dynamics, pressure relief, orthotics, assistive equipment and compensatory strategies.[25]

ROLE OF REHABILITATION IN PALLIATIVE CARE

At first glance it would appear that the two fields of rehabilitation and palliative care are divergent. Rehabilitation, in the traditional sense, focuses on the restoration of function lost either through illness, trauma or intervention. Acutely, patients may be cared for in a hospital setting and then transitioned to outpatient services. The expectation is that even with alterations in physical functioning, the patient should reestablish the premorbid level of activity. In contrast, in palliative medicine, the patient is presumed to be in a terminal phase of either an acute or chronic illness. Restoration of physical and cognitive functioning may occur, but is not the overall objective. The goal of palliation becomes assessing symptoms related to the disease state or its subsequent treatment, i.e. pain, dyspnea, asthenia, fatigue, cachexia, somnolence, delirium, depression, constipation; and instituting an appropriate intervention. As an internist, the palliative expert also attempts to maintain a homeostatic balance for the body. Unique to palliative medicine has been the arena of close, dynamic interplay with patients and their families. Whereas most physicians typically distance themselves from talking about dying, coping with illness, and the incorporation of family into this process, the palliative care physician sees this as a prerequisite in the total care of the patient. Discussion of end-of-life issues is viewed merely as a completion of this task.

The role of the cancer rehabilitationist has been modified. Without a clear understanding of the patient's prior health, disease process, prognosis, anticipated limitations based on pharmacological intervention, surgery, radiation and lastly family and economic supports, the rehabilitationist is unable to completely care for the patient. Therefore, the rehabilitationist dons – in limited fashion – the cloak of the palliative care physician. The goal, however, is maintaining function in the immediate future and preparing for possible future decline. Maintenance of the patient's autonomy in functioning, whether transferring to a chair or to the toilet, is attempted. A close collaboration between both disciplines is essential. In a study of 239 hospice patients, Yoshioka[31] demonstrated that functional improvement occurred in 27 percent of patients. In another study by Montagnini et al.[32] 18 out of 100 palliative care patients took part in a physical therapy program. In this group, 90 percent had ongoing deconditioning and pain. Montagnini found that 56 percent of those undergoing physical therapy demonstrated functional improvement.[32]

The complementary roles of physical medicine and palliative care medicine should be further investigated. Indeed, both disciplines 'enable the dying person to live until he dies, at his own maximum potential performing to the limit of his physical and mental capacity with control and independence whenever possible'.[33]

CONCLUSION

In general, researchers have yet to look at the overall dynamic of patients with cancer. When a patient presents for initial evaluation to a physician, the overall health and background of the patient is evaluated. Initial presenting complaint, general past medical health, concurrent medical comorbidities such as cardiopulmonary and endocrine disease are typically investigated. Emphasis should also be on how patients function in the home, within the family unit, at work, financially, emotionally – all of these are essential to determine what resources patients will draw upon to combat their illness. If there is no motivation or impetus to get better; if there is a poor support network, negative sense of self-worth, spiritual conflict or inability to work in trusting union with healthcare workers, the patient is at a marked disadvantage. Correlations have been shown with mood, affect, depression and the state of one's immune functioning.

Likewise, if a sound relationship of concern, compassion, and investment is not shared by the physician or conveyed in word or action to the patient, medical treatment will not be successful. In terminal disease, the idealistic goal is cure. Cure, however, may not be medically available at this time – despite the best of our scientific endeavors and research protocols. The goal, therefore, is simply and clearly explaining to the patient their disease process; options of optimal care; the true risks and disabilities inherently possible in current treatment regimens; and the promise by healthcare providers of attempting to physically do as little harm as possible in seeking a physical cure wherever possible. When attempts at treatment are exhausted, healthcare workers need to maintain a symptom-relieving role while providing ongoing educational and emotional support to the patient and caregiver.

Key learning points

- Palliative medicine and rehabilitation medicine both aim to restore function. The patient is viewed as a complex individual.

- To understand the patient's psychologic, physical, medical, and spiritual dimensions requires an interactive team approach by physician(s), advanced practice nurses, hospital/clinical nursing, psychologist, chaplain, social work and case manager.

- Physical activity may improve immunological function, cardiorespiratory status, motor ability, and endurance. It may relieve stress and improve symptoms of asthenia, fatigue, dyspnea, anorexia, and constipation.

- Family support is essential in the patient's ongoing medical care and successful transition from hospital to home or hospice setting.

- The goal of both rehabilitation medicine and palliative medicine is restoring autonomy (informed decision making) back to the patient and allowing mental and spiritual clarity.

REFERENCES

1 Sliwa JA, Marciniak C. Physical rehabilitation of the cancer patient [review]. *Cancer Treat Res* 1999; **100**: 75–89.
2 Watson PG. Cancer rehabilitation: an overview. *Semin Oncol Nurs* 1992; **8**: 167–73.
3 DeLisa JA. A history of cancer rehabilitation. *Cancer* 2001; **92**: 970–4.
4 Dietz JH. Rehabilitation of the cancer patient. *Med Clin North Am* 1969; **53**: 607–24.
5 O'Toole DM, Goden AM. Evaluating cancer patients for rehabilitation potential. *West J Med* 1991; **155**: 384–7.
6 Karnofsky. Performance Status Scale Definitions Rating (%) Criteria. Available at: www.hospicepatients.org/karnofsky.html (accessed 18 June 2006).
7 Functional Independence Measure. Available at: www.medfriendly.com/functionalindependencemeasure.html (accessed 18 June 2006).
8 Marciniak CM, James JA, Spill G, *et al.* Functional outcome following rehabilitation of the cancer patient. *Arch Phys Med Rehabil* 1996; **77**: 54–7.
9 Muller EA. 1970; Influence of training and of inactivity on muscle strength. *Arch Phys Med Rehabil* **51**: 449.
10 Gogin PP, Schneider VS, LeBlaner AD, *et al.* Bed rest effect on extremity muscle torque in healthy men. *Arch Phys Med Rehabil* 1988; **69**: 1030–2.

11 Dietrich JE, Whedon GD, Shon E. Effects of immobilization upon various metabolic and physiologic functions of normal men. *Am J Med* 1948; **4**: 3.
12 Hyatt KH, Kamenetsky LG, Smith WM. Extravascular dehydration as an etiologic factor in post-recumbency orthostasis. *Perosp Med* 1969; **40**: 644–50.
13 Taylor HL, Henschel A, Brozek J, *et al.* Effects of bedrest on cardiovascular function and work performance. *J Appl Physiol* 1949; **2**: 223.
14 Bolin RH. Sensory deprivation: an overview. *Nurs Forum* 1974; **13**: 241–58.
15 Allman RM, Laprade CA, Noel LB, *et al.* Pressure sores among hospitalized patients. *Ann Intern Med* 1986; **105**: 337–42.
16 Posner JB. *Intracranial Metastases in Neurologic Complications of Cancer.* Philadelphia: FA Davis, 1995; 77–110.
17 Rozenthal JM. Nervous system complications in cancer in current therapy. In: Earlen P, Brain M, eds. *Hematology/Oncology*, Vol. 3. New York: BC Decker, 1998; 314–19.
18 Cairncross JG, Kim J-H, Posner JB. Radiation therapy for brain metastases. *Ann Neurol* 1980; **7**: 529–41.
19 Young DF, Posner JP, Chu F, *et al.* Rapid course radiation therapy of cerebral metastases: results and complications. *Cancer* 1974; **4**: 1069–76.
20 Huang ME, Cifer DX, Marcus LK. Functional outcome following brain tumor and acute stroke: a comparative analysis. *Arch Phys Med Rehabil* 1998; **79**: 1386–90.
21 O'Dell MS, Barr K, Spanier P, Warnick R. Functional outcome of inpatient rehabilitation in persons with brain tumors. *Arch Phys Med Rehabil* 1998; **79**: 1530–4.
22 Sherer M, Meyers CA, Bergloff P. Efficacy of post acute brain injury rehabilitation for patients with primary malignant brain tumors. *Cancer* 2001; **92**(4 Suppl): 1049–52.
23 Posner J. *Neurologic Complications of Cancer.* Philadelphia: FA Davis, 1995: 118.
24 Cheville A. Rehabilitation of patients with advanced cancer. *Cancer* 2001; **92**(4 Suppl): 1039–48.
25 Santiago-Palma J, Payne R. Palliative care and rehabilitation. *Cancer* 2001; **92**(4 Suppl): 1049–52.
26 Winningham, ML. Strategies for managing cancer related fatigue syndrome: a rehabilitation approach. *Cancer* 2001; **92**: 988–97.
27 Deuster PA, Curale AM. Exercise-induced changes in populations of peripheral blood mononuclear cells. *Med Sci Sports Exerc* 1987; **20**: 276–80.
28 Easson AM, Hinshaw DB, Johnson DL. The role of tube feeding and total parenteral nutrition in advanced illness. *J Am College Surg* 2002; **194**: 225–8.
29 Olson E, Cristian A. The role of rehabilitation medicine and palliative care in the treatment of patients with end-stage disease. *Phys Med Rehabil Clin North Am* 2005; **16**: 285–305.
30 Abrahm JL. Update in palliative medicine and end of life care. *Annu Rev Med* 2003; **54**: 53–72.
31 Yoshioka H. Rehabilitation for the terminal cancer patient. *Am J Phys Med Rehabil* 1994; **73**: 199–206.
32 Montagnini M, Lodhi M, Born W. The utilization of physical therapy in a palliative care unit. *J Palliat Med* 2003; **6**: 11–17.
33 Saunders C. Foreword. In: Doyle D, Hanks G, MacDonald N, eds. *Oxford Textbook of Palliative Medicine*, 2nd ed. Oxford: Oxford University Press, 1998: v–ix.

94

Integrative and alternative medicine and palliative medicine

NANCY C RUSSELL, LORENZO COHEN

DEFINITION AND TYPES OF TRADITIONAL AND COMPLEMENTARY THERAPIES

Traditional medicine is defined by the World Health Organization (WHO) as health practices, approaches, knowledge, and beliefs incorporating plant, animal and mineral based medicines, spiritual therapies, manual techniques and exercises singularly or in combination to treat, diagnose, and prevent illnesses or maintain wellbeing.[1] Complementary/alternative medicine (CAM) is defined by the US National Center for Complementary and Alternative Medicine (NCCAM) as a group of diverse medical and healthcare systems, practices, and products that are not presently considered as part of conventional medicine. *Complementary medicine*, as defined by NCCAM, combines mainstream medical therapies with CAM therapies for which there is some high-quality scientific evidence of safety and effectiveness. *Alternative medicine*, however, is typically defined as a treatment modality for which there is no scientific evidence of efficacy and it is used *in place of* conventional, mainstream medicine.[2]

To integrate complementary medicine with conventional medicine, it must be practiced with the knowledgeable awareness of the conventional healthcare professional. The complementary medicine practitioner should be aware of and knowledgeable about the conventional treatments and at the least there is an open communication between the two practitioners. When this occurs, patients receive complementary treatment modalities using an integrative medicine approach versus simply receiving two different treatment modalities (conventional and complementary).

Complementary therapies have been subdivided into five subsections:[2]

- *Alternative medical systems* that have evolved independently and sometimes earlier than conventional Western medicine, e.g. traditional Chinese medicine (herbal and acupuncture), homeopathy, and Ayurveda (Indian-based medicine).
- *Biologically based approaches* such as nutrition, herbal/plant, animal/mineral, or other products.
- *Body-manipulative systems* such as chiropractic and massage.
- *Energy-based therapies* that seek to affect proposed energy fields of individuals through electromagnetic waves or the energy of individual practitioners, e.g. yoga, tai chi, qigong, Reiki, Healing Touch.
- *Mind-body approaches* such as meditation, prayer, support groups, guided imagery, music therapy, art therapy, and other behavioral techniques.

In palliative care settings, complementary/integrative medicines (CIM) may be used for managing symptoms, increasing wellness (quality of life, reported sense of wellbeing), and improving treatment efficacy.

In this chapter we will describe the use and need for complementary therapies, assessments of their effectiveness, quality assurance, evidence-based internet resources, standards of care, and the role of the healthcare professional in advising patients about their use. Although we will highlight some findings from previously published reviews of their effectiveness for patients with cancer, we will not provide comprehensive reviews of specific modalities. Rather, we will focus on some guidelines and evidence-based internet resources that can assist healthcare professionals in their advice to patients and families.

USE OF COMPLEMENTARY THERAPIES

The WHO estimates that up to 80 percent of people in developing countries rely on traditional medicines for their primary healthcare. People in more developed countries also seek out these medicines and practices assuming that they are effective and may be safer than allopathic medicine because they are natural.[3] A 1997 survey of US adults found CAM use (excluding self-prayer) varied from 32 percent to 54 percent among the sociodemographic groups surveyed.[4] A 2002 survey by the US Centers for Disease Control and Prevention (CDC) found that 36 percent of adults had used CAM therapies (non-prayer) during the past 12 months.[5]

An estimated 48–69 percent of US patients with cancer use CAM therapies[6,7] and percentages increase if spiritual practices are included.[7] Complementary therapies are used in 70 percent of all oncology departments engaged in palliative care in Britain[8,9] and by 28 percent of advanced cancer/palliative care patients in a Canadian community and hospital setting.[10] A survey of five clinics within a US comprehensive cancer care center found that CAM therapies were used by 68.7 percent of patients (excluding psychotherapy and spiritual practices) and were 11.6 times more likely to be used by patients with distant or unstaged disease (95 percent confidence interval [CI] 1.5 to 92.8).[7] A later survey in the breast and gynecological clinics within that same center found that CAM therapies, (defined as herbs, supplements, and mega doses of vitamins) were used by 48 percent of patients. Again, statistically significant differences existed by disease status with CAM therapies used by 38 percent of newly diagnosed patients, 49 percent of those with recurrence or relapse, and 55 percent of those in remission ($\chi^2 = 9.34$, $P = 0.009$).[6]

Whether or not patients use CAM therapies for treatment of cancer or its effects, they may use them for other chronic conditions such as arthritis. CAM therapies were currently being used by 69 percent of patients attending six university-based primary care clinics for osteoarthritis, rheumatoid arthritis, or fibromyalgia.[11]

NEED FOR COMPLEMENTARY THERAPIES

Conventional medical approaches have powerful pharmaceutical medicines for managing problems within palliative care settings. Yet all drugs have limitations and a medicine for one set of problems often has side effects that aggravate other problems. Pain and related problems, for example, can be pharmaceutically managed with opioids, corticosteroids, nonsteroidal anti-inflammatory drugs (NSAIDs), and psychotropic medications. However, this pharmaceutical management often comes at a price in terms of both financial costs and physiological side effects.[12,13] Any approach or therapy that can lower the doses needed or delay the start of these drugs would be beneficial.

EFFECTIVENESS OF COMPLEMENTARY THERAPIES

Assessing the effectiveness of complementary therapies requires the same standards of research methodology as conventional therapies. Yet, popular pressure may rush some of these therapies into full-scale phase III clinical trials before the proper preclinical research and dose-finding studies have prepared the basis for a scientifically sound well-designed trial. Conducting a phase III clinical trial with too small a dose may yield results of noneffectiveness when, in fact, other doses or regimens might have been found to be effective.[14]

Although the randomized, double blind, placebo controlled trial is considered the gold standard for clinical research, it is especially challenging for many of these therapies. Randomization may affect recruitment of subjects if those who are eligible already have strong biases in favor of either the standard or the alternative complementary therapy. Healthcare practitioners may have biases in favor of certain treatments or ideas about which groups might benefit the most. Disguising nonpharmaceutical therapies is not as simple as disguising pharmaceuticals with tablet coatings. Some herbal therapies may have associated tastes, textures, or smells that are part of their effectiveness and difficult to either disguise or duplicate. Disguising acupuncture, exercise, or mind-body approaches with sham treatments is difficult to do without adding some effects. Most complementary therapies require trained practitioners who would have difficulty providing a sham therapy while untrained practitioners might have difficulty providing a convincing sham therapy. If a sham therapy is to be provided, the information provided to the patient during the informed consent process must be honest without exposing the sham procedure. In comparisons between unconventional and standard treatments this document must again be honest without biasing the patient in favor of either procedure. Blinding of therapies to both the patient and the practitioner can be especially challenging.[15,16]

The number and variety of complementary therapies limits the extent to which any one review of the evidence can do justice to all therapies; nevertheless, several reviews have been published. Ernst reviewed nine complementary therapies used in palliative cancer care for which there were some scientific data: acupuncture, aromatherapy, enzyme therapy, homeopathy, hypnotherapy, massage, reflexology, relaxation, and spiritual (energy) healing. He concluded that acupuncture could be effective for reducing nausea and vomiting after chemotherapy, although he called for more rigorous clinical trials.[8***] His conclusion is consistent with a US National Institutes of Health consensus statement.[17***]

For most other therapies, Ernst reported encouraging, but not compelling evidence and again stated a need for more trials with rigorous designs. He noted a few herbs with palliative care possibilities: St John's wort and kava for mood regulation, ginger for nausea, and valerian for sleep problems. However, these had not had adequate testing in patients with cancer at the time of his review.[8***] Subsequent reviews of these herbs by the collaborative review organization, Natural Standard, found each of them to be effective.[18***] However, important contraindications need to be observed when prescribing these herbs; in particular, St John's wort, as it increases metabolism of certain drugs, and kava, which has been found to have toxicities in people with previous liver problems.[18–20] Newell and colleagues[21] reviewed psychological therapies for cancer patients and concluded that interventions involving self-practice and hypnosis for managing nausea and vomiting could be recommended, but further research was suggested to examine the benefits of relaxation training and guided imagery. Further research was also warranted to examine the benefits of relaxation and guided imagery for managing general nausea, anxiety, quality of life, and overall physical symptoms.[21***] Natural Standard also concluded that guided imagery could improve quality of life and sense of comfort, but that further research was needed for firm conclusions. Meditation to relieve anxiety had some reported benefits, but better designed studies were needed. Numerous studies have showed evidence that relaxation techniques may moderately reduce anxiety and insomnia, but again studies with better designs were needed.[18***]

Wendy Weiger and colleagues reviewed CAM therapies commonly used by patients with cancer.[22***] They concluded that the direction of evidence suggested effectiveness for several types of therapies: energy-based, body manipulative, and mind-body, and specifically, acupuncture, to relieve chemotherapy-related nausea and exercise to improve physical function, psychological state, and physical symptoms in patients receiving conventional therapy. Mind-body therapies indicating effectiveness included various forms of individual and group therapy, relaxation, imagery, hypnosis, and meditation. These could alleviate emotional distress and certain physical symptoms of disease and side effects of conventional treatment including cancer-related pain.[22***]

Weiger *et al.* found good evidence for the use of massage to relieve anxiety, nausea (related to bone marrow transplantation), and lymphedema (manual lymph drainage).[22***] Natural Standard's review of massage, however, found the studies concerning anxiety and cancer-related pain to be inconclusive. They did find evidence of benefit for the massage known as 'manual lymphatic drainage' when combined with elastic sleeves or bandaging for patients with arm edema after breast cancer surgery.[18***] They found no evidence that the usual practices of massage promoted cancer although, of course, it should not be done directly on tumors and care must be exercised in patients who have bony metastases, are prone to bleeding, or have just had radiation or surgery.[18] One study (not noted in that review) has identified metastasis associated with massage, but it followed deliberate attempts immediately after breast cancer surgery to enhance dye uptake into sentinel lymph nodes for diagnostic purposes.[23*,24*,25*]

The only herbal product included in the Weiger review was PC-SPES, a combination of eight herbs: *Isatis indigotica* (da qing ye), *Glycyrrhiza glabra* (licorice), *Panax pseudoginseng* (san qi), *Ganoderma lucidum* (ling zhi), *Scutellaria baicalensis* (Chinese skullcap), *Chrysanthemum morifolium* (chrysanthemum), *Rabdosia rubescens*, and *Serenoa repens* (saw palmetto). Although beneficial and adverse effects had been demonstrated in randomized controlled trials, these effects were largely attributed to contamination with estrogen. Nevertheless, reviewers noted several *in vitro* effects that could not be attributed entirely to estrogen.[22***]

QUALITY ASSURANCE

Widely reported contamination of PC-SPES and other products has highlighted the need for quality assurance within the herbal industry. The US Food and Drug Administration and the WHO, in consultation with major producers, have proposed guidelines for good manufacturing practices (GMPs). However, actual regulation of herbal processing and shipping involves complex issues since most herbs are classified as foods that cannot be regulated in the same manner as drugs. Nevertheless, GMPs are being supported by some major producers and independent nongovernmental groups such as the American Botanical Council,[26,27] and results of independent laboratory testing are available. ConsumerLab (www.consumerLab.com), for example, tests products according to recognized standards of quality, ingredients claimed on labels, purity, and biological availability. Lists of brands that have passed their tests may be accessed for free, but names of those that have failed require a subscription.[28]

To responsibly suggest or even accept the use of readily available herbal supplements, behavioral techniques, or alternative modalities such as acupuncture and massage for symptom control, clinicians must have access to routinely updated authoritative evidence-based reviews. These reviews must consider the preponderance of evidence from all known well-designed studies and meta-analyses rather than isolated individual studies. Comprehensive reviews must include information concerning safety, specific indications for use, potential interactions, dosing, frequency, and quality of different brands. Clinicians in previous decades would have sought such information within large reference volumes in libraries. Today's clinicians may more easily access the latest comprehensive reviews through the internet, but they must also be able to quickly filter through many resources to find those that are most reliable.

EVIDENCE–BASED INTERNET REVIEWS

The rapidity with which a comprehensive review can become out of date and the ease of internet publishing have fostered the growth of comprehensive scientific review organizations that provide electronic access to their reviews. An assessment of websites with reviews of CAM therapies for patients with cancer was published in 2004 by Schmidt and Ernst.[29] They used eight popular search engines to search for the terms 'complementary' or 'alternative medicine' and 'cancer' and identified the first 50 websites that appeared on at least three engines. Their final list of 32 websites was evaluated for

- quality based upon a Sandvik score of 0–5 points as 'poor', 6–10 points as 'medium' and 11–14 points as 'excellent'
- reliability based on whether it displayed the Health on the Net (HON) code
- risk to patients based on an overall score and type of CAM discussed (curative, preventative, or palliative).

Each website was also scored based upon discouraging the use of conventional medicine or clinician's advice, and providing commercial details. Ten websites received a score of 12 or better. Seven of these top 10 websites were sponsored by either government or academic institutions and three were sponsored by individuals or private businesses.[29]

For recommendation to the health professionals reading this chapter, we evaluated 15 websites: the 10 websites recognized by Schmidt and Ernst (Quackwatch;[30] Oxford University's Bandolier;[31] the National Cancer Institute [NCI] Fact Sheets;[32] Rosenthal Center of Columbia University;[33] Holistic online;[34] International Health News – yourhealthbase;[35] Oncolink sponsored by the Abramson Cancer Center of the University of Pennsylvania;[36] University of Virginia Medical Center;[37] NCI Office of Cancer Complementary and Alternative Medicine [OCCAM] PDQ summaries;[38] and The University of Texas MD Anderson Cancer Center Complementary/Integrative Medicine Education Resources [CIMER][25]) plus five others that were not identified by Schmidt and Ernst as being in the top 32 websites: American Cancer Society,[39] Memorial Sloan–Kettering Cancer Center,[19] the Cochrane Review Organization,[40] Natural Standard,[18] and Natural Medicines Comprehensive Database.[20]

Eight of these 15 complementary/alternative websites provide generally reliable information for patients and the general public, but are not adequate for health professionals. Quackwatch[30] has a predominantly negative bias consistent with its mission to 'combat health related frauds'. NCI Fact Sheets[32] provide authoritative summaries of reviews for patients and the general public, but lack specific citations. Holistic online[34] provides generally positive information about an extensive set of herbs and other therapies (both alternative and conventional), but it does not provide professional documentation or descriptions of their review process. The Rosenthal Center at Columbia University provides the herbal database of abstracts, HerbMedPro,[33] but no systematic reviews of therapies. The University of Virginia Medical Center[37] describes opportunities for research at their center, but no reviews or study results. The University of Pennsylvania's Oncolink[36] provides brief synopses and frequently asked questions about complementary therapies. International Health News[35] provides summaries of individual articles. At the time of the Schmidt and Ernst review, the American Cancer Society[39] provided summaries of reviews, but these are no longer available.

Seven remaining websites provide valuable resources for healthcare professionals. Natural Medicines Comprehensive Database (www.naturaldatabase.com) provides the largest number of evidence-based reviews of complementary therapies (over 1000). The majority of its authors and editors are doctors of pharmacy and their reviews include scientific names, uses, safety, effectiveness, mechanisms of action, adverse reactions, interactions, dosage and administration. Full access requires an individual or institutional subscription.[20] It has received top ratings in comparative evaluations for answering questions about herbal and dietary supplements.[41–43] However, these one to two page reviews do not provide background or indepth assessments of the evidence on which their conclusions are based.

The oldest and most comprehensive of the scientific review organizations for conventional therapies is the Cochrane Review Organization (www.cochrane.org). Founded in 1993 as an international nonprofit independent organization, it now provides over 2000 systematic reviews and has recently added the complementary therapies of massage, acupuncture, and chiropractic. Its review process includes searches of multiple bibliographic databases by professional librarians. At least two blinded independent reviewers evaluate studies according to standard sets of questions with discrepancies resolved through conferences with attempts to contact authors for resolution of remaining questions. A statistician and an editorial board join with reviewers for development and summation of final conclusions. Abstracts of Cochrane reviews are free, but completed reviews require either individual or institutional subscription.[40,44]

Indepth analyses and commentaries about recent systematic reviews and meta-analyses of some complementary therapies found in searches of the *Cochrane Library* and PubMed are a feature of *Bandolier*, a monthly journal about evidence-based healthcare produced by scientists at

Oxford University (www.jr2.ox.ac.uk/bandolier).[31] Modeling itself upon the Cochrane organization, Natural Standard (www.naturalstandard.com) formed a multidisciplinary, multi-institutional initiative dedicated to the review of complementary and alternative therapies. It follows a similar process to build indepth evidence and consensus-based analysis of scientific data in addition to historical and folkloric perspectives. It now provides several hundred authoritative reviews. Access requires subscription, but some institutions with subscriptions have also purchased summaries of reviews for public access.[18]

The NCI Office of Cancer Complementary and Alternative Medicine (OCCAM) has reviewed about a dozen complementary therapies (www3.cancer.gov/occam). These 'PDQ' cancer information summaries provide extensive details and citations for health professionals including background, history of development, proposed mechanisms of action, and relevant laboratory, animal and clinical studies.[38] Memorial Sloan–Kettering Cancer Center (www.mskcc.org/mskcc/html/11571.cfm) provides over a hundred evidence-based reviews. These are written either by an oncology-trained pharmacist with expertise in botanicals or a cancer nutrition specialist with secondary reviews by at least two other editors or panel advisors.[19] The University of Texas MD Anderson Cancer Center's website for complementary/integrative medicine (www.mdanderson.org/cimer) provides over 80 reviews that include indepth assessments of the background and evidence by their own staff plus purchased summaries of some of the previously described reviews by Natural Standard and the *Cochrane Library* and access to all reviews by the NCI OCCAM and Memorial Sloan–Kettering. Their own methodology includes searches by library personnel, reviews by an epidemiologist and secondary reviews by appropriate faculty members or outside advisors.[25]

Searching these seven websites may be efficiently accomplished by physicians or delegated to appropriate clinic personnel. Patients or caregivers can then be given specific recommendations, printed summaries, or the names of these or other prescreened websites. Questions generated from this information can then be brought back for discussion with the physician or other clinic professional.

Although the NCI, the American Cancer Society and the MD Anderson Cancer Center websites also provide links to other reliable websites, patients or caregivers may wish to investigate independently. If so, they should be encouraged to look for websites that subscribe to the principles of the Health on the Net Foundation and carry its 'Honcode' seal. This nongovernmental organization is supported by the State of Geneva in Switzerland, the Swiss Institute of Bioinformatics and the University Hospitals of Geneva. It screens websites for compliance with its eight principles of authority: medically trained and qualified professionals, support of the patient/site visitor and his or her physician, confidentiality, clear references to source data, claims supported by appropriate and balanced evidence, transparency of authorship, transparency of ownership, and honesty in advertising and editorial policy.[45] The Honcode is displayed by two of the above seven websites for healthcare professionals: the NCI and the MD Anderson Cancer Center.

STANDARDS OF CARE

As some complementary therapies have demonstrated evidence of effectiveness, they may have become accepted standards of practice in some areas. Accordingly, it is wise to keep an open mind and to consult with other professional colleagues such as physical therapists, registered dieticians, and psychologists before making quick judgments that may be recognized as inadequate by knowledgeable patients and caregivers. Certain types of massage, nutritional guidelines, and behavioral techniques for example, are now accepted standards of care for certain conditions.

ROLE OF THE PALLIATIVE CARE PROVIDER

Deciding whether to recommend a complementary therapy or warn against its use may not even be an option for the healthcare provider if patients are already using it without the physician's knowledge. The percentage of patients using complementary therapies in cancer centers without telling their physicians has varied from 38 percent to 60 percent.[6,7] For this reason, physicians, nurse practitioners and other palliative care professionals must strive to maintain an inquiring, but nonjudgmental attitude toward patients concerning complementary therapies. Their role is to assist the patient in relieving their symptoms with the best of conventional and/or complementary resources rather than dismissing their efforts. General role playing in such situations has been described in articles[46] and internet videos.[25] The ultimate goal is to understand a patient's motivations and ensure that the approach they choose is safe and potentially worth the investment when there is an associated cost with little evidence for efficacy.

Key learning points

- Important distinctions exist between *alternative* medicines with little evidence of effectiveness that may be used in place of conventional treatments for cancer and *complementary* medicines with some evidence of effectiveness that may be used in addition to conventional treatments for cancer and its side effects. To *integrate* complementary treatments with conventional treatments requires the knowledgeable awareness of the conventional practitioner based upon open dialog with the patient.

- Many patients with cancer engage in some type of CAM modality at some point in the treatment trajectory, but especially when disease is advanced.

- Some CAM treatments may be beneficial, some may cause harm on their own or due to negative interactions with conventional medicine, and others may have no benefit.

- Cancer patients are typically well-informed medical consumers, but they may gather information about CAM from both reputable and questionable sources. Accordingly, it is the responsibility of healthcare professionals to become as informed as possible in this new and expanding area.

- Today's healthcare professionals and patients have powerful new tools and professional societies that have developed for evaluating the potential of proposed complementary therapies for palliative care needs. Working together, healthcare professionals and patients can make educated decisions about what to incorporate and what to avoid at different stages of the cancer treatment trajectory.

- Appropriate discussions about CAM in the palliative care setting will increase an open dialog about this important topic, optimize patient healing and comfort, and ensure that patients are provided safe and effective care.

REFERENCES

1   World Health Organization. Traditional medicine. 2003; Available at: www.who.int/mediacentre/factsheets/fs134/en/ (accessed October 26, 2004).

✱ 2   National Center for Complementary/Alternative Medicine of the National Institutes of Health. What is complementary and alternative medicine? Available at: http://nccam.nih.gov/health/whatiscam/ (accessed October 3, 2005).

3   World Health Organization. New WHO guidelines to promote proper use of alternative medicines. 2004; Available at: www.who.int/mediacentre/news/releases/2004/pr44/en/ (accessed October 26, 2004).

● 4   Eisenberg DM, Davis RB, Ettner SL, *et al.* Trends in alternative medicine use in the United States, 1990–1997: results of a follow-up national survey. *JAMA* 1998; **280**: 1569–75.

5   Barnes PM, Powell-Griner E, McFann K, Nahin RL. Complementary and Alternative Medicine Use Among Adults: United States, 2002. Advance Date From Vital and Health Statistics 2004; (343).

6   Navo MA, Phan J, Vaughan C, *et al.* An assessment of the utilization of complementary and alternative medication in women with gynecologic or breast malignancies. *J Clin Oncol* 2004; **22**: 671–7.

● 7   Richardson MA, Sanders T, Palmer JL, *et al.* Complementary/alternative medicine use in a comprehensive cancer center and the implications for oncology. *J Clin Oncol* 2000; **18**: 2505–14.

◆ 8   Ernst E. Complementary therapies in palliative cancer care. *Cancer* 2001; **91**: 2181–5.

9   White P. Complementary medicine treatment of cancer: a survey of provision. *Complement Ther Med* 1998; **6**: 10–13.

10   Oneschuk D, Hanson J, Bruera E. Complementary therapy use: a survey of community- and hospital-based patients with advanced cancer. *Palliat Med* 2000; **14**: 432–4.

11   Herman CJ, Allen P, Hunt WC, *et al.* Use of complementary therapies among primary care clinic patients with arthritis. *Prevent Chronic Dis* 2004; **1**: A12.

12   Raj PP. *Practical Management of Pain*, 2nd ed. St. Louis: CV Mosby, 1992.

13   Oneschuk D, Bruera E. The 'dark side' of adjuvant analgesic drugs. *Prog Palliat Care* 1997; **5**: 5–13.

14   National Center for Complementary and Alternative Medicine. Guidance on designing clinical trials of CAM therapies: determining dose ranges. 5 December 2003; Available at: http://nccam.nih.gov/research/policies/guideonct.htm (accessed May 20, 2004).

15   Jonas WB, Linde K. Conducting and evaluating clinical research on complementary and alternative medicine. In: Gallin JI, ed. *Principles and Practice of Clinical Research.* San Diego: Academic Press, 2002: 401–26.

16   Margolin A, Avants SK, Kleber HD. Investigating alternative medicine therapies in randomized controlled trials. *JAMA* 1998; **280**: 1626–8.

◆ 17   NIH Consensus Development Panel on Acupuncture. Acupuncture. *JAMA* 1998; **280**: 1518–24.

18   Basch E, Ulbricht C, Chief Editors. Natural Standard. 1918; Available at: www.naturalstandard.com (accessed September 17, 2004).

19   Memorial Sloan-Kettering Cancer Center. About Herbs. Available at: www.mskcc.org/mskcc/html/11571.cfm (accessed September 17, 2004).

20   Jellin JM, Editor in Chief. Natural Medicines Comprehensive Database. Available at: www.naturaldatabase.com (accessed September 17, 2004).

◆ 21   Newell SA, Sanson-Fisher RW, Savolainen NJ. Systematic Review of Psychological Therapies for cancer patients: overview and recommendations for future research. *J Natl Cancer Inst* 2002; **94**: 558–84.

◆ 22   Weiger WA, Smith M, Boon H, *et al.* Advising patients who seek complementary and alternative medical therapies for cancer. *Ann Intern Med* 2002; **137**: 889–903. Erratum in: *Ann Intern Med* 2003; **139**: 155.

23   Rosser RJ. Sentinel lymph nodes and postinjection massage: It is premature to reject caution. *J Am Coll Surg* 2001; **193**: 338.

24   Rosser RJ. A point of view: Trauma is the cause of occult micrometastatic breast cancer in sentinel axillary lymph nodes. *Breast J* 2000; **6**: 209–12.

25   The University of Texas MD Anderson Cancer Center. Complementary/Integrative Medicine Education Resources (CIMER). Reviews updated approximately every two years; Available at: www.mdanderson.org/cimer (accessed September 17, 2004).

26   Blumenthal M, Watts D. FDA issues proposed GMPs for dietary supplements. *HerbalGram: The Journal of the American Botanical Council* 2003; **58**: 62–5, 80.

27   Blumenthal M. American Botanical Council. Available at: www.herbalgram.org (accessed December 6, 2004).

28   ConsumerLab. About ConsumerLab. Available at: www.consumerlab.com/aboutcl.asp (accessed September 17, 2004).

◆ 29 Schmidt K, Ernst E. Assessing websites on complementary and alternative medicine for cancer. *Ann Oncol* 2004; **15**: 733–42.

30 Barrett, S. Quackwatch. Available at: www.quackwatch.org (accessed September 17, 2004).

31 Oxford University. Bandolier: evidence based thinking about health issues. Available at: www.jr2.ox.ac.uk/bandolier/booth/booths/altmed.html (accessed December 6, 2004).

32 National Cancer Institute. Fact Sheets. Available at: http://cis.nci.nih.gov/fact/ (accessed November 9, 2004).

33 Rosenthal Center for Complementary and Alternative Medicine. HerbMedPro. Available at: http://rosenthal.hs.columbia.edu (accessed September 17, 2004).

34 Mathew J, Chief Editor & Founder. HolisticHealth.Com. Available at: http://holisticonline.com/hol_about.htm (accessed November 9, 2004).

35 Larsen H, Editor. International Health News. Available at: www.yourhealthbase.com (accessed November 9, 2004).

36 Abramson Cancer Center of the University of Pennsylvania. Oncolink. Available at www.oncolink.com/templates/treatment/t (accessed September 17, 2004).

37 University of Virginia. Center for the study of complementary and alternative therapies (CSCAT). Available at: www.healthsystem.virginia.edu/internet/cscat/ (accessed September 17, 2004).

38 NCI Office of Cancer Complementary & Alternative Medicine (OCCAM). CAM Information. Available at: www3.cancer.gov/occam/information.html (accessed September 17, 2004).

39 American Cancer Society. Complementary and Alternative Therapies. Available at: www.cancer.org/docroot/eto/eto_5.asp?sitearea=eto (accessed November 30, 2004).

✱ 40 Cochrane Collaboration Steering Group. The Cochrane Collection. Available at: www.cochrane.org (accessed December 6, 2004).

41 Chambliss WG, Hufford CD, Flagg ML, Glisson JK. Assessment of the quality of reference books on botanical dietary supplements. *J Am Pharm Assoc* 2002; **42**: 723–34.

42 Walker JB. Evaluation of the ability of seven herbal resources to answer questions about herbal products asked in drug information centers. *Pharmacotherapy* 2002; **22**: 1611–15.

43 Sweet BV, Gay WE, Leady MA, Stumpf JL. Usefulness of herbal and dietary supplement references. *Ann Pharmacother* 2003; **37**: 494–9.

44 Dickersin K, Manheimer E. The Cochrane collaboration: evaluation of health care and services using systematic reviews of the results of randomized controlled trials. *Clin Obstet Gynecol* 1998; **41**: 315–31.

✱ 45 Health on the Net Foundation. About Health on the Net. 20 March 1996; Available at: www.hon.ch/global/ (accessed September 17, 2004).

46 Cassileth B. Enhancing doctor-patient communication. *J Clin Oncol* 2001; **19**(18s): 61s–63s.

95

Human immunodeficiency virus and palliative care

ROBERT E HIRSCHTICK, JAMIE H VON ROENN

INTRODUCTION

Therapeutic advances in recent years have extended the survival of patients infected with the human immunodeficiency virus (HIV) in the developed world.[1*] In affluent countries, HIV infection has become a chronic, treatable condition, similar in many ways to congestive heart failure. However, there is still considerable morbidity and mortality associated with HIV infection.[2] Moreover, as with congestive heart failure, the trajectory of late-stage illness does not proceed steadily downward but rather follows an irregular course of sudden valleys and surprising peaks.[3,4]

Many of the issues faced by people with advanced HIV infection fall within the traditional purview of hospice and palliative care. For example, the palliative care consultation service of a large urban hospital reported the following issues in patients with acquired immune deficiency syndrome (AIDS): pain in 40 percent, psychosocial issues in 31 percent, nausea and/or vomiting in 14 percent, and interpersonal conflicts in 13 percent.[5] However, there are many unique aspects involved in the palliative care of HIV-infected individuals, and HIV/AIDS remains largely a socially unacceptable disease. Infected patients may be shunned by family or friends and suffer physical and emotional isolation as a result.[6] The young age at death of HIV-infected patients may exact a toll upon healthcare providers. The presence of a homosexual partner may exacerbate friction with family members, especially when major healthcare decisions need to be made. The patient may have a history of past or current narcotic abuse, which can challenge not only

the prescribing expertise of practitioners but also the limits of their compassion. Finally, many HIV-infected patients, owing to social, cultural, or economic considerations, may be reluctant or unable to access support services and medical resources, including hospice and palliative care programs. For example, African Americans now comprise the largest group of HIV-infected persons in the USA.[2] However, they are less likely to use hospice and palliative care services than are European Americans.[7] Moreover, physicians are less likely to have discussions about end-of-life issues with African American AIDS patients than they are with European American AIDS patients.[8]

SYMPTOM BURDEN

A significant symptom burden is associated with HIV infection throughout the trajectory of disease, although it is greatest in patients with advanced and/or refractory HIV infection.[4,5,9] The high prevalence of pain and other symptoms in patients with AIDS has been documented since the onset of the epidemic. The etiology of some of the most common symptoms has changed over the course of the epidemic, but the overall prevalence has not. Without the use of highly active antiretroviral therapy (HAART), opportunistic infections account for many symptoms: headaches with cryptococcal meningitis, wasting and abdominal pain with mycobacterium avium complex infection, and blindness from cytomegalovirus retinitis, to name but a few. The contribution of opportunistic infections to pain and other symptoms in patients with AIDS has diminished over time as HIV therapy, where available, has become more effective and the frequency of these infections has decreased.

In the pre-HAART era, the most common symptoms in patients with AIDS included weight loss, pain, anorexia, depression, anxiety, cough, dyspnea, fatigue, and diarrhea.[4,5,9] More recent data (1996) from 3000 US patients reported the following as the 10 most common symptoms: constitutional symptoms (fever, sweats, chills) – 51 percent, diarrhea – 51 percent, nausea and anorexia – 50 percent, numbness and tingling/neuropathic pain in the hands and feet – 49 percent, headaches – 39 percent, weight loss – 37 percent, vaginal symptoms – 36 percent, sinus symptoms – 35 percent, visual disturbances – 32 percent, and cough or shortness of breath – 30 percent.[10] Currently, the median number of symptoms in patients with advanced HIV infection is 4, with a range of 0–25 in patients in a palliative care setting.[9]

PAIN

Pain frequently complicates the course of HIV infection. Often underdiagnosed and undertreated, pain is now more frequently a result of chronic HIV infection and/or medication toxicities than opportunistic infection in the developed world. One longitudinal study found that over a 2-year period, almost 90 percent of AIDS patients experienced pain and almost 70 percent experienced continuous pain.[11] Peripheral neuropathy, headache, and abdominal pain are the most common pain syndromes.[11]

Neuropathy

Peripheral polyneuropathy develops in about a third to half of patients with AIDS.[10,12,13] The predominant symptoms are pain, paresthesias, and numbness involving the feet and lower legs. The two most common causes of neuropathy are medication-induced and HIV-induced. These two conditions are indistinguishable clinically. The severity of distal sensory neuropathy induced by HIV is worse in late-stage disease.[14] The antiretroviral medications stavudine (D4T) and didanosine (DDI) are the medications most often associated with painful peripheral neuropathy. Pain may improve or stabilize after discontinuation of these medications but frequently it persists.

Management of peripheral neuropathy in the setting of HIV is similar to that of peripheral neuropathy in general. Gabapentin is the most commonly used medication. It appears to be effective in this setting but most experience is anecdotal. A daily dose of ⩾600 mg is required for efficacy.[15***] In a placebo-controlled trial involving diabetics, gabapentin at 900–3600 mg per day was significantly more effective than placebo in reducing pain intensity and quality of life. Dizziness (in 20 percent of subjects) and sleepiness (in 23 percent) were the most common adverse effects.[16**]

Gabapentin is more effective in reducing pain than in reducing numbness.

Lamotrigine has been studied as a treatment for HIV-associated neuropathy. Simpson *et al.* found that 11 weeks of lamotrigine was more effective than placebo in reducing neuropathic pain.[17] However, there was no benefit relative to placebo in patients who were no longer taking neurotoxic antiretroviral therapy. Hence, lamotrigine may have less relevance in end-of-life care, when neurotoxic antiretroviral therapy would likely be discontinued. Rash occurred in 14 percent of lamotrigine-treated patients, which was not significantly greater than placebo.

Tricyclic antidepressants are inexpensive medications often used for neuropathic pain. However, their frequent adverse effects limit their utility. A controlled trial of amitriptyline showed no benefit and more adverse effects compared with placebo.[18**] Topical capsaicin has also been demonstrated to be ineffective for this indication.[19]

FATIGUE

Fatigue, a highly prevalent symptom in patients with HIV infection, interferes with normal function and quality of life. Leading physiological factors contributing to fatigue in patients with HIV infection include anemia, deconditioning, muscle wasting, involuntary weight loss, hypogonadism, and opportunistic infection. General considerations for the evaluation and treatment of fatigue are outlined in Box 95.1.

Box 95.1 General considerations for the evaluation and treatment of fatigue

Assessment

- Severity, duration, impact
- Muscle weakness, wasting, somnolence
- Impaired cognitive function, altered mood

Potential etiologies

- Antiretroviral medications
- Other medications
- Opportunistic infection
- Anemia
- Depression/anxiety disorder
- Cachexia/wasting
- Major organ failure
- Dehydration

- Substance abuse
- Sleep disorder
- Endocrine abnormality
- Deconditioning
- Chronic pain

Anemia is a well-documented, reversible cause of fatigue. Randomized controlled trials have demonstrated significant improvement in overall quality of life in association with an increase in hematocrit.[20–22] Although health professionals frequently wait until the hemoglobin is 8 g/dL or less to intervene, studies have demonstrated that the incremental increases in quality of life with treatment are highest when hemoglobin is in the range of 11–13 g/dL.[23] The increase in hematocrit has been associated with improvements in energy, activity, and functional level and overall quality of life.

Fatigue has frequently been associated with depression and is a hallmark of major depressive disorders. But treatment of depression, in and of itself, in patients with cancer has not been shown to reverse fatigue.[24**] No similar data are available in the setting of HIV infection. Hormonal abnormalities, such as hypothyroidism and hypogonadism, are readily reversible causes of fatigue. Hypogonadism is the most common endocrine abnormality in patients with HIV infection, with low testosterone concentrations currently identified in about 15 percent of HIV-infected men in countries where HAART is available.[25] Changes in exercise or activity pattern, particularly associated with infections or opportunistic infection-related deconditioning, results in decreased activity and performance status, and are associated with fatigue regardless of the underlying cause of the deconditioning.

The first step in treatment is the identification of reversible factors that may contribute to fatigue. Common contributing factors, in addition to those above, include pain, sleep disorders, medications, and opportunistic infection. Both pharmacological and nonpharmacological interventions have been evaluated for the treatment of fatigue. Nonpharmacological interventions include exercise programs and maintenance of optimal levels of activity; restorative therapies; sleep therapy; and psychosocial interventions, including stress management, relaxation, and support groups.

The potential utility of psychostimulants for the treatment of HIV-related fatigue is supported by the results of a limited number of trials. A randomized, double-blind, placebo-controlled trial of methylphenidate (up to 60 mg daily), pemoline (150 mg/day), or placebo in patients with AIDS-related fatigue demonstrated an improvement in fatigue with treatment.[26**] Of methylphenidate-, pemoline-, and placebo-treated patients, 41 percent, 36 percent, and 15 percent, respectively, demonstrated improvement in fatigue on self-reported rating scales. Corticosteroids are thought to provide a boost in energy for patients with advanced malignancy, though it is unclear what their role and/or adverse effects might be in patients with chronic viral infection.

GASTROINTESTINAL SYMPTOMS

Diarrhea

Diarrhea is much less common since the introduction of HAART. However, it remains a chronic problem, reported by 28 percent of HIV-infected individuals who are receiving HAART.[27] Prior to the availability of effective anti-HIV therapy, infection was the most common cause of diarrhea. Now most cases are noninfectious, usually medication related.[28,29*] In one reported cohort, infection was responsible for 53 percent of cases of chronic diarrhea prior to the availability of HAART. Two years later, after HAART became available, the prevalence of chronic diarrhea was unchanged but infection accounted for only 13 percent of case.[29] Many antiretroviral agents, particularly protease inhibitors, cause diarrhea. The most common infectious causes are cytomegalovirus (CMV), cryptosporidiosis, *Clostridium difficile*, and *Giardia*. The patient's CD4 lymphocyte count (T cell count) is useful in determining the likelihood of certain pathogens. For example, CMV colitis, *Mycobacterium avium* complex (MAC), and microsporidiosis tend to occur only in patients with CD4 lymphocyte counts lower than 100/mm^3.

The initial approach to diarrhea in a palliative care situation is to discontinue potential medication culprits (e.g. protease inhibitors) and/or initiate nonspecific anti-diarrhea therapy such as loperamide. If fever or abdominal pain is present or if initial symptomatic therapy is unsuccessful, stool studies for ova and parasites, culture and sensitivity for bacterial pathogens, cryptosporidiosis, *C. difficile*, and mycobacteria are warranted. Upper and lower endoscopy with biopsies would be the next step. An extensive workup of this nature would be expected to yield a specific etiological diagnosis in two-thirds of patients.[30,31] Such a workup may not be appropriate in a palliative situation. If the diagnostic workup fails to identify a specific etiology, antimotility agents, such as loperamide, atropine/diphenoxylate, or tincture of opium can be quite helpful. High doses may be necessary. Subcutaneous octreotide is an effective albeit expensive treatment.[32] Changing or discontinuing antiretroviral agents may also be helpful.

Nausea

Virtually every anti-HIV medication has the potential to cause nausea. Zidovudine and the protease inhibitors are the worst offenders in this regard. Switching anti-HIV medications is the preferred option. In the patient with end-stage infection, stopping anti-HIV therapy altogether is an appropriate step. We have seen many patients who perked up considerably after HAART was discontinued, but only for a period of weeks to a few months.

Oral and esophageal symptoms

Oral candidiasis (thrush) is frequently seen in late stage infection.[33] It typically appears as white 'cottage cheese'-like plaques on buccal, pharyngeal, or lingual mucosa. Less often it manifests as patchy erythema. It may be asymptomatic but frequently is associated with oral discomfort and difficulty swallowing.[34]

Esophageal candidiasis is the most common cause of dysphagia. Concomitant oral thrush is present in approximately 80 percent of cases.[35] Empirical therapy with oral fluconazole is appropriate for dysphagia, even in the absence of oral thrush. Oral fluconazole is an effective treatment with a 90 percent response rate.[36**] Extensive use of this drug has fostered the development of resistant strains, particularly in individuals with end-stage AIDS.[37] If fluconazole proves unsuccessful, there may be value in trying oral voriconazole[38] or oral amphotericin suspension.[39] Although the unfavorable side effect profile of IV amphotericin B generally makes it unsuitable in the palliative care setting, once weekly dosing may be effective and well tolerated in the management of recalcitrant oral and esophageal candidiasis.

Odynophagia (painful swallowing) is usually caused by CMV, herpes simplex virus (HSV), or idiopathic esophageal ulcers.[40] The first two conditions are treated with anti-CMV therapy (e.g. ganciclovir or valganciclovir) and anti-HSV therapy (aciclovir or valaciclovir), respectively. The last condition responds to treatment with oral corticosteroids.

INVOLUNTARY WEIGHT LOSS AND WASTING

Involuntary weight loss, even as little as 5 percent of pre-morbid weight, portends a poor prognosis for persons with HIV infection.[41] Weight loss is still common even in the era of HAART.[42] In one cohort of HIV-infected subjects, the majority of them receiving HAART, 18 percent of subjects lost >10 percent of body weight and 21 percent lost greater than 5 percent of body weight. In the Multicenter AIDS Cohort (MACS), an ongoing study of 5622 homosexual and bisexual men at four US sites, the proportion of AIDS diagnoses in which wasting was present increased from 5 percent in the period between 1988 and 1990 to 18.9 percent in the time period 1996–99.[43] Whether or not lipodystrophy (a syndrome of central adiposity and peripheral lipoatrophy) is being misdiagnosed as the wasting syndrome is unclear from current data but needs additional study.

The assessment of patients with HIV-related wasting includes evaluation for opportunistic infections, degree of HIV control, gonadal function, potential adverse effects of medications, gastrointestinal function, symptoms that interfere with oral intake, and psychosocial or financial factors

that might contribute to weight loss. Many HIV medications have gastrointestinal side effects.

Endocrine disturbances, particularly gonadal dysfunction, contribute to HIV-related weight loss. Early in the epidemic, and potentially currently, in the absence of HAART, as many as 50 percent of men with AIDS were hypogonadal. With the availability of HAART, the incidence has dropped to about 15 percent.[25] Loss of lean body mass and decreased functional status are highly correlated with androgen concentrations in HIV-infected men with hypogonadism and wasting.[44***,45,46] Testosterone therapy in both hypogonadal and eugonadal men increases lean body mass.[44***] A recent meta-analysis of the use of testosterone therapy for the HIV wasting syndrome concluded that testosterone improves lean body mass and weight to a small degree, with the greatest effect seen when testosterone is delivered intramuscularly.[44***]

Anorexia is an important contributor to HIV-related weight loss and was the primary target of early interventions for wasting. Megestrol acetate, a synthetic, orally active progestational agent, has been used widely as an appetite stimulant in patients with advanced cancer.[47**,48**] In patients with AIDS-associated weight loss, treatment with 800 mg/day of megestrol acetate, as compared to placebo, leads to significant improvement in weight, overall sense of wellbeing, appetite, and caloric intake.[49**,50**] Although generally well tolerated, megestrol acetate may lead to a variety of adverse endocrinological effects. Megestrol acetate, similar to glucocorticoids, suppresses the pituitary adrenal axis and may cause reversible adrenal suppression, diabetes mellitus, and a steroid withdrawal syndrome.[51,52] In addition, across a broad range of doses, megestrol acetate reduces serum testosterone to castrate levels.[53]

Studies of megestrol acetate for the treatment of cachexia have consistently demonstrated improvement in appetite and weight gain.[47–50] The composition of this weight gain, however, as evaluated by dual energy X-ray absorptiometry, tritiated body water methodologies, or bioimpedance analysis (BIA), is primarily fat mass without a significant increase in lean tissue or edema.[48,54] Dronabinol (delta-9-tetrahydrocannabinol) was first evaluated as an orexigenic agent in patients with cancer-related anorexia and cachexia. A subsequent multicenter, randomized, double-blind, placebo-controlled study of dronabinol, as compared with placebo, demonstrated improved appetite, as measured by a visual analog scale ($P = 0.01$) and improved mood ($P = 0.005$).[55**] There was no significant increase in weight. The dronabinol dose was reduced to 2.5 mg once daily in 18 percent of patients due to central nervous system toxicity. A four-arm, randomized, pharmacokinetic study evaluated the use of single-agent dronabinol, megestrol acetate, or combination therapy. The addition of dronabinol to megestrol acetate provided no added benefit compared with megestrol acetate treatment alone.[56]

Thalidomide is an inhibitor of tumor necrosis factor (TNF) production by monocytes in vitro. Three placebo-controlled trials of thalidomide in patients with

HIV-associated weight loss have demonstrated weight gain with treatment.[57**,58**,59**] In the largest of these trials, thalidomide 100 mg daily for 8 weeks produced a significant weight gain (+1.7 kg vs. placebo), about half of which was lean body mass. Anabolic agents offer the potential to improve weight and body composition, ideally by replenishing lean body mass. Two oral anabolic agents, oxandrolone and oxymetholone, have been evaluated in placebo-controlled trials for treatment of HIV wasting.[60**] Oxandrolone led to a sustained increase in weight (mean +1.8 kg) over 14 weeks, while oxymetholone-treated patients gained a mean of 3 kg over 16 weeks.

Resistance training also can increase lean body mass, 1.4 to 2.1 kg, in asymptomatic HIV-infected men receiving HAART and in eugonadal men with AIDS wasting.[61,62] More dramatic improvements in lean body mass are observed from combination treatment with exercise and an anabolic agent. A randomized controlled trial of testosterone and resistance training stimulated a 4.6 kg gain in lean body mass,[63**] whereas treatment with supraphysiological doses of nandrolone and resistance training resulted in a net weight gain of 2.9 kg.[64]

Growth hormone increases protein synthesis and has anticatabolic, protein-sparing effects. A randomized placebo-controlled study of recombinant growth hormone 0.1 μg/kg per day subcutaneously in patients with AIDS-related weight loss demonstrated increased weight (+1.6 kg; $P < 0.0001$) and lean body mass (+3 kg; $P < 0.001$) and decreased body fat (−1.7 kg; $P < 0.0001$).[65**] Paton et al. evaluated the protein-sparing effects of recombinant human growth hormone in HIV-infected subjects with acute opportunistic infections compared with placebo. Improvement in weight and lean body mass was observed in the treated subjects.[66] This suggests the potential short-term use of growth hormone to prevent or attenuate opportunistic infection-associated wasting. Optimal therapeutic schedules and dosing of growth hormone are unclear, and its cost has limited its use to some degree.

Weight loss remains a clinically and prognostically significant issue for HIV-infected individuals. There is now a large body of knowledge to support the benefits of nutritional counseling, dietary supplements, appetite stimulants, anabolic agents, and an exercise prescription for the treatment of HIV-related weight loss.

DRUG INTERACTIONS

There are many potential drug interactions in the palliative care of HIV-infected individuals. In this regard, the protease inhibitors (PI) and non-nucleoside reverse transcriptase inhibitors (NNRTI) are the most problematic. For example, the PI ritonavir is a potent inhibitor of CYP3A4 enzyme of the hepatic cytochrome P450 enzyme system. As a result, ritonavir significantly slows the metabolism of several palliative medications. Ritonavir therapy increases plasma levels and prolongs the duration of activity of benzodiazepines (in particular, midazolam and triazolam), bupropion, and ergot derivatives. These medications should not be used in combination with ritonavir. Furthermore, ritonavir decreases plasma levels of methadone, fentanyl, codeine, and hydrocodone. Increased dosages of these medications may be needed when used concomitantly with ritonavir. Ritonavir is the PI most likely to interact with other medications. Among the remaining PIs, nelfinavir, fosamprenavir, and indinavir are less likely to interact with other drugs. Saquinavir is least likely.[67] Ritonavir is frequently used in a fixed dose combination capsule with another PI, lopinavir (Kaletra). The NNRTIs efavirenz and nevirapine reduce plasma levels of methadone by 35–50 percent. An increase in methadone dosage of approximately 20 percent is required to prevent narcotic withdrawal symptoms when efavirenz is added to a stable methadone regimen. The NNRTI delavirdine increases plasma levels of methadone and amfetamines (see Tables 95.1 and 95.2).

Alternative therapies are commonly used by people infected with HIV. There is an interaction between St John's

Table 95.1 *Palliative drugs that should not be used concurrently with anti-HIV drugs*

HIV medication	Drugs that should not be coadministered
Protease inhibitors	Midazolam, triazolam, ergot derivatives, bupropion
Non-nucleoside reverse transcriptase inhibitors	
Delavirdine	Alprazolam, midazolam, triazolam, phenytoin, carbamazepine

HIV, human immunodeficiency virus.

Table 95.2 *Palliative drugs that may require dosage adjustment when given concurrently with anti-HIV drugs*

HIV medication	Drugs requiring dosage adjustment
Protease inhibitors	Methadone, fentanyl, tramadol, propoxyphene, clonazepam, carbamazepine, nefazodone, SSRI antidepressants, tricyclic antidepressants, amfetamines, dronabinol, risperidone, diazepam, zolpidem, dexamethasone, phenytoin
Non-nucleoside reverse transcriptase inhibitors	
Delavirdine	Methadone, amfetamines
Efavirenz	Methadone, carbamazepine, sertraline
Nevirapine	Methadone

HIV, human immunodeficiency virus; SSRI, selective serotonin reuptake inhibitor.

wort and the PI indinavir. St John's wort induces CYP3A4 and decreases plasma levels of indinavir.[67] Similarly, St John's wort can affect the metabolism of NNRTIs. Thus, St John's wort should not be taken by patients who are taking PIs or NNRTIs.

PROGNOSIS

HIV infection and AIDS have become chronic conditions in countries where HAART is available. Without effective antiretroviral therapy, the median survival following an AIDS-defining condition is less than 2 years.[68] Now with HAART, it is hoped, and expected, that people with AIDS will live for decades.[1] Rates of HIV-associated death have fallen by 80 percent in the USA as a result of HAART.[1,2] Since even patients with advanced immunodeficiency may respond to HAART,[69, 70**] no patient, regardless of how ill they might appear, should be given a poor prognosis until they have received treatment if it is available.

These improvements have been remarkable. Yet death rates from HIV in the USA have leveled off although AIDS remains the fifth leading cause of death in people aged 24–44 years.[2] African Americans are disproportionately infected. The combination of longer life expectancy plus 40 000 new infections annually in the USA has yielded an increasing prevalence of the disease.[2]

The modes of AIDS-related death have changed for patients treated with HAART. Although opportunistic infections continue to be the primary cause of death in the developing world, they are much less frequent and are no longer the leading causes of HIV-associated death in countries where HAART is routinely prescribed. Rather, chronic liver disease is now the most common cause of death in people infected with HIV.[71] This is in large part due to coinfection with hepatitis C virus (HCV). It is estimated that 30–40 percent of HIV-infected individuals are also infected with HCV.[72] In coinfected individuals, almost half of deaths are due to liver disease. Coinfection with HIV and HCV appears to accelerate the course of both.[73***]

RECOGNITION OF END-STAGE DISEASE

Recognizing the potential for dramatic improvement in health with HAART for patients with previously untreated, advanced HIV disease, how does one recognize the patient who is no longer appropriate for life-sustaining therapy? Virological, clinical characteristics, and comorbidities provide useful information. Patients with a history of nonadherence to antiretroviral therapy regimens, inability to obtain HAART, and/or highly resistant HIV infection fare poorly. Underlying liver disease, particularly cirrhosis and/or active hepatitis interfering with the ability to deliver effective antiretroviral therapy safely, also poses a significant risk for patients' overall longevity.

Refractory malignancy, with or without adequate control of HIV infection, predicts a poor prognosis, as it does in the general population. Similarly, end-stage liver disease, generally secondary to hepatitis C virus, carries a poor prognosis. For patients whose prognosis is defined by a secondary illness or uncontrolled, refractory HIV infection, withdrawal of HIV medications should at least be considered and discussed at length with the patient. The balance between the potential benefit from HAART versus the burden of continuing to take the medications should be weighed in the context of the patient's goals and comorbidities. As is the case for all patients with chronic and/or progressive illness, constant reassessment of goals, toxicities of therapy, and definitions of quality of life need repeated evaluation and discussion.

Key learning points

- HIV-associated death rates have fallen in developed countries.

- The symptom burden of HIV-infected people remains high, averaging four symptoms per person.

- Anti-HIV medications frequently cause symptoms.

- Fatigue is common and often responds to pharmacotherapy.

- Weight loss is common and often responds to pharmacotherapy.

- Nausea and diarrhea are common and may require discontinuation of anti-HIV therapy.

- Anti-HIV medications frequently interact with palliative medications.

REFERENCES

● 1 Palella FJ, Delaney KM, Moorman AC, *et al.* Declining morbidity and mortality among patients with advanced human immunodeficiency virus infection. *N Engl J Med* 1998; **338**: 853–60.

2 Centers for Disease Control and Prevention. *HIV/AIDS Surveillance Report, 2002.* Atlanta: CDC, 2002. Also available at http://www.cdc.gov/hiv/stats/hasrlink.htm (accessed March 8, 2006).

3 Lynn J. Serving patients who may die soon and their families. *JAMA* 2001; **285**: 925–32.

4 Selwyn PA, Forstein M. Overcoming the false dichotomy of curative vs palliative care for late-stage HIV/AIDS. *JAMA* 2003; **290**: 806–14.

5 Selwyn PA, Rivard M, Kappell D, *et al.* Palliative care for AIDS at a large urban teaching hospital: program description and preliminary outcomes. *J Palliat Med* 2003; **6**: 461–74.

6 Scannell K. *Death of the Good Doctor. Lessons from the Heart of the AIDS Epidemic.* San Francisco, CA: Cleis Press, Inc, 1999.

7   Crawley L, Payne R, Bolden J, *et al.* Palliative and end-of-life care in the African American community. *JAMA* 2000; **284**: 2518–21.

8   Curtis JR, Patrick DL, Aldwell E, *et al.* The quality of patient-doctor communication about end-of-life care: a study of patients with advanced AIDS and their primary care clinicians. *AIDS* 1999; **13**: 1123–31.

9   Selwyn PA, Rivard M. Palliative care for AIDS: challenges and opportunities in the era of highly active anti-retroviral therapy. *J Palliat Med* 2003; **6**: 475–87.

10 Mathews W, McCutcheon JA, Asch S, *et al.* National estimates of HIV-related symptom prevalence from the HIV Cost and Services Utilization Study. *Med Care* 2000; **38**: 750–62.

11 Frich LM, Borgbjerg FM. Pain and pain treatment in AIDS patients: a longitudinal study. *J Pain Symptom Manage* 2000; **19**: 339–47.

12 Schiffito G, McDermott MP, McArthur JC, *et al.* Incidence and risk factors for HIV-associated distal sensory polyneuropathy. *Neurology* 2002; **58**: 1764–8.

13 Hewitt DJ, McDonald M, Portenoy RK, *et al.* Pain syndromes and etiologies in ambulatory AIDS patients. *Pain* 1997; **70**: 117–23.

14 Simpson DM, Haidich A-B, Schifitto GB, *et al.* Severity of HIV-associated neuropathy is associated with plasma HIV-1 RNA levels. *AIDS* 2002; **16**: 407–12.

15 Mendell JR, Sahenk Z. Painful sensory neuropathy. *N Engl J Med* 2003; **348**: 1243–55.

16 Backonja M, Beydoun A, Edwards KR, *et al.* Gabapentin for the symptomatic treatment of painful neuropathy in patients with diabetes mellitus: a randomized controlled trial. *JAMA* 1998; **280**: 1831–6.

17 Simpson DM, McArthur JC, Olney R, *et al.* Lamotrigine for HIV-associated painful sensory neuropathies: a placebo-controlled trial. *Neurology* 2003; **60**: 1508–14.

18 Kieburtz K, Simpson D, Yiannoutsos C, *et al.* A randomized trial of amitriptyline and mexiletine for painful neuropathy in HIV infection. AIDS Clinical Trial Group 242 Protocol Team. *Neurology* 1998; **51**: 1682–8.

19 Paice JA, Ferrans CE, Lashley FR, *et al.* Topical capsaicin in the management of HIV-associated peripheral neuropathy. *J Pain Symptom Manage* 2000; **19**: 45–52.

20 Abrams DI, Steinhart C, Frascino R. Epoetin alfa therapy for anaemia in HIV-infected patients: impact on quality of life. *Int J STD AIDS* 2000; **11**: 659–65.

21 Grossman H, Bowers P, Leitz G. Once-weekly epoetin alfa (Procrit®) corrects hemoglobin and improves quality of life as effectively as three-times-weekly dosing in HIV+ patients [poster ThPeB7381]. In: *Proceedings of the XIV International AIDS Conference (Barcelona)*. Stockholm: International AIDS Society, 2002.

22 Saag MS, Levine AM, Leitz GJ, Bowers PJ. Once-weekly epoetin alfa increases hemoglobin and improves quality of life in anemic HIV+ patients [poster]. In: *Proceedings of the 39th Annual Meeting of the Infectious Diseases Society of American (San Francisco)*. Alexandria, VA: Infectious Diseases Society of America, 2001.

23 Crawford J, Cella D, Cleeland CS, *et al.* Relationship between changes in hemoglobin level and quality of life during chemotherapy in anemic cancer patients receiving epoetin alfa therapy. *Cancer* 2002; **95**: 888–95.

24 Morrow GR, Hickok JT, Raubertas RF, *et al.* Effect of an SSRI antidepressant on fatigue and depression in 738 cancer patients treated with chemotherapy: a URCC CCOP study [abstract 1531]. *Proc Amer Soc Clin Oncol* 2001; **20**: 384a.

25 Berger D, Muurshainen N, Witten B, *et al.* Hypogonadism and wasting in the era of HAART in HIV-infected patients. Program and Abstracts of the XII World AIDS Conference, June–July 1998, Geneva, Switzerland [abstract 32174].

26 Breitbart W, Rosenfeld B, Kaim M, Funesti-Esch J. A randomized, double-blind, placebo-controlled trial of psychostimulants for the treatment of fatigue in ambulatory patients with human immunodeficiency virus disease. *Arch Intern Med* 2001; **161**: 411–20.

27 Knox TA, Spiegelman D, Skinner SC, Gorbach S. Diarrhea and abnormalities of gastrointestinal function in a cohort of men and women with HIV infection. *Am J Gastroenterol* 2000; **95**: 3482–9.

● 28 Monkemuller KE, Call SA, Lazenby AJ, Wilcox CM. Declining prevalence of opportunistic gastrointestinal disease in the era of combination antiretroviral therapy. *Am J Gastroenterol* 2000; **95**: 457–62.

29 Call SA, Heudebert G, Saag M, Wilcox CM. The changing etiology of chronic diarrhea in HIV-infected patients with CD4 cell counts less than 200 cells/mm³. *Am J Gastroenterol* 2000; **95**: 3142–6.

30 Kartalija M, Sande MA. Diarrhea and AIDS in the era of highly active antiretroviral therapy. *Clin Infect Dis* 1999; **28**: 701–7.

31 Wilcox CM, Rabeneck L, Friedman S. AGA technical review: malnutrition and cachexia, chronic diarrhea, and hepatobiliary disease in patients with human immunodeficiency virus infection. *Gastroenterology* 1996; **111**: 1724–52.

32 Simon DM, Cello JP, Valenzuela J, *et al.* Multicenter trial of octreotide in patients with refractory acquired immuno-deficiency syndrome-associated diarrhea. *Gastroenterology* 1995; **108**: 1753–60.

33 Ball SC. Oroesophageal candidiasis in a patient with AIDS. *AIDS Reader* 2004; **14**: 289–90, 292.

◆ 34 Vazquez JA, Sobel JD. Mucosal candidiasis. *Infect Dis Clin North America* 2002; **16**: 793–820.

35 Wilcox CM, Straub RF, Clark WS. Prospective evaluation of oropharyngeal findings in human immunodeficiency virus-infected patients with esophageal ulceration. *Am J Gastroenterol* 1995; **90**: 1938–41.

36 Phillips P, DeBeule K, Frechette G, *et al.* A double-blind comparison of itraconazole oral solution and fluconazole capsules for the treatment of oropharyngeal candidiasis in patients with AIDS. *Clin Infect Dis* 1998; **26**: 1368–73.

37 Maenza JR, Keruly JC, Moore RD, *et al.* Risk factors for fluconazole-resistant candidiasis in human immunodeficiency virus-infected patients. *J Infect Dis* 1996; **173**: 219–25.

38 Ruhnke M, Schmidt-Westhausen A, Trautmann M. In vitro activities of voriconazole (UK-109, 496) against fluconazole-susceptible and –resistant *Candida albicans* isolates from oral cavities of patients with human immunodeficiency virus infection. *Antimicrob Agents Chemother* 1997; **41**: 575–7.

39 Nguyen MT, Weiss PJ, LaBarre RC, Wallace MR. Orally administered amphotericin B in the treatment of oral candidiasis in HIV-infected patients caused by azole-resistant *Candida albicans*. *J Acquir Immune Defic Syndr* 1996; **10**: 1745–7.

40 Wilcox CM, Straub RF, Alexander LN, Clark WS. Etiology of esophageal disease in human immunodeficiency virus-infected

patients who fail antifungal therapy. *Am J Med* 1996; **101**: 599–604.

41 Tang AM, Forrester J, Spiegelman D, *et al*. Weight loss and survival in HIV-positive patients in the era of highly active antiretroviral therapy. *J Acquir Immune Defic Syndr* 2002; **31**: 230–6.

42 Wanke C, Silva M, Knox T, Forrester J, Speigelman D, Gorbach S. Weight loss and wasting remain common complications in individuals infected with HIV in the era of highly active antiretroviral therapy. *Clin Infect Dis* 2000; **31**: 803–5.

43 Smit E, Skolasky RL, Dobs AS, *et al*. Changes in the incidence and predictors of wasting syndrome related to human immunodeficiency virus infection, 1987–1999. *Am J Epidemiol* 2002; **156**: 211–18.

44 Kong A, Edmonds P. Testosterone therapy in HIV wasting syndrome: systematic review and meta-analysis. *Lancet* 2002; **2**: 692–9.

45 Roubenoff R, Wilson IB. Effect of resistance training on self-reported physical functioning in HIV infection. *Med Sci Sports Exerc* 2001; **33**: 1811–17.

46 Schroeder ET, Terk M, Sattler FR. Androgen therapy improves muscle mass and strength but not muscle quality: results from two studies. *Am J Physiol Endocrinol Metab* 2003; **285**: E16–E24.

● 47 Loprinzi CL, Ellison NM, Schaid DJ, *et al*. Controlled trial of megestrol acetate for the treatment of cancer anorexia and cachexia. *J Natl Cancer Inst* 1990; **82**: 1127–32.

48 Loprinzi CL, Michalak JC, Schaid DJ, *et al*. Phase III evaluation of four doses of megestrol acetate as therapy for patients with cancer anorexia and/or cachexia. *J Clin Oncol* 1993; **11**: 762–7.

49 Von Roenn JH, Armstrong D, Kotler DP, *et al*. Megestrol acetate in patients with AIDS related cachexia. *Ann Internal Med* 1994; **121**: 393–9.

50 Oster MH, Enders SR, Samuels SJ, *et al*. Megestrol acetate in patients with AIDS and cachexia. *Ann Intern Med* 1994; **121**: 400–8.

51 Mann M, Koller E, Murgo A, *et al*. Glucocorticoidlike activity of megestrol. *Arch Intern Med* 1997; **157**: 1651–6.

52 Loprinzi CL, Jensen MD, Jiang NS, Schaid DJ. Effect of megestrol acetate on the human pituitary-adrenal axis. *Mayo Clin Proc* 1992; **67**: 1160–2.

53 Engelson ES, Pi-Sunyer FX, Kotler DP. Effects of megestrol acetate therapy on body composition and circulating testosterone concentration in patients with AIDS. *AIDS* 1995; **9**: 1107–8.

54 Eubanks V, Koppersmith N, Wooldridge N, *et al*. Effects of megestrol acetate on weight gain, body composition, and pulmonary function in patients with cystic fibrosis. *J Pediatr* 2002; **140**: 439–44.

55 Plasse TF, Gorter RW, Krasnow SH, *et al*. Recent clinical experience with dronabinol. *Pharmacol Biochm Behav* 1991; **40**: 695–700.

56 Timpone JG, Wright DJ, Li N, *et al*. The safety and pharmacokinetics of single-agent and combination therapy with megestrol acetate and dronabinol for the treatment of HIV wasting syndrome. *AIDS Res Hum Retroviruses* 1997; **13**: 305–15.

57 Kaplan G, Thomas S, Fierer DS, *et al*. Thalidomide for the treatment of AIDS-associated wasting. *AIDS Res Hum Retroviruses* 2000; **16**: 1345–55.

58 Reyes-Teran G, Sierra-Madero JG, Martinez del Cerro V, *et al*. Effects of thalidomide on HIV-associated wasting syndrome: a randomized, double-blind, placebo-controlled clinical trial. *AIDS* 1996; **10**: 1501–7.

59 Klausner JD, Makonkawkeyoon S, Akarasewi P, *et al*. The effect of thalidomide on the pathogenesis of human immunodeficiency virus Type 1 and *M. tuberculosis* infection. *J Acquir Immune Defic Syndr Hum Retrovirol* 1996; **11**: 247–57.

60 Hengge UR, Stocks KR, Wiehler H, *et al*. Double-blind, randomized, placebo-controlled phase III trial of oxymetholone for the treatment of HIV wasting. *AIDS* 2003; **17**: 699–710.

61 Roubenoff R, McDermott A, Weiss L, *et al*. Short-term progressive resistance training increases strength and lean body mass in adults infected with human immunodeficiency virus. *AIDS* 1999; **13**: 231–9.

62 Yarasheski KE, Tebas P, Stanerson B, *et al*. Resistance exercise training reduces hypertriglyceridernia in HIV-infected men treated with antiviral therapy. *J Appl Physiol* 2001; **90**: 133–8.

63 Bhasin S, Storer T, Javanbakht M, *et al*. Testosterone replacement and resistance exercise in HIV-infected men with weight loss and low testosterone levels. *JAMA* 2000; **283**: 763–70.

64 Sattler F, Jaque S, Schroeder E, *et al*. Effects of pharmacological doses of nandrolone decanoate and progressive resistance training in immunodeficient patients infected with human immunodeficiency virus. *J Clin Endocrinol Metab* 1999; **84**: 1268–76.

● 65 Schambelan M, Mulligan K, Grunfeld C, *et al*. Recombinant human growth hormone in patients with HIV-associated wasting. *Ann Intern Med* 1996; **125**: 873–82.

66 Paton N, Newton P, Sharpstone D, *et al*. Short-term growth hormone administration at the time of opportunistic infection in HIV-positive people. *AIDS* 1999; **13**: 1195–202.

◆ 67 Piscitelli SD, Gallicano KD. Interactions among drugs for HIV and opportunistic infections. *N Engl J Med* 2001; **344**: 984–96.

68 National Center for HIV, STD, and TB Prevention. AIDS case surveillance data. Available at: www.cdc.gov/hiv (accessed February 4, 2005).

69 Goodman E. Living with AIDS: the Lazarus Syndrome. *Baltimore Sun*, March 18, 1997, p. 9A.

● 70 Staszewski S, Morales-Ramirez J, Tashima KT, *et al*. Efavirenz plus zidovudine and lamivudine, efavirenz plus indinavir, and indinavir plus zidovudine and lamivudine in the treatment of HIV-1 infection in adults. *N Engl J Med* 1999; **341**: 1865–73.

71 Bica I, McGovern B, Dhar R, *et al*. Increasing mortality due to end-stage liver disease in patients with human immunodeficiency virus infection. *Clin Infect Dis* 2001; **32**: 492–7.

72 Monga HK, Rodriguez-Barradas MC, Breaux K, *et al*. Hepatitis C virus infection-related morbidity and mortality among patients with human immunodeficiency virus infection. *Clin Infect Dis* 2001; **33**: 240–7.

◆ 73 Sulkowski MS, Thomas DL. Hepatitis C in the HIV-infected person. *Ann Intern Med* 2003; **138**: 197–207.

96

Neurological diseases

RACHEL BURMAN

INTRODUCTION

This chapter will focus on the palliative care of adults with the more common progressive neurodegenerative diseases and their carers, and stroke will also be considered in some detail. More detailed discussion of palliative care in children can be found in Chapter 98, and of neoplasms – radiotherapy and chemotherapy – in Chapters 91 and 92, respectively. Studies have supported the application of the principles of specialist palliative care to the care of people with neurological disorders for some time. Saunders et al. described the first successful inclusion of patients with a neurodegenerative disorder (amyotrophic lateral sclerosis [ALS]) in a palliative care service back in 1981.[1] O'Brien et al. later researched the role of specialist services for these ALS patients and their carers and confirmed its relevance.[2] Addington-Hall and McCarthy demonstrated that data from the 'Regional study of care for the dying' showed dying from cancer was not much different from dying of chronic obstructive pulmonary disease (COPD), congestive heart failure, or stroke.[3] Furthermore they were able to demonstrate that people dying from congestive cardiac failure, COPD, and stroke had unmet health and social care needs in the last year of life.[4] Epidemiological data analyzed by Higginson in 1997 showed that only a quarter of all deaths dealt with by healthcare professionals on a daily basis in the UK are due to cancer.[5]

Neurologists have also endorsed the relevance of palliative care to people with neurological conditions. The American Association of Neurology issued a statement in 1996 saying that neurologists have a duty to provide adequate palliative care to their patients.[6] There is also a palliative care research group as part of the World Federation of Neurology. More recently the Multiple Sclerosis Society of Great Britain has funded a 3-year project to look at the palliative care needs of people severely affected by multiple sclerosis; this is still ongoing. There is no room for complacency when studies in the Netherlands report 5 percent of patients with multiple sclerosis and 20 percent of patients with ALS request and die by either physician-assisted suicide or euthanasia.[7,8] The disease progression of these neurodegenerative disorders cannot be significantly altered, it is therefore all the more important that appropriate palliation of the attendant symptoms and psychological distress is given.

STROKE

Stroke is a heterogeneous collection of conditions. It may be as a result of intracerebral bleeding or infarction of an area of the brain or it can occur following a subarachnoid hemorrhage. Rarer causes include vasculitis and venous sinus thrombosis. The prevalence of stroke varies in different populations and differs also with age and ethnicity. The Framingham study in the USA estimated the annual age-adjusted incidence for women was 4.5/1000 and for men 6/1000.[9] Of these, 60 percent are atherothrombotic infarctions, 23 percent cardiac embolisms, 7 percent subarachnoid hemorrhage, 7 percent intracerebral hemorrhage. Brain infarction may be due to emboli from the heart, aorta, or major brain supplying arteries. Hemodynamic changes due to severe stenosis or occlusions may cause infarctions as can the microangiopathy of hypertension and diabetes.

The typical clinical manifestations of stroke are hemiparesis, visual loss, hypesthesia, diplopia, hemianopia, or loss of consciousness. The therapeutic options for stroke patients include admission to a specialist stroke unit for management of imbalanced hemostasis and prevention of secondary infections, etc., administration of aspirin or in selected cases, thrombolysis. Thrombolysis improves mortality and morbidity by up to 30 percent, whereas aspirin improves these by only 1–5 percent.[10] The long-term prognosis of stroke is also poor. There are several predictors of functional recovery after stroke: age, previous stroke, consciousness at onset, urinary continence.[11] Only 25 percent of stroke patients survive without major disability; 20–50 percent of all patients experience some kind of disability with 20–25 percent of patients developing poststroke dementia and 10–30 percent dying within a year of experiencing a stroke.[11] Of these, many will die suddenly making it more difficult to predict the number or indeed which patients and families might best be helped by palliative care. A study of palliative day care in England showed that human immunodeficiency virus (HIV)/acquired immune deficiency syndrome (AIDS), ALS and stroke were the three second most important diagnoses after cancer which require palliative care.[12] Also a secondary analysis of the Regional Study of Care for the Dying undertaken in England found that 65 percent of bereaved relatives reported stroke patients as experiencing pain in the last year of life while 51 percent experienced confusion, 56 percent urinary incontinence and 56 percent depressed mood. Pain control was reported as inadequate.[4]

Palliative care challenges

SYMPTOM CONTROL – PAIN

The pain requirements of patients prior to sustaining a stroke should not be overlooked particularly when there are communication difficulties following the stroke. The direct result of the stroke may cause several pain problems. Around 30 percent of stroke patients experience poststroke headache. Up to 70 percent of such patients experience 'shoulder–hand syndrome', the upper limb has reduced movement and therefore becomes stiff, this in turn leads to hand swelling and the hand appears blue, clammy, and hot. A neuropathic central poststroke pain occurs in 8 percent of patients. It is not particularly responsive to opioids but it shows some response to amitriptyline.[13*] Another study of central pain showed lamotrigine to be effective.[14*]

PSYCHOSOCIAL CARE – DEPRESSION AND ANXIETY

Poststroke depression is reported as a common occurrence. In a Scandinavian study, minor depression was diagnosed in 14 percent of patients and 26 percent of the patients experienced major depression. The only independent predictors of poststroke depression were found to be a premorbid history of depression and dependency in daily living following stroke. Relatives caring for such patients in the community report that they would have liked more support and those stroke patients who died in hospital are reported as requiring more psychological support in one study.[4] This would suggest a role for palliative care in supporting these patients and their families.

ADVANCE PLANNING/END-OF-LIFE CARE – FEEDING

The dysphagia which necessitates artificial feeding of stroke patients is in itself a poor prognostic indicator.[15] Whether to provide artificial nutrition to patients with such a poor prognosis is an important consideration. Following a stroke, 30 percent of conscious patients have an impaired swallow on the day after the stroke, 16 percent at 1 week and 2 percent at 1 month.[16] Poor nutrition may predispose to muscle weakness and fatigue which will impair rehabilitation, it will also predispose the patient to pressure area sores. Hence, persistent dysphagia may require the insertion of a nasogastric tube or percutaneous gastrostomy. The relative risks and benefits of these two procedures were looked at in a randomized controlled trial. Greater mortality and decreased nutritional intake was demonstrated in the nasogastric group. However, the median survival rate post-insertion of a percutaneous gastrostomy was found to be only 53 days. The International Stroke Trials Collaboration FOOD Trial data have now been published and recently reported that it cannot support the early parenteral feeding of people following a stroke.[17**] The input of specialists in palliative care with their experience of end-of-life decision making may be helpful as this issue engenders strong feelings among families and friends of stroke patients.[18]

NEURODEGENERATIVE DISEASES

Multiple sclerosis

Multiple sclerosis is the most common of the demyelinating diseases which share the pathological features of focal areas of degeneration of the myelin sheath that surrounds nervous tissue. It is the most common cause of chronic disability in young adults. The process of demyelination is associated with inflammation and then gliosis. Evidence suggests this is a T-cell–mediated inflammatory process experienced by genetically susceptible people in the presence of particular environmental factors. The pathological plaques are discrete areas of scarring which are scattered throughout the central nervous system in different locations at different times. This leads to a wide range of clinical signs and symptoms.[19] It particularly affects the brain stem, optic nerves, and spinal cord. In Britain and northern Europe its prevalence is about 80–100 per 1 000 000 population. It is roughly twice as common in females as in males and the mean age of onset is around 30 years, with a range of 20–50 years. Multiple sclerosis has a variable disease trajectory. About 25 percent of people affected have relatively benign disease with mild exacerbations from which they make a complete recovery. Unfortunately, 10 percent of patients develop a rapidly progressive (primary) illness which leads to severe disability relatively quickly.[20]

In most patients the disease follows a relapsing and remitting course with variable degrees of recovery, at least initially, before a progressive (secondary) deterioration ensues; 80–90 percent of people will convert to secondary progressive multiple sclerosis within 20–25 years of diagnosis. The median survival from onset is 28 years for men and 33 years for women, with overall life expectancy being 7 years less than would be expected; death is most often as a result of infection. During this time an ever increasing burden of disability and symptoms is accrued with the inevitable impact on the person's quality of life.

There is no cure for multiple sclerosis at present. Acute relapses often respond to corticosteroids, most often administered intravenously for 3–5 days. Trials have shown immunomodulating therapies interferon-β1a, interferon-β1b and glatiramer acetate reduce both the frequency of acute attacks and the accumulations of plaques within the central nervous system .[21*]

Amyotrophic lateral sclerosis

This is the most common degenerative disorder of the motor neuron system in adults with 1.5–2/100 000 per year. Most people are diagnosed after the age of 40 with a mean age of onset around the late fifties.[22] For most the cause is unknown. There is a family history in only 5 percent of cases, of these 20 percent have a gene mutation of the superoxide dismutase (SOD1) gene on chromosome 21. Amyotrophic lateral sclerosis is characterized by involvement of upper and lower motor neurons. This manifests itself clinically with fasciculations and slowly progressive paresis of the voluntary muscles coupled with hyperreflexia and spasticity (see also Box 96.1).

The sensory system is normal with sparing of eye movements and sphincters in the vast majority of patients. The average prognosis is 3–4 years although there is considerable variation. About 20–30 percent of patients present with bulbar symptoms of slurred speech and difficulty in swallowing.[23] Ten percent of patients live more than 10 years. Cognitive function is usually intact although dementia is present in around 2 percent of patients. There are no disease-specific drug treatments for ALS. Riluzole, an antiglutamate agent has been shown to prolong life by approximately 3 months.[24*]

Parkinson disease

Parkinson disease is a progressive neurodegenerative disorder which results from the loss of pigmented neurons from the substantia nigra. The idiopathic form is assumed when no cause of symptomatic parkinsonism is found such as the side effects of neuroleptic medication. The diagnosis is made on the symptoms of bradykinesia occurring with cogwheel rigidity with or without a resting, pill-rolling tremor[25] in the presence of positive response to levodopa or other dopaminergic therapies. The dyskinesias may respond to levodopa/dopaminergic therapies, but these in themselves cause problems in the longer term. A number of additional symptoms of Parkinson disease cannot be relieved by the drug therapies (Box 96.2).

Younger patients do better than older patients with an expectation of a prognosis of 20–30 years when their motor manifestations are controlled by drugs and neurosurgical procedures such as deep brain stimulation. In particular, older patients may, 5–10 years following diagnosis, begin to experience more and more difficulty with problems that are not only related to drug-induced on–off periods but also to neuropsychiatric problems.[26] Hallucinations and cognitive decline often herald the onset of diffuse Lewy body disease or dementia with Lewy bodies.[27] Depression is more common

---

Box 96.1 Symptoms of amyotrophic lateral sclerosis

Direct symptoms

- Atrophy ± weakness
- Spasticity
- Dyspnea
- Dysphagia
- Dysarthria

Indirect symptoms

- Sleep disturbance
- Thick secretions
- Drooling
- Constipation
- Pain

Box 96.2 Parkinson disease

Bradykinesia ± tremor/rigidity

Additional features

- Bladder symptoms – hypomimia (mask-like face)
- Constipation – seborrhea
- Pain – shuffling gait
- Cognitive disturbance – freezing episodes
- Psychiatric problems – bulbar symptoms
- Postural imbalance – stooped posture

in older patients and complicates at least 20 percent of patients, rising with increasing age of onset.

Huntington disease

This is a genetically transmitted neurodegenerative disease which affects movement, personality and cognitive ability. It is an autosomal dominant condition which affects female and male patients equally. The prevalence of the disorder is 5–10 per 100 000 population.[28] There is a juvenile variant which may present before the age of 20 but most people present with the condition around the age of 40. Voluntary and involuntary movement deteriorates during the disease trajectory. Cognitive impairment is usually apparent at the onset of the choreoathetotic movements which occur. These predominantly affect the upper limbs and may also involve the mouth and face. The orofacial movements may interfere with mastication, speech, and swallowing. While the cognitive features appear with the movement disorder, mood disturbance often predates this. The most common mental disturbances are depression, mania, or hypomania. There may also be violent outbursts of antisocial behavior or frank psychosis. Predictive testing of risk individuals as well as prenatal screening is now possible. This is because of the discovery in 1993 of the Huntington mutation on gene IT-15 of chromosome 4.[29] Interestingly, as little as 18 percent of at-risk individuals have participated in predictive testing programs.[30]

Palliative care challenges

SYMPTOM CONTROL

Pain

Around 50 percent of people with multiple sclerosis[31] and up to 75 percent of people with ALS[2] experience pain, although there is no evidence of sensory involvement in the ALS patients.[32] Musculoskeletal pain is often overlooked in patients with neurodegenerative disorders. It may be the result of immobility in combination with muscle weakness. It is also the result of spasticity, gait disturbance, and poor sitting posture. Joint pain may be exacerbated by the loss of a protective muscle sheath or abnormal tone. Appropriate involvement of physiotherapists and occupational therapists in conjunction with nonsteroidal anti-inflammatory drugs (NSAIDs) can be beneficial. In immobile patients there may be pain secondary to 'skin pressure', continuous pressure on pressure areas. The pain caused if these areas actually breakdown is very difficult to control.

Neuropathic pain is described by patients with both ALS and multiple sclerosis; it is described as being burning or shooting in nature. Patients often also describe altered sensations particularly in the lower limbs. These can be likened to insects crawling over the skin. This is as a result of nerve damage and the pain responds to neuropathic agents such as amitriptyline and newer agents such as gabapentin or pregabalin. A recent paper concluded that the combination of an opioid and gabapentin is more effective than either agent on its own.[33**] The use of nonpharmacological interventions such as transcutaneous electrical nerve stimulation has been reported to be of benefit on occasions. In multiple sclerosis the formation of plaques on sensory nerves can lead to pseudoradicular pain syndromes such as facial pain which mimics the condition *tic douloureux*. Many patients experience more than one if not all of these different pain problems and the involvement of a palliative care specialist who is experienced in taking a complete and holistic pain history can be appropriate and helpful.

Spasticity

All the neurodegenerative disorders can result in muscle cramps, spasms, and spasticity. It is however, the most typical and debilitating of MS symptoms. It reflects the degree of corticospinal tract involvement. Spasticity increases fatigue and immobility. Care must be taken in treating spasticity in a person who is still able to weight bear and therefore carry out activities such as transferring. The extensor spasm they are experiencing in their lower limbs may be the reason they can still carry out these activities as it compensates for the loss of strength. Spasticity is also associated with flexor spasm triggered by touch or movement. These can be extremely painful. Any number of preventable stressors such as cold, a full bladder, stretching, over exertion, and infection can initiate spasms and should be avoided.[34] Simple measures such as leg warmers and positioning should be tried but almost inevitably pharmacological management becomes essential.

Oral baclofen, diazepam, dantrolene and tizanidine are all agents that are equally effective at controlling muscle spasm.[35***] They all have different mechanisms of action and so can be alternated or combined and titrated against clinical effect. All these drugs can be sedating and cause weakness. Baclofen is associated more often with nausea, benzodiazepines with delirium and dantrolene with hepatitis. If only a few muscle groups are affected then local injection of botulinum toxin may be helpful but only in combination with adequate post-injection physiotherapy. Baclofen can be delivered continuously to severely affected individuals via an intrathecal pump situated subcutaneously. Palliative care is characterized by the systematic and meticulous monitoring of symptoms and their pharmacological management. This expertise could be of benefit to this group of patients.

SECRETIONS

Salivary drooling

The inability to swallow one's own saliva may be the result of a specific bulbar palsy such as occurs most commonly in ALS or it may just be the product of a generally deteriorating swallow as may occur with any of the neurodegenerative disorders. Whatever the etiology, it is a very embarrassing symptom which causes local soreness and excoriation. Drug therapy is aimed at reducing the amount of saliva produced.

Anticholinergic medication such as hyoscine hydrobromide administered either sublingually or transdermally may be of benefit. Other medications such as glycopyrronium bromide or amitriptyline can also be useful. Radiotherapy has been tried in refractory cases and botulinum B toxin injections into the salivary glands are being researched.[36]

Thick mucous secretions

This is a problem most often found in patients with ALS. They produce large amounts of viscid secretions which they are unable to cough up because of their reduced respiratory effort. This can cause distress and airway compromise if they become retained in the pharynx. It is particularly of concern if there is the possibility of the use of noninvasive positive pressure ventilation (NIPPV) as these secretions may be forced back into the lungs during this therapy and cause an increase risk of chest infection. The use of humidified air is sometimes helpful in loosening secretions. Anticholinergic drugs may reduce the amount of such secretions but in turn make them more tenacious. Mucolytic enzymes such as acetylcysteine have been tried via the nebulized or oral route. There may have to be very careful balancing between the control of salivary drooling and thick pharyngeal mucous secretions in patients with ALS.

CONSTIPATION

Bowel and bladder involvement in the late stages of neurodegenerative disorders is inevitable. It is the result of poor gut mobility. Constipation may also be exacerbated by poor dietary intake, limited mobility and decreased intake of fluid for fear of urinary incontinence. Bulking agents should be avoided, the use of stool softening aperients is important. Movicol is preferable to lactulose as it is iso-osmolar and does not cause the same degree of associated flatulence and bloating. Stimulants such as senna or sodium picosulfate may be required. Rigorous bowel management including occasional suppositories is crucial to avoid impaction. Enemata and manual evacuation become necessary otherwise and in extreme circumstances the formation of a colostomy has been necessary.

BREATHLESSNESS

See section on noninvasive positive pressure ventilation below.

PSYCHOSOCIAL CARE

Advance planning – parenteral feeding

Most patients with a neurodegenerative disorder will have a functioning gastrointestinal tract but they will also develop a degree of dysphagia. One study indicated up to 87 percent of people with ALS will have a swallowing deficit of some severity.[32] The problems with initiating or coordinating a swallow are often compounded by the presence of excessive saliva, weight loss, and a lack of interest in food. Fear of

choking can also contribute to decreased oral intake. It is important that regular assessment of both oral intake and swallow function are undertaken. This should be done by a multiprofessional team involving speech and language therapists, dietetic specialists, and occupational therapists, and there is also a role for a palliative care specialist.

The goal is to maintain nutrition by the oral route for as long as possible. This period may be extended by appropriate eating aids, neck positioning, and oral food supplements. However it is important to be aware of the optimal timing for any placement of a tube to initiate parenteral feeding.[37] If a patient becomes too emaciated and weak they are less able to withstand the procedure to place a permanent feeding tube. The deterioration of respiratory function, which most commonly accompanies ALS, is also a major factor because if a person's respiratory function has deteriorated too far they will not be able to tolerate the placement of a percutaneous endoscopic gastrostomy and the necessary anesthetic. They will have to then undergo a radiologically inserted gastrostomy instead. Those patients who are too weak for either procedure will only be able to tolerate the insertion of a nasogastric tube. They may indeed be too unwell and weak for any parenteral feeding to be appropriate. There are obvious ethical dilemmas involved in this decision making .[38] The provision of nutrition to a loved one is a fundamental part of providing care for that person and the inability to do this can have a very distressing effect on the families of these patients.[39]

Whereas it may be obvious with a patient who has entered the terminal phase of their illness that to proceed with artificial hydration and nutrition is inappropriate, it is a more difficult decision in those with only a limited prognosis. A number of factors should be considered apart from the individual's ability to undergo a placement procedure. There are practical issues about the community and carer support that may or may not be available. There may be strong cultural or other beliefs of the patient and their family to consider. Of paramount importance is whether the benefits of starting feeding outweigh the anticipated burdens. These include the likelihood of any complications either of the procedure or post-procedure such as pain, hemorrhage, or an infection. The possibility that the patient is at risk of regurgitation and aspiration or indeed the probable prolongation of prognosis, which is not universally or always regarded by a patient as an advantage. Advance planning and discussion with or without the writing of a formal advance directive ensures that the wishes of the patient are known. (See Chapter 109 for further details of advance directives.) This further ensures that any decision is made in the patient's best interests as it can take into account the patient's own assessment of their quality of life, wellbeing, and spiritual or religious beliefs. A specialist in palliative care has appropriate experience to be able to helpfully facilitate this highly individual set of considerations.

Noninvasive positive pressure ventilation

Neurodegenerative disorders often lead to hypoventilation, initially experienced at night. This is a particular feature of

ALS. Symptoms of hypoventilation have been successfully treated with NIPPV. These include daytime fatigue and somnolence, depression and anxiety, morning headache, reduced appetite and weight loss, disturbed sleep, and nightmares.[40] Dyspnea is a problem for up to 85 percent of patients with ALS,[32] and NIPPV has been shown to alleviate these symptoms successfully. It has also been shown to extend a person's prognosis. This extended prognosis is, however, in the face of continuing and ongoing disability. Significantly, carer burden has also been shown to increase. Patients with predominantly bulbar ALS are less likely to benefit from NIPPV. One study showed that two-thirds of patients unable to tolerate NIPPV had bulbar symptoms and were less likely to be able to protect their airway.[41] It is important that people embarking on the use of NIPPV know that the symptoms of breathlessness can also be palliated by the use of benzodiazepines[42] and opioid drugs[43] and that NIPPV does not preclude the use of these. A discussion should take place detailing the progressive nature of the respiratory muscle weakness and also the tendency to ventilator dependence. It is best practice to refer all these patients using NIPPV to local community palliative care teams for local support as this inevitable deterioration takes place. The involvement of a palliative care healthcare professional in the whole of the discussion and decision-making process is therefore very important.

Key learning points

- It would appear there is a role for the needs-focused approach of palliative care in the management of people affected by neurodegenerative disorders.

- There is a need for symptom control, psychosocial support, and help with advance planning and end-of-life decision making.

- There are particular challenges working with people who have an unpredictable disease course of uncertain length.

- There will be learning needs for palliative care team members.

- These patients are prone to fatigue and communication difficulties, which affects their ability to participate in psychosocial support and counseling.

- Cognitive complications of neurodegenerative disorders raise issues around competency in decision making and advance planning.

- Finally, there are particular treatment options and decisions such as percutaneous endoscopic gastrostomy feeding and starting NIPPV. These require a specific multiprofessional assessment, which should usefully include specialist palliative care.

REFERENCES

◆ 1 Saunders C, Walsh TD, Smith M. Hospice care in motor neuron disease. In: Saunders C, Summers DH, Teller N, eds. *Hospice: The Living Idea.* London: Arnold, 1981: 126–47.

◆ 2 O'Brien T, Kelly M, Saunders C. Motor neurone disease: a hospice perspective. *BMJ* 1992; **304**: 471–3.

● 3 Addington-Hall JM, McCarthy M. The regional study of care for the dying: methods and sample characteristics. *Palliat Med* 1995; **9**: 27–35.

● 4 Addington-Hall JM, Lay M, Altmann D, McCarthy M. Symptom control, communication with healthcare professionals, and hospital care of stroke patients in the last year of life as reported by surviving family, friends and officials. *Stroke* 1995; **26**: 2242–8.

◆ 5 Higginson IJ. Healthcare needs assessment: palliative and terminal care. In: Stevens A, Raferty J, eds. *Healthcare Needs Assessment, 2nd Series.* Oxford: Radcliffe Medical Press, 1997.

6 The American Academy of Neurology. Ethics and Humanities Subcommittee. Palliative care in neurology. *Neurology* 1996; **46**: 870–2.

● 7 Van der Wal G, Onwuteaka-Philipsen BD. Cases of euthanasia and assisted suicide reported to the public prosecutor in North Holland over 10 years. *BMJ* 1996; **312**: 612–13.

● 8 Veldink JH, Wokke JH, Van der Wal G, *et al.* Euthanasia and physician assisted suicide among patients with amyotrophic lateral sclerosis in the Netherlands. *N Engl J Med* 2002; **346**: 1638–44.

◆ 9 Barker WH, Mullooly JP. Stroke in a defined elderly population, 1967–1985 – a less lethal and disabling but no less common disease. *Stroke* 1997; **28**: 284–90.

◆ 10 Hankey GJ, Warlow CP. Treatment and secondary prevention of stroke: evidence, costs and effects on individuals and populations. *Lancet* 1999; **354**: 1457–63.

◆ 11 Kwakkel G, Wagenaar RC, Kollen BJ, Lankhorst GJ. Predicting disability in stroke – a critical review of the literature. *Age Ageing* 1996 **25**: 479–89.

● 12 Higginson IJ Hearn J, Myers K, *et al.* Palliative day care: what do services do? Palliative Day Care Project Group. *Palliat Med* 2000; **14**: 277–86.

◆ 13 Leijon G, Boivie J. Central post-stroke pain – a controlled trial of amitriptyline and carbamazepine. *Pain* 1989; **36**: 27–36.

◆ 14 Vestergaard K, Andersen G, Gottrup H, *et al.* Lamotrigine for central poststroke pain. *Neurology* 2001; **56**: 184–90.

◆ 15 Gordon C, Laughton Hewer R, Wade DT. Dysphagia in acute stroke. *BMJ* 1987; **295**: 411–14.

16 Barer DH. The natural history and functional consequences of dysphagia after hemispheric stroke. *J Neurol Neurosurg Psychiatry* 1989; **52**: 236–41.

● 17 Dennis MS, Lewis SC, Warlow C; FOOD Trial Collaboration. Effect of timing and method of enteral tube feeding for dysphagic stroke patients (FOOD): a multicentre randomised controlled trial. *Lancet* 2005; **365**: 764–72.

18 British Medical Association discussion document. *Withholding and Withdrawing Life-prolonging Medical Treatment: Guidance for decision making.* London: BMJ Books, 1999.

19 McDonald WI, Ron MA. Multiple sclerosis: the disease and its manifestations. *Phil Trans R Soc Lond B* 1999; **54**: 1615–22.

◆ 20 Lublin FD, Reingold SC. The National Multiple Sclerosis Society (USA) advisory committee on Clinical Trials of new agents in multiple sclerosis. Defining the clinical course of multiple sclerosis: results of an international survey. *Neurology* 1996; **46**: 907–11.

◆ 21 Neilley LK, Goodin DS, Goodkin DE, Hauser SL. Side effect profile of interferon beta-1b multiple sclerosis: results of an open label trial. *Neurology* 1996; **46**: 991–4.

22 Borasio GD, Miller RG. Clinical characteristics and management of ALS. *Semin Neurol* 2001; **21**:155–66.

◆ 23 Li TM, Alberman E, Swash M. Clinical associations of 560 cases of motor neuron disease. *J Neurol Neurosurg Psychiatry* 1990; **51**: 778–84.

● 24 Lacomblez L, Bensimon G, Leigh PN, *et al.* (for the amyotrophic lateral sclerosis Riluzole study Group II). Dose ranging study of riluzole in amyotrophic lateral sclerosis. *Lancet* 1996; **347**: 1425–31.

25 Yahr MD, Clough CG. Parkinson's disease. In: Yhar MD, ed. *Houston Merritt Memorial Volume.* New York: Raven Press, 1983.

26 Hardie RJ, Lees AJ, Stern GM. On-off fluctuations. A clinical and neuropharmacological study. *Brain* 1984; **107**: 487–506.

✱ 27 McKeith I, Glasko D, Kosaka K, *et al.* Consensus guidelines for the clinical and pathological diagnosis of dementia with Lewy bodies. *Neurology* 1996; **47**: 1113–24.

28 Conneally PM. Huntington's disease: genetics and epidemiology. *Am J Hum Genet* 1984; **36**: 506–26.

● 29 Huntington's Disease Collaborative Research Group. A novel gene containing a trinucleotide repeat that is expanded and unstable on Huntington's disease chromosomes. *Cell* 1993; **72**: 971–8.

● 30 Adam S, Wiggins S, Bloch M, *et al.* Five year study of prenatal testing for Huntington's disease, demand, attitudes, and psychological assessment. *J Med Genet* 1993; **30**: 549–6.

31 Moulin DE. Pain in multiple sclerosis. *Neurol Clin* 1989; **7**: 321–31.

32 Oliver D. The quality of care and symptom control – the effects on the terminal phase of ALS/MND. *J Neurol Sci* 1996; **139**(Suppl): 134–6.

● 33 Gilron I, Bailey JM, Dongsheng T *et al.* Morphine, gabapentin, or their combination for neuropathic pain. *N Engl J Med* 2005; **352**: 1324–34.

34 Mitchell G. Update on multiple sclerosis therapy. *Med Clin North Am* 1993; **77**: 231–49.

● 35 Shakespear DT, Young CA, Boggild M. Anti-spasticity agents for multiple sclerosis. *Cochrane Library* 2000: Issue 4.

36 Newall AR, Orser R, Hunt M. The control of oral secretions in ALS/MND. *J Neurol Sci* 1996; **139** (Suppl): 43–4.

● 37 Mazzini L, Corra T, Zaccala M, *et al.* Percutaneous endoscopic gastrostomy and enteral nutrition in amyotrophic lateral sclerosis, *J Neurol* 1995; **242**: 695–8.

38 Huang Z-B, Ahronheim JC. Nutrition and hydration in terminally ill patients. *Clin Geriatr Med* 2000; **16**: 313–25.

39 Holden CM. Anorexia in the terminally ill cancer patient: the emotional impact on the patient and the family. *Hosp J* 1991; **7**: 73–84.

◆ 40 Schlamp V, Karg O, Abel A, *et al.* Non-invasive intermittent home mechanical ventilation as a palliative treatment in amyotrophic lateral sclerosis: *Nervenarzt* 1998; **69**: 1074–82.

● 41 Aboussouan LS, Khan SU, Meeker DP, *et al.* Effect of non-invasive positive pressure ventilation on survival in amyotrophic lateral sclerosis. *Ann Intern Med* 1999; **127**: 450–3.

● 42 Woodcock A, Gross E, Geddes D. Drug treatment of breathlessness: contrasting effects of diazepam and promethazine in pink puffers. *BMJ* 1981; **283**: 343–6.

◆ 43 Bruera E, Macmillan K, MacDonald RN. Effects of morphine on dyspnea of terminal cancer patients. *J Pain Symptom Manage* 1990; **5**: 341–4.

97

End-stage congestive heart failure

EDWARD R DUNCAN, AJAY M SHAH, MARK T KEARNEY

INTRODUCTION

Most chronic cardiac disorders result in the common end-point of left, right or biventricular dysfunction. This is true whether or not the root cause is valvular, ischemic, congenital, or metabolic. Therefore this chapter will focus on the management of end-stage heart failure.

Traditionally palliative care specialists have concentrated their efforts on patients with malignant disease. However, it is now well established that patients with end-stage cardiac disease have a similar prognosis and symptoms as those with cancer. Moreover, there is growing evidence supporting the need for increased involvement of palliative care services in the management of these patients. Despite this, only a small minority of patients who die of cardiac failure received palliative care support compared with the majority of those with neoplastic disease. Consonant with this, heart failure patients make up only 1–2 percent of total hospice admissions in the UK.[1]

The prevalence of terminal chronic heart failure is rising due to the aging population and improved survival of patients with occlusive coronary artery disease. This has helped focus the attention of physicians across specialities on the care needs of this large group of patients. Greater input from palliative medicine specialists will be necessary if these needs are to be met.

DEFINITION AND CLASSIFICATION

The term 'congestive heart failure' (CHF) describes the complex syndrome of signs and symptoms resulting from ventricular dysfunction and the ensuing reduced cardiac output. The stages of heart failure are most commonly defined using the New York Heart Association (NYHA) criteria. However, another staging model has been proposed by the American Heart Association (AHA; Table 97.1). This better reflects the underlying pathophysiology and progressive

Table 97.1 *Comparison of the models proposed by the New York Heart Association and the American Heart Association for the staging of heart failure*

New York Heart Association	NYHA class I: patients with cardiac disease but with unlimited physical activity	NYHA class II: patients with cardiac disease resulting in slight limitation of physical activity	NYHA class III: patients with cardiac disease resulting in marked limitation of physical activity. Mild activity causes symptoms	NYHA class IV: patients with cardiac disease and are unable to do any physical activity without symptoms. May be symptomatic at rest
American Heart Association	Stage A: patients at high risk of heart failure but without cardiac dysfunction	Stage B: patients with structural heart disease 'in situ' but no symptoms	Stage C: patients with structural heart disease with previous or current symptoms	Stage D: patients with refractory symptoms that require special intervention such as hospice care or positive inotropes

nature of the disease and is analogous to models of neoplastic disease.

CLINICAL COURSE AND EPIDEMIOLOGY

Left ventricular dysfunction is often a progressive problem. An insult to the myocardium, such as an ischemic event, can result in a gradual decline toward ventricular failure irrespective of etiology. Only rarely does left ventricular function actually improve, e.g. after valve replacement surgery. In response to insults such as increased pressure load or loss of muscle mass from myocardial infarction, the ventricle undergoes 'remodeling', whereby both structural and biochemical changes occur. Activation of the sympathetic nervous system and the renin–angiotensin–aldosterone axis are initially probably adaptive, but in the long-term cause progressive worsening of cardiac function and heart failure through multiple mechanisms.[2] Medical therapies (such as angiotensin converting enzyme [ACE] inhibitors) can slow this process, but eventually worsening left ventricular function leads to the onset of symptoms. The common etiologies of cardiac failure include ischemic heart disease (~70 percent), hypertensive heart disease (~15 percent) and valvular heart disease (~5 percent).[3] Cardiomyopathies and congenital heart disease are less common but remain significant and affect a younger population. Nutritional deficiencies (e.g. beri-beri) contribute to cardiac failure in the developing world.

The prevalence of left ventricular dysfunction is increasing as improved management of myocardial infarction and ischemic heart disease prolong survival.[4] Medical therapies for cardiac failure have also improved prognosis but the underlying pathological process is usually only delayed and not reversed. In 2000, the incidence of first admission to hospital with a primary diagnosis of cardiac failure was 1–2 per 1000 population,[5] with a prevalence of up to 2 percent among a northern European population. Heart failure is also much more common in older people. In the UK, the incidence increases in an exponential fashion with age from 1.7 per 1000 population in those aged 55–64 to 16.8 per 1000 in those aged >85.[6] Older people with cardiac failure often have multiple associated comorbidities, e.g. reduced mobility, cognitive impairment, or depression. Physicians must therefore also be adept at managing these issues.

PROGNOSIS AND MODE OF DEATH

Historically, palliative medicine developed within hospices to care for those patients who were terminally ill with cancer. It is now argued that its remit be extended, as studies show that heart failure is associated with symptoms and a prognosis as poor as the majority of soft tissue tumors.[7] Indeed, 1-year mortality following a first admission to hospital with a diagnosis of heart failure remains greater than 25 percent.[8] This is despite evidence that for the first time demonstrates a fall in annual mortality rates. A large Swedish study showed a reduction in 1-year mortality of up to 10 percent between 1993 and 2000. However, this improvement was seen in young patients (age <64) who only represented 8 percent of the study cohort. Annual mortality in older patients (age >75) fell by just 3 percent. These reductions in mortality coincided with widespread introduction of ACE inhibitors in the 1990s as well as improved management of underlying disease processes. Further improvement in prognosis after 2000 would be expected due to increased use of β blockers and other interventions. However, the overall impact on heart failure deaths has been relatively small and the prognosis in chronic heart failure remains poor.

A barrier to the integration of palliative care services in the management of terminal heart failure is prognosis. Many cardiologists feel it is important to be able to recognize when a patient is entering their last months of life before thinking about referral to palliative care services. This is extremely difficult in those with heart failure. The course of this disease is erratic with long periods of chronic illness and decline interspersed with acute and severe exacerbations from which patients can make a surprising recovery (Fig. 97.1). Up to half of heart failure patients die suddenly and unexpectedly[9]

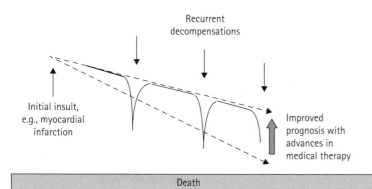

Figure 97.1 *Life trajectory of a patient with heart failure. Following an initial insult to the myocardium, patients experience a chronic decline in function with acute decompensations that require hospitalization. Death is often sudden and unexpected. Both prognosis and the rate of decline have improved with advances in heart failure management.*

and these are often those who are the least symptomatic. Most deaths are from cardiovascular causes (intractable heart failure, myocardial infarction). Only a minority (~10 percent) die from noncardiovascular causes.[10]

Multiple studies have shown factors that predict high or low mortality among groups of patients with CHF. Unfortunately they are poor predictors of death for each individual patient. These factors include low ejection fraction,[11] functional capacity (whether measured by NYHA class or 6-minute walk test),[12] elevated B-type natriuretic peptide,[13] intolerance of ACE inhibitors,[14] or worsening renal function.[12] At present it is necessary to use such indicators of prognosis in advanced heart failure, however they remain inadequate. The Study to Understand Prognoses and Preferences for Outcomes and Risks of Treatment (SUPPORT) demonstrated the failings of guidelines for determining prognosis in CHF. Guidelines based on those supplied by the National Hospice Organization in the USA failed to identify CHF patients with a prognosis of less than 6 months. Narrowing the inclusion criteria dramatically cut sensitivity excluding many that did subsequently die.[15] The current AHA guidelines recommend hospice care to ease patient suffering as an 'end-of-life consideration' but do not advise when to implement it.[16] The European Society of Cardiology recommends palliation in persistent NYHA class IV heart failure despite optimum therapy where no long-term treatment is available.[17]

Once a strategy for determining the terminal stages of heart failure has been found, it will be easier to ensure timely palliative care input and a move away from invasive treatments. Some centers are exploring combined care, where palliative medicine expertise is combined with standard cardiology care in multidisciplinary clinics. Such a strategy does not require that a point in time be identified where the patient 'becomes palliative'.

SYMPTOMS

Heart failure and malignant conditions share many features including distressing symptoms, poor quality of life, and gradual debilitation. Palliative care physicians are experienced at treating these symptoms albeit in different circumstances. Interestingly, the level of symptoms experienced by patients is not proportional to their degree of ventricular dysfunction, and patients with extremely poor ventricular function can remain remarkably asymptomatic for a long period of time.

Characteristic symptoms of CHF include shortness of breath, fatigue, and ankle swelling, but others include depression, poor quality sleep, confusion, short-term memory loss, dizziness, and nausea.[18] As would be expected, the most commonly reported symptom is breathlessness, present in up to 90 percent of patients.[19] Breathlessness presents either on exertion or at rest, as orthopnea, or nocturnal dyspnea.

Fatigue is also prevalent (69 percent) and exaggerated by ankle edema, weight gain/loss, and depression. Depression is very common and yet underdiagnosed and undertreated in those with cardiac failure. Up to 48 percent of nonhospitalized patients with NYHA class II or worse are depressed (Beck Depression Inventory score >10) and rates of major depression correspond to those seen in patients with other chronic diseases.[20] Depression has also been linked to increased mortality, increased rates of rehospitalization and worsening quality of life in those with heart failure.[21] Despite this only 7 percent of patients receive antidepressants.[20]

Many patients also experience pain in the last 6 months of life (up to 75 percent).[19] Chest and joint pains have been reported as common, but often the cause of pain is not specified. In elderly patients pain may relate to comorbidity rather than to left ventricular failure itself. SUPPORT reported that severe pain in the last 3 days of life occurs at comparable frequencies in heart failure and a number of cancers.[22]

Cardiac cachexia is a well-recognized complication of CHF arising in approximately 10–15 percent of patients with CHF.[23,24] It is characterized by a poor prognosis and a severe wasting process that particularly affects skeletal muscle and promotes exercise intolerance with marked breathlessness and fatigue at low workloads.[25]

MEDICAL MANAGEMENT

Patients with severe and end-stage heart failure benefit from both standard medical therapy and palliative care, and both of these approaches should be integrated and continued until the terminal stages of the illness. Early discontinuation of regular medical treatments is not recommended due to difficulties in predicting death, and because these treatments are proved to reduce symptoms and increase time out of hospital.

A number of drug therapies are recommended for routine use by the AHA in most patients with left ventricular dysfunction. These include an ACE inhibitor, a β adrenergic blocker, and a diuretic.[16]*** Large trials have demonstrated reduced hospitalization rates and clear prognostic benefits of ACE inhibitors,[14]** β blockers[26]** and the aldosterone antagonist spironolactone.[14,26,27]** Both ACE inhibitors and diuretics maintain euvolemia, thus improving symptoms, especially breathlessness and weight gain. β Blockers provide prognostic and symptomatic benefit.[28] This benefit is seen in older patients[29] and in all classes of heart failure.[30] There is however a lack of strong evidence to guide prescription of β blockers in end-stage heart failure. Anecdotally it has been described that they are poorly tolerated and make patients feel worse in the short term. Where patients have symptoms attributable to β blockers, tapering down the dose or stopping the drug may be appropriate. More recently angiotensin receptor blocking agents have been demonstrated to reduce hospital admissions and improve prognosis when used both alone and in combination with ACE inhibitors.[31**]

Among patients with refractory heart failure (AHA stage D) use of diuretic infusions or continuous outpatient support with inotropes may achieve hospital discharge in those patients proving to be inotrope-dependent in hospital.[32*] Furthermore, there is evidence supporting use of intermittent inotropic support in an outpatient population for relief of refractory heart failure symptoms.[33] However, concerns have been raised that despite beneficial effects on symptoms, the outpatient use of inotropes may be associated with a shortened life expectancy.[34,35] This risk may prove to be acceptable to highly symptomatic patients with end-stage heart failure. It must also be noted that most of the evidence regarding use of outpatient inotropic support is anecdotal or gleaned from small studies and that further research is required in this area.

Cardiac surgery for ventricular dysfunction in the form of cardiac transplantation is an established treatment for end-stage heart failure but the majority of patients are not candidates due to age, other comorbidity or shortage of donor organs. An increasing number of patients with severe cardiac dysfunction and severe symptoms are now receiving electrophysiological devices in the form of implanted cardiac defibrillators, biventricular pacemakers or devices that combine both functions.   *CRT*

Cardiac damage results in dyssynchronous and inefficient cardiac contraction. Biventricular pacing resynchronizes the left and right ventricles thereby increasing cardiac output. Cardiac resynchronization improves exercise tolerance, quality of life and reduces hospitalization.[36**] In terminally ill patients, these devices should be treated like any simpler pacemaker implant. Defibrillator implantation improves prognosis in those with significant left ventricular impairment (ejection fraction <30 percent) after myocardial infarction.[37**] Furthermore the combination of biventricular pacing and defibrillator capability in a single device has additional prognostic benefits when compared to biventricular pacing alone in NYHA class III/IV heart failure.[38**] Concerns have however been raised over the psychological impact of defibrillator insertion, and evidence exists that suggests increased levels of anxiety and depression in this group of patients compared to the general cardiac population.[39] It is likely that the presence of a defibrillator in a patient with end-stage disease will also have a significant and detrimental psychological impact. It is therefore essential for patients to be adequately advised prior to defibrillator implantation of the indications, contraindications, and consequences of this procedure. Furthermore, situations where the device might be turned off should be discussed at this time. This will help avoid surprises near the end of life. Implantable defibrillators are becoming increasingly common and the results of recent trials suggest this trend will continue. Physicians working in the hospice setting with heart failure patients will need to be aware of these devices and their management (see Box 97.1).

Box 97.1 Implantable defibrillators: key practical points

- The use of implantable defibrillators is increasing

- Those touching a patient with an implantable defibrillator at the time of a shock will not receive a shock

- Defibrillators can be activated or deactivated at the bedside using a programming device. As defibrillators become increasingly common, more hospitals outside major centers will become equipped to program them. Alternatively, representatives of the manufacturer can be contacted. Defibrillators must be deactivated before removal

- Patients with implantable defibrillators require psychological support before and after insertion. The device can be misperceived as life saving and acts as a focus of attention for patients with end-stage disease and their relatives

- There is little published evidence regarding management of defibrillator devices in those patients entering terminal stages of their illness where defibrillation may be unacceptable

- The situations when deactivation of a device would be appropriate must be discussed clearly with the patient when the device is implanted

---

PALLIATIVE CARE IN TERMINAL CARDIAC FAILURE

A consensus conference convened in the USA in 2003 to define the then current state of 'palliative and supportive care in advanced heart failure' acknowledged that symptom palliation in advanced heart failure had simply not been studied.[40***] There is a dearth of data supporting the use of treatments that are extremely well established in palliative care in other disease states.

This is emphasized in the management of breathlessness in cardiac failure. Despite opioids being of irrefutable value in the treatment of acute left ventricular failure and malignancy, there is only anecdotal evidence supporting their use in chronic heart failure. There are no large trial data to reinforce this.[40,41] Further beneficial effects of opioids could include relief of anxiety and pain. There is also no clear role for domiciliary oxygen therapy in end-stage heart failure, as no conclusive evidence exists showing oxygen therapy relieves the sensation of breathlessness, despite reducing hypoxia.[42***]

The experience of palliative care physicians in other disease states must therefore be applied in cardiac failure to manage the many familiar symptoms until the necessary research has been completed. Patients with cardiac failure are poorly informed about the course of their illness and the purpose of their medications. They often mistake symptoms of their underlying heart failure for side effects of their medication.[18] This occurs because of poor education of patients at and following diagnosis, compounded by barriers to good communication such as fatigue, hypoxia, and confusion. Patients need and want to be better informed regarding their condition and management.[43] The evolution of specialist multidisciplinary heart failure services, in particular the arrival of specialist heart failure nurses, should start to address this, and may help to integrate specialist cardiology and palliative services.

Patients with severe heart failure report having to rely heavily on family and friends for help performing activities of daily living. This provokes feelings of 'being a burden'. Poor mobility and an inability to leave the house promote isolation. Qualitative studies suggest the majority of patients with severe heart failure have thought about death and find it difficult to discuss with those close to them.[43] Access to psychological support, counseling and social services therefore could be of great benefit.

'Best practice' in the terminal stages of heart failure remains unclear. The SUPPORT study gives insight into current practice and highlights how palliative care input is needed. Patients with CHF are more likely to die in hospital than those with a malignancy,[22] with only 3 percent dying in a hospice despite almost 50 percent preferring comfort care rather than life-extending care. Heart failure patients also experienced higher incidence of invasive life-sustaining treatments (including cardiopulmonary resuscitation, ventilation, and nasogastric feeding) during their last 3 days than those patients with lung or colon cancer.[44] Furthermore, those who received 'do not resuscitate' orders take longer to do so than those with cancer and often continue to receive invasive treatments.

Among patients with CHF admitted to hospital in NYHA Class IV it is reported that only 25 percent discussed their resuscitation preference with a physician[45] despite the majority being conscious and able to communicate during their last days. Around 25 percent did not want to be resuscitated in the event of a cardiac arrest. The SUPPORT study emphasizes the need for palliation in CHF patients, that the patients themselves are aware of their poor prognosis and that a large number would welcome care aimed specifically at maintaining comfort. The problem of predicting death in CHF remains.

CONCLUSIONS

Patients with severe cardiac failure represent a highly symptomatic population with a poor overall prognosis who would benefit from palliative care support. Further research is needed to validate existing palliative treatments for use in cardiac disease, but this should not stop these patients receiving appropriate care. Greater communication is required between the specialities involved to ensure adequate and timely integration of palliative care services into the management of these patients.

Key learning points

- The incidence of congestive cardiac failure is increasing. It is predominantly a disease of older people.

- The symptoms and prognosis of patients with cardiac failure are similar to those of patients with terminal malignant disease.

- There is a lack of research into symptom alleviation in terminal cardiac disease. The experience of palliative care specialists in other disease states must be used at present.

- Breathlessness, fatigue, and pain are the most commonly reported symptoms. Depression is also common.

- Routine medical therapy (including ACE inhibitors, β blockers and diuretics) has a role in reducing symptoms and hospital admissions.

- The incidence of implantable defibrillators is increasing.

- Congestive cardiac failure patients need to be better informed regarding their disease and their prognosis, and thus be more capable of making end-of-life decisions.

REFERENCES

1   Eve A, Higginson IJ. Minimum dataset activity for hospice and hospital palliative care services in the UK 1997/98. *Palliat Med* 2000; **14**: 395–404.

2   Jessup M, Brozena S. Heart failure. *N Engl J Med* 2003; **348**: 2007–18.

3   McMurray JJ, Stewart S. Epidemiology, aetiology, and prognosis of heart failure. *Heart* 2000; **83**: 596–602.

4   Kearney MT, Marber M. Trends in incidence and prognosis of heart failure; You always pass failure on the way to success. *Eur Heart J* 2004; **25**: 283–4.

5   Stewart S, MacIntyre K, MacLeod MM, *et al.* Trends in hospitalization for heart failure in Scotland, 1990–1996. An epidemic that has reached its peak? *Eur Heart J* 2001; **22**: 209–17.

6   Cowie MR, Wood DA, Coats AJ, *et al.* Incidence and aetiology of heart failure; a population-based study. *Eur Heart J* 1999; **20**: 421–8.

7   Stewart S, MacIntyre K, Hole DJ, *et al.* More 'malignant' than cancer? Five-year survival following a first admission for heart failure. *Eur J Heart Fail* 2001; **3**: 315–22.

8   Schaufelberger M, Swedberg K, Koster M, *et al.* Decreasing one-year mortality and hospitalization rates for heart failure in

Sweden; Data from the Swedish Hospital Discharge Registry 1988 to 2000. *Eur Heart J* 2004; **25**: 300–7.

9 Uretsky BF, Sheahan RG. Primary prevention of sudden cardiac death in heart failure: will the solution be shocking? *J Am Coll Cardiol* 1997; **30**: 1589–97.

● 10 Poole-Wilson PA, Uretsky BF, Thygesen K, *et al*. Mode of death in heart failure: findings from the ATLAS trial. *Heart* 2003; **89**: 42–8.

11 Vasan RS, Larson MG, Benjamin EJ, *et al*. Congestive heart failure in subjects with normal versus reduced left ventricular ejection fraction: prevalence and mortality in a population-based cohort. *J Am Coll Cardiol* 1999; **33**: 1948–55.

12 Cowburn PJ, Cleland JG, Coats AJ, Komajda M. Risk stratification in chronic heart failure. *Eur Heart J* 1998; **19**: 696–710.

13 Gwechenberger M, Hulsmann M, Berger R, *et al*. Interleukin-6 and B-type natriuretic peptide are independent predictors for worsening of heart failure in patients with progressive congestive heart failure. *J Heart Lung Transplant* 2004; **23**: 839–44.

14 Garg R, Yusuf S. Overview of randomized trials of angiotensin-converting enzyme inhibitors on mortality and morbidity in patients with heart failure. Collaborative Group on ACE Inhibitor Trials. *JAMA* 1995; **273**: 1450–6.

● 15 Fox E, Landrum-McNiff K, Zhong Z, *et al*. Evaluation of prognostic criteria for determining hospice eligibility in patients with advanced lung, heart, or liver disease. SUPPORT Investigators. Study to Understand Prognoses and Preferences for Outcomes and Risks of Treatments. *JAMA* 1999; **282**: 1638–45.

✱ 16 Hunt SA, Baker DW, Chin MH, *et al*. ACC/AHA guidelines for the evaluation and management of chronic heart failure in the adult: executive summary. *J Heart Lung Transplant* 2002; **21**: 189–203.

✱ 17 Remme WJ, Swedberg K. Comprehensive guidelines for the diagnosis and treatment of chronic heart failure. Task force for the diagnosis and treatment of chronic heart failure of the European Society of Cardiology. *Eur J Heart Fail* 2002; **4**: 11–22.

18 Rogers A, Addington-Hall JM, McCoy AS, *et al*. A qualitative study of chronic heart failure patients' understanding of their symptoms and drug therapy. *Eur J Heart Fail* 2002; **4**: 283–7.

19 Nordgren L, Sorensen S. Symptoms experienced in the last six months of life in patients with end-stage heart failure. *Eur J Cardiovasc Nurs* 2003; **2**: 213–17.

20 Gottlieb SS, Khatta M, Friedmann E, *et al*. The influence of age, gender, and race on the prevalence of depression in heart failure patients. *J Am Coll Cardiol* 2004; **43**: 1542–9.

21 Jiang W, Alexander J, Christopher E, *et al*. Relationship of depression to increased risk of mortality and rehospitalization in patients with congestive heart failure. *Arch Intern Med* 2001; **161**: 1849–56.

22 Lynn J, Teno JM, Phillips RS, *et al*. Perceptions by family members of the dying experience of older and seriously ill patients. SUPPORT Investigators. Study to Understand Prognoses and Preferences for Outcomes and Risks of Treatments. *Ann Intern Med* 1997; **126**: 97–106.

23 Anker SD, Ponikowski P, Varney S, *et al*. Wasting as independent risk factor for mortality in chronic heart failure. *Lancet* 1997; **349**: 1050–3.

24 Davos CH, Doehner W, Rauchhaus M, *et al*. Body mass and survival in patients with chronic heart failure without cachexia: the importance of obesity. *J Card Fail* 2003; **9**: 29–35.

25 Coats AJ. Origin of symptoms in patients with cachexia with special reference to weakness and shortness of breath. *Int J Cardiol* 2002; **85**: 133–9.

26 Krum H, Roecker EB, Mohacsi P, *et al*. Effects of initiating carvedilol in patients with severe chronic heart failure: results from the COPERNICUS Study. *JAMA* 2003; **289**: 712–18.

27 Pitt B, Zannad F, Remme WJ, *et al*. The effect of spironolactone on morbidity and mortality in patients with severe heart failure. Randomized Aldactone Evaluation Study Investigators. *N Engl J Med* 1999; **341**: 709–17.

28 Packer M, Fowler MB, Roecker EB *et al*. Effect of carvedilol on the morbidity of patients with severe chronic heart failure: results of the carvedilol prospective randomized cumulative survival (COPERNICUS) study. *Circulation* 2002; **106**: 2194–9.

29 Dulin BR, Haas SJ, Abraham WT, Krum H. Do elderly systolic heart failure patients benefit from beta blockers to the same extent as the non-elderly? Meta-analysis of >12 000 patients in large-scale clinical trials. *Am J Cardiol* 2005; **95**: 896–8.

30 Hjalmarson A, Goldstein S, Fagerberg B, *et al*. Effects of controlled-release metoprolol on total mortality, hospitalizations, and well-being in patients with heart failure: the Metoprolol CR/XL Randomized Intervention Trial in congestive heart failure (MERIT-HF). MERIT-HF Study Group. *JAMA* 2000; **283**: 1295–302.

31 Pfeffer MA, Swedberg K, Granger CB, *et al*. Effects of candesartan on mortality and morbidity in patients with chronic heart failure: the CHARM-Overall programme. *Lancet* 2003; **362**: 759–66.

32 Hershberger RE, Nauman D, Walker TL, *et al*. Care processes and clinical outcomes of continuous outpatient support with inotropes (COSI. in patients with refractory endstage heart failure. *J Card Fail* 2003; **9**: 180–7.

33 Lopez-Candales A, Vora T, Gibbons W, *et al*. Symptomatic improvement in patients treated with intermittent infusion of inotropes: a double-blind placebo controlled pilot study. *J Med* 2002; **33**: 129–46.

34 Elis A, Bental T, Kimchi O, *et al*. Intermittent dobutamine treatment in patients with chronic refractory congestive heart failure: a randomized, double-blind, placebo-controlled study. *Clin Pharmacol Ther* 1998; **63**: 682–5.

35 Oliva F, Latini R, Politi A, *et al*. Intermittent 6-month low-dose dobutamine infusion in severe heart failure: DICE multicenter trial. *Am Heart J* 1999; **138**(2 Pt 1): 247–53.

36 Abraham WT, Fisher WG, Smith AL, *et al*. Cardiac resynchronization in chronic heart failure. *N Engl J Med* 2002; **346**: 1845–53.

37 Moss AJ, Zareba W, Hall WJ, *et al*. Prophylactic implantation of a defibrillator in patients with myocardial infarction and reduced ejection fraction. *N Engl J Med* 2002; **346**: 877–83.

38 Bristow MR, Saxon LA, Boehmer J, *et al*. Cardiac-resynchronization therapy with or without an implantable defibrillator in advanced chronic heart failure. *N Engl J Med* 2004; **350**: 2140–50.

39 Sears SF Jr, Conti JB. Quality of life and psychological functioning of ICD patients. *Heart* 2002; **87**: 488–93.

◆ 40 Goodlin SJ, Hauptman PJ, Arnold R, *et al*. Consensus statement: palliative and supportive care in advanced heart failure. *J Card Fail* 2004; **10**: 200–9.

41 Johnson MJ, McDonagh TA, Harkness A, *et al*. Morphine for the relief of breathlessness in patients with chronic heart failure – a pilot study. *Eur J Heart Fail* 2002; **4**: 753–6.

◆ 42 Booth S, Wade R, Johnson M, *et al*. The use of oxygen in the palliation of breathlessness. A report of the expert working group of the Scientific Committee of the Association of Palliative Medicine. *Respir Med* 2004; **98**: 66–77.

43 Horne G, Payne S. Removing the boundaries: palliative care for patients with heart failure. *Palliat Med* 2004; **18**: 291–6.

44 Tanvetyanon T, Leighton JC. Life-sustaining treatments in patients who died of chronic congestive heart failure compared with metastatic cancer. *Crit Care Med* 2003; **31**: 60–4.

45 Krumholz HM, Phillips RS, Hamel MB, *et al*. Resuscitation preferences among patients with severe congestive heart failure: results from the SUPPORT project. Study to Understand Prognoses and Preferences for Outcomes and Risks of Treatments. *Circulation* 1998; **98**: 648–55.

98

Palliative care for children

FINELLA CRAIG, ANN GOLDMAN

INTRODUCTION

The death of a child is one of the biggest tragedies that can happen to a family. In the developed world, the plans and expectations of a parent barely acknowledge the possibility that their child might die. Society has become unfamiliar and uncomfortable with death in childhood, leaving many, including professionals, ill equipped, both emotionally and by a lack of experience, to provide support during the child's illness and after death. Consequently, many families will feel alone and unsupported while experiencing a grief and distress that is intense and longlasting.

Children and families need experienced professionals to support and guide them through their child's illness and death and through the bereavement process. In the UK, care is often shared between the primary care team, based in the local community (which includes the family doctor, children's community nurses, and the local hospital) and disease-specific specialist teams (e.g. oncology, neurology teams) based at a tertiary hospital. Although the management of symptoms can be similar in adults and children, the palliative journey and the difficulties encountered are often very different.

In this chapter we have drawn on our experience to emphasize some of the specific issues of pediatric palliative care that are relevant to children in any area of the world. We hope professionals will find this a useful tool when working with children and families.

CHILDREN NEEDING PALLIATIVE CARE

Children with life-limiting illness can be considered in four broad groups, each with different palliative care needs:[1]

- Life-threatening conditions where curative treatment may be possible but can fail. Palliative care is needed in times of prognostic uncertainty or when cure becomes impossible. Cancer is an example.
- Conditions where premature death is inevitable but where life can be prolonged by periods of intensive treatment. Cystic fibrosis and acquired immune deficiency syndrome (AIDS) fit this pattern.
- Progressive conditions where treatment is entirely palliative and may extend over many years. Neuro-degenerative diseases and many inborn errors of metabolism are examples.
- Irreversible but nonprogressive conditions causing severe disability, such as severe cerebral palsy. These can lead to a susceptibility to health complications and the likelihood of premature death.

The range of life-limiting conditions that affect children is wide, with many conditions rare, specific to the pediatric population and with a protracted course. The number of children requiring palliative care is relatively small. In the UK, the annual mortality for children and adolescents (0–19 years) with life-limiting conditions is 1.5–1.9 per 10 000 and the prevalence of children requiring palliative care is 12–17 per 10 000.[1] In a health district with a child population of 50 000, in any 1 year there will be 60–85 children known to have a life-limiting condition, of whom 8 are likely to die: 3 from cancer, 2 from heart disease, and 3 from other conditions.[1] With such relatively small numbers, pediatric palliative care is unlikely to be a priority when there are limited resources available, yet it can be difficult for any one professional to develop adequate experience and expertise.

PROVIDING SERVICES FOR THE FAMILY

An essential requirement of palliative care is that children receive good care for their underlying condition as well as expert palliative care support, wherever they choose to be. Most children and families prefer to spend as much time as possible at home and it is essential that the primary healthcare team be actively involved in care provision. Most primary healthcare teams, however, will have limited experience of caring for children with life-limiting illness and are unlikely to have any specialist knowledge of the underlying condition. In contrast, many families will become experts in the disease and its management.

Most children with palliative care needs have a number of different teams and professionals involved in their care. For example, a child with cerebral palsy may see a neurologist, a gastroenterologist, the local pediatrician, and family doctor, in addition to attending a child development clinic and having input from education and respite and social services. With each professional doing his or her own bit, there is a risk that care is poorly coordinated with no one person addressing the overall needs of the child and family. For some children care may focus around inpatient or outpatient hospital management. Families may build close relationships with hospital staff, placing considerable trust in a few professionals with experience in their child's particular disorder and questioning the advice of others. It is easy for the primary healthcare team to feel superfluous and marginalized, making it difficult to define their role. For other disorders, frequent hospital contact is unnecessary and there is no clearly identified specialist team. This can lead to the contrasting situation of a child with long-term illness being cared for at home by the family, with very little or no hospital input. Here the primary healthcare team may at times be overwhelmed and feel abandoned and unsupported by hospital services.

It is essential that for every child with a life-limiting diagnosis, one person from the group of professionals involved be identified to act as a key worker for the child and family, facilitating good communication and coordinating professional care. This ensures that all the family's needs are being met, without overlap or gaps developing, and minimizes the chance of any part of the team becoming marginalized. In most situations the professional who fulfills this role most effectively is a nurse.

ORGANIZATION OF SERVICES

Pediatric palliative care is an evolving specialty and still defining and researching the clinical care children need and the best way to provide services. Globally, there has been a steady increase in the number of specialist pediatric palliative care medical and nursing posts and in the number of children's hospices and community-based teams providing pediatric palliative care. However, no one model of care will fit all countries and all localities and care continues to be provided by a variety of professionals with different backgrounds and experiences. To ensure that children and families receive appropriate support it is essential that their needs be considered individually, in the context of the illness and of what is available locally.

One established model of pediatric palliative care is for children with cancer. Here the child's care is likely to be shared between a children's cancer center some distance from where they live, their local pediatric department, and care at home. Pediatric oncology outreach nurse specialists are usually hospital based but go out into the community. They offer expertise and experience in symptom management, as well as psychosocial support. When the child is at home they liaise closely with the local pediatric community nurses and primary healthcare teams, who in turn provide most of the ongoing medical and nursing care for the child. Second, children with other life-limiting diseases, especially those with a prolonged course where care is mainly home based, have traditionally had less well-structured provisions for care. However in the UK, an increasing number of districts have now developed multidisciplinary teams of local professionals (e.g. community pediatrician, nurse, social worker, and psychologist) who devote part of their time to providing palliative care support for these children.

A third model of care is that provided by the increasing number of children's hospices.[2,3] Here, care is provided by a multidisciplinary team of professionals with experience and expertise in pediatric palliative care, often working closely with local community and hospital based services. Unlike adult palliative care, relatively few children die in hospices, so a major role is in the provision of respite care, particularly for children with prolonged illnesses and considerable nursing needs. Children with cancer tend to be referred to hospices less frequently than those with nonmalignant disease, perhaps because the need for respite care is not as great. In addition to providing respite care many children's hospices have developed considerable experience and expertise in palliative symptom management. Some have particular expertise in rare disorders, such as Batten disease and muscular dystrophy. A fourth model for palliative care is the specialist palliative care team based in a tertiary pediatric center. These teams see sufficient numbers of patients to develop considerable palliative care expertise and liaise closely with the primary healthcare team and local pediatric services providing most of the ongoing care.

As there is no single model of service provision, the service available to children and families remains, to some extent, dependent on geographical location and the underlying condition. Some children may not have access to any of the service models discussed above, whereas others may access a children's hospice, locally based palliative care services, and palliative care services coordinated from a tertiary center. It is essential that whatever the local set-up, the allocation of a key worker with a specific remit for palliative care should ensure that families are neither neglected nor the focus of inappropriate or uncoordinated help. The key worker needs know what services are available locally, be able to access existing services and be able to identify and find ways to supplement gaps in service provision.

PALLIATIVE CARE NEEDS

For children dying from cancer the point at which treatment becomes symptom directed rather than curative is often clear – usually when all realistic attempts at curative treatment have been exhausted. For many other children with life-limiting diseases, however, there is no clear transition point. One of the big challenges of pediatric palliative care is to balance aggressive disease-specific management aiming to prolong life with symptom-directed management and quality of life. It is essential that palliative care is provided alongside good care of the underlying disease. Parents and professionals need to recognize which takes priority at different times, as this will influence their choices, for example in where they choose to be and how the symptoms should be managed.

Choosing the location of care

Ideally, families and children should be given a choice as to where they will be cared for, although limited resources may prohibit this. Many families will choose different places at different times, so it is important that they are given some flexibility to move between home, hospital, and hospice as they choose, without their care being compromised. If there is a possibility that their child may benefit from medical interventions, such as intravenous antibiotics, many families will choose to be in hospital. When death seems inevitable most families will choose to be at home.[4] Families need to be given a realistic idea of the support that is available and what to expect with regard to the needs of their child as they deteriorate, to enable them to make informed choices regarding where they want to be. Those who are at home must have access to advice and support 24 hours a day.

Parents bear a heavy responsibility for nursing and personal care of their child, especially when they are at home, and most take on the burdens willingly. However, while viewing parents as part of the caring team, it is important to acknowledge their need for support themselves, as well as the needs of siblings. The needs of the professionals caring for the child on a day-to-day should also be considered, as they may need access to specialist palliative care advice and support, especially if they have limited experience themselves.

Empowering children and families

The greatest fear for most parents is that their child will suffer distressing symptoms which neither they nor the professionals supporting them will be able to relieve. It is essential to provide families with detailed and honest information about their child's current symptoms and any others that may be anticipated, especially if there are concerns about the possibility of sudden distressing symptoms, such as convulsions, acute agitation, or bleeding. As death approaches parents will need and value further information, including what signs might suggest that death is imminent and the possible modes of death. Although professionals can sometimes be reluctant to undertake such frank discussion, families who know what to expect and have a clear plan of what to do are likely to feel more in control, and more confident and less anxious.

Advanced planning is a vital component of good palliative care. As well as discussing anticipated symptoms, an appropriate management plan should be drawn up for each possible scenario. Both the parents and the sick child need to take an active part in planning a practical and acceptable regimen of care. The team should ensure that appropriate drugs are prescribed and available, with suitable doses via accessible routes being calculated ahead of time so that medication can be given as soon as it is needed. If the child is at home, the medication doses and the route of administration should be such that the parents will be able to give the drugs themselves, although there should always be a professional available whom they can contact for additional support.

SYMPTOM MANAGEMENT

The symptoms experienced, the principles of symptom management and the drugs used in palliative care are often similar in pediatric and adult practice. The main differences lie in the disorders encountered, the assessment of symptoms, the routes of administration, and the doses used.

Many of the symptoms encountered in pediatric palliative care are common to a variety of illnesses. However when a child has a rare disorder it may be difficult to anticipate which particular problems will develop as the disease progresses. It is always worth seeking advice from professionals with disease-specific expertise as well as contacting parent help groups for rare illnesses as these may offer additional information and practical advice.

Patterns of symptoms

As in adult palliative care, the pattern of symptoms experienced is dependent on the underlying condition. Some children, such as those with cancer, usually have a relatively short final illness lasting only weeks or months, with pain from tumor invasion as a predominant symptom. Others, such as those with neurodegenerative disease, will have a more protracted illness, with progressive impairment of intellect, communication, and mobility over a number of years and with seizures, excessive secretions, and recurrent pneumonia as predominant features.

Assessment of symptoms

As in adults, thorough assessment of any symptom is essential before developing a plan of management. Since the experience of pain and other symptoms is subjective, ideally the children should provide this information themselves. However, their ability to do so will vary in relation to their level of understanding, experience, and communication skills. In preverbal children and those with severe developmental delay this can be particularly challenging.[5]

A variety of approaches are usually necessary to build up a more complete picture of a child's symptoms. Much can be gained from observing a child's behavior and comparing it to a time when symptoms were absent or different. Parents are particularly adept at this and their opinions should be sought and respected. When it comes to listening to the child, a range of assessment tools for different ages and developmental levels are available, but these were developed more specifically for acute pain. They include body charts, pictures of faces and visual analog scales.[6] Play specialists can also help to uncover a child's symptoms with the use of toys, puppets, art, and music. The team should remember that psychological and social factors affecting the child and family are often significant and are an important part of the assessment (Box 98.1).

A holistic approach

A holistic approach to symptom management is essential. Unresolved social, psychological, or spiritual concerns are likely to have a detrimental impact on the symptom experience. Children, like adults, have hopes and expectations for the future and mourn these losses. Many are aware of what they will not achieve in this life and need to explore a continued identity in the future, perhaps the reassurance that they will not be forgotten by their parents or the possibility of a spiritual continuity. Like adults, they may have tasks they want to achieve before death and business affairs to deal with, such as who will have their possessions and who will look after their pets.

For both parents and children, a fear of what the symptom means may lead to underreporting of symptoms, or unnecessary anxiety about relatively small problems. They must be given an opportunity to discuss what the symptom means to them, as this may highlight specific anxieties or misunderstandings that need to be addressed. Explaining the reason for the symptom and discussing a logical stepwise approach to management can also be helpful, reassuring the child and family that the situation is not out of control.

Basic principles

Simple measures for symptom management should always be considered, either on their own or alongside drug therapy. The value of maintaining a calm environment and care

---

Box 98.1 Assessing a child's pain

Watch the child:

Nonspecific, but often enlightening

Behavioral changes

- Crying, screaming, irritable, aggressive, head banging
- Clinging, quiet, withdrawn, frightened look, reluctant to move

Physiological changes

- Increased heart rate/respiratory rate/blood pressure
- Decreased saturations, change in color, sweating

Ask the child:

Difficult, dependent on age/developmental level/ contributory factors

Use play, puppets, drawings, music (play specialists)

Specific assessment tools:

- Over 3 years – FACES scales (e.g. Bieri, Wong, Baker, Oucher)[7,8]
- School age – Visual analog scale (straight line, ± numbers); color body chart (different colors for different pains)
- Older child – Any of the above; numerical rating scales; direct questioning

Ask the parents:

They know their child best, but they may lack confidence in their own assessment

Consider contributory factors:

Coping skills of the child and family

Past experience of the child and family

Anxiety and emotional distress levels in the child and family

Meaning of the pain and underlying disease to the child and family

---

over positioning should not be underestimated, as well as distraction, imagery and relaxation techniques, play, art and music therapy.

Where medication is necessary, the preferences of the child and family need to be taken into account. Many find that taking a lot of medication is difficult, so complex regimens may not be possible. It is important to find the most acceptable route for the child and to be flexible to changing situations. The key issues in deciding on routes of administration are as follows:

- The oral route is often preferable.
- Long-acting preparations are more convenient and less intrusive.
- The child should be allowed to choose between liquids and whole or crushed tablets.
- As a child's condition deteriorates the treatment plan often has to be simplified, routes of administration altered and priority given to those drugs that contribute most to the child's comfort.
- Although rectal drugs are not popular in some countries, they can have a role. Some children prefer these to using any needles and they may be helpful in the final hours when the child's level of consciousness has deteriorated.
- If parenteral drugs are needed they are usually given by continuous subcutaneous infusion, not as bolus doses. Alternatively, an intravenous line can be used if it is already in place.
- Intramuscular drugs are painful and not necessary.

Many of the drugs used in palliative care have not been recommended formally for use in children but a body of clinical experience has developed in the absence of many trials or extensive pharmacokinetic data.[9] Doses of drugs for children are usually calculated according to their weight. In general neonates tend to need reduced doses relative to their size, whereas infants and young children may need comparatively higher doses and at shorter intervals than adults. Our recommendation is that drug dose is determined using a standard pediatric formulary. In the UK this includes *Medicines for Children* produced by the Royal College of Paediatrics and Child Health[10] or the *BNF for Children* (*BNF* is the *British National Formulary*).

Pain

After thorough assessment of pain a treatment regimen can be planned. This should consider the likely cause of the pain and whether this can be relieved by specific measures (e.g. radiotherapy for an isolated bony metastasis, antibiotics for a urinary tract infection). Symptomatic relief can be addressed by combining pharmacological, psychological, and practical approaches. Although analgesics often form the backbone to a plan, this combined approach is more likely to be successful.

The World Health Organization ladder of analgesia is widely adopted for children, although recent evidence has shed some doubt on the routine use of codeine. Up to 10 percent of the UK population may be poor metabolizers of the drug (to morphine) rendering it of little or no benefit to them, and there may be very low efficacy in infants due to their immature enzyme systems.[11]

STRONG OPIOIDS

These are used extensively in managing pain in pediatric palliative care (see also Chapter 50). When prescribing strong opioids for children, the following points should be borne in mind:

- Long-acting morphine preparations are effective and particularly convenient.
- Families should also have a short-acting preparation for breakthrough pain.
- Where oral administration is difficult or impossible transdermal patches such as fentanyl or buprenorphine should be considered.[12*]
- If oral or transdermal routes are not appropriate, morphine or diamorphine can be given via subcutaneous or intravenous infusion.
- Some children may have sudden onset of severe pain, needing breakthrough analgesia with a faster onset of action than oral morphine. Fentanyl lozenges can fulfill this role, although it may not be possible to use them in very young children or those with severe neurological impairment.[13*]
- Studies of the pharmacokinetics of oral opioids and their metabolites suggest that in young children metabolism is more rapid than in adults and they may require relatively higher doses for analgesia. Neonates and children under 6 months old, however, require a lower starting dose of opioids because of their reduced metabolism and increased sensitivity.[10]

Side effects of opioids

Many doctors lack experience of using strong opioids in children and exercise undue caution, prescribing doses that are too low or too infrequent. Respiratory depression with strong opioids is not usually a problem in children with severe pain and the side effects from opioids tend to be less marked than in adults. Nausea and vomiting, for example, are rare and routine antiemetics are not needed. Constipation is probably the most common side effect of opioids and regular laxatives should always be prescribed. For some children relatively mild laxatives such as lactulose may be sufficient, but the majority will require a stimulant in addition to a softener.

Some children are initially quite sleepy on starting opioids and parents should be warned about this or they may fear that the child's disease has suddenly progressed and that death is imminent. The drowsiness usually resolves within a few days. Itching with morphine may occur and may respond to antihistamines. If either the somnolence or the pruritus remain troublesome, switching to fentanyl or hydromorphone (or a combination of the two) is usually effective.[14*]

Parental concerns over opioids

Parents may be reluctant for their child to have strong opioids. It is important to establish exactly what their concerns are, particularly as children may be aware of their parents' reluctance and may consequently underreport their pain. Parents may be anxious about the side effects, in which case it will be helpful to reassure them that these too can be treated. They may also be worried that if opioids are started 'too early' there will be nothing left for later. It is important to explain to parents and children that there is no upper dose limit to strong opioids and that gaining good pain control early is the best way of optimizing the long-term management of pain.

Another difficulty for parents is the feeling that by agreeing to start opioids they are acknowledging that their child is really going to die. They may even be concerned that this step represents them giving up hope – something they would find unacceptable. This clearly requires sensitive discussion and support. It may be helpful to explain that death is unlikely to be imminent, and to gently encourage them to focus again on the immediate needs of the child. With this, in the vast majority of cases, their perception will change such that their child can again receive the analgesia that he or she requires.

MUSCULOSKELETAL PAIN

Nonsteroidal anti-inflammatory drugs are often helpful for musculoskeletal pains, especially in children with nonmalignant disease. However, some caution is needed in children with cancer who have bone marrow infiltration because of the increased risk of bleeding. Bisphosphonates may also be used for bony pain in a variety of diseases, such as malignant disease and osteogenesis imperfecta. Oral chemotherapy should also be considered in children with malignant disease.

HEADACHES

Headaches from central nervous system leukemia respond well to intrathecal methotrexate. Headaches from raised intracranial pressure, associated with progressive brain tumors, are best managed with gradually increasing analgesics. Although steroids may seem helpful initially, the symptoms will inevitably recur as the tumor increases in size and a spiral of increasing steroid doses will then develop. The side effects of steroids in children almost always outweigh the benefits.[15] There is an increase in appetite (at a time when feeding may be difficult), dramatically changed appearance and often marked mood swings. Both parents and the children find these distressing.

OTHER FORMS OF PAIN

Neuropathic pain can often be helped by antiepileptic and antidepressant drugs. As with adults, there may be a role for methadone or ketamine. For severe pain unresponsive to these drugs, epidurals and nerve blocks should be considered. Painful dystonia or muscle spasms may improve with diazepam, baclofen, or trihexyphenidyl.

Gastroesophageal reflux should always be considered in children having episodes of pain associated with abnormal posturing, as reflux can mimic dystonia and often occurs alongside neurodevelopmental abnormalities. Physiotherapists and occupational therapists may also be able to help with pain management using exercises, positioning, and physical aids.

Feeding

The neurological impairment in children with neurodegenerative diseases and brain tumors often leads to difficulty with chewing and swallowing, to the extent that they are unable to tolerate an oral diet. Others, such as those with cancers, respiratory and cardiac disease, lose their appetite as the disease progresses. This can be one of the most difficult symptoms for parents to cope with as the inability to feed and to nourish their child often makes them feel they are failing in a basic parental role.

Assisted feeding, via a nasogastric tube or gastrostomy, is often appropriate for children with slowly progressive diseases. However, it is unlikely to be appropriate for children in the end stages of a rapidly progressive illness. In this situation nutritional goals aimed at restoring health should become secondary to comfort and enjoyment. It is often helpful to explain to parents that their child's deteriorating appetite is part of the dying process and that giving sufficient volumes of feed to achieve nutritional goals will not only be difficult, but may make their child feel more unwell and could precipitate vomiting. As long as the risk of aspiration is small, parents should be encouraged to allow their child to eat small amounts of foods they enjoy whenever they feel like it. They should be dissuaded from putting large plates of food in front of their child with the expectation that they should try to eat it, as this is likely to result in failure and disappointment for both the child and the parents.

Nausea and vomiting

Nausea and vomiting are frequent problems in a variety of diseases. Children with conditions that compromise oxygenation of the gastrointestinal tract, such as cardiac and respiratory diseases, can be very sensitive to the volume of feed given. Overfeeding can also be a precipitating factor, as parents often want to give extra nutrition to a child who is unwell or underweight. For some children, therefore, reducing the volume of feed given at any one time can cause significant improvement.

Gastrointestinal reflux should also be considered as a cause of vomiting, particularly in children with neurological impairment. A trial of antireflux medication may be appropriate. As in adults, antiemetics should be selected according to their site of action and the presumed cause of vomiting. Hyoscine patches and rectal medications are probably used more frequently in pediatrics than in adult palliative care, to avoid the need for subcutaneous or intravenous administration in children who cannot tolerate drugs enterally, especially those with a relatively long disease course.

Seizures

Watching a child have a seizure is extremely frightening for parents and they should always be warned and advised about management if there is any possibility that this may happen. Children with neurodegenerative diseases often develop seizures as part of their ongoing disease and will already be taking long-term anticonvulsants. These can be adjusted when the pattern of seizures changes.

Sudden acute onset of seizures can be treated with rectal diazepam or, if the child or parents prefer, buccal midazolam. This has now been extensively studied in children and found to be at least as effective as rectal diazepam, well tolerated and highly acceptable to families.[16*] If the buccal preparation is not available, the intravenous preparation can be used buccally. Repeated severe or continuous seizures in a terminally ill child can be treated at home with a continuous subcutaneous infusion of midazolam, adding phenobarbital if necessary.

Agitation and anxiety

As with adults, agitation and anxiety may occur as a consequence of unresolved fears and distress. Children, especially, are often given limited information and excluded from conversations and discussions about their illness. Rather than protecting them, this can increase anxiety as limited or conflicting information makes it harder for them to make sense of what is happening. In addition, they will need to use their imagination to fill in the gaps and this can be so much more frightening than reality. Children must be given opportunities to seek information, clarify misconceptions and receive support. Medications, such as benzodiazepines, haloperidol, and levomepromazine should only be used as an adjunct to this.

Respiratory symptoms

Dyspnea, cough, and excess secretions can all cause distress to children and anxiety for their parents. If the underlying cause of the symptom can be relieved, even temporarily, this may be appropriate. Palliative radiotherapy, for example, can bring good symptomatic relief to some children with malignant disease in the chest.

Where treatment of the underlying cause is unlikely to be beneficial, symptom relief can be addressed by combining drugs with practical and supportive approaches. Fear is often an important element in dyspnea, so reassurance and management of anxiety may help to relieve symptoms. Simple practical measures such as finding the optimum position, using a fan and relaxation exercises may all help. The sensation of breathlessness can be relieved with opioid drugs and small doses of sedatives, such as diazepam or midazolam, are often helpful in relieving the associated anxiety.

Children with chronic chest diseases causing gradually increasing hypoxemia may suffer from headaches, nausea, daytime drowsiness, and poor-quality sleep. Intermittent oxygen may help relieve these symptoms and can be given relatively easily at home. Children with dyspnea in the later stages of malignant disease do not usually find oxygen helpful. Excess secretions are often a problem for children with chronic neurodegenerative diseases as they become less able to cough and swallow. This may also occur in other terminally ill children as they approach death. Oral glycopyrronium bromide, or hyoscine hydrobromide (given transdermally or subcutaneously) can help to reduce the secretions. Altering the child's position often provides temporary relief, but suction equipment is not usually helpful in the long term.

Anemia and bleeding

The treatment of anemia in the late stages of a child's life should be directed toward relief of symptoms rather than the level of hemoglobin. Transfusions are only helpful if they make the child feel better and it should be explained to the child and family that there is likely to come a point in the illness where they will stop finding transfusions beneficial. Blood counts are not routinely indicated but are sometimes helpful to support a clinical decision to transfuse.

Florid bleeding (e.g. severe hemoptysis or hematemesis) is extremely frightening for a child, distressing for the carers and may leave the family with unforgettable painful memories. If this is a serious risk, such as in liver disease, emergency drugs should be readily available and include an appropriate analgesic and sedative, such as diamorphine and midazolam. Correct dosage should be calculated ahead of time and the drugs and syringes immediately accessible. In an emergency parents can give these drugs by the buccal route, but must be shown in advance how to administer them.

Many children with malignant diseases have widespread bone marrow infiltration and low platelet counts. Although petechiae and minor gum bleeding are common, serious bleeding is unusual. Minor gum/nose bleeding can be managed with tranexamic acid, either orally or by direct application to the bleeding point. Platelet transfusions are usually confined to bleeding that is severe or interferes with the quality of life. They are rarely justified solely on the basis of a low platelet count. A child with an established history of bleeding throughout the illness, however, may appropriately be treated with regular platelet transfusions.

SUPPORT FOR THE CHILD AND FAMILY

Support for the child and family begins at the time of diagnosis and continues as the illness progresses, through the

Box 98.2 Predicting how well a family will cope

Positive

- Cohesive family
- Supportive family
- Flexible approach
- Open communication in family
- Open communication with staff
- Good record with past stress

Negative

- Over-involved family
- Unconnected family
- Rigid approach
- Closed communication in family
- Closed communication with staff
- Poor record with past stress
- Previous parental psychopathology
- Concurrent stresses (e.g. single parent, parental strife, financial problems)

child's death and into bereavement. All the family – the sick child, the parents, siblings, and the wider family – will be affected by the illness and need support, both as a family unit and as individuals. A flexible approach, with time to listen and build up relationships, is important.

Although all families will suffer emotional distress the majority possess considerable strength and resilience and do find ways to continue to function effectively from day to day. A number of factors have been identified which can help predict a family's capacity to cope, and this knowledge can be helpful in identifying families who may be at extra risk and need particular support (Box 98.2). It is important to be aware of families and family members who have language difficulties or a different cultural approach to illness and death.

At diagnosis

The time of diagnosis of a life-threatening illness is one of great turmoil for the family. This is when their bereavement begins. The way in which the diagnosis is given has a powerful impact and forms the foundation for communication in the future. The family's expectations and pattern of life are disrupted and, especially if frequent hospital admissions are involved, many practical difficulties arise in day-to-day living. It can be easy for the parents and other

children to feel overwhelmed, helpless, and out of control. Parents have a great need for information at this time and may value written information, contact with other parents in similar situations and links with self-help groups. The sick children face the trauma of being in hospital and the experience of unpleasant and frightening investigations and treatment. They may be particularly confused as explanations of what is happening may be delayed while parents themselves are just learning about the illness. Some parents may be reluctant to discuss the diagnosis with their children and need encouragement and help to do so.

As the disease progresses

As the illness progresses the family have to live with the underlying conflict of maintaining some hope and semblance of day-to-day life despite persistent uncertainty. The parents may develop depression, anxiety, and sleep disturbance although they are often reluctant to speak of these problems unless asked specifically. Marital discord and loss of libido are also common. Parents may find it difficult to maintain discipline and boundaries for the sick child and to balance their time and emotions between the sick child and well siblings.[17] If frequent hospital admissions are involved there are practical difficulties of travel, separation, and finance. If the child has heavy nursing needs, with physical disability and/or developmental delay, the burdens of care can be considerable. Parents may have little time to themselves or to devote to well brothers and sisters, so the opportunity for some respite care for the sick child, either at home or away from home, becomes essential.[1,18] Trying to encourage as normal a life as possible – maintaining friendships, education, and outside activities – within the confines of the illness is a continual but important struggle. Children usually want to attend school as much as possible, so as the illness progresses extra support, special facilities and home education may need to be introduced.

Most families use some avoidance and denial as part of their coping strategy, including avoiding discussion and reminders of the illness. This is normal behavior that helps protect them from extremes of emotion. It allows them to live with the illness and function day-to-day, while coming to understand and recognize the situation gradually. This needs to be recognized and respected, as frequent discussions about the disease at this time may prove burdensome rather than supportive. In addition to this, parents often want health professionals to maintain some hope as long as their child is alive. This has to be expressed in the context of honest information about the progression of the disease and it can prove challenging to get the balance right for each individual family.[19]

The final stages

Eventually it becomes clearer that not only is death inevitable but that the time of death is becoming quite close. This may be apparent from gradual deterioration in a long progressive illness or occur more abruptly such as after a relapse in cancer. The emotional impact at this time can be dramatic for parents, particularly for those who have held a very positive and 'fighting' approach throughout treatment. For others it is just a confirmation of what they have dreaded and known was inevitable all along. Sometimes there is a sense of relief that the uncertainty and suffering will soon be over, alongside the distress and sadness. The sense of relief can be very confusing for parents as they can interpret this as wishing their child dead, which, of course, is not what they want.

In addition to being given information and the opportunity to discuss their child's care, parents need an opportunity to explore their own feelings and express their emotions. They may be able to talk to each other openly and offer each other support, but more often they will cope in different ways and find the whole experience so physically and emotionally exhausting that they have little strength left to offer support either to each other or to their other children. Both the parents and well siblings can find it helpful to talk to someone outside the immediate family during this time.[19,20]

Many parents have never seen anyone die and will value the opportunity of talking about what may happen at the moment of death. They also appreciate information about the practical details of what to do after their child has died. Most will have been anticipating the funeral in their mind and are relieved to be able to acknowledge this and make some plans before the child has died.

An important issue for parents at this time is what to discuss with the child who is sick and with their other children. A natural reaction is to protect their children from the fear of death and many parents feel they can only do this by not allowing the child to know that they are going to die. However, it is clear that children understand and learn about their illness and its implications whether the parents and the professionals encourage it or not.[21] It is important to provide opportunities for the sick child to seek the information they want in order to make sense of what is happening and to discuss what is actually on his or her mind. Parents (and health professionals) can be surprised by the nature of the child's fears: rather than being scared of death *per se* it is more common that they are scared of situations that they can be genuinely reassured about. Even when parents are very open with their children, it is not unusual for the *children* to 'protect' their *parents* by keeping their worries to themselves, so a trusted professional may be the most appropriate person with whom a child can talk freely. Open discussion with children, particularly when death is a real possibility, can be a daunting prospect and very difficult to establish in practice.

Communicating with children must take into consideration their level of understanding about illness and the concept of death.[21,22] It also will be influenced by the child's previous experiences, the family's style of communication,

and their own personal defenses. Some approaches to helping families toward a more open and honest pattern of communication include:

- shifting the emphasis from 'telling' to 'listening'
- helping them identify the child's indirect cues as well as obvious questions
- discovering the child's fears and fantasies
- maintaining the child's trust through honesty
- building up the whole picture gradually
- explaining that communication need not rely on talking – drawings, stories, and play are often more effective and easier for children.[23,24]

It can be equally difficult for the parents to discuss the seriousness of the situation with their other children. Siblings may feel isolated and left out by their parents and, noticing the differential treatment they are receiving, can come to resent their sick brother or sister. They may feel less worthy and develop low self-esteem as a result. This is less likely if they have opportunities to talk about their feelings and are given honest answers to their questions about what is happening. They also benefit from being involved in the day to day care of their brother or sister, by having a role in planning and attending the funeral and by being allowed to keep some of their sibling's possessions.[25,26]

The bereaved family

The grief suffered after the loss of a child has been described as the most painful, enduring and difficult to survive and is associated with a high risk of pathological grief. Parents lose not only the child they have loved, but their hopes for the future and their confidence in themselves as parents. It puts an additional stress on their own relationship and alters the whole family structure. The brothers and sisters who are grieving may continue to feel isolated and neglected as their parents can spare little time or emotion for them.

Ideally the professionals who know the family well and have been involved throughout the sick child's life should continue to be available through the bereavement. Grief is likely to continue over many years and its depth and persistence is often underestimated. Parents value continuing contact with professionals who have known their child and the opportunity to talk about the child and their grief when others in the community expect them to 'have come to terms with it'.[19] This support, initially more frequent and gradually decreasing, helps facilitate the normal tasks of mourning. Help can be offered for brothers and sisters and information provided about appropriate literature, telephone helplines, and support organizations. Most families will not need formal counseling but it is important to be able to recognize when there are signs of abnormal grief that may require referral for specialist help.

CONCLUSIONS

Helping to care for a child and family with a life-threatening illness is rarely easy. It presents many challenges both in terms of the professional tasks that may be required and to our own emotional resources. Families greatly value professionals who stay alongside them throughout their journey, offering practical help and support in an almost intolerable situation. Parents will have a lasting memory of their child's death and as professionals we have the opportunity to help make these memories as good as they can be.

Key learning points

- The numbers of children receiving palliative care are small compared with the adult population and many of the diseases encountered are rare.

- Parents are usually the main carers and a family-oriented approach is essential.

- Professionals providing day-to-day care may have limited experience of the underlying disease, yet it is essential that palliative care is delivered alongside good disease-specific management.

- A key worker must be allocated to coordinate the care, which is often provided by professionals from a number of different organizations.

- When talking to children it is essential to be sensitive to their level of understanding, previous experience, and communication ability.

- The principles of symptom management are similar in adults and children, but the assessment of symptoms, the doses of medication, and the routes by which medication is given are often different.

- The death of a child raises specific issues in bereavement and appropriate support for families and professionals must be provided.

REFERENCES

- 1 ACT/RCPCH. *A Guide to the Development of Children's Palliative Care Services*. Update of a Report by the Association for Children with life-threatening or Terminal conditions and their families (ACT) and the Royal College of Paediatrics and Child Health (RCPCH). Bristol: ACT/RCPCH, 2003.
- 2 Association for Children with life threatening or Terminal conditions and their families. *ACTPACK – Children's Hospices*. Bristol: ACT, 1998.
- 3 Dominica F. The role of the hospice for the dying child. *Br J Hosp Med* 1996; **38**: 334–43.
- 4 Goldman A, ed. *Care of the Dying Child*. Oxford: Oxford University Press, 1994.

- 5 Hunt A, Mastroyannopoulou K, Goldman A, Seers K. Not knowing – the problem of pain in children with severe neurological impairment. *Int J Nurs Stud* 2003; **40**: 171–83.
- 6 Mathews JR, McGrath PJ, Pigeon H. Assessment and measurement of pain in children. In: Schechter NL, Berde CB, Yaster M, eds. *Pain in Infants, Children and Adolescents*. Baltimore: Williams & Wilkins, 1993: 97–112.
- 7 Franck LS, Greenberg CS, Stevens B. Pain assessment in infants and children. *Pediatr Clin North Am*. 2000; **47**: 487–512.
- 8 Hain RD. Pain scales in children: a review. *Palliat Med* 1997; **11**: 341–50.
- 9 McGrath P, Brown S, Collins J. Paediatric palliative medicine. In: Doyle D, Hanks G, Cherny NI, Calman K, eds. *Oxford Textbook of Palliative Medicine*, 3rd ed. Oxford: Oxford University Press 2004: 775–97.
- 10 Royal College of Paediatrics and Child Health. *Medicines for Children*, 2nd ed. London: RCPCH, 2003.
- 11 William DG, Hatch DJ, Howard RF. Codeine phosphate in paediatric medicine. *Br J Anaesth* 2001; **86**: 413–21.
- 12 Hunt A, Goldman A, Devine T, Phillips M; FEN-GBR-14 Study Group. Transdermal fentanyl for pain relief in a paediatric palliative care population. *Palliat Med* 2001;15:405–12.
- 13 Wheeler M, Birmingham PK, Dsida RM, *et al*. Uptake pharmacokinetics of the fentanyl oralet in children scheduled for central venous access removal. *Paediatr Anaesth* 2002; **12**: 594–9.
- 14 Goodarzi M. Comparison of epidural morphine, hydromorphone and fentanyl for postoperative pain control in children undergoing orthopaedic surgery. *Paediatr Anaesth* 1999; **9**: 419–22.
- 15 Watterson G, Goldman A, Michalski A. Corticosteroids in the palliative phase of paediatric brain tumours. *Arch Dis Child* 2002; 86(Suppl 1): A76.
- 16 Scott RC, Besag FM, Neville BG. Buccal midazolam and rectal midazolam for treatment of prolonged seizures in childhood and adolescence: a randomised trial. *Lancet* 1999; **353**: 623–6.
- 17 Bluebond-Langner M. *In the Shadow of Illness: Parents and Siblings of the Chronically Ill Child*. Princeton: Princeton University Press, 1996.
- 18 Miller S. Respite care for children who have complex health care needs. *Paediatr Nurs* 2002; 14; 33–7.
- 19 Laakso H, Paunonen-Ilmonen M. Mothers' experience of social support following the death of a child. *J Clin Nurs* 2002; **11**: 176–85.
- 20 Martin TL, Doka KJ. *Men Don't Cry . . . Women Do: Transcending Gender Stereotypes of Grief*. Philadelphia: Brunner/Mazel, 2000.
- 21 Bluebond-Langner M. *The Private Worlds of Dying Children*. Princeton: Princeton University Press, 1978.
- 22 Stevens M. Psychological adaptation of the dying child. In: Doyle D, Hanks G, Cherny NI, Calman K, eds. *Oxford Textbook of Palliative Medicine*, 3rd ed. Oxford: Oxford University Press 2004: 799–806.
- 23 Wellings T. Drawings by dying and bereaved children. *Paediatr Nurs* 2001; **13**: 30–6.
- 24 List of age appropriate books: www.winstonswish.org.uk
- 25 Foster C, Eiser C, Oades P, *et al*. Treatment demands and differential treatment of patients with cystic fibrosis and their siblings. *Child Care Health Dev* 2001; **27**: 349–64.
- 26 Pettle Michael SA, Lansdown RG. Adjustment to death of a sibling. *Arch Dis Child* 1986; **61**: 278–83.

99

Chronic obstructive pulmonary disease

J RANDALL CURTIS, GRAEME ROCKER

INTRODUCTION

Chronic obstructive pulmonary disease (COPD), or chronic obstructive airways disease, is a leading cause of morbidity and mortality worldwide and age-adjusted mortality continues to increase whereas mortality from other leading causes of death, including cardiovascular disease and cancer, has decreased.[1,2] Among patients with life-limiting illnesses such as COPD, there are documented shortcomings in our current provision of end-of-life care.[3] There has been growing recognition of the importance of improving the quality of palliative care for patients with COPD, as evidenced by the appearance of sections on palliative care in the recent American Thoracic Society/European Respiratory Society (ATS/ERS; www.thoracic.org/copd) and Canadian Thoracic Society COPD guidelines released in 2004.[4] This chapter will examine the important aspects of providing high quality palliative care for patients with COPD.

The focus of the chapter is on the specific issues of providing high quality 'end-of-life' care to patients with COPD as well as high quality palliative care. Since end-of-life care for patients with COPD often occurs in the setting of an acute exacerbation of their chronic disease, good quality end-of-life care requires communication with patients *prior* to the acute exacerbation to be sure they receive the care they want. Therefore, the first section to follow will review the problems with current end-of-life care for patients with COPD; and the second section will review issues concerning prognostication for patients with COPD. The third section explores issues around communication about end-of-life care that are unique or particularly important for patients with COPD. Since palliative care can also be viewed more broadly to refer to the care intended to palliate symptoms

and maximize quality of life, much of the care provided to patients with severe COPD is in fact palliative care focused on symptom management and improving or maintaining quality of life. Therefore, the fourth section will cover some of the issues regarding symptom management and quality of life unique to the patient with severe COPD.

IDENTIFYING THE PROBLEM WITH END-OF-LIFE CARE FOR PATIENTS WITH COPD

The landmark study called SUPPORT (the Study to Understand Prognosis and Preferences for Outcomes and Treatments) enrolled seriously ill, hospitalized patients with one of six life-limiting illnesses that included COPD. The SUPPORT study found that compared with patients with lung cancer, patients with COPD were much more likely to die in the intensive care unit, on mechanical ventilation, and with dyspnea.[5*] These differences in the kind of care occurred despite the fact that most patients with COPD preferred a course of care that focused on comfort, rather than prolonging life. In fact, the SUPPORT investigators found that patients with lung cancer and patients with COPD were equally likely to prefer not to be intubated and not to receive cardiopulmonary resuscitation (CPR).[5] In addition, a study in Britain also found that patients with COPD were much more less likely to die at home and much less likely to receive palliative care services than patients with lung cancer.[6*] These differences seem likely to be due in part to the difficulty physicians have in prognosticating for patients with COPD and especially for identifying with confidence those patients who are likely to die within 6 months. This fact was demonstrated using the SUPPORT prognostic model showing that 5 days prior to death, the prognostic model predicted that a patient with lung cancer had a less than 10 percent chance of surviving 6 months, whereas for patients with COPD the model predicted a more than 50 percent chance of surviving 6 months.[5] Nonetheless, despite these difficulties in prognostication, it remains the responsibility of physicians caring for patients with severe COPD to address issues of end-of-life care to provide the best possible care for these patients at the end of their lives.

Although reasons that patients with COPD receive less palliative care than those with lung cancer are not entirely clear, prior studies show that only a small proportion of patients with moderate to severe COPD have discussed treatment preferences and end-of-life care issues with their physicians and the vast majority of these patients believe their physicians do not understand their preferences for end-of-life care.[7,8] A recent study suggested that only a third of patients with oxygen-dependent COPD had discussed end-of-life care with their physicians and there were important aspects of end-of-life care that less than 10 percent of physicians discussed with their patients.[9*] Patients with COPD are more likely than patients with cancer or AIDS to express concern about the lack of education that they receive about their disease, treatment, prognosis, and advance care planning.[10*] It is likely that at least part of the reason that patients with COPD may receive less palliative care is that patient–physician communication about end-of-life care occurs less often, is more difficult to conduct for patients with a less certain prognosis, or some combination of both. It is also possible that since patients with cancer and patients with COPD are often cared for by different specialists, there may be differences in attitudes, skill, or experience among these different specialists.

PROGNOSTICATION FOR PATIENTS WITH COPD

Since one of the barriers to providing high quality palliative care to patients with COPD is the difficulty in making an accurate prognosis for these patients, it is important for those providing palliative care to these patients to be familiar with the data that do exist. Table 99.1 outlines the prognostic factors for patients with COPD during acute exacerbations and when they are stable and the studies identifying these factors are discussed below.

Acute exacerbations of COPD requiring hospitalization

The SUPPORT study published outcomes of 1016 patients admitted to five US hospitals with hypercapnia complicating acute exacerbations of COPD (AECOPD).[3*] The average age of patients was 70 years, 51.5 percent were male, and 78.1 percent had >2 significant comorbid illnesses.

Table 99.1 *Independent predictors of increased mortality in the SUPPORT (at 6 months) and BTS (at 3 months) trials*

	SUPPORT	BTS
Acute physiology score (APACHE)	✓	NR
Impaired performance status	✓	✓
Low BMI	✓	NR
Increased age	✓	✓
Increased heart rate	✓	NR
Poor oxygenation	✓ (low Pao_2/Fio_2)	✓ (low Sao_2)
Low albumin	✓	NR
Low pH	✓	✓
Leg edema	✓ (reduces mortality)	✓ (increases mortality)
Assisted ventilation	NR	✓

NR, not reported; BMI, body mass index; APACHE, Acute Physiology, Age, and Chronic Health Evaluation.

The mortality for the index admission was 11 percent rising to 20 percent at 60 days, 33 percent at 180 days, and 43 percent at 1 year. The median survival for these patients was approximately 2 years. Six-month mortality was higher for those patients readmitted two or more times (36 percent) than for patients not readmitted (21 percent). The SUPPORT study data were collated between 1989 and 1994 from only five US centers before widespread use of noninvasive mechanical ventilation (NIV) for AECOPD complicated by hypercapnia,[11] which may limit generalizability of these findings. Another study to look at outcomes of AECOPD comes from the UK using a British Thoracic Society (BTS) clinical audit.[12*] The BTS study reported on data collated from 1400 admissions between 1997 and 2001 of whom only 13 percent of eligible patients received some form of ventilatory support. The predictors of 3-month mortality included age, comorbidities, and the severity of the exacerbation.[12]

Other recent studies of more than 100 patients with AECOPD reported index hospital admission mortality rates of 11–24 percent.[13–16*] Higher mortality rates have been reported in patients using long-term oxygen (50 percent index admission mortality in a Spanish study)[17*] and patients who could not be weaned after 3 weeks of mechanical ventilation (68 percent 2-year mortality).[18*]

Age is one of the most consistent predictors of death for patients admitted with AECOPD. Relative to patients in the BTS study <65 years old, the odds (95 percent confidence intervals [CI]) of death at 3 months for patients aged 75–79 years and >80 years were 2.2 (1.3 to 1.7) and 3.0 (1.8 to 4.9), respectively.[12*] In other follow-up studies of 270 and 362 patients, age and presence of comorbidities were consistent predictors of death beyond successful discharge.[16,19*] Other factors that predict survival in some but not all studies include the severity of the initial respiratory acidosis.

The BTS study showed that a presenting $pH < 7.26$ increased the relative risk of mortality at 3 months (relative to $pH > 7.35$) to 3.8 (95 percent CI 2.7 to 5.4), but this was not found in SUPPORT. For a patient bed bound before admission, one study found that the risk of death increased by a factor of 20.[12*] Finally, in the BTS study, a presenting $Sa_{O_2} < 86$ percent increased the mortality risk by a factor of 2.3 (95 percent CI 1.6 to 3.2) relative to an $Sa_{O_2} > 92$ percent.[12] Most recently, in recognition that single indicators of disease severity are not in themselves sufficiently powerful as predictors of death in COPD, Celli and colleagues have described a multidimensional tool (the BODE index) that integrates measures of the body mass index (B), the degree of airflow obstruction (O), dyspnea scores (D), and exercise capacity (E).[20*] As a multidimensional score it proved more accurate in mortality predictions in a validation cohort of 625 patients than the forced expiratory volume in 1 second (FEV_1) alone, both for deaths from all causes and for deaths related to respiratory disease.[20] Whether the BODE index will prove useful in clinical practice and for both men and women with COPD is not yet determined.

Predictors of survival in stable COPD

Initial FEV_1 and age were the most important predictors of survival among 985 COPD patients followed for 3 years.[21*] In a retrospective study of 400 patients with COPD in Holland, low body mass index (BMI), age and low Pa_{O_2} were significant independent predictors of increased mortality.[21] Weight gain through nutritional therapy with or without anabolic steroids had a positive impact on survival in a prospective study of 203 patients.[22*] A low BMI was also associated with an increased mortality risk (relative risk 7.11, 95 percent CI 2.97 to 17.05) in the Copenhagen City Heart Study that enrolled 2132 subjects with airflow obstruction and followed them for 17 years[23*] and in a recent UK prospective cohort study of 137 elderly patients with COPD.[24*]

Readmission rates

In SUPPORT 900 patients survived to index discharge, of whom 446 or 50 percent were readmitted 754 times over the next 6 months: 28 percent of patients were readmitted once, 13 percent twice, and 9 percent three times or more. Of the 416 patients who died with COPD, 15–25 percent of their last 6 months was spent in hospital.[25*] Canadian data also demonstrate that the majority of patients with COPD die in hospital.[26*] Of the 1400 BTS study patients, 34 percent were readmitted within 3 months of the index hospitalization.[12*] The following factors were the major independent predictors of hospital readmission: previous admission (odds ratio [OR] 2.5, 95 percent CI 2.0 to 3.2); lower percent-predicted FEV_1 (1.8, 1.4 to 2.3) and more than five medications at the time of readmission (2.7, 2.0 to 3.7).[12]

In summary, despite the increasing amount of prognostic data to help clinicians identify patients with severe COPD at high risk of death, these data do not provide clinicians with an easy way to identify with certainty those patients with a prognosis of less than 6 months. Since the hospice benefit in the USA is based on a prediction of a prognosis of less than 6 months, clinicians will need to use their clinical judgment to identify patients likely to benefit from hospice care and they will, in our opinion, need to be willing to accept a higher degree of uncertainty in this prognosis than is often seen for patients with metastatic cancer.

COMMUNICATION ABOUT END-OF-LIFE CARE WITH PATIENTS WITH COPD

Communication about end-of-life care is a particularly important component of caring for the patient with severe COPD because these patients are at high risk for an acute exacerbation of their disease that may result in respiratory failure of rapid onset. For this reason, discussions about patient preferences in the event of acute respiratory failure and for circumstances in which they would not want life-sustaining therapies started or continued are important topics for discussion for patients, their physicians, and their families.

Prior research shows that the majority of patients with severe COPD report that their physicians have not end-of-life care with them.[7–9*] A recent study of patients with oxygen-dependent COPD suggested that there were aspects of discussing end-of-life care, such as prognosis and what dying might be like, that are rarely discussed. When these discussions occur, patients rate the quality of these discussions relatively poorly.[9*] These studies suggest physicians need to be aware of the barriers to communication about end-of-life care and should work to improve the ways they discuss this issue. Another report from this study suggests that the barriers to communication about end-of-life for patients with COPD are diverse and patient specific.[27*] Two barriers were endorsed by more than 50 percent of patients including, 'I'd rather concentrate on staying alive than talk about death' and 'I'm not sure which physician will be taking care of me if I get very sick'. The former suggests that physicians must be skilled in talking about this difficult subject with patients who would rather not talk about it. It may be helpful in these situations to acknowledge that this is a difficult topic for discussion but an important one for patients and physicians to address. The second barrier suggests that discussions of continuity may be an important aspect to encouraging these discussions.

When discussing mechanical ventilation for 'end-stage COPD', 41 percent of Canadian respirologists responding to a survey reported that the majority of these discussions take place in the intensive care unit (ICU) and only 23 percent in the clinic or office.[28*] Often these discussions occur late in the disease trajectory. For example, 84 percent of physicians wait until dyspnea is severe and 75 percent of physicians wait until the FEV_1 is <30 percent predicted. When discussing mechanical ventilation almost all physicians spontaneously mention intubation (96.8 percent) but far fewer physicians discuss aspects of weaning, sleeping, or eating. Some discourage mechanical ventilation in a setting of alcohol abuse, severe depression, and smoking.[28] The authors wrote, 'At the very least, this observation suggests that physicians should question their beliefs and biases when making end of life recommendations'.[28] Physicians need to be aware that the way they frame discussions influences choices patients make.[29]

There has been increasing dissatisfaction with advance directives over the past two decades. A number of studies have suggested that advance directives do not influence the treatments that patients receive[30–32**] and do not change end-of-life decision making.[33–35*] However, in the setting of good communication between patients, families, and physicians, advance directives may be an important component to end-of-life care and may be especially useful among patients with COPD who have strong feelings about the situations in which they would want to forego CPR or, particularly relevant for COPD, mechanical ventilation for acute respiratory failure. This is a topic that should be discussed with all patients with severe COPD. For patients who have experienced mechanical ventilation in the past, this offers physicians an opportunity to use their prior experience as a reference point for discussing potential future episodes of acute respiratory failure and circumstance under which they would not want mechanical ventilation. Patients' prior experiences with mechanical ventilation or with relatives or friends who have required life support can be important facilitators to patient–physician communication about treatment preferences and end-of-life care.[27*]

It is important to realize that depression may modify patients' treatment preferences. Depression is common among patients with COPD[36–39*] and a recent study suggests that patients with depressive symptoms are more likely to choose to forego CPR that those without depressive symptoms.[40*] As noted below, depression can be treated in patients with COPD and if depression improves, treatment preferences should be revisited.

Based on the prognostic information described in the preceding section and on clinical experience, there is an emerging profile of patients for whom discussions about treatment preferences or end-of-life care are especially important.[41] This profile includes patients with FEV_1 <30 percent predicted, those with more than one admission in the last year, those patients who are becoming increasingly dependent on others, those with left heart failure or other comorbidities, older patients, depressed patients, or the unmarried patient with advanced COPD. Any one of these factors should trigger a clinician to consider initiating a discussion of treatment preferences for life-sustaining treatments and end-of-life care. The presence of more than

one of these prognostic indicators should be clear criteria for having such a discussion with the patient.

PALLIATING SYMPTOMS AND MAXIMIZING QUALITY OF LIFE

The majority of treatments available for patients with COPD are palliative in the sense that the majority of these treatments are focused exclusively on palliating symptoms and maximizing quality of life. The few exceptions include long-term oxygen therapy,[42,43**] lung transplantation,[44*] and, perhaps in highly selected patients, lung volume reduction surgery.[45**] Otherwise, most treatments are provided with the goal of palliative care. As a consequence, these therapies should generally be started with the understanding that the patient and clinician will reassess whether they are serving the goal of palliating symptoms or improving or maintaining quality of life without causing adverse effects. This review will not attempt to summarize all aspects of management of COPD, but will attempt to cover some of the unique features of managing symptoms, particularly dyspnea, for patients with severe COPD. In addition, this review will cover some of the treatments shown to improve health-related quality of life among patients with severe COPD. Health-related quality of life is an important outcome measure for the provision of high quality palliative care and there have been considerable advances in the measurement and reporting of health-related quality of life as an outcome measure for patients with chronic lung diseases.[46]

Bronchodilators

Inhaled bronchodilator therapy is a mainstay of treatment for dyspnea among patients with COPD. There is some evidence that for most patients, the combination of a β agonist and quaternary anticholinergic agent such as ipratropium provides a better degree of bronchodilatation and reduction in acute exacerbations than either agent alone.[47*] There is also recent evidence that patients with severe COPD may benefit with a long-acting quaternary anticholinergic such as tiotroprium.[48**] The data for use of long-acting β agonist therapy in the stable COPD population are less clear, although there may be some benefit of these agents.[48]

Systemic therapies targeting bronchodilation are less successful. Theophylline is used much less commonly today than 20 years ago because it has relatively weak bronchodilatory effects and can have significant systemic side effects. Nonetheless, there may be some patients with severe COPD who have received maximal inhaled bronchodilator therapy and remain symptomatic. A study by Kirsten and colleagues suggests that patients with severe COPD on theophylline have worsening dyspnea and exercise tolerance when the drug is stopped.[49**] In addition, a trial by Mahler and colleagues suggests patients with severe COPD may have decreased symptoms of dyspnea even without any improvement in exercise tolerance.[50**] Therefore, patients who remain symptomatic after maximal inhaled bronchodilator therapy may benefit from a trial of theophylline.

Corticosteroids

There are precious few data that systemic corticosteroids are beneficial long term in the setting of chronic, stable COPD. The recent GOLD statements on COPD recommend that systemic steroids not be used in this setting due to the significant side effects and lack of compelling data suggesting significant benefit.[1] Inhaled corticosteroids certainly have much less adverse effects, but the data that they benefit patients with chronic stable severe COPD are also limited. A randomized trial by Burges and colleagues (the 'ISOLDE trial') did suggest that patients with moderate or severe COPD have a very small but statistically significant benefit in health-related quality of life with a slightly slower decline over several years than patients randomized to placebo.[51**] The patients receiving inhaled corticosteroids also had a small reduction in the number of exacerbations compared to those receiving placebo suggesting that the number of patients one needed to treat to eliminate 1 exacerbation per year was only 3. Therefore, inhaled corticosteroids are a reasonable adjunct treatment for patients with severe COPD especially if they have frequent exacerbations.

Oxygen

Oxygen therapy is an important component of treatment for patients who meet criteria used in two large randomized controlled trials of oxygen. These trials used the following criteria in determining eligibility for enrollment in the study:

- PaO_2 ≤55 or oxygen saturation <88 percent or
- PaO_2 56–60 or oxygen saturation of 88 percent

  and one of the following criteria as evidence of end organ damage from chronic hypoxia:

  – hematocrit >45 percent
  – evidence of right heart strain by electrocardiogram (EKG)
  – peripheral edema.

These studies, in combination, showed that oxygen therapy improves survival and quality of life for patients who met eligibility criteria and also suggest that the closer patients come to 24 hour a day use, the more benefit they obtain.[42,43**] However, it is important for clinicians to realize that patients who are terminally ill, but do not meet the strict oxygenation criteria above still qualify for oxygen therapy on the basis of their terminal illness and many of these patients may benefit from oxygen therapy.

Noninvasive positive pressure ventilation

Noninvasive positive pressure ventilation has been evaluated for the management of chronic respiratory failure (generally defined as an increased $PaCO_2$) in patients with severe COPD. There have been several small randomized trials that have suggested that in highly select patients with COPD, noninvasive positive pressure ventilation during the night can improve symptoms and health-related quality of life.[52–55**] However, clinical experience suggests that most patients with severe COPD and chronic respiratory failure will not tolerate NIV at home. A consensus conference suggests considering a trial of noninvasive positive pressure ventilation for patients with COPD and chronic respiratory failure if patients meet the following criteria:

- documented obstructive lung disease optimally treated
- persistent daytime symptoms
- chronic respiratory failure defined as:
  – $PaCO_2$ ≥55
  or
  – PCO_2 50–54 and nocturnal desaturation (≤88 percent for 5 consecutive minutes on 2 L/min O_2)
  or
  – $PaCO_2$ 50–54 and two or more hospitalizations for COPD in 12 months.[56]

Opiates

Opiates are an important part of the armamentarium for the treatment of dyspnea in the patient with severe COPD maximally treated with bronchodilators and other therapies; however, it is important to acknowledge that the benefit achieved with these agents is relatively modest. There have been a number of randomized trials and a recent meta-analysis that suggest that oral opiates reduce the sensation of dyspnea although are associated with some side effects.[57***] For example, a recent randomized trial of sustained release morphine for 4 days showed reduced dyspnea scores but increased constipation despite laxative treatment.[58] The meta-analysis also suggests that while oral and parental opiates can reduce the sensation of dyspnea, there are inadequate data to conclude that nebulized opiates are effective. Opioids are an important therapeutic option for patients with dyspnea that persists despite maximal bronchodilator therapy. They should be considered not only in end-of-life situations, but also in stable patients whenever breathlessness is severe in COPD and continues despite maximal bronchodilator therapy. However, clinicians should assess the benefit of this therapy and the burden of side effects for each individual patient.

Other pharmacologic agents for dyspnea

A number of small studies have examined the role of other oral agents including benzodiazepines, phenothiazines, and buspirone. These studies, recently reviewed in two reviews of treatment of dyspnea in severe COPD, were either negative or inconclusive, suggesting that these agents should not be routinely used for dyspnea in patients with COPD.[59,60**]

Although antidepressants are not routinely used for the treatment of dypnea in patients with COPD, it is important to note that depression is very common among patients with COPD.[36–39*] Antidepressants can significantly improve mood in patients with COPD and depression and, in addition, in these patients with depression, antidepressants can also improve physical symptoms including dyspnea.[61**]

Nonpharmacological treatments

There are a number of nonpharmacological approaches that can have an important effect on dyspnea and other symptoms as well as quality of life. An example of such approaches includes pulmonary rehabilitation. Although different pulmonary rehabilitation programs include different components, randomized trials have clearly shown that pulmonary rehabilitation can improve dyspnea, exercise tolerance, and health-related quality of life.[62–64**] Important components of this nonpharmacological therapy include teaching patients breathing techniques and teaching nonpharmacological methods such as the use of fans and relaxation techniques that may help reduce sensations of anxiety and increase the perception of control when patients feel dyspneic.

Another important treatment option for patients with severe COPD is referral to hospice. Hospice programs may be able to offer patients with COPD tremendous amounts of psychologic, emotional, and spiritual support in their final months as well as intensive symptom assessment and management above what a hospital or office-based physician can offer. Hospice is underutilized by patients with COPD in part because of the difficulty prognosticating for these patients.[6] However, there are many patients with severe COPD for whom a physician may have reasonable confidence that the patient is likely to die within 6 months. If patients improve, they can be taken off the hospice benefit without penalty and still be eligible to return to hospice if they deteriorate again.

Caregiver burden

Few studies have reported measures of caregiver burden for the families of patients with COPD. One randomized, controlled, multicenter trial involved 1966 patients in the USA and included patients with COPD. Compared with usual care, a team-managed, home-based primary care model significantly reduced caregiver burden and improved caregiver health-related quality of life.[65**] In a

Canadian multicenter study of patients with COPD, patients reported that reducing burdens on their loved ones was the aspect of care that they considered needed most attention.[66*]

In summary, palliative care is an important and large component of the treatment of patients with severe COPD. Physicians caring for such patients must be familiar with the treatments that can palliate patients' symptoms and improve or slow the decline in their quality of life. In addition, communication about end-of-life care is an important aspect of care for all these patients.

Key learning points

- Patients with COPD were much more likely to die in the intensive care unit, on mechanical ventilation, and with dyspnea and are less likely to receive palliative care than patients with lung cancer despite the fact that most patients with COPD prefer a course of care that focused on comfort, rather than prolonging life.

- Only a third of patients with oxygen-dependent COPD have discussed end-of-life care with their physicians and there were important aspects of end-of-life care that less than 10 percent of physicians discussed with their patients. Furthermore, patients with COPD are more likely than other patients to express concern about the lack of education that they receive about their disease, treatment, prognosis, and advance care planning.

- Despite increasing amount of prognostic data to help clinicians identify patients with severe COPD at high risk of death, these data do not provide clinicians with an easy way to identify with certainty those patients with a prognosis of less than 6 months. Clinicians will need to use their clinical judgment to identify patients likely to benefit from hospice care and they will, in our opinion, need to be willing to accept a higher degree of uncertainty in this prognosis than is often seen for patients with metastatic cancer.

- There is an emerging profile of patients for whom discussions about treatment preferences or end-of-life care are especially important and this profile includes patients with FEV_1 <30 percent predicted, those with more than one hospital admission in the last year, those patients who are becoming increasingly dependent on others, those with left heart failure or other comorbidities, the elderly, the depressed, or the unmarried patient with advanced COPD. Any one of these factors should trigger a clinician to consider initiating a discussion of treatment preferences for life-sustaining treatments and end-of-life care and the presence of more than one of these prognostic indicators should be clear criteria for having such a discussion with the patient.

- The foundation of treatment of dyspnea in severe COPD includes bronchodilators and oxygen. Opiates are also useful, although benefits may be limited by side effects for some patients. Corticosteroids and other pharmacological agents are of less certain benefit for stable patients. Nonpharmacological therapies are important adjuncts for treatment in this population and pulmonary rehabilitation programs are one option for providing these therapies to patients.

REFERENCES

* 1 Pauwels RA, Buist AS, Calverley CR, Hurd SS, on behalf of the GOLD Scientific Committee. Global strategy for the diagnosis, management, and prevention of Chronic Obstructive Pulmonary Disease, NHLBI/WHO Workshop Summary. *Am J Respir Crit Care Med* 2001; **163**: 1256–76.

2 Mannino DM. COPD: epidemiology, prevalence, morbidity and mortality, and disease heterogeneity. *Chest* 2002; **121**: S121–S126.

● 3 The SUPPORT Principal Investigators. A controlled trial to improve care for seriously ill hospitalized patients: The study to understand prognoses and preferences for outcomes and risks of treatments (SUPPORT). *JAMA* 1996; **274**: 1591–8.

* 4 O'Donnell DE, Aaron S, Bourbeau J, *et al.* State of the Art Compendium: Canadian Thoracic Society recommendations for the management of chronic obstructive pulmonary disease. *Can Respir J* 2004; **11**(Suppl B): 7B–59B.

● 5 Claessens MT, Lynn J, Zhong Z, *et al.* Dying with lung cancer or chronic obstructive pulmonary disease: Insights from SUPPORT. *J Am Geriatr Soc* 2000; **48**: S146–S153.

● 6 Gore JM, Brophy CJ, Greenstone MA. How do we care for patients with end stage chronic obstructive pulmonary disease (COPD)? A comparison of palliative care and quality of life in COPD and lung cancer. *Thorax* 2000; **55**: 1000–6.

● 7 Heffner JE, Fahy B, Hilling L, Barbieri C. Outcomes of advance directive education of pulmonary rehabilitation patients. *Am J Respir Crit Care Med* 1997; **155**: 1055–9.

8 Heffner JE, Fahy B, Hilling L, Barbieri C. Attitudes regarding advance directives among patients in pulmonary rehabilitation. *Am J Respir Crit Care Med* 1996; **154**: 1735–40.

● 9 Curtis JR, Engelberg RA, Nielsen EL, Au DH, Patrick DL. Patient-physician communication about end-of-life care for patients with severe COPD. *Eur Respir J* 2004; **24**: 200–5.

● 10 Curtis JR, Wenrich MD, Carline JD, *et al.* Patients' perspectives on physicians' skills at end-of-life care: Differences between patients with COPD, cancer, and AIDS. *Chest* 2002; **122**: 356–62.

11 Plant PK, Owen JL, Elliott MW. Non-invasive ventilation in acute exacerbations of chronic obstructive pulmonary disease: long term survival and predictors of in-hospital outcome. *Thorax* 2001; **56**: 708–12.

12 Roberts CM, Lowe D, Bucknall CE, *et al.* Clinical audit indicators of outcome following admission to hospital with acute exacerbation of chronic obstructive pulmonary disease. *Thorax* 2002; **57**: 137–41.

13 Moran JL, Green JV, Homan SD, *et al.* Acute exacerbations of chronic obstructive pulmonary disease and mechanical ventilation: a reevaluation. *Crit Care Med* 1998; **26**: 71–8.

14 Nevins ML, Epstein SK. Predictors of outcome for patients with COPD requiring invasive mechanical ventilation. *Chest* 2001; **119**: 1840–9.

15 Esteban A, Anzueto A, Frutos F, *et al.* Characteristics and outcomes in adult patients receiving mechanical ventilation: a 28-day international study. *JAMA* 2002; **287**: 345–55.

16 Seneff MG, Wagner DP, Wagner RP, *et al.* Hospital and 1-year survival of patients admitted to intensive care units with acute exacerbation of chronic obstructive pulmonary disease. *JAMA* 1995; **274**: 1852–7.

17 Anon JM, Garcia de Lorenzo A, Zarazaga A, *et al.* Mechanical ventilation of patients on long-term oxygen therapy with acute exacerbations of chronic obstructive pulmonary disease: prognosis and cost-utility analysis. *Intensive Care Med* 1999; **25**: 452–7.

18 Nava S, Rubini F, Zanotti E, *et al.* Survival and prediction of successful ventilator weaning in COPD patients requiring mechanical ventilation for more than 21 days. *Eur Respir J* 1994; **7**: 1645–52.

19 Antonelli Incalzi R, Fuso L, De Rosa M, *et al.* Co-morbidity contributes to predict mortality of patients with chronic obstructive pulmonary disease. *Eur Respir J* 1997; **10**: 2794–800.

20 Celli BR, Cote CG, Marin JM, *et al.* The body-mass index, airflow obstruction, dyspnea, and exercise capacity index in chronic obstructive pulmonary disease. *N Engl J Med* 2004; **350**: 1005–12.

21 Anthonisen NR, Wright EC, Hodgkin JE. Prognosis in chronic obstructive pulmonary disease. *Am Rev Respir Dis* 1986; **133**: 14–20.

22 Schols AM, Slangen J, Volovics L, Wouters EF. Weight loss is a reversible factor in the prognosis of chronic obstructive pulmonary disease. *Am J Respir Crit Care Med* 1998; **157**: 1791–7.

23 Landbo C, Prescott E, Lange P, *et al.* Prognostic value of nutritional status in chronic obstructive pulmonary disease. *Am J Respir Crit Care Med* 1999; **160**: 1856–61.

24 Yohannes AM, Baldwin RC, Connolly M. Mortality predictors in disabling chronic obstructive pulmonary disease in old age. *Age Ageing* 2002; **31**: 137–40.

25 Ferrer M, Alonso J, Morera J, *et al.* Chronic obstructive pulmonary disease stage and health-related quality of life. The Quality of Life of Chronic Obstructive Pulmonary Disease Study Group. *Ann Intern Med* 1997; **127**: 1072–9.

26 Heyland DK, Lavery JV, Tranmer JE, *et al.* Dying in Canada: is it an institutionalized, technologically supported experience? *J Palliat Care* 2000; **16**(Suppl): S10–S16.

27 Knauft ME, Nielsen EL, Engelberg RA, *et al.* Barriers and facilitators to communication about end-of-life care for patients with COPD. *Chest* 2005; **127**: 1886–8.

28 McNeely PD, Hebert PC, Dales RE, *et al.* Deciding about mechanical ventilation in end-stage chronic obstructive pulmonary disease: how respirologists perceive their role. *Can Med Assoc J* 1997; **156**: 177–83.

29   Sullivan KE, Hebert PC, Logan J, et al. What do physicians tell patients with end-stage COPD about intubation and mechanical ventilation? Chest 1996; 109: 258–64.

30   Schneiderman LJ, Kronick R, Kaplan RM, et al. Effects of offering advance directives on medical treatment and costs. Ann Intern Med 1992; 117: 599–606.

31   Danis M, Mutran E, Garrett JM. A prospective study of the impact of patient preferences on life-sustaining treatment and hospital cost. Crit Care Med 1996; 24: 1811–17.

32   Danis M, Southerland LI, Garrett JM, et al. A prospective study of advance directives for life-sustaining care. N Engl J Med 1991; 324: 882–8.

33   Teno JM, Lynn J, Connors AFJ, et al. The illusion of end-of-life savings with advance directives. J Am Geriatr Soc 1997; 45: 513–18.

34   Teno JM, Lynn J, Wegner N, et al. Advance directives for seriously ill hospitalized patients: effectiveness with the Patient Self-Determination Act and the SUPPORT Intervention. J Am Geriatr Soc 1997; 45: 500–7.

35   Teno JM, Licks S, Lynn J, et al. Do advance directives provide instructions that direct care? J Am Geriatr Soc 1997; 45: 508–12.

36   McSweeny A, Heaton R, Grant I, et al. Chronic obstructive pulmonary disease; socioemotional adjustment and life quality. Chest 1980; 77: 309–11.

37   Prigatano GP, Wright EC, Levin D. Quality of life and its predictors in patients with mild hypoxemia and chronic obstructive pulmonary disease. Arch Intern Med 1984; 144: 1613–19.

38   Light RW, Merrill EJ, Despars JA, et al. Prevalence of depression and anxiety in patients with COPD. Chest 1985; 87: 35–8.

39   Engstrom CP, Persson LO, Larsson S, et al. Functional status and well being in chronic obstructive pulmonary disease with regard to clinical parameters and smoking: a descriptive and comparative study. Thorax 1996; 51: 825–30.

40   Stapleton R, Nielsen EL, Engelberg RA, et al. Association of depression and life-sustaining treatment preferences in patients with chronic obstructive pulmonary disease. Chest 2005; 127: 328–34.

41   Hansen-Flaschen J. Chronic obstructive pulmonary disease: the last year of life. Respir Care 2004; 49: 90–7; discussion 97–8.

● 42   Medical Research Council Working Party. Long term domiciliary oxygen therapy in chronic hypoxic cor pulmonale complicating chronic bronchitis and emphysema. Lancet 1981; 1: 681–6.

● 43   Nocturnal Oxygen Therapy Trial Group. Continuous or nocturnal oxygen therapy in hypoxemic chronic obstructive lung disease. Ann Intern Med 1980; 93: 391–8.

44   Ramsey SD, Patrick DL, Albert RK, et al. The cost-effectiveness of lung transplantation. A pilot study. Chest 1995; 108: 1594–601.

● 45   Fishman A, Martinez F, Naunheim K, et al. A randomized trial comparing lung-volume-reduction surgery with medical therapy for severe emphysema. N Engl J Med 2003; 348: 2059–73.

46   Curtis JR, Martin DP, Martin TM. Patient-assessed health outcomes in chronic lung disease: What are they, how do they help us, and where do we go from here? Am J Respir Crit Care Med 1997; 156: 1032–9.

47   Friedman M, Serby CW, Menjoge SS, et al. Pharmacoeconomic evaluation of a combination of ipratropium plus albuterol compared with ipratropium alone and albuterol alone in COPD. Chest 1999; 115: 635–41.

48   Tashkin DP, Cooper CB. The role of long-acting bronchodilators in the management of stable COPD. Chest 2004; 125: 249–59.

49   Kirsten DK, Wegner RE, Jorres RA, Magnussen H. Effects of theophylline withdrawal in severe chronic obstructive pulmonary disease. Chest 1993; 104: 1101–17.

50   Mahler DA, Matthay RA, Snyder PE, et al. Sustained-release theophylline reduces dyspnea in nonreversible obstructive airway disease. Am Rev Respir Dis 1985; 131: 22–5.

● 51   Burges PS, Calverley PMA, Jones PW, et al. Randomised, double blind, placebo controlled study of fluticasone porpionate in patients with moderate to severe chronic obstructive pulmonary disease: the ISOLDE trial. BMJ 2000; 320: 1297–303.

52   Meecham Jones DJ, Paul EA, Jones PW, Wedzicha JA. Nasal pressure support ventilation plus oxygen compared with oxygen therapy alone in hypercapnic COPD. Am J Respir Crit Care Med 1995; 152: 538–44.

53   Garrod R, Mikelsons C, Paul EA, Wedzicha JA. Randomized controlled trial of domiciliary noninvasive positive pressure ventilation and physical training in severe chronic obstructive pulmonary disease. Am J Respir Crit Care Med 2000; 162: 1335–41.

54   Krachman SL, Quaranta AJ, Berger TJ, et al. Effects of noninvasive positive pressure ventilation on gas exchange and sleep in COPD patients. Chest 1997; 112: 623–8.

55   Casanova C, Celli BR, Tost L, et al. Long-term controlled trial of nocturnal nasal positive pressure ventilation in patients with severe COPD. Chest 2000; 118: 1582–90.

✱ 56   Consensus Conference. Clinical indications for non-invasive positive ventilation in chronic respiratory failure due to restrictive lung disease, COPD, and nocturnal hypoventilation – a consensus conference report. Chest 1999; 116: 521–34.

◆ 57   Jennings AL, Davies AN, Higgins JP, et al. A systematic review of the use of opioids in the management of dyspnoea. Thorax 2002; 57: 939–44.

● 58   Abernethy AP, Currow DC, Frith P, et al. Randomised, double blind, placebo controlled crossover trial of sustained release morphine for the management of refractory dyspnoea. BMJ 2003; 327: 523–8.

59   Manning HL. Dyspnea treatment. Respir Care 2000; 45: 1342–50; discussion 1350–4.

60   Runo JR, Ely EW. Treating dyspnea in a patient with advanced chronic obstructive pulmonary disease. West J Med 2001; 175: 197–201.

61   Borson S, McDonald GJ, Gayle T, et al. Improvement in mood, physical symptoms, and function with nortriptyline for depression in patients with chronic obstructive pulmonary disease. Psychosomatics 1992; 33: 190–201.

● 62   Ries AL, Kaplan RM, Limberg TM, Prewitt LM. Effects of pulmonary rehabilitation on physiologic and psychosocial outcomes in patients with chronic obstructive pulmonary disease. Ann Intern Med 1995; 122: 823–32.

● 63 Wijkstra PJ, Van Altena RV, Kraan J, *et al.* Quality of life in patients with chronic obstructive pulmonary disease after rehabilitation at home. *Eur Respir J* 1994; **7**: 269–73.

64 Wijkstra PJ, Ten Vergert EM, van Altena R, *et al.* Long term benefits of rehabilitation at home on quality of life and exercise tolerance in patients with chronic obstructive pulmonary disease. *Thorax* 1995; **50**: 824–8.

65 Hughes SL, Weaver FM, Giobbie-Hurder A, *et al.* Effectiveness of team-managed home-based primary care: a randomized multicenter trial. *JAMA* 2000; **284**: 2877–85.

66 Rocker G, Heyland D, Groll D, *et al.* Meeting the needs of patients with end stage COPD: A Multicenter study. *Am J Respir Crit Care Med* 2004; **169**: A50.

100

Other infectious diseases: malaria, rabies, tuberculosis

SUE MARSDEN

INTRODUCTION

Malaria, rabies, and tuberculosis are diseases from which people die in the developing world.[1–8] These are diseases associated with poverty, and therefore are not usually seen as diseases creating palliative care issues for the developed world. Hence they have received little attention in this regard. Nonetheless, each year some 3 million people die worldwide from tuberculosis, 2 million from malaria, and about 40 000–100 000 die from rabies;[1–8] these are conservative estimates. These three infectious diseases, and others, are all preventable or treatable and clearly public health interventions are critically important in this respect. However, while deaths are occurring with unrelieved symptoms and distress as happens daily, management of patients dying with these diseases demands the application of palliative care principles.

MALARIA

Malaria is a life-threatening parasitic disease caused by the genus *Plasmodium*, transmitted by female mosquitoes of the genus *Anopheles*.[1,2,9] Although malaria has been essentially eliminated from many countries with temperate climates, 40 percent of the world's population, mostly those living in the developing countries, remain at risk. Today, in tropical and subtropical countries malaria causes acute illnesses in 300–500 million people and is responsible for approximately 2 million deaths each year.[1,2,10] Most of these deaths are in young children with 90 percent of deaths due to malaria

occurring in sub-Saharan Africa.[2] It is estimated that an African child dies from malaria every 30 seconds.[2]

Etiology and pathogenesis

Malaria in humans is caused by one of four species of *Plasmodium*: *P. falciparum*, *P. vivax*, *P. ovale*, and *P. malariae*.[1,2] *P. falciparum* causes the highest mortality and is the most common causative organism in sub-Saharan Africa.[1,2,9] *P. vivax* is more widely distributed and causes mild recurrent disease if the first episode is not treated adequately. *P. ovale* is rare and can also cause recurrent disease.[2] *P. malariae* has scattered distribution, mainly in Africa and can live in asymptomatic hosts for decades or cause acute illness.[2] It has been associated with membranoproliferative glomerulonephritis and nephrotic syndrome in children.[2,11]

LIFE CYCLE OF THE MALARIAL PARASITE[1,2]

Plasmodium sporozoites are transmitted to humans from the salivary gland of the female *Anopheles* mosquito by injection under the skin. The life cycle in the human host, summarized in Box 100.1, results in some merozoites differentiating into gametocytes. These can then be transferred from an infected human to a biting mosquito. The parasite completes its sexual cycle within the mosquito forming new sporozoites, which are then available to infect another human. *P. vivax* and *P. ovale* can remain dormant in liver parenchyma for months or years and are responsible for recurrent malaria if treatment has not intervened.

Box 100.1 Life cycle of *Plasmodium* in humans[1,2]

Exo-erythrocytic and asymptomatic phase of infection

1 Sporozoites reach the blood stream and travel to the liver

2 Hepatocytes are infected and the asexual sporozoites multiply to a form called schizont containing thousands of merozoites

3 After 6–16 days merozoites are liberated into the bloodstream

Erythrocytic phase

4 The merozoites invade the red blood cells

5 In the red blood cells they turn into ring forms, trophozoites, and degrade hemoglobin

6 Once more, this time within red blood cells, the parasite forms squizonts, which multiply and lyse the red blood cells

7 Thousands of merozoites are liberated into the blood stream infecting new red blood cells

8 This process continues with repetitive cycles of red blood cells invasion and lysis resulting in hemolytic anemia

9 Some merozoites differentiate into gametocytes, the form acquired by female mosquitoes after biting an infected human

PATHOGENESIS

P. falciparum infection is more severe with a higher mortality and thus most likely to be implicated when a patient requires palliative care. It is the only *Plasmodium* causing microvascular disease.[12] As the parasites mature the infected red blood cells adhere to the endothelial cells in capillaries and post-capillary venules of, significantly, the brain and kidneys but also other organs.[1,13–15] This sequestration leads to a functional microvascular obstruction.[16,17] Cytokines, e.g. tumor necrosis factor α (TNFα), contribute to the process.[1,18,19]

In addition, there is consumption of glucose and production of lactate by the parasite as well as the hypoglycemic effects of TNFα.[1] These contribute to glucose deprivation, lactate excess, and acidemia at a tissue level. There is lysis of red blood cells leading to acute anemia, as the schizont stage parasites mature. Chronic anemia occurs from lysis and the effect of TNFα.[1,20]

In contrast, *P. vivax* and *P. ovale* do not cause sequestration and hence do not cause the microvascular complications in brain, kidneys, and lungs. However, sickle hemoglobin, which can provide some protection against severe *P. falciparum* does not protect against those parasites that do not sequester.[1,21]

Prevention

Cooperative public health initiatives aimed at controlling mosquito populations and reducing transmission are critical in preventing malaria, e.g. the World Health Organization (WHO) Roll Back Malaria global partnership.[9]

Clinical manifestations

The incubation period after an infectious bite is 8–14 days except for *P. malariae*, which may be 18–42 days.[9] The presentation of uncomplicated malaria is variable and mimics many other infectious diseases.[2] Fever is common and may initially be persistent rather than tertian.[3] Most commonly there may be general malaise, headache, backache, chills, episodic sweating, and sometimes vomiting and abdominal pain.[22] In young children there may be nonspecific irritability, refusal to eat, and vomiting. Anemia, jaundice, hepatomegaly, and splenomegaly may follow.

As malaria can mimic a number of other acute illnesses, it is crucial to have a high index of suspicion.[2,3] It should always be considered in the differential diagnosis of acute febrile illness in endemic areas or in people traveling to these areas. Unless *P. falciparum* infection is diagnosed and treated promptly, deterioration can occur at an alarming rate, especially in children.[3] Severe malaria may develop with its attendant morbidity and mortality.[3,23,24] Severe malaria may present with:[2,3]

- CNS dysfunction – clinical manifestations may vary from confusion, delirium, obtundation to seizures and deep coma. Unrousable coma, not attributable to any other cause in a patient with falciparum malaria is defined by the WHO as cerebral malaria
- Hypoglycemia
- Acidosis
- Acute renal failure
- Abnormal bleeding
- Pulmonary edema
- Hyperparasitemia – this occurs where more than 5 percent of red blood cells are infected

Diagnosis

Microscopic examination of thick and thin blood smears for the parasites is highly sensitive, specific, and economical.[2,3] The thin smear allows identification of the *Plasmodium* species. Rapid diagnostic tests are available, which detect antigens by immunochromatography. They are easy to perform and quick but their sensitivity varies.

Due to the rapid evolution and high mortality of severe malaria it is crucial to make a rapid diagnosis. Treatment may need to be initiated before laboratory tests are available. For practical purposes and in the environment where severe malaria occurs this is justified and often necessary.[2]

Treatment

Severe malaria should, if at all possible, be treated aggressively with appropriate antimalarial medications together with general supportive measures and management of organ failures in an intensive care unit.[3] Antimalarial medications include quinine (WHO recommended drug of choice), quinidine, artesunate, artemether, artemisinin and chloroquine, although the last is of limited use due to drug resistance.[3,24–28]

Even with prompt treatment with an effective antimalarial drug, cerebral malaria has an estimated fatality rate for hospital admissions of 20–50 percent.[2] Sadly, patients often present late and are misdiagnosed. Also, in the environments where severe malaria usually occurs intensive medical support measures and/or appropriate medications are not available.

Symptom management

As part of the management of malaria, meticulous attention must be paid to all symptoms and emotional support of the patient and family. When it is recognized that treatment aimed at aggressive disease is not possible or is futile, palliative care principles clearly must continue and assume the primary focus of care.[2]

CENTRAL NERVOUS SYSTEM SYMPTOMS[2*]

Delirium

In the earlier stages of the disease trajectory attempts must be made to treat any potentially reversible causes of delirium, e.g. dehydration, hypoglycemia, urinary retention, fever. Otherwise the following are important:

- *Environment.* General comfort support measures as always include attention to the physical environment, noise level, presence of family, and quiet music if possible.
- *Medications.* Antipsychotics, e.g. haloperidol 2–5 mg every 6 hours and 2–5 mg every 1 hour prn. Rapid titration may be necessary with initial doses given more frequently. Alternative medications are chlorpromazine and levomepromazine.
- *Sedation.* As well as antipsychotics, the patient may require sedation. Diazepam, lorazepam, and midazolam if available should be considered.

Convulsions

Seizure activity requires the use of anticonvulsants, e.g. diazepam 10–20 mg intravenously (IV), rectally (PR) or intramuscularly (IM); midazolam 5–10 mg IM/IV/SC or phenobarbital 200 mg SC/IM.

Coma

It is essential to pay careful attention to physical care to maintain skin integrity and maintain hygiene.

PAIN

Severe pain may be the result of increased muscle tone and spasm. Baclofen 5–10 mg SC/IM or diazepam 5–10 mg IM/IV may be given. Opioids may also be required.

FEVER

Fever may be alleviated with oral acetaminophen (paracetamol) in the early stages and may be given rectally if necessary.

OTHER ASPECTS

In addition to good symptom management and personal care of the patient, provision of emotional and spiritual support to the patient and family are important. This can be particularly poignant as the disease presenting earlier is curable and as many of the patients are so young. Both the patient and the family also require clear explanation as to the nature of the disease, prognosis, and symptoms that are being experienced and their management.

RABIES

Rabies is a fatal acute encephalomyelitis and remains one of the most common viral causes of death in developing countries.[4,5,29] It has 100 percent mortality in previously unvaccinated patients who, without palliation have agonizing deaths.[4,5]

Reliable data on the incidence of rabies in humans are scarce. Estimates of the incidence, worldwide, range from 40 000 to 100 000 annually, the vast majority in developing countries.[4–6,30] It is estimated that some 10 million people receive postexposure treatments annually, following bites from animals suspected to have rabies. Unfortunately most are treated with vaccines carrying a high risk of neurological complications. The incidence of human rabies in developed countries is very low, e.g. one to two cases annually in the 1990s in the USA. Some island nations are reported to be rabies free. Most cases in developed countries are from bites from rabid wild animals, e.g. bats, foxes, and raccoons. In developing countries bites from domestic and feral animals, usually dogs, are responsible.[5,6,30] Transmission between humans has only been documented as a result of corneal transplant.[4–6,29]

Etiology and pathogenesis[4–6]

Rabies is caused by a *Lyssavirus*, a bullet-shaped, negative-stranded RNA virus, a member of the *Rhabdoviridae* family. It is transmitted via the saliva of infected animals, being introduced by bites, scratches, licks on broken skin, and contact with mucous membranes. After entry through a breach in the skin or mucous membrane the virus replicates in muscle cells, and infects the muscle spindle and subsequently the nerve innervating the spindle. Further replication occurs within these neurons and virus rapidly spreads centrally toward the central nervous system. Virus is present within dorsal root ganglia within 72 hours of inoculation.

Rabies infection appears to require local viral replication, perhaps to reach a critical load, before nervous system infection occurs.[4,5] Thus, if anti-rabies immunoglobulin and active immunization are given in time, virus may be prevented from spread to the nervous system and disease prevented. Once virus has entered the peripheral nerve, however, disease is inevitable. After spreading to the spinal cord, the virus spreads throughout the central nervous system and then centrifugally out to the rest of the body via peripheral nerves. High concentration of virus in saliva results from shedding from sensory nerve endings in the oral mucosa as well as replication in salivary glands. The brain in rabies shows an encephalic picture and the spinal cord shows severe inflammation and necrosis.

Prevention[5,6]

The control of animal rabies is central to the prevention of human disease. Unfortunately, few countries have been able to achieve this. Prophylaxis for domestic animals and humans at high risk together with postexposure treatment for exposed humans is the basis of control. Dramatic decreases in human cases have been reported recently in China, Thailand, Sri Lanka, and Latin America, This follows the implementation of programs for improved postexposure treatment of humans and the vaccination of dogs, with also encouraging trends in the Philippines.[31] However, in many developing countries the cost of these programs and the cost of controlling feral dog populations remain obstacles and may not achieve political priority.

PREEXPOSURE PROPHYLAXIS[5,6,31]

Preexposure prophylaxis (PEP) is usually confined to people at high risk of rabies exposure, e.g. veterinarians and laboratory workers. Those caring for patients with rabies should ideally be vaccinated, but in the underresourced settings that rabies usually occurs this is prohibitively expensive and vaccination is unlikely to occur. Transmission to healthcare workers has *not* been reported and remains a theoretical risk when normal universal infection control measures are observed. This may, of course be difficult if a patient has uncontrolled aggressive and violent delirium.

The recommended PEP involves a series of three intramuscular or intradermal injections given on days 0, 7, and 21 or 28 with a booster every 2–3 years.

Postexposure treatment[6,31,32]

- *First aid*. The most effective mechanism to protect against rabies following a suspicious bite is to vigorously wash and flush the wound with soap and water. Ethanol, iodine or povidone-iodine solution should be applied.
- *Anti-rabies immunoglobulin*. This should ideally be applied on the day of the bite (day 0) but can be applied up to day 7. Human immunoglobulin, if available should be used or alternatively equine, following a skin test. The immunoglobulin is infiltrated in and around the wound.
- *Vaccination*. This is recommended following a bite from an animal in which rabies is a possibility but may be discontinued if the animal remains healthy for 10 days or is proved at autopsy to be negative for rabies. Purified vero-cell vaccine (PVCV) or purified duck embryo (PDEV) vaccines are used. There are various vaccination schedules. Reduced intradermal regimens have been found to be effective and less expensive.

Obstacles to treatment

Although postexposure treatment is available there remain real and heart-rending obstacles to obtaining this. Many patients do not seek treatment through ignorance, fear, folk beliefs, and overwhelming poverty. Education programs are making inroads in some places. An example of this is the national program of the Department of Health in the Philippines encouraging pet owners to have dogs vaccinated and to seek vaccination following a suspicious bite.[5] However, overwhelming poverty and political motivation remain worldwide issues in the eradication of rabies as with many global health problems.

Clinical manifestations (Table 100.1)[4,5,29]

The incubation period for rabies may be from a few days to several years. The average incubation period is 20–90 days. The time of onset of symptoms depends on:

- the severity of the wound, i.e. the depth, size, or multiplicity
- clothing protection at the site of bite
- the site of wound in relation to the brain, i.e. patients with facial bites develop symptoms earlier.

The early clinical features are nonspecific influenzalike symptoms and localized paresthesia, pain, and pruritus at the bite site. The later clinical presentation evolves into two forms: the encephalitic (furious) form (in about 80 percent of patients) or the paralytic (dumb) form.

'FURIOUS' RABIES

The features of encephalitic rabies are typically described as hydrophobia – representing an exaggerated irritant reflex of the respiratory tract with laryngeal spasm – episodic hyperactivity, seizures, aerophobia, hyperventilation, and

Table 100.1 *Clinical stages and symptoms of rabies*[5]

Stage	Time period	Symptoms
Incubation period	<30 days (25%) 30–90 days (50%) 90 days–1year (20%) >1 year (5%)	
Prodromal symptoms	2–10 days	At bite site: paresthesia, pain and pruritus General: fever, malaise nausea, vomiting

Acute disease
Furious (80%)
	2–7 days	Hydrophobia
		Aerophobia
		Dysphagia
		Delirium with:
		  aggression
		  disorientation
		  hallucinations
		  terror
		  hyperexcitement
		  hypervigilance
		  confusion
		Autonomic dysfunction with:
		  hypersalivation
		  sweating
		  priapism
		Seizures

Dumb (20%)	2–7 days	Ascending flaccid paralysis

autonomic dysfunction with papillary dilatation, increased salivation, sweating, and occasionally priapism. However, the feature of rabies that is often most distressing for patients, families and carers is delirium. The features that predominate are aggression, disorientation, hallucinations, overwhelming terror, hyperexcitability, hypervigilance, and confusion.

'DUMB' RABIES

Paralytic rabies is characterized by ascending paralysis resembling Guillain–Barré syndrome.

Outcome

Whatever the initial symptom complex, cardiac arrhythmias and coma intervene and death is inevitable within a few days. Most patients die within 72 hours of the onset of clinical symptoms.

Symptom management

DELIRIUM[5,33,34*]

As in any palliative care situation the first priority is good symptom management. This in turn allows personal care of the patient and psychosocial and spiritual issues for the patient and family to be addressed. There are few other situations where this is as true as in need for control of the delirium associated with rabies. Rabies patients without appropriate medication often die alone in a locked and barred room, physically restrained, agitated, terrified, paranoid, and with classic hydrophobia and aerophobia. The delirium can be managed with:

- Haloperidol 5 mg given hourly subcutaneously (SC) or IM titrated to the desired effect (with a minimum of three doses), followed by regular four hourly injections.
- Levomepromazine 25–100 mg every 4–6 hours SC or chlorpromazine 50–100 mg every 4–6 hours IM may be considered as alternatives.
- It may be necessary to add sedation with a benzodiazepine, e.g. diazepam or midazolam.

HYDROPHOBIA AND AEROPHOBIA

These do not respond to haloperidol as shown in a recent unpublished study (Starfish Palliative Care Program, San Lazaro Hospital, Manila, Republic of Philippines, personal communication, November 2004, March 2005, July 2005). Hydrophobia describes, in fact the exaggerated reflex of the respiratory tract with laryngeal spasm[4] and is not a 'phobic' symptom as such. It is more likely to respond to antispasmodics such as diazepam (Starfish Palliative Care Program, personal communication, November 2004, March 2005, July 2005).

SECRETIONS

These have been successfully controlled with diphenhydramine 50–100 mg every 4–6 hours.[5,33,34*] Alternatives that may be considered, if available, are glycopyrrolate or hyoscine butylbromide. Hyoscine hydrobromide should not be used as it may aggravate agitation.

SEIZURE ACTIVITY

This will require the use of anticonvulsants, e.g. benzodiazepines, such as diazepam or midazolam, or phenobarbital.

NAUSEA AND VOMITING

Antidopaminergic antipsychotics such as haloperidol and levomepromazine are effective antiemetics. If these are not being used to control delirium then other antiemetics such as metoclopramide may be considered.

FEVER

This is usually a more significant symptom in the prodromal phase and can be managed with paracetamol.

Physical environment

The room in which the patient is cared for should be clean, pleasant, as quiet as possible, and free of draughts. Seating should be available for family.

Family support and communication ([5,33,34] and Starfish Palliative Care Program, personal communication, November 2004, March 2005, July 2005)

When symptom control is achieved patient and family can communicate, say their goodbyes, and deal with as much unfinished business as possible in the short remaining time. Staff have an important role in supporting and facilitating this. To support the family the following are important:

- Space should be provided close to the patient for the family to rest, talk, and receive support and information.
- Honest gentle communication concerning the imminence of death should be provided. Emotional support is necessary for the family who are experiencing a sudden loss, often of the family breadwinner. Any practical advice concerning social support services available is important. Most often the family is from a very poor socioeconomic background.
- Discussion and education concerning transmission of disease and indications for postexposure vaccination. Families need information that the disease is spread by saliva introduced into a wound or mucous membrane. It is not transmitted through touching intact skin. Thus families need reassurance that it is safe to sit with their dying loved one and that careful contact will not transmit the disease. Postexposure vaccination is recommended for:
  - sexual partners, due to the possibility of transmission through saliva
  - others considered at risk, e.g. a contact who has been bitten by the patient or exposed to the saliva of the patient.
- When a rabies patient's symptoms are well controlled the family may decide to take their loved one home (reference 5 and Starfish Palliative Care Program, personal communication, November 2004, March 2005, July 2005). This may be for purely important economic reasons. It is cheaper to transport a live person than a dead body. It also has obvious emotional and social benefits for patient and family. Families need careful counseling and practical support for this to occur.

Carer education and support[5]

All healthcare professionals and other carers involved in caring for rabies patients need education regarding:

- The facts concerning rabies transmission. In most developing countries PEP is prohibitively expensive. However, as mentioned above, transmission to healthcare workers has *not* been reported and remains theoretical and unlikely if normal care and universal infection control rules are followed. Staff attending to patients' personal care should ideally wear protective gown, gloves, and goggles. If good symptom control is achieved the risk of being bitten or spat at by a patient is minimized.
- The principles of palliative care, emphasizing the pivotal role of good symptom control with *appropriate, adequate, regular* medication.

TUBERCULOSIS

Tuberculosis is an infectious disease caused by mycobacteria. The histology characteristically consists of granulomas.[7] Infection usually occurs following inhalation of infectious particles into the lungs.[7,8] It then spreads via blood stream, lymphatics, airways, or direct extension. Pulmonary tuberculosis is the most common form of the disease constituting 80 percent of tuberculosis infections in developing countries. However, any organ or part of the body can be affected.

Mycobacterium tuberculosis infects nearly 2 billion people worldwide and causes 3 million deaths a year.[7] These occur mostly in developing countries and mainly in the age group of 15–49 years.[8] Tuberculosis is associated with overcrowding, poverty, malnutrition, alcohol abuse, and an increase in the rate of human immunodeficiency virus (HIV)/acquired immune deficiency syndrome (AIDS) infection.[7,8] In developed countries tuberculosis had been steadily decreasing until the mid-1980s. With the AIDS epidemic this decrement has ceased or reversed and is again concentrated in underprivileged and low socioeconomic communities in these countries.[7,35,36]

Pathogenesis and transmission[7,8]

The usual causative organism is *M. tuberculosis*, an aerobic, nonspore-forming acid-fast bacillus, but occasionally *M. bovine* can also be the cause. Microorganisms are expelled into the air in tiny droplets from an infected patient with pulmonary tuberculosis. These dry rapidly, becoming droplet nuclei that harbor the microorganisms and may remain suspended in air for several hours. *M. tuberculosis* can remain alive for up to several hours, and even up to 3 years in a closed environment. A close contact may inhale the droplet nuclei, following which bacterial multiplication begins in the terminal airspaces. Initially the focus is subpleural – in the mid-lung zone. Macrophages ingest the bacteria and an initial pulmonary Ghon focus is formed. Macrophages may be carried by the lymphatics to regional lymph nodes, where they form the primary complex, and sometimes to distant lymph nodes. However, in an immunocompromised host they are not retained in the lymph nodes and may spread through the blood stream to other organs. The primary complex itself may progress causing bronchial collapse, erosion of the bronchus and further distal spread, pneumonia and cavitation or lympho-hematogenous dissemination, resulting in miliary tuberculosis.

Development of tuberculosis is usually arrested at the primary stage by the host's immune system. Hence healthy well-nourished individuals with an intact immune system do not usually develop the disease, whereas those with a compromised immune system, e.g. due to malnutrition or HIV infection, are very likely to develop tuberculosis following mycobacterium exposure. Determinants of infection occurring are: closeness of contact and infectiousness of the source. Patients with positive smears, i.e. direct microscopy positive, are highly infectious. Those with positive findings only on culture, i.e. direct microscopy negative, are less infectious.

Tuberculosis morbidity in a given population, however, is determined by two factors, the risk of infection (e.g. as in overcrowding) and the risk of developing active disease once infected (e.g. as where immune deficiency exists).

Clinical presentation and diagnosis[7,8,37]

In the presence of nonspecific symptoms tuberculosis should always be suspected if occurring in the environment previously described. This is especially so where there are associated sputum-positive family or contacts.

PULMONARY TUBERCULOSIS

The respiratory symptoms of pulmonary tuberculosis may be cough, sputum, which may be bloodstained, dysnea, and chest wall and pleuritic pain.[7,8] Generalized symptoms include weight loss, anorexia, fatigue cachexia, night sweats, and fever.[7,8] Diagnosis is made by direct microscopy of sputum smears using Ziehl–Neelsen stain (wherever possible three specimens are collected), sputum culture, and radiography.[7,8]

COMPLICATIONS[8]

Complications of pulmonary tuberculosis include hemoptysis, acute respiratory distress (due to pleural effusion, lung collapse, pneumothorax or cardiopulmonary insufficiency due to cor pulmonale), and bronchiectasis and/or pulmonary fibrosis.

EXTRAPULMONARY TUBERCULOSIS

Tuberculosis lymphadenitis and pleuritis are the two most common.[7,8] Others are: meningitis, pericarditis, peritonitis, and urogenital and skeletal tuberculosis.[7,8] The specific symptoms will depend on the organ involved, e.g. chest pain in pleuritis and lymphadenitis, bone pain in skeletal tuberculosis and delirium, and seizure activity, headache, vomiting, meningism, focal signs, and coma in tuberculosis meningitis.

TUBERCULIN SKIN TESTS

These reflect exposure to M. tuberculosis and have little value in diagnosing clinical disease where tuberculosis is common. Especially in adults, a positive test is infrequently followed by disease and a negative test does not exclude disease. It may be useful in young children who have been in contact with infectious persons recently. The tine test is usually used for screening and contact tracing in children while the Mantoux test is preferred for diagnosis. The diagnosis of tuberculosis in children may be difficult and the WHO has developed clear criteria in this respect.[8]

Tuberculosis treatment[7,8]

The cornerstone of treatment of tuberculosis is appropriate chemotherapy. The usual antituberculosis drugs used are isoniazid, rifampicin, pyrazinamide, ethambutol, and streptomycin. For successful treatment it is essential that the medications are taken:

- in appropriate combination
- in the correct dosage
- regularly
- for a sufficient period to prevent relapse, i.e. for at least 6 months.

Unfortunately these criteria are often not met in environments of poverty and overcrowding,[35,38] and patient ignorance of the importance of continued treatment. Inadequately treated tuberculosis can be worse than not treating at all due to the emergence of drug-resistant organisms.[8] Therefore education and counseling of patients, their families and communities and public health measures are critical in the management of tuberculosis.

The implementation of the highly cost effective Directly Observed Treatment Short Course (DOTS)[8*] in 1991 has resulted in cure rates of 95 percent even in some of the poorest countries. The DOTS strategy uses four different drugs given over 6–8 months, with medications taken under direct observation of healthcare workers who continually monitor patients during the course.

Unfortunately in recent years there has been an alarming emergence of multidrug-resistant (MDR) tuberculosis organisms in some populations. These can develop when incorrect medications or wrong combinations are given or drugs are not taken for long enough.[8] It is estimated that some 50 million people worldwide are already infected with MDR tuberculosis. The WHO and its international partners have formed the DOTS-plus working group in an attempt to address this problem.[8,39–48]

Tuberculosis prevention[8,49–51]

Bacille Calmette Guérin (BCG) vaccination, using live attenuated vaccine from a strain of *M. bovis*, is used for prevention of tuberculosis throughout much of the world. Although evidence is conflicting it is suggested that BCG vaccination of children will result in 60–80 percent decrease in the incidence of tuberculosis in a population.

Chemoprophylaxis is used to treat those at risk of developing tuberculosis, usually using isoniazid.[8,37] It is used for contacts of smear-positive patients and those with depressed immunity in a population where tuberculosis is prevalent.[8]

Palliative care

Tuberculosis is treatable and every effort should be made to treat and cure the disease even in extremely sick patients.[8] However, when this is no longer achievable, applying palliative care principles is paramount. The focus must include attention to physical, emotional, spiritual, social, and educational needs of the patient and family.

Symptom management

Most patients dying from tuberculosis have respiratory and nonspecific symptoms (Box 100.2).[8]

Box 100.2 Symptoms in dying patients with pulmonary tuberculosis

Respiratory symptoms

- Dyspnea
- Cough
- Hemoptysis
- Thoracic pain
- Terminal secretions

General symptoms

- Fatigue
- Cachexia
- Night sweats
- Fever

RESPIRATORY SYMPTOMS

Dyspnea
- Treat any reversible aspect
  - Pleural effusion: drain if feasible.
  - Associated obstructive airways disease: optimal use of bronchodilators and steroids.

- General symptomatic measures
  - Supplemental oxygen in the presence of hypoxia.
  - Air flow using fans or simply open window.
  - Opioids: these reduce the subjective sensation of breathlessness.[52*] If the patient is opioid naïve a starting dose of oral morphine 5–10 mg every 4 hours or 2.5–5 mg SC every 4 hours with additional as needed doses available for exacerbations. Patients will still have tachypnea and this needs to be explained to families with reassurance that this in itself is not distressing.[52]
  - Benzodiazepines: where there are significant anxiety episodes benzodiazepines could be considered, e.g. lorazepam 1 mg prn or diazepam 5–10 mg prn.

Cough
A dry cough is always present in these patients. As the disease progresses it may become purulent and blood stained. Opioids may be useful, e.g. morphine 5–10 mg every 4 hours prn. Inhaled cromoglicate may be useful.

Hemoptysis
Hemoptysis can be a very distressing symptom for both patient and family especially when massive, when it can be the terminal event. The following should be considered:

- In the earlier stages tranexamic acid 500 mg three times daily, if available, should be considered.
- Dark linen and towels, if available, can reduce the visual impact.
- If massive bleeding and associated choking are possibilities, a short-acting benzodiazepine such as midazolam or lorazepam should be available. In the home situation a preloaded syringe, e.g. of midazolam 5–10 mg, should be made available.

Respiratory secretions
As the patient becomes more unresponsive and secretions accumulate it is important to counsel the family that the noisy breathing is not distressing for the patient and represents pooling of secretions. It does not indicate that the patient is choking.[52] Medications that may be used to reduce secretions are glycopyrrolate 0.4 mg SC every 4 hours or hyoscine butylbromide 10–20 mg SC every 4–6 hours. Hyoscine hydrobromide should be used with caution as it may cause or aggravate agitation.

NONSPECIFIC SYMPTOMS

Fatigue and cachexia
Fatigue and cachexia are among the most common and severe symptoms in tuberculosis. Pain and clinical depression may contribute to fatigue and should be appropriately managed. Antidepressants and psychostimulants, e.g. methylphenidate should be considered.

Patients with anemia may benefit from blood transfusion. Food intake *per se* is unlikely to resolve the severe weight loss related to tuberculosis as cachexia is a syndrome resulting from metabolic abnormalities. However, it may be that cachexia syndrome has been confused with malnutrition in the environment where these patients are dying. Encouraging and extraordinary results have been seen where patients have merely been fed adequately (Starfish Palliative Care Program, personal communication, November 2004, March 2005, July 2005). However, in the presence of true cachexia syndrome the social value of meals remains important even where the patient is able to take very little. Families need counseling that cachexia is a metabolic consequence of advanced disease.

Night sweats and fever

These are common and unpleasant. Hydration needs to be maintained. Fever can be managed with acetaminophen or nonsteroidal anti-inflammatory medications.

PAIN

Pain is often underreported and under-treated due to reluctance to use analgesics in the presence of dyspnea. Thoracic and skeletal pain is managed with the usual principles of initially using regular nonopioids, e.g. acetaminophen and a nonsteroidal anti-inflammatory, moving to opioids as necessary.

OTHER SYMPTOMS

Less common extrapulmonary tuberculosis presentations require symptom management depending on the site. For example tuberculosis meningitis may result in delirium, seizure activity, and coma requiring appropriate attention to these symptoms.

Physical care[8]

Dying tuberculosis patients are inevitably wasted, dependent and often bed bound. They require meticulous attention to skin care and bodily functions to prevent pressure areas and skin excoriation, and tears.

Emotional, spiritual, and social needs

The very diagnosis of tuberculosis without the knowledge that it is incurable and the patient is now dying will have evoked many emotional issues including fear, grief, anger, and despair. Patients are often in the most productive part of their lives and may be parents and breadwinners. As well as fears for themselves they may have fears for future support of their families, a sense of uselessness as well as the stigma attached to the diagnosis.

Patients may see their disease and fate as punishment and this may be inextricably intertwined with spiritual and religious beliefs. Emotional and spiritual counseling and support for both patient and family are thus important. Patients and families may become socially isolated as a result of the diagnosis. The diagnosis has important personal and financial implications. The despair resulting may be compounded by the impoverished, underresourced environments in which patients die from tuberculosis, where the above mentioned suggestions made for symptom management of the dying patient are unavailable and/or unaffordable.

These factors, and the public health issue of ensuring that families and contacts are treated and monitored, emphasizes the inextricable interconnection between public health medicine and palliative care in the management of tuberculosis in developing countries.

Key learning points

- Malaria, rabies, and tuberculosis are treatable or preventable diseases that together result in millions of deaths with uncontrolled symptoms in the developing world.

- When it is clear that no disease-orientated treatment is available or no longer possible, palliation of symptoms is paramount. This must not be seen as an excuse to reduce attempts to aggressively treat tuberculosis and malaria if at all possible.

- Patients dying of these diseases are often young and in their most productive years. The families' despair and grief needs emotional and social support.

- Public health and palliative care are inextricably linked in the management of these patients, their families, and communities.

REFERENCES

1   Krogstad DJ. Plasmodium species (malaria). In: Mandell GL, Bennett JE, Dolin R, eds. *Mandell, Douglas and Bennett's Principles and Practice of Infectious Disease*, 5th ed. New York: Churchill Livingstone, 2000: 2817–31.

● ✱ 2   Villegas MV, Teano R, Zuluaga T, Wenk R. Malaria. In: Bruera E, De Lima L, Wenk R, Farr W, eds. *Palliative Care in the Developing World: Principles and Practice*. Houston: IAHPC Press, 2004: 207–14.

◆ 3   World Health Organization. *Management of Severe Malaria. A Practical Handbook*, 2nd ed. Geneva: WHO, 2000. Available at: http://mosquito.who.int/docs/hbsm_toc.htm (accessed October 13, 2005).

4   Bleck TP, Ruprecht CE. Rabies virus. In: Mandell GL, Bennett JE, Dolin R, eds. *Mandell, Douglas and Bennett's Principles and Practice of Infectious Disease*, 5th ed. New York: Churchill Livingstone, 2000: 1811–20.

● ✱ 5   Marsden SC. Rabies. In: Bruera E, De Lima L, Wenk R, Farr W, eds. *Palliative Care in the Developing World: Principles and Practice*. Houston: IAHPC Press, 2004: 217–26.

6   World Health Organization. Media Centre Fact Sheet No 99. Rabies September 2005. www.who.int/mediacentre/factsheets/fs099/en (accessed October 22, 2005).

7   Hass DW. Mycobacterium tuberculosis. In: Mandell GL, Bennett JE, Dolin R, eds. *Mandell, Douglas and Bennett's Principles and Practice of Infectious Disease*, 5th ed. New York: Churchill Livingstone, 2000: 2576–615.

● * 8   Clemens E. Tuberculosis. In: Bruera E, De Lima L, Wenk R, Farr W, eds. *Palliative Care in the Developing World: Principles and Practice*. Houston: IAHPC Press, 2004: 187–205.

9   World Health Organization. Roll Back Malaria Information sheet. Geneva: WHO www.rbm.who.int/cmc_upload/0/000/015/372.RBMInfosheet_1.htm (accessed October 22, 2005).

◆ 10 Phillips RS. Current status of malaria and potential for control. *Clin Microbiol Rev* 2001; **14**: 208–26.

11 Kibukamusoke JW, Hutt MSR, Wilks NE. The nephrotic syndrome in Uganda and its association with quartan malaria. *Q J Med* 1967; **36**: 393–408.

12 Miller LH, Good MF, Milon G. Malaria pathogenesis. *Science* 1994; **264**: 1878–83.

13 Aikawa M, Iseki M, Barnwell JW, *et al.* The pathology of human cerebral malaria. *Am J Trop Med Hyg* 1990; **43**: 30–7.

14 Aikawa M, Rabbege JR, Udeinya IJ, *et al.* Electron microscopy of knobs in Plasmodium falciparum-infected erythrocytes. *J Parasitol* 1983; **69**: 435–7.

15 Riganti M, Pongponiratn E, Tegoshi T, *et al.* Human cerebral malaria in Thailand: a clinicopathological correlation. *Immunol Lett* 1990; **25**: 199–205.

16 Turner G. Cerebral malaria. *Brain Pathol* 1997; 7: 569–82.

17 Warrell DA, Molyneux ME, Beales PF, eds. *Severe and Complicated Malaria. Trans R Soc Trop Med Hyg* 1990; **84**: 1–65.

18 Grau GE, Tafor TE, Molyneux ME, *et al.* Tumour necrosis factor and disease severity in children with falciparum malaria. *N Engl J Med* 1989; **320**: 1586–91.

19 Kwiatkowski D, Hill AV, Sambou I, *et al.* TNF concentration in fatal cerebral, non-fatal cerebral, and uncomplicated *Plasmodium falciparum* malaria. *Lancet* 1990; **336**: 1201–4.

20 Barnwell JW. Cyto-adherence and sequestration in falci-parum malaria. *Exp Parasitol* 1989; **69**: 407–12.

21 Friedman JM. Erythrocytic mechanism of sickle cell resistance to malaria. *Proc Natl Acad Sci USA* 1978; **75**: 1994–7.

22 Warrell DA. Clinical features of malaria. In: Gilles HM, Warrell DA, eds. *Bruce-Chwatt's Essential Malariology*, 3rd ed. London: Arnold, 1993: 35–49.

23 Jaffar S, Boele van Hensbroek M, Palmer A, *et al.* Predictors of fatal outcome following cerebral malaria. *Am J Trop Med Hyg* 1997; **57**: 20–4.

◆ 24 World Health Organization. Communicable disease cluster. Severe Falciparum malaria: prognostic indices in adults. *Trans R Soc Trop Med Hyg* 2000; **94**: 11–18.

◆ 25 White NJ. The treatment of malaria. *N Engl J Med* 1996; **335**: 800–6.

26 Warrell DA, Looaseesuwan S, Warrell MJ, *et al.* Dexamethasone proves deleterious in cerebral malaria: A double blind clinical trial in 100 comatose patients. *N Engl J Med* 1982; **306**: 313–18.

27 Tsai YL, Kregstad DJ. The resurgence of malaria. In: Scheld WM, Craig WA, Hughes JM, eds. *Emerging Infections 2*. Washington DC: American Society for Microbiology, 1998: 195–212.

28 White NI, Warrell DA. The management of severe malaria. In: Wernsdorfer WH, McGregor IA, eds. *Principles and Practice of Malariology, Volume 1*. London: Churchill Livingstone, 1988: 865–88.

◆ 29 Jackson AC, Warrell MJ, Rupprecht CE, *et al.* Rabies in humans. *Clin Infect Dis* 2003; **36**: 60–3.

30 World Health Organization. *WHO Expert Consultation on Rabies (2004: Geneva, Switzerland)*. Technical Report Series 931. Geneva: World Health Organization, 2005. www.who.int/rabies/931/en/print.html via www.who.int/csr/en/ (accessed October 22, 2005).

31 Republic of Philippines, Department of Health. *Guidelines on Rabies Prevention and Control*. Manila: Department of Health, 2002: 1–17.

◆ 32 World Health Organization. Recommendations on Rabies Post-Exposure Treatment and the Correct Techniques of Intradermal Immunization against Rabies. WHO/EMC/ZOO/96.6 whqlibdoc.who.int/hq/1996/WHO EMC ZOO 96.6.pdf via www.who.int/csr/en/ (accessed October 22, 2005).

33 Dizon MOM, Belandres Jr DC, Marsden SC, *et al.* Palliative care in rabies. In: Abstracts, Posters, 14th International Congress on Care of the Terminally Ill. *J Palliat Care* 2002; **18**: 229.

34 Marsden SC. Palliative care in rabies in Manila. Poster, abstract. In: *5th Asia Pacific Hospice Conference Program and Abstracts*. Osaka: Conference Organizing Committee, 2003: 207.

35 Farmer PE. *Infections and Inequalities. The Modern Plagues*, 2nd ed. Berkeley: University of California Press, 2001.

36 Farmer PE. *Pathologies of Power: Health, Human Rights, and the New War on the Poor*. Berkeley: University of California Press, 2002.

37 Davies PDO, Ormerod P, eds. *Case Presentations in Clinical Tuberculosis*. London: Arnold, 1999.

38 Farmer PE. Hidden epidemics of tuberculosis. In: *Infectious Disease and Social Inequalities: From Hemispheric Insecurity to Global Cooperation*. A Working Paper of the Latin American Program of the Woodrow Wilson International Center for Scholars. Washington DC: Wilson Center, 1999: 31–55.

39 World Health Organization. *Tuberculosis. Drug-and Multidrug-resistant Tuberculosis*. Geneva: WHO. www.who.int/tb/dots/dotsplus/en/ via www.who.int/tb/en (accessed October 22, 2005).

40 Farmer PE, Kim J, Mitnick C, Timperi R. Responding to outbreaks of multidrug-resistant tuberculosis: introducing 'DOTS-Plus'. In: Reichman LB, Hershfield ES, eds. *Tuberculosis: A Comprehensive International Approach*, 2nd ed. New York: Marcell Dekker, 1999: 447–69.

41 Farmer PE, Shin SS, Bayona J, *et al.* Making DOTS-Plus work. In: Bastain I, Portaels F, eds. *Multidrug Resistant Tuberculosis*. Dordrecht, Netherlands: Kluwer Academic Publishers, 2000: 285–306.

42 Shin SS, Bayona J, Farmer PE. DOTS and DOTS-Plus: Not the only answer. In: Davies PDO, ed. *Clinical Tuberculosis*, 3rd ed. London: Arnold, 2003: 211–23.

43 Becerra MC, Freeman J, Bayona J, *et al.* Using treatment failure under effective direct observed short-course chemotherapy programs to identify patients with multi-drug-resistant tuberculosis. *Int J Tuberc Lung Dis* 2000; **4**: 108–14.

44 Farmer PE, Bayone J, Becerra M, *et al.* The dilemma of MDR-TB in the global era. *Int J Tuberc Lung Dis* 1998; **2**: 869–76.

45 Farmer, PE, Furin JJ, Bayona J, *et al.* Management of MDR-TB in resource-poor countries. *Int J Tuberc Lung Dis* 1999; **3**: 643–5.

46 Farmer PE, Furn JJ, Shin SS. Managing multidrug-resistant tuberculosis. *J Respir Dis* 2000; **21**: 53–6.

47 Farmer PE, Kim JY. Community-based approaches to the control of multidrug-resistant tuberculosis. Introducing 'DOTS-plus'. *BMJ* 1998; **317**: 671–4.

48 Garrett L. *The Coming Plague: Newly Emerging Diseases in a World out of Balance.* New York: Farrar, Strauss and Giroux, 1994.

49 Murray C, Styblo, Rouillon A. Tuberculosis. In: Jamison DT, Mosley WH, Measham AR, Bodadella JL, eds. *Disease Control Priorities in Developing Countries.* Oxford: Oxford University Press, 1993: 233–59.

50 Clemens JD, Chung JH, Feinstein AR. The BCG controversy. A methodological and statistical reappraisal. *JAMA* 1989; **249**: 2362–9.

51 Fine PEM. The BCG story; lessons from the past and implications for the future. *Rev Infect Dis* 1989; **11**: 353–9.

52 Driver LC, Bruera E, eds. *The M.D. Anderson Symptom Control and Palliative Care Handbook*, 2nd ed. Houston: The University of Texas MD Anderson Cancer Center, 2002.

101

Practical aspects of palliative care delivery in the developing world

ROBERTO WENK, LILIANA DE LIMA

INTRODUCTION

The *World Health Report*, published by the World Health Organization (WHO), indicates that almost 57 million deaths occurred worldwide in 2001. The vast majority of these deaths occurred in developing countries, where over three-fourths of the people in the world live. Infectious diseases such as human immunodeficiency virus (HIV) infection, malaria, tuberculosis, and respiratory infections caused over half of the cumulative deaths in developing countries.[1]

With the exception of the USA, developed countries registered a decline or no change in population during the last decade, and 99 percent of population growth took place in the developing countries. If this trend continues, by 2050, industrialized nations will record a population increase of only 4 percent, whereas the population in developing countries will expand by 55 percent. For example, countries in western Asia are expected to gain about 186 million people by 2050.[1] Overall, the world population will reach approximately 9 billion by mid century. Developing countries will face the burden of this population growth, which will result in greater demand for healthcare services. With limited funding, inadequate infrastructure, and limited access to preventive and curative measures, more individuals will require palliative care services.

The developing world varies greatly from country to country and region to region. A limited number of excellent facilities are available in developing countries, with the latest technology and medications and capable of delivering care similar to that of the developed countries, but the majority of the population does not have access to these institutions and are cared for in facilities with limited resources.

Healthcare initiatives in the developing world must deal with poverty, inadequate infrastructure, poor administrative systems, limited access to medications, bureaucratic and inefficient processes related to the production, importation and distribution of medications, restrictive laws and regulations related to the prescribing of opioids, insufficient support from national health authorities, low level of political will to establish palliative care programs,[2–4] and limited education for healthcare providers.[5] An additional barrier to the implementation of palliative care programs in developing countries is that the majority of healthcare spending, both public and private, goes toward curative efforts.

Patients in resource-poor settings pose challenges which need to be taken into account when developing palliative care programs and strategies. Many palliative care initiatives in these countries have developed as islands of excellence but they are not well integrated into the national health systems and have limited impact. Palliative care is still not included in the mainstream of care and tends to be delegated to a secondary role. This has resulted in the development and implementation of different models of care. Care is provided by local programs and teams with structural and operational differences shaped by the needs and limitations of each setting rather than by following a set of consistent guidelines. Programs are adapted to their environment and most survive using resources in unique ways.[6] Sadly, there is evidence that the quality of care during the dying process is poor and that many patients suffer unnecessary pain and symptoms.[7]

To adapt to these limitations and the needs of the population, it is imperative that palliative care workers adopt practical measures to provide cost-effective and efficient care to the patients. These include strategies to build and improve capacity, adopting low-cost treatment measures, developing data management procedures to establish mechanisms for quality control, and identifying sources of funding to cover the costs of the palliative care services. This chapter describes these strategies and provides some examples of settings where they have been successful in improving the delivery of palliative care.

CAPACITY-BUILDING STRATEGIES

Capacity strengthening is crucial for effective palliative care programs with the ability to reach the majority of the population in need. Many initiatives have been successful largely as a result of the capacity-building strategies adopted by program leaders, which have positively influenced the willingness of policy makers to incorporate palliative care in the healthcare agendas. Some of the programs implemented in developed countries that have shown significant results may be applicable to and adapted by developing countries. Initiatives such as the Programa de Cuidados Paliativos del Servicio Extremeño de Salud in Spain, have been successful by adopting a basic structure that relies on full regional coverage through mobile teams consisting of a doctor, a nurse, and a psychologist, who visit patients either at home or in any of the public hospitals of the region. The program requires centralized coordination as a way to monitor progress and activities and to measure outcomes.[8]

As a result of these capacity-building strategies, several important governmental as well as nongovernmental palliative care initiatives have emerged in recent years in developing countries. But even with these improvements, there are still enormous gaps to be bridged to bring palliative care to those in need of it.

Community health approach in home care

Given the extent of the problem in developing countries where healthcare resources are severely limited, a community health approach that relies extensively on home-based care and community involvement in the provision of care and support is the most cost-effective approach. The community health approach requires development of teams and networking with actions and tasks carried out by community members; a high level of population coverage; and periodic evaluations to improve the quality and performance of programs providing palliative care in patients' homes. In some countries, for diseases such as HIV/acquired immune deficiency syndrome (AIDS) and cancer these palliative care activities are integrated with the ongoing activities of other healthcare providers.

In Kerala, India, neighborhood network palliative care programs have shown exceptionally good success rates.

More than 50 percent coverage for all severely ill patients seems to have been achieved within 2 years of initiation of the project and the district where it was first launched now has an estimated coverage of more than 70 percent. Involving the local community in all stages, from planning to monitoring, has ensured sustainability of the project. Neighborhood groups find the resources to deliver care locally: 80 percent of the funds for programs are raised locally. The groups' advocacy role also results in generating support from local government.[9]

In Africa, several model programs are demonstrating the beneficial integration of hospice-, community-, and home-based care for people with cancer and HIV/AIDS.[10,11] For example, the South Coast Hospice in KwaZulu-Natal, South Africa, developed an integrated care program in which patients with HIV/AIDS are referred to teams of nurses and trained community caregivers who care for them in their own homes.[12] The program has halved average patient stays at the local hospital, and extended care provided at home costs less than a 2-day stay in the hospital.[13] Hospice Uganda has been successful in implementing a hospice model which has become part of Uganda's national healthcare policy. Hospice Uganda has been particularly successful in improving access to morphine by establishing a cost-effective distribution system of inexpensive morphine sulfate preparations.[14]

Volunteers

In settings where human resources are limited, the use of volunteers for home-based care programs has proved to be useful and practical. Volunteers play an essential role in palliative care, and more so in developing countries where limited funds hinder the capacity to hire human resources for end-of-life care.[15,16] Patients in developing countries who are diagnosed with terminal diseases are usually sent home to die with little or no treatment recommendations. By carrying out many of the tasks of the palliative care providers, volunteers from the community become an important and crucial source of support for such patients and their families and when available, to the palliative care team.[17] In this process family members are empowered to the highest possible degree to ensure continuity of treatment.

Volunteers in palliative care have proved to be efficient in two main areas: direct patient care (feeding, hygiene, administration of medication, patient evaluation, helping in domestic chores such as shopping for food, cleaning house, cooking, etc.) and providing administrative support to the program (administrative and secretarial tasks). Individuals who are interested in undertaking volunteer work in palliative care need to be carefully selected, trained, and taught about the chores and tasks that they will be helping with. Some of the practical aspects in volunteer programs which have proved to be effective in the

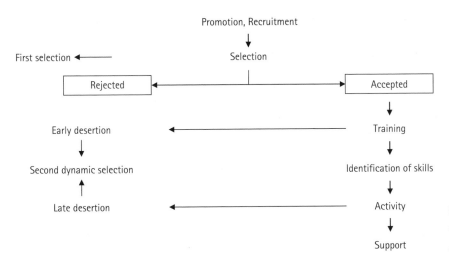

Figure 101.1 *Process to initiate and maintain a volunteer program in palliative care.*

Programa Argentino de Medicina Paliativa – Fundacion FEMEBA (PAMPFF) include:

- *Selection.* Careful selection guidelines are aimed to match the required personal skills[18,19] with the needs of the patient, the family, and the program.
- *Dropouts.* The program found that 10 percent of volunteers who fulfilled the selection criteria dropped out during the training. Fifteen percent of volunteers who completed the training dropped out after starting the work. A strategy was designed to solve this problem and early and late dropouts were significantly reduced after including a description of the volunteer tasks, and stories of other volunteers' experiences, and an initial interview with a psychologist before training.
- *Training:* A comprehensive training program for volunteers is a practical way to maximize their role and to prevent dropout. PAMPFF's training program is based on other successful initiatives, and includes bedside training and spending time with the palliative care team before being sent out into the community.[20] Figure 101.1 shows the steps to initiate and maintain a volunteer program in palliative care designed by the PAMPFF group.[21]

Volunteers need to feel that they have the support of the program, the patient, and the family. Much of the work done by volunteers is based on mutual trust, and in order for volunteers to feel comfortable in their role and perform their tasks they need to know that their work is crucial and needed.

Distant care

An additional barrier to the implementation of palliative care programs in developing countries is that a majority of healthcare spending, both public and private, goes toward curative efforts; hospitals in urban areas often account for more than 80 percent of total healthcare costs. However, the majority of the population in the developing world continues to live in rural areas.[22] This means that inexpensive and effective healthcare strategies need to be put in place to improve the access and delivery of care to the rural populations. One of these strategies is 'distant care'. In settings where the provision of care in distant areas is not possible, distant care programs, through a main care provider, have proved to be a useful and practical approach.

Most palliative care teams or units in developing countries are based in large and medium urban areas[23] and terminally ill patients living in small cities and rural areas need to travel long distances to receive palliative care. This becomes even more difficult when patients are frail and unable to travel for follow-up visits. Additional difficulties patients may face when having to travel to cities to see a doctor include not having access to a car, having to travel slowly and uncomfortably by bus, living in areas with no access to public transportation, or inability to afford the transportation fees.[24]

As in other regions of the world, some teams have solved this problem with the help of trained volunteers who do home visits, during which they perform basic care tasks and provide practical support to the main caregiver.[25] However, this is not always possible as not all volunteers are willing to travel to rural areas or have access to the required resources to perform such visits. To improve the care for such patient groups, some teams in developing countries have implemented the practical strategy of 'distant care', which is carried out through a main caregiver and without an initial clinical evaluation of the patient.[26]

The PAMPFF implements distant care as follows:

1 When a patient is unable to attend an initial doctor evaluation, a relative seeks help by contacting the palliative care group or care provider.
2 The relative is then informed about 'distant care' and its limitations, including the risks involved.
3 If acceptable to them, the relative is asked to identify the main caregiver in the family.
4 The main caregiver then provides information about the patient, his/her clinical situation using an assessment form which combines elements of the Edmonton Symptom Assessment Scale (ESAS)[27,28**] and the Memorial Symptom Assessment System (MSAS).[29**] Figure 101.2

shows the assessment form used by the PAMPFF which includes items from these scales, and has proved to be useful in the palliative care program.

5   Based on existing information about frequent syndromes in palliative care and using the information provided by the main caregiver, a presumptive diagnosis of the patient's condition is made.

6   If needed, medications are prescribed for pain and symptom control, following the WHO[30***] guidelines and other recommendations in the literature.

7   The main caregiver receives verbal and written instructions on the administration of medications, symptom evaluation, diet and hydration, hygiene and other important tasks.

8   The main caregiver is given a phone number that they can call to consult the team at any time and they are asked to report the patient's situation once a week.

9   Patients may be hospitalized in public institutions for severe or refractory symptoms or if the main caregiver is unable to continue providing the necessary care.

A pilot study measured the effectiveness of the distant care model[26*] and indicated that it is significantly correct and helpful. The data showed that the presumptive diagnosis was incorrect in 10 percent of the cases, and the majority of the main caregivers reported being very satisfied with the level of care provided.

Diagnosing and treating a patient without clinical assessment entails a risk but the benefits of providing comfort and relief of suffering greatly surpass this risk. Distant care fulfills both the medical responsibility of caring for people with the available resources and the therapeutic obligation of providing treatment with a favorable benefit/burden ratio.[31]

COST-EFFECTIVE TREATMENT STRATEGIES

The WHO and several professional and scientific organizations have promoted public health policies and made recommendation to national governments to implement pain relief and palliative care as components of cancer and AIDS care.[6,30***,32***,33] A large body of knowledge has emerged on the assessment and management of the physical and psychosocial problems that occur in patients who develop cancer and other progressive incurable illnesses. However, the overwhelming majority of the available written material refers to the delivery of palliative care using resources mostly available in developed countries which may not be available in developing countries or may not be applicable to the conditions and diseases that occur in the patient population. In addition, there are socioeconomic and cultural issues that pose particular challenges for the healthcare team. By motivating and empowering health care providers to develop their own treatment protocols and by enabling the implementation of appropriate knowledge in the field of palliative care, both the quality of life and the quality of death of terminally ill people can be improved significantly.[25]

Some treatment strategies and inexpensive technologies have been successfully adopted and implemented in the developing world. A few of these include:

- *Proctoclysis.* This is a simple and inexpensive alternative method of hydration, which may be helpful when resources are limited. A small nasogastric tube is inserted in the rectum for hydration, daily or every other day. It uses the colon's intrinsic ability to absorb normal saline or tap water. Assessments of comfort showed that this technique is well tolerated and that family members can successfully administer proctoclysis at home.[34*] This method may be especially helpful in situations in which technical difficulties make intravenous or subcutaneous infusion difficult or expensive. Such settings may include developing countries, a rural setting, or when nursing care is limited.

- *Edmonton injector.* The Edmonton injector is a simple, nondisposable, low-cost device, which was originally designed in Argentina. It permits patients to self-administer injections of opioids, metoclopramide, or other drugs intermittently into a subcutaneously inserted needle. A bag containing 50–100 mL of medication allows pharmacists to prepare the medication from powder at a minimal cost. A simple mechanical movement safely allows patients to inject medication. The device does not need batteries and requires little training for use by patients and families. The cost of this treatment is less than US$1.00 per day and the device is not patented, thus enabling groups in developing countries to manufacture their own devices.[35*] Unfortunately, in some countries this injector is not available or has not been approved by the local healthcare authorities, mostly due to its extremely low cost which makes it unattractive to manufacturers.

- *Methadone.* A synthetic opioid and N-methyl-D-aspartate (NMDA) antagonist, methadone is a potent analgesic for treating cancer pain. Its characteristics include excellent absorption, high lipid solubility, high potency, long half-life, lack of known metabolites, decreased opioid cross-tolerance, and low cost which makes it suitable for developing countries.[36***,37**]

- *Thalidomide.* This drug has been available for approximately 50 years but its beneficial effect in large research studies has not been established. In some pilot studies it has been found to be effective in reducing anorexia, chronic nausea, fatigue, and insomnia in patients with advanced cancer.[38*] It has also been found to have analgesic effects in patients with neuropathic pain related to leprosy reactions and aphthous ulcers related to HIV. The drug is not patent protected and therefore it could be readily available at a minimal cost to developing countries. Unfortunately, there has been no major research on this agent and further studies need to be conducted to determine the potential beneficial uses in cachexia, fatigue, and other symptoms related to advanced cancer.

AVAILABILITY AND ACCESS TO OPIOID ANALGESICS

Pain relief is the cornerstone of palliative care and adequate access to and availability of opioid analgesics to all patients in need are crucial.[39,40] Many countries have reported an improvement in the availability of different weak and strong opioid analgesics but the high prices relative to the monthly salary constitutes a barrier to access.[41*] A recent study among developing and developed nations demonstrated that the median cost of opioid medication was twice as high in developing countries as it is in developed countries. In US dollars, a 30-day prescription was US$112 in developing countries compared with US $53 in developed countries. Cost as percent of gross national product (GNP) per capita per month was 10-fold higher in developing countries where patients have to spend more than a third of their salary to cover pain therapy. Median cost was 31 percent of GNP per capita per month in the developing countries compared with 3 percent of GNP per capita per month in the developed countries. Half of opioid preparations cost more than 33 percent of monthly GNP per capita in developing countries compared with only 4 percent in developed countries. And there are fewer programs to offset medication costs in developing countries. Only one of the five developing nations (20 percent) in the study had a subsidization program or socialized medicine compared with four of seven (57 percent) of the developed nations.[42*] Probable reasons for the high prices are relative small markets, red tape, bureaucratic procedures, and tax burdens. Thus, large overheads are needed to cover the costs of production, distribution, and sales. Government-imposed caps on the prices of opioids is not a good solution as this could risk the availability of medications, especially in countries with small markets where the operating costs for the pharmaceutical industry are not compensated for the limited sales. In some countries the only solution is for the healthcare system to subsidize the opioid analgesics.

Unfortunately the problem of accessibility does not seem to be a priority for international institutions working to improve pain relief. It is crucial that these organizations initiate claims and requests to governments, the pharmaceutical industry, and healthcare providers, to help address and solve this problem. Several hospice and palliative care programs have adopted cost-effective strategies to produce and distribute inexpensive morphine. These include establishing links with local pharmaceutical companies willing to produce the opioid as immediate-release tablets and compound preparations (made by a pharmacist according to the national pharmacopoeia as per a patient's needs), or generic preparations of the following:

- For oral use: aqueous solutions of morphine (6 mg/mL), oxycodone (3 mg/mL) or methadone (10 mg/mL).
- For subcutaneous use: micropore cold sterilized aqueous solutions of morphine or oxycodone (10 mg/mL) The same can be done with dexamethasone, metoclopramide, hyoscine, haloperidol.

INFORMATION DISSEMINATION AND DATA MANAGEMENT

Data collection and analysis are critical in palliative care for understanding the current levels of quality and ways to measure improvement in care. Also, information facilitates the caring process, especially when several disciplines and different services participate.[43***] Unfortunately, only limited information regarding end-of-life care is available in developing countries, and to our knowledge, no national government systematically collects information on quality end-of-life care of its patients.

In countries with financial limitations it is difficult to secure the support of professional data managers to develop and maintain a system designed to meet the needs of the program. This can lead to the quite opposite situations of either collecting large amounts of useless data or nothing at all. To establish a cost-effective program, it is important to identify the crucial information that needs to be collected and then develop a data management system based on the needs and existing resources.[44,45] Several palliative care programs have adopted data collection systems with successful results.[46] One such initiative was developed by the PAMPFF which includes data collection forms and a database based on the Minimum Data Set from the National Council for Palliative Care in the UK.[47] The information is collected in two categories:

- *General information.* This includes basic demographic indicators, religious affiliation, health insurance, main caregiver information, diagnosis, prescribed medications and treatments, addictions, other diseases, other medications currently in use, anatomical diagram for registration of pain and the Edmonton Labeled Visual Information System (ELVIS).[48**]
- *Process of care.* This includes information on sources of referral, evolution and prognosis of clinical disorders including assessments using tools such as ESAS,[28**] Edmonton Comfort Assessment Form (ECAF), Confusion Assessment Method (CAM)[49*] or Mini-Mental State Examination (MMSE),[50*] and other conditions such as hydration, bowel movements, hospitalization between consultations, opioid routes and doses, adjuvant drugs, diagnostic and therapeutic practices.

The database was created using the Microsoft Access 2000® software, which has proved to be flexible, safe, and comprehensive. The information is retrieved easily and can be exported to other software applications. Figure 101.2 shows the basic form which has been used in the PAMPFF and may be used for data collection. The form can be completed by volunteers or professionals, and the information may be provided by the patient or the main caregiver. Figure 101.3 shows the steps followed to load data and retrieve information.

Date ___/___/___ Patient .... ID #..............................

☐ Patient consultation
☐ Main caregiver consultation
☐ Patient ☎ consultation
☐ Main caregiver ☎ consultation
☐ Team ☎ call

☐ Outpatient
☐ Inpatient
☐ Patient in Hospital

Admissions within consultations
☐ NO ☐ YES ___ times, __ days

ECOG
☐ Zero
☐ One
☐ Two
☐ Three
☐ Four

PAIN			
APPETITE			
NAUSEA/VOMITING			
SHORTNESS OF BREATH			
FATIGUE			
DROWSINESS			
DIFFICULTY SLEEPING			
ANGUISH			
SADNESS			

☐ NO ☐ YES ☐ ?	Delirium	☐ NO ☐ YES ☐ ?	Skin lesions/pruritus	A n a l g e s i c s
☐ NO ☐ YES ☐ ?	Limb swelling	☐ NO ☐ YES ☐ ?	Problems with urination	
☐ NO ☐ YES ☐ ?	Dry/painful mouth	☐ NO ☐ YES ☐ ?	Cough	
☐ NO ☐ YES ☐ ?	Difficulty swallowing	☐ NO ☐ YES ☐ ?	Fever	
☐ NO ☐ YES ☐ ?	Diarrhea	☐ NO ☐ YES ☐ ?	Bleeding	
OTHER				
Days without bowel movement ? 0 1 2 3 4 5 6 7 8 9 10				

....

Adjuvants ....
Psychoactive drugs...
Interventions/prescriptions ....
To be reviewed ....

Figure 101.2 *The PAMPFF assessment form. Note: a body diagram is on the back of the form. The four categories for symptom intensity are in Spanish.*

FUNDING STRATEGIES

With a few exceptions, palliative care in developing countries is neither recognized as a discipline nor is it incorporated within health systems. As a result there is no budgetary allocation through public funds[51] and palliative care programs are unable to receive reimbursement for services rendered through health insurance programs. Palliative care workers in developing countries are forced to work *pro bono* or in other areas and dedicate the remaining hours to palliative care. Programs are forced to look for funding through private pay, donations, and charity from the community in order to cover the cost of operations and the provision of services. Long-term financing of palliative care is a big challenge and the mechanisms to finance and sustain the services vary depending on the structure of the team or program.

Thus, palliative care programs in developing countries usually develop with community support; are based in donated houses, churches or community institutions; provide

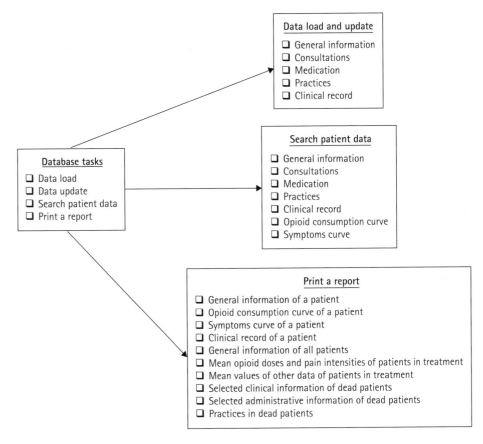

Figure 101.3 *Database working scheme.*

services through volunteer work; and raise funds for non-volunteer professional fees, medication, and supplies from local charity, religious orders, neighborhood groups, donations, and sometimes from contracts with local purchasers. These funding mechanisms have proved to be effective in sustaining palliative care services in small towns and where there is a relatively small population base.[52] As patients share similar needs, and the amount of resources needed to run the services is small, it can be offered by locals who establish partnerships with other individuals and institutions which have the capacity to raise and/or provide money. Hospital-based programs delivering care through multidisciplinary teams face tougher challenges to fund their activities. They are more complex, require a larger infrastructure, and more staff members.

Some countries have adopted funding mechanisms which combine efforts from the program and the institution. This joint funding collaboration has worked well in the PAMPFF and it has provided additional benefits to the program, such as full responsibility over budgetary allocation and the identification of funding sources outside the healthcare system. Both strategies have proved to be practical and safeguard the programs from the pressures and limitations of the healthcare system. Palliative care programs and initiatives in developing countries need to identify sources and activities capable of generating funds to support the operational

costs of the program. PAMPFF had implemented teaching and educational activities, which require registration fees and generate additional revenue. These have proved to be a substantial source of funding for the program.

Many other alternatives exist and programs in each country need to evaluate the resources in the community and their needs to develop and implement successful resource-generating strategies. Long-term survival depends on the ability to confront critical economic and human resource situations which interfere with the smooth development of the activity. Economic autonomy requires dedication and labor, but guarantees sustainability.

CONCLUSION

Developing countries face two socioeconomic challenges that may delay the development of palliative care initiatives. First, the need to constantly adapt to legal, political, economic, and social changes reduces the demand for modifications in the healthcare system.[40*] Second, most of the economic growth registered by developing nations is still not enough to satisfy the social needs of the population. These factors pose financial, organizational, and educational barriers to the development of palliative care. However, the drive to reduce these barriers and generate feasible programs will result in the development of practical strategies such as the ones described in this chapter. The provision of palliative care is far from homogeneous and many developing nations have designed and implemented effective and successful strategies which have proved to help patients and families live a better quality of life until the end.

Many of these strategies are not acceptable under the standards of care in developed nations, but a flexible approach is needed to be able to help those in need. Home-based care may be the only feasible option for adequate access to palliative care in areas with limited resources. Effective palliative care for patients and families should rely on the development of home-based palliative care integrated within the existing healthcare system. Countries should plan to bridge the current gaps by building on their existing strengths and optimizing available resources. Low-cost and high-coverage approaches and national policies to promote accessibility and drug availability are key components. An understanding of the palliative care needs of a community will help establish broad support from the local people and the health authorities in each country. The support that palliative care workers in developed nations may provide to their colleagues in developing countries includes the empowerment to generate their own models of care, strengthen their capacity to reach patients and provide care, development of inexpensive medications, and design and application of research to evaluate the effectiveness of their treatment protocols.

Key learning points

- During the last decade 99 percent of population growth took place in developing countries. If this trend continues, by 2050 the population in developing countries will expand by 55 percent. This will result in greater demand for healthcare services. With limited funding, inadequate infrastructure and limited access to preventive and curative measures, more individuals will require palliative care services.

- Developing countries face several limitations which challenge the development of palliative care. To adapt to these limitations and the needs of the population, it is imperative that palliative care workers adopt practical measures to provide cost effective and efficient palliative care to the patients. These include strategies to build and improve capacity, low-cost treatment measures, data management procedures to establish mechanisms for quality control, and identifying sources of funding to cover the costs of the palliative care services.

- Volunteers play an essential role in palliative care, and more so in developing countries where limited funding hinders the capacity to hire human resource for end-of-life care. By carrying out many of the tasks of the palliative care providers, volunteers from the community become an important and crucial source of support for the patient and the family, and when available, to the palliative care team. In this process family members are empowered to their highest degree possible to ensure continuity of treatment.

- In some developing countries where it is not possible to treat patients in distant rural areas, some teams have implemented a practical strategy called 'distant care' which is carried out through a main caregiver and without initial clinical evaluation of the patient. Data show that the distant care model is significantly accurate and helpful, and the majority of the main caregivers have reported being very satisfied with the level of care provided.

- The overwhelming majority of published material refers to the delivery of palliative care using resources mostly available in developed countries which may not be available in developing countries or may not be applicable to the conditions and diseases that occur in that patient population. There are alternative treatment strategies and inexpensive technologies that have been successfully adopted and implemented in the developing world, such as proctoclysis, Edmonton injector, methadone, and thalidomide.

- Many countries report an improvement in the availability of different weak and strong opioid analgesics but their high prices relative to the monthly salaries constitute a barrier to access. The problem of limited access to opioids needs to be addressed by international organizations working to improve pain relief. In the mean time, the provision of opioids needs to be subsidized by governments or through preparation of low-cost opioids.

- Data collection and analysis are critical in palliative care to understand the current levels of quality and ways to measure improvement in care. The amount of information available in developing countries in end-of-life care is limited and to the authors' knowledge none of the national governments systematically collect information on quality end-of-life care of their palliative population.

- With a few exceptions, palliative care in developing countries is neither recognized as a discipline nor is it incorporated within the health system. This results in no budgetary allocation through public funds and the inability to receive reimbursement for services rendered through health insurance programs. Palliative care workers in developing countries are forced to work *pro bono* or in other areas and dedicate the remaining hours to palliative care. Programs are forced to look for funding through private pay, donations, and charity from the community to cover the cost of operations and the provision of services.

- Palliative care programs and initiatives in developing countries need to identify sources and activities capable of generating funds to support the operational costs of the program. Long-term survival is dependent on the ability to confront critical economic and human resource situations which interfere with the smooth development of the activity. Economic autonomy requires dedication and labor but guarantees sustainability.

REFERENCES

1 World Health Organization. *The World Health Report 2002: Reducing Risks, Promoting Healthy Life.* Geneva: WHO, 2002.

2 De Lima L, Hamzah E. Socioeconomic, cultural and political issues in palliative care. In: Bruera E, De Lima L, Wenk R, Farr W, eds. *Palliative Care in the Developing World: Principles and Practice.* Houston: IAHPC Press, 2004.

3 Rajagopal MR, Mazza D, Lipman AG, eds. *Pain and Palliative Care in the Developing World and Marginalized Populations: A Global Challenge.* Binghampton, NY: Haworth Press, 2003.

4 World Health Organization. *Cancer Control Program: Policies and Managerial Guidelines.* Geneva: WHO, 2002.

5 Heber D. New themes in palliative care: book review. *Soc Sci Med* 1993; **48**: 1301–3.

6 Bruera E. Palliative care programs in Latin America. *Palliat Med* 1992; **6**: 182–4.

7 Field D, James N. Where and how people die. In: Clark D, ed. *The Future for Palliative Care: Issues of Policy and Practice.* Philadelphia: Open University Press, 1996.

8 Servicio Extremeño de Salud. *Programa Marco de Cuidados Paliativos.* Junta de Extremadura, Consejeria de Sanidad y Consumo: Mérida, España, 2004.

9 Kumar S. Palliative care can be delivered through neighbourhood networks. *BMJ* 2004; **329**: 1184.

10 Hardman M. Models of community-based HIV care. *S Afr J HIV Med* 2001; **4**: 12–13.

11 World Health Organization – Programme on Cancer Control and Department of HIV/AIDS. *A Community Health Approach to Palliative Care for HIV/AIDS and Cancer Patients in Africa.* Geneva: WHO, 2004.

12 Campbell L. Audit of referral of AIDS patients from hospital to an integrated community-based home care programme in Kwazulu-Natal, South Africa. *S Afr J HIV Med* 2001: 9–11.

13 Diana Fund. *Palliative Care Initiative.* The Diana, Princess of Wales, Memorial Fund Promotional Information, 2001.

14 Merriman A. Uganda: current status of palliative care. *J Pain Symptom Manage* 2002; **24**: 252–6.

15 Claxton-Oldfield S, Jefferies J, Fawcet C, *et al.* Palliative care volunteers: why do they do it? *J Palliat Care* 2004; **20**: 78–84.

16 Seibold D, Rossi S, Berteotti C, Soprych S, McQuillan L. Volunteer involvement in a hospice care program. *Am J Hosp Care* 1987; **4**: 43–55.

17 Patchner M, Finn M. Volunteers: the life-line of hospice. *Omega* 1987; **18**: 135.

18 Lamb D, de St. Aubin T, Foster M. Characteristics of most effective and least effective hospice volunteers. *Am J Hosp Care* 1985; **2**: 42–5.

19 Black B, Kovacs P. Direct care and indirect care hospice volunteers: motivations, acceptance, satisfaction, and length of service. *Journal of Volunteers Administration* 1996; **14**: 21–32.

20 National Hospice Organization; Bates IJ, Brand KE, eds. *Volunteer Training Curriculum.* Arlington: NHO, 1990.

21 Jaime E, Wenk R. Diseño y Aplicación de un Programa de Voluntariado en Cuidados Paliativos. In: Bruera E, De Lima L, eds. *Cuidados Paliativos: Guias para el Manejo Clinico,* 2nd ed. International Association for Hospice and Palliative Care y Organización Panamericana de la Salud. Washington: OPS, 2004.

22 World Health Organization. *Cities and the Population issue.* 44th World Health Assembly, Technical Discussion 7, background document, Geneva 1991.

23 Torres I. Determinants of quality of advanced cancer care in Latin America: a look at five countries [doctoral dissertation]. Houston: University of Texas, School of Public Health, 2004.

24 Stajduhar K, Davies B. Death at home: Challenges for families and directions for the future. *J Palliat Care* 1998; **14**: 8–14.

25 Wenk R. Developing countries WHO Cancer Pain Relief Program: a patient care model. *J Pain Symptom Manage* 1991; **3**: 40–3.

26 Wenk R, Monti C, Bertolino M. Asistencia a distancia: mejor o peor que nada? *Medicina Paliativa* 2003; **10**: 136–41.

27 Guidelines for using the Edmonton Symptom Assessment System (ESAS). Available at www.palliative.org/PC/ClinicalInfo/ AssessmentTools/esas.pdf (accessed August 28, 2005).

28 Bruera E, MacDonald S. Audit methods: The Edmonton System Assessment Scale. In: Higginson I, ed. *Clinical Audit in Palliative Care.* Oxford: Radcliffe Medical Press, 1993.

29 Lobchuk ML. The Memorial Symptom Assessment Scale: modified for use in understanding family caregivers of cancer patient's symptom experiences. *J Pain Symptom Manage* 2003; **26**: 644–54.

30 World Health Organization – technical report series 804. *Cancer Pain Relief and Palliative Care.* Geneva: WHO, 1990.

31 Randall F, Downie RS. *Palliative Care Ethics: A Companion for all Specialties.* Oxford: Oxford University Press, 1999.

32 World Health Organization/UNAIDS. *Key Elements in HIV/AIDS Care and Support.* Geneva: UNAIDS, 2000.

33 Institute of Medicine National Research Council. *Improving Palliative Care for Cancer.* Foley K, Gelband H, eds. Washington: National Academy Press, 2001.

34 Bruera A, Pruvost M, Schoeller T, *et al.* Proctoclysis for hydration of terminally ill cancer patients. *J Pain Symptom Manage* 1998; **15**: 4.

35 Pruvost M, De la Colina OE, Monasterolo NA. Edmonton Injector: Use in Cordoba, Argentina. *J Pain Symptom Manage* 1996; **12**: 6.

36 Davis MP, Walsh D. Methadone for relief of cancer pain: a review of pharmacokinectics, pharmacodynamics, drug interactions and protocols of administration. *Support Care Cancer* 2001; **9**: 2.

37 Bruera E, Palmer JL, Bosnjak S, *et al.* Methadone versus morphine as a first line strong opioid for cancer pain: a randomized, double blind study. *J Clin Oncol* 2004; **22**: 1.

38 Bruera E, Neumann CM, Pituskin E, *et al.* Thalidomide in patients with cachexia due to terminal cancer: Preliminary report. *Ann Oncol* 1999; **10**: 1.

✱ 39   World Health Organization. *Achieving Balance in National Opioids Control Policy: Guidelines for Assessment.* Geneva: WHO, 2000.

◆ 40   Joranson DE. Improving availability of opioid pain medications: Testing the principle of balance in Latin America. Innovations in End-of-Life Care. 2003; 5. Available at: www.edc.org/lastacts (accessed August 28, 2005).

● 41   Wenk R, Bertolino M, Pussetto J. High costs of opioids in developing countries: an availability barrier that can be overcome. *J Pain Symptom Manage* 2000; **20**: 81–2.

● 42   De Lima L, Sweeney C, Palmer JL, Bruera E. Potent analgesics are more expensive for patients in developing countries: a comparative study. *J Pain Palliat Care Pharmacother* 2004; **18**: 1.

◆ 43   Radbruch L, Sabatowski R, Loick G, et al. MIDOS–Validierung eines minimalen Dokumentationssystems für die Palliativmedizin. *Der Schmerz* 2000; **14**: 231–9.

44   Standing Senate Committee on Social Affairs and Technology: Recommendation II. In: Quality end of life care: The right of every Canadian: Final report of the Subcommittee to update Of Life and Death. Ottawa: Senate of Canada, 2000.

✱ 45   Wenk R, Bertolino M, Minatel M. Recopilación, registro y analisis de información en Cuidados Paliativos. *Medicina Paliativa* 2004; **11**: 102–6.

46   Herrera E, Cáceres FL, Rocafort J, et al. Las tecnologías de la información y comunicación (TICs) son pilar fundamental del proyecto de desarrollo de la sanidad en la Comunidad Autónoma de Extremadura. *Revista Esalud* 2004; 1. Available at: www.revistaesalud.com/revistaesalud/index.php (accessed August 28, 2005).

✱ 47   National Council for Palliative Care, Hospice Information Service. Minimum Data Set for Specialist Palliative Care Services (version 1.2). London: National Council Palliative Care. 1996; Available at: www.ncpc.org.uk/policy_unit/ mds/data_manual.html (accessed December 30, 2005).

✱ 48   Walker P, Nordell C, Cace, et al. Impact of the Edmonton Labeled Visual Information System on physician recall of metastatic cancer patient histories: a randomized controlled trial. *J Pain Symptom Manage* 2001; **21**: 4–11.

✱ 49   Inouye S, van Dyck C, Alessi C, et al. Clarifying confusion: The Confusion Assessment Method. *Ann Intern Med* 1990; **113**: 941–8.

✱ 50   Folstein MF, Folstein SE, McHugh P. Mini-Mental State: a practical guide for grading the cognitive state of patients for the clinician. *J Psychiatr Res* 1975; **12**: 189–98.

● 51   Wenk R, Bertolino M. Developing countries: Palliative care status 2002. *J Pain Symptom Manage* 2002; **24**: 166–9.

◆ 52   Wenk R. Developing countries: status of cancer pain and palliative care. *J Pain Symptom Manage* 1993; **8**: 385–7.

102

Prognostic indicators of survival

MARCO MALTONI, AUGUSTO T CARACENI, CATERINA MODONESI

INTRODUCTION

Experts in the field of palliative care may argue that it is such a valid therapeutic option at any stage of chronic, debilitating diseases, that it should be recommended and administered in any situation. From this perspective, survival prognosis predictions would not have any impact on clinical practice, but promote palliative medicine purely as 'end-of-life' care. On the other hand, although a 'palliative approach' is clearly desirable along the entire course of chronic-degenerative diseases, it is also reasonable to consider life expectation as being one of the useful parameters for defining the most adequate proposal in terms of choices relating to therapeutic and support programs. Box 102.1 shows the reasons why survival prognosis prediction could be useful.

Box 102.1 Reasons for making a prognosis prediction

To help:

- oncological specialists understand when chemotherapeutic treatment is inappropriate and becomes futile[1*,2]

- other specialist doctors or general practitioners understand the most timely moment to direct a patient to a palliative care programme[3*]

- palliative care doctors choose the most suitable palliative treatment intensity

- palliative care doctors understand whether the patient's condition is such that he or she is eligible for state reimbursement, when this is linked to determined life-expectancy conditions[4]

- researchers in identifying a precise population in which the results of therapeutic action can be assessed and compared with those obtained in other populations

- clinicians in communicating with both patients and their families

- both patients and their families take part in clinical choices

- both patients and their families deal with practical issues which depend on life-expectancy

- patients deal with the existential and spiritual issues of life

---

Prognostic information, however, is probabilistic, and individual variations are such that the therapeutic choice for each individual patient should only be made after taking many other physical, psychologic, and spiritual variables into consideration.

GENERAL PROGNOSIS

The proportion of patients with cancer assisted in palliative care programs exceeds 80 percent in all major case studies.[5*] This is due to the fact that, in its advanced stage, the course of neoplastic disease is foreseeable and, therefore, appropriate assistance can be planned. General prognosis in cancer is related to diagnosis, stage of the disease,

Cancer disease

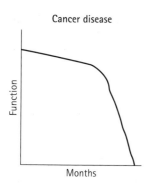

Organ failure

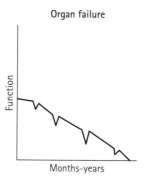

Frailty

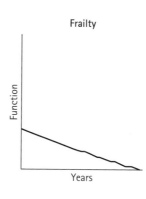

Figure 102.1   *Different trajectories of functional decline approaching death in three clinical situations. Modified from Lunney et al.[7]*

and – partially – to the impact of therapies. During the early stages of solid and hematological malignant diseases, the outcome doctors aim for is cure. In disseminated advanced solid cancers, the only possible objective outcome is to prolong survival, and there is heterogeneity with respect to prognosis, revealed by strongly differing survival medians among different tumors.[6]

In noncancer diseases, prognostic assessment and the patient's subsequent introduction to hospice programs are more problematic, as the disease trajectories are more difficult to forecast, and there is greater variability in individual prognosis (Fig. 102.1).

PROGNOSIS IN PATIENTS WITH ADVANCED CANCER

In addition to the early and the metastatic stages of cancer disease, is it possible to identify a third situation ('far advanced cancer disease' or 'terminal cancer phase') for which survival prognosis indicators could be defined? And, if this phase does exist, is it formed by a homogeneous population or does it incorporate various types of patient?

A weak point in all studies carried out on prognostic indicators in advanced stages of cancer is the investigated population, or, better, the 'inception cohort'. Its definition would allow homogeneous recruitment at a fixed and uniform point in time along the natural history of the disease. Some authors have included all patients who entered hospices or palliative care programs in their studies on prognostic indicators;[8,9*,10*,11*] other have attempted to standardize and code the population's 'terminality' criteria;[12*,13*,14*] whereas still others have elaborated specific criteria to define when patients with different cancers could be considered in a terminal phase.[15*]

The problematic issues in the methodology of studies on prognostic indicators are shown in Box 102.2.

Clinically, 90 days can be considered as the most relevant period of time used to define the terminal phase, even though the median survival of patients in most hospice programs is approximately 30–45 days.[16]

Box 102.2   Weak points in the methodology of studies on prognostic indicators

- Identification of the inception cohort

- Retrospective cohorts

- Heterogeneous population sampling and setting

- Limited use of multivariate statistical analyses

- Brief description of the statistical method and insufficient information about the recruitment method and sampling procedures

- Extremely limited use of the training and testing sample method

- Inadequate ratio between the number of variables studied and number of patients enrolled

- Lack of a systematic procedure, heterogeneity, and selection of the variables studied

- Little attention paid to variables which are currently becoming more important, such as comorbidity

---

PROGNOSTIC INDICATORS IN PATIENTS WITH TERMINAL CANCER

Prognostic indicators in oncology patients referred to palliative care programs have generally been studied using a set of observations on prognostic variables in series of patients, then assessing the outcome for each patient. After this, researchers generally use statistical models to evaluate the link between predictors and outcomes. Information about the prognostic predictivity of different indicators can be gathered from both original studies and systematic reviews of literature. Although such revisions were merely qualitative in the past,[17] they have recently been conducted according to evidence-based medicine directives[18***,19***,20***,21***] (Table 102.1).

Prognostic indicators

CLINICAL PREDICTION OF SURVIVAL

The Clinical Prediction of Survival (CPS), or the carer's clinical judgment of the possible course of the patient's illness, was the first indicator whose prognostic predictivity was assessed.[22*] It proved able to maintain its prognostic importance in a multivariate analysis.[13*]

One often emphasized fact is that CPS is inaccurate, and that the CPS exceeds actual survival (AS) by a factor ranging from 1.08 to 5.3. Error percentages range from 30 percent to 78 percent, with the rate of optimistic errors out of total errors from 12 percent to 88 percent[19***] generally equal to or higher than 60 percent. A recently published, systematic review confirmed the over-optimism of CPS: median CPS 42 days, median AS 29 days on eight evaluable studies with 1563 patients. Although agreement between CPS and AS was considered poor (weighted κ 0.369), the two were highly significantly associated after log transformation (Spearman rank correlation 0.60, $P < 0.001$).[20***] To define CPS as being accurate, much depends on the definition of accuracy which, in turn, depends on how the clinical estimate is expressed and the error defined. Both definitions are heterogeneous in published studies. In most studies, CPS is calculated temporally, that is, it is expressed numerically in terms of the time each individual patient can be expected to live, and then compared with the same patient's AS.[10*,22*,23*,24*]

Other methods have also been used to express prediction. For example a method gives a minimum and maximum estimate of predicted survival,[25*,26*] another estimates that the patient will still be alive after a given period of time from the prediction,[27*] another includes the patient in a range of lengths of estimated survival,[14*,28*] yet another provides the smallest range that would include 90 percent of deaths of similar patients.[29*]

The error definition used in the studies has been very inconsistent: 100 percent error for overestimation and underestimation (CPS = 2 AS or AS = 2 CPS),[12*,22*,24*,29*] 33 percent deviation from CPS and AS,[30*] AS over or under the maximum or minimum CPS limit,[25*] CPS correlations with various periods of AS.[10*,27*] Two issues need to be considered related to this heterogeneity. First, the modifications in accuracy due to either variations in the measuring units in defining the error or variability in the survey methods are apparent rather than real. Second, the percentage deviations between CPS and AS that are statistically significant and recorded as errors may actually be clinically irrelevant.

When making individual prognosis, however, clinicians should consider a range of factors which limit the CPS. It has been suggested that CPS is affected by the 'horizon effect', implying that the closer the moment of death, the more accurate the prediction.[9*,28*] Other authors do not confirm this hypothesis,[10*,25*] however, and others still stress there is greater accuracy in the long or short compared to the medium term.[14*] It appears that repeated predictions improve their predictive ability.[9*,22*,25*] The continuous involvement of the physician along the course of disease of the patient appears to lower CPS reliability.[30*]

As far as the prediction variability is concerned, Maltoni et al. demonstrated that the correlation coefficient between CPS and AS is 0.78 ($P < 0.01$) for oncologists with experience in palliative care and 0.45 ($P = 0.01$) for less experienced oncologists.[24] Christakis and Lamont reported that nononcologist specialists are three times more pessimistic than general physicians, and that more experienced physicians are more accurate.[30*] Llobera et al. indicate a higher accuracy among oncologists rather than among general physicians.[31*] Other studies have failed to demonstrate any significant differences among the various disciplines[16,22*,23*] or professional roles.[27*] A small study revealed high accuracy in nurse auxiliaries during the last days of the patients' lives.[9*] The accuracy achieved by specialist palliative care professionals appears to have improved over the years whereas that of referrers to palliative care services has apparently remained the same.[16]

Other features of CPS deserve further investigation, including whether two prognosticators are better than one,[32] and whether patients' characteristics are relevant. One study showed less over-optimism for cancer than for noncancer patients.[30*] CPS is best used if integrated with other, more objective and reproducible prognostic indicators, also resulting from multivariate analyses.[13*,33*,34*]

PERFORMANCE STATUS

Performance status (PS) has been studied in great depth, and undoubtedly proved to be an independent prognostic parameter.[18***] It has been assessed using different scales and according to various survey approaches, such as the Karnofsky Performance Status (KPS),[12*,24*,25*,35*,36*] Activities of Daily Living (ADL),[37*] Eastern Cooperative Oncology Group (ECOG) PS,[38*,39*] and a tailored version of KPS for palliative settings, namely the Palliative Performance Scale (PPS).[40*]

The KPS is the most widely used scale in palliative care studies. Low KPS values are tightly linked to short survival rates, although high values do not necessarily indicate longer survival, since values may drop extremely quickly at any time due to a patient's rapid, unexpected, deterioration. Although initial studies of KPS showed good interrater reliability, later studies registered some controversial data.

PHYSICAL SIGNS AND SYMPTOMS, AND PSYCHOLOGICAL FACTORS

Several signs and symptoms have been integrated with both CPS and PS to increase their prognostic capability. In 1988, after having identified PS as significant prognostic indicator

Table 102.1 *Comparison of systematic reviews on prognostic indicator studies*

Author, year	No. of studies/No. of patients	Criteria selection of studies/PFs examined
Viganò *et al.*, 2000,[18]	22/7089	Examined 18 clinical-biologic possible predictors evaluated in at least three studies (of the 136 assessed)
Chow *et al.*, 2001,[19]	CPS: 12/2920 PFs: 18/6158	Biochemical and molecular markers were not studied
Glare *et al.*, 2003,[20]	8/1591	CPS only
Maltoni *et al.*, 2004,[21]	Four systematic reviews CPS: 16/3079 Signs and symptoms: 21/7621 Biological factors: 9/2919 Prognostic scores: 8/1954	Only studies with a median population survival of ≤ 90 days

*, strength of recommendation.
CPS, Clinical Prediction of Survival; PFs, prognostic factors.

in their series of 1592 hospice patients, Reuben *et al.* found that 5 out of 14 evaluated symptoms retained their prognostic value which was independent at the multivariate analysis.[36*] The symptoms linked to survival included shortness of breath, dry mouth, eating problems or anorexia, trouble swallowing, and weight loss. Four out of these five symptoms were related to the nutritional state of the patient, so a 'terminal cancer syndrome' hypothesis was formulated (characterized by a reduction in the functional state of the patient, and symptoms of the cancer anorexia-cachexia syndrome [CACS]), independent of both the original location and metastatic spread of the disease.

In a vast majority of the studies in which the signs and symptoms of CACS were tested, they appeared significant for a correlation with worse prognosis, in univariate or multivariate analyses.[12*,36*,37*,41*,42*] A negative prognostic

Results	Level of study evidence and/or strength of recommendation shown	Formal meta-analysis	Comment
Prognostic factors categorized according to their relationship with prognosis: probably non-associated possibly associated definitely associated The latter were: low performance status; CPS cognitive impairment; anorexia dyspnea; xerostomia; weight loss; dysphagia	No	No	Clinical prediction should be considered as one of the criteria, and used together with other factors
CPS used alone: D* Use of aggregates of PFs including CPS: B* PFs: performance status; anorexia; weight loss; dysphagia; cognitive failure; CPS	Yes	No	The study used evidence criteria which were more sound for clinical trials than prognostic studies
Agreement between CPS and AS poor (κ 0.36), but the two were highly significantly associated after log transformation (Spearman rank correlation 0.60, $P < 0.001$)	Yes	No	Median CPS 42 (28–84) days Median AS 29 (13–62) days Clinicians overestimate survival, but predictions are correlated with survival; predictions have discriminatory ability, even if they are miscalibrated
Recommendations on PFs: Use of CPS indicated, but together with other PFs (A*) Performance status (B*) Some cancer anorexia-cachexia symptoms (weight loss, anorexia, dysphagia, xerostomia)(B*) Cognitive failure (B*) Dyspnea (B*) Leukocytosis (B*) Lymphocytopenia (B*) C-Reactive protein (B*) Prognostic score (A*)	Yes	No	Specific assessment methods of the quality for prognostic studies were chosen

correlation has also been reported for asthenia.[15*,31*] Other symptoms for which a correlation with negative prognosis has definitely been shown are cognitive failure[10*,41*,43*] and dyspnea.[12*,36*,44*]

A series of other psychosocial factors or factors linked to the original disease have only sporadically shown prognostic predictivity. For example, these (age, sex, race, marital status, education and income, socioeconomic factors and possibility of psychosocial support; type, histology and stage of cancer) were included in univariate analysis, but not confirmed in multivariate analysis, or studied in populations with illnesses at a less advanced stage.[45*,46*]

Some authors have drawn attention to a link between quality of life and survival in palliative care populations,[31*,42*] whereas others consider the quality of life less important than organic and physical factors.[27*] Some recent data suggest that the prognostic value of quality of life multidimensional evaluation tools should be ascribed to subscales referring to physical symptoms.[45*,46*] A recent study of two independent cohorts of 248 and 756 patients showed that physical health-related quality of life indicators should be focused to gather prognostic evidence.[47*]

BIOLOGICAL FACTORS

The prognostic value of some biological factors, particularly if linked to the patient's nutritional state, has been demonstrated in population settings, which cannot always be extrapolated to those included in palliative care programs. These include albumin and prealbumin levels, Nutritional Index (NI), Prognostic Nutritional Index (PNI), and Prognostic Inflammatory and Nutritional Index (PINI).[48] Among those factors which are directly or indirectly linked to a patient's nutritional state, lymphocytopenia has proven to be important in populations included in palliative care programmes.[13*,49*] A poor prognostic correlation has also been demonstrated for leukocytosis,[13*,49*] and high levels of C-reactive protein.[50*,51*] Less convincing evidence is there for increased levels of bilirubin[38*] and vitamin B_{12},[50*] and low pseudocholinesterase levels.[49*]

Some studies of heterogeneous populations of patients have given prognostic importance to hemoglobin, levels of sodium and calcium, some enzymes, and proteinuria.

Strengthening of prognostic accuracy achieved by the combined use of CPS and other prognostic factors

Some studies have aimed to verify the increase in prognostic accuracy from the combined use of CPS and other prognostic factors. Morita et al.[8*] reported that the prognostic accuracy of physicians before and after the combined use of clinical judgment and an instrument comprising more objective parameters improved as follows:

- Number of cases with a difference between AS and CPS of 28 days or longer – from 42 percent to 23 percent, $P < 0.01$.
- Number of patients with an AS either twice as long or half as long as CPS – from 49 percent to 37 percent, $P = 0.05$.
- Number of cases with serious errors of prognostication, i.e. patients who represented both the previous situations – from 27 percent to 16 percent, $P = 0.028$.

Furthermore, in the previously mentioned review by Glare et al.,[20***] it emerged that for all the KPS categories identified (<40, 40–50, >50), R^2 values obtained in 981 patients for CPS alone, other prognostic factors alone, and CPS plus other prognostic factors, were as follows, respectively: KPS < 40: 0.46, 0.25, 0.50; KPS 40–50: 0.35, 0.15, 0.38; and KPS > 50: 0.24, 0.08, 0.27.

Finally, even when used in a slightly different population consisting of seriously ill hospitalized adults, the combination of the Study to Understand Prognosis and Preferences for Outcomes and Treatments (SUPPORT) model with physicians' estimates improved both predictive accuracy (receiver operating characteristic [ROC] curve area = 0.82) and the capacity to identify patients with a higher probability of survival or death.[33*]

Prognostic indicators combined in prognostic models

PROGNOSTIC SCORES

The prognostic scores studied in only those populations included in palliative care programs have been reported here. A systematic review[21***] identified eight works on the development of prognostic scores in cancer patient populations in palliative care programs, with a median survival inferior than or equal to 90 days. In four of these works, the prognostic score was built: Poor Prognostic Indicator,[10*] Palliative Prognostic Score,[13*] Palliative Prognostic Index,[41*] and Terminal Cancer Prognostic Score.[52*] Validation on an independent population was supplied for the Palliative Prognostic (PaP) Score in three works,[11*,34*,43*] whereas Morita et al. validated the Palliative Prognostic Index (PPI) in the original work.[41*] Another score was recently developed, following the period examined by the quoted review: the Prognostic Scale.[53*]

The PaP Score is based on factors identified in an Italian prospective multicenter study of 540 patients with advanced cancer, with a median survival of 32 days (1–355).[13*] The final model obtained by means of a backward selection procedure is shown in Table 102.2. Three risk groups were formed, and patients were fairly well distributed between the three groups. The survival curves are shown in Figure 102.2. The PaP Score was also tested on a population of noncancer patients, where it retained its predictive ability.[54*] The peculiarity of the PaP Score is that it can be used 'together with' rather than 'instead of' the clinical judgment of the physician, since it includes the CPS.

The PPI comprises the Palliative Performance Scale, oral intake, edema, dyspnea at rest, and delirium.[41*] It has been shown that PPI improves the predictive ability of physicians with experience in palliative care.[8*] The Prognostic Scale was also validated, and demonstrated that, like different PS values, differing degrees of severity of the symptoms impacted survival differently too.[53*]

PROGNOSIS IN NONCANCER PATIENTS

Chronic degenerative diseases are more common among older people, and the average age is increasing at a considerable rate in more developed Western countries. Changes in disease patterns including a chronic course, multiorgan insufficiency and polymorbidity are linked to the general aging pattern of the population. The subjective problems older people have are similar to those of patients with advanced cancer. A series of problems specific to noncancer diseases hinders prognostic assessment. Since the progressive functional decline can regress repeatedly, it is more difficult to define this as a prognostic indicator for noncancer patients. The 'typical' terminal phase in some noncancer diseases is difficult to identify, and sometimes even does not exist.[7*]

Patients' access to hospices can be limited by the fact that, in some countries, reimbursements are only granted if the said patients can produce certification specifying 'a life expectancy of 6 months or less, should the disease take its usual course'. The National Hospice Organization (NHO) prognostic guidelines may be useful in predicting prognosis in noncancer patients.[4] Excessively restrictive eligibility criteria may lead to a risk that sensitivity decreases, thus preventing many patients who would be entitled to hospice programs from accessing them. Considering the peculiar course of noncancer diseases, it is advisable that the judgment regarding prognosis be periodically reviewed, and modified if necessary.

Similar to what has happened with terminal cancer patients, specific studies of selected populations of non-cancer patients in hospice programs may help to better identify targeted features and prognostic indicators, although this issue is still controversial.[55*] However, some indicators, that is, the 'general prognostic indicators' and the 'specific prognostic indicators', can be found in these patients, too.

General prognostic indicators in noncancer diseases

IMPAIRED FUNCTIONAL STATUS

A recent reduction in functional status has been shown to have prognostic value, when evaluated as KPS or ADL,

Table 102.2 *Palliative Prognostic Score (PaP Score)*

Prognostic factor		Partial score
Dyspnea	Absent	0
	Present	1
Anorexia	Absent	0
	Present	1.5
Karnofsky Performance Status (KPS)	≥50	0
	30–40	0
	10–20	2.5
Clinical Prediction of Survival (CPS) (weeks)	>12	0
	11–12	2.0
	9–10	2.5
	7–8	2.5
	5–6	4.5
	3–4	6.0
	1–2	8.5
Total white blood cell (WBC) count (cell/mm³)	Normal (4800–8500)	0
	High (8501–11000)	0.5
	Very high (>11000)	1.5
Lymphocyte percentage (%)	Normal (20.0–40.0)	0
	Low (12.0–19.9)	1.0
	Very low (0–11.9)	2.5

PaP Score = Dyspnea score + anorexia score + KPS score + CPS score + Total WBC count score + lymphocyte percentage score.

Risk groups	Total score
A: 30-day survival probability >70%	0–5.5
B: 30-day survival probability 30–70%	5.6–11.0
C: 30-day survival probability <30%	11.1–17.5

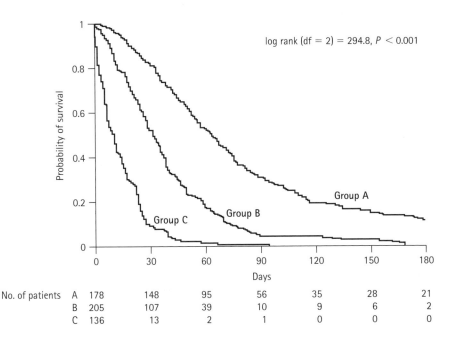

log rank (df = 2) = 294.8, $P < 0.001$

No. of patients								
	A	178	148	95	56	35	28	21
	B	205	107	39	10	9	6	2
	C	136	13	2	1	0	0	0

Figure 102.2 *Survival curves of patients in palliative care programs in an Italian multicenter study. Groups identified according to the Palliative Prognostic (PaP) Score value. Modified from Pirovano et al.[13]*

in several studies of older people, and various diseases, including heart disease, lung disease, dementia, coma, and stroke.[4,55*,56]

ALTERATIONS IN NUTRITIONAL STATUS

Alterations in nutritional status have also proved to have prognostic value for heart disease, pulmonary disease, dementia, human immunodeficiency virus (HIV) disease, liver disease, renal disease, stroke and coma, and end stage amyotrophic lateral sclerosis in patients with swallowing difficulties without gastrostomy feeding.[4,55*,56]

Specific prognostic indicators in noncancer diseases

HEART DISEASE

In the absence of a precipitating factor which can be treated, survival usually ranges from 6 months to 4 years. Functional status described according to the New York Heart Association Classification (NYHA) is the most important prognostic factor: class IV, namely, symptoms of congestive heart failure at rest, despite optimal treatment with diuretics and vasodilators, is correlated with the worst prognosis.

Factors which contribute to poorer prognoses include a left ventricular ejection fraction of 20 percent or less, aging, intractability of underlying heart disease, dilated cardiomyopathy, uncontrolled arrhythmia, contractility changes over time, high cardiothoracic ratio measured on a standard chest radiograph, and oxygen consumption.[4,55*,56,57*,58*]

LUNG DISEASE

Making a prognostic prediction for lung diseases at an advanced stage is extremely difficult. The 5-year survival was shown to be 45 percent in a study on hospitalized patients with chronic obstructive pulmonary disease.[59*] Negative prognostic indicators have been identified: low forced expiratory volume at one second (FEV_1) (less than 30 percent), repeated episodes of respiratory failure, presence of cor pulmonale, hypoxemia, dyspnea at rest unresponsive to therapies, and low functional status.[4,55*,56]

DEMENTIA

The mean survival rate of patients with dementia ranges from 5 to 8 years, and the 'advanced' stage of the disease may last 2 years. Difficulty in formulating a prognosis is one of the obstacles for those hospices who accept patients with dementia.[60*] In hospice programs, such patients have a significantly higher survival rate than patients with other diseases (35 percent >6 months).[5*] The prognostic indicators that are considered are functional status measured with Functional Assessment Staging (FAST). Stage 7 FAST patients presented a mean survival of 6.9 months and a median survival of 4 months.[61*] Other factors include type

of dementia (vascular dementia appears to lead to death more rapidly than Alzheimer disease), age, gender, severity of dementing illness (inability to walk without assistance), presence of medical complications.[56*]

HIV DISEASE

Mortality due to acquired immune deficiency syndrome (AIDS) dropped considerably from the early 1990s to 1997, when it leveled off. The median survival rate increased from 11 months in 1984 to 46 months in 1995.[62*] The advent of Highly Active AntiRetroviral Therapy (HAART), together with the treatment of opportunistic infections and symptom palliation, altered the prognostic of a disease which invariably led to death in a few months to a more a prolonged one.

Late-stage HIV disease definition could, however, be applied to patients with long standing, symptomatic HIV disease, with severe immunosuppression, cumulative morbidity, and failure or inability to tolerate antiretroviral therapy.[63] Consequently, the importance of some of the traditional prognostic indicators used (CD4 cell count, viral load, certain opportunistic infections) may lessen.[7*,64*] These factors should thus be integrated with more recent ones, such as a noncompliance or nonreaction to HAART, functional deficits (impaired ability to conduct routine activities, cognitive impairment) and/or the existence of other life-threatening conditions predictive of short-term mortality: weight loss and neurological abnormalities.[63]

AMYOTROPHIC LATERAL SCLEROSIS

Palliative care in amyotrophic lateral sclerosis (ALS) begins with how the patient is informed of the diagnosis, and continues to prevent both the 'choking to death' and the 'locked-in syndrome' in an intensive care unit after intubation and artificial ventilation'.[65] The NHO criteria enable clinicians to predict a survival of ≤6 months for ALS hospice patients. They include critically impaired breathing or rapid progression and life-threatening complications, or rapid progression and critical nutritional impairment.[4] These criteria were present in only 5 of the 97 ALS patients enrolled on a hospice program, of which 91 percent had a survival of less than 6 months. The same work force aimed to update the criteria, and suggested adding forced vital capacity (FVC) of less than 30 percent, or an FVC < 60 percent with a steady decline over past 2–3 months, and either two other respiratory indicators or one respiratory and one nutritional indicator.[66*]

LIVER DISEASE

Prognostic indicators that are additively negative in end-stage cirrhosis are laboratory indicators of severely altered liver functionality, and clinical indicators of end-stage liver disease (ascites refractory to therapies, spontaneous bacterial peritonitis, hepatorenal syndrome, hepatic encephalopathy refractory to therapies, recurrent variceal bleeding).[55*] Other factors have also been reported, including malnutrition, muscle wasting, active alcoholism, hepatocellular carcinoma, HBsAg positivity.[4]

RENAL DISEASE

The Core Curriculum in Nephrology Palliative Care[67] has reported that end-stage renal disease (ESRD) patients in dialysis survive a quarter the time of age-matched patients without renal disease, with an annual mortality rate of 23 percent. The NHO examines different situations, such as ESRD, acute and chronic renal failure, with chronic ambulatory peritoneal dialysis (CAPD).[4] Laboratory criteria for renal failure, clinical signs and symptoms associated with renal failure, and comorbid complications that predict early mortality in hospital and patients with acute renal failure are given.

STROKE AND COMA

Predictors of early mortality during the acute phase immediately following the acute episode have been identified:

- coma beyond 3 days' duration (associated with any four of the following: abnormal brain stem response, absent verbal response, absent withdrawal response to pain, high serum creatinine level, age >70)
- severe dysphagia
- certain computed tomography (CT) or magnetic resonance imaging (MRI) findings.

Some clinical factors are correlated with poor survival once the patient has entered the chronic stage: age, poor functional and nutritional status, post-stroke dementia, medical complications.[4]

CONCLUSIONS

Awareness of prognostic indicators may help physicians who do not feel particularly confident about making a prognosis, find it difficult and stressful to make predictions, and believe that patients' expectations of the prognostic ability of their carers are excessive.[68*] As far as communication of the prognostic in the frame of the physician–patient relationship is concerned, ethical, cultural, religious and psychological issues should be considered by doctors, to avoid causing a severely ill patient even more suffering: although there is a patient's right to be informed there is no patient's duty to be informed.

Therefore, appropriate use of life-expectancy prognostication, to improve and personalize the treatment of patients in the advanced and terminal stages of the disease, can only be achieved if it forms part of a multidisciplinary palliative care program, which still considers the individual value of the patient's remaining lifetime invaluable.

Key learning points

- Awareness of the prognostic survival indicators helps clinicians in the difficult decision-making process, and may lead to better communication with both patients and their families. Prognostication has only a probabilistic value, which should be carefully considered when examining the possible course of each individual patient's illness.

- Trajectories of noncancer chronic disease make prognosis prediction for these diseases more complex compared with the palliative phase of cancer.

- Prognostic indicators in palliative care patients differ from those for the early and advanced stages.

- Clinical Prediction of Survival is an independent prognostic indicator in palliative care cancer patients. However, as its accuracy is conditioned by a number of restrictions, and it should only be used in conjunction with other, more objective, prognostic indicators.

- The following indicators have definitely shown independent prognostic ability: Performance Status, signs and symptoms of CACS, delirium, dyspnea.

- Clinical Prediction of Survival and other prognostic indicators may be included in simple models or prognostic scores. The prognostic ability of the score increases when it is used 'together with' rather than 'instead of' clinical judgment.

- Prognostic indicators can also be found in noncancer diseases. Some of them are common to more than one disease (functional status and nutritional status), whereas others are specific to individual diseases.

- The main aim of prognostication is to personalize the treatment of patients when dealing with the severest stage of their disease, while simultaneously continuing to fully consider the individual value of the patient's remaining lifetime.

REFERENCES

1 Earle CC, Neville BA, Landrum MB, *et al.* Trends in the aggressiveness of cancer care near the end of life. *J Clin Oncol* 2004; **22**: 315–21.

2 Earle CC, Park ER, Lai B, *et al.* Identifying potential indicators of the quality of end-of-life cancer care from administrative data. *J Clin Oncol* 2003; **21**: 1133–8.

3 Lamont EB, Christakis NA. Physician factors in the timing of cancer patient referral to hospice palliative care. *Cancer* 2002; **94**: 2733–7.

* 4 Standards and Accreditation Committee, Medical Guidelines Task Force of the National Hospice Organization. *Medical Guidelines for Determining Prognosis in Selected Non-Cancer*

Diseases, 2nd edn. Arlington VA: National Hospice
Organization, 1996.

● 5   Christakis N, Escarce JJ. Survival of Medicare patients after
enrollment in hospice programs. *N Engl J Med* 1996; **335**:
172–8.

◆ 6   Lamont EB, Christakis NA. Complexities in prognostication in
advanced cancer. *JAMA* 2003; **290**: 98–104.

● 7   Lunney JR, Lynn J, Foley D, *et al.* Patterns of functional
decline at the end of life. *JAMA* 2003; **289**: 2387–92.

8   Morita T, Tsunoda J, Inoue S, Chihara S. Improved accuracy
of physicians' survival prediction for terminally ill cancer
patients using the Palliative Prognostic Index. *Palliat Med*
2001; **15**: 419–24.

9   Oxenham D, Cornbleet MA. Accuracy of prediction of survival
by different professional groups in a hospice. *Palliat Med*
1998; **12**: 117–18.

● 10   Bruera E, Miller MJ, Kuehn N, *et al.* Estimate of survival of
patients admitted to a Palliative Care Unit: a prospective
study. *J Pain Symptom Manage* 1992; **7**: 82–6.

11   Glare P, Virik K. Independent prospective validation of the
PaP Score in terminally ill patients referred to a hospital-
based palliative medicine consultation service. *J Pain
Symptom Manage* 2001; **22**: 891–8.

● 12   Maltoni M, Pirovano M, Scarpi E, *et al.* Prediction of survival
of patients terminally ill with cancer. Results of an Italian
prospective multicentric study. *Cancer* 1995; **75**: 2613–22.

● 13   Pirovano M, Maltoni M, Nanni O, *et al.* A new Palliative
Prognostic Score (PaP Score). A first step for the staging of
terminally ill cancer patients. *J Pain Symptom Manage* 1999;
17: 231–9.

14   Viganò A, Dorgan M, Bruera E, Suarez-Almazor ME. The
relative accuracy of the Clinical Estimation of the duration of
life for patients with end of life cancer. *Cancer* 1999; **86**:
170–6.

● 15   Viganò A, Bruera E, Jhangri GS, *et al.* Clinical survival
predictors in patients with advanced cancer. *Arch Intern Med*
2000; **160**: 861–8.

16   Glare P, Christakis N. Predicting survival in patients with
advanced disease. In: Doyle D, Hanks G, Cherny N, Calman K,
eds. *Oxford Textbook of Palliative Medicine*, 3rd edn. Oxford:
Oxford University Press, 2004: 29–42.

17   Den Daas N. Estimating length of survival in end-stage
cancer: a review of the literature. *J Pain Symptom Manage*
1995; **10**: 548–55.

◆ 18   Viganò A, Dorgan M, Buckingham J, *et al.* Survival prediction
in terminal cancer patients: a systematic review of the
literature. *Palliat Med* 2000; **14**: 363–74.

◆ 19   Chow E, Harth T, Hruby G, *et al.* How accurate are physicians'
clinical predictions of survival and the available prognostic
tools in estimating survival times in terminally ill cancer
patients? A systematic review. *Clin Oncol* 2001; **13**: 209–18.

◆ 20   Glare P, Virik K, Jones M, *et al.* A systematic review of
physicians' survival predictions in terminally ill cancer
patients. *BMJ* 2003; **327**: 195–200.

✱ 21   Maltoni M, Caraceni A, Brunelli C, *et al.* Prognostic factors
in advanced cancer patients: evidence-based clinical
recommendations – a study by the Steering Committee of
the European Association for Palliative Care. *J Clin Oncol*
2005; **23**: 6240–8.

● 22   Parkes CM. Accuracy of predictions of survival in later stages
of cancer. *BMJ* 1972; **2**: 29–31.

23   Heyse-Moore LH, Johnson-Bell VE. Can doctors accurately
predict the life-expectancy of patients with terminal cancer?
Palliat Med 1987; **1**: 165–6.

24   Maltoni M, Nanni O, Derni S, *et al.* Clinical prediction of
survival is more accurate than the Karnofsky Performance
Status in estimating life span of terminally-ill cancer
patients. *Eur J Cancer* 1994; **30**: 764–6.

25   Evans C, McCarthy M. Prognostic uncertainty in terminal care:
can the Karnofsky Index help? *Lancet* 1985; **251**: 1204–6.

26   Higginson IJ, Costantini M. Accuracy of prognosis estimates
by four palliative care teams: a prospective cohort study.
BMC Palliat Care 2002; **1**: 1–5.

27   Addington-Hall JM, Mac Donald LD, Anderson HR. Can the
Spitzer Quality of Life Index help to reduce uncertainty in
terminal care? *Br J Cancer* 1990; **62**: 695–9.

28   Mackillop WJ, Quirt CF. Measuring the accuracy of prognostic
judgements in oncology. *J Clin Epidemiol* 1997; **50**: 21–9.

29   Forster LE, Lynn J. Predicting life span for applicants to
inpatient hospice. *Arch Intern Med* 1988; **148**: 2540–3.

30   Christakis NA, Lamont EB. Extent and determinants of error
in doctors' prognoses in terminally ill patients: prospective
cohort study. *BMJ* 2000; **320**: 469–73.

31   Llobera J, Esteva M, Rifa J, *et al.* Terminal cancer. Duration
and prediction of survival time. *Eur J Cancer* 2000; **36**:
2036–43.

◆ 32   Christakis NA. *Death Foretold. Prophecy and Prognosis in
Medical Care.* Chicago: University Chicago Press, 1999.

● 33   Knaus WA, Harrell FE, Lynn J, *et al.* The SUPPORT prognostic
model: objective estimates of survival for seriously ill
hospitalized adults. *Ann Intern Med* 1995; **122**: 191–203.

34   Maltoni M, Nanni O, Pirovano M, *et al.* Successful validation
of the Palliative Prognostic Score in terminally ill cancer
patients. *J Pain Symptom Manage* 1999; **17**: 240–7.

35   Mor V, Laliberte L, Morris JN, Wiemann M. The Karnofsky
Performance Status Scale: an examination of its reliability
and validity in a research setting. *Cancer* 1984; **53**: 2004–7.

● 36   Reuben DB, Mor V, Hiris J. Clinical symptoms and length of
survival in patients with terminal cancer. *Arch Intern Med*
1988; **148**: 1586–91.

37   Schonwetter RS, Robinson BE, Ramirez G. Prognostic factors
for survival in terminal lung cancer patients. *J Gen Intern
Med* 1994; **9**: 366–71.

38   Rosenthal MA, Gebski VJ, Kefford RF, Stuart-Harris RC.
Prediction of life-expectancy in hospice patients: identification
of novel prognostic factors. *Palliat Med* 1993; **7**: 199–204.

39   Allard P, Dionne A, Patvin D. Factors associated with length
of survival among 1081 terminally ill cancer patients. *J Palliat
Care* 1995; **11**: 20–4.

40   Morita T, Tsunoda J, Inoue S, Chihara S. Survival prediction of
terminally ill cancer patients by clinical symptoms: development
of a simple indicator. *Jpn J Clin Oncol* 1999; **29**: 156–9.

● 41   Morita T, Tsunoda J, Inoue S, Chihara S. The Palliative
Prognostic Index: a scoring system for survival prediction of
terminally ill cancer patients. *Support Care Cancer* 1999; **7**:
128–33.

42   Tamburini M, Brunelli C, Rosso S, Ventafridda V. Prognostic
value of quality of life scores in terminal cancer patients.
J Pain Symptom Manage 1996; **11**: 32–41.

43   Caraceni A, Nanni O, Maltoni M, *et al.* Impact of delirium on
short term prognosis of advanced cancer patients. *Cancer*
2000; **89**: 1145–9.

44 Hardy JR, Turner R, Saunders M, A'Hern R. Prediction of survival in a hospital-based continuing care unit. *Eur J Cancer* 1994; **30** (A): 284–8.

45 Earlam S, Glover C, Fordy C *et al.* Relation between tumor size, quality of life, and survival in patients with colorectal liver metastases. *J Clin Oncol* 1996; **14**: 171–5.

46 Chang V T, Thaler HT, Polyak TA, *et al.* Quality of life and survival. The role of multidimensional symptom assessment. *Cancer* 1998; **83**: 173–9.

47 Vigano A, Donaldson N, Higginson IJ, *et al.* Quality of life and survival prediction in terminal cancer patients. *Cancer* 2004; **101**: 1090–8.

48 Maltoni M, Amadori D. Prognosis in advanced cancer. *Hematol Oncol Clin North Am* 2002; **16**: 715–29.

49 Maltoni M., Pirovano M, Nanni O, *et al.* Biological indices predictive of survival in 519 terminally ill cancer patients. *J Pain Symptom Manage* 1997; **13**: 1–9.

50 Geissbuhler P, Mermillod B, Rapin CH. Elevated serum vitamin B12 associated with CRP as a predictive factor of mortality in palliative care cancer patients: a prospective study over five years. *J Pain Symptom Manage* 2000; **20**: 93–103.

51 McMillan DC, Elahi MM, Sattar N, *et al.* Measurement of the systemic inflammatory response predicts cancer-specific and non-cancer survival in patients with cancer. *Nutr Cancer* 2001; **41**: 64–9.

● 52 Yun HY, Heo Ds, Heo BY, *et al.* Development of terminal cancer prognostic score as an index in terminally ill cancer patients. *Oncol Rep* 2001; **8**: 795–800.

● 53 Chuang RB, Hu WY, Chiu TY, Chen CY. Prediction of survival in terminal cancer patients in Taiwan: constructing a Prognostic Scale. *J Pain Symptom Manage* 2004; **28**: 115–22.

54 Glare P, Eychmueller S, Virik K. The use of the Palliative Prognostic Score in patients with diagnoses other than cancer. *J Pain Symptom Manage* 2003; **26**: 883–5.

55 Fox E, Landrum-Mc Niff K, *et al.* Evaluation of prognostic criteria for determining hospice eligibility in patients with advanced lung, heart, or liver disease. *JAMA* 1999; **282**: 1638–45.

◆ 56 Schonwetter RS, Chirag RJ. Survival estimation in non cancer patients with advanced disease. In: Portenoy RK, Bruera E, eds. *Topics in Palliative Care,* Vol 4. Oxford: Oxford University Press, 2000: 55–74.

57 Vranckx P, Van Cleemput J. Prognostic assessment of end-stage cardiac failure. *Acta Cardiol* 1998; **53**: 121–5.

58 Jaagosild P, Dawson NV, Thomas C, *et al.* Outcome of acute exacerbation of severe congestive heart failure: quality of life, resource use, and survival. SUPPORT Investigators. The Study to Understand Prognosis and Preferences for Outcomes and Risks of Treatment. *Arch Intern Med* 1998; **158**: 1081–9.

59 Vestbo J, Prescott E, Lange P, *et al.* Vital prognosis after hospitalization for COPD: a random population sample. *Respir Med* 1998; **92**: 772–6.

60 Hanrahan P, Luchins DJ. Access to hospice programs in end-stage dementia: a national survey of hospice programs. *J Am Geriatr Soc* 1995; **43**: 56–9.

✱ 61 Luchins DJ, Hanrahan P, Murphy K. Criteria for enrolling dementia patients in hospice. *J Am Geriatr Soc* 1997; **45**: 1054–9.

62 Lee LM, Karon JM, Selik R, *et al.* Survival after AIDS diagnosis in adolescents and adults during the treatment era, United States, 1984–1997. *JAMA* 2001; **285**: 1308–15.

◆ 63 Selwyin PA, Forstein M. Overcoming the false dichotomy of curative vs palliative care for late-stage HIV/AIDS. *JAMA* 2003; **290**: 806–14.

64 Gerard L, Flandre P, Raguin G, *et al.* Life expectancy in hospitalized patients with AIDS: prognostic factors on admission. *J Palliat Care* 1996; **12**: 26–30.

◆ 65 Borasio GD, Voltz R. Palliative care in amyotrophic lateral sclerosis. *J Neurol* 1997; **244** (Suppl 4): S11–S17.

✱ 66 McCluskey L, Houseman G. Medicare hospice referral criteria for patients with amyotrophic lateral sclerosis: a need for improvement. *J Palliat Med* 2004; **7**: 47–53.

67 Moss AH, Holley JL, Davison S, *et al.* Core curriculum in Nephrology. Palliative Care. *Am J Kidney Dis* 2004; **43**: 172–3.

68 Christakis NA, Iwashyna TJ. Attitude and self-reported practice regarding prognostication in a national sample of internists. *Arch Intern Med* 1998; **158**: 2389–95.

103

Palliative sedation

NATHAN I CHERNY

INTRODUCTION

Sedation in the context of palliative medicine is the monitored use of medications intended to induce varying degrees of unconsciousness to induce a state of decreased or absent awareness (unconsciousness) in order to relieve the burden of otherwise intractable suffering. The intent is to provide adequate relief of distress.[1]

Sedation is controversial insofar as it diminishes capacity: capacity to interact, to function, and, in some cases to live. In the context of a field of endeavor committed to helping the ill and suffering to live better, there is a potential contradiction of purpose. Sedation for the relief of suffering touches at the most basic conflict of palliative medicine: are we doing 'enough' or are we doing 'too much'. This issue exemplifies the tensions in achieving the dual goals of palliative care: first, to relieve suffering and, second to do so in such a manner so as to preserve the moral sensibilities of the patient, the professional carers, and concerned family and friends.

Sedation is used in palliative care in several settings:

- transient controlled sedation
- sedation in the management of refractory symptoms at the end of life
- emergency sedation
- respite sedation
- sedation for psychological or existential suffering.

Each of these will be discussed, describing the context of application, and practical and ethical considerations.

TRANSIENT CONTROLLED SEDATION

Transient controlled sedation is routinely and uncontroversially used to manage the severe pain and anxiety associated with noxious procedures. Sedation enables patients to endure interventions that would otherwise be intolerable. The depth of sedation required is influenced by the nature of the noxious stimulus, the level of relief achieved by other concurrent approaches, and individual patient factors. When these techniques are well applied, reports of pain and suffering are infrequent. Since these patients are expected to recover, careful attention is paid to maintaining adequate ventilation, hydration, and nutrition.

Occasionally transient sedation will be needed for a self-limiting severe exacerbation of pain.[2] In the full anticipation that this will be a reversible intervention of last resort, close monitoring of respiratory and homodynamic stability is essential. In one case report this was achieved with midazolam administered by a patient controlled analgesia device.[2]

SEDATION IN THE MANAGEMENT OF REFRACTORY SYMPTOMS AT THE END OF LIFE (PALLIATIVE SEDATION)

At the end of life the goals of care may shift and the relief of suffering may predominate over other considerations relating to functional capacity. In this setting, the designation of a symptom as 'refractory' may justify the use of induced sedation, particularly since this is the only option that is capable of providing the necessary relief with certainty and speed. Various names have been applied to the issue of sedation in this setting: terminal sedation, palliative sedation. Though no single term has achieved universal support, of these options, palliative sedation is generally preferred.[3–6]

Symptoms at the end of life

Among patients with advanced cancer, clinical experience suggests that optimal palliative care can effectively manage the symptoms of most cancer patients during most of the course of the disease. Physical and psychological symptoms cannot be eliminated, but are usually relieved enough to adequately temper the suffering of the patient and family.[7–12] This phase may be referred to as the ambulatory phase of advanced cancer.

As the disease progresses and the end of life approaches, patients commonly suffer more physical and psychological symptoms (including pain) and it often becomes more difficult to achieve adequate relief.[13–16] For some patients, the degree of suffering related to these symptoms may be intolerable. Despite intensified efforts to manage such problems, some patients do not achieve adequate relief and they continue to suffer from inadequately controlled symptoms that may be termed 'refractory'.

Refractory symptoms at the end of life

The term 'refractory' can be applied to symptoms that cannot be adequately controlled despite aggressive efforts to identify a tolerable therapy that does not compromise consciousness. The diagnostic criteria for the designation of a refractory symptom include that the clinician must perceive that further invasive and noninvasive interventions are either (i) incapable of providing adequate relief, (ii) associated with excessive and intolerable acute or chronic morbidity, or (iii) unlikely to provide relief within a tolerable time-frame. The implication of this designation is that the pain will not be adequately relieved with routine measures and that sedation may be needed to attain adequate relief.

EPIDEMIOLOGY OF REFRACTORY SYMPTOMS AT THE END OF LIFE

The prevalence of refractory pain at the end of life remains somewhat controversial.[17–20] The use of sedation in the management of refractory symptoms has been evaluated in several studies over the past 10 years[19,21–24] (Table 103.1).

In a study of homecare patients treated by the palliative care service of the Italian National Cancer Institute, Ventafridda et al. found that 63 of 120 terminally ill patients developed otherwise unendurable symptoms which required deep sedation for adequate relief.[19] In almost half of these cases the underlying problem was severe pain. In a retrospective survey of 100 patients who died in an inpatient palliative care ward, Fainsinger et al.[21] found that 16 patients required sedation for adequate symptom control prior to death, 6 for pain; an additional 2 patients who may have benefited from sedation died with severe uncontrolled pain. Stone et al.[23] compared two palliative care services in London, England and retrospectively looked at 115 patients. They found that 30 patients (26 percent) were prescribed sedatives. The commoner reasons were agitated delirium, mental anguish, pain, and dyspnea.

Survey data show that 5–35 percent of patients in hospice programs describe their pain as 'severe' in the last week of life and that 25 percent describe their shortness of breath as 'unbearable'.[28]

Sedation at the end of life as a clinical dilemma

Persistent severe pain at the end of life challenges the clinician clinically, emotionally and morally and contributes to the onerous nature of clinical decision making in this setting. It is useful to recognize both the clinical and the ethical dimensions of this dilemma. From a moral perspective, there is a major dilemma related to nonmalfeasance. Clinicians want neither to subject severely distressed patients to therapies that provide inadequate relief or excessive morbidity, nor to sacrifice conscious function when viable alternatives remain unexplored.

Table 103.1 *Surveys of the use of sedation in the management of refractory symptoms*

Authors(s)	Year	N	Place	Percentage sedated for refractory symptoms
Ventafridda et al.[19]	1990	120	Home	52
Fainsinger et al.[21]	1991	100	Hospital	16
Morita et al.[22]	1996	143	Hospice	43
Stone et al.[23]	1997	115	IP and home	26
Fainsinger et al.[24]	1998	76	IP hospice	30
Chiu et al.[25]	2001	251	IP palliative care	28
Muller-Busch et al.[26]	2002	548	IP palliative care	14
Morita[27]	2004		Multicenter	<10–50

The clinical corollary of this moral dilemma is the need to distinguished a 'refractory' pain state from 'the difficult situation', which could potentially respond within a tolerable time-frame to noninvasive or invasive interventions and yield adequate relief and preserved consciousness without excessive adverse effects. The challenge inherent in this decision making requires that patients with unrelieved symptoms undergo repeated evaluation prior to progressive application of routine therapies.

Case conference approach to decision making

Since individual clinician bias can influence decision making,[29,30] a case conference approach is prudent when assessing a challenging case. This conference may involve oncologists, palliative care physicians, specialists from other fields relevant to the prevailing symptom control problem, nurses, social workers, and others. The discussion attempts to clarify the remaining therapeutic options and the goals of care.

Clearly, it is critical that clinicians who are expert in symptom control be involved in the patient evaluation. When local expertise is limited, telephone consultation with physicians who are expert in palliative medicine is strongly encouraged.

CLINICAL PRACTICE

Preconditions and guidelines

In a thoughtful review, Wein[31] described a set of nine clinical preconditions for the consideration of sedation in the management of refractory symptoms:

- The illness must be irreversible and advance to death imminent.
- The symptoms need be determined to be untreatable and refractory by other means.
- The goals of care must be clear.
- Informed consent from the patient (direct, living will, advanced directives), or by proxy, must be obtained.
- Corroborative consultation should be sought.
- Staff should be involved and informed as appropriate.
- The family should be involved as guided by the patient's wishes and clinical condition.
- Full documentation of clinical condition and medication.
- Agreement must be undertaken that cardiopulmonary resuscitation (CPR) will not be initiated.

A clinical practice guideline has been published in Canada.[32] The purpose of the guide is to establish ethically acceptable criteria and guidelines for the use of palliative sedation as a form of treatment for intractable pain and symptoms associated with acute or chronic morbidity in the palliative care setting. The guideline defines palliative

sedation and refractory symptoms, states the rational for the use of sedation, and sets criteria for its application. In this guideline the basic criteria for considering the use of palliative sedation include the following: (i) a terminal disease exists, (ii) the patient/client suffers from a refractory symptom/s, (iii) in all but the most unusual circumstances, death must be imminent (within days), and (iv) a 'do not resuscitate' order must be in effect. If the criteria are met, then a 5-step process is set in progress:

1 The attending physician shall ensure the patient is assessed by a physician expert in symptom management.
2 The attending physician, based on the recommendation and advice from a physician expert in symptom management, shall consult directly with the patient and family and as appropriate with the other care providers regarding the option of palliative sedation.
3 If the option of palliative sedation is selected by the patient or 'agent' as identified within the Personal Directives Act, the attending physician or physician expert shall ensure the discussion by which the appropriate consent was obtained is documented on the health record.
4 Once consent is obtained for palliative sedation, the physician expert in symptom management will arrange for palliative sedation and appropriate monitoring of the patient.
5 The existing criteria and rationale used to determine the patient is a candidate for palliative sedation and the consultation process between the attending physician, palliative care consultants, patient and family will be documented on the health record.

It is important to note that this guideline explicitly indicates that expertise in the area of pain or symptom management is required by the healthcare disciplines implementing palliative sedation.

Discussing sedation with the patient and their family members

If the clinician perceives that there is no treatment capable of providing adequate relief of intolerable symptoms without compromising interactional function, or that the patient would be unable to tolerate specific therapeutic interventions, refractoriness to standard approaches should be acknowledged. In this situation, the clinician should explain that, by virtue of the severity of the problem and the limitations of the available techniques, the goal of providing the needed relief without the use of drugs that may impair conscious state is probably not possible.

The offer of sedation as an available therapeutic option is often received as an empathic acknowledgment of the severity of the degree of patient suffering. The enhanced patient trust in the commitment of the clinician to the relief of suffering may, in itself, influence decision making, particularly if there are other tasks or life issues that need to be completed before a state of diminished function develops. Indeed, patients can, and often do, decline sedation, acknowledging that symptoms will be unrelieved but secure in the knowledge that if the situation becomes intolerable this decision can be rescinded. Alternatively, the patient can assert comfort as the paramount consideration and accept the initiation of sedation.

With the hope and knowledge that it may be possible to achieve adequate relief without compromising interactional function, the patient who equally prioritizes comfort and function may elect to pursue only those approaches with modest morbidity, despite a relatively low or indeterminate likelihood of success. As the goals of prolonging survival and optimizing function become increasingly unachievable, priorities often shift. When comfort is the overriding goal of care, and the principal intent of any further intervention is to achieve lasting relief, there may be no tolerable time-frame for exploring other therapeutic options. In this situation, interventions of low or indeterminate likelihood of success are often rejected in favor of more certain approaches, even if they may involve impairment of cognitive function, or possibly foreshortened duration of survival.

This situation becomes more complicated when the clinician is less certain that the available approaches will fail. Therapeutic decision making is strongly influenced by the patient's readiness to accept the risk of morbidity and enduring discomfort until adequate relief is achieved. As always, patient evaluation of therapeutic options requires a candid disclosure of the therapeutic options, including information regarding the likelihood of benefit, the procedural morbidity, the risks of side effects, and the likely time to achieve relief. If these are acceptable to the patient, then further trials of standard therapies should be pursued. If the patient requires relief and either the procedural morbidity, the risks of adverse effects or the likely time to achieve relief are unacceptable, then refractoriness should be acknowledged and sedation should be offered.

These decisions are usually made by consensus between the clinicians, the patient and the patient's family. The process of this decision making is predicated on an understanding of the goals of care for the individual patient. These goals can generally be grouped into three broad categories: (i) prolonging survival, (ii) optimizing comfort (physical, psychological, and existential), and (iii) optimizing function. The processes of goal prioritization and informed decision making require candid discussion that clarifies the prevailing clinical predicament and presents the alternative therapeutic options. Other relevant considerations, including existential, ethical, religious, and familial concerns, may benefit from the participation of a religious counselor, social worker or clinical ethics specialist.

With the patient's consent, it is prudent to involve the family in these discussions. They suffer with the patient and will survive with the memories, pain and the potential for guilt at not having been effective advocates for their loved one: either because the patient died in unrelieved pain or remorseful that the patient may have been sedated when other options were not given a fair chance. If it is agreed that sedation is the most humane and appropriate way to control symptoms, it is advisable to ask the patient and family members if they have any specific goals that need to be met prior to starting sedation or if they would appreciate a chaplain/spiritual support prior to starting sedation.

Discussing sedation with the ancillary staff members

Involvement of ancillary staff such as social workers, primary care nurse, psychologist and other health professionals is a point that cannot be adequately emphasized. Just as cancer is a family illness, so is its management a team effort. Information about who the patient is comes from many sources; the patient and family will find support and connect with different personalities; team involvement allows support for its members, prevents burn-out and helps monitor counter-transference issues.[31]

Consent and 'do not resuscitate' status

Consent to the use of sedation acknowledges the primacy of comfort as the dominant goal of care. The initiation of CPR at the time of death is almost always futile in this situation,[33–35] and furthermore, is inconsistent with the agreed goals of care.[33,35] Sedating pharmacotherapy for refractory symptoms at the end of life should not be initiated until a discussion about CPR has taken place with the patient, or, if appropriate, with the patient's proxy, and there is agreement that CPR will not be initiated.

Drug selection

The published literature describing the use of sedation in the management of refractory symptoms at the end of life is anecdotal and refers to the use of opioids, neuroleptics, benzodiazepines, barbiturates, and propofol.

OPIOIDS

In the management of pain, an attempt is usually made to first escalate the opioid dose. Although some patients will benefit from this intervention, inadequate sedation, or the development of neuroexcitatory side effects, such as myoclonus or agitated delirium, often necessitate the addition of a second agent.[36–38]

MIDAZOLAM

In general midazolam is the most commonly used agent.[22,24,39–45] This benzodiazepine has a relatively short

half-life and therefore, for the purposes of palliative sedation, generally needs to be administered by continuous
infusion. The short half-life also allows for rapid dose titration. A subcutaneous or intravenous line can be used. A
starting dose of midazolam 1 mg/h by continuous infusion
is suggested. This dose may need to be titrated rapidly to
effect. In most cases, doses of between 1 mg/h and 7 mg/h
are required. Some suggest using a higher dose of sedative
initially to obtain sedation as soon as possible. Once deep
sedation is induced, the dose should be lowered until the
lowest effective dose to maintain sedation has been found.
Reassessment of the patient is required on a regular basis.
Rarely, benzodiazepine drugs can cause a paradoxical agitation, and an alternative strategy is required.

BARBITURATES

Greene[46] reported experience in the management of refractory physical symptoms using barbiturates alone among 17
imminently dying terminally ill patients suffering from
persistent physical symptoms. Amobarbital (9 cases) or
thiopental (8 cases) were used and adequate symptom
relief was achieved in all cases. The median survival of
these patients after initiation of the infusion was 23 hours
(range 2 hours to 4 days). Although most of the patients
maintained interactional function for a time, all patients
died in their sleep. This approach has been endorsed by
Truog et al.,[47] who also described the potential utility of
barbiturates for terminal agitation or terminal anguish.

METHOTRIMEPRAZINE

Methotrimeprazine is an antipsychotic phenothiazine
which can be administered orally or parenterally (intravenously [IV], subcutaneously [SC], or intramuscularly
[IM]). Parenterally, it is often used to provide sedation in
the management of refractory symptoms at the end of
life.[48,49] In addition to its sedative properties, it is also
moderately analgesic. Parenteral dosing is conventionally
started at 6.25 mg every 8 hours and every 1 hour prn for
breakthrough agitation. If necessary, the dose may be
increased to 12.5 mg or 25 mg every 8 hours and every
1 hour prn for breakthrough agitation. Orthostatic hypotension is a common adverse effect and this medication is best
avoided for ambulatory patients.

CHLORPROMAZINE

Chlorpromazine is an antipsychotic phenothiazine which
can be administered orally, parenterally (IV or IM), and
rectally. It has been used to provide sedation in the setting
of agitated delirium and refractory dyspnea at the end of
life.[50] In this published experience, the median rectal dose
was 25 mg every 4–12 hours and the median IV dose was
12.5 mg every 4–12 hours.[50] It is a relatively cost effective
option that can be easily used in the home.[51]

PROPOFOL

The published experience in the use of propofol for sedation in this setting is anecdotal.[42,52–55] In the rare event that
other agents have been unable to provide adequate relief its
anesthetic properties may be particularly useful to provide
sedation. Propofol is very similar to the short-acting barbiturates but it has a short duration of action and a rapid
onset. These characteristics make it relatively easy to
titrate.[53] In one report the patient was started on a loading
dose of 20 mg, followed by an infusion of 50–70 mg/h.[54]

Drug administration

The management of sedating pharmacotherapy for refractory symptoms in patients with advanced cancer demands a
high level of clinical vigilance. Irrespective of the agent
selected, administration initially requires dose titration to
achieve adequate relief, followed subsequently by provision
of ongoing therapy to ensure maintenance of effect. The
depth of sedation that is required to achieve adequate relief is
highly variable. In some situations, patients may require only
light sedation to achieve adequate relief, in other situations,
particularly at the end of life, deep sedation may be required.

Regular, 'around the clock' administration can be maintained by continuous infusion or intermittent bolus. The
route of administration can be IV, SC, or rectal. In some
situations drugs can be administered via a stoma or gastrostomy. In all cases, provision for emergency bolus therapy to manage breakthrough symptoms is recommended.

Patient monitoring

Once adequate relief is achieved the parameters for patient
monitoring and the role of further dose titration is determined by the goal of care:

- *When the goal of care is to ensure comfort until death for an
  imminently dying patient.* In this setting the only salient
  parameters for ongoing observation are those pertaining
  to comfort. Symptoms should be assessed until death;
  observations of pulse, blood pressure, and temperature
  do not contribute to the goals of care and can be
  discontinued. Respiratory rate is monitored primarily to
  ensure the absence of respiratory distress and tachypnea.
  Since downward titration of drug doses places the patient
  at risk for recurrent distress, in most instances it is not
  recommended even as the patient approaches death.
- *If the patient wishes to be less sedated and dying is not
  imminent.* In this context comfort, the level of sedation
  and routine physiological parameters such as heart rate
  blood pressure and oxygen saturation are monitored. In
  these cases, the drug should be administered by the lowest
  effective dose that provides adequate comfort. The depth
  of sedation necessary to control symptoms varies greatly.
  For some patients, a state of 'conscious sedation', in which

they retain the ability to respond to verbal stimuli, may provide adequate relief without total loss of interactive function.[22,41,45,46] Some authors have suggested that doses can be titrated down to reestablish lucidity after an agreed interval or for preplanned family interactions.[22,46,47] This, of course, is a potentially unstable situation, and the possibility that lucidity may not be promptly restored or that death may ensue as doses are again escalated should be explained to both the patient and family.

Nutrition and hydration when patients are sedated

Contrary to the assertions of Quill et al.[56,57] and Orentlicher et al.[58] the discontinuation of hydration and nutrition are *not* essential elements to the administration of sedation in the management of refractory symptoms at the end of life. While there is wide consensus that invasive forms of enteral or parenteral nutrition are not essential aspects of care for patients who lose the ability to eat and drink at the end of life,[59] no consensus exists regarding the withholding of hydration. Available data do not support the assertion that it is 'typical'[58] or essential to the approach of 'terminal sedation'.[56,60]

Opinions and practices vary. This variability reflects the heterogeneity of attitudes of the involved clinicians, ethicists, the patient, family and local norms of good clinical and ethical practice.[39] Individual patients, family members and clinicians may regard the continuation of hydration as a non-burdensome humane supportive intervention that represents (and may actually constitute) one means of reducing suffering.[60,61] Alternatively, hydration may be viewed as a superfluous impediment to inevitable death that does not contribute to patient comfort or the prevailing goals of care and that can be appropriately withdrawn.[62] Often, the patient will request relief of suffering and give no direction regarding supportive measures. In this circumstance the family and healthcare providers must reach consensus as to what constitutes a morally and personally acceptable approach based on the ethical principles of beneficence, nonmalfeasance, and respect for personhood.

In cases where there are religious or culturally based reservations regarding the discontinuation of nutritional support, it should be maintained unless there is evidence of direct patient harm by the intervention.

EMERGENCY SEDATION

The context

In some cases, patients who are in an immediately preterminal stage will present with overwhelming symptoms as they are dying. In these situations emergency decisions will need to be made without recourse to a case conference or even cross consultation. This may occur in the setting of a dying patient with sudden onset severe dyspnea,[63] agitated delirium,[64] massive bleeding, or pain. Care planning that anticipates potential emergencies and plans responses can help reduce the stress of emergency decision making in situations such as these.

Planning

Contingency plans for the management of catastrophic situations should be discussed with the patient and with family members. If the patient is at home, sedating medications should be prepared and a clear plan for emergency administration should be discussed. In situations in which family members or other carers at home feel that they would be unable to administer emergency medications, consideration should be given to inpatient care.

Administration

As in the previous scenario, midazolam is recommended as the drug of choice. Initial sedation can be achieved with a bolus of 2.5 mg SC/IV which can be repeated after 5 minutes if adequate sedation is not achieved. Once the patient is calm an SC or IV infusion can be used. In the patient who is in an immediately preterminal stage the only salient parameters for ongoing observation are those pertaining to comfort. Symptoms should be assessed until death; observations of pulse blood pressure and temperature are superfluous. Respiratory rate is monitored primarily to ensure the absence of respiratory distress and tachypnea.

RESPITE SEDATION

The context

In many instances, the notion of refractoriness is relative. Among patients who are not imminently dying, severe emotional and physical fatigue influence the patient's perception of the intolerability of symptoms or of further attempts to alleviate them. Since this may be a reversible phenomenon, sedation is often presented initially as a respite option to provide relief and rest, with a planned restoration of lucidity after an agreed interval. After such respite, some patients will be sufficiently rested to consider further trials of symptomatic therapy.[22]

Administration

There are critical differences in the monitoring of sedation in this setting. In addition to the level of sedation it is essential to monitor routine physiological parameters such as heart rate blood pressure and oxygen saturation. In these cases, the sedating agent should be administered by the lowest effective dose that provides adequate comfort. Despite all of these pre-cautions, sedation of this sort is a potentially unstable situation, and the possibility that lucidity may not be promptly restored or that death is among the risks involved, should be explained to both the patient and family.

SEDATION FOR PSYCHOLOGICAL OR EXISTENTIAL SUFFERING

The context

Patients approaching the end of life often suffer from existential issues including hopelessness, futility, meaninglessness, disappointment, remorse, death anxiety, and disruption of personal identity.[65–69] If life is perceived to offer, at best, comfort in the setting of fading potency or, at worst, ongoing physical and emotional distress as days pass slowly until death, anticipation of the future may be associated with feelings of hopelessness, futility, or meaninglessness such that the patient sees no value in continuing to live.[67,69–74] Death anxiety is common among cancer patients; surveys have shown that 50–80 percent of terminally ill patients have concerns or troubling thoughts about death, and that only a minority achieve an untroubled acceptance of death.[70,75,76] Together, these symptoms have been labeled a 'demoralization syndrome'.[77] In a Japanese report, 1 of 240 patients received sedation for the relief of severe existential distress alone, but a further 19 patients who received sedation for other symptoms described their lives as meaningless.[78]

Specific consideration in this situation

Sedation in the management of refractory psychological symptoms and existential diastases is different. By the nature of the symptoms being addressed it is much more difficult to establish that they are truly refractory: the severity of distress of some of these symptoms may be very dynamic and idiosyncratic, the standard treatments have low intrinsic morbidity and for some, like existential distress, there are no well established strategies. Additionally, the presence of these symptoms does not necessarily indicate a far advanced state of physiological deterioration. This factor, compounded with the observations that psychological distress and the desire for death may be very variable[74] and that psychological adaptation and coping is common,[79] cast doubt over the issue of proportionality.

The dilemma

These situations present a major dilemma insofar as it is neither desirable to subject patients with refractory psychological or existential suffering to protracted trials of therapies that provide inadequate relief, nor to sedate patients when viable alternatives remain unexplored. In this setting, as with physical symptoms, refractory psychological or existential distress must be distinguished from 'difficult' problems which have been resistant to relief thus far but which could potentially respond within a tolerable time-frame.

Published guidelines

Guidelines to assist in this situation have been published:[80–82]

- This approach should be reserved for patients in the advanced stages of a terminal illness with a documented 'do not resuscitate' order.
- The designation of such symptoms as refractory should only be done following a period of repeated assessment by clinicians skilled in psychological care who have established a relationship with the patient and his or her family along with trials of routine approaches for anxiety,[79] depression,[79] and existential distress[83–87].
- The evaluation should be made in the context of a case conference since individual clinician bias or burnout can influence decision making.[1,88,89]
- In the rare situations that this strategy is indeed appropriate and proportionate to the situation, it should be initiated on a respite basis with planned downward titration after a pre-agreed interval. It has been reported that respite sedation can break a cycle of anxiety, distress, and catastrophizing that precipitates requests of this kind. Only after repeated trials of respite sedation with intensive intermittent therapy should continuous sedation be considered.

ETHICAL CONSIDERATIONS

Sedation to relieve otherwise intolerable suffering for patients who are dying as normative practice

There is no distinct ethical problem in the use of sedation to relieve otherwise intolerable suffering for patients who are dying. Rather, the decision making and application of this therapeutic option represents a continuum of good clinical practice. Good clinical practice is predicated on careful patient evaluation (as previously described) which incorporates assessment of current goals of care. Since all medical treatments involve risks and benefits, each potential option must be evaluated for its potential to achieve the goals of care. Where risks of treatment are involved, the risks must be proportionate to the gravity of the clinical indication. In these deliberations, clinician considerations are guided by an understanding of the goals of care and must be within accepted medical guidelines of beneficence and nonmalfeasance. Finally, the penultimate decision to act on these considerations depends on informed consent or advanced directive of the patient. In this clinical context, the decision to offer the use of sedation to relieve intolerable suffering to terminally ill patients presents no new ethical problem.[88,90]

As with any other high risk clinical practice, potential for nonbeneficent abuse exists. Wein has described prerequisites to ensuring that sedation of imminently dying remains on an ethically sound footing:[31] appropriate patient selection; candor and consent; cross-consolation; documentation; knowledge of medications and illness; and a commitment to titrate and monitor. Despite the potential for shortening life, this approach has been endorsed as acceptable normative practice by legal precedent.[91] In the 1957 English case of *R v Adams*, Justice Devlin wrote in his judgment:

> If the first purpose of medicine, the restoration of health, can no longer be achieved, there is still much for a doctor to do, and he is entitled to do all that is proper and necessary to relieve pain and suffering, even if the measures he takes may incidentally shorten life.

He justified this approach rejecting the notion that this is a special defense, but rather by endorsing the clinical pragmatist approach that[92]

> The cause of death is the illness or the injury, and the proper medical treatment that is administered and that has an incidental effect on determining the exact moment of death is not the cause in any sensible use of the term.

This approach was lent further support by the recent decision of the Supreme Court of the United States that rejected a constitutional right that encompasses assisted suicide but endorsed the use of sedation as an extreme form of palliative care in the management of refractory symptoms at the end of life.[93]

Potential for abuse

Undoubtedly the use of sedation in the relief of symptoms at the end of life is potentially open to abuse. Indeed, some physicians administer doses of medication, ostensibly to relieve symptoms but with a covert intention of hastening the patient's death. Data from the Netherlands indicated that administration of sedating medication, ostensibly to relieve distress but with manifest intent of hastening death, is commonplace.[94,95] In a recent survey of Dutch physicians who had used sedation at the end of life, hastening of death was partly the intention of the physician in 47 percent (95% CI, 41 percent to 54 percent) of cases and the explicit intention in 17 percent (95% CI, 13 percent to 22 percent) of cases.[96] Research in Australia[97,98] and the USA[99,100] indicates that this practice is not uncommon. An Australian survey of 683 general surgeons found that 36 percent had given drugs in doses that they perceived to be greater than those required to relieve symptoms with the intention of hastening death.[101] Similar practices, albeit much less common, were reported in a survey of end-of-life care practices in six European countries.[102]

These duplicitous practices represent an unacceptable deviation from normative ethical clinical practice. Infrastructural guidelines are necessary to avoid deceitful practices of this kind.

Distinction from 'slow euthanasia'

Some authors argue that although sedation in the relief of uncontrolled symptoms may be justifiable, the concurrent discontinuation of nutrition and hydration does not contribute to patient comfort and almost certainly hastens death by starvation and dehydration. Consequently, they argue, sedation for the management of refractory symptoms is practically the same as 'slow euthanasia'.[61,103–105] This proposition is argued both by opponents to euthanasia, who are concerned about harmful aspects of the practice of forgoing nutrition and hydration,[61,103–106] and also by proponents of elective death who argue that if these acts are morally equivalent, then the more rapid mode of elective death, such as euthanasia or assisted suicide, is more humane and dignified.[56,57]

Another concern is that since sedation may hasten the death of the patient, the plea of no moral responsibility for foreseen, inevitable untoward outcomes is at best, spurious, or at worst dishonest.[107] This relates to the so called 'doctrine of double effect' which will be discussed in the subsequent section. While we absolutely reject the appropriateness of the term 'slow euthanasia' we feel that it important to address this charge.

With regard to the first concern, it is important to reassert that, contrary to the assertions of Quill[56,57] and Orentlicher,[58] the discontinuation of hydration and nutrition is *not* an essential element to the administration of sedation in the management of refractory symptoms (see Ethical issues regarding nutrition and hydration below). Furthermore, there are no data to support the assertion that it is 'typical'.[108] We hold that sedation in the management of refractory symptoms is distinct from euthanasia insofar as:

- the intent of the intervention is to provide symptom relief not to end the life of the suffering patient
- the intervention is proportionate to the prevailing symptom, its severity and the prevailing goals of care
- finally, and most importantly, unlike euthanasia or assisted suicide, the death of the patient is not a criterion for the success of the treatment.

Distinction from euthanasia

Euthanasia refers to the deliberate termination of the life of a patient by active intervention, at the request of the patient in the setting of otherwise uncontrolled suffering. This is distinct from physician-assisted suicide, where the physician provides the means of suicide and instruction to a patient to facilitate successful suicide. The use of sedation to relieve otherwise unendurable symptoms at the end of life falls under the rubric of 'the provision of a potentially lethal medication for a patient with a narrow therapeutic index'. Clearly this situation may result in the inadvertent foreshortening of the patient's life either by direct action of the drug or as an adverse effect (such as aspiration). The use of sedation in this setting is critically distinct from euthanasia for three fundamental reasons: first, the intent of the intervention is to provide symptom relief, secondly the intervention is proportionate to the prevailing symptom, its severity and the prevailing goals of care and, finally, and most importantly, the death of the patient is not a criterion for the success of the treatment.

The doctrine of double effect

In cases where a contemplated action has both good effects and bad effects the doctrine provides an approach to answer the question: Do the means justify the end? According to 'double effect ethics', an action is permissible if it is not wrong in itself and it does not require that one directly intends the bad result. Double effect ethics assumes the integrity of the physician and unambiguous intent and motive. Classically five criteria have been described to evaluate the validity of a double effect claim:[109]

- The action is either morally good or is morally neutral.
- The undesired yet foreseen untoward result is not directly intended.
- The good effect is not a direct result of the foreseen untoward effect.
- The good effect is 'proportionate to' the untoward effect.
- There is no other way to achieve the desired ends without the untoward effect.

The 'doctrine of double effect' is problematic insofar as it does not always apply to the use of sedation in the management of refractory symptoms. When sedation is used to relieve otherwise refractory pain and suffering at the end of life, the intention is to relieve otherwise unendurable suffering. The untoward consequences that are foreseen include the possibility of foreshortened survival and the definite loss of interactional function. Since the death of the patient at the end of a long and difficult illness is not always perceived as untoward, there is a significant problem with the application of the double-effect justification. Indeed, in Jewish tradition, there is a blessing for a 'timely' death, *Baruch Dayan Ha Emet* (Blessed is the Supreme Judge). Thus, to call the potential for foreshortened survival a 'bad outcome' may, in some cases, be inaccurate (at best) or dishonest (at worst).

Since the moral justification of sedation by double effect requires that clinicians make unequivocal claims regarding the undesirability of the possibility of the patient's death, it is often inappropriate.[107] Indeed, it undermines the essential element of clinician credibility. This view regarding the 'double effect' justification for the use of sedation is supported by other critics who have claimed that, at worst it has become a meaningless mantra recited by cynical surreptitious practitioners of euthanasia cloaked as palliative care clinicians.[105]

It is prudent and appropriate to emphasize that there is no clear evidence that the use of sedation in the relief of refractory symptoms at the end of life foreshortens survival. Three studies have addressed this issue in the setting of hospice care.[23,25,110] Three other studies have addressed this issue on the management of patients with terminal dyspnea after withdrawal of mechanical ventilation.[111–113] In the latter setting, the studies found no correlation between level of sedation, dose of sedatives, and duration of survival until death.

Ethical issues regarding nutrition and hydration when patients are sedated

Although sedation is clearly beneficent in terms of providing relief of otherwise intolerable suffering, the beneficence of withdrawal of nutrition and hydration in the already sedated and comfortable patient is not self-evident, and indeed it may be perceived as harmful. This debate has both medical and ethical dimensions.

Medically, there are few data to support the clinical benefit of hydration or artificial nutrition in the imminently dying, or to suggest that it prolongs life or contributes to comfort.[114–116] Ethically, the withdrawal of potentially death deferring treatments (such as hydration) among dying patients is, for some, controversial.[60,61] For reasons of clarity, the issue of sedation must be distinguished from the distinct and separate issue of hydration.

Opinions and practices vary. This variability reflects the heterogeneity of attitudes of the involved clinicians, ethicists, the patient, family and local norms of good clinical and ethical practice.[39] Individual patient's, family members, and clinicians may regard the continuation of hydration as a non-burdensome humane supportive intervention that represents (and may actually constitute) one means of reducing suffering.[60,61] Alternatively, hydration may be viewed as a superfluous impediment to inevitable death, that does not contribute to patient comfort or the prevailing goals of care and that can be appropriately withdrawn.[62] Often, the patient will request relief of suffering and give no direction regarding supportive measures. In this circumstance the family and healthcare providers must reach consensus as to what constitutes a morally and personally acceptable approach based on the ethical principles of beneficence, nonmalfeasance, and respect for personhood.

In cases where there are religious or culturally based reservations regarding the discontinuation of nutritional support, it should be maintained unless there is evidence of direct patient harm by the intervention.

CONCLUSIONS

Sedation is a critically important therapeutic tool of last resort. It enables the clinician to provide relief from intolerable distress when other options are not adequately effective. Because sedation undermines the capacity to interact, it must be used judiciously. Clear indications and guidelines for use are necessary to prevent abuse of this approach to facilitate the deliberate killing of patients, which while benevolently intended, may have untoward sociological and ethical consequences for palliative care clinicians and the image of palliative medicine as a profession.

Key learning points

- At the end of life, all patients have the right to the adequate relief of physical symptoms.

- There is need to ensure that appropriate infrastructural measures are addressed to enhance the likelihood that this right will be fulfilled.

- Symptoms at the end of life must be assessed.

- The adequacy of symptom relief is determined by the patient.

- Inadequately received symptoms in dying patients must be relieved to the patient's satisfaction.

- Symptoms that are difficult to control must be evaluated by clinicians expert in symptom control at the end of life.

- When a symptom is refractory to normal palliative approaches, and only sedation can provide the needed relief, this should be available to patients (with appropriate infrastructural guidelines to prevent the inappropriate application of this approach).

REFERENCES

● ◆ ✱ 1   Cherny NI, Portenoy RK. Sedation in the management of refractory symptoms: guidelines for evaluation and treatment. *J Palliat Care* 1994; **10**: 31–8.

2   del Rosario MA, Martin AS, Ortega JJ, Feria M. Temporary sedation with midazolam for control of severe incident pain. *J Pain Symptom Manage* 2001; **21**: 439–42.

3   Rousseau PC. Palliative sedation. *Am J Hosp Palliat Care* 2002; **19**: 295–7.

4   Jackson WC. Palliative sedation vs. terminal sedation: what's in a name? *Am J Hosp Palliat Care* 2002; **19**: 81–2.

5   Beel A, McClement SE, Harlos M. Palliative sedation therapy: a review of definitions and usage. *Int J Palliat Nurs* 2002; **8**: 190–9.

◆ 6   Cowan JD, Walsh D. Terminal sedation in palliative medicine – definition and review of the literature. *Support Care Cancer* 2001; **9**: 403–7.

7   Mercadante S. Pain treatment and outcomes for patients with advanced cancer who receive follow-up care at home [see comments]. *Cancer* 1999; **85**: 1849–58.

8   Salisbury C, Bosanquet N, Wilkinson EK, *et al.* The impact of different models of specialist palliative care on patients' quality of life: a systematic literature review. *Palliat Med* 1999; **13**: 3–17.

9   Higginson IJ, Wade AM, McCarthy M. Effectiveness of two palliative support teams. *J Public Health Med* 1992; **14**: 50–6.

10   Higginson IJ, McGregor AM. The impact of palliative medicine? [editorial]. *Palliat Med* 1999; **13**: 285–98.

11   Peruselli C, Di Giulio P, Toscani F, *et al.* Home palliative care for terminal cancer patients: a survey on the final week of life. *Palliat Med* 1999; **13**: 233–41.

12   Higginson IJ, Hearn J. A multicenter evaluation of cancer pain control by palliative care teams. *J Pain Symptom Manage* 1997; **14**: 29–35.

13   Conill C, Verger E, Henriquez I, *et al.* Symptom prevalence in the last week of life. *J Pain Symptom Manage* 1997; **14**: 328–31.

14   Storey P. Symptom control in advanced cancer. *Semin Oncol* 1994; **21**: 748–53.

15   Lichter I, Hunt E. The last 48 hours of life. *J Palliat Care* 1990; **6**: 7–15.

16   Johanson GA. Symptom character and prevalence during cancer patients' last days of life. *Am J Hosp Palliat Care* 1991; **8**: 6–8, 18.

17   Enck RE. Drug-induced terminal sedation for symptom control. *Am J Hosp Palliat Care* 1991; **8**: 3–5.

18   Roy DJ. Need they sleep before they die? *J Palliat Care* 1990; **6**: 3–4.

● 19   Ventafridda V, Ripamonti C, De Conno F, *et al.* Symptom prevalence and control during cancer patients' last days of life. *J Palliat Care* 1990; **6**: 7–11.

20   Mount B. A final crescendo of pain? *J Palliat Care* 1990; **6**: 5–6.

21   Fainsinger R, Miller MJ, Bruera E, *et al.* Symptom control during the last week of life on a palliative care unit. *J Palliat Care* 1991; **7**: 5–11.

22   Morita T, Inoue S, Chihara S. Sedation for symptom control in Japan: the importance of intermittent use and communication with family members. *J Pain Symptom Manage* 1996; **12**: 32–8.

23   Stone P, Phillips C, Spruyt O, Waight C. A comparison of the use of sedatives in a hospital support team and in a hospice. *Palliat Med* 1997; **11**: 140–4.

24   Fainsinger RL, Landman W, Hoskings M, Bruera E. Sedation for uncontrolled symptoms in a South African hospice. *J Pain Symptom Manage* 1998; **16**: 145–52.

25   Chiu TY, Hu WY, Lue BH, *et al.* Sedation for refractory symptoms of terminal cancer patients in Taiwan. *J Pain Symptom Manage* 2001; **21**: 467–72.

26   Muller-Busch HC, Andres I, Jehser T. Sedation in palliative care – a critical analysis of 7 years experience. *BMC Palliat Care* 2003; **2**: 2.

27   Morita T. Differences in physician-reported practice in palliative sedation therapy. *Support Care Cancer* 2004; **12**: 584–92.

28   Coyle N. The last four weeks of life. *Am J Nurs* 1990; **90**: 75–6, 78.

29   Feldman HA, McKinlay JB, Potter DA, *et al.* Nonmedical influences on medical decision making: an experimental technique using videotapes, factorial design, and survey sampling. *Health Serv Res* 1997; **32**: 343–66.

30   Christakis NA, Asch DA. Biases in how physicians choose to withdraw life support. *Lancet* 1993; **342**: 642–6.

◆ ✳ 31   Wein S. Sedation in the imminently dying patient. *Oncology (Huntingt)* 2000; **14**: 585–92; discussion 592, 597–8, 601.

✳ 32   Braun TC, Hagen NA, Clark T. Development of a clinical practice guideline for palliative sedation. *J Palliat Med* 2003; **6**: 345–50.

33   Haines IE, Zalcberg J, Buchanan JD. Not-for-resuscitation orders in cancer patients – principles of decision-making. *Med J Aust* 1990; **153**: 225–9.

34   Rosner F, Kark PR, Bennett AJ, *et al.* Medical futility. Committee on Bioethical Issues of the Medical Society of the State of New York. *N Y State J Med* 1992; **92**: 485–8.

35   Marik PE, Zaloga GP. CPR in terminally ill patients? *Resuscitation* 2001; **49**: 99–103.

36   Portenoy RK. Continuous intravenous infusion of opioid drugs. *Med Clin North Am* 1987; **71**: 233–41.

37   Potter JM, Reid DB, Shaw RJ, *et al.* Myoclonus associated with treatment with high doses of morphine: the role of supplemental drugs [see comments]. *BMJ* 1989; **299**: 150–3.

38   Dunlop RJ. Excitatory phenomena associated with high dose opioids. *Curr Ther* 1989; **30**: 121–3.

39   Chater S, Viola R, Paterson J, Jarvis V. Sedation for intractable distress in the dying – a survey of experts. *Palliat Med* 1998; **12**: 255–69.

40   Nordt SP, Clark RF. Midazolam: a review of therapeutic uses and toxicity. *J Emerg Med* 1997; **15**: 357–65.

41   Burke AL. Palliative care: an update on 'terminal restlessness'. *Med J Aust* 1997; **166**: 39–42.

42   Collins P. Prolonged sedation with midazolam or propofol [letter; comment]. *Crit Care Med* 1997; **25**: 556–7.

43   Johanson GA. Midazolam in terminal care. *Am J Hosp Palliat Care* 1993; **10**: 13–14.

44   Power D, Kearney M. Management of the final 24 hours. *Ir Med J* 1992; **85**: 93–5.

45   Burke AL, Diamond PL, Hulbert J, *et al.* Terminal restlessness – its management and the role of midazolam [see comments]. *Med J Aust* 1991; **155**: 485–7.

46   Greene WR, Davis WH. Titrated intravenous barbiturates in the control of symptoms in patients with terminal cancer. *South Med J* 1991; **84**: 332–7.

● 47   Truog RD, Berde CB, Mitchell C, Grier HE. Barbiturates in the care of the terminally ill. *N Engl J Med* 1992; **327**: 1678–82.

48   Oliver DJ. The use of methotrimeprazine in terminal care. *Br J Clin Pract* 1985; **39**: 339–40.

49   O'Neill J, Fountain A. Levomepromazine (methotrimeprazine) and the last 48 hours. *Hosp Med* 1999; **60**: 568–70.

50   McIver B, Walsh D, Nelson K. The use of chlorpromazine for symptom control in dying cancer patients. *J Pain Symptom Manage* 1994; **9**: 341–5.

51   LeGrand SB. Dyspnea: the continuing challenge of palliative management. *Curr Opin Oncol* 2002; **14**: 394–8.

52   Tobias JD. Propofol sedation for terminal care in a pediatric patient. *Clin Pediatr (Phila)* 1997; **36**: 291–3.

53   Krakauer EL, Penson RT, Truog RD, King LA, Chabner BA, Lynch TJ, Jr. Sedation for intractable distress of a dying patient: acute palliative care and the principle of double effect. *Oncologist* 2000; **5**: 53–62.

54   Mercadante S, De Conno F, Ripamonti C. Propofol in terminal care. *J Pain Symptom Manage* 1995; **10**: 639–42.

55   Moyle J. The use of propofol in palliative medicine. *J Pain Symptom Manage* 1995; **10**: 643–6.

56   Quill TE, Lo B, Brock DW. Palliative options of last resort: a comparison of voluntarily stopping eating and drinking, terminal sedation, physician-assisted suicide, and voluntary active euthanasia. *JAMA* 1997; **278**: 2099–104.

◆ 57   Quill TE, Byock IR. Responding to intractable terminal suffering: the role of terminal sedation and voluntary refusal of food and fluids. ACP-ASIM End-of-Life Care Consensus Panel. American College of Physicians-American Society of Internal Medicine. *Ann Intern Med* 2000; **132**: 408–14.

58   Orentlicher D, Caplan A. The Pain Relief Promotion Act of 1999: a serious threat to palliative care. *J Am Acad Psychiatry Law* 1999; **27**: 527–39; discussion 540–5.

59   Bozzetti F, Amadori D, Bruera E, *et al.* Guidelines on artificial nutrition versus hydration in terminal cancer patients. European Association for Palliative Care. *Nutrition* 1996; **12**: 163–7.

60   Jansen LA, Sulmasy DP. Sedation, alimentation, hydration, and equivocation: careful conversation about care at the end of life. *Ann Intern Med* 2002; **136**: 845–9.

61   Craig GM. On withholding artificial hydration and nutrition from terminally ill sedated patients. The debate continues [published erratum appears in *J Med Ethics* 1996; **22**: 361]. *J Med Ethics* 1996; **22**: 147–53.

62   Ashby M, Stoffell B. Artificial hydration and alimentation at the end of life: a reply to Craig. *J Med Ethics* 1995; **21**: 135–40.

63   Campbell ML. Terminal dyspnea and respiratory distress. *Crit Care Clin* 2004; **20**: 403–17, viii–ix.

64   Kress JP, Hall JB. Delirium and sedation. *Crit Care Clin* 2004; **20**: 419–33, ix.

65   Cassell EJ. The nature of suffering and the goals of medicine. *N Engl J Med* 1982; **306**: 639–45.

66   Moberg DO, Brusek PM. Spiritual well-being: a neglected subject in quality of life research. *Soc Indicators Res* 1978; **5**: 303–23.

67   Yalom ID. *Existential Psychotherapy*. New York: Basic Books, 1980.

68   Kissane DW. Psychospiritual and existential distress. The challenge for palliative care. *Aust Fam Physician* 2000; **29**: 1022–5.

69   Ellis JB, Smith PC. Spiritual well-being, social desirability and reasons for living: is there a connection? *Int J Soc Psychiatry* 1991; **37**: 57–63.

70   Bolmsjo I. Existential issues in palliative care – interviews with cancer patients. *J Palliat Care* 2000; **16**: 20–4.

71   Breitbart W, Rosenfeld B, Pessin H, *et al.* Depression, hopelessness, and desire for hastened death in terminally ill patients with cancer. *JAMA* 2000; **284**: 2907–11.

72   Breitbart W, Rosenfeld BD. Physician-assisted suicide: the influence of psychosocial issues. *Cancer Causes Control* 1999; **6**: 146–61.

73   Chochinov HM, Tataryn D, Clinch JJ, Dudgeon D. Will to live in the terminally ill. *Lancet* 1999; **354**: 816–19.

74   Chochinov HM, Wilson KG, Enns M, *et al.* Desire for death in the terminally ill. *Am J Psychiatry* 1995; **152**: 1185–91.

75   Neubauer BJ, Lai JY. Death anxiety and attitudes toward hospice care. *Psychol Rep* 1988; **63**: 195–8.

76   Stedeford A. Couples facing death. I–Psychosocial aspects. *Br Med J (Clin Res Ed)* 1981; **283**: 1033–6.

77 Kissane DW, Clarke DM, Street AF. Demoralization syndrome – a relevant psychiatric diagnosis for palliative care. *J Palliat Care* 2001; **17**: 12–21.

78 Morita T, Tsunoda J, Inoue S, Chihara S. Terminal sedation for existential distress. *Am J Hosp Palliat Care* 2000; **17**: 189–95.

79 Breitbart W, Chochinov HM, Passik SD. Psychiatric aspects of palliative care. In: Doyle D, Hanks GW, MacDonald N, eds. *Oxford Textbook of Palliative Medicine*, 2nd ed. Oxford: Oxford University Press, 1998: 933–54.

∗ 80 Cherny NI. Commentary: sedation in response to refractory existential distress: walking the fine line. *J Pain Symptom Manage* 1998; **16**: 404–6.

∗ 81 Rousseau P. Existential suffering and palliative sedation: a brief commentary with a proposal for clinical guidelines. *Am J Hosp Palliat Care* 2001; **18**: 151–3.

82 Rousseau P. Careful conversation about care at the end of life. *Ann Intern Med* 2002; **137**: 1008–10; author reply 1008–10.

83 Kissane DW, Bloch S, Miach P, *et al.* Cognitive-existential group therapy for patients with primary breast cancer – techniques and themes. *Psychooncology* 1997; **6**: 25–33.

84 Georgesen J, Dungan JM. Managing spiritual distress in patients with advanced cancer pain. *Cancer Nurs* 1996; **19**: 376–83.

85 Millison MB. Spirituality and the caregiver. Developing an underutilized facet of care. *Am J Hosp Care* 1988; **5**: 37–44.

86 Stepnick A, Perry T. Preventing spiritual distress in the dying client. *J Psychosoc Nurs Ment Health Serv* 1992; **30**: 17–24.

87 Speck PW. Spiritual issues in palliative care. In: Doyle D, Hanks GW, MacDonald N, eds. *Oxford Textbook of Palliative Medicine*, 2nd ed. Oxford: Oxford University Press, 1998: 804–14.

88 Fins JJ, Bacchetta MD, Miller FG. Clinical pragmatism: A method of moral problem solving. *Kennedy Inst Ethics J* 1997; **7**: 129–45. 1997; **7**: 129–45.

∗ 89 Cherny NI, Coyle N, Foley KM. The treatment of suffering when patients request elective death. *J Palliat Care* 1994; **10**: 71–9.

90 Miller FG, Fins JJ, Bacchetta MD. Clinical pragmatism: John Dewey and clinical ethics. *J Contemp Health Law Policy* 1996; **13**: 27–51.

91 Gevers S. Terminal sedation: a legal approach. *Eur J Health Law* 2003; **10**: 359–67.

92 Devlin P. *Easing the Passing*. London: Bodley Head, 1985.

◆ 93 Burt RA. The Supreme Court speaks – not assisted suicide but a constitutional right to palliative care. *N Engl J Med* 1997; **337**: 1234–6.

94 van der Maas PJ, van Delden JJ, Pijnenborg L. Euthanasia and other medical decisions concerning the end of life. An investigation performed upon request of the Commission of Inquiry into the Medical Practice concerning Euthanasia. *Health Policy* 1992; **21**: vi–x, 1–262.

95 van der Maas PJ, van der Wal G, Haverkate I, *et al.* Euthanasia, physician-assisted suicide, and other medical practices involving the end of life in the Netherlands, 1990–1995. *N Engl J Med* 1996; **335**: 1699–705.

96 Rietjens JA, van der Heide A, Vrakking AM, *et al.* Physician reports of terminal sedation without hydration or nutrition for patients nearing death in the Netherlands. *Ann Intern Med* 2004; **141**: 178–85.

97 Kuhse H, Singer P, Baume P, Clark M, Rickard M. End-of-life decisions in Australian medical practice. *Med J Aust* 1997; **166**: 191–6.

98 Stevens CA, Hassan R. Management of death, dying and euthanasia: attitudes and practices of medical practitioners in South Australia. *Arch Intern Med* 1994; **154**: 575–84.

99 Willems DL, Daniels ER, van der Wal G, *et al.* Attitudes and practices concerning the end of life: a comparison between physicians from the United States and from The Netherlands [In Process Citation]. *Arch Intern Med* 2000; **160**: 63–8.

100 Meier DE, Emmons CA, Wallenstein S, *et al.* A national survey of physician-assisted suicide and euthanasia in the United States [see comments]. *N Engl J Med* 1998; **338**: 1193–201.

101 Douglas CD, Kerridge IH, Rainbird KJ, *et al.* The intention to hasten death: a survey of attitudes and practices of surgeons in Australia. *Med J Aust* 2001; **175**: 511–15.

102 van der Heide A, Deliens L, Faisst K, *et al.* End-of-life decision-making in six European countries: descriptive study. *Lancet* 2003; **362**: 345–50.

103 Craig GM. On withholding nutrition and hydration in the terminally ill: has palliative medicine gone too far? *J Med Ethics* 1994; **20**: 139–43; discussion 144–5.

104 Craig G. Is sedation without hydration or nourishment in terminal care lawful? *Med Leg J* 1994; **62**(Pt 4): 198–201.

105 Orentlicher D. The Supreme Court and physician-assisted suicide – rejecting assisted suicide but embracing euthanasia. *N Engl J Med* 1997; **337**: 1236–9.

106 Brody H. Causing, intending, and assisting death. *J Clin Ethics* 1993; **4**: 112–17.

107 Quill TE, Dresser R, Brock DW. The rule of double effect – a critique of its role in end-of-life decision making. *N Engl J Med* 1997; **337**: 1768–71.

108 Sulmasy DP, Ury WA, Ahronheim JC, *et al.* Palliative treatment of last resort and assisted suicide. *Ann Intern Med* 2000; **133**: 562–3.

109 Boyle J. Medical ethics and double effect: the case of terminal sedation. *Theor Med Bioeth* 2004; **25**: 51–60.

110 Sykes N, Thorns A. Sedative use in the last week of life and the implications for end-of-life decision making. *Arch Intern Med* 2003; **163**: 341–4.

111 Daly BJ, Thomas D, Dyer MA. Procedures used in withdrawal of mechanical ventilation [see comments]. *Am J Crit Care* 1996; **5**: 331–8.

112 Campbell ML, Bizek KS, Thill M. Patient responses during rapid terminal weaning from mechanical ventilation: a prospective study [see comments]. *Crit Care Med* 1999; **27**: 73–7.

113 Wilson WC, Smedira NG, Fink C, *et al.* Ordering and administration of sedatives and analgesics during the withholding and withdrawal of life support from critically ill patients [see comments]. *JAMA* 1992; **267**: 949–53.

114 Ahronheim JC. Nutrition and hydration in the terminal patient. *Clin Geriatr Med* 1996; **12**: 379–91.

115 Barber MD, Fearon KC, Delmore G, Loprinzi CL. Should cancer patients with incurable disease receive parenteral or enteral nutritional support? *Eur J Cancer* 1998; **34**: 279–85.

116 Koshuta MA, Schmitz PJ, Lynn J. Development of an institutional policy on artificial hydration and nutrition. *Kennedy Inst Ethics J* 1991; **1**: 133–9; discussion 139–40.

PART 16

Interdisciplinary issues

104

Physical and occupational therapy in palliative care

PAMELA R MASSEY, EILEEN S DONOVAN

Against our confidence in mastery and control, we need to remember that old age and dying are not problems to be solved but human experiences that must be faced. In the years ahead, we will be judged as a people by our willingness to stand by one another, not only in the rare event of natural disaster but also in the everyday care of those who gave us life and to whom we owe so much.

We [must] emphasize ... the singular importance of seeking to serve the life the patient still has...

Leon R Kass (2005)[1]

INTRODUCTION

With the current overall survival rate at 50 percent, cancer is now a chronic disease and joins the ranks of the other major chronic conditions (cardiovascular disease, lung disease, and dementia) that account for end of life.[2] According to the President's Council on Bioethics report, 'the most common trajectory toward death (in the United States) ... is a lengthy period of debility, frailty and dementia lasting not months but years.'[3] Treatment for any of these life-threatening diseases, especially in those who are elderly, results in a variety of medical problems, complex functional changes, and significantly compromised quality of life.[4-6] People with cancer and other serious illnesses need comprehensive care designed to relieve symptoms of pain, fatigue, and weakness during all phases of their disease including pretreatment, treatment, post treatment, recurrence, and end-of-life phases.[7] To provide that level of comprehensive care requires a team of health professionals who can address both curative care and palliative care issues regardless of where the patient is on the life–death continuum. However, the World Health Organization (WHO) has recognized that it is unrealistic to expect that the emerging needs for palliative care can be met by just expending the workforce of specialists in palliative care. WHO suggests that expanding the knowledge and skills of health professionals in general is the answer to addressing the increasing healthcare needs as individuals live longer.[8] The key to increasing the numbers of health professionals who can improve function and quality of life for seriously ill people and their families is to enhance the awareness and skills of physical therapists and occupational therapists so they feel confident in working with palliative patients and their families.

The roles that physical and occupational therapy play in comprehensive healthcare fit naturally into a palliative care model. Both physical and occupational therapy are professions that are dedicated to the maximization of a person's functional abilities to allow that person to perform tasks and roles that are important to them. Although both professions have somewhat different approaches to the achievement of their mission, there is considerable overlap and collaboration between the two disciplines is common. As defined by the World Federation of Occupational Therapists (WFOT), 'the primary role of occupational therapy is to enable people to participate in the activities of everyday life and occupational therapists do so by enabling people to do things that will enhance their ability to participate or by modifying the environment to better support participation.'[9] The World Confederation for Physical Therapy

(WCPT) has identified a number of roles for physical therapists including:

- preventing disability and deformity
- educating/training disabled people to move around
- promoting self-care
- education, training, and transferring skills to other local staff and families
- acting as an expert resource.[10]

While physical therapy and occupational therapy are traditionally viewed as rehabilitation interventions, providing rehabilitation services for terminally ill patients is not a new concept. In 1969, Dietz described categories of rehabilitation services of benefit to persons with cancer as restorative, supportive, and palliative. Dietz defined the palliative setting as one in which there is increasing disability to be expected from progressing disease with an associated decrease in functional capacity, but where appropriate provision of treatment would eliminate some of the anticipated complications (i.e. bedsores, contracture, problems in personal hygiene, and emotional deterioration secondary to inactivity and depression).[11] The benefits of physiotherapy in palliative care were recognized in the UK in 1978. Shank described the physiotherapist's role in *relief of discomfort and pain* through the use of massage, exercise, supportive positioning, splinting, and chest physiotherapy and in *maintenance/improvement in function* with assistive devices, exercise, and retraining. She concluded that the retention of an element of independence could provide the patient with valuable hope

and reduced anxiety.[12] Physical therapists in the USA had historically provided terminally ill patients with therapeutic measures such as massage, heat and hydrotherapy. However, with the inception of the hospice movement, physical therapists took on the additional roles of educator to patient, family and other health professionals, as well as becoming a functioning member of the patient treatment team.[13] About the same time occupational therapists advocated that good end-of-life care included not only the management of symptoms but also the assistance to make the best of every day. In 1983, Tigges and Sherman described the role of occupational therapists in fostering hospice patients' independence in occupational roles of self-care, work and leisure as important interventions in coping with feelings of isolation and loss of independence (Box 104.1).[14]

WHEN TO MAKE REFERRALS

It is well recognized in developed nations that people are living longer and the types of disease they are dying from are chronic diseases that are often associated with musculoskeletal disorders and disabilities. Heart disease, stroke, pulmonary failure, and cancer are recognized as the main causes of death, but comorbid conditions such as arthritis, dementia, and osteoporosis are also contributing to increased disability and the need for additional care.[15] In a study published in the *Journal of the American Medical Association* clinicians examined the patterns of functional decline at end of life for four types of illness trajectories (cancer death, organ failure death, sudden death, and frailty) and concluded that; 'End of life care must also serve those who become increasingly frail even without a life threatening illness'.[16]* Additionally, research from WHO indicates that palliative care interventions such as good pain relief, communication, information, and coordinated care from skilled professionals are effective in reducing symptoms and suffering, and that these experiences do not differ widely by disease or across countries.[15] The decision of when to begin physical and occupational therapy for the palliative care patient is often based upon the need to manage symptoms early in the course of the disease, reduce the burden on caregivers, or improve the quality of life of the patient.

Early referrals for symptom management

The use of palliative care interventions is applicable early in the course of an illness (not just at the end-of-life stage) to manage distressing clinical complications. Physicians may not consider the benefit of physical and occupational therapy early in the course of cancer, cardiovascular or respiratory diseases; but preventive interventions offered by these rehabilitation specialists may prevent pain and functional loss during the end-of-life phase of these diseases. Gerber

---

Box 104.1 Role of physical/occupational therapy in palliative care

- Help patient/caregivers determine which activities and roles they can realistically perform

- Enable the patient to take an active part in establishing goals and treatment priorities

- Apply physical/occupational therapy interventions to minimize symptoms and optimize functional abilities

- Assist the patient to find meaning with their available range of activity and occupation considering the interplay between physical, psychological, social, and vocational domains of function

- Instruct patient and caregivers regarding methods to maximize function within limits of energy, safety, and capabilities

- Enhance quality of life at the end of life for the patient and their family

noted that referrals to rehabilitation professionals for cancer patients usually target either specific impairments at anatomical level (i.e. loss of range of motion or lymphedema) or problems with mobility. However, she recommends earlier referrals to prevent predictable problems associated with medical treatment, such as skin care and exercise to manage connective tissue side effects from radiation.[7]

Multiple studies have demonstrated that the benefits of exercise include improvement in mood, sleep patterns, fitness, lipid profile, strength, functional activity, fatigue and pain levels.[7] Exercise can prevent loss of strength and functional abilities often associated with lack of activity or disuse in the cancer population.[17***] In a study of 155 androgen-deprived patients with prostate cancer, resistive exercise was effective in reducing fatigue and improving fitness and health-related quality of life.[18**] Even in the bone marrow transplant populations, Demeo has shown that exercises can be done safely immediately following high-dose chemotherapy and can effectively reduce fatigue, maintain physical performance and improve hemoglobin levels.[19*,20**,21*]

Reduce burden of caregivers

The delivery of rehabilitation services by physical and occupational therapists within a palliative care framework is appropriate in all healthcare settings including hospitals, outpatient, community, home and special palliative units.[22] Lynn observed 'Living with serious illness through to death can be an extraordinarily important phase of life for patient and loved ones, but only if the dying person is comfortable, assured of the resources needed for daily living, and respected.'[23] However, as noted in the Rand White Paper 'Living well at the end of life', the current US model, including hospice, does not serve the seriously ill populations well; addressing the healthcare delivery systems is critical to meeting the needs of these individuals and their families.[2] The number of therapists involved in palliative care in the USA is growing but is still not sufficient to meet the increased demand. Likewise, the WHO acknowledges that some developed countries conduct rehabilitation programs in nursing homes (the Netherlands and USA), but in most countries the provision of quality end-of-life care is hampered by shortages of staff with palliative care skills.[15]

In most countries, older people live at home despite their gradual functional decline. With aging populations and an associated decline in numbers of younger people to function as caregivers, the strain on older caregivers (i.e. family members) is increased. Although palliative care is often preferred to 'medical care' by patients at end of life, healthcare systems often do not provide palliative or comfort care and funding for end-of-life care is usually limited. This places further burdens on families.

An analysis of relevant studies by WHO indicates that most people (75 percent) would prefer to die at home and would prefer home care at the end of life.[15] In a study of 340 seriously ill patients, items that were consistently rated as very important at end of life by more than 70 percent of the patients included the desire not to be a burden to family and to society.[24*] However, maintaining the individual in the home setting can place extraordinary burdens on the caregiver who is usually a family member. Care at home, which can include carrying out activities of daily living such a bathing, dressing, and toileting, involves a level of intimacy and degree of physical effort often not anticipated by family members. 'Long term care for seriously ill relatives is unpaid and unsupported work that may damage the health, wellbeing and financial security of caregivers themselves'.[15] Physical and occupational therapists can teach caregivers how to provide this intimate care, how to move and assist the patient in a safe manner, and how to modify the home environment to minimize these burdens.

Improve quality of life for the person

Quality of life has different meanings for different persons. For the measurement of quality of life to be considered valid, the definition of quality of life must be determined by what the individual identifies it to be at a given point in time.[25] Calman proposed a model for assessment of quality of life in which it is defined as the difference (at a particular period in time) between the hopes and expectations of the individual and their present experience.[26] The gap between hopes and realities may be narrowed by improving patients' function through treatment or by reducing their expectations through better understanding of the limitations imposed by their disease. Using this model, improving quality of life for the palliative care patient is a dynamic process that must continually address the ongoing changes in the gap of hope and reality as their disease progresses. Physical therapists and occupational therapists, by the nature of their therapeutic and educational interventions, can and often do assist the seriously ill patient to manage the gap between hope and reality.

Nolen and Mock noted that, in addition to the importance of having control over traditional activities of daily living (bathing, dressing, and eating), having functional control over healthcare decision making and fulfillment or role expectations are equally important to patients at the end of life.[27] Occupational therapists can tailor treatments and goals to allow patients to continue to carry out meaningful activities and fulfill self-identified important life roles. Yoshioka demonstrated the importance of patient control over healthcare decisions in his study of 301 cancer patients who received rehabilitation therapy during their last 6 months of life.[28*] Although mobility and self-care scores improved with therapy for all participants, the patients and families who received the greatest benefit were those who more actively participated in their rehabilitation and helped to direct their care.

Improvement in quality of life with physical and occupational therapy interventions has been shown to be beneficial even in the last days of life (Box 104.2). In a study of 56 cancer patients in Switzerland, the benefits of physical therapy were noted up right up to the last 24 hours before death;[29] 79 percent of the patients received beneficial respiratory management techniques during the 24 hours preceding death and 55 percent received beneficial interventions aimed at improving self care during the 8 days that preceded their death.

Box 104.2 When physical or occupational therapy is appropriate for palliative patients

- Any patient with a serious illness can benefit from therapy services

- Physical/occupational therapy can provide specialized treatment of pain, discomfort, and functional loss at any stage of illness

- Referral is encouraged early in the patient's care to prevent predicable morbidities but can be received at any time, including during and after curative treatment

- Therapy services can be provided in hospitals, nursing homes, community settings, the patient's home and the hospice/palliative care unit

---

GUIDE FOR PHYSICAL/OCCUPATIONAL THERAPY IN PALLIATIVE CARE

Therapeutic goals

The goals of rehabilitation interventions in supportive care, chronic relapsing disease, and end-of-life care are similar:

- maintain the patient's optimal function within the limits of their ability and the time frame available
- address symptoms of pain, limited cardiopulmonary capacity, strength, and range of motion as they interfere with patient comfort and function
- reduce caregiver burden via education and training
- increase caregiver competence/confidence in physical management of the patient.

Goals should be realistic and take into consideration many interrelated factors such as age, stage/type of disease, social/economic factors and cognitive abilities. The process of setting the appropriate goals is as important as the goals themselves. Although any type of patient should collaborate in the development of rehabilitation goals, it is especially helpful for patients in the palliative setting as the process provides a therapeutic outcome of allowing the patient continued control in directing his or her care. Therapists in the palliative care setting can encourage patients to explore what is truly important to them at that point in their life. Collaborative goal setting also provides an ideal opportunity for assisting patients in reframing unrealistic goals to match their current medical condition, if necessary.

Therapists' specialized skills

Physical and occupational therapists involved in the care of patients with progressive, debilitating illness or age associated decline must demonstrate not only well-developed clinical skills, but also the ability to communicate effectively, facilitate team interactions, and innovate extemporaneously. They must be sensitive to the emotional needs of the patient and family, as well as the needs of their fellow team members. In more ways than in any other rehabilitation treatment situation, the wants and needs of this patient population drive the treatment plan. The palliative care therapist must be able to establish a treatment plan focused on comfort and quality of life rather than on recovery of normal function.

In the healthcare culture where there is often a general discomfort around the topic of death, physical and occupational therapists traditionally focus on rehabilitation for living. However, in the palliative care setting, therapists must be able to manage their own fears and feelings about serious illness and death to effectively support the patients and their families who are facing those issues.[30] Trump advises that to be effective in the palliative care setting, therapists may need to address and sometimes share in patients' and families' intense emotions.[31] Furthermore, when death does occur the therapist must have appropriate methods for bringing about professional and personal closure to prevent emotional burnout. Foles *et al.* outlines a series of professional and personal activities that promote emotional wellbeing for the therapist, including attending a wake, funeral, or memorial service that allows the therapist to say goodbye to the patient and family.[32] Professional reflection on the outcomes of the therapy provided and reliance on one's own personal/spiritual beliefs and values are essential skills for therapists working in palliative care (Box 104.3).

Box 104.3 Special skills required for therapists working in palliative care

- Effective communication skills: active listening, empathy, and intuition

- Problem-solving skills and creative approaches to individual needs

- Ability to form compassionate bonds with emotional detachment

- Ability to accept death as a reality but never take away hope

Potential benefits – therapeutic interventions to optimize function

Physical and occupational therapists specialize in addressing physical function. Though functional decline may be inevitable in terminal illness and some chronic disease, there are many interventions that can assist in prolonging functional abilities. 'Optimizing levels of function in meaningful activities, occupational roles and in functional mobility for as long as possible is one of the benefits that therapy offers the patient. . . .'[33]

An objective assessment of function, routinely done on all patients, allows implementation of rehabilitation measures to slow, prevent or remediate performance problems. Physicians and nurses typically evaluate function, in persons with cancer, using the Karnovsky, Eastern Cooperative Oncology Group (ECOG) or similar rating scales. These scales are not always true indicators of a person's actual physical abilities as the ratings are usually based on cursory observation of the patient in an artificial environment (a clinic visit) in which they are 'stimulated . . . by the environment, anxiety and expectations.'[34] In a small study of patients with nonsmall cell lung cancer at the Jewish General Hospital in Montreal, Dalzell et al. compared ECOG performance status ratings (PS) with a global functional score composed of three objective measures of performance. They found that 'PS evaluation persistently underestimated the degree of functional disability as measured by the objective measures.'[35*] Cashy and Cella compared the results of PS assessment of lung cancer patients performed by the physician versus the patient's self assessment of their function and found that physicians, in general, rated the patients as performing better than the patients rated themselves.[36*]

A better indicator of the patient's actual functional abilities are objective tests of observed performance in which time or distance is measured. Functional performance tests such as 6-minute walk, 50-foot fastest speed, timed sit to stand and others have been compared between groups (i.e. cancer, HIV, AIDS and low back pain). Although all groups show overall decreased performance from normal, the cancer patient group was the lowest performing group.[37*] Lee et al. evaluated the self-reported fatigue measures and objective functional performance of individuals with lymphoma and recommended that physical performance measures be used in addition to self-reported measures when evaluating outcomes of rehabilitation.[38*] The 6-minute walk has also been used in studies of heart failure and shows promise as an easier to perform alternative to a multistaged exercise test.[39]

MAINTAINING FUNCTIONAL MOBILITY

Decline in functional mobility may be due to any number(s) of impairments. Often an individual impairment is not sufficient to interfere with function, but the additive effect of multiple mild impairments overcomes the patient's ability to compensate and results in functional loss. An example might be a cancer patient with mild dyspnea and marginal hemoglobin who must now alter his gait pattern to reduce pain of one limb during the stance phase. The energy cost of his abnormal gait pattern is higher than that of normal gait. This patient might be able to compensate for one or even two of his impairments, but is unable to overcome the combination of the three. Reducing the pain of weight bearing on a limb through use of gait training with an appropriate assistive device and teaching pursed lip breathing might restore this patient's independent ambulation.

Ambulatory aids vary in their ease of use and utility for given gait requirements. Crutches, canes, and walkers come in many different weights, designs and with multiple accessories such as wheels, brakes, seats, and platform attachments. Selection of the appropriate device is based on the type of assistance needed (weight relief, balance deficits, etc.), the recommended gait pattern, the overall physical and cognitive abilities of the patient and the setting in which the device will be used (out of doors, over carpet, smooth surfaces, etc.). The energy cost of using different devices differs. The amount of energy required to walk with a standard walker is significantly higher than with a rolling walker, and may require excessive cardiac work for any patient with serious illness.[18**,19*,20**,21*,39,40***] But the rolling walker may not provide the required stability for safe ambulation for an individual patient. Certain gait patterns are more energy costly than others. For instance nonweight-bearing gait is significantly more energy costly than touch down gait and requires significantly higher cardiac work.[41] Improperly adjusted ambulatory aids can be dangerous at worst and inefficient at best. Among the problems that can be seen with poorly fitted devices are:

- an inability to effectively transmit weight through the device
- dangerous or painful alterations in posture to accommodate the height of the device.

Prescription for and training in the use of a gait device should be done by a physical therapist.[42]

At some point in the course of chronic debilitating illness, the individual may need greater assistance to maintain their functional mobility. Like ambulatory devices, wheelchairs also come in many sizes, weights, and configurations and with many options. One size does not fit all. Poorly fitted wheelchairs can cause pain, contribute to skin breakdown, increase the work of sit-to-stand transfers, decrease rolling stability etc. Width and depth of the seat, height from the floor, height of the back, position of the axle, types of armrests and footrests, material of frame, and seating surface must all be taken into consideration. Patients may desire powered mobility but have not given thought to how they will get the device into and out of their home or transport it in their vehicle. For other patients, powered mobility may make the difference between dependence and modified independence in the home and between community integration and isolation. Therapists prescribe specific wheelchairs based on the size and needs of each individual patient and how it will improve their functional ability as well as their quality of life.

MAINTAINING MEANINGFUL ACTIVITIES AND OCCUPATIONAL ROLES

'The quality of life and control over one's life to the end of that life are essential to the maintenance of dignity and self-respect.'[43] Occupational therapists assist the patient and family in maintaining quality of life in the areas of self-care, work, and leisure by:

- enabling patients to select and continue meaningful occupation within their physical ability
- prescribing and training in assistive devices or equipment to reduce the time or effort to perform activities of daily living (ADLs) or leisure activities
- teaching energy conservation techniques to counteract fatigue
- modifying the environment to facilitate continued participation in meaningful social and occupational activities
- preventing isolation by helping patients continue their social role.

Picard and Magno advocate that occupational therapists can address the patient's need for meaning in life even if that life is measured in days. Occupational therapists can help the terminally ill patient answer the painful question: What do I do tomorrow while I am waiting to die?[44] Approaching the patient from both a biomedical and biosocial model, occupational therapists encourage the patient to determine what is important to them and enable the patient to continue to exert control of their life as much as possible.[14]

Working with the patient and the family in the home setting, occupational therapists make recommendations for home modifications, which will allow continued independence in self-care, work, and play. For example, installing a ramp to allow wheelchair access to the outdoor might encourage a gardener to return to a meaningful occupation or modifying the kitchen table might encourage the homemaker to maintain her supervision of meal preparations. Additionally, the therapist can introduce any number of assistive devices and/or adapted techniques that facilitate the performance of basic and instrumental activities of daily living. Long handled bathing sponges, tub/shower benches and hand held showers can reduce the energy cost and increase the safety of bathing. Dressing sticks, reachers, button hooks, sock aids, etc. can facilitate dressing. There are many other devices to increase ability and/or reduce energy cost of activities. Occupational therapists are familiar with these devices and where to obtain them.

In institutional settings, the use of therapeutic groups can be beneficial in assisting the patient to make major life transitions. Modifying old occupational roles and transitioning to new roles is part of the therapeutic process as function declines. Dawson described the use of occupational therapy groups in a hospice setting that created a safe and supportive environment designed to assist patients in adjusting and adapting to their changing roles.[45]

In summary, rehabilitation interventions by physical and occupational therapists may not restore a palliative patient to a previous functional level but may rather provide a reasonable degree of independence and quality of life during their final days.

Potential benefits – therapeutic interventions for symptom management

During rehabilitation of terminally ill patients, there is a delicate balance between maintaining optimal function and providing comfort relief. At some point, the focus on function will diminish and the efforts on comfort will increase until death.[46] Some impairments that are consistently encountered in patients with chronic or end-of-life disease are pain, dyspnea, skin breakdown, edema, weakness, loss of coordination, loss of soft tissue or joint mobility and impaired cognition. Any or all of these impairments can have a negative impact on patient function, but they may also cause discomfort and distress in and of themselves.[4]

PAIN MANAGEMENT

Pain is a frequently cited and much feared symptom of cancer and other chronic illnesses. Although pharmacological therapies are used effectively in many cases, nonpharmacological interventions can be important adjuncts, depending on the etiology of the pain. The inadequacy of training regarding the comprehensive management of cancer pain was the focus of a study (the Network Project) which determined that existing educational programs for health professionals put little emphasis on integrating psychosocial and rehabilitation issues in managing cancer pain.[47*] Too often pain is assessed while the patient is at rest. Determining the patient's incident pain levels during their basic or desired activities is important. Patients who fear movement-associated pain will limit their movement and eventually limit their ability to move. In evaluating patient pain, the therapists must also take into consideration cultural bias, diminished capacity to report pain, special needs of older patients and the complexity of some pain syndromes.[48]

Patients with advanced cancer may have painful bone metastases. Other causes of musculoskeletal pain may be related to soft tissue tightness, postural changes and arthritis or other comorbid conditions. Interventions such as orthotics, weight relief strategies, ambulatory aids, assistive devices, instruction in specific movement patterns, and correction of faulty posture or abnormal gait may afford relief.

Neuropathic pain can be severe and interfere with function. This type of pain may due to amputation of limb or breast, nerve impingement, chemotherapy or diabetic induced neuropathy, or other nerve disruptions. Interventions such as thermal modalities, electrical stimulation, photostimulation, and massage can be useful components of a management plan for neuropathic pain. Finally, training in relaxation techniques such as guided imagery or progressive relaxation exercise assist the patient in managing pain.

RESPIRATORY MANAGEMENT

Dyspnea is a common symptom in advanced cancer as well as in heart failure, chronic obstructive pulmonary disease (COPD) and other chronic illnesses. The causes of dyspnea are myriad and in most cases, more than one mechanism is involved.[49] The reader is referred to Chapter 69 for indepth discussion of dyspnea. Positioning, respiratory muscle training, aerobic/strength training, stretching, airway clearance techniques, and education in breathing techniques (e.g. pursed lip breathing, etc.) are all methods which rehabilitation professionals are trained to perform on patients with pulmonary impairments.

When dyspnea is due to mechanical restriction of the thorax (e.g. postural changes, shortening of intercostal muscles etc.), specific manual techniques to improve thoracic mobility may improve the patient's ability to effectively ventilate. Dyspnea can also be due to respiratory muscle weakness or fatigue. 'Clear evidence reveals that specific respiratory muscle training improves inspiratory and expiratory strength and decreases symptomatic reports of ventilatory load perception – how difficult it seems to breathe.'[50] Weiner et al. demonstrated a decrease in dyspnea and an increase in exercise capacity in patients with congestive heart failure who participated in specific inspiratory muscle training exercises.[51*] Sanchez Riera et al. described similar results in patients with severe COPD.[52**] Cahalin described decreased dyspnea and improvement in maximum inspiratory and expiratory pressure following inspiratory muscle training in patients with advanced heart failure awaiting transplantation.[39] Bredin et al. studied breathlessness in patients with lung cancer.[53**] Their intervention group received advice and support on managing breathlessness, training in breathing control techniques, relaxation and distraction as well as other information and support. Their control group received standard management and treatment. They found that although overall survival was not significantly different between groups, the intervention group reported significant improvement in breathlessness at best as well as improvement in activity levels. No objective functional performance measures were included in the study. For patients who can tolerate cardiovascular endurance training, Carrieri Kohlman et al. noted a decrease in dyspnea, associated anxiety and distress, along with an improvement in exercise performance in those patients who performed 12 treadmill walking sessions followed by an unsupervised walking program.[54**]

Therapists can also use breathing retraining to reduce dyspnea. Education regarding effective use of accessory muscles, positioning to optimize muscle length tension, pursed lip breathing, prolonged exhalation, timing breaths with activities, and other techniques have been widely used in lung disease populations. Cahalin states 'body position is an important principle to include in the treatment of people with heart failure.'[39] The position of the patient can alter the work of breathing. Respiratory airflow resistance and breathlessness increased when a group of patients with left ventricular failure were placed in supine position.[55*] In patients with inspiratory muscle weakness, positioning in Fowlers can reduce resistance to diaphragmatic excursion by maximizing the assistance of gravity.[50] Positioning patients in sidelying with the diseased lung superior improved oxygenation in some studies.[56] Positioning also can help prevent the accumulation of secretions or assist in the mobilization of secretions. Patients often have difficulty clearing secretions due to pain or weakness. Positioning, postural drainage, assisted cough and alternative cough techniques (e.g. huffing), or the use of airway clearance devices such as the Flutter® or Acapella™ may be of benefit.[57*] Patients with severe weakness of abdominal musculature (e.g. spinal cord compression) may benefit from application of an abdominal binder.

SKIN MANAGEMENT

Skin breakdown can be a significant problem for many patients and the potential for skin compromise increases as the patient becomes increasingly ill or less mobile. Loss of skin integrity (due to trauma, pressure, shear force injuries) as well as impaired skin health (due to edema, nutritional deficiencies, and impaired circulation) can contribute to the skin breakdown. Physical and occupational therapists can use several methods to address causes of skin breakdown. Positioning to reduce pressure, selection of appropriate seating/bed surfaces, teaching of weight shifts, and prescription of properly fitted wheelchairs all contribute to effective skin management. For patients who are confined to bed, it is important to avoid extended periods of time with both the head and knees in an elevated position as that increases the risk of sacral decubitus. Therapists can instruct the patient and caregivers on safe alternative positions and an effective schedule for turning to prevent skin breakdown, functional training in bathing and hygiene, improving the patient's skills in bed mobility, transfers and, if possible, gait can also have a positive effect.[58] Proper transfer training is important to prevent shearing forces which produce skin burns or tears.

EDEMA MANAGEMENT

Edema can be caused by a number of conditions (venous or lymphatic obstruction, renal failure, right heart failure, hypoalbuminemia, and others). The reader is referred to Chapter 83 for an in-depth discussion of lymphedema. Regardless of the cause, swelling may be painful, can interfere with functional mobility and contribute to skin compromise. Management of edema depends in part on the etiology of the swelling.

For patients with lymphedema complex decongestive therapy may be beneficial. Complex decongestive therapy includes manual lymphatic drainage (a very specific form of massage), lymphatic exercises, and bandaging with short stretch bandages. This form of therapy has long been used in Europe and Australia but is gaining increased acceptance in the USA as the number of trained clinicians increases and research has supported its efficacy. In a review of treatment approaches for arm edema in breast cancer patients, Erickson et al. concluded that a program of complex decongestive therapy consisting of manual lymphatic massage, exercise, and compression wrapping was effective in treating lymphedema related to breast cancer.[59***] In 2005 a Cochrane review of studies of physical therapy for managing lymphedema identified 195 studies out of which only 10 were randomized clinical trials.[60***] Of those 10, data were included from only three studies as the other seven were unavailable or otherwise ineligible for inclusion. None of the three studies included evaluated the same interventions nor had any of the three studies been replicated. The Cochrane group concluded that there was weak evidence to support the use of compression bandaging with compression hosiery over compression hosiery alone. In their discussion the authors commented that although it is evident that improvement can be obtained it is unclear which treatments are most effective and yield sustained improvement. Both reviews identified the need for well-designed clinical research to identify the best approach to manage lymphedema.

In addition, many references on management of lymphedema caution against the use of massage and other manual techniques in the presence of active disease.[61] The therapist must determine the relative risks of intervention versus the benefits of treatment. In a patient with painful swelling due to lymphatic obstruction from advanced disease, for whom cure is no longer a possibility, lymphatic drainage and bandaging may provide comfort relief and be entirely justified. The use of off-the-shelf compression garments, bicycle shorts or low stretch bandaging may help alleviate the discomfort of edema. Scrotal edema is a frequently encountered problem and may occur with or without extremity edema. It is painful and often interferes with sitting, transfers, and gait. Commercially available scrotal supports are usually too small to accommodate a very swollen scrotum but, with a sewing machine, can be modified to provide the compression necessary to alleviate pain. Due to costs, rapid changes in limb dimensions, and length of time required for ordering, fabrication, and delivery, custom garments are usually not indicated.

MANAGEMENT OF WEAKNESS/FATIGUE

Many patients complain of weakness and attribute to it their declining functional performance. Patients may use the term 'weakness' to describe lack of stamina, specific motor weakness, or asthenia. Physical evaluation can help differentiate between generalized muscle weakness, cardiopulmonary impairment, specific muscle weakness, steroid myopathy, cancer-related fatigue or other contributing issues. Exercise prescription will depend on the evaluation finding and will be specific to the problem. There are multiple studies to support the use of exercise as an intervention in cancer, lung disease and other diseases.[62***,63**,64*,65**,66**] Even assisted exercise for the extremely weak can be beneficial in optimizing a person's functional abilities. In the case of specific muscle weakness, braces or splints to assist with function and/or protect joint or muscle integrity may be recommended. Additionally, training patients in the use of energy conservation techniques can assist in management of fatigue.

MANAGEMENT OF SKELETAL COMPLICATIONS

Bone lesions are often seen in patients with advanced cancer, especially lung, breast, kidney, or prostate disease. Persons with multiple myeloma, osteoporosis, or those patients who have been on steroids are also subject to fracture. Management of pathologic fractures is difficult and requires a multidisciplinary approach to control pain and preserve functional mobility. Prevention of fractures should be a focus of management of any patients at risk. Many of these patients are at risk for spinal cord or root compression with resultant functional loss. Early identification of lesions at risk for fracture might allow prophylactic surgical fixation, protective bracing or weight relief to prevent an actual break. Strengthening exercises, gait training, and orthotics are all effective measures to reduce the risk of falls (Box 104.4).

Box 104.4 Types of orthoses and benefits

Ankle foot orthosis

- Assist in clearing the toes in swing phase of gait
- Maintains stability of the ankle in stance (avoid inversion or eversion injuries)

Knee orthosis

- Unload a painful arthritic knee joint
- Prevent hyperextension of the knee when hamstrings are weak or joint capsule is lax
- Assist in stabilizing knee if quadriceps are weak

Spinal orthosis

- Limits movement of spinal segments
- Relieves pressure on nerve roots
- Facilitates patient mobility

In summary, physical and occupational interventions for the palliative care patient are varied, multifaceted, and designed to address both the maintenance of function and the reduction of symptoms. As noted in the manual from the National Institute of Clinical Excellence on supportive and palliative care in cancer (UK), there is a growing body of evidence that supports the effectiveness of many combinations of rehabilitation intervention but more detailed studies are needed to understand the relative effectiveness of these interventions (Boxes 104.5 and 104.6). [67]***

Box 104.5 Physical therapy interventions in palliative care

- Functional mobility training

- Therapeutic exercises

- Dyspnea management

- Positioning for skin care, comfort, and function

- Lymphedema control

- Orthotics

- Therapeutic modalities (heat, cold, massage, electrical)

- Caregiver instruction and training

Box 104.6 Occupational therapy interventions in palliative care

- Engagement in meaningful activities that reflect valued roles

- ADL training/adapted techniques

- Energy conservation techniques/fatigue management

- Assessment/training in use of assistive devices and modification of environment

- Group activities (emotional and social benefits)

- Orthotics

- Positioning for skin care, comfort, and function

- Caregiver instruction and training

CONCLUSIONS/FUTURE ISSUES

Disability is defined by cultures – disability does not define people but how disability is viewed is determined by the society in which one lives. What might be considered a disability in one society or culture may not be viewed as such in another. Likewise, the definition of *independence* may vary depending on the stakeholder. Governments may see independence as increasing self-reliance and reducing the burden on the state whereas healthcare professionals focus on the individual's ability to carry out self-care activities independently. For disabled people, independence may be viewed in terms of personal autonomy and the ability to take control of one's life.[9]

For the person who is at the end of life, independence or lack of disability may be defined as the ability to continue to live one's life with dignity, exerting control over one's care and maintaining functional independence in self care activities as far as reasonably possible. Physical and occupational therapy can facilitate the patient's function at a minimum level of dependence regardless of life expectancy and improve the quality of survival at the end of life, so the patient's life can be as comfortable and productive as possible. Research is still needed to understand which interventions will achieve the best outcomes and what is the optimal time for interventions over the continuum of the life–death cycle. However, there is little doubt that quality of life and the quality of the death experience are enhanced when physical and occupational therapists are part of a team of health professions supporting the palliative care patient and their family.

Key learning points

- Rehabilitation interventions should be an integral part of palliative care.

- Physical and occupational therapy enhance function and quality of life for seriously ill people and their families, and address their psychological and spiritual needs through meaningful activities.

- Improved care results in meaningful and hopeful end of life.

- Referrals should be made early in the disease to provide symptom management, reduce the caregiver's burden and improve the patient's quality of life.

- Goals of physical and occupational therapy for palliative patients are based upon what is most important to them at the time of evaluation and are continually revised as their priorities change over the trajectory of their disease.

- Therapists use specialized skills to enhance communication, form compassionate bonds, and set goals which are realistic but do not take away hope.

- The measurement of function should be performance based and use objective measures.

- Therapists can provide a wide range of interventions to improve/maintain function and reduce symptoms such pain, edema, dyspnea, weakness, fatigue, skin breakdown, and other musculoskeletal complications.

ACKNOWLEDGMENTS

Thanks to Pam Lathem OTR, Mack Ivy OTR, Marvin Nuval PT, and the rest of the caring and committed physical and occupational therapists in the Rehabilitation Services department, University of Texas M D Anderson Cancer Center. Special thanks to Kelly Esslinger for manuscript support.

REFERENCES

1   Kass LR. Lingering longer: who will care? *Washington Post* September 29, 2005: Section A: 23.

∗ 2   Lynn J, Adamson DM. *Living Well at the End of Life: Adapting Health Care to Serious Chronic Illness in Old Age.* Santa Monica, CA: RAND White Paper, 2003.

● 3   The President's Council on Bioethics. Taking care: ethical care giving in our aging society. *Taking Care* 2005: 8–116.

4   Cheville A. American Cancer Society. Cancer rehabilitation in the new millennium: rehabilitation of patients with advanced cancer. *Cancer* 2001; **92**: 1039–48.

5   Boyd KJ, Murray SA, Kendall M, *et al.* Living with advanced heart failure: a prospective, community based study of patients and their careers. *Eur J Heart Fail* 2004; **6**: 585–9.

6   Horne G, Payne S. Removing the boundaries: palliative care for patients with heart failure. *Palliat Med* 2004; **18**: 291–6.

7   Gerber L. American Cancer Society. Cancer Rehabilitation in the New Millennium: cancer rehabilitation into the future. *Cancer* 2001; **92**:975–9.

∗ 8   World Health Organization–Europe. *Palliative Care. The Solid Facts.* Geneva: WHO, 2004: 7–32.

9   World Federation of Occupational Therapists [homepage on the internet]. Australia: World Federation of Occupational Therapist; c2002 Available at: www.wfot.org.au/WFOT_information/default.cfm (updated October 4, 2005; accessed October 4, 2005).

10   World Confederation for Physical Therapy. Primary health care and community based rehabilitation: implications for physical therapy based on a survey of WCPT's member organizations and a literature review. UK: WCPT, WCPT Briefing Paper 1. 2003; **1**: 1–33.

● 11   Dietz J. Rehabilitation of the cancer patient. *Med Clin North Am* 1969; **53**: 607–24.

● 12   Shanks R. Physiotherapy in palliative care. *Physiotherapy* 1982; **68**: 405–7.

13   Toot J. Physical therapy and hospice – concept and practice. *J Phys Ther* 1984; **64**: 665–71.

14   Tigges KN, Sherman LM. The treatment of the hospice patient: from occupational history to occupational role. *Am J Occup Ther* 1983; **37**: 235–38.

15   Davies E, Higginson I, eds. World Health Organization – Europe. *Better Palliative Care for Older People.* Geneva: WHO, 2004: 6–37.

● 16   Lunney JR, Lynn J, Foley D, *et al.* Patterns of functional decline at the end of life. *JAMA* 2003; **289**: 2387–92.

◆ 17   Fialka-Moser V, Crevenna R, Korpan M, Quittan M. Cancer rehabilitation – particularly with aspects on physical impairments. *J Rehabil Med* 2003; **35**: 153–62.

18   Segal RJ, Reid RD, Courneya KS, *et al.* Resistance exercise in men receiving androgen deprivation therapy for prostate cancer. *J Clin Oncol* 2003; **21**: 1653–9.

● 19   Demeo FC, Tilmann MHM, Bertz H, *et al.* Aerobic exercise in the rehabilitation of cancer patients after high dose chemotherapy and autologous peripheral stem cell transplant. *Cancer* 1997; **79**: 1717–22.

20   Demeo FC, Stieglitz RD, Novelli-Fisher U, *et al.* Effects of physical activity on the fatigue and psychologic status of cancer patients during chemotherapy. *Cancer* 1999; **85**: 2273–7.

21   Demeo F, Schwartz, Fietz, *et al.* Effects of endurance training on the physical performance of patients with hematological malignancies during chemotherapy. *Support Care Cancer* 2003; **11**: 623–7.

22   Tookman AJ, Hopkins K, Scharpen-von-Heussen. Rehabilitation in palliative medicine. In: Doyle D, Hanks G, Cherny N, Calman K, eds. *Oxford Textbook of Palliative Medicine,* 2nd ed. New York: Oxford University Press, 1998: 1022–30.

23   Lynn J. Serving patients who may die soon and their families: the role of hospice and other services. *JAMA* 2001; **285**: 925–32.

● 24   Steinhauser K, Christakis N, Clipp E, McNeilly M, *et al.* Factors considered important at the end of life by patients, family, physicians and other care providers. *JAMA* 2000; **284**: 2476–82.

25   O'Boyle CA, Waldron D. Quality of life issues in palliative medicine. *J Neurol* 1997; **244**: 18–25.

● 26   Calman KC. Quality of life in cancer patients – an hypothesis. *J Med Ethics* 1984; **10**: 124–7.

27   Nolan MT, Mock V. A conceptual framework for end-of-life care: a reconsideration of factors influencing the integrity of the human person. *J Prof Nurs* 2004; **20**: 351–60.

● 28   Yoshioka H. Rehabilitation for the terminal cancer patient. *Am J Phys Med Rehabil* 1994; **73**: 199–206.

29   Marcant D, Rapin CH. Role of the physiotherapist in palliative care. *J Pain Symptom Manage* 1993; **8**: 68–71.

30   Hayes C. General medicine and surgery. In: Hopkins H, Smith H, eds. *Willard and Spachman's Occupational Therapy*, 5th ed. Philadelphia: JB Lippincott Co, 1978: 437.

31   Trump SM. Occupational therapy and hospice: a natural fit. *OT Practice* 2001; **6**: 7–11.

32   Foles D, Tigges K, Weisman T. Occupational therapy in hospice home care: student tutorial. *Am J Occup Ther* 1986; **40**: 623–28.

33   Pizzi M, Briggs R. Occupational and physical therapy in hospice: the facilitation of meaning, quality of life, and well being. *Topics Geriatr Rehabil* 2004; **20**: 120–30.

34   Winningham ML, Donovan ES. Fatigue and oncology rehabilitation: an historical perspective. In: Winningham ML and Barton-Burke M, eds. *Fatigue in Cancer: A Multidimensional Approach.* Sadbury: Jones and Bartlett, 2000: 263–76.

35   Dalzell MA, Kreisman H, Small D, MacDonald N. Is performance status related to functional capacity in patients with non small cell lung cancer (NSCLC). *J Clin Oncol* 2004; **22**(14 Suppl): 7224.

36   Cashy J, Cella D. Discrepancy analysis of patient vs physician assessments of performance status in patients with advanced lung cancer [abstract]. *J Clin Oncol* 2005; **23**(16 Suppl): Abs No 8103.

● 37 Simmonds MJ. Physical function in patients with cancer: psychometric characteristics and clinical usefulness of a physical performance test battery. *J Pain Symptom Manage* 2002; **24**: 404–14.

38 Lee JQ, Simmonds MJ, Wang XS, Novy DM. Differences in physical performance in men and women with and without lymphoma. *Arch Phys Med Rehabil* 2003; **84**: 1747–52.

39 Cahalin LP. Exercise training in heart failure: inpatient and outpatient considerations. *AACN Clinical Issues: Advanced Practice in Acute and Critical Care* 1998; **9**: 225–243.

◆ 40 Courneya KS. Exercise in cancer survivors: an overview of research. *Official Journal of the American College of Sports Medicine* 2003; **35**: 1846–52.

41 Donovan ES. What the rehabilitation therapies can do. In: Winningham ML, Barton-Burke M, eds. *Fatigue in Cancer: A Multidimensional Approach.* Sadbury: Jones and Bartlett, 2000: 303–22.

42 Donovan E, Lathem P. Rehabilitation issues. In: Fieler V, Hanson P, eds. *Oncology Nursing in the Home.* Pittsburgh: Oncology Nursing Press, 2000: 127–36.

43 Pizzi MA. Occupational therapy in hospice care (hospice, locus of control, occupation, quality of life). *Am J Occup Ther* 1984; **38**: 252–7.

● 44 Picard HB, Magno JB. The role of occupational therapy in hospice care. *Am J Occup Ther* 1982; **36**: 597–8.

45 Dawson S. The role of occupational therapy groups in an Australian hospice. *Am J Hosp Palliat Care* 1993; **July/August**: 13–17.

46 Santiago-Palma J, Payne R; American Cancer Society. Cancer Rehabilitation in the New Millennium: palliative care and rehabilitation. *Cancer* 2001; **92**: 1049–52.

● 47 Breitbart W, Rosenfeld B, Passik SD. The network project: a multidisciplinary cancer education and training in pain management, rehabilitation, and psychosocial issues. *J Pain Symptom Manage* 1998; **15**: 18–26.

48 Ferrell B, Jacobson JA, Irick N. Issues of importance: maintaining comfort and compassion for patients in pain. *ONS News* 2004; **19**: 15–6.

49 Manning HL, Schwartzstein RM. Mechanisms of disease: pathophysiology of dyspnea. *N Engl J Med* 1995; **323**: 1547–53.

50 Tecklin JS. The patient with ventilatory pump dysfunction/ failure – preferred practice pattern 6E. In: Irwin S, Tecklin JS, eds. *Cardiopulmonary Physical Therapy: A Guide to Practice.* St Louis: Mosby, 2004: 344–71.

51 Weiner P, Waizman J, Magadle R, *et al.* Effect of specific inspiratory muscle training on dyspnea and exercise tolerance in congestive heart failure [abstract translated from Hebrew]. *Harefuah* 1999; **136**: 774–7.

52 Sanchez Riera H, Montemayor Rubio T, Ortega Ruiz F, *et al.* Inspiratory muscle training in patients with COPD: effect on dyspnea, exercise performance and quality of life. *Chest* 2001; **120**: 748–56.

53 Bredin M, Corner J, Krishnasamy M, *et al.* Multicentre randomized controlled trial of nursing intervention for breathlessness in patients with lung cancer. *BMJ* 1999; **318**: 901–4.

54 Carrieri Kohlman V, Gormley J, Douglas M, *et al.* Exercise training decreases dyspnea and the distress and anxiety associated with it: monitoring alone may be as effective as coaching. *Chest* 1996; **110**: 1526–35.

55 Yap JCH, Moore DM, Cleland JGF, Pride NB. Effect of supine position on respiratory mechanics in chronic left ventricular failure. *Am J Respir Crit Care Med* 2000; **162**: 1285–91.

56 Malone DJ, Adler J. The patient with respiratory failure-preferred practice pattern 6F. In: Irwin S, Tecklin JS, eds. *Cardiopulmonary Physical Therapy: A Guide to Practice.* St Louis: Mosby, 2004: 372–99.

57 Volsko TA, DiFiore JM, Chatburn RL. Performance comparison of two oscillating positive expiratory pressure devices: acapella versus flutter. *Respir Care* 2003; **48**: 124–30.

58 Froiland KG. Wound care of the advanced cancer patient. *Hematol Oncol Clin North Am* 2002; **16**: 627–39.

◆ 59 Erickson VS, Pearson ML, Ganz PA, *et al.* Arm edema in breast cancer patients. *J Natl Cancer Inst* 2001; **93**: 96–111.

◆ 60 Badger C, Preston N, Seers K, Mortimer P. Physical therapies for reducing and controlling lymphedema of the limbs. *Cochrane Database Syst Rev* 2005: CD003141.

61 Weissleder H, Schuchhardt C, eds. *Lymphedema, Diagnosis and Therapy*, 3rd ed. Germany: Viavital, 2001.

◆ 62 Stricker CT, Drake D, Hoyer KA, Mock V. Evidence-based practice for fatigue management in adults with cancer: exercise as an intervention. *Oncol Nurs Forum* 2004; **31**: 963–75.

63 Berglund G, Bolund C, Gustafsson UL, Sjoden PO. One-year follow-up of the 'starting again' group rehabilitation programme for cancer patients. *Eur J Cancer* 1994; **30A**: 1744–51.

64 Holley S, Borger D. Energy for living with cancer: preliminary findings of a cancer rehabilitation group intervention study. *Oncol Nurs Forum* 2001; **28**: 1393–6.

65 Mock V, Burke MD, Sheehan P, *et al.* A nursing rehabilitation program for women with breast cancer receiving adjuvant chemotherapy [including commentary by Foltz AT]. *Oncol Nurs Forum* 1994; **21**: 899–908.

66 Mock V, Dow KH, Meares CJ, *et al.* Effects of exercise on fatigue, physical functioning and emotional distress during radiation therapy for breast cancer. *Oncol Nurs Forum* 1997; **24**: 991–1000.

◆ 67 Gysels M, Higginson IJ. Improving supportive and palliative care for adults with cancer: Research Evidence. National Institute for Clinical Excellence, 2004. Available at www.nice.org.uk/pdf/csgspresearchevidence.pdf (accessed February 10, 2006).

105

Staff stress and burnout in palliative care

MARY L S VACHON

INTRODUCTION

Working in palliative care can be both challenging and stressful. What happens when clinicians become stressed and/or burnout? This chapter will provide an overview of stress and burnout in palliative care, discuss the extent of the problem, identify the factors associated with stress and burnout, and review some approaches to avoiding and dealing with these issues in palliative care.

DEFINITION OF TERMS

Stress

The concept of stress has been used to cover a number of divergent dimensions ranging from stimuli or stressors that lead to changes in the organism, to the outcome of such stimuli, and the emotional state or experience accompanying a changing social or personal situation.[1] Much of the current interest in the subject can be dated to the research of Hans Selye, who in 1936[2] articulated his biological concept of stress as the 'General Adaptation Syndrome', a set of non-specific physiological reactions to various noxious environmental agents.[3]

Antonovsky[4] sees stress as evolving from exposure to stressors. He distinguishes between stressors and routine stimuli. A routine stimulus is seen as being one to which the person can respond more or less automatically. A stressor is a demand made by the internal or external environment of an organism that upsets its homeostasis, restoration of which depends on a nonautomatic and not readily available energy-expending action. A routine stimulus can become a stressor under certain circumstances. Whether a stimulus is a stressor depends on the meaning of the stimulus to the person at that point in time and on the repertoire of coping mechanisms readily available. In Antonovsky's model, 'stress' refers to the strain that remains 'in response to the failure to manage tensions well and to overcome stressors'.[4 (p. 10)]

Stress can be observed at the physiological, psychological, and behavioral levels of analysis.[5–7] It is an ongoing process affected by individual personality factors and environmental variables. The individual is constantly responding to and interacting with the environment and whether the stress is a benefit or a harm to the individual depends greatly on the individual's cognitive appraisal of the stress and subsequent coping process. More recently, the European Agency for Safety and Health at Work,[8] has stated that:

> There is increasing consensus around defining work-related stress in terms of the 'interactions' between employee and (exposure to hazards in) their work environment. Within this model stress can be said to be experienced when the demands from the work environment exceed the employee's ability to cope with (or control) them.

Burnout

The term burnout is generally credited to Freudenberger.[9,10] Burnout has been characterized as 'the progressive loss of idealism, energy and purpose experienced by people in the helping professions as a result of the conditions of their work'.[11] (p. 14) 'The root cause of burnout lies in people's need to believe that their life is meaningful, and that the things they do – and consequently they themselves – are important and significant'.[12] (p. 633)

Christina Maslach, who developed the Maslach Burnout Inventory,[13] the most commonly used instrument to measure burnout, has reviewed research in the field of burnout over the past 25 years.[14] (p. 398)

> What has emerged from all this research is a conceptualization of job burnout as a psychological syndrome in response to chronic interpersonal stressors on the job. The three key dimensions of this response are an overwhelming exhaustion, feelings of cynicism and detachment from the job, and a sense of ineffectiveness and lack of accomplishment. The exhaustion component represents the basic individual stress dimension of burnout. It refers to feelings of being overextended and depleted of one's emotional and physical resources. The cynicism (or depersonalization) component represents the interpersonal context dimension of burnout. It refers to a negative, callous, or excessively detached response to various aspects of the job. The component of reduced efficacy or accomplishment represents the self-evaluation dimension of burnout. It refers to feelings of incompetence and a lack of achievement and productivity at work.

A MODEL OF BURNOUT AND OCCUPATIONAL STRESS

In reviewing the research, Maslach *et al.*[14] note previous research in occupational stress focused on the person–environment fit model.[15] More recent research focuses on the degree of match or mismatch between the person and six domains of the job environment. The greater the gap or mismatch between the person and the environment, the greater the likelihood of burnout. The greater the match or fit, the greater the likelihood of engagement with work. Mismatches arise when the process of establishing a psychological contract leaves critical issues unresolved, or when the working relationship changes to something that the person finds unacceptable. Six areas of work life come together in a framework that encompasses the major organizational antecedents of burnout: workload, control, reward, community, fairness, and values.

Burnout arises from chronic mismatches between people and their work settings in some or all of these areas. Preliminary evidence suggests that the area of values may play a central mediating role for the other areas. Alternatively, people may vary in the extent to which each of the six areas is important to them. Some people may place a higher weight on rewards than on values, or people may be prepared to tolerate a mismatch regarding workload if they receive praise, good pay, and have good relationships with colleagues. The palliative care literature will be reviewed using this framework.

STRESS AND BURNOUT IN PALLIATIVE CARE VERSUS OTHER SPECIALTIES

A review of the literature of stress in palliative care over the past quarter century[16] found many studies reported that staff working in palliative care had either less burnout and stress than other professionals or that they experienced no more stress than other healthcare professionals working with seriously ill and/or dying persons.

That stress in palliative care may be less than in other specialties does not negate the stress that does occur. The use of drugs, alcohol, and suicidal ideation of hospice medical directors and matrons was identified.[17] Hospice nurses were more anxious, with associated psychosomatic complaints than hospital nurses, although the latter were more dissatisfied with their jobs. High levels of mental ill health were predicted by a lack of social support and involvement in work and high workload.[18] Hospice nurses were found to be higher on the death and dying dimension of the Nursing Stress Scale and were slightly more depressed than medical/surgical or intensive care unit nurses.[19]

More recent studies confirm that palliative care specialists in the UK experience less stress and burnout than their oncology colleagues.[20] In a questionnaire sent to all consultant nonsurgical oncologists in the UK, the stress and stressors of medical oncologists, clinical oncologists, and palliative care specialists were assessed. Clinical oncologists were more likely to experience burnout. Palliative care specialists generally reported the lowest mean percentage of items rated as contributing 'quite a bit' or 'a lot' to overall job stress. The estimated prevalence of psychiatric disorder was 28 percent, similar to that of British junior house officers. The percentage of clinicians reporting high levels of exhaustion on the Maslach Burnout Inventory was similar to that of the normative sample (31 percent vs. 33 percent).[21] One-third of cancer clinicians and the normative sample reported low personal accomplishment. Significantly fewer of the UK cancer clinicians reported high levels of depersonalization compared to the US sample (23 percent vs. 33 percent, $P < 0.0001$). British palliative care nurses[22] also experienced lower burnout than expected.

Compared with oncology staff in Canada[23] and the USA,[24] the stress of the UK palliative care staff stands in marked contrast. European samples tend to have lower levels of exhaustion and cynicism compared with similar North American samples,[14] perhaps because of cultural values or it may be that American jobs are more stressful. A more recent study of senior house officers in UK hospices[25] found median stress score as measured on a visual analog scale was 55 mm (range 0–98 mm). Five respondents (22 percent) scored for identifiable psychological distress on the General Health Questionnaire (GHQ).[26] More senior British physicians also report stress,[27] which appeared to be equal to or greater than that of the oncologists and palliative care specialists. Up to a third of consultants and nearly half of general practitioners (GPs) showed symptoms of stress that was serious enough to affect their health and impair their ability to provide high-quality care to patients. Much of this stress was due to excessive workload and lack of control over their workload and work environment. Other factors include inadequate resources for the job and sharing the emotional distress and suffering of patients.

A large study of 11 000 employees from 19 National Health Service (NHS) trusts found that 26.8 percent of health service workers reported significant levels of minor psychiatric disorders. This compared with 17.8 percent of the general population.[28] In a Canadian study of staff employed by Cancer Care Ontario,[23] physician exhaustion was much higher (53.3 percent) than reported in the UK study; 48.8 percent of physicians reported low feelings of personal accomplishment. The feelings of depersonalization in the Canadian group were similar to the UK sample (22.1 percent) of physicians. These figures are comparable to a study in which 46 percent of physicians surveyed by the Canadian Medical Association said they were burned out and emotionally exhausted. They attributed their burnout to the bureaucratic health system and fewer physicians to handle patients with complex problems.[29]

VARIABLES ASSOCIATED WITH STRESS AND BURNOUT

Demographic variables

Younger caregivers report more stressors, more manifestations of stress, and fewer coping strategies.[5] Burnout is associated with being under the age of 55 years;[20] being of age 55 years or less is an independent risk factor for burnout.[30] Increased job satisfaction is associated with older age.[31,32]

Female physicians experience more role strain than males[33] and are more likely to report suicidal ideation.[34] However, female physicians report greater job satisfaction and greater wellbeing than matched controls.[35] The latter finding was replicated in the Physician Work Life Study (N = 5704).[36] Women were more likely to report satisfaction with their specialty and with patient and colleague relationships, but less likely to be satisfied with autonomy, relationships with community, pay, and resources. There is some evidence that female physicians may be more at risk of mental health problems.[37] In the Physician Work Life Study,[36] women were 1.6 times more likely to report burnout than men. The odds increased by 12–15 percent for each additional 5 hours worked per week over 40 hours. Lack of workplace control predicted burnout in women but not in men. Women with young children who received support

for balancing their lives from their partner, significant other, and colleagues were 40 percent less likely to report burnout.

In a large study of almost 2000 British family practitioners,[35] male physicians had higher anxiety scores than the norms and had less job satisfaction and drank more alcohol than their female counterparts. Dealing with death and dying was not a major source of stress; however it was associated with excess alcohol use, especially for female physicians.[38] Being single was an independent risk factor for burnout in the study of consultants in the UK.[30]

Job–home interaction

A model of burnout was tested in a study comparing burnout in two large samples of physicians in the USA (N = 1824) and the Netherlands (N = 1435).[39] Half the burnout was explained for both samples. Older physicians in the USA felt they had more control than did younger physicians. The study found an adverse impact of academic practice on work control and work–home interference in the USA. American male physicians described significantly more work control than female physicians, a sex difference not seen in the Netherlands. For both countries, work control was correlated with job stress and satisfaction, whereas work–home interference was associated with work hours, children, stress, (dis)satisfaction, and burnout. The UK study[20] also found job characteristics associated with burnout included 'being overloaded and its effect on home life'.

Occupational variables

WORKLOAD

When palliative care specialists were compared with clinical and radiation oncologists, problems with 'feeling overloaded and its effects on home life' were found to be significantly greater for the medical and clinical oncologists than for the palliative care specialists. Depersonalization and high GHQ scores were also associated with being overloaded.[20] Senior house officers in UK hospices[25] described their posts as stressful. A palliative care physician acknowledged that workload may be self-induced. He said, 'Lots of us feeling overloaded and overworked create it ourselves. We start dancing to a tune that you're called to play by yourself.'[5]

Hospice staff initially prided themselves on having the time to spend with patients that was conducive to the best patient care. Current issues with managed care, the nursing shortage, and fiscal restraint has changed this in many settings.[40] Direct patient care activities have an impact on stress through a heavy workload of complex care, a shortage of staff, and a lack of competence.[41] Nurses working with critically ill and dying children in Hong Kong and Greece felt unable to provide quality care because of the shortage in nursing personnel. This added to their stress.[42]

However, in a study of hospice nurses in the UK, Payne[22] found that despite workload being a frequently reported stressor it was not related to burnout.

CONTROL

Research suggests that restructuring high-demand, low-control jobs may enhance productivity and reduce disability costs.[43] Physicians' studies report low levels of satisfaction from not having adequate resources to perform their role.[20] In a study comparing general internists with internal medicine subspecialists and family practitioners, higher satisfaction for general internists was associated with less time pressure during office visits, fewer work hours, and fewer patients with complex psychosocial problems.[32] Seale and Cartwright[44] found 43 percent of GP respondents needed more time to give to dying patients, around one third had trouble coping with their own emotional responses to dying patients and these GPs seemed most likely to have difficulty communicating with patients who were dying and their relatives.

Recent practices in hospice led by fiscal constraints have raised increasing concern. Nurses are sometimes expected to perform procedures in the community without adequate supervision and training. When people are expected to assume responsibility with inadequate training, they have difficulty functioning.[45,40]

Nurses report being in situations both in the hospital and in the community where they feel responsible for alleviating the pain of a palliative care patient, yet do not have a physician willing to order the medication they feel will be sufficient to control pain. In addition, with earlier discharge of sicker patients, nurses with limited experience may be expected to care for seriously ill palliative care patients in their home, without access to physicians skilled in effective palliative care and symptom management.[45] Dr Neil MacDonald[46] testified before a Senate subcommittee on end-of-life care in Canada that in a study of Quebec oncologists and palliative care physicians, their opinion was that the big problem in managing cancer pain was the reluctance on the part of physicians to use opioids and the misunderstanding of patients about the use of pain medications. A nurse said that when she reported that a dying patient was in severe pain and she felt that he needed to have his medication increased, the physician asked who he was treating – the patient or the nurse?[47]

Problems of control may also involve issues of personal safety. Nurses working in a hospice in South Africa were uncomfortable going into some settings, particularly at night. As a group they explored with administration the option of refusing to go into some areas. The hospice provided them with cell phones. Brainstorming together, the nurses suggested working with the police to alert the police when the nurses were going into a potentially dangerous situation. The nurses asked the police to accompany them if they were really uncomfortable visiting certain areas but felt they should visit for the sake of the patient.[40]

REWARD

Issues related to funding have been a problem for many programs.[38] Participants in an Australian study[48] reported that economic pressures resulted in less staff support, competition between services for funding, inadequate funding to provide services in areas of need, lack of support for psychosocial needs including bereavement care, and experienced staff leaving palliative care. Nurses in a Canadian study[49] reported difficulty with resource allocation issues, but the majority of their concerns were related to their inability to provide quality care because of financial constraints and staffing cutbacks.[47]

COMMUNITY

Team communication problems have been a significant part of hospice palliative care since the early days of the specialty[16] and continue to the present time.[25,41] In the European Union, the recognition that there were communication problems between palliative care mobile teams (PCMTs) and hospital staff, led to a program of intervention, discussed below.[50]

Team issues have been documented in numerous studies and across many cultures.[5,16,41,42] In a group of 33 nurses from three midwestern cities[51] predictors of free-floating anxiety in hospice nurses included the degree of staff support and staff participation in decision making, as well as the final relationship between the patient and the nurse. Since the early days of hospices, caregivers have reported problems with timely referrals[5] and these issues continue with the development of the specialty of palliative care. Field[52] surveyed GPs in the UK working with dying patients and found that while relationships between the GPs and the district nurses with whom they worked were good, the relationships with hospitals were generally satisfactory, but rarely more than that, and there were negative comments about the provision of information from hospitals to both patients and GPs. An issue of contemporary relevance was the tension over the role of hospice and specialist terminal care services. General practitioners appreciate calling on specialist care but do not want to surrender care to the 'experts' as the GPs feel they have the best social knowledge of the patient and family. They resented hospices that were not willing to involve the GP and team as partners but wanted to deliver care on their terms. The GPs also expressed concern that the involvement of specialist providers of palliative care can have detrimental consequences for the generalist expertise of GPs (and community nurses) by deskilling them. Conflict also exists between the district nurses and the Macmillan nurses.[53]

A more recent study[54] in Wales showed significant enthusiasm among consultant physicians, 94 percent of whom would consider referring patients with nonmalignant disease to a specialist palliative care service. The physicians thought that a system of shared care and responsibility would be a means of addressing concerns regarding the lack of disease-specific expertise within the palliative care team. In Spain problems with the system also exist.[55] Half of physicians and

60 percent of nurses surveyed reported that caring for terminally ill patients at home made them feel frustrated. The 'system' was the main cause of frustration; frequently mentioned issues were bureaucracy (particularly with regard to access to narcotic analgesics) and the isolation of primary healthcare professionals, especially in rural areas. Women, younger caregivers, and those who had attended fewer patients in the past year were more likely to report feelings of frustration.

In the USA, the problem continues with timely referral.[56] Given the documented deficiencies in end-of life care,[57] it is to be hoped that the philosophy of palliative care could be incorporated into end-of-life care for increasing numbers of people. However, Byock[58] writes of the tensions between the 'loyalists' who have generally been associated with the hospice movement and the 'progressives' who 'tend to be caring, committed clinicians and administrators, often based in hospitals, nursing homes, or home health, who have awakened to the need to improve care for the dying in their own systems and are earnestly trying to do just that'.[53 (pp. 155–6)] Payne[22] found that dealing with death and dying, inadequate preparation, and workload were slightly more of a problem than were conflicts with doctors, conflicts with other nurses, lack of support, and uncertainty concerning treatment. However, conflict with staff contributed to both the emotional exhaustion and depersonalization subscales of the Maslach Burnout Inventory. Palliative care workers in rural Australia spoke of the difficulty involved in being expected to work beyond normal working hours and of the lack of anonymity in a small rural community.[47,59]

FAIRNESS

The issue of rivalries between hospice and other settings of care and between hospice programs has long been an issue.[5,40] Rivalries are encountered as programs try to determine with which agencies, if any, they will have preferred partner arrangements. Other settings have developed palliative care programs in an apparent move to avoid referral to hospices, and to gain access to funding that might be made available for dying persons.[40] In addition there are financial barriers that include reimbursement systems that provide only for the options of cure or certain death.[60,61]

> Patients without a care provider; unwilling to forego beneficial palliative chemotherapy, radiation, or surgery; or with a prognosis that was not absolutely certain to be six months or less, were caught in the middle. This part of the path felt treacherous; we had no trail markers, no compass, and darkness was about to fall.[61 (p. 27)]

VALUES

In *Crossing Over: Narratives of Palliative Care*, describing the experience of palliative care in two settings in the USA and Canada, Barnard *et al.*[62] state:

> palliative care is whole-person care not only in the sense that the whole person of the patient (body, mind, spirit) is the object of care, but also in that the whole person of the caregiver is involved. Palliative care is, par excellence, care that is given through the medium of a human relationship.[62 (p. 5)]

A study of nurses in a European academic palliative care setting (N = 14)[63] was undertaken to gain insight into the fact that many nurses were leaving feeling frustrated by the far-reaching medical orientation on the ward and feeling unable to provide the care they wanted to give. This study challenges whether or not the assumptions of Barnard are completely generalizable at this point in time. The majority of nurses in this study had a model described as *striving to adopt a well-organized and purposeful approach* (N = 12) compared with the small group of nurses who were described as *striving to increase the wellbeing of patients* (N = 2). The pattern of the first group involved: adopting an academic attitude; developing a professional attitude; striving to remain objective; being task oriented; avoiding emotional stress; and embracing a practitioner-focused perspective. In contrast, the second group was described as: adopting a humble attitude; giving attention to patients and their experiences; being available; valuing a caring attitude; remaining attentive and thoughtful and trying to accept and cope with emotional strain. The authors quote James and Field[64] who said that by marginalizing the originating ethics of palliative care, the heart and soul of care are endangered. 'Expert' values based on medical technologies and psychosocial skills replace the compassionate help by which death is no longer a truth to confront but a process that has to be managed as efficiently as possible. The nurses were encouraged to acquire knowledge and skills, while developing moral qualities necessary to care for those who are dying were not addressed. They responded less to problems because their moral values were endangered, but mainly because they conflicted with their professional norms and established rules. In contrast Webster and Kristjanson's[48] Australian study of caregivers in palliative care found the work allowed caregivers to bring personal values to the workplace and encouraged personal growth.

ISSUES OF DEATH AND DYING

While the literature has been somewhat divided as to whether or not the care of the dying is a major stressor in hospice palliative care,[5,16] recent research in the burnout area has focused explicitly on emotion–work variables (e.g. requirement to display or suppress emotions on the job, requirements to be emotionally empathic) and has found these emotional factors do account for additional variance in burnout scores over and above job stressors.[14] Factors associated with burnout in Ramirez *et al.*'s study[20] included 'dealing with patients' suffering'. Depersonalization was associated 'dealing with patients' suffering' as well as low levels of satisfaction from 'dealing well with patients and relatives'. Low personal accomplishment was associated with stress from 'being involved with treatment toxicity and errors' and low levels of satisfaction from 'dealing well with patients and relatives' and from 'having professional status and esteem'.[20] [(p. 1268)] The most problematic stressor reported by UK hospice nurses was 'death and dying',[22] although in a North American study these were of much less concern.[51]

COPING

When close to 600 caregivers of the critically ill, dying, and bereaved were interviewed and asked what enabled them to continue working in the field, the top five coping mechanisms identified were: a sense of competence, control or pleasure in one's work (13 percent); team philosophy, building and support (11 percent); control over aspects of practice (10 percent); lifestyle management (9 percent); and a personal philosophy of illness, death, and one's role in life (9 percent).[5] Other studies have looked at sources of satisfaction in the work of palliative care staff. These include: dealing well with patients and relatives,[20] having professional status and esteem, deriving intellectual satisfaction, having adequate resources to perform one's role,[20] helping patients and families find meaning in suffering,[62,65] and having good relationships with colleagues.[66*] Palliative care has been described as a way of living. Vitality – the capacity to live and develop which is associated with energy, life, animation, and importance – is the core meaning of palliative care. The way of living involves unity with self, being touched to the heart, and personal meaning.[48]

Job engagement is conceptualized as being the opposite of burnout. It involves energy, involvement, and efficacy. Engagement involves the individual's relationship with work. It involves a sustainable workload, feelings of choice and control, appropriate recognition and reward, a supportive work community, fairness and justice, and meaningful and valued work. Engagement is also characterized by high levels of activation and pleasure.[14] Engagement is defined as a persistent, positive-affective-motivational state of fulfillment in employees that is characterized by vigor, dedication, and absorption.[14] Clearly many caregivers are engaged in their work in palliative care.

It is also important, however, to have time for one's self and family. In the study comparing physicians in the Netherlands and the USA[39] there were remarkable benefits of home support on stress reduction in the latter country.

STUDIES OF INTERVENTION

Despite a variety of articles describing intervention with palliative care staff, there have been few studies documenting the efficacy of intervention in this or other groups. A recent meta-analysis of 48 occupational stress-reducing interventions (N = 3736 participants)[67***] categorized the studies as: cognitive–behavioral interventions, relaxation techniques, multimodal programs (emphasizing both active and passive coping skills), and organization-focused

interventions. A small but significant overall effect was found. Cognitive–behavioral and multimodal interventions had a moderate effect, a small effect was found for relaxation and the effect size for organization-focused intervention was nonsignificant. Cognitive–behavioral interventions appeared to be effective in improving perceived quality of work life, enhancing psychological resources and responses, and reducing complaints. Multimodal programs showed similar effects; however, they appeared to be ineffective in increasing psychological resources and responses. The authors note that there is a marginally significant effect of job status on treatment outcome – those who appeared to have more job control had a better response to the interventions. The authors urge caution here because job status was inferred. They suggest the relatively large effect of cognitive–behavioral interventions in those with higher job control may be because employees profit most when they are provided with individual coping skills in a job that allows them to use these skills. The lack of effect of organization-focused interventions was attributed to a variety of factors.

van Staa et al.[41*] describe an intervention in a new palliative care unit in the Netherlands which may shed some light on the above findings. A carefully designed training program and staff support activities were meant to enhance personal growth, to give emotional support, and to deal with death and bereavement issues. The interventions did not involve mutual collaboration, practical problems, managerial and communication skills, and the skills needed to deliver complex palliative care. There was a cultural difference between the external consultants who embraced a relational therapeutic worldview and the hospice staff who came from a rational technical hospital environment. The former approach involves complete trust and openness in order to work. Not all staff members were convinced of the value of the nondirective approach. In addition a therapeutic group is fundamentally different from a group that has to work together after the session. The authors suggest that future leaders should focus on content as well as process issues. They also suggest that adequate resources, a supportive management structure, an extensive educational training program, and attention to individual needs should accompany support groups. These issues have been identified earlier[5,16] so it is worth noting that they still exist.[53]

Fallowfield et al.[68**] recently showed improvement in the communication skills of oncologists, which the authors hypothesized as leading to personally and professionally more rewarding consultations; the consultation can have a significant impact on clinical care and patients' and physicians' wellbeing.

STUDIES IN PROCESS

Medland et al.[66*] describe an intervention with 150 members of the multidisciplinary team in the oncology department at Northwestern Memorial Hospital. The program aims to decrease absenteeism and enhance community to create a meaningful and rewarding work environment. The program targets both individual and organizational issues. Research has not yet been conducted but staff retention has improved. Plans are underway to measure the effectiveness of the program through 'increased overall patient satisfaction, psychosocial patient satisfaction, and spiritual patient satisfaction scores'. The level of staff psychosocial wellness, as evidenced by follow-up human services surveys, is planned for the future. Most importantly, staff will be monitored for changes in behavior reflecting use of positive coping strategies and constructive self-care behaviors.

EDUCATIONAL INTERVENTIONS

Another model for shifting established patterns is being conducted in the European Union with a goal of improving the interaction between PCMTs and the hospital staff with whom they interact.[50*] In this model, recognizing the full range of convictions held by individuals in a hospital setting, the concept of palliative care/terminal care has been bolstered by the concept of *continuous care*. Continuous care tends to *articulate* curative and palliative procedures focusing on the holistic care of patients and their family. 'Promoting the integration of continuous care in the hospital' intends to identify the challenges in integrating continuous care through an inventory and analysis of the activity of PCMTs in several countries of Europe. Competencies for PCMTs have been derived, and based on these, a pilot three phase educational programme with PCMTs undertaken and evaluated.[p.4]

Meier *et al.*[69] recently proposed an approach to physician awareness which involves identifying and working with emotions that may affect patient care. This involves looking at physician, situational, and patient risk factors that can lead to physician feelings and thus influence patient care. The steps include:

- Identify the factors that predispose to emotions that might affect patient care
- Monitor for signs (behavioral) and symptoms (feelings) of emotions
- Name and accept the emotion
- Identify possible sources of the emotion
- Respond constructively to the emotion
  - Step back from the situation to gain perspective
  - Identify behaviors resulting from the feeling
  - Consider implications and consequences of behaviors
  - Think through alternative outcomes for patients according to different behaviors
  - Consult a trusted professional colleague.

CONCLUSIONS

Palliative care is both stressful and rewarding. Although previous studies have shown that work in palliative care is not more stressful, and may be less stressful than other specialties, the increase in workload in recent years may well serve to increase the stress experienced by staff. Current work on coping holds exciting promise to change the culture of the field and to decrease team stress – which has been identified since the early days of the movement.

Key learning points

- Stress and burnout are generally less of a problem in palliative care than in other areas of healthcare, but nonetheless there are stressors and issues of concern.

- Burnout is associated with the degree of match or mismatch between the person and six domains of the job environment. The greater the gap or mismatch between the person and the environment, the greater the likelihood of burnout. The greater the match or fit the greater the likelihood of engagement with work.

- Workload, control, reward, community, fairness, and values and emotion-work variables are the primary domains of work associated with burnout. Individuals vary with respect to which are most important,

- Burnout levels are often higher in North America than in other countries for a variety of cultural reasons, however, there is some indication that burnout levels are increasing in many other countries. Palliative care staff may be experiencing increasing burnout as a result of work variables.

- Job engagement is the opposite of burnout. There is much in the literature to show that palliative care staff are engaged in their work.

- The research on the effectiveness of intervention in palliative care is still limited. A recent meta-analysis of occupational stress-reducing interventions showed that cognitive–behavioral and multimodal interventions had a moderate effect, and the effect size for organization-focused interventions was nonsignificant. Communication skills programs and educational interventions hold some promise but much research is yet to be done.

REFERENCES

1   Levine S, Scotch NA. *Social Stress*. Chicago: Aldine, 1973.
2   Selye H. *Stress without Distress*. Philadelphia: Lippincott, 1974.
3   Selye H. *The Stress of Life*. New York: McGraw-Hill, 1956.

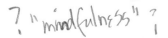
? "mindfulness" ?

4   Antonovsky A. *Health, Stress and Coping.* San Francisco: Jossey-Bass, 1979.

5   Vachon MLS. *Occupational Stress in the Care of the Critically Ill, the Dying and the Bereaved.* New York: Hemisphere Press, 1987.

6   Lazarus RS, Cohen J. Psychological stress and adaptation: Some unresolved issues. In: H. Selye, ed. *Selye's Guide to Stress Research,* Vol 1. New York: Von Nostrand Reinhold, 1980: 90–117.

7   Lazarus R, Launier R. Stress related transactions between person and environment. In: Pervin L, Lewis M, eds. *Perspectives in International Psychology.* New York: Plenum, 1978: 287–327.

8   European Agency for Safety and Health at Work. Safety at Work. Available at: http://agency.osha.eu.int/publications/factsheets/8/en/facts8_en.pdf (2000) (accessed December 15, 2005).

9   Freudenberger HJ. Staff burnout. *J Soc Issues* 1974; **30**: 159–65.

10 Freudenberger HJ, Richelson G. *Burn Out: the High Cost of High Achievement.* New York: Anchor Press, 1980.

11 Edelwich J, Brodsky A. *Burn-Out: Stages of Disillusionment in the Helping Professions.* New York: Springer, 1980.

12 Pines AM. Burnout: an existential perspective. In: Schaufeli W, Maslach C, Marek T, eds. *Professional Burnout.* Washington, DC: Taylor and Francis, 1993.

13 Maslach C, Jackson SE. *The Maslach Burnout Inventory (Manual),* 2nd ed. Palo Alto, CA: Consulting Psychologists Press, 1986.

14 Maslach C, Schaufeli WB, Leiter MP. Job burnout. *Annu Rev Psychol* 2001; **52**: 397–422.

15 French JRP, Rodgers W, Cobb S. Adjustment as person-environment fit. In: Coelho GV, Hamburg DA, Adams E, eds. *Coping and Adaptation.* New York: Basic Books, 1974: 316–33.

16 Vachon MLS. Staff stress in palliative/hospice care: a review. *Palliat Med* 1995; **9**: 91–122.

17 Finlay IG. Sources of stress in hospice medical directors and matrons. *Palliat Med* 1990; **4**: 5–9.

18 Cooper CL, Mitchell S. Nursing the critically ill and dying. *Hum Relat* 1990; **43**: 297–311.

19 Bene B, Foxall MJ. Death anxiety and job stress in hospice and medical-surgical nurses. *Hosp J* 1991; **7**: 25–41.

20 Ramirez AJ, Graham J, Richards MA, *et al.* Burnout and psychiatric disorder among cancer clinicians. *Br J Cancer* 1995; **71**: 1263–9.

21 Maslach C, Jackson SE. Burnout in health professions: a social psychological analysis. In: Sanders GS, Suls J, eds. *Social Psychology of Health and Illness.* London: Erlbaum, 1982.

22 Payne N. Occupational stressors and coping as determinants of burnout in female hospice nurses. *J Adv Nurs* 2001; **33**: 396–405.

23 Grunfeld E, Whelan TJ, Zitzelsberger L, *et al.* Cancer care workers in Ontario: prevalence of burnout, job stress and job satisfaction. *CMAJ* 2000; **163**: 166–9.

24 Kash KM, Holland JC, Breitbart W, *et al.* Stress and burnout in oncology. *Oncology* 2000; **14**: 1621–37.

25 Lloyd Williams M. Senior house officers' experience of a six month post in a hospice. *Med Educ* 2002; **36**: 45–8.

26 Goldberg D, Williams P. *A User's Guide to the General Health Questionnaire.* Windsor, Berkshire: NFER-Nelson, 1988.

27 Beecham L. BMA warns of stress suffered by senior doctors. *BMJ* 2000; **321**: 56.

28 Wall TD, Bolden RI, Borrill CS, *et al.* Minor psychiatric disorder in NHS trust staff: occupational and gender differences. *Br J Psychiatry* 1997; **171**: 519–23.

29 Manisses Communication Group. In case you haven't heard . . . 46% of Canadian physicans report burnout. *Mental Health Weekly* 2003; **13**: 8.

30 Ramirez AJ, Graham J, Richards MA, *et al.* Mental health of hospital consultants: the effect of stress and satisfaction at work. *Lancet* 1996; **347**: 724–8.

31 Beck-Friis B, Strang P, Sjödén P-O. Caring for severely ill cancer patients: a comparison of working conditions in hospital-based home care and in hospital. *Support Care Cancer* 1993; **1**: 145–51.

32 Wetterneck TB,, Linzer M, McMurray JE, *et al.* Worklife and satisfaction of general internists. *Arch Intern Med* 2002; **162**: 649–56.

33 Heim E. Job stressors and coping in health professions. *Psychother Psychosom* 1991; **55**: 90–9.

34 Cassels D. Tarnished images. *Survey 1993: The Medical Post National Survey of Canadian Doctors.* Toronto: Maclean Hunter Limited, 1993: 8,12.

35 Cooper CL, Rout U, Faragher B. Mental health, job satisfaction, and job stress among general practitioners. *BMJ* 1989; **298**: 366–70.

36 McMurray JE, Linzer M, Konrad TR, *et al.,* for the SGIM Career Satisfaction Study Group. The work lives of women physicians: results from the physician work life study. *J Gen Intern Med* 2000; **15**: 372–80.

37 Graham J, Ramirez AJ, Cull A, *et al.* Job stress and satisfaction among palliative physicians: A CRC/ICRF Study. *Palliat Med* 1996; **10**: 185–94.

38 Vachon MLS. Staff stress and burnout. In: Berger AM, Portenoy RK, Weissman DE, eds. *Palliative Care and Supportive Oncology.* Philadelphia: Lippincott Williams & Wilkins. 2002: 831–48.

39 Association of Professors of Medicine (Linzer M, Visser MR, Oort FJ, Smets EMA, McMurray JE, de Haes HCJM for the Society of General Internal Medicine (SGIM) Career Satisfaction Study Group [CSSG]). Predicting and preventing physician burnout: results from the United States and the Netherlands. *Am J Med* 2001; **111**: 170–5.

40 Vachon MLS. The nurse's role: the world of palliative care nursing. In: Ferrell B, Coyle N, eds. *The Oxford Textbook of Palliative Nursing.* New York: Oxford University Press, 2001: 647–62.

41 van Staa AL, Visser A, van der Zouwe N. Caring for caregivers: experiences and evaluation of interventions for a palliative care team. *Patient Educ Couns* 2000; **41**: 93–105.

42 Papadatou D, Martinson IM, Chung P, Man MN. Caring for dying children: a comparative study of nurses' experiences in Greece and Hong Kong. *Cancer Nurs* 2001; **24**: 402–12.

43 Yandrick RM. High demand low control. *Behav Healthc Tomorrow* 1997; **6**: 41–4.

44 Seale C, Cartwright A. *The Year Before Death.* Aldershot: Avebury, 1994.

45 Coyle N. Focus on the nurse: ethical dilemmas with highly symptomatic patients dying at home. *Hosp J* 1997; **12**: 33–41.

46 MacDonald N. Testimony before The Subcommittee to Update 'Of Life and Death' of the Standing Senate Committee on

Social Affairs, Science and Technology, Ottawa, Ontario, March 28, 2000.

◆ 47   Vachon MLS. The experience of the nurse in end-of-life care in the 21st century. In: Ferrell B, Coyle N, eds. *The Oxford Textbook of Palliative Nursing*. New York: Oxford University Press, 2nd ed. (in press).

48   Webster J, Kristjanson LJ. 'But isn't it depressing?' The Vitality of palliative care. *J Palliat Care* 2002; **18**: 15–24.

49   Oberle K, Hughes D. Doctors' and nurses' perceptions of ethical problems in end-of-life decisions. *J Adv Nurs* 2001; **33**: 707–15.

50   European Commission. *Promoting the Development and Integration of Palliative Care Mobile Support Teams in the Hospital*. Brussels: Directorate-General for Research Food Quality and Safety, 2004.

51   Dean RA. Occupational stress in hospice care: causes and coping strategies. *Am J Hosp Palliat Care* 1998; **15**: 151–4.

52   Field D. Special not different: general practitioners' accounts of their care of dying people. *Soc Sci Med* 1998; **46**:1111–20.

◆ 53   Vachon MLS. Stress of caregivers. In: Doyle D, Hanks G, Cherny N, Calman K, eds. *Oxford Textbook of Palliative Medicine*, 3rd ed. Oxford: Oxford University Press, 2004: 992–1004.

54   Dharmasena HP, Forbes K. Palliative care for patients with non-malignant disease: will hospital physicians refer? *Palliat Med* 2001; **15**: 413–18.

55   Porta M, Busquet X, Jariod M. Attitudes and views of physicians and nurses towards cancer patients dying at home. *Palliat Med* 1997; **11**: 116–26.

56   Boling A, Lynn J. Hospice: current practice, future possibilities. *Hosp J* 1998; **13**: 29–32.

57   Field M, Cassel CK. *Approaching Death: Improving Care at the End of Life*. Washington DC: Institute of Medicine, National Academies Press, 1997.

● 58   Byock I. Hospice and palliative care: a parting of the ways or a path to the future? *J Palliat Med* 1998; **1**: 165–76.

59   McConigley R, Kristjanson, LJ, Morgan A. Palliative care nursing in Western Australia. *Int J Palliat Care Nurs.* 2000; **6**: 80–90.

60   Lynn J, O'Mara A. Reliable, high quality, efficient end-of-life care for cancer patients: Economic issues and barriers. In: Foley K, Gelband H, eds. *Improving Palliative Care for Cancer: Summary and Recommendations*. Washington, DC: National Academies Press, 2001: 67–95.

61   Whedon MB. Revisiting the road not taken: integrating palliative care into oncology nursing. *Clin J Onc Nurs* 2002; **6**: 27–33.

62   Barnard D, Towers A, Boston P, Lambrinidou Y. *Crossing Over: Narratives of Palliative Care*. New York: Oxford, 2000.

● 63   Georges JJ, Grypdonck M, De Casterle BD. Being a palliative care nurse in an academic hospital: a qualitative study about nurses' perceptions of palliative care nursing. *J Clin Nurs* 2002:**11**: 785–93.

64   James N, Field D. The routinization of hospice: charisma and bureaucracy. *Soc Sci Med* 1992; **34**: 1363–75.

65   Kearney M. *A Place of Healing: Working with Suffering in Living and Dying*. Oxford: Oxford University Press, 2000.

66   Medland J, Howard-Ruben, Whitaker E. Fostering psychosocial wellness in oncology nurses: addressing burnout and social support in the workplace. *Oncol Nurs Forum* 2004; **31**: 47–54.

◆ 67   van der Klink JJL, Blonk RWB, Schene AH, van Dijk FJH. The benefits of intervention for work-related stress. *Am J Public Health* 2001; **91**: 270–6.

● 68   Fallowfield L, Jenkins V, Farewell V, *et al.* Efficacy of a Cancer Research UK communication skills training model for oncologists: a randomized controlled trial. *Lancet* 2002; **359**: 650–6.

● 69   Meier DE, Back AL, Morrison RS. The inner life of physicians and the care of the seriously ill. *JAMA* 2002; **286**: 3007–14.

106

Communication in palliative care

JOSEPHINE M CLAYTON, MARTIN H N TATTERSALL

INTRODUCTION

When physicians communicate effectively they are more likely to understand and address the issues that are important for the individual patient, and patients are more likely to understand their medical problems and treatment options.[1] Moreover effective communication can reduce patient anxiety and distress[2] and improve satisfaction with the consultation.[3] Good communication in a palliative care setting is paramount. While communication in palliative care shares many of the general features of physician–patient communication in other settings, the fear and uncertainty associated with a life-limiting illness adds a greater emotional element to the interaction and thus communication may assume an even greater significance. Indeed optimal communication has been identified by patients and their families as one of the more important aspects of medical care at the end of life.[4–7]

This chapter reviews research findings relevant to communication in palliative medicine. The main focus is on physician–patient and physician–carer communication, with particular emphasis on meeting the information needs of palliative care patients and their carers.

COMPONENTS OF GOOD PHYSICIAN–PATIENT COMMUNICATION

Several components of good quality communication between physicians and patients with advanced progressive illnesses have been discussed in the literature. A good physician–patient relationship is the cornerstone to effective communication in this setting.[8,9] Attributes of a good physician–patient relationship include mutual trust, care, respect, honesty, empathy, support, and partnership, as well as the patients' confidence in their physicians' professional competence.[10,11] In general it is recommended that a physician should create an atmosphere where the patient is treated as a 'whole person' and feels that the physician is interested in and sensitive to their problems and feelings.[1] Even brief expressions of empathy may reduce patient anxiety.[12**]

Facilitation of information exchange

Prior to imparting information, it is recommended that physicians actively listen to the patient and elicit their full list of concerns.[1,13,14] The extent to which patients' concerns have been disclosed and resolved has been found to be associated with the likelihood of subsequent depression and anxiety.[15] When physicians elicit 'patients' perceptions of the problems and reactions, and the impact on their daily lives, patients feel more satisfied and comply better with offered advice and medication'.[16] Physicians cannot assume that patients will volunteer all of their concerns. Studies in palliative care and oncology settings show that a substantial number of patients' concerns remain undisclosed in practice.[17,18] For example, Heaven and Maguire[17] found that hospice patients had on average seven concerns, but only three of these were disclosed to hospice nurses. The patients in this study 'showed a strong bias towards disclosing physical concerns' and 'concerns about the future, appearance and loss of independence were withheld more than 80 percent of the time'. Patients may be reluctant to disclose their psychosocial and other more sensitive concerns and believe these are an inevitable part of their illness, for which nothing can be done.[14] Furthermore, patients may perceive their concerns to be embarrassing or abnormal and/or be concerned about burdening their health professionals, whom they see as busy people. Therefore physicians and nurses need to encourage patients to disclose their psychosocial and other sensitive concerns. They also need to acknowledge and respond empathically when such concerns are raised.[19] However, health professionals may feel ill-equipped to elicit and deal with patients' psychosocial problems.[20]

INFORMATION NEEDS OF PALLIATIVE CARE PATIENTS

Patients use information for various purposes:

- to understand their illness and treatment options[21,22]
- gain realistic expectations[23]
- make plans and priorities for the future[22]
- care for themselves[21]
- participate in treatment decisions[22]
- provide a sense of autonomy and control[21]
- as a way of coping with a serious illness.[24]

In developed countries numerous studies have documented that the majority of English-speaking patients with serious illnesses prefer to be fully informed about a variety of topics including diagnosis, prognosis, and treatment options.[25–27] However, not all patients want extensive information about their illness or prognosis.[28,29] Furthermore, patients' information needs may be strongly influenced by their countries' culture and also by the different cultures within countries. Patients from some cultures may prefer nondisclosure, especially when life expectancy is short.[30,31] However, the evidence for this is conflicting with other studies suggesting that the majority of people from certain non-Western countries still want to be fully informed about their diagnosis and prognosis.[32–34] Other factors may influence patients' preferences for information. Higher levels of information tend to be desired by patients who are younger,[25,35,36] female,[25] come from a higher socioeconomic background,[37,38] and are better educated.[35] Patients may also desire less detailed information over time as their illness progresses.[26,39]

Little is known about the specific information needs of patients referred to a specialist palliative care service or of terminally ill patients in general. Kutner et al.[27] examined the information needs and concerns of patients who met the criteria for outpatient hospice enrollment in the USA. Qualitative interviews with 22 participants identified seven key issues including: 'change in functional status or activity level; role change; symptoms, especially pain; stress of the illness on family members; loss of control; financial burden; and conflict between wanting to know what is going on and fearing bad news.'

These data were used to develop a questionnaire which was then administered to a second population of 56 patients. More than 80 percent of participants in the survey wanted

Table 106.1 *Kutner et al.'s[27] findings regarding preferences of terminally ill patients for information (N = 56)*

Specific type of information	Proportion of patients wanting this information (%)
Changes in disease status	98
What treatment will accomplish	88
Side effects of treatment	84
Expected course of disease	80
What treatments are available	77
If pain will be relieved	77
If dignity will be respected	77
Likelihood of cure	71
Effectiveness of treatment for others	71
The specific name of the disease	71
Options if treatment does not work	70
Effect of illness on daily life	64
If will be able to eat	64
If will be in pain in future	64
Who will provide follow-up care	64
Life expectancy	59
What to do if unable to care for self	54
What to tell family	50
More about resuscitation/CPR	41
How will pay for care	34
About getting help at home	32
How to write a will	30

CPR, cardiopulmonary resuscitation.

their physicians to be honest (100 percent) but they also wanted their physicians to be optimistic (91 percent). Participants' preferences for some specific types of information are shown in Table 106.1. The expressed information needs and concerns were not associated with any identifiable patient characteristics. The authors conclude that physicians and other health professionals

> should be aware of the diversity of needs and concerns of the terminally ill and should routinely identify, negotiate and address specific individual needs and expectations.

Further research is needed to explore the specific information needs of palliative care patients from different cultural backgrounds.

Incurable cancer and palliative care patients' preferences for information about prognosis and dying

Physicians are challenged to deliver information relevant to prognosis and dying. Yet having a physician who is willing to talk about dying and who is sensitive to when to discuss this issue has been identified by patients and their families as one of the more important needs at the end of life.[5,6] There may be reticence to discuss dying for fear that this could be contrary to the patients' wishes or best interests. Finding a balance between honesty and hope can be difficult to achieve. Nevertheless open conversation about death and dying can bring considerable relief to patients and their families. Furthermore, feedback from Western patients suggests that open and supportive communication, rather than nondisclosure, may be most hope giving to patients.[40]

Surveys of Western patients with advanced cancer[41] and other far progressive life-limiting illnesses[9] suggest that most patients want prognostic and end-of-life information but prefer to negotiate the level of detail and timing of this information.[41] Qualitative studies of dying patients and their families, from Western countries, have identified various important elements in health professionals' communication about prognosis and end-of-life issues, including: the need for honesty,[6,39] clear straightforward language,[6,39] showing empathy and compassion,[6,39] willingness to discuss dying but being sensitive to when the patient is ready to hear this information,[6,39] pacing information so it can be assimilated,[39] encouraging questions,[6] and assuring patients that they will not be abandoned as their illness progresses.[39]

Little is known about patients from non-Western countries preferences for style of prognostic and end-of-life communication. Further research is needed in this area.

Specific information needs of carers of palliative care patients

The support of families, both before and after the death of a patient, is an integral component of palliative care.[42] Families need information to enable them to care for their dying relative[39,43–45] and prepare for their own future after a patient's death.[5] Family members need information about a patient's illness to be mentally prepared, organize their daily life, and to be a source of information to others.[46]

Research findings suggest that caregivers of palliative care patients may have distinct information needs from the patient,[39,44,47] particularly regarding prognosis and end-of-life issues. The caregiver may need more detailed information than the patient about the dying process in order to provide care.[47] The importance of open discussion and consistent information being given to patients and caregivers has been highlighted, particularly in studies conducted in Western countries.[39,47] However, it may not be possible to meet the information needs of both the patient and their family without having individual discussions. This allows the health professional to explore individual concerns and information needs without the barrier of patient/carer protectiveness.

Patients' preferences for family members to be informed and/or influence the information they receive

The issue of confidentiality and sensitively obtaining the patient's permission prior to talking with the caregiver has

been emphasized in literature from Western countries.[39,47] It cannot be assumed that patients are close to their families or want them to be fully informed.[39,48] On the other hand patients from some cultural backgrounds may prefer disclosure negotiated through the family, when the prognosis is poor.[31,32]

Importance of establishing individual patients' and carers' information needs

Together the above findings stress the importance of establishing individual patients' information needs and patients' preferences regarding how much and how information should be shared within the family. Moreover the information needs of a patient's carer(s) may differ from the patient. Furthermore needs may change over time. An essential component of good communication is to ensure that patients and their families receive information at the level of detail that they desire, and to provide opportunities for them to discuss their fears and concerns about the future.

CURRENT PRACTICE IN INFORMATION PROVISION IN PALLIATIVE CARE AND ONCOLOGY

Physicians' information disclosure to patients

Patients with far advanced progressive illnesses may not be adequately informed of their situation or treatment options by their physicians in general medical and oncology settings in Western countries.[49–52] For example, an Australian study[49] in patients with advanced cancer found that while most of the 118 participating patients were informed about the aim of anticancer treatment (85 percent), 25 percent of patients were not told that their cancer was incurable. Only 44 percent of patients were told about alternatives to anticancer treatment such as supportive care and 36 percent of patients were informed about how such treatments would affect their quality of life. Greater levels of information disclosure were not associated with increased anxiety. Actual communication about other topics such as health-related quality of life issues, pain, and other symptoms may be less than ideal[53–55] and physicians may not recognize or respond to patients' subtle hints or cues for information.[56,57] Moreover, in general medical settings end-of-life conversations often do not occur or are conducted poorly.[51**,58*]

Little is known about what is actually discussed during palliative medicine physician consultations. We have audiotaped consultations between 18 different palliative medicine physicians and 270 different patients/carers and we will be coding these audiotapes specifically with regard to prognostic and end-of-life communication. The analysis of these data is in progress.

Although studies of actual communication are limited, some survey data are available. A study by Lamont and Christakis[59] reveals that physicians may not provide their best estimate of survival even when asked by terminally ill patients. One reason for this may be that physicians' survival estimates in terminally ill patients are often wrong and are usually overoptimistic.[60***] However, physicians may also lack confidence in communicating survival predictions or may fear that such information will cause the patient to lose hope.

There is evidence of cultural differences among health professionals in their attitudes towards truth disclosure to patients with life-limiting illnesses, with a tendency towards nondisclosure in certain non-Western cultures.[61–63] For example, Bruera et al.[64] surveyed 182 palliative care physicians from different regions and found that only 26 percent of European physicians and 18 percent of South American physicians, compared with 93 percent of Canadian physicians, thought that the majority of their patients would want to know about their terminal prognosis, ($P < 0.001$).

Patients' misunderstanding of information and the consequences of this

Several studies have shown that patients with cancer and other life-limiting conditions frequently have misunderstandings about their illness, prognosis, and goals of treatment.[51**,52,65–67] For example, Gattellari et al.[66] found that 17 percent of 244 cancer patients with metastatic disease believed their cancer was localized and incorrectly believed their treatment was given with curative intent.

When patients are not adequately informed of their prognosis they are more likely to choose aggressive treatments, which will probably not extend their life and may compromise its quality.[52] The et al.[68] showed that patients may subsequently regret such decisions. Chochinov et al.[69] found that depression was almost three times greater in 200 patients with advanced cancer who did not acknowledge their prognosis, compared with those who had partial or complete understanding ($P = 0.029$).

Summary of limitations in current practice with regards to information provision to palliative care and oncology patients and their carers

Overall these findings suggest that there are significant gaps in providing information and addressing the concerns of patients with life-limiting illnesses and their families. Interventions are needed to help patients express their concerns and have their information needs met. While less is known about the current practice in information provision specifically in palliative care consultations, such interventions may also be useful in a palliative care setting.

INTERVENTIONS TO HELP MEET PATIENTS' INFORMATION NEEDS AND PROMOTE INVOLVEMENT IN THE CONSULTATION

Interventions targeted at both health professionals and patients have been developed with the aim of (i) helping patients meet their information needs and (ii) encouraging patient participation during medical consultations. Interventions directed at health professionals primarily involve communication skills training. In addition a number of practical aids have been suggested to improve communication and/or help patients to assimilate information and achieve their information preferences.

Communication skills training for health professionals

Health professional communication skills do not reliably improve with experience alone. A randomized controlled trial of a 3-day residential communication skills course for oncologists found that course participants used more focused and open questions, greater expressions of empathy, more appropriate responses to patients cues and less leading questions at immediate[70**] and 12 months[71**] follow-up. Provision of written feedback alone to participants had little effect on objective communication outcomes.[70**]

Communication skills training modules specific to a palliative care setting, with greater emphasis on discussing prognosis and end-of-life issues, are needed.

Provision of audiotapes or written summaries of consultations

One simple intervention that has been investigated is the provision of audiotape recordings or written summaries of the consultation. A systematic review in the oncology setting was conducted by Scott et al.[72***] Trials consistently found that most people who received the audiotapes or written summaries of their consultations valued them. Improved recall of the consultation in those patients provided with an audiotape or letter was found in five out of nine studies. Patients who received an audiotape or letter were more satisfied with the information received in four out of seven studies. The only study[73**] to compare the impact of audiotapes versus summary letters found that patients preferred audiotapes to letters.

McHugh et al.[74**] found that patients who were informed of a poor prognosis at their initial oncology consultation and received an audiotape of the consultation had less improvement in psychological distress at 6 months follow-up than those who did not receive the tape. Therefore, Scott et al.[72***] advised caution in the use of interventions 'to reinforce bad news when alternative interventions such as counselling may be more appropriate'. This may be a concern for palliative care settings where nearly all patients have a poor prognosis. However, this result was found in only one study at the point of initial diagnosis.

Only one study[75**] was conducted in the setting of a 'pain and symptom clinic' for patients with advanced cancer. In this small study (60 patients) from the USA, patients who received the tape were significantly more satisfied with the consultation and recalled significantly more information given during the consultation. Patients who received the audiotape rated it highly and it was also valued by family and friends. The authors point out that most patients in this study[75**] were receiving advice about control of physical symptoms rather than bad news. Further research is needed to assess the value of audiotape provision to palliative care patients and their families and the potential for adverse psychological effects if the audiotape includes discussion of end-of-life issues or other sensitive information.

Provision of information in written, audiovisual, or electronic format

Information leaflets about individual palliative care services and palliative care topics, such as bereavement, are commonly provided.[76] Patient education materials designed to teach patients about management of pain and other symptoms have also been developed. There are few research data regarding the effectiveness of providing information in written formats to patients in a palliative care setting. However, a survey in the UK found that '64 percent of leaflets could be understood by only an estimated 40 percent of the population'.[77]

Question prompt lists

Studies of cancer and palliative care patients' views have emphasized the importance for patients of having the opportunity to ask questions of their clinicians.[6,78] Other studies have found improved health outcomes when patients are encouraged to ask questions during general medical consultations.[79***,80**] Some health professionals encourage patients to write down their questions and bring them to medical appointments, but patients may not know what questions to ask or how to articulate their concerns.[81]

Butow et al.[82**] explored the use of a question prompt list given to cancer patients before their initial consultation with oncologists. A question prompt list is a structured list containing examples of questions for the patient to ask their physician if they wish. It is designed to encourage patient participation during a medical consultation and to assist patients in acquiring information that is suited to their needs and at their own pace. This simple and inexpensive intervention has been found to promote question asking about prognosis in three separate studies[82**,83**,84**] in the oncology setting. In the most recent of these studies,[84**]

provided the oncologist specifically addressed questions in the question prompt list during the consultation, those patients who received the prompt list were significantly less anxious immediately after the consultation and had better recall and significantly shorter consultations.

We have developed and piloted a question prompt list for patients being referred to a palliative care team.[85*] In order to identify suitable questions for inclusion in the question prompt list we conducted a series of focus groups and individual interviews with palliative care patients, their carers, and palliative care health professionals. A wide range of issues emerged for inclusion in the question prompt list including questions about: the palliative care service, physical symptoms and treatment, lifestyle and quality of life, the illness and what to expect in the future, support, if you are concerned about your professional care, for carers, and end-of-life issues. All participants felt the question prompt list, in booklet form, could be a useful tool. Of 23 patients in the pilot study, 22 agreed the question prompt list was helpful, contained useful questions, was easy to understand and would be useful in the future. State anxiety decreased after receiving the booklet and seeing the physician in 16 out of 19 patients. Participants in the pilot study endorsed the inclusion of end-of-life issues in the question prompt list, despite some reservations expressed about this by health professionals in the individual interviews. We have recently completed recruitment for a randomized controlled trial of the question prompt list in 174 patients seeing one of 15 palliative care clinicians in 10 different palliative care centers. Analysis of the results of this study is in progress. The question prompt list for palliative care patients and their families, including 112 sample questions in a booklet form, can be downloaded from www.psych.usyd.edu.au/mpru/communication_tools.html

SUMMARY

Communication is an essential component of the care of palliative care patients and their families. Most patients and their families have high needs for information, but not all patients want detailed information about their condition at all stages of their illness. There is evidence of significant gaps in information provision and addressing concerns of patients. Less is known about the specific information needs of palliative care patients and their carers and whether or not these needs are met. Discussing prognosis and end-of-life issues is particularly important but challenging in palliative care. Little research evidence is available about what information palliative care patients and their carers want and how they feel this information should be portrayed. Most relevant research regarding physician–patient communication in this setting has been conducted in Western countries. Further research is needed to evaluate the needs of patients and their families from different cultural backgrounds.

Interventions may be needed to facilitate discussion of prognosis and end-of-life issues plus help palliative care patients and their carers meet their general needs for information. Communication skills training for physicians has been found to improve communication. Some tools such as question prompt lists and audiotaping the consultation are helpful in promoting question asking, and/or patient satisfaction and recall of information. Question prompt lists seem to particularly promote question asking about prognosis and may be useful in facilitating discussion about other sensitive topics such as end-of-life issues. Further research is needed in order to optimize communication with palliative care patients and their carers.

Key learning points

- Communication has been identified by patients and their families as one of the most important aspects of medical care at the end of life.

- Most patients and their families, at least in Western countries, have high needs for information, but not all patients want detailed information about their condition at all stages of their illness.

- There is evidence of significant gaps in information provision and addressing concerns of patients with far-advanced progressive illnesses in general medical and oncology settings. Less is known about the specific information needs of palliative care patients and their carers and whether or not these needs are met.

- Communication skills training for physicians has been found to improve communication.

- Other practical tools such as question prompt lists and audiotaping the consultation are helpful in promoting question asking, and/or patient satisfaction and recall of information. Question prompt lists seem to particularly promote question asking about prognosis and may be useful in facilitating discussion about other sensitive topics such as end-of-life issues.

REFERENCES

1   Maguire P, Pitceathly C. Key communication skills and how to acquire them. *BMJ* 2002; **325**: 697–700.

2   Roberts CS, Cox CE, Reintgen DS, *et al.* Influence of physician communication on newly diagnosed breast patients' psychologic adjustment and decision-making. *Cancer* 1994; **74**: 336–41.

3   Kaplan SH, Ware JE. The patients' role in healthcare and quality assessment. In: Goldfield N, Nash DB, eds. *Providing Quality Care: Future Challenges.* Ann Arbor, MI: Health Administration Press, 1995: 25–7.

4   Curtis JR, Wenrich MD, Carline JD, *et al.* Understanding physicians' skills at providing end-of-life care perspectives of patients, families, and health care workers. *J Gen Intern Med* 2001; **16**: 41–9.

5   Steinhauser KE, Clipp EC, McNeilly M, *et al.* In search of a good death: observations of patients, families, and providers. *Ann Intern Med* 2000; **132**: 825–32.

6   Wenrich MD, Curtis JR, Shannon SE, *et al.* Communicating with dying patients within the spectrum of medical care from terminal diagnosis to death. *Arch Intern Med* 2001; **161**: 868–74.

7   Tong E, McGraw SA, Dobihal E, *et al.* What is a good death? Minority and non-minority perspectives. *J Palliat Care* 2003; **19**: 168–75.

8   Wenrich MD, Curtis JR, Ambrozy DA, *et al.* Dying patients' need for emotional support and personalized care from physicians: perspectives of patients with terminal illness, families, and health care providers. *J Pain Symptom Manage* 2003; **25**: 236–46.

9   Steinhauser KE, Christakis NA, Clipp EC, *et al.* Factors considered important at the end of life by patients, family, physicians, and other care providers. *JAMA* 2000; **284**: 2476–82.

10 Henman MJ, Butow PN, Brown RF, *et al.* Lay constructions of decision-making in cancer. *Psychooncology* 2002; **11**: 295–306.

11 Wright EB, Holcombe C, Salmon P. Doctors' communication of trust, care, and respect in breast cancer: qualitative study. *BMJ* 2004; **328**: 864–7.

12 Fogarty LA, Curbow BA, Wingard JR, *et al.* Can 40 seconds of compassion reduce patient anxiety? *J Clin Oncol* 1999; **17**: 371–9.

13 Makoul G. Essential elements of communication in medical encounters: The Kalamazoo consensus statement. *Acad Med* 2001; **76**: 390–3.

14 Arora NK. Interacting with cancer patients: the significance of physicians' communication behaviour. *Soc Sci Med* 2003; **57**: 791–806.

15 Parle M, Jones B, Maguire P. Maladaptive coping and affective disorders among cancer patients. *Psychol Med* 1996; **26**: 735–44.

16 Maguire P. Improving communication with cancer patients. *Eur J Cancer* 2000; **35**: 2058–65.

17 Heaven CM, Maguire P. Disclosure of concerns by hospice patients and their identification by nurses. *Palliat Med* 1997; **11**: 283–90.

18 Stewart F, Walker A, Maguire P. *Psychiatric and Social Morbidity in Women Treated for Cancer of the Cervix.* Report to the Cancer Research Campaign, UK. 1988.

19 Maguire P, Faulkner A, Booth K, *et al.* Helping cancer patients disclose their concerns. *Eur J Cancer* 1996; **32A**: 78–81.

20 Fallowfield L, Lipkin M, Hall A. Teaching senior oncologists communication skills: results from phase I of a comprehensive longitudinal program in the United Kingdom. *J Clin Oncol* 1998; **16**: 1961–8.

21 Ream E, Richardson A. The role of information in patients' adaptation to chemotherapy and radiotherapy: a review of the literature. *Eur J Cancer Care* 1996; **5**: 132–8.

22 Hinds C, Streater A, Mood D. Functions and preferred methods of receiving information related to radiotherapy: perceptions of patients with cancer. *Cancer Nurs* 1995; **18**: 374–84.

23 Mills M, Davies HTO, Macrae WA. Care of dying patients in hospital. *BMJ* 1994; **309**: 583–6.

24 van der Molen B. Relating information needs to the cancer experience: 1. Information as a key coping strategy. *Eur J Cancer Care* 1999; **8**: 238–44.

25 Jenkins V, Fallowfield L, Saul J. Information needs of patients with cancer: results from a large study in UK cancer centres. *Br J Cancer* 2001; **84**: 48–51.

26 Butow PN, Maclean M, Dunn SM, *et al.* The dynamics of change: cancer patients' preferences for information, involvement and support. *Ann Oncol* 1997; **8**: 857–63.

● 27 Kutner JS, Steiner JF, Corbett KK, *et al.* Information needs in terminal illness. *Soc Sci Med* 1999; **48**: 1341–52.

28 Leydon GM, Boulton M, Moynihan C, *et al.* Cancer patients' information needs and information seeking behaviour: in depth interview study. *BMJ* 2000; **320**: 909–13.

29 Friis LS, Elverdam B, Schmidt KG. The patient's perspective: a qualitative study of acute myeloid leukaemia patients' need for information and their information-seeking behaviour. *Support Care Cancer* 2003; **11**: 162–70.

30 Huang X, Butow PN, Meiser M, *et al.* Communicating in a multi-cultural society: The needs of Chinese cancer patients in Australia. *Aust N Z J Med* 1999; **29**: 207–13.

31 Goldstein D, Thewes B, Butow P. Communicating in a multicultural society II: Greek community attitudes towards cancer in Australia. *Intern Med J* 2002; **32**: 289–96.

32 Kai I, Ohi G, Yano E, Kobayashi Y, *et al.* Communication between patients and physicians about terminal care: a survey in Japan. *Soc Sci Med* 1993; **36**: 1151–9.

33 Fielding R, Hung J. Preferences for information and involvement in decisions during cancer care among a Hong Kong Chinese population. *Psychooncology* 1996; **5**: 321–9.

34 Yun YH, Lee CG, Kim SY, *et al.* The attitudes of cancer patients and their families toward the disclosure of terminal illness. *J Clin Oncol* 2004; **22**: 307–14.

35 Cassileth BR, Zupkis RV, Sutton-Smith K, March V. Information and participation preferences among cancer patients. *Ann Intern Med* 1980; **92**: 832–6.

36 Blanchard CG, Labrecque MS, Ruckdeschel JC, Blanchard EB. Information and decision-making preferences of hospitalized adult cancer patients. *Soc Sci Med* 1988; **27**: 1139–45.

37 Meredith C, Symonds P, Webster L, *et al.* Information needs of cancer patients in west Scotland: cross sectional survey of patients' view. *BMJ* 1996; **313**: 724–6.

38 Jones R, Pearson J, McGregor S, *et al.* Cross sectional survey of patients' satisfaction with information about cancer. *BMJ* 1999; **319**: 1247–8.

● 39 Kirk P, Kirk I, Kristjanson LJ. What do patients receiving palliative care for cancer and their families want to be told? A Canadian and Australian qualitative study. *BMJ* 2004; **328**: 1343–7.

40 Sardell AN, Trierweiler SJ. Disclosing the cancer diagnosis. Procedures that influence patient hopefulness. *Cancer* 1993; **72**: 3355–65.

● 41 Hagerty RG, Butow PN, Ellis PA, *et al.* Cancer patient preferences for communication of prognosis in the metastatic setting. *J Clin Oncol* 2004; **22**: 1721–30.

42 World Health Organization. *National Cancer Control Guidelines: Policies and Managerial Guidelines.* Geneva: World Health Organization, 2002.

43 Rose KE. A qualitative analysis of the information needs of informal carers of terminally ill cancer patients. *J Clin Nurs* 1999; **8**: 81–8.

44 Grbich C, Parker D, Maddocks I. Communication and information needs of care-givers of adult family members at diagnosis and during treatment of terminal cancer. *Prog Palliat Care* 2000; **8**: 345–50.

45 Wilkes L, White K, O'Riordan L. Empowerment through information: supporting rural families of oncology patients in palliative care. *Aust J Rural Health* 2000; **8**: 41–6.

46 Friedrichsen MJ. Justification for information and knowledge: perceptions of family members in palliative home care in Sweden. *Palliat Support Care* 2003; **1**: 239–45.

47 Clayton JM, Butow PN, Tattersall MHN. The needs of terminally ill cancer patients versus those of their caregivers for information regarding prognosis and end-of-life issues. *Cancer* 2005; **103**: 1957–64.

48 Benson J, Britten N. Respecting the autonomy of cancer patients when talking with their families: qualitative analysis of semistructured interviews with patients. *BMJ* 1996; **313**: 729–31.

● 49 Gattellari M, Voigt KJ, Butow PN, *et al.* When the treatment goal is not cure: are cancer patients equipped to make informed decisions? *J Clin Oncol* 2002; **20**: 503–13.

50 Koedoot CG, Oort FJ, de Haan RJ, *et al.* The content and amount of information given by medical oncologists when telling patients with advanced cancer what their treatment options are. palliative chemotherapy and watchful-waiting. *Eur J Cancer* 2004; **40**: 225–35.

● 51 SUPPORT Principal Investigators. A controlled trial to improve care for the seriously ill hospitalised patients: the Study to Understand Prognoses and Preferences for Outcomes and Risks of Treatment (SUPPORT). *JAMA* 1995; **274**:1591–8.

● 52 Weeks JC, Cook EF, O'Day SJ, *et al.* Relationship between cancer patients' predictions of prognosis and their treatment preferences. *JAMA* 1998; **279**: 1709–14.

● 53 Detmar SB, Muller MJ, Wever LD, *et al.* The patient-physician relationship. Patient-physician communication during outpatient palliative treatment visits: an observational study. *JAMA* 2002; **285**: 1351–7.

54 Rogers MS, Todd CJ. The 'right kind' of pain: talking about symptoms in outpatient oncology consultations. *Palliat Med* 2000; **14**: 299–307.

55 Berry DL, Wilkie DJ, Thomas CR, *et al.* Clinicians communication with patients experiencing cancer pain. *Cancer Investig* 2003; **21**: 374–81.

56 Maguire P, Booth K, Elliott C, *et al.* Helping health professionals involved in cancer care acquire key interviewing skills-the impact of workshops. *Eur J Cancer* 1996; 32A: 1486–9.

57 Butow PN, Brown RF, Cogar S, *et al.* Oncologists' reactions to cancer patients' verbal cues. *Psychooncology* 2002; **11**: 47–58.

58 Hofmann JC, Wenger NS, Davis RB, *et al.* Patient preferences for communication with physicians about end-of-life decisions. *Ann Intern Med* 1997; **127**: 1–12.

59 Lamont EB, Christakis NA. Prognostic disclosure to patients with cancer near the end of life. *Ann Intern Med* 2001; **134**: 1096–105.

◆ 60 Glare P, Virik K, Jones M, *et al.* A systematic review of physicians' survival predictions in terminally ill cancer patients. *BMJ* 2003; **327**: 195–201.

61 Tan TK, Teo FC, Wong K, Lim HL. Cancer: to tell or not to tell? *Singapore Med J* 1993; **34**: 202–3.

62 Georgaki S, Kalaidopoulou O, Liarmakopoulos I, Mystakidou K. Nurses' attitudes toward truthful communication with patients with cancer. A Greek Study. *Cancer Nurs* 2002; **25**: 436–41.

63 Harris JJ, Shao J, Sugarman J. Disclosure of cancer diagnosis and prognosis in Northern Tanzania. *Soc Sci Med* 2003; **56**: 905–13.

64 Bruera E, Neumann CM, Mazzocato C, *et al.* Attitudes and beliefs of palliative care physicians regarding communication with terminally ill cancer patients. *Palliat Med* 2000; **14**: 287–98.

65 Mackillop WJ, Stewart WE, Ginsburg AD, *et al.* Cancer patients' perception of their disease and its treatment. *Br J Cancer* 1988; **58**: 355–8.

66 Gattellari M, Butow PN, Tattersall MHN, *et al.* Misunderstanding in cancer patients; Why shoot the messenger. *Ann Oncol* 1999; **10**: 39–46.

67 Chan A, Woodruff RK. Communicating with patients with advanced cancer. *J Palliat Care* 1997; **13**: 29–33.

68 The AM, Hak T, Koeter G, *et al.* Collusion in doctor-patient communication about imminent death: an ethnographic study. *BMJ* 2001; **321**: 1376–81.

69 Chochinov HM, Tataryn DJ, Wilson KG, *et al.* Prognostic awareness and the terminally ill. *Psychosomatics* 2000; **41**: 500–4.

● 70 Fallowfield L, Jenkins V, Farewell V, *et al.* Efficacy of a Cancer Research UK communication skills training model for oncologists: a randomised controlled trial. *Lancet* 2002; **359**: 650–6.

71 Fallowfield L, Jenkins V, Farewell V, *et al.* Enduring impact of communication skills training: results of a 12-month follow-up. *Br J Cancer* 2003; **89**: 1445–9.

◆ 72 Scott JT, Entwistle VA, Sowden AJ, *et al.* Recordings or summaries of consultations for people with cancer. *Cochrane Database Syst Rev* 2003; **2**: CD001539.

73 Tattersall MH, Butow PN, Griffin AM, *et al.* The take-home message: patients prefer consultation audiotapes to summary letters. *J Clin Oncol* 1994; **12**: 1305–11.

74 McHugh P, Lewis S, Ford S, *et al.* The efficacy of audiotapes in promoting psychological well-being in cancer patients: a randomised, controlled trial. *Br J Cancer* 1995; **71**: 388–92.

75 Bruera E, Pituskin E, Calder K, *et al.* The addition of an audiocassette recording of a consultation to written recommendations for patients with advanced cancer: a randomized, controlled trial. *Cancer* 1999; **86**: 2420–5.

76 Fallowfield L. Communication with the patient and family in palliative medicine. In Doyle D, Hanks G, Cherny N, Calman K, eds. *Oxford Textbook of Palliative Medicine*, 3rd ed. Oxford: Oxford University Press, 2004: 101–7.

77 Payne S, Large S, Jarrett N, *et al.* Written information given to patients and families by palliative care units: a national survey. *Lancet* 2000; **355**: 1792.

78 Lobb EA, Kenny DT, Butow PN, *et al.* Women's preferences for discussion of prognosis in early breast cancer. *Health Expect* 2001; **4**: 48–57.

79 Kaplan SH, Greenfield S, Ware JE Jr. Assessing the effects of physician-patient interactions on the outcomes of chronic disease. *Med Care* 1989; **27**: S110–S127.

80 Thompson SC, Nanni LM, Schwankovsky L, *et al.* Patient-oriented interviews to improve communication in a medical office visit. *Health Psychol* 1990; **9**: 390–404.

81 Neufeld KR, Degner LF, Dick JA. A nursing intervention strategy to foster patient involvement in treatment decisions. *Oncol Nurs Forum* 1993; **20**: 631–5.

82 Butow PN, Dunn SM, Tattersall MH, *et al.* Patient participation in the cancer consultation: evaluation of a question prompt sheet. *Ann Oncol* 1994; **5**: 199–204.

83 Brown R, Butow PN, Boyer MJ, *et al.* Promoting patient participation in the cancer consultation: evaluation of a prompt sheet and coaching in question-asking. *Br J Cancer* 1999; **80**: 242–8.

84 Brown RF, Butow PN, Dunn SM, Tattersall MH. Promoting patient participation and shortening cancer consultations: a randomised trial. *Br J Cancer* 2001; **85**: 273–9.

● 85 Clayton J, Butow P, Tattersall M, *et al.* Asking questions can help: development and preliminary evaluation of a question prompt list for palliative care patients. *Br J Cancer* 2003; **89**: 2069–77.

107

Spiritual care

SUSAN STRANG, PETER STRANG

THE INTERSECTION BETWEEN RELIGION AND MEDICINE

People in all phases of their lives have to struggle with existential and spiritual issues, but these come to a head when a person is afflicted with a severe illness.[1–3] When a cure is no longer an alternative, the focus of care-related efforts must move from curative to palliative care. Within palliative care, emphasis is not only on physical, mental and social factors, but also on the importance of the existential/spiritual dimension,[4–6] since spirituality intersects with medicine at the juncture of suffering.[7] When facing death, existential anxiety is activated: 'Why me and why now?', 'What was the meaning of my life and is there any meaning or purpose left to live for?', 'What will happen to me and my family?', 'Is there an existence beyond death?', 'Has God abandoned me?'. For the physician and the staff, knowledge about their patients' beliefs is essential, as some patients may explicitly base decisions about life-sustaining interventions on their spiritual or religious beliefs.[8] Other patients may not bring up spiritual concerns but still are troubled by them, and in that way spiritual issues will affect the overall wellbeing.

The division into four dimensions – physical–mental–social and spiritual – is useful to understand all dimensions of palliative care. Still, it is a didactic oversimplification, as few, if any, experiences are unidimensional. For example, body pain is primarily a physical problem, but it has definite mental, social, and spiritual impact in the form of mood disturbances[9] and impaired social functioning,[10] and pain might also trigger existential suffering.[11] The 'empty nest syndrome' is definitely a social issue, an important event in life when the last child leaves home. Still, it is also a psychological challenge and not at least an existential boundary situation: it is a turning point in life, reminding us of the shortness of life. In such ways the dimensions are intertwined. The reverse is also true: existential suffering, e.g. death anxiety or existential guilt, may manifest itself in physical pain without obvious underlying pathology,[11] anxiety, or social withdrawal (Case 107.1).[9]

Case 107.1

'A young man recently diagnosed with cancer of the testes (with suspected metastasis to the retro peritoneal glands). Severe back pain, requiring spinal administration of analgesics. Great anxiety over living and dying. Once the man spoke to understanding personnel about the excellent prognosis, and learned that he could have his sperm frozen and become a father despite the treatment, the pain disappeared and the spinal catheter could be removed.' Source: reference 11.

In this case, existential anxiety reinforced an existing physical pain, and once the patient was supported in his existential crisis he experienced a substantial pain reduction.

It is sometimes difficult to distinguish between the emotional and existential/spiritual dimensions and, in fact, sometimes they overlap. The external manifestation might be similar, but the underlying cause is different and, therefore, the treatment and support should be tailored considering the nature of the problem. As an example, anxiety that manifests itself in the form of restlessness and sleep difficulties should be handled differently, depending on the cause, which could be physical (unrelieved pain or dyspnea), mental, social (e.g. economic problems, divorce) or spiritual (religious guilt). Still, the division into four dimensions is useful for the sake of clarity.

SPIRITUAL NEEDS

There are no exact definitions with regard to spiritual needs, as different people emphasize different facets or interpretations of this construct.[4,12–15] In healthcare contexts, spiritual care normally includes religion and general spirituality, but less often existential issues as defined within existentialism. These aspects, though, are central to life for all people, even atheists.[16] It is impossible to draw a dividing line between the concepts. Instead, key words defining the core of each concept are more useful (Box 107.1).

Box 107.1 Key words for spirituality, religion and existentialism

Spirituality
- Meaning
- Transcendence
- Higher power/source of energy
- Relationship
- Religious dimension

Religion
- God
- Worship
- Rituals
- Social manifestations

Existentialism
- Freedom
- Isolation
- Meaning/meaninglessness
- Death

Spirituality

Today, most authors in healthcare present a holistic view of the concept of 'spirituality' that is partly distinguished from and broader than religion.[4,17–20] McCurdy stresses that spirituality deals with 'our need and capacity for relationship to whatever or whoever gives meaning, purpose, and direction to our lives'.[21] Spirituality generally comprises the following

domains, although there is great overlapping: meaning, transcendence, energy, relationships, and religious dimensions.

Religion

Religion can be, but does not have to be, an important part of a person's spirituality. In religion there is always a deity, a God. Religion joins together individuals who share the same beliefs, traditions, rituals, and worshipful acts within some kind of social institution.[22,23] In scientific terms a *substantial* definition describes what religion 'is': the Holy texts, symbols, congregation etc. whereas *functional* definitions focus on what religion 'does': e.g. offers a frame of interpretation for death, the dualism between evil and good, suffering.[24]

Existentialism

Existentialism is a philosophical movement advocated by philosophers with different backgrounds, such as Kierkegaard, Heidegger, Jaspers, Frankl, and Sartre. A clinically useful way of summarizing the existential domains has been provided by Yalom and is described below.[16]

Freedom forces us to be responsible for our lives, but by forcing us to make choices it also creates existential anxiety. Unethical choices are linked to existential guilt. Such guilt might be activated at the end of life. The person feels uneasy and is in need of 'making good'. Therefore it has clinical consequences (Case 107.2).

Case 107.2

The elderly female patient suffered from several distressing symptoms, including pelvic pain, but she refused help. Efforts to persuade her failed when the staff tried to explain the problem in medical terms. When an empathetic staff member at last came to understand that the patient considered her illness to be a punishment for a previous decision, they were able to help her: She had had an abortion when she was young, and now she felt that justice was being made, she suffered from cancer 'there' (in her genitals), consequently, she had refused help. After counseling she realized that she had been punishing herself her entire adult life. When she was allowed to put it in her own words in an accepting environment, she realized that she had been punishing herself enough through the years. This was a relief for her and she accepted now medical help for her cancer symptoms.

Meaninglessness versus meaning is another existentialistic dimension that is central both in existentialism and in general spirituality and religion.[25] Meaninglessness is the

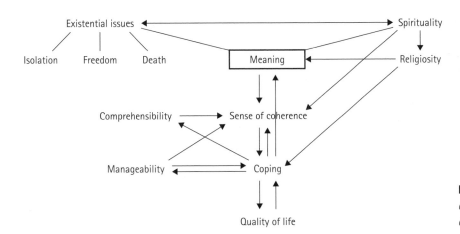

Figure 107.1 *An attempt to relate different concepts where meaning issues are central.*

basic condition that forces us to search for meaning or to create meaning.[16] Some existential philosophers with a religious background such as Frankl would not agree, but emphasize that there is an inherent meaning to be found and that man can also create meaning.[26] Clinically, meaning issues have raised much attention during recent years, as meaning seems to be the strongest predictor of quality of life in palliative care settings.[27–29] Meaning is also strongly connected to concepts such as meaning-based coping[30] and sense of coherence (Fig. 107.1).[31]

Isolation refers to an unbridgeable gulf between oneself and any other being; each of us must enter existence alone and must depart from it alone. This kind of isolation may be revealed in critical transitions, e.g. when facing one's death.[32] The concept of existential isolation is therefore relevant to palliative care. It is important to realize that existential isolation cannot be resolved, but closeness and relationships make it possible to endure the burden (Case 107.3).

Case 107.3

A 50-year-old woman with breast cancer admitted to palliative care: 'I was calm, may be in shock when my doctor explained that my breast cancer had spread to my back and my lungs. However, when I left his office that day I realized that now I was facing a great loneliness, the greatest of them all. Yes, I had my family and my friends and of course they were there for me, but still I was very lonely. They would never understand what I really felt then.'

The reality of *death* creates death anxiety, which has its roots in the fear of definite separation and, in anxiety about annihilation. In the clinical setting the impending separation seems especially painful to encounter.[1] However, as claimed by existential philosophers, when death becomes a close reality, life may also become more real and intense. Heidegger describes this as a more 'authentic' mode of life.[33] People

value basic things in life such as family, relationships, and nature. The closeness of death may also make it easier to choose between important and unimportant things. However, in the terminal phase anger and demoralization may be more prominent features.[34]

RELIGIOUS PSYCHOLOGY: MODELS FOR UNDERSTANDING RELIGION

Psychology might seem superfluous for the religious believer but it can partially explain for more secularized persons which needs are satisfied by religious practice. The simplest answer would be: religious needs, an important fact, as man is religious or spiritually inclined by nature: every known culture has had a religion. An alternative way of describing it, as suggested by religion psychologists, would be: religious, cognitive, emotional, social, and political needs.[35]

Religion provides direction and meaning to a person's life and it provides him or her with tools to handle the eternal questions. In that sense, religion satisfies a *cognitive* or intellectual need. Moreover, it offers support, comfort, and security when facing suffering and death and in that way this Divine presence fulfills a deep *emotional* need. A living God who is merciful and allows close contact in prayers and rituals can be the most powerful help for the existential emptiness and meaninglessness that people may experience at times, especially in boundary situations. Furthermore, a congregation is a social institution with close interpersonal relations and within this community, a common faith creates a sense of togetherness with all believers around the world. Thus, religion provides a strong *social* structure in a fragile situation. In some societies, religion even works in concert with *political* needs and motives, e.g. in the liberation theology.

Although religion is much more than the sum of these separate facets, and a believer would probably not discuss them in these terms, this analysis may still explain why religion, in fact, fulfills many important needs. Still, the 'longing for essence in existence' is not possible to describe in analytical terms.

Religious coping

When discussing the psychology of religion, coping is an important issue. General research on coping with cancer started in the 1970s with important studies by Weisman.[36] In the 1980s Lazarus and Folkman emphasized the stress-appraisal-response model[37] and in the 1990s Folkman also emphasized that meaning-based coping was important as a complement to the above-mentioned model.[30] Inclusion of meaning in coping theories adds an existential facet to coping and brings this type of coping close to religious coping.

Specific religious coping has been studied, e.g. by Pargament who states that prayers and reading the Bible are important tools for such forms of coping.[38] Also ceremonies, symbols, rituals, meditation, religious literature, and religious mystic experiences are useful mediators of religious coping. For example, a believer may find consolation in comparing his or her life situation with the situation of biblical persons, and well-known rituals may create structure in a chaotic situation. It has also been suggested that religious belief systems are helpful to resolve grief.[39] Religious coping, at its best, may provide the suffering person with hope and a sense of control despite a chaotic situation. Other positive aspects include a sense of purpose, meaning, and acceptance. Although rituals and other forms of religious coping often have a positive effect for believers, negative outcomes are also possible, according to Pargament.

HOSPITAL CHAPLAINS

The role of the hospital chaplain has changed over time, and today hospital chaplaincy has contact with various patient groups in crisis, regardless of their faith or lack of faith.[40] The hospital chaplaincy has an important role helping people who are facing life-threatening illness. As Steinhauser showed in a comprehensive study of severely ill patients, doctors, relatives, hospital chaplains and other staff, the wishes of patients and doctors do not always coincide: 'Whereas physicians tend to focus on physical aspects, patients and families tend to view the end of life with broader psychosocial and spiritual meaning'.[41]

It is of great importance that both hospital chaplains and healthcare staff are well informed of each other's areas of competence, considering that traumatic crises and existential crises are intimately connected. Such knowledge is especially important when deciding how to offer help in acute existential crises and how to develop relevant spiritual support in healthcare. Existential support is always needed in existential crises, but sometimes medical help is also beneficial.

Although spiritual support is regarded as important,[42,43] it is not usually offered by healthcare staff due to their lack of knowledge and guidance about how to support patients with these questions.[44,45] However, hospital and hospice chaplains possess such professional knowledge. Nevertheless, there may not be apparent routines for effective teamwork or referral, despite the fact that a majority of doctors and nurses feel that ideally a chaplain should address such issues.[44] Modern healthcare still feels lost when faced with the existential dimension because of its 'unscientific character', and chooses to focus on the medical/technical aspects[46] or clear-cut psychosocial issues. Nonetheless, people seek help and support, and questions still remain such as: 'What needs does a severely ill person have?', 'What kind of support is wanted in a partially secularized society?'. Consequently, what is the role of hospital chaplaincy?[47] It is important to bear in mind that the first questions a person who faces severe illness poses are of an existential nature: 'Why me, and why now?', 'Where is the justice?', 'Will I die?', and 'If I will not be cured, is there any meaning left?'.

What questions do patients pose to the hospital chaplains?

Recent studies show that patients do not contact the hospital chaplain primarily to discuss spiritual or religious questions. Instead the most frequently posed questions seem to be of a general existential character and are concerned with meaning-related issues, with illness, death and dying, and with their love for and care of their family.[40,48,49] These types of questions seem to be of great importance to all individuals, regardless of their religious inclination or faith.[16,50] Hospital chaplaincy is a unique resource; they are educated and have extensive training in listening, supporting and counseling others with these kind of issues.

Teamwork

Although chaplains and community-based clergy bear the primary responsibility for spiritual care, to a certain extent basic support can be provided by any member of the healthcare team.[51] The hospital chaplain's core profession is to offer deeper soul care (pastoral psychotherapy), to support the staff and to handle religious and symbolic issues.[52] However, even if staff have the privilege of using the unique competence of the hospital chaplaincy, this does not mean that the staff can deny their own situation-bound responsibility for existential or spiritual questions. Not all patients want to meet a chaplain, and hospital chaplains are not always available when acute existential crises emerge. Therefore, healthcare staff will encounter existential crises and need to handle them when they occur, since patients often have a great deal of confidence in them, and they are 'there' and available.

The central purpose of spiritual support for healthcare staff is to see and to acknowledge the patient[45,53] to listen actively to 'why-questions', questions about justice, anxiety, the vulnerability of life and, about death and dying, without providing definite answers. In a simplified way, with reference to psychotherapeutic experiences, it could be said that the *process* of listening is more important than the actual *content*, as the patients need to find and formulate their own answers. This kind of spiritual support should, however, not be too deep or theological in nature. Instead, some of the talks might indicate the need for an additional contact with a hospital chaplain, a psychologist or with a social counselor.[52]

Many times, it is just enough to be a fellow human being, supporting the patient and his or her family through closeness, openness, friendship and engagement. This can be done by simple means, e.g. by offering a glass of water, letting the patient listen to his or her favorite music, and by just 'being there'. Existence is, to a considerable degree, about relations, to others and to the world.[54] By being there, performing everyday tasks, by validating the patient, they feel acknowledged for what they are. When a staff member does not share the same faith, there might be difficulties in offering explicit religious help. In such instances, the staff member should contact the hospital chaplaincy or ask another staff member for assistance. This is especially important in the multicultural societies of today.

RELIGIOUS STUDIES

What impact does religion have on health, survival, coping or wellbeing? How does one measure religion and is it possible to create a high scientific standard?[55] There are difficulties when measuring and operationalizing religion[56] and also a skepticism to mix-up religion with medical treatment.[57,58] Still, systematic reviews have shown that religion seems to have a positive influence on health and that it also provides tools for manageability and wellbeing during periods of illness.[59–63] Efforts have been made to summarize data. For instance, a meta-analysis has been performed on data from 42 independent studies examining the association of a measure of religious involvement and all-cause mortality. It concluded that religious involvement was significantly associated with lower mortality, indicating that people practicing or involved in religious involvement were more likely to be alive at a follow-up time than people lower in religious involvement.[64]

There is a disagreement among researchers about the definition of religion and how to measure it. Does religious membership always imply religious beliefs or religious participation? When measuring 'religiousness', do we measure the 'believers' or the 'belongers', those devoting much time to prayer or those who are merely the church participants? Several sophisticated religious scales have been devised, but still there are no commonly accepted measurement tools, probably due to the indistinct subject.[65]

The believer–belonger division of religiosity has also been conceptualized as intrinsic and extrinsic. Individuals with an intrinsic religiosity view every aspects of their lives, even illness, within the context of their religion and the religiosity is closely integrated in their daily lives. In contrast, for individuals with extreme extrinsic religiosity, religion is not an integrated part of their lives, but it may still offer security, sociability and status.[66] When facing an existential crisis the support from the congregation may still be of great help for extrinsics, whereas lack of an intrinsic belief might become a burden on a more religious level.

CULTURAL ASPECTS

In palliative care settings, spiritual care is sometimes synonymous with providing Christian soul care. In the multicultural society of today it is important to not forget other religions. Most religions offer hope in one way or another: hope for an eternal life in some form, hope for resurrection (Christianity), hope in living through the lives of one's children (Judaism), hope for rebirth and belief in karma (Eastern traditions).[67] To provide spiritual care on equal terms, healthcare needs to have good contacts with representatives of several religions, to provide holistic care for the patient. For example, in the Islamic tradition, there are five important cornerstones to the religion often unknown for Christians: the Islamic confession; the five daily prayers; the 'Ramadan' (fasting for a month each year); 'Zakat', i.e. a special form of taxes of 2.5% that one should give to poor people; and pilgrimage: when once in a lifetime a Muslim should make a pilgrimage to Mecca, if possible.[68] Certain rituals should be followed when a person is dying and there are also rituals and strict rules for taking care of the dead body. When facing death such issues may create substantial suffering if not addressed in a proper way. In a similar way there are rituals and rules for other major religions; therefore contact with representatives of respective religions is advisable.

Christianity, Judaism, and Islam have common roots and therefore may be easier for westerners to comprehend. Eastern cultures and religions are often less well-known in healthcare. As exemplified in a qualitative study of eight family caregivers, both family and caregivers may move between modern medicine, traditional/folk medicine, supernatural healing rites, religious performances, and home remedies in their search for a cure.[69]

TO PRACTICE SPIRITUAL CARE

The interest in spiritual issues has increased in recent decades.[42,63,70,71] However, the interest has seldom been translated into support and is still seldom practiced. The medical staff are often insecure in dealing with existential and spiritual care.[72,73] Once healthcare staff acknowledge the impact of spiritual care, and are willing to offer support, when needed, how do they practice it? The guidelines described below are mainly empirically based and with few exceptions formally tested. Still, they can be used as a basis when evaluating spiritual needs and providing support in a clinical setting.

General spiritual care

Kissane advocates grief therapy in palliative care.[6] In short, the doctor or the therapist should allow the patient to talk about his or her life and all the painful losses. The therapist should not try to comfort or minimize the problems, but listen empathetically and focus on acceptance. Perhaps everything in life did not turn out right, but much in life was of great value. When a person reaches to acceptance, he feels a relief. Kissane also suggests that the therapist should focus on transcendence: when the physical situation cannot be changed any longer, one's attitude still can be modified. To transcend, i.e. to accept that one is a part of something bigger may feel comforting: to be a part of a Holy creation with a personal God (a religious form of transcendence); to be part of nature and everything living (a more secularized form of transcendence); to feel comfort in the fact that generations come and generations go and I am part of that cycle; to have a faith in a life after death and perhaps once again meet family and friends on the other side of death.

There are some other models in spiritual care that have recently developed. Rousseau stresses that physicians, together with other members of the team, are obliged to provide support in addressing spiritual concerns by listening and discussing spiritual issues, demonstrating empathy and engaging in a patient's search for meaning, thus breaking through the rigid boundaries of medical care.[74] According to Rousseau, the specific interventions that alleviate spiritual distress include: controlling physical symptoms; providing a supportive presence; encouraging life review to assist in recognizing purpose, value, and meaning; exploring issues of guilt, remorse, forgiveness, and reconciliation; abetting and facilitating religious expression; reframing goals into short-term endeavors that can be accomplished, and encouraging use of meditation, guided imagery, music, reading, poetry, and art that focuses on healing rather than cure.[74]

Greenstein and Breitbart have developed a meaning-centered group psychotherapy for patients with cancer based on the concept of the search for meaning. The goal of the intervention is to help patients focus on what has been meaningful and can still be meaningful in their lives and to encourage dying patients to find meaning in living until their death. The groups meet for eight sessions and possible sources of meaning are explored, including responsibility to others, creativity, transcendence, and ascertaining one's values and priorities.[75]

Both models focus on meaning-issues and transcendence and have great support in literature. Other similar approaches were proposed earlier, e.g. by Frankl who developed logotherapy (logos = meaning). Logotherapy focuses on finding meaning or creating meaning and Frankl distinguishes between three forms of meaning:[76]

- Creative meaning (what one accomplishes)
- Experiential meaning – what one takes from the world in terms of encounters and experiences
- Attitudinal meaning – one's stand toward suffering, toward a fate that one cannot change.

In a similar fashion, Antonovsky's concept – sense of coherence – consists of three facets: comprehensibility, manageability, and meaningfulness, but it is mainly focused on the latter aspect.[31] To focus on meaning and meaningful events is possible also for ordinary staff working with palliative care. In all stages of life, good relations, experiences and hope create meaning and this is also true for end-of-life care. Through practical measures staff can facilitate good relations, e.g. by allowing family members to stay overnight when a patient is experiencing hardship. Also dying patients enjoy positive experiences: music, flowers, beautiful environments. By focusing hope on realistic goals the staff may increase meaningfulness in fragile situations, e.g. hope for a symptom-free weekend when grandchildren come for a visit.

Another model/advise to help physicians who feel uncomfortable discussing spiritual concerns, has been offered by Lo et al.:[8]

> First, some patients may explicitly base decisions about life-sustaining interventions on their spiritual or religious beliefs. Physicians need to explore those beliefs to help patients think through their preferences regarding specific interventions.
>
> Second, other patients may not bring up spiritual or religious concerns but are troubled by them. Physicians should identify such concerns and listen to them empathetically, without trying to alleviate the patient's spiritual suffering or offering premature reassurance.
>
> Third, some patients or families may have religious reasons for insisting on life-sustaining interventions that physicians advise against. The physician should listen and try to understand the patient's viewpoint. Listening respectfully does not require the physician to agree with the patient or misrepresent his or her own views. Patients and families who feel that the physician understands them and cares about them may be more willing to consider the physician's views on prognosis and treatment. By responding to patients' spiritual and religious concerns and needs, physicians may help them find comfort and closure near the end of life.

As a help for healthcare staff, Puchalski has developed a spiritual assessment tool, FICA. It is meant to be a guide for healthcare providers regarding how to start the spiritual history and what to listen for:[55]

F – Faith and belief. Do you consider yourself spiritual or religious? (If not, what gives you meaning?).

I – Importance. What importance does your faith or belief have in your life?
C – Community. Are you a part of a spiritual or religious community?
A – Address/Action in care. What needs to be done with the information?

THE FUNCTION OF RITUALS

Spiritual needs can be met by traditional religious acts such as rituals, prayers, and worship.[77] These rituals may provide meaning to everyday life and help patients through hardships such as pain, illness and personal disasters. These needs are influenced by ethnic and cultural backgrounds.[3,78,79] Every culture in the world has some kind of rites and rituals to highlight important events in people's lives. 'Transition rites', e.g. when a child is born, weddings and funerals, are typical examples. The rituals are characterized by a predetermined form of group behavior which is internalized by the participants. Rituals, especially in association with dying and death, play a large role in the process of mourning, both on an individual and on a collective level. Besides being an official announcement of a death, funeral rituals provide an opportunity to try to find meaning through funeral oration, songs, and sacral music, all of which might appeal to inner feelings, giving them an appropriate means of expression. In that way, they help to create control in the chaos. Within healthcare it is important that the staff create space for and recognize the importance of the dimensions of rituals of dying and death, as active planning and participation in rituals might have a positive function in the mourning process.[80]

SPECIFIC SPIRITUAL/RELIGIOUS (CHRISTIAN) CARE

Soul care is facing great and varying challenges today. The task to help and support people in acute crisis is becoming more and more important as the individual person is getting more vulnerable today in existential boundary situations. To facilitate the handling of existential crises, people need room for encounter, reflection, and for the exploration of one's own life, especially when encountering suffering and death. During different times in history, different aspects of soul care have been stressed and today general counseling with a psychotherapeutic approach is not uncommon.

So in what aspects does soul care differ from psychotherapeutic counseling? In short, a psychotherapist focuses on emotional aspects, interpersonal relations and inner conflicts. The therapist approaches the patient in an objective fashion and follows a certain theory or plan of action. In Sweden, the members of the hospital chaplaincy normally have education in psychology and counseling, but in contrast with psychotherapists, chaplains are not only representing themselves, but also God and the church. They aim at integrating the patient narrative into a religious frame of interpretation and use the symbolic language of the church as well as rituals. The difference can be exemplified in the following way. A patient realizes that he has an incurable disease and asks: 'What is it like to be dying, how will it be for me?'. A psychotherapist would respond: 'Would you like to tell me more about this, what are your feelings, how are you relating to this issue yourself?' and so on, but he would never offer an explicit answer. In soul care, the chaplain may start with similar questions to comprehend the whole situation, but then also talk about the heavenly promise, God's eternal love that never abandons a person in need. In such ways a chaplain may offer spiritual comfort by offering a religious frame of interpretation.

In Sweden, Owe Wikström, a chaplain and also a prominent professor of psychology of religion has summarized four dimensions of Christian soul care in the following way:[35]

- *Care and understanding.* The first issue of soul care is not to change or cure, but to show respect, care and, understanding for a fellow being.
- *Consideration/presence of mind.* Soul care should focus on existential and spiritual aspects, the individual experiences of being a part of something beyond the physical world, and on the moral aspects of one's own life.
- *Interpretation.* Soul care is aiming at integrating private experiences and an all-embracing Christian interpretation of life. The person providing soul care uses their theological knowledge and experience. Here lies a significant difference between the (psycho)therapist and the chaplain.
- *Deepening.* The interpretation leads to a further deepening, where the chaplain tries to help a fellow being mature in their belief. This deepening comprises *experiences* of God, in contrast with intellectual opinions about religion. The deepening also leads to a longing for goodness, and for spiritual growth and spiritual sources.[35]

FUTURE ISSUES

The growing awareness of spiritual issues must have consequences for future care. The physical and the psychosocial aspects should be integrated with existential awareness, as the life-and-death issues are existential rather than psychological. Therefore, existential and spiritual aspects, e.g. the nature of existential crisis should be integrated already in basic education in order to supplement psychological theories.

Both students and staff should realize that spiritual care is not necessarily synonymous with religious support. Consequently, both staff and hospital church should be involved and work as a team.[52] Religious issues should exclusively be handled by hospital chaplaincy, whereas both staff and hospital chaplaincy should be prepared to support in existential crisis of more general nature. Meaning is the core concept and has been proved to be a central predictor to quality of life.[29] Therefore staff should have a good theoretical basis and training in supporting in meaning-based questions in order to facilitate quality of life of the patients.

Key learning points

- When facing death, existential anxiety is activated and here spirituality and existential issues intersect with medicine at the juncture of suffering.

- In healthcare contexts, spiritual care normally includes religion and general spirituality, but also general more philosophical existential issues should be considered.

- Intrinsic religious belief might fulfill several significant needs: namely religious, cognitive, emotional, social, political ones.

- Hospital chaplaincy is a unique resource; the members have extensive training in listening, supporting and counseling others, especially in religious crises. Still, the most frequently posed questions seem to be of a general existential character.

- Basic spiritual support can to an certain extent be provided by any member of the healthcare team but presupposes a basic knowledge and training.

- Useful examples of models in spiritual care are Kissane's grief therapy, Breitbart's meaning-centered group psychotherapy, Puchalski's spiritual assessment tool.

- Rituals may provide meaning to everyday life and help patients through suffering and in the mourning process.

REFERENCES

1 Adelbratt S, Strang P. Death anxiety in brain tumour patients and their spouses. *Palliat Med* 2000; **14**: 499–507.

2 Hall BA. Patterns of spirituality in persons with advanced HIV disease. *Res Nurs Health* 1998; **21**: 143–53.

3 Moadel A, Morgan C, Fatone A, et al. Seeking meaning and hope: self reported spiritual and existential needs among an ethically-diverse cancer patient population. *Psychooncology* 1999: 378–85.

◆ ✱ 4 Wright M. Hospice care and models of spirituality. *Eur J Palliat Care* 2004; **11**: 74–8.

✱ 5 Kellehear A. Spirituality and palliative care: a model of needs. *Palliat Med* 2000; **14**: 149–55.

✱ 6 Kissane DW. Models of psychological response to suffering. *Prog Palliat Care* 1998; **6**: 197–204.

7 Barnes L, Plotinikoff G, Fox K, Pendleton S. Spirituality, religion, and pediatrics: intersecting worlds of healing. *Pediatrics* 2000; **106**: 899–908.

✱ 8 Lo B, Ruston D, Kates L, et al. Discussing religious and spiritual issues at the end of life: a practical guide for physicians. *JAMA* 2002; **287**: 749–54.

◆ 9 Strang P. Cancer pain – a provoker of emotional, social and existential distress. *Acta Oncol* 1998; **37**(7–8): 641–4.

10 Strang P. Emotional and social aspects of cancer pain. *Acta Oncol* 1992; **31**: 323–6.

11 Strang P, Strang S, Hultborn R, Arnér S. Existential pain – an entity, a provocation or a challenge? *J Pain Symptom Manage* 2004; **27**: 241–50.

12 Aldridge D. *Spirituality, Healing and Medicine*. London: Jessica Kingsley, 2000.

13 Coyle J. Spirituality and health: towards a framework for exploring the relationship between spirituality and health. *J Adv Nurs* 2002; **37**: 587–97.

14 Narayanasamy A. Nurses' awareness and educational preparation in meeting their patients' spiritual needs. *Nurse Educ Today* 1993; **13**: 196–201.

15 Piles CL. Providing spiritual care. *Nurse Educ Today* 1990; **15**: 36–41.

16 Yalom I. *Existential Psychotherapy*. New York: Basic Books, 1980.

17 Daaleman T, VandeCreek L. Placing religion and spirituality in end-of-life care. *JAMA* 2000; **284**: 2514–17.

18 Price J, Stevens HO, LaBarre MC. Spiritual caregiving in nursing practice. *J Psychosoc Nurs* 1995; **33**: 5–9.

19 Speck P. Spiritual issues in palliative care. In: Doyle D, Hanks G, MacDonald N, eds. *Oxford Textbook of Palliative Medicine*, 2nd ed. New York: Oxford University Press, 1998.

20 Colleen S, Rosenfeld B, Breitbart W. Effect of spiritual well-being on end of life despair in terminally ill cancer patients. *Lancet* 2003; **361**: 1603–7.

21 McCurdy D. Personhood, spirituality, and hope in the care of human beings with dementia. *J Clin Ethics* 1998; **9**: 81–91.

22 King M, Dein S. The spiritual variable in psychiatric research. *Psychol Med* 1998; **28**: 1259–62.

23 Burton LA. The spiritual dimension of palliative care. *Semin Oncol Nurs* 1998; **14**: 121–8.

24 Geels A, Wikström O. *Den religiösa människan* [in Swedish, author's translation: The religious human being], 3rd ed. Falkenberg: Natur och Kultur, 1999.

25 Ferrell B, Smith S, Juarez G, Melancon C. Meaning of illness and spirituality in ovarian cancer survivors. *Oncol Nurs Forum* 2003; **30**: 249–57.

26 Frankl V. *Man's Search for Meaning*. London: Hodder and Stoughton, 1987.

27 Cohen S, Mount BM, Thomas J, Mount L. Existential well-being is an important determinant of quality of life. *Cancer* 1999; **77**: 576–86.

28 Cohen SR, Mount BM, Strobel MG, Bui F. The McGill Quality of Life Questionnaire: a measure of quality of life appropriate for people with advanced disease. A preliminary study of validity and acceptability. *Palliat Med* 1995; **9**: 207–19.

29 Axelsson B, Sjöden P. Quality of life of cancer patients and their spouses in palliative home care. *Palliat Med* 1998; **12**: 29–39.

● 30 Folkman S. Positive psychological states and coping with severe stress. *Soc Sci Med* 1997; **45**: 1207–21.

31 Antonovsky A. *Unravelling the Mystery of Health: How People Manage Stress and Stay Well*. San Francisco: Jossey-Bass, 1987.

32 Jaspers K. *Existenzphilosophie*. Frankfurt: a.M, 1937.

33 Heidegger M. *Sein und Zeit* [Being and time]. Tubingen: Max Nienmeyer, 1928.

✱ 34 Kissane D, Kelly B. Demoralization, depression and desire for death: problems with the Dutch guidelines for euthanasia of the mentally ill. *Aust N Z J Psychiatry* 2000; **34**: 325–33.

35 Wikström O. *Den outgrundliga människan. Livsfrågor, psykoterapi och självavård* [in Swedish, author's translation: The inscrutable mankind – eternal questions, psychotherapy and soul care], 2nd ed. Borås: Natur och Kultur, 1999.

36 Weisman A. *Coping with Cancer*. San Francisco: McGraw-Hill, 1979.

✱ 37 Lazarus R, Folkman S. *Stress Appraisal and Coping*. New York: Springer, 1982.

✱ 38 Pargament K. *The Psychology of Religion and Coping. Theory, Research and Practice*. New York: Guilford, 1997.

39 Walsh K, King M, Jones L, *et al*. Spiritual beliefs may affect outcome of bereavement: prospective study. *BMJ* 2002; **324**: 1551.

● 40 Wright M. Spiritual care in hospice and hospital: findings from a survey in England and Wales. *Palliat Med* 2001; **14**: 229–42.

● 41 Steinhauser K, Christakis N, Clipp E, *et al*. Factors considered important at the end of life by patients, family, physicians, and other care providers. *JAMA* 2000; **284**: 2476–82.

● 42 King DE, Bushwick B. Beliefs and attitudes of hospital inpatients about faith healing and prayer. *J Fam Pract* 1994; **39**: 349–52.

● 43 Strang S, Strang P. Spiritual thoughts, coping and 'sense of coherence' in brain tumour patients and their spouses. *Palliat Med* 2001; **15**: 127–34.

● 44 Kristeller J, Zumbrun C, Scilling R. 'I would if I could': How oncologists and oncology nurses address spiritual distress in cancer patients. *Psychooncology* 1999; **8**: 451–8.

● 45 Strang S, Strang P, Ternestedt B. Existential support in brain tumour patients and their spouses. *Support Care Cancer* 2001; **9**: 625–33.

● 46 Vandecreek L. Professional chaplaincy: an absent profession? *J Pastoral Care* 1999; **53**: 417–32.

◆ 47 Weaver A, Flannelly L, Flannelly K, *et al*. A 10-year review of research on chaplains and community-based clergy in 3 primary oncology nursing journals: 1990–1999. *Cancer Nurs* 2001; **24**: 335–40.

● 48 Strang S, Strang P. Questions posed to hospital chaplains by palliative care patients. *J Palliat Med* 2002; **5**: 857–64.

● 49 Klemm P, Miller MA, Fernsler J. Demands of illness in people treated for colorectal cancer. *Oncol Nurs Forum* 2000; **27**: 633–9.

● 50 Fry P. The unique contribution of key existential factors to the prediction of psychological well-being of older adults following spousal loss. *Gerontologist* 2001; **41**: 69–81.

● 51 Flannelly K, Weaver A, Handzo G. A three-year study of chaplains' professional activities at Memorial Sloan-Kettering Cancer Center in New York city. *Psychooncology* 2003; **12**: 760–8.

● 52 Strang S, Strang P. Spiritual support for palliative care patients – a duty for hospital chaplains and/or health care staff? *Supportive Palliat Cancer Care* (In press).

53 Mount B. Healing and palliative care: charting our way forward. *Palliat Med* 2003; **17**: 657–8.

54 Strasser F, Strasser A. *Existential Time-limited Therapy. The Wheel of Existence*. New York: Wiley, 1997.

● 55 Post SG, Puchalski CM, Larson DB. Physicians and patient spirituality: professional boundaries, competency, and ethics. *Ann Intern Med* 2000; **132**: 578–83.

◆ 56 Dein S, Stygall J. Does being religious help or hinder to cope with chronic illness? A critical literature review. *Palliat Med* 1997; **11**: 291–8.

57 Sloan R, Bagiella E, Powell T. Religion, spirituality and medicine. *Lancet* 1999; **20**: 664–7.

◆ 58 Oman D KJ, Strawbridge WJ, Cohen RD. Religious attendance and cause of death over 31 years. *Int J Psychiatry Med* 2002; **32**: 69–89.

◆ 59 Matthews D, McCullough M, Larson D, Koenig H, Swyers J, Milano M. Religious commitment and health status: a review of the research and implications for family medicine. *Arch Fam Med* 1998; **7**: 118–24.

● 60 Koenig H, Pargament KI, Nielsen J. Religious coping and health status in medically ill hospitalized older adults. *J Nerv Ment Dis* 1998; **186**: 513–21.

◆ 61 Larson DB, Pattison EM, Blazer DG, *et al*. Systematic analysis of research on religious variables in four major psychiatric journals, 1978–1982. *Am J Psychiatry* 1986; **14**: 329–34.

62 Levin J. How religion influences morbidity and health: reflections on natural history, salutogenesis and host resistance. *Soc Sci Med* 1996; **43**: 849–64.

63 Levin J, Larson DB, Puchalski CM. Religion and spirituality in medicine: research and education. *JAMA* 1997; **278**: 792–3.

◆ 64 McCullough M, Hoyt W, Larson D, *et al*. Religious involvement and mortality: a meta-analytic review. *Health Psychol* 2000; **19**: 211–22.

● 65 Thoresen C, Harris A. Spirituality and health: what's the evidence and what's needed? *Ann Behav Med* 2002; **24**: 3–13.

● 66 Fehring R, Miller J, Shaw C. Spiritual well-being, religiosity, hope, depression, and other mood states in elderly people coping with cancer. *Oncol Nurs Forum* 1997; **24**: 663–71.

✱ 67 Puchalski C. Spiritual care. In: Berger A, Portenoy R, Weissman DE, eds. *Principles and Practice of Palliative Care and Supportive Oncology*. Philadelphia: Lippincott Williams Wilkins, 2002: 799–812.

68 DeMarinis V. *Tvärkulturell vård i livets slutskede* [in Swedish, author's translation: Transcultural care at the end-of-life]. Lund: Studentlitteratur, 1998.

● 69 Nilmanat K, Street A. Search for a cure: narratives of Thai family caregivers living with a person with AIDS. *Soc Sci Med* 2004: 1003–10.

● 70 Holland JC, Passik S, Kash KM, *et al*. The role of religious and spiritual beliefs in coping with malignant melanoma. *Psychooncology* 1999; **8**: 14–26.

71 Koenig HG, Idler E, Kasl S, *et al*. Religion, spirituality, and medicine. A rebuttal to sceptics. *Int J Psychiatry Med* 1999; **29**: 123–31.

● 72 Kuupelomäki M. Spiritual support for terminally ill patients: nursing staff assessments. *J Clin Nurs* 2001; **10**: 660–70.

73 Larson E, Witham L. Leading scientists still reject God. *Nature* 1998; **394**: 313.

✱ 74 Rousseau P. Spirituality and the dying patient. *J Clin Oncol* 2000; **18**: 2000-2.

✱ 75 Greenstein M, Breitbart W. Cancer and the experience of meaning: a group psychotherapy program for people with cancer. *Am J Psychother* 2000; **54**: 486-500.

✱ 76 Frankl V. *The Will to Meaning: Foundations and Applications of Logotherapy.* New York: World Publishing, 1969.

● 77 Labun E. Spiritual care: an element in nursing planning. *J Adv Nurs* 1998; **13**: 314-20.

● 78 Ashworth P. Spiritual care: a challenge in multicultural critical care. *Intensive Crit Care Nurs* 1999; **15**: 63-4.

✱ 79 Morita T, Tsunoda J, Inoue S, Chichara S. An exploratory factor analysis of existential suffering in Japanese terminally ill cancer patients. *Psychooncology* 2000; **9**: 164-8.

80 Stifoss-Hanssen H. Ritualer vid dödsfall [in Swedish]. In: Kaasa S, ed. *Palliativ behandling och vård:* Studentlitteratur; 2001: 100-7.

Family care

LINDA J KRISTJANSON

INTRODUCTION

A fundamental tenet of good palliative care is the importance of attention and support to the family.[1] This principle of care is supported by empirical evidence that demonstrates that a terminal illness in a relative has a marked effect on family members.[2–5*] Families provide practical care and hold vigil with the patient as they attempt to offer emotional support and reassurance. Family members usually feel unprepared for this caregiver role because they lack specific knowledge, skills, and understanding of about how to best provide support. They therefore look to health professionals for information, practical advice, and emotional sustenance to help them cope with the feelings of loss and helplessness.[3,6] As they witness and participate in the patient's care, they make judgments about the quality of care that the patient and they receive.[7***] They often view themselves as the patient's care advocate and may experience remorse if they believe that they did not achieve the best possible care for their loved one. Recognition of the weighty impact of the illness on the family member's psychological and physical health has led them to be branded 'hidden patients'.[7***]

This chapter synthesizes current empirical findings related to the care needs of families in palliative care. The definition of 'family' is discussed and the prime needs of family members are described with a focus on how the palliative care team might best support families to sustain their supportive role and manage the impact of the illness on their own physical and emotional health.

DEFINING THE FAMILY

The World Health Organization[1] refers to the family as the 'unit of care' and affirms the importance of family care as part of a palliative approach. In the context of the impact of a terminal illness, the definition of who constitutes the family needs to be necessarily broad and inclusive. For example, the Canadian Palliative Care Association's[8] definition of family is:

> those closest to the patient in knowledge care and affection. This includes the biological family, the family of acquisition (related by marriage/contract), and the family of choice and friends (not related biologically, by marriage/contract).

According to this definition, families may include different individuals who may or may not be related through blood or legal ties.[7***] Families may include immediate relatives, a larger network of extended family members, neighbors, and friends.

Failure to recognize the distinct characteristics or membership of families may exclude some family members who may be in need of support. This error may be more common when families do not fit a traditional definition of family (e.g. blended families, families who live geographically apart).[9***,10,11**] Therefore, supportive palliative care to families begins with a careful and open consideration of who constitutes the family. From a clinical perspective, the most practical approach to defining the family affected by the patient's illness is to permit the patient and his or her family members to define the family.

THE FAMILY'S NEEDS

The literature related to families' needs has been classified into four categories: pain management, information needs, needs for physical help with care, and assistance to manage family communication and family functioning.

Family pain management

Family members who observe poorly managed symptoms such as pain, dyspnea, and appetite problems, experience considerable distress and a type of 'vicarious suffering', especially if they feel poorly prepared to respond. In particular, pain management is consistently identified by family caregivers as their leading concern related to care of a relative with advanced disease and is a particular worry for those who provide care at home.[12*,13*,14*] Poorly managed pain may prompt fears about disease progression, and is emotionally and physically exhausting for both patient and family members who witness the distress.[14*] If family caregivers are unable to relieve the patient's suffering they may experience guilt and distress and feelings of helplessness.[15*]

Family members who are not educated in palliative care pain management practices may hold a number of attitudes and beliefs about pain medication that prevent good pain relief. For example, family members may have fears that the patient will become addicted to opioids, may experience respiratory depression because of these strong medications or may 'use up' the medication early in their illness and therefore have no access to pain relief later when the pain is more severe.[14*] Family caregivers who are unfamiliar with pain management medications may over-medicate or under-medicate patients with opioids, resulting in medical complications and increased suffering.[14*] When family caregivers do not feel confident and knowledgeable about pain management, patients are more likely to require hospital admission and more frequent medical interventions and need more respite care.[16*]

An intervention study was undertaken recently to test a family pain education program for family caregivers of patients with end-stage cancer.[17***] Ninety-two family members were randomized to either the family pain education program or standard care. The education program was delivered in the family's home via four 1-hour sessions. Family caregivers were provided with a comfort diary to record the patient's pain and their treatment approaches, a video demonstrating how to safely move the patient without causing discomfort, and an education booklet outlining information about safe use of medications. The results indicated that family caregivers who received the pain education program had more positive attitudes toward pain management, were more knowledgeable about pain management approaches and used medications more effectively in providing pain relief to the patient. Palliative care teams therefore need to ensure that family caregivers have the information they require when providing pain relief to the patient.[17***] Further research is needed to develop family-oriented interventions specific to the concerns families may experience in relation to other symptoms (e.g. dyspnea, fatigue). The capacity of the family to respond to patient distress is a central component of care.

Information needs

Family members consistently report difficulties accessing information.[7***,18***] Health professionals may overload families with large amounts of information or may provide information in small amounts in an effort not to overwhelm them with too much detail.[18***,19*,20*] Families are reluctant to bother busy health professionals with questions about care because they believe that health professionals are primarily responsible to the patient and that family concerns are tangential.[3,7***] The perceived unimportance of communication with the family is reinforced by the lack of time and space for this type of exchange.[18***,21***] The pace of busy work schedules may also limit time spent with families and health professionals may wrongly assume that the patient/family has understood the information conveyed.[22] In some instances, health professionals may avoid information sharing with families because they lack comfort in knowing how to communicate difficult/bad news.[22,23]

One of the most effective ways of assisting families is to provide them with liberal amounts of well-timed, simple information that helps them cope with the care challenges they face.[24] Families require information about how to provide comfort care, how to communicate within the family, how to pace their own energies, and when to call for assistance.[3]

Home care nurses are reported to be a valuable source of information[3,18***,25] and families value 24-hour access to information.[26*] In rural communities, the nurse has been reported to be particularly important to families. Nurses are often the most accessible and specific in providing information regarding how to provide care and support[18***,27] Use of a family conference has also been reported by family members to be a helpful source of information and an opportunity to clarify questions.[26*] Practical information to help families anticipate the next steps of the patient's illness is also beneficial.[24] This information allows families to 'stay in front' of symptoms, know what to expect and not be caught in a moment of crisis unprepared for deterioration in the patient's condition.

One of the particular fears that families report is a worry about how to manage care at the time of death.[18***,24,28,29] Families also appreciate knowing the common signs that indicate that death may be approaching.[28,29] Information given in a calm, specific, and reassuring manner can help families to feel prepared and able to manage. This information helps them to prepare psychologically for the patient's death and allows time to call family members who may wish to be present.[18***,24]

A recent study by Kirk and colleagues[30*] involved interviews with 38 palliative cancer patients and 36 family members to ascertain their experiences of the information disclosure process. Their results indicated that the process of information sharing was as important as the content. The timing, management, and delivery of information by the healthcare team all need to be carefully considered. The most important content areas were information about prognosis and hope. All patients, regardless of ethnic/cultural background, wanted information about their illness, and almost all were willing to share this fully with their families. All family members thought it important that the patient be aware of the diagnosis. As the illness progressed both patients and family members reported that information needs changed and there was greater divergence between the patient's and family's needs. At the palliative phase of an illness many patients reported not wanting as much detail as they had asked for initially, and some requested that their family member speak with the healthcare professionals on their own. These findings point to the importance of the quality of the relationship between health professionals and patients and families and the need for sensitive and individualized information exchange.[18***]

Physical care needs

Families who provide care to a patient with a terminal diagnosis experience many physical demands and practical needs, which may be underestimated.[31*,32*] Family members may need to assume duties that the ill person cannot undertake, and may experience practical problems associated with transportation to treatments, child care, and unrelenting work demands.[7***] Buehler[33] undertook a longitudinal study of families caring for patients with advanced cancer in rural communities and documented a lack of available resources. This lack of support may occur, in part, because family caregivers are viewed as resources rather than as recipients of care.[11***]

In instances when the family caregiver is an older person and has health problems of his or her own, the demands of caregiving can be extremely taxing.[18***,34,35] However, family members may stretch their efforts beyond their usual limits because of a sense of duty to care for the patient. The additive effect of these burdens and strains may be notable[11***] with this type of over-functioning resulting in caregiver fatigue.[36] There is a risk that signs of caregiver fatigue may be missed or underestimated by clinicians who observe family members briefly and intermittently.[7***]

Respite services can be helpful to families in sustaining their caregiving energies. These services may take the form of external (hospital/hospice based) care whereby patients are admitted if they have intractable symptoms, they are imminently dying and home is not the desired place of death, and/or to allow the family to rest.[24] In other instances, provision of home respite may allow families time to be relieved of caregiving duties for a short period of time.[18***] Bramwell and colleagues[37*] surveyed caregivers' needs for overnight respite. They found that 73 percent of caregivers received less than 4 hours of sleep and as a result were more vulnerable to exhaustion. Further, 70 percent of all caregivers surveyed indicated that they would use an overnight

respite service. The researchers recommended further investigation of the relationship between carer exhaustion and early hospital admission and whether or not night respite would prevent hospital admission.

A recent study evaluated a community-based night respite service for terminally ill cancer patients and reported positive outcomes.[38**] Care aides were trained to provide night respite support and 53 patients received this support over an 11-month time period. Families who indicated moderate-to-severe levels of carer fatigue were identified as urgent candidates for night respite support. Almost 70 percent of patients who died were able to die at home, compared with 50 percent of patients who died at home without this service. Family carers reported that this assistance helped them to manage the patient at home. Costs associated with home deaths and the night respite service were much less than was the case for patients admitted to an inpatient facility for end-stage care.[38**]

In summary, the practical, physical challenges associated with providing care and support have notable effects on the physical and emotional wellbeing of family caregivers.[7***,39] Without adequate family interventions and targeted support, the burden placed on families may limit their abilities to provide good quality patient care.[40]

Family communication and family functioning issues

A family's ability to support a patient emotionally and practically depend to a large extent on the amount and quality of social and health professional support the family itself receives.[32] Poor communication causes more suffering to patients with cancer and their families than any other problem – with the exception of unrelieved pain.[41] Communication is essential to healthy family functioning, and families who have limited communication skills are less able to manage stressful situations.[42] Some family members may be open and clear in their exchanges about the illness, treatment decisions, fears, and doubts. Others may be reserved in their expressions of feelings, holding back worries, regrets, and uncertainty.[7***]

Families usually rely on a patients to relay information about the illness, which helps them understand the plan of care and subsequent phases of the disease. Families may feel uncertain or frustrated if they lack this information, especially if the patients assume the role of information gatekeeper in an effort to shield family members. This protective behavior is common when parents have cancer and are cautious about sharing information with their children.[43*,44*] Information shielding can also occur in reverse when family members attempt to shelter the patient from what they perceive to be unsettling information. Relationship strains may occur, contributing to conflict, anxiety, and poor communication within the family.[7***]

Families who communicated effectively prior to the illness have been found to cope more effectively during the illness than those with histories of less functional communication.[45] Questions to explore early with the family about how they communicate may allow the health professional to be alert to difficulties and help the family to talk through how they are going to share information and discuss concerns in a way that might avoid conflict and communication mistakes.[18***]

Emotional needs of family members include a need for support to help them manage issues of loss, uncertainty about the patient's illness and eventual death, communication difficulties within the family, and their own psychological distress.[46] Research to delineate the coping strategies most helpful to families reveals that the strategy labeled 'taking one day at a time' has been used to manage uncertainty.[47*] Acceptance, rationalization, and social support were also identified as useful coping strategies that family members used to cope with changes in the patient's condition.[11***,46] Offering families some of these approaches can be helpful in reminding them about how to cope, how to reach out for assistance, and how to compartmentalize the stresses they face into more manageable parts.[24]

Family members who witness a traumatic illness or death may be at risk for a more complicated bereavement reaction.[48*] Therefore, caring for the family during the palliative phase of an illness is a preventive health strategy that may place them in a better position to deal with this crisis and integrate the loss in a way that maintains their own health.[49] Those who have experienced a difficult death or observed a patient's unrelieved suffering may require special support to contend with difficult memories and feelings of regret.[7***]

SOCIAL AND FINANCIAL PRESSURES

The social and financial pressures that families encounter in response to the challenges of the patient's illness have also been well documented and may place additional strain on the family. One study conducted in the USA reported that many caregivers of terminally ill patients with moderate or high care needs reported spending 10 percent of their household income on healthcare costs and that they or their families had to sell assets, take out a loan or mortgage, or obtain an additional job to meet healthcare costs.[50] The economic impact of day-to-day family involvement in living with cancer can be profound, especially due to the unavailability of support services in many geographical areas.[51] Findings from the few cost-estimate studies indicate that families find themselves responsible for purchasing medications and home care supplies, for renting equipment, and for paying for transportation and respite services.[52]

In Canada, the financial costs associated with the move from institutional care to home care has been shown to be borne by recipients and their carers.[53] Many of these costs

would be absorbed by the government if the recipients were in hospital, especially expenses related to medical equipment, special meals, renovations to accommodate disabilities, repairs and maintenance of the care setting, and in some instances prescription and nonprescription drugs. Australian data reported by Schofield et al.[54] confirms that caring commitments may mean that some carers are unable to work, or have to work fewer hours or in a lower paid job with financial consequences. The 'Caring Costs' study confirmed the low-income levels of most carers as two-thirds listed a government pension or benefit as a main source of income.[55]

Although these findings do not diminish the fact that the role of family caregiving can be rewarding, these studies alert us to the potential negative effects of caring over time. These studies confirm that families may have significant unmet needs related to their caregiving roles despite the significant, yet often invisible, contribution that they make to society and to the healthcare economy.

CONCLUSION

The physical and psychological distress of families during the patient's illness and in the bereavement period is clearly reported. Palliative care providers who view the needs of all family members as important are better able to assess and identify supports for those in need of assistance. In the palliative phase of an illness, attention to families who may be psychologically vulnerable, lack resources, or have concomitant health issues and concerns constitutes good preventive family care. However, there have been few intervention studies focused on reducing negative aspects of family caregiving. Harding and Higginson[56***] have called for evaluation studies focused on the family caregiving population with attention to cost-effective allocation of resources. This recommendation warrants attention and should direct future family studies in palliative care research.

Key learning points

- The most practical approach to defining the family is to permit the patient and the family members to define the family.

- Pain management is consistently identified by family caregivers as their key concern.

- Family caregivers experience both physical and emotional health strains.

- One of the most effective ways of assisting families is to offer liberal amounts of well timed, simple information.

- Families will require information about how to provide pain relief and comfort care, how to communicate within the family, how to pace their own energies, and when to call for assistance.

- Use of targeted respite may assist family caregivers to maintain their caregiving role and allow the patient to remain at home longer.

- Family members need support to help them cope with issues of loss, uncertainty about the patient's illness, the possible death of their relative, communication issues within the family, and their own psychological distress.

- Family members who have witnessed a difficult death or unrelieved patient suffering may be in particular need in the bereavement period.

- Social and financial strains associated with family caregiving may be notable.

REFERENCES

1   World Health Organization. Palliative care, 2003. Available at: www.who.int/hiv/topics/palliative/care/en (accessed May 30, 2004).

2   Ferrell BR. The family. In: Doyle C, Hanks GWC, McDonald N, eds. *Oxford Textbook of Palliative Medicine*, 2nd ed. Oxford: Oxford University Press, 1998: 909–17.

3   Hudson PL, Aranda S, Kristjanson LJ. Meeting the supportive needs of family caregivers in palliative care: Challenges for health professionals. *J Palliat Med* 2004; **7**: 19–25.

4   Andershed B, Ternestedt B. Involvement of relatives in the care of the dying in different care cultures: Involvement in the dark or in the light? *Cancer Nurs* 1998; **21**: 106–16.

5   Kristjanson LJ, Sloan JA, Dudgeon DJ, Adaskin E. Family members' perceptions of palliative cancer care: predictors of family functioning and family members' health. *J Palliat Care* 1996; **12**: 10–20.

6   Hudson P, Aranda S, Kristjanson LJ. Information provision for palliative care families. *Eur J Palliat Care* 2004; **11**: 153–7.

◆ 7   Kristjanson LJ, Aoun S. Palliative care for families: remembering the hidden patients. *Can J Psychiatry* 2004; **49**: 359–65.

8   Canadian Palliative Care Association. *Standards for Palliative Care Provision*. Ottawa: Canadian Palliative Care Association, 1998.

◆ 9   Kristjanson LJ, Ashcroft T. The family's cancer journey: A literature review. *Cancer Nurs* 1994; **17**: 1–17.

10 Kristjanson LJ, Davis S. The impact of cancer on the family. In: Porock D, Palmer D, eds. *Cancer of the Gastrointestinal Tract*. London: Whurr Publishers, 2004: 51–68.

◆ 11 Leis A, Kristjanson LJ, Koop P, Laizner A. Family health and the palliative care trajectory: a research agenda. *Can J Clin Oncol* 1997; **1**: 352–60.

12 Bucher JA, Trostle GB, Moore M. Family reports of cancer pain, pain relieve and prescription access. *Cancer Pract* 1999; **7**: 71–7.

13 Ferrell BR. Pain observed: the experience of pain from the family caregiver's perspectives. *Clin Geriatr Med* 2001; **17**: 595–608.

14 Oldham L, Kristjanson LJ. Development of a pain management program for family caregivers of advanced cancer patients at home. *Int J Palliat Nurs* 2004; **10**: 91–9.

15 Ferrell B, Rhiner M, Cohen MZ, Grant M. Pain as a metaphor for illness. Part I: Impact of cancer pain on family caregivers. *Oncol Nurs Forum* 1991; **18**: 1303–9.

16 Ferrell B, Taylor EJ, Grant M, *et al.* Pain management at home, *Cancer* 1993; **16**: 169–78.

17 Oldham L, Kristjanson LJ. Pain management education for family carers of people living with advanced cancer in the community. *ACCNS J Comm Nurses* 2004; **9**: 13–15.

◆ 18 Kristjanson LJ. Caring for families of people with cancer: evidence and interventions. *Cancer Forum* 2004; 28: 123–7.

● 19 Northouse PG, Northouse LL. Communication and cancer: Issues confronting patients, health professionals, and family members. *J Psychosoc Oncol* 1998; **5**: 17–45.

● 20 Northouse LL, Golden-Peters H. Cancer and the family: Strategies to assist spouses. *Semin Oncol Nurs* 1993; **9**: 74–82.

● 21 Northouse L. The impact of cancer on the family: An overview. *Int J Psychiatr Med* 1984; **14**: 215–42.

22 Andershed B, Ternestedt B. Development of a theoretical framework describing relatives' involvement in palliative care. *J Adv Nurs* 2001; **24**: 554–62.

23 Bottorff JL, Gogag M, Engelberg-Lotzkar M. Comforting: Exploring the work of cancer nurses. *J Adv Nurs* 1995; **22**: 1077–84.

24 Kristjanson LJ, Hudson P, Oldham L. Working with families in palliative care. In: Aranda S, O'Connor M, eds. *Palliative Care Nursing: A Guide to Practice*, 2nd ed. Melbourne: AUSMED publications, 2003.

25 Hull MM. Hospice nurses. Caring support for caregiving families. *Cancer Nurs* 1991; **14**: 63–70.

● 26 Kristjanson LJ. Quality of terminal care: Salient indicators identified by families. *J Palliat Care* 1989; **5**: 21–8.

27 Rose K. A qualitative analysis of the information needs of informal carers of terminally ill cancer patients. *J Clin Nurs* 1999; **8**: 81–8.

28 Grbich C, Parker D, Maddocks I. Communication and information needs of care-givers of adult family members at diagnosis and during treatment of terminal cancer. *Prog Palliat Care* 2000; **8**: 345–50.

29 Vachon M. Psychosocial needs of patients and families. *J Palliat Care* 1998; **14**: 49–56.

● 30 Kirk P, Kirk I, Kristjanson LJ. What do palliative cancer patients and their families want to be told? A Canadian and Australian qualitative study. *BMJ* 2004; **328**: 1343.

31 Meyers JL, Gray LN. The relationships between family primary caregiver characteristics and satisfaction with hospice care, quality of life, and burden. *Oncol Nurs Forum* 2001; **28**: 73–82.

32 Emanuel EJ, Fairclough DL, Slutsman J, *et al.* Assistance from family members, friends, paid caregivers, and volunteers in the care of terminally ill patients. *N Engl J Med* 1999; **341**: 956–63.

● 33 Buehler JA, Lee HJ. Exploration of home care resources for rural families with cancer. *Cancer Nurs* 1992; **15**: 299–308.

34 Cobbs EL. Health of older women. *Med Clin North Am* 1998; **82**: 127–44.

35 Given BA, Given CW. Health promotion for family caregivers of chronically ill elders. *Annu Rev Nurs Res* 1998; **16**: 197–217.

36   Yang C, Kirschling JM. Exploration of factors related to direct care and outcomes of caregiving: caregivers of terminally ill older person. *Cancer Nurs* 1992; **15**: 173–81.

37   Bramwell L, MacKenzie J, Laschinger H, Cameron N. Need for overnight respite for primary caregivers of hospice clients. *Cancer Nurs* 1995; **18**: 337–43.

● 38   Kristjanson LJ, Cousins K, White K, *et al.* Evaluation of a night respite community palliative care service. *Int J Palliat Nurs* 2004; **10**: 84–90.

39   Hudson P. The educational needs of lay carers. *Eur J Palliat Care* 1998; **5**: 183–6.

40   Pasacreta JV, McCorkle R. Cancer care: impact of interventions on caregiver outcomes. *Annu Rev Nurs Res* 2000; **18**: 127–48.

41   Stedeford A. Couples facing death: unsatisfactory communication. *BMJ* 1981; **2**: 1098.

42   Kemp C. *Terminal Illness: A Guide to Nursing Care.* Toronto: JB Lippincott Company, 1995: 75–88.

● 43   Kristjanson LJ, Chalmers K, Taylor-Brown J, *et al.* Information needs of adolescent children of women with breast cancer. *Oncol Nurs Forum* 2004; **31**: 111–20.

44   Chalmers K, Kristjanson LJ, Taylor-Brown J, *et al.* Perceptions of the role of the school in providing information and support to adolescent children of women with breast cancer. *J Adv Nurs* 2000; **31**: 1430–8.

45   Kissane DW, Bloch S. Family grief. *Br J Psychiatry* 1994; **164**: 728–40.

46   Hull MM. Coping strategies of family caregivers in hospice home care. *Oncol Nurs Forum* 1992; **19**: 1179–87.

47   Higginson IJ, Wade AM, McCarthy M. Effectiveness of two palliative support teams. *J Public Health Med* 1992; **14**: 50–6.

48   Kristjanson LJ, Nikoletti S, Porock D, *et al.* Congruence between patients' and family caregivers' perceptions of symptom distress in patients with terminal cancer. *J Palliat Care* 1998; **14**: 24–30.

49   Kellehear A. *Health Promoting Palliative Care.* Melbourne: Oxford University Press, 1999.

50   Emanuel E, Fairclough D, Slutsman J, Emanuel L. Understanding economic and other burdens of terminal illness: the experience of patients and their caregivers. *Ann Intern Med* 2000; **132**: 451–9.

51   McCorkle R, Pasacreta J. Enhancing caregiver outcomes in palliative care. *Cancer Control* 2001: **8**: 36–45.

52   Given BA, Given GW, Stommel M. Family and out-of-pocket costs for women with breast cancer. *Cancer Pract* 1994; **2**: 189–93.

53   Morris M, Robinson J, Simpson J, *et al.* The changing nature of home care and its impact on women's vulnerability to poverty. Canadian Research Institute for the Advancement of Women, 1999. See: http://publications.gc.ca/contro/quickPublicSearch (accessed December 18, 2005).

54   Schofield H, Murphy B, Nankervis J, Singh B. Family carers: women and men, adult offspring, partners and parents. *J Fam Stud* 1997; **3**: 149–68.

55   Carers Association of Australia. *Caring Costs: A Survey of Tax Issues and Health and Disability Related Costs for Carer Families.* Canberra: Carers Association of Australia, 1997.

◆ 56   Harding R, Higginson I. What is the best way to help caregivers in cancer and palliative care? A systematic literature review of interventions and their effectiveness. *Palliat Med* 2003; **17**: 63–74.

A transcultural perspective of advance directives in palliative care

DONNA S ZHUKOVSKY

DEFINITIONS

Advance directives are closely related to the concept of patient autonomy, a highly valued tenet of Western medicine.[1] Autonomy, intrinsic to patient self-determination, is contingent upon informed consent and informed refusal of medically indicated treatments. The goal of advanced directives is to afford the individual an element of control over future healthcare decisions in the event that he or she loses the capacity to participate in medical decision making.[2] It is important to note that while patient autonomy is a significant factor in medical decision making, other ethical principles such as beneficence and distributive justice must also be considered with each treatment decision.[3] Two main types of advance directive exist:

- Instructional documents, more commonly known as living wills or directives, that specify wishes for future health states.
- Documents that designate a surrogate decision maker, variously called healthcare proxy, medical power of attorney, or durable power of attorney forms.

In addition, the majority of states in the USA offer a more limited type of advance directive, in the form of out-of-hospital 'Do Not Resuscitate' (DNR) orders.[4*]

In today's healthcare climate, living wills have evolved from specifying treatment refusal to indicating types of treatment the patient would accept or decline in specified healthcare states or conditions, such as terminal diseases, or in irreversible conditions that ultimately become fatal without the use of life-sustaining treatments. For healthcare proxies, the role of the surrogate decision maker as initially proposed is to make recommendations based on substituted judgment, i.e. what the patient would have wanted if able to express him or herself, and if not known, on best interests of the patient, as guided by patient values.[5]

Instructional directives and proxy documents are complementary, as one cannot presuppose all future states of incapacity or illness that may occur. Neither type comes into effect unless the individual is in a state of incapacity related to decision making for the question at hand.[6] Decision making capacity is a medical determination for the relevant decision and not synonymous with competency, which is legally determined. However, the two terms are often used interchangeably. Not well understood is that the goal of advance directives is to facilitate patient autonomy for medically sound treatment choices, and does not support demands for interventions considered to be medically futile or otherwise inappropriate.[2] Regular review of advance directives is recommended, especially with changes in life status such as marriage, childbirth, divorce, or death of a spouse, as well as with significant changes in medical status, to ensure consistency with a patient's goals of care.

LEGAL ISSUES

From a legal perspective, advance directives may be statutory or advisory in nature. Statutory documents, designed to protect physicians who follow patients' wishes from liability, are based on legal criteria codified in state law. US states will frequently honor statutory documents of other states. Although nonstatutory instructional documents do not always conform to state statutes, they, too, are legally binding if clear evidence of the patient's wishes is documented, as common law affords competent individuals the right to accept or refuse treatment, including life-sustaining interventions.[6] The state of New York distinguishes artificial nutrition and hydration from other treatment choices, placing this treatment choice in a separate category from other medical interventions. Surrogates are unable to make decisions about artificial nutrition and hydration, unless the agent reasonably knows the patient's wishes, as explicitly expressed beforehand.[7]

Regarding children, few states in the USA have statutes regulating the implementation of directives on behalf of minors and even fewer address the implementation of DNR orders in the school setting.[8] Recently, the state of West Virginia implemented the West Virginia Health Care Decisions Act, granting mature minors the legal ability to execute written advance directives and make end-of-life decisions.[9] There are limited guidelines for determination of mature minor status. However, the literature suggests that minors 15 years of age or older should be presumed competent to provide consent for major health decisions in the absence of evidence to the contrary. Adolescents between the ages of 11 and 14 are in a transition period, with many capable of competent consent. For those who have not yet realized full decision making capacity, and for children younger than 11, gradual, escalating involvement in decision making to facilitate skill development and confidence for future decisions is recommended. Although the majority of states in the USA do not specifically address end-of-life decision making for mature minors, the literature increasingly supports the role of pediatric assent in medical decision making, including for end-of-life care decisions such as treatment discontinuation and advance care planning, as consistent with the child's decision making capacity and willingness to participate.[10–13] Among healthcare professionals, it remains controversial if mature minors should have primary authority for consent that is in conflict with parental opinion or if all decisions should be made in consideration of the provider, patient, and family relationship, with parents having primary authority for consent.[9] Despite lack of specific legislation regarding the mature minor doctrine in most states, there have not been any successful lawsuits against physicians who have honored the consent of mature minors 15 years of age or older, in absence of parental consent, for more than 40 years.

HISTORY AND EXAMPLES OF ADVANCE DIRECTIVES

Historically, the earliest instructional directives in the USA date back to 1968 when the living will was developed to support the widespread belief that 'heroic' levels of technological intervention were not medically indicated if the patient's prognosis was 'hopeless'.[6] Highly technological care had become prominent at the end-of-life subsequent to the introduction of closed chest massage in 1960, precluding the need for open thoracotomy and direct cardiac massage during cardiac resuscitation. However, instructional directives did not come into common usage until the 1970s with the development of hospital policies regulating the withholding of cardiopulmonary resuscitation (CPR), in the form of DNR orders.[14] In 1974, the American Medical Association suggested that decision DNR be entered into the patient's medical record and communicated to the attending staff.[15] Two years later, a working group of the Harvard School of Public Health prepared a statement to support hospitals in their development of policies regarding the decision making process for the use of CPR. Their discussion centered upon the medical appropriateness of CPR for patients with irreversible, irreparable illness whose death was anticipated imminently, defined as a period of 2 weeks or less and the right of competent patients to provide informed acceptance or rejection of treatment. Key features of the process included determination of medical appropriateness of a DNR order by the primary physician after discussion with other clinicians involved in the patient's care, as well as with a senior physician not involved in the patient's care, and informed choice of the competent patient or with agreement of all appropriate family members for the incompetent patient. Additional steps included physician responsibility of informing family members of competent patients, after obtaining permission to do so and documenting details of the steps above in the patient's medical record, together with discussions that took place with family members upon their appraisal of the decision.[14]

Over time, the scope of instructional directives has broadened from treatment limitation to that of preferred treatment choices. Several preformatted documents have been developed that allow the patient to indicate preferences for various treatments in the context of different medical conditions. One or these, the Medical Directive, was developed in 1989 by Emanuel and Emanuel to overcome some of the limitations of early forms of instructional directives, namely, failure to accommodate positive requests for treatment, vague language affording multiple interpretations of terms used in the directive, lack of flexibility for unforeseen clinical situations and poor patient–physician communication. Composed of five sections, the Medical Directive includes an introduction, which emphasizes the importance of personal values and goals in the decision-making process and of communicating values and goals of care with the patient's family, friends, and physicians, a section containing four illness scenarios designed to elicit preferences for medical care with regard to specific life-sustaining medical treatments given different outcomes, a section for the designation of a proxy decision maker, a section for organ donation, and lastly, a personal statement.[16]

At approximately the same time that the Medical Directive was proposed, Doukas and McCullough introduced the Values History into the literature, a two-part instrument that elicits patient values about terminal medical care and therapy-specific directives.[17] Like the Medical Directive, the Values History was structured to facilitate patient–physician communication and provides for designation of surrogate decision maker and consent for organ donation. Additionally, it allows for autopsy consent and for a trial of selected treatment interventions, as an intermediate option to intervention or nonintervention. Subsequent study of this document exploring the relation between values and stated preferences for individuals in the outpatient setting indicates that respondents (N = 118, mean age 39 years, 61 percent female, 68 percent married) preferred quality of life to longevity and identified general communication issues, family burden, and physician-compliance factors as meaningful psychological values. Family burden considerations were highly relevant to the decision-making process.[18*] Five Wishes is another well-known advance planning instrument that is available in English and in Spanish versions through a nonprofit organization called Aging with Dignity.[19] Caring Conversations, consisting of a 16-page workbook, living will and durable power of attorney forms, is available from the Center for Practical Bioethics.[20]

EFFICACY OF ADVANCE DIRECTIVES

For advance directives to be effective, they must impact on care provided in a direction consistent with patient preferences. Requisite components for successful use of living wills include awareness of their existence, provision of information adequate to facilitate informed consent and informed refusal of medical treatments for future medical states based on personal values and goals of care, documentation of treatment choices in unambiguous terms, communication of choices to surrogate decision makers and healthcare clinicians and utilization of this information by surrogate decision makers and physicians when the individual is in the specified condition. To support the use of advance directives, the US Congress passed the Patient Self-Determination Act (PSDA) in 1990, requiring that all patients be asked about the existence of advance directives at the time of registration or admission to a healthcare facility, as a prerequisite for federal funding.[21] The Joint Commission on Accreditation of Health Care Organizations further recommended that such healthcare facilities have available a process facilitating completion of advance care directives, for those patients who so choose.[6]

Despite strong advocacy for advance directives from members of the medical, ethical, legal, and lay communities, they have not made a significant impact on medical care for most patients.[22,23] In most settings, less than 20 percent of patients have formal advance directives and even fewer have provided copies to their physicians.[24,25,26*,27*,28,29*] Family members, surrogate decision makers, and physicians are frequently unaware that the individual has an advance directive and are unlikely to predict patient preferences accurately more often than by chance alone,[30] often believing the patient's prior wishes to be for more intervention than the patient had chosen.[31] Furthermore, physicians frequently do not follow patients' known treatment preferences,[32] as demonstrated by the Study to Understand Prognoses and Preferences for Outcomes and Risks of Treatments (SUPPORT), a major multisite intervention of over 9000 seriously ill patients,[6,30*] and other studies.[33*]

Numerous reasons have been cited for the failure of advance directives to extend patient autonomy into periods of incapacity for medical decision making, many of which relate to the emotional distress inherent in discussing end-of-life issues. Patients and physicians are often reluctant to initiate advance care planning, waiting for the other to take the lead and/or delaying until the individual is seriously ill and/or no longer has decision-making capacity. Data from a cross-sectional descriptive survey of randomly selected primary care patients and physicians in the USA indicated that differences in opinion about the timing of such discussions and who should initiate them also plays a role. Patients felt the discussion should take place earlier in the physician–patient relationship and disease course than did physicians, with the majority of patients believing that discussions should take place in the outpatient setting while they are still healthy. More patients than physicians believed the discussion should occur with the diagnosis of a life-threatening illness (90 percent vs. 60 percent, respectively). While the majority of both groups believed it was the physician's role to initiate discussion of advance directives, patients believed so more often than physicians.[34*] Of those who complete advance directives, many do so with minimal or no physician involvement, raising the question of adequate informed consent and refusal. Communication between patients, physicians, family members and other healthcare surrogates is often suboptimal, resulting in overly optimistic estimates of prognosis by all involved.[35] The latter has the potential to influence patient decision making, as data from SUPPORT indicate that perceived prognosis may influence patient preference for life-extending versus comfort-focused care.[36*] Compounding inaccurate estimates of prognosis is a focus on isolated DNR decisions, leading to patient fears of abandonment. Lack of specificity of many instructional documents and limited awareness of patient directives and their content by relevant parties contribute to their limited impact on end-of-life care.[6,37,38*] For some individuals, advance directives may be considered irrelevant due to the presence of involved family[39*] or may not be culturally congruent with end-of-life care.[40]

Given their overall lack of influence on patient care, some authors have recommended that living wills be abandoned in favor of medical powers of attorney for those individuals who want control over future decisions. Arguments against use of surrogate decision makers include the limited execution of formal healthcare proxy documents, infrequent and incomplete discussions with family members about end-of-life care preferences and limited concordance of proxy decision maker choices with patients, resulting in failure to extend patient wishes into the future. Furthermore, the emotional and financial burden of caring for patients with advanced disease may present potential conflicts of interest for the proxy decision maker, especially if a family member or significant other, and is psychologically stressful.[41]

Fins and his group[42] make a cogent case that the act of being selected as an individual's proxy is at least as important to the individual as articulating the patient's known preferences, despite the lack of congruence frequently seen in patient–proxy decisions. They posit that the patient effectively achieves self-determination by a combination of *substantive* moral authority, based on knowledge of the patient's wishes and *procedural* moral authority, empowerment of the proxy by the act of being chosen to use interpretative discretion to assess the current situation and make judgments, even if they counter the patient's previously expressed wishes. An empirical study of 50 patient–proxy pairs and 52 individuals who had acted as proxies for individuals who had died provides initial support for their hypothesis. Variables such as disease trajectory, clarity of prognosis, quality of instructions, and instructional valence ('do everything' vs. 'do nothing') influenced the degree to which proxies adhered to the patient's initial instructions.[42*] Additional points offered in support of surrogate decision-making documents include simplicity, little change from current practice and legislative support designating proxies for incompetent individuals that already exists in some states.[22]

To date, advance directives have not significantly altered end-of-life care for the majority of individuals. However, the widespread variation of their prevalence and of the aggressiveness of end-of-life care suggests that advance directives may yet play a role in influencing patient care. The best known example is the Oregon experience, where a state-wide effort to enhance public knowledge about end-of-life care options has resulted in high rates of advance care planning, with family members of 68 percent of decedents reporting that a living will had been executed.[43*] Physician Orders for Life-Sustaining Treatment (POLST), a more specialized application of advance directives, has been in use across the continuum of care settings at the ElderPlace (a Program for All-Inclusive Care for the Elderly), Portland, Oregon site since 1994. In a preprinted and signed doctor's order form, competent individuals or their surrogates specify treatment instructions in the event of serious illness including orders for treatment preferences related to CPR, level of medical intervention desired, antibiotic use, and artificial administration of fluid and nutrition. Use of POLST has resulted in a high level of consistency with treatment preferences (84–94 percent), but less so for desired level of intervention (46 percent).[44] A survey of living will completion rates by nursing home residents in California,

Massachusetts, New York, and Ohio further supports their potential impact on end-of-life decision making. Completion rates ranged from 2.1 percent in California to 32.5 percent in Ohio. The difference in completion rates was only partly explained by previously noted associations with race, suggesting a potential to influence advance directive use by interventions.[25*] Hickey has suggested that adoption and enforcement by all states of the uniform Health Care Decisions Act, recognition of a physician's ethical duty to assist patients in advance directive formulation and routine third-party payor reimbursement to physicians for their role in patients' advance care planning will lead to increased completion and compliance with patient directives.[23]

Pollack suggests listing simplified advance directives on Medicare cards as a means of enhancing advance directive completion, as well as availability at time of need.[45]

CULTURAL LESSONS FROM THE USA

A series of studies by Blackhall and colleagues evaluating 800 older adults residing in the USA has illuminated the role that ethnicity plays in attitudes toward patient autonomy, use of life-sustaining technology and knowledge of, attitude toward, and possession of advance directives. As a group, Korean Americans and Mexican Americans favored models of family-centered decision making over those based on patient autonomy, which are preferred by African Americans and European Americans. Korean Americans and Mexican Americans were less likely to believe that a diagnosis of metastatic cancer or of a terminal prognosis should be disclosed to the patient or that the patient should decide about use of life-sustaining technology than African Americans or European Americans. Whereas Korean Americans and Mexican Americans were most likely to favor the use of life-sustaining technology, unlike Mexican Americans, Korean Americans did not want such technology used for themselves. As Mexican Americans became more acculturated to the US lifestyle, they were more likely to prefer the patient autonomy model.[46] Of the four groups evaluated, European Americans were the least likely to endorse a favorable attitude toward life support and the least likely to want life-sustaining technologies for themselves. African Americans, despite their generally negative perception of life support, were the most likely to favor personal use of life-prolonging technology.[47*] Knowledge about advance care directives was lowest for African Americans (12 percent) and Korean Americans (13 percent), intermediate for Mexican Americans (47 percent) and highest for European Americans (69 percent), $P < 0.001$. For those with knowledge of advance directives, possession rates were low overall, at 0 percent, 2 percent, 10 percent, and 28 percent for Korean Americans, African Americans, Mexican Americans and European Americans, respectively. After controlling for ethnicity and socioeconomic status, factors associated with possession of advance directives were personal experience with illness and more years of schooling. Factors associated with lack of advance directives were a negative attitude toward advance directives and government-assisted insurance.[48*]

Possible explanations of differences between ethnic groups in this work are elicited from ethnographic data. The apparent conflict in the expressed Korean American preference for use of life-sustaining technology in general, but not on an individual basis, relates to the concept of hyodo or filial piety, where family obligation is to prolong the life of their relative as long as possible. In this system of family-centered decision making, honoring family wishes takes precedence over patient autonomy as the 'right thing to do', analogous to the European concept of virtue. For Mexican Americans, the dichotomy between positive beliefs toward life support in general versus negative preference for personal use was not seen, perhaps due to the perception that the physician would not offer life-sustaining technology if the situation was truly hopeless. For African Americans, lack of trust in physicians on multiple levels associated with a greater wish for more prolonged life support was a more common theme than for other groups, along with the acknowledgment that it was acceptable to withhold or withdraw life support under some circumstances. European Americans based their negative views of life-sustaining technology largely on two factors: fear of cognitive impairment and of becoming a burden to family members.[46,47*,48] Like Korean Americans and Mexican Americans, the Navajo view of disclosure of negative information was unfavorable. The traditionally held Navajo concept of hozho, which combines the concepts of beauty, goodness, order, harmony, and everything that is positive or ideal, together with the belief that thought and language have the power to shape reality and control events, leads to ethical concerns that advance care planning is in violation of traditional Navajo culture.[49*] Clearly, differences in the value placed on patient autonomy influence perceptions of advance directives and their utility.

Similar attitudes and barriers to advance care planning have been found by other investigators.[39*,50*] For African Americans, numerous studies indicate that as a group, African Americans are less likely to discuss treatment preferences before death, to complete a living will or medical power of attorney or to have a DNR order before death and are more likely to prefer life-prolonging therapies than Caucasian Americans.[25,27*,31*,51*,52] Physician preferences for end-of-life treatment choices follow the same pattern by race as patient preferences.[53*] Content analysis of community-based focus groups exploring African American perspectives on end-of-life care planning and decision making revealed six explanatory themes as possible mediators of differences between the groups: death is not an option, religiosity and end-of-life care planning is a paradox, the healthcare system is a microcosm of societal and historical events, a 'trusted' family member or friend is the contract for life-and-death options, ethnically relevant initiatives are essential to increase advance directives participation, and people are people.[54*] However, trust, frequently cited as a factor associated with negative attitudes to advance care planning and treatment limitations for the African American community, was not consistently found to be a contributing variable across studies.[27*,31]

CULTURAL PERSPECTIVES OUTSIDE THE USA

Europe

Advance directives are used even less commonly outside the USA. In a thoughtful treatise, Sanchez-Gonzalez evaluated the use of advance directives from a transcultural perspective, looking at the relative importance of different values from the perspective of the three prevailing ethical traditions in Europe: Anglo Saxon, northern (or central) European and Mediterranean.[1] To varying degrees in different parts of Europe, there is greater importance placed on virtue over (individual) rights, stoicism over consumerism, rationalism over empiricism, statism over citizens' initiative, and justice over autonomy. Consequently, family and physician contribution to medical decision making in many parts of Europe is greater than in the USA, where patient autonomy prevails. Confidence in family and physician virtue allows for decisions from a shared set of communitarian beliefs and values. Additionally, a strong emphasis on stoicism, with happiness determined by inner states of spirit and in relationships with others independent of material goods and other adversities and an aspiration to understand the universal nature of things, has led to distrust of the individual ego and of consumerism. The dominance of rationalism, with efforts to establish norms that have some universal and substantive content, as well as several of the concepts discussed above, has led to placing the common good over individual liberty in continental Europe. Consequently, best interest is favored over substituted judgment, unlike the USA, where substituted judgment is the more valued standard for surrogate decision making.[1] Interestingly, for incompetent patients without advance directives, Emanuel and Emanuel have suggested an end-of-life decision-making process that is guided by preferences of local communities of patients,[55] consistent with many of the European values noted above. Ultimately, Gonzalez concluded that autonomy has a transcultural value that must be balanced with other principles.[1]

China

China consists of many different cultures. Overall, traditional views value interdependency of family members, obligations, responsibilities to others, and the common good over individual self-determination.[56*] Dying at home in the main hall, the most sacred place in the house, holds special significance as it denotes a full life and is crucial to bringing good fortune to living family members and to the spirit of the deceased. The spirits of those unable to die at home are barred from entering the home by the 'door god' and are unable to bring wellbeing to living descendants. To that end, dying patients are sometimes intubated to allow transfer home, where they are then extubated.[57,58*] In one retrospective study of 177 consecutive deaths of clinical trial patients hospitalized at a Chinese cancer center, 20 percent were transferred home to die. For more than 90 percent, death occurred within 24 hours of arriving home. Conversations about death universally were held with the family, but physicians rarely informed patients of the futility of CPR, often at the request of the family. While almost two-thirds of the overall population and 60 percent of those taken home to die had signed DNR orders, in only one instance was it signed by the patient. Physicians did not resuscitate 13 patients without a DNR order, but did attempt to resuscitate 30 patients with a DNR order, typically due to family insistence.[58] Similarly negative attitudes toward resuscitation were held by nonassimilated Chinese seniors living in Toronto, Canada, despite an indifferent or negative attitude toward advance directives. The 40 participants in this qualitative study based their decisions on the interrelated concepts of hope, suffering and the burden, the future, emotional harmony, the life cycle, respect for doctors and the family, values that are consistent with Buddhist, Confucianist, and Taoist beliefs.[56] In contrast, the majority of 43 older Chinese patients attending a daycare centre in Singapore, but born in Hong Kong or in the People's Republic of China, favored the use of aggressive life support measures. They also favored disclosure of the diagnosis and prognosis of a terminal illness, but were unaware of the Singapore Advanced Medical Directive Act, enacted in 1996. Of note is that the latter does not provide for a surrogate decision maker once patients are no longer competent to communicate treatment wishes.[59*,60*] In Taiwan, the Hospice Palliative Act, passed in May 2000, allows a competent person to provide signed informed consent for DNR status in the event of terminal cancer.[61*]

Japan

In Japan, an individual's death is considered a personal and private matter, as well as a familial, communal and social matter.[62] Traditionally, disclosure of diagnosis and prognosis of terminal illness has been to family members and not to the individual in question. When disclosure to patients or to families occurs, a significant minority prefers that it takes place nonverbally, an unfamiliar concept to most physicians practicing in the USA. Surrogate decision making is more common and attitudes toward advance directives and foregoing of life-sustaining therapy are less favorable

than is seen in Western medicine. However, recent surveys suggest a shift toward Western practices, with a growing preference for disclosure to those in a terminal situation, increasing use of advance directives, and expressed preferences for foregoing of life-sustaining therapy in terminal situations. For Japanese Americans, preference for disclosure is inversely related to degree of acculturation, as is the desire for informing the patient using words and direct patient participation in decision making.[62,63*,64*,65*]

The Japanese Society for Dying with Dignity (JSDD) has the largest membership in Japan of organizations assisting individuals with the completion of advance directives, which carry no legal status in Japan.[66*] Results of a population-based study indicate that disclosure of diagnosis and prognosis and expression of end-of-life treatment preferences were the most useful purposes of advance directives. Oral and written advance directives were both satisfactory. Family members, spouses, and relatives were considered to be the most suitable surrogate decision makers, with loose interpretation of directives by family and physicians being permissible. Preferences for advance directives was associated with awareness of living wills, experience with their use, preferences for end-of-life treatment, preferences for disclosure and intent of creating a living will.[64]

For those who complete written advance directives with the assistance of JSDD, a survey of family members and guardians of 1626 deceased individuals indicates a high rate of use, with presentation of the document to their physician by 64 percent, most often for patients with cancer. Care was perceived as congruent with the directive by 94 percent.[66] However, other studies suggest that following advance directives was not a priority for many physicians caring for patients at the end of life. Among the reasons cited for overriding patient wishes were family wishes to sustain a patient life, high possibility of recovery, and performing CPR to allow the patient's family time to arrive at the bedside.[67*,68*,69]

ROLE OF ADVANCE DIRECTIVES IN END-OF-LIFE DECISION MAKING

In the USA, advance directives are a direct outcome of the emphasis placed on patient autonomy, allowing for informed consent and informed refusal of medically appropriate care options. Successful use of advance directives is a process contingent on awareness of their existence, integration of the patient's values and goals into an informed decision making process, documentation and effective communication of advance directive content to the patient's family, friends and physicians and execution under the appropriate medical circumstances. However, despite strong endorsement of advance directives by Congress, the Joint

Commission on Accreditation of Health Care Organizations and multiple medical societies including the American Medical Association and the lay public, they have not played a major role in healthcare decisions for the majority of patients and families. Focused initiatives such as POLST have successfully resulted in increased rates of advance directive completion, as well as care congruent with the individual's expressed wishes. Reasons cited for the failure of advance directives to take root more globally include generalized lack of awareness of advance directives, the difficulty in talking about emotionally charged issues, patients and physicians each expecting the other to take the lead in initiating advance directive discussions, the perception of the USA as a death-denying culture, the increasingly fragmented nature of medical care in the USA and costs associated with the time needed to guide the patient through the decision-making process.

Although varied, the prevalence of advance directive use is even lower outside the dominant culture in the USA and among different cultural groups in the USA. Differences in commonly held values underlie their less frequent use, with less emphasis placed on patient autonomy. Strong prohibitions against disclosure of diagnosis and terminal prognosis to the patient further limit discussions related to goals of care and informed decision making, requisite to advance care planning. Family-centered models of decision making typically prevail. Notwithstanding, trends toward increased disclosure and advance care planning are being seen throughout the world, paralleling changes seen in the USA over the past 30 years.

CONCLUSIONS

The provision of medically appropriate care congruent with the individual's goals and values, the basis for advance care planning, remains a moral imperative. Lessons from the history of advance directives in the USA and elsewhere suggest the need for strategic changes to more effectively achieve optimal advance care planning. Heightened physician awareness of and sensitivity to differences between cultures, diversity within cultures and of widespread differences in personal values and goals, would likely result in a more effective medical decision-making process for future medical conditions. Offering truth is a useful strategy that respects the integrity of both professionals and patients. If declined, the patient has chosen informed refusal and may then delegate truth telling and decision making to specified individuals or to family members. Such an approach is consistent with the convenantal (interpretative) approach of proxy decision-making favored by patients and proxies when the prognosis was poor, as noted in Fins et al.'s study.[42] Fundamental to successful advance care planning is expert communication skills integrated with caring and compassion.

Key learning points

- Advance directives relate to the concept of patient autonomy for advance care planning.

- Advance directives are contingent upon informed consent and informed refusal of *medically appropriate* treatments as relate to the patient's values and goals of care.

- Instructional directives and documents designating surrogate decision makers are the two main types of advance directives.

- Patients want physicians to take the lead in initiating discussions of advance directives.

- Family-centered decision making is of greater value than patient autonomy in some cultures and for some patients.

- Offering truth is a strategy that respects professional integrity and patient/family values from a transcultural perspective.

- Establishing advance directives that identify surrogate decision makers may be more effective than the current emphasis on instructional directives.

- Expert communication skills are integral to advance care planning.

REFERENCES

● 1 Sanchez-Gonzales MA. Advance directives outside the USA: are they the best solution everywhere? *Theor Med* 1997; **18**: 283–301.

◆ 2 Decisions near the end of life. Council on Ethical and Judicial Affairs, American Medical Association. *JAMA* 1992; **267**: 2229–33.

3 Danis M, Southerland LI, Garrett JM, et al. A prospective study of advance directives for life-sustaining care. Reply. *N Engl J Med* 1991; **324**: 1255–6.

4 Sabatino CP. Survey of state EMS-ENR laws and protocols. *J Law Med Ethics* 1999; **27**: 297–315.

5 Emanuel LL. What makes a directive valid? *Hastings Cent Rep* 1994; **24**(Suppl): S27–S29.

◆ 6 Emanuel LL. Advance directives. In: Berger AM, Portenoy RK, Weissman DE, eds. *Principles and Practice of Palliative Care and Supportive Oncology*. Philadelphia: Lippincott, Williams and Wilkins, 2002: 861–79.

◆ 7 Nolde D. The New York State health care proxy law and the issue of artificial hydration and nutrition. *J N Y State Nurs Assoc* 2003/2004; **Fall/Winter**: 22–7.

8 Costante CC. Managing DNR requests in the school setting. *J School Nurs* 1998; **14**: 49–55.

9 Badzek L, Kanosky S. Mature minors and end-of-life decision making: A new development in their legal right to participation. *J Nurs Law* 2002; **8**: 23–9.

10 Hilden JM, Himelstein BP, Freyer DR, *et al.* End-of-life care: Special issues in pediatric oncology. In: Foley KM, Gelband H, eds. *Improving Palliative Care for Cancer.* Washington, DC: National Academy Press, 2001: 161–98.

11 A call for change: Recommendations to improve the care of children living with life-threatening conditions. Children's International Project on Palliative/Hospice Services (ChIPPS) Administrative Policy Workgroup of the National Hospice and Palliative Care Organization. 2001; Alexandria, Virginia. www.nhpco./files./public/ChIPPSCallforChange.pdf (accessed September 6, 2005).

12 Committee on Bioethics. Informed consent, parental permission and assent in pediatric practice. *Pediatrics* 1995; **95**: 314–17.

13 Weir RF, Peter C. Affirming the decisions adolescents make about life and death. *Hastings Cent Rep* 1997; **2**: 29–40.

✱ 14 Rabkin MT, Gillerman G, Rice NR. Orders not to resuscitate. *N Engl J Med* 1976; **295**: 364–9.

✱ 15 Standards for cardiopulmonary resuscitation (CPR) and emergency cardiac care (ECC). V. medicolegal considerations and recommendations. *JAMA* 1974; **227(Suppl)**: 864–6.

16 Emanuel LL, Emanuel EJ. The medical directive – a new comprehensive advance care document. *JAMA* 1989; **262**: 3288–93.

17 Doukas DJ, McCullough LB. The values history: The evaluation of the patient's values and advance directives. *J Family Pract* 1991; **32**: 1–6.

18 Doukas DJ, Gorenflo DW. Analyzing the values history: An evaluation of patient medical values and advance directives. *J Clin Ethics* 1993; **4**: 41–5.

19 Aging with dignity. www.agingwithdignity.org (accessed October 9, 2005).

20 Center for Practical Bioethics. Caring Conversations. Available at: www.practicalbioethics.org/mbc-cc.htm (accessed September 6, 2005).

21 The Federal Patient Self-Determination Act, Omnibus Budget Reconciliation Act of 1990, Pub. L. No. 101–508, § 4206, 104 Stat. 1388–115 (codified at 42 U.S.C.A., § 1395cc(f) (2004).

22 Fagerlin A, Schneider CE. Enough: The failure of the living will. *Hastings Cent Rep* 2004; **34**: 30–42.

◆ 23 Hickey DP. The disutility of advance directives: we know the problems, but are there solutions? *J Health Law* 2003; **36**: 455–73.

24 Emanuel LL. Advance directives for medical care: Reply. *N Engl J Med* 1991; **325**: 1256.

25 Kiely DK, Mitchell SL, Marlow A, *et al.* Racial and state differences in the designation of advance directives in nursing home residents. *J Am Geriatr Soc* 2001; **49**: 1346–52.

26 Hanson L, Rodgman E. The use of living wills at the end of life: A national study. *Arch Intern Med* 1996; **156**: 1018–22.

27 McKinley ED, Garrett J, Evans AT, Danis M. Differences in end-of-life decision making among black and white ambulatory cancer patients. *J Gen Intern Med* 1996; **11**: 651–6.

28 Vital and Health Statistics. National Mortality Followback Survey: 1986 summary, United States, Series 20, No. 19, US Department of Health and Human Services, Publication No. (PHS) 92–1856, 1992.

29 Klinkenberg M, Willelms DL, Onwuteaka-Philipsen BD, *et al.* Preferences in end-of-life care of older persons: After-death interviews with proxy respondents. *Soc Sci Med* 2004; **59**: 2467–77.

30 Covinsky KE, Fuller JD, Yaffe K, *et al.* Communication and decision-making in seriously ill patients: Findings of the SUPPORT Project. *J Am Geriatr Soc* 2000; **48**: S187–S193.

31 Phipps E, True G, Harris D, *et al.* Approaching the end of life: Attitudes, preferences, and behaviors of African American and white patients and their family caregivers. *J Clin Oncol* 2003; **21**: 549–54.

32 Orentlicher D. The illusion of patient choice in end-of-life decisions. *JAMA* 1992; **267**: 2101–4.

33 Danis J, Southerland LI, Garrett JM, *et al.* A prospective study of advance directives for life-sustaining care. *N Engl J Med* 1991; **324**: 882–8.

34 Johnston SC, Pfeifer MP, McNutt R. The discussion about advance directives: Patient and physician opinions regarding when and how it should be conducted. *Arch Intern Med* 1995; **155**: 1025–30.

35 Lamont EB, Christakis N. Prognostic disclosure to patients near the end of life. *Ann Intern Med* 2001; **134**: 1096–105.

36 Weeks JC, Cook EF, O'Day SJ, *et al.* Relationship between cancer patients' predictions of prognosis and their treatment preferences. *JAMA* 1998; **279**: 1709–14.

37 Morrison RS, Morrison EW, Glickman DF. Physician reluctance to discuss advance directives. *Arch Intern Med* 1994; **154**: 2311–18.

38 Tulsky JA, Fischer GS, Rose MR. Opening the black box: How do physicians communicate about advance directives? *Ann Intern Med* 1998; **129**: 441–9.

39 Morrison SR, Zayas L, Mulvihill M, *et al.* Barriers to completion of health care proxies: An examination of ethnic differences. *Arch Intern Med* 1998; **158**: 2493–7.

40 Pacquiao D. Addressing cultural incongruities of advance directives. *Bioethics Forum* 2001; **17**: 27–31.

41 Emanuel EJ, Emanuel LL. Proxy decision making for incompetent patients: an ethical and empirical analysis. *JAMA* 1992; **267**: 2067–71.

● 42 Fins JJ, Maltby BS, Friedmann E, *et al.* Contracts, convenants and advance care planning: An empirical study of the moral obligations of patient and proxy. *J Pain Symptom Manage* 2005: **29**: 55–68.

43 Tolle SW, Tilden VP, Rosenfeld AG, Hickman SE. Family reports of barriers to optimal care of the dying. *Nurs Res* 2000; **49**: 310–17.

44 Lee MA, Brummel-Smith K, Meyer J, *et al.* Physician orders for life-sustaining treatment (POLST): Outcomes in a PACE Program. *J Am Geriatr Soc* 2000; **48**: 1219–25.

45 Pollack S. A new approach to advance directives. *Crit Care Med* 2000; **28**: 3146–8.

● 46 Blackhall L, Murphy ST, Frank G, *et al.* Ethnicity and attitudes toward patient autonomy. *JAMA* 1995; **274**: 820–5.

◆ 47 Blackhall LJ, Frank G, Murphy ST, *et al.* Ethnicity and attitudes towards life sustaining technology. *Soc Sci Med* 1999; **48**: 1779–89.

48 Murphy ST, Palmer AJM, Azen S, *et al.* Ethnicity and advance care directives. *J Law Med Ethics* 1996; **24**: 108–17.

49 Carrese JA, Rhodes LA. Western bioethics on the Navajo reservation: Benefit or harm? *JAMA* 1995; **274**: 826–9.

50 Perkins HS, Geppert CMA, Gonzales A, *et al.* Cross-cultural similarities and differences in attitudes about advance care planning. *J Gen Intern Med* 2002; **17**: 48–57.

51 Hopp FP, Duffy SA. Racial variations in end-of-life care. *J Am Geriatr Soc* 2000; **48**: 658–63.

52 Shepardson LB, Gordon HS, Ibrahim SA, *et al.* Racial variation in the use of Do-Not-Resuscitate orders. *J Gen Intern Med* 1999; **14**: 15–20.

53 Mebane EW, Oman RF, Kroonen LT, Goldstein MK. The influence of physician race, age and gender on physician attitudes toward advance care directives and preferences for end-of-life decision-making. *J Am Geriatr Soc* 1999; **47**: 579–91.

54 Waters CM. Understanding and supporting African Americans' Perspectives of end-of-life care planning and decision making. *Qual Health Res* 2001; **11**: 385–98.

55 Emanuel LL, Emanuel EJ. Decisions at the end of life: Guided by communities of patients. *Hastings Cent Rep* 1993; **23**: 6–14.

56 Bowman KW, Singer PA. Chinese seniors' perspectives on end-of-life decisions. *Soc Sci Med* 2001; **53**: 455–64.

◆ 57 Tang ST. Meanings of dying at home for Chinese patients in Taiwan with terminal cancer. *Cancer Nurs* 2000; **23**: 367–70.

58 Liu JM, Lin WC, Chen YM, *et al.* The status of the do-not-resuscitate order in Chinese clinical trial patients in a cancer centre. *J Med Ethics* 1999; **25**: 309–14.

59 Low JA, Ng WC, Yap KB, Chan KM. End-of-life issues – preferences and choices of a group of elderly Chinese subjects attending a day care centre in Singapore. *Ann Acad Med Singapore* 2000; **29**: 50–6.

60 Leng TK, Sy SLH. Advance medical directives in Singapore. *Med Law Rev* 1997; **5**: 63–101.

61 Chao CC. Physcians' attitudes toward DNR of terminally ill cancer patients in Taiwan. *J Nurs Res* 2002; **10**: 161–7.

62 Kimura R. Death and dying in Japan. *Kennedy Inst Ethics J* 1996; **6**: 374–8.

63 Matsumura S, Bito S, Liu H, *et al.* Acculturation of attitudes toward end-of-life care. A cross-cultural survey of Japanese Americans and Japanese. *J Gen Intern Med* 2002; **17**: 531–9.

64 Akabayashi A, Slingsby BT, Kai I. Perspectives on advance directives in Japanese society: a population-based questionnaire survey. *BMC Med Ethics* 2003; **4**: 5.

65 Asai A, Fukuhara S. Attitudes of Japanese and Japanese-American physicians towards life-sustaining treatment. *Lancet* 1995; **346**: 356–9.

66 Masuda Y, Fetters MD, Shimokata H, *et al.* Outcomes of written living wills in Japan – A survey of deceased ones' families. *Bioethics Forum* 2001; **17**: 41–52.

67 Masuda Y, Fetters MD, Hattori A, *et al.* Physicians' reports on the impact of living wills at the end of life in Japan. *J Med Ethics* 2003; **29**: 248–52.

68 Asai A, Mkura Y, Tanabe N, *et al.* Advance directives and other medical decisions concerning the end of life in cancer patients in Japan. *Eur J Cancer* 2998; **34**: 1582–6.

69 Asai A, Fukuhara S, Inoshita O, *et al.* Medical decisions concerning the end of life: a discussion with Japanese physicians. *J Med Ethics* 1997; **23**: 323–7.

Bereavement

VICTORIA H RAVEIS

INTRODUCTION

Although bereavement and loss are familiar occurrences in palliative care, an appreciation of what constitutes grief and an understanding of the special circumstances of bereavement in the palliative care setting may aid clinicians in attending to the needs of families facing the impending loss of a loved one. Bereavement refers to a loss through death of someone significant. A universal occurrence, it also is a particularly potent and stressful life event. Bereavement can predispose people to physical and mental illness, precipitate illness and death, and aggravate existing illness.[1***,2] Death represents a multifaceted challenge for the survivors. They must adapt to the social and economic readjustments emerging from the death and come to terms with changes in self-identity resulting from their loss, while dealing with the psychological and physiological reactions engendered by their loss. Mourning is the expression of grief and represents the process of coming to terms with this loss.[3***]

BEREAVEMENT IN PALLIATIVE CARE

The terminal period of an illness can be an extremely stressful time for the families of dying patients. Although bereavement is usually the specific event that precipitates the grieving process, for deaths that occur in the context of palliative care, a variety of circumstances occurring prior to the death are likely to impact survivors' grief.

Illness-related losses need to be mourned

When death is preceded by a chronic illness, grieving is inexorably tied up with mourning the losses experienced during the course of an illness. These losses include altered relationships, changes in lifestyle, the forfeit of future dreams that will never be realized, as well as losses related to illness-induced changes (e.g. progressive debilitation, increasing dependence, and excessive pain).[4]

Caregiving demands may complicate recovery from bereavement

Families are commonly involved in the provision of emotional and practical assistance to their ill family members in palliative care situations. While the benefits to the patient of familial caregiving are readily apparent, this care provision is not without cost to the care providers. Financial stress, neglect of their own health, physical and psychological exhaustion from providing care, and the social isolation resulting from restricting outside activities to carry out caregiving responsibilities, are some of the routine consequences endured by families providing illness-related support and care.[5] In addition, during the final illness period, families often direct all their energy and attention toward tending to the patient, delaying or inhibiting any advance psychological preparation for the impending death.[6] The multiple stresses and demands that the illness and its treatment have imposed on the survivors increase their risk for morbid bereavement outcomes.[5*,7*]

Anticipatory grief

Palliative care situations enable families to be forewarned about an impending death, permitting their preparation for the impending loss. Anticipatory grief refers to the process whereby survivors rehearse the bereaved role and initiate working through the emotional changes associated with a death.[4] It is generally thought that anticipatory grief mitigates the intensity of the grief reaction following the actual death, leaving the survivor less vulnerable to maladaptive reactions. However, the evidence on the adaptive value of being forewarned that a death will occur is inconsistent.[8] Some investigations have shown that bereaved who have had opportunity for anticipatory grief adjust better to their loss,[9*,10*] while other research has not demonstrated any benefit.[11*,12***] One factor that may mitigate any advantage derived from advance forewarning of the death is the circumstances leading up to the death. A long and protracted illness, or one marked by intensive caregiving demands, may impede the bereaved individual's ability to initiate preparations for the death and deplete personal resources for coping with the impending loss.[13*] Another risk factor is the development of premature grief, whereby family members socially and emotionally withdraw from the dying patient in advance of the death. This can result in the bereaved experiencing guilt after the death over having abandoned their dying relative.[2]

Experiencing death

In Western society, dying is 'medicalized' and the family is generally distanced from death.[14] Death in a home setting is unfamiliar. With the provision of palliative care, families are intimately exposed to the dying process. Anticipating its occurrence and the resultant responsibility associated with this event can induce considerable distress and anxiety. Families worry that they will be unable to address their relative's potential suffering at the end and express concern that they will be unable to cope with the challenges of being 'in charge' during this dying event.[6]

OVERVIEW OF THE GRIEF PROCESS

Freud's seminal essay on 'Mourning and melancholia'[15] provided the foundation for contemporary understanding of grief and bereavement. His work conceptualized mourning as a prolonged inner struggle to adapt to and accept an irreversible loss. Grief therapists have delineated four tasks that define the mourning process.[3***] The bereaved needs to: (i) accept the reality of the loss (i.e. face the reality that the person is dead, will not return and that reunion is impossible); (ii) acknowledge and work through the emotional and behavioral pain associated with the loss; (iii) adjust to an environment in which the deceased is missing (for the

widowed this involves coming to terms with living alone, facing an empty house, and managing finances alone); and (iv) withdraw emotional energy from the deceased and reinvest it in other relationships. These tasks are not necessarily performed in sequence. Overlap and revisiting of tasks can occur. The clinical evidence remains equivocal as to whether all these tasks need to be accomplished.[16***,17***]

The dual process model of coping with bereavement[18] represents an integrative approach to describing the ways bereaved individuals come to terms with a significant loss. It posits that the bereaved undertake both loss-oriented and restoration-oriented coping. Loss-orientation refers to dealing with or processing some aspect of the loss experience itself, particularly relating to the deceased. This is analogous to grief work. Restoration-orientation focuses on the secondary sources of stress that the bereaved need to deal with, such as changes in financial status or social loneliness, e.g. the bereavement tasks outlined above.[16***,17***] However, the dual process model introduces a third concept – oscillation. Coping with bereavement is posited to be a dynamic process, one in which individuals confront their loss some of the time and at other times avoid such confrontation. Oscillation is necessary to provide a balance to this process and prevent the adverse mental and physical costs arising with unremitted grieving.

Bereavement specialists and cross-cultural researchers[14,19,20*] have increasingly noted that understanding of the grief process has been strongly influenced by Western thought. Its applicability to non-Western societies merits reflection, given the fundamental world-view differences in how death is perceived in different cultures. For example, in Asian cultures, through practices such as ancestor worship, death represents a transition to a different state in which deceased relatives remain important participants in the world of the living and communication is still considered possible.[21*] Proponents of the dual process model stress that it accommodates individual, situational, and cultural variations in coping with bereavement.[18]

PHASES OF GRIEF

Immediately following a death, bereaved individuals are usually in a state of shock. They feel numb and experience disbelief over the event, even when the death has been anticipated, as in palliative care.[22] During this period, cognitions may be impacted. The bereaved may experience a sense of confusion and have difficulty concentrating.[3***,23***] During the acute mourning period, these initial grief responses give way to intense feelings of loss and longing for the deceased. It is not uncommon for the bereaved to feel a sense of the deceased's presence or to experience auditory or visual hallucinations about the deceased.[3***] The bereaved may also exhibit restless behavior, revisit places that relate to the deceased, and treasure or revere objects that belonged to the deceased.[3***,24***] As the realization of the loss becomes more evident, the bereaved may engage in frequent crying spells, have difficulty sleeping, withdraw from other people, show little interest in outside activities, and experience a loss of appetite.[3***,9*,23***] Individuals who are grieving can experience a variety of psychological and physiological reactions of varying intensity and duration.[1***,3***,9*] The most commonly expressed emotions include shock, numbness, sadness, anxiety, loneliness, fatigue, anger, relief, and guilt. Bereaved individuals often report somatic complaints as well, such as weakness, lethargy, loss of appetite, tightness in the throat or chest, shortness of breath, and sleeplessness.

DURATION OF GRIEF

Although there is considerable variability in the rate at which individuals adjust to bereavement, the clinical and epidemiological literature support that in Western societies most bereaved return to a normal level of functioning 1–2 years after their loss.[1***,2,16***] Grief-related distress is generally highest in the first year following the loss, although elevated rates of distress can persist for more than 2 years. Societal mores can influence grief duration. For example, Taiwanese cultural ideology proscribes 'one man per lifetime' and widows are expected to grieve for the rest of their lives.[21*]

NORMAL AND PATHOLOGICAL GRIEF

Lindemann's landmark study of bereavement,[25*] following the Coconut Grove nightclub fire, focused attention on the intensity and duration of expressed grief. This work also introduced the distinction between normal and pathological grief as important dimensions in understanding the grief process. Grief that is chronic, persistent, intense, inhibited, or delayed is regarded as pathological or complicated.[9*] However, an understanding of what constitutes normal grief is heavily influenced by Western conceptions of death and dying and does not accommodate different cultural and ideological perspectives.[19] While there is consensus that grief is universally experienced, response to loss is culturally bound. Wailing, unrestrained crying, self-mutilation, or prostration may be common and acceptable means of expressing grief in some societies,[14] but regarded as indicative of an intense or severe grief reaction by other cultural groups.

VULNERABILITY FACTORS FOR ADVERSE GRIEF REACTIONS

The clinical and research literature on bereavement suggests a constellation of situational and individual factors that can affect the course and outcome of the grieving process.[1***,9*,26***,27***] A number of these factors are commonly present in palliative care situations.

Protracted illness

Bereaved relatives whose loved one suffered a long, lingering illness actually adjust more poorly to bereavement than those whose loved one died after a short illness.[28,29*] This outcome may reflect the impact of providing informal support and care during an extended illness and the stresses of having lived with a protracted illness course.[6,13*,30*]

Disease course

Terminal conditions that impact patients' functioning and quality of life, such as severe, chronic pain, are difficult for family members to witness. Their distress is exacerbated when they also feel helpless in alleviating or managing these conditions,[30*] further increasing their risk of severe grief reactions.[9*]

Stigmatized death

When death is from an illness that is stigmatized or associated with unhealthy or socially unacceptable lifestyles, such as alcoholism or drug abuse, the family may be less open about the cause of death or the circumstances leading up to the event. As a consequence, the naturally occurring support systems available to the bereaved may be less forthcoming. The family may also experience conflicting emotions or encounter difficulty resolving their feelings about the deceased. In communicable illnesses such as human immunodeficiency virus (HIV)/acquired immune deficiency syndrome (AIDS), the bereaved may be infected as well or may be dealing with multiple deaths or advanced disease of other family members.[31]

Nature of the loss

The death of a spouse is considered to be one of the most stressful life events, although the loss of a child is regarded as particularly problematic for the survivor to resolve.[1***] A high level of dependency or an ambivalent relationship (feelings of love/hate, need/resentment) between the deceased and the bereaved often culminates in a severe grief reaction and difficulty in accepting and resolving the loss.[32*]

Life circumstances

Vulnerability to poor adjustment is increased by the occurrence of additional severe stresses concurrent to the bereavement, such as multiple losses or life changes.[26***] Deficits in social support or restricted social resources can also contribute to adverse grief outcomes. Limited financial resources prior to the death or declining income as a consequence of the death can precipitate problems in grieving. Widowhood can have especially adverse economic, social, and psychological ramifications for older adults and bereavement reactions may be severe.[13*]

Individual characteristics

The bereaved individual's preexisting physical health condition, history of substance abuse, and/or premorbid mental illness[32*] can contribute to adverse bereavement outcomes. Personality characteristics, such as low self-esteem or a low internal sense of control are also associated with increased distress after the death. In Western societies, men are at higher risk for bereavement related mortality; women experience more affective distress.

HEALTH CONSEQUENCES OF BEREAVEMENT

Bereavement can predispose people to physical and mental illness, precipitate suicide and death, and aggravate existing health conditions.[1***,2,33] In Western societies, the recently bereaved have been shown to display an increased incidence of depressive symptoms and somatic complaints, as well as changes in their endocrine, immune, and cardiovascular systems. Although most individuals eventually return to a normal level of functioning, bereaved individuals have higher rates of utilization of medical and mental health care services (i.e. increased hospitalizations, prescribed drug use, and physician and mental health clinician visits) compared with nonbereaved samples.[24***,34*] Bereavement is not a transient life crisis. It can have enduring negative consequences for some individuals. Some bereaved individuals, in an attempt to cope with their grief, intensely engage in behaviors that can be injurious to their health, such as alcohol or substance abuse.[35*,36*]

PRINCIPLES OF BEREAVEMENT SUPPORT IN PALLIATIVE CARE

There are five broad principles of bereavement support that apply in the palliative care setting: (i) view the patient and family as one unit of care, (ii) enable open discussion of illness and death-related concerns, (iii) provide emotional support, (iv) facilitate practical assistance, and (v) respect cultural, ethnic, and religious practices.

View patient and family as one unit of care

Palliative care offers the healthcare practitioner multiple opportunities to attend to the wellbeing of affected family members prior to the patient's death.[37*,38*] The terminal illness period is stressful to the family. Patients and families should be viewed as one unit of care. Attending to the informational, emotional, and practical support needs of the family may make the dying experience less stressful for the family, facilitate their grieving, and reduce their risk of adverse bereavement outcomes.[39***] As a secondary benefit, addressing family members' needs during this period can facilitate their remaining engaged in the patient's care provision.

Enable open discussion of illness and death related concerns

Attending to families' concerns about the patient's condition and care, and providing reassurance that appropriate therapeutic and ameliorative measures are being utilized, can comfort families and reduce later recriminations. Enabling open communication and discussion of emerging concerns can avert the development of future regrets, facilitating families' grieving process.[13*]

Provide emotional support

Supporting survivors in their grief during the terminal phase of the illness is also important in facilitating adjustment after the death. In palliative care, most families are aware of the nature of their relative's condition and its prognosis. Families can experience anger, sadness, regret, resentment or guilt regarding the illness, the consequent burdens they are required to assume, and the impending death. They may also feel isolated and alone. Families need to be given permission to express their feelings and be reassured that these feelings are normal.[13*]

A family's contact with the palliative care team often ceases with the patient's death. For many families this is a significant loss. Its impact can be lessened by a condolence card or brief sympathy call from a member of the care team. Anniversaries of the death or important family events are also times when grief is intensified.[24***] A follow-up note or call from the palliative team on these occasions may be beneficial.

Facilitate practical assistance

Families often become very involved in the dying patient's care, neglecting their own health and setting unreasonable expectations of what they personally should accomplish. It is common for families to be fearful about leaving the patient for any length of time, curtailing outside activities and cutting themselves off from their broader social network. The palliative care team may need to encourage them to respect and attend to their own needs.[13*] Assisting the family with arranging for respite services, or suggesting ways to mobilize other network members, with the goal of reducing the care burden on the family, are means of facilitating needed practical assistance. Families may also require assistance in ensuring that issues related to the dying patient's finances and legal matters are attended to and that procedures for adhering to the patient's preferences for care at end of life are established (e.g. advance directives, healthcare proxy).

Respect cultural, ethnic, and religious practices

Bereavement takes place within a social context in which rituals and customs provide for the sanctioned public articulation of private distress.[1]*** When individuals are prevented from performing such activities, their grief can become complicated and their mourning prolonged.[40]* Institutional policies that limit children's visiting rights, restrict the number of visitors in a room, or bar the performance of special services and ceremonies can impede families from carrying out specific practices required at death. Terminal illness provides forewarning of the death. This affords the palliative care team an opportunity to become aware of and address any particular needs and requirements associated with specific mourning customs and rituals.

BEREAVEMENT RESOURCES, PROGRAMS, AND TREATMENTS

There is a plethora of supportive and treatment programs that have been developed to assist bereaved individuals through their grieving process. Efforts to establish evidence-based practice guidelines regarding the content, format, timing and targeting of bereavement services have been hampered by variations in the format and content of the bereavement services, small sample sizes, and the limited number of rigorously designed evaluation trials.[39]***,[41]***,[42]***,[43]***,[44]***

Most evidence-based reviews have not explicitly distinguished between bereavement services that are initiated or delivered during the terminal phase of the illness and services that begin after the death.[41]***,[43]***,[44]*** However, recent best practice guidance offered by the National Institute of Clinical Excellence on Supportive and Palliative Care[39]*** supports the value of initiating theory-based bereavement care during the terminal phase of an illness for those in need. Additional recommendations are to implement an ongoing assessment plan to enable the identification of those at risk and the matching of services to their needs.

Supportive services

Bereavement-related supportive services are provided in a variety of treatment modalities and venues. Hospice and palliative care settings routinely make available one or more

types of bereavement support services to affected family members. Community groups, churches, and charitable organizations, such as Cruse Bereavement Care in the UK, also sponsor a range of services. Some programs are delivered by mental health clinicians; others use trained volunteers supported by professionals, such as the 'Widow-to-Widow' program in the USA. Supportive counseling, delivered individually or through a group session, helps to normalize the bereaved individual's experiences while also supporting their grief. Peer support and self-help groups involve bereaved individuals offering friendship and empathy of shared status. The duration of these various bereavement services can range from a single session or meeting to ongoing programs that are initiated during the terminal illness period and continued after the death. Although the clinical evidence base is inconclusive,[41]*** participant satisfaction is high and clinical and anecdotal reports document the efficacy of these types of services in reducing bereavement distress, supporting grief, and facilitating mourning.[1]***,[2]

Preventive intervention programs

Consensus is stronger regarding the utility of theory-based bereavement interventions developed for individuals at high-risk for complicated or pathological grief or other adverse bereavement outcomes.[9],[39]***,[41]***,[44]***,[45]*** Palliative care settings provide the opportunity to initiate delivery of preventive interventions during the terminal phase of the illness, providing targeted support and counseling to individuals at increased risk[39]*** with the goal of reducing their risk factors and increasing protective factors.[45]*** Screening tools such as the Index of Bereavement Risk[9]* are helpful in identifying individuals at 'high risk'. Using appropriate assessments ensures that this type of resource is delivered to those who will derive the maximum benefit.[46]*

Psychotherapeutic interventions

Most bereaved individuals will not require psychotherapy or specialized grief therapy.[3]*** However, persistent depressive or somatic symptoms that do not lessen in intensity over time; prolonged social withdrawal; expressed difficulty adjusting to the loss; and/or engaging in health-endangering behavior, such as drug or alcohol abuse, are triggers for referral to a mental health professional for evaluation.[1]***,[2]

Pharmacological therapies

Pharmacological treatment may be appropriate in some circumstances. Antidepressants, tranquilizers, and sedatives are prescribed to lessen the intensity of a variety of persistent and severe bereavement-related reactions (e.g. depression, anxiety, sleeplessness) that impair functioning and exacerbate the bereaved individual's distress. While it may be clinically indicated to intervene pharmacologically to remediate intense bereavement-related reactions, such treatments warrant discretion.[1***] A review of case–control studies demonstrated a beneficial effect for pharmacological treatment of depression and sleep quality. However, these benefits persisted only while the subjects received the medication and there was no demonstrated impact on their resolution of grief.[41***]

CONCLUSIONS

Although there may be considerable individual variation in the experience and expression of grief, grieving is a normal response to a significant loss. Understanding of the grief process has been substantially influenced by Western thought. Consequently, clinicians should be careful to not ascribe pathological or abnormal labels to mourning responses when the cultural meaning or appropriateness of these actions are not well understood. Although the cognitive and emotional responses abate over time, some bereaved are at increased risk for psychological and physical health consequences following their loss. Clinicians involved in palliative care are in contact with families at a point of heightened vulnerability. The provision of emotional support and compassionate care by the healthcare team during this stressful period may facilitate families' grieving process and reduce adverse bereavement consequences.

Grief specialists[45***] advise, supported by clinical evidence,[41***,43***,44***] that preventive interventions are not necessary for most bereaved individuals. Consensus opinion is that such an approach may do more harm than good, impeding the activation of the bereaved individual's natural support systems and disrupting the pattern of the normal grieving.[43***,44***] Only a small proportion of individuals experience grief reactions of such severity or chronicity that necessitate professional intervention. An understanding and appreciation of grief and the individual and situational factors that may complicate mourning will aid clinicians in determining when professional intervention is indicated. As Raphael et al.[45***(p. 587)] succinctly state: 'There can be no justification for routine intervention for bereaved persons in terms of therapeutic modalities – either psychotherapeutic or pharmacological – because grief is not a disease'.

Key learning points

- Grief is expressed with a constellation of psychological and physiological reactions.

- Grieving is a process comprised of numbness, searching and pining, depression and recovery.

- Normal grief and mourning practices reflect cultural and ideological belief systems.

- Bereavement can predispose some people to physical and mental illness and precipitate death.

- Benefits of anticipatory grief are mitigated by care provision, illness duration, and cause of death.

- Patients and families should be viewed as a unit of care.

- Attending to carers' needs during the terminal phase of illness can forestall adverse outcomes.

- Facilitating culturally appropriate death rites and mourning practices benefits the bereaved.

REFERENCES

◆ 1 Osterweis M, Solomon F, Green M, eds. *Bereavement: Reactions, Consequences, and Care.* A report of the Institute of Medicine, National Academy of Sciences. Washington, DC: National Academy Press, 1984.

2 Zisook S. Understanding and managing bereavement in palliative care. In: Chochinov HM, Breitbart W, eds. *Handbook of Psychiatry in Palliative Medicine.* New York: Oxford University Press, 2000: 321–34.

◆ 3 Worden JW. *Grief Counseling and Grief Therapy: A Handbook for the Mental Health Practitioner,* 2nd ed. New York: Springer, 1991.

4 Rando TA. Understanding and facilitating anticipatory grief in the loved ones of the dying. In: Rando TA, ed. *Loss and Anticipatory Grief.* Lexington, MA: Lexington Books, 1986: 97–130.

5 Raveis VH, Karus D, Siegel K. Correlates of depressive symptomatology among adult daughter caregivers to a parent with cancer. *Cancer* 1998; **83**: 1652–63.

6 Raveis VH. Psychosocial impact of spousal caregiving at the end-of-life: challenges and consequences. *Gerontologist* 2004; **44**(Special Issue 1): 191–2.

7 Schulz R, Beach SR, Lind B, *et al.* Involvement in caregiving and adjustment to death of a spouse: Findings from the Caregiver Health Effects Study. *JAMA* 2001; **285**: 3123–9.

8 Siegel K, Weinstein L. Anticipatory grief reconsidered. *J Psychosoc Oncol* 1984–85; **1**: 61–73.

9 Parkes CM, Weiss RS. *Recovery From Bereavement.* New York: Basic Books, 1983.

10 Vachon MLS, Rogers J, Lyall WA, *et al.* Predictors and correlates of adaptation to conjugal bereavement. *Am J Psychiatry* 1982; **139**: 998–1002.

11 Dessonville-Hill C, Thompson LW, Gallagher D. The role of anticipatory bereavement in older women's adjustment to widowhood. *Gerontologist* 1988; **28**: 792–6.

12 Maddison D, Walker WL. Factors affecting the outcome of conjugal bereavement. *Br J Psychiatry* 1967; **113**: 1057–67.

13 Raveis VH. Facilitating older spouses adjustment to widowhood: A preventive intervention program. *Soc Work Health Care* 1999; **29**: 12–32.

14 Laungani P, Young B. Conclusions 1; Implications for practice and policy. In: Parkes CM, Pittu L, Young B, eds. *Death and*

Bereavement Across Cultures. London: Routledge, 1997: 218–32.

● 15 Freud S. Mourning and melancholia. In: Strachey J, ed. *The Standard Edition of Complete Psychological Work of Sigmund Freud.* London: Hogarth Press, 1957 [Original work published 1917].

◆ 16 Bonanno GA, Kaltman S. The varieties of grief experience. *Clin Psychol Rev* 2001; **21**: 705–34.

17 Wortman CB, Silver RC. The myths of coping with loss revisited. In: Stroebe MS, Hansson RO, Stroebe W, Schut H, eds. *Handbook of Bereavement Research: Consequences, Coping, and Cure.* Washington, DC: American Psychological Association, 2001: 405–29.

● 18 Stroebe M, Schut H. The dual process model of coping with bereavement: rationale and description. *Death Stud* 1999; **23**: 197–24.

19 Rosenblatt PC. Cross-cultural variation in the experience, expression, and understanding of grief. In: Irish DP, Lundquist KF, Nelson VJ, eds. *Ethnic Variations in Dying, Death and Grief: Diversity in Universality.* Philadelphia: Taylor and Francis, 1993: 13–19.

20 Klass D. Continuing bonds in the resolution of grief in Japan and North American. *Am Behav Sci* 2001; **44**: 742–63.

21 Hsu MT, Kahn DL, Lee WL. Recovery through reconnection: A cultural design for family bereavement in Taiwan. *Death Stud* 2004; **28**: 761–86.

22 Ravies VH. Psychosocial impact of spousal caregiving at the end-of-life: challenges and consequences. *Gerontologist* 2004; **44**(Special Issue 1): 191–20.

◆ 23 Shuchter SR. *Dimensions of Grief: Adjusting to the Death of a Spouse.* San Francisco: Jossey-Bass Publishers, 1986.

◆ 24 Raphael B. *The Anatomy of Bereavement.* New York: Basic Books, 1983.

● 25 Lindemann E. Symptomatology and management of acute grief. *Am J Psychiatry* 1944; **101**: 141–8.

◆ 26 Sanders C. *Grief: The Mourning After Dealing With Adult Bereavement.* New York: John Wiley and Sons, 1989.

27 Stroebe W, Schut H. Risk factors in bereavement outcome: a methodological and empirical review. In: Stroebe MS, Hansson RO, Stroebe W, Schut H, eds. *Handbook of Bereavement Research: Consequences, Coping, and Cure.* Washington, DC: American Psychological Association, 2001: 349–71.

28 Sanders CM. Effects of sudden vs. chronic illness death on bereavement outcome. *Omega* 1982–83; **12**: 227–41.

29 Gerber I, Weiner A, Battin D, Arkin AM. Brief therapy to the aged bereaved. In: Schoenberg B, Gerber I, Wiener A, et al, eds. *Bereavement: Its Psychosocial Aspects.* New York: Columbia University Press, 1975: 310–33.

30 Vachon MLS, Freedman K, Formo A, *et al.* Correlates of enduring distress patterns following bereavement: Social network, life situation and personality. *Psychol Med* 1982; **12**: 783–8.

31 Raveis VH, Siegel K. Impact of caregiving on informal or familial caregivers. *AIDS Patient Care* 1991; **5**: 39–43.

32 Kelly B, Edwards P, Synott R, *et al.* Predictors of bereavement outcome for family carers of cancer patients. *Psychooncology* 1999; **8**: 237–49.

33 Rozenzweig A, Prigerson H, Miller MD, Reynolds CF. Bereavement and late-life depression: Grief and its complications in the elderly. *Annu Rev Med* 1997; **48**: 421–8.

34 McHorney CA, Mor V. Predictors of bereavement depression and its health services consequences. *Med Care* 1988; **26**: 882–93.

35 Stroebe W. *Social Psychology and Health*, 2nd ed. Buckingham: Open University Press, 2000.

36 Zisook S, Shuchter SR, Mulvihill M. Alcohol, cigarette and medication use during the first year of widowhood. *Psychiatr Ann* 1990; **20**: 318–26.

37 Raveis VH, Pretter S. Existential plight of adult daughters following their mother's breast cancer diagnosis. *Psychooncology* 2005; **14**: 49–60.

38 Koffman JS, Higginson I. Fit to care: a comparison of informal caregivers of first-generation Black Caribbeans and White dependants with advanced progressive disease in the UK. *Health Soc Care Comm* 2003; **11**: 528–36.

◆ 39 Gysels M, Higginson IJ. *Guidance on Cancer Services: Improving Supportive and Palliative Care for Adults With Cancer, Research Evidence.* National Institute for Clinical Excellence: King's College London. www.nice.org.uk/page.aspx?o=110011 (accessed June 29, 2005).

40 Firth S. Approaches to death in Hindu and Sikh communities in Britain. In: Dickenson D, Johnson M, Katz JS, eds. *Death, Dying and Bereavement.* London: Sage Publications, 2000: 28–34.

41 Forte A, Hill M, Pazder R, Feudtner C. Bereavement care interventions: a systematic review. *BMC Palliat Care* 2004; **3**: 3.

◆ 42 Harding R, Higginson IJ. What is the best way to help caregivers in cancer and palliative care? A systematic literature review of interventions and their effectiveness. *Palliat Med* 2003; **17**: 64–74.

◆ 43 Schut H, Stroebe MS, van den Bout J, Terheggen M. The efficacy of bereavement interventions: Determining who benefits. In: Stroebe MS, Hansson RO, Stroebe W, Schut H, eds. *Handbook of Bereavement Research: Consequences, Coping, and Cure.* Washington, DC: American Psychological Association, 2001: 705–37.

◆ 44 Stroebe W, Schut H, Stroebe MS. Grief work, disclosure and counseling: do they help the bereaved? *Clin Psychol Rev* 2005; **25**: 395–414.

45 Raphael B, Minkov C, Dobson M. Psychotherapeutic and pharmacological intervention for bereaved persons. In: Stroebe MS, Hansson RO, Stroebe W, Schut H, eds. *Handbook of Bereavement Research: Consequences, Coping, and Cure.* Washington, DC: American Psychological Association, 2001: 587–612.

46 Payne SA, Relf M. The assessment of need for bereavement follow-up in palliative and hospice care. *Palliat Med* 1994; **8**: 291–7.

Children of palliative care patients

ESTELA BEALE

INTRODUCTION

Children of palliative care patients present unique challenges for the palliative care professional. This group of children represents a hidden high-risk group whose needs are often minimized or overlooked by overwhelmed parents and are unknown to most of the medical staff. The reasons for the neglect of this population vary. There is a common belief among parents and caretakers that children are generally adaptive and that they will adjust to their circumstances. Also, parents and caretakers sometimes voice the belief that children, particularly younger ones, do not really understand what is going on and, therefore, it is best not to discuss the situation with them.[1–5] In all of these cases, the children who are about to lose a parent often do not receive the information and attention they need at this critical time. Thus, it is important that members of palliative care teams be aware of the needs of these children and provide appropriate intervention.

Many factors must be taken into consideration in determining the best way to help a child cope with their parent's terminal condition and adjust to the idea and subsequent reality of the parent's death. However, the short-term and long-term bereavement process of these children may be considerably mitigated by early intervention during the parent's terminal phase. Effective intervention must be appropriate to the developmental age of the child. Other critical factors that strongly influence children at this time are their relationship to the well parent, family characteristics, and the stability of their home and social environment.

This chapter focuses on children of parents with terminal cancer. A patient with terminal cancer presents the palliative care professional with a unique set of situations that can create severe distress in children, including dramatic fluctuations of the patient's symptoms due to the cancer treatment or the course of palliative medication, and the potential of an extensive terminal phase with increasingly alarming physical and mental deterioration. Communicating the bad news of a cancer diagnosis is difficult enough for doctors, so it is not surprising that parents dying of cancer, who are coming to terms with the existential issues surrounding dying, are often at a loss as to when, how, and what to tell their children about cancer and death.[6–9] It often falls to a member of the palliative care team to advise and assist the parents in comforting and communicating with the children at this critical time.

The research and clinical experience of a wide range of medical professionals from many countries and cultures is providing a foundation to assist us in developing effective interventions for children of palliative care patients. This chapter reviews the research concerning the main issues that affect these children and the types of intervention that appear most promising.

FACTORS INFLUENCING A CHILD'S RESPONSE TO A TERMINALLY ILL PARENT

Developmental age

Throughout the past several decades, developmental theorists have tried to understand the impact of parental loss on a young child. Attachment theory was first espoused by Bowlby[10] who, in groundbreaking research, demonstrated that when primates are separated from the mother early in life their reaction escalates from a state of protest to marasmus and death. Since then other researchers have confirmed the instinctual roots of attachment, which assures the safety of infants who use intuitive behaviors to engage their caretakers and to guarantee their caretaker's presence and attentiveness. Internalization of primary caretakers is a process that becomes established by the time a child is 2 or 3 years of age. Once this process of internalization is accomplished, the child can sustain prolonged separations yet retain the memory of the parent. For the child to be able to obtain optimal emotional, social, and psychosexual maturity, a predictable, caring environment is required.

Separation from the primary caretaker produces anxiety, which is manifested differently depending on the child's developmental stage, and is exacerbated by a terminal illness. Specific adverse reactions at this age tend to be bodily, such as sleeping and feeding difficulties, constipation, and bedwetting.[11] However, there is still much discussion about whether or not such young children are capable of mourning.[12,13] By 5 years of age, most children can distinguish between a short separation and death. At this point some characteristics of personality are most likely established. In addition, a variety of other factors will now influence the child's development, such as the relationship to the well parent, the family structure, and the child's general social circumstances, as well as genetic makeup. These children often become overprotective of the well parent and may withhold showing them any signs of distress. At the death of the parent, it is characteristic of this age group for there to be increased activity, often resulting in behavioral problems.[11] Several lines of research indicate that children from 5 to 11 years should be informed that the parent is terminally ill and told what to expect.[14–22]

Developmental factors also shape the adolescent's response to the terminal illness of a parent. Support by health professionals, coping strategies, and the adolescent's own mastery of adaptive tasks are posed by the terminal phase of the parent's illness.[23] Open communication between parents and children is of utmost importance.[24] Often the parent's illness creates the need for greater assistance in the home that clashes with the adolescent's developmental tasks of withdrawing and achieving emotional independence from the parents. An adolescent's inconsistent behavior and mood swings typically become exaggerated under the stress of a parent's illness. The adolescent's advanced cognitive abilities may lead to more intense grief than younger children due to their increased ability to comprehend the enduring consequences of death. Some adolescents experience prolonged emotional disturbance during the parent's illness and for several years after the parent's death. These adolescents tend to exhibit severe depression, or alcohol and/or drug abuse, or refusal to attend school, and oftentimes suicidal ideation.[24–29]

Researchers who have used development-derived age categories to study the impact of development on children's response to terminal illness and death of a parent have reported the emergence of behavior patterns. Further clarification of such patterns could help the clinician determine more effective age-specific interventions.[24,28,29]

Situational factors

Situational factors that can affect a child's response and adjustment to the death of a parent have been gaining attention among researchers. Raveis et al.[30] provided a comprehensive review of these studies and conceptualized situational factors into three broad domains: background characteristics, factors associated with the parent's death, and attributes of the family environment.

Background characteristics include the background of the child, the parents, and the family. The most commonly studied characteristics include the age and gender of the child and the gender of the deceased parent. Less studied characteristics include birth order, family size, and the presence of siblings. Factors associated with the parent's death include length of illness, advance knowledge of the impending death, and the degree to which the child was aware that the parent would die. Particularly in the terminal illness period, factors that appear to impact the child's grief process include stress, alterations in lifestyle, the absence or withdrawal of the ill parent, changes in the household activities, and economic stress of the family due to a prolonged illness. The primary attribute of the family environment is the surviving parent's distress level and adjustment to the death. The ability of the surviving parent to care for the child at this time is critical.[30–33] In a longitudinal study of 25 preadolescent children living on a kibbutz who had lost their fathers in the Arab–Israeli war of 1973, Elizur and Kaffman found that pretraumatic family and environmental factors were significant determinants of the duration and severity of bereavement.[14] Their findings demonstrated that childhood bereavement symptoms tend to become exacerbated when the stress of the loss is compounded by pertinent child, family, and situational factors. In most cases, the combination of several factors determined the intensity of the bereavement response rather than the exclusive influence of any single factor. The results suggested that the child's emotional response during the early months of bereavement is largely determined by pretraumatic antecedent variables, whereas posttraumatic factors became more influential during the years following bereavement. This study points out the importance of the availability of a supportive, stable family environment as well as the accessibility of professional intervention.

Kranzler et al.[20] reported on the acute bereavement reactions of a cohort of preschool-aged children who experienced the death of their mother or father. The aims of the study were to describe the children's acute state, to examine developmental influences that might impact on their vulnerability, and to identify important outcome mediators. The study supported both the importance of preexisting relationships in the family, and the effects of ongoing adversity, especially depression in the surviving parent. It also provided acute bereavement data that support the retrospectively determined findings of Harris et al.[34] and Breier et al.[35] who concluded that although the death of a parent creates a vulnerability, ongoing provoking agents, particularly inadequate parenting after the loss, increases the child's risk. The surviving parent's ability to cope with his or her own grief and capacity to respond to the emotional and other needs of their young children is critical. The young child's sensitivity to deficits in parental caretaking may create a particular vulnerability to parental loss.

For school-age children, the social environment can also play a significant role in the child's adjustment to the death of a parent. By the time a child is 10 years old, he or she has usually developed a social network that includes relationships with teachers, classmates, and friends outside school. A study by Lowton and Higginson[37] provides suggestions for creating a healthy social environment for a grieving child. The surviving parent or caretaker should meet with the child's teachers and parents of his or her friends to make sure they are aware of the situation so that they will understand any marked changes in the child's behavior and provide the support needed when they are unavailable. In addition, they should know that although the child needs to grieve, he also needs to reestablish normal relationships with friends and classmates.[37] Given the amount of time a child spends in school each day, teachers and classmates can play a major role in the child's bereavement process. The teacher can provide a safe place for the child to express their feelings.[38] For most children, loss and fear go hand in hand, and the fearful child cannot concentrate in school. The key to a teacher helping a grieving child is the appreciation that recovery from loss requires the reshaping of existing relationships with family members, classmates and teachers. In dealing with loss in the classroom, the teacher should pay close attention to the child's mood, their play themes, stories, and drawings. The better the teacher can understand the child's feelings, the easier it will be to comfort and support them. Each child who has experienced loss should be free to communicate his or her pain and bewilderment only when they are ready to do so. By being attentive, sensitive, and supportive, a teacher can become an important emotional bridge for a child at times of loss.[39] The teacher can also help the child's classmates to communicate messages of condolence and to understand the changes in their classmate's behavior. It is important that children understand that their grieving friend may act differently, may withdraw, or seem angry, but that this does not mean that these changes will last. The teacher should explain to children that their regular friendship may be an important source of support for their grieving classmate.[40] A healthy social environment, in and outside school, provides a grieving child with opportunities to reestablish relationships and to feel a much needed sense of connection and normalcy.

Communication

Studies by Waechter and others provide support for the belief that giving a child opportunities to discuss their fears does not heighten anxiety. Also, providing the child with understanding and with acceptance of their feelings and conveyance of permission to discuss any aspect of the parent's illness can decrease feelings of isolation and alienation, and dispel the sense that the illness is too terrible to discuss.[17–19] Waechter points out the striking dichotomy between the child's degree of awareness of the prognosis, as inferred from his or her imaginative stories, and the parent's belief about the child's degree of awareness of the parent's prognosis.[19] This dichotomy suggests that knowledge is communicated to the child by the changes that they encounter in their total environment after the diagnosis is made, and by their perceptiveness of various nonverbal clues. This disparity presages a deepening isolation that is exacerbated when the child becomes aware of the evasiveness that meets expressions of his or her concern.

Hilden et al.[21] found that when given the opportunity to communicate, children can conquer their fears as well as express their love in the terminal phase of a parent's illness, and that honesty is indeed the best policy with children of all ages. In this way, the reality of the situation, no matter how awful it is, can be shared in an open manner. Trying to protect children from knowledge about what is really happening often confuses the child even more than circumstances alone and escalates concerns about events that are beyond their control. A study conducted by Pfeffer et al.[22] reported that the children in their sample were likely either denying or reluctant to acknowledge problems in the emotional domains assessed, for reasons that were directly or indirectly related to the loss of their parent. For example, they may have been reluctant to acknowledge their own feelings of depression for fear that doing so would upset other family members.

However, reports of bereaved parents regarding their children's psychological distress and symptoms of depression revealed lower incidences than found in the children's reports of their own distress and psychiatric symptomatology. Bereaved parents may be so overwhelmed by their own grief and mourning that they are not fully aware of the level of distress of their children, or they may not be able to cope with their children's psychologically distressed states. There should be no curtain of silence drawn around the child's worst fears.[16,18,33,41,42]

Children who are forewarned of the imminence and inevitability of death have lower levels of anxiety than those who are not, even children within the same family. The practitioner needs to be aware that some children may need specialized help in recovering from depressive and other symptoms that are associated with bereavement. An editorial by Kroll et al.[15] cites several studies specifically related to parents dying of cancer. These studies reiterate the importance of communication between parents and children and provide support for the claim that parents underestimate the impact of a terminal illness on their children. The results suggest that emotional restraint in the surviving parent made it difficult for the child to express feelings, which led to a sense of intensified loneliness, and increased anxiety and confusion.[32] Elizur and Kaffman[14] and Kranzler *et al.*[20] found that the ability of bereaved children to report grieving emotions correlated significantly with improved functioning.

SHORT-TERM AND LONG-TERM EFFECTS OF CHILDHOOD BEREAVEMENT

There has been some progress in assessing the short-term effects of the bereavement process in children. The most consistent finding in the literature is the association between parental bereavement and depression. The results of several studies cited in a meta-analysis by Lutzke *et al.*[43] compared bereaved children 1–12 months after a parent's death with a comparable nonbereaved sample of children or adolescents. These investigations revealed higher rates of depression in the bereaved children.[20,44,45] The differences were more striking in the studies that assessed overall negative affects such as sadness, crying, or moodiness than those assessing symptoms more typical of clinical depression. Other studies revealed a relationship between anxiety withdrawal and childhood bereavement, particularly among adolescents 1–6 months after a parent's death.[46–49] Studies of bereaved children 1–2 years after parental death have shown small to moderate differences of self-esteem and academic success between bereaved and nonbereaved children.[47,50,51]

Studies regarding the long-term effect of childhood parental loss have been inconsistent or inconclusive.[45,48] The evidence from many of these studies provide mixed evidence for the changes in psychological symptoms of bereaved children over time.[43] Some of the studies indicate a significant difference in depression and suicide in adults bereaved in childhood,[52–54] whereas other studies show no significant difference in this group.[55–57]

There are several reasons for the lack of consistent results and agreement among researchers studying the short-term and long-term effects of bereavement on children. These range from the use of nonrepresentative samples of bereaved children to small sample sizes to the use of a wide range of methods for data collection. which makes it difficult to compare otherwise similar studies.

INTERVENTIONS FOR THE CHILDREN OF PALLIATIVE CARE PATIENTS

A study by Sivesind and Beale[58**] showed a high percentage of children of a terminally ill parent sought reassurance, and most of them considered themselves to be caregivers of their dying parent. Faced with the parent's obvious deterioration and fear of the parent's death, a strong wish to do everything possible to keep the parent alive was triggered. It also appeared that while the child was lost in frenetic activity he or she was not faced with as much anxiety and grief as might otherwise occur or as might be expected.

In contrast to the standard account of developmental stages, small children demonstrated a remarkable awareness of the parent's medical condition and its implications.[59***] Disruptive behavior alternated with some desperate attempts to be helpful. The helpfulness was always associated with the wish to help the parent get better. These findings are consistent with the findings of Siegel *et al.*[60*] The latency age group tended to present academic difficulties, which the parents tended to relate to the disruptions caused by the cancer. Among children whose families were secure, this provided enough stability for the children to free themselves from the worries of the illness and continue with their day-to-day life. Those in situations where financial or family problems prevailed felt much more at sea and the potential loss was one more assault to throw them into a state of helplessness. The children from this group attached themselves to the therapist, recognizing him or her as one trustworthy person in their life. Results of this study suggest that children with dying parents manifest significant distress as well as a greater understanding of their parent's illness than is usually suspected. Three types of intervention were found to be useful: normalization for both patient and family (50 percent), expressive-supportive counseling (100 percent), and occasional cognitive reframing (35 percent).

In an article by Black,[11***] the author states that:

> Children are rarely prepared for the death of a parent or a sibling, and yet we know from studies of bereaved adults that mourning is aided by a foreknowledge of the imminence and inevitability of death.[42] Children who are forewarned have lower levels of anxiety than those who are not, even within the same family.[41]

After the death of the parent, she suggests that young children in particular may need to see the dead parent, but that it does not have to be the well parent who accompanies the child during this viewing. This could be done by a member of the care team whom the child feels comfortable with. A controlled trial of family therapy with children bereaved of a parent showed that the post-bereavement morbidity of 40 percent at 1 year could be reduced to 20 percent by six sessions of family meetings.

These meetings focused on helping the family share their mourning with each other and encouraging communication about the dead parent.[61**,62*] The author believes that preventive counseling is properly the responsibility of the primary care team, utilizing the resources of bereavement counseling services as necessary. Finally, the practitioner needs to be aware of the small number of children who may need more specialized help in recovering from depressive or other symptoms that may be associated with bereavement.

Christ[29*] developed a psychoeducational intervention to facilitate the adjustment of children to the terminal illness and subsequent death of a parent. The intervention emphasized a parent-guidance approach.[63*] As part of this intervention, a telephone supportive intervention was also developed as a control condition.

> A social worker telephoned the well parent every four to eight weeks. The goal of this intervention was to maintain contact with the well parent between psychological evaluations, to provide referrals to community based therapists or support groups when such a referral was requested, or to appropriate hospital personnel when questions such as uncertainty about planned treatment procedures, billing, or untoward reactions of the ill parent were raised by the well parent. Since the data generated by this intervention were insufficient for qualitative analyses, only data from families who participated in the psycho-educational intervention were used for the qualitative arm of the analyses.

On the basis of clinical experience, the interventions started during the terminal illness. The researchers found that the family member's responses differed substantially during the terminal stage of the illness from responses following the death. 'This clinical experience was confirmed by the quantitative analyses of depression and anxiety measures that indicated that children were significantly more anxious and depressed during the pre-death period than at the end of the reconstitution stage'.[60*,63*]

A typical psychoeducational parent-guidance intervention spanned about 14 months and included six or more 60–90-minute therapeutic interviews during the terminal stage of the illness and six or more after the death. The therapeutic engagement was emphasized during the second interview. It was the family's option to include the patient in these interviews. At each meeting, ways of handling problems with the children were discussed. A separate interview was then done with each child. This was followed by an informing interview with the parent in which the parent was given an assessment of the children's adaptation to the illness. A family interview that included the well parent and all of the children in that family was then done and was followed by two or more biweekly to monthly parent interviews. Beginning 2–4 weeks after the death of the parent, a similar schedule of interviews was followed. Additional child and/or family interviews were scheduled as requested.

After the final interview, the social worker initiated bimonthly to monthly telephone contacts with the surviving parent until the final post-death psychological assessment was completed about 14 months after the death of the parent. Additional telephone contacts were scheduled if significant family crises emerged either during the psychologist's final assessment or during the social worker's final telephone contact. Finally, if necessary, individual parent, child and/or family sessions were offered.

Dr Paula Rauch is the founder of a parent-guidance program at Massachusetts General Hospital called 'Parenting at a Challenging Time' (PACT). The program provides individual and group parenting support by child psychiatrists and psychologists for patients with cancer, and their spouses and children. Of the program Dr Rauch says, 'I tell parents – because it's true – that they are the experts on their children. My role is to be a co-pilot navigating with them the unfamiliar waters of a life threatening illness.' Through lessons learned from this program for adults with cancer, Dr Rauch has developed a series of guiding principles for supporting children and parents facing cancer.[64***]

Hahn et al.[33**] developed a parent-guidance model of communicating the parent's terminal illness to children to try to positively affect the children's adjustment process to the terminal illness and death of a parent due to cancer. The specific goals of the intervention were to facilitate the competency of the parents and increase communication among the family members about the illness and impending death. The intervention consisted of 3 hours of providing information, advice, and communication training to both parents. The authors report that this model seems promising and points to the importance of a standardized intervention program for children with a terminally ill parent.

CONCLUSIONS

Several themes emerge from these studies and are relevant to both the short-term and the long-term care of children who experience the death of a parent from cancer. Healthcare professionals who intervene should be aware of these themes:

- Previous family history affects the child's bereavement process.
- A child's increased anxiety is directly correlated with a lack of information about their parent's cancer diagnosis.
- Anxiety increases when information is available but there is no opportunity for discussion with the child.
- Children of parents with cancer are at a higher risk of psychological disturbance.
- A large percentage of bereaved children experience a major depressive disorder in adulthood.
- Meeting with a mental health professional provides an avenue for supportive discussions, which in turn model for the family how discussions can be conducted to clarify issues, dispel fears, bring people together, or plan for the future.

It is important to remember that making recommendations to families in such a situation is difficult. There is no clear-cut solution for dealing with a family's reaction to terminal cancer. When a parent is dying of cancer, discussions among parents, children, and all other adult caretakers are important. However, these discussions are part of a process that should begin when the patient is first aware of their terminal condition. This may coincide with their referral to a palliative care team. The mental health professional should contact the family at this entry point and establish a connection. An assessment of the parent's adaptation to the illness, and of the family and other support systems is important. The children should be assessed independently to determine developmental age, level of information, adaptation to the critical situation, understanding of facts and wishes and fantasies about the future. Finally, the interventions have to take place before despair or resignation sets in so there is enough motivation to accomplish a higher level of communication and possibly resolution of conflicts before death is imminent.

Interventions for children of palliative care patients and their families have two different aspects: (i) the structure of the meeting (or the form) and (ii) the content. The structure determines where the meeting takes place, when it happens, who is present, and how long it takes. The site should be comfortable, quiet, and relatively private so there are no distractions or interruptions. The family and the professional should meet when the patient first enters the palliative care service. Ideally, the ill parent should be conscious and have enough energy to be able to connect with the children as well as to continue participating in whatever limited way in their lives. Time should be sufficient for the discussion so that the meeting is not ended prematurely. The professional acts as a consultant to the family by promoting disclosure, clarifying the goals of the meeting, and eliciting information from the different participants, especially the children.

The content of the meeting is determined by the discussion, which is not arbitrarily confined to this situation but uses this time to revisit events. It is of primary importance to explore the information, speculations, and conclusions that the children have reached so far. This provides a springboard for clarifications, more information, and beginning a discussion of the ill parent's prognosis. When this is new information to a child, he or she will need time to react and possibly talk about feelings. It is also important to pay attention to the child's tolerance for information and pace the discussion based on the child's ability to absorb. The child may not want to hear or continue the discussion. The challenge is to know how much to push without assaulting the child with unwelcome facts and when to back-off and wait.

This discussion is personal, intimate, and private, requiring a great deal of acceptance and support. The professional will model this through empathetic statements and reassurance. This is a time when the expressions of love, regret for the truncated life, gratitude, and reassurance of unending memory will solidify the bonds and, paradoxically, facilitate the ability to let go. As this is a very personal, intimate subject, parents are ideally the ones to have this conversation with the child. However, parents are so often burdened with the weight of the illness and all of their other responsibilities that they are not able to take on this task. As previously stated, the two parents, or just the well parent with a professional assistant, may create the optimal situation to clarify issues, provide reassurance, intensify trust and attachment, and prepare the child for the final farewell.

ISSUES FOR THE FUTURE

The research studies, theories, intervention strategies, and guidelines discussed above are providing a body of knowledge and clinical experience from which we will be able to develop more effective intervention strategies for the children of palliative care patients.

Many difficulties are associated with framing these types of study – the large number of variables involved, the difficulty of determining appropriate control groups, small sample sizes, etc. However, there is general agreement among investigators from different countries and cultures that early intervention for children of palliative care patients holds great hope for positively affecting these children's bereavement process and ultimately their adjustment into adulthood to their childhood experience of losing a parent. Much more research is needed in this area.

Key learning points

- Previous family history and social circumstances affects the child's bereavement process.

- A child's increased anxiety is directly correlated with a lack of information about his or her parent's cancer diagnosis.

- Anxiety increases when information is available but there is no opportunity for discussion with the child.

- Children of parents with cancer are at a higher risk of psychological disturbances.

- A large percentage of bereaved children experience a major depressive disorder in adulthood.

- Meeting with a mental health professional provides an avenue for supportive discussions, which in turn model for the family how discussions can be conducted to clarify issues, dispel fears, bring people together, or plan for the future.

- The reactions of the healthy parent to the spouse's illness are critical to the children's and the patient's adaptation to the illness and to the loss.

REFERENCES

1   Chesterfield P. Communicating with dying children. *Nurs Stand* 1992; **6**: 30–2.

2   Kastenbaum R. The child's understanding of death: How does it develop? In: Grollman E, ed. *Explaining Death to Children*. Boston: Beacon Press, 1967; 89–108.

3   Pettle SA, Britten CM. Talking with children about death and dying. *Child Care Health Dev* 1995: 395–404.

4   Spinetta JJ. The dying child's awareness of death: a review. *Psychol Bull* 1974; **81**: 256–60.

5 Stambrook M, Parker KCH. The development of the concept of death in childhood: a review of the literature. *Merrill Palmer Q* 1987; **33**: 133–57.

6 Buckman R. Breaking bad news: why is it still so difficult? *Br Med J (Clin Res Ed)* 1984; **288**: 1597–9.

7 Butow PN, Brown RF, Cogar S, *et al.* Oncologists' reactions to cancer patients' verbal cues. *Psychooncology* 2002; **11**: 447–58.

8 Fallowfield L, Jenkins V. Effective communication skills are the key to good cancer care. *Eur J Cancer* 1999; **35**: 1592–7.

9 Maguire P. Improving communication with cancer patients. *Eur J Cancer* 1999; **35**: 1415–22.

◆ 10 Bowlby J. *Attachment and Loss: Sadness and Depression*, Vol. 3. London: Hogarth Press, 1980.

11 Black D. Coping with loss: bereavement in childhood, *BMJ* 1998; **316**: 931–3.

12 Wolfenstein M. How is mourning possible? *Psychoanal Study Child* 1966; **21**: 93–123.

13 Kliman G. Death in the family – its impact on children, Terry Friedman Klein Memorial Lecture. Leonia, NJ: Behavioral Sciences Tape Library, 1974.

14 Elizur E, Kaffman M. Factors influencing the severity of childhood bereavement reactions. *Am J Orthopsychiatry* 1983; **53**: 668–76.

15 Kroll L, Barnes J, Jones AL, Stein A. Cancer in parents: telling children [editorial]. *BMJ* 1998; **316**: 880.

16 Sourkes BM. Views of the deepening shade: psychological aspects of life-threatening illness. *Am J Hosp Care* 1987; **4**: 22–9.

17 Sourkes BM. The child with a life-threatening illness. In: Brandell J, ed. *Countertransference in Psychotherapy With Children and Adolescents*. New York: Jason Aronson, 1992: 267–84.

18 Sourkes BM. The broken heart: anticipatory grief in the child facing death. *J Palliat Care* 1996; **12**: 56–9.

19 Waechter EH. Children's awareness of fatal illness. *Am J Nurs* 1971; **7**: 1168–72.

20 Kranzler EM, Shaffer D, Wasserman G, *et al.* Early childhood bereavement. *J Am Acad Child Adolesc Psychiatry* 1990; **29**: 513–20.

21 Hilden JM, Watterson J, Chrastek J. Tell the children. *J Clin Oncol* 2000; **18**: 3193–95.

22 Pfeffer CR, Karus D, Siegel K, *et al.* Child survivors of parental death from cancer or suicide: depressive and behavioral outcomes. *Psychooncology* 2000; **9**: 1–10.

23 Blos P. *On Adolescence*. New York: Macmillan, 1962.

24 Christ GH, Siegel K, Christ AE. Adolescent grief: 'It never hit me . . . until it actually happened.' *JAMA* 2002; **288**: 1269–78.

25 Clark D, Pynoos R, Gobel A. Mechanisms and processes of adolescent bereavement. In: Haggerty RJ, Sherrod LR, Garmezy N, Rutter M, eds. *Stress, Risk and Resilience in Children and Adolescents: Processes, Mechanisms, and Interventions*. New York: Cambridge University Press, 1994: 100–46.

● 26 Christ GH, Siegel K, Mesagno FP, Langosch D. A preventive intervention program for bereaved children: problems of implementation. *Am J Orthopsychiatry* 1991; **61**: 168–78.

● 27 Christ GH, Siegel K, Sperber D. Impact of parent terminal cancer on adolescents. *Am J Orthopsychiatry* 1994; **64**: 604–13.

● 28 Christ GH. Impact of development on children's mourning. *Cancer Pract* 2000; **8**: 72–81.

◆ 29 Christ GH. *Healing Children's Grief: Surviving a Parent's Death From Cancer*. Oxford University Press, 2000.

30 Raveis VH, Siegel K, Karus, D. Children's psychological distress following the death of a parent. *J Youth Adolesc* 1999; **28**: 165–80.

● 31 Buxbaum L. When a parent dies from cancer. *Clin J Oncol Nurs* 2001; **5**: 135–40.

32 Baker JE, Sedney MA, Gross E. Psychological tasks for bereaved children. *Am J Orthopsychiatry* 1992; **61**: 105–16.

33 Hahn D, Kaats E, Stutterheim A, *et al.* Facilitation of children's adjustment to the terminal illness and death of a parent due to cancer [abstract]. *Eur J Cancer* 1997; **33**: 339.

34 Harris T, Brown GW, Bifulco A. Loss of parent in childhood and adult psychiatric disorder: the role of lack of adequate parental care. *Psychol Med* 1986; **16**: 641–59.

35 Breier A, Kelsoe JR Jr, Kirwin PD, *et al.* Early parental loss and development of adult psychopathology. *Arch Gen Psychiatry* 1988; **45**: 987–93.

36 Webb NB. *Helping Bereaved Children: a Handbook for Practitioners*. New York: Guilford Press, 1993.

37 Lowton K, Higginson I. Bereavement in the classroom. *Eur J Palliat Care* 2004; **11**: 28–31.

38 Deaton RL, Berkan WA. *Planning and Managing Death Issues in the Schools: A Handbook*. Westport, CT: Greenwood Publishing Group, 1995.

39 Rowling L, Holland J. Grief and school communities: the impact of social context, a comparison between Australia and England. *Death Stud* 2000; **24**: 35–50.

40 Lowton K, Higginson I, Shipman C. Evaluation of an intervention to reduce the impact of childhood bereavement at school. *J Interprof Care* 2001; **15**: 397–8.

41 Rosenheim E, Reicher R. Informing children about a parent's terminal illness. *J Child Psychol Psychiatry* 1985; **36**: 995–8.

42 Parkes CM. *Bereavement: Studies of Grief in Adult Life*. Harmondsworth: Penguin, 1986.

43 Lutzke JR, Ayers TX, Sandler IN, Barr A. Risks and interventions for the parentally bereaved child. In: Wolchik S, Sandler IN, eds. *Handbook of Children's Coping: Linking Theory and Intervention*. New York: Plenum Press, 1997; 215–43.

44 van Eerdewegh MM, Bieri MD, Parilla RH, Clayton PJ. The bereaved child [abstract]. *Br J Psychiatry* 1982; **140**: 23–29.

◆ 45 Worden W. *Children and Grief: When a Parent Dies*. New York: Guilford Press, 1996.

46 Saucier JF, Ambert AM. Adolescents' perception of self and of immediate environment by parental marital status: a controlled study. *Can J Psychiatry* 1986; **31**: 505–12.

47 Heatherington E. Effects of paternal absence on personality development in adolescent daughters, *Dev Psychol* 1972; **7**: 313.

48 Worden JW, Silvermann PR. Parental death and the adjustment of school-age children. *Omega J Death Dying* 1996; **33**: 91–102.

49 Felner RD, Stolberg AL, Cowen EL. Crisis events and the school mental health referral patterns of young children. *J Consult Clin Psychol* 1975; **43**: 305–10.

50 Partridge S, Kotler T. Self-esteem and adjustment in adolescents from bereaved, divorced, and intact families: family type versus family environment. *Aust J Psychol* 1987; **39**: 223–34.

51 Sandler IN, West SG, Baca L, *et al.* Linking empirically based theory and evaluation: the family bereavement program. *Am J Comm Psychol* 1992; **20**: 491–521.

52 Adams-Greenly M, Moynihan R. Helping the children of fatally ill parents. *Am J Orthopsychiatry* 1983; **53**: 219–29.

53   Barnes GE, Prosen H. Parental death and depression. *J Abnorm Psychol* 1985; **94**: 64–9.

54   Zall DS. The long term effects of childhood bereavement: impact on roles as mothers. *Omega* 1994; **29**: 219–30.

55   Hallstrom T. The relationships of childhood socio-demographic factors and early parental loss to major depression in adult life. *Acta Psychiatr Scand* 1987; **75**: 212–16.

56   Kendler KS, Neale MC, Kessler RC, *et al.* Childhood parental loss and adult psychopathology in women. A twin study perspective. *Arch Gen Psychiatry* 1992; **49**: 109–16.

● 57   Siegel K, Raveis V, Karus D. Patterns of communication with children when a parent has cancer. In: Cooper C, Baider L, Kaplan De-Nour, eds. *Cancer and the Family*. New York: John Wiley & Sons, 1996; 109–28.

58   Sivesind DM, Beale E. Children of terminally ill cancer patients: findings of psychosocial assessment and counseling, 2002 *ASCO Annual Meetings* 2002, Abstract No: 1441.

◆ 59   Matthews GB. Children's conceptions of illness and death. In: Kopelman LM, Moskop JC, eds. *Children and Health Care: Moral and Social Issues*. Boston: Kluwer Academic Publishers, 1989; 133–46.

60   Siegel K, Karus D, Raveis V. Adjustment of children facing the death of a parent due to cancer. *J Am Acad Child Adolesc Psychiatry* 1996; **35**: 442–50.

61   Black D, Urbanowicz MA. Family intervention with bereaved children. *Psychol Psychiatry* 1987; **28**: 467.

● 62   Weller RA, Weller EB, Fristad MA, Bowes JM. Depression in recently bereaved prepubertal children. *Am J Psychiatry* 1991; **148**: 1536–40.

63   Siegel K, Mesagno FP, Karus D, *et al.* Psychosocial adjustment of children with a terminally ill parent. *J Am Acad Child Adolesc Psychiatry* 1992; **31**: 327–33.

64   Rauch P. Comment: Supporting the child within the family. *J Clin Ethics* 2000; **11**: 169–70.

Index

Page numbers in **bold** denote figures and tables. All entries refer to palliative medicine/care unless otherwise stated.